U0189348

Dorland's Pocket Medical Dictionary

道兰医学英汉速查手册

·原书第30版·

原著　Dorland

主审　邓忠良　陈仲强

主译　陈萧霖

中国科学技术出版社

·北　京·

图书在版编目（CIP）数据

道兰医学英汉速查手册 : 原书第 30 版 / (美) 道兰 (Dorland) 原著 ; 陈萧霖主译 .
— 北京 : 中国科学技术出版社, 2024.10
书名原文 : Dorland's Pocket Medical Dictionary, 30E
ISBN 978-7-5046-9219-1

Ⅰ . ①道… Ⅱ . ①道… ②陈… Ⅲ . ①医学—名词术语—英、汉 Ⅳ . ① R-61

中国版本图书馆 CIP 数据核字（2021）第 197227 号

著作权合同登记号：01-2021-6335

策划编辑　刘　阳　焦健姿
责任编辑　史慧勤
装帧设计　佳木水轩
责任印制　徐　飞

出　　版　中国科学技术出版社
发　　行　中国科学技术出版社有限公司
地　　址　北京市海淀区中关村南大街 16 号
邮　　编　100081
发行电话　010-62173865
传　　真　010-62179148
网　　址　http://www.cspbooks.com.cn

开　　本　889mm×1194mm　1/32
字　　数　2509 千字
印　　张　36
版　　次　2024 年 10 月第 1 版
印　　次　2024 年 10 月第 1 次印刷
印　　刷　北京盛通印刷股份有限公司
书　　号　ISBN 978-7-5046-9219-1 / R·3281
定　　价　298.00 元

Elsevier (Singapore) Pte Ltd.

3 Killiney Road, #08-01 Winsland House I, Singapore 239519

Tel: (65) 6349-0200; Fax: (65) 6733-1817

Dorland's Pocket Medical Dictionary, 30E

Copyright © 2019 by Elsevier, Inc. All rights reserved.

Previous editions copyrighted © 2013, 2009, 2004, 2001, 1995, 1989, 1982, 1977, 1968, 1959, 1953, 1946, 1942, 1938, 1934, 1930, 1926, 1922, 1919, 1917, 1915, 1913, 1911, 1909, 1906, 1903, 1900, 1899, 1898 by Sunders, an imprint of Elsevier Inc.

Copyright renewed 1987, 1974, 1970, 1966, 1962, 1958, 1954, 1950, 1947, 1945, 1943, 1941, 1939 by Saunders, an imprint of Elsevier Inc.

ISBN-13: 978-0-323-55493-0

注　意

本译本由中国科学技术出版社完成。相关从业及研究人员必须凭借其自身经验和知识对文中描述的信息数据、方法策略、搭配组合、实验操作进行评估和使用。由于医学科学发展迅速，临床诊断和给药剂量尤其需要经过独立验证。在法律允许的最大范围内，爱思唯尔、译文的原文作者、原文编辑及原文内容提供者均不对译文或因产品责任、疏忽或其他操作造成的人身及（或）财产伤害及（或）损失承担责任，亦不对由于使用文中提到的方法、产品、说明或思想而导致的人身及（或）财产伤害及（或）损失承担责任。

译者名单

主　审　邓忠良　重庆医科大学附属第二医院

　　　　陈仲强　北京大学第三医院 北京大学国际医院

主　译　陈萧霖　重庆医科大学附属第二医院

副主译　牛宏涛　中日友好医院 / 国家呼吸医学中心

　　　　朱成佩　首都医科大学附属北京佑安医院

　　　　杨安力　中山大学肿瘤防治中心

　　　　王彬丞　上海市第一人民医院

　　　　张靖雪　北京大学医学部

　　　　黄庆霞　复旦大学生命科学学院

秘　书　黄庆霞　复旦大学生命科学学院

译　者　（以姓氏笔画为序）

　　　　于冰心　首都医科大学附属北京友谊医院

　　　　王　珍　浙江大学医学院

　　　　王　媛　中国医学科学院北京协和医院

　　　　王智强　重庆市渝北区人民医院

　　　　韦雨策　北京协和医学院 中国医学科学院肿瘤医院

　　　　任士萌　郑州大学第一附属医院

　　　　刘　瑞　重庆医科大学附属第二医院

　　　　刘国都　中山大学中山医学院

　　　　闫卫新　广州中医药大学第一附属医院

　　　　苏颖杭　广州中医药大学第一附属医院

　　　　李玉龙　北京市和平里医院

　　　　李红雯　山东第一医科大学附属省立医院

李淑娥　重庆医科大学附属第二医院

杨　旭　重庆医科大学附属第二医院

杨　倩　西安市中心医院

杨远航　重庆医科大学附属第二医院

吴　桐　华中科技大学同济医学院附属同济医院

吴美容　福建医科大学附属第二医院

张力天　南方医科大学皮肤病医院

范天晴　中南大学湘雅二医院

林　路　重庆医科大学附属第二医院

金　昭　北京大学肿瘤医院

赵　悦　复旦大学附属肿瘤医院

赵国江　北京大学第三医院

赵柄骅　中山大学中山医学院

姜　薇　中山大学肿瘤防治中心

姚胜勇　重庆医科大学附属第二医院秀山分院

原　昊　北京大学第三医院

郭　政　Vanderbilt University Medical Center（范德比尔特大学医学中心）

郭佳佳　中山大学肿瘤防治中心

唐嘉萱　Osaka University（大阪大学）

彭书杰　深圳大学总医院

彭茂桓　北京大学人民医院

谭波涛　重庆医科大学附属第二医院

熊　乐　上海交通大学医学院附属仁济医院

潘亚静　首都医科大学宣武医院

内容提要

医学是研究人体各种疾病或病变的一门学科，它的研究、发展和普及对整个人类社会的发展至关重要。2019 年 12 月至今，因 COVID-19 大流行的出现，人类健康面临空前挑战，"人类命运共同体"受到各国认同，为守护人类健康，医学相关知识、经验的国际化交流显得尤为重要。

Dorland's Illustrated Medical Dictionary 是具有较高权威及良好实用性的一部医学词典，自首版问世以来，已有 120 余年的历史，之后多次再版，已成为许多医学院校师生、医务工作者的医学词典首选。此次中国科学技术出版社获得授权翻译出版的 *Dorland's Pocket Medical Dictionary , 30E* 是 *Dorland's Illustrated Medical Dictionary* 的简明版。纵观全书，虽为简明版本，但其内容涵盖各医学学科，收录 36000 余个词条及 200 余幅图解，较前一版新增了 2000 余个词条及 30 余幅图解。其特点是深入浅出，易懂易记，易携带和查阅，是一部极具价值的案头医学词典。

补充说明

本书彩色配图"人体结构与功能详解"已更新至网络，读者可扫描右侧二维码，关注出版社医学官方微信"焦点医学"，后台回复"9787504692191"，即可获取。

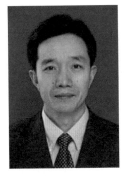

主任医师，教授，博士研究生导师，重庆医科大学附属第二医院副院长。国际内镜脊柱外科学会（ISESS）执行委员，中国中西医结合学会骨科微创专业委员会副主任委员兼脊柱内镜学组组长，中国康复医学会脊柱脊髓专业委员会脊柱脊髓基础研究学组副主任委员，教育部临床实践分教指委委员。

邓忠良

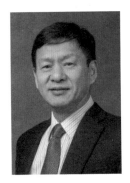

主任医师，教授，博士研究生导师。北京大学国际医院院长，原北京大学第三医院院长、骨科副主任。中国医疗保健国际交流促进会骨科分会副主任委员，中国医师协会骨科医师分会常委，中国医院协会专家委员会副主任委员，海峡两岸医药卫生交流协会副会长、首届骨科学会主任委员，中国残疾人康复协会脊髓损伤专业委员会副主任委员。

陈仲强

主译简介

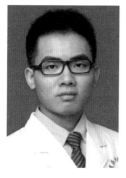

陈萧霖

博士后，讲师、主治医师，重庆医科大学第二医院骨科脊柱外科。AO脊柱会员，《局解手术学》审稿人，主持/参与国家自然科学基金、北京市自然科学基金、北大－清华生命中心、重庆市教委及国家大创等课题。发表论文10余篇，主编专著2部，主译3部。

原书前言

自 1898 年 *Dorland's Pocket Medical Dictionary* 首次以 *American Pocket Medical Dictionary* 为名问世至今，我们一直致力于实现初版时设立的目标：为医疗从业人员、学生及其他医疗领域相关人士提供简洁精准而又权威全面的医疗词典参考。随着医学领域的扩大和医学用语的增长，再版的挑战越来越大，但本书的这一宗旨从未改变。经过一如既往仔细的核查，我们推出了全新第 30 版。

全新版本，我们对词典的格式进行了重新设计，以提高其携带的便捷性同时又保证内容的全面性和易读性。上一版中增加的插图部分广受读者好评，本版再次增加了插图数量以便读者阅读。为适应医学词汇的发展，我们对词汇条目进行了增添和修正，如我们引入了 *Terminologia Anatomica* 和 DSM-Ⅴ中更新的条目。本次修订，我们将词典主体部分的多数词汇组合元素进行了删减，并将其统一归入医学术语结合形式一栏中，减少重复，增加读者检索的便捷。解剖附图在本版中得以保留，其中包含插图及与之结合的手绘图。

以人名命名的词条依旧以无属格（'s）的形式呈现，在表达方式上保持一致，同时反映出其实际应用的常规形式，但并非每个条目都如此，例如一些只有一个正确形式或惯用法的单词，如 *Apgar score* 和 *Down Syndrome*。

医学在不断进步发展，而 *Dorland's Pocket Medical Dictionary* 的目标始终如一：提供重要医学术语的正确、精准的信息，成为读者值得信赖的伙伴。

Sean T. Webb
Chief Lexicographer

译者前言

　　我们组织了协和、北医、重医、中山等多所院校的教师、医生及医学博士进行第30版的翻译工作，译者团队年轻且严谨。我们精心准备，仔细参阅了大量医学参考资料及医学词典，认真翻译了整部词典，全部译名采用国内惯用规范医学词汇，为广大读者呈现每个词条的正确、清晰释义。经讨论，确定书名为《道兰医学英汉速查手册（原书第30版）》，因为"词典"往往会被束之高阁，希望"速查手册"能增进读者开卷使用。

　　我要感谢所有参译人员，特别感谢重庆医科大学附属第二医院邓忠良教授和北京大学第三医院陈仲强教授对整体翻译工作给予的指导与审核，感谢牛宏涛、朱成佩、杨安力、王彬丞、张靖雪和黄庆霞的分工协作，并对中国科学技术出版社为该词典的出版所做的大量工作表示感谢！

　　尽管我们在翻译过程中做了很大努力，但由于该词典覆盖广泛，加之中外术语规范及语言表述习惯有所不同，书中可能遗有疏漏及不妥之处。在此我们衷心希望广大读者不吝赐教，以便日后更新版本时修订。

陈萧霖

于重庆秀山

快速使用指南

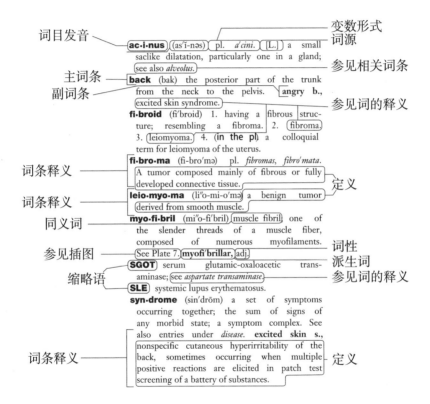

词目发音 —— 变数形式

词源

ac·i·nus (as′ĭ-nəs) pl. *a′cini.* [L.] a small saclike dilatation, particularly one in a gland; see also *alveolus.* —— 参见相关词条

主词条 —— **back** (bak) the posterior part of the trunk
副词条 —— from the neck to the pelvis. **angry b.,** excited skin syndrome. —— 参见词的释义

fi·broid (fi′broid) 1. having a fibrous structure; resembling a fibroma. 2. fibroma. 3. leiomyoma. 4. (in the pl) a colloquial term for leiomyoma of the uterus.

词条释义 —— **fi·bro·ma** (fi-bro′mə) pl. *fibromas, fibro′mata.* A tumor composed mainly of fibrous or fully developed connective tissue. —— 定义

词条释义 —— **leio·myo·ma** (li″o-mi-o′mə) a benign tumor derived from smooth muscle.

同义词 —— **myo·fi·bril** (mi″o-fi′bril) muscle fibril, one of the slender threads of a muscle fiber, composed of numerous myofilaments.
参见插图 —— See Plate 7. **myofi′brillar,** adj. —— 词性
派生词

缩略语 —— **SGOT** serum glutamic-oxaloacetic transaminase; see *aspartate transaminase.* —— 参见词的释义

SLE systemic lupus erythematosus.

syn·drome (sin′drōm) a set of symptoms occurring together; the sum of signs of any morbid state; a symptom complex. See also entries under *disease.* **excited skin s.,**
词条释义 —— nonspecific cutaneous hyperirritability of the back, sometimes occurring when multiple positive reactions are elicited in patch test screening of a battery of substances. —— 定义

使用说明

主词条和副词条的安排

本词典中，词条均以主词条和副词条的形式列出。词条若包括两个或两个以上单词则为副词条，位于主词条下方，主词条常为名词，如 *Addison disease*，*collagen disease*，*Raynaud's disease* 都以副词条的形式归入主词条 disease 中。特定的酸如 *sulfuric acid*（硫酸）和酶如 *acetyl-CoA carboxylase*（乙酰辅酶 A 羧化酶）不适用于本规则，这些词条以主词条的形式列于首个单词下方。

由两个及以上单词组成的化学物质以副词条的形式出现在其中第一个单词词条的下方，如 *sodium chloride* 就以 *sodium* 的副词条形式列出，*ferric chloride* 以 *ferric* 作为主词条。

在副词条中，主词条以缩写形式出现，例如 *humoral i.* 为 *immunity* 的副词条。副词条若为复数形式，以其中的主词条加符号（*'s*）表示。如位于主词条 *body* 下方的副词条 *Aschoff b's* 表示 *Aschoff bodies*，*Ketone b's* 表示 *Ketone bodies*。不规则复数则以完整拼写形式列出，如 *vasa afferentia* 作为 *vas* 的副词条以完整拼写列于其下。

每个词条的其他词性形式（通常为形容词）以加粗字体在主词条后列出，其重音标记也一并给出，词性缩写跟随其后，如 allele...alle'lic, adj., allergen...allergen'ic, adj.。同样，不规则复数形式和拉丁词的复数形式分别以其独自的复数形式列出，如 epiphysis...pl. epi' physes。但有时这些单词也可以以单独的主词条形式出现，如 viscera *viscus* 的复数形式。为了节省空间，本版中我们将词条的组合词元素 [如 gangli(o)，- esis] 统一归入 "医学术语组合形式" 中。

词的音节划分

本词典基于主词条的发音方式进行音节划分，以原点作为分节点将各音节分开，但单个元音位于词条的开头或结尾时不进行单独划分。由于一个单词可能存在不同发音方式，其音节划分形式可能不仅限于本词典中列出的形式。

发 音

本词典中所有主词条的发音均在词条后括号内以音标拼写注出。音标注出单词最常见的发音方式而未列出其他发音方式，但也有例外。为了使用方便，词条的音标注音均以最简明的变音符号呈现。音标中唯一用到的特殊符号是 ə，非重读央元音，如单词 sofa 中末尾的元音字母 a。当元音字母同 r 组成非重读音节时，以非重读央元音表示其中元音的发音，如 sulfur 和 other 的倒数第二个元音字母。

基本发音规则如下。未加记号的元音，其音节发音为长音。未加记号的元音在其音节中以辅音结尾，其元音为短音。长元音在一音节中以辅音结尾，其元音以长音符号标出，即 ā、ē、ī、ō、ū。短元音结尾的音节以短音符号标出，ă、ĕ、ĭ、ŏ、ŭ。

在多音节单词中，词的主重音以重音符号（′）标出，次重音以次重音符号（″）标出，非重音音节以"-"连接。单音节词没有重音符号，除非它们是复合词的一部分，在这种情况下，除连词和其他小词外每个单词都有一个重音标记，以保证清晰。

许多外来词、专有名词和人名的母语发音难以直接用简化音标表示出，只能尽可能以接近它们原发音的英语发音注出。

发音参考

元音
（短音和长音的规则见上）

ə	sofa	ě	met	ǒ	got	oi	boil
ā	mate	ī	bite	ū	fuel	ōō	boom
ă	bat	ĭ	bit	ŭ	but	ŏŏ	book
ē	beam	ō	home	aw	all	ou	fowl

辅音

b	book	m	mouse	ch	chin
d	dog	n	new	ks	six
f	fog	p	park	kw	quote
g	get	r	rat	ng	sing
h	heat	s	sigh	sh	should
j	jewel, gem	t	tin	th	thin, than
k	cart, pick	w	wood	zh	measure
l	look	z	size, phase		

以人名命名的医学术语形式

近年来，以人名命名的医学术语倾向于使用其无属格形式（即，无 's），但这一趋势并非完全普遍，医学术语的属格形式也常见。在本书中，为了保证前后一致，我们均将词条以无属格的形式呈现，仅个别（如法律类）的单词例外，其中包含较多非医学词汇，使用上以其属格形式更为普遍。

缩略语表

a.	artery (L. *arteria*)	动脉	L.	Latin	拉丁语
adj.	adjective	形容词	l.	ligament (L.*ligamentum*)	韧带
ant.	anterior	前面的	lat.	lateral	侧面的
cf.	compare (L.*confer*)	比较	m.	muscle (L.*musculus*)	肌肉
e.g.	For example(L. *exempli gratia*)	例如	n.	nerve (L.*nervus*)	神经
Fr.	French	法语	pl.	plural	复数
gen.	genitive	属格，属格的	post.	posterior	后面的
Ger.	German	德语	q.v.	which see (L.*quod vide*)	参见
Gr.	Greek	希腊语	sing.	singular	单数
i.e.	that is (L.*id est*)	即，那就是	sup.	superior	上面的
inf.	inferior	下面的	v.	vein (L.*vena*)	静脉

医学术语组合形式

　　以下为医学词汇中常见的构词成分。从附加于构词成分的破折号可以看出，它并非一个完整的单词，如果破折号在构词成分之前，则表示它通常作为单词后缀出现，如果构词成分的前后都有破折号，则它通常出现在其他两个构词成分之间。相近的构词成分通常以括号的形式列在同一词条中：如 carbo(n)- 既可表示 carbo-(*carbohydrate*)，也可表示 carbon-(*carbonuria*)。在每种构词成分后的第一项信息是词源，[Gr.] 为希腊语词语，而 [L.] 为拉丁语词语，有时两种词源会同时给出。在词源中出现破折号表示它在该语言中不作为独立的单词出现。随后，有时将在括号中列出理解该构词成分所需的额外信息。接下来列出的为该构词成分的一个或多个含义，且有时会引用同义的构词成分。在每一个词条的最后，将列出该构词成分在复合英语派生词中应用的实例。

a-¹ *a-* [Gr.]（*n* is added before words beginning with a vowel）不，无，缺。例：*a*metria

a-² *a-* [L.] 离。例：*a*vulsio

ab- *ab* [L.] 离开，脱离。Cf. apo-。例：*ab*ducent

abdomin- *abdomen, abdominis* [L.] 腹。例：*abdomin*ohysterectomy

abs- *abs* [L.] ab 的变体。例：*abs*cess

ac- 参见 ad-。例：*ac*cretion

acanth- *akantha* [Gr.] 棘状的。例：acanthocyte

acar- *akari* [Gr.] 螨。例：*acar*odermatitis

acet- *acetum* [L.] 醋，乙酰。例：*acet*ic acid

acid- *acidus* [L.] 酸。例：*acid*uric

acou- *akouō* [Gr.] 听，听觉。例：acoustic。（也拼作 acu-）

acr- *akron* [Gr.] 肢端，末端。例：*acr*omegaly

act- *ago, actus* [L.] 促使，行动。例：re*act*ion

actin- *aktis, aktinos* [Gr.] 光线，放射线。Cf. radi-。例：*Actin*obacillus

acu- 参见 acou-。例：dys*acu*sis

ad- *ad* [L.]（*d* changes to *c, f, g, p, s,* or *t* before words beginning with those consonants）近，向，增加。例：*ad*renal

-ad¹ *-ad* [L.] 向，至。例：cephal*ad*

-ad² *-as, ados* [Gr.] 族，起源，相关。例：trichomon*ad*

aden- *adēn* [Gr.] 腺。Cf. gland-。例：*aden*oma

adip- *adeps, adipis* [L.] 脂肪。Cf. lip- 和 stear-。例：*adip*ocellular

adren- *adren* [Gr.] 肾上腺。Cf. gland-。例：*adren*al

aer- *aēr* [Gr.] 气。例：an*aer*obiosis

af- 参见 ad-。例：*af*ferent

ag- 参见 ad-。例：agglutinant

-agogue *agōgos* [Gr.] 促，利，促进剂。例：galactagogue

-agra *agra* [Gr.] 疼痛发作。例：podagra

-al[1] *-alis* [L.] 具有……的特性。例：arterial, diarrheal

-al[2] *-alia* [L.] 行为，过程。例：denial

alb- *albus* [L.] 白。Cf. leuk-。例：albiduria

algesi- *algēsis* [Gr.] 痛。例：analgesia, algesimeter

-algia *algia* [Gr.] 痛。例：neuralgia

algo- *algos [Gr.]* 痛。例：algophobia

all- *allos* [Gr.] 其他，不同。例：allergy

allant- *allas, allantos* [Gr.] 香肠。例：allantiasis, allantoid

alle- *allēlōn* [Gr.] 对偶，与另一方关系。例：allelic

alve- *alveus* [L.] 沟，槽，腔。例：alveolar

ambi- *ambi-* [L.]（*i* is dropped before words beginning with a vowel）两，双。例：ambidextrous

ambly- *amblys* [Gr.] 钝，弱。例：amblyopia

ambo- *ambo* [L.] 双。例：amboceptor

ameb- *amoibē* [Gr.] 变。例：ameboid

amni- *amnion* [Gr.] 羊膜。例：amniocentesis

amphi- *amphi* [Gr.]（*i* may be dropped before words beginning with a vowel）两侧。例：amphicentric

ampho- *amphō* [Gr.] 双，两。例：amphoteric

amygdal- *amygdalē* [Gr.] 杏仁。

例：amygdalin, amygdaloid

amyl- *amylon* [Gr.] 淀粉。例：amyluria

an[1] 参见 a-[1]。例：aniridia

an[2] 参见 ana-。例：anode

ana- *ana* [Gr.]（韵母 *a* 在以元音开头的单词之前去掉）向上，重回到。例：anabolism

ancyl- 参见 ankyl-。例：ancylostomiasis

andr- *anēr, andros* [Gr.] 男，雄。例：androgen

angi- *angeion* [Gr.] 血管。Cf. vas-。例：angioma

anis- *anisos* [Gr.] 不相等的，不均匀的。例：anisocoria

ankyl- *ankylos* [Gr.] 弯曲。例：ankylosis。（也拼作 ancyl-）

anomal- *an ō malos* [Gr.] 不规则。例：anomaly

ant- 参见 anti-。例：antacid

ante- *ante* [L.] 前。例：anteflexion

anthrac- *anthrax* [Gr.] 炭。例：anthracosilicosis

anthrop- *anthrōpos* [Gr.] 人类学。例：anthropomorphism

anti- *anti* [Gr.]（*i* may be dropped before words beginning with a vowel）反。Cf. contra. 例：antipruritic

antr- *antron* [Gr.] 腔，空洞。例：antrocele

ap- 参见 ad-。例：appendage

aph- *haptō, haph-* [Gr.] 触觉。例：dysaphia。（参见 hapt-）

apic- *apex* [L.] 顶，尖。例：apicoectomy

apo- *apo* [Gr.]（*o* may be dropped before words beginning with a vowel）脱，离。Cf. ab-。例：apolipoprotein

appendic- *appendix, appendicis* [L.] 附件，阑尾。例：

appendicitis

arachn- *arachnē* [Gr.] 蜘蛛，蛛网膜。例：arachnodactyly

arch- *archē* [Gr.] 开始，起源。例：archenteron

arteri- *arteria* [Gr.]（*i* 有时会被删掉）动脉，气管。例：periarteritis

arteriol- *arteriola*, dim. of *arteria* [L.] 小动脉，微动脉。例：arteriolopathy

arthr- *arthron* [Gr.] 关节。Cf. articul-。例：synarthrosis

articul- *articulus* [L.] 关节。Cf. arthr-。例：disarticulation

as- 参见 ad-。例：assimilation

-ase *ase* 在酶的命名中使用。例：transaminase

-asis *asis* [Gr.] 状态。例：hypochondriasis

asthen- *asthenēs [Gr.]* 无力，虚弱。例：asthenocoria

astr- *astron* [Gr.] 星。例：astrocyte

at- 参见 ad-。例：attenuate

atel- *atelēs* [Gr.] 不全。例：atelocardia

ather- *athērē* [Gr.] 粥样。例：atherosclerosis

atlant- *atlas, atlantos* [Gr.] 寰椎。例：atlantoaxial

atm- *atmos* [Gr.] 蒸汽。例：atmosphere

atri- *atrium* [L.] 心房。例：atrioventricular

atroph- *atrophia* [Gr.] 萎缩。例：atrophoderma

atto- *atto* [Danish] 十八。例：attometer

audi- *audire* [L.] 听。例：audiometry

aur- *auris* [L.] 耳朵。Cf. ot-。例：aural

aut- *autos* [Gr.] 自身。例：*aut*oimmunity

aux- *auxō* [Gr.] 增加。例：*aux*otrophic

ax- *axōn* [Gr.] 或 *axis* [L.] 轴。例：*ax*olemma

axon- *axōn* [Gr.] 轴。例：*axon*opathy

ba- *bainō, ba-* [Gr.] 行，走，站。例：a*bas*ia

bacill- *bacillus* [L.] 杆状。Cf. bacter-. 例：actino*bacill*osis

bacter- *bactērion* [Gr.] 杆状。Cf. bacill-. 例：*bacter*iophage

balan- balanos [Gr.] 龟头。例：*balan*itis

ball- *ballō, bol-* [Gr.] 投掷。例：*ball*ismus。（参见 bol-）

bar- *baros* [Gr.] 重，压。例：*bar*osinusitis

bas- 参见 basi-。例：*bas*ophil

basi- *basis* [Gr.] 碱。例：*basi*hyoid

bath(y)- *bathys* [Gr.] 深。例：*bath*rhodopsin, *bathy*pnea

bi¹ *bios* [Gr.] 生命。Cf. vit-. 例：aero*bi*c

bi² *bi-* [L.]（an *n* may be added before words beginning with a vowel）两，双。例：*bi*cornuate。（参见 di-¹）

bil- *bilis* [L.] 胆汁。Cf. chol-. 例：*bil*iary

bin- 参见 bi-²。例：*Bin*ocular

bio- *bios* [Gr.] 生命。例：*bio*logy

bis- *bis* [L.] 两个，两次。例：*bis*ferious

blast- *blastos* [Gr.] 胚，母细胞。Cf. germ-. 例：*blast*oma, mono*blast*

blenn- *blenna* [Gr.] 黏液。例：*blenn*orrhea

blep- *blepō* [Gr.] 看。例：

mono*blep*sia

blephar- blepharon [Gr.]（来自 blepō；参见 blep-）睑。Cf. cili-. 例：*blephar*itis

bol- 参见 ball-。例：em*bol*ism

brachi- *brachiōn* [Gr.] 臂。例：*brachi*ocephalic

brachy- *brachys* [Gr.] 短。例：*brachy*dactyly

brady- *bradys* [Gr.] 慢。例：*brady*cardia

brevi- *brevis* [Gr.] 短。例：*brevi*collis

brom- *brōmos* [Gr.] 臭。例：*brom*hidrosis

bronch- *bronchos* [Gr.] 气管。例：*bronch*oscopy

bronchiol- *bronchiolus*, dim. of *bronchus* [Gr.] 细支气管。例：*bronchiol*ectasis

bry- *bryō* [Gr.] 生命。例：em*bry*onic

bucc- *bucca* [L.] 颊。例：*bucc*oclusion

bulb- *bulbus* [L.] 球部。例：*bulb*ospiral

butyr- *boutyron* [Gr.] 奶酪，黄油（因丁酸的气味像变质的黄油而得名）。例：*butyr*ophenone

cac- *kakos* [Gr.] 坏。Cf. mal-. 例：*cac*ogeusia。（参见 dys-）

calc-¹ *calx, calcis* [L.]（cf. lith-）钙或钙盐，石灰石。例：*calc*ipexy

calc-² *calx, calcis* [L.] 跟骨。例：*calc*aneodynia

calor- *calor* [L.] 热。Cf. therm-. 例：*calor*imeter

campt- *camptos* [Gr.] 弯曲。例：*campt*odactyly

cancr- *cancer, cancri* [L.] 癌。Cf. carcin-. 例：*cancr*oid。（也拼作 chancr-）

canth- *kanthos* [Gr.] 异质的。例：

例：*canth*oplasty

capit- *caput, capitis* [L.] 头部。Cf. cephal-. 例：de*capit*ation

capn- *kapnos* [Gr.] 烟。例：*capn*ography

caps- *capsa* [L.]（来自 capio；参见 cept-）容器。例：*caps*ule

carbo(n)- *carbo, carbonis* [L.] 碳。例：*carbo*hydrate, *carbon*ic acid

carcin- *karkinos* [Gr.] 癌。Cf. cancr-. 例：*carcin*oma

cardi- *kardia* [Gr.] 心。例：lipo*cardi*ac

cari- *caries* [L.] 龋，腐烂。例：*cari*ogenesis

cary- 参见 kary-。例：Eu*cary*otae

cata- *kata* [Gr.]（final *a* is dropped before words beginning with a vowel）下，负。例：*cata*crotism, *cat*ion

caud- *cauda* [L.] 尾。例：*caud*ad

cav- *cavus* [L.] 洞，腔，中空的。Cf. coel-. 例：con*cav*e

cec- *caecus* [L.] 盲。例：*cec*otomy

cel-¹ 参见 -cele。例：varico*cel*ectomy

cel-² 参见 coel-。例：a*cel*omate

cel-³ 参见 celi-。例：*cel*itis

-cele¹ *kēlē* [Gr.] 肿瘤，疝。例：gastro*cele*

-cele² *koilos* [Gr.] 洞，腔，中空的。例：rhino*cele*

celi- *koilia* [Gr.] 肚，腹。例：*celi*otomy

cell- *cella* [L.] 房，细胞。Cf. cyt-. 例：*cell*ular

cement- *caementum* [L.] 骨质。例：*cement*oblast

cen- *koinos* [Gr.] 普通。例：*cen*esthesia

cente- *kenteō* [Gr.] 穿刺。Cf. punct-. 例：entero*centesis*

centi- *centum* [L.] 百分之一。Cf. hect-. [通常，在公制单位中，如该单位表示米的分数（如 centimeter，decimeter，millimeter），则起源于拉丁语；如该单位表示米的倍数（如 hectometer，decameter，kilometer），则起源于希腊语] 例：*centi*meter, *centi*pede

centr- *kentron* [Gr.] 或 *centrum* [L.] 中心。例：*centri*fugal, *centro*mere

cephal- *kephalē* [Gr.] 头。Cf. capit-. 例：en*cephal*itis, *cephalo*centesis

cept- *capio, -cipientis, -ceptus* [L.] 接收，收到。例：re*cept*or

cer- *kēros* [Gr.] 或 *cera* [L.] 蜡。例：*cero*plasty, *cer*umen

cerat- *keras, keratos* [Gr.] 角。例：*cerat*oid 。（也拼作 kerat-）

cerc- *kerkos* [Gr.] 尾。例：Oncho*cerca*

cerebell- *cerebellum* [L.] 小脑。例：*cerebell*ifugal

cerebr- *cerebrum* [L.] 脑。例：*cerebro*spinal

cervic- *cervix, cervicis* [L.] 颈。Cf. trachel-. 例：*cervic*itis

chancr- 参见 cancr-。例：*chancr*oid

cheil- *cheilos* [Gr.] 唇。Cf. labi-. 例：*cheilo*schisis

cheir- *cheir* [Gr.] 手。Cf. man-. 例：macro*cheir*ia 。（也拼作 chir-）

chem- *chēmeia* [Gr.] 化学。例：*chem*istry, *chemo*therapy

chir- 参见 cheir-。例：*chir*opractic

chlor- *chlōros* [Gr.] 绿。例：*chlor*ophyll

choan- *choanē* [Gr.] 漏斗。例：*choan*omastigote

chol- *cholē* [Gr.] 胆汁。Cf. bil-. 例：*chol*angitis

choledoch- *cholē* [Gr.] 总胆管。例：*choledoch*oplasty

chondr- *chondros* [Gr.] 软骨。例：*chondr*omalacia

chondri- *chondrion* [Gr.] 颗粒。例：mito*chondri*a

chord- *chordē* [Gr.] 腱，带。例：peri*chord*al

chore- *choreia* [Gr.] 舞蹈。例：*chore*oathetosis

chori- *chorion* [Gr.] 膜。例：*chorio*carcinoma

chro- *chrōs* [Gr.] 颜色。例：poly*chro*matic

chron- *chronos* [Gr.] 时。例：syn*chron*ous

chrys- *chrysos* [Gr.] 金。例：*chrys*otherapy

chy- *cheō, chy-* [Gr.] 倾，注。例：ec*chy*mosis

chyl- *chylos* [Gr.] 乳糜。例：*chyl*iform, *chylo*pericardium

-cid(e) *caedo, -cisus* [L.] 切，杀。例：fungi*cide*, germi*cid*al

cili- *cilium* [L.] 眼睑，睫。Cf. blephar-. 例：*cili*ary

cine- 参见 kine-。例：acro*cine*sis

-cipient 参见 cept-。例：ex*cipient*

circum- *circum* [L.] 环，周。Cf. peri-. 例：*circum*ferential

cirs- *kirsos* [Gr.] 静脉曲张。例：*cirs*oid

cis- *cis* [L.] 顺。例：*cis*platin

-cis- *caedo, -cisus* [L.] 切。例：ex*cis*ion

-clast *klaō* [Gr.] 破。例：osteo*clast*

cleid- *kleis, kleidos* [Gr.] 锁骨。例：*cleid*ocranial

-cleisis *kleiein* [Gr.] 闭。例：colpo*cleisis*

clin- *klinō* [Gr.] 弯曲，倾斜。例：*clin*ocephaly

clus- *claudo, -clusus* [L.] 关，合。例：maloc*clus*ion

cnid- *knidē* [Gr.] 荨麻。例：*Cnid*aria

co- 参见 con-[1]。例：*co*hesion

cocc- *kokkos* [Gr.] 球菌。例：gono*cocc*us

coel- *koilos* [Gr.] 腔，穴，孔。Cf. cav-. 例：*coel*ozoic 。（也拼作 cel-）

-coele 参见 coel-。例：blasto*coele*

coen- 参见 cen-。例：*Coen*urus

coin- 参见 cen-。例：*coin*osite

col[1] 参见 colon-。例：*col*ic

col[2] 参见 con-[1]。例：*col*lapse

colon- *kalon* [Gr.] 结肠。例：*colon*ic

colp- *kolpos* [Gr.] 阴道。Cf. sin- and vagin-. 例：*colp*itis

com- 参见 con-[1]。例：*com*mensal

con-[1] *con-* [L.]（becomes co- before vowels or h; col- before l; com- before b, m, or p; cor- before r）总，合。Cf. syn-. 例：*con*traction

con-[2] *kōnos* [Gr.] 锥，锥体。例：*con*oid

coni- *konis* [Gr.] 尘。例：*coni*ofibrosis

contra- *contra* [L.] 相反，反对。Cf. anti-. 例：*contra*indication

copr- *kopros* [Gr.] 粪。Cf. sterc-. 例：*copr*ophilia

cor-[1] *korē* [Gr.] 瞳孔。例：iso*cor*ia

cor-[2] 参见 con-[1]。例：

*cor*relation

cord- 参见 chord-。例：
*cord*otomy

corpor- *corpus, corporis* [L.] 体。
Cf. som(at)-. 例：intra*corpor*eal

cortic- *cortex, corticis* [L.] 皮质。
例：*cortic*osterone

cost- *costa* [L.] 肋。Cf. pleur-.
例：inter*cost*al

counter- 参见 contra-。例：
*counter*traction

crani- *kranion* [Gr.] 或 *cranium*
[L.] 颅骨。例：peri*crani*um

-crasia *krasis* [Gr.] 混合。例：
dys*crasia*

creat- *kreas, kreato-* [Gr.] 肉。
例：*creat*ine

-crescence *cresco, crescentis,*
cretus [L.] 生长。例：
ex*crescence*

cret-1 *cerno, cretus* [L.] 辨别，
分开。Cf. crin-. 例：dis*cret*e

cret-2 参见 -crescence。例：
ac*cret*ion

crin- *krinō* [Gr.] 分泌。Cf. cret-
1. 例：endo*crin*ology

crur- *crus, cruris* [L.] 胫。例：
talo*crur*al

cry- *kryos* [Gr.] 冷，冷冻。例：
*cry*esthesia。(参见：crym-)

crym- *krymos* [Gr.] 冻。例：
*crym*odynia。(参见：cry-)

crypt- *kryptō* [Gr.] 隐，隐窝。
例：*crypt*orchidism

cult- *colo, cultus* [L.] 护理，培
养。例：*cult*ure

cune- *cuneus* [L.] 楔状，楔骨。
Cf. sphen-. 例：*cune*iform

cut- *cutis* [L.] 皮肤。Cf.
derm(at)-. 例：sub*cut*aneous

cyan- *kyanos* [Gr.] 青紫，绀，
蓝，氰。例：*cyan*ophil

cycl- *kyklos* [Gr.] 环，圆形。
例：*cycl*ophoria

-cyesis *kyēsis* [Gr.] 妊娠。例：
pseudo*cyesis*

cymb- *kymbē* [Gr.] 舟形。例：
*cymb*ocephaly

cyn- *kyōn, kynos* [Gr.] 犬。例：
*cyn*ophobia

cyst- *kystis* [Gr.] 囊，胞。Cf.
vesic-. 例：*cyst*algia

cyt- *kytos* [Gr.] 细胞。Cf. cell-.
例：*cyt*otaxis

dacry- *dakry* [Gr.] 泪。例：
*dacry*ocyst

dactyl- *daktylos* [Gr.] 指，趾。
Cf. digit-. 例：hexa*dactyl*y

de- *de* [L.] 脱掉，去掉。例：
*de*composition

deca- *deka* [Gr.] 十，表示公
制中的倍数。Cf. deci-. 例：
*deca*gram

deci- *decem* [L.] 十，表示公制
分数(十分之一)。Cf. deca-. 例：
*deci*bel, *deci*liter

dendr- *dendron* [Gr.] 树。例：
*dendr*ite

dent- *dens, dentis* [L.] 牙。Cf.
odont-. 例：inter*dent*al

deoxy- (化学前缀，表示比参
考物质少含一个氧原子的化合
物)脱氧

derm(at)- *derma, dermatos* [Gr.]
皮肤。Cf. cut-. 例：endo*derm*,
*dermat*itis

-desis *desis* [Gr.] 固定，固定
术。例：arthro*desis*

desm- *desmos* [Gr.] 带，索。
例：syn*desm*oplasty

desoxy- 参见 deoxy-。

deut(er)- *deuteros* [Gr.] 第二，
次，亚。例：*deuter*anopia,
*deut*an

dextr- *dexter, dextr-* [L.] 右。
例：ambi*dextr*ous

di-1 *di* [Gr.] 二，双，两。例：
*di*morphism。(参见 bi-2)

di-2 参见 dia-。例：*di*uresis

di-3 参见 dis-。例：*di*vergent

dia- *dia* [Gr.] (*a* is dropped
before words beginning with a
vowel) 通过，横过，分离。
Cf. per-. 例：*Dia*gnosis

diaz- (表示化合物包含该基
团)—N═N— 重氮基

dicty- *diktyon* [Gr.] 网，网状结
构。例：*dicty*otene

didym- *didymos* [Gr.] 双。Cf.
gemin-. 例：epi*didym*al

digit- *digitus* [L.] 指，趾。Cf.
dactyl-. 例：*digit*ation

diplo- *diploos* [Gr.] 双，二。
例：*diplo*myelia

dips- *dipsa* [Gr.] 口渴。例：
poly*dips*ia, *dips*ogen

dis- [L.] (*s* may be dropped
before a word beginning with a
consonant) 分离，除去，无。
例：*dis*location

disc- *diskos* [Gr.] 或 *discus* [L.]
盘。例：*disc*oplacenta。(也拼
作 disk-)

dolich- *dolichos* [Gr.] 长。例：
*dolich*ocephalic

dors- *dorsum* [L.] 背，背侧。
例：*dors*oventral

drom- *dromos* [Gr.] 传导，走，
行。例：*drom*ograph

-ducent 参见 duct-。例：
ad*ducent*

-duct *duco, ducentis, ductus* [L.]
导管。例：ovi*duct*

dur- *durus* [L.] 硬。Cf. scler-. 例：
in*dur*ation

dynam- *dynamis* [Gr.] 力，
动力。例：*dynam*ometer,
thermo*dynam*ics

dys- *dys-* [Gr.] 异常，困难。Cf.
mal-. 例：*dys*trophic。(参见
cac-)

e- *e* [L.] 离，外。Cf. ec-1 and

ex-. 例：emission

ec-¹ *ek* [Gr.] 在外。Cf. e- and ex-. 例：eccentric

ec-² *oikos* [Gr.] 家。例：*eco*tropic

-ech- *echō* [Gr.] 有，拿着，成为。例：syn*ech*otomy

echin- *echinos* [Gr.] 棘，刺。例：*echin*ococcus

ect- *ektos* [Gr.] 外。Cf. extra-. 例：*ect*oderm. (参见 exo-)

ectr- *ektrōsis* [Gr.] 先天缺损。例：*ectr*odactyly

ede- *oideō* [Gr.] 肿，水肿。例：*ede*matous

ef- 参见 ex-。例：*ef*florescent

elast- *elasticus* [L.] 弹性，弹性蛋白。例：*elast*ofibroma

electro- *ēlectron* [Gr.] 电。例：*electro*therapy

em- 参见 en-。例：*em*bolism, *em*pathy

-em- *haima* [Gr.] 血。例：an*em*ia。[参见 hem(at)-]

-emesis *emein* [Gr.] 呕吐。例：hyper*emesis*

en- *en* [Gr.] (*n* changes to *m* before *b, m, p,* or *ph*) 在……之内，在……之中。Cf. in-¹. 例：*en*arthrosis

encephal- *enkephalos* [Gr.] 脑。例：*encephal*opathy

end- *endon* [Gr.] 内。Cf. intra-. 例：*end*angitis. (参见 eso-)

ent- *entos* [Gr.] 内。例：*ent*optic

enter- *enteron* [Gr.] 肠。例：dys*enter*y

entom- *entomon* [Gr.] 昆虫。例：*entom*ology

epi- *epi* [Gr.] (*i* is dropped before words beginning with a vowel) 上，外面。例：*epi*glottis, *ep*axial

epipl- *epiploon* [Gr.] 网膜。例：

gastro*epipl*oic

episi- *epision* [Gr.] 阴部，外阴。例：*episi*otomy

erg- *ergon* [Gr.] 工作，劳动，行为。例：*en*ergy

erot- *erōs, erōtos* [Gr.] 性，色情。例：*erot*omania

erythr- *rythros* [Gr.] 红。Cf. rub(r)-. 例：*erythr*ocyte

-esis *sis* [Gr.] 状态。例：hypophon*esis*

eso- *esō* [Gr.] 内。Cf. intra-. 例：*eso*gastritis. (参见 end-)

esthe- *aisthanomai, aisthē-* [Gr.] 感觉。Cf. sens-. 例：an*esthe*sia

etio- *aitia* [Gr.] 原因。例：*etio*logy

eu- *eu* [Gr.] 好，正常。例：*eu*pepsia

eury- *eurys* [Gr.] 宽，广。例：*eury*cephalic

ex- *ex* [Gr.] 或 *ex* [L.] 向外。Cf. e- and ec-¹. 例：*ex*cretion

exo- *exō* [Gr.] 外。Cf. extra-. 例：*exo*skeleton. (参见 ect-)

extra- *extra* [L.] 外，在……外面，额外。Cf. ect- and exo-. 例：*extra*cellular。(也拼作 extro-)

extro- 参见 extra-。例：*extro*vert

faci- *facies* [L.] 面。Cf. prosop-. 例：*faci*olingual

-facient *facio, facientis, factus, -fectus* [L.] 促成。Cf. poie-. 例：cale*facient*

-fact- 参见 -facient。例：arti*fact*

fasci- *fascia* [L.] 筋膜。例：*fasci*otomy

febr- *febris* [L.] 热。Cf. pyr-. 例：*febr*icity

-fect- 参见 -facient。例：de*fect*ive

femor- *femur* [L.] 股，股骨。

例：*femor*ocele

-ferent *fero, ferentis, latus* [L.] 带来，拿来。Cf. phor-. 例：ef*ferent*

-ferous *ferre* [L.] 产生……的，含有……的。例：lacti*ferous*

ferr- *ferrum* [L.] 铁。例：*ferro*protein

fet- *fetus* [L.] 胎儿。例：*fet*oscope

fibr- *fibra* [L.] 纤维。Cf. in-³. 例：chondro*fibr*oma

fil- *filum* [L.] 丝。例：*fil*iform

fiss- *findo, fissus* [L.] 裂，分裂。Cf. schis-. 例：*fiss*ion

flagell- *flagellum* [L.] 鞭。例：*flagell*ation

flav- *flavus* [L.] 黄。Cf. xanth-. 例：ribo*flav*in。(参见 lute-)

-flect- *flecto, flexus* [L.] 弯曲。例：de*flect*ion

-flex- 参见 -flect-。例：re*flex*ometer

flu- *fluo, fluxus* [L.] 流动。Cf. rhe-. 例：*flu*id

flux- 参见 flu-。例：de*flux*ion

for- *foro* [L.] 孔，口。例：im*for*ate

-form *forma* [L.] 形状。Cf. -oid. 例：cruci*form*

fract- *frango, fractus* [L.] 部分，破碎。例：re*fract*ion

front- *frons, frontis* [L.] 前，前额。例：naso*front*al

-fug(e) *fugio* [L.] 退，驱除。例：vermi*fuge*, centri*fug*al

funct- *fungor, functus* [L.] 功能，机能。例：*funct*ion

fund- *fundo, fusus* [L.] 灌，注。例：in*fund*ibulum。

fus-¹ 参见 fund-。例：dif*fus*ion

fus-² *fusus* [L.] 梭。例：*fus*ocellular

galact- *gala, galactos* [Gr.] 乳。Cf. lact-. 例：*galact*orrhea

gam- *gamos* [Gr.] 婚配。例：*gam*ete

gangli- *ganglion* [Gr.] 神经节。例：*gangli*itis

gastr- *gastēr, gastros* [Gr.] 胃。例：cholangio*gastr*ostomy

ge- *gē* [Gr.] 土，地。例：*ge*ophagia

gelat- *gelo, gelatus* [L.] 冻，凝固。例：*gelat*in

gemin- *geminus* [L.] 两，双。Cf. didym-. 例：quadri*gemin*al

gen-¹ *gignomai, gen-, gon-* [Gr.] 起源，发生。例：endo*gen*ous

gen-² *gennaō* [Gr.] 生殖，起源。例：cyto*gen*ic

-genesis *gen* [Gr.] 生殖，形成。例：patho*genesis*

geni- *geneion* [Gr.] 颏，下巴。例：*geni*al

genit- *genitalis* [L.] 生殖。例：*genit*ourinary

-genous *gen* [Gr.] 产生，形成。例：andro*genous*

ger- *gēras* [Gr.] 老年。例：*ger*oderma

germ- *germen, germinis* [L.] 胚，芽。Cf. blast-. 例：*germ*inal

geront- *gerōn, gerontos* [Gr.] 老年人。例：*geront*ology

gest- *gero, gerentis, gestus* [L.] 妊娠。例：con*gest*ion

gingiv- *gingiva* [L.] 龈。例：*gingiv*itis

gland- *glans, glandis* [L.] 腺。Cf. aden-. 例：uni*gland*ular

gli- *glia* [Gr.] 胶质。例：neuro*glia*, *gli*oma

glomerul- *glomerulus*, dim. of *glomus* [L.] 小球，肾小球。例：*glomerul*onephritis

gloss- *glōssa* [Gr.] 舌。Cf.

lingu-. 例：tricho*gloss*ia

glott- *glōtta* [Gr.] 舌头。Cf. lingu-. 例：*glott*al

gluc- 参见 glyc(y)-。例：*gluc*ophore

glutin- *gluten, glutinis* [L.] 胶。例：ag*glutin*ation

glyc(y)- *glykys* [Gr.] 糖原，葡萄糖。例：*glyc*emia, *glycy*rrhiza。（也拼作 gluc-）

gnath- *gnathos* [Gr.] 颌。例：ortho*gnath*ous

gno- *gignōsō, gnō-* [Gr.] 认知，辨别。例：dia*gno*sis

gon-¹ *gonē* [Gr.] 后代，种子，生殖器官。例：*gon*ocyte, *gon*orrhea

gon-² *gony* [Gr.] 膝。例：*gon*arthritis

gonad- *gonas, gonadis* [L.] 性腺。例：*gonad*ectomy

goni- *gōnia* [Gr.] 角。例：*goni*ometer, *goni*otomy

grad- *gradior* [L.] 行，走。例：retro*grad*e

-gram *gramma* [Gr.] 标记，图。例：cardio*gram*

gran- *granum* [L.] 谷，颗粒。例：lipo*granu*loma

graph- *graphō* [Gr.] 描记，记录。例：angio*graph*y

grav- *gravis* [L.] 重。例：multi*grav*ida

gymn- *gymnos* [Gr.] 裸。例：*gymn*astics

gyn(ec)- *gynē, gynaikos* [Gr.] 女性，雌性。例：andro*gyn*y，*gyn*ecologic

gyr- *gyros* [Gr.] 脑回，环。例：*gyr*ospasm

haem(at)- 参见 hem(at)-。例：*Haem*aphysalis

hamart- *hamartia* [Gr.] 缺陷，错构瘤。例：*hamart*oma

hapl- *haploos* [Gr.] 单一，单独。例：*hapl*otype

hapt- *haptō* [Gr.] 接触，结合。例：*hapt*ics

hect- *hekaton* [Gr.] 百。Cf. centi-. 例：*hect*ogram

hel- *hēlos* [Gr.] 甲，鸡眼，胼胝。例：*hel*oma

helc- *helkos* [Gr.] 溃疡。例：kerato*helc*osis

helic- *helix, helikos* [Gr.] 螺旋。例：*helic*otrema

hem(at)- *haima, haimatos* [Gr.] 血。Cf. sanguin-. 例：*hem*angioma, *hemat*ocele。（参见 -em-）[也拼作 haem(at)-]

hemi- *hēmi* [Gr.] 半。Cf. semi-. 例：*hemi*ageusia

hepat(ic)- *hēpar, hēpatos* [Gr.] 肝。例：*hepat*ocele, *hepatic*olithotomy

hept(a)- *hepta* [Gr.] 七。Cf. sept-². 例：*hepta*chromic, *hept*ose

hered- *heres, beredis* [L.] 遗传。例：*hered*itary

herpet- *herpo, herpet-* [Gr.] 爬。例：*herpet*ic

heter- *heteros* [Gr.] 异，杂。例：*heter*ochromia

hex- *echō, hech-* [Gr.] (hech- added to s becomes hex-) 有，是。例：cach*ex*ia

hex(a)- *hex* [Gr.] 六。Cf. sex-¹. 例：*hex*ose, *hexa*dactyly

hidr- *hidros* [Gr.] 汗。例：hyper*hidr*osis

hipp- *hippos* [Gr.] 马。例：*hippo*campus

hist- *histos* [Gr.] 组织。例：*hist*ocompatibility

hod- *hodos* [Gr.] 路。例：*hod*oneuromere。（参见 -od- 和 -ode¹）

hol- *holos* [Gr.] 全部，完全。例：*hol*osystolic

hom- *homos* [Gr.] 相同。例：*hom*ograft

home- *homoios* [Gr.] 类似。例：*home*ostasis

horm- *ormē* [Gr.] 冲动，脉冲。例：*horm*one

hyal- *hyalos* [Gr.] 玻璃。例：*hyal*oplasm

hydat- *hydōr, hydatos* [Gr.] 水。例：*hydat*id

hydr- *hydōr, hydr-* [Gr.] 水。例：achlor*hydr*ia。（参见 lymph-）

hygr- *hygros* [Gr.] 湿。例：*hygr*ometry

hymen- *hymēn* [Gr.] 膜。例：*Hymen*optera, *hymen*ology

hyp- 参见 hypo-。例：*hyp*axial

hyper- *hyper* [Gr.] 在……之上。Cf. super-。例：*hyper*trophy

hypn- *hypnos* [Gr.] 睡眠。例：*hypn*otic

hypo- *hypo* [Gr.]（o is dropped before words beginning with a vowel）在……之下。Cf. sub-。例：*hypo*calcemia

hyps- *hypsos* [Gr.] 高。例：*hyps*arrhythmia

hyster- *hystera* [Gr.] 子宫。Cf. uter-。例：*hyster*opexy。（参见 metr-²）

-ia *ia* [Gr.] 状态。例：aphas*ia*

iatr- *iatros* [Gr.] 医师。例：pedi*atr*ician

ichthy- *ichthys* [Gr.] 鱼。例：*ichthy*osis

icter- *ikteros* [Gr.] 黄疸。例：*icter*ohepatitis

id- *eidos* [Gr.] 形状，型。例：homin*id*, dermatophyt*id*

idi- *idios* [Gr.] 自体，特异。例：*idi*osyncrasy

il-¹ 参见 in-¹。例：*il*lumination

il-² 参见 in-²。例：*il*legible

ile- 参见 ili-。（ile- 常用于指代小肠的回肠部分）。例：*ile*ostomy

ili- *ilium (ileum)* [L.] 髂骨。（ili- 常用于指代髋关节外上部的髂骨部分）。例：*ili*ofemoral

im-¹ 参见 in-¹。例：*im*mersion

im-² 参见 in-²。例：*im*perforate

in-¹ *in* [L.]（n changes to *l* before *l*, *m* before *b*, *m*, or *p*, and *r* before *r*）在。Cf. en-。例：*in*sertion

in-² *in-* [L.]（n changes to *l* before *l*, *m* before *b*, *m*, or *p*, and *r* before *r*）无，没有。Cf. a-。例：*in*compatible

in-³ *is, inos* [Gr.] 素。Cf. fibr-。例：*in*otropic

infra- *infra* [L.] 下方，低于。例：*infra*orbital

insul- *insula* [L.] 岛。例：*insul*in

inter- *inter* [L.] 间，相互。例：*inter*costal

intra- *intra* [L.] 内，内部。Cf. end- and eso-。例：*intra*venous

intro- *intro* [L.] 在内。例：*intro*spection

ipsi- *ipse* [L.] 相同。例：*ipsi*lateral

ir-¹ 参见 in-¹。例：*ir*radiation

ir-² 参见 in-²。例：*ir*reducible

irid- *iris, iridos* [Gr.] 虹膜。例：*irid*ocyclitis

is- *isos* [Gr.] 相等，同种。例：*is*otope

isch- *ischein* [Gr.] 抑制。例：*isch*emia

ischi- *ischion* [Gr.] 髋，坐骨。例：*ischi*opubic

-ism *-ismos* [Gr.] 情况，状态，……主义。例：vegetarian*ism*, thigmotrop*ism*, alcohol*ism*

-itis *-itis* [Gr.] 炎。例：dermat*itis*, phleb*itis*

-ize *-izein* [Gr.] 动词形后缀。使……成为。例：cauter*ize*, oxid*ize*

jact- *iacio, iactus* [L.] 投掷。例：*jact*itation

-ject *iacio, -iectus* [L.] 投掷。例：in*ject*ion

jejun- *ieiunus* [L.] 空。例：gastro*jejun*ostomy

jug- *iugum* [L.] 联合，接合。例：con*jug*ation

junct- *iungo, junctus* [L.] 联合，接合。例：con*junct*iva

juxta- *juxta* [L.] 接近。例：*juxta*glomerular

kak- *kakos* [Gr.] 不良，有病的。例：*kak*odyl

kary- *karyon* [Gr.] 核。Cf. nucle-。例：mega*kary*ocyte。（也拼作 cary-）

kata- *kata* [Gr.] 下，向下。例：*kata*didymus

kerat- *keras, keratos* [Gr.] 角。例：*kerat*olysis（也拼作 cerat-）

ket- C＝O 酮基。表示拥有羰基。例：*ket*oacidosis

kilo- *chilioi* [Gr.] 千。表示公制中的倍数。Cf. milli-。例：*kilo*gram

kine- *kineō* [Gr.] 运动。例：*kine*scope。（也拼作 cine-）

-kinesis *kineō* [Gr.] 运动，活动。例：hyper*kinesis*

klept- *kleptein* [Gr.] 偷窃。例：*klept*omania

koil- *koilos* [Gr.] 凹，中空。例：*koil*onychia

labi- *labium* [L.] 唇。Cf. cheil-。例：*labi*omental

lact- *lac, lactis* [L.] 乳。Cf. galact-。例：*lact*iferous

lal- *laleō* [Gr.] 言语。例：
glosso*lal*ia

lapar- *lapara* [Gr.] 腹。例：
*lapar*otomy

laryng- *larynx, laryngos* [Gr.]
喉。例：*laryng*ectomy

lat- *fero, latus* [L.] 拿出，带出。
参见 -ferent。例：trans*lat*ion

later- *latus, lateris* [L.] 侧，旁。
例：ventro*later*al

lecith- *lekithos* [Gr.] 卵黄。例：
iso*lecith*al

leio- *leios* [Gr.] 平滑。例：
*leio*myoma

-lemma *lemma* [Gr.] 膜。例：
axo*lemma*

lent- *lens, lentis* [L.] 晶状体。
Cf. phac-. 例：*lent*iconus

lep- *lambanō, lēp* [Gr.] 拿，取，
抓。例：cata*lep*sy

lept- *leptos* [Gr.] 细长的。例：
*lept*omeninges

leuc- 参见 leuk-。例：*leuc*ine

leuk- *leukos* [Gr.] 白。Cf. alb-.
例：*leuk*orrhea。(也拼作 leuc-)

lev- *laevus* [L.] 左。例：
*lev*ocardia, *lev*orotatory

lien- *lien* [L.] 脾脏。Cf. splen-.
例：gastro*lien*al

lig- *ligo* [L.] 韧带。例：*lig*ature

lingu- *lingua* [L.] 舌。Cf. gloss-.
例：sub*lingu*al

lip- *lipos* [Gr.] 脂，脂肪。Cf.
adip-. 例：glyco*lip*id

lith- *lithos* [Gr.] 石。Cf. calc-^{1}.
例：nephro*lith*otomy

loc- *locus* [L.] 地点。Cf. top-. 例：
*loc*omotion

log- *legō, log-* [Gr.] 言语。例：
*log*orrhea, embryo*log*y

loph- *lophos* [Gr.] 脊，丛。例：
*loph*otrichous

lumb- *lumbus* [L.] 腰。例：

*lumb*ago

lute- *luteus* [L.] 黄。Cf. xanth-.
例：*lute*oma。(参见 flav-)

lymph- *lympha* [Gr.] 淋巴。例：
*lymph*adenopathy。(参见 hydr-)

lyo- *lyō* [Gr.] 溶解。Cf. solut-.
例：*lyo*philization

lys- *lysis* [Gr.] 溶化。例：
kerato*lys*is, *lys*ogen

macr- *makros* [Gr.] 长，大。
例：*macr*omyeloblast

mal- *malus* [L.] 坏，不良。Cf.
cac- and dys-. 例：*mal*formation

malac- *malakos* [Gr.] 软化。例：
osteo*malac*ia

mamm- *mamma* [L.] 乳房。Cf.
mast-. 例：sub*mamm*ary

man- *manus* [L.] 手。Cf. cheir-.
例：*man*ipulation

mani- *mania* [Gr.] 精神异常，
躁狂。例：klepto*mani*a

mast- *mastos* [Gr.] 乳房。Cf.
mamm-. 例：hyper*mast*ia

mechan- *mēchanē* [Gr.] 机械。
例：*mechan*oreceptor

medi- *medius* [L.] 中间。Cf.
mes-. 例：*medi*olateral

mega- *megas* [Gr.] 巨，大。例：
*mega*colon, *mega*volt。(参见
megal-)

megal- *megas, megalou* [Gr.] 巨，
大。例：acro*megal*y

mel-^{1} *melos* [Gr.] 肢。例：
sym*mel*ia

mel-^{2} *mēlon* [Gr.] 颊。例：
*mel*oplasty

melan- *melas, melanos* [Gr.] 黑。
例：*melan*ocyte

men- *mēn* [Gr.] 月。例：
dys*men*orrhea

mening- *mēninx, mēningos* [Gr.]
脑膜，脊膜。例：*mening*itis

ment- *mens, mentis* [L.] 颏。Cf.
phren-, psych-, and thym-^{2}. 例：

de*ment*ia

mer-^{1} *meros* [Gr.] part 部分。
例：poly*mer*ic

mer-^{2} *mēros* [Gr.] 股。例：
*mer*algia

mes- *mesos* [Gr.] 正中。Cf.
medi-. 例：*mes*oderm

mesi- *mesos* [Gr.] 近中。例：
*mesi*odens

meta- *meta* [Gr.] (*a* is dropped
before words beginning with
a vowel) 后，旁，次。例：
*meta*carpal, *met*encephalon

-meter *metron* [Gr.] 计量。例：
dia*meter*

metr-^{1} *metron* [Gr.] 测量。例：
audio*metr*y

metr-^{2} *metra* [Gr.] 子宫。Cf.
uter-. 例：endo*metr*itis。(参见
hyster-)

mi- *meiōn* [Gr.] 小。例：*mi*osis

micr- *mikros* [Gr.] 微，小。
也表示公制分数（百万分之
一）。例：photo*micr*ograph,
*micr*ogram

milli- *mille* [L.] 千。也表示公
制分数（千分之一）。Cf. kilo-.
例：*milli*gram, *milli*pede

-mimetic *mimētikos* [Gr.] 模拟，
相似。例：sympatho*mimetic*

mis- *misos* [Gr.] 厌恶，憎恨。
例：*mis*ogamy

miss- 参见 -mittent。例：
intro*miss*ion

mit- *mitos* [Gr.] 线，丝。例：
*mit*ochondria

-mittent *mitto, mittentis, missus*
[L.] 送。例：inter*mittent*

mne- *mimnēskō, mnē-* [Gr.] 记
忆。例：amnesia

mon- *monos* [Gr.] 单一。例：
*mon*oplegia

morph- *morphē* [Gr.] 形态。例：
poly*morph*onuclear

mot- *moveo, motus* [L.] 动，运动。例：vaso*mot*or

muc- *mucus* [L.] 黏液。例：*muci*lage, *muc*ogingival, *muc*oprotein

multi- *multus* [L.] 多。例：*multi*para

my- *mys, myos* [Gr.] 肌肉。例：leio*my*oma

-myces *mykēs, mykētos* [Gr.] 霉菌。例：Strepto*myces*

myc(et)- 参见 -myces。例：strepto*myc*in, *myc*etoma

myel- *myelos* [Gr.] 脊髓。例：polio*myel*itis

myring- *myringa* [L.] 鼓膜。例：*myring*otomy

myx- *myxa* [Gr.] 黏液。例：*myx*edema

nan- *nanos* [Gr.] 矮，小。也表示公制中的分数(十亿分之一)。例：*nan*ophthalmos, *nan*ometer

narc- *narkē* [Gr.] 麻痹。例：*narc*olepsy

nas- *nasus* [L.] 鼻。Cf. rhin-. 例：*nas*opalatine

ne- *neos* [Gr.] 新。例：*ne*onate

necr- *nekros* [Gr.] 尸体。例：*necr*ophilia

nemat- *nēma, nēmatos* [Gr.] 线。例：*nemat*ocide

nephel- *nephelē* [Gr.] 云，雾，浑浊。例：*nephel*ometer

nephr- *nephros* [Gr.] 肾。Cf. ren-. 例：para*nephr*ic

neur- *neuron* [Gr.] 神经。例：*neur*algia

neutr- *neuter* [Gr.] 中。例：*neutr*ophil

nev- *naevus* [L.] 痣。例：*nev*olipoma

noci- *noceo* [L.] 伤害。例：*noci*ceptor

nod- *nodus* [L.] 结节。例：*nod*osity

nom- *nomos* [Gr.] (from *nemō* deal out, distribute) 法规，惯例。例：taxo*nom*y

non-¹ *non* [L.] 不，无。例：*non*disjunction

non-² *nona* [L.] 九。例：*non*apeptide

norm- *norma* [L.] 规则，规定。例：*norm*otensive

nos- *nosos* [Gr.] 疾病。例：*nos*ology

not- *nōton* [Gr.] 后。例：*not*ochord

nucle- *nucleus* [L.] (from *nux, nucis* nut) 核。Cf. kary-. 例：*nucle*ocapsid

nutri- *nutrio* [L.] 营养。例：mal*nutri*tion

nyct- *nyx, nyctos* [Gr.] 夜。例：*nyct*ophobia

nymph- *nymphē* [Gr.] 新娘。例：*nymph*omania, *nymph*otomy

ob- *ob* [L.] (*b* changes to *c* before words beginning with that consonant) 抗，对，靠。例：*ob*tusion

oc- 参见 ob-。例：*oc*clude

oct- *oktō* [Gr.] 或 *octo* [L.] 八。例：*oct*igravida

ocul- *oculus* [L.] 眼。Cf. ophthalm-. 例：*ocul*omotor

-od 参见 ode¹。例：esthes*od*ic

-ode¹ *hodos* [Gr.] 路。例：cath*ode*。(参见 hod-)

-ode² 参见 -oid。例：nemat*ode*

odont- *odous, odontos* [Gr.] 牙。Cf. dent-. 例：orth*odont*ia

odyn- *odynē* [Gr.] 痛苦。例：gastr*odyn*ia, *odyn*ophagia

-oid *eidos* [Gr.] 像……的。Cf. -form. 例：hy*oid*

-ol 参见 ole-。例：cholester*ol*

ole- *oleum* [L.] 油。例：*ole*oresin

olig- *oligos* [Gr.] 低，少。Cf. pauci-. 例：*olig*ospermia

om- *ōmos* [Gr.] 肩。例：*om*oclavicular

-oma *ōma* [Gr.] 名词形后缀。瘤。例：hepat*oma*, carcin*oma*

omphal- *omphalos* [Gr.] 脐。例：*omphal*ectomy

-on *iōn* [Gr.] 离子。例：neutr*on*

onc-¹ *onkos* [Gr.] 大量。例：*onc*ogenesis

onc-² *onkos* [Gr.] 钩，刺。例：*onc*osphere

onch- 参见 onc-²。例：*Onch*ocerca

oneir- *oneiros* [Gr.] 梦。例：*oneir*ism

onych- *onyx, onychos* [Gr.] 爪，甲。例：an*onych*ia

oo- *ōon* [Gr.] 卵。Cf. ov-. 例：*oo*genesis

oophor- *ōophoros* [Gr.] 卵巢。Cf. ovari-. 例：*oophor*ectomy

op- *hōraō, op-* [Gr.] 视力。例：heter*op*sia

ophthalm- *ophthalmos* [Gr.] 眼。Cf. ocul-. 例：ex*ophthalm*os

opisth- *opisthen* [Gr.] 后。例：*opisth*otonos

opt- *hōraō, op-* [Gr.] 可见的，视觉。例：*opt*ics

or- *os, oris* [L.] 嘴。Cf. stom(at)-. 例：intra*or*al

orb- *orbis* [L.] 环。例：sub*orb*ital

orchi- *orchis* [Gr.] 睾丸。Cf. test-. 例：*orchi*opathy

organ- *organon* [Gr.] 器官，机构。例：*organ*omegaly

orth- *orthos* [Gr.] 正。例：*orth*opedics

oscill- *oscillare* [L.] 振动，摇摆。例：*oscill*opsia

-osis *-osis* [Gr.] 名词形后缀。病，病态。例：dermat*osis*, acid*osis*

osm-¹ *osmē* [Gr.] 气味。例：*osm*ophore

osm-² *ōsmos* [Gr.] 冲动。例：*osm*oregulation

oss- *os, ossis* [L.] 骨。Cf. ost(e)-.例：*oss*iferous

ost(e)- *osteon* [Gr.] 骨。Cf. oss-.例：en*ost*osis, *oste*oarthritis

-ostomy *stoma* [Gr.] 造口术。例：col*ostomy*

ot- *ous, ōtos* [Gr.] 耳。Cf. aur-.例：par*ot*id, *ot*otoxic

ov- *ovum* [L.] 卵。Cf. oo-.例：syn*ov*ia, *ov*ovegetarian

ovari- *ovarium* [L.] 卵巢。Cf. oophor-.例：*ovari*opexy

oxy- *oxys* [Gr.]（有时会去掉 y，常表示与氧气有关；氧，氧化）尖锐。例：*oxy*cephalic, *ox*idation

pachy- *pachys* [Gr.] 厚。例：*pachy*derma

pag- *pēgnymi, pag-* [Gr.] 固定。例：thoraco*pag*us

palat- *palatum* [L.] 腭。例：*palat*orrhaphy

pale- *palaios* [Gr.] 旧。例：*pale*ocortex

pali(n)- *palin* [Gr.] 向后。例：*palin*opsia

pan- *pan* [Gr.] 全。例：*Pan*demic

pancreat- *pankréas* [Gr.] 胰。例：*pancreat*ic

par-¹ *pario* [L.] 生育。例：primi*par*a

par-² 参见 para-。例：*par*occipital

para- *para* [Gr.] (final *a* is sometimes dropped before words beginning with a vowel) 旁，外。例：*para*cervical, *para*oral, *par*amnesia

pariet- *paries, parietis* [L.] 墙。例：*pariet*ofrontal

part- *pario, partus* [L.] 生育。例：*part*urition

path- *pathos* [Gr.] 患病。例：psycho*path*ic, cardio*path*y

pauci- *paucus* [L.] 少。Cf. olig-.例：*pauci*synaptic

pec- *pēgnymi, pēg-* [Gr.] (*pēk-* before *t*) 固定。例：amylo*pec*tin。(参见 pex-)

ped-¹ *pais, paidos* [Gr.] 儿童。例：*ped*iatrics

ped-² *pes, pedis* [L.] 足。例：*ped*orthics, *ped*ometer

pell- *pellis* [L.] 皮，皮肤。例：*pell*agra

-pellent *pello, pellentis, pulsus* [L.] 驱，赶。例：chemore*pellent*

pen- *penomai* [Gr.] 缺乏。例：neutro*pen*ia

pend- *pendeo* [L.] 挂。例：ap*pend*ix

pent(a)- *pente* [Gr.] 五。Cf. quint-.例：*pent*ose, *penta*gastrin

peps- *peptō, peps-* [Gr.] 消化。例：eu*peps*ia

pept- *peptō* [Gr.] 消化。例：dys*pept*ic

per- *per* [L.] 穿过。Cf. dia-.例：*per*oral

peri- *peri* [Gr.] 环绕。Cf. circum-.例：*peri*phery

pero- *pēros* [Gr.] 残疾的。例：*pero*melia

pet- *peto* [L.] 寻找。例：centri*pet*al

pex- *pēgnymi, pēg-* [Gr.] (*pēg-* added to *s* becomes *pēx-*) 固定。例：hepato*pexy*

pha- *phēmi, pha-* [Gr.] 说。例：dys*pha*sia

phac- *phakos* [Gr.] 晶状体。Cf. lent-.例：*phac*osclerosis。(也拼作 phak-)

phag- *phagein* [Gr.] 吃。例：dys*phag*ia

phak- 参见 phac-。例：*phak*itis

phalang- *phalanx, phalangos* [Gr.] 指骨，趾骨。例：*phalang*ectomy

phall- *phallos* [Gr.] 阴茎。例：*phall*oplasty

pharmac- *pharmakon* [Gr.] 药学。例：*pharmac*ognosy

pharyng- *pharynx, pharyng-* [Gr.] 咽。例：*pharyng*ocele

-phas- *phasis* [Gr.] 言语。例：a*phas*ia

phe- *phaios* [Gr.] 嗜铬的。例：*phe*ochrome

phen- *phainō, phan-* [Gr.] 表现。例：phos*phen*e, *phen*ocopy

pher- *pherō, phor-* [Gr.] 支持。例：*peri*phery

phil- *phileō* [Gr.] 亲和力，嗜。例：eosino*phil*ia

phleb- *phleps, phlebos* [Gr.] 静脉。Cf. ven-.例：*peri*phlebitis

phleg- *phlogō, phlog-* [Gr.] 发炎。例：*phleg*mon

phlog- 参见 phleg-。例：*phlog*ogenic

phob- *phobos* [Gr.] 恐惧。例：claustro*phob*ia

phon- *phōne* [Gr.] 声，音。例：*phon*ocardiography

phor- 参见 pher-。Cf. -ferent.例：exo*phor*ia

-phoresis *fóresi* [Gr.] 移动。例：electro*phoresis*

phos- 参见 phot-。例：

*phos*phorus

phot- *phōs, phōtos* [Gr.] 光。例：
*phot*ophobia

phrag- *phrassō, phrag-* [Gr.]
隔开，阻止。Cf. sept-¹. 例：
dia*phrag*m

phrax- *phrassō, phrag-* [Gr.]
(*phrag-* added to *s* becomes
phrax-) 隔开，阻止。例：
salpingem*phrax*is

phren- *phrēn* [Gr.] 精神，意志。
Cf. ment-. 例：*phren*oplegia，
*phren*otropic。(参见 psych- 或
thym-²)

phthi- *phthinō* [Gr.] 腐蚀。例：
*phthi*sis

phy- *phyō* [Gr.] 产生。例：
osteo*phy*te

phyc- *phykos* [Gr.] 海藻。例：
*phyc*omycosis

phyl- *phylon* [Gr.] 种族，类别。
例：*phyl*ogeny

phylac- *phylax* [Gr.] 保卫。例：
pro*phylac*tic

phyll- *phyllon* [Gr.] 叶。例：
chloro*phyll*

phys- *physaō* [Gr.] 充气，积气。
例：*phys*ometra

physe- *physaō, physē* [Gr.] 充气，
积气。例：em*physe*ma

physi- *physis* [Gr.] 本质。例：
*physi*ology

phyt- *phyton* [Gr.] 植物。例：
*phyt*obezoar, dermato*phyt*e

pico- *picco* [It.] 兆分之一

picr- *pikr* [Gr.] 苦。例：*picr*ic

-piesis *piesis* [Gr.] 压。例：
aniso*piesis*

pil- *pilus* [L.] 毛发。例：
e*pil*ation

pituit- *pituita* [L.] 黏液。例：
*pituit*ary

placent- *placenta* [L.] {from
plakous [Gr.]} 胎盘。例：

extra*placent*al

plas- *plassō* [Gr.] 成形，塑形。
例：rhino*plas*ty

platy- *platy-* [Gr.] 扁，平。例：
*platy*podia

pleg- *plēssō, pleg-* [Gr.] 瘫痪。
例：di*pleg*ia

pleo- *pleiōn* [Gr.] 多。例：
*pleo*morphism, *pleio*tropy。(也
拼作 pleio-)

plet- *pleo, -pletus* [L.] 多。例：
*plet*hora

pleur- *pleura* [Gr.] 胸膜。Cf.
cost-. 例：*pleur*algia

plex- *plēssō, plēg-* [Gr.] (*plēg-*
added to *s* becomes *plēx-*) 瘫痪。
例：apo*plex*y

plic- *plico* [L.] 褶，襞。例：
com*plic*ation, *plic*ate

pluri- *plus, pluris* [L.] 多。例：
*pluri*glandular

pne- *pneuma, pneumatos* [Gr.] 呼
吸。例：ortho*pne*a

pneum(at)- *pneuma, pneumatos*
[Gr.] 呼吸。例：*pneum*arthrosis,
*pneumat*ocele

pneumo(n)- *pneumōn* [Gr.]
肺。Cf. pulmo(n)-. 例：
*pneumo*enteritis, *pneumon*otomy

pod- *pous, podos* [Gr.] 足。例：
*pod*iatry

poie- *poieō* [Gr.] 产生。Cf.
-facient. 例：sarco*poie*tic

poikil- *poikilos* [Gr.] 有斑点的。
例：*poikil*oderma

pol- *polos* [Gr.] 轴，极。例：
uni*pol*ar

poli- *polios* [Gr.] 灰。例：
*poli*omyelopathy

poly- *polys* [Gr.] 多。例：
*poly*spermy

pont- *pons, pontis* [L.] 脑桥。
例：*pont*ocerebellar

por-¹ *poros* [Gr.] 管道。例：

*por*adenitis

por-² *pōros* [Gr.] 胼胝，老茧。
例：*por*okeratosis

-pos- *posis* [Gr.] 饮。例：
hyper*pos*ia

posit- *pono, positus* [L.] 放，置。
例：re*posit*or

post- *post* [L.] 后。例：
*post*natal, *post*renal

pre- *prae* [L.] 前。例：*pre*natal,
*pre*vesical

presby- *presbys* [Gr.] 老人。例：
*presby*opia

press- *premo, pressus* [L.] 压。
例：*press*oreceptive

pro- *pro* [Gr.] 或 *pro* [L.]
在……之前。例：*pro*hormone,
*pro*labium, *pro*lapse

proct- *prōktos* [Gr.] 肛门。Cf.
rect-. 例：*proct*ology

pros- *prosō* [Gr.] 前。例：
*pros*odemic

prosop- *prosōpon* [Gr.] 面。Cf.
faci-. 例：*prosop*agnosia

prot- *prōtos* [Gr.] 首先。例：
*prot*oplasm

psamm- *psammos* [Gr.] 沙。例：
*psamm*oma

pseud- *pseudēs* [Gr.] 假。例：
*pseud*oparaplegia

psych- *psychē* [Gr.] 精
神，心理。Cf. ment-. 例：
*psych*osomatic。(参见 phren- 或
thym-²)

psychr- *psychros* [Gr.] 冷。例：
*psychr*algia

pto- *piptō, ptō* [Gr.] 下垂。例：
nephro*pto*sis

ptyal- *ptyalon* [Gr.] 涎，唾液。
例：*ptyal*ism

pub- *pubes* [L.] 成年的，成
年人。例：ischio*pub*ic（参见
puber-)

puber- *puber* [L.] 成年的，成年

人。例：puberty

pulmo(n)- *pulmo, pulmonis* [L.] 肺。Cf. pneumo(n)-。例：cardio*pulmon*ary

puls- *pello, pellentis, pulus* [L.] 驱，赶，推进。例：pro*puls*ion

punct- *pungo, punctus* [L.] 穿，刺。Cf. cente-。例：*punct*iform

pupill- *pupilla* [L.] 瞳孔，女孩。例：*pupill*ometry

pur- *pus, puris* [L.] 脓。Cf. py-。例：sup*pur*ation

py- *pyon* [Gr.] 脓。Cf. pur-。例：spondylo*py*osis

pyel- *pyelos* [Gr.] 肾盂。例：nephro*pyel*itis

pyg- *pygē* [Gr.] 臀。例：*pyg*algia

pykn- *pyknos* [Gr.] 浓厚，浓缩。例：*pykn*omorphous。(参见 pycn-)

pyl- *pylē* [Gr.] 门，开口，通路。例：*pyl*ephlebitis

pyr- *pyr* [Gr.] 火。Cf. febr-。例：*pyr*ogen

quadr- *quadr-* [L.] 四。Cf. tetr(a)-。例：*quadr*igeminal

quasi- *quasi* [L.] 类似，似乎。例：*quasi*dominance

quint- *quintus* [L.] 第五。Cf. pent(a)-。例：*quint*uplet

rachi- *rachis* [Gr.] 脊柱。Cf. spin-。例：*rachi*odynia (也拼作 rhachi-)

radi- *radius* [L.] 辐射，放射。Cf. actin-。例：ir*radi*ation, *radi*ocarpal

re- *re-* [L.] 再，又。例：*re*traction

rect- *rectum* [L.] 直肠。Cf. proct-。例：*rect*ocele

ren- *renes* [L.] 肾。Cf. nephr-。例：ad*ren*al, *ren*ography

ret- *rete* [L.] 网。例：*ret*iform

retr- *retro* [L.] 后。例：*retr*odeviation

rhabd- *rhabdos* [Gr.] 杆状。例：*rhabd*omyolysis

rhag- *rhēgnymi, rhag-* [Gr.] 突然发作。例：hemor*rhag*ic

rhaph- *rhaphē* [Gr.] 缝。例：arterior*rhaph*y

rhe- *rheos* [Gr.] 流。Cf. flu-。例：diar*rhe*al

rhex- *rhēgnymi, rhēg-* [Gr.] (*rhēg-* added to *s* becomes *rhēx-*) 突然出现。例：metror*rhex*is

rhin- *rhis, rhinos* [Gr.] 鼻。Cf. nas-。例：*rhin*oplasty

rhiz- *rhiza* [Gr.] 根。例：*rhiz*otomy

rhod- *rhodon* [Gr.] 玫瑰 (色)，红。例：*rhod*opsin

rhytid- *rhytis, rhytidos* [Gr.] 皱纹。例：*rhytid*ectomy

rot- *rota* [L.] 轮。例：*rot*ation

rub(r)- *ruber, rubri* [L.] 红。Cf. erythr-。例：bili*rub*in, *rub*rospinal

sacchar- *sakcharon* [Gr.] 糖。例：*sacchar*ide

sacr- *sacrum* [L.] 骶 (骨)。例：*sacr*algia

salping- *salpinx, salpingos* [Gr.] 管。例：*salping*itis

sangui(n)- *sanguis, sanguinis* [L.] 血。Cf. hem(at)-。例：*sangui*facient, *sangui*neous

sapr- *sapros* [Gr.] 腐败。例：*sapr*ophyte

sarc- *sarx, sarkos* [Gr.] 肌，肉。例：*sarc*oma

scaph- *skaphē* [Gr.] 舟状。例：*scaph*ocephaly

scat- *skōr, skatos* [Gr.] 粪。例：*scat*ology

schis- *schizō, schid-* [Gr.] (*schid-* before *t* or added to *s* becomes

schis-) 裂。Cf. fiss-。例：*schis*tocyte，thoraco*schis*is。(也拼作 schiz-)

schiz- 参见 schis-。例：*schiz*onychia

scirrh- *skirrhos* [Gr.] 硬。例：*scirrh*ous

scler- *sklēros* [Gr.] 硬。Cf. dur-。例：*scler*osis

scoli- *skolios* [Gr.] 弯曲。例：*scoli*okyphosis

scop- *skopeō* [Gr.] 看，视。例：endo*scop*e

scot- *skotos* [Gr.] 黑，暗。例：*scot*ophobia

sect- *seco, sectus* [L.] 切。Cf. tom-。例：*sect*ion

semi- *semi* [L.] 半。Cf. hemi-。例：*semi*flexion

sens- *sentio, sensus* [L.] 感觉，知觉。Cf. esthe-。例：*sens*ory

sep- *sepō* [Gr.] 腐烂。例：*sep*sis

sept-¹ *saepio, saeptus* [L.] 隔 Cf. phrag-。例：*sept*onasal

sept-² *septum* [L.] 七。Cf. hept(a)-。例：*sept*uplet

ser- *serum* [L.] 血清。例：*ser*osynovitis

sex-¹ *sex* [L.] 六。Cf. hex(a)-。例：*sex*tuplet

sex-² *sexus* [L.] 性。例：*sex*duction

sial- *sialon* [Gr.] 唾液，涎。例：*sial*adenitis

sider- *sidēros* [Gr.] 铁。例：*sider*oblast

sin- *sinus* [L.] 窦。Cf. colp-。例：*sin*obronchitis

sinistr- *sinister* [L.] 左。例：*sinistr*ocerebral

-sis *-sis* [Gr.] 状态。例：amebia*sis*，psycho*sis*，diagno*sis*

sit- *sitos* [Gr.] 食物。例：parasi*tic*

solut- *solvo, solventis, solutus* [L.] 溶解，分离。Cf. lyo-。例：dissolution

-solvent 参见 solut-。例：resolvent

som(at)- *sōma, somatos* [Gr.] 体，身体。Cf. corpor-。例：psychosomatic, chromosome

somn- *somnus* [L.] 睡眠。例：somnambulism

spas- *spaō, spas-* [Gr.] 痉挛。例：spasm, spastic

spectr- *spectrum* [L.] 光谱。例：microspectroscope

sperm(at)- *sperma, spermatos* [Gr.] 种子，精子。例：spermicide, spermatozoon

spers- *spargo, -spersus* [L.] 分散。例：dispersion

sphen- *sphēn* [Gr.] 楔形。Cf. cune-。例：sphenoid

spher- *sphaira* [Gr.] 圆形的，球状的。例：hemisphere

sphygm- *sphygmos* [Gr.] 脉搏的。例：sphygmomanometer

spin- *spina* [L.] 脊柱。Cf. rachi-。例：spinocerebellar

spir- *speira* [Gr.] 螺旋。例：spirochete

spir(at)- *spiro, spiratus* [L.] 呼吸。例：spirometry, respiratory

splanchn- *splanchna* [Gr.] 内脏。例：neurosplanchnic

splen- *splēn* [Gr.] 脾。Cf. lien-。例：splenomegaly

spondyl- *spondylos* [Gr.] 脊椎。例：spondylolisthesis

spongi- *spongia* [L.] 海绵。例：spongioblastoma

spor- *sporos* [Gr.] 孢子，芽孢。例：sporocyst, zoospore

squam- *squama* [L.] 疤痕。例：desquamation

sta- *histēmi, sta-* [Gr.] 停。例：hemostasis

stal- *stellō, stal-* [Gr.] 送。例：peristalsis。(参见 -stol-)

staphyl- *staphylē* [Gr.] 葡萄状。例：staphylococcus, staphyline

stear- *stear, steatos* [Gr.] 脂，脂肪。Cf. adip-。例：stearate。(参见 lip-)

steat- 参见 stear-。例：steatorrhea

sten- *stenos* [Gr.] 狭小。例：stenothorax

ster- *stereos* [Gr.] 固体，实体。例：cholesterol

sterc- *stercus* [L.] 粪。Cf. copr-。例：stercoroma

stereo- *stereo* [Gr.] 固体，立体。例：stereotactic

stern- *sternon* [Gr.] 胸骨。例：sternalgia, sternoschisis

steth- *stēthos* [Gr.] 胸。例：stethoscope

sthen- *sthenos* [Gr.] 力，力量。例：asthenia

-stol- *stellō, stol-* [Gr.] 送。例：diastole

stom(at)- *stoma, stomatos* [Gr.] 口，口腔。Cf. or-。例：anastomosis, stomatalgia

-stomy *stoma* [Gr.] 造口术，吻合术。例：ileostomy

strep(h)- *strephō, strep-* (before *t*) [Gr.] 链状，链球菌。Cf. tors-。例：strephosymbolia, streptomycin (参见 stroph-)

strict- *stringo, stringentis, strictus* [L.] 拉紧，压缩（而造成疼痛）。例：constriction

-stringent 参见 strict-。例：astringent

stroph- *strephō, stroph-* [Gr.] 扭，斜，旋。Cf. tors-。例：diastrophic。(参见 strep(h)-)

struct- *struo, structus* [L.] 堆积。例：obstruction

styl- *stilus* [L.] 茎状，茎突。例：stylohyoid

sub- *sub* [L.] (*b* changes to *f* and *p* before words beginning with those con- sonants) 下，次。Cf. hypo-。例：sublingual

suf- 参见 sub-。例：suffusion

sup- 参见 sub-。例：suppository

super- *super* [L.] 上，外。Cf. hyper-。例：supermotility

supra- *supra* [L.] 上，在上。例：supraduction

sy- 参见 syn-。例：systole

sym- 参见 syn-。例：symbiosis, symmetry, sympathetic, symphysis

syn- (*n* disappears before *s*, changes to *l* before *l*, and changes to *m* before *b, m, p,* and *ph*) 连，联合，共同。Cf. con-。例：Synarthrosis

syndesm- *syndes* [Gr.] 结缔组织，韧带。例：syndesmophyte

syring- *syrinx, syringos* [Gr.] 管，瘘。例：syringocystadenoma

ta- 参见 ton-。例：ectasia

tac- *tassō, tag-* [Gr.] (*tag-* changes to *tak-,* which becomes *tac-,* before *t*) 指令，安排。例：atactiform

tach(y)- *tachys* [Gr.] 快速，急。例：tachography, tachycardia

tact- *tango, tactus* [L.] 触，接触。例：contact

taenia- *taenia* [L.] 丝带，绦虫。例：taeniafuge。(也拼作 tenia-)

tars- *tarsos* [Gr.] 睑板，跗骨。例：tarsorrhaphy, tarsoclasis

taut- *tautos* [Gr.] 相同，同一。例：tautomerism

tax- *tassō, tag-* [Gr.] (*tag-* added to *s* becomes *tax-*) 排列，类别。例：ataxia

tect- 参见 teg-。例：protective

teg- *tego, tectus* [L.] 覆盖。例：integument

tel- *telos* [Gr.] 末端。例：telomere

tele- *tēle* [Gr.] 远距离。例：teleceptor

tempor- *tempus, temporis* [L.] 时间。例：temporomandibular

tend(in)- *tendo, tendines* [L.] 腱。例：tendovaginal, tendinitis

ten(ont)- *tenōn, tenontos* [Gr.] (from *teinō* stretch) 腱。例：tenodynia, tenontology

tens- *tendo, tensus* [L.] 伸展。Cf. ton-. 例：extensor

terat- *teras, teratos* [Gr.] 畸形。例：teratoma

ter(ti)- *ter* [L.] 三次。Cf. tri-. 例：ternary, tertigravida

test- *testis* [L.] 睾丸。Cf. orchi-. 例：testitis

tetr(a)- *tetra-* [Gr.] 四。Cf. quadr-. 例：tetradactyly

thanat- *thanatos* [Gr.] 死。例：thanatophobia

the- *tithēmi, thē-* [Gr.] 放，置。例：synthesis

thec- *thēkē* [Gr.] 膜。例：thecostegnosis

thel(e)- *thēlē* [Gr.] 乳头。例：thelerethism, theleplasty

therap- *therapeia* [Gr.] 治疗。例：chemotherapy

therm- *thermē* [Gr.] 热。Cf. calor-. 例：diathermy

thi- *theion* [Gr.] 硫。例：thiol, thiocyanate

thigm- *thigma* [Gr.] 触。例：thigmotaxis

thorac- *thōrax, thōrakos* [Gr.] 胸。例：thoracoplasty

-thrix 参见 trich-。例：monilethrix

thromb- *thrombos* [Gr.] 血栓，凝块。例：thrombocytopenia

thym-¹ *thymos* [Gr.] 胸腺，凝块。例：thymoma

thym-² *thymos* [Gr.] 精神，心灵。Cf. ment-. 例：dysthymia, thymoleptic。（参见 phren- 和 psych-）

thyr- *thyreos* [Gr.] [shaped like a door (*thyra*)] 保护。例：thyroid

-tme- *temnō, tmē-* [Gr.] 切。例：axonotmesis

toc- *tokos* [Gr.] 分娩，生育。例：dystocia。（也拼作 tok）

tom- *temnō, tom-* [Gr.] 切，割。Cf. sect-. 例：appendectomy, tomography

ton- *teino, ton-, ta-* [Gr.] 张力，紧张，强直。Cf. tens-. 例：peritoneum

top- *topos* [Gr.] 局部，部位。Cf. loc-. 例：topesthesia, isotope

tors- *torqueo, torsus* [L.] 扭曲，弯曲。Cf. strep(h)- and stroph-. 例：torsion

tox(ic)- *toxikon* [Gr.]（from *toxon* bow）毒。例：toxemia, toxicology

trache- *tracheia* [Gr.] 气管。例：tracheotomy

trachel- *trachēlos* [Gr.] 颈，项。Cf. cervic-. 例：trachelopexy

tract- *traho, tractus* [L.] 拖，拉。例：protraction

trans- *trans* [L.] 穿过，经过。例：transaortic, transfection

traumat- *trauma, traumatos* [Gr.] 创伤。例：traumatic

trepo- *trepō* [Gr.] 旋转，转动。例：trepopnea, treponema

tri- *treis, tria* [Gr.] 或 *tri-* [L.] 三。Cf. ter(ti)-. 例：trilaminar

trich- *thrix, trichos* [Gr.] 发。例：trichobezoar

trip- *tribō* [Gr.] 摩擦。例：lithotripsy

trop- *trepō, trop-* [Gr.] 转，反应。例：sitotropism

troph- *trepō, troph-* [Gr.] 营养。例：atrophy

tub- *tubus* [L.] 管。例：tuboplasty

tuber- *tuber* [L.] 结节，肿块。例：tubercle

tympan- *tympanon* [Gr.] 鼓，鼓膜。例：tympanocentesis

typ- *typos* [Gr.] (from *typto* strike) 类型。例：atypical

typh- *typhos* [Gr.] 伤寒。例：typhus

tyr- *tyros* [Gr.] 酪，干酪。例：tyromatosis

ul-¹ *oulē* [Gr.] 瘢痕。例：ulerythema

ul-² *oulon* [Gr.] 牙龈。例：ulotomy

-ulose 酮

ultra- *ultra* [L.] 外。例：ultrastructure

uni- *unus* [L.] 单，一。例：unilateral

ur- *ouron* [Gr.] 尿。例：polyuria

uran- *ouran* [Gr.] 腭。例：brachyuranic

-uresis *ourēsis* [Gr.] 排尿。例：enuresis

ureter- *ourētēr* [Gr.] 输尿管。例：ureterography

urethr- *ourēthra* [Gr.] 尿道。例：urethropexy

-uria *ouria* [Gr.] 尿。例：albinuria

uter- *uterus* [L.] 子宫。Cf. hyster- and metr-². 例：uterorectal

vacc- *vacca* [L.] 接种，牛痘接种。例：vaccine

vagin- *vagina* [L.] 阴道，鞘。例：invagination, vaginitis

varic- *varix, varicis* [L.] 静脉曲张。例：varicocele

vas- *vas* [L.] 血管，脉管。Cf. angi-. 例：vascular

ven- *vena* [L.] 静脉。Cf. phleb-. 例：venopressor

ventr- *venter* [L.] 腹侧。例：ventrofixation, ventriculotomy

vers- 参见 vert-。例：inversion

vert- *verto, versus* [L.] 转。例：diverticulum

vesic- *vesica* [L.] 膀胱，泡。Cf. cyst-. 例：vesicovaginal

video- *video* [L.] 看。例：videolaparoscopy

viscer- *viscus, visceris* [L.] 内脏。例：visceromotor

vit- *vita* [L.] 生命。Cf. bi-[1]. 例：devitalize

vivi- *vivus* [L.] 获得。例：viviparous

vuls- *vello, vulsus* [L.] 牵拉，痉挛。例：convulsion

xanth- *xanthos* [Gr.] 黄。Cf. flav- and lute-. 例：xanthochromia

xen- *xenos* [Gr.] 外来的，异物。例：xenograft

xer- *xēros* [Gr.] 干燥。例：xeroderma

xiph- *xiphos* [Gr.] 剑，剑突。例：xiphocostal

-yl- *hyle* [Gr.] 物质。例：carboxyl

zo- *zoē* [Gr.] 生命，或 *zōon* [Gr.] 动物。例：microzoon

zyg- *zygon* [Gr.] 轭，结合。例：zygapophysis

zym- *zymē* [Gr.] 酶，发酵。例：enzyme

目　录

A

A　accommodation 适应，调节；adenine or adenosine 腺苷酸或腺苷；alanine 丙氨酸；ampere 安培；anode 阳极；anterior 前面的

A　absorbance 吸光度；见 activity (3)；area 面积；mass number 质量数

A₂　aortic second sound 主动脉瓣第二音

Å　angstrom 埃的符号

a　accommodation 调节，适应；atto- 阿托

a.　[L.] an′num (year) 年；a′qua (water) 水；arte′ria (artery) 动脉

a　见 activity (2)

α　(alpha, the first letter of the Greek alphabet) 阿尔法（希腊字母表的第一个字母）；heavy chain of IgA 重链免疫球蛋白；α chain of hemoglobin 血红蛋白 α 链

α-　前缀 (1) the position of a substituting atom or group in a chemical compound 取代原子或基团在化合物中的位置；(2) the specific rotation of an optically active compound 旋光化合物的比旋光度；(3) the orientation of an exocyclic atom or group 环外原子或基团的定向；(4) a plasma protein migrating with the α band in electrophoresis 电泳中沿 α 带迁移的血浆蛋白；(5) first in a series of related entities or chemical compounds 相关化合物系列中的一种

AA　achievement age 成就年龄；Alcoholics Anonymous 嗜酒者互诫协会；amino acid 氨基酸

A̅A̅　ana (of each), used in prescription writing ana 各处方用语

aa.　[L.] arte′riae (arteries) 动脉

AAA　American Association of Anatomists 美国解剖学家协会

AAAA　American Academy of Anesthesiologist Assistants 美国麻醉师助理学会

AAAAI　American Academy of Allergy Asthma and Immunology 美国过敏性哮喘与免疫学会

AAAS　American Association for the Advancement of Science 美国科学发展协会

AAB　American Association of Bioanalysts 美国生物分析师协会

AABB　American Association of Blood Banks 美国血库协会

AAC　abnormal anterior coaptation 异常前联合

AACA　American Association of Clinical Anatomists 美国临床解剖学家协会

AACAP　American Academy of Child and Adolescent Psychiatry 美国儿童与青少年精神病学会

AACC　American Association for Clinical Chemistry 美国临床化学协会

AACE　American Association of Clinical EndoCrinologists 美国临床内分泌学家协会

AACH　American Academy on Communication in Healthcare 美国医疗通信学会

AACN　American Association of Colleges of Nursing 美国护理学院协会；American Association of Critical-Care Nurses 美国危重病人护理协会

AAD　American Academy of Dermatology 美国皮肤病学会

AADS　American Association of Dental Schools 美国牙科学校协会

AAE　American Association of Endodontists 美国牙髓病学家协会

AAEP　American Association of Equine Practitioners 美国马术从业者协会

AAFP　American Academy of Family Physicians 美国家庭医师学会

AAGP　American Association for Geriatric Psychiatry 美国老年精神病学会

AAHA　American Animal Hospital Association 美国动物医院协会

AAHC　American Association of Healthcare Consultants 美国医疗顾问协会；Association of Academic Health Centers 学术健康中心协会；American Accreditation HealthCare Commission, Inc. 美国认证医疗委员会

AAHD　American Association of Hospital Dentists 美国医院牙科医师协会

AAHE　Association for the Advancement of Health Education 卫生教育发展协会

AAHPER　American Alliance for Health, Physical Education, Recreation and Dance 美国健康、体育、娱乐和舞蹈联盟

AAHS　American Association for Hand Surgery 美国手外科协会

AAHSL　Association of Academic Health Sciences Libraries 学术健康科学图书馆协会

AAI　American Association of Immunologists 美国免疫学家协会

AAID　American Academy of Implant Dentistry 美国植牙学会

AALNC　American Association of Legal Nurse Consultants 美国法律护士顾问协会

AAMA　American Association of Medical Assistants 美国医疗护理协会

AAMC　American Association of Medical Colleges 美国医学院协会

AAMFT　American Association for Marriage and Family Therapy 美国婚姻家庭治疗协会

AAMI　Association for the Advancement of Medical Instrumentation 医疗器械进步协会

AAMP　American Academy of Maxillofacial Prosthetics 美国上颌面修复学会；American

Association of Medical Personnel 美国医务人员协会

AAMT American Association for Medical Transcription 美国医学转录协会

AAN American Academy of Neurology 美国神经病学学会；American Academy of Nursing 美国护理学会

AANA American Association of Nurse Anesthetists 美国护士麻醉师协会

AANN American Association of Neuroscience Nurses 美国神经科学护士协会

AANP American Association of Nurse Practitioners 美国执业护士协会；American Association of Naturopathic Physicians 美国自然疗法医师协会；American Association of Neuropathologists 美国执业护士协会

AAO American Academy of Ophthalmology 美国眼科协会；American Academy of Optometry 美国视力测定协会；American Academy of Osteopathy 美国骨病协会；American Academy of Otolaryngology 美国耳鼻咽喉科学会；American Association of Orthodontists 美国牙齿矫正医师协会

AAOHN American Association of Occupational Health Nurses 美国职业健康护士协会

AAO-HNS American Academy of Otolaryngology–Head and Neck Surgery 美国耳鼻咽喉学会头颈外科

AAOM American Academy of Oral Medicine 美国口腔医学会；American Association of Oriental Medicine 美国中医学会；American Association of Orthopaedic Medicine 美国骨科医学协会

AAOMR American Academy of Oral and Maxillofacial Radiology 美国口腔和颌面放射学会

AAOMS American Association of Oral and Maxillofacial Surgery 美国口腔颌面外科协会

AAOP American Academy of Oral Pathology 美国口腔病理学会

AAOS American Academy of Orthopaedic Surgeons 美国骨科医师学会

AAP American Academy of Pediatrics 美国儿科学会；American Academy of Pedodontics 美国儿童牙科学会；American Academy of Periodontology 美国牙周病学会；American Academy of Psychotherapists 美国心理治疗师学会；American Association of Pathologists 美国病理学家协会；Association of American Physicians 美国医师协会

AAPA American Academy of Physician Assistants 美国助理医师学会；American Association of Pathologists' Assistants 美国病理学家协会

AAPCC American Association of Poison Control Centers 美国毒物控制中心协会

AAPD American Academy of Pediatric Dentists 美国儿科牙医学会

AAPHD American Association of Public Health Dentistry 美国公共卫生牙科协会

AAPHP American Association of Public Health Physicians 美国公共卫生医师协会

AAPM American Academy of Pain Medicine 美国疼痛学会；American Association of Physicists in Medicine 美国医学物理学家协会

AAPM&R American Academy of Physical Medicine and Rehabilitation 美国物理医学与康复学会

AAPS American Association of Pharmaceutical Scientists 美国药学科学家协会；American Association of Plastic SurGeons 美国整形外科医师协会；Association of American Physicians and Surgeons 美国内科和外科医生协会

AARC American Association for Respiratory Care 美国呼吸治疗协会

AART American Association for Rehabilitation Therapy 美国康复疗法协会

AAS 1. abuse assessment screening 滥用评估筛选；2. American Analgesia Society 美国镇痛学会；3. anabolic-androgenic steroid 促合成代谢的雄激素类固醇

AAST American Association for the Surgery of Trauma 美国创伤外科协会

AATA American Art Therapy Association 美国艺术治疗协会

AATS American Association for Thoracic Surgery 美国胸外科协会

AB [L.] Ar′tium Baccalau′reus (Bachelor of Arts) 文学士

Ab antibody 抗体

ab [L.] preposition *from* 介词，从

ab- word element [L.], *from* 构词成分，从；*off* 离开；*away from* 远离

ABA American Burn Association 美国烧伤协会

abac·a·vir (ə-bak′ə-vir) a nucleoside analogue reverse transcriptase inhibitor used as the sulfate salt as an antiretroviral in the treatment of human immunodeficiency virus infection 阿巴卡韦

abar·og·no·sis (a″bar-əg-no′sis) baragnosis 压觉缺失，辨重不能

ab·ar·thro·sis (ab″ahr-thro′sis) abarticulation 可动关节

ab·ar·tic·u·la·tion (ab″ahr-tik″u-la′shən)1. synovial joint 滑膜关节；2. dislocation of a joint 关节脱位

aba·sia (ə-ba′zhə) inability to walk 步行不能；**aba′sic, abat′ic** adj. a.-asta′sia, astasia-abasia 步行不能的；a.atac′tica, abasia with uncertain movements, due to a defect of coordination 共济失调；**choreic a.,** abasia due to chorea of the legs 舞蹈病性步行不能；**paralytic a.,** abasia due to paralysis of leg muscles 麻痹性步行不能，由于腿部肌肉麻

痹而失去知觉；**paroxysmal trepidant a., spastic a.**, abasia due to spastic stiffening of the legs on attempting to stand 阵发震颤性步行不能；**a. tre′pidans**, abasia due to trembling of the legs 震颤性步行不能

ABAT American Board of Applied Toxicology 美国应用毒理学委员会

ab·a·ta·cept (ab″ə-ta′sept) a synthetic recombinant protein that acts as an inhibitor of T-cell activation; used in the treatment of moderate to severe rheumatoid arthritis unresponsive to other medications 阿巴西普

abate·ment (ə-bāt′mənt) decrease in severity of a pain or symptom 减少，减轻（痛或症状）

ABC argon beam coagulator 氩气刀；aspiration biopsy cytology 针吸活检细胞学

ab·cix·i·mab (ab-sik′sĭ-mab) a human-murine monoclonal antibody Fab fragment that inhibits the aggregation of platelets, used as an antithrombotic in percutaneous transluminal coronary angioplasty 阿昔单抗；抗原综合片段

ABCP American Board of Cardiovascular Perfusion 美国心血管灌注委员会

ab·do·men (ab′də-mən) (ab-do′mən) that part of the body lying between the thorax and the pelvis, and containing the abdominal cavity and viscera 腹（部）身体位于胸腔和盆腔之间的部分；**acute a.**, an acute intra-abdominal condition of abrupt onset, usually associated with pain due to inflammation, perforation, obstruction, infarction, or rupture of abdominal organs, and usually requiring emergency surgical intervention 急腹症；**carinate a., navicular a.**, 见 scaphoid a.；**a. obsti′pum**, congenital shortness of the rectus abdominis muscle. 曲腹（腹直肌先天性短缩）；**scaphoid a.**, one whose anterior wall is hollowed, occurring in children with cerebral disease 舟状腹 **surgical a.**, 见 acute a.

ab·dom·i·nal (ab-dom′ĭ-nəl) pertaining to the abdomen 腹的

ab·dom·i·no·cen·te·sis (ab-dom″ĭ-no-sente′sis) surgical puncture of the abdomen 腹腔穿刺术

ab·dom·i·no·cys·tic (ab-dom″ĭ-no-sis′tik) pertaining to the abdomen and gallbladder 腹胆囊的

ab·dom·i·no·hys·ter·ec·to·my (ab-dom″ino-his″tər-ek′tə-me) hysterectomy through an abdominal incision 剖腹子宫切除术，腹式子宫切除术

ab·dom·i·no·hys·ter·ot·o·my (ab-dom″ĭnohis″tər-ot′ə-me) abdominal hysterotomy 剖腹子宫切开术，腹式子宫切开术

ab·dom·i·no·vag·i·nal (ab-dom″ĭ-no-vaj′ĭnəl) pertaining to the abdomen and vagina 腹阴道的

ab·dom·i·no·ves·i·cal (ab-dom″ĭ-no-ves′ĭkəl) 1. abdominocystic 腹胆囊的；2. pertaining to or connecting the abdominal cavity and urinary bladder 属于或连接腹腔和膀胱的

ab·du·cens (ab-doo′sənz) [L.] abducent 外展的

ab·du·cent (ab-doo′sənt) serving to abduct a part 外展的一部分

ab·duct (ab-dukt′) to draw away from the median plane, or (the digits) from the axial line of a limb （外）展；**abdu′cent** adj. （外）展的

ab·duc·tion (ab-duk′shən) the act of abducting; the state of being abducted 外展的动作或状态

ab·duc·tor (ab-duk′tor) that which abducts 展肌，另见 muscle 下词条和图 6

ab·er·ran·cy (ab-er′ən-se) 见 aberration (3)

ab·er·rant (ă-ber′ənt) (ab′ər-ənt) wandering or deviating from the usual or normal course 违反常规的；反常的

ab·er·ra·tio (ab″ər-a′she-o) [L.] 见 aberration (1)

ab·er·ra·tion (ab″ər-a′shən) 1. deviation from the normal or usual 离，偏差；2. unequal refraction or focalization of a lens 光行差；3. in cardiology, aberrant conduction （心脏中）异常传导的；**chromatic a.**, unequal refraction of light rays of different wavelength, producing a blurred image with fringes of color 色象差；**chromosome a.**, an irregularity in the number or structure of chromosomes, usually a gain, loss, exchange, or alteration of sequence of genetic material, which often alters embryonic development 染色体畸变；**intraventricular a.**, aberrant conduction within the ventricles of an impulse generated in the supraventricular region, excluding abnormalities due to fixed organic defects in conduction 心室内差异性传导；**mental a.**, any pathological deviation from normal mental activity, usually limited to a circumscribed deviation in an otherwise adapted individual 精神错乱

abeta·lipo·pro·tein·emia (a-ba″tə-lip″opro″te-ne′me-ə) an autosomal recessive disorder affecting the transfer of lipid to apolipoprotein (apo) B, marked by lack of apo B–containing lipoproteins (chylomicrons, VLDLs, and LDLs) in blood and by acanthocytosis, hypocholesterolemia, progressive ataxia, atypical retinitis pigmentosa, and intestinal lipid malabsorption 无 β- 脂蛋白血症

ABGC American Board of Genetic Counseling 美国遗传咨询委员会

abi·os·is (a″bi-o′sis) absence of life 无生命；生命力缺损；**abiot′ic** adj. 无生命的；生命力缺损的

abi·ot·ro·phy (a″bi-ot′rə-fe) progressive loss of vitality of certain tissues, leading to disorders 某些组织的活力逐渐丧失，导致疾病；applied to degenerative hereditary diseases of late onset, e.g.,

Huntington chorea 适用于晚发性退行性遗传病，如亨廷顿舞蹈症

abir·at·er·one (ab″ir-at′ər-ōn) a 17 α -hydroxylase inhibitor used in the treatment of metastatic castration-resistant prostate cancer 阿比特龙

ab·late (ab-lāt′) to remove, especially by cutting; to extirpate 消除，尤指切除

ab·la·tion (ab-la′shən) 1. separation or detachment; extirpation; eradication 脱离；2. removal or destruction, especially by cutting 部分切除术；**transurethral needle a. (TUNA)**, production of localized necrotic lesions of the prostate using radiofrequency energy delivered through interstitial needles inserted via the urethra into the prostate; used in the treatment of benign prostatic hyperplasia 经尿道针刺消融术

able·pha·ria (a″blĕ-far′e-ə) cryptophthalmos 无睑畸形；**ableph′arous** adj. 无睑畸形的

ABMG American Board of Medical Genetics 美国医学遗传学会

ABMS American Board of Medical Specialties 美国医学专业委员会

ab·nor·mal (ab-nor′məl) not normal; contrary to the usual structure, position, condition, behavior, or rule 异常的，反常的

ab·nor·mal·i·ty (ab″nor-mal′ĭ-te) 1. the state of being abnormal 反常，异常；2. a malformation 畸形

abo·bot·u·li·num·tox·in A (ab″o-boch″u-li′nəm-tok″sin) a preparation of botulinum toxin type A, used to treat cervical dystonia and glabellar lines A 型肉毒杆菌毒素

ABOHN American Board for Occupational Health Nurses 美国职业健康护士委员会

ab·orad (ab-or′ad) directed away from the mouth 离口

ab·oral (ab-or′əl) opposite to, away from, or remote from the mouth 离口的，远口的

abort (ə-bort′) 1. to arrest prematurely a disease or developmental process 过早地阻止疾病或发育过程；2. to cause, undergo, or experience abortion 使流产；3. to become checked in development 在发展中阻止

abor·ti·fa·cient (ə-bor″tĭ-fa′shənt) 1. causing abortion 堕胎的；2. an agent that induces abortion 堕胎药

abor·tion (ə-bor′shən) 1. expulsion from the uterus of the products of conception before the fetus is viable 流产；2. premature stoppage of a natural or a pathological process 顿挫；**artificial a.**, 见 induced a.; **complete a.**, one in which all the products of conception are expelled from the uterus and identified 完全流产；**habitual a.**, spontaneous abortion occurring in three or more successive pregnancies, at about the same level

of development 习惯性流产；**incomplete a.**, that with retention of parts of the products of conception 不全流产；**induced a.**, that brought on intentionally by medication or instrumentation 人工流产；**inevitable a.**, a condition in which vaginal bleeding has been profuse, the cervix has become dilated, and abortion will invariably occur 难免流产；**infected a.**, that associated with infection of the genital tract 感染性流产；**missed a.**, retention in the uterus of an abortus that has been dead for at least eight weeks 过期流产；**septic a.**, that associated with serious infection of the uterus leading to generalized infection 脓毒性流产；**spontaneous a.**, that occurring naturally 自发性流产；**therapeutic a.**, that induced for medical considerations 治疗性流产；**threatened a.**, a condition in which vaginal bleeding is less than in inevitable abortion, the cervix is not dilated, and abortion may or may not occur 先兆流产

abor·tive (ə-bor′tiv) 1. incompletely developed 不全发育的；2. 见 abortifacient (1); 3. cutting short the course of a disease 缩短病程

abor·tus (ə-bor′təs) a fetus weighing less than 500 g or having completed less than 20 weeks' gestational age at the time of expulsion from the uterus, having no chance of survival 流产胎儿（体重小于500g 或胎龄小于 20 周）

ABPANC American Board of Perianesthesia Nursing Certification 美国麻醉护理认证委员会

abra·sion (ə-bra′zhən) 1. a rubbing or scraping off through unusual or abnormal action 磨损，磨耗；另见 planing；2. a rubbed or scraped area on skin or mucous membrane 擦伤

abra·sive (ə-bra′siv) 1. causing abrasion 磨损的；2. an agent that produces abrasion 产生磨损的药剂

ab·re·ac·tion (ab″re-ak′shən) the reliving of an experience in such a way that previously repressed emotions associated with it are released 疏泄，精神发泄

ab·rup·tio (ab-rup′she-o) [L.] separation 分离，分开；**a. placen′tae**, premature detachment of the placenta 胎盘早期脱离

ab·scess (ab′ses) a localized collection of pus within tissues, organs, or confined spaces 脓肿；**amebic a.**, one caused by *Entamoeba histolytica*, usually occurring in the liver but also in the lungs, brain, and spleen 阿米巴脓肿；**alveolar a.**, 见 apical a. (2); **apical a.**, 1. an abscess at the apex of an organ 尖端脓肿；2. a suppurative inflammatory reaction involving the tissues surrounding the apical portion of a tooth, occurring in acute and chronic forms 牙槽脓肿；**appendiceal a.**, **appendicular a.**, one resulting from perforation of an acutely inflamed appendix 阑尾脓肿；**Bartholin a.**, acute infection of the excretory duct of a Bartholin gland 巴氏腺囊肿；**Bezold a.**, one deep in the neck as a complication of acute mastoiditis 贝佐尔德脓肿 ; **brain a.,** one affecting the brain as a result of extension of an infection (e.g., otitis media) from an adjacent area, or through bloodborne infection. 脑脓肿 ; **Brodie a.,** a roughly spherical region of bone destruction, filled with pus or connective tissue, usually in the metaphyseal region of long bones and caused by *Staphylococcus aureus* or *S. albus* 布罗迪脓肿 ; **cold a.,** 1. one of slow development and with little inflammation 冷脓肿 ; 2. tuberculous a. 结核性脓肿 ; **collar button a.,** a superficial abscess connected with a deeper one by a fistulous tract 哑铃形脓肿 ; **diffuse a.,** a collection of pus not enclosed by a capsule 弥漫性脓肿 ; **gas a.,** one containing gas, caused by gas-forming bacteria such as *Clostridium perfringens* 气脓肿 ; **miliary a.,** any of a group of small multiple abscesses 粟粒状脓肿 ; **Pautrier a.,** 见 *microabsces* 下一条 ; **perianal a.,** one beneath the skin of the anus and the anal canal 肛周脓肿 ; **periodontal a.,** a localized collection of pus in the periodontal tissue 牙周脓肿 ; **peritonsillar a.,** one in the connective tissue of the tonsil capsule, from suppuration of the tonsil 扁桃体周脓肿 ; **phlegmonous a.,** one associated with acute inflammation of the subcutaneous connective tissue 蜂窝织炎脓肿 ; **ring a.,** a ring-shaped purulent infiltration at the periphery of the cornea 环形脓肿 ; **septicemic a.,** one due to septicemia 败血症性脓肿 ; **stitch a.,** one developed around a stitch or suture 缝线脓肿 ; **thecal a.,** one arising in a sheath, as in a tendon sheath 腱鞘脓肿 ; **tuberculous a.,** one due to infection with tubercle bacilli 结核性脓肿 ; **vitreous a.,** an abscess of the vitreous humor, resulting from infection, trauma, or foreign body 玻璃体脓肿 ; **wandering a.,** one that burrows into tissues and finally points at a distance from the site of origin 游走性脓肿 ; **Welch a.,** 见 gas a.

ab·scis·sa (*x*) (ab-sis'ə) the horizontal line in a graph along which are plotted the units of one of the factors considered in the study 横坐标

ab·scis·sion (ab-sĭ'zhən) removal by cutting 切除

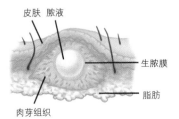

皮肤　脓液

生脓膜

脂肪

肉芽组织

▲ 脓肿（**abscess**）的横截面

ab·scop·al (ab-sko'pəl) pertaining to the effect on nonirradiated tissue resulting from irradiation of other tissue of the organism 远位的，用于修饰因辐照生物体组织而对非辐照组织的影响

Ab·sid·ia (ab-sid'e-ə) a genus of fungi of the order Mucorales, commonly found as environmental contaminants. *A. corymbi'fera* can cause mucormycosis 犁头霉属

ab·so·lute (ab'sə-loot) free from limitations; unlimited 不受限制的 ; uncombined 未结合的

ab·sorb (ab-sorb') 1. to take in or assimilate, as to take up substances into or across tissues, e.g., the skin or intestine 吸收，物质通过组织（例如皮肤，肠壁）进行吸收 ; 2. to react with radiation energy so as to attenuate it 对辐射线的反应进行而使之衰减 ; 3. to retain specific wavelengths of radiation incident upon a substance, either raising its temperature or changing the energy state of its molecules 保持放射线在其放射的物质的特色波长或提高其被放射物质的温度或者是改变其物质分子的能量状态

ab·sorb·able (ab-sorb'ə-bəl) capable of being absorbed 能被吸收的

ab·sor·bance (ab-sor'bəns) 1. in analytical chemistry, a measure of the light that a solution does not transmit compared to a pure solution 分析化学中指吸光度 ; 2. in radiology, a measure of the ability of a medium to absorb radiation, expressed as the logarithm of the ratio of the intensity of the radiation entering the medium to that leaving it 放射学中指吸收率（一种介质吸收放射能力的量度）

ab·sor·be·fa·cient (ab-sor"bə-fa'shənt) 1. causing or promoting absorption 引起或促进吸收 ; 2. 见 absorbent (3)

ab·sor·bent (ab-sor'bənt) 1. able to take in, or suck up and incorporate 能吸收的 ; 2. a tissue structure involved in absorption 吸收剂 ; 3. a substance that absorbs or promotes absorption 吸收作用

ab·sorp·tion (ab-sorp'shən) 1. the uptake of substances into or across tissues 吸收 ; 2. in psychology, devotion of thought to one object or activity only 心理学上的精神集中在某一物体或某一行动 ; 3. in radiology, uptake of energy by matter with which radiation interacts 放射学上指与辐射相互作用的物质对能量的吸收 ; 4. in chemistry, the penetration of a substance within the inner structure of another 化学上指一种物质在另一种物质内部结构中的渗透 ; **intestinal a.,** the uptake from the intestinal lumen of fluids, solutes, proteins, fats, and other nutrients into the intestinal epithelial cells, blood, lymph, or interstitial fluids 肠吸收

ab·sorp·tive (ab-sorp'tiv) capable of absorbing; absorbent; pertaining to absorption 能吸收的 ; 与

吸收有关的

ab·sorp·tiv·i·ty (ab″sorp-tiv′ĭ-te) a measure of the amount of light absorbed by a solution 吸光率，吸光度

ab·sti·nence (ab′sti-nəns) a refraining from the use of or indulgence in food, stimulants, or sexual activity 节制，禁戒

ab·strac·tion (ab-strak′shən) 1. the withdrawal of any ingredient from a compound 抽出，提取；2. malocclusion in which the occlusal plane is farther from the eye–ear plane, causing lengthening of the face 拉长；cf. *attraction* (2)

Ab·stral (ab′strəl) trademark for a preparation of fentanyl citrate 芬太尼

abu·lia (ə-boo′le-ə) 1. loss or deficiency of will power, initiative, or drive 意志缺失；2. akinetic mutism that is less than total 无动性缄默；**abu′lic** adj. 意志缺失的，无动性缄默的

abuse (ə-būs′) misuse, maltreatment, or excessive use 滥用，误用；**child a.,** 见 *battered-child syndrome*；**drug a.,** 见 substance a.; **physical a.,** any act resulting in a nonaccidental physical injury 肉 体 的 摧残；**psychoactive substance a.,** 见 substance a.; **sexual a.,** assault or other crime of a sexual nature, which need not be physical. Acts of a sexual nature are considered abuse if performed with minors or nonconsenting adults 性 虐 待；**substance a.,** use of a substance that modifies mood or behavior in a manner characterized by a maladaptive pattern of use（精神性）药物滥用，另见 *dependence* 下的词条 *substance dependence*

abut·ment (ə-but′mənt) a supporting structure to sustain lateral or horizontal pressure, as the anchorage tooth for a fixed or removable partial denture 桥基，基牙

AC acromioclavicular 肩 锁 的；air conduction 空气传导；alternating current 交替气流；anodal closure 阳极通电；aortic closure 主动脉闭锁

a.c. [L.] an′te ci′bum (before meals) 饭前

ACA 1. Affordable Care Act 平价医疗法案；2. American Chiropractic Association 美国脊椎按摩协会；3. American College of Apothecaries 美国药剂师学会；4. American Council on Alcoholism 美 国 酗 酒 委 员 会；5. American Counseling Association 美国咨询协会

ACAAI American College of Allergy, Asthma and Immunology 美国过敏、哮喘和免疫学学院

a·ca·i (aw-saw′ē) a grapelike fruit harvested from acai palm trees; used as an alternative treatment for a variety of health conditions and to support in weight loss 来源于一种棕榈树上的葡萄柚状果实，巴西莓

ACAM American College for Advancement in Medicine 美国医学高等专科学校

acamp·sia (ə-kamp′se-ə) rigidity of a part or limb 屈挠不能

acan·tha (ə-kan′thə) 1. spine (1) 棘；2. a spinous process of a vertebra 棘突

acan·tha·me·bi·a·sis (ə-kan″thə-me-bi′ə-sis) infection with *Acanthamoeba castellanii* 棘 阿 米巴病

Acan·tha·moe·ba (ə-kan″thə-me′bə) a genus of free-living ameboid protozoa (order Amoebida) found usually in fresh water or moist soil. Some species, including *A. astronyx'is, A. castella'nii, A. culbertso'ni, A. hatchet'ti, A. poly'phaga,* and *A. rhyso'des,* may occur as human pathogens 棘 阿 米巴属

acan·thes·the·sia (ə-kan″thes-the′zhə) perverted sensation of a sharp point pricking the body 针刺感

acan·thi·on (ə-kan′the-on) a point at the tip of the anterior nasal spine 鼻前棘点

Acan·tho·ceph·a·la (ə-kan″tho-sef′ə-lə) a phylum of elongate, mostly cylindrical organisms (thorny-headed worms) parasitic in the intestines of all classes of vertebrates; in some classifications, considered to be a class of the phylum Nemathelminthes 棘头门，棘头纲

Acan·tho·ceph·a·lus (ə-kan″tho-sef′ə-ləs) a genus of parasitic worms (phylum Acanthocephala) 棘头虫

acan·tho·cyte (ə-kan′tho-sīt) a spiculed erythrocyte with spiny protoplasmic projections of varying lengths distributed irregularly over its surface, as is seen in abetalipoproteinemia 棘 红 细胞，棘细胞

acan·tho·cy·to·sis (ə-kan″tho-si-to′sis) the presence in the blood of acanthocytes, characteristic of abetalipoproteinemia and sometimes used synonymously 棘红细胞增多症

acan·thol·y·sis (ak″an-thol′ĭ-sis) dissolution of the intercellular bridges of the stratum spinosum of the epidermis 皮肤棘层松解；**acantholyt′ic** adj. 皮肤棘层松解的

ac·an·tho·ma (ak″an-tho′mə) pl. *acanthomas, acantho'mata.* A tumor composed of epidermal or squamous cells 棘皮瘤

Acan·tho·phis (ə-kan′tho-fis) a genus of snakes of the family Elapidae. *A. antarc'ticus* is the death adder of Australia and New Guinea 棘蛇属

ac·an·tho·sis (ak″an-tho′sis) diffuse hyperplasia and thickening of the stratum spinosum of the epidermis 棘皮症；**acantholyt′ic** adj. 棘皮症的；**a. ni′gricans,** diffuse velvety acanthosis with dark pigmentation, chiefly in the axillae; in adults, one form is often associated with an internal carcinoma (*malignant a. nigricans*), and another form is benign, nevoid, and more or less generalized. A benign juvenile form is called *pseudoacanthosis nigricans* 黑棘皮症

acan·thro·cy·to·sis (ə-kan″thro-si-to′sis) acanthocytosis 棘红细胞（增多）

acar·bose (a′kahr-bōs) an α -glucosidase inhibitor used in treatment of type 2 diabetes mellitus 阿卡波糖

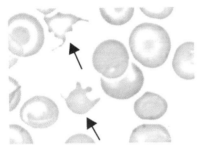

▲ 棘红细胞（**acanthocytes**）（箭示）

acar·dia (a-kahr′de-ə) congenital absence of the heart 无心（畸形）

acar·di·us (a-kahr′de-əs) an imperfectly formed free twin fetus, lacking a heart and other body parts 未完全成形的游离双胎，缺少心脏和其他身体部位

ac·a·ri·a·sis (ak″ə-ri′ə-sis) infestation with mites 螨病．又称 *acarinosis*

acar·i·cide (ə-kar′ĭ-sīd) 1. destructive to mites 杀螨的；2. an agent that destroys mites 杀螨药

ac·a·rid (ak′ə-rid) a tick or mite of the order Acarina 螨，粉螨，壁虱

acar·i·di·a·sis (ə-kar″ĭ-di′ə-sis) acariasis 螨病，壁虱病

Ac·a·ri·na (ak″ə-ri′nə) an order of arthropods (class Arachnida), including mites and ticks 螨目，壁虱目

ac·a·ro·der·ma·ti·tis (ak″ə-ro-dur″mə-ti′tis) any skin inflammation caused by mites (acarids) 螨性皮炎；*a. urticarioi′des*, grain itch 荨麻疹样螨性皮炎

ac·a·rol·o·gy (ak″ə-rol′ə-je) the scientific study of mites and ticks 螨（类）学

Ac·a·rus (ak′ə-rəs) a genus of small mites, frequent causes of skin diseases such as itch or mange 螨，壁虱；*A. folliculo′rum, Demodex folliculorum* 毛囊脂螨；*A. si′ro*, a mite that causes vanillism in vanilla pod handlers 引起香兰子中毒的西卡罗螨

acat·a·la·sia (a″kat-ə-la′zhə) a rare hereditary disease seen mostly in Japan and Switzerland, marked by absence of catalase; it may be associated with infections of oral structures. Called also *acatalasemia* 过氧化氢酶缺乏（症）

acau·date (a-kaw′dāt) lacking a tail 无尾的

ACC American College of Cardiology 美国心脏病学会

ACCA American College of Cardiovascular Administrators 美国心血管管理学院

ac·cel·er·a·tor (ak-sel′ər-a″tər) [L.] 1. an agent or apparatus that increases the rate at which something occurs or progresses 加速剂，加速器；2. any nerve or muscle that hastens the performance of a function 加速神经，加速肌；3. any of a group of chemicals used in the vulcanization of rubber or other polymerization reactions 化学催化剂；**serum prothrombin conversion a. (SPCA)**, coagulation factor Ⅶ. 血清凝血酶原转变加速素；**serum thrombotic a.**, a factor in serum that has procoagulant properties and the ability to induce blood coagulation 血清凝血加速素

ac·cep·tor (ak-sep′tər) a substance that unites with another substance; specifically, one that unites with hydrogen or oxygen in an oxidoreduction reaction and so enables the reaction to proceed 受体，受器，受者

ac·ces·sion·al (ak-sesh′ən-əl) pertaining to that which has been added or acquired 附加的

ac·ces·so·ry (ak-ses′ə-re) supplementary; affording aid to another similar and generally more important thing 副的，辅助性的

ac·ci·den·tal (ak″sĭ-den′təl) 1. occurring by chance, unexpectedly, or unintentionally 意外的；2. nonessential; not innate or intrinsic 不必要的，非固有的

ac·cli·ma·tion (ak″lĭ-ma′shən) the process of becoming accustomed to a new environment 服水土，水土适应，气候适应

ACCME Accreditation Council for Continuing Medical Education 继续医学教育评审委员会

ac·com·mo·da·tion (A) (a) (ə-kom″ə-da′shən) adjustment, especially of the eye for seeing objects at various distances 调节；**negative a.**, adjustment of the eye for focusing at long distances by relaxation of the ciliary muscle 负（性）调节，视远调节；**positive a.**, adjustment of the eye for focusing at short distances by contraction of the ciliary muscle 正（性）调节，近视调节

ac·com·mo·da·tive (ə-kom′ə-da″tiv) pertaining to, of the nature of, or affecting accommodation 适应的，调节的

ac·couche·ment (ah-koosh-maw′) [Fr.] 1. childbirth 生产；2. delivery 分娩；**a. forcé**, (for-sa′) rapid forcible delivery by one of several methods; originally, rapid dilatation of the cervix with the hands, followed by version and extraction of the fetus 强促分娩，强迫分娩，催促生产

ACCP American College of Chest Physicians 美国胸科医师学会; American College of Clinical Pharmacology 美国临床药理学学院; American College of Clinical Pharmacy 美国临床药学院

ac·cre·men·ti·tion (ak″rə-men-tish′ən) growth by addition of similar tissue 增生

ac·cre·tion (ə-kre′shən) 1. growth by addition of material 增积（加）; 2. accumulation 增积（物）; 3. adherence of parts normally separated 粘连

ACCSCT Accrediting Commission of Career Schools and Colleges of Technology 职业技术学院认证委员会

ac·e·bu·to·lol (as″ə-bu′tə-lol) a cardioselective β₁-adrenergic blocking agent with intrinsic sympathomimetic activity; used as the hydrochloride salt in the treatment of hypertension, angina pectoris, and arrhythmias 醋丁酰心安

acel·lu·lar (a-sel′u-lər) not cellular in structure 无细胞的，非细胞组成的

ace·lo·mate (a-se′lə-māt) having no coelom or body cavity 无体腔的

ACEN Academy of Canadian Executive Nurses (Canada) 加拿大执行护士学会

acen·tric (a-sen′trik) 1. not central; not located in the center 离心的; 2. lacking a centromere, so that the chromosome will not survive cell divisions 无中心粒的

ACEP American College of Emergency Physicians 美国急救医师协会

aceph·a·lous (a-sef′ə-ləs) headless 无头的

aceph·a·lus (a-sef′ə-ləs) a headless fetus 无头畸胎

acer·vu·line (ə-sur′vu-līn) aggregated; heaped up; said of certain glands 堆积的，集合的

ac·e·tab·u·lar (as″ə-tab′u-lər) pertaining to the acetabulum 髋臼的

ac·e·tab·u·lec·to·my (as″ə-tab″u-lek′tə-me) excision of the acetabulum 髋臼切除术

ac·e·tab·u·lo·plas·ty (as″ə-tab′u-lo-plas″te) plastic repair of the acetabulum 髋臼成形术

ac·e·tab·u·lum (as″ə-tab′u-ləm) pl. *aceta'bula* [L.] the cup-shaped cavity on the lateral surface of the coxal bone, receiving the head of the femur 髋臼; **acetab′ular** *adj.* 髋臼的

ac·e·tal (as′ə-təl) 1. any of a class of organic compounds formed by combination of an aldehyde molecule and two alcohol molecules 缩醛类的; 2. $CH_3CH(OC_2H_5)_2$, a colorless, volatile liquid used as a solvent and in cosmetics 醛缩醇，乙缩醛

ac·et·al·de·hyde (as″ət-al′də-hīd″) a colorless, volatile, flammable liquid used in the manufacture of acetic acid, perfumes, and flavors; it is also an intermediate in the metabolism of alcohol. It can cause irritation of mucous membranes, pneumonia, headache, and unconsciousness 乙醛

ace·ta·min·o·phen (ə-se″tə-min′ə-fen) an analgesic and antipyretic with effects similar to aspirin's but only weakly antiinflammatory 对乙酰氨基酚

ac·e·tate (as′ə-tāt) any salt of acetic acid 乙酸盐

ac·et·a·zol·a·mide (as″et-ə-zol′ə-mīd) a renal carbonic anhydrase inhibitor with uses that include treatment of glaucoma, epilepsy, familial periodic paralysis, acute mountain sickness, and uric acid renal calculi 乙酰唑胺

Ace-test (as′ə-test) trademark for a reagent tablet containing sodium nitroprusside, aminoacetic acid, dibasic sodium phosphate, and lactose, turning purple in the presence of ketone bodies in urine, blood, plasma, or serum, the intensity of the color reaction indicative of the acetoacetate or acetone concentration 丙酮检出试剂

ace·tic (ə-se′tik) (ə-set′ik) pertaining to vinegar or its acid; sour 醋酸的，醋的

ace·tic ac·id (ə-se′tik) the two-carbon carboxylic acid, the characteristic component of vinegar; used as a solvent, menstruum, and pharmaceutic necessity. *Glacial a. a.* (anhydrous acetic acid) is used as a solvent, vesicant and caustic, and pharmaceutical necessity 乙酸，醋酸

ace·to·ace·tic ac·id (ə-se″to-ə-se′tik) β-ketobutyric acid, one of the ketone bodies produced in the liver and occurring in excess in the blood and urine in ketosis 乙酰乙酸

Ace·to·bac·te·ra·ceae (ə-se″to-bak″tər-a′se-e) a family of aerobic, gram-negative, acetic acid–producing bacteria of the order Rhodospirillales 醋杆菌科

ac·e·to·hex·a·mide (as″ə-to-hek′sə-mīd) an oral hypoglycemic used in the treatment of type 2 diabetes mellitus 醋磺环己脲

ac·e·to·hy·drox·am·ic ac·id (as″ə-to-hi″droksam′ik) an inhibitor of bacterial urease used in the prophylaxis and treatment of certain renal calculi and the treatment of urinary tract infections caused by urease-producing bacteria 醋羟胺酸

ac·e·tone (as′ə-tōn) a flammable, colorless, volatile liquid with a characteristic odor, which is a solvent and antiseptic and is one of the ketone bodies produced in ketoacidosis 丙酮

ace·to·ni·trile (as″ə-to-ni′trīl) a colorless liquid with an etherlike odor used as an extractant, solvent, and intermediate; ingestion or inhalation yields cyanide as a metabolic product 乙腈，氰化甲烷

ac·e·ton·uria (as″ə-to-nu′re-ə) ketonuria 丙酮尿

ace·tous (as′ə-təs) pertaining to, producing, or resembling acetic acid 醋（酸）的

ac·e·tract (as′ə-trakt) an extract of a medicinal herb prepared using acetic acid as the solvent 醋浸剂

ac·e·tyl (as′ə-təl) (as′ə-tēl″) (ə-se′təl) the monovalent radical CH₃CO—, a combining form of acetic acid 乙酰（基）

acet·y·la·tion (ə-set″ə-la′shən) introduction of an acetyl radical into an organic molecule 乙酰化作用

acet·y·la·tor (ə-set″ə-la′tər) an organism capable of metabolic acetylation; in humans, acetylator status (fast or slow) is determined by the rate of acetylation of sulfamethazine 乙酰化个体

ac·e·tyl·cho·line (ACh) (as″ə-təl-) (as″ə-tēlko′lēn) the acetic acid ester of choline, which is a neurotransmitter at cholinergic synapses in the central, sympathetic, and parasympathetic nervous systems; used in the form of the chloride salt as a miotic 乙酰胆碱

ac·e·tyl·cho·lin·es·ter·ase (AChE) (as″ə-təl-) (as″ə-tēl-ko″lī-nes′tə-rās) an enzyme present in the central nervous system, particularly in nervous tissue, muscle, and red cells, that catalyzes the hydrolysis of acetylcholine to choline and acetic acid 乙酰胆碱酯酶

ac·e·tyl-CoA car·box·yl·ase (as′ə-təl-) (as″ə-tēl′ko·a′ kahr-bok′sə-lās) a ligase that catalyzes the rate-limiting step in the synthesis of fatty acids from acetyl groups 乙酰辅酶A 羧化酶

ac·e·tyl co·en·zyme A (as″ē-tīl′ ko-en′zīm) an important intermediate in the tricarboxylic acid cycle and the chief precursor of lipids and steroids; it is formed by the attachment to coenzyme A of an acetyl group during the oxidation of carbohydrates, fatty acids, or amino acids 乙酰辅酶A。又称 *acetyl CoA*

ac·e·tyl·cys·te·ine (as″ə-təl-) (as″ə-tēl-sis′te-ēn) a derivative of cysteine used as a mucolytic in various bronchopulmonary disorders and as an antidote to acetaminophen poisoning 乙酰半胱氨酸

acet·y·lene (ə-set′ə-lēn) HC≡CH, a colorless, volatile, explosive gas, the simplest alkyne (unsaturated, triple-bonded hydrocarbon) 乙炔

N-**ac·e·tyl·ga·lac·to·sa·mine** (as″ə-təl-) (as″ə-tēl-gal″ak-tōs′ə-mēn) the acetyl derivative of galactosamine; it is a component of structural glycosaminoglycans, glycolipids, and membrane glycoproteins N- 乙酰半乳糖胺

N-**ac·e·tyl·glu·co·sa·mine** (as″ə-təl-) (as″ə-tēl″gloo-kōs′ə-mēn) the acetyl derivative of glucosamine; it is a component of structural glycosaminoglycans, glycolipids, and membrane glycoproteins N- 乙酰葡（萄）糖胺

N-**ac·e·tyl·neu·ra·min·ic ac·id** (as″ə-təl-) (as″ə-tēl-noor″ə-min′ik) the acetyl derivative of the amino sugar neuraminic acid; it occurs in many glycoproteins, glycolipids, and polysaccharides N-乙酰神经氨（糖）酸，唾液酸

ac·e·tyl·sal·i·cyl·ic ac·id (ASA) (ə-se′təlsal″ə-sil′ik) aspirin 乙酰水杨酸

ac·e·tyl·trans·fer·ase (as″ə-təl-) (as″ə-tēltrans′fər-ās) any of a group of enzymes that catalyze the transfer of an acetyl group from one substance to another 乙酰转移酶

ACFAS American College of Foot and Ankle Surgeons 美国足踝外科医师学会

ACG American College of Gastroenterology 美国胃肠病学会；angiocardiography 心血管造影术；apexcardiogram 心尖搏动图

AcG accelerator globulin (coagulation factor V) 促凝血球蛋白

ACGIH American Conference of Governmental Industrial Hygienists 美国政府工业卫生学家会议

ACh acetylcholine 乙酰胆碱

ACHA American College Health Association 美国大学健康协会

ach·a·la·sia (ak″ə-la′zhə) failure of smooth muscle fibers of the gastrointestinal tract to relax at a junction of one part with another, especially failure of the lower esophageal sphincter to relax with swallowing due to degeneration of ganglion cells in the wall of the organ. The thoracic esophagus also loses its normal peristaltic activity and becomes dilated 弛缓不能，失弛缓性

Ach·a·ti·na (ak″ə-ti′nə) a genus of very large land snails, including *A. fuli'ca,* which serves as an intermediate host of *Angiostrongylus cantonensis* 玛瑙螺属

ACHE American College of Healthcare ExecuTives 美国医疗管理学院；American Council for Headache Education 美国头痛教育委员会

AChE acetylcholinesterase 乙酰胆碱酯酶

ache (āk) 1. a continuous, fixed pain, as distinguished from twinges 持续，固定的疼痛，区别于刺痛；2. to suffer such pain. 遭受这种疼痛

achei·ria (ə-ki′re-ə) 1. congenital absence of one or both hands 无手（畸形）；2. lack of sensation of the hands or a feeling of their absence 无手感觉症

achil·lo·dy·nia (ə-kil″o-din′e-ə) pain in the Achilles tendon 跟腱痛

ach·il·lor·rha·phy (ak″ī-lor′ə-fe) suturing of the Achilles tendon 跟腱缝合术

achil·lo·te·not·o·my (ə-kil″o-tə-not′ə-me) surgical division of the Achilles tendon 跟腱切除术

achlor·hy·dria (a″klor-hi′dre-ə) absence of

A

hydrochloric acid from gastric secretions 盐酸缺乏；
achlorhy′dric *adj.* 盐酸缺乏的

ACHNE Association of Community Health Nursing Educators 社区卫生护理教育工作者协会

acho·lia (a-ko′le-ə) lack of bile, such as with atresia or absence of secretion 无胆汁（症）；**acho′lic** *adj.* 无胆汁症的

acho·lu·ric (a″ko-lu′rik) not characterized by choluria 无胆色素尿的

achon·dro·gen·e·sis (a-kon″dro-jen′ə-sis) a genetically heterogeneous, invariably lethal, hereditary disorder characterized by hypoplasia of bone, micromelia, enlarged head, shortened trunk, and deficient or absent ossification of the lower spine and pubis 软骨成长不全

achon·dro·pla·sia (a-kon″dro-pla′zhə) an autosomal dominant disorder of epiphyseal chondroblastic growth and maturation, caused by mutation of a fibroblast growth factor receptor; characterized by dwarfism with short limbs, narrow trunk, large head with frontal bossing and midface hypoplasia, lordosis, and trident hand 软骨发育不全；**achondroplas′tic** *adj.* 软骨发育不全的

achres·tic (ə-kres′tik) not using some normal tool or process, as the inability of those with achrestic anemia to utilize vitamin B$_{12}$ 利用不能的，失利用性的

achro·ma·sia (ak″ro-ma′zhə) 1. hypopigmentation 色素缺乏；2. 见 achromatosis (2)

achro·mat (ak′ro-mat) 1. an achromatic objective 消色差透镜；2. monochromat 全色盲者

achro·mat·ic (ak″ro-mat′ik) 1. producing no discoloration 无色的；2. staining with difficulty 不易染色的；3. refracting light without decomposing it into its component colors 消色差的，不分光的；4. 见 monochromatic (2)

achro·ma·to·phil (ak″ro-mat′o-fil) 1. not easily stainable 不易染色的；2. an organism or tissue that does not stain easily 不易染色的机体或组织

achro·ma·top·sia (a-kro″mə-top′se-ə) monochromatic vision 全色盲，色盲

achro·ma·to·sis (ə-kro″mə-to′sis) 1. hypopigmentation 色素缺乏；2. lack of staining power in a cell or tissue 染色性缺乏

achro·ma·tous (ə-kro′mə-tus) colorless 无色的

achro·ma·tu·ria (ə-kro″mə-tu′re-ə) the excretion of colorless urine 无色尿

achro·mia (ə-kro′me-ə) hypopigmentation 色素缺乏，无色性；**achro′mic** *adj.* 色素缺乏，无色性的

achy·lia (ə-ki′le-ə) absence of hydrochloric acid and pepsinogens (pepsin) in the gastric juice 胃液缺乏

acic·u·lar (ə-sik′u-lər) needle-shaped 针形的

ac·id (as′id) 1. sour 酸 的；2. a chemical compound that dissociates in solution, releasing hydrogen ions and lowering the solution pH (a proton donor). An acidic solution has a pH below 7.0. Cf. *base* (3). For particular acids, see the specific names 酸；**amino a.,** 见 *amino acid*；**carboxylic a.,** any organic compound containing the carboxy group (—COOH), including amino and fatty acids 羧基酸；**a. citrate dextrose (ACD),** anticoagulant citrate dextrose solution 枸橼酸葡萄糖；**fatty a.,** 见下 *F*；**haloid a.,** an acid that contains no oxygen in the molecule but is composed of hydrogen and a halogen element 卤酸；**hydroxy a.,** an organic acid that contains an additional hydroxyl group 羟基酸；**inorganic a.,** any acid containing no carbon atoms 无机酸；**nucleic a.,** 见下 *N*；**obeticholic a.,** a semisynthetic bile acid analogue; used in the treatment of primary biliary cholangitis (PBC) 奥贝胆酸；**organic a.,** an acid containing one or more carbon atoms; often specifically a carboxylic acid 有机酸

ac·id al·pha-glu·co·si·dase (as′id al′fə glooko′sĭ-dās) acid maltase 酸性麦芽糖酶

Ac·id·ami·no·coc·ca·ceae (as″id-ə-me″nokok-a′se-e) a family of anaerobic, gramnegative bacteria of the order Clostridiales 氨基酸球菌

ac·i·de·mia (as″ĭ-de′me-ə) increased acidity of the blood. For those characterized by increased concentration of a specific acid, see at the acid 酸血症；**organic a.,** increased concentration of one or more organic acids in the blood 有机酸血症

acid-fast (as′id-fast) not readily decolorized by acids after staining 耐酸的，抗酸的

ac·id α-glu·co·si·dase (as′id gloo-ko′sĭ-dās) acid maltase 酸性麦芽糖酶

acid·ic (ə-sid′ik) of or pertaining to an acid 酸的；acid-forming 成酸的

acid·i·fi·a·ble (ə-sid′ə-fi″ə-bəl) capable of being made acid 可酸化的，能变酸的

acid·i·fied (ə-sid′ĭ-fīd) having been made acid 酸化

acid·i·fi·er (ə-sid′ĭ-fi″ər) an agent that causes acidity; a substance used to increase gastric acidity 酸化剂

acid·i·ty (ə-sid′ĭ-te) the quality of being acid; the power to unite with positively charged ions or with basic substances 酸化

ac·id li·pase (as″id li′pās) 1. cholesterol esterase 胆固醇酯酶；2. a lipase with an acid pH optimum 酸性 pH 时最佳的脂肪酶

ac·id mal·tase (as′id mawl′tās) a hydrolase that catalyzes the degradation of glycogen to glucose in the lysosomes; deficiency of enzyme activity results in glycogen storage disease, type Ⅱ 1,4 - α - 葡萄糖苷酶

acid·o·phil (ə-sid′o-fil″) 1. a structure, cell,

or other histologic element staining readily with acid dyes 嗜酸细胞，嗜酸组织；2. one of the hormone-producing acidophilic cells of the anterior pituitary lobe, including corticotrophs, lactotrophs, lipotrophs, and somatotrophs 垂体嗜酸性细胞；3. an organism that grows well in highly acid media 嗜酸；4. acidophilic 嗜酸性的

ac·i·do·phil·ic (as″ĭ-do-fil′ik) 1. readily stained with acid dyes 嗜酸的；2. growing in highly acid media; said of microorganisms 嗜酸菌

ac·i·do·sis (as″ĭ-do′sis) 1. the accumulation of acid and hydrogen ions or depletion of the alkaline reserve (bicarbonate content) in the blood and body tissues, decreasing the pH 酸中毒；2. a pathologic condition resulting from this process 酸中毒的病理过程. Cf. *alkalosis*；**acido′sic, acidot′ic** *adj.* **compensated a.**, a condition in which the compensatory mechanisms have returned the pH toward normal 代偿性酸中毒；**diabetic a.**, 见 *ketoacidosis* 下词条；**hypercapnic a.**, respiratory a 血碳酸过多性酸中毒；**hyperchloremic a.**, metabolic acidosis accompanied by elevated plasma chloride 血氯过多性酸中毒；**lactic a.**, a metabolic acidosis occurring as a result of excess lactic acid in the blood, due to conditions causing impaired cellular respiration 乳酸酸中毒；**metabolic a., nonrespiratory a.**, a disturbance in which the acid-base status shifts toward the acid because of loss of base or retention of noncarbonic, or fixed (nonvolatile), acids 代谢性酸中毒；**renal hyperchloremia a., renal tubular a. (RTA)**, metabolic acidosis resulting from impairment of renal function 肾性高氯血症酸中毒；**respiratory a.**, acidosis due to excess retention of carbon dioxide in the body 呼吸性酸中毒；**starvation a.**, metabolic acidosis due to accumulation of ketone bodies that may accompany a caloric deficit 饥饿性酸中毒；**uremic a.**, metabolic acidosis seen in chronic renal disease when the ability to excrete acid is decreased 尿毒症性酸中毒

ac·id phos·pha·tase (as′id fos′fə-tās) a hydrolase found in mammalian liver, spleen, bone marrow, plasma and formed blood elements, and prostate gland, catalyzing the cleavage of orthophosphate from orthophosphoric monoesters under acid conditions; determination of its activity in serum is an important diagnostic test 酸性磷酸酶

acid·u·lat·ed (ə-sid′u-lāt″ed) rendered acid in reaction 酸化的

acid·u·lous (ə-sid′u-ləs) somewhat acid 微酸的，具有酸味的

ac·id·u·ria (as″ĭ-du′re-ə) excess of acid in the urine. For those characterized by increased concentration of a specific acid, see at the acid 尿酸症；or-

ganic a., excessive excretion of one or more organic acids in the urine 器质性尿酸症

ac·id·uric (as″ĭ-doo′rik) capable of growing in extremely acid media; said of bacteria 耐酸的

ac·i·nar (as′ĭ-nər) pertaining to or affecting one or more acini 腺泡的。又称 *acinous*；**acin′ic**

Ac·i·net·o·bac·ter (as″ĭ-net″o-bak′tər) a genus of bacteria (family Moraxellaceae), consisting of aerobic, gram-negative, paired coccobacilli, it is widely distributed in nature and part of the normal mammalian flora, but can cause severe primary infections in compromised hosts 不动杆菌

acin·i·form (ə-sin′ĭ-form) shaped like an acinus, or grape 腺泡状的，葡萄状的

acin·i·tis (as″ĭ-ni′tis) inflammation of the acini of a gland 腺泡炎

ac·i·nose (as′ĭ-nōs) made up of acini 由腺泡组成的

ac·i·nus (as′ĭ-nəs) pl. *a′cini* [L.] a small saclike dilation, particularly one in a gland; see also *alveolus* 腺泡；**liver a.**, the smallest functional unit of the liver, a diamond-shaped mass of liver parenchyma that is supplied by terminal branches of the portal vein and hepatic artery and drained by a terminal branch of the bile duct 肝腺泡；**pancreatic a.**, one of the secretory units of the exocrine pancreas, where pancreatic juice is produced 胰腺泡；**pulmonary a.**, terminal respiratory unit 肺泡；**thyroid acini**, 见 *follicle* 下词条

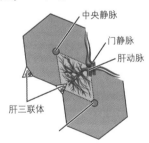

中央静脉
门静脉
肝动脉
肝三联体

▲ 肝腺泡（liver acinus）：肝小叶由六边形（实线）表示；肝腺泡以菱形（虚线）表示

ac·i·tret·in (as″e-tret′in) a second generation retinoid used in treatment of severe psoriasis 阿维 A

ACLA American Clinical Laboratory Association 美国临床实验室协会

acla·sis (ak′lə-sis) pathologic continuity of structure, as in multiple exostoses 续连症，骨软骨划分不清；**diaphyseal a.**, multiple exostoses 骨干性续连症

ac·me (ak′me) the critical stage or crisis of a disease（疾病的）极期

ACMG American College of Medical Genetics 美国医学遗传学学院

ACMT American College of Medical Toxicology 美国医学毒理学学院

ACN American College of Nutrition 美国营养学会

ac·ne (ak'ne) an inflammatory disease of the skin; often specifically, *acne vulgaris* 痤疮，粉刺；**bromide a.**, a type caused by ingestion of bromide compounds, one of the most common manifestations of bromine intoxication; it does not include comedo formation 溴（化物）痤疮；**common a.**, 见 a. vulgaris.；**a. congloba'ta, conglobate a.**, severe acne with many comedones, marked by suppuration, cysts, sinuses, and scarring 聚合性痤疮；**contact a.**, acne produced by contact with a chemical, such as in cosmetic or grooming agents or in industry 接触性痤疮；**cosmetic a.**, contact acne on the chin and cheeks as a reaction to facial cosmetics 美容性痤疮；**cystic a.**, acne with cysts that contain keratin and sebum 囊肿痤疮；**a. deter'gicans**, aggravation of acne lesions by frequent or severe washing with soaps or rough cloths 去垢剂刺性痤疮；**excoriated a.**, a superficial type seen most often in girls and young women, caused by the neurotic habit of picking and squeezing tiny (or nonexistent) facial lesions; it produces secondary lesions that can leave scars 剥脱性痤疮；**a. ful'minans**, a severe form seen in teenage males, with sudden onset of fever and eruption of highly inflammatory, tender, ulcerative, crusted lesions on the back, chest, and face 暴发性痤疮；**halogen a.**, that caused by ingestion of salts of bromine, chlorine, or iodine, such as in cold remedies, sedatives, analgesics, and vitamin supplements 卤素痤疮；**a. indura'ta**, a progression of papular acne with deep, destructive lesions that may leave scars 硬结性痤疮；**keloid a., keloidal a., a. keloida'lis**, development of hard follicular plaques along the posterior hairline, which fuse to form a thick, sclerotic band across the occiput 瘢瘤性痤疮；**a. mecha'nica, mechanical a.**, aggravation of acne lesions by mechanical factors such as rubbing or stretching, as by chin straps, clothing, back packs, casts, or car seats 机械性痤疮；**nodulocystic a.**, severe cystic acne, usually seen in young men, with subcutaneous nodules that may become inflamed and leave scars 结节囊肿性痤疮；**occupational a.**, contact acne caused by exposure to industrial chemicals, such as oils, tars, waxes, or chlorinated hydrocarbons 职业性痤疮；**papular a.**, acne vulgaris with formation of papules 丘疹性痤疮；**pomade a.**, contact acne in blacks who groom their scalp and facial hair with greasy lubricants, marked by closed comedones 香膏性痤疮；**premenstrual a.**, acne that appears shortly before menses (or occasionally after them) 月经前痤疮；**tropical a.**, a severe type seen in hot, humid climates, with nodular, cystic, and pustular lesions chiefly on the back, buttocks, and thighs 热带痤疮；**a. venena'ta**, 见 contact a.；**a. vulga'ris**, chronic acne, usually seen in adolescence, with comedones, papules, nodules, and pustules on the face, neck, and upper part of the trunk 普通粉刺

ac·ne·gen·ic (ak"ne-jen'ik) producing acne 痤疮的，致痤疮的

ACNM American College of Nurse-Midwives 美国护士助产士学会

ACNP American College of Nurse Practitioners 美国护士执业协会

acoe·lo·mate (a-se'lo-māt) without a coelom or body cavity 无体腔；an animal lacking a body cavity 无体腔动物

ACOEM American College of Occupational and Environmental Medicine 美国职业与环境医学院

ACOG American College of Obstetricians and Gynecologists 美国妇产科学会

ac·o·nite (ak'ə-nīt) a poisonous substance from the dried tuberous root of *Aconitum napellus*, which contains aconitine and related alkaloids and causes potentially fatal ventricular fibrillation and respiratory paralysis. It is used in Chinese herbal medicine and homeopathy as an analgesic, antiinflammatory, and cardiac tonic 乌头

acon·i·tine (ə-kon'ĭ-tin) a poisonous alkaloid, the active principle of aconite 乌头碱

aco·rea (ə-kor'e-ə) absence of the pupil 无瞳孔（畸形）

aco·ria (ə-kor'e-ə) excessive ingestion of food, not from hunger but due to loss of the sensation of satiety 贪食，不饱症

ACOS American College of Osteopathic Surgeons 美国骨病外科医师学会

acous·tic (ə-koos'tik) relating to sound or hearing 听的，声学的

acous·tics (ə-koos'tiks) the science of sound or of hearing 声学

acous·to·gram (ə-koos'to-gram) the graphic tracing of the curves of sounds produced by motion of a joint 关节音图

ACP acid phosphatase 酸性磷酸酶；Alliance of Cardiovascular Professionals 心血管专业人员联盟；American College of Physicians 美国医师学会；American College of Psychiatrists 美国精神病学学院

ACPM American College of Preventive Medicine 美国预防医学学院

ACPS acrocephalopolysyndactyly 尖头多并指

畸形

ac·quired (ə-kwīrd′) incurred as a result of factors acting from or originating outside the organism; not inherited 后天的

ac·qui·si·tion (ak″wĭ-zĭ′shən) in psychology, the period in learning during which progressive increments in response strength can be measured. Also, the process involved in such learning 获得，掌握，学识，习得

ACR American College of Radiology 美国放射学会 ; American College of Rheumatology 美国风湿病学会

ac·ral (ak′rəl) pertaining to or affecting a limb or other extremity 肢端的

Ac·re·mo·ni·um (ak″rə-mo′ne-əm) a genus of imperfect fungi rarely isolated from human infection. *A. falcifor′me, A. kilien′se,* and *A. reci′fei* are agents of eumycotic mycetoma 支顶孢属

ac·ri·dine (ak′rĭ-dēn) an alkaloid from anthracene used in the synthesis of dyes and drugs 吖啶

ac·ri·vas·tine (ak′rĭ-vas′tēn) an antihistamine used in treatment of seasonal allergic rhinitis 阿伐斯汀

ac·ro·ag·no·sis (ak″ro-ag-no′sis) lack of sensory recognition of a limb; lack of acrognosis 肢体感觉缺乏

ac·ro·an·es·the·sia (ak″ro-an″es-the′zhə) anesthesia of the limbs 肢麻木

ac·ro·ar·thri·tis (ak″ro-ahr-thri′tis) arthritis of the limbs 肢关节炎

ac·ro·blast (ak′ro-blast) Golgi material in the spermatid from which the acrosome develops 原顶体，初尖体

ac·ro·brachy·ceph·a·ly (ak″ro-brak″ĭ-sef′ə-le) abnormal height of the skull, with shortness of its anteroposterior dimension 扁头畸形 ; **acrobrachy-cephal′ic** *adj.*

ac·ro·cen·tric (ak″ro-sen′trik) having the centromere toward one end of the replicating chromosome so that one arm is much longer than the other 近端着丝的

ac·ro·ceph·a·lo·poly·syn·dac·ty·ly (ACPS) (ak″ro-sef″ə-lo-pol″e-sin-dak′tə-le) any of a group of hereditary disorders characterized by acrocephaly, syndactyly, and polydactyly, sometimes with additional anomalies. Type II is *Carpenter syndrome* 尖头并指（趾），多指（趾）畸形

ac·ro·ceph·a·lo·syn·dac·ty·ly (ak″ro-sef″ə-lo-sin-dak′tə-le) any of a group of hereditary disorders in which craniostenosis is associated with acrocephaly and syndactyly. Type I is *Apert syndrome*, type III is *Saethre-Chotzen syndrome*, and type V is *Pfeiffer syndrome* 尖头并指（趾）畸形

ac·ro·ceph·a·ly (ak″ro-sef′ə-le) increased height of the skull due to premature closure of multiple sutures, with the forehead generally broad and flattened; however, sometimes used interchangeably with oxycephaly to denote any abnormally tall skull 尖头畸形

ac·ro·chor·don (ak″ro-kor′dən) skin tag; a small pedunculated growth, occurring principally on the head, neck, upper chest, or axilla of older women 软垂疣

ac·ro·ci·ne·sis (ak″ro-si-ne′sis) excessive motility; abnormal freedom of movement 运动过多 ; **acrocinet′ic** *adj.*

ac·ro·con·trac·ture (ak″ro-kən-trak′chər) contracture of the muscles of the hand or foot 肢挛缩

ac·ro·cy·a·no·sis (ak″ro-si″ə-no′sis) cyanosis of the limbs with discoloration of the skin of digits, wrists, and ankles, and profuse sweating and coldness of digits 手足发绀

ac·ro·der·ma·ti·tis (ak″ro-dur′mə-ti′tis) inflammation of the skin of the hands and feet 肢皮炎 ; **a. chro′nica atro′phicans**, chronic inflammation of the skin, usually of limbs, leading to sclerosis and atrophy of the skin, caused by the spirochete *Borrelia burgdorferi* 慢性萎缩性肢皮炎 ; **a. con-ti′nua**, a variant of pustular psoriasis, with chronic inflammation of limbs that in some cases becomes generalized 持续性肢皮炎 ; **a. enteropa′thica**, a hereditary disorder due to defective zinc uptake, with a vesiculopustulous dermatitis preferentially located around orifices and on the head, elbows, knees, hands, and feet, associated with gastrointestinal disturbances, chiefly manifested by diarrhea, and total alopecia 肠病性肢皮炎 ; **Hallopeau a.**, 见 a. continua. ; **infantile a., papular a. of childhood,** Gianotti-Crosti syndrome 婴儿肢皮炎

ac·ro·der·ma·to·sis (ak″ro-dur′mə-to′sis) pl. *acrodermato′ses.* Any disease of the skin of the limbs 肢皮病

ac·ro·dol·i·cho·me·lia (ak″ro-dol″ĭ-ko-me′le-ə) abnormal length of the hands and feet 手足过长

ac·ro·dyn·ia (ak″ro-din′e-ə) a disease of early childhood marked by pain and swelling in, and pink coloration of, the fingers and toes and by listlessness, irritability, failure to thrive, profuse perspiration, and sometimes scarlet coloration of the cheeks and tip of the nose. Most cases are toxic neuropathies caused by exposure to mercury 肢痛症

ac·ro·es·the·sia (ak″ro-es-the′zhə) 1. exaggerated sensitiveness 感觉过敏 ; 2. pain in the limbs 肢痛

ac·rog·no·sis (ak″rog-no′sis) sensory recognition of the limbs and of the different portions of each limb in relation to each other 肢体感

ac·ro·hy·po·ther·my (ak″ro-hi′po-thur″me) abnormal coldness of the hands and feet 手足温度过低，手足厥冷

ac·ro·ker·a·to·sis (ak″ro-ker′ə-to′sis) a condition in which there are horny growths on the skin of the limbs 肢端角化症

ac·ro·ki·ne·sia (ak″ro-kĭ-ne′zhə) acrocinesis 运动过度 ; **acrokinet′ic** *adj.* 运动过度的

acro·le·in (ak-ro′le-in) a volatile, highly toxic liquid, produced industrially and also one of the degradation products of cyclophosphamide 丙烯醛

ac·ro·meg·a·ly (ak″ro-meg′ə-le) abnormal enlargement of limbs, caused by hypersecretion of growth hormone after maturity 肢端肥大症

ac·ro·meta·gen·e·sis (ak″ro-met″ə-jen′ə-sis) undue growth of the limbs 四肢发育过度

ac·ro·mic·ria (ak″ro-mik′re-ə) hypoplasia of the limbs and digits, nose, and jaws 肢端过小症

acro·mio·cla·vic·u·lar (ə-kro″me-o-klə-vik′ulər) pertaining to the acromion and clavicle 肩（峰）锁（骨）的

acro·mi·on (ə-kro′me-on) the lateral extension of the spine of the scapula, forming the highest point of the shoulder 肩峰 ; **acro′mial** *adj.*

acro·mio·nec·to·my (ə-kro″me-o-nek′tə-me) resection of the acromion 肩峰切除术

acro·mio·plas·ty (ə-kro′me-o-plas″te) surgical removal of the anterior hook of the acromion to relieve mechanical compression of the rotator cuff during movement of the glenohumeral joint 肩峰成形术

acrom·pha·lus (ə-krom′fə-ləs) 1. bulging of the navel; sometimes a sign of umbilical hernia 脐膨出 ; 2. the center of the navel 脐心

ac·ro·myo·to·nia (ak″ro-mi″o-to′ne-ə) contracture of the hand or foot resulting in spastic deformity 肢体强直

ac·ro·neu·ro·sis (ak″ro-noo-o-ro′sis) any neuropathy of the limbs 肢体神经（功能）病，肢体神经官能症

ac·ro·os·te·ol·y·sis (ak″ro-os″te-ol′ĭ-sis) osteolysis involving the distal phalanges of the fingers and toes 肢端骨质溶解

ac·ro·pachy (ak′ro-pak″e) clubbing of the fingers and toes 杵状指（趾）

ac·ro·pachy·der·ma (ak″ro-pak″ĭ-dur″mə) thickening of the skin of the limbs, as seen in acromegaly and pachydermoperiostitis 肢厚皮病

ac·ro·pa·ral·y·sis (ak″ro-pə-ral″ĭ-sis) paralysis of limbs 肢麻痹，肢瘫痪

ac·ro·par·es·the·sia (ak″ro-par″es-the′zhə) 1. paresthesia of the digits 肢端感觉异常 ; 2. a disease marked by attacks of tingling, numbness, and

stiffness chiefly in the fingers, hands, and forearms, sometimes with pain, skin pallor, or slight cyanosis 肢端麻痹症

ac·ro·pa·thol·o·gy (ak″ro-pə-thol′ə-je) pathology of diseases of limbs （四）肢病理学

acrop·a·thy (ă-krop′ə-the) any disease of limbs 四肢病

ac·ro·pho·bia (ak″ro-fo′be-ə) irrational fear of heights 高处恐怖症，高空恐怖症

ac·ro·pus·tu·lo·sis (ak″ro-pus″tu-lo′sis) pustulosis of the extremities. A congenital form (*infantile a.*) is characterized by recurring episodes of small pruritic pustules on the hands and feet followed by remission 肢体脓疱病

ac·ro·scle·ro·der·ma (ak″ro-skler″o-dur″mə) acrosclerosis 肢硬皮病，指（趾）硬皮病

ac·ro·scle·ro·sis (ak″ro-sklə-ro′sis) a combination of Raynaud disease and scleroderma of the distal limbs, especially digits, the neck, and often the nose 肢端硬皮病

ac·ro·so·mal (ak″ro-so′məl) pertaining to the acrosome 顶体的

ac·ro·some (ak′ro-sōm) the caplike, membrane-bound structure covering the anterior portion of the head of a spermatozoon; it contains enzymes for penetrating the oocyte 顶体

ac·ro·spi·ro·ma (ak″ro-spi-ro′mə) a benign adnexal tumor of the distal portion of a sweat gland 顶端螺旋瘤

ac·ro·tism (ak′ro-tiz-əm) absence or imperceptibility of the pulse 无脉，脉搏微弱 ; **acrot′ic** *adj.* 无脉的

acryl·a·mide (ə-kril′ə-mīd) a vinyl monomer used in the production of polymers with many industrial and research uses; the monomeric form is a neurotoxin 丙烯酰胺

acryl·ic (ə-kril′ik) pertaining to or containing polymers of acrylic acid, methacrylic acid, or acrylonitrile; see also under *resin* 丙烯酸的

acryl·ic ac·id (ə-kril′ik) a readily polymerizing liquid used as a monomer for acrylic polymers 丙烯酸

ac·ry·lo·ni·trile (ak″rə-lo-ni′trīl) a colorless halogenated hydrocarbon used in the making of plastics and as a pesticide; its vapors are irritant to the respiratory tract and eyes, can cause systemic poisoning, and are carcinogenic 丙烯腈

ACS American Cancer Society 美国癌症协会 ; American Chemical Society 美国化学学会 ; American College of Surgeons 美国外科医学会

ACSM American College of Sports Medicine 美国运动医学院

ACTA American Cardiology Technologists Association 美国心脏病学技术专家协会

ACTE Association for Career and Technical Education 职业技术教育协会

Ac·tem·ra (ak-tem′rə) trademark for a preparation of tocilizumab 托珠单抗

ACTH adrenocorticotropic hormone 促肾上腺皮质激素；见 *corticotropin*

ac·tin (ak′tin) a structural protein present in all eukaryotic cells, important both as a component of the cytoskeleton and for its role in cell motility, existing as a globular monomer (*G-actin*) and as long fibers (*F-actin*). In combination with myosin it is responsible for muscular contraction 肌动蛋白

act·ing out (ak′ting out) the expression of unconscious feelings and fantasies in behavior; reacting to present situations as if they were the original situation that gave rise to the feelings and fantasies 潜意识显露，舒放

ac·tin·ic (ak-tin′ik) producing chemical action; said of rays of light beyond the violet end of the spectrum 光化性的

ac·tin·i·um (Ac) (ak-tin′e-əm) a rare, soft, silvery white, metallic radioactive element; at. no. 89, at. wt. 227 锕

ac·ti·no·bac·il·lo·sis (ak″tĭ-no-bas″ĭ-lo′sis) an actinomycosis-like disease of domestic animals and occasionally humans, caused by *Actinobacillus lignieresii*, in which the bacilli form radiating structures in the tissues 放线杆菌病

Ac·ti·no·ba·cil·lus (ak″tĭ-no-bə-sil′us) a genus of gram-negative, nonmotile, coccoid or rod-shaped bacteria that cause actinobacillosis in domestic animals and occasionally humans; *A. ure′ae* is a cause of ozena 放线杆菌属

Ac·ti·no·bac·te·ria (ak″tĭ-no-bak-tēr′e-ə) 1. a morphologically and physiologically diverse phylum of bacteria, containing a large number of medically important organisms 放线菌门；2. the sole class of bacteria of this phylum; it is divided into several subclasses 放线菌

Ac·ti·no·bac·te·ri·dae (ak″tĭ-no-bak-tēr′ĭ-de) a large, diverse subclass of bacteria of the class Actinobacteria 放线菌亚纲

Ac·ti·no·ba·cu·lum (ak″tĭ-no-bak′u-ləm) a genus of gram-positive, anaerobic or facultatively anaerobic, rod-shaped bacteria of the family Actinomycetaceae. *A. schaa′lii*, *A. massi′liae*, and *A. urina′le* cause urinary tract infections 放线棒菌属

ac·ti·no·der·ma·ti·tis (ak″tĭ-no-dur″mə-ti′tis) radiodermatitis X 线皮炎

Ac·ti·no·ma·du·ra (ak″tĭ-no-mə-door′ə) a genus of bacteria (family Thermomonosporaceae). *A. madu′rae* causes actinomycotic mycetoma in which granules in the discharged pus are white; *A.*

pelletie′ri causes actinomycotic mycetoma in which granules are red 马杜拉放线菌属

Ac·ti·no·my·ces (ak″tĭ-no-mi′sēz) a genus of bacteria (family Actinomycetaceae) 放线菌属；*A. israe′lii*, a species parasitic in the mouth, proliferating in necrotic tissue; it is the etiologic agent of human actinomycosis and can cause actinomycotic mycetoma 衣氏放线菌；*A. naeslun′dii*, an anaerobic species that is a normal inhabitant of the oral cavity and a cause of human actinomycosis and periodontal disease 内氏放线菌

Ac·ti·no·my·ce·ta·ceae (ak″tĭ-no-mi″sə-ta′se-e) a family of gram-positive bacteria of the suborder Actinomycineae (order Actinomycetales) 放线菌科

Ac·ti·no·my·ce·ta·les (ak″tĭ-no-mi″sə-ta′lēz) an order of bacteria of the subclass Actinobacteridae made up of elongated cells having a tendency to branch 放线菌目

ac·ti·no·my·cete (ak″tĭ-no-mi′sēt) any bacterium of the order Actinomycetales 放线菌类；**nocardioform a′s,** a morphological group of actinomycetes characterized by a mycelium that breaks up into bacillary or coccal forms; all genera in this group are gram-positive and aerobic 诺卡氏菌形放线菌

ac·ti·no·my·cin (ak″tĭ-no-mi′sin) a family of antibiotics from various species of *Streptomyces*, which are active against bacteria and fungi; it includes the antineoplastic agent dactinomycin (actinomycin D) 放线菌素

Ac·ti·no·my·ci·neae (ak″tĭ-no-mi-sin′e-e) suborder of bacteria of the order Actinomycetales 放线菌亚目

ac·ti·no·my·co·sis (ak″tĭ-no-mi-ko′sis) an infectious disease caused by *Actinomyces*; marked by swelling and abscesses in the head and neck region and sometimes in the peritoneum, or in the lung due to aspiration 放线菌病；**actinomycot′ic** *adj.* 放线菌病的

ac·ti·no·ther·a·py (ak″tĭ-no-ther′ə-pe) phototherapy 放射疗法

ac·tion (ak′shən) the accomplishment of an effect, whether mechanical or chemical, or the effect so produced 作用，动作；**ball-valve a.,** the intermittent obstruction caused by a free or partially attached foreign body in a tubular or cavitary structure, as by a foreign body in a bronchus, a stone in a bile duct, or a tumor in the cardiac atrium 球瓣作用；**cumulative a.,** action of increased intensity, as the sudden and markedly increased action of a drug after administration of several doses, due to the accumulation of the drug in the body 累积作用；**reflex a.,** a response, often involuntary, resulting from passage of excitation potential from a receptor to a muscle or gland over a reflex arc 反射作用

ac·ti·va·tion (ak″tĭ-va′shən) 1. the act or process of rendering active 活 化 ; 2. the transformation of a proenzyme into an active enzyme by the action of a kinase or another enzyme 激活 ; 3. the process by which the central nervous system is stimulated into activity through the mediation of the reticular activating system 中枢神经系统激发过程 ; 4. the deliberate induction of a pattern of electrical activity in the brain 脑内电活动的诱导 ; **allosteric a.**, increase in enzyme activity by binding of an effector at an allosteric site that affects binding or turnover at the catalytic site 变构活化 ; **contact a.**, initiation of the intrinsic pathway of coagulation through interaction of coagulation factor Ⅻ with various electronegative surfaces 接触活化 ; **lymphocyte a.**, stimulation of lymphocytes by antigen or mitogens resulting in macromolecular synthesis (RNA, protein, and DNA) and production of lymphokines, followed by proliferation and differentiation of the progeny into various effector and memory cells 淋巴细胞活化

ac·ti·va·tor (ak′tĭ-va″tər) 1. a substance that combines with an enzyme to increase its catalytic activity (酶) 活化剂 ; 2. a substance that stimulates the development of a specific structure in the embryo 促使胚胎特定结构发育的物质 ; 3. a chemical or other form of energy that causes another substance to become reactive or that induces a chemical reaction 能使另一种物质发生反应或引起化学反应的化学物质或其他形式的能量 ; **plasminogen a.**, any of a group of substances that have the ability to cleave plasminogen and convert it into the active form plasmin 纤溶酶原激活药 ; **prothrombin a.**, any one of the substances in the extrinsic or intrinsic pathways of coagulation 凝血酶原激活剂 ; **single chain urokinasetype plasminogen a. (scu-PA)**, prourokinase 单链血浆酶原尿激酶激活剂 ; **tissue plasminogen a. (TPA) (t-PA), t-plasminogen a.**, an endopeptidase synthesized by endothelial cells that binds to fibrin clots and catalyzes the cleavage of plasminogen to the active form plasmin. t-PA produced by recombinant technology is used for therapeutic thrombolysis 组织型纤溶酶原激活物 ; **u-plasminogen a., urokinase.**, **urinary plasminogen a.**, 尿激酶型纤溶酶原激活物

ac·tive (ak′tiv) characterized by action; not passive; not expectant 活动的；积极的；主动的

ac·tive ro·bot·ics (ăk′tiv rō″bŏd′icks) the practice of using computer-assisted robotic devices in surgery to increase the accuracy of procedures and implantation 使用计算机辅助的机器人以提高外科手术中操作的精确度

ac·ti·vin (ak′tĭ-vin) any of several polypeptide growth and differentiation factors, members of the transforming growth factor-β family, that stimulate the secretion of follicle-stimulating hormone, play roles in neuroendocrine regulation, modulate production of other hormones, and affect gonadal functions 苯丙酸诺龙

ac·tiv·i·ty (ak-tiv′ĭ-te) 1. the quality or process of exerting energy or of accomplishing an effect 活性，活力 ; 2. a thermodynamic quantity that represents the effective concentration of a solute in a nonideal solution. Symbol a. 热动力度 ; 3. the number of disintegrations per unit time of a radioactive material. Symbol A. 放射活性 ; 4. the presence of recordable electrical energy in a muscle or nerve (*electrical a.*) 脑电和肌电描记 ; 5. 见 optical a.; **end-plate a.**, spontaneous activity recorded close to motor end plates in normal muscle 终板活动 ; **enzyme a.**, the catalytic effect exerted by an enzyme, expressed as units per milligram of enzyme (*specific a.*) or as molecules of substrate transformed per minute per molecule of enzyme (*molecular a.*) 酶活力 ; **intrinsic sympathomimetic a. (ISA)**, the ability of a β-blocker to stimulate β-adrenergic receptors weakly during β-blockade 内源性拟交感活动 ; **optical a.**, the ability of a chemical compound to rotate the plane of polarization of plane-polarized light 旋光度

ac·to·my·o·sin (ak″to-mi′o-sin) the complex of actin and myosin occurring in muscle fibers 肌动球蛋白

acu·i·ty (ə-ku′ĭ-te) clarity or clearness, especially of vision 清晰度

acu·mi·nate (ə-ku′mĭ-nāt) sharp-pointed 尖的

acu·point (ak′u-point) any of the specific sites for needle insertion in acupuncture; also used in other therapies, including acupressure and moxibustion. Most are areas of high electrical conductance on the body surface 穴位，针灸穴位

acu·pres·sure (ak′u-presh″ər) the use of pressure applied, usually with the hands, at acupoints in order to release muscular tension for therapeutic purposes 指压法

acu·punc·ture (ak′u-punk″chər) a traditional Chinese practice of piercing specific areas of the body (acupoints) along peripheral nerves with fine needles to relieve pain, to induce surgical anesthesia, and for therapeutic purposes. Other means of stimulating the acupoints, including lasers, ultrasound, and electricity, may also be used 针灸 ; **Korean hand a.**, a type in which the hand is considered to be a representation of the entire body, and stimulation of specific points on the hand is used to obtain effects in distant areas of the body 韩国手针刺术

acus (a′kəs) a needle or needle-like process 针或针样突

acute (ə-kūt′) having severe symptoms and a short course 急性的

ACVIM American College of Veterinary Internal Medicine 全美兽医内科医学院

ACVP American College of Veterinary Pathologists 美国兽医病理学家学院

acy·a·not·ic (a-si″ə-not′ik) characterized by absence of cyanosis 不发绀的

acy·clo·vir (a-si′klo-vēr) a synthetic purine nucleoside with selective activity against most human herpesviruses, particularly types 1 and 2; used as the base or the sodium salt in the treatment of genital and mucocutaneous herpesvirus infections 阿昔洛韦

acyl (a′səl) an organic radical derived from an organic acid by removal of the hydroxyl group from the carboxyl group 酰基

ac·yl·ase (a′sə-lās) 见 amidase (1)

ac·yl-CoA de·hy·dro·gen·ase (a′səl ko-a′de-hi′dro-jən-ās) any of several enzymes that catalyze the oxidation of acyl coenzyme A thioesters as a step in the degradation of fatty acids. Individual enzymes are specific for certain ranges of acyl chain lengths: *long-chain a.-CoA d. (LCAD), medium-chain a.-CoA d. (MCAD)*, and *short-chain a.-CoA d. (SCAD)* 酰基辅酶 A 脱氢酶

ac·yl co·en·zyme A (a′səl ko-en′zīm) acyl CoA; a thiol ester of a carboxylic acid, particularly a long-chain fatty acid, and coenzyme A; its formation is the first step in fatty acid oxidation 酰基辅酶 A

ac·yl·glyc·er·ol (a″səl-glis′ər-ol) glyceride 甘油酯

N-**ac·yl·sphin·go·sine** (a″səl-sfing′gosēn) ceramide *N*- 酰基鞘氨醇

ac·yl·trans·fer·ase (a″səl-trans′fər-ās) any of a group of enzymes that catalyze the transfer of an acyl group from one substance to another 酰基转移酶

acys·tia (a-sis′te-ə) congenital absence of the bladder 无膀胱（畸形）

AD [L.] au′ris dex′tra (right ear) 右耳

ad [L.] preposition, *to* 向，至

ADA adenosine deaminase 腺苷脱氨酶；American Dental Association 美国牙科协会；American Diabetes Association 美国糖尿病协会；American Dietetic Association 美国饮食协会；Americans with Disabilities Act 美国残疾人法案；Australian Dental Association 澳大利亚牙科协会

ADAA American Dental Assistants Association 美国牙科助理协会

adac·ty·ly (a-dak′tə-le) congenital absence of fingers or toes 无指（趾）；**adac′tylous** *adj.*

ada·lim·u·mab (a″də-lim′u-mab) a recombinant human IgG1 monoclonal antibody that binds to and blocks the action of tumor necrosis factor α, used to alleviate the signs and symptoms of and inhibit the progression of structural damage in rheumatoid arthritis; administered subcutaneously 阿达木单抗

ad·a·man·tine (ad″ə-man′tin) pertaining to the enamel of the teeth 釉质的

ad·a·man·ti·no·ma (ad″ə-man″tĭ-no′mə) ameloblastoma 成釉（上皮）瘤

ad·a·man·to·blast (ad″ə-man′to-blast) ameloblast 成釉细胞

ad·a·man·to·ma (ad″ə-man-to′mə) ameloblastoma 成釉细胞瘤

adap·a·lene (ə-dap′ə-lēn) a synthetic analogue of retinoic acid used topically in the treatment of acne vulgaris 阿达帕林（用于治疗普通粉刺）

ad·ap·ta·tion (ad″ap-ta′shən) 1. the adjustment of an organism to its environment, or the process by which it enhances such fitness 机体对环境的适应或提高这种适应的过程；2. the normal adjustment of the eye to variations in intensity of light 眼依光线强度进行自我调节的正常能力；3. the decline in the frequency of firing of a neuron, particularly of a receptor, under conditions of constant stimulation 神经元，特别是感受神经器在持续刺激下冲动发动频率的减低；4. in dentistry 牙科学指：(*a*) the proper fitting of a denture 义齿的适应，(*b*) the degree of proximity and interlocking of restorative material to a tooth preparation 修复材料对牙体制备的密合性和连接程度，(*c*) the exact adjustment of bands to teeth 带环密牙的精密调整；5. in microbiology, the adjustment of bacterial physiology to a new environment 微生物学上指细菌针对新环境所作生理机制的调整；**color a.**, 1. changes in visual perception of color with prolonged stimulation 色适应；2. adjustment of vision to degree of brightness or color tone of illumination 视力调节；**dark a.**, adaptation of the eye to vision in the dark or in reduced illumination 暗适应；**genetic a.**, the natural selection of the progeny of a mutant better adapted to a new environment 遗传适应；**light a.**, adaptation of the eye to vision in the sunlight or in bright illumination (photopia), with reduction in the concentration of the photosensitive pigments of the eye 光适应；**phenotypic a.**, a change in the properties of an organism in response to genetic mutation or to a change in the environment 表型适应

ad·ap·tom·e·ter (ad″ap-tom′ə-tər) an instrument for measuring the time required for retinal adaptation, i.e., for regeneration of the visual purple; used in detecting night blindness, vitamin A deficiency, and retinitis pigmentosa 适应计；**color a.**, an instrument to demonstrate adaptation of the eye to color or light 彩色适应计

ADCC antibody-dependent cell-mediated cytotoxicity 抗体依赖的细胞介导的细胞毒性

ADD attention defificit disorder 注意力缺陷紊乱

ad·der (ad′ər) 1. *Vipera berus* 极北蝰；2. any of many venomous snakes of the family Viperidae, such as the puff adder and European viper 蝰蛇科动物的统称；**death a.**, *Acanthophis antarcticus*, an extremely venomous elapid snake of Australia and New Guinea with a short, stout body and a tail with a spine at the tip 死亡蝰蛇；**puff a.**, *Bitis arietans*, an extremely venomous, brightly colored viperine snake found in Africa and Arabia; when annoyed, it inflates its body and hisses loudly 鼓腹巨蝰

ad·dic·tion (ə-dik′shən) 1. the state of being given up to some habit or compulsion 瘾；2. strong physiological and psychological dependence on a drug or other psychoactive substance 成瘾

ad·di·son·ism (ad′ĭ-sən-iz″əm) addisonian syndrome 类青铜色皮病。又称 *Addison disease*

ad·duct[1] (ə-dukt′) to draw toward the median plane or (in the digits) toward the axial line of a limb 收，内收

ad·duct[2] (ă′dukt) inclusion complex 加合物

ad·duc·tion (ə-duk′shən) the act of adducting; the state being adducted 收（作用），内收（作用）

ad·duc·tor (ə-duk′tər) [L.] that which adducts, as the adductor muscle 内收肌

ad·e·nal·gia (ad″ə-nal′jə) pain in a gland 腺痛

aden·drit·ic (a″den-drit′ik) lacking dendrites 无树突的

ad·e·nec·to·my (ad″ə-nek′tə-me) excision of a gland 腺切除术

ad·en·ec·to·pia (ad″ə-nek-to′pe-ə) malposition or displacement of a gland 腺异位

ade·nia (ə-de′ne-ə) chronic enlargement of the lymphatic glands, as in lymphoma 淋巴腺增生病，假白血病

ad·e·nine (A) (ad′ə-nēn) a purine base; in plant and animal cells usually occurring complexed with ribose or deoxyribose to form adenosine and deoxyadenosine, components of nucleic acids, nucleotides, and coenzymes. A preparation is used to improve the preservation of whole blood 腺嘌呤 **a. arabinoside,** vidarabine 阿糖腺苷

ad·e·ni·tis (ad″ə-ni′tis) inflammation of a gland 腺炎；**Bartholin a.**, inflammation of the greater vestibular glands (Bartholin glands) resulting from acute infection of the gland 前庭大腺炎；**cervical a.**, 见 *lymphadenopathy* 下词条；**mesenteric a.**, 见 *lymphadenitis* 下词条；**vestibular a.**, chronic inflammation of the lesser vestibular glands with small, painful ulcerations of the mucosa of the vestibule of the vagina 前庭腺炎

ad·e·no·ac·an·tho·ma (ad″ə-no-ak″an-tho′mə) adenocarcinoma in which some of the cells exhibit squamous differentiation 腺棘皮癌

ad·e·no·am·e·lo·blas·to·ma (ad″ə-no-ə-mel″oblas-to′mə) adenomatoid odontogenic tumor 腺性成釉细胞瘤

ad·e·no·blast (ad′ə-no-blast″) an embryonic cell that gives rise to glandular tissue 成腺细胞

ad·e·no·car·ci·no·ma (ad″ə-no-kahr″sĭ-no′mə) carcinoma derived from glandular tissue or in which the tumor cells form recognizable glandular structures 腺癌；**acinar a.**, 1. 见 *carcinoma* 下词条；2. the most common neoplasm of the prostate, usually arising in the peripheral acini 最常见的前列腺肿瘤；**acinic cell a., acinous a.**, 见 *carcinoma* 下词条；**bronchogenic a.**, the usual type of adenocarcinoma of the lung 小腺泡状腺癌；cf. *bronchioloalveolar carcinoma*; **clear cell a.**, a rare malignant tumor of the female genital tract, containing tubules or small cysts; it may occur in the ovary, uterus, cervix, or vagina. One form has been linked to in utero exposure to diethylstilbestrol 透明细胞腺癌；**ductal a. of the prostate,** adenocarcinoma of columnar epithelium in the peripheral prostatic ducts; it may project into the urethra 前列腺管状腺癌；**endometrioid a.**, the most common form of endometrioid carcinoma, containing tumor cells differentiated into glandular tissue with little or no stroma 子宫内膜样腺癌；**gastric a.**, any of a group of common stomach cancers, usually located in the antrum; it occurs particularly in Japan, Iceland, Chile, and Finland and may be linked to certain dietary substances such as nitrosamines and benzopyrene 胃腺癌；**a. of the lung,** a type of bronchogenic carcinoma made up of cuboidal or columnar cells in a discrete mass, usually at the periphery of the lungs 肺腺癌；**papillary a., polypoid a.**, that in which the tumor elements are arranged as finger-like processes or as a solid spherical nodule projecting from an epithelial surface 乳头状腺癌；**a. of the prostate,** 见 acinar a. (2)

ad·e·no·cele (ad′ə-no-sēl″) cystadenoma 腺囊肿

ad·e·no·cel·lu·li·tis (ad″ə-no-sel″u-li′tis) inflammation of a gland and the tissue around it 腺蜂窝织炎

ad·e·no·cys·tic (ad″ə-no-sis′tik) having both glandular (adenoid) and cystic elements 腺囊性的

ad·e·no·cys·to·ma (ad″ə-no-sis-to′mə) cystadenoma 囊腺瘤

ad·e·no·cyte (ad′ə-no-sīt″) a mature secretory cell of a gland 腺细胞

ad·e·no·fi·bro·ma (ad″ə-no-fi-bro′mə) a tumor composed of connective tissue containing glandular structures 腺纤维瘤

ad·e·nog·e·nous (ad″ə-noj′ə-nəs) originating from glandular tissue 腺原的

ad·e·nog·ra·phy (ad″ə-nog′rə-fe) radiography of the glands 腺放射造影术；**adenograph′ic** *adj.*

ad·e·no·hy·poph·y·sec·to·my (ad″ə-no-hipof″ĭ-sek′tə-me) excision or ablation of the anterior pituitary lobe 腺垂体切除术

ad·e·no·hy·poph·y·sis (ad″ə-no-hi-pof′ĭ-sis) the anterior (glandular) lobe of the pituitary gland; it secretes the anterior pituitary hormones such as growth hormone, thyrotropin, and others 腺垂体前叶；**adenohypophys′eal** *adj.*

ad·e·noid (ad′ə-noid) 1. pharyngeal tonsil 咽扁桃体；2. pertaining to a pharyngeal tonsil 咽扁桃体的；3. resembling a gland 腺样的；4. (*in the pl.*) the pharyngeal tonsils; used particularly when they are hypertrophied 咽扁桃体肥大

ad·e·noid·i·tis (ad″ə-noid-i′tis) inflammation of the adenoids 增殖腺炎

ad·e·no·li·po·ma (ad″ə-no-lĭ-po′mə) a tumor composed of both glandular and fatty tissue elements 腺脂瘤

ad·e·no·lym·pho·ma (ad″ə-no-lim-fo′mə) a benign parotid gland tumor characterized by cystic spaces lined by tall columnar eosinophilic epithelial cells, overlying a lymphoid tissue–containing stroma 腺淋巴瘤

ad·e·no·ma (ad″ə-no′mə) a benign epithelial tumor in which the cells form recognizable glandular structures or in which the cells are derived from glandular epithelium 腺瘤；**adrenocortical a.**, a benign tumor of the adrenal cortex, usually small and unilateral; most types cause endocrine symptoms 肾上腺皮质腺瘤；**basal cell a.**, a benign, encapsulated, slow-growing, painless salivary gland tumor of intercalated or reserve cell origin, occurring mainly in males, in the parotid gland or upper lip; *solid, canalicular, trabecular-tubular*, and *membranous* types can be distinguished histologically 基底细胞腺瘤；**bile duct a.**, a small firm white nodule with multiple bile ducts embedded in a fibrous stroma 胆管腺瘤；**bronchial a's**, tumors of low-grade malignancy situated in the submucosal tissues of large bronchi; sometimes composed of well-differentiated cells and usually circumscribed, with two histologic forms: carcinoid and cylindroma 支气管腺瘤；**carcinoma ex pleomorphic a.**, 见 *carcinoma* 下词条；**chromophobe a., chromophobic a.**, 见 null-cell a.；**corticotroph a.**, a pituitary adenoma made up predominantly of corticotrophs and secreting excess corticotropin 促肾上腺皮质激素分泌；**endocrine-active a.**, 见 functioning a.；

endocrine-inactive a., 见 nonfunctioning a.；**follicular a.**, adenoma of the thyroid in which the cells are arranged in the form of follicles 滤泡性腺瘤；**functional a., functioning a.**, a pituitary adenoma that secretes excessive amounts of a hormone 功能性腺瘤；**glycoprotein a.**, a pituitary adenoma that causes excessive secretion of one of the three glycoprotein hormones (follicle-stimulating hormone, luteinizing hormone, and thyrotropin) 糖蛋白腺瘤；**gonadotrope a., gonadotroph a.**, a pituitary adenoma made up of gonadotroph-like cells that secrete excessive amounts of folliclestimulating hormone or luteinizing hormone, causing precocious puberty, visual disturbances, or hypogonadism 促性腺素腺瘤；**growth hormone–secreting a.**, a pituitary adenoma made up of somatotroph-like cells that secrete excessive amounts of growth hormone, causing gigantism in children or acromegaly in adults 生长激素分泌腺瘤；**hepatocellular a.**, a benign circumscribed tumor of the liver, usually in the right lobe, growing in a sheetlike fashion; it may be highly vascular with a tendency to hemorrhage and with areas of necrosis 肝细胞腺瘤；**Hürthle cell a.**, 见 *tumor* 下词条；**liver cell a.**, 见 hepatocellular a.；**macrofollicular a.**, a follicular adenoma composed of large follicles filled with colloid and lined with flat epithelium 大滤泡型腺瘤；**microfollicular a.**, a follicular adenoma with small, closely packed follicles lined with epithelium 小滤泡型腺瘤；**mixed-cell a.**, a pituitary adenoma containing more than one cell type, usually making it plurihormonal 混合细胞腺瘤；**monomorphic a.**, any of a group of benign salivary gland tumors that lack connective tissue changes and are each predominantly composed of a single cell type 单形性腺瘤；**nipple a.**, a benign lesion of the breast, clinically resembling Paget disease of the breast, consisting of ductal and stromal proliferation beneath the nipple; it presents as a mass, ulceration, or erosion, with a serous or bloody discharge 乳头腺瘤；**nonfunctional a., nonfunctioning a.**, a pituitary adenoma that does not secrete excessive amounts of any hormone; many null-cell adenomas are of this type 无功能腺瘤；**null-cell a.**, a pituitary adenoma whose cells give negative results on tests for staining and hormone secretion, although some may contain functioning cells and be associated with a hyperpituitary state 无细胞腺瘤；**oncocytic a., oxyphilic a.**, 1. oncocytoma. 大嗜酸性粒细胞腺瘤；2. Hürthle cell adenoma Hürthle 细胞腺瘤；**papillary a.**, 见 nipple a.；**papillary cystic a.**, papillary cystadenoma 乳头状囊腺瘤；**pituitary a.**, a benign neoplasm of the anterior pituitary gland 垂体腺瘤；见 *functional a.* and *nonfunctional a.*；

pleomorphic a., a benign, slow-growing epithelial tumor of the salivary gland, usually of the parotid gland, sometimes serving as a locus for development of a malignant epithelial neoplasm (*malignant pleomorphic a.*) 多形性腺瘤 ; **plurihormonal a.**, an endocrine-active adenoma that secretes two or more hormones, usually growth hormone and one or more of the glycoprotein types 多激素腺瘤 ; **prolactin cell a.**, **prolactinsecreting a.**, prolactinoma 催乳素瘤 ; **sebaceous a.**, **a. seba′ceum**, 1. 见 *hyperplasia* 下词条 ; 2. a widely used misnomer for a hamartoma on the face seen with tuberous sclerosis 皮脂腺腺瘤 ; **thyrotrope a.**, **thyrotroph a.**, a pituitary adenoma made up of thyrotroph- like cells that secrete excess thyrotropin and cause hyperthyroidism 促甲状腺素细胞腺瘤 ; **trabecular a.**, a follicular adenoma whose cells are closely packed to form cords or trabeculae, with only a few small follicles 柱状腺瘤 ; **tubular a.**, 管状腺瘤, 1. an adenoma whose cells are arranged in tubules 腺瘤细胞管状排列，形成结肠瘤样息肉，某些乳腺纤维腺瘤和男性细胞瘤 ; 2. 见 androblastoma (1); 3. the most common type of adenomatous polyp of the colon, with tubules highly variable in size and often occurring singly 结肠腺瘤样息肉的最常见类型 ; **villous a.**, an uncommon type of adenomatous polyp of the colon that is large, soft, and papillary and often premalignant 绒毛状腺瘤

ad·e·no·ma·la·cia (ad″ə-no-mə-la′shə) abnormal softening of a gland 腺软化

ad·e·no·ma·toid (ad″ə-no′mə-toid) resembling adenoma 腺瘤样的

ad·e·no·ma·to·sis (ad″ə-no-mə-to′sis) the development of numerous adenomatous growths 腺瘤病

ad·e·nom·a·tous (ad″ə-nom′ə-təs) 1. pertaining to an adenoma 腺瘤的 ; 2. pertaining to nodular hyperplasia of a gland 腺瘤结节的

ad·e·no·meg·a·ly (ad″ə-no-meg′ə-le) enlargement of a gland 腺肿大

ad·e·no·mere (ad′ə-no-mēr″) the blind terminal portion of a developing gland, becoming the functional portion of the organ 腺节

ad·e·no·myo·fi·bro·ma (ad″ə-no-mi″o-fibro′mə) a fibroma containing both glandular and muscular elements 腺肌纤维瘤

ad·e·no·my·o·ma (ad″ə-no-mi-o′mə) 1. a benign tumor consisting of smooth muscle and glandular elements 腺肌瘤 ; 2. 见 *adenomyosis*

ad·e·no·my·o·ma·to·sis (ad″ə-no-mi″ə-mə-to′sis) the formation of multiple adenomyomatous nodules in the tissues around or in the uterus 腺肌瘤病

ad·e·no·myo·me·tri·tis (ad″ə-no-mi″o-mə-tri′tis) an inflammatory lesion of the endometrium, which may lead to adenomyosis 子宫腺肌炎

ad·e·no·myo·sar·co·ma (ad″ə-no-mi″o-sahrko′mə) a mixed mesodermal tumor containing striated muscle cells 腺肉瘤

ad·e·no·my·o·sis (ad″ə-no-mi-o′sis) benign ingrowth of the endometrium into the uterine musculature, sometimes with hypertrophy of the latter; if the lesion forms a circumscribed tumorlike nodule, it is called *adenomyoma* 子宫内膜异位

ad·e·nop·a·thy (ad″ə-nop′ə-the) lymphadenopathy 腺肿大，淋巴结增大，淋巴结病

ad·e·no·phar·yn·gi·tis (ad″ə-no-far″in-ji′tis) inflammation of the adenoids and pharynx, usually involving the tonsils 咽扁桃体炎

ad·e·no·sar·co·ma (ad″ə-no-sahr-ko′mə) a mixed tumor composed of both glandular and sarcomatous elements 腺肉瘤

ad·e·no·scle·ro·sis (ad″ə-no-sklĕ-ro′sis) hardening of a gland 腺硬化

aden·o·sine (A) (ə-den′o-sēn) a purine nucleoside consisting of adenine and ribose; a component of RNA. It is also a cardiac depressant and vasodilator used as an antiarrhythmic and as an adjunct in myocardial perfusion imaging in patients incapable of exercising adequately to undergo an exercise stress test 腺苷 ; **cyclic a. monophosphate (3′,5′-AMP) (cAMP) (cyclic AMP)**, a cyclic nucleotide, adenosine 3′,5′-cyclic monophosphate, that serves as an intracellular, and sometimes extracellular, "second messenger" mediating the action of many peptide or amine hormones 环腺苷酸 ; **a. diphosphate (ADP)**, a nucleotide, the 5′-pyrophosphate of adenosine, involved in energy metabolism; it is produced by the hydrolysis of adenosine triphosphate (ATP) and converted back to ATP by the metabolic processes oxidative phosphorylation and substrate-level phosphorylation 二磷酸腺苷 ; **a. monophosphate (AMP)**, adenylic acid; a nucleotide, the 5′-phosphate of adenosine, involved in energy metabolism and nucleotide synthesis 磷酸腺苷 ; **a. triphosphate (ATP)**, a nucleotide, the 5′-triphosphate of adenosine, involved in energy metabolism and required for RNA synthesis; it occurs in all cells and is used to store energy in the form of high-energy phosphate bonds. The free energy derived from its hydrolysis is used to drive metabolic reactions, to transport molecules against concentration gradients, and to produce mechanical motion 三磷酸腺苷

aden·o·sine de·am·i·nase (ADA) (ə-den′osēn de-am′ĭ-nās) an enzyme that catalyzes the hydrolytic deamination of adenosine to form inosine, a reaction of purine metabolism. Enzyme activity is absent in many individuals with severe combined immunodeficiency 腺苷脱氨酶

aden·o·sine·tri·phos·pha·tase (ə-den″osēn-tri-fos′fə-tās) an enzyme that catalyzes the hydrolysis of ATP to ADP, driving processes such as muscle contraction, maintenance of concentration gradients, membrane transport, and regulation of ion concentrations 腺苷三磷酸酶

ad·e·no·sis (ad″ə-no′sis) 1. any disease of the glands 腺的任何病变；2. the abnormal development of glandular tissue 腺组织的异常发生或形成；**mammary sclerosing a., sclerosing a.** of breast, a form of disease of the breast characterized by multiple firm tender nodules, fibrous tissue, mastodynia, and sometimes small cysts 乳房硬化腺病

ad·e·no·squa·mous (ad″ə-no-skwa′məs) having both glandular (adenoid) and squamous elements 腺鳞癌

aden·o·syl·co·ba·la·min (AdoCbl) (ə-den″osəl-ko-bal′ə-min) one of two metabolically active forms of cobalamin synthesized upon ingestion of vitamin B_{12}; it is the predominant form in the liver 腺苷钴胺素

ad·e·no·tome (ad′ə-no-tōm″) an instrument for excision of adenoids 增殖腺刀

Ad·e·no·vi·ri·dae (ad″ə-no-vir′ĭ-de) the adenoviruses: a family of DNA viruses that have narrow host ranges; the genus *Mastadenovirus* infects humans 腺病毒科

ad·e·no·vi·rus (ad′ə-no-vi″rəs) any virus belonging to the family Adenoviridae 腺病毒；**adenovi′ral** *adj.* **mammalian a's,** 乳腺病毒，见 *Mastadenovirus*

ad·e·nyl (ad′ə-nəl) 1. the radical of adenine 腺嘌呤基；2. sometimes (incorrectly) used for *adenylyl* 有时被误用为 adenylyl

aden·yl·ate (ə-den′ə-lāt) the dissociated form of adenylic acid 腺嘌呤核苷酸

aden·yl·ate ki·nase (ə-den′ə-lāt ki′nās) an enzyme that catalyzes the conversion of two molecules of ADP to AMP and ATP; it occurs predominantly in muscle, providing energy for muscle contraction 腺苷酸激酶

ad·e·nyl cy·clase (ad′ə-nəl si′klās) an enzyme that catalyzes the conversion of adenosine triphosphate (ATP) to cyclic adenosine monophosphate (cAMP) and inorganic pyrophosphate (PPi). It is activated by the attachment of a hormone or neurotransmitter to a specific membranebound receptor 腺苷酸环化酶

ad·e·nyl·ic ac·id (ad″ə-nil′ik) phosphorylated adenosine, usually adenosine monophosphate 腺苷酸

aden·yl·yl (ad′ə-nəl-əl) the radical of adenosine

monophosphate with one OH ion removed 腺嘌呤核苷酰基

ad·e·qua·cy (ad′ə-kwə-se) the state of being sufficient for a specific purpose 适当，充足；**velopharyngeal a.,** sufficient functional closure of the velum against the postpharyngeal wall so that air and hence sound cannot enter the nasopharyngeal and nasal cavities 咽腭闭合良好

Ad·e·san (ă duh′săn) trademark for a preparation of candesartan cilexetil 坎地沙坦西酯的商标

ADH antidiuretic hormone 抗利尿激素

ADHA American Dental Hygienists' Association 美国牙科保健师协会

ad·her·ence (ad-hēr′əns) the act or condition of sticking to something 黏附；**adher′ent** *adj.*；**immune a.,** the adherence of antigen-antibody complexes or cells coated with antibody or complement to cells bearing complement receptors or Fc receptors. It is a sensitive detector of complement-fixing antibody 免疫黏附

ad·he·sion (ad-he′zhən) 1. the property of remaining in close proximity 粘连，黏着；2. the stable joining of parts to one another, which may occur abnormally 几部分相互稳固的结合；3. a fibrous band or structure by which parts abnormally adhere 把各部分异常地粘连在一起的纤维带或纤维组织；**interthalamic a.,** a band of gray matter joining the thalami; it develops as a secondary adhesion and may be absent 丘脑间黏合；**primary a.,** healing by first intention 原发性粘连；**secondary a.,** healing by second intention 继发性粘连

ad·he·si·ot·o·my (ad-he″ze-ot′ə-me) surgical division of adhesions 粘连切离术

ad·he·sive (ad-he′siv) 1. sticky; tenacious 粘着的；2. a substance that causes close adherence of adjoining surfaces 黏合剂

adi·a·do·cho·ki·ne·sia (ə-di″ə-do″ko-kī-ne′zhə) a dyskinesia consisting of inability to perform the rapid alternating movements of diadochokinesia 轮替动作不能

adi·a·pho·ria (a″di-ə-for′e-ə) nonresponse to stimuli as a result of previous exposure to similar stimuli 无反应，无活动；另见 *period* 下词条 *refractory period*

adi·a·spi·ro·my·co·sis (ad″e-ə-spi″ro-mi-ko′sis) a pulmonary disease of many species of rodents and occasionally of humans, due to inhalation of spores of the fungi *Emmonsia parva* and *E. crescens*, and marked by large spherules (adiaspores) in the lungs 大孢子菌病

adi·a·spore (ad′e-ə-spor″) a spore produced by the soil fungi *Emmonsia parva* and *E. crescens* 不育大孢子；见 *adiaspiromycosis*

A

ad·i·po·cele (ad'ĭ-po-sēl″) a hernia containing fat or fatty tissue 脂肪疝

ad·i·po·cel·lu·lar (ad″ĭ-po-sel'u-lər) composed of fat and connective tissue 脂肪结缔组织的

ad·i·po·cere (ad'ĭ-po-sēr″) a waxy substance formed during decomposition of dead animal bodies, consisting mainly of insoluble salts of fatty acids 尸蜡；**adipocer'atous** adj.

ad·i·po·cyte (ad'ĭ-po-sīt) fat cell 脂肪细胞

ad·i·po·cy·to·kine (ad″ĭ-po-si'to-kīn) a general term for any of a number of bioactive factors, synthesized and secreted by adipose tissue, that modulate the physiological function of other tissues 脂肪细胞因子

ad·i·po·fi·bro·ma (ad″ĭ-po-fī-brō'mə) tumor composed of fat and fibrous or connective tissue 脂肪纤维瘤

ad·i·po·gen·ic (ad″ĭ-po-jen'ik) lipogenic 脂肪形成的

ad·i·po·ki·ne·sis (ad″ĭ-po-kĭ-ne'sis) the mobilization of fat in the body 脂肪移动；**adipokinet'ic** adj.

ad·i·pol·y·sis (ad″ĭ-pol'ĭ-sis) lipolysis 脂肪水解；**adipolyt'ic** adj.

ad·i·po·ne·cro·sis (ad″ĭ-po-nə-kro'sis) necrosis of fatty tissue 脂肪坏死

ad·i·po·nec·tin (ad-ĭ-po-nek'tin) an adipocytokine important in insulin resistance and energy homeostasis; plasma and adipose tissue levels are reduced in diabetic and obese persons 脂连蛋白

ad·i·po·pex·is (ad″ĭ-po-pek'sis) the fixation or storing of fats 积脂；**adipopec'tic** adj.

ad·i·pose (ad'ĭ-pōs) 1. fatty 肥胖；2. the fat present in the cells of adipose tissue 脂肪

ad·i·po·sis (ad″ĭ-po'sis) 1. obesity 肥胖症；2. fatty change in an organ or tissue 积脂病；**a. doloro'sa**, a disease, usually of women, marked by painful fatty swellings and nerve lesions; pulmonary complications may be fatal 痛性肥胖病；**a. hepa'ti-ca**, fatty change of the liver 脂肪肝

ad·i·po·si·tis (ad″ĭ-po-si'tis) panniculitis 脂膜炎

ad·i·pos·i·ty (ad″ĭ-pos'ĭ-te) obesity 肥胖

ad·i·po·su·ria (ad″ĭ-po-su're-ə) lipiduria 脂肪尿

adip·sia (ə-dip'se-ə) absence of thirst, or abnormal avoidance of drinking 渴感缺乏

ad·i·tus (ad'ĭ-təs) pl. *a'ditus* [L.] in anatomic nomenclature, an opening or entrance 入口，口

ad·just·ment (ə-just'mənt) 1. the act or process of modification of physical parts made in response to changing conditions 调节；2. in psychology, the relative degree of harmony between an individual's needs and the requirements of the environment 调整；3. in chiropractic, any of various manual and mechanical interventions, most often applied to the spine, in which controlled and directed forces are applied to a joint to correct structural dysfunction and restore normal nerve function 调节器

ad·ju·vant (aj'ə-vənt) (ă-joo'vənt) 1. assisting or aiding 辅助的；2. a substance that aids another, such as an auxiliary remedy 辅药；3. a nonspecific stimulator of the immune response 佐剂，在免疫学上，免疫反应的非特异性刺激物；**aluminum a.**, an aluminum-containing compound, such as aluminum hydroxide or alum, that by combining with soluble antigen forms a precipitate; slow release of the antigen from the precipitate on injection causes a strong, prolonged antibody response 铝佐剂；**Freund a.**, a water-in-oil emulsion incorporating antigen, in the aqueous phase, into lightweight paraffin oil with the aid of an emulsifying agent. On injection, this mixture (*Freund incomplete a.*) induces strong persistent antibody formation. The addition of killed, dried mycobacteria, e.g., *Mycobacterium butyricum*, to the oil phase (*Freund complete a.*) elicits cell-mediated immunity (delayed hypersensitivity), as well as humoral antibody formation 弗氏佐剂

ad·ju·van·tic·i·ty (aj″ə-vən-tis'ĭ-te) (ă-joo″vən-tis'ĭ-te) the ability to modify the immune response 佐剂性，免疫佐剂性

ad·ner·val (ad-nur'vəl) 1. situated near a nerve 近神经的；2. toward a nerve, said of electric current that passes through muscle toward the entrance point of a nerve 向神经的。又称 *adneural*

ad·nexa (ad-nek'sə) [L., pl.] appendages 附件；**a. o'culi**, the eyelids, lacrimal apparatus, and other eye appendages 眼附件；**skin a.**, 皮肤附件，见 *appendage* 下词条；**a. u'teri**, uterine appendages 子宫附件

ad·nex·al (ad-nek'səl) pertaining to adnexa 附件的

ADNI Alzheimer Disease Neuroimaging Initiative 老年痴呆症神经成像计划

AdoCbl adenosylcobalamin 腺苷钴胺素

ad·o·les·cence (ad″o-les'əns) the period between puberty and the completion of physical growth, roughly from 11 to 19 years of age 青春期；**adoles'cent** adj.

ad·or·al (ad-or'əl) toward or near the mouth 向口的，近口的

ADP adenosine diphosphate 二磷酸腺苷

ad·re·nal (ə-dre'nəl) 1. paranephric 肾上腺素的；2. suprarenal gland 肾上腺；3. pertaining to a suprarenal gland 肾旁

Adren·a·lin (ə-dren'ə-lin) trademark for preparations of epinephrine 肾上腺素

adren·a·line (ə-dren'ə-lin) epinephrine 肾上腺素

adren·a·lin·uria (ə-dren″ə-lin-u′re-ə) the presence of epinephrine in the urine 肾上腺素尿

adren·al·ism (ə-dren′əl-iz-əm) any disorder of adrenal function, whether decreased or increased 肾上腺功能障碍

adre·na·li·tis (ə-dre″nəl-i′tis) inflammation of the suprarenal glands 肾上腺炎

ad·ren·er·gic (ad″ren-ur′jik) 1. activated by, characteristic of, or secreting epinephrine or related substances, particularly the sympathetic nerve fibers that liberate norepinephrine at a synapse when a nerve impulse passes 肾上腺素能的；2. any agent that produces such an effect 拟肾上腺素药。另见 *receptor* 下词条

adre·no·cep·tor (ə-dre″no-sep′tər) adrenergic receptor 肾上腺素能受体；**adrenocep′tive** *adj.*

adre·no·cor·ti·cal (ə-dre″no-kor′tĭ-kəl) pertaining to or arising from the adrenal cortex 肾上腺皮质的

adre·no·cor·ti·co·hy·per·pla·sia (ə-dre″nokor″tĭ-ko-hi″pər-pla′zhə) adrenal cortical hyperplasia 肾上腺皮质增生

adre·no·cor·ti·coid (ə-dre″no-kor′tĭ-koid″) corticosteroid 肾上腺皮质激素

adre·no·cor·ti·co·mi·met·ic (ə-dre″nokor″tĭ-ko-mi-met′ik) having effects similar to those of hormones of the adrenal cortex 类皮质激素的

adre·no·cor·ti·co·trophic (ə-dre″no-kor″tĭko-tro′fik) adrenocorticotropic 促肾上腺皮质激素

adre·no·cor·ti·co·troph·in (ə-dre″no-kor″tĭkotro′fin) corticotropin 促肾上腺皮质激素的

adre·no·cor·ti·co·trop·ic (ə-dre″no-kor″tĭkotro′pik) having a stimulating effect on the adrenal cortex 促肾上腺皮质的

adre·no·dox·in (ə-dre″no-dok′sin) an ironsulfur protein of the adrenal cortex that serves as an electron carrier in the biosynthesis of adrenal steroids from cholesterol 肾上腺皮质铁氧还蛋白

adre·no·leu·ko·dys·tro·phy (ə-dre″noloo″ ko-dis′trə-fe) an X-linked disorder of childhood, characterized by diffuse abnormality of the cerebral white matter with severe dementia and progressive adrenal dysfunction 肾上腺脑白质营养不良

adre·no·lyt·ic (ə-dre″no-lit′ik) inhibiting the action of the adrenergic nerves, or the response to epinephrine 抗肾上腺素的

adre·no·med·ul·lary (ə-dre″no-med′u-lar″e) pertaining to or originating in the adrenal medulla 肾上腺髓质

adre·no·meg·a·ly (ə-dre″no-meg′ə-le) enlargement of one or both of the suprarenal glands 肾上腺（肿）大

adre·no·mi·met·ic (ə-dre″no-mi-met′ik) sympathomimetic 类肾上腺素能作用的

adre·no·my·elo·neu·rop·a·thy (ə-dre″nomi″ə-lo-nu o-rop′ə-the) a phenotypic variant of adrenoleukodystrophy manifested primarily by spinal cord degeneration and peripheral neuropathy 肾上腺脊髓神经病

adre·no·re·cep·tor (ə-dre″no-re-sep′tər) adrenergic receptor 肾上腺素能受体

adre·no·tox·in (ə-dre″no-tok′sin) any substance that is toxic to the suprarenal glands 肾上腺毒素

Adri·a·my·cin (a″dre-ə-mi′sin) trademark for preparations of doxorubicin hydrochloride 阿霉素

ad·sorb (ad-sorb′) to attract and retain other material on the surface; to conduct the process of adsorption 吸附，吸引

ad·sor·bent (ad-sor′bənt) 1. pertaining to or characterized by adsorption 吸附的；2. a substance that attracts other materials or particles to its surface by adsorption 吸附剂

ad·sorp·tion (ad-sorp′shən) the action of a substance in attracting and holding other materials or particles on its surface 吸附

ADTA American Dance Therapy Association 美国舞蹈治疗协会

ad·tor·sion (ad-tor′shən) intorsion 内旋（眼）

adult (ə-dult′) having attained full growth or maturity, or an organism that has done so 成年，成人；成虫，成体

adul·ter·a·tion (ə-dul″tər-a′shən) addition of an impure, cheap, or unnecessary ingredient to cheat, cheapen, or falsify a preparation; in legal terminology, incorrect labeling, including dosage not in accordance with the label 掺杂，掺假

ad·vance di·rec·tive (ăd-văns də′ rĕc-tiv) instruction about a person's wishes, goals, and values regarding what will be done in case the person becomes incapable of making decisions about medical care 预前指示。又称 *living will*, *durable power of attorney for health care*, and sometimes *advance health care directive or health care advance directive*

ad·vance·ment (ad-vans′mənt) 1. surgical detachment, as of a muscle or tendon, followed by reattachment at a point farther forward than the original position 前徙术；2. the surgical moving forward of the mandible in the correction of jaw deformity 一种下颌骨向前移来矫正下颌畸形的外科手术

ad·ven·ti·tia (ad″ven-tish′e-ə) 1. the outer coat of various tubular structures 管状结构的外层；2. tunica adventitia 外膜

ad·ven·ti·tial (ad″ven-tish′əl) pertaining to the tunica adventitia 外膜的

ad·ven·ti·tious (ad″ven-tish′əs) 1. accidental or acquired; not natural or hereditary 偶发的，后天的，

获得的 ; 2. found out of the normal or usual place 异位的 ; 3. adventitial 外膜的

ad·ver·sive (ad-vur′siv) opposite 相反的 ; as the turning to one side in an adverse seizure 在癫痫旋转性发作时转向一侧

adys·pla·sia (a″dis-pla′zhə) severe dysplasia in which an organ or part is shrunken and sometimes ectopic, and initially appears to be absent 发育不良

A-E, AE above-elbow 肘上 ; 见 *amputation* 下词条

AED automatic external defibrillator 自动体外除颤器

Ae·des (a-e′dēz) a genus of mosquitoes, including approximately 600 species; some are vectors of disease, others are pests. It includes *A. aegyp′ti,* a vector of yellow fever and dengue 伊蚊属

AEDF absent end diastolic flow 舒张末期血流消失

aer·a·tion (ār-a′shən) 1. the exchange of carbon dioxide for oxygen by the blood in the lungs 换气 ; 2. the charging of a liquid with air or gas 充 气, 曝气

aero·al·ler·gen (ār″o-al′ər-jən) an airborne particle capable of producing an allergic reaction 气源性致敏原

aer·obe (ār′ōb) a microorganism that lives and grows in the presence of free oxygen 需 氧 菌 ; **facultative a.,** one that can live in the presence or absence of oxygen 兼性需氧菌 ; **obligate a.,** one that requires oxygen for growth 专性需氧菌

aer·o·bic (ār-o′bik) 1. having molecular oxygen present 有氧的 ; 2. growing, living, or occurring in the presence of molecular oxygen 好氧的 ; 3. requiring oxygen for respiration 需氧的 ; 4. designed to increase oxygen consumption by the body 增强心肺功能的

aero·bi·ol·o·gy (ār″o-bi-ol′ə-je) the study of the distribution of microorganisms by the air 空气微生物学

aero·bi·o·sis (ār″o-bi-o′sis) life in the presence of molecular oxygen 需氧生活

aero·cele (ār′o-sēl) pneumatocele (1) 气肿 ; **epidural a.,** a collection of air between the dura mater and the wall of the vertebral column 硬膜外气肿

Aero·coc·ca·ceae (ār″o-kŏ-ka′se-e) a family of gram-positive cocci of the order Lactobacillales, occurring singly or in pairs, tetrads, or short chains 气球菌科

Aero·coc·cus (ār″o-kok′əs) a genus of aerobic, gram-positive cocci of the family Aerococcaceae. *A. vi′ridans,* a part of the normal skin flora, is an opportunistic pathogen 气球菌属

subcutaneous emphysema 皮下气肿

aer·odon·tal·gia (ār″o-don-tal′jə) 1. pain in the teeth due to lowered atmospheric pressure at high altitudes 航空性牙痛 ; 2. barodontalgia 气压性牙痛

aero·gen (ār′o-jen) a gas-producing bacterium 产气菌

Aero·mo·nas (ār″o-mo′nəs) a genus of schizomycetes usually found in water, some being pathogenic for fish, amphibians, reptiles, and humans 气单胞菌属

aero·peri·to·nia (ār″o-per″ĭ-to′ne-ə) pneumoperitoneum 气腹

aero·pha·gia (ār″o-fa′jə) excessive swallowing of air, usually an unconscious process associated with anxiety 吞气症

aero·phil·ic (ār″o-fil′ik) requiring air for proper growth 嗜气的, 需气的

aero·si·nus·itis (ār″o-si″nəs-i′tis) barosinusitis 航空性鼻窦炎

aer·o·sol (ār′o-sol) a colloid system in which solid or liquid particles are suspended in a gas, especially a suspension of a drug or other substance to be dispensed in a fine spray or mist 悬 浮 微 粒, 气溶胶

aero·tax·is (ār″o-tak′sis) movement of an organism in response to the presence of molecular oxygen 向氧性, 向气性

aer·oti·tis (ār″o-ti′tis) barotitis 航空耳炎

aero·tol·er·ant (ār″o-tol′ər-ənt) surviving and growing in small amounts of air; said of anaerobic microorganisms 空气耐受

aero·tym·pa·nal (ār″o-tim′pə-nəl) pertaining to or involving the air and the tympanum 空气鼓室的

aes- for words beginning thus, see those beginning *es-, et-.* 参见 es-,et-

Aescu·la·pi·us (es″ku-la′pe-əs) [L.] the god of healing in Roman mythology 罗马神话中的医神 ; 另见 *caduceus* and *staff* 下词条

a·fa·ti·nib (ă-fə′-tĭ-nĭb) an inhibitor of the protein tyrosine kinase, used as an antineoplastic to treat tumors with certain *EGFR* mutations; administered orally in tablet formulation 阿法替尼

afe·brile (a-feb′ril) without fever 无热的, 不发热的

af·fect (af′ekt) the external expression of emotion attached to ideas or mental representations of objects 情感, 感情 ; **affec′tive** *adj*; **pseudobulbar a.,** frequent, involuntary, uncontrollable episodes of laughing or crying secondary to certain neurologic disorders 假性延髓情绪

af·fer·ent (af′ər-ənt) 1. conveying toward a center 传入的, 输入的 ; 2. something that so conducts, such as a fiber or nerve 传导物

af·fin·i·ty (ə-fin′ĭ-te) 1. attraction; a tendency to seek out or unite with another object or substance 亲和力; 2. in chemistry, the tendency of two substances to form strong or weak chemical bonds forming molecules or complexes 化学亲和力; 3. in immunology, the thermodynamic bond strength of an antigen-antibody complex 免疫亲和力 Cf. *avidity*

afi·brin·o·gen·emia (a″fi-brin″o-jə-ne′me-ə) deficiency or absence of fibrinogen (coagulation factor Ⅰ) in the blood 纤维蛋白原缺乏血症; **congenital a.**, a rare autosomal recessive hemorrhagic coagulation disorder characterized by complete incoagulability of the blood 先天性纤维蛋白原缺乏血症

A·fin·i·tor (ə-fin′ĭ-tor) trademark for a preparation of everolimus 依维莫司

af·la·tox·in (af′lə-tok″sin) a toxin produced by the fungus *Aspergillus*, which infects peanuts, corn, cottonseed, and other plants; it has been implicated as a cause of hepatic carcinoma 黄曲霉毒素

a·flib·er·cept (ə-flĭb′-er-sept) a recombinant fusion protein that combines vascular endothelial growth factor receptors and IgG to inhibit growth factors and decrease vascular permeability in retinal and oncologic conditions; administered by injection into the eye or the vein 阿柏西普

AFP alpha fetoprotein 甲胎蛋白

af·ter·birth (af′tər-bərth) the placenta and membranes delivered from the uterus after childbirth 胞衣

af·ter·de·po·lar·iza·tion (af″tər-de-po″lər-ĭza′shən) a depolarizing afterpotential, frequently one of a series, sometimes occurring in tissues not normally excitable. It may occur before (*early a.*) or after (*delayed a.*) full repolarization 后去极化

af·ter·im·age (af′tər-im″əj) a retinal impression remaining after cessation of the stimulus causing it 后像

af·ter·load (af′tər-lōd″) the force against which cardiac muscle shortens: in isolated muscle, the force resisting shortening after the muscle is stimulated to contract; in the intact heart, the pressure against which the ventricle ejects blood 后负荷

af·ter·pains (af′tər-pānz) cramplike pains following the birth of a child, due to uterine contractions 产后痛

af·ter·po·ten·tial (af″tər-po-ten′shəl) the small action potential generated following termination of the spike or main potential; it has negative and (paradoxically named) positive phases, the latter being in fact more negative than the resting potential 后电位

af·ter·taste (af′tər-tāst) a taste continuing after the substance producing it has been removed 后味,余味

AFX atypical fibroxanthoma. 非典型纤维黄(色)瘤

AG atrial gallop 心房性奔马律

Ag antigen; silver (L. [*argen'tum*]) 抗原, 银

AGA American Gastroenterological Association 美国胃肠协会

aga·lac·tia (a″gə-lak′she-ə) absence or failure of secretion of milk 泌乳缺乏, 无乳

agam·ma·glob·u·lin·emia (a-gam″ə-glob″ulĭ-ne′me-ə) absence of all classes of immunoglobulins in the blood 无丙种球蛋白血症。另见 *hypogammaglobulinemia*。**X-linked a.**, an X-linked disorder characterized by absence of circulating B lymphocytes, plasma cells, or germinal centers in lymphoid tissues, very low levels of circulating immunoglobulins, susceptibility to bacterial infection, and symptoms resembling rheumatoid arthritis; apparently due to failure of pre-B cells to differentiate into mature B cells X连锁无丙种球蛋白血症

agan·gli·on·ic (a-gang″gle-on′ik) pertaining to or characterized by the absence of ganglion cells 无神经节细胞的

agan·gli·on·o·sis (a-gang″gle-on-o′sis) congenital absence of parasympathetic ganglion cells 无神经节细胞症

agar (ag′ahr) a dried hydrophilic, colloidal substance extracted from various species of red algae; used in solid culture media for bacteria and other microorganisms, as a bulk laxative, in making emulsions, and as a supporting medium in procedures such as immunodiffusion and electrophoresis 琼脂

Agar·i·ca·les (ə-gar″ĭ-ka′lēz) a large order of fungi that includes edible and toxic mushrooms 蘑菇目

Agar·i·cus (ə-gar′ĭ-kəs) a genus of mushrooms containing the common edible cultivated species *A. bispo'rus* (button mushroom) and *A. campes'tris* (field mushroom) and numerous species causing gastrointestinal irritation 落叶松蕈

agas·tric (a-gas′trik) having no alimentary canal 无胃的, 无消化道的

age (āj) 1. the duration, or the measure of time, of the existence of a person or object 年龄, 时期; 2. the measure of an attribute relative to the chronologic age of an average normal individual 智龄; **achievement a.**, the age of a person expressed as the chronologic age of a normal person showing the same proficiency in study 智力成就年龄; **bone a.**, osseous development shown radiographically, stated in terms of the chronologic age at which the development is ordinarily attained 骨龄 ; **chronologic a.**, the measure of time elapsed since a person's birth 时序年龄，实足年龄 ; **fertilization a.**, the age of a conceptus defined by the time elapsed since fertilization 受精龄 ; **gestational a.**, the age of a conceptus or pregnancy; in human clinical practice, timed from onset of the last normal menstrual period. Elsewhere the onset may be timed from estrus, coitus, artificial insemination, vaginal plug formation, fertilization, or implantation 孕龄 ; **mental a.**, the age level of mental ability of a person as gauged by standard intelligence tests 智力年龄

agen·e·sia (a″jə-ne′zhə) 1. imperfect development 发育不全 ; 2. sterility or impotence 无生殖力

agen·e·sis (a-jen′ə-sis) absence of an organ, particularly that due to nonappearance of its primordium in the embryo 发育不全 ; **gonadal a.**, complete failure of gonadal development, as in *Turner syndrome* 生殖腺发育不全 ; **nuclear a.**, Möbius syndrome 核发育不全

agen·i·tal·ism (a-jen′ĭ-təl-iz″əm) 1. absence of the genitals 生殖缺失 ; 2. a condition caused by failure to secrete gonadal hormones 生殖腺功能缺失

ageno·so·mia (a-jen″o-so′me-ə) congenital absence or imperfect development of the genitals and eventration of the lower part of the abdomen 无生殖器，生殖器发育不全

agent (a′jənt) something capable of producing an effect 剂，物，动因 ; **adrenergic blocking a.**, one that inhibits the response to sympathetic impulses by blocking the alpha (*alpha-adrenergic blocking a.*) or beta (*beta-adrenergic blocking a.*) receptor sites of effector organs 肾上腺素能阻滞剂 ; **adrenergic neuron blocking a.**, a substance that inhibits the release of norepinephrine from postganglionic adrenergic nerve endings 肾上腺素能神经元阻滞剂 ; **alkylating a.**, a cytotoxic agent, e.g., a nitrogen mustard, that is highly reactive and can donate an alkyl group to another compound. Alkylating agents inhibit cell division by reacting with DNA and are used as antineoplastic agents 烷化剂 ; **blocking a.**, an agent that inhibits a biological action, such as movement of an ion across the cell membrane, passage of a neural impulse, or interaction with a specific receptor 阻滞剂 ; **calcium channel blocking a.**, any of a class of drugs that inhibit the influx of calcium ions across the cell membrane or inhibit the mobilization of calcium from intracellular stores; used in the treatment of angina, cardiac arrhythmias, and hypertension 钙通道阻滞剂 ; **chelating a.**, 1. a compound that combines with metal ions to form stable ring structures 以两个或两个以上配价与金属离子结合形成稳定的环状结构的化合物 ; 2. a substance used to reduce the concentration of free metal ion in solution by complexing it 通过络合来减低溶液中游离金属离子浓度的物质 ; **cholinergic blocking a.**, a substance that blocks or inactivates acetylcholine 胆碱能阻滞剂 ; **emulsifying a.**, emulsifier 乳化剂 ; **ganglionic blocking a.**, one that blocks nerve impulses at autonomic ganglial synapses 神经节阻滞剂 ; **inotropic a.**, any of a class of agents affecting the force of muscle contraction, particularly a drug affecting the force of cardiac contraction; positive inotropic agents increase, and negative inotropic agents decrease the force of cardiac muscle contraction 正性肌力药 ; **luting a.**, 见 *lute* (1) ; **neuromuscular blocking a.**, a compound that causes paralysis of skeletal muscle by blocking neural transmission at the neuromuscular junction 神经肌肉阻滞剂 ; **nonsteroidal antiinflammatory a.**, 见 *drug* 下词条 ; **A. Orange**, a herbicide containing 2,4,5-T and 2,4-D and the contaminant dioxin; it is suspected of being carcinogenic and teratogenic 出莠剂，落叶剂 ; **oxidizing a.**, a substance capable of accepting electrons from another substance, thereby oxidizing the second substance and itself becoming reduced 氧化剂 ; **potassium channel blocking a.**, any of a class of antiarrhythmic agents that inhibit the movement of potassium ions through the potassium channels, thus prolonging repolarization of the cell membrane 钾通道阻滞剂 ; **progestational a.**, progestin: any of a group of hormones secreted by the corpus luteum and placenta and, in small amounts, by the adrenal cortex, including progesterone; they induce the formation of a secretory endometrium. Agents having progestational activity are also produced synthetically 促孕剂 ; **psychoactive a.**, 见 *substance* 下词条 ; **reducing a.**, a substance that acts as an electron donor in a chemical redox reaction 还原剂 ; **sclerosing a.**, sclerosant; a chemical irritant injected into a vein in sclerotherapy 硬化剂 ; **sodium channel blocking a.**, any of a class of antiarrhythmic agents that prevent ectopic beats by acting on partially inactivated sodium channels to inhibit abnormal depolarizations 钠通道阻滞剂 ; **surface-active a.**, a substance that exerts a change on the surface properties of a liquid, especially one that reduces its surface tension, as a detergent 表面活性剂 ; **wetting a.**, a substance that lowers the surface tension of water to promote wetting 湿润剂

ageu·sia (ə-goo′zhə) absence of the sense of taste 味觉缺失 ; **ageu′sic** *adj.*

ag·ger (aj′er) pl. **ag′geres** [L.] an eminence or elevation 堤，丘 ; **a. na′si**, a ridgelike elevation midway between the anterior extremity of the middle nasal concha and the inner surface of the dorsum of the nose 鼻中隔

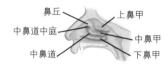

鼻丘　上鼻甲
中鼻道中庭　　中鼻甲
中鼻道　　下鼻甲

▲　鼻丘（**agger nasi**），位于鼻侧壁中间的前面，位于中庭的上方

ag·glu·ti·nant　(ə-gloo′tĭ-nənt) 1. promoting union by adhesion 黏合的 ; 2. a tenacious or gluey substance that holds parts together during the healing process 黏合剂

ag·glu·ti·na·tion　(ə-gloo″tĭ-na′shən) 1. the action of an agglutinant substance 黏合 ; 2. the process of union in wound healing 愈合 ; 3. the clumping together in suspension of antigen-bearing cells, microorganisms, or particles in the presence of specific antibodies(agglutinins) 凝集 ; **agglu′tinative** *adj.* 黏合的，愈合的，凝集的 ; **cross a.,** the agglutination of particulate antigen by antibody raised against a different but related antigen 交叉凝集 ; 另见 *group a.*; **group a.,** agglutination of members of a group of biologically related organisms or corpuscles by an agglutinin specific for that group 群凝集 ; **intravascular a.,** clumping of particulate elements within the blood vessels; used conventionally to denote red blood cell aggregation 血管内凝集

ag·glu·ti·nin　(ə-gloo′tĭ-nin) 1. antibody that aggregates a particulate antigen, e.g., bacteria, following combination with the homologous antigen 凝集类 ; 2. any substance other than antibody, e.g., lectin, that is capable of agglutinating particles 凝集素。又称 *agglutinator*。**anti-Rh a.,** an agglutinin not normally present in human plasma, which may be produced in an Rh⁻ mother carrying an Rh⁺ fetus or after transfusion of Rh⁺ blood into an Rh⁻ patient 抗 Rh 凝集剂 ; **chief a.,** 见 major a.; **cold a.,** one that agglutinates erythrocytes or bacteria more efficiently at temperatures below 37℃ than at 37℃ 冷凝集素 ; **group a.,** one that has a specific action on a particular group of microorganisms 类属凝集素 ; **H a.,** one that is specific for flagellar antigens of the motile strain of a microorganism 鞭毛凝集素 ; **immune a.,** any agglutinating antibody 免疫凝集素 ; **incomplete a.,** one that at appropriate concentrations fails to agglutinate the homologous antigen 不完全性凝集素 ; **leukocyte a.,** one that is directed against neutrophilic and other leukocytes 白细胞凝集素 ; **major a.,** that present at highest titer in an antiserum 主凝集素 ; **minor a., partial a.,** one that is present in agglutinative serum and acts on organisms and cells that are closely related to the specific antigen, but in a lower dilution 副凝集素 ; **warm a.,** one more reactive at 37 ℃ than at lower temperatures 温热凝集素

ag·glu·tin·o·gen　(ag″loo-tin′o-jen) 1. any substance that, acting as an antigen, stimulates the production of agglutinin 凝集（素）原 ; 2. the particulate antigen used in conducting agglutination tests 凝集试验用的颗粒抗原

ag·glu·ti·no·phil·ic　(ə-gloo″tĭ-no-fil′ik) agglutinating easily 易凝集的

ag·gre·gate¹　(ag′rə-gāt) to crowd or cluster together 集合，聚集

ag·gre·gate²　(ag′rə-gət) 1. crowded or clustered together 成群的 ; 2. a mass or assemblage 聚合的

ag·gre·ga·tion　(ag″rə-ga′shən) 1. massing or clumping of materials or people together 集合，凝集 ; 2. a clumped mass of material 集合物，凝集物 ; **familial a.,** the occurrence of more cases of a given disorder in close relatives of a person with the disorder than in control families 家族性聚集 ; **platelet a.,** a clumping together of platelets induced by various agents (e.g., thrombin) as part of the mechanism leading to thrombus formation 血小板聚集

ag·gres·sion　(ə-gresh′ən) behavior leading to self-assertion; it may arise from innate drives and/or a response to frustration, and may be manifested by destructive and attacking behavior, by hostility and obstructionism, or by a selfexpressive drive to mastery 攻击

ag·gres·sive　(ə-gres′iv) 1. characterized by aggression 侵略的 ; 2. rapidly spreading and invasive, as a tumor 侵袭性的 ; 3. characterized by or pertaining to intensive or vigorous treatment 与加强治疗有关的

ag·ing　(āj′ing) the gradual structural changes that occur with the passage of time, that are not due to disease or accident, and that eventually lead to death 老化，衰老

ag·i·ta·tion　(aj″ĭ-ta′shən) excessive, purposeless cognitive and motor activity or restlessness, usually associated with a state of tension or anxiety 激动，激越。又称 *psychomotor a.*

aglos·sia　(a-glos′e-ə) congenital absence of the tongue 无舌

agly·ce·mia　(a″gli-se′me-ə) absence of sugar from the blood 血糖缺乏

agly·con　(a-gli′kon) the noncarbohydrate group of a glycoside molecule 苷元，糖苷配基

agly·cone　(a-gli′kōn) aglycon 苷元，糖苷配基

ag·na·thia　(ag-na′the-ə) a congenital anomaly

characterized by absence of the lower jaw 无颌畸形； **agnath′ic, agnath′ous** adj.

ag·ni (ug-ne′) [Sanskrit] in ayurveda, the digestive and metabolic energy created by the doshas that transforms nourishment into forms (ojas) that are used by the body and mind 阿耆尼，在阿育吠陀中，三大能量产生的消化和代谢能量，将营养转化为身体和精神所使用的形式（活力素）

ag·no·gen·ic (ag″no-jen′ik) idiopathic 原因不明的

ag·no·sia (ag-no′zhə) inability to recognize the import of sensory impressions; the varieties correspond with several senses and are distinguished as *auditory (acoustic), gustatory, olfactory, tactile,* and *visual* 失认（症）；**environmental a.,** inability to orient oneself to a familiar environment, although one may be able to locate it on a map or picture, owing to a lesion in the right temporal or occipital lobe 环境失认；**face a., facial a.,** prosopagnosia 面容失认；**finger a.,** loss of ability to indicate one's own or another's fingers 手指认识不能；**time a.,** loss of comprehension of the succession and duration of events 时间认识不能；**visual a.,** inability to recognize familiar objects by sight, usually due to a lesion in one of the visual association areas 视觉认识不能

ago·na·dism (a-go′nad-iz″əm) the condition of being without sex glands 无性腺症；**agonad′al** adj.

ag·o·nal (ag′ə-nəl) pertaining to or occurring just before death 濒死的

ag·o·nist (ag′ə-nist) 1. one involved in a struggle or competition 斗争或竞争的人；2. agonistic muscle 解剖学上的主动肌；3. in pharmacology, a drug that has an affinity for and stimulates physiologic activity at cell receptors normally stimulated by naturally occurring substances 药理学上的激动剂，兴奋剂

ag·o·nis·tic (ag″ə-nis′tik) pertaining to a struggle or competition; as an agonistic muscle, counteracted by an antagonistic muscle 竞争的

ag·o·ra·pho·bia (ag″ə-rə-fo′be-ə) intense, irrational fear of open spaces, characterized by marked fear of venturing out alone or of being in public places where escape would be difficult or help might be unavailable; sometimes occurring in association with panic attacks 广场恐怖症，广场恐惧症

agram·ma·tism (a-gram′ə-tiz-əm) inability to speak grammatically because of brain injury or disease, usually with simplified sentence structure and errors in tense, number, and gender 语法缺失（症）

agran·u·lar (a-gran′u-lər) lacking granules 无颗粒的

agran·u·lo·cyte (a-gran′u-lo-sīt″) nongranular leukocyte 无粒白细胞

agran·u·lo·cy·to·sis (a-gran″u-lo-si-to′sis) a symptom complex characterized by decreased granulocytes and by lesions of the throat, other mucous membranes, gastrointestinal tract, and skin; most cases are complications of drug therapy, radiation, or exposure to chemicals 粒细胞缺乏症

agran·u·lo·plas·tic (a-gran″u-lo-plas′tik) forming nongranular cells only; not forming granular cells 只形成无粒细胞的，不形成粒细胞的

agraph·ia (ə-graf′e-ə) impairment or loss of the ability to write 失写（症）；**agraph′ic** adj.

Ag·ri·flu (ă-grŭ-floo) trademark name for an influenza virus vaccine for subtypes A and B 甲型和乙型流感病毒疫苗的商标名称

AGS American Geriatrics Society 美国老年医学协会

AGT antiglobulin test 抗球蛋白试验

agy·ria (a-ji′re-ə) a malformation in which the convolutions of the cerebral cortex are not fully formed, so that the brain surface is smooth 无脑回畸形；**agyr′ic** adj.

AHA acetohydroxamic acid 醋羟胺酸；American Heart Association 美国心脏协会；American Hospital Association 美国医院协会

AHCA American Health Care Association 美国卫生保健协会

AHDI Association for Healthcare Documentation Integrity 卫生保健文档完整性协会

AHEAD Addiction Health Evaluation and Disease Management 成瘾健康评估和疾病管理

AHF antihemophilic factor (coagulation factor Ⅷ) 抗血友病因子

AHG antihemophilic globulin (coagulation factor Ⅷ) 抗血友病球蛋白

AHIMA American Health Information Management Association 美国健康信息管理协会

AHNA American Holistic Nurses Association 美国全体护士协会

AI aortic insufficiency 主动脉瓣关闭不全；artificial insemination 人工授精

AICC anti-inhibitor coagulant complex 促凝剂复合物抗凝剂

AICD activation-induced cell death 激活诱导性细胞死亡；automatic implantable cardioverter-defibrillator 自动可植入复律除颤仪

AID donor insemination (artificial insemination by donor) 供者人工授精

aid (ād) help or assistance; by extension, applied to any device by which a function can be improved or augmented, as a hearing aid 帮助，助理，辅助；**first a.,** the initial emergency care and treatment of an injured or ill person before definitive medical and surgical management can be secured 急救；**hear-**

ing a., a device that amplifies sound to help deaf persons hear, often specifically a device worn on the body 助听器 ; **pharmaceutical a.,** 药物佐剂，见 *necessity* 下词条

AIDS acquired immunodeficiency syndrome 获得性免疫缺陷综合征 ; 艾滋病

AIH American Institute of Homeopathy 美国顺势疗法研究所 ; artificial insemination by husband 同配授精

AIHA American Industrial Hygiene Association 美国工业卫生协会 ; American International Health Alliance 美国国际卫生联盟 ; autoimmune hemolytic anemia 自身免疫性溶血性贫血

AIIC Association des Infiirmières et Infiirmiers du Canada 加拿大医务室协会

AILA argon ion laser atheroablation 氩离子激光治疗

ai·lu·ro·pho·bia (i-loor″o-fo′be-ə) irrational fear of cats 恐猫症

ain·hum (i′num) (ān′hum) (Port. īn′yoom) [Port.] a disease in which formation of a linear constriction around a digit, particularly the fifth toe, leads to spontaneous amputation of the distal part of the digit 箍趾病，自发性断趾病

AIP acute intermittent porphyria 急性间歇性卟啉病

AIR American Institutes for Research 美国研究协会

air (ār) the gaseous mixture that makes up the atmosphere 气，空气 ; **alveolar a.,** 肺泡气，见 *gas* 下词条 ; **residual a.,** 余气，见 *volume* 下词条 ; **tidal a.,** 潮气，见 *volume* 下词条

air·borne (ār′born) suspended in, transported by, or spread by air 空气传播的

air·sick·ness (ār′sik-nis) motion sickness due to travel by airplane 晕机

air·way (ār′wa) 1. the passage by which air enters and leaves the lungs 气道 ; 2. a device for securing unobstructed respiration 导气管 ; **conducting a.,** the upper and lower airways considered together 上下导气管 ; **esophageal obturator a.,** a tube inserted into the esophagus to maintain airway patency in unconscious persons for positivepressure ventilation through the attached face mask 食管填充器导气管 ; **laryngeal mask a.,** a device for maintaining a patent airway without tracheal intubation, consisting of a tube connected to an oval inflatable cuff that seals the larynx 导气罩 ; **lower a.,** the airway from the inferior end of the larynx to the ends of the terminal bronchioles 下喉导气管 ; **nasopharyngeal a.,** a tube inserted through a nostril, across the floor of the nose, and through the nasopharynx so that the tongue does not block air flow in an unconscious

person 鼻咽导气管 ; **oropharyngeal a.,** a tube inserted through the mouth and pharynx so that the tongue does not block air flow in an unconscious person 口咽导气管 ; **upper a.,** the airway from the nares and lips to the larynx 上导气管

AIUM American Institute of Ultrasound in Medicine 美国超声医学研究所

AJCC American Joint Committee on Cancer 美国癌症联合委员会

Ajel·lo·my·ces (a″jə-lo-mi′sēz) a genus of fungi of the family Ajellomycetaceae. *A. capsula′tus* is the teleomorph of *Histoplasma capsulatum; A. dermati′tidis* is the teleomorph of *Blastomyces dermatitidis* 阿耶罗菌属

A-K, AK above-knee 膝盖上，截肢下 ; 见 *amputation* 下词条 *transfemoral amputation*

ak·a·this·ia (ak″ə-thī′zhə) a condition marked by motor restlessness, ranging from anxiety to an inability to lie or sit quietly or to sleep, a common extrapyramidal side effect of neuroleptic drugs 静坐不能

aki·ne·sia (a″kī-ne′zhə) absence, poverty, or loss of control of voluntary muscle movements 运动不能 ; **a. al′gera,** a condition characterized by generalized pain associated with movement of any kind 痛性运动不能

akin·es·the·sia (ə-kin″es-the′zhə) absence orloss of movement sense (kinesthesia) 运动感觉缺失

aki·net·ic (a-kī-net′ik) pertaining to, characterized by, or causing akinesia 运动不能的

Al aluminum 元素铝的化学符号

ALA American Laryngological Association 美国喉科学会 ; American Lung Association 美国肺脏学会 ; aminolevulinic acid 氨乙酰丙酸

Ala alanine 丙氨酸

ala (a′lə) pl. *a′lae* [L.] a winglike process 翼，翼膜 ; **a′lar** adj.; **a. na′si,** wing of nose: the flaring cartilaginous expansion forming the outer side of each of the nares 鼻翼

alac·ta·sia (a″lak-ta′zhə) malabsorption of lactose due to deficiency of lactase 乳糖吸收不良 ; 见 lactase *deficiency*

al·a·nine (Ala, A) (al′ə-nēn) a nonessential amino acid occurring in proteins and also free in plasma 丙氨酸 ; **β-a.,** an amino acid not found in proteins but occurring free and in some peptides; it is a precursor of acetyl CoA and an intermediate in uracil and cytosine catabolism β-丙氨酸

al·a·nine ami·no·trans·fer·ase (al′ə-nēn ə-me″no-trans′fər-ās) alanine transaminase 谷丙转氨酶，丙氨酸转氨酶

al·a·nine trans·am·i·nase (al′ə-nēn transam′ī-nās) an enzyme normally present in serum and body tissues, especially in the liver; it is released into the serum as a result of tissue injury; hence the concentration in the serum may be increased in patients with acute damage to hepatic cells 丙氨酸转氨酶

alar (a'lər) pertaining to an ala, or wing 翼的

alate (a'lāt) having wings; winged 有翼的

alat·ro·flox·a·cin (ə-lat″ro-flok'sə-sin) a broad-spectrum antibacterial that is the prodrug of trovafloxacin, to which it is rapidly converted after intravenous infusion; used as the mesylate salt 阿拉曲沙星，一种广谱抗生素

al·ba (al'bə) [L.] white 白，白色

al·be·do (al-be'do) [L.] whiteness 白色；**a. re′tinae,** paleness of the retina due to edema caused by transudation of fluid from the retinal capillaries 视网膜水肿

al·ben·da·zole (al-ben'də-zōl) a broad-spectrum anthelmintic used against many helminths and in the treatment of hydatid disease and neurocysticercosis 阿苯达唑，丙硫咪唑

al·bi·cans (al'bĭ-kanz) [L.] white 白色的

al·bi·du·ria (al″bĭ-du're-ə) the discharge of white or pale urine 乳糜尿。又称 *albinuria*

al·bi·nism (al'bĭ-niz-əm) a group of genetic abnormalities of melanin synthesis causing reduction or absence of melanin in the eyes and skin. It may affect the eyes only (*ocular albinism*) or eyes, hair, and skin (*oculocutaneous albinism*) 白化病；**albinot′ic** *adj.*; **ocular a.,** X-linked albinism that affects primarily the eyes, with pigment of the hair and skin being normal or only slightly diluted. It is characterized by reduced visual acuity, retinal hypopigmentation, nystagmus, strabismus, photophobia, and hypoplasia of the fovea 眼白化病；**oculocutaneous a. (OCA),** autosomal recessive albinism that affects the skin, hair, and eyes. There are several types (OCA1–OCA4), varying in incidence and in genetic, biochemical, and clinical characteristics; all of them are marked by reduced or absent pigment of the hair, skin, and eyes, foveal hypoplasia, photophobia, nystagmus, and decreased visual acuity 眼皮肤白化病

al·bi·no (al-bi'no) a person affected with albinism 白化体

al·bi·noid·ism (al-bĭ-noid'iz-əm) defective pigmentation of ocular or oculocutaneous structures, but without the eye defects seen in albinism 不完全白化病

al·bu·gin·ea (al″bu-jin'e-ə) tunica albuginea, particularly of the testis 白膜

al·bu·min (al-bu'min) 1. any protein that is soluble in water and also in moderately concentrated salt solutions 白蛋白；2. the major plasma protein, responsible for much of the plasma colloidal osmotic pressure and serving as a transport protein for large organic anions (e.g., fatty acids, bilirubin, some drugs) and for some hormones when their specific binding globulins are saturated 清蛋白；**albu′minous** *adj.*; **egg a.,** albumin of egg whites 卵清蛋白；**a. human,** a preparation of human serum albumin, used as a plasma volume expander and to increase bilirubin binding in hyperbilirubinemia 人血清白蛋白；**iodinated I 125 a.,** a radiopharmaceutical used in blood and plasma volume, circulation time, and cardiac output determinations, consisting of albumin human labeled with iodine-125 放射碘（碘 ^{125}）人血清蛋白；**iodinated I 131 a.,** a radiopharmaceutical used in blood pool imaging and plasma volume determinations, consisting of albumin human labeled with iodine-131 放射碘（碘 ^{131}）人血清清蛋白；**serum a.,** albumin; (2) 血清白蛋白

al·bu·mi·no·cho·lia (al-bu″mĭ-no-ko'le-ə) the presence of albumin in the bile 蛋白胆汁症

al·bu·mi·noid (al-bu'mĭ-noid″) 1. resembling albumin 白蛋白样的；2. a scleroprotein 纤维蛋白；3. an albumin-like substance, such as a scleroprotein 硬蛋白

al·bu·mi·nop·ty·sis (al-bu″mĭ-nop'tĭ-sis) albumin in the sputum 白蛋白分解

al·bu·min·uria (al″bu-mĭ-nu're-ə) presence in the urine of serum albumin, the most common kind of proteinuria 蛋白尿；**albuminu′ric** *adj.*

al·bu·ter·ol (al-bu'tər-ol) a β_2-adrenergic receptor agonist used as the base or sulfate salt in a bronchodilator 舒喘宁，沙丁胺醇

al·caf·ta·dine (al-kaf'tədēn) a topical antihistamine (H$_1$-receptor antagonist) used in the treatment of allergic conjunctivitis 阿卡他定

Al·ca·li·ge·na·ceae (al″kə-lij″ə-na'se-e) a family of gram-negative, aerobic, rod-shaped bacteria of the order Burkholderiales 产碱菌科

Al·ca·li·ge·nes (al″kə-lij′ə-nēz) a widespread genus of gram-negative, rod-shaped bacteria of the family Alcaligenaceae, found in the intestines and as part of the normal skin flora, and occasionally the cause of opportunistic infections. *A. faeca′lis* causes nosocomial septicemia 产碱杆菌属

al·clo·met·a·sone (al-klo-met′ə-sōn″) a synthetic corticosteroid used topically in the dipropionate form for the relief of inflammation and pruritus 阿氯米松

al·co·hol (al'kə-hol) 1. any of a class of organic compounds containing the hydroxyl (—OH) functional group except those in which the OH group is attached to an aromatic ring (*phenols*). Alcohols are classified as *primary, secondary,* or *tertiary* according to whether the carbon atom to which the OH group is attached is bonded to one, two, or three other carbon atoms and as *monohydric, dihydric,* or *trihydric* according to whether they contain one, two, or three OH groups; the latter two are called *diols* and *triols,* respectively 醇; 2. ethanol 酒精; 3. a pharmaceutical preparation of ethanol, used as a disinfectant, solvent, and preservative; applied topically as a rubefacient, disinfectant, astringent, hemostatic, and coolant; and used internally in sclerotherapy and in the treatment of pain, of spasticity, and of poisoning by methyl alcohol or ethylene glycol 酒精制剂; **absolute a.,** 见 dehydrated a.; **benzyl a.,** a colorless liquid used as a bacteriostatic in solutions for injection and topically as a local anesthetic 苯甲醇; **cetostearyl a.,** a mixture of stearyl alcohol and cetyl alcohol used as an emulsifier 鲸脂醇; **cetyl a.,** a solid alcohol used as an emulsifying and stiffening agent 鲸蜡醇; **dehydrated a.,** an extremely hygroscopic, transparent, colorless, volatile liquid, 100 percent strength ethanol; used as a solvent and injected into nerves and ganglia for relief of pain 无水乙醇; **denatured a.,** ethanol rendered unfit for internal use by addition of methanol or acetone 变性醇; **ethyl a., grain a.,** ethanol 乙醇; **isopropyl a.,** a transparent, colorless, volatile liquid, used as a solvent and disinfectant, and as a topical antiseptic 异丙醇; **isopropyl rubbing a.,** a preparation containing between 68 and 72 percent isopropyl alcohol in water, used as a rubefacient 擦洗异丙醇; **methyl a.,** a clear, colorless, flammable liquid, CH_3OH, used as a solvent. Ingestion may cause blindness or death 甲醇; **polyvinyl a.,** a water-soluble synthetic polymer used as a viscosity-increasing agent in pharmaceuticals and as a lubricant and protectant in ophthalmic preparations 聚乙烯醇; ***n*-propyl a.,** a colorless liquid with an alcohol-like odor; used as a solvent 正丙醇; **rubbing a.,** a preparation of acetone, the alcohol denaturant methyl isobutyl ketone, and 68.5 to 71.5 percent ethanol; used as a rubefacient 擦洗乙醇; **stearyl a.,** a solid alcohol prepared from stearic acid and used as an emollient and emulsifier 十八烷醇; **wood a.,** methanol 木精, 木甲醇

al·co·hol   de·hy·dro·gen·ase (ADH) (alʹkə-hol de-hiʹdro-jən-ās) an enzyme that catalyzes the reversible oxidation of primary or secondary alcohols to aldehydes; the reaction is the first step in the metabolism of alcohols by the liver 醇脱氢酶

al·co·hol·ic (al″kə-holʹik) 1. pertaining to or containing alcohol 醇的; 2. a person suffering from alcoholism 嗜酒者

al·co·hol·ism (alʹkə-hol-iz-əm) a disorder marked by a pathological pattern of alcohol use that causes serious impairment in social or occupational functioning. It includes both alcohol abuse and alcohol dependence 酒精中毒, 醇中毒

al·co·hol·y·sis (al″kə-holʹĭ-sis) decomposition of a compound due to the incorporation and splitting of alcohol 醇解

al·cu·ro·ni·um (al-ku-roʹne-əm) a nondepolarizing skeletal muscle relaxant used as the chloride salt 阿库氯铵

al·dar·ic   ac·id (al-darʹik) a dicarboxylic acid resulting from oxidation of both terminal groups of an aldose to carboxyl groups 糖二酸

ALDC afferent lymph dendritic cell 传入淋巴树突状细胞

al·de·hyde (alʹdə-hīd) 1. any of a class of organic compounds containing the group —CHO, i.e., one with a carbonyl group (C — O) located at one end of the carbon chain 醛; 2. a suffix used to denote a compound occurring in aldehyde conformation 用于表示醛构象中的化合物的后缀; 3. acetaldehyde 乙醛

al·de·hyde-ly·ase (al″də-hīd-liʹās) any of a group of lyases that catalyze the cleavage of a C—C bond in a molecule having a carbonyl group and a hydroxyl group to form two molecules, each an aldehyde or ketone 醛裂解酶

al·de·hyde re·duc·tase (alʹdə-hīd re-dukʹ tās) an enzyme that catalyzes the reduction of aldoses; in one form of galactosemia, its catalysis of reduction of excess galactose in the lens of the eye results in cataract formation 醛还原酶

al·des·leu·kin (al″dəs-looʹkin) a recombinant interleukin-2 product used as an antineoplastic and biological response modifier 阿地白介素

al·di·carb (alʹdĭ-kahrb) a carbamate pesticide used as an insecticide; in some countries, also used as a rodenticide 氨基甲酸酯类农药

al·do·lase (alʹdo-lās) 1. aldehyde-lyase 醛缩酶; 2. an enzyme that acts as a catalyst in the production of dihydroxyacetone phosphate and glyceraldehyde phosphate from fructose 1,6-bisphosphate. It occurs in several isozymes, one of which is deficient in hereditary fructose intolerance 果糖1,6-二磷酸醛缩酶

al·don·ic ac·id (al-donʹik) a carboxylic acid resulting from oxidation of the aldehyde group of an aldose to a carboxyl group 糖酸

al·dose (alʹdōs) one of two subgroups of monosaccharides, being those containing an aldehyde group (—CHO) 醛糖

al·dos·ter·one (al-dosʹtər-ōn) the major mineralocorticoid hormone secreted by the adrenal cortex. It promotes the retention of sodium and bicarbonate, the excretion of potassium and hydrogen ions, and the secondary retention of water. Large excesses can invoke plasma volume expansion, edema, and hypertension 醛固酮

al·dos·ter·on·ism (al-dos′tə-ro-niz″əm) hyperaldosteronism; an abnormality of electrolyte balance caused by excessive secretion of aldosterone 醛固酮增多症; **primary a.,** that due to oversecretion of aldosterone by an adrenal adenoma, marked by hypokalemia, alkalosis, muscular weakness, polyuria, polydipsia, and hypertension 原发性醛固酮增多症; **pseudoprimary a.,** signs and symptoms identical to those of primary aldosteronism but caused by factors other than excessive aldosterone secretion 假原发性醛固酮增多症; **secondary a.,** that due to extra-adrenal stimulation of aldosterone secretion, usually associated with edematous states such as the nephrotic syndrome, cirrhosis, heart failure, or malignant hypertension 继发性醛固酮增多症

al·dos·ter·o·no·ma (al″do-ster″o-no′mə) a tumor, usually an adenoma, of the adrenal cortex that secretes aldosterone, causing primary aldosteronism 醛固酮瘤

al·drin (al′drin) a chlorinated hydrocarbon insecticide, closely related to dieldrin; ingestion or skin contact causes neurotoxic reactions that can be fatal 艾氏剂, 氯甲桥萘

alec·i·thal (a-les′ĭ-thəl) without yolk; applied to eggs with very little yolk 无卵黄

al·em·tuz·u·mab (al″əm-tuz′u-mab″) a recombinant monoclonal antibody directed against the CD antigen CD52; used as an antineoplastic in the treatment of chronic lymphocytic leukemia 阿仑单抗

alen·dro·nate (ə-len′dro-nāt) a bisphosphonate calcium-regulating agent used in the form of the sodium salt to inhibit the resorption of bone in the treatment of osteitis deformans, osteoporosis, and hypercalcemia related to malignancy 阿仑膦酸钠, 一种双膦酸盐化合钙调节剂

aleu·ke·mia (a″loo-ke′me-ə) 1. leukopenia 白细胞减少; 2. aleukemic leukemia 白细胞缺乏性白血病

aleu·ke·mic (a″loo-ke′mik) pertaining to or characterized by leukopenia 白细胞缺乏的

aleu·kia (a-loo′ke-ə) leukopenia 白细胞缺乏症

aleu·ko·cy·to·sis (a-loo″ko-si-to′sis) leukopenia 白细胞减少

alex·ia (a-lek′se-ə) a form of receptive aphasia in which ability to understand written language is lost as a result of a cerebral lesion 失读（症）; **alex′ic** *adj.*; **cortical a.,** a form of sensory aphasia due to lesions of the left gyrus angularis 皮质性失读症;

motor a., alexia in which the patient understands written or printed material but cannot read it aloud 运动性失读症; **musical a.,** loss of the ability to read music 读乐谱不能; **optical a.,** alexia 视觉性失读症; **subcortical a.,** alexia due to interruption of the connection between the optic center and the parietal lobe, including the gyrus angularis of the dominant hemisphere 皮质下性失读

aley·dig·ism (a-li′dig-iz″əm) absence of androgen secretion by Leydig cells 莱迪希细胞功能缺失

al·fa·cal·ci·dol (al″fə-kal′sĭ-dol) a synthetic analogue of calcitriol, used in the treatment of hypocalcemia, hypophosphatemia, rickets, and osteodystrophy associated with various medical conditions 阿法骨化醇

al·fen·ta·nil (al-fen′tə-nil) an opioid analgesic of rapid onset and short duration derived from fentanyl, used as the hydrochloride salt in the induction of general anesthesia and as an adjunct in general, regional, and local anesthesia 阿芬太尼

ALG antilymphocyte globulin 抗淋巴细胞球蛋白

al·ge·sia (al-je′ze-ə) 1. pain sense 痛觉; 2. excessive sensitivity to pain, a type of hyperesthesia 痛觉过敏; **alge′sic, alget′ic** *adj.*

al·ge·sim·e·ter (al″jə-sim′ə-tər) an instrument for measuring sensitiveness to pain 痛觉计, 痛觉仪

al·ge·sio·gen·ic (al-je″ze-o-jen′ik) dolorific 产生疼痛的

al·ges·the·sia (al″jes-the′zhə) 1. pain sense 痛觉; 2. any painful sensation 痛情绪

al·gid (al′jid) chilly or cold 寒冷的, 冷的

al·gi·nate (al′jĭ-nāt) a salt of alginic acid 藻酸盐; water-soluble alginates are useful as materials for dental impressions 水溶性藻酸盐可用作牙科印模材料

al·gin·ic ac·id (al-jin′ik) a hydrophilic colloidal carbohydrate obtained from seaweed, used as a tablet binder and emulsifying agent 藻酸

al·glu·cer·ase (al-gloo′sər-ās″) a form of β-glucocerebrosidase used to replace glucocerebrosidase (glucosylceramidase) in the treatment of the adult form of Gaucher disease 阿糖脑苷酶, 一种用于替换人体内的葡糖脑苷脂酶, 用于治疗成年戈谢病的 β-葡糖脑苷脂酶

al·go·dys·tro·phy (al″go-dis′trə-fe) complex regional pain syndrome type 1 痛性营养障碍

al·go·gen·ic (al-go-jen′ik) algesiogenic 产生疼痛的

al·go·pho·bia (al″go-fo′be-ə) irrational fear of pain 疼痛恐怖症

al·go·rithm (al′gə-rith-əm) 算法 1. a step-by-step method of solving a problem or making decisions, as in making a diagnosis 做出判断时,

解决问题或做出决定循序渐进的方法；2. an established mechanical procedure for solving certain mathematical problems 用于解决某些数学问题的既定机械程序

a·li·as·ing (a′le-əs-ing) 混淆现象 1. introduction of an artifact or error in sampling of a periodic signal when the sampling frequency is too low to capture the signal properly 当采样频率过低而不能正确捕获信号时，周期性信号采样中混入伪影或误差；2. in pulsed Doppler ultrasonography, an artifact occurring when the velocity of the sampled object is too great for the Doppler frequency to be determined by the system 在脉冲多普勒超声技术中，当采样对象的速度过大系统无法确定多普勒频率时，会产生一种伪影；3. an artifact occurring in magnetic resonance imaging when a part being examined is larger than the field of view; an image of the area outside the field of view appears as an artifact inside the field of view 在磁共振成像中，当被测部件大于视场时所产生的伪影，视场外部区域的图像显示为视场内的一个伪影

al·i·cy·clic (al″ĭ-sik′lik) having the properties of both aliphatic and cyclic substances 脂环族的

ali·form (al′ĭ-form) shaped like a wing 翼状的

al·i·men·ta·ry (al″ə-men′tər-e) pertaining to food or nutritive material, or to the organs of digestion 消化器官的，营养的

al·i·men·ta·tion (al″ə-men-ta′shən) giving or receiving of nourishment 营养；**rectal a.**, feeding by injection of nutriment into the rectum 直肠营养法；**total parenteral a.**, 全肠外营养法，见 *nutrition* 下词条

ali·na·sal (al′ĭ-na′səl) pertaining to either ala of the nose 鼻翼的

al·i·phat·ic (al″ĭ-fat′ik) pertaining to any member of one of the two major groups of organic compounds, those with a straight or branched chain structure 脂肪族的

al·is·ki·ren (al″is-ki′rən) a direct renin inhibitor, interfering with the renin-angiotensinaldosterone system; used as a. hemifumarate in the treatment of hypertension 阿利吉仑，一种直接抑制肾素、干扰肾素 - 血管紧张素 - 醛固酮系统，用于治疗高血压的药物

ali·sphe·noid (al-ĭ-sfe′noid) 1. pertaining to the greater wing of the sphenoid bone 蝶骨大翼的；2. a cartilage of the fetal chondrocranium on either side of the basisphenoid; later in development it forms the greater part of the greater wing of sphenoid 蝶骨大翼软骨的，在胎儿软骨颅基蝶骨两侧的软骨；在发育的后期，它形成蝶骨大翼的大部分

al·i·tret·i·noin (al″ĭ-tret′ĭ-noin″) a topical antineoplastic used in the treatment of AIDS-related cutaneous Kaposi sarcoma 阿利维 A 酸，一种外用抗肿瘤药物，用于治疗与艾滋病有关的皮肤卡波西肉瘤

aliz·a·rin (ə-liz′ə-rin) a red crystalline dye prepared synthetically or obtained from madder; its compounds are used as indicators 茜素，一种合成或从茜草中得到的红色结晶染料，可以作为指示剂

al·ka·le·mia (al″kə-le′me-ə) increased pH (abnormal alkalinity) of the blood 碱血症

al·ka·li (al′kə-li) any of a class of compounds with pH greater than 7.0, which form soluble soaps with fatty acids, turn red litmus blue, and form soluble carbonates, e.g., hydroxides or carbonates of sodium or potassium 碱

al·ka·line (al′kə-līn) (-lin) 1. having the reactions of an alkali 碱性的；2. having a pH greater than 7.0 碱的

al·ka·line hy·drol·y·sis (al′kə-līn hi-drol′ə-sis) a process of using water, heat, and potassium hydroxide to dispose of a dead body; used as an alternative to traditional cremation 碱性水解，一种利用水、热和氢氧化钾处理尸体的过程；作为传统火葬的替代品。又称 *biocremation*

al·ka·line phos·pha·tase (ALP) (al′kə-līn) (-lin fos′fə-tās) an enzyme that catalyzes the cleavage of orthophosphate from orthophosphoric monoesters under alkaline conditions. Differing forms of the enzyme occur in normal and malignant tissues. The activity in serum is useful in the clinical diagnosis of many illnesses. Deficient bone enzyme activity, an autosomal recessive trait, causes hypophosphatasia 碱性磷酸酶，一种在碱性条件下催化正磷酸单酯裂解为正磷酸盐的酶，以不同形式存在于正常组织和恶性组织中，其血清活性对多种疾病的临床诊断具有重要意义，骨中酶活性不足是一种常染色体隐性遗传特征，可导致低磷血症；**leukocyte a. p. (LAP),** the isozyme of alkaline phosphatase occurring in the leukocytes, specifically in the neutrophils; LAP activity is used in the differential diagnosis of neutrophilia, being lowered in chronic myelogenous leukemia and elevated in a variety of other disorders 白细胞碱性磷酸酶，白细胞（尤其是中性粒细胞）中碱性磷酸酶的同工酶，LAP 活性用于中性粒细胞增多症的鉴别诊断，在慢性粒细胞白血病中降低，但在其他疾病中活性升高

al·ka·lin·uria (al″kə-lĭ-nu′re-ə) an alkaline condition of the urine 碱性尿

al·ka·liz·er (al′kə-li″zər) an agent that neutralizes acids or causes alkalinization 碱化剂

al·ka·loid (al′kə-loid″) any of a group of organic basic substances found in plants, many of which are pharmacologically active, e.g., atropine, caffeine, morphine, nicotine, quinine, and strychnine 生物碱，一组存在于植物中，许多具有药理活性的有机物质，如阿托品、咖啡碱、吗啡、尼古丁、奎宁和士的宁；**vinca a's,** alkaloids produced by the common periwinkle plant (*Vinca rosea*); two, vincristine and vinblastine, are used as antineoplastic agents 长春花属植物产生的生物碱，其中长春新碱和长春碱是抗肿瘤药物

al·ka·lo·sis (al″kə-lo′sis) a pathologic condition due to accumulation of base in, or loss of acid from, the body 碱中毒。Cf. *acidosis.* **alkalot′ic** *adj.*; **altitude a.,** increased alkalinity in blood and tissues due to exposure to high altitudes 高原反应性碱中毒；**compensated a.,** a form in which compensatory mechanisms have returned the pH toward normal 代偿性碱中毒；**hypochloremic a.,** metabolic alkalosis marked by hypochloremia together with hyponatremia and hypokalemia, resulting from the loss of sodium chloride and hydrochloric acid due to prolonged vomiting 低氯性碱中毒；**hypokalemic a.,** metabolic alkalosis associated with a low serum potassium level 低钾性碱中毒；**metabolic a.,** a disturbance in which the acid-base status shifts toward the alkaline side because of retention of base or loss of noncarbonic, or fixed (nonvolatile), acids 代谢性碱中毒；**respiratory a.,** a state due to excess loss of carbon dioxide from the body, usually as a result of hyperventilation 呼吸性碱中毒

al·kane (al′kān) any of a class of saturated hydrocarbons with a straight or branched chain structure, of the general formula C_nH_{2n+2} 烷烃

al·kap·ton·uria (al-kap″to-nu′re-ə) an autosomal recessive aminoacidopathy with accumulation of homogentisic acid in urine (causing urine to darken on standing), ochronosis, and arthritis 尿黑酸尿症，一种常染色体隐性氨基酸缺陷病，尿黑酸在尿液中蓄积（引起站立时小便变黑），并有褐皮病和关节炎症状；**alkaptonu′ric** *adj.*

al·kyl (al′kəl) the monovalent radical formed when an aliphatic hydrocarbon loses one hydrogen atom 烷基，烃基

al·kyl·a·tion (al″kə-la′shən) the substitution of an alkyl group for an active hydrogen atom in an organic compound 烷基化，烷化

ALL acute lymphoblastic leukemia 急性淋巴细胞白血病

al·la·ches·the·sia (al″ə-kes-the′zhə) allesthesia 异位感觉

al·lan·ti·a·sis (al″an-ti′ə-sis) sausage poisoning; botulism from improperly prepared sausages 腊肠中毒，不新鲜的香肠引起的肉毒中毒

al·lan·to·cho·ri·on (ə-lan″to-kor′e-on) a compound membrane formed by fusion of the allantois and chorion 尿囊绒膜

al·lan·to·ic (al″an-to′ik) pertaining to the allantois 尿囊的

al·lan·toid (ə-lan′toid) 1. resembling the allantois 像尿囊的；2. sausage-shaped 腊肠状的

al·lan·toi·do·an·gi·op·a·gous (al″ən-toi″doan″je-op′ə-gəs) joined by the vessels of the umbilical cord, as some twins 脐血管相连接的

al·lan·to·in (ə-lan′to-in) a crystalline substance found in allantoic fluid, fetal urine, and many plants and produced synthetically; used topically as an astringent and keratolytic 尿囊素，一种在尿囊液、胎儿尿和许多植物中发现并人工合成的结晶状物质；可外用作收敛剂和角质剥脱剂

al·lan·to·is (ə-lan′to-is) a ventral outgrowth of the embryos of reptiles, birds, and mammals. In humans, it is vestigial except that its blood vessels give rise to those of the umbilical cord 尿囊

al·lele (ə-lēl′) one of two or more alternative forms of a gene occurring at a particular chromosomal locus; they determine alternative characters in inheritance 等位基因；**allel′ic** *adj.*; **hypomorphic a.,** a mutant allele whose effect is subnormal expression of a normal phenotype 亚效等位基因；**multiple a's,** alleles of which there are more than two alternative forms possible at any one locus 复等位基因；**null a., silent a.,** an allele that codes for a nonfunctional or undetectable product 无效等位基因

al·le·lo·tax·is (ə-le″lo-tak′sis) development of an organ from several embryonic structures 异源发生

al·ler·gen (al′ər-jən) an antigenic substance capable of producing immediate hypersensitivity (allergy) 过敏原；**allergen′ic** *adj.*

al·ler·gy (al′ər-je) a hypersensitive state acquired through exposure to a particular allergen, reexposure bringing to light an altered capacity to react 变态反应，超敏反应，过敏性反应。见 *hypersensitivity*; **aller′gic** *adj.*; **atopic a.,** atopy 特应性变态反应；**bacterial a.,** specific hypersensitivity to a particular bacterial antigen 细菌性超敏反应；**bronchial a.,** atopic asthma; see asthma 支气管过敏反应；**cold a.,** a condition manifested by local and systemic reactions, mediated by histamine, which is released from mast cells and basophils as a result of exposure to cold 冷过敏；**contact a.,** 见 *dermatitis* 下词条；**delayed a.,** 见 *hypersensitivity* 下词条；**drug a.,** an allergic reaction occurring as the result of unusual sensitivity to a drug 药物过敏反应；**food a., gastrointestinal a.,** allergy produced by ingested antigens in food, having a variety of skin, gastrointestinal, and respiratory manifestations 食物过敏反应；**hereditary a.,** atopy 遗传性变态反应；**immediate a.,** 见 *hypersensitivity* 下词条；**latent a.,**

allergy not manifested by symptoms but detectable by tests 潜伏性变态反应；**physical a.**, a condition in which the patient is sensitive to the effects of physical agents, such as heat, cold, light, etc 物理性变态反应；**pollen a.**, hay fever 花粉性过敏反应；**polyvalent a.**, 见 *pathergy* (2); **spontaneous a.**, atopy 自发性变态反应

al·les·the·sia (al″es-the′zhə) the experiencing of a sensation, e.g., pain or touch, as occurring at a point remote from where the stimulus actually is applied 异处感觉

al·le·thrin (al′ə-thrin) a synthetic analogue of the natural insecticide pyrethrin, used as an insecticide 丙烯菊酯，一种天然杀虫剂除虫菊酯的合成类似物，用作杀虫剂

al·li·cin (al′ĭ-sin) an oily substance, extracted from garlic, which has antibacterial activity 蒜素，从大蒜中提取的一种油性物质，具有抗菌活性

al·lo·an·ti·body (al″o-an′tĭ-bod″e) isoantibody 同种抗体

al·lo·an·ti·gen (al″o-an′tĭ-jən) an antigen present in allelic forms encoded at the same gene locus in different individuals of the same species 同种抗原

al·lo·chi·ria (al″o-ki′re-ə) dyschiria in which if one limb is stimulated the sensation is referred to the opposite side 感觉定侧不能；**allochi′ral** *adj.*

al·lo·cor·tex (al″o-kor′teks) the older, original part of the cerebral cortex, comprising the archicortex and the paleocortex 异皮质，大脑皮层较老的、原始的部分，包括古皮质和旧皮质

Al·lo·der·ma·nys·sus (al″o-dur′mə-nis′əs) a genus of blood-sucking mites; *A. sanguineus* is a parasite of mice and a vector of *Rickettsia akari*, the cause of rickettsialpox 异刺皮螨属，吸血螨属的一种，寄生于鼠，媒介传播小蛛立克次氏体，导致立克次体痘

al·lo·dyn·ia (al″o-din′e-ə) pain produced by a non-noxious stimulus 触痛；痛觉超敏

al·lo·erot·i·cism (al″o-ə-rot′ĭ-siz-əm) 1. sexual feeling directed to another person 对于其他人产生爱欲的感觉；2. a state of maturity characterized both by direction of erotic energies to another and also by the ability to form a love relationship with that other 一种成熟的状态，其特征是可以爱另一个人，并与另一个人建立爱的关系；**alloerot′ic** *adj.*

al·lo·ge·ne·ic (al″o-jə-ne′ik) 同种异型的 1. having cell types that are antigenically distinct 同一类型的细胞，具有不同的抗原；2. in transplantation biology, denoting individuals (or tissues) that are of the same species but antigenically distinct 在移植生物学中，指同种但抗原完全不同的个体（或组织）。Cf. *syngeneic* and *xenogeneic*. Spelled also

allogenic

al·lo·graft (al′o-graft) a graft between individuals of the same species, but of different genotypes 同种异体移植。又称 *homograft*

al·lo·group (al′o-groop) an allotype linkage group, especially of allotypes for the four IgG subclasses, which are closely linked and inherited as a unit 同种异型组

al·lo·im·mune (al″o-ĭ-mūn′) specifically immune to an allogeneic antigen 同种异体免疫

al·lo·im·mu·ni·za·tion (al″o-im″u-nĭ-za′shən) an immune response generated in an individual or strain of one species by an alloantigen from a different individual or strain of the same species 同种异体免疫反应

al·lom·er·ism (ə-lom′ər-iz-əm) change in chemical constitution without change in crystalline form 同晶异质性，化学成分的变化而不改变结晶形态

al·lo·mor·phism (al″o-mor′fiz-əm) change in crystalline form without change in chemical constitution 同质异晶性，晶体形态的变化而不改变化学成分

al·lop·a·thy (al-op′ə-the) that system of therapeutics in which diseases are treated by producing a condition incompatible with or antagonistic to the condition to be cured or alleviated 对抗疗法，一种治疗方法，通过产生一种与要治愈或减轻的病症不相容或对立的病症来治疗疾病。Cf. *homeopathy*. **allopath′ic** *adj.*

al·lo·pla·sia (al″o-pla′zhə) heteroplasia 发育异常

al·lo·plast (al′o-plast) an inert foreign body used for implantation into tissue 异体移植物

al·lo·plas·tic (al″o-plas′tik) 1. pertaining to an alloplast 骨代移植；2. pertaining to or characterized by alloplasty 异体移植

al·lo·plas·ty (al′o-plas″te) in psychoanalytic theory, adaptation by alteration of the environment 在精神分析理论中，通过改变环境来适应

al·lo·pur·i·nol (al″o-pūr′ĭ-nol) an isomer of hypoxanthine, capable of inhibiting xanthine oxidase and thus of reducing serum and urinary levels of uric acid; used in prophylaxis and treatment of hyperuricemia and uric acid nephropathy and prophylaxis of renal calculus recurrence 别嘌呤醇，一种次黄嘌呤的异构体，能够抑制黄嘌呤氧化酶，从而降低血清和尿中尿酸水平，用于预防和治疗高尿酸血症和尿酸肾病并预防肾结石复发

al·lo·re·ac·tive (al″o-re-ak′tiv) pertaining to the immune response in reaction to a transplanted allograft 同种反应性

al·lo·rhyth·mia (al″o-rith′me-ə) irregularity of the

heart beat or pulse that recurs regularly 节律异常 ; **allorhyth′mic** *adj.*

all or none (awl or nun) the heart muscle, under whatever stimulation, will contract to the fullest extent or not at all; in other muscles and in nerves, stimulation of a fiber causes an action potential to travel over the entire fiber, or not to travel at all 全或无, 心肌在任意刺激下不收缩或者直接收缩到最大程度, 在其他肌肉和神经中, 对神经纤维的刺激会导致动作电位在整个纤维上传导或者根本不传导

al·lo·sen·si·ti·za·tion (al″o-sen″sĭ-ti-za′shən) sensitization to alloantigens (isoantigens), as to Rh antigens during pregnancy 同种致敏作用

al·lo·some (al′o-sōm) a foreign constituent of the cytoplasm that has entered from outside the cell 异染色体, 在胞质中, 由细胞外进入胞质的外来成分

al·lo·sta·sis (al″o-sta′sis) (ə-los′tə-sis) an organism's maintenance of physical or psychological stability by constant adaptation to changing internal and external conditions 稳态, 有机体通过不断适应不断调整内部和外部条件而保持生理或心理稳定 ; **allostat′ic** *adj.*

al·lo·ster·ic (al″o-ster′ik) pertaining to allostery 变构的

al·lo·ster·ism (al′o-ster″iz-əm) allostery 变构状态

al·lo·ste·ry (al′o-ster″e) the condition in which binding of a substrate, product, or other effector to a subunit of a multi-subunit enzyme at a site (allosteric site) other than the functional site alters its conformation and functional properties 变构性, 底物、产物或其他效应器与多亚基酶的一个亚基（变构位点）上的一个非功能位点（变构位点）结合而改变其构象和功能特性的状态

al·lo·tope (al′o-tōp) a site on the constant or nonvarying portion of an antibody molecule that can be recognized by a combining site of other antibodies 同种异型位, 抗体分子上的一个位点, 位于抗体分子的恒定部分上, 可由其他抗体的结合位点识别

al·lo·trans·plan·ta·tion (al″o-trans-planta′shən) allogeneic transplantation 同种移植术, （同种）异基因移植

al·lo·tro·pic (al″o-tro′pik) 1. exhibiting allotropism 同素异形的 ; 2. concerned with others; said of a type of personality that is more preoccupied with others than with oneself 关心他人, 指一种比自己更关心于他人的性格

al·lot·ro·pism (ə-lot′rə-piz″əm) existence of an element in two or more distinct forms, e.g., graphite and diamond 同素异形现象

al·lo·type (al′o-tīp) any of several allelic variants of a protein that are characterized by antigenic differences 同种异型, 一种以抗原差异为特征的等位基因变异 ; **alloty′pic** *adj.*

al·lox·an (ə-lok′san) an oxidized product of uric acid that tends to destroy the islet cells of the pancreas, thus producing diabetes (*alloxan diabetes*) 四氧嘧啶, 尿酸的氧化产物, 可破坏胰岛细胞, 导致糖尿病

al·lyl (al′əl) a univalent radical, —CH_2=$CHCH_2$ 烯丙基

al·mo·trip·tan (al″mo-trip′tan) a selective serotonin receptor agonist used as the malate salt in the acute treatment of migraine 阿莫曲坦, 一种选择性 5 羟色胺受体激动剂, 苹果酸盐可用于偏头痛的急性治疗

al·oe (al′o) 1. a succulent plant, of the genus *Aloe*. 芦荟属的一种肉质植物 ; 2. the dried juice of leaves of various species of *Aloe*, used in various dermatologic and cosmetic preparations 芦荟叶的干汁, 用于各种皮肤和化妆品制剂中 ; **aloet′ic** *adj.*

al·o·pe·cia (al″o-pe′shə) baldness; absence of hair from skin areas where it is normally present 脱发 ; **alope′cic** *adj.*; **androgenetic a.**, a progressive, diffuse, symmetric loss of scalp hair, believed due to a combination of genetic predisposition and increased response of hair follicles to androgens, in men beginning around age 30 with hair loss from the vertex and frontoparietal regions (*male pattern a.* or *male pattern baldness*), and in women beginning later with less severe hair loss in the frontocentral area of the scalp (*female pattern a.* or *female pattern baldness*) 雄激素性脱发 ; **a. area′ta**, hair loss, usually reversible, in sharply defined areas, usually involving the beard or scalp 斑秃 ; **cicatricial a.**, irreversible loss of hair associated with scarring, usually on the scalp 瘢痕性脱发 ; **female pattern a.**, 见 *androgenetic a.*; **male pattern a.**, 见 *androgenetic a.*; **a. tota′lis**, loss of hair from the entire scalp 完全脱发 ; **traction a.**, traumatic alopecia due to continuous or prolonged traction on the hair 牵引性脱发 ; **traumatic a.**, hair loss caused by injury to the hair follicles in a given area, as by rubbing, traction, or a chemical agent 创伤性脱发 ; **a. universa′lis**, loss of hair from the entire body 全身毛发脱落

ALOX arachidonate lipoxygenase 花生四烯酸脂氧合酶

ALP alkaline phosphatase 碱性磷酸（酯）酶

al·pha (al′fə) α, the first letter of the Greek alphabet α, 希腊字母的第一个 ; 另见 α-

al·pha₂ -an·ti·plas·min (al′fə an″tĭ-plaz′min) α_2-纤溶酶抑制剂 ; 见 *antiplasmin*

al·pha₁ -an·ti·tryp·sin (al′fə an″tĭ-trip′sin) a plasma α_1-globulin produced primarily in the liver;

it inhibits the activity of elastase, cathepsin G, trypsin, and other proteolytic enzymes. Deficiency is associated with development of emphysema α₁-胰蛋白酶抑制剂

al·pha fe·to·pro·tein (al′fə fe″to-pro′tēn) a plasma protein produced by the fetal liver, yolk sac, and gastrointestinal tract and also by hepatocellular carcinoma, germ cell neoplasms, other cancers, and some benign hepatic diseases in adults. The serum AFP level is used to monitor the effectiveness of cancer treatment, and the amniotic fluid AFP level is used in the prenatal diagnosis of neural tube defects 甲胎蛋白

al·pha·lyt·ic (al′fə-lit′ik) 1. blocking α-adrenergic receptors 阻滞 α 肾上腺素受体; 2. α-blocker α 受体阻滞剂

al·pha₂ -mac·ro·glob·u·lin (al′fə mak′ro-glob″u-lin) α₂-macroglobulin α₂- 巨球蛋白

al·pha·mi·met·ic (al′fə-mi-met′ik) 1. stimulating or mimicking stimulation of α-adrenergic receptors 拟 α- 肾上腺素能的; 2. an alpha-adrenergic agent α- 肾上腺素能药物的

Al·pha·pap·il·lo·ma·vi·rus (al″fə-pap″ĭlo′mə-vi″rəs) a genus of viruses of the family Papillomaviridae that contains several of the human papillomaviruses α 乳头瘤病毒

Al·pha·pro·teo·bac·te·ria (al″fə-pro″te-obak-tēr′e-ə) a class of bacteria of the Proteobacteria α 变形菌纲

Al·pha·vi·rus (al′fə-vi″rəs) a genus of viruses of the family Togaviridae, including eastern, western, and Venezuelan equine encephalitis viruses, and others that cause denguelike illnesses in parts of Africa 甲病毒属

al·pra·zo·lam (al-pra′zo-lam) a short-acting benzodiazepine used as an antianxiety agent 阿普唑仑，一种短效苯二氮平类药物，用作抗焦虑剂

al·pros·ta·dil (al-pros′tə-dil) name for prostaglandin E₁ when used pharmaceutically as a vasodilator and platelet aggregation inhibitor; used for the treatment of patent ductus arteriosus and the diagnosis and treatment of impotence 前列地尔，用作血管扩张剂和抗血小板聚集药物时称作前列腺素 E₁；用于治疗动脉导管未闭及阳痿的诊断和治疗

ALPSA anterior labral periosteal sleeve avulsion 前盂唇及骨膜套袖状撕裂

ALS amyotrophic lateral sclerosis 肌萎缩侧索硬化; antilymphocyte serum 抗淋巴细胞血清

Al·ta·ve·ra (al″tə-ver′ə) trademark for a combination preparation of levonorgestrel and ethinyl estradiol 左炔诺孕酮与乙基雌二醇联用制剂的商标

al·te·plase (al′tə-plās) a tissue plasminogen activator produced by recombinant DNA technology; used in fibrinolytic therapy for acute myocardial infarction and as a thrombolytic in the treatment of acute ischemic stroke and pulmonary embolism 阿替普酶，重组 DNA 技术生产的组织纤溶酶原激活剂，用于急性心肌梗死的纤溶治疗和急性缺血性脑卒中及肺栓塞的溶栓治疗

al·ter·nans (awl-tur′nanz) [L.] 1. alternating; 见 *pulsus alternans*; 2. alternation 交替; **electrical a.,** alternating variations in the amplitude of specific electrocardiographic waves over successive cardiac cycles 电 交 替; **mechanical a.,** alternation of the heart, particularly in contrast to electrical alternans 机械交替; **pul′sus a.,** 见 *pulsus* 下词条; **total a.,** pulsus alternans in which alternating beats are so weak as to be undetected, causing apparent halving of the pulse rate 完全交替

Al·ter·na·ria (awl″tər-nar′e-ə) a genus of anamorphic fungi; *A. alterna′ta* and other species are common allergens, causing a variety of respiratory diseases as well as cutaneous, corneal, and peritoneal infections 链格孢属

al·ter·nar·i·o·sis (awl″tər-nar-e-o′sis) infection by species of *Alternaria* 链格孢病

al·ter·nate (awl′tər-nət) 1. following in turns 交替; 2. pertaining to every other one in a series 系列中的每一个的; 3. occurring in place of another 代替他人发生的; acting as a substitute 充当替代品

al·ter·nat·ing (awl′tər-nāt′ing) 1. occurring in regular succession 有规律地连续发生; 2. alternately direct and reversed 直接和反向交替

al·ter·na·tion (awl″tər-na′shən) the succession of two opposing or different events in turn 交替; **a. of generations,** the regular alternation of two or more different forms or of different modes of reproduction in the life cycle; sometimes specifically the alternating formation of diploid and haploid generations 世代交替; **a. of the heart,** mechanical alternans; alternating variation in the intensity of the heartbeat or pulse over successive cardiac cycles of regular rhythm 心脏交替，机械交替

al·ter·no·bar·ic (awl-tər″no-bar′ik) pertaining to alternating or changing barometric pressures 气压变化的

al·tret·amine (al-tret′ə-mēn) an antineoplastic agent used in the palliative treatment of ovarian cancer 六甲蜜胺，一种用于卵巢癌姑息治疗的抗肿瘤药物

al·um (al′əm) 明矾 1. a local astringent and styptic, prepared as an ammonium (*ammonium a.*) or potassium (*potassium a.*) compound; also used as an adjuvant in adsorbed vaccines and toxoids 一种制备为胺或钾

化合物的局部止血剂，也用作吸附疫苗和类毒素的佐剂；2. any member of a class of double sulfates formed on this type 该类型的任意一种双硫酸盐

alu·mi·na (ə-loo′mĭ-nə) 1. aluminum oxide 氧化铝；2. (in pharmaceuticals) aluminum hydroxide 氢氧化铝（药品中）; **hydrated a.,** aluminum hydroxide 氢氧化铝

alu·mi·no·sis (ə-loo″mĭ-no′sis) pneumoconiosis due to the presence of aluminum-bearing dust in the lungs 铝尘肺，由于肺中存在含铝尘埃而引起的肺尘埃沉着病

alu·mi·num (Al) (ə-loo′mĭ-nəm) an extremely light, silvery white, lustrous, malleable, ductile metallic element, abundant in the earth's crust; at. no. 13, at. wt. 26.982 铝；**a. acetate,** a salt prepared by the reaction of aluminum hydroxide and acetic acid; used in solution as an astringent 醋酸铝；**basic a. carbonate,** 碱式碳酸铝，见 gel 下词条；**a. chloride,** a topical astringent and anhidrotic 三氧化铝；**a. chlorohydrate,** the hydrate of aluminum chloride hydroxide, astringent and anhidrotic; used as an antiperspirant and as an anhidrotic in the treatment of hyperhidrosis 氯羟化铝；**a. hydroxide,** Al(OH)₃, used as an antacid, and as an adjuvant in adsorbed vaccines and toxoids 氢氧化铝；另见 gel 下词条；**a. oxide,** Al₂O₃, occurring naturally as various minerals such as corundum; used in the production of abrasives, refractories, ceramics, catalysts, to strengthen dental ceramics, and in chromatography 氧化铝；**a. phosphate,** an aluminum salt used as an adjuvant in adsorbed vaccines and toxoids, with calcium sulfate and sodium silicate in dental cements, and as an antacid 磷酸铝；**a. subacetate,** a basic acetate ester derivative used topically as an astringent 乙酸铝；**a. sulfate,** an astringent, used topically as a local antiperspirant; also used in the preparation of aluminum subacetate topical solution 硫酸铝

al·ve·o·lar (al-ve′ə-lər) pertaining to an alveolus 肺泡的

al·ve·o·late (al-ve′ə-lāt) marked by honeycomb-like pits 蜂窝状的

al·ve·o·li·tis (al″ve-o-li′tis) inflammation of a dental or pulmonary alveolus 牙槽炎或肺泡炎；**allergic a., extrinsic allergic a.,** hypersensitivity pneumonitis 过敏性肺炎

al·ve·o·lo·cap·il·lary (al-ve″ə-lo-kap′ĭ-lar″e) pertaining to the pulmonary alveoli and capillaries 肺泡毛细血管

al·ve·o·lo·cla·sia (al-ve″ə-lo-kla′zhə) disintegration or resorption of the inner wall of a tooth alveolus 牙槽破坏

al·ve·o·lo·den·tal (al-ve″ə-lo-den′təl) pertaining to a tooth and its alveolus 牙和牙槽的

al·ve·o·lo·plas·ty (al-ve′ə-lo-plas″te) surgical alteration of the shape and condition of the alveolar process, in preparation for denture construction 牙槽骨修整术

al·ve·o·lus (al-ve′ə-ləs) pl. alve′oli [L.] a small saclike dilatation 囊状的小扩张；另见 acinus; **dental a.,** tooth socket; one of the cavities of the jaw, in which the roots of the teeth are embedded 牙槽；**pulmonary alveoli,** small outpocketings of the alveolar ducts and sacs and terminal bronchioles through whose walls the exchange of carbon dioxide and oxygen takes place between the alveolar air and capillary blood；见图 25 肺泡

al·ve·us (al′ve-əs) pl. al′vei [L.] a canal or trough 海马槽

alym·pho·cy·to·sis (a-lim″fo-si-to′sis) deficiency or absence of lymphocytes from the blood; lymphopenia 淋巴细胞缺乏

alym·pho·pla·sia (a-lim-fo-pla′zhə) failure of development of lymphoid tissue 淋巴组织发育不良

AM [L.] Ar′tium Magis′ter (Master of Arts) 文学硕士

Am americium 镅

AMA Aerospace Medical Association 航空航天医学协会；American Medical Association 美国医学协会；Australian Medical Association 澳大利亚医学协会

ama (ah′mə) [Sanskrit] in ayurveda, physical and mental toxins that are produced by poor digestion and living habits and accumulate and clog the channels of the body 毒素，在阿育吠陀中，指由消化不良和生活习惯产生的毒素，聚集并堵塞身体的通道

am·a·crine (am′ə-krēn) 1. without long processes 无长突细胞；2. 见 cell 下词条

amal·gam (ə-mal′gəm) an alloy of two or more metals, one of which is mercury 汞齐

amal·ga·ma·tion (ə-mal′gə-ma′shən) 汞齐化，见 trituration (3)

Am·a·ni·ta (am″ə-ni′tə) a genus of poisonous mushrooms including several deadly species, notably A. phalloi′des, which causes delayed gastrointestinal symptoms followed by a brief period of improvement and culminating in hepatic and renal failure. Several other species contain toxins that cause transient central nervous system excitation 蛤蟆菌属菌类

aman·ta·dine (ə-man′tə-dēn) an antiviral compound used as the hydrochloride salt to treat influenza A; also used as an antidyskinetic in the treatment of parkinsonism and drug-induced extrapyramidal reactions 金刚烷胺，一种用作治疗甲型流感的抗病毒盐酸盐化合物；也是用于治

疗帕金森病和药物引起的锥体外系反应的抗运动障碍药物

amas·tia (ə-mas′te-ə) congenital absence of one or both mammary glands 无乳房

amas·ti·gote (ə-mas′tĭ-gōt) a morphologic stage in the life cycle of trypanosomatid protozoa; the oval or round cell has a nucleus, kinetoplast, and basal body but neither an undulating membrane nor an external flagellum 无鞭毛体，锥形虫生活史的形态学阶段，为卵圆形或圆形细胞，有细胞核、着丝粒和基体，但无波状膜、外鞭毛

am·a·tox·in (am′ə-tok″sin) any in a group of lethally hepatotoxic, bicyclic, octapeptide compounds found in *Amanita*, particularly *A. phalloides*, and several other genera of poisonous mushrooms 毒伞肽

am·au·ro·sis (am″aw-ro′sis) 黑矇 1. blindness 失明；2. blindness in which there is no apparent lesion of the eye 无眼部明显损害的失明；**amaurot′ic** *adj.*; **Leber congenital a.**, an autosomal recessive retinal disorder characterized by severe or complete loss of vision that becomes apparent early in infancy, absent or attenuated electroretinogram responses, inattention to visual stimuli, sluggish pupillary responses, and roving eye movements 先天性黑矇，一种常染色体隐性视网膜疾病，特征为严重或完全失明，于婴儿期早期较明显，视网膜电图反应缺失或减弱，对视觉刺激不反应，瞳孔反应迟缓，眼球运动不稳定

am·be·no·ni·um (am″bə-no′ne-əm) a cholinesterase inhibitor; the chloride salt is used to treat symptoms of muscular weakness and fatigue in myasthenia gravis 安贝氯铵，胆碱酯酶抑制剂，氯盐用于治疗重症肌无力的肌肉无力和疲劳症状

am·bi·dex·trous (am″bī-dek′strəs) able to use either hand with equal dexterity 双手灵巧的

am·bi·lat·er·al (am″bī-lat′ər-əl) pertaining to or affecting both sides 两侧的

am·bi·le·vous (am″bī-le′vəs) unable to use either hand with dexterity 双手不利的

am·bi·o·pia (am″be-o′pe-ə) diplopia 复视

am·bi·sex·u·al (am″bī-sek′shoo-əl) 1. 疑性别的，见 bisexual (1,2); 2. having the capability to become either sex, as the undifferentiated gonads in embryonic development 能够成为任意一种性别的，如胚胎发育中的未分化性腺; 3. denoting sexual characteristics common to both sexes, e.g., pubic hair 两性共有的性特征的

am·biv·a·lence (am-biv′ə-ləns) simultaneous existence of conflicting attitudes, emotions, ideas, or wishes toward the same object 矛盾心态; **ambiv′alent** *adj.*

Am·bly·om·ma (am″ble-om′ə) a genus of hard-bodied ticks with about 100 species; they transmit Rocky Mountain spotted fever, tick paralysis, and a variety of animal diseases 花蜱属

am·bly·o·pia (am″ble-o′pe-ə) dimness of vision without detectable organic lesion of the eye 弱视; **amblyop′ic** *adj.*; **a. ex anop′sia**, that resulting from long disuse 废用性弱视; **color a.**, dimness of color vision due to toxic or other influences 色弱; **nocturnal a.**, abnormal dimness of vision at night 夜盲; **nutritional a.**, scotomata due to poor nutrition; seen in alcoholics and patients with severe nutritional deprivation or vitamin B₁₂ deficiency, as in pernicious anemia 营养性弱视; **toxic a.**, that due to poisoning, as from alcohol or tobacco 中毒性弱视

am·blyo·scope (am″ble-o-skōp″) an instrument for training an amblyopic eye to take part in vision and for increasing fusion of the eyes 弱视镜

am·bo (am′bo) ambon 关节盂缘

am·bo·cep·tor (am′bo-sep″tər) hemolysin, particularly its double receptors, the one combining with the blood cell, the other with complement 溶血素，特别指溶血素的两个受体，一个与血细胞结合，另一个与补体结合

am·bon (am′bon) the fibrocartilaginous ring forming the edge of the socket in which the head of a long bone is lodged 关节盂缘

am·brox·ol (ăm-brox′əl) as a hydrochloride salt, the active secretolytic ingredient in medications; its mucolytic and expectorant properties thin or decrease mucus to treat respiratory diseases; administered orally and sometimes by injection 氨溴索，其盐酸盐为活性药物成分，溶痰、祛痰作用良好，黏液稀薄或减少，可治疗呼吸道疾病，口服，有时注射

am·bu·la·to·ry (am′bu-lə-tor″e) 1. walking or able to walk; not confined to bed 行走，能走动的; 2. of a condition or a procedure, not requiring admission to a hospital 无需住院的。又称 ambulant

am·cin·o·nide (am-sin′ə-nīd″) a synthetic corticosteroid used topically for the relief of inflammation and pruritus in corticosteroidresponsive dermatoses 安西缩松，一种外用的人工合成皮质类固醇，用于减轻皮质类固醇反应性皮肤病的炎症和瘙痒

am·di·no·cil·lin (am-de′no-sil″in) a semisynthetic penicillin effective against many gramnegative bacteria and used in the treatment of urinary tract infections 美西林，一种半合成青霉素，对许多革兰阴性细菌有效，用于治疗尿路感染

ame·ba (ə-me′bə) pl. *ame′bae*, *amebas* [L.] a minute protozoan (class Rhizopoda, subphylum Sarcodina), occurring as a single-celled nucleated mass of protoplasm that changes shape by extending

A

cytoplasmic processes (pseudopodia), by means of which it moves about and absorbs food; most amebae are free-living but some parasitize humans 阿米巴；**ame′bic** *adj.*

ame·bi·a·sis (am″e-bi′ə-sis) infection with amebae, especially *Entamoeba histolytica* 阿米巴病；**a. cu′tis,** painful ulcers or verrucous plaques on the skin, seen in persons with active intestinal or hepatic amebiasis 皮肤阿米巴病；**hepatic a.,** amebic hepatitis 肝阿米巴病；**intestinal a.,** amebic dysentery 肠阿米巴病；**pulmonary a.,** infection of the thoracic space secondary to intestinal amebiasis, with amebic liver abscesses 肺阿米巴病

ame·bi·cide (ə-me′bĭ-sīd) an agent that kills amebae 抗阿米巴药；**amebici′dal** *adj.*

ame·bo·cyte (ə-me′bo-sīt″) ameboid cell 阿米巴样细胞

ame·boid (ə-me′boid) resembling an ameba in form or movement 阿米巴样的

am·e·bo·ma (am″e-bo′mə) a tumor-like mass caused by granulomatous reaction in the intestines in amebiasis 阿米巴瘤

ame·bu·la (ə-me′bu-lə) the motile ameboid stage of spores of certain sporozoa 变形虫样孢子

amel·a·not·ic (a″mel-ə-not′ik) pertaining to or characterized by the absence of melanin 无黑色素的

ame·lia (ə-me′le-ə) congenital absence of a limb or limbs 无肢畸形，先天性无肢

amel·i·fi·ca·tion (ə-mel″ĭ-fĭ-ka′shən) the development of enamel cells into enamel 釉质化，牙釉质细胞发育成牙釉质

am·e·lo·blast (am′ə-lo-blast″) a cell that takes part in forming dental enamel 成釉细胞

am·e·lo·blas·tic (am″ĕlo-blas′tik) pertaining to ameloblasts or to an ameloblastoma 成釉细胞的，成釉细胞瘤的

am·e·lo·blas·to·ma (am″ə-lo-blas-to′mə) a usually benign but locally invasive neoplasm consisting of tissue characteristic of the enamel organ but not differentiating to the point of enamel formation; often classifed on the basis of histologic appearance and sometimes classified as *multicystic* versus *unicystic* 成釉细胞瘤；**melanotic a.,** melanotic neuro-ectodermal tumor. 黑色素性成釉细胞瘤；**pituitary a.,** craniopharyngioma 垂体性成釉细胞瘤

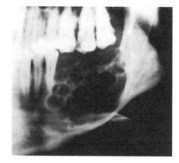

▲ 下颌骨左侧多囊性成釉细胞瘤（**ameloblastoma**）

am·e·lo·den·ti·nal (am″ə-lo-den′tĭ-nəl) pertaining to the enamel and dentin of a tooth 牙釉质和牙本质的

am·e·lo·gen·e·sis (am″ə-lo-jen′ə-sis) the formation of dental enamel 釉质发生；**a. imperfec′ta,** a hereditary condition resulting in defective development of dental enamel, marked by a brown color of the teeth; due to improper differentiation of the ameloblasts 釉质发育不全

am·e·lo·gen·in (am″ə-lo-jen′in) any of several proteins secreted by ameloblasts and forming the organic matrix of tooth enamel 釉原蛋白

am·e·lus (am′ə-ləs) an individual exhibiting amelia 无（缺）肢畸胎

amen·or·rhea (ə-men″o-re′ə) absence or abnormal stoppage of the menses 闭经，月经不调；**amenorrhe′al** *adj.*; **primary a.,** failure of menstruation to occur at puberty 原发性闭经；**secondary a.,** cessation of menstruation after it has once been established at puberty 继发性闭经

amen·sal·ism (a-men′səl-iz-əm) symbiosis in which one population (or individual) is adversely affected and the other is unaffected 偏害共生，一种种群（或个体）受到不利影响而另一种群（或个体）不受影响的共生现象

am·er·ic·i·um (Am) (am″ər-is′e-əm) a silvery white, synthetic, transuranium element; at. no. 95, at. wt. 243 镅

ame·tria (a-me′tre-ə) congenital absence of the uterus 无子宫（畸形）

ame·tro·pia (am″ə-tro′pe-ə) a condition of the eye in which images fail to come to a proper focus on the retina, due to a discrepancy between the size and refractive powers of the eye 屈光不正；**ametrop′ic** *adj.*

AMI acute myocardial infarction 急性心肌梗死；Association of Medical Illustrators 医学插图画家协会

AMIA American Medical Informatics Association 美国医学信息学会

amic·u·lum (ə-mik′u-ləm) pl. *ami'cula* [L.] a dense surrounding coat of white fibers, as the sheath of the inferior olive and of the dentate nucleus 一种密集的白色纤维包围层，如下橄榄的鞘和齿状核的鞘

am·i·dase (am′ĭ-dās) 酰胺酶 1. any of a group of enzymes that catalyze the cleavage of carbon–nitrogen bonds in amides 一组催化酰胺碳氮键断裂的酶；2. an enzyme that catalyzes the cleavage of the carbon–nitrogen bond of a monocarboxylic acid amide to form a monocarboxylic acid and ammonia 能够催化单羧酸酰胺的碳氮键裂解，形成单羧酸和氨的酶

am·ide (am′īd) any compound derived from ammonia by substitution of an acid radical for hydrogen, or from an acid by replacing the –OH group by – NH_2 酰胺

am·i·dine (am′ĭ-dēn″) any compound containing the amidino RC(=NH)–NH_2 group 脒

am·i·dine·ly·ase (am′ĭ-dēn lī′ās) an enzyme that catalyzes the removal of an amidino group, as from argininosuccinate to form fumarate and arginine 脒裂解酶

am·i·do·li·gase (ə-me″do-) (am″ĭ-do-li′gās) any of a group of enzymes that catalyze the transfer of the amide nitrogen from glutamine to an acceptor molecule 酰胺连接酶

am·i·fos·tine (am″ĭ-fos′tēn) a chemoprotectant used to prevent renal toxicity in cisplatin chemotherapy 氨磷汀，一种化学保护剂，用于预防顺铂化疗中的肾毒性

am·i·ka·cin (am″ĭ-ka′sin) a semisynthetic aminoglycoside antibiotic derived from kanamycin, used as the sulfate salt in the treatment of a wide range of infections due to aerobic gram-negative bacilli 阿米卡星，一种从卡那霉素中提取的半合成氨基糖苷类抗生素，硫酸盐可用于治疗好氧性革兰阴性杆菌引起的广泛感染

amil·o·ride (ə-mil′ə-rīd) a potassium-sparing diuretic used as the hydrochloride salt in the treatment of edema and hypertension and in the prevention and treatment of hypokalemia 阿米洛利，一种保钾利尿药，盐酸盐用于治疗水肿和高血压以及预防和治疗低钾血症

am·il·ox·ate (am″il-ok′sāt) an absorber of ultraviolet B radiation, used topically as a sunscreen 阿米沙酯，一种吸收紫外线 B 辐射的物质，可外用作防晒霜

amim·ia (a-mim′e-ə) loss of the power of expression by the use of signs or gestures 表情不能

am·i·na·tion (am″ĭ-na′shən) the creation of an amine, either by addition of an amino group to an organic acceptor compound or by reduction of a nitro compound 氨基化

amine (ə-mēn′) (am′in) an organic compound containing nitrogen; any of a group of compounds formed from ammonia by replacement of one or more hydrogen atoms by organic radicals 胺；**biogenic a's,** amines synthesized by plants and animals and frequently involved in signaling, e.g., neurotransmitters such as acetylcholine, catecholamines, and serotonin 生物胺；**sympathomimetic a's,** amines that mimic the actions of the sympathetic nervous system, comprising the catecholamines and drugs that mimic their actions 交感神经兴奋胺

am·in·er·gic (am″ĭ-nur′jik) activated by, characteristic of, or secreting one of the biogenic amines 胺能的

ami·no (ə-me′no) (am′ĭ-no″) the monovalent radical NH_2, when not united with an acid radical 氨基

ami·no ac·id (ə-me′no) one of a class of organic compounds containing the amino (NH_2) and the carboxyl (COOH) groups; they occur naturally in plant and animal tissue and form the chief constituents of protein 氨基酸；**branchedchain a. a's,** leucine, isoleucine, and valine 支链氨基酸；**essential a. a's,** the nine α-amino acids that cannot be synthesized by humans but must be obtained from the diet 必需氨基酸；**nonessential a. a's,** the eleven α-amino acids that can be synthesized by humans and are not specifically required in the diet 非必需氨基酸

ami·no·ac·id·emia (ə-me″no-as″ĭ-de′me-ə) an excess of amino acids in the blood 高氨酸血（症）

ami·no·ac·i·dop·a·thy (ə-me″no-as″ĭ-dop′ə-the) any of a group of disorders due to a defect in an enzymatic step in the metabolic pathway of one or more amino acids or in a protein mediator necessary for transport of certain amino acids into or out of cells 氨基酸代谢病

ami·no·ac·i·du·ria (ə-me″no-as″ĭ-du′re-ə) an excess of amino acids in the urine 氨基酸尿

ami·no·acy·lase (ə-me″no-a′sĭ-lās) an enzyme that catalyzes the hydrolytic cleavage of the acyl group from acylated l-amino acids 酰化氨基酸水解酶

ami·no·ben·zo·ate (ə-me″no-ben′zo-āt) *p*-aminobenzoate, any salt or ester of *p*-aminobenzoic acid; the potassium salt is used as an antifibrotic in some dermatologic disorders, and various esters are used as topical sunscreens 氨基苯甲酸酯，钾盐在一些皮肤病中被用作抗纤维化剂，而各种酯类化合物被用作局部防晒剂

***p*-ami·no·ben·zo·ic ac·id (PABA)** (ə-me″nobenzo′ik) a substance required for folic acid synthesis by many organisms; it also absorbs ultraviolet light (UVB rays) and is used as a topical sunscreen 对氨基苯甲酸。又称 *aminobenzoic acid*

γ-ami·no·bu·ty·rate (ə-me″no-bu′tə-rāt) the anion of γ-aminobutyric acid γ- 氨基丁酸的阴离子

γ-ami·no·bu·tyr·ic ac·id (GABA) (ə-me″nobu-tēr′ik) the principal inhibitory neurotransmitter in the brain but also occurring in several extraneural tissues, including kidney and pancreatic islet beta cells. Released from presynaptic cells upon depolarization, it modulates membrane chloride permeability and inhibits postsynaptic cell firing γ-氨基丁酸

ε-ami·no·ca·pro·ic ac·id (ə-me″no-kə-pro′ik) a nonessential amino acid that is an inhibitor of plasmin and of plasminogen activators and, indirectly, of fibrinolysis; used for treatment (as *aminocaproic acid*) of acute bleeding syndromes due to fibrinolysis and for the prevention and treatment of postsurgical hemorrhage ε - 氨基己酸

ami·no·glu·teth·i·mide (ə-me″no-gloo-teth′ĭ-mīd) an inhibitor of cholesterol metabolism, thereby reducing adrenocortical steroid synthesis; used in the treatment of Cushing syndrome. It also inhibits estrogen production from androgens in peripheral tissue 氨鲁米特，一种胆固醇代谢抑制剂，减少肾上腺皮质类固醇的合成，用于治疗库欣综合征。它还能抑制外周组织利用雄激素产生雌激素

ami·no·gly·co·side (ə-me″no-gli′ko-sīd) any of a group of antibacterial antibiotics (e.g., streptomycin, gentamicin) derived from various bacterial species, especially species of *Streptomyces*, or produced synthetically; they interfere with the function of bacterial ribosomes 氨基糖苷类

p-ami·no·hip·pu·rate (ə-me″no-hip′u-rāt) a salt, conjugate base, or ester of *p*-aminohippuric acid; the sodium salt is used to measure effective renal plasma flow and to determine the functional capacity of the tubular excretory mechanism 对氨基马尿酸盐（酯、根）

p-ami·no·hip·pu·ric ac·id (PAH, PAHA) (ə-me″no-hī-pūr′ik) the glycine amide of *p*-aminobenzoic acid, which is filtered by the renal glomeruli and secreted into the urine by the proximal tubules 对氨基马尿酸。另见 *p-aminohippurate*

ami·no·lev·u·lin·ate (ə-me″no-lev″u-lin′āt) the conjugate base of aminolevulinic acid 氨基酮戊酸盐（酯、根）

ami·no·lev·u·lin·ic ac·id (ALA) (ə-me″nolev″u-lin′ik) δ -aminolevulinic acid; an intermediate in the synthesis of heme; blood and urinary levels are increased in lead poisoning, and urinary levels are increased in some porphyrias. The hydrochloride salt is used as a topical photosensitizer in the treatment of nonhyperkeratotic actinic keratoses 氨乙酰丙酸

am·i·nol·y·sis (am″ə-nol′ə-sis) reaction with an amine, resulting in the addition of (or substitution by) an imino group –NH– 氨解反应，与胺发生反应，导致亚胺基 –NH– 的引入

6-ami·no·pen·i·cil·lan·ic ac·id (ə-me″nopen″ĭ-səl-an′ik) the active nucleus common to all penicillins; it may be substituted at the 6-amino position to form the semisynthetic penicillins 6- 氨基青霉烷酸

p-ami·no·phe·nol (ə-me″no-fe′nol) a dye intermediate and photographic developer and the parent compound of acetaminophen; it is a potent allergen that causes dermatitis, asthma, and methemoglobinemia 对氨基苯酚

am·i·noph·yl·line (am″ĭ-nof′ə-lin) a salt of theophylline, used as a bronchodilator and as an antidote to dipyridamole toxicity 氨茶碱，一种茶碱盐，用作支气管扩张剂和双嘧达莫毒性的解毒剂

ami·no·quin·o·line (ə-me″no-kwin′o-lēn) a heterocyclic compound derived from quinoline by the addition of an amino group 氨基喹啉，一种杂环化合物，由喹啉加上一个氨基得到；the *4-aminoquinoline* and *8-aminoquinoline* derivatives constitute classes of antimalarials 4- 氨基喹啉衍生物和 8- 氨基喹啉衍生物是抗疟药物的两大类

ami·no·sa·lic·y·late (ə-me″no-sə-lis′ə-lāt) any salt of *p*-aminosalicylic acid; they are antibacterials effective against mycobacteria, and the sodium salt is used as a tuberculostatic 对氨基水杨酸钠

ami·no·sal·i·cyl·ic ac·id (ə-me″no-sal-ĭ-sil′ik) official pharmaceutical name for *p*-aminosalicylic acid 对氨基水杨酸的官方药品名

5-ami·no·sal·i·cyl·ic ac·id (5-ASA) (ə- me″no-sal-ĭ-sil′ik) mesalamine 5- 氨基水杨酸

p-ami·no·sal·i·cyl·ic ac·id (PAS, PASA) (ə-me″no-sal-ĭ-sil′ik) an analogue of *p*-aminobenzoic acid (PABA) with antibacterial properties; used to inhibit growth and multiplication of the tubercle bacillus 对氨基水杨酸

ami·no·trans·fer·ase (ə-me″no-trans′fər-ās) transaminase 转氨酶

am·in·uria (am″ĭ-nu′re-ə) an excess of amines in the urine 胺尿症

ami·o·da·rone (ə-me′o-də-rōn″) a potassium channel blocking agent used as the hydrochloride salt in the treatment of ventricular arrhythmias 胺碘酮，一种钾离子通道阻滞剂，盐酸盐可用于治疗

室性心律失常

ami·to·sis (am″ĭ-to′sis) direct cell division, i.e., the cell divides by simple cleavage of the nucleus without formation of spireme spindle figures or chromosomes 无丝分裂; **amitot′ic** *adj.*

am·i·trip·ty·line (am″ĭ-trip′tə-lēn) a tricyclic antidepressant with sedative effects; also used in treating enuresis, chronic pain, peptic ulcer, and bulimia nervosa 阿米替林，一种具有镇静作用的三环类抗抑郁药，也用于治疗遗尿、慢性疼痛、消化性溃疡和神经性贪食症

AML acute myelogenous leukemia 急性髓性白血病

am·lex·a·nox (am-lek′sə-noks″) a topical antiulcer agent used in the treatment of recurrent aphthous stomatitis 氨来咕诺，一种外用抗溃疡药物，用于治疗复发性口腔溃疡

am·lo·di·pine (am-lo′dĭ-pēn) a calcium channel blocking agent used as the besylate salt in the treatment of hypertension and chronic stable and vasospastic angina 氨氯地平，一种钙离子通道阻滞剂，苯磺酸盐用于治疗高血压和慢性稳定型血管痉挛型心绞痛

am·me·ter (am′me-tər) an instrument for measuring in amperes or subdivisions of amperes the strength of a current flowing in a circuit 电流计

am·mo·nia (ə-mōn′yə) a colorless alkaline gas with a pungent odor and acrid taste, NH_3. Ammonia labeled with ^{13}N is used in positron emission tomography of the cardiovascular system, brain, and liver 氨

am·mo·ni·um (ə-mo′ne-əm) the hypothetical radical, NH_4, forming salts analogous to those of the alkaline metals 铵; **a. carbonate**, a mixture of ammonium bicarbonate (NH_4HCO_3) and ammonium carbamate ($NH_2CO_2NH_4$), used as a stimulant, as in smelling salts, and as an expectorant 碳酸铵; **a. chloride**, a systemic and urinary acidifying agent and diuretic, also used orally as an expectorant 氯化铵; **a. lactate**, lactic acid neutralized with ammonium hydroxide, applied topically in the treatment of ichthyosis vulgaris and xerosis 乳酸铵

am·mo·ni·uria (ə-mo″ne-u′re-ə) hyperammonuria 铵尿症

am·mo·nol·y·sis (am″o-nol′ĭ-sis) a process analogous to hydrolysis, but in which ammonia takes the place of water 氨解作用，一种类似水解的过程，但在此过程中氨取代了水

am·ne·sia (am-ne′zhə) pathologic impairment of memory 健忘（病）; **anterograde a.**, amnesia for events occurring subsequent to the episode precipitating the disorder 顺行性遗忘（病）; **dissociative a.**, a dissociative disorder characterized by a sudden loss of memory for important personal information and which is not due to the direct effects of a psychogenic substance or a general medical condition 解离性失忆症; **psychogenic a.**, 心因性遗忘，见 dissociative a.; **retrograde a.**, amnesia for events occurring prior to the episode precipitating the disorder 逆行性遗忘; **transient global a.**, a temporary episode of short-term memory loss without other neurological impairment 短暂性全面性遗忘; **visual a.**, alexia 视性失语

am·ne·sic (am-ne′sik) affected with or characterized by amnesia 失去记忆的

am·nes·tic (am-nes′tik) 1. amnesic 失去记忆的; 2. causing amnesia 导致失去记忆的

am·nio·cele (am′ne-o-sēl) omphalocele 脐疝

am·nio·cen·te·sis (am″ne-o-sen-te′sis) surgical transabdominal or transcervical penetration of the uterus for aspiration of amniotic fluid 羊膜穿刺术

am·nio·gen·e·sis (am″ne-o-jen′ə-sis) the development of the amnion 羊膜形成

am·nio·in·fu·sion (am″ne-o-in-fu′zhən) introduction of solutions into the amnion 羊膜腔灌注

am·ni·on (am′ne-on) bag of waters; the extraembryonic membrane of birds, reptiles, and mammals, which lines the chorion and contains the fetus and the amniotic fluid 羊膜; **amnion′ic, amniot′ic** *adj.*; **a. nodo′sum**, a nodular condition of the fetal surface of the amnion, usually appearing near the insertion of the cord 羊膜结节

am·ni·or·rhex·is (am″ne-o-rek′sis) rupture of the amnion 羊膜破裂

am·nio·scope (am′ne-o-skōp″) an endoscope passed through the uterine cervix to visualize the fetus and amniotic fluid 羊膜镜

am·ni·ote (am′ne-ōt) any member of the group of vertebrates that develop an amnion, including reptiles, birds, and mammals 羊膜动物

am·ni·ot·ic (am″ne-ot′ik) pertaining to or developing an amnion 羊膜的

am·ni·ot·o·my (am″ne-ot′ə-me) surgical rupture of the fetal membranes to induce labor 人工破膜

amo·bar·bi·tal (am″o-bahr′bĭ-təl) an intermediate-acting hypnotic and sedative; also used as the sodium salt 异戊巴比妥，一种中间作用的催眠药和镇静剂

Amoe·ba (a-me′bə) a genus of amebae 阿米巴属

amorph (a′morf) silent allele 无效等位基因

amor·phia (ə-mor′fe-ə) the fact or quality of being amorphous 无定形

amor·pho·syn·the·sis (a-mor″fo-sin′thə-sis) defective perception of somatic sensations from one side of the body, which may be accompanied by generalized faulty awareness of spatial relationships and is often a sign of a parietal lobe lesion 形体综合不能，身体一侧对躯体感觉的感知有缺陷，并可能伴随着对空间关系的普遍错误认知，通常是顶叶病变的迹象

amor·phous (ə-mor′fəs) 1. having no definite form; shapeless 无 定 形 ; 2. having no specific orientation of atoms 非 晶 质 ; 3. in pharmacy, not crystallized 非结晶的

amox·a·pine (ə-mok′sə-pēn) a tricyclic antidepressant of the dibenzoxazepine class 阿莫沙平，一种二苯氧氮平类的三环类抗抑郁药

amox·i·cil·lin (ə-mok′sĭ-sil′in) a semisynthetic derivative of ampicillin effective against a broad spectrum of gram-positive and gram-negative bacteria 阿莫西林，氨苄西林的一种半合成衍生物，对广泛的革兰阳性菌和革兰阴性菌均有效

AMP adenosine monophosphate 腺 苷 一 磷 酸 ; ″3′,5′-AMP, cyclic AMP, cyclic adenosine monophosphate 环腺苷酸

am·pere (A) (am′pēr) the base SI unit of electric current strength, defined in terms of the force of attraction between two parallel conductors carrying current 安培

am·phet·a·mine (am-fet′ə-mēn″) 1. a sympathomimetic amine with a stimulating effect on the central and peripheral nervous systems, used in the treatment of narcolepsy and attention-deficit/hyperactivity disorder, usually as the sulfate or aspartate salt. Abuse may lead to dependence 安非他明，一种对中枢和外周神经系统都有刺激作用的拟交感神经胺，用于治疗嗜睡和注意力缺陷／多动障碍，通常为硫酸盐或天冬氨酸盐，滥用可能导致依赖 ; 2. any drug closely related to amphetamine and having similar actions, e.g., methamphetamine 与安非他明密切相关并具有类似作用的药物，如甲基苯丙胺

am·phi·ar·thro·sis (am″fe-ahr-thro′sis) a joint permitting little motion, the opposed surfaces being connected by disks of fibrocartilage, as between vertebrae, or interosseous ligaments, as between the distal tibia and fibula 微动关节

Am·phib·ia (am-fib′e-ə) a class of vertebrates, including frogs, toads, newts, and salamanders, capable of living both on land and in water 两栖纲

am·phi·bol·ic (am″fĭ-bol′ik) uncertain or vacillating 摇摆不定的

am·phi·cen·tric (am″fĭ-sen′trik) beginning and ending in the same vessel 起止同源的

am·phi·di·ar·thro·sis (am″fĭ-di″ahr-thro′sis) a joint having the nature of both ginglymus and arthrodia, as that of the lower jaw 一种关节兼有屈戍关节和滑动关节的特点，如下颌 ; **amphiarthro′dial** *adj.*

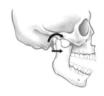

▲ 双关节畸形（**amphidiarthrosis**），以颞下颌关节为例。箭头表示运动的滑动部件（滑动关节）和铰链部件（屈戍关节）

am·phit·ri·chous (am-fit′rĭ-kəs) having flagella at each end 两端鞭毛的

am·pho·cyte (am′fo-sīt) a cell staining with either acid or basic dyes 双染细胞，能用酸性和碱性染料染色的细胞

am·pho·lyte (am′fo-līt) amphoteric electrolyte 两性电解质

am·pho·phil (am′fo-fil) 1. a cell that stains readily with acid or basic dyes 易被酸性或碱性染料染色的细胞 ; 2. amphophilic 两性的

am·pho·phil·ic (am-fo-fil′ik) staining with either acid or basic dyes 两染性的，可以被酸性或碱性染料染色的

am·phor·ic (am-for′ik) pertaining to a bottle; resembling the sound made by blowing across the neck of a bottle 空瓮音的

am·pho·ter·ic (am-fə-ter′ik) having opposite characters; capable of acting as both an acid and a base; capable of neutralizing either bases or acids 有酸碱两性的，有对立的性质，能同时作为酸和碱，中和碱或酸的

am·pho·ter·i·cin B (am″fə-ter′ĭ-sin) an antibiotic derived from strains of *Streptomyces nodosus*; effective against a wide range of fungi and some species of *Leishmania* 两性霉素 B，从结节链霉菌中提取的抗生素，对多种真菌和利什曼原虫有效

am·phot·o·ny (am-fot′ə-ne) tonicity of the sympathetic and parasympathetic nervous systems 双重神经过敏，交感神经和副交感神经系统的紧张度

am·pi·cil·lin (am″pĭ-sil′in) a semisynthetic, acidresistant, penicillinase-sensitive penicillin used as an antibacterial against many gram-negative and gram-positive bacteria; also used as the sodium salt 氨苄青霉素，一种半合成的、耐酸的、对青霉素酶敏感的青霉素，用作对许多革兰阴性菌和革兰阳性菌的抗菌药物；其钠盐也用作药物

am·pli·fi·ca·tion (am″plĭ-fĭ-ka′shən) the act or result of increasing in number, size, power, or other variable, such as the increase of an auditory or visual stimulus as a means of improving its perception 放大；在数量、大小、力量或其他变量上增加的

行为或结果，如增加听觉或视觉刺激以改善其知觉；**DNA a.,** 1. an in vitro nucleic acid amplification technique in which a DNA segment is amplified DNA 扩增，一种 DNA 片段的体外核酸扩增技术；2. in vivo gene amplification 体内基因的扩增；**gene a.,** 1. selective replication of a specific gene or genes disproportionate to their representation in the parent molecule 特定基因或与其在母体分子表现不相称的基因的选择性复制；2. sometimes, in vitro nucleic acid amplification, even though the sequence amplified may not correspond precisely to a gene 有时体外核酸扩增，扩增的序列可能与基因并不完全对应；**nucleic acid a.,** increase in the number of copies of a specific nucleic acid sequence, either DNA or RNA; usually used to denote any of various in vitro techniques employed to aid detection of a nucleic acid sequence of interest 增加特定核酸序列 (DNA 或 RNA) 的拷贝数；通常用于表示任何一种帮助检测目的核酸序列的体外技术

am·pli·tude (am′plə-tood) 1. largeness, fullness, wideness in range or extent 广阔；2. in a phenomenon that occurs in waves, the maximal deviation of a wave from the baseline 振幅；**a. of accommodation,** amount of accommodative power of the eye (眼的) 调节幅度

am·pren·a·vir (am-pren′ə-vir) an HIV protease inhibitor used in the treatment of HIV-1 infection 安普那韦，一种用于治疗 HIV-1 感染的 HIV 蛋白酶抑制剂

am·pule (am′pūl) a small glass or plastic container capable of being sealed so as to preserve its contents in a sterile condition; used principally for sterile parenteral solutions 安瓿，可密封的小玻璃或塑料容器，以便在无菌条件下保存其内物质；主要用于盛装无菌注射药物溶液

am·pul·la (am-pul′ə) pl. *ampul′lae* [L.] a flask-like dilatation of a tubular structure, especially of the expanded ends of the semicircular canals of the ear 壶腹；**ampul′lar** *adj.*; **a. ductus deferens,** the enlarged and tortuous outer end of the ductus deferens in the penis 输精管壶腹；**hepatopancreatic a., a. hepatopancrea′tica,** the dilatation formed by junction of the common bile and the pancreatic ducts proximal to their opening into the lumen of the duodenum 肝胰壶腹；**ampul′lae membrana′-ceae,** membranous ampullae: the dilatations at one end of each of the three semicircular ducts, anterior, lateral, and posterior 膜壶腹；**ampul′lae os′seae,** the dilatations at one of the ends of the semicircular canals, anterior, lateral, and posterior 骨壶腹；**phrenic a.,** a dilatation seen transiently at the lower end of the esophagus during swallowing, consequent to longitudinal esophageal muscle contraction and physiologic herniation of gastric cardia above the respiratory diaphragm 膈壶腹；**rectal a., a. rec′ti,** the dilated portion of the rectum just proximal to the anal canal 直肠壶腹；**a. of Thoma,** one of the small terminal expansions of an interlobar artery in the pulp of the spleen 托马壶腹；**a. of uterine tube,** the thin-walled, almost muscle-free, midregion of the uterine tube; its mucosa is greatly plicated 输卵管壶腹；**a. of Vater,** 见 **a. hepatopancreatica**

am·pu·ta·tion (am″pu-ta′shən) removal of a limb or other appendage of the body 离断，截肢术；**aboveelbow (A-E) a.,** amputation of the upper limb between the elbow and the shoulder 上臂截肢；**aboveknee (A-K) a.,** 见 transfemoral a.; **below-elbow (B-E) a.,** amputation of the upper limb between the wrist and the elbow 肘下截肢；**below-knee (B-K) a.,** 见 transtibial a.; **Chopart a.,** amputation of the foot by a midtarsal disarticulation 截肢，因跗中关节脱位而导致的足部截肢；**closed a.,** amputation in which flaps are made from the skin and superficial fascia and sutured over the end of the bone 闭合性截肢，皮瓣由皮肤和浅筋膜制成并缝合在骨头末端的截肢；**a. in contiguity,** amputation at a joint 关节截肢；**a. in continuity,** amputation of a limb elsewhere than at a joint 不连续截肢；**double-flap a.,** closed amputation in which two flaps are formed 形成的两皮瓣的闭合性截肢；**Dupuytren a.,** amputation of the arm at the glenohumeral joint 盂肱关节的截肢，手臂盂肱关节的截肢；**flap a.,** closed a. 皮瓣截肢；**flapless a.,** guillotine a. 无皮瓣截肢；**Gritti-Stokes a.,** amputation of the leg through the knee, using an oval anterior flap 截肢，用卵圆形前部皮瓣从膝盖处截去腿；**guillotine a.,** one performed rapidly by a circular sweep of the knife and a cut of the saw, the entire cross-section being left open for dressing 斩断术；**Hey a.,** amputation of the foot between the tarsus and metatarsus 截肢，跗骨和跖骨之间的足部截肢；**interpelviabdominal a.,** amputation of the thigh with excision of the lateral half of the pelvis 腹盆部分截肢，截肢大腿，切除骨盆的上半部分；**interscapulothoracic a.,** amputation of the arm with excision of the lateral portion of the shoulder girdle 肩胸间截肢，肩胛带外侧部分进行手臂截肢；**Larrey a.,** amputation at the glenohumeral joint 截肢，盂肱关节截肢；**Lisfranc a.,** 截肢 1. Dupuytren a. 截肢；2. amputation of the foot between the metatarsus and tarsus 跖骨和跗骨之间的足部截肢；**oblique a.,** oval a. 斜截肢；**open a.,** guillotine a. 开放切断术；**oval a.,** one in which the incision consists of two reversed spirals 卵圆形截肢，一种切口由两个反向螺旋组成；**Pirogoff a.,** amputation of the foot at the ankle, part of the calcaneus being left in the stump 截肢，足踝部截肢，部分跟骨留在残肢内；**pulp a.**, pulpotomy 牙髓切断术；**racket a.**, one in which there is a single longitudinal incision continuous below with a spiral incision on either side of the limb 球拍形截肢，两侧肢体从一连续向下的纵向切口与螺旋切口截去；**root a.**, removal of one or more roots from a multirooted tooth, leaving at least one root to support the crown; when only the apex of a root is involved, it is called *apicoectomy* 截根术；**spontaneous a.**, loss of a part without surgical intervention, as in diabetes mellitus 糖尿病在没有手术治疗的情况下失去肢体；**Stokes a.**, Gritti-Stokes a. 截肢；**subperiosteal a.**, one in which the cut end of the bone is covered by periosteal flaps 骨膜下切断；**Syme a.**, disarticulation of the foot with removal of both malleoli 截肢，足部脱臼后去除两踝；**Teale a.**, amputation with short and long rectangular flaps 蒂尔氏截肢术，从长短矩形皮瓣的截肢；**transfemoral a.**, aboveknee (A-K) a.; amputation of the lower limb between the knee and the hip 截肢膝盖和臀部之间的下肢截肢；**transtibial a.**, below-knee (B-K) a.; amputation of the lower limb between the ankle and the knee 踝关节和膝盖之间的下肢截肢

am·ri·none (am′rĭ-nōn) inamrinone 氨力农

AMRL Aerospace Medical Research Laboratories 航空航天医学研究所

AMSA American Medical Students Association 美国医学生协会；amsacrine 安吖啶

am·sa·crine (am′sə-krēn) an antineoplastic that inhibits DNA synthesis 安吖啶，一种抑制 DNA 合成的抗肿瘤药物；used to treat some forms of leukemia 用于治疗某些类型的白血病

AMSN Academy of Medical-Surgical Nurses 外科医学护士学会

AMT American Medical Technologists 美国医疗技术人员

AMTA American Music Therapy Association 美国音乐治疗协会

amu atomic mass unit 原子质量单位

amu·sia (ə-mu′ze-ə) a form of auditory agnosia in which the patient has lost the ability to recognize or produce music 失乐感（症），一种听觉失认症，病人失去辨认或产生音乐的能力

AMWA American Medical Women's Association 美国医学妇女协会；American Medical Writers Association 美国医学作家协会

amy·elin·ic (a-mi″ə-lin′ik) unmyelinated 无髓鞘的

amyg·da·la (ə-mig′də-lə) 1. almond 扁桃仁；2. an almond-shaped structure 扁桃仁状结构；3. corpus amygdaloideum 杏仁核

amyg·da·lin (ə-mig′də-lin) a glycoside found in bitter almonds and other members of the same family 苦杏仁苷，苦杏仁中的一种糖苷，存在于苦杏仁和其他同科植物中；it is split enzymatically into glucose, benzaldehyde, and hydrocyanic acid 酶解得到葡萄糖、苯甲醛和氢氰酸；另见 *Laetrile* and *laetrile*

amyg·da·line (ə-mig′də-lēn) 1. like an almond 扁桃仁样的；2. tonsillar 扁桃体的

amyg·da·loid (ə-mig′də-loid) resembling an almond or tonsil 扁桃仁样的

am·yl (am′əl) the radical $-C_5H_{11}$ 戊基；**a. nitrite**, a volatile, flammable liquid with a pungent ethereal odor. It is administered by inhalation for the treatment of cyanide poisoning, producing methemoglobin, which binds cyanide, and as a diagnostic aid in tests of reserve cardiac function and diagnosis of certain heart murmurs. It is abused to produce euphoria and as a sexual stimulant 亚硝酸戊酯

am·y·la·ceous (am″ə-la′shəs) composed of or resembling starch 淀粉组成的，淀粉状的

am·y·lase (am′ə-lās) an enzyme that catalyzes the hydrolysis of starch into simpler compounds. The α-*a's* occur in animals and include pancreatic and salivary amylase; the β-*a's* occur in higher plants 淀粉酶

am·y·lo-1,6-glu·co·si·dase (am″ə-lo-glooko′sī-dās) a hydrolase that catalyzes the cleavage of terminal α-1,6-glucoside linkages in glycogen and similar molecules; deficiency causes glycogen storage disease, type Ⅲ 淀粉 -1,6- 葡萄苷酶

am·y·loid (am′ə-loid) 1. starchlike; amylaceous 淀粉状的；2. the pathologic, extracellular, waxy, amorphous substance deposited in amyloidosis, being composed of fibrils in bundles or in a meshwork of polypeptide chains 淀粉样变性物质的；**AA a.**, a pathological fibrillar low-molecular-weight protein formed by cleavage of serum amyloid A (SAA) protein. It is deposited in the tissues secondary to chronic inflammatory conditions; see *secondary amyloidosis*, under *amyloidosis* AA 淀粉样蛋白；**Aβ a.**, an abnormal peptide found in aggregates in the cerebrovascular walls and the cores of the plaques in Alzheimer disease; it is derived from amyloid precursor protein Aβ 淀粉样蛋白；**AL a.**, a pathological fibrillar low-molecular-weight protein derived from circulating monoclonal immunoglobulin light chains, usually λ chains; it may be composed of whole chains, fragments, or both. It is deposited in the tissues in primary amyloidosis (q.v.) AL 淀粉样蛋白

am·y·loi·do·sis (am″ə-loi-do′sis) a group of conditions caused by accumulation of amyloid in organs and tissues, which compromises their function. Associated disease states may be inflammatory, hereditary, or neoplastic, and deposition can be local, generalized, or systemic. The most widely used classification is based on the chemistry of the amyloid fibrils and includes primary (AL), secondary (AA), and familial forms 淀粉样变性，由淀粉样物质积聚于组织器官，并损害相关功能而导致的一组病理学改变。相关疾病可能为炎性、遗传性或肿瘤性的。积聚部位可以是局限性、广泛性或系统性的。最常用的分类是基于淀粉样纤维的化学本质，将其分为原发性淀粉样变性（AL）、继发性淀粉样变性（AA）和家族性淀粉样变性；**AA a.,** secondary a. 继发性淀粉样变性；**a. of aging,** senile a. 老年性淀粉样变性；**AL a., primary a.** 原发性淀粉样变性；**ATTR a.,** the most common form of familial amyloidosis (q.v.), associated with mutations of the gene encoding transthyretin 家族性淀粉样变性中最常见的形式 (q.v.)，与编码甲状腺素转载蛋白的基因突变有关；**cutaneous a.,** a type localized to the skin, usually with pruritus; it may be a primary condition or part of a secondary amyloidosis 皮肤淀粉样变性，变性局限于皮肤的一种淀粉样变性，通常伴有瘙痒；可能是原发性的表现或继发性淀粉样变性的部分表现；**familial hemodialysis-associated a.,** that occurring in patients on long-term hemodialysis, caused by the deposition of beta$_2$- microglobulin, which cannot be removed from the blood by hemodialysis, in the joints, synovial membranes, and tendon sheaths. Manifestations include carpal tunnel syndrome and arthritis 家族性透析相关性淀粉样变性，发生于长期透析的患者，是 β_2 微球蛋白无法通过透析排出，沉积于关节、滑膜和腱鞘所致。临床表现包括腕管综合征和关节炎；**hereditary a.,** any inherited form of amyloidosis; usually used to denote any of various systemic autosomal dominant disorders of amyloid deposition that involve the nervous system. The most common form, ATTR amyloidosis, is associated with mutations of the transthyretin protein, but rare mutations of other proteins can also be a cause. The term can also, less commonly, be said to include several types of secondary amyloidosis in which the deposition is associated with an inherited disease (e.g., familial Mediterranean fever). Subclassifications are based on clinical presentation and biochemical composition of the fibrils deposited; originally they were distinguished on the basis of kinship. Called also heredofamilial a. and familial a. See also *familial amyloid polyneuropathy,* under *polyneuropathy* 遗传性淀粉样变性，通常表示淀粉样物质沉积并累及神经系统的各种常染色体显性遗传疾病。其中，ATTR 淀粉样变性最常见，是由甲状腺素转运蛋白突变所致，但其他蛋白的罕见突变也可导致。在较少见的情况下，本词也

可表示几种与遗传因素有关的继发性淀粉样变性（如家族性地中海热）。又称家族遗传性淀粉样变性和家族性淀粉样变性。参见 polyneuropathy 下的 familial amyloid polyneuropathy; **lichen a.,** the most common form of cutaneous amyloidosis, with translucent papules symmetrically distributed on shins, thighs, and occasionally elsewhere 苔藓样淀粉样变；**primary a.,** a systemic form in which the deposited fibrillar material is AL amyloid; it may be due to either aberrant synthesis or processing of immunoglobulin light chains. It is associated with tumors or dyscrasias of immunoglobulin-producing plasma cells and involves some combination of the skin and subcutaneous tissue, nerves, liver, spleen, heart, kidney, intestine, and tongue. Called also *AL a.* 沉积的纤维物质为 AL 淀粉样物质的一类系统性淀粉样变性；可能是由免疫球蛋白轻链的异常合成或加工所致。与肿瘤或浆细胞失调有关，可合并有皮肤、皮下组织、神经、肝、脾、心脏、肾脏、小肠和舌的病变。又称 AL 淀粉样变性；**reactive a.,** secondary a. 继发性淀粉样变性；**renal a.,** amyloid deposits in the kidneys; in the primary type the fibrils are mainly AL amyloid, and in secondary types they are AA amyloid. Secondary types may accompany inflammatory disorders, chronic infectious diseases, or neoplastic diseases 肾脏中发生的淀粉样物质沉积；原发性主要为 AL 淀粉样物质，继发性主要为 AA 淀粉样物质。继发性淀粉样变性可能继发于炎性疾病、慢性感染性疾病和肿瘤性疾病；**secondary a.,** that in which AA amyloid is deposited, and which occurs secondary to a chronic inflammatory condition, either infectious or noninfectious. It usually involves the liver, spleen, and kidneys 淀粉样物质沉积所致的一类淀粉样变性，继发于感染性或非感染性的慢性炎症。通常累及肝、脾、肾脏；**senile a.,** amyloidosis seen in the elderly, usually involving the heart, brain, pancreas, or spleen, typically due to the deposition of transthyretin 老年发生的淀粉样变性，通常累及心脏、脑、胰、脾，最典型的为甲状腺素转运蛋白沉积所致。又称 *a. of aging*

am·y·lo·pec·tin (am″ə-lo-pek′tin) a highly branched, water-insoluble glucan; the insoluble constituent of starch; the soluble constituent is amylose 支链淀粉

am·y·lo·pec·ti·no·sis (am″ə-lo-pek″tĭ-no′sis) glycogen storage disease, type Ⅳ 糖原贮积症Ⅳ型

am·y·lor·rhea (am″ə-lo-re′ə) presence of excessive starch in the stools 淀粉便，粪便中含过多淀粉

am·y·lose (am′ə-lōs) a linear, water-soluble glucan; the soluble constituent of starch, as opposed to amylopectin 直链淀粉

am·y·lu·ria (am″əl-u′re-ə) an excess of starch in the urine 淀粉尿，尿液中含过多淀粉

amyo·pla·sia (a-mi″o-pla′zhə) lack of muscle formation or development 肌发育不良 ; **a. conge′nita,** generalized lack in the newborn of muscular development and growth, with contracture and deformity at most joints 先天性肌发育不良

amyo·sta·sia (a-mi″o-sta′zhə) a tremor of the muscles 肌震颤

amyo·to·nia (a″mi-o-to′ne-ə) atonic condition of the muscles 肌张力不全

amy·ot·ro·phy (a″mi-ot′rə-fe) muscular atrophy 肌萎缩 ; **amyotro′phic** adj.; **diabetic a.,** a painful condition, associated with diabetes, with progressive wasting and weakening of muscles, usually limited to the muscles of the pelvic girdle and thigh 糖尿病性肌萎缩，伴有进行性肌肉丢失，通常局限于骨盆和大腿肌肉 ; **neuralgic a.,** atrophy and paralysis of the muscles of the pectoral girdle, with pain across the shoulder and upper arm 神经痛性肌萎缩，肩胛带肌肉发生萎缩和瘫痪，伴有肩部及上肢疼痛

amyx·ia (ə-mik′se-ə) absence of mucus 黏液缺乏

An anode 阳极

ANA American Neurological Association 美国神经学会 ; American Nurses Association 美国护士协会 ; antinuclear antibodies 抗核抗体

ana (an′ah) [Gr.] so much of each 各若干

ana·bi·o·sis (an″ə-bi-o′sis) restoration of the vital processes after their apparent cessation 复苏，在生命体征消失后重新恢复的过程 ; bringing back to consciousness 苏醒 ; **anabiot′ic** adj.

anab·o·lism (ə-nab′ə-liz″əm) the constructive process by which living cells convert simple substances into more complex compounds, especially into living matter 合成代谢，细胞将简单物质转化为复杂化合物，特别是生物组成物质 ; **anabol′ic** adj.

anab·o·lite (ə-nab′ə-līt″) any product of anabolism 合成代谢产物

an·acid·i·ty (an″ə-sid′ĭ-te) lack of normal acidity 酸缺乏 ; **gastric a.,** achlorhydria 胃酸缺乏

ana·cli·sis (an″ə-kli′sis) physical and emotional dependence on another for protection and gratification 依赖心理，为了获得保护或满足而对他人产生躯体上或情感上的依赖

ana·clit·ic (an″ə-klit′ik) 1. pertaining to anaclisis 依赖心理的 ; 2. exhibiting excessive emotional dependency 表现出过多的情感依赖

ana·crot·ic (an″ə-krot′ik) 1. pertaining to the ascending limb of a pulse tracing 脉象的上升支 ; 2. characterized by a notch, i.e., two waveforms in the ascending limb of the pulse tracing 有切迹，如脉象上升支的两个波形

anac·ro·tism (ə-nak′rə-tiz-əm) the presence of an anacrotic pulse 存在脉象上升支的现象

an·adre·nal·ism (an″ə-dre′nəl-iz-əm) absence or failure of adrenal function 肾上腺功能缺失

an·aer·obe (an′ə-rōb) an organism that lives and grows in the absence of molecular oxygen 厌氧菌 ; **facultative a.,** one that can live and grow with or without molecular oxygen 兼性厌氧菌 ; **obligate a.,** one that can grow only in the complete absence of molecular oxygen; some are killed by oxygen 专性厌氧菌

an·aer·o·bic (an″ə-ro′bik) 1. lacking molecular oxygen 无氧的 ; 2. growing, living, or occurring in the absence of molecular oxygen; pertaining to an anaerobe 厌氧的

an·aer·o·bi·o·sis (an″ə-ro″bi-o′sis) metabolic processes occurring in the absence of molecular oxygen 厌氧生活

an·aero·gen·ic (an″aero-ro-jen′ik) 1. producing little or no gas 不产气的 ; 2. suppressing the formation of gas by gas-producing bacteria 抑制产气性细菌的产气过程

anagen (an′ə-jen) the first phase of the hair cycle, during which synthesis of hair takes place 毛发生长期，毛发生长循环的第一阶段

an·ag·re·lide (an-ag′rə-līd) an agent used to reduce elevated platelet counts and the risk of thrombosis in the treatment of hemorrhagic thrombocythemia; used as the hydrochloride salt 阿那格雷

an·a·kin·ra (an″ə-kin′rə) a recombinant form of the human interleukin-1 receptor antagonist, used as an antiinflammatory in the treatment of rheumatoid arthritis 阿那白滞素

an·aku·sis (an″ə-koo′sis) total deafness 全聋

anal (a′nəl) relating to the anus 肛门的

an·al·bu·min·emia (an″al-bu″mĭ-ne′me-ə) absence or deficiency of serum albumins 无白蛋白血症

ana·lep·tic (an″ə-lep′tik) 1. stimulating, invigorating, or restorative 兴奋的，刺激的，恢复的 ; 2. a drug that acts as a central nervous system stimulant, such as caffeine 苏醒药

an·al·ge·sia (an″əl-je′ze-ə) 1. absence of sensibility to pain 痛觉缺失 ; 2. the relief of pain without loss of consciousness 镇痛 ; **continuous epidural a.,** continuous injection of an anesthetic solution into the sacral and lumbar plexuses within the epidural space to relieve the pain of childbirth; also used in general surgery to block the pain pathways below the navel 连续性硬膜外镇痛 ; **epidural a.,** analgesia induced by introduction of the analgesic agent into the epidural space of the vertebral canal 硬膜外镇痛；**infiltration a.,** paralysis of the nerve endings at the site of operation by subcutaneous injection of an anesthetic 浸润镇痛；**paretic a.,** loss of the sense of pain accompanied by partial paralysis 麻痹止痛法；**relative a.,** in dental anesthesia, a maintained level of conscious sedation, short of general anesthesia, in which the pain threshold is elevated; usually induced by inhalation of nitrous oxide and oxygen 相对性镇痛，在牙科麻醉中，维持在清醒镇静的状态，痛阈提高，但麻醉程度弱于全身麻醉；通常由吸入笑气和氧气诱导麻醉；**spinal a.,** analgesia produced by injection of an opioid into the subarachnoid space around the spinal cord 脊髓镇痛

an·al·ge·sic　(an″əl-je′zik) 1. relieving pain 镇痛的；2. pertaining to analgesia 痛觉缺失的；3. an agent that relieves pain without causing loss of consciousness 镇痛药；**narcotic a.,** opioid a. 麻醉性镇痛药；**nonsteroidal antiinflammatory a. (NSAIA),** 非甾体类镇痛抗炎药，见 *drug* 下词条；**opioid a.,** any of a class of compounds that bind with the opioid receptors in the central nervous system to block the perception of pain or affect the emotional response to pain, including opium and its derivatives 阿片类镇痛药

an·al·gia　(an-al′jə) 见 analgesia；**anal′gic adj.**

anal·o·gous　(ə-nal′ə-gəs) resembling or similar in some respects, as in function or appearance, but not in origin or development 相似的，在某些方面相似（如功能或形态），但不同源

ana·logue　(an′ə-log) 1. a part or organ having the same function as another, but of different evolutionary origin 同功结构或器官；2. a chemical compound having a structure similar to that of another but differing from it in respect to a certain component; it may have a similar or opposite action metabolically（化学）类似物

anal·o·gy　(ə-nal′ə-je) the quality of being analogous; resemblance or similarity in function or appearance, but not in origin or development 相似性

anal·y·sand　(ə-nal′ĭ-sand) one who is being psychoanalyzed 接受精神分析者

anal·y·sis　(ə-nal′ĭ-sis) pl. *anal′yses* 1. separation into component parts; the act of determining the component parts of a substance 分析，将整体分成各组成部分，或确定某种物质的组成成分；2. psychoanalysis 精神分析；**analyt′ic, analyt′ical adj.; bite a.,** 见 occlusal a；**blood gas a.,** the laboratory determination of the pH and the partial pressures and concentrations of oxygen and carbon dioxide in the blood 血气分析；**gasometric a.,** analysis by measurement of the gas evolved 气体分析；

gravimetric a., quantitative analysis in which the analyte or a derivative is determined by weighing after purification 重量分析；**occlusal a.,** study of the relations of the occlusal surfaces of opposing teeth 咬合分析，研究对应牙齿的咬合关系；**pulsechase a.,** a method for examining a cellular process occurring over time by successively exposing the cells to a radioactive compound (pulse) and then to the same compound in nonradioactive form (chase) 脉冲追踪分析；**qualitative a.,** chemical analysis in which the presence or absence of certain compounds in a specimen is determined 定性分析；**quantitative a.,** determination of the proportionate quantities of the constituents of a compound 定量分析；**spectroscopic a., spectrum a.,** that done by determining the wavelength(s) at which electromagnetic energy is absorbed by the sample 光谱分析；**transactional a.,** a type of psychotherapy based on an understanding of the interactions (transactions) between patient and therapist and between patient and others in the environment 交互分析，一种精神治疗方法，通过使患者理解与治疗师及其他人互动的意义来进行治疗；**vector a.,** analysis of a moving force to determine both its magnitude and its direction, e.g., analysis of the scalar electrocardiogram to determine the magnitude and direction of the electromotive force for one complete cycle of the heart 矢量分析

ana·lyte　(an′ə-lit) a substance undergoing analysis. 被分析物

ana·ly·zer　(an′ə-li″zer) 1. a device used in the analysis of the physical or chemical characteristics of a sample or system 分析仪；2. a device that transmits only plane polarized light 检偏器；3. a nervous receptor together with its central connections, by means of which sensitivity to stimulations is differentiated 一类神经受体及其中枢联结，通过其可使对刺激的敏感性差异化

an·am·ne·sis　(an″am-ne′sis) [Gr.] 1. recollection 记忆；2. a patient case history, particularly using the patient's recollections 既往病史，特指患者回忆的部分；3. immunologic memory 免疫记忆

an·am·nes·tic　(an″am-nes′tik) 1. pertaining to anamnesis 记忆的；2. aiding the memory 辅助记忆的

ana·morph　(an′ə-morf″) the state of a fungus in which reproduction is asexual; as opposed to teleomorph. 另见 fungus 下的 *anamorphic fungi*（真菌）无性型

ana·phase　(an′ə-fāz) the stage of cell division following metaphase, in which the chromatids lined up on the spindle move to the poles (anaphase A), followed by elongation of the cell and further separation of the poles (anaphase B) 细胞分裂后期

ana·phia (ə-na′fe-ə) tactile anesthesia 触觉缺失

ana·pho·ria (an″ə-for′e-ə) a tendency for the visual axes of both eyes to divert above the horizontal plane 上隐斜视，双眼视轴有向上偏斜的倾向

an·aph·ro·dis·iac (an″af-ro-diz′e-ak) 1. repressing sexual desire 抑制性欲的；2. a drug that represses sexual desire 性欲抑制药

ana·phy·lac·to·gen·e·sis (an″ə-fə-lak″tojen′ə-sis) the production of anaphylaxis 过敏反应发生 **ana-phylactogen′ic** adj 过敏反应发生的

ana·phy·lac·toid (an″ə-fə-lak′toid) resembling anaphylaxis 过敏反应样的

ana·phyl·a·tox·in (an″ə-fil′ə-tok″sin) a substance that is produced in blood serum during complement fixation and serves as a mediator of inflammation by inducing mast cell degranulation and histamine release; on injection into animals, it causes anaphylactic shock 过敏毒素

ana·phy·lax·is (an″ə-fə-lak′sis) a type I hypersensitivity reaction in which exposure of a sensitized individual to a specific antigen or hapten results in urticaria, pruritus, and angioedema, followed by vascular collapse and shock and often accompanied by life-threatening respiratory distress 过敏反应，Ⅰ型超敏反应; **anaphylac′tic** adj. 过敏反应的; active a., that produced by injection of a foreign protein 主动性过敏反应，由注射外源性蛋白后产生; antiserum a., 见 passive a.; passive a., that resulting in a normal person from injection of serum of a sensitized person 被动性过敏反应，由正常人注射敏感者的血清后产生; passive cutaneous a., PCA; localized anaphylaxis passively transferred by intradermal injection of an antibody and, after a latent period (about 24 to 72 hours), intravenous injection of the homologous antigen and Evans blue dye; blueing of the skin at the site of the intradermal injection is evidence of the permeability reaction. Used in studies of antibodies causing immediate hypersensitivity reaction 被动性皮下过敏反应; reverse a., that following injection of antigen, succeeded by injection of antiserum 反转性过敏反应，注射抗原后再注射抗血清后产生

ana·pla·sia (an″ə-pla′zhə) dedifferentiation; loss of differentiation of cells and of their orientation to one another and to their axial framework and blood vessels, a characteristic of tumor tissue 间变，细胞去分化并失去转分化能力，为肿瘤组织的特性; **anaplas′tic** adj.

Ana·plas·ma (an″ə-plaz′mə) a genus of gramnegative, tick-borne bacteria of the family Anaplasma-

taceae that are parasitic in cells of the hematopoietic system and associated tissues. Most cause veterinary infections, but *A. phagocyto′philum* causes human granulocytic anaplasmosis 无形体属

Ana·plas·ma·ta·ce·ae (an″ə-plaz″mə-ta′se-e) a family of bacteria of the order Rickettsiales that are parasitic in cells of the blood and hematopoietic system 无形体科

ana·plas·mo·sis (an″ə-plaz-mo′sis) infection with organisms of the genus *Anaplasma* 无浆体病; **human granulocytic a.**, infection with *Anaplasma phagocytophilum*, transmitted by ticks of the genus Ixodes. It affects primarily neutrophils, is characterized by flulike symptoms with leukopenia and thrombocytopenia, and ranges in severity from asymptomatic to fatal 人粒细胞无形体病

an·apoph·y·sis (an″ə-pof′ĭ-sis) an accessory vertebral process 副突

anap·tic (ə-nap′tik) marked by anaphia 触觉缺失的

an·ar·thria (an-ahr′thre-ə) severe dysarthria resulting in speechlessness 构音不全

anas·to·mo·sis (ə-nas″tə-mo′sis) pl. *anastomo′ses* [Gr.] 1. a connection between two vessels or other tubular structures 吻合，两根血管或其他管腔结构的连接; 2. surgical, traumatic, or pathological formation of an opening between two normally distinct spaces or organs 手术、创伤或病理改变造成两个空间或器官的连通; **anastomot′ic** adj. 吻合的，连通的; arteriovenous a., 1. one that directly interconnects the arterial and venous systems and acts as a shunt to bypass the capillary bed 动静脉吻合; 2. 见 arteriovenous shunt (2); crucial a., an arterial anastomosis in the upper part of the thigh 十字形吻合，大腿上部的一处动脉吻合; end-to-end a., the surgical joining together of two tubular structures that have been cut perpendicular to their length 端—端吻合; end-to-side a., an anastomosis connecting the end of one tubular structure with the side of a larger one 端—侧吻合; heterocladic a., an anastomosis between branches of different arteries 异支吻合; homocladic a., one between two branches of the same artery 同支吻合; ileoanal pull-through a., anastomosis of an ileoanal reservoir to the anal canal by means of a short conduit of ileum pulled through the rectal cuff and sutured to the anus, allowing continent elimination of feces following colectomy 将回肠的一条短管拉过直肠袖口，与肛门缝合，由此进行回肠肛门与肛管的吻合术，将回肠短导管穿过直肠袖口并缝合到肛门，使结肠切除术后粪便从此排出; intestinal a., establishment of a communication between two formerly distant portions of the intestine 肠吻合; a.

of Riolan, anastomosis of the superior and inferior mesenteric arteries 肠系膜上、下动脉的吻合; **Roux-en-Y a.,** any Y-shaped anastomosis in which the small intestine is included Roux-en-Y 吻合, 任何包括小肠的 Y 形吻合

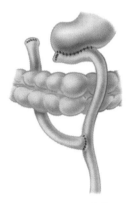

▲　Roux-en-Y 吻合

anas·tro·zole (ə-nas′trə-zōl) an antineoplastic used for treatment of advanced breast carcinoma in postmenopausal women 阿那曲唑

anat. anatomy 解剖学

ana·tom·ic (an″ə-tom′ik) anatomical 解剖学的

ana·tom·i·cal (an″ə-tom′ĭ-kəl) pertaining to anatomy, or to the structure of an organism 解剖学的

anat·o·my (ə-nat′ə-me) the science of the structure of living organisms 解剖学; **applied a.,** anatomy as applied to diagnosis and treatment 应用解剖学; **clinical a.,** anatomy as applied to clinical practice 临床解剖学; **comparative a.,** comparison of the structure of different animals and plants, one with another 比较解剖学; **developmental a.,** the field of study concerned with the changes that cells, tissues, organs, and the body as a whole undergo from fertilization of a secondary oocyte to the resulting offspring; it includes both prenatal and postnatal development 发育解剖学; **gross a.,** that dealing with structures visible with the unaided eye 大体解剖学; **histologic a.,** histology 组织解剖学, 组织学; **homologic a.,** the study of the related parts of the body in different animals 同源解剖学; **macroscopic a.,** 见 gross a.; **microscopic a.,** histology 微观解剖学, 组织学; **morbid a., pathological a.,** anatomic pathology 病理解剖学, 解剖病理学; **physiological a.,** the study of the organs with respect to their normal functions 生理解剖学; **radiological a.,** the study of the anatomy of tissues based on their visualization on x-ray films 放射解剖学; **special**

a., the study of particular organs or parts 特定解剖学, 研究特定的器官或结构; **topographic a.,** the study of parts in their relation to surrounding parts 局部解剖学; **x-ray a.,** 见 radiological a.

ana·tro·pia (an″ə-tro′pe-ə) upward deviation of the visual axis of one eye when the other eye is fixing 上隐斜视, 当一眼固定, 另一眼视轴偏向上偏斜; **anatrop′ic** adj.

ANCC American Nurses Credentialing Center 美国护士资格认证协会

an·chor·age (ang′kər-əj) 1. fixation, e.g., surgical fixation of a displaced viscus or, in operative dentistry, fixation of fillings or of artificial crowns or bridges 固定, 如脏器移位的外科固定, 或口腔手术中填料、人工牙冠、桥体的固定; 2. in orthodontics, the nature and degree of resistance to displacement offered by an anatomical unit when force is applied to cause movement during a procedure（口腔正畸学）支抗, 当施力移动牙齿时, 该解剖单位会产生阻止移位的反作用力, 这种性质及其程度称为支抗

an·cip·i·tal (an-sip′ĭ-təl) two-edged or two-headed 有两边的, 有两头的

an·co·ne·al (ang-ko′ne-əl) cubital 肘的

an·co·ni·tis (ang″ko-ni′tis) inflammation of the elbow joint 肘关节炎

An·cy·los·to·ma (an″sĭ-los′tə-mə) a genus of hookworms (family Ancylostomatidae). *A. brasilien′se* and *A. cani′num* normally infest cats and dogs but can cause cutaneous larva migrans in humans. *A. duodena′le* is the common European or Old World hookworm, parasitic in the small intestine of humans and the usual cause of hookworm disease 钩虫属

an·cy·los·to·mi·a·sis (an″sĭ-lo″sto-mi′ə-sis) hookworm disease caused by a species of *Ancylostoma* 钩虫病

an·cy·roid (an′sə-roid) anchor-shaped 锚形的

an·dro·blas·to·ma (an″dro-blas-to′mə) 1. a rare benign tumor of the testis histologically resembling the fetal testis; there are three varieties: diffuse stromal, mixed (stromal and epithelial), and tubular (epithelial). The epithelial elements contain Sertoli cells, which may produce estrogen and thus cause feminization 睾丸母细胞瘤; 2. a rare ovarian tumor characterized by both Sertoli and Leydig cells, usually occurring in young women; it secretes testosterone and usually causes masculinization and hirsutism 卵巢睾丸母细胞瘤

an·dro·gen (an′dro-jən) any substance, e.g., testosterone, that promotes masculinization 雄激素, 任何促进雄性化的物质; **adrenal a's,** the 19-carbon steroids synthesized by the adrenal cortex that

A

function as weak steroids or steroid precursors; e.g., dehydroepiandrosterone 肾上腺雄激素

an·dro·gen·e·sis (an″dro-jen′ə-sis) development of a zygote that contains only paternal chromosomes, as after fertilization of an oocyte whose chromosomes are absent or inactivated 孤雄生殖

an·dro·ge·net·ic (an″dro-jə-net′ik) caused by androgens 雄激素源性的

an·dro·gen·ic (an″dro-jen′ik) 1. producing masculine characteristics 产生雄性特征的；2. pertaining to an androgen 雄激素的

an·drog·y·ny (an-droj′ĭ-ne) 1. the state of having both male and female characteristics or features 雌雄同体；2. the state of being neither distinctly masculine nor distinctly feminine 既不明显雄性化，也不明显雌性化；androg′ynous adj. 雌雄同体的

an·droid (an′droid) resembling a man 人形的

an·dro·pause (an′dro-pawz) a variable complex of symptoms, including decreased Leydig cell numbers and androgen production, occurring in men after middle age, purported to be analogous to menopause in women 男性更年期

an·dro·phil·ia (an′-dro-fil′e-ə) sexual attraction to adult males or masculinity 对成年男性或男性化特征的性偏好

an·dro·stane (an′dro-stān) the hydrocarbon nucleus, $C_{19}H_{32}$, from which androgens are derived 雄固烷，雄激素的母环系统，所有雄激素均为其衍生物

an·dro·stane·di·ol (an″dro-stān-di′ol) (-stān′de-ol) an androgen implicated in the regulation of gonadotropin secretion; *a. glucuronide*, a metabolite of dihydroxytestosterone formed in the peripheral tissues, is used to estimate peripheral androgen activity 雄固烷二醇

an·dro·stene (an′dro-stēn) a cyclic hydrocarbon, $C_{19}H_{30}$, forming the nucleus of testosterone and certain other androgens 雄甾烯

an·dro·stene·di·ol (an″dro-stēn-di′ol) (-stēn′de-ol) a testosterone metabolite that may contribute to gonadotropin secretion 雄甾烯二醇

an·dro·stene·di·one (an″dro-stēn-di′ōn) (-stēn′de-ōn) an androgenic steroid produced by the testis, adrenal cortex, and ovary; converted metabolically to testosterone and other androgens 雄甾烯二酮

an·dros·ter·one (an-dros′tər-ōn) an androgen degradation product that in some species exerts weak androgenlike effects 雄酮

an·ec·do·tal (an″ek-do′təl) based on case histories rather than on controlled clinical trials 轶事证据的，基于病史而非对照临床试验

an·echo·ic (an-ə-ko′ik) 1. without echoes; said of a chamber for measuring the effects of sound 无回声的；2. sonolucent（超声）透声的

an·ec·ta·sis (an-ek′tə-sis) congenital atelectasis due to developmental immaturity 原发性肺不张，由发育不成熟导致的先天性肺不张

an·e·jac·u·la·tion (an″e-jak″u-la′shən) failure of ejaculation of semen from the urinary meatus in sexual intercourse 不射精症

ane·mia (ə-ne′me-ə) reduction below normal of the number of erythrocytes, quantity of hemoglobin, or volume of packed red cells in the blood; a symptom of various diseases and disorders 贫血；ane′mic adj.; achrestic a., any of various types of megaloblastic anemia resembling pernicious anemia but unresponsive to therapy with vitamin B_{12} 利用不良性贫血，所有与恶性贫血类似但对维生素 B_{12} 治疗无效的巨幼细胞贫血；aplastic a., a diverse group of anemias characterized by bone marrow suppression with replacement of the hematopoietic cells by fat, which causes pancytopenia, often accompanied by granulocytopenia and thrombocytopenia 再生障碍性贫血，由骨髓抑制造成，造血细胞被脂肪替代，导致全血细胞减少，通常伴有粒细胞减少和血小板减少；aregenerative a., anemia characterized by bone marrow failure, so that functional marrow cells are regenerated slowly or not at all 再生障碍性贫血，由骨髓衰竭造成，有功能的骨髓细胞再生缓慢或停止；autoimmune hemolytic a., AIHA; a general term covering a large group of anemias involving autoantibodies against red cell antigens; they may be idiopathic or may have any of a number of causes, including autoimmune disease, hematologic neoplasms, viral infections, or immunodeficiency disorders 自身免疫性溶血性贫血；congenital hypoplastic a., 1. 见 Diamond-Blackfan a.；2. 见 Fanconi a.；congenital nonspherocytic hemolytic a., any of a heterogeneous group of inherited anemias characterized by shortened red cell survival, lack of spherocytosis, and normal osmotic fragility with erythrocyte membrane defects, multiple intracellular enzyme deficiencies or other defects, or unstable hemoglobins 先天性非球形细胞性溶血性贫血；Cooley a., thalassemia major 贫血，地中海贫血的主要类型；Diamond-Blackfan a., a genetically and clinically diverse congenital anemia, often associated with other congenital anomalies; characterized by deficiency of red cell precursors in an otherwise normally cellular bone marrow, and unresponsive to hematinics 先天性纯红细胞再生障碍性贫血，一组遗传和临床上有差异性的先天性贫血，通常伴有其他先天异常；特征为骨髓中缺乏红细胞前

体，对补血药无反应；**drug-induced immune hemolytic a.**, immune hemolytic anemia produced by drugs, classified as the *penicillin type*, in which the drug induces the formation of specific antibodies; the *methyldopa type*, in which the drug induces the formation of anti-Rh antibodies; and the *stibophen type*, in which circulating drug-antibody complexes bind to red cells 药物诱导免疫复合物溶血性贫血；**Fanconi a.**, an autosomal recessive disorder of chromosome fragility, due to mutation in a cluster of genes involved in DNA repair; it is characterized by some combination of pancytopenia, bone marrow hypoplasia, skin pigmentation changes, congenital anomalies of the musculoskeletal and genitourinary systems, and a predisposition to cancer Fanconi 贫血，与染色体脆性有关的一种常染色体隐性疾病，由一组关于 DNA 修复的基因发生突变所致；特征为全血细胞减少、骨髓发育不全、皮肤色素改变、肌肉骨骼和泌尿生殖系统的先天异常，具有癌症易感性；**hemolytic a.**, any of a group of acute or chronic anemias, inherited or acquired, characterized by shortened survival of mature erythrocytes and inability of bone marrow to compensate for the decreased life span 溶血性贫血；**hereditary iron-loading a.**,　　见 hereditary sideroblastic a.；**hereditary sideroachrestic a.**, 见 hereditary sideroblastic a.；**hereditary sideroblastic a.**, an X-linked anemia characterized by ringed sideroblasts, hypochromic, microcytic erythrocytes, poikilocytosis, weakness, and later by iron overload 遗传性铁粒幼细胞贫血；**hookworm a.**, hypochromic microcytic anemia resulting from infection with *Ancylostoma* or *Necator* 钩虫性贫血；另见 *disease* 下词条；**hypochromic a.**, that characterized by a disproportionate reduction of red cell hemoglobin and an increased area of central pallor in the red cells 低色素性贫血；**hypoplastic a.**, that due to varying degrees of erythrocytic hypoplasia without leukopenia or thrombocytopenia 再生不良性贫血；**iron deficiency a.**, a form characterized by low or absent iron stores, low serum iron concentration, low transferrin saturation, elevated transferrin, low hemoglobin concentration or hematocrit, and hypochromic, microcytic red blood cells 缺铁性贫血；**macrocytic a.**, a group of anemias of varying etiologies, marked by larger than normal red cells, absence of the customary central area of pallor, and an increased mean corpuscular volume and mean corpuscular hemoglobin 巨细胞性贫血；**Mediterranean a.**, thalassemia major 地中海贫血，珠蛋白生成障碍性贫血；**megaloblastic a.**, any anemia characterized by megaloblasts in the bone marrow, such as pernicious a. 巨幼细胞贫血；**microcytic a.**, that marked by decrease in size of the red cells 小细胞性贫血；**myelopathic a.**, **myelophthisic a.**, leukoerythroblastosis 骨髓病性贫血；**normochromic a.**, anemia in which the hemoglobin content of the red cells as measured by the MCHC is in the normal range 正常色素性贫血；**normocytic a.**, that marked by a proportionate decrease in the hemoglobin content, the packed red cell volume, and the number of erythrocytes per cubic millimeter of blood 正常细胞性贫血；**pernicious a.**, megaloblastic anemia, most commonly affecting older adults, due to failure of the gastric mucosa to secrete adequate and potent intrinsic factor, resulting in malabsorption of vitamin B_{12} 恶性贫血；**polar a.**, an anemic condition that occurs during exposure to low temperature; initially microcytic, but subsequently becoming normocytic 极地贫血，低温环境下发生的贫血，开始为小细胞性，随后转变为正常细胞性；**pure red cell a.**, anemia characterized by absence of red cell precursors in the bone marrow; the congenital form is *Diamond-Blackfan a.* 纯红细胞再生障碍性贫血；**refractory normoblastic a.**, 难治性正幼细胞性贫血，见 refractory sideroblastic a.；**refractory sideroblastic a.**, a sideroblastic anemia clinically similar to the hereditary sideroblastic form but occurring in adults and often only slowly progressive. It is unresponsive to hematinics or to withdrawal of toxic agents or drugs and may be preleukemic 难治性铁粒幼细胞性贫血；**sickle cell a.**, a hereditary hemolytic anemia seen primarily in those of West African descent; it is an autosomal recessive disorder caused by mutation of the gene encoding the β-globin chain of hemoglobin, resulting in hemoglobin S with its reduced solubility in the deoxygenated form, leading to abnormal erythrocytes (*sickle cells*) in the blood. Homozygous individuals have the full-blown syndrome with accelerated hemolysis, increased blood viscosity and vasoocclusion, arthralgias, acute attacks of abdominal pain, and ulcerations of the lower limbs; some have periodic attacks of *sickle cell crises*. The heterozygous condition is called *sickle cell trait* and is usually asymptomatic 镰状细胞贫血；**sideroachrestic a.**, 见 sideroblastic a.；**sideroblastic a.**, any of a group of anemias that may have diverse clinical manifestations; commonly characterized by large numbers of ringed sideroblasts in the bone marrow, ineffective erythropoiesis, variable proportions of hypochromic erythrocytes in the peripheral blood, and usually increased levels of tissue iron 铁粒幼细胞贫血；**sideropenic a.**, a group of anemias marked by low levels of iron in the plasma; it includes iron deficiency anemia and the anemia of chronic disorders 缺铁性贫血，包括了狭义的缺

铁性贫血和慢性疾病造成的贫血；**spur cell a.,** anemia in which the red cells have a bizarre spiculated shape and are destroyed prematurely, primarily in the spleen; it is an acquired form occurring in severe liver disease and represents an abnormality in the cholesterol content of the red cell membrane 棘刺红细胞症；**toxic hemolytic a.,** that due to toxic agents, including drugs, bacterial lysins, and snake venoms 中毒性溶血性贫血

an·en·ceph·a·ly (an″ən-sef′ə-le) congenital absence of the cranial vault, with the cerebral hemispheres completely missing or reduced to small masses 无脑畸形；**anencephal′ic** adj. 无脑畸形的

an·er·gy (an′ər-je) 1. extreme lack of energy 缺乏精力；2. diminished reactivity to one or more specific antigens（免疫）无反应性，对一或多种特定抗原失去反应；**aner′gic** adj. 缺乏精力的；（免疫）无反应性的

an·eryth·ro·pla·sia (an″ə-rith″ro-pla′zhə) absence of erythrocyte formation 红细胞发生不能；**anerythroplas′tic** adj. 红细胞发生不能的

an·eryth·ro·poi·e·sis (an″ə-rith″ro-poi-e′sis) deficient production of erythrocytes 红细胞发生不全

an·es·the·sia (an″es-the′zhə) 1. loss of sensation, usually by damage to a nerve or receptor 感觉缺失，通常由神经或受体损伤导致；2. loss of the ability to feel pain, caused by administration of a drug or other medical intervention 麻醉；**basal a.,** narcosis produced by preliminary medication so that the inhalation of anesthetic necessary to produce surgical anesthesia is greatly reduced 基础麻醉；**block a.,** 阻滞麻醉，见 regional a.；**bulbar a.,** that due to a lesion of the pons 延髓麻醉；**caudal a.,** 见 block 下词条；**closed circuit a.,** that produced by continuous rebreathing of a small amount of anesthetic gas in a closed system with an apparatus for removing carbon dioxide 紧闭循环式麻醉，通过闭路的呼吸支持系统，持续吸入少量麻醉气体以达到麻醉效果；**crossed a.,** 交叉性感觉缺失，见 hemianesthesia 下词条；**a. doloro′sa,** pain in an area or region that is anesthetic 痛性感觉缺失，麻木部位的疼痛感；**electric a.,** that induced by passage of an electric current 电麻醉；**endotracheal a.,** that produced by introduction of a gaseous mixture through a tube inserted into the trachea 气管内麻醉；**epidural a.,** 硬膜外阻滞，见 block 下词条；**general a.,** a state of unconsciousness and insusceptibility to pain, produced by administration of anesthetic agents by inhalation, intravenously, intramuscularly, rectally, or via the gastrointestinal tract 全身麻醉；**infiltration a.,** local anesthesia produced by injection of the anesthetic solution in the area of terminal nerve endings 浸润麻醉；**inhalation a.,** that produced by the inhalation of vapors of a volatile liquid or gaseous anesthetic agent 吸入麻醉；**insufflation a.,** that produced by blowing a mixture of gases or vapors into the respiratory tract through a tube 吹入麻醉，通过管道将混合气体吹入呼吸道以达到麻醉效果；**local a.,** that produced in a limited area, as by injection of a local anesthetic or by freezing with ethyl chloride 局部麻醉；**lumbar epidural a.,** that produced by injection of the anesthetic into the epidural space at the second or third lumbar interspace 腰椎硬膜外麻醉；**muscular a.,** loss or lack of muscle sense 肌肉麻醉；**open a.,** general inhalation anesthesia using a cone, without significant rebreathing of exhaled gases 开放式麻醉，使用锥状物进行全身吸入麻醉，无大量重吸入和呼出气体；**peripheral a.,** that due to changes in the peripheral nerves 外周麻醉；**regional a.,** insensibility of a part induced by interrupting the sensory nerve conductivity of that region of the body; it may be produced by either *field block* or *nerve block* (see under *block*) 区域麻醉；**sacral a.,** spinal anesthesia by injection of anesthetic into the sacral canal and about the sacral nerves 骶管麻醉；**saddle block a.,** 鞍状阻滞麻醉，见 *block* 下词条；**spinal a.,** 1. regional anesthesia by injection of a local anesthetic into the subarachnoid space around the spinal cord 脊椎麻醉；2. loss of sensation due to a spinal lesion 脊椎麻醉；**surgical a.,** that degree of anesthesia at which operation may safely be performed 外科麻醉；**tactile a.,** loss or impairment of the sense of touch 触觉缺失；**topical a.,** that produced by application of a local anesthetic directly to the area involved, as to the oral mucosa or the cornea 表面麻醉；**transsacral a.,** 见 sacral a.

an·es·the·si·ol·o·gy (an″əs-the″ze-ol′ə-je) the branch of medicine that studies anesthesia and anesthetics 麻醉学

an·es·thet·ic (an″əs-thet′ik) 1. characterized by anesthesia; numb 感觉缺失的；2. pertaining to or producing anesthesia 麻醉的；3. an agent that produces anesthesia 麻醉药；**local a.,** an agent, e.g., lidocaine, procaine, or tetracaine, that produces anesthesia by paralyzing sensory nerve endings or nerve fibers at the site of application. The conduction of nerve impulses is blocked by stopping the entry of sodium into nerve cells 局部麻醉药；**topical a.,** a local anesthetic applied directly to the area to be anesthetized, usually the mucous membranes or the skin 表面麻醉药

anes·the·tist (ə-nes′thə-tist) a nurse or technician

trained to administer anesthetics 麻醉师

an·e·to·der·ma (an″ə-to-dur′mə) localized elas-tolysis producing circumscribed areas of soft, thin, wrinkled skin that often protrude in small outpouch-ings 皮肤松垂

an·eu·ploi·dy (an′u-ploi″de) any deviation from an exact multiple of the haploid number of chromo-somes, whether fewer or more 非整倍性

an·eu·rysm (an′u-riz″əm) a sac formed by local-ized dilatation of the wall of an artery, a vein, or the heart 动脉瘤; **aneurys′mal** *adj.* 动脉瘤的; **aortic a.,** aneurysm of the aorta 主动脉瘤; **arteriosclerotic a.,** an aneurysm arising in a large artery, usually the abdominal aorta, as a result of weakening of the wall in severe atherosclerosis 动脉硬化性动脉瘤; **arteriovenous a.,** abnormal communication be-tween an artery and a vein in which the blood flows directly into a neighboring vein or is carried into the vein by a connecting sac 动静脉瘤，动静脉之间的异常连接，从此处动脉血流可直接或通过连接囊进入静脉; **atherosclerotic a.,** 粥样硬化性动脉瘤，见 arteriosclerotic a.; **berry a.,** a small saccular aneurysm of a cerebral artery, usually at the junction of vessels in the circle of Willis, having a narrow opening into the artery 颅内小动脉瘤; **compound a.,** one in which some layers of the vessel wall are ruptured and others are only dilated 复合性动脉瘤，血管壁的某些层发生破裂而其他层仅扩张的一种动脉瘤; **dissecting a.,** one resulting from hemorrhage that causes longitudinal splitting of the arterial wall, producing a tear in the intima and es-tablishing communication with the lumen; it usually affects the aorta (*aortic dissection*) 夹层动脉瘤; **false a.,** 1. one in which the entire wall is injured and the blood is retained in the surrounding tissues; a sac communicating with the artery (or heart) is eventually formed 假性动脉瘤，血管全壁损伤，血液滞留于周围组织中，与血管（心脏）相通的囊腔形成周围组织中; 2. pseudoaneurysm 假性动脉瘤; **infected a.,** one produced by growth of mi-croorganisms in the vessel wall, or infection arising within a preexisting arteriosclerotic aneurysm 感染性动脉瘤; **mycotic a.,** 1. an infected aneurysm resulting from infective endocarditis 真菌性动脉瘤; 2. occasionally, any aneurysm resulting from an infectious cause 有时指所有感染因素引起的动脉瘤; **racemose a.,** dilatation and tortuous length-ening of the blood vessels 蔓状动脉瘤; **saccular a., sacculated a.,** a distended sac affecting only part of the arterial circumference 囊状动脉瘤; **vari-cose a.,** one in which an intervening sac connects the artery with contiguous veins 静脉曲张性动脉瘤

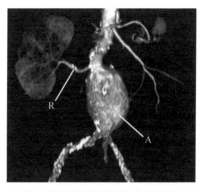

▲ 轴向增强计算机断层扫描显示了肾旁主动脉瘤（aortic aneurysm）与其他结构的关系（A），其中包括近端的右肾动脉（R）和远端的主动脉分叉

an·eu·rys·mo·plas·ty (an″u-riz′mo-plas″te) plas-tic repair of the affected artery in the treatment of aneurysm 动脉瘤成形术

an·eu·rys·mor·rha·phy (an″u-riz-mor′ə-fe) su-ture of an aneurysm 动脉瘤缝闭术

ANF antinuclear antibody (antinuclear factor) 抗核抗体; American Nurses' Foundation 美国护士协会

an·gi·as·the·nia (an″je-əs-the′ne-ə) loss of tone in the vascular system 脉管无力，脉管系统听诊不到任何声音

an·gi·ec·ta·sis (an″je-ek′tə-sis) gross dilatation and often lengthening of a blood or lymph vessel 脉管扩张; **angiectat′ic** *adj.*

an·gi·ec·to·my (an″je-ek′tə-me) excision or resec-tion of a vessel 血管切除术

an·gi·ec·to·pia (an″je-ek-to′pe-ə) abnormal posi-tion or course of a vessel 血管异位

an·gi·i·tis (an″je-i′tis) pl. **angii′tides** Vasculitis 脉管炎; **allergic granulomatous a.,** Churg-Strauss syndrome 过敏性肉芽肿性脉管炎综合征

an·gi·na (an-ji′nə) (an′jĭ-nə) 1. a. pectoris 心绞痛; 2. spasmodic, choking, or suffocating pain 咽峡炎; **an′ginal** *adj.* 心绞痛的; 咽峡炎的; **a. of effort,** stable a. pectoris 劳累型心绞痛; 见 *a. pectoris*; **herpes a., a. herpe′tica,** herpangina 疱疹性咽峡炎; **intestinal a.,** cramping abdominal pain shortly after a meal, lasting one to three hours, due to ischemia of the smooth muscle of the bowel 肠绞痛; **a. in-ver′sa,** 见 Prinzmetal a.; **Ludwig a.,** a severe form of cellulitis of the submaxillary space and secondary involvement of the sublingual and submental spaces, usually from infection or a penetrating injury to the floor of the mouth 咽峡炎; **a. pec′toris,** paroxysmal pain in the chest, often radiating to the arms, particularly the left, usually due to interference with the supply of oxygen to the heart muscle, and precipitated by excitement or effort. It is subdivided into *stable* and *unstable a. pectoris* based on the predictability of the frequency, duration, and causative factors for attacks 心绞痛；**Prinzmetal a.**, a variant of angina pectoris in which the attacks occur during rest, exercise capacity is well preserved, and attacks are associated electrocardiographically with elevation of the ST segment 变异型心绞痛；**pseudomembranous a.**, necrotizing ulcerative gingivostomatitis 坏死性溃疡性龈口炎；**silent a.**, an episode of coronary insufficiency in which no pain is experienced 无症状性心肌缺血或沉默性心绞痛；**variant a. pectoris**, 见 Prinzmetal a.

an·gio·blast (an′je-o-blast″) 1. the embryonic mesenchymal tissue from which blood cells and blood vessels arise; 2. an individual vessel-forming cell 成血管细胞；**angioblas′tic** *adj.* 成血管细胞的

an·gio·blas·to·ma (an″je-o-blas-to′mə) 1. hemangioblastoma 成血管细胞瘤；2. angioblastic meningioma 脑膜成血管细胞瘤

an·gio·car·di·og·ra·phy (an″je-o-kahr″deog′rə-fe) radiography of the heart and great vessels after introduction of an opaque contrast medium into a blood vessel or a cardiac chamber 心血管造影术；**equilibrium radionuclide a.**, a form of radionuclide angiocardiography in which images are taken at specific phases of the cardiac cycle over a series of several hundred cycles, with image recording set, or gated, by the occurrence of specific electrocardiographic waveforms 均衡性放射性核素心血管造影术；**first pass radionuclide a.**, a form of radionuclide angiocardiography in which a rapid sequence of images is taken immediately after administration of a bolus of radioactive material to record only the initial transit through the central circulation 首过性放射性核素心血管造影术；**radionuclide a.**, a form in which the contrast material is a radionuclide, usually a compound of technetium 99m 放射性核素心血管造影术

an·gio·car·dio·ki·net·ic (an″je-o-kahr″de-okī-net′ik) affecting the movements of the heart and blood vessels; also, an agent that affects such movements 心血管动力学的

an·gio·car·di·tis (an″je-o-kahr-di′tis) inflammation of the heart and blood vessels 血管心脏炎

an·gio·cen·tric (an″je-o-sen′trik) pertaining to lesions originating in blood vessels 血管中心性的，指病变起源于血管

an·gio·dys·pla·sia (an″je-o-dis-pla′zhə) small

vascular abnormalities, such as of the intestinal tract 血管发育异常

an·gio·ede·ma (an″je-o-ə-de′mə) a vascular reaction in the deep dermis or subcutaneous or submucosal tissues; localized edema is caused by dilatation and increased permeability of the capillaries, with development of giant wheals 血管性水肿；**hereditary a.**, an autosomal dominant disorder of C1 inhibitor, causing uncontrolled activation of the classical complement pathway; there are recurrent episodes of edema of the skin and upper respiratory and gastrointestinal tracts with increased levels of several vasoactive mediators of anaphylaxis. It may follow minor trauma, sudden changes in environmental temperature, or sudden emotional stress 遗传性血管性水肿

an·gio·en·do·the·li·o·ma (an″je-o-en″dothe″le-o′mə) hemangioendothelioma 血管内皮细胞瘤

an·gio·en·do·the·lio·ma·to·sis (an″je-oen″dothe″le-o-mə-to′sis) intravascular proliferation of tumors derived from endothelial cells 反应性血管内皮瘤病

an·gio·fi·bro·ma (an″je-o-fi-bro′mə) a lesion characterized by fibrous tissue and vascular proliferation 血管纤维瘤；**juvenile nasopharyngeal a.**, a benign tumor of the nasopharynx composed of fibrous connective tissue with abundant endothelium-lined vascular spaces, usually occurring during puberty in boys; nasal obstruction may become total, with adenoid speech, discomfort in swallowing, and auditory tube obstruction 幼年型鼻咽血管纤维瘤

an·gio·fol·lic·u·lar (an″je-o-fŏ-lik′u-lər) pertaining to a lymphoid follicle and its blood vessels 血管滤泡性的

an·gio·gen·e·sis (an″je-o-jen′ə-sis) vasculogenesis; development of blood vessels either in the embryo or in the form of neovascularization or revascularization 血管发生

an·gio·gen·ic (an″je-o-jen′ik) 1. pertaining to angiogenesis 血管发生的；2. of vascular origin 血管源性的

an·gi·og·ra·phy (an″je-og′rə-fe) radiography of the blood vessels after introduction of a contrast medium 血管造影术；**angiograph′ic** *adj.* 血管造影术的；**computed tomography a. (CTA)**, a minimally invasive form of angiography in which contrast material is injected intravenously through a small needle or cannula and images of the vascular system are produced by computed tomography 计算机断层血管造影；**digital subtraction a.**, an angiographic technique that produces images by subtracting background structures and enhancing the contrast of those areas that change in density between a preliminary "mask" image and subsequent images 数字减影血管造影；**magnetic resonance a. (MRA),** a form of magnetic resonance imaging used to study blood vessels and blood flow 磁共振血管造影

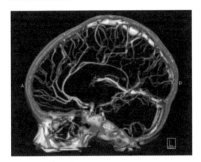

▲ 用于选择性脑血管成像的计算机断层血管造影（CTA）

an·gio·he·mo·phil·ia (an″je-o-he′mo-fil′e-ə) von Willebrand disease 血管性血友病

an·gio·hy·a·li·no·sis (an″je-o-hi″ə-li-no′sis) hyaline degeneration of the walls of blood vessels. 血管透明变性

an·gi·oid (an′je-oid) resembling blood vessels 血管样的

an·gio·ker·a·to·ma (an″je-o-ker″ə-to′mə) a skin disease in which telangiectases or warty growths occur in groups, together with epidermal thickening 血管角化瘤；**a. circumscrip′tum,** a rare form with discrete papules and nodules usually localized to a small area on the leg or trunk in children 局限性血管角化瘤

an·gio·ki·net·ic (an″je-o-kī-net′ik) vasomotor 血管舒缩的

an·gio·leio·my·o·ma (an″je-o-li″o-mi-o′mə) a leiomyoma arising from vascular smooth muscle, usually a solitary nodular, sometimes painful, subcutaneous tumor on the lower limb, particularly in middle-aged women 血管平滑肌瘤。又称 *angiomyoma*

an·gio·lipo·leio·my·o·ma (an″je-o-lip″o-li-omi-o′mə) a benign tumor composed of blood vessel, adipose tissue, and smooth muscle elements, such as occurs in the kidney in association with tuberous sclerosis, where it is usually called *angiomyolipoma* 血管平滑肌脂肪瘤

an·gio·li·po·ma (an″je-o-li-po′mə) an often painful lipoma containing clusters of thin-walled proliferating blood vessels 血管脂肪瘤

an·gi·ol·o·gy (an″je-ol′ə-je) the study of the vessels of the body; also, the sum of knowledge relating to the blood and lymph vessels 脉管学

an·gi·ol·y·sis (an″je-ol′ĭ-sis) retrogression or obliteration of blood vessels, as in embryologic development 血管破坏

an·gi·o·ma (an″je-o′mə) a tumor whose cells tend to form blood vessels (hemangioma) or lymph vessels (lymphangioma); a tumor made up of blood vessels or lymph vessels 血管瘤；**angiom′atous** *adj.* 血管瘤的；**a. caverno′sum, cavernous a.,** 海绵状血管瘤，见 *hemangioma* 下词条；**cherry a.,** a bright red, circumscribed, round angioma with many vascular loops, seen mainly in the elderly on the trunk or sometimes elsewhere, due to a telangiectatic vascular disturbance 樱桃样血管瘤，老年性血管瘤；**senile a.,** 见 cherry a.；**a. serpigino′sum,** a skin disease marked by tiny red vascular points arranged in rings on the skin 匐行性血管瘤；**spider a.,** a telangiectasis caused by dilatation and ramification of superficial cutaneous arteries, appearing as a bright red central area with branching rays looking like the legs of a spider; it may appear spontaneously or be associated with pregnancy or liver disease 蜘蛛痣

an·gi·o·ma·to·sis (an″je-o-mə-to′sis) a diseased state of the vessels with formation of multiple angiomas 血管瘤病；**bacillary a.,** a condition seen in patients with the acquired immunodeficiency syndrome, with varying characteristics ranging from erythematous angiomatous skin lesions to more widespread disease, believed to be an opportunistic infection by a rickettsia 杆状血管瘤病；**cerebroretinal a.,** von Hippel-Lindau disease 脑视网膜血管瘤病，又称冯希佩尔 - 林道综合征；**encephalofacial a., encephalotrigeminal a.,** Sturge-Weber syndrome 脑面血管瘤病，斯德奇 - 韦伯综合征；**a. of retina,** von Hippel disease 视网膜血管瘤病；**retinocerebral a.,** von Hippel-Lindau disease 视网膜脑血管瘤病

an·gio·myo·li·po·ma (an″je-o-mi″o-lĭ-po′mə) a benign tumor containing vascular, adipose, and muscle elements, occurring most often as a renal tumor with smooth muscle elements (more correctly called *angiolipoleiomyoma*), usually in association with tuberous sclerosis, and considered to be a hamartoma 血管平滑肌脂肪瘤

an·gio·myo·sar·co·ma (an″je-o-mi″o-sahrko′mə) a tumor composed of elements of angioma, myoma, and sarcoma 血管平滑肌肉瘤

an·gio·neu·rop·a·thy (an″je-o-noo-rop′ə-the) 1. angiopathic neuropathy 血管源性神经病；2. any neuropathy affecting the blood vessels; a disorder of the vasomotor system, as angiospasm or vasomotor paralysis 任何影响血管的神经病，血管舒缩功能

失调，造成血管痉挛或麻痹；**angioneuropath′ic, angioneurot′ic** *adj.* 血管源性神经病的；血管神经病的

an·gio·no·ma (an″je-o-no′mə) ulceration of blood vessels 血管溃疡

an·gio·pa·ral·y·sis (an″je-o-pə-ral′ə-sis) vasomotor paralysis 血管麻痹

an·gio·pa·re·sis (an″je-o-pə-re′sis) vasoparesis 血管不全麻痹

an·gi·op·a·thy (an-je-op′ə-the) any disease of the vessels 血管病；**angiopath′ic** *adj.* 血管病的

an·gio·plas·ty (an′je-o-plas″te) an angiographic procedure for elimination of areas of narrowing in the blood vessels 血管成形术；**balloon a.**, inflation and deflation of a balloon catheter inside an artery, stretching the intima and leaving a ragged interior surface, triggering a healing response and breaking up of plaque 球囊血管成形术；**percutaneous transluminal a.**, a type of balloon angioplasty in which the catheter is inserted through the skin and through the lumen of the vessel to the site of the narrowing 经皮腔内血管成形术；**percutaneous transluminal coronary a. (PTCA)**, percutaneous transluminal angioplasty to enlarge the lumen of a sclerotic coronary artery 经皮腔内冠状动脉成形术

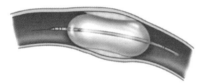

▲ 球囊血管成形术（**balloon angioplasty**），使用扩张的球囊压迫血管狭窄处

an·gio·poi·e·sis (an″je-o-poi-e′sis) angiogenesis 血管形成；**angiopoiet′ic** *adj.*

an·gio·pres·sure (an′je-o-presh″ər) the application of pressure to a blood vessel to control hemorrhage 血管压迫法

an·gi·or·rha·phy (an″je-or′ə-fe) suture of a vessel or vessels 血管缝合术

an·gio·sar·co·ma (an″je-o-sahr-ko′mə) a malignant neoplasm arising from vascular endothelial cells; the term may be used generally or may denote a subtype, such as hemangiosarcoma 血管肉瘤；**hepatic a.**, a malignant liver tumor characterized by dilated sinusoids with hypertrophied or necrotic hepatocytes that leave vascular channels lined by malignant cells; it usually affects older men and has been linked to exposure to toxins 肝血管肉瘤

an·gio·scle·ro·sis (an″je-o-sklĕ-ro′sis) hardening of the walls of blood vessels 血管硬化；**angioscle-**

rot′ic *adj.* 血管硬化的

an·gio·scope (an′je-o-skōp″) see angioscopy 血管镜

an·gi·os·co·py (an″ge-os′kə-pe) 1. use of a fiber-optic angioscope to visualize the lumen of a blood vessel 血管镜检查，使用光纤血管镜观察血管腔；2. visualization of capillary blood vessels with a special microscope (angioscope) 血管镜检查，使用特制的显微镜观察毛细血管

an·gio·sco·to·ma (an″je-o-sko-to′mə) a centrocecal scotoma caused by shadows of the retinal blood vessels 血管暗点

an·gio·sco·tom·e·try (an″je-o-sko-tom′ə-tre) the plotting or mapping of an angioscotoma; done particularly in diagnosing glaucoma 血管暗点测量法

an·gio·spasm (an′je-o-spaz″əm) vasospasm 血管痉挛；**angiospas′tic** *adj.* 血管痉挛的

an·gio·ste·no·sis (an″je-o-stə-no′sis) narrowing of the caliber of a vessel 血管狭窄

an·gio·stron·gy·li·a·sis (an″je-o-stron″jī-li′ə-sis) infection with *Angiostrongylus cantonensis* 广州管圆线虫病

An·gio·stron·gy·lus (an″je-o-stron′jī-ləs) a genus of nematode parasites. *A. cantonen′sis* causes eosinophilic meningitis and *A. costaricen′sis* is associated with abdominal pain, vomiting, and a lower right quadrant mass 管圆线虫属

an·gio·te·lec·ta·sis (an″je-o-tə-lek′tə-sis) pl. *angiotelec′tases*. Dilatation of the minute arteries and veins 血管扩张

an·gio·ten·sin (an″je-o-ten′sin) a decapeptide hormone (a. Ⅰ) formed from the plasma glycoprotein angiotensinogen by renin secreted by the juxtaglomerular apparatus. It is in turn hydrolyzed by a peptidase in the lungs to form an octapeptide (a. Ⅱ), which is a powerful vasopressor and stimulator of aldosterone secretion by the adrenal cortex. This is in turn hydrolyzed to form a heptapeptide (a. Ⅲ), which has less vasopressor activity but more adrenal cortex–stimulating activity 血管紧张素

an·gio·ten·sin·ase (an″je-o-ten′sin-ās) any of a group of plasma or tissue peptidases that cleave and inactivate angiotensin 血管紧张素酶

an·gio·ten·sin-con·vert·ing en·zyme (an″je-o-ten′sin kən-vurt′ing en′zīm) 血管紧张素转化酶，见 *peptidyldipeptidase A*

an·gio·ten·sin·o·gen (an″je-o-ten-sin′o-jen) a serum α₂-globulin secreted in the liver that, on hydrolysis by renin, gives rise to angiotensin 血管紧张素原

an·gio·tome (an′je-o-tōm″) one of the segments of the vascular system of the embryo 血管节，胚胎脉管系统中的一个节段

an·gio·ton·ic (an″je-o-ton′ik) increasing vascular tension 血管紧张的

an·gio·tro·phic (an″je-o-tro′fik) vasotrophic 血管营养的

an·gle (ang′gəl) 1. the point at which two intersecting borders or surfaces converge 角，两条线或两个平面的相交处；2. the degree of divergence of two intersecting lines or planes 角度，两条相交线或两个相交平面的偏离程度；**acromial a.**, the subcutaneous bony point at which the lateral border becomes continuous with the spine of the scapula 肩峰角；**axial a.**, any line angle parallel with the long axis of a tooth 轴角，所有与牙齿长轴平行的线所成角度；**cardiodiaphragmatic a.**, that formed by the junction of the shadows of the heart and respiratory diaphragm in posteroanterior radiographs of the chest 心膈角；**costovertebral a.**, that formed on either side of the vertebral column between the last rib and the lumbar vertebrae 肋脊角；**a. of eye**, canthus 眦；**filtration a.**, 见 iridocorneal a.；**iridial a., iridocorneal a., a. of iris**, a narrow recess between the sclerocorneal junction and the attached margin of the iris, marking the periphery of the anterior chamber of the eye; it is the principal exit site for the aqueous fluid 虹膜角，虹膜角膜角；**line a.**, an angle formed by the junction of two planes; in dentistry, the junction of two surfaces of a tooth or of two walls of a tooth cavity 线角，两个平面相交所成的角；在口腔医学中，指牙齿两面或龋洞、髓腔内壁的相交处；**Louis a., Ludwig a.**, 见 sternal a.；**optic a.**, 见 visual a.；**point a.**, one formed by the junction of three planes; in dentistry, the junction of three surfaces of a tooth, or of three walls of a tooth cavity 点角；**a. of pubis**, 见 subpubic a.；**sternal a.**, the angle between the sternum and manubrium 胸骨角；**subpubic a.**, that formed by the conjoined rami of the ischial and pubic bones 耻骨下角；**tooth a's**, those formed by two or more tooth surfaces 牙角，两个或多个牙齿表面所成的角；**venous a.**, the angle formed by junction of the internal jugular and subclavian veins 静脉角；**visual a.**, the angle formed between two lines extending from the nodal point of the eye to the extremities of the object seen 视角，由眼节点到被视物的连线所成的角；**YY a.**, that between the radius fixus and the line joining the lambda and inion 人字点、枕外隆突点的连线与固定半径所产生的角

ang·strom (Å) (ang′strəm) a unit of length used for atomic dimensions and light wavelengths; it is nominally equivalent to 10^{-10} meter 埃用于量度波长和原子间的距离，等于 10^{-10}m

an·gu·lar (ang′gu-lər) sharply bent; having corners or angles 角的

an·gu·la·tion (ang″gu-la′shən) 1. formation of a sharp obstructive bend, as in the intestine, ureter, or similar tubes 成角，形成锐利的转角，造成肠、输尿管等管道的阻塞；2. deviation from a straight line, as in a badly set bone 成角，偏离正常的直线，如骨移位

an·gu·lus (ang′gu-ləs) pl. *an′guli* [L.] angle; used for a triangular area or the angle of a particular structure or part of the body 角，用于三角形区域或特定构造、人体结构的角

an·he·do·nia (an″he-do′ne-ə) inability to experience pleasure in normally pleasurable acts 兴趣缺失

an·hi·dro·sis (an″hi-dro′sis) absence or deficiency of sweating 无汗

an·hi·drot·ic (an″hi-drot′ik) 1. promoting anhidrosis 止汗的；2. an agent that suppresses sweating 止汗药

an·hy·dre·mia (an″hi-dre′me-ə) deficiency of water in the blood 缺水血症，血液中水分缺乏。Cf. *dehydration* and *hypovolemia*

an·hy·dride (an-hi′drīd) any compound derived from a substance, especially an acid, by abstraction of a molecule of water 酸酐；**chromic a.**, chromic acid 铬酐；**phthalic a.**, a reactive low-molecular-weight compound with various industrial uses; it causes skin irritation and its fumes cause hypersensitivity pneumonitis 邻苯二甲酸酐

ANIA American Nursing Informatics Association 美国护理信息学会

an·ic·ter·ic (an″ik-ter′ik) not associated with jaundice 无黄疸的

an·i·lide (an′ĭ-līd) any compound formed from aniline by substituting a radical for the hydrogen of NH_2 酰苯胺

an·i·line (an′ĭ-lin) the parent substance of colors or dyes derived from coal tar; it is an important cause of serious industrial poisoning associated with bone marrow depression as well as methemoglobinemia, and high doses or prolonged exposure may be carcinogenic 苯胺

an·i·lin·ism (an′ĭ-lin-iz-əm) poisoning by exposure to aniline 苯胺中毒。又称 *anilism*

anil·i·ty (ə-nil′ĭ-te) 1. the state of existing as or like an old woman 老妪，或像老妪的；2. senility 老年

an·i·ma (an′ĭ-mə) [L.] 1. the soul 灵魂；2. in jungian terminology, the unconscious, or inner being, of the individual, as opposed to the personality presented to the world (persona); by extension, used to denote the more feminine soul or feminine component of a man's personality 在荣格心理学派中，

指个体的非意识性部分或内在，与人格的外在表现相对；可延伸指男性人格中女性化的部分；cf. *animus*

an·i·mal (anʹī-məl) 1. a living organism having sensation and the power of voluntary movement and requiring for its existence oxygen and organic food; animals constitute one of the six kingdoms of living organisms 动物；2. of or pertaining to such an organism 动物的；**control a.**, an untreated animal otherwise identical in all respects to one that is used for purposes of experimentation, used for checking results of treatment 对照动物；**hyperphagic a.**, an experimental animal in which the cells of the ventromedial nucleus of the hypothalamus have been destroyed, abolishing its awareness of the point at which it should stop eating; excessive eating and savageness characterize such an animal 食欲亢进动物，实验动物的下丘脑腹正中核被损毁，使其无法产生停止进食的意识；**spinal a.**, one whose spinal cord has been severed, cutting off communication with the brain 脊髓横断动物

an·i·mus (anʹī-məs) [L.] 1. disposition 意　图；2. ill will, hostility; animosity 敌 意；3. in jungian psychology, the masculine aspect of a woman's soul or inner being 在荣格心理学派中，指女性灵魂或内在中男性化的部分；cf. *anima* (2)

an·ion (anʹi-on) a negatively charged ion 阴离子；**anion'ic** *adj.*

an·ion·ot·ro·py (an″e-on-otʹrə-pe) a type of tautomerism in which the migrating group is a negative ion rather than the more usual hydrogen ion 阴离子转移。Cf. prototropy

an·irid·ia (anʺī-ridʹe-ə) congenital absence of the iris 无虹膜，先天性虹膜缺失

an·i·sa·ki·a·sis (anʹī-sə-kiʹə-sis) infection with the third-stage larvae of the roundworm *Anisakis marina*, which burrow into the stomach wall, producing an eosinophilic granulomatous mass. Infection is acquired by eating undercooked marine fish 异尖线虫病

An·i·sa·kis (anʺī-saʹkis) a genus of nematodes that parasitize the stomachs of marine mammals and birds 异尖线虫

an·is·ei·ko·nia (anʺis-i-koʹne-ə) inequality of the retinal images of the two eyes 物像不等症，双眼视网膜所成物像不等

o-**an·i·si·dine** (ə-nisʹī-dēn) a yellow to red oily aromatic amine used as an intermediate in the manufacture of azo dyes; it is an irritant and carcinogen 邻氨基苯甲醚

an·is·in·di·one (anʺis-in-diʹōn) an indanedione anticoagulant 茴茚二酮

an·iso·chro·mat·ic (an-iʺso-kro-matʹik) not of the same color throughout 色素不均的

an·iso·co·ria (an-iʺso-korʹe-ə) inequality in size of the pupils of the eyes 瞳孔大小不等

an·iso·cy·to·sis (an-iʺso-si-toʹsis) presence in the blood of erythrocytes showing excessive variations in size 红细胞大小不等，红细胞大小不等症

an·iso·gam·ete (an-iʺso-gamʹēt) a gamete differing in size or structure from the one with which it unites 异配子；**anisogamet'ic** *adj.*

an·isog·a·my (anʺi-sogʹə-me) in the most restrictive sense, fertilization of a large motile female gamete by a small motile male gamete; often used more generally for the sexual union of two dissimilar gametes (heterogamy), particularly in lower organisms 异配生殖；**anisog'amous** *adj.*

an·iso·kary·o·sis (an-iʺso-kar'e-oʹsis) inequality in the size of the nuclei of cells 细胞核大小不等

an·iso·me·tro·pia (an-iʺso-mə-troʹpe-ə) inequality in refractive power of the two eyes 屈光参差；**anisometrop'ic** *adj.*

an·iso·pi·esis (an-iʺso-pi-eʹsis) variation or inequality in the blood pressure as registered in different parts of the body 各部位血压不等

an·iso·poi·ki·lo·cy·to·sis (an-iʺso-poiʺkī-losi-toʹsis) the presence in the blood of erythrocytes of varying sizes and abnormal shapes（大小）不均性红细胞异形症

an·iso·spore (an-iʹso-spor″) 1. an anisogamete of organisms reproducing by spores 由孢子繁殖的有机体的异形孢子；2. an asexual spore produced by heterosporous organisms 由异孢子生物产生的无性孢子

an·isos·then·ic (an-iʺsos-thenʹik) not having equal power; said of muscles 力量不等的

an·iso·ton·ic (an-iʺso-tonʹik) 1. varying in tonicity or tension 张力不等的；2. having different osmotic pressure; not isotonic 渗透压不等的

an·iso·tro·pic (an-iʺso-troʹpik) 1. having unlike properties in different directions 各 向 异 性 的；2. doubly refracting, or having a double polarizing power 双折射的，具有双偏振能力的

an·iso·tro·py (anʺi-sotʹrə-pe) the quality of being anisotropic 各向异性

an·is·trep·lase (an-is-trepʹlās) a thrombolytic agent used to clear coronary vessel occlusions associated with myocardial infarction 链激酶激活复合物

an·i·su·ria (anʺi-suʹre-ə) alternating oliguria and polyuria 尿量不等，交替少尿或多尿

an·kle (angʹkəl) 1. 见 tarsus (1)；2. by extension, the joint between the leg and foot, or the region of the leg and foot including and immediately adjacent to this joint 踝关节

an·ky·lo·bleph·a·ron (ang″kə-lo-blef′ə-ron) adhesion of the ciliary edges of the eyelids to each other 睑缘粘连

an·ky·lo·glos·sia (ang″kə-lo-glos′e-ə) tonguetie 舌系带短缩；a. supe′rior, extensive adhesion of the tongue to the palate, associated with deformities of the hands and feet 舌上颚黏连，与手足畸形相关

an·ky·losed (ang′kə-lōzd) fused or obliterated, as an ankylosed joint 关节强直的

an·ky·lo·sis (ang″kə-lo′sis) pl. *ankylo′ses* [Gr.] immobility and consolidation of a joint due to disease, injury, or surgical procedure 关节强直；**ankylot′ic** *adj.*；**artificial a.**, arthrodesis 人造关节强直，关节固定术；**bony a.**, union of the bones of a joint by proliferation of bone cells, resulting in complete immobility; true a. 骨强直；**extracapsular a.**, that due to rigidity of structures outside the joint capsule 关节囊外强直；**false a.**, 假性关节强直，见 fibrous a.；**fibrous a.**, reduced joint mobility due to proliferation of fibrous tissue 纤维性关节强直；**intracapsular a.**, that due to disease, injury, or surgery within the joint capsule 关节囊内强直

an·ky·rin (ang′kə-rin) a membrane protein of erythrocytes and brain that anchors spectrin to the plasma membrane at the sites of ion channels 锚蛋白

an·ky·roid (ang′kĭ-roid) hook-shaped 钩样的

an·lage (ahn-lah′gə) (an′lāj) pl. *anla′gen* [Ger.] primordium 原基

ANNA American Nephrology Nurses' Association 美国肾脏护理协会

an·neal (ə-nēl′) 1. to toughen, temper, or soften a material, as a metal, by controlled heating and cooling（金属）退火；2. in molecular biology, to cause the association or reassociation of single-stranded nucleic acids so that double-stranded molecules are formed, often by heating and cooling 分子生物学中，通过加热和冷却使单链核酸配对或重新配对成为双链分子

an·nec·tent (ə-nek′tənt) connecting; joining together 连接的，过渡的

an·ne·lid (an′ə-lid) any member of Annelida 环节动物

An·ne·li·da (ə-nel′ĭ-də) a phylum of metazoan invertebrates, the segmented worms, including leeches 环节动物门

an·nu·lar (an′u-lər) ring-shaped 环形的

an·nu·lo·aor·tic (an″u-lo-a-or′tĭk) pertaining to the aorta and the fibrous ring of the heart at the aortic orifice 指主动脉及心脏内主动脉瓣纤维环相关的

an·nu·lo·plas·ty (an′u-lo-plas″te) plastic repair of a cardiac valve 心脏瓣膜成形术

an·nu·lor·rha·phy (an″u-lor′ə-fe) closure of a hernial ring or defect by sutures 环形缝合术

an·nu·lus (an′u-ləs) pl. *an′nuli* [L.] anulus 环形物

an·ode (an′ōd) the electrode at which oxidation occurs and to which anions are attracted 阳极；**ano′dal** *adj.*

an·odon·tia (an″o-don′shə) congenital absence of some or all of the teeth 无齿症

an·o·dyne (an′o-dīn) 1. relieving pain 止痛的；2. a medicine that eases pain 止痛药

anom·a·lad (ə-nom′ə-lad) 见 sequence (2)

anom·a·ly (ə-nom′ə-le) marked deviation from normal, especially as a result of congenital or hereditary defects 异常，尤其指先天或遗传缺陷导致；**anom′alous** *adj.*；**Alder a.**, an autosomal dominant condition in which leukocytes of the myelocytic series, and sometimes all leukocytes, contain coarse azurophilic granules 黏多糖病性白细胞异常，为常染色体显性遗传病，髓系中的白细胞或有时是所有白细胞内含有粗糙的嗜天青颗粒；**Axenfeld a.**, a developmental anomaly consisting of posterior embryotoxon and iris processes to the Schwalbe ring Axenfald 异常，具有角膜后胚胎环及突向 Schwalbe 环的虹膜条带；**congenital a.**, a developmental anomaly present at birth 先天性异常；**developmental a.**, 1. a structural abnormality of any type 任何类型的结构异常；2. a defect resulting from imperfect embryonic development 胚胎发育异常引起的缺陷；**Ebstein a.**, a malformation of the right atrioventricular valve, usually associated with an atrial septal defect 埃布斯坦综合征，右心房室瓣畸形，常与房间隔缺损有关；**May-Hegglin a.**, an autosomal dominant disorder of blood cell morphology, characterized by RNA-containing cytoplasmic inclusions (similar to Döhle bodies) in granulocytes, by large, poorly granulated platelets, and by thrombocytopenia Döhle 小体白细胞异常综合征，常染色体显性遗传病，红细胞形态异常，粒细胞内有含 RNA 成分胞浆包涵体，血小板体积大且颗粒少，且有血小板减少症；**Pelger-Huët a.**, a hereditary or acquired defect in which the nuclei of neutrophils and eosinophils appear rodlike, spherical, or dumbbell-shaped; the nuclear structure is coarse and lumpy Pelger-Huët 异常，一种遗传性或获得性缺陷，中性粒细胞及嗜酸粒细胞细胞核呈棒状、球状或哑铃状，核结构粗糙不平；**Peters a.**, congenital corneal central opacity associated with a posterior defect in Descemet membrane and endothelium, sometimes with adhesions of the cornea, iris, and lens and often associated with other ocular or systemic anomalies; usually sporadic Peters 异常，为先天性角膜混浊伴角膜后弹力层膜

及角膜内皮缺陷，有时伴角膜，虹膜和晶状体黏连及其他眼部及全身异常，常为散发

an·o·mer (an′o-mər) either of a pair of cyclic stereoisomers (designated α or β) of a sugar or glycoside, differing only in configuration at the reducing carbon atom 端基差向异构体; **anomer′ic** adj.

ano·mia (ə-no′me-ə) anomic aphasia 命名性失语症

ano·mic (ə-no′mik) lacking a name 无名的

an·onych·ia (an″o-nik′e-ə) congenital absence of a nail or nails 无甲，甲缺如

Anoph·e·les (ə-nof′ə-lēz) a widely distributed genus of mosquitoes, comprising over 300 species, many of which are vectors of malaria; some are vectors of *Wuchereria bancrofti* 疟蚊属

an·oph·thal·mia (an″of-thal′me-ə) a developmental anomaly characterized by complete absence of the eyes (rare) or by the presence of vestigial eyes 无眼症

ano·plas·ty (a′no-plas″te) plastic or reparative surgery of the anus 肛门成形术

an·or·chia (an-or′ke-ə) congenital absence of one or both testes in a male 无睾症

an·or·chic (an-or′kik) 见 anorchia

an·or·chid (an-or′kid) lacking testes or not having testes in the scrotum 无睾丸的

an·or·chid·ism (an-or′kĭd-iz″əm) 见 anorchia

an·or·chism (an-or′kiz-əm) 见 anorchia

ano·rec·tic (an″o-rek′tik)1. pertaining to anorexia 厌食，神经性厌食; 2. an agent that diminishes the appetite 食欲减退药物

an·orex·ia (an″o-rek′se-ə) lack or loss of appetite for food 厌食; **a. nervo′sa**, an eating disorder usually occurring in adolescent girls, characterized by refusal to maintain a normal minimal body weight, fear of gaining weight or becoming obese, disturbance of body image, undue reliance on body weight or shape for selfevaluation, and amenorrhea. The two subtypes include one characterized by dieting and exercise alone and one also characterized by binge eating and purging 神经性厌食

ano·rex·i·gen·ic (an″o-rek″sĭ-jen′ik) 1. producing anorexia 使厌食的; 2. an agent that diminishes or controls the appetite 食欲减退药

an·or·gas·mia (an″or-gaz′me-ə) inability or failure to experience orgasm 性快感障碍; **anorgas′mic** adj.

an·or·thog·ra·phy (an″or-thog′rə-fe) agraphia 运动性失写症

an·or·tho·pia (an″or-tho′pe-ə) asymmetrical or distorted vision 斜视

ano·sig·moid·os·co·py (a″no-sig″moid-os′kə-pe) endoscopic examination of the anus, rectum, and sigmoid colon 直肠乙状结肠镜检查; **anosigmoidoscop′ic** adj.

an·os·mia (an-oz′me-ə) lack of sense of smell 嗅觉缺乏; **anosmat′ic anos′mic** adj.

ano·sog·no·sia (an-o″sog-no′zhə) unawareness or denial of a neurological deficit, such as hemiplegia 病感失认（症）; **anosogno′sic** adj.

an·os·to·sis (an-os-to′sis) defective formation of bone 骨发育不全

an·otia (an-o′shə) congenital absence of one or both external ears 无耳畸形

an·ovar·ism (an-o′vər-iz-əm) absence of the ovaries 无卵巢畸形

an·ov·u·lar (an-ov′u-lər) anovulatory 不排卵的

an·ov·u·la·tion (an″ov-u-la′shən) absence of ovulation 无排卵

an·ov·u·la·to·ry (an-ov′u-lə-tor″e) not accompanied by discharge of an oocyte 无排卵的

anox·ia (ə-nok′se-ə) a total lack of oxygen; often used interchangeably with *hypoxia* to indicate a reduced oxygen supply to tissues 缺氧; **anox′ic** adj; altitude a., 高空缺氧，见 *sickness* 下词条; anemic a., that due to decrease in amount of hemoglobin or number of erythrocytes in the blood 贫血性缺氧; anoxic a., that due to interference with the oxygen supply 乏氧性缺氧; histotoxic a., severe histotoxic hypoxia 组织毒性缺氧

ANP atrial natriuretic peptide 心房钠尿肽

ANPD Association for Nursing Professional Development 护理专业发展协会

ANRC American National Red Cross 美国全国红十字会

an·sa (an′sə) pl. *an′sae* [L.] a looplike structure 一种环形结构; **a. cervica′lis**, a nerve loop in the neck that supplies the infrahyoid muscles 颈襻; **a. lenticula′ris**, a small nerve fiber tract arising in the globus pallidus and joining the anterior part of the ventral thalamic nucleus 豆状核襻; **a. nephro′ni**, Henle loop 髓襻; **a. peduncula′ris**, a complex grouping of nerve fibers connecting the amygdaloid nucleus, piriform area, and anterior hypothalamus, and various thalamic nuclei 脑脚襻; **a. subcla′via**, **a. of Vieussens**, nerve filaments passing around the subclavian artery to form a loop connecting the middle and inferior cervical ganglia 锁骨下襻

an·ser·ine (an′sər-īn) pertaining to or like a goose 鹅肌肽

ant·ac·id (ant-as′id) counteracting acidity; an agent that so acts 抗酸药

an·tag·o·nism (an-tag′ə-niz″əm) opposition or contrariety between similar things, as between muscles, medicines, or organisms 相反状态，对立状态;

cf. *antibiosis*

an·tag·o·nist (an-tag′ə-nist) 1. a substance that tends to nullify the action of another, as a drug that binds to a cell receptor without eliciting a biological response, blocking binding of substances that could elicit such responses 拮抗剂；2. antagonistic muscle 拮 抗 肌；3. a tooth in one jaw that articulates with one in the other jaw 与一侧牙颌内某牙齿相连接的对侧牙颌内的牙齿；**antagonis′tic** *adj.*；α**-adrenergic a.**, alphaadrenergic blocking agent α-肾上腺素能拮抗剂；见 *adrenergic blocking agent*；β**-adrenergic a.**, beta-adrenergic blocking agent β- 肾 上 腺 素 能 拮 抗 剂；见 *adrenergic blocking agent*；**folic acid a.**, an antimetabolite, e.g., methotrexate, that interferes with DNA replication and cell division by inhibiting the enzyme dihydrofolate reductase; used in cancer chemotherapy 叶 酸 拮 抗 剂；**H₁ receptor a.**, any of a large number of agents that block the action of histamine by competitive binding to the H₁ receptor; they also have sedative, anticholinergic, and antiemetic effects and are used for the relief of allergic symptoms, as antiemetics, as antivertigo agents, and as antidyskinetics in parkinsonism H₁ 受体拮抗剂；**H₂ receptor a.**, an agent that blocks the action of histamine by competitive binding to the H₂ receptor; used to inhibit acid secretion in the treatment of peptic ulcer H₂ 受体拮抗剂

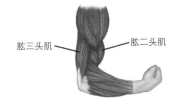

肱三头肌　　　　　　肱二头肌

▲　拮抗肌（**antagonist**）。肱三头肌在肘部伸展前臂，而它的拮抗肌肱二头肌负责弯曲肘部

ant·al·gic (ant-al′jik) 1. counteracting or avoiding pain, as a posture or gait assumed so as to lessen pain 抵消或防止疼痛的，形容减轻疼痛的体位或步态；2. analgesic 止痛的

ant·arth·rit·ic (ant″ahr-thrit′ik) antiarthritic 抗关节炎的

an·te·bra·chi·um (an″te-bra′ke-əm) the forearm 前臂；**antebra′chial** *adj.*

an·te·ce·dent (an″te-se′dənt) a precursor 前 体；**plasma thromboplastin a. (PTA)**, coagulation factor XI 血浆促凝血酶原激酶前体，凝血因子 XI

an·te·flex·ion (an-te-flek′shən) forward curvature of an organ or part, so that its top is turned anteri-

orly, such as the normal forward curvature of the uterus 前屈

an·te·grade (an′tĭ-grād) anterograde 顺行性的

an·te mor·tem (an′te mor′təm) [L.] before death 死前

an·te·mor·tem (an″te-mor′təm) [L.] occurring before death 临死前的

an·ten·na (an-ten′ə) pl. *anten′nae*. Either of the two lateral appendages on the anterior segment of the head of arthropods 触角

an·te·par·tal (an″te-pahr′təl) 见 *antepartum*

an·te·par·tum (an″te-pahr′təm) occurring before parturition, or childbirth, with reference to the mother 产前

an·te·ri·or (an-tēr′e-ər) situated at or directed toward the front; opposite of posterior 前面的

an·tero·clu·sion (an″tər-o-kloo′zhən) mesiocclusion 前咬合

an·tero·col·lis (an″tər-o-kol′is) abnormal forward flexion of the head and neck associated with increased tonicity of the anterior cervical muscles in cervical dystonia 前屈颈，指头颈部异常的向前弯曲，与颈前部肌肉肌张力升高有关

an·tero·grade (an′tər-o-grād″) extending or moving anteriorly 顺行性的

an·tero·lat·er·al (an″tər-o-lat′ər-əl) situated anteriorly and to one side 前外侧的

an·tero·pos·te·ri·or (an″tər-o-pos-tēr′e-ər) directed from the front toward the back 前后的

an·te·ver·sion (an″te-vur′zhən) the tipping forward of an entire organ or part 器官整个或部分前倾

ant·hel·min·tic (ant″həl-min′tik) 1. vermifugal; destructive to worms 驱除蠕虫的；2. vermicide or vermifuge; an agent destructive to worms 杀蠕虫药

an·thra·cene (an′thrə-sēn) a crystalline hydrocarbon derived from coal tar and used in the manufacture of anthracene dyes 蒽

an·thra·cene·di·one (an″thrə-sēn-di′ōn) any of a class of derivatives of anthraquinone, some of which have antineoplastic properties 蒽二酮

an·thra·coid (an′thrə-koid) resembling anthrax or a carbuncle 类炭疽的

an·thra·co·ne·cro·sis (an″thrə-ko-nə-kro′sis) degeneration of tissue into a black mass 坏疽

an·thra·co·sil·i·co·sis (an″thrə-ko-sil″ĭ-ko′sis) anthracosis combined with silicosis 碳矽末沉着症

an·thra·co·sis (an-thrə-ko′sis) 1. pneumoconiosis, usually asymptomatic, due to deposition of anthracite coal dust in the lungs 炭 末 沉 着 病；2. blackening of lung tissue by the deposition of inhaled carbon, with little or no cellular reaction; the presence of carbon particles is of little or no pathologic significance 煤肺病；Cf. coal workers' pneumoconiosis

an·thra·cy·cline (an″thrə-si′klēn) a class of antineoplastic antibiotics produced by *Streptomyces peucetius* and *S. coeruleorubidus*, including daunomycin and doxorubicin 蒽环素

an·thra·lin (an′thrə-lin) an anthraquinone derivative used topically in psoriasis 蒽林

an·thra·quin·one (an″thrə-kwin′ōn) 1. the 9,10 quinone derivative of anthracene, used in dye manufacture 蒽醌；2. any of the derivatives of this compound, some of which are dyes. They occur in aloes, cascara sagrada, senna, and rhubarb and are cathartic 蒽醌类衍生物

an·thrax (an′thraks) an often fatal infectious disease of ruminants due to ingestion of spores of *Bacillus anthracis* in soil; acquired by humans through contact with contaminated wool or other animal products or by inhalation of airborne spores 炭疽；**cutaneous a.**, that due to inoculation of *Bacillus anthracis* into superficial wounds or abrasions of the skin, producing a black crusted pustule on a broad zone of edema; it may progress to a systemic condition 皮肤炭疽；**gastrointestinal a.**, anthrax involving the gastrointestinal tract, caused by ingestion of poorly cooked meat contaminated by *Bacillus anthracis* spores; bowel obstruction, hemorrhage, and necrosis may result 胃肠炭疽；**inhalational a.**, a highly fatal form due to inhalation of dust containing anthrax spores, which are transported by alveolar pneumocytes to regional lymph nodes, where they germinate; it is primarily an occupational disease in persons handling wools and fleeces 吸入性炭疽；**intestinal a.,** 见 gastrointestinal a. **pulmonary a.,** 见 inhalational a.

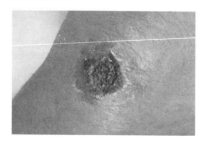

▲ 皮肤炭疽（**cutaneous anthrax**）病损

an·thro·po·cen·tric (an″thrə-po-sen′trik) with a human bias; considering human beings the center of the universe 以人类为中心的

an·thro·poid (an′thrə-poid) resembling a human being, as an anthropoid ape 类人的

An·thro·poi·dea (an″thrə-poi′de-ə) a suborder of Primates, including monkeys, apes, and humans 类人猿亚目

an·thro·pom·e·try (an″thrə-pom′ə-tre) the science dealing with measurement of the size, weight, and proportions of the human body 人体测量学；**anthropomet′ric** adj.

an·thro·po·mor·phism (an″thrə-po-mor′fiz-əm) the attribution of human characteristics to nonhuman objects 拟人论

an·thro·po·phil·ic (an″thrə-po-fil′ik) preferring humans to other animals; said of parasites such as fungi or mosquitoes 嗜人血的

an·ti·abor·ti·fa·cient (an″te-ə-bor″tĭ-fa′shənt) an agent that prevents abortion or promotes pregnancy 促受孕药

an·ti·ad·re·ner·gic (an″te-ad″rə-nur′jik) 1. sympatholytic; opposing the effects of impulses conveyed by adrenergic postganglionic fibers of the sympathetic nervous system 抗交感神经的；2. an agent that so acts 抗肾上腺素能药

an·ti·ag·glu·ti·nin (an″te-ə-gloo′tĭ-nin) a substance that opposes the action of an agglutinin 抗凝集素

an·ti·ame·bic (an″te-ə-me′bik) destroying or suppressing the growth of amebas, or an agent that does this 抗阿米巴的，抗阿米巴药

an·ti·ana·phy·lax·is (an″te-an-ə-fə-lak′sis) a condition in which the anaphylaxis reaction does not occur because of free antigens in the blood; the state of desensitization to antigens 抗过敏性

an·ti·an·dro·gen (an″te-an′drə-jən) any substance capable of inhibiting the biological effects of androgens 抗雄激素物质

an·ti·ane·mic (an″te-ə-ne′mik) counteracting anemia, or an agent that does this 抗贫血的，抗贫血药

an·ti·an·gi·nal (an″te-an-ji′nəl) preventing or alleviating angina, or an agent that does this 抗心绞痛的，抗心绞痛药

an·ti·an·ti·body (an″te-an′tĭ-bod″e) an immunoglobulin formed in the body after administration of antibody acting as immunogen, and which interacts with the latter 抗抗体

an·ti·an·xi·e·ty (an″te-ang-zi′ə-te) anxiolytic; reducing anxiety 抗焦虑的

an·ti·ar·rhyth·mic (an″te-ə-rith′mik) 1. preventing or alleviating cardiac arrhythmias 抗心律失常的；2. an agent that so acts 抗心律失常药

an·ti·ar·thrit·ic (an″te-ahr-thrit′ik) alleviating arthritis, or an agent that so acts 抗关节炎的，抗关节炎药

an·ti·asth·mat·ic (an″te-az-mat′ik) providing

relief of asthma, or an agent that does this 平喘的，平喘药

an·ti·bac·te·ri·al (an″te-) (an″ti-bak-tēr′e-əl) 1. destroying or suppressing growth or reproduction of bacteria 抗菌的；2. an agent that so acts 抗菌药

an·ti·bi·o·gram (ăn″tee-bī′ō-grăm) the susceptibility profile of a microorganism exposed to a battery of antimicrobial agents 抗菌谱

an·ti·bi·o·sis (an″te-) (an″ti-bi-o′sis) an association between two organisms that is detrimental to one of them, or between one organism and an antibiotic produced by another 抗生作用

an·ti·bi·ot·ic (an″te-) (an″ti-bi-ot′ik) a chemical substance, usually produced by a microorganism or semisynthetically, having the capacity to kill or inhibit growth of other microorganisms; those sufficiently nontoxic to the host are used to treat infectious diseases 抗生素，**broad-spectrum a.**, one effective against a wide range of bacteria 广谱抗生素；**β-lactam a.**, any of a group of antibiotics, including the cephalosporins and the penicillins, whose chemical structure contains a β -lactam ring; they inhibit synthesis of the bacterial peptidoglycan wall β- 内酰胺类抗生素

an·ti·body (Ab) (an′tĭ-bod″e) an immunoglobulin molecule that reacts with a specific antigen that induced its synthesis and with similar molecules; classified according to mode of action as agglutinin, bacteriolysin, hemolysin, opsonin, or precipitin. Antibodies are synthesized by B lymphocytes that have been activated by the binding of an antigen to a cell-surface receptor 抗体。见 *immunoglobulin*；**antimitochondrial a's,** circulating antibodies directed against inner mitochondrial antigens seen in almost all patients with primary biliary cirrhosis 抗线粒体抗体；**antinuclear a's (ANA),** autoantibodies directed against components of the cell nucleus, e.g., DNA, RNA, and histones 抗核抗体；**antiphospholipid a's,** a group of antibodies against phosphorylated polysaccharide esters of fatty acids, thought to be markers of a hypercoagulable state of the blood; included are anticardiolipin antibodies and lupus anticoagulant 抗磷脂抗体；**antireceptor a's,** autoantibodies against cell-surface receptors, e.g., those directed against β_2-adrenergic receptors in some patients with allergic disorders 抗受体抗体；**antisperm a. (ASA),** any of various surface-bound antibodies found on sperm after infection, trauma to the testes, or vasectomy; they interfere with the fertilization process or result in nonviable zygotes 抗精子抗体；**antithyroglobulin a's,** those directed against thyroglobulin, demonstrable in about one-third of patients with thyroiditis,

Graves disease, and thyroid carcinoma 抗甲状腺球蛋白抗体；**blocking a.,** 1. one (usually IgG) that reacts preferentially with an antigen, preventing it from reacting with a cytotropic antibody (IgE), and producing a hypersensitivity reaction 封闭性抗体；2. 见 incomplete a.；**complement-fixing a.,** one that activates complement when reacted with antigen: IgM and IgG fix complement by the classical pathway; IgA, by the alternative pathway 补体结合抗体；**complete a.,** one that reacts with the antigen in saline, producing an agglutination or precipitation reaction 完全抗体；**cross-reacting a.,** an antibody that combines with an antigen other than the one that induced its production 交叉反应性抗体；**cytophilic a.,** 见 cytotropic a.；**cytotoxic a.,** any specific antibody directed against cellular antigens that, when bound to the antigen, activates the complement pathway or activates killer cells, resulting in cell lysis 细胞毒性抗体；**cytotropic a.,** any of a class of antibodies that attach to tissue cells through their Fc segments to induce the release of histamine and other vasoconstrictive amines important in immediate hypersensitivity reactions 嗜细胞性抗体；**Donath-Landsteiner a.,** an IgG antibody directed against the P blood group antigen; it binds to red cells at low temperatures and induces complement-mediated lysis on warming, and is responsible for hemolysis in paroxysmal cold hemoglobinuria Donath-Landsteiner 抗体，是一种抗 P 血型抗原 IgG，低温下与红细胞结合并在升温时诱导补体介导的溶血，在阵发性冷血红蛋白尿中引起溶血；**Forssman a.,** a heterophile antibody directed against the Forssman antigen Forssman 抗体，一种针对 Forssman 抗原的嗜异性抗体；**heteroclitic a.,** antibody produced in response to immunization with one antigen but having a higher affinity for a second antigen that was not present during immunization 变态抗体；**heterogenetic a., heterophil a., heterophile a.,** antibody directed against heterophile antigens; heterophile sheep erythrocyte agglutinins appear in the serum of patients with infectious mononucleosis 异嗜性抗体；**immune a.,** one induced by immunization or by transfusion incompatibility, in contrast to natural antibodies 免疫抗体；**incomplete a.,** 1. antibody that binds to erythrocytes or bacteria but does not produce agglutination 与红细胞或细菌结合但不产生凝集作用的抗体；2. a univalent antibody fragment, e.g., Fab fragment 单价抗体片段，例如 Fab 片段；**indium-111 antimyosin a.,** a monoclonal antibody against myosin, labeled with indium 111; it binds selectively to irreversibly damaged myocytes and is used in infarct avid scintigraphy 111In- 抗肌球蛋白抗体；**mono-**

clonal a's, chemically and immunologically homogeneous antibodies produced by hybridomas, used as laboratory reagents in radioimmunoassays, ELISA, and immunofluorescence assays 单克隆抗体; **natural a's,** ones that react with antigens to which the individual has had no known exposure 天然抗体; **neutralizing a.,** one that, on mixture with the homologous infectious agent, reduces the infectious titer 中和抗体; **OKT3 monoclonal a.,** a mouse monoclonal antibody directed against T3 lymphocytes and used to prevent or treat organ rejection after transplantation 抗 CD3 抗体; **panel-reactive a. (PRA),** 1. the percentage of such antibody in the recipient's blood 此类抗体在受者血液中的百分比; 2. the preexisting antibody against HLA antigens in the serum of a potential allograft recipient; it reacts with a specific antigen in a panel of leukocytes, with a higher percentage indicating a higher risk of a positive crossmatch 群体反应性抗体, 即同种异体移植受者血清中预先存在的抗 HLA 抗原抗体, 与白细胞特定抗原反应, 其百分比越高表明交叉配型阳性风险越高; **P-K a's, Prausnitz-Küstner a's,** cytotropic antibodies of the immunoglobulin class IgE, responsible for cutaneous anaphylaxis P-K 抗体, 与皮肤过敏相关的嗜细胞性 IgE 抗体; **protective a.,** one responsible for immunity to an infectious agent observed in passive immunity 保护性抗体; **Rh a's,** those directed against the antigen (Rh factor) of human erythrocytes. Not normally present, they may be produced when Rh-negative persons receive Rh-positive blood by transfusion or when an Rh-negative person is pregnant with an Rh-positive fetus 抗人红细胞 Rh 抗原抗体; **saline a.,** 见 complete a.

an·ti·car·io·gen·ic (an″te-) (an″ti-kar″e-ojen′ik) effective in suppressing caries production 防龋齿的

an·ti·cho·le·litho·gen·ic (an″te-) (an″tiko″lə-lith″o-jen′ik) 1. preventing the formation of gallstones 抗胆结石的; 2. an agent that so acts 抗胆结石药

an·ti·cho·les·ter·emic (an″te-) (an″ti-kə-les″tər-e′mik) promoting a reduction of cholesterol levels in the blood; also, any agent that so acts 降血脂的, 降血脂药

an·ti·cho·lin·er·gic (an″te-) (an″ti-ko″linur′jik) parasympatholytic; blocking the passage of impulses through the parasympathetic nerves; also, an agent that so acts 抗副交感神经的, 抗副交感神经药

an·ti·cho·lin·es·ter·ase (an″te-) (an″tiko″lin-es-′tər-ās) cholinesterase inhibitor 抗胆碱酯酶剂

an·ti·clin·al (an″te-) (an″ti-kli′nəl) sloping or inclined in opposite directions 背斜的, 对向倾斜的

an·ti·co·ag·u·lant (an″te-) (an″ti-ko-ag′ulənt) act-ing to suppress, delay, or nullify blood coagulation, or an agent that does this 抗凝血的, 或抗凝血物质; **circulating a.,** a substance in the blood that inhibits normal blood clotting and may cause a hemorrhagic syndrome 循环抗凝物; **lupus a.,** a circulating anticoagulant that inhibits the conversion of prothrombin to thrombin; it paradoxically increases the risk of thromboembolism and is seen in some cases of systemic lupus erythematosus 狼疮抗凝物

an·ti·co·ag·u·la·tion (an″te-) (an″ti-ko-ag″u-la′shən) 1. the prevention of coagulation 防止凝血; 2. the use of drugs to render the blood sufficiently incoagulable to discourage thrombosis 抗凝药物使用

an·ti·co·don (an″te-) (an″ti-ko′don) a triplet of nucleotides in transfer RNA that is complementary to the codon in messenger RNA that specifies the amino acid 反密码子

an·ti·com·ple·ment (an″te-) (an″ti-kom′plə-mənt) a substance that counteracts a complement 抗补体物质

an·ti·con·vul·sant (an″te-) (an″ti-kənvul′sənt) inhibiting convulsions, or an agent that does this 抗惊厥的, 抗惊厥药

an·ti·con·vul·sive (an″te-) (an″ti-kən-vul′siv) 抗惊厥的, 见 anticonvulsant

an·ti·cus (an-ti′kəs) [L.] anterior 前方的

an·ti-D antibody against D antigen, the most immunogenic of the Rh factors. Commercial preparations of anti-D, Rh$_0$(D) immune globulin, are administered to Rh-negative women following the birth of an Rh-positive baby in order to prevent maternal alloimmunization against the D antigen, which could cause erythroblastosis fetalis in a subsequent pregnancy. Called also anti-Rh$_0$ 抗 D 抗原抗体

an·ti·de·pres·sant (an″te-) (an″ti-de-pres′ənt) preventing or relieving depression; also, an agent that so acts 预防或缓解抑郁; 抗抑郁药; **tricyclic a.,** any of a class of drugs with a particular tricyclic structure and potentiating catecholamine action; used for the treatment of depression 三环类抗抑郁药, 具有特定三环结构和增强儿茶酚胺作用的一类药物; 用于治疗抑郁

an·ti·di·a·bet·ic (an″te-) (an″ti-di″ə-bet′ik) 1. preventing or alleviating diabetes 预防或减轻糖尿病; 2. an agent that so acts 降糖药

an·ti·di·ar·rhe·al (an″te-) (an″ti-di″ə-re′əl) counteracting diarrhea, or an agent that so acts 抵抗腹泻, 止泻药

an·ti·di·uret·ic (an″te-) (an″ti-di″u-ret′ik) 1. pertaining to or causing suppression of urine 抗利尿的; 2. an agent that so acts 抗利尿药

an·ti·dote (an′tĭ-dōt) an agent that counteracts

a poison 解毒剂，可用于拮抗毒物的药物；**an-tido′tal** *adj.*; **chemical a.**, one that neutralizes the poison by changing its chemical nature 通过改变毒物的化学结构而中和毒性的解毒剂；**mechanical a.**, one that prevents absorption of the poison 可防止毒物吸收的解毒剂；**physiologic a.**, one that counteracts the effects of the poison by producing opposing physiologic effects 通过产生相反的生理效应来抵消毒药作用的解毒剂

an·ti·drom·ic (an″te-drom′ik) conducting impulses in a direction opposite to the normal 逆向的，逆行的，以与正常方向相反的方向进行冲击

an·ti·dys·ki·net·ic (an″te-) (an″ti-dis″kĭnet′ik) relieving or preventing dyskinesia, or an agent that so acts 缓解或预防运动障碍，或具有缓解或预防运动障碍作用的药物

an·ti·emet·ic (an″te-ə-met′ik) preventing or alleviating nausea and vomiting; also, an agent that so acts 止吐药

an·ti·es·tro·gen (an″te-es′trə-jen) a substance capable of inhibiting the biological effects of estrogens 具有抑制雌激素生理效应作用的物质；**antiestro-gen′ic** *adj.*

an·ti·feb·rile (an″te-) (an″ti-feb′ril) 退热药，见 antipyretic (1)

an·ti·fi·bri·nol·y·sin (an″te-) (an″ti-fi″brĭnol′ĭ-sin) antiplasmin 抗纤维蛋白溶解剂

an·ti·fi·bri·no·lyt·ic (an″te-) (an″ti-fi″brĭ-nolit′ik) inhibiting or preventing fibrinolysis, or an agent that does this 抗纤维蛋白溶解的，抗纤维蛋白溶解药

an·ti·fi·brot·ic (an″te-) (an″ti-fi-brot′ik) causing regression of fibrosis, or an agent that so acts 导致纤维化消退，或具有导致纤维化消退作用的药物

an·ti·fi·lar·i·al (an″te-) (an″ti-fĭ-lar′e-əl) suppressing or killing filaria; also, an agent that does this 抑制或杀灭丝虫；以及具有抑制或杀灭丝虫作用的药物

an·ti·flat·u·lent (an″te-) (an″ti-flat′u-lənt) relieving or preventing flatulence, or an agent that does this 缓解或预防腹胀，或具有缓解或预防腹胀作用的药物

an·ti·fun·gal (an″te-) (an″ti-fung′gəl) destroying fungi, or suppressing their reproduction or growth; effective against fungal infections 抗真菌的

an·ti·ga·lac·tic (an″te-) (an″ti-gə-lak′tik) 1. diminishing or stopping secretion of milk 减少或阻止乳汁分泌；2. an agent with this effect 具有减少或阻止乳汁分泌作用的药物

an·ti·gen (Ag) (an′tĭ-jən) any substance capable of inducing a specific immune response and of reacting with the products of that response, i.e., with specific antibody or specifically sensitized T lym-phocytes, or both 抗原，能引起特异性免疫反应并能与该反应产物进行反应的某种物质，例如，可与特异性抗体或特异性致敏 T 淋巴细胞发生反应，或与两者均可反应；**antigen′ic** *adj.*; **blood group a′s**, erythrocyte surface antigens whose antigenic differences determine blood groups 血型抗原；**cancer a. 125 (CA 125)**, a surface glycoprotein associated with müllerian epithelial tissue; elevated serum levels are often associated with epithelial ovarian carcinomas, particularly with nonmucinous tumors, but are also seen in some other malignant and various benign pelvic disorders 一种与 Müllerian 上皮组织相关的表面糖蛋白；其血清水平升高通常与上皮性卵巢癌有关，尤其是与非黏液性肿瘤相关，亦可见于其他某些恶性疾病和多种良性盆腔疾病；**capsular a.**, one found in the capsule of a microorganism 一种可见于微生物荚膜的抗原；**carcinoembryonic a. (CEA)**, a cancer-specific glycoprotein antigen of colon carcinoma, also present in many adenocarcinomas of endodermal origin and in normal gastrointestinal tissues of human embryos 癌胚抗原，结肠癌的一种特异性糖蛋白抗原，亦存在于许多内胚层起源性腺癌和人类胚胎的正常胃肠道组织中；**CD a.**, any of a number of cell surface markers expressed by leukocytes and used to distinguish cell lineages, developmental stages, and functional subsets; such markers can be identified by monoclonal antibodies 白细胞分化抗原，白细胞表达的细胞表面标志物之一，可用于区分细胞谱系、发育阶段和功能亚群；这些标记物可由单克隆抗体识别；**class I a′s,**, major histocompatibility antigens found on every cell except erythrocytes, recognized during graft rejection, and involved in MHC restriction 一种可见于除红细胞外所有细胞的主要组织相容性抗原，该抗原可在移植物排斥反应中识别，该抗原涉及主要组织相容性复合体限制性（MHC 限制性）；**class II a′s**, major histocompatibility antigens found only on immunocompetent cells, primarily B lymphocytes and macrophages 一种仅见于免疫活性细胞的主要组织相容性抗原，该类抗原主要见于 B 淋巴细胞和巨噬细胞；**common acute lymphoblastic leukemia a. (CALLA)**, a tumor-associated antigen occurring on lymphoblasts in about 80 percent of patients with acute lymphoblastic leukemia (ALL) and in 40–50 percent of patients with blastic phase chronic myelogenous leukemia (CML) 一种肿瘤相关性抗原，该抗原可见于约 80% 急性淋巴细胞白血病患者的淋巴母细胞，和 40% ～ 50% 急变期慢性粒细胞白血病患者；**complete a.**, one that both stimulates an immune response and reacts with the products of that response 完全抗原，一种既能激发免疫反应又能与该反应

产物进行反应的抗原；**conjugated a.,** one produced by coupling a hapten to a protein carrier molecule through covalent bonds; when it induces immunization, the resultant immune response is directed against both the hapten and the carrier 一种通过共价键将半抗原与蛋白质载体分子偶联而产生的抗原；当其诱发免疫反应时，产生的免疫反应既针对半抗原又针对蛋白质载体；**D a.,** a red cell antigen of the Rh blood group system, important in the development of isoimmunization in Rh-negative persons exposed to the blood of Rh-positive persons 一种 Rh 血型系统的红细胞抗原，对暴露于 Rh 阳性血液的 Rh 阴性个体的同种免疫发育有重要作用；**E a.,** a red cell antigen of the Rh blood group system 一种 Rh 血型系统的红细胞抗原；**flagellar a.,** H antigen H 抗原；**Forssman a.,** a heterogenetic antigen inducing the production of antisheep hemolysin, occurring in various unrelated species, mainly in the organs but not in the erythrocytes (guinea pig, horse), but sometimes only in the erythrocytes (sheep), and occasionally in both (chicken) 一种可引发产生抗绵羊溶血素的异种抗原，该抗原存在于多种相互无亲缘关系的物种，主要见于其内脏器官而非红细胞（豚鼠、马），有时可仅见于其红细胞（羊），偶尔可同时见于其内脏器官和红细胞（鸡）；**H a.,** 1. a bacterial flagellar antigen important in the serologic classification of enteric bacilli 一种细菌鞭毛抗原，该抗原在肠杆菌的血清学分类中起重要作用；2. the precursor of the A and B blood group antigens; normal type O individuals lack the enzyme to convert it to A or B antigens A、B 血型抗原的前体物质；正常 O 型血个体缺乏可将其转换为 A 或 B 抗原的酶；**hepatitis B core a. (HBcAg),** an antigen of the DNA core of the hepatitis B virus, indicating the presence of replicating hepatitis B virus 乙型肝炎核心抗原，乙型肝炎的 DNA 核心抗原，该抗原阳性表明存在乙型肝炎病毒复制；**hepatitis B e a. (HBeAg),** an antigen of hepatitis B virus sometimes present in the blood during acute infection, usually disappearing afterward but sometimes persisting in chronic disease 乙型肝炎 e 抗原，乙型肝炎病毒的抗原之一，它在急性感染期存在于血液中，通常于急性感染期过后消失，然而有时可在慢性疾病中持续存在；**hepatitis B surface a. (HBsAg),** a surface coat lipoprotein antigen of the hepatitis B virus, peaking with the first appearance of clinical disease symptoms. Tests for serum HBsAg are used in the diagnosis of acute or chronic hepatitis B and in testing blood products for infectivity 乙型肝炎表面抗原，乙型肝炎病毒的一种表面包被脂蛋白抗原，该抗原在首次出现临床症状时达到峰值。血清乙型肝炎表面抗原检测可用于诊断急性或慢性

乙型肝炎以及检测血制品的传染性；**heterogenetic a.,** heterophile a. 异嗜性抗原；**heterologous a.,** an antigen that reacts with an antibody that is not the one that induced its formation 可与非其诱导产生的抗体进行反应的抗原；**heterophil a.,** heterophile a., an antigen common to more than one species and whose species distribution is unrelated to its phylogenetic distribution (viz., Forssman antigen, lens protein, certain caseins, etc.) 多个物种共有的抗原，且该抗原的物种分布与其系统发育分布无关（即 Forssman 抗原、晶状体蛋白、某些酪蛋白等）；**histocompatibility a's,** genetically determined isoantigens found on the surface of nucleated cells of most tissues, which incite an immune response when grafted onto a genetically different individual and thus determine compatibility of tissues in transplantation 组织相容性抗原，一种基因决定的同种抗原，该抗原可见于多数组织的有核细胞表面，在组织移植至某个基因不同的个体时，该基因可激发免疫反应，并由此决定移植过程中的组织相容性；**HLA a's,** human leukocyte antigens 人白细胞抗原；**homologous a.,** 1. the antigen inducing antibody formation 可诱导抗体形成的抗原；2. isoantigen 同种抗原；**human leukocyte a's,** histocompatibility antigens (glycoproteins) on the surface of nucleated cells (including circulating and tissue cells) determined by a region on chromosome 6 bearing several genetic loci, designated HLA-A, -B, -C, -DP, -DQ, -DR, -MB, -MT, and -Te. They are important in cross-matching procedures and are partially responsible for the rejection of transplanted tissues when donor and recipient HLA antigens do not match 有核细胞（包括循环细胞和组织细胞）表面的组织相容性抗原（糖蛋白），该类抗原由 6 号染色体的某个区域决定，该区域有数个基因位点，分别称为 HLA-A、HLA-B、HLA-C、HLA-DP、HLA-DQ、HLA-DR、HLA-MB、HLA-MT 和 HLA-Te。该类抗原在交叉配型过程中具有重要意义，并且是供、受体的人白细胞抗原（HLA）配型不相符时发生移植组织排异反应的部分原因；**H-Y a.,** a histocompatibility antigen of the cell membrane, determined by a locus on the Y chromosome; it is a mediator of testicular organization (hence, sexual differentiation) in the male 一种细胞膜的组织相容性抗原，该抗原由 Y 染色体的某基因位点决定；该抗原是男性睾丸组织发生的影响因素之一（因而亦是性别分化的影响因素之一）；**Ia a's,** one of the histocompatibility antigens governed by the I region of the major histocompatibility complex, located principally on B lymphocytes, macrophages, accessory cells, and granulocyte precursors 组织相容性抗原之一，该抗原受主要组织相容性复合物 I 区控制，主要位

于 B 淋巴细胞、巨噬细胞、辅助细胞和粒细胞前体；Inv group a's，见 Km a's ；isogeneic a., an antigen carried by an individual and capable of eliciting an immune response in genetically different individuals of the same species, but not in an individual bearing it 某个体携带的抗原，可在同一物种不同基因型的个体中引发免疫反应，而不会在携带该抗原的个体自身引发免疫反应；K a., a surface antigen occurring on the bacterial capsule 存在于细菌荚膜的一种表面抗原；Km a's, the three alloantigens found in the constant region of the κ light chains of immunoglobulins 可见于免疫球蛋白 κ 轻链恒定区的三种同异型抗原；Ly a's, Lyt a's, antigenic cell-surface markers of subpopulations of T lymphocytes, classified as Ly 1, 2, and 3; they are associated with helper and suppressor activities of T lymphocytes T 淋巴细胞亚群的抗原性细胞表面标记物，可分为 Ly 1、2 和 3 三类；该类抗原与 T 淋巴细胞的辅助和抑制活性有关；mumps skin test a., a sterile suspension of mumps virus; used as a dermal reactivity indicator 流行性腮腺炎病毒的无菌悬液；可用作皮肤反应性指标；O a., one occurring in the lipopolysaccharide layer of the wall of gram-negative bacteria 一种存在于革兰阴性菌细胞壁脂多糖层的抗原；oncofetal a., 见 carcinoembryonic a.; organ-specific a., any antigen occurring only in a particular organ and serving to distinguish it from other organs; it may be limited to an organ of a single species or be characteristic of the same organ in many species 器官特异性抗原；partial a., hapten 半抗原；private a's, antigens of the low frequency blood groups, probably differing from ordinary blood group systems only in their incidence 低频率血型的抗原，该类抗原可能只在其发生率上不同于普通血型系统；prostatespecific a. (PSA), an endopeptidase secreted by the epithelial cells of the prostate gland; serum levels are elevated in benign prostatic hyperplasia and prostate cancer 前列腺特异性抗原，前列腺上皮细胞分泌的一种肽链内切酶；其血清水平升高可见于良性前列腺增生和前列腺癌；public a's, antigens of the high frequency blood groups, so called because they are found in almost all persons tested 高频率血型的抗原，该命名是由于此类抗原可见于几乎所有受检个体；self-a., autoantigen 自身抗原；T a., 1. tumor antigen, any of several coded for by the viral genome, and associated with transformation of infected cells by certain DNA tumor viruses 肿瘤抗原，该抗原由病毒基因组编码，与某些 DNA 肿瘤病毒对受感染细胞的转化有关；2. 见 CD a.; 3. an antigen present on human erythrocytes that is exposed by treatment with neuraminidase or contact with certain bacteria 一种存在于人

红细胞的抗原，该抗原可经神经氨酸酶治疗或接触某些细菌而暴露；T-dependent a., one requiring the presence of helper cells to stimulate antibody production by B cells 胸腺依赖性抗原，一种需要辅助性 T 细胞存在以刺激 B 细胞产生抗体的抗原；T-independent a., one able to trigger B cells to produce antibodies without the presence of T cells 胸腺非依赖性抗原，一种无须辅助性 T 细胞存在、可独立刺激 B 细胞产生抗体的抗原；tumor a., 见 1. T a. (1); 2. tumor-specific a. 肿瘤特异性抗原；3. 见 tumor-associated a.; tumor-associated a. (TAA), one associated with tumor cells; it may also be present normally under specific conditions, in specific organs, or at lower levels 肿瘤相关性抗原，与肿瘤细胞有关的抗原；该抗原亦可在某些特定情况下在某些器官正常存在或以较低水平存在；tumor-specific a. (TSA), any cell-surface antigen of a tumor that does not occur on normal cells of the same origin 肿瘤特异性抗原，一种肿瘤细胞表面抗原，该抗原不存在于其同源的正常细胞；Vi a., a K antigen of *Salmonella typhi* originally thought responsible for virulence 伤寒沙门菌的一种 K 抗原，该抗原最初认为是细菌产生毒力的原因

an·ti·gen·emia (an″tĭ-jə-ne′me-ə) the presence of antigen (e.g., hepatitis B surface antigen) in the blood 抗原（例如，乙型肝炎表面抗原）存在于血液中；**antigene′mic** *adj.*

an·ti·gen·ic (an-tĭ-jen′ik) having the properties of an antigen 具有抗原性质的

an·ti·ge·nic·i·ty (an″tĭ-jə-nis′ĭ-te) the capacity to stimulate the production of antibodies or the capacity to react with an antibody 抗原性

an·ti·glau·co·ma (an″te-) (an″tĭ-glawko′mə) preventing or alleviating glaucoma 预防或减轻青光眼

an·ti·glob·u·lin (an′tĭ-glob″u-lin) an antibody directed against gamma globulin, as used in the antiglobulin test 一种针对丙种球蛋白的抗体，可用于抗球蛋白试验

an·ti·he·lix (an″te-he′liks) the prominent semicircular ridge on the lateral aspect of the auricle of the external ear, anteroinferior to the helix 对耳轮，对耳轮是外耳廓侧面突出的半圆形峭，位于耳轮的前下方；spelled also *anthelix* 又写作 anthelix

an·ti·he·mol·y·sin (an″te-) (an″ti-he-mol′ə-sin) any agent that opposes the action of a hemolysin 抗溶血剂

an·ti·he·mo·phil·ic (an″te-) (an″ti-he″mofil′ik) counteracting hemophilia, or an agent that so acts 抗血友病，或具有抗血友病作用的药物

an·ti·hem·or·rhag·ic (an″te-) (an″ti-hem″oraj′ik) exerting a hemostatic effect; counteracting hemorrhage, or an agent that does this 止血的，止血药

an·ti·his·ta·mine (an″te-) (an″ti-his′tə-mēn) an

agent that counteracts the action of histamine; usually used for agents blocking H_1 receptors (H_1 receptor antagonists) and used to treat allergic reactions and as components of cough and cold preparations. Agents blocking H_2 receptors, used to inhibit gastric secretion in peptic ulcer, are usually called H_2 receptor antagonists 抗组胺药

an·ti·his·ta·min·ic (an″te-) (an″ti-his-tə-min′ik) 1. counteracting the effect of histamine 抗组胺作用；2. antihistamine 抗组胺药物

an·ti·hy·per·cho·les·ter·ol·emic (an″te-) (an″ti-hi″pər-kə-les″tər-ol-e′mik) effective against hypercholesterolemia, or an agent with this quality 有效治疗高胆固醇血症，或具有抗高胆固醇血症作用的药物

an·ti·hy·per·gly·ce·mic (an″te-) (an″ti-hi″pər-gli-se′mik) counteracting high levels of glucose in the blood, or an agent that so acts 抗高血糖，降糖药

an·ti·hy·per·ka·le·mic (an″te-) (an″ti-hi″pər-kə-le′mik) effective in decreasing or preventing an excessively high blood level of potassium, or an agent that so acts 有效降低血钾水平或防止血钾过高，或具有降低血钾作用的药物

an·ti·hy·per·lip·i·de·mic (an″te-) (an″ti-hi″pər-lip″ĭ-de′mik) promoting a reduction of lipid levels in the blood, or an agent that so acts 促进血脂水平降低，降脂药

an·ti·hy·per·lipo·pro·tein·emic (an″te-) (an″ti-hi″pər-lip″o-pro″tēn-e′mik) promoting a reduction of lipoprotein levels in the blood, or an agent that does this 促进血液中脂蛋白水平降低，或有降低血脂蛋白作用的药物

an·ti·hy·per·ten·sive (an″te-) (an″ti-hi″pərten′siv) counteracting high blood pressure, or an agent that does this 抗高血压的，降压药

an·ti·hy·po·gly·ce·mic (an″te-) (an″ti-hi″po-gli-se′mik) counteracting hypoglycemia, or an agent that so acts 抗低血糖，或具有抗低血糖作用的药物

an·ti·hy·po·ten·sive (an″te-) (an″ti-hi″poten′siv) counteracting low blood pressure, or an agent that so acts 抗低血压，升压药

an·ti·in·fec·tive (an″ti-in-fek′tiv) counteracting infection, or an agent that does this 抗感染，抗感染药物

an·ti·in·flam·ma·to·ry (an″ti-in-flam′ə-tor″e) counteracting or suppressing inflammation；also, an agent that so acts 对抗或抑制炎症，抗炎药

an·ti·leu·ko·cyt·ic (an″te-) (an″ti-loo″kosit′ik) destructive to white blood cells (leukocytes) 对白细胞有破坏作用的

an·ti·li·pe·mic (an″te-) (an″ti-lĭ-pe′mik) antihyperlipidemic 促进血脂水平降低，降脂药

an·ti·lith·ic (an″te-) (an″ti-lith′ik) preventing the formation of calculi, or an agent that so acts 预防结石形成，或具有防结石形成作用的药物

an·ti·ly·sis (an″te-) (an″ti-li′sis) inhibition of lysis 抗溶解

an·ti·lyt·ic (an″te-) (an″ti-lit′ik) 1. pertaining to antilysis 与抗溶解有关；2. inhibiting or preventing lysis 抑制或预防溶解

an·ti·ma·lar·i·al (an″te-) (an″ti-mə-lar′e-əl) therapeutically effective against malaria, or an agent with this quality 可有效治疗疟疾的，抗疟药

an·ti·mere (an′tĭ-mēr) one of the opposite corresponding parts of an organism that are symmetrical with respect to the longitudinal axis of its body 相对于自身纵轴对称的生物体，其相对的对称部位之一

an·ti·me·tab·o·lite (an″te-) (an″ti-mə-tab′olīt) a substance bearing a close structural resemblance to one required for normal physiological functioning, and exerting its effect by interfering with the utilization of the essential metabolite 抗代谢药物，该物质在结构上与正常生理功能所需物质极为相似，并通过干扰必需代谢物的利用而发挥作用

an·ti·met·he·mo·glo·bin·emic (an″te-) (an″ti-met-he″mo-glo″bĭ-ne′mik) 1. promoting reduction of methemoglobin levels in the blood 促进血中高铁血红蛋白水平降低；2. an agent that so acts. 具有降低血中高铁血红蛋白水平作用的药物

an·ti·me·tro·pia (an″te-) (an″ti-mə-tro′pe-ə) hyperopia of one eye, with myopia in the other 屈光参差，一眼远视而另一眼近视

an·ti·mi·cro·bi·al (an″te-) (an″ti-mikro′be-əl) 1. killing microorganisms or suppressing their multiplication or growth 杀灭微生物，或抑制其繁殖或生长；2. an agent with such effects 具有杀灭或抑制微生物作用的药物

an·ti·mo·ny (Sb) (an′tĭ-mo″ne) a crystalline, bluish metalloid element；at. no. 51, at. wt. 121.760, forming various medicinal and poisonous salts. Ingestion of antimony compounds, and rarely industrial exposure to them, may produce symptoms similar to those of acute arsenic poisoning. *A. potassium tartrate* and *a. sodium tartrate* have been used as antischistosomals 锑，一种结晶、带蓝色的类金属元素；原子序数 51，相对原子质量 121.760，可形成多种药用和有毒性的盐类。摄入锑的化合物或发生罕见的工业暴露，可能导致出现类似急性砷中毒的症状。酒石酸锑钾和酒石酸锑钠已用作抗血吸虫剂；**antimo′nial** *adj.*

an·ti·mus·ca·rin·ic (an″te-) (an″ti-mus′kə-rin′ik) 1. acting against the toxic effects of muscarine 抗毒蕈碱的毒性作用；2. blocking the muscarinic receptors 阻断毒蕈碱受体；3. an agent having either such action 具有抗毒蕈碱毒性或阻断毒蕈碱受体作用的药物

an·ti·my·as·then·ic (an″te-) (an″ti-mi′əsthen′ik) counteracting or relieving muscular weakness in myasthenia gravis, or an agent that so acts 消除或减轻重症肌无力的肌无力症状，抗肌无力药物

an·ti·my·co·bac·ter·ial (ăn-tē″mī-cō-băcteer-ēəl) a drug that acts as an antiinfective against mycobacterium 抗结核药物

an·ti·my·cot·ic (an″ti-mi-kot′ik) antifungal 抗真菌的，抗真菌药物

an·ti·nau·se·ant (an″te-) (an″ti-naw′ze-ənt) preventing or relieving nausea, or an agent that so acts 预防或减轻恶心，具有预防或减轻恶心作用的药物；另见 *antiemetic*

an·ti·neo·plas·tic (an″te-) (an″ti-ne″o-plas′tik) 1. inhibiting or preventing development of neoplasms; checking maturation and proliferation of malignant cells 抑制或预防肿瘤发展；抑制恶性细胞的成熟和繁殖；2. an agent that so acts 抗肿瘤药物

an·tin·ion (an-tin′e-on) the frontal pole of the head 头部额极；the median frontal point farthest from the inion 距枕骨隆突最远的前正中点

an·ti·no·ci·cep·tive (an″te-) (an″ti-no″sīsep′tiv) reducing sensitivity to painful stimuli 降低对疼痛刺激的敏感度

an·ti·nu·cle·ar (an″te-) (an″ti-noo′kle-ər) destructive to or reactive with components of the cell nucleus 对细胞核组分有破坏性或可与之反应的

an·ti·ox·i·dant (an″te-ok″sī-dənt) preventing or delaying oxidation, or a substance or agent that so acts 抗氧化，预防或延缓氧化，抗氧化剂

an·ti·par·al·lel (an″te-) (an″ti-par′ə-lel) denoting molecules arranged side by side but in opposite directions 反向平行，表示分子方向相反并排列

an·ti·par·a·sit·ic (an″te-) (an″ti-par″ə-sit′ik) destructive to parasites, or an agent that does this 杀灭寄生虫，抗寄生虫药物

an·ti·par·kin·so·ni·an (an″te-) (an″ tipahr″kin-so′ne-ən) effective in treatment of parkinsonism, or an agent with this quality 可有效治疗帕金森综合征的，抗帕金森综合征药物

an·ti·per·i·stal·sis (an″te-) (an″ti-per″īstawl′sis) reversed peristalsis 逆蠕动

an·ti·per·i·stal·tic (an″te-) (an″ti-per″īstawl′tik) 1. pertaining to or causing antiperistalsis 与逆蠕动相关或造成逆蠕动；2. diminishing peristalsis；or an agent that so acts 减少蠕动，抗蠕动药物

an·ti·per·spir·ant (an″te-) (an″ti-pur′spər-ant) inhibiting or preventing perspiration, or an agent that does this 抑制或预防出汗，止汗剂

an·ti·plas·min (an″te-) (an″ti-plaz′min) a sub-stance in the blood that inhibits plasmin. The most important is α2-*a.*, which forms stable complexes with free plasmin, is crosslinked to fibrin by factor XIII, and inhibits the binding of plasminogen to fibrin；deficiency results in tendency to severe bleeding, including hemarthrosis 抗纤溶酶，血中抑制纤溶酶的物质，最重要的是 α2 纤溶酶，其可与游离纤溶酶形成稳定复合物，通过凝血因子 XIII 与纤维蛋白交联，可抑制纤溶酶原和纤维蛋白的结合；抗纤溶酶缺乏可导致包括关节腔积血在内的严重的出血倾向

an·ti·plas·tic (an″te-) (an″ti-plas′tik) 1. unfavorable to healing 不易愈合的；2. an agent that sup-presses formation of blood or other cells 抑制血细胞或其他细胞形成的药物

an·ti·port (an′tī-port) a mechanism of coupling the transport of two compounds across a membrane in opposite directions 一种将两种化合物以相反方向在膜上耦合传输的机制

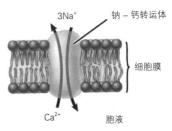

▲ 逆向运输（antiport）：钠－钙转运体。Na⁺ 的电化学梯度用于将 Ca²⁺ 泵出细胞，从而调节细胞内 Ca²⁺ 的水平

anti·pro·ges·tin (an″te-) (an″ti-pro-jes′tin) a substance that inhibits the formation, transport, or action of progestational agents 抑制孕激素生成、运输或发挥作用的物质

an·ti·pro·throm·bin (an″te-) (an″ti-prothrom′bin) 1. directed against prothrombin 抗凝血酶原；2. an anticoagulant that retards the conversion of pro-thrombin into thrombin 能延缓凝血酶原转化为凝血酶的抗凝剂

an·ti·pro·to·zo·al (an″te-) (an″ti-pro-tə-zo′əl) lethal to protozoa, or checking their growth or reproduction；also, an agent that so acts 杀灭原虫或抑制其生长或繁殖；抗原虫药物

an·ti·pru·rit·ic (an″te-) (an″ti-proo-rit′ik) preventing or relieving itching, or an agent that does this 预防或缓解瘙痒，止痒药

an·ti·pso·ri·at·ic (an″te-) (an″ti-sor″e-at′ik) effective against psoriasis, or an agent that so acts 可有效治疗银屑病的，抗银屑病药物

an·ti·psy·chot·ic (an″te-) (an″ti-si-kot′ik) effective in the treatment of psychotic disorders; also, an agent that so acts 可有效治疗精神疾病的，抗精神疾病药物

an·ti·py·ret·ic (an″te-) (an″ti-pi-ret′ik) 1. relieving or reducing fever 退热；2. an agent that so acts 退热药

an·ti·py·rine (an″te-pi-rēn) an analgesic used as a component of topical solutions for decongestion and analgesia in acute otitis media 安替比林，一种止痛药，可用于急性中耳炎减轻充血和止痛的局部用药；另见 *dichloralphenazone*

an·ti·py·rot·ic (an″te-) (an″ti-pi-rot′ik) 1. effective in the treatment of burns 可有效治疗烧伤的；2. an agent with this quality 治疗烧伤的药物

an·ti·ret·ro·vi·ral (an″te-) (an″ti-ret′ro-vi″rəl) effective against retroviruses, or an agent with this quality 可有效抗逆转录病毒的，抗逆转录病毒药物

an·ti·rheu·mat·ic (an″te-) (an″ti-roo-mat′ik) 1. relieving or preventing rheumatism 缓解或预防风湿性疾病；2. an agent that so acts 抗风湿药物

an·ti·rick·ett·si·al (an″te-) (an″ti-rĭ-ket′se-əl) 1. effective against rickettsiae 可有效抗立克次体的；2. an agent having this quality 抗立克次体药物

an·ti·schis·to·so·mal (an″te-) (an″ti-shis″to-so′məl) 1. suppressing or killing schistosomes 抑制或杀灭血吸虫；2. an agent that so acts 抗血吸虫药物

an·ti·scor·bu·tic (an″te-) (an″ti-skor-bu′tik) effective in the prevention or relief of scurvy 可有效预防或缓解坏血病

an·ti·se·cre·to·ry (an″te-) (an″ti-sə-kre′to-re) 1. secretoinhibitory; inhibiting or diminishing secretions, especially in the stomach 抑制分泌的；抑制或减少分泌，尤其是胃液分泌；2. an agent that so acts 抗分泌药物

an·ti·sense (an″te-) (an′ti-sens) referring to the strand of a double-stranded molecule that does not directly encode the product (the *sense strand*) but is complementary to it 反义链，是指双联分子中不直接编码基因产物（即有义链）而与有义链互补的单链

an·ti·sep·sis (an″tĭ-sep′sis) 1. the prevention of sepsis by antiseptic means 通过抗菌手段预防败血症；2. any procedure that reduces to a significant degree the microbial flora of skin or mucous membranes 任何能够很大程度减少皮肤或黏膜微生物菌群的程序

an·ti·sep·tic (an″tĭ-sep′tik) 1. pertaining to antisepsis 与防腐有关的；2. preventing decay or putrefaction 防止腐败或腐烂；3. a substance that inhibits the growth and development of microorganisms without necessarily killing them 能够抑制微

生物生长发育而无需杀灭微生物的物质

an·ti·se·rum (an″tĭ-se′rəm) a serum containing antibody(ies), obtained from an animal immunized either by injection of antigen or by infection with microorganisms containing antigen 抗血清，一种含有多克隆抗体的血清，可从已受免疫的动物体中获得，动物体可经注射抗原或感染携带抗原的微生物而免疫

an·ti·si·al·a·gogue (an″te-) (an″ti-si-al′ə-gog) counteracting saliva formation; also, an agent that does this 抗唾液生成，止涎药；**antisialagog′ic** *adj.*

an·ti·so·cial (an″te-) (an″ti-so′shəl) 1. denoting behavior that violates the rights of others, societal mores, or the law 表示侵犯他人权利、违反社会习俗或法律的行为；2. denoting the specific personality traits seen in antisocial personality disorder 表示反社会人格障碍所具有的特定人格特征

an·ti·spas·mod·ic (an″te-) (an″ti-spazmod′ik) 1. preventing or relieving spasms 预防或缓解肌肉痉挛；2. an agent that so acts 解痉药

an·ti·spas·tic (an″te-) (an″ti-spas′tik) antispasmodic with specific reference to skeletal muscle 特指缓解骨骼肌痉挛，缓解骨骼肌痉挛的药物

an·ti·sym·pa·thet·ic (an″te-) (an″ti-sim″pə-thet′ik) sympatholytic 阻滞交感神经的

an·ti·the·nar (an″te-the′nar) placed opposite to the palm or sole 小鱼际

an·ti·throm·bin (an″te-throm′bin) any naturally occurring or therapeutically administered substance that neutralizes the action of thrombin and thus limits or restricts blood coagulation 抗凝血酶，任何天然存在或治疗性使用的物质，其能够中和凝血酶的作用，并由此限制血液凝固过程；a. Ⅰ, fibrin, referring to its capacity to adsorb thrombin and thus neutralize it 纤维蛋白，其能够吸附凝血酶，从而中和其作用；a. Ⅲ, a plasma α_2-globulin of the serpin family that inactivates thrombin and also inhibits certain coagulation factors and kallikrein. Inherited deficiency is associated with recurrent deep vein thrombosis and pulmonary emboli; the complications are prevented and treated with a preparation of antithrombin Ⅲ from pooled human plasma 一种隶属于丝氨酸蛋白酶抑制剂家族的血浆 α_2 球蛋白，可灭活凝血酶，并抑制某些凝血因子和激肽释放酶作用。该物质的遗传性缺陷与复发性深静脉血栓形成和肺栓塞有关；上述并发症可由人群血浆中获得的抗凝血酶Ⅲ预防和治疗

an·ti·throm·bo·plas·tin (an″te-) (an″tithrom″bo-plas′tin) any agent or substance that prevents or interferes with the interaction of blood coagulation factors as they generate prothrombinase 任何能够在凝血酶原酶产生期间阻止或干扰凝血因子间相

互作用的药物

an·ti·throm·bot·ic (an″te-) (an″ti-throm·bot′ik) 1. preventing or interfering with the formation of thrombi 预防或干扰血栓形成；2. an agent that so acts 抗栓药

an·ti·thy·roid (an″te-thi′roid) counteracting thyroid functioning, especially in its synthesis of thyroid hormones 抗甲状腺功能，尤其是抵抗其合成甲状腺激素的功能

an·ti·tox·in (an″tĭ-tok′sin) antibody produced in response to a toxin of bacterial (usually an exotoxin), animal (zootoxin), or plant (phytotoxin) origin, which neutralizes the effects of the toxin 针对细菌毒素（通常是外源性毒素）、动物毒素或植物毒素产生的抗体，该类抗体可中和毒素作用；**an′titoxic** adj; **botulism a.**, an equine antitoxin against toxins of the types A and B and/or E strains of Clostridium botulinum 肉毒杆菌抗毒素，一种抗肉毒杆菌 A、B 和（或）E 型菌株毒素的马抗毒素；**diphtheria a.**, equine antitoxin from horses immunized against diphtheria toxin or the toxoid 白喉抗毒素，一种由对白喉毒素或类毒素免疫的马血清中获得的马抗毒素；**equine a.**, an antitoxin derived from the blood of healthy horses immunized against a specific bacterial toxin 一类从对特定细菌毒素免疫的健康的马血清中获得的抗毒素；**tetanus a.**, equine antitoxin from horses that have been immunized against tetanus toxin or toxoid 破伤风抗毒素，一种由对破伤风毒素或类毒素免疫的马血清中获得的马抗毒素

an·ti·tra·gus (an″te-tra′gəs) a projection on the ear opposite the tragus 对耳屏

an·ti·trich·o·mo·nal (an″te-trik″omo′nəl) effective against Trichomonas; also, an agent having such effects 抗毛滴虫的，抗毛滴虫药物

an·ti·try·pan·o·so·mal (an″te-) (an″ti-trĭpan″ə-so′məl) 1. killing or suppressing trypanosomes 杀灭或抑制锥虫；2. an agent that so acts 抗锥虫药物

α₁-an·ti·tryp·sin (an″tĭ-trip′sin) alpha₁-antitrypsin α₁ 抗胰蛋白酶

an·ti·tu·ber·cu·lar (an″te-) (an″ti-toobur′ku-lər) 1. therapeutically effective against tuberculosis 可有效治疗结核的；2. an agent with this characteristic 抗结核药物

an·ti·tu·ber·cu·lin (an″te-too-bur′ku-lin) an antibody developed after injection of tuberculin into the body 体内注射结核菌素后产生的抗体

an·ti·tus·sive (an″te-) (an″ti-tus′iv) effective against cough, or an agent with this quality 可有效对抗咳嗽的，止咳药

an·ti·ul·cer·a·tive (an″te-ul′sə-ra″tiv) (an″-teul′sər-ə-tiv) preventing ulcers or promoting their healing, or an agent that so acts 预防溃疡或促进溃疡愈合，抗溃疡药物

an·ti·uro·lith·ic (an″te-u″ro-lith′ik) 1. preventing the formation of urinary calculi 预防泌尿系结石形成；2. an agent that so acts 抗尿路结石药物

an·ti·ven·in (an″te-) (an″ti-ven′in) an antitoxin against animal venom 抗蛇毒素，一种抗动物毒液的抗毒素；**black widow spider a.**, a. (Latrodectus mactans) 黑寡妇蜘蛛抗毒素；**a. (Crotalidae) polyvalent**, a serum containing specific venomneutralizing globulins, produced by immunizing horses with venoms of the fer-de-lance and the western, eastern, and tropical rattlesnakes, used for treatment of envenomation by most pit vipers throughout the world 多价蝮蛇科抗蛇毒素，一种包含某些毒液中和球蛋白的血清，该抗毒素由经矛头蛇、膝部、东部和热带响尾蛇免疫的马产生，该抗毒素可用于治疗世界上绝大多数蝮蛇咬伤；**a. (Latrodectus mactans)**, a serum containing specific venomneutralizing globulins, prepared by immunizing horses against venom of the black widow spider (L. mactans) 球蛛科寇蛛属抗蛇毒素，一种包含某些毒素中和球蛋白的血清，该抗蛇毒素由经黑寡妇蜘蛛毒液免疫的马产生；**a. (Micrurus fulvius)**, **North American coral snake a.**, a serum containing specific venom-neutralizing globulins, produced by immunization of horses with venom of the eastern coral snake (M. fulvius) 东部珊瑚蛇抗蛇毒素，北美珊瑚蛇抗毒素，一种包含某些毒液中和球蛋白的血清，由经东部珊瑚蛇毒液免疫的马产生；**polyvalent crotaline a.**, a. (Crotalidae) polyvalent 多价蝮蛇科抗蛇毒素

an·ti·vi·ral (an″te-) (an″ti-vi′rəl) destroying viruses or suppressing their replication, or an agent that so acts 杀灭病毒或抑制病毒复制，抗病毒药物

an·tri·tis (an-tri′tis) inflammation of an antrum, such as the pyloric antrum or maxillary antrum (sinus) 窦腔炎症，例如幽门窦或上颌窦

an·tro·cele (an′tro-sēl) cystic accumulation of fluid in the maxillary antrum 上颌窦囊性积液

an·tro·na·sal (an″tro-na′zəl) pertaining to the maxillary antrum and nasal fossa 与上颌窦和鼻腔有关的

an·tro·scope (an′trə-skōp″) an instrument for inspecting the maxillary antrum (sinus) 上颌窦镜

an·tros·to·my (an-tros′tə-me) the operation of making an opening into an antrum for purposes of drainage 窦造口术，对窦腔进行造口以便引流的手术

an·trot·o·my (an-trot′ə-me) antrostomy 窦切开术

an·trum (an′trəm) pl. an′tra, antrums [L.] a cavity or chamber 腔 或 室；**an′tral** adj; **cardiac a.**, the short conical portion of the esophagus below the respiratory diaphragm, its base being continuous with the cardiac orifice of the stomach 贲门窦，横膈膜下食道的短圆锥形部分，其底部与胃的贲门部相连；**frontal a.**, 额窦，见 *sinus* 下词条；**mastoid a.**, **a. mastoi′deum**, an air space in the mastoid portion of the temporal bone communicating with the tympanic cavity and the mastoid cells 乳突窦或鼓窦，颞骨乳突部分的气腔，其与鼓室和乳突细胞相通；**maxillary a.**, 上颌窦，见 *sinus* 下词条；**pyloric a.**, **a. pylo′ricum**, the dilated portion of the pyloric part of the stomach, between the body of the stomach and the pyloric canal 幽门窦，胃幽门部的扩张部分，位于胃体和幽门管之间；**tympanic a.**, 见 mastoid a.

ANUG acute necrotizing ulcerative gingivitis 急性坏死性溃疡性龈炎

anu·lus (an′u-ləs) pl. *a′nuli* [L.] a small ring or encircling structure; spelled also *annulus* 小的环或环状结构；又写作 annulus；**a. fibro′sus**, 1. fibrous ring of heart: one of the dense fibrous rings that surround the right and left atrioventricular (tricuspid and mitral) orifices and to which are attached the atrial and ventricular muscle fibers 心脏纤维环：环绕左右房室口（二尖瓣和三尖瓣）的致密纤维环，其上附有心房和心室的肌纤维；2. fibrous ring of intervertebral disk: the circumferential ringlike portion of an intervertebral disk 椎间盘纤维环：椎间盘的环状部分；**a. of spermatozoon**, an electron-dense body at the caudal end of the neck of a spermatozoon 精子颈部尾端的电子密体结构

an·ure·sis (an″u-re′sis) 1. retention of urine in the bladder 尿潴留；2. anuria 无尿；**anuret′ic** *adj.*

an·uria (an-u′re-ə) complete suppression of urine formation and excretion 无尿，尿液的形成和排泄完全受到抑制；**anu′ric** *adj.*

anus (a′nəs) pl.*a′ni* [L.] the opening of the rectum on the body surface; the distal orifice of the alimentary canal 肛门；**imperforate a.**, persistence of the anal epithelial plug so that the anus is closed, either completely or partially 肛门闭锁

an·vil (an′vil) incus 砧骨

an·xi·e·ty (ang-zi′ə-te) a feeling of apprehension, uncertainty, and fear without apparent stimulus, associated with physiological changes (tachycardia, sweating, tremor, etc.) 焦虑，一种在无明显刺激时出现的担忧、不确定、恐惧感，常伴有生理性改变（心动过速、出汗、颤抖等）；**separation a.**, apprehension due to removal of significant persons or familiar surroundings, common in infants 12 to 24 months old 分离焦虑，因离开重要的人物或熟悉的环境而产生的焦虑，常见于 12—24 月龄的婴幼儿；见 *disorder* 下词条

anx·io·lyt·ic (ang″ze-o-lit′ik) 1. antianxiety 抗焦虑的；2. an antianxiety agent 抗焦虑药物

AOA American Optometric Association 美国视光协会；American Orthopaedic Association 美国矫形外科协会；American Orthopsychiatric Association 美国行为精神病学协会；American Osteopathic Association 美国骨病协会

AONE American Organization of Nurse Executives 美国护理管理者组织

AOPA American Orthotics and Prosthetics Association 美国矫形学与修复学协会

AORN Association of Perioperative Registered Nurses (formerly the Association of Operating Room Nurses) 围术期注册护士协会（此前为"手术室护士协会"）

aor·ta (a-or′tə) pl. *aor′tae*, aortas [L.] the great artery arising from the left ventricle, being the main trunk from which the systemic arterial system proceeds; it arises from the left ventricle of the heart, passes upward (*ascending a.*), bends over (*aortic arch*), and then proceeds downward (*descending a.*); the latter is subdivided into an upper thoracic plexus and a lower abdominal plexus. At about the level of the fourth lumbar vertebra, it divides into the two common iliac arteries 主动脉，起源于左心室，是体循环动脉系统的主干；主动脉起自左心室，先上行（升主动脉），再转向（主动脉弓），再向下行（降主动脉）；降主动脉可进一步划分为胸主动脉和腹主动脉。在大约第四腰椎水平，腹主动脉又进一步分为左、右髂总动脉。见图 15。**aor′tal, aor′tic**；**overriding a.**, a congenital anomaly occurring in tetralogy of Fallot, in which the aorta is displaced to the right so that it appears to arise from both ventricles and straddles the ventricular septal defect 主动脉骑跨，属于法洛四联症的先天性畸形之一，该疾病中主动脉向右移位，导致其看似同时起自两侧心室并骑跨于室间隔缺损上方

aor·ti·co·pul·mo·nary (a-or″tĭ-ko-pool′monar″e) pertaining to or lying between the aorta and pulmonary artery 属于或位于主动脉和肺动脉之间的

aor·ti·tis (a″or-ti′tis) inflammation of the aorta 主动脉炎

aor·tog·ra·phy (a″or-tog′rə-fe) radiography of the aorta after introduction into it of a contrast material 主动脉造影

aor·top·a·thy (a″or-top′ə-the) any disease of the aorta 主动脉病，主动脉的任何疾病

aor·to·plas·ty (a-or′to-plas″te) surgical repair of the aorta 主动脉成形术，主动脉修复手术

aor·tor·rha·phy (a″or-tor′ə-fe) suture of the aorta 主动脉缝合术

aor·to·scle·ro·sis (a-or″to-sklə-ro′sis) sclerosis of the aorta 主动脉硬化

aor·tot·o·my (a″or-tot′ə-me) incision of the aorta

主动脉切开术

AOS American Ophthalmological Society 美国眼科学学会; American Otological Society 美国耳科学学会

AOTA American Occupational Therapy Association 美国职业治疗协会

AP action potential 动作电位; angina pectoris 心绞痛; anterior pituitary (gland) 垂体前叶 (腺垂体); anteroposterior 前后的; arterial pressure 动脉压

APA American Pharmaceutical Association 美国制药协会; American Podiatric Association 美国足病协会; American Psychiatric Association 美国精神病学学会; American Psychological Assocation 美国心理学学会

apal·les·the·sia (ə-pal″es-the′zhə) pallanesthesia 振动觉缺失

APAP Association of Physician Assistant Programs 医师助理计划协会

apa·reu·nia (a″pə-roo′ne-ə) impossibility of sexual intercourse 性交不能症

ap·a·thy (ap′ə-the) lack of feeling or emotion 情感淡漠，缺乏感觉或情绪; indifference 冷漠。**apathet′ic** adj。

APC atrial premature complex 房性期前收缩; activated proteinC 活化蛋白 C

APD atrial premature depolarization 心房过早去极化 (见 complex 下 atrial premature complex); pamidronate 帕米膦酸二钠

apel·lous (a-pel′əs) 1. skinless 无 皮 肤 的; not covered with skin 无皮肤覆盖的; not cicatrized (said of a wound) (指伤口) 未愈合的; 2. having no prepuce 无阴茎包皮

aper·i·stal·sis (a-per″ĭ-stawl′sis) absence of usual peristalsis 蠕动停止

ap·er·tog·na·thia (ə-pur″tog-na′the-ə) open bite 开𬌗

ap·er·tu·ra (ap″ər-too′rə) pl. apertu′rae [L.] opening 口、孔

ap·er·ture (ap′ər-chər) opening 口、孔; **piriform a.**, the anterior end of the bony nasal opening, connecting the external nose with the skull 梨状孔，鼻骨开口的前端，连接外鼻和颅骨

apex (a′peks) pl. apexes, a′pices [L.] tip; the pointed end of a conical part; the top of a body, organ, or part 尖; 圆锥部分的尖端; 身体、器官或某个部分的顶部; **a. of lung,** the rounded upper extremity of either lung 肺尖，肺的钝圆上端; **root a.,** the terminal end of the root of the tooth 牙根尖，齿根的末端

apex·car·dio·gram (a″peks-kahr′de-o-gram) the record produced by apexcardiography 心尖心动图

apex·car·di·og·ra·phy (a″peks-kahr″deog′rə-fe) a method of graphically recording the pulsations of the anterior chest wall over the apex of the heart 心尖心动描记法，一种用图像记录心尖上方前胸壁搏动的方法

APHA American Public Health Association 美国公共卫生协会

APhA American Pharmacists Association 美国药剂师协会

apha·gia (ə-fa′jə) refusal or inability to swallow 吞咽不能，拒绝或无法吞咽

apha·kia (ə-fa′ke-ə) absence of the lens of an eye, occurring congenitally or as a result of trauma or surgery 无晶状体，可见于先天性畸形或创伤或手术后; **apha′cic apha′kic** adj.

apha·lan·gia (a-fə-lan′jə) absence of fingers or toes 无指 (趾) 畸形

apha·sia (ə-fa′zhə) defect or loss of the power of expression by speech, writing, or signs, or of comprehending spoken or written language, due to injury or disease of the brain centers 失语症，由于大脑中枢的损伤或疾病，语言、书写或符号表达能力的缺陷或丧失，或理解口头或书面语言能力的丧失。另见 agrammatism, dysphasia, and paraphasia; **apha′sic** adj.; **amnesic a., amnestic a.,** defective recall of specific names of objects or other words, with intact abilities of comprehension and repetition 遗忘性失语，对物体或其他词语的特定名称的记忆存在缺陷，但理解和复述能力完好; **anomic a.,** that in which recall of names is faulty 命名性失语，对名称的记忆存在缺陷; **auditory a.,** a form of receptive aphasia in which sounds are heard but convey no meaning to the mind, due to disease of the auditory center of the brain 听觉性失语，感觉性失语的一种，由于大脑听觉中枢的疾病，患者能听到声音，但却不能理解声音的内容; **Broca a.,** 见 motor a.; **conduction a.,** aphasia believed to be due to a lesion of the path between sensory and motor speech centers; spoken language is comprehended normally but words cannot be repeated correctly 传导性失语，由感觉性和运动性语言中枢之间传导通路的损伤而导致的失语症; 对口语的理解能力正常，而无法正确复述听到的内容; **expressive a.,** 见 motor a.; **fluent a.,** a type of receptive aphasia in which speech is well articulated and grammatically correct but is lacking in content 流利性失语，感觉性失语的一种，其患者说话时表述清晰，语法正确，但缺少实际内容; **global a.,** total aphasia involving all the functions involved in speech or communication 完全性失语，语言或交流中涉及的所有能力全部丧失; **jargon a.,** that with utterance of meaningless phrases, either neologisms or incoherently arranged known words 杂乱性失语，混杂新词或语无伦次的词语组合，讲话内容为大量无意义的短语; **mixed a.,** 见 global a.;

motor a., Broca or nonfluent aphasia; that in which the ability to speak and write is impaired, due to a lesion in the insula and surrounding operculum 运动性失语，Broca 失语或非流利性失语；由于脑岛及其周围岛盖的病变，患者说话和书写能力受损；**nominal a.**，见 anomic a.；**nonfluent a.**，见 motor a.；**receptive a.**, inability to understand written, spoken, or tactile speech symbols, due to disease of the auditory and visual word centers 感觉性失语，由于听觉和视觉语言中枢的病变，无法理解书面、口头或触觉语言符号；**sensory a.**，见 receptive a.；**total a.**，见 global a.；**visual a.**, alexia 失读症；**Wernicke a.**, receptive a. 感觉性失语

apha·si·ol·o·gy (ə-fa″ze-ol′ə-je) the scientific study of aphasia and the specific neurologic lesions producing it 失语症学，研究失语症及导致失语症的神经系统病变的学科

aph·e·re·sis (af-ə-re′sis) withdrawal of blood from a donor, with a portion (plasma, leukocytes, platelets, etc.) being separated and retained and the remainder retransfused into the donor. It includes leukapheresis, plasmapheresis, thrombocytapheresis, etc 分离性输血，从献血者体内抽取血液，将其中一部分（血浆、白细胞、血小板等）分离并保留，其余部分再回输至献血者体内。分离性输血包括白细胞提取法、血浆置换、血小板提取法等

APHL Association of Public Health Laboratories 公共卫生实验室协会

apho·nia (a-fo′ne-ə) loss of voice; inability to produce vocal sounds 失声，发音不能

aphot·ic (a-fot′ik) without light; totally dark 无光的，完全黑暗的

aphra·sia (ə-fra′zhə) inability to speak 组句不能

aph·ro·dis·iac (af″ro-diz′e-ak) 1. arousing sexual desire 激发性欲的；2. a drug that arouses sexual desire 催欲药

aph·tha (af′thə) pl. **aph′thae** [L.] a small ulcer, such as the round lesion with a grayish exudate surrounded by a red halo in recurrent aphthous stomatitis 口疮，一种小溃疡，例如复发性阿弗他口炎中的圆形病变，伴有灰色渗出物，病灶周围带有红色晕圈；**Bednar aphthae,** symmetric excoriation of the posterior hard palate in infants Badnar 口疮，婴儿硬腭后部的对称性表皮剥脱；**contagious aphthae,** foot-and-mouth disease 口蹄疫

aph·tho·sis (af-tho′sis) a condition marked by the presence of aphthae 口疮病

aph·thous (af′thəs) pertaining to, characterized by, or affected with aphthae 口疮的，以口疮为特征的，受口疮影响的

Aph·tho·vi·rus (af′tho-vi″rəs) a genus of viruses of the family Picornaviridae that cause foot-and-mouth disease 口蹄疫病毒，可引起口蹄疫的微小病毒

科的一个属支

ap·i·cal (ap′ĭ-kəl) pertaining to or located at an apex 属于或位于顶点的

ap·i·ca·lis (ap″ĭ-ka′lis) [L.] apical 属于或位于顶点的

api·cec·to·my (a″pĭ-sek′tə-me) excision of the apex of the petrous portion of the temporal bone 岩尖切除术，颞骨岩部尖部切除术

api·ci·tis (a″pĭ-si′tis) inflammation of an apex, of the lung or the root of a tooth 根尖炎，肺尖或牙根尖炎症

api·co·ec·to·my (a″pĭ-ko-ek′tə-me) excision of the apical portion of the root of a tooth through an opening in overlying tissues of the jaw 根尖切除术，通过下颌骨组织上的开口切除牙根的顶端部分

a·pix·a·ban (ŭ-pix′-ŭ-băn) a factor Xa inhibitor used for the prevention of thrombosis; administered orally 阿哌沙班，凝血因子 Xa 抑制剂，用于预防血栓形成，通常口服

ap·la·nat·ic (ap″lə-nat′ik) correcting spherical aberration, as an aplanatic lens 等光程的，消球面差的

apla·sia (ə-pla′zhə) lack of development of an organ or tissue（器官或组织）发育不全，先天萎缩；**aplas′tic** adj.；**a. cu′tis conge′nita,** localized failure of development of skin, most commonly of the scalp; the defects are usually covered by a thin translucent membrane or scar tissue, or may be raw, ulcerated, or covered by granulation tissue; usually lethal 先天性皮肤发育不全，局部皮肤发育不全，最常见于头皮；此类缺陷常由薄透明膜、瘢痕组织覆盖，亦可能表现为破损的、溃烂的、或由肉芽组织覆盖；该疾病通常可致死

APLS antiphospholipid antibody syndrome 抗磷脂抗体综合征

ap·nea (ap′ne-ə) cessation of breathing 呼吸暂停，窒息；**apne′ic** adj.；**central sleep a.,** sleep apnea from failure of stimulation by medullary respiratory centers 中枢性睡眠呼吸暂停，髓质呼吸中枢无法正常刺激呼吸运动导致的呼吸暂停；**obstructive sleep a.,** sleep apnea from collapse or obstruction of the airway during sleep, such as in the obese 阻塞性呼吸暂停，睡眠期间气道塌陷或阻塞导致的呼吸暂停，可见于肥胖患者；**sleep a.,** transient attacks of apnea during sleep, resulting in acidosis and pulmonary arteriolar vasoconstriction and hypertension 睡眠呼吸暂停，睡眠期间呼吸暂停的短暂发作，可导致酸中毒和肺小动脉收缩及肺动脉高压

ap·neu·sis (ap-noo′sis) sustained effort for inhalation unrelieved by exhalation 长吸式呼吸，持续吸气且不因呼气而缓解；**apneu′stic** adj.

apo·chro·mat (ap″o-kro′mat) an apochromatic objective 复消色差物镜

apo·chro·mat·ic (ap″o-kro-mat′ik) free from chromatic and spherical aberrations 无色差和球面像差的

apo·crine (ap′o-krin) exhibiting that type of glandular secretion in which the free end of the secreting cell is cast off along with the secretory products accumulated therein (e.g., mammary and sweat glands) 顶浆分泌的，一种腺体分泌方式，该方式中分泌细胞的游离端与其内积累的分泌产物一同脱落（如乳腺细胞，汗腺细胞）

apo·en·zyme (ap″o-en′zīm) the protein component of an enzyme separable from the prosthetic group (coenzyme) but requiring the presence of the prosthetic group to form the functioning compound (holoenzyme) 酶蛋白/脱辅基酶蛋白，酶的蛋白质组分，可从辅基（辅酶）中分离出来，但需要辅基的存在才能形成具有功能的化合物（全酶）

ap·o·fer·ri·tin (ap″o-fer′ĭ-tin) an apoprotein that can bind many atoms of iron per molecule, forming ferritin, the intracellular storage form of iron 脱铁铁蛋白，一种载脂蛋白，每分子脱铁铁蛋白可结合许多铁原子形成铁蛋白，铁蛋白即铁在细胞内的储存形式

apo·lar (a-po′lər) having neither poles nor processes; without polarity 无极的，无突的，无极性的

apo·lipo·pro·tein (ap″o-lip″o-pro′tēn) any of the protein constituents of lipoproteins, grouped by function in four classes, A, B, C, and E 载脂蛋白，脂蛋白的一种蛋白质组分，按功能划分为 4 类 A、B、C 和 E

ap·o·neu·ror·rha·phy (ap″o-noo-ror′ə-fe) suture of an aponeurosis 腱膜缝合术

ap·o·neu·ro·sis (ap″o-noo-ro′sis) pl. *aponeuro'ses* [Gr.] a sheetlike tendinous expansion, mainly serving to connect a muscle with the parts it moves 腱膜，腱片状扩张结构，主要用于连接肌肉及其带动运动的部分；**aponeurot′ic** *adj.*；**extensor a.**, 伸肌腱膜，见 *expansion* 下词条；**apoph·y·sis** (ə-pof′ə-sis) pl. *apoph'yses* [Gr.] any outgrowth or swelling, especially a bony outgrowth that has never been entirely separated from the bone of which it forms a part, such as a process, tubercle, or tuber 骨突，任何外生结构或肿胀，尤指未和骨骼完全分离的外生骨赘，其可形成一个突起、结节或隆起；**apophys′eal** *adj.*

apoph·y·si·tis (ə-pof″ə-si′tis) inflammation of an apophysis 骨突炎；**traction a.**, damage to an apophysis caused by chronic traction of a tendon at its insertion, occurring commonly during periods of rapid growth in childhood and adolescence 牵引性骨突炎，肌腱插入时长时间牵引导致的骨突损伤，常见于儿童和青少年的快速生长时期

ap·o·plec·ti·form (ap″o-plek′tĭ-form) resembling apoplexy 卒中样的，类中风的

ap·o·plexy (ap′o-plek″se) stroke syndrome 卒中，中风；**adrenal a.**, sudden massive hemorrhage into the adrenal (suprarenal) gland, occurring in Waterhouse-Friderichsen syndrome 肾上腺卒中，肾上腺突发大量出血，可见于沃 - 弗综合征

apo·pro·tein (ap″o-pro′tēn) the protein moiety of a molecule or complex, as of a lipoprotein 脱辅基蛋白，分子或复合物的蛋白质部分，例如脂蛋白中的载脂蛋白

ap·op·to·sis (ap″op-to′sis) (ap″o-to′sis) a pattern of cell death affecting single cells, marked by shrinkage of the cell, condensation of chromatin, and fragmentation of the cell into membrane-bound bodies that are eliminated by phagocytosis. Often used synonymously with *programmed cell death* 凋亡，一种影响单细胞的细胞死亡模式，其特征是细胞收缩、染色质凝集、细胞碎裂成膜结合体，后通过吞噬作用消除。常与"程序性细胞死亡"同义；**apoptot′ic** *adj.*

apo·re·pres·sor (ap″o-re-pres′ər) an inactive form of a repressor, requiring binding of a corepressor to become a functional repressor 辅阻遏蛋白，阻遏物的非活性形式，需要与辅阻遏物结合才能形成功能性阻遏物

apoth·e·cary (ə-poth′ə-kar″e) pharmacist 药剂师

APP abdominal perfusion pressure 腹腔灌注压；amyloid precursor protein 淀粉样前体蛋白

ap·pa·ra·tus (ap″ə-rā′təs) pl.*appara'tus, apparatuses* [L.] a number of parts acting together to perform a special function 仪器，设备，许多部件共同工作以实现某个特殊的功能；**branchial a.**, 见 pharyngeal a.；**Golgi a.**, 高尔基体，见 *complex* 下词条；**juxtaglomerular a.**, 肾小球旁器，见 *cell* 下词条；**Kirschner a.**, a wire and stirrup apparatus for applying skeletal traction in leg fractures 克氏针，一种用于腿部骨折患者骨骼牵引的钢丝和马镫形装置；**lacrimal a., a. lacrima′lis**, the lacrimal gland and ducts and associated structures 泪器，泪腺、导管及相关结构；**pharyngeal a.**, the pharyngeal arches, pouches, and grooves considered as a unit 咽器，鳃弓、鳃囊及鳃槽等的总称；**subneural a.**, 见 *cleft* 下词条；**vestibular a.**, the structures of the inner ear concerned with stimuli of equilibrium, including the semicircular canals, saccule, and utricle 前庭器，内耳结构中与平衡有关的部分，包括半规管、球囊和椭圆囊

ap·pen·dage (ə-pen′dəj) a subordinate portion of a structure, or an outgrowth, such as a tail 附属物，某结构的从属部分或外生物，例如尾巴；**epiploic a's**, 肠脂垂，见 *appendix* 下词条；**a's of eye**, adnexa oculi 眼附属器；**skin a's**, the hair, nails, sebaceous glands, sweat glands, and mammary glands 皮肤附属器，包括毛发、指（趾）甲、皮脂腺、汗腺和乳腺；**uterine a's**, the ovaries, uterine tubes, and uterine ligaments 子宫附件，包括卵巢、输卵管和子宫韧带

ap·pen·dec·to·my (ap″en-dek′tə-me) excision of the vermiform appendix 阑尾切除术

ap·pen·dic·e·al (ap″en-dis′e-əl) pertaining to an appendix 阑尾的，属于阑尾的

ap·pen·di·ci·tis (ə-pen″dĭ-si′tis) inflammation of the vermiform appendix 阑尾炎；**acute a.**, appendicitis of acute onset, requiring prompt surgery, and usually marked by pain in the right lower abdominal quadrant, referred rebound tenderness, overlying muscle spasm, and cutaneous hyperesthesia 急性阑尾炎，阑尾炎急性发作通常需要立即手术，该疾病特点常包括右下腹疼痛、压痛、反跳痛、肌肉痉挛和皮肤感觉过敏；**chronic a.**, 慢性阑尾炎；1. that characterized by fibrotic thickening of the organ wall due to previous acute inflammation 由于既往急性阑尾炎导致的器官外壁纤维化增厚 2. formerly, chronic or recurrent pain in the appendiceal area, without evidence of acute inflammation. 阑尾区既往存在慢性或反复性疼痛，无明显急性阑尾炎征象；**fulminating a.**, that marked by sudden onset and usually death 暴发性阑尾炎，该疾病特点包括突然发作和常可致死；**gangrenous a.**, that complicated by gangrene of the organ, due to interference of blood supply 坏疽性阑尾炎，阑尾炎并发血供受阻导致的器官坏疽；**obstructive a.**, a common form with obstruction of the lumen, usually by a fecalith 梗阻性阑尾炎，伴有阑尾腔内阻塞的阑尾炎，常由粪石引起

ap·pen·di·cos·to·my (ə-pen″dĭ-kos′tə-me) surgical creation of an opening into the vermiform appendix to irrigate or drain the large bowel 阑尾造口术，利用外科手术的方式在阑尾腔体开口以便冲洗肠道或引流肠内容物

ap·pen·di·co·ves·i·cos·to·my (ə-pen″dĭko-ves″ĭkos′tə-me) surgical transference of the isolated appendix so that it can be used as a conduit for urinary diversion from the bladder to the skin in children with cloacal exstrophy or neurogenic bladder, making a route for insertion of a catheter 可控制阑尾输出道尿流改道术，将阑尾作为尿流改道、尿液自膀胱到体表皮肤的输出道，从而创建出可插入尿管的通道，该术式用于患有泄殖腔外翻或神经源性膀胱的患儿

ap·pen·dic·u·lar (ap″en-dik′u-lər) 1. pertaining to the vermiform appendix 阑尾的；2. pertaining to an appendage 附件的，附属的

ap·pen·dix (ə-pen′diks) pl. *appen′dices, appen′dixes* [L.] 1. a supplementary, accessory, or dependent part attached to a main structure 附件；2. 见 vermiform a.；**epiploic appendices**, small peritoneum-covered tabs of fat attached in rows along the taeniae coli 肠脂垂，由腹膜覆盖的小块脂肪沿结肠带成行排列；**vermiform a.**, a wormlike diverticulum of the cecum 阑尾，盲肠的虫样憩室

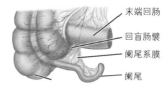

末端回肠
回盲肠襞
阑尾系膜
阑尾

▲ 阑尾（**vermiform appendix**) 及其邻近结构

ap·per·cep·tion (ap″ər-sep′shən) the process of receiving, appreciating, and interpreting sensory impressions 接收、欣赏和理解感官印象的过程

ap·pe·stat (ap′ə-stat) the brain center (probably in the hypothalamus) concerned with controlling the appetite 食欲中枢，负责控制食欲的大脑中枢（可能位于下丘脑）

ap·pla·na·tion (ap″lə-na′shən) undue flatness, as of the cornea （过度）扁平，例如角膜扁平

ap·pla·nom·e·ter (ap″lə-nom′ĕ-tər) applanation tonometer 压平式眼压计

ap·pli·ance (ə-pli′əns) in dentistry, a device used to provide a function or therapeutic effect 装置，矫正器，牙科中用于提供某种特殊功能或治疗效果的装置；**fixed a.**, one attached to the teeth by cement or an adhesive material 固定矫治器，用粘固剂或粘合材料固定于牙齿上的矫正器；**orthodontic a.**, braces; an appliance either fixed to the teeth or removable, that applies force to the teeth and their supporting structures to produce changes in their relationship to each other and to control their growth and development 正畸矫治器，一种可固定或可拆卸的牙齿矫正器，可向牙齿及其支撑结构施力，以改变其位置关系并控制其生长发育

ap·po·si·tion (ap″ə-zish′ən) juxtaposition; the placing of things in proximity; specifically, the deposition of successive layers upon those already present, as in cell walls 并置，并列；接合，对合，对位；外积，外加，在原有层次上逐层连续累积，如细胞壁中；**apposi′tional** *adj.*

ap·pre·hen·sion (ap″re-hen′shən) 1. perception and understanding 感知和理解；2. anticipatory fear or anxiety 预期的恐惧或焦虑

ap·proach (ə-prōch′) in surgery, the specific procedures by which an organ or part is exposed 进路，外科手术中暴露某个器官或部位的特殊解剖步骤

ap·prox·i·ma·tion (ə-prok″sĭ-ma′shən) 1. the act

or process of bringing into proximity or apposition 接近，逼近，使……接近的过程；2. a numerical value of limited accuracy 近似值

ap·ra·clon·i·dine (ap″rə-klon′ĭ-dēn) an α₂-adrenergic receptor agonist used as the hydrochloride salt to reduce intraocular pressure in the treatment of open-angle glaucoma and ocular hypertension 阿可乐定，一种 α₂ 受体激动剂，其盐酸盐形式可用于开角型青光眼和高眼压症患者降低眼内压

aprac·tag·no·sia (ə-prak″tag-no′zhə) a type of agnosia marked by inability to use objects or perform skilled motor activities 空间关系失认症，失认症的一种，其特征是无法使用物件或进行熟练的运动活动

aprax·ia (ə-prak′se-ə) loss of ability to carry out familiar purposeful movements in the absence of motor or sensory impairment, especially inability to use objects correctly 失用症，在无运动或感觉系统损伤的情况下，无法进行熟悉的有目的的运动，尤其是无法正确使用物件；**amnestic a.,** loss of ability to carry out a movement on command due to inability to remember the command 遗忘性失用症，由于无法记住命令而表现为丧失按照命令进行动作的能力；**Cogan oculomotor a., congenital oculomotor a.,** an absence or defect of horizontal eye movements so that the head must turn and the eyes exhibit nystagmus in attempts to see an object off to one side 先天性动眼神经失用症，眼球水平运动的缺失或缺陷，使得眼睛在试图看向一侧物体时头部必须转动且出现眼球震颤；**gait a., a. of gait,** a disorder of gait and equilibrium caused by a lesion in the frontal lobe, commonly seen in elderly persons and those with Alzheimer disease; the person walks with a broad-based gait, taking short steps and placing the feet flat on the ground 步态失用症，额叶病变导致的步态和平衡紊乱，常见于老年人和阿尔茨海默症患者；此类患者走路时双腿间距较宽，步幅较小，拖步行走，双脚着地困难；**ideational a.,** 见 sensory a.；**motor a.,** impairment of skilled movements not explained by weakness of the affected parts, the patient appearing clumsy rather than weak 运动性失用症，不能以受损肢体的虚弱的能力受损，且该症状不能以受损肢体的虚弱来解释，患者表现为笨拙而非虚弱；**sensory a.,** loss of ability to use an object due to lack of perception of its purpose 观念性失用症，感觉性失用症，由于对物体的用途缺乏认知而导致丧失使用该物体的能力

ap·ro·bar·bi·tal (ap″ro-bahr′bĭ-təl) an intermediate-acting barbiturate, used as a sedative and hypnotic 烯丙异丙巴比妥，一种中效巴妥酸盐，可用作镇静剂和催眠药

apro·ti·nin (ap″ro-ti′nin) an inhibitor of proteo-lytic enzymes used to reduce perioperative blood loss in patients undergoing cardiopulmonary bypass during coronary artery bypass graft 抑肽酶，一种蛋白水解酶抑制剂，用于减少冠状动脉旁路移植术患者围术期失血

APS American Pain Society 美国疼痛学会；American Physiological Society 美国生理学学会

APSF Anesthesia Patient Safety Foundation 麻醉患者安全基金会

APTA American Physical Therapy Association 美国物理治疗协会

APTT aPTT activated partial thromboplastin time 活化部分凝血活酶时间

ap·ty·a·lism (ap-ti′ə-liz-əm) deficiency or absence of saliva 唾液缺乏

APUD [*a*mine *p*recursor *u*ptake (and) *d*ecarboxylation] 胺前体吸收（和）脱羧，见 cell 下词条

apud·o·ma (a″pəd-o′mə) a tumor derived from APUD cells 胺前体摄取脱羧细胞瘤，起源自胺前体吸收（和）脱羧细胞的肿瘤

apy·ret·ic (a″pi-ret′ik) afebrile 无热的，不发热的

apy·rex·ia (a″pi-rek′se-ə) absence of fever. 无热期，热歇期

AQ achievement quotient 成就商数

Aq. dest. [L.] a′qua destilla′ta (distilled water) 同 a′qua destilla′ta 蒸馏水

aq·ua (ah′kwə) (ak′wə) [L.] water 水

aq·ua·pho·bia (ak″wə-fo′be-ə) irrational fear of water 恐水症，病态恐水

aqua·po·rin (ak″wə-po′rin) any of a family of proteins found in the plasma membrane that permit passage of water and very small solutes 水通道蛋白，水孔蛋白。该蛋白属于位于细胞膜上的一个蛋白家族，其作用是允许水分子和非常小的溶质分子通过。又称 *water channel*

aq·ue·duct (ak′wə-dukt″) any canal or passage 导管，水管，沟渠；**cerebral a.,** a narrow channel in the midbrain connecting the third and fourth ventricles 中脑水管，中脑中连接第三脑室和第四脑室的狭窄通道；**cochlear a.,** a small canal that interconnects the scala tympani with the subarachnoid space 蜗水管，连接鼓阶和蛛网膜下腔的细小管道；**a. of Sylvius, ventricular a.,** 见 cerebral a.

aque·ous (a′kwe-əs) 1. watery 水 的；prepared with water 用水制备的；2. 见 *humor* 下词条

AR alarm reaction 警戒反应；aortic regurgitation 主动脉瓣返流；artificial respiration 人工呼吸

Ar argon 氩

ARA anorectal angle 肛直角

ara-A adenine arabinoside 阿糖腺苷；见 *vidarabine*

ara-C cytarabine 阿糖胞苷

arach·ic ac·id (ə-rak′ik) arachidic acid 花生酸

ar·a·chid·ic ac·id (ar″ə-kid′ik) a saturated 20-carbon fatty acid occurring in peanut and other vegetable oils and fish oils 花生酸，一种饱和 20 碳脂肪酸，存在于花生及其他植物油、鱼油中

arach·i·don·ic ac·id (ə-rak″ĭ-don′ik) a polyunsaturated 20-carbon essential fatty acid occurring in animal fats and formed by biosynthesis from linoleic acid; it is a precursor to leukotrienes, prostaglandins, and thromboxane 花生四烯酸，一种多不饱和 20 碳必需脂肪酸，存在于动物脂肪中，由亚油酸经生物合成形成；该物质是白三烯、前列腺素和血栓素等的前体

Arach·ni·da (ə-rak′nĭ-də) a class of the Arthropoda, including the spiders, scorpions, ticks, and mites 蛛形纲，节肢动物门下的一纲，包括蜘蛛、蝎子、蜱和螨等

arach·no·dac·ty·ly (ə-rak″no-dak′tə-le) extreme length and slenderness of fingers and toes 蜘蛛样指（趾），趾指细长

arach·noid (ə-rak′noid) 1. resembling a spider's web 蛛网样的；2. a delicate membrane interposed between the dura mater and the pia mater, separated from the latter by the subarachnoid space 蛛网膜，硬脑（嵴）膜和软脑（嵴）膜之间的一层薄膜，蛛网膜与软脑（嵴）膜分离，其间形成蛛网膜下腔；**a. mater**, 蛛网膜，见 arachnoid (2)

arach·noi·dal (ar″ak-noi′dəl) pertaining to the arachnoid 蛛网膜的

arach·noi·dea ma·ter (ar″ak-noi′de-ə ma′tər) (mah′tcr) 蛛网膜，见 arachnoid (2)

arach·noid·i·tis (ə-rak″noid-i′tis) inflammation of the arachnoidea mater 蛛网膜炎

arach·no·pho·bia (ə-rak″no-fo′be-ə) irrational fear of spiders 蜘蛛恐惧症，对蜘蛛的病态性恐惧

ar·bor (ahr′bər) pl. **ar′bores** [L.] a treelike structure or part 树状结构或部分；**a. vi′tae**, 1. (of cerebellum) treelike outlines seen in a median section of the cerebellum 小脑活树，小脑中间部分的一种树状轮廓；2. (of uterus) palmate folds（子宫）棕榈襞；3. the tree *Thuja occidentalis*; its leafy twigs contain the medicinal substance thuja but can be poisonous 侧柏树；其多叶的枝条含有药用物质侧柏，但其可能具有毒性

ar·bo·res·cent (ahr″bə-res′ənt) branching like a tree 树样分支的

ar·bo·ri·za·tion (ahr″bə-rī-za′shən) a collection of branches, as the branching terminus of a nerve-cell process（树状）分支，如神经细胞胞突的分支末梢

ar·bo·vi·rus (ahr′bo-vi″rəs) a term used by epidemiologists to refer to any of numerous viruses that replicate in blood-feeding arthropods such as mosquitoes and ticks and are transmitted to humans by biting 虫媒病毒，流行病学术语，指在蚊子和蜱虫等吸血节肢动物中复制并通过叮咬传播人类的众多病毒中的任何一种；**arbovi′ral** *adj.*

ar·but·amine (ahr-bu′tə-mēn″) a synthetic catecholamine used as a diagnostic aid in cardiac stress testing in patients unable to exercise sufficiently for the test; administered as the hydrochloride salt 阿布他明，一种合成儿茶酚胺，用于心脏负荷试验中无法负荷该运动量的患者的辅助诊断，所用药物为其盐酸盐形式

ARC AIDS-related complex 艾滋病相关综合征；American Red Cross 美国红十字会；anomalous retinal correspondence 异常视网膜对应

arc (ahrk) 1. a structure or projected path having a curved outline 弧；2. a visible electrical discharge taking the outline of an arc 电弧；3. in neurophysiology, the pathway of neural reactions 神经生物学中神经反应的路径；**reflex a.**, the neural arc used in a reflex action; an impulse travels centrally over afferent fibers to a nerve center, and the response travels outward to an effector organ or part over efferent fibers 反射弧，冲动通过传入纤维集中传递至神经中枢，而产生的反应信息通过传出纤维向外传递至效应器官或组织

ARCA American Rehabilitation Counseling Association 美国康复咨询协会

Ar·ca·no·bac·te·ri·um (ahr-ka″no-baktēr′e-əm) a genus of rod-shaped, gram-positive bacteria of the family Actinomycetaceae. *A. haemoly′ticus* causes human infection, characterized in adolescents by pharyngitis and a scarlatiniform rash 隐秘杆菌属，放线菌科下的一个杆状革兰阳性菌属。溶血隐秘杆菌可导致人类感染，多表现为青少年咽炎和猩红热

ARCD alcohol-related cognitive disorder 酒精相关认知障碍

arch (ahrch) a structure of bowlike or curved outline 弓，曲线形或弧形的结构；**a. of aorta**, the curving portion between the ascending aorta and the descending aorta, giving rise to the brachiocephalic trunk, the left common carotid artery, and the left subclavian artery 主动脉弓，升主动脉和降主动脉之间的弯曲部分，其上发出头臂干、左颈总动脉和左锁骨下动脉；**aortic a.**, 1. a. of aorta 主动脉弓；2. any of a group of paired vessels arching from the ventral to the dorsal aorta through the branchial arches of fishes and the pharyngeal arches of amniote embryos. In mammalian development, arches 1 and 2 disappear; 3 joins the common to the internal carotid artery; 4 becomes the arch of the aorta and joins the aorta and subclavian artery; 5 disappears; 6 forms the pulmonary arteries and, until birth, the ductus arteriosus 动脉弓，动脉弧，任何一组由腹主动脉经鱼类鳃弓和脊椎动物胚胎咽弓到背主动脉的成对血管。

在哺乳动物的发育过程中，弓Ⅰ和弓Ⅱ消失；弓Ⅲ连接颈总动脉和颈内动脉；弓Ⅳ形成主动脉弓，连接主动脉和锁骨下动脉；弓Ⅴ消失；弓Ⅵ形成肺动脉和出生之前的动脉导管；**branchial a's,** paired arched columns that bear the gills in lower aquatic vertebrates and which, in embryos of higher vertebrates, become modified into structures of the head and neck. In human embryos, called *pharyngeal a's* 鳃弓，成对的柱状弓形隆起，在低等水生脊柱动物中具有鳃，在高等脊椎动物的胚胎中，参与颜面和颈部构成；**cervical aortic a.,** a rare anomaly in which the aortic arch has an unusually superior location 颈位主动脉弓，一种主动脉弓异常高位的罕见异常；**dental a.,** the curving structure formed by the teeth in their normal position; the *inferior dental a.* is formed by the mandibular teeth, the *superior dental a.* by the maxillary teeth 牙弓，牙齿位于正常结构时排列形成的弧形结构称为牙弓；下颌牙形成下牙弓，上颌牙形成上牙弓；**double aortic a.,** a congenital anomaly in which the aorta divides into two branches that embrace the trachea and esophagus and reunite to form the descending aorta 双主动脉弓，一种先天发育异常，主动脉分成两大分支，行经器官和食管后重新汇合形成降主动脉；**a's of foot,** the longitudinal and transverse arches of the foot 足弓，足的纵弓和横弓；**lingual a.,** a wire appliance that conforms to the lingual aspect of the dental arch, used to promote or prevent movement of the teeth in orthodontic work 舌弓，一种遵照牙弓舌侧制定的钢丝器具，用于正畸中促进或防止牙齿移动；**mandibular a.,** 1. the first pharyngeal arch, from which are developed the bone of the lower jaw, malleus, and incus 第一咽弓，由此发育形成下颌骨、锤骨和砧骨；2. inferior dental a. 下颌弓；**maxillary a.,** 1. 见 palatal a. 2. superior dental a. 上颌弓；见 *dental a.*；**neural a.,** the primordium of the vertebral arch; one of the cartilaginous structures surrounding the embryonic spinal cord 神经弓，椎弓的始基，环绕胚胎脊髓的软骨结构之一；**open pubic a.,** a congenital anomaly in which the pubic arch is not fused, the bodies of the pubic bones being spread apart 开放性耻骨弓，耻骨弓未融合、耻骨体分离的先天畸形；**oral a.,** one formed by the roof of the mouth from the teeth (or residual dental arch) on one side to those on the other 口弓，硬腭弓，由口腔顶部形成的自一侧牙齿（或牙残弓）至另一侧牙齿的弓形结构；**palatal a.,** the arch formed by the roof of the mouth from the teeth on one side of the maxilla to the teeth on the other or, if the teeth are missing, from the residual dental arch on one side to that on the other 硬腭弓，由口腔顶部形成的自上颌牙（或牙齿缺失后的牙残弓）至另一侧牙齿（或牙残弓）的弓形结构；**palatoglossal a.,** the anterior of the two folds of mucous membrane on either side of the oropharynx, enclosing the palatoglossal muscle 腭舌弓，口咽两侧黏膜皱襞的前部，其上附有腭舌

肌；**palatopharyngeal a.,** the posterior of the two folds of mucous membrane on either side of the oropharynx, enclosing the palatopharyngeal muscle 腭咽弓，口咽两侧黏膜皱襞的后部，其上附有腭咽肌；**palmar a's,** four arches in the palm: the *deep palmar arterial a.* formed by anastomosis of the terminal part of the radial artery with the deep branch of the ulnar, its accompanying *deep venous palmar a.,* and the *superficial palmar arterial a.* formed by anastomosis of the terminal part of the ulnar artery with the superficial palmar branch of the radial and its accompanying *superficial venous palmar a.* 掌弓，手掌有四条弓：掌深弓由桡动脉终末支和尺动脉的掌深支吻合形成，其伴行掌深静脉弓；掌浅动脉弓由尺动脉终末支和桡动脉掌浅支吻合形成，伴行掌浅静脉弓；**pharyngeal a's,** the branchial arches in the human embryo 鳃弓，咽弓；**plantar a.,** 1. the arch in the foot formed by anastomosis of the lateral plantar artery with the deep plantar branch of the dorsal artery 足底外侧动脉和足背动脉足底深支吻合形成的足底动脉弓；2. the deep venous arch that accompanies the plantar arterial arch 伴行足底动脉弓的足底深静脉弓；3. the hollow on the sole of the foot 足弓，足底凹陷；**pubic a.,** the arch formed by the conjoined rami of the ischial and pubic bones on two sides of the body 耻骨弓，由两侧坐骨和耻骨的连接支构成；**pulmonary a's,** the most caudal of the aortic arches; they become the pulmonary arteries 肺动脉弓，主动脉弓的最尾部；后形成肺动脉；**residual dental a.,** the curved contour of the ridge remaining after tooth removal 牙残弓，剩余牙槽嵴弓，去除牙齿后剩余牙槽嵴形成的曲线轮廓；**right aortic a.,** a congenital anomaly in which the aorta is displaced to the right and passes behind the esophagus, thus forming a vascular ring that may cause compression of the trachea and esophagus 右位主动脉弓，一种先天性畸形，主动脉移位至右侧并行经食管后方，从而形成一个血管环，可能导致压迫气管和食管；**supraorbital a.,** the curved margin of the frontal bone forming the upper boundary of the orbit 眶上弓，额骨的弯曲边缘形成的眶上边界；**tarsal a's,** two arches of the median palpebral artery, one of which supplies the upper eyelid, the other the lower 睑动脉弓，睑正中动脉的两个血管弓，其一供应上眼睑，另一者供应下眼睑；**tendinous a.,** a linear thickening of fascia over some part of a muscle 腱弓，在肌肉某处的线状筋膜增厚；**vertebral a.,** the bony arch on the posterior aspect of a vertebra, composed of the laminae and pedicles 椎弓，脊椎后部的骨弓，由椎板和椎弓根构成；**zygomatic a.,** one formed by processes of zygomatic and temporal bones 颧（骨）弓，由颧骨和颞骨的突出部分构成

Ar·chaea (ahr-ke′ə) one of the two large divisions into which prokaryotes are grouped; they are genetically distinct from the Bacteria, most live in extreme environments, and none are human pathogens 古细菌，原核生物的两大分支之一；它们在基因上与细菌不同，大多生活于极端环境中，其中没有可感染人类的病原体

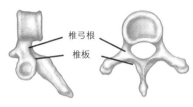

▲ 椎弓（vertebral arch），由一对椎弓根和一对椎板组成

ar·chaeo·cer·e·bel·lum (ahr″ke-o-ser″ə-bel′əm) archicerebellum 古小脑，原小脑

ar·chaeo·cor·tex (ahr″ke-o-kor′teks) archicortex 古皮质，原皮质

arch·en·ceph·a·lon (ahrk″ən-sef′ə-lon) the primordial brain from which the midbrain and forebrain develop 原脑，发育为中脑和前脑的原始大脑

arch·en·ter·on (ahrk-en′tər-on) the primordial digestive cavity of those embryonic forms whose blastula becomes a gastrula by invagination 原肠，胚胎时期的原始消化腔，胚胎的囊胚通过内陷变成胃腔

ar·che·type (ahr′kə-tīp) an ideal, original, or standard type or form 原型，原始型，一种理想的、原始的或标准的类型或形式

ar·chi·cer·e·bel·lum (ahr″kĭ-ser″ə-bel′əm) the phylogenetically old part of the cerebellum, viz., the flocculonodular node and the lingula 古小脑，原小脑，小脑系统进化上出现最早的部分，即绒球小结和小舌

ar·chi·cor·tex (ahr″kĭ-kor′teks) that part of the cerebral cortex (pallium) that with the paleocortex develops in association with the olfactory system and is phylogenetically older than the neocortex and lacks its layered structure 原皮质，古皮质。古皮质和旧皮质的发育均与嗅觉系统相关，这两者在种系发生上较新皮质古老，且缺乏分层结构。

ar·chi·neph·ron (ahr″kĭ-nef′ron) a unit of the pronephros 原肾，前肾的一个单位

ar·chi·pal·li·um (ahr″kĭ-pal′e-əm) archicortex 原皮质，古皮质

ar·ci·form (ahr′sĭ-form) arcuate 弓形的，弓状的

Arc·to·staph·y·los (ahrk″to-staf′ə-lōs) a genus of North American evergreens; A. uva-ur′si is uva ursi (q.v.) 熊果属，北美常绿植物的属支之一；熊果

ar·cu·ate (ahr′ku-āt) arc-shaped; arranged in arches 弓形的；弓状排列的

ar·cu·a·tion (ahr-ku-a′shən) a curvature, especially an abnormal curvature 曲线，弯曲，尤指异常的曲线

ar·cus (ahr′kəs) pl. 复 数 形 式 *ar′cus* [L.] arch; bow 弓；**a. aor′tae**, aortic arch 主 动 脉 弓；**a. cor′neae, a. juveni′lis, a. seni′lis**, a white or gray opaque ring in the margin of the cornea, sometimes present at birth, but usually occurring bilaterally in persons of 50 years or older as a result of cholesterol deposits in or hyalinosis of the corneal stroma 角膜弓／老人环，青年环，老年环。角膜边缘的白色或灰色的不透明环，部分患者出生时即存在此现象，但其通常发生于50岁以上人群，且多为双侧出现，该现象是由于胆固醇沉积于角膜基质或角膜基质透明变性

ar·de·par·in (ahr-de-par′in) a low-molecular-weight heparin used as the sodium salt in the prophylaxis of deep vein thrombosis and pulmonary thromboembolism after knee replacement surgery 阿地肝素，一种低分子肝素，其钠盐形式用于膝关节置换术后预防深静脉血栓形成和肺血栓栓塞

ARDMS American Registry of Diagnostic Medical Sonographers 美国注册诊断医疗超声医师协会

ARDS acute respiratory distress syndrome 急性呼吸窘迫综合征；adult respiratory distress syndrome 成人呼吸窘迫综合征

ar·ea (ār′e-ə) pl. *a′reae, areas* [L.] a limited space; in anatomy, a specific surface or functional region 有限的空间；解剖学中特定的表面或功能区域；**association a's**, areas of the cerebral cortex (excluding primary areas) connected with each other and with the neothalamus; they are responsible for higher mental and emotional processes, including memory, learning, etc. 联合区，大脑皮质（不包括主要区域）相互连接和与下丘脑相连的区域；该区域负责更高级的思维和情感过程，包括记忆、学习等；**auditory a's**, two contiguous areas of the temporal lobe in the region of the anterior transverse temporal gyrus 听觉区，颞叶的两个相邻区域，位于前颞横回区域；**Broca motor speech a.**, an area comprising parts of the opercular and triangular portions of the inferior frontal gyrus; injury to this area may result in motor aphasia Broca 运动言语区或布洛卡运动言语区，大脑皮质汇总以其六种细胞层次的排列不同而与其余部分相区别的区域；通过对每个区域进行编号来标识；**Brod-mann a's**, areas of the cerebral cortex distinguished by differences in arrangement of their six cellular layers; identified by numbering each area 布罗德曼分区；**embryonic a.**, see under *disc*. 参见 disc **germinal a.**, embryonic disc 胚盘；**hypophysio-tropic a.**, the hypothalamic component containing neurons that secrete hormones that regulate adenohypophysial cells 促垂体区，下丘脑的组成部分，其中包含某种神经元，其可分泌激素调节腺垂体细胞；**Kiesselbach a.,** one on the anterior part of the nasal septum above the intermaxillary bone, richly supplied with capillaries, and a common site of nosebleed 基塞尔巴氏区，上颌间骨上方、鼻中隔前下部区域，毛细血管丰富，是鼻出血的常见区域；**motor a.,** any area of the cerebral cortex primarily involved in stimulating muscle contractions, often specifically the primary somatomotor area 运动区，大脑皮质中主要参与刺激肌肉收缩的区域，尤指主要的躯体运动区域；**prefrontal a.,** the cortex of the frontal lobe immediately in front of the premotor cortex, concerned chiefly with associative functions 额前区，紧靠运动前区前方的额叶皮质，主要与联想功能有关；**premotor a.,** the motor cortex of the frontal lobe immediately in front of the precentral gyrus 运动前区，紧邻中央前回前方的额叶皮质；**primary a's,** areas of the cerebral cortex comprising the motor and sensory regions 大脑皮质的部分区域，包括运动区和感觉区；cf. *association a's*；**primary somatomotor a.,** an area in the posterior part of the frontal lobe just anterior to the central sulcus; different regions control motor activity of specific parts of the body 第 I 躯体运动区，位于额叶后部、紧邻中央沟前方；不同区域控制身体特定部位的运动活动；**a. subcallo′sa, subcallosal a.,** a small area of cortex on the medial surface of each cerebral hemisphere 胼胝体下区，大脑半球内侧表面的一小部分皮质区；**a. of superficial cardiac dullness,** a triangular area of dullness observed on percussion of the chest, corresponding to the area of the heart not covered by lung tissue 心脏浊音区，胸部叩诊时可观察到的一个三角形浊音区，对应心脏被肺组织覆盖的区域；**thymus-dependent a.,** any of the areas of the peripheral lymphoid organs populated by T lymphocytes, e.g., the paracortex in lymph nodes, the centers of the malpighian corpuscle of the spleen, and the internodal zone of Peyer patches 胸腺依赖区，周围淋巴器官中主要由 T 淋巴细胞构成的区域，例如淋巴结的副皮质区，脾的马氏皮基氏体（马氏小体）的中心区，和派尔集合淋巴结的结间区；**thymus-independent a.,** any of the areas of the peripheral lymphoid organs populated by B lymphocytes, e.g., the spleen lymph nodules and the lymph nodes 非胸腺依赖区，周围淋巴器官中主要由 B 淋巴细胞构成的区域，例如脾淋巴小结和淋巴结；**vocal a.,** rima glottidis 声门区，声门裂；**watershed a.,** any of several areas over the convexities of the cerebral or cerebellar hemispheres; at times of prolonged systemic hypotension they are particularly susceptible to infarction 分水岭区，大脑或小脑半球突起的数个区域；长时间低血压时该区域极易发生梗死；**Wernicke a., Wernicke second motor speech a.,** originally a term denoting a language center on the posterior part of the superior temporal gyrus, now used to include also the supramarginal and angular gyri 韦尼克区，韦尼克第二运动言语区，原指颞上回后部的语言中枢，现亦包括缘上回和角回

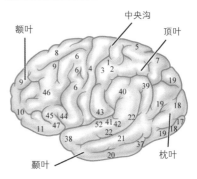

▲ 大脑半球侧面观，显示某些 Brodmann（Brodmann areas）分区

are·flex·ia (a″re-flek′se-ə) absence of reflexes 无反射，反射消失；**detrusor a.,** failure of the detrusor urinae muscle to respond to stimuli, resulting in failure to empty the bladder completely on urination 逼尿肌无反射，逼尿肌对刺激无反应，导致排尿时无法完全排空膀胱

are·gen·er·a·tive (a″re-jen′ər-ə-tiv) characterized by absence of regeneration 再生障碍的

Are·na·vi·ri·dae (ə-re″nə-vir′ĭ-de) the arenaviruses, a family of RNA viruses containing just one genus, *Arenavirus* 沙粒病毒科，RNA 病毒的一个科，只包含一个属即沙粒病毒属

Are·na·vi·rus (ə-re″nə-vi′rəs) the single genus of the family Arenaviridae, including several that cause hemorrhagic fevers and the viruses of the Tacaribe complex. The natural hosts are rodents 沙粒病毒属，沙粒病毒科的唯一属支，包含数种可导致出血热毒和塔卡里伯病毒群。该病毒的自然宿主为啮齿动物

are·na·vi·rus (ə-re″nə-vi″rəs) any virus of the family Arenaviridae 沙粒病毒，沙粒病毒科的任何病毒

are·o·la (ə-re′o-lə) pl. *are′olae* [L.] 1. any minute space or interstice in a tissue 小区，细隙：组织中任何微小的空间或空隙；2. a circular area of different color surrounding a central point, as that surrounding the nipple of the breast 晕，围绕中心

点周围的不同颜色的环形区，如围绕乳头的乳晕；**are′olar** *adj.*

Arg arginine 精氨酸

Ar·gas (ahr′gəs) a genus of ticks (family Argasidae), parasitic in poultry and other birds and sometimes humans 锐缘蜱属 / 隐喙蜱属，蜱科的一个属支（隐喙蜱科 / 软蜱科），寄生于家禽和其他鸟类，有时亦可寄生于人类

ar·ga·sid (ahr′gə-sid) 1. a tick of the family Argasidae 隐喙蜱，属于隐喙蜱科 2. pertaining to a tick of the genus *Argas*. 隐喙蜱属的

Ar·gas·i·dae (ahr-gas′ĭ-de) a family of arthropods (superfamily Ixodoidea) made up of the soft-bodied ticks 隐喙蜱科，节肢动物（蜱总科）的一个科，由软（体）蜱组成

ar·gat·ro·ban (ahr-gat′ro-ban″) an anticoagulant used in the prophylaxis and treatment of heparin-induced thrombocytopenia 阿加曲班，一种抗凝剂，可用于预防和治疗肝素诱导性血小板减少症

ar·gen·taf·fin (ahr-jen′tə-fin) staining with silver and chromium salts 嗜银的，可被银盐和铬盐染色；另见 *cell* 下词条

ar·gen·taf·fi·no·ma (ahr″jən-taf″ĭ-no′mə) carcinoid tumor 嗜银细胞瘤，一种类癌肿瘤

ar·gi·nase (ahr′jĭ-nās) an enzyme existing primarily in the liver, which hydrolyzes arginine to form urea and ornithine in the urea cycle 精氨酸酶，该酶主要存在于肝脏，在尿素循环中可水解精氨酸形成尿素和鸟氨酸

ar·gi·nine (Arg) (R) (ahr′jĭ-nēn) a nonessential amino acid occurring in proteins and involved in the urea cycle, which converts ammonia to urea, and in the synthesis of creatine. Preparations of the base or the glutamate or hydrochloride salt are used in the treatment of hyperammonemia and as a diagnostic aid in the assessment of pituitary function 精氨酸，一种非必须氨基酸，存在于蛋白质中，参与将氨转化为尿素的尿素循环和肌酐的合成。该物质的碱类或谷氨酸盐或盐酸盐制剂可用于治疗高氨血症，可用于垂体功能评估的辅助诊断

ar·gi·ni·no·suc·ci·nate (ahr″jĭ-ne″no-suk′sīnāt) the anionic form of argininosuccinic acid 精氨（基）琥珀酸，精氨（基）琥珀酸的阴离子形式

ar·gi·ni·no·suc·cin·ate syn·thase (ahr″jīne″-no-suk″sī-nāt sin′thās) an enzyme that catalyzes the condensation of citrulline and aspartate, a step in the hepatic urea cycle; deficiency causes citrullinemia 精氨（基）琥珀酸合成酶，一种可催化瓜氨酸和天冬氨酸缩合的酶，该反应过程是肝脏尿素循环的步骤之一；精氨（基）琥珀酸合成酶的缺乏可导致瓜氨酸血症

ar·gi·ni·no·suc·cin·ic ac·id (ASA) (ahr″jīne″-no-suk-sin′ik) an amino acid formed in the urea

cycle 精氨（基）琥珀酸，一种在尿素循环中生成的氨基酸

ar·gi·ni·no·suc·cin·ic ac·id·uria (ahr″jī-ne″no-suk-sin″ik as″ī-du′re-ə) 1. an inherited aminoacidopathy due to a urea cycle enzyme deficiency, characterized by excessive levels of argininosuccinic acid in the blood and urine; there are neonatal and late-onset forms, whose symptoms vary widely in severity and include intellectual disability, seizures, ataxia, splenomegaly, and brittle hair 精氨（基）琥珀酸尿，一种由尿素循环中某种酶缺乏导致的遗传性氨基酸病，其特征是血液和尿液中精氨（基）琥珀酸含量过高；该疾病分为新生儿型和晚发型，两种类型的症状在严重程度上有很大差异，该疾病的主要症状包括智力障碍、癫痫、共济失调、脾大和脆发；2. excretion in the urine of argininosuccinic acid 精氨（基）琥珀酸经尿液排泄

ar·gon (Ar) (ahr′gon) a colorless, odorless chemical element of the noble gas group; at. no. 18, at. wt. 39.948 氩，一种无色无味的稀有气体化学元素，原子序数 18，相对原子质量 39.948

ar·gyr·ia (ahr-jir′e-ə) poisoning by silver or its salts; chronic argyria is marked by a permanent ash gray discoloration of the skin, conjunctivae, and internal organs 银质沉着病，因银或银盐而中毒；慢性银质沉着病的特征是皮肤、结膜和内脏器官永久性变为灰白色

ar·gy·ro·phil (ahr′jə-ro-fil) (ahr-ji′rofil) capable of binding silver salts 嗜银的，可与银盐结合的

ARHP Association of Rheumatology Health Professionals 美国风湿病卫生专业人员协会

ari·bo·fla·vin·o·sis (a-ri″bo-fla″vĭ-no′sis) deficiency of riboflavin in the diet, marked by angular cheilosis, nasolabial lesions, optic changes, and seborrheic dermatitis 核黄素缺乏症，饮食中核黄素缺乏的疾病，主要表现为口角干裂、鼻唇部病变、视力改变和脂溢性皮炎

ARIN Association for Radiologic and Imaging Nursing 美国放射与影像护理协会

ar·i·pip·ra·zole (ar″ī-pip′rə-zōl) an antipsychotic used in the treatment of schizophrenia and bipolar disorder 阿立哌唑，用于治疗精神分裂症和双相情感障碍的一种抗精神病药物

ARJ anorectal junction 肛门直肠交界

arm (ahrm) 1. brachium; the part of the upper limb from the shoulder to the elbow 臂；上肢从肩到肘的部分；2. in common usage, the entire upper limb 通常指整个上肢；3. a slender part or extension that projects from a main structure 从主体结构中伸出的细长部分或延伸部分；**chromosome a.**, either of the two segments of a chromosome separated by the centromere 染色体臂，由着丝粒分开

的染色体两段中的任意一段

Ar·mil·li·fer (ahr-mil′ĭ-fər) a genus of wormlike endoparasites of reptiles; the larvae of *A. armilla′tus* and *A. monilifor′mis* are occasionally found in humans 蛇舌状虫属，洞头虫，虫状内寄生爬行动物的一个属支；腕带蛇舌状虫和串珠蛇舌状虫偶尔可在人类中发现

arm·pit (ahrm′pit) the externally visible part of the axilla 腋窝，腋窝的外部可见部分

ARN Association of Rehabilitation Nurses 美国康复护士协会；acute retinal necrosis 急性视网膜坏死

ar·ni·ca (ahr′nĭ-kə) the dried flower heads of the composite-flowered species *Arnica montana*; preparations are used topically for contusions, sprains, and superficial wounds, and as a counterirritant 山金车属，蒙大拿山金车属菊科植物的干花头；其制剂可局部用于挫伤、扭伤和表浅伤口，并且可作为抗刺激制剂

aro·ma·tase (ə-ro′mə-tās) an enzyme activity in the endoplasmic reticulum that catalyzes the conversion of testosterone to the aromatic compound estradiol 芳香化酶，其酶活性可在内质网中催化睾酮转化为芳香化合物雌二醇

aro·ma·ther·a·py (ə-ro′mə-ther″ə-pe) the therapeutic use of essential oils extracted from plants by steam distillation or expression; used by inhalation, introduced internally, or applied topically 芳香疗法，治疗性应用从植物中通过蒸汽蒸馏或压榨术提取的精油；应用方法包括吸入、内服或局部应用

ar·o·mat·ic (ar″o-mat′ik) 1. having a spicy odor 芳香的，有芳香气味的；2. in chemistry, denoting a compound containing a ring system stabilized by a closed circle of conjugated double bonds or nonbonding electron pairs, e.g., benzene or naphthalene 芳香族的，化学中指含环系的化合物，由共轭双键的闭环或非键合电子对促进稳定，例如苯和萘

arous·al (ə-rou′zəl) 1. a state of responsiveness to sensory stimulation or excitability 觉醒，对感觉刺激有反应的状态；2. the act or state of waking from or as if from sleep 从睡眠中醒来或类似从睡眠中醒来的行为或状态；3. the act of stimulating to readiness or to action 激起、激发，刺激准备或行动的行为；**sexual a.**, physical and psychological responses to mental or physical erotic stimulation 性唤醒，性觉醒，对精神或肉体性刺激的生理和心理反应

ar·rec·tor (ə-rek′tər) pl. *arrecto′res* [L.] raising, or that which raises 直立或能直立的物体；an arrector muscle 立毛肌

ar·rest (ə-rest′) cessation or stoppage, as of a function or a disease process 功能或疾病进程的

中止或停止；**cardiac a.**, sudden cessation of the pumping function of the heart with disappearance of arterial blood pressure, connoting either ventricular fibrillation or ventricular standstill 心搏骤停，心脏泵血功能突然中止，表现为动脉血压下降，意味着心室颤动或心室停顿；**developmental a.**, a temporary or permanent cessation of development 发育停止，发育阻滞，发育过程暂时性或永久性中止；**epiphyseal a.**, premature interruption of longitudinal growth of bone by fusion of the epiphysis and diaphysis 骨骺闭合，骨骺生长停止，骨骺与骨干融合导致骨骼纵向生长永久性中断；**maturation a.**, interruption of the process of development, as of blood cells, before the final stage is reached（血细胞的）成熟停止，血细胞的发育成熟过程在到达最后阶段之前发生中断；**sinus a.**, a pause in the normal cardiac rhythm due to a momentary failure of the sinus node to initiate an impulse, lasting for an interval that is not an exact multiple of the normal cardiac cycle 窦性停搏，由于窦房结一时无法产生冲动而导致的正常窦性心律的停顿，停顿时间不是正常心动周期的整数倍

ar·rhe·no·blas·to·ma (ə-re″no-blas-to′mə) 卵巢男性细胞瘤，见 androblastoma (2)

ar·rhin·ia (ə-rin′e-ə) congenital absence of the nose 无鼻畸形，先天性鼻缺失

ar·rhyth·mia (ə-rith′me-ə) variation from the normal rhythm of the heartbeat, encompassing abnormalities of rate, regularity, site of impulse origin, and sequence of activation. **arrhyth′mic** *adj.* 心律失常，与正常心跳节律有所不同；包括心率、心律、冲动起源部位和激活顺序上的异常 **nonphasic a.**, a form of sinus arrhythmia in which the irregularity is not linked to the phases of respiration. 非时相性心律失常，窦性心律失常的一种，其心律不齐与呼吸时相无关 **sinus a.**, the physiologic cyclic variation in heart rate related to vagal impulses to the sinoatrial node; it is common, particularly in children, and is not abnormal. 窦性心律失常，心率的生理性周期性变化，与窦房结迷走神经冲动有关；属于常见现象，在儿童中尤为常见，并非异常征象

ar·rhyth·mo·gen·esis (ə-rith″mo-jen′ə-sis) the development of an arrhythmia 心律失常形成

ar·rhyth·mo·gen·ic (ə-rith″mo-jen′ik) producing or promoting arrhythmia 产生或促进心律失常的

ARRS American Roentgen Ray Society 美国伦琴射线放射学会

ARRT American Registry of Radiologic Technologists 美国放射医学专家注册处

ar·se·nic (As) (ahr′sə-nik) a metalloid element; at. no. 33, at. wt. 74.922. Acute arsenic poisoning is marked by skin rashes, vomiting, diarrhea, abdominal pain, muscular cramps, and swelling of the eyelids, feet, and hands; it may result in shock and death. Chronic poisoning, due to ingestion of small amounts of arsenic over long periods, is marked by skin pigmentation accompanied by scaling, hyperkeratosis of palms and soles, transverse lines on the fingernails, headache, peripheral neuropathy, and confusion 砷，一种准金属元素；原子序数 33，相对原子质量 74.922。急性砷中毒主要表现为皮疹、呕吐、腹泻、腹痛、肌肉痉挛以及眼睑和手足肿胀；急性砷中毒可能导致休克和死亡。长期摄入微量砷元素导致的慢性中毒主要表现为皮肤色素沉着伴有鳞片样改变、手掌足底角化过度、指甲横纹、头痛、周围神经病变和神志不清；**a. trioxide**, an oxidized form of arsenic used in weed killers and rodenticides; also used as an antineoplastic in the treatment of acute promyelocytic leukemia 三氧化二砷，砷的一种氧化形式，用于除草剂和灭鼠剂；亦可用作抗肿瘤药物治疗急性早幼粒细胞白血病；**ar·sine** (ahr′sēn) any member of a group of volatile arsenical bases; the typical is AsH3, a carcinogenic and very poisonous gas; some of its compounds have been used in warfare 胂，挥发性的含砷基团；典型者为三氧化砷，一种有致癌作用和强烈毒性的气体；该物质组成的某些复合物曾用于战争

ART Accredited Record Technician 审定记录技师；assisted reproductive technology 辅助生殖技术；automated reagin test 自动反应素试验

Ar·te·mi·sia (ahr″tə-mis′e-ə) [L.] a genus of composite-flowered plants. *A. absin′thium* is common wormwood and *A. vulga′ris* (mugwort) is the source of moxa and is also used orally 蒿属，苦艾属，菊科植物的一个属支。中亚艾蒿是常见的苦艾，北艾（艾蒿）是针灸用艾绒的原料，亦可口服

ar·ter·al·gia (ahr″tər-al′jə) pain emanating from an artery, such as headache from an inflamed temporal artery 动脉痛，从动脉发出的疼痛，例如由发炎的颞动脉引起的头痛

ar·te·ria (ahr-tēr′e-ə) pl. *arte′riae* [L.] artery 动脉；**a. luso′ria**, an abnormally situated retroesophageal vessel, usually the subclavian artery from the aortic arch 畸形动脉（尤指锁骨下的），一种位置异常的食管后动脉，通常是主动脉弓发出的锁骨下动脉

ar·te·ri·al (ahr-tēr′e-əl) pertaining to an artery or to the arteries 动脉的

ar·te·ri·ec·ta·sis (ahr-tēr″e-ek′tə-sis) dilatation and, usually, lengthening of an artery 动脉扩张，动脉扩张并常变长

ar·te·ri·og·ra·phy (ahr″tēr-e-og′rə-fe) angiography of arteries 动脉影术；**catheter a.**, radiography of vessels after introduction of contrast material through a catheter inserted into an artery 经导管动脉造影术，经导管插入动脉、注入造影剂后进行的血管造影；**selective a.**, radiography of a specific vessel, which is opacified by a medium introduced directly into it, usually via a catheter 选择性动脉造影术，对某个特定血管的造影，通常是经导管向该血管直接注入某种介质而使其变得不透明

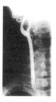

▲ 右颈总动脉及其分叉发出颈内动脉和颈外动脉部分的动脉造影（**arteriography**），呈前后向投影

ar·te·ri·o·la (ahr-tēr″e-o′lə) pl.*arterio′lae* [L.] arteriole 微动脉，小动脉

ar·te·ri·ole (ahr-tēr′e-ōl) a minute arterial branch 微动脉，小动脉，一种微小的动脉分支；**arterio′lar** *adj.*；**afferent glomerular a.**, a branch of an interlobular artery that goes to a renal glomerulus 入球小动脉，小叶间动脉的分支，通向肾小球；**efferent glomerular a.**, one arising from a renal glomerulus, breaking up into capillaries to supply renal tubules 出球小动脉，起自肾小球，分支成毛细血管以供应肾小管；**postglomerular a.**，球后动脉，见 efferent glomerular a.；**precapillary a.**, arterial capillary 毛细血管前微动脉，动脉毛细血管；**preglomerular a.**，见 afferent glomerular a.；**straight a's of kidney**, branches of the arcuate arteries of the kidney arising from the efferent glomerular arterioles and passing down to the renal pyramids 肾直小动脉，肾弓状动脉的分支，起自出球小动脉，下至肾锥体

ar·te·rio·lith (ahr-tēr′e-o-lith″) a chalky concretion in an artery 动脉石，动脉中的白色凝固物

ar·te·rio·lo·ne·cro·sis (ahr-tēr″e-o-lo-nə-kro′sis) necrosis or destruction of arterioles 小动脉坏死

ar·te·ri·o·lop·a·thy (ahr-tēr′e-o-lop′ə-the) any disease of the arterioles 小动脉病

ar·te·rio·lo·scle·ro·sis (ahr-tēr″e-o″lo-skla-ro′sis) sclerosis and thickening of the walls of arterioles. The hyaline form may be associated with nephrosclerosis, the hyperplastic with malignant hypertension, nephrosclerosis, and scleroderma. 小动脉硬化，小动脉壁硬化增厚。小动脉玻璃样变可能与肾硬化有关，增生性病变可能与恶性高血压、肾硬化和硬皮病有关；**arteriolosclerot′ic** *adj.*

ar·te·rio·mo·tor (ahr-tēr″e-o-mo′tər) involving or

causing dilation or constriction of arteries 涉及或导致动脉收缩的

ar·te·ri·op·a·thy (ahr-tēr″e-op′ə-the) any disease of an artery 动脉病；**hypertensive a.**, widespread involvement of arterioles and small arteries, associated with arterial hypertension, and characterized by hypertrophy of the tunica media 高血压性动脉病，广泛累及微动脉和小动脉，与动脉性高血压有关，其特征为动脉中膜肥厚

ar·te·rio·plas·ty (ahr-tēr′e-o-plas″te) surgical repair or reconstruction of an artery 动脉成形术，对动脉进行修补或重建的外科手术；applied especially to the Matas operation for aneurysm 尤指治疗动脉瘤的 Matas 手术

ar·te·ri·or·rha·phy (ahr-tēr″e-or′ə-fe) suture of an artery 动脉缝合术

ar·te·ri·or·rhex·is (ahr-tēr″e-o-rek′sis) rupture of an artery 动脉破裂

ar·te·rio·scle·ro·sis (ahr-tēr″e-o-sklə-ro′sis) a group of diseases characterized by thickening and loss of elasticity of the arterial walls, occurring in three forms: atherosclerosis, Mönckeberg arteriosclerosis, and arteriolosclerosis 动脉硬化，特征为动脉壁增厚和弹性丧失的一组疾病，有三种发生形式：动脉粥样硬化，动脉中层钙化（Mönckeberg 动脉硬化）和小动脉硬化，**arteriosclerot′ic adj.**；**Mönckeberg a.**, arteriosclerosis with extensive deposits of calcium in the middle coat of the artery 动脉中层钙化（Mönckeberg 动脉硬化），动脉硬化伴有动脉中层大量钙质沉积；**a. obli′terans**, that in which proliferation of the intima of the small vessels has caused complete obliteration of the lumen of the artery 闭塞性动脉硬化，小血管内膜增生导致动脉管腔完全闭塞；**peripheral a.**, arteriosclerosis of the limbs 周围动脉硬化，四肢血管动脉硬化

ar·te·rio·ste·no·sis (ahr-tēr″e-o-stə-no′sis)constriction of an artery 动脉狭窄

ar·te·rio·ve·nous (ahr-tēr″e-o-ve′nəs) both arterial and venous 动静脉的；pertaining to or affecting an artery and a vein 属于或影响某支动静脉的

ar·ter·i·tis (ahr″tə-ri′tis) pl. *arteri′tides*. Inflammation of an artery 动脉炎；**aortic arch a.**, 主动脉弓动脉炎，见 Takayasu a.；**brachiocephalic a.**, **a. brachiocepha′lica**, 头臂干动脉炎，无脉症，见 Takayasu a.；**coronary a.**, inflammation of the coronary arteries 冠状动脉炎；**cranial a.**, 颅动脉炎，见 giant cell a.；**giant cell a.**, a chronic vascular disease of unknown origin, usually in the carotid arterial system, occurring in the elderly; it is characterized by severe headache, fever, and proliferative inflammation, often with giant cells and granulomas. Ocular involvement may cause blindness 巨细胞动脉炎，一种起源不明的慢性血管疾病，通常发生于颈动脉系统，常见于老年人；其特征是严重头痛、发热和增生性炎症，常伴有巨细胞和肉芽肿。眼部受累可能导致失明；**rheumatic a.**, generalized inflammation of arterioles and arterial capillaries occurring in rheumatic fever 风湿性动脉炎，风湿热患者发生的小动脉和动脉毛细血管的广泛炎症；**Takayasu a.**, pulseless disease; progressive obliteration of the brachiocephalic trunk and left subclavian and left common carotid arteries, leading to loss of pulse in arms and carotids and to ischemia of brain, eyes, face, and arms 动脉炎，无脉症；头臂干、左锁骨下动脉和左颈总动脉的进行性闭塞，导致上肢和颈动脉搏动消失和大脑、眼、面和上肢缺血；**temporal a.**, 颞动脉炎，见 giant cell a.

ar·te·ry (ahr′tə-re) a vessel through which the blood passes away from the heart to the various parts of the body, in the systemic circulation carrying oxygenated blood 动脉，血液通过该血管由心脏流向全身各部分，体循环系负责运输含氧量高的血液；**accessory obturator a.**, a name given to the obturator artery when it arises from the inferior epigastric instead of the internal iliac artery 副闭孔动脉，当闭孔动脉起源于腹壁下动脉而非髂内动脉时被称为副闭孔动脉。又称 *arteria obturatoria accessoria*；**accompanying a. of sciatic nerve**, a. to sciatic nerve 坐骨神经伴行动脉；**acromiothoracic a.**, 见 thoracoacromial a.；**a. of Adamkiewicz**, an unusually large anterior segmental medullary artery arising from an intersegmental branch of the aorta, varying from the lower thoracic to the upper lumbar level, and traveling posteriorly to supply the

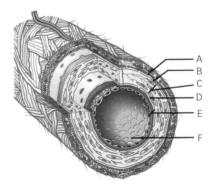

▲ 一个较大的肌性动脉（mnscular artery）的组织分层：A. 外膜（绿色）；B. 外弹力膜（黄色）；C. 中膜（粉色）；D. 内弹力膜（黄色）；E. 内膜（蓝色）；F. 管腔

spinal cord by anastomosing with the anterior spinal artery 根髓大动脉，一种管径异常粗大的前根髓动脉，起源于主动脉的节间动脉分支，其起源部位可由下胸段至上腰段不等，其走行于椎管后方，通过与脊髓前动脉吻合来供应脊髓血供。又称 *arteria radicularis magna*；**alveolar a's, anterior superior**, *origin*, infraorbital artery; *branches*, dental and peridental branches; *distribution*, incisor and canine regions of upper jaw, maxillary sinus 上牙槽前动脉，起源于眶下动脉，分支包括牙支和牙周支，分布于上颌的切牙和尖牙区以及上颌窦。又称 *arteriae alveolares superiores anteriores*；**alveolar a., inferior**, *origin*, maxillary artery; *branches*, dental, peridental, mental, and mylohyoid branches; *distribution*, lower jaw, lower lip, and chin 下牙槽动脉，起源于上颌动脉，分支包括牙支、牙周支、脑支和下颌舌骨肌支，分布于下颌、下唇和颏部。又称 *arteria alveolaris inferior*；**alveolar a., posterior superior**, origin, maxillary artery; *branches*, dental and peridental branches; *distribution*, molar and premolar regions of upper jaw, maxillary sinus 上牙槽后动脉，起源于上颌动脉，分支包括牙支和牙周支，分布于上颌的磨牙和前磨牙区以及上颌窦。又称 *arteria alveolaris posterior superior*；**angular a.**, *origin*, facial artery; *branches*, none; *distribution*, lacrimal sac, lower eyelid, nose 内眦动脉，起源于面动脉，无分支，分布于泪囊、下眼睑和鼻部。又称 *arteria angularis*；**a. of angular gyrus**, *origin*, terminal part of middle cerebral artery; *branches*, none; *distribution*, temporal, parietal, and occipital lobes 角回动脉，起源于大脑中动脉的终末部分，无分支，分布于颞叶、顶叶和枕叶。又称 *arteria gyrus angularis*；**anterior choroidal a.**, *origin*, internal carotid or sometimes middle cerebral artery; *branches*, many small branches; *distribution*, interior of brain, including choroid plexus of lateral ventricle and adjacent parts 脉络膜前动脉，起源于颈内动脉，有时亦可起源于大脑中动脉，分支包括许多细小分支，分布于大脑内面、侧脑室及其邻近部分的脉络丛。又称 *arteria choroidea anterior*；**anterior interventricular a.**, left anterior descending coronary a. 前室间动脉，冠状动脉左前降支；**appendicular a.**, *origin*, ileocolic artery; *branches*, none; *distribution*, vermiform appendix 阑尾动脉，起源于回结肠动脉，无分支，分布于阑尾。又称 *arteria appendicularis*；**arcuate a. of foot**, *origin*, dorsalis pedis artery; *branches*, deep plantar branch and dorsal metatarsal arteries; *distribution*, foot, toes 足弓状动脉，起源于足背动脉，分支包括足底深支和跖背动脉，分布于足和脚趾。又称 *arteria arcuata pedis*；**arcuate a's of kidney**, *origin*, interlobar artery; *branches*, interlobular artery and straight arterioles;

distribution, parenchyma of kidney 肾弓状动脉，起源于叶间动脉，分支包括小叶间动脉和直小动脉，分布于肾实质。又称 *arteriae arcuatae renis*；**arcuate a's of uterus**, branches of the uterine artery that run circumferentially in the uterine wall as anterior and posterior groups, anastomosing across the midline both anteriorly and posteriorly, and giving rise to radial arteries that supply deeper layers 子宫弓状动脉，子宫动脉的分支，分为前后两组在子宫壁内环圈存在，在子宫前后两侧的中线上相互吻合，发出放射状动脉以供应更深层次的子宫壁组织；**ascending pharyngeal a.**, *origin*, external carotid artery; *branches*, posterior meningeal, pharyngeal, and inferior tympanic; *distribution*, pharynx, soft palate, ear, meninges 咽升动脉，起源于颈外动脉，分支包括脑膜后支、咽支和鼓室下支，分布于咽部、软腭、耳和脑膜。又称 *arteria pharyngea ascendens*；**atrioventricular nodal a.**, a branch of the right coronary artery usually arising opposite the origin of the posterior interventricular artery and inserting into the atrioventricular node 房室结动脉，右冠状动脉的分支，通常发自后室间动脉的对侧位置，流向房室结；**auricular a's, anterior**, the anterior auricular branches of the superficial temporal artery, supplying the lateral aspect of the pinna and the external acoustic meatus 耳前动脉，颞浅动脉的耳前支，供应耳廓和外耳道的侧面；**auricular a., deep**, *origin*, maxillary artery; *branches*, none; *distribution*, skin of auditory canal, tympanic membrane, temporomandibular joint 耳深动脉，起源于上颌动脉，分布于耳道皮肤、鼓膜和颞下颌关节。又称 *arteria auricularis profunda*；**auricular a., posterior**, *origin*, external carotid artery; *branches*, auricular and occipital branches, stylomastoid artery; *distribution*, middle ear, mastoid cells, auricle, parotid gland, digastric and other muscles 耳后动脉，起源于颈外动脉，分支包括耳支、枕支和茎乳动脉，分布于中耳、乳突细胞、耳廓、腮腺、二腹肌和其他肌肉等。又称 *arteria auricularis posterior*；**axillary a.**, *origin*, continuation of subclavian artery; *branches*, subscapular branches, and superior thoracic, thoracoacromial, lateral thoracic, subscapular, and anterior and posterior circumflex humeral arteries; *distribution*, upper limb, axilla, chest, shoulder 腋动脉，起源于锁骨下动脉的直接延续，分支包括肩胛下动脉、胸上动脉、胸肩峰动脉、胸外侧动脉、旋肱前动脉和旋肱后动脉，分布于上肢、腋窝、胸部和肩部。又称 *arteria axillaris*；**basilar a.**, *origin*, from junction of right and left vertebral arteries; *branches*, pontine, anterior inferior cerebellar, mesencephalic, superior cerebellar, and posterior cerebral arteries; *distribution*, brainstem, internal ear, cerebellum, posterior cerebrum 基底动脉，起源于左右两侧椎动脉的汇合处，分支包括脑桥动脉、小脑前下动脉、中脑动脉、小脑上动脉和大脑后动脉，分布于内耳、小脑和大脑后部。又称 *arteria basilaris*；**brachial a.**, *origin*, continuation of axillary artery; *branches*, profunda brachii, nutrient of humerus, superior ulnar collateral, inferior ulnar collateral, radial, and ulnar arteries; *distribution*, shoulder, arm, forearm, hand 肱动脉，起源于腋动脉的直接延续，分支包括肱深动脉、肱骨滋养动脉、尺侧上副动脉、尺侧下副动脉、桡动脉和尺动脉，分布于肩部、上臂、前臂和手。又称 *arteria brachialis*；**brachial a., superficial**, an occasional vessel that arises from high bifurcation of the brachial artery and assumes a more superficial course than usual 浅肱动脉，一种发自肱动脉的高位分叉处的偶发动脉，其走行较通常更为表浅。又称 *arteria brachialis superficialis*；**bronchial a's**, branches arising from the descending thoracic aorta to supply the bronchi and lower trachea, and passing along the posterior sides of the bronchi to ramify about the respiratory bronchioles; distributed also to adjacent lymph nodes, pulmonary vessels, and pericardium, and to part of the esophagus 支气管动脉，是由胸主动脉发出的分支，供应支气管和气管下段，并沿支气管后侧走行、环绕呼吸性细支气管分布；亦分布于邻近淋巴结、肺血管、心包和部分食管；**buccal a.**, *origin*, maxillary artery; *branches*, none; *distribution*, buccinator muscle, mucous membrane of mouth 颊动脉，起源于上颌动脉，无分支，分布于颊肌和口腔黏膜。又称 *arteria buccalis*；**bulbourethral a., a. of bulb of penis**, *origin*, internal pudendal artery; *branches*, none; *distribution*, bulbourethral gland, bulb of penis 尿道球腺动脉，起源于阴部内动脉，无分支，分布于尿道球腺和尿道球部。又称 *arteria bulbi penis*；**a. of bulb of vestibule**, *origin*, internal pudendal artery; *branches*, none; *distribution*, bulb of vestibule of vagina, greater vestibular glands 前庭球腺动脉，起源于阴部内动脉，无分支，分布于阴道前庭球和前庭大腺。又称 *arteria bulbi vestibuli*；**callosomarginal a.**, *origin*, anterior cerebral artery; *branches*, anteromedial frontal, intermediomedial frontal, posteromedial frontal, cingular, and paracentral branches; *distribution*, medial and superolateral surfaces of cerebral hemisphere 胼胝体缘动脉，起源于大脑前动脉，分支包括前内侧额叶支、中内侧额叶支、后内侧额叶支、扣带回支和旁中心支，分布于大脑半球的内侧和上外侧表面。又称 *arteria calloso marginalis*；**capsular a's**, the branches of renal artery supplying the renal capsule 肾包膜动脉，供应肾包膜的肾动脉分支；**caroticotympanic a's**, branches of the petrous part of the internal carotid artery that supply the tympanic cavity 颈鼓动脉，颈内动脉岩段的分支，供应鼓室。又称 *arteriae caroticotympanicae*；**carotid a., common**, origin, brachiocephalic trunk (right), aortic arch (left); *branches*, external and internal carotid arteries; *distribution*, see *external carotid a.* and *internal carotid a* 颈总动脉，起源于头臂干（右侧）或主动脉弓（左侧），分支包括颈内动脉和颈外动脉，分布见 external carotid a. 和 internal carotid a。又称 *arteria carotis communis*；**carotid a., external**, *origin*, common carotid; *branches*, superior thyroid, ascending pharyngeal, lingual, facial, sternocleidomastoid, occipital, posterior auricular, superficial temporal, maxillary; *distribution*, neck, face, skull 颈外动脉，起源于颈总动脉，分支包括甲状腺上动脉、咽升动脉、舌动脉、面动脉、胸锁乳突肌支、枕动脉、耳后动脉、颞浅动脉和上颌动脉等，分布于颈部、面部和颅骨。又称 *arteria carotis externa*；**carotid a., internal**, *origin*, common carotid; divided into four parts: cervical, petrous, cavernous, and cerebral; *branches*, numerous, including caroticotympanic arteries; tentorial basal, tentorial marginal, meningeal, and cavernous branches; and inferior hypophysial artery; ophthalmic, superior hypophysial, posterior communicating, anterior choroidal, anterior cerebral, and middle cerebral arteries; *distribution*, middle ear, brain, pituitary gland, orbit, choroid plexus 颈内动脉，起源于颈总动脉，分为四部分：颈段、岩段、海绵窦段和颅内段；分支众多，包括颈鼓动脉、小脑幕底支、小脑幕缘支、脑膜支和海绵窦支、垂体下动脉、眼动脉、垂体上动脉、后交通动脉、脉络膜前动脉、大脑前动脉和大脑中动脉；分布于中耳、脑部、垂体腺、眶部和脉络膜。又称 *arteria carotis interna*；**caudal a., median sacral a.** 尾正中动脉，骶正中动脉；**a. of caudate lobe**, either of two branches, one from the right and one from the left branch of the hepatic artery proper, supplying twigs to the caudate lobe of the liver 尾状叶动脉，肝固有动脉的左右侧分支中的一支，供应肝尾状叶。又称 *arteria lobi caudati*；**cecal a., anterior**, *origin*, ileocolic; *branches*, none; *distribution*, cecum 盲肠前动脉，起源于回结肠动脉，无分支，分布于盲肠。又称 *arteria caecalis anterior*；**cecal a., posterior**, *origin*, ileocolic; *branches*, none; *distribution*, cecum 盲肠后动脉，起源于回结肠动脉，无分支，分布于盲肠。又称 *arteria caecalis posterior*；**central a's, anterolateral**, *origin*, sphenoid part of middle cerebral artery; *branches*; proximal lateral and distal lateral sets of branches; *distribution*, anterior lenticular and caudate nuclei and internal capsule of brain 前外侧中央动脉，起源于大脑中动脉蝶窦段，分支包括

外侧近端支和外侧远端支，分布于豆状核前部、尾状核和内囊。又称 arteriae centrales anterolaterales。**central a's, anteromedial,** *origin,* anterior communicating artery and anterior cerebral artery; *branches,* none; *distribution,* anterior and medial corpus striatum 前内侧中央动脉，起源于前交通动脉和大脑前动脉，无分支，分布于纹状体前部和内侧。又称 arteriae centrales anteromediales; **central a., long,** distal medial striate a. 长中央动脉，远端内侧纹状动脉; **central a's, posterolateral,** *origin,* posterior cerebral artery; *branches,* none; *distribution,* cerebral peduncle, posterior thalamus, colliculi, medial geniculate and pineal bodies. The group includes the thalamogeniculate artery and the peduncular and posterior medial and lateral choroidal branches 后外侧中央动脉，起源于大脑后动脉，无分支，分布于大脑脚、丘脑后部、上下丘、内侧膝状体和松果体。该组动脉包括丘脑膝状体动脉、大脑脚支、后内侧和后外侧脉络膜支。又称 arteriae centrales posterolaterales; **central a's, posteromedial, from posterior cerebral a.,** *origin,* posterior cerebral artery; *branches,* none; *distribution,* anterior thalamus, lateral wall of third ventricle, and globus pallidus of lentiform nucleus 后内侧中央动脉（起自大脑后动脉），起源于大脑后动脉，无分支，分布于丘脑前部、第三脑室侧壁和豆状核的苍白球。又称 arteriae centrales posteromediales arteriae cerebri posterioris; **central a's, posteromedial, from posterior communicating a.,** *origin,* posterior communicating artery; *branches,* anterior and posterior branches; *distribution,* medial thalamic surface and walls of third ventricle 后内侧中央动脉（起自后交通动脉），起源于后交通动脉，分支包括前、后两支，分布于丘脑内部表层和第三脑室壁。又称 arteriae centrales posteromediales arteriae communicantis posterioris; **central a's, short,** the anteromedial central arteries, excepting the long central artery (distal medial striate artery) 短中央动脉，前内侧中央动脉中除去长中央动脉（远端内侧纹状动脉）以外的部分; **central a. of retina, central retinal a.,** *origin,* ophthalmic artery; *branches,* superior and inferior nasal, and superior and inferior temporal; *distribution,* courses within dural sheath and then pierces and runs within optic nerve to retina 视网膜中央动脉，起源于眼动脉，分支包括上鼻支、下鼻支、颞上支和颞下支，走行于硬膜鞘内，后又穿出硬膜鞘，并入视神经中到达视网膜。又称 arteria centralis retinae; **a. of central sulcus,** *origin,* superior terminal branch of middle cerebral artery; *branches,* none; *distribution,* cortex on either side of central sulcus 中央沟动脉，起源于大脑中动脉的上终末支，无分支，分布于中央沟两侧皮质。又称 arteria sulci centralis; **cerebellar a., anterior inferior,** *origin,* basilar artery; *branches,* labyrinthine artery (usually); *distribution,* anterolateral inferior part of cerebellum, lower and lateral parts of pons, and sometimes upper part of medulla oblongata 小脑前下动脉，起源于基底动脉，分支通常包括迷路动脉，分布于小脑的前外侧下半部以及脑桥下部和外侧，有时亦分布于延髓上半部。又称 arteria inferior anterior cerebelli; **cerebellar a., posterior inferior,** *origin,* vertebral artery; *branches,* medial, lateral, and cerebellar tonsillar branches, choroidal branch to fourth ventricle, posterior spinal artery; *distribution,* lower and medial cerebellum, medulla 小脑后下动脉，起源于椎动脉，分支包括内侧支、外侧支、小脑扁桃体支、发至第四脑室的脉络膜支和脊髓后动脉，分布于小脑下部和内侧以及延髓。又称 arteria inferior posterior cerebelli; **cerebellar a., superior,** *origin,* basilar artery; *branches,* lateral and medial branches; *distribution,* upper cerebellum, midbrain, pineal body, choroid plexus of third ventricle 小脑上动脉，起源于基底动脉，分支包括内侧支和外侧支，分布于小脑上部、中脑、松果体、第三脑室脉络丛。又称 arteria superior cerebelli; **cerebral a., anterior,** *origin,* internal carotid artery; *branches, (precommunicating part, A1)* anteromedial central arteries; *(postcommunicating part, A2–5)* distal medial striate, medial frontobasal, polar frontal, callosomarginal (and its branches), and pericallosal (and its branches) arteries; *distribution,* orbital, frontal, and parietal cortex, corpus callosum, diencephalon, corpus striatum, internal capsule, and choroid plexus of lateral ventricle 大脑前动脉，起源于颈内动脉；分支包括（前交通段，A1 段）前内侧中央动脉、（后交通段，A2~A5 段）远端内侧纹状动脉、额叶底内侧动脉、额极动脉、胼胝体缘动脉（及其分支）和胼胝体周围动脉（及其分支）；分布于眶部、额叶和顶叶皮质、胼胝体、间脑、纹状体、内囊和侧脑室脉络丛。又称 arteria cerebri anterior; **cerebral a., middle,** the larger terminal branch of the internal carotid artery. It begins as single vessel *(sphenoid part, M1)* and branches at the limen insulae, usually into inferior and superior cortical branches distributing below and above the sylvian fissure, respectively. The branches run first in the sylvian fissure *(insular part, P2),* through the inner aspects of the opercula *(opercular part, P3),* and end along the lateral surface of the cerebral hemisphere *(cortical part, P4).* *Branches,* anterolateral central, polar temporal, and insular arteries, anterior temporal, middle temporal, posterior temporal, and temporo-occipital branches, artery to angular gyrus, lateral frontobasal, prefrontal, anterior parietal, and posterior parietal arteries, and arteries of precentral, central, and postcentral sulci; *distribution*, orbital, frontal, parietal, and temporal cortex, corpus striatum, internal capsule 大脑中动脉，颈内动脉较大的终末支。该动脉起初为单支血管（蝶骨段，M1 段），进而在岛阈处分支，通常分为颈上支和颈下支，分别分布于大脑外侧裂的上、下侧。其分支起初走行于大脑侧裂中（岛叶段，M2 段），进而穿过岛盖内侧面（岛盖段，M3 段），继而沿大脑半球外侧面走行（皮质段，M4 段）。其分支包括前外侧中央动脉、额极动脉、岛叶动脉、颞叶前动脉、颞叶中动脉、颞叶后动脉、颞枕动脉、角回动脉、额叶底内侧动脉、额叶前动脉、顶叶前动脉、顶叶后动脉、前中央沟动脉、中央沟动脉和后中央沟动脉。分布于眶部、额叶、顶叶和颞叶皮质，纹状体，和内囊。又称 *arteria cerebri media*；**cerebral a., posterior**, *origin*, terminal bifurcation of basilar artery; *branches (precommunicating part, P1)*, posteromedial central, short circumferential, thalamoperforating, and collicular arteries; *(postcommunicating part, P2)*, posterolateral central and thalamogeniculate arteries, and medial and lateral posterior choroidal and peduncular branches; *(lateral occipital artery, P3)*, anterior, intermediate, and posterior temporal arteries; *(medial occipital artery, P4)*, parietal, parietooccipital, calcarine, and occipitotemporal branches, and dorsal branch to corpus callosum; *distribution*, occipital and temporal cortex, diencephalon, midbrain, choroid plexus of lateral and third ventricles, and visual area of cerebral cortex and other structures associated with the visual pathway 大脑后动脉，起源于基底动脉的末端分叉处；分支包括（前交通段，P1 段）后内侧中央动脉、短旋动脉、丘脑穿通动脉和上下丘动脉，（后交通段，P2 段）后外侧中央动脉、丘脑膝状体动脉、内侧和后外侧脉络膜支和脑脚支，（枕叶外侧动脉，P3 段）颞叶前、中、后动脉，（枕叶内侧动脉，P4 段）顶叶支、顶枕支、距状皮层支、枕颞支和胼胝体背侧支；分布于枕颞叶皮质、间脑、中脑、侧脑室和第三脑室脉络丛、大脑皮质视觉区和其他与视觉通路相关的结构。又称 *arteria cerebri posterior*；**cervical a., ascending**, *origin*, inferior thyroid artery or directly from thyrocervical trunk; *branches*, spinal branches; *distribution*, muscles of neck, vertebrae, vertebral canal 颈升动脉，起源于甲状腺下动脉或直接起源于甲状颈干，分支包括脊支，分布于颈部肌肉、椎骨、椎管。又称 *arteria cervicalis profunda*；**cervical a., deep**, *origin*, costocervical trunk; *branches*; none; *distribution*, deep neck muscles 颈深动脉，起源于肋颈干，无分支，分布于颈深肌。又称 *arteria cervicalis profunda*；**ciliary a's, anterior**, *origin*, muscular arteries; *branches*,

episcleral and anterior conjunctival arteries; *distribution*, iris, conjunctiva 睫状前动脉，起源于肌动脉，分支包括结膜上动脉和结膜前动脉，分布于虹膜和结膜。又称 *arteriae ciliares anteriores*；**ciliary a's, long posterior**, *origin*, ophthalmic artery; *branches*, none; *distribution*, iris, ciliary processes 睫状后长动脉，起源于眼动脉，无分支，分布于虹膜和睫状突。又称 *arteriae ciliares posteriores longae*；**ciliary a's, short posterior**, *origin*, ophthalmic artery; *branches*, none; *distribution*, choroid coat of eye 睫状后短动脉，起源于眼动脉，无分支，分布于眼脉络膜。又称 *arteriae ciliares posteriores breves*；**circumflex a.**, the circumflex branch of the left coronary artery, which curves around to the back of the left ventricle in the coronary sulcus, supplying the left ventricle and left atrium 回旋动脉，左冠状动脉回旋支，沿冠状沟弯曲走行至左心室后部，供应左心室和左心房；**circumflex femoral a., lateral**, *origin*, deep femoral artery; *branches*, ascending, descending, and transverse branches; *distribution*, hip joint, thigh muscles 旋股外侧动脉，起源于股深动脉，分支包括升支、降支和横支，分布于髋关节和大腿肌肉。又称 *arteria circumflexa femoris lateralis*；**circumflex femoral a., medial**, *origin*, deep femoral artery; *branches*, deep, superficial, ascending, transverse, and acetabular branches; *distribution*, hip joint, thigh muscles 旋股内侧动脉，起源于股深动脉，分支包括深支、浅支、升支、横支和髋臼支，分布于髋关节和大腿肌肉。又称 *arteria circumflexa femoris medialis*；**circumflex fibular a.**, the fibular circumflex branch of the posterior tibial artery, which winds laterally around the neck of the fibula, helping supply the soleus muscle and contributing to the anastomosis around the knee joint 旋腓骨颈动脉，胫后动脉的旋腓骨颈支，绕血管环绕腓骨颈外侧，协助供应比目鱼肌，参与膝关节周围的血管吻合；**circumflex humeral a., anterior**, *origin*, axillary artery; *branches*, none; *distribution*, glenohumeral joint and head of humerus, long tendon of biceps, tendon of pectoralis major muscle 旋肱前动脉，起源于腋动脉，无分支，分布于盂肱关节、肱骨头、肱二头肌长头腱和胸大肌肌腱。又称 *arteria circumflexa humeri anterior*；**circumflex humeral a., posterior**, *origin*, axillary artery; *branches*, none; *distribution*, deltoid, glenohumeral joint, teres minor and triceps muscles 旋肱后动脉，起源于腋动脉，无分支，分布于三角肌、盂肱关节、小圆肌和肱三头肌。又称 *arteria circumflexa humeri posterior*；**circumflex iliac a., deep**, *origin*, external iliac artery; *branches*, ascending branches; *distribution*, iliac region, abdominal wall, inguinal region 旋髂深动脉，起源于髂外动脉，分支包括

升支，分布于髂骨区、腹壁和腹股沟区。又称 *arteria circumflexa ilium profunda*；**circumflex iliac a.**, *superficial*, *origin*, femoral artery; *branches*, none; *distribution*, inguinal region, abdominal wall 旋髂浅动脉，起源于股动脉，无分支，分布于腹股沟区和腹壁。又称 *arteria circumflexa ilium superficialis*；**circumflex scapular a.**, *origin*, subscapular artery; *branches*, none; *distribution*, inferolateral muscles of the scapula 旋肩胛动脉，起源于肩胛下动脉，无分支，分布于肩胛骨下外侧肌肉。又称 *arteria circumflexa scapulae*；**coccygeal a.**, median sacral a. 尾骨动脉，骶正中动脉；**cochlear a.**, *common*, *origin*, labyrinthine artery; *branches*, vestibulocochlear, proper cochlear, and spiral modiolar arteries; *distribution*, cochlea and vestibules 耳蜗总动脉，起源于迷路动脉，分支包括前庭耳蜗动脉、耳蜗固有动脉和耳蜗螺旋动脉，分布于耳蜗和前庭。又称 *arteria cochlearis communis*；**cochlear a.**, *proper*, *origin*, common cochlear artery; *branches*, none; *distribution*, cochlea 耳蜗固有动脉，起源于耳蜗总动脉，无分支，分布于耳蜗。又称 *arteria cochlearis propria*；**colic a.**, *accessory superior*, middle colic a. 结肠上副动脉，中结肠动脉；**colic a.**, *inferior right*, 右下结肠动脉，见 ileocolic a.；**colic a.**, *left*, *origin*, inferior mesenteric artery; *branches*, none; *distribution*, descending colon 左结肠动脉，起源于肠系膜下动脉，无分支，分布于降结肠。又称 *arteria colica sinistra*；**colic a.**, *middle*, *origin*, superior mesenteric artery; *branches*, none; *distribution*, transverse colon 中结肠动脉，起源于肠系膜上动脉，无分支，分布于横结肠。又称 *arteria colica media*；**colic a.**, *right*, *origin*, superior mesenteric artery; *branches*, none; *distribution*, ascending colon 右结肠动脉，起源于肠系膜上动脉，无分支，分布于升结肠。又称 *arteria colica dextra*；**collateral a.**, *medial*, *origin*, profunda brachii artery; *branches*, none; *distribution*, triceps muscle, elbow joint 尺侧副动脉，起源于肱深动脉，无分支，分布于肱三头肌和肘关节。又称 *arteria collateralis media*；**collateral a.**, *radial*, *origin*, profunda brachii artery; *branches*, none; *distribution*, brachioradialis and brachialis muscles 桡侧副动脉，起源于肱深动脉，无分支，分布于肱桡肌和肱肌。又称 *arteria collateralis radialis*；**collicular a.**, *origin*, posterior cerebral artery; *branches*, none; *distribution*, corpora quadrigemina of the tectum of the midbrain 丘动脉，四叠体动脉，起源于大脑后动脉，无分支，分布于中脑顶盖的四叠体。又称 *arteria collicularis*；**communicating a.**, *anterior*, *origin*, anterior cerebral artery; *branches*, anteromedial central arteries; *distribution*, establishes connection between the right and left anterior cerebral arteries 前交通动脉，

起源于大脑前动脉，分支包括前内侧中央动脉，其作用在于建立左右两侧大脑前动脉的连接。又称 *arteria communicans anterior*；**communicating a.**, *posterior*, establishes connection between internal carotid and posterior cerebral arteries; *branches*, posteromedial central, thalamotuberal, and mammillary arteries, artery of tuber cinereum, and branches to the optic chiasm, oculomotor nerve, and hypothalamus 后交通动脉，建立颈内动脉和大脑后动脉的联系，其分支包括后内侧中央动脉、丘脑结节动脉、乳头体动脉、灰结节动脉以及供应视交叉、动眼神经和下丘脑的分支。又称 *arteria communicans posterior*；**conducting a's**, arterial trunks characterized by large size and elasticity, such as the aorta, subclavian and common carotid arteries, and brachiocephalic and pulmonary trunks 大动脉，以其管径粗大及其血管壁弹性为特征的动脉干，如主动脉、锁骨下动脉、颈总动脉、头臂干和肺动脉干等；**conjunctival a's**, *anterior*, *origin*, anterior ciliary arteries; *branches*, none; *distribution*, conjunctiva 结膜前动脉，起源于睫状前动脉，无分支，分布于结膜。又称 *arteriae conjunctivales anteriores*；**conjunctival a's**, *posterior*, *origin*, medial palpebral arteries; *branches*, none; *distribution*, lacrimal caruncle, conjunctiva 结膜后动脉，起源于睑内侧动脉，无分支，分布于泪阜和结膜。又称 *arteriae conjunctivales posteriores*；**corkscrew a's**, small arteries in the macular area of the retina that appear markedly tortuous 黄斑螺旋状动脉，视网膜黄斑区的细小动脉，走行异常弯曲；**coronary a.**, *left*, *origin*, left aortic sinus; *branches*, anterior interventricular and circumflex branches; *distribution*, left ventricle, left atrium 左冠状动脉，起源于左主动脉窦，分支包括前室间支和回旋支，分布于左心室和左心房。又称 *arteria coronaria sinistra*；**coronary a.**, *left anterior descending*, the anterior interventricular branch of the left coronary artery, which runs to the apex of the heart in the anterior interventricular sulcus, supplying the ventricles and most of the interventricular septum 冠状动脉左前降支，左冠状动脉发出的前室间支，沿前室间沟走行至心尖部，供应心室和大部分室间隔区域；**coronary a.**, *posterior descending*, the posterior interventricular branch of the right coronary artery, which runs toward the apex of the heart in the posterior interventricular sulcus, supplying the diaphragmatic surface of the ventricles and part of the interventricular septum 冠状动脉后降支，右冠状动脉发出的后室间支，沿后室间沟走行至心尖部，供应心室横膈膜面和部分室间隔区域；**coronary a.**, *right*, *origin*, right aortic sinus; *branches*, conus artery and atrial, atrioventricular node, intermediate atrial, posterior interventricular, right marginal, and sinoatrial node branches; *distribution*, right ventricle, right atrium 右冠状动脉，起源于右主动脉窦，分支包括动脉圆锥支、心房支、房室结支、右房中间支、后室间支、右缘支和窦房结支，分布于右心室和右心房。又称 *arteria coronaria dextra*; **cortical radiate a's of kidney**, interlobular a's of kidney 肾皮质放射状动脉，肾的小叶间动脉；**cremasteric a.**, *origin*, inferior epigastric artery; *branches*, none; *distribution*, cremaster muscle, coverings of spermatic cord 提睾肌动脉，起源于腹壁下动脉，无分支，分布于提睾肌，即精索外被。又称 *arteria cremasterica*; **cystic a.**, *origin*, right branch of hepatic artery proper; *branches*, none; *distribution*, gallbladder 胆囊动脉，起源于肝固有动脉右支，无分支，分布于胆囊。又称 *arteria cystica*; **deep a. of arm**, profunda brachii a. 肱深动脉；**deep a. of clitoris**, *origin*, internal pudendal artery; *branches*, none; *distribution*, clitoris 阴蒂深动脉，起源于阴部内动脉，无分支，分布于阴蒂。又称 *arteria profunda clitoridis*; **deep lingual a.**, *origin*, lingual artery; *branches*, none; *distribution*, tongue 舌深动脉，起源于舌动脉，无分支，分布于舌部。又称 *arteria profunda linguae*; **deep a. of penis**, *origin*, internal pudendal artery; *branches*, none; *distribution*, corpus cavernosum of penis 阴茎深动脉，起源于阴部内动脉，无分支，分布于阴茎海绵体。又称 *arteria profunda penis*; **deep a. of thigh**, deep femoral a. 股深动脉；**deferential a.**, a. of ductus deferens 输精管动脉；**digital a's, collateral**, proper palmar digital a's 指掌侧固有动脉；**digital a's of foot, common**, plantar metatarsal a's 趾足底总动脉；**digital a's of foot, dorsal**, dorsal metatarsal arteries; *branches*, none; *distribution*, dorsum of toes 趾背动脉，起源于跖背动脉，无分支，分布于足趾背侧。又称 *arteriae digitales dorsales pedis*; **digital a's of hand, dorsal**, *origin*, dorsal metacarpal arteries; *branches*, none; *distribution*, dorsum of fingers 指背动脉，起源于掌背动脉，无分支，分布于手指背侧。又称 *arteriae digitales dorsales manus*; **distributing a's**, most of the arteries except the conducting arteries; of muscular type, they extend from the large vessels to the arterioles 分配动脉，中动脉，除大动脉之外的多数动脉，肌性动脉由大动脉延伸至小动脉；**dorsal a. of clitoris**, *origin*, internal pudendal artery; *branches*, none; *distribution*, clitoris 阴蒂背动脉，起源于阴部内动脉，无分支，分布于阴蒂。又称 *arteria dorsalis clitoridis*; **dorsal a. of foot**, 见 dorsalis pedis a; **dorsal a. of nose**, dorsal nasal a. 鼻背动脉；**dorsal a. of penis**, *origin*, internal pudendal artery; *branches*, none; *distribution*, glans, corona, and prepuce of penis 阴茎背动脉，起源于阴部

内动脉，无分支，分布于阴茎头、冠和包皮。又称 *arteria dorsalis penis*; **dorsalis pedis a.**, *origin*, continuation of anterior tibial artery; *branches*, lateral and medial tarsal, arcuate, and deep plantar arteries; *distribution*, foot, toes 足背动脉，是胫前动脉的直接延续，分支包括内、外侧跗骨动脉、弓状动脉和足底深动脉，分布于足和足趾。又称 *arteria dorsalis pedis*; **a. to ductus deferens**, *origin*, umbilical artery; *branches*, ureteral artery; *distribution*, ureter, ductus deferens, seminal vesicles, testes 输精管动脉，起源于脐动脉，分支包括输尿管动脉，分布于尿道、输精管、精囊和睾丸。又称 *arteria ductus deferentis*; **elastic a's**, 见 conducting a's.; **end a.**, one that undergoes progressive branching without development of channels connecting with other arteries, so that if occluded it cannot supply sufficient blood to the tissue depending on it 末梢动脉，终动脉，一种已经不断分支且目前未与其他动脉血管建立联系通道的小动脉，若此动脉发生闭塞则无法向依赖该血管的组织提供足够血供；**epigastric a., inferior**, *origin*, external iliac artery; *branches*, pubic branch, cremasteric artery, artery of round ligament of uterus; *distribution*, abdominal wall 腹壁下动脉，起源于髂外动脉，分支包括耻骨支、提睾肌动脉和子宫圆韧带动脉，分布于腹壁。又称 *arteria epigastrica inferior*; **epigastric a., superficial**, *origin*, femoral artery; *branches*, none; *distribution*, abdominal wall, inguinal region 腹壁浅动脉，起源于股动脉，无分支，分布于腹壁和腹股沟区。又称 *arteria epigastrica superficialis*; **epigastric a., superior**, *origin*, internal thoracic artery; *branches*, none; *distribution*, abdominal wall, respiratory diaphragm 腹壁上动脉，起源于胸廓内动脉，无分支，分布于腹壁和横膈。又称 *arteria epigastrica superior*; **episcleral a's**, *origin*, anterior ciliary arteries; *branches*, none; *distribution*, iris, ciliary processes 巩膜上动脉，起源于睫状前动脉，无分支，分布于虹膜和睫状突。又称 *arteriae episclerales*; **ethmoidal a., anterior**, *origin*, ophthalmic artery; *branches*, anterior meningeal, anterior septal, and anterior lateral nasal branches; *distribution*, dura mater, nose, frontal sinus, anterior ethmoidal cells 筛前动脉，起源于眼动脉，分支包括脑膜前部、鼻中隔前部和鼻部前外侧分支，分布于硬脑膜、鼻部、额窦和筛前细胞。又称 *arteria ethmoidalis anterior*; **ethmoidal a., posterior**, *origin*, ophthalmic artery; *branches*, meningeal and septal and lateral nasal branches; *distribution*, posterior ethmoidal cells, dura mater, nose 筛后动脉，起源于眼动脉，分支包括脑膜支、鼻中隔支和鼻外侧支，分布于筛后细胞、硬脑膜和鼻部。又称 *arteria ethmoidalis posterior*; **facial a.**, *origin*, external carotid artery; *branches*, ascending palatine, tonsillar, submental, inferior labial, superior labial, septal, lateral nasal, angular, glandular; *distribution*, face, tonsil, palate, submandibular gland 面动脉，起源于颈外动脉，分支包括上颚、扁桃体、颏下、下唇、上唇、鼻中隔、鼻外侧、口角、腺体等，分布于面部、扁桃体、颚和颌下腺等。又称 *arteria facialis*；**fallopian a.**，输卵管动脉，见 uterine a.；**femoral a.**，*origin*, continuation of external iliac; *branches*, superficial epigastric, superficial circumflex iliac, external pudendal, deep femoral, descending genicular; *distribution*, lower abdominal wall, external genitalia, lower extremity NOTENOTE: The portion of the femoral artery proximal to the branching of the deep femoral is sometimes referred to as the *common femoral a.*, and its continuation as the *superficial femoral a.* 股动脉，是髂外动脉的直接延续，分支包括腹壁前动脉、旋髂浅动脉、阴部外动脉、股深动脉和膝降动脉，分布于腹壁下部、外生殖器和下肢。又称 *arteria femoralis*。注意：股动脉上近股深动脉分叉处有时可称为股总动脉，其直接延续段称为股浅动脉；**femoral a., common,** 见 *femoral a.*；**femoral a., deep,** *origin*, femoral artery; *branches*, medial and lateral circumflex arteries of thigh, perforating arteries; *distribution*, thigh muscles, hip joint, gluteal muscles, femur 股深动脉，起源于股动脉，分支包括旋股内侧动脉和旋股外侧动脉，以及穿通动脉，分布于大腿肌肉、髋关节、臀部肌肉和股骨。又称 *arteria profunda femoris*；**femoral a., superficial,** 股浅动脉，见 *femoral a.*；**femoral nutrient a's,** *origin*, third perforating artery; *branches*, none; *distribution*, femur 股骨滋养动脉，起源于第三穿通动脉，无分支，分布于股骨。又称 *arteriae nutriciae femoris* **fibular a.,**；见 peroneal a.；**fibular nutrient a.,** *origin*, fibular artery; *branches*, none; *distribution*, fibula 腓骨滋养动脉，起源于腓动脉，无分支，分布于腓骨。又称 *arteria nutricia fibulae*；**frontobasal a., lateral,** *origin*, middle cerebral artery; *branches*, none; *distribution*, cortex of lateroinferior frontal lobe 额叶底外侧动脉，起源于大脑中动脉，无分支，分布于额叶外下部皮质。又称 *arteria frontobasalis lateralis*；**frontobasal a., medial,** *origin*, anterior cerebral artery; *branches*, none; *distribution*, cortex of medioinferior frontal lobe 额叶底内侧动脉，起源于大脑前动脉，无分支，分布于额叶内下部皮质。又称 *arteria frontobasalis medialis*；**frontopolar a.,** polar frontal a. 额极动脉；**funicular a.,** 见 testicular a.；**gastric a., left,** *origin*, celiac trunk; *branches*, esophageal branches; *distribution*, esophagus, lesser curvature of stomach 胃左动脉，起源于腹腔干，分支包括食管支，分布于食管、胃小弯。又称 *arteria gas-*

trica sinistra；**gastric a., posterior,** *origin*, splenic artery; *branches*, none; *distribution*, posterior gastric wall 胃后动脉，起源于脾动脉，无分支，分布于胃后壁。又称 *arteria gastrica posterior*；**gastric a., right,** *origin*, common hepatic artery; *branches*, none; *distribution*, lesser curvature of stomach 胃右动脉，起源于肝总动脉，无分支，分布于胃小弯。又称 *arteria gastrica dextra*；**gastric a's, short,** *origin*, splenic artery; *branches*, none; *distribution*, upper part of stomach. 胃短动脉，起源于脾动脉，无分支，分布于胃上半部。又称 *arteriae gastricae breves*；**gastroduodenal a.,** *origin*, common hepatic artery; *branches*, supraduodenal and posterior superior pancreaticoduodenal arteries; *distribution*, stomach, duodenum, pancreas, greater omentum 胃十二指肠动脉，起源于肝总动脉，分支包括十二指肠上动脉和胰十二指肠上后动脉，分布于胃、十二指肠、胰腺和大网膜。又称 *arteria gastroduodenalis*；**gastroepiploic a., left,** left gastro-omental a. 胃网膜左动脉；**gastroepiploic a., right,** right gastro-omental a. 胃网膜右动脉；**gastro-omental a., left,** *origin*, splenic artery; *branches*, gastric, omental branches; *distribution*, stomach, greater omentum 胃网膜左动脉，起源于脾动脉，分支包括胃支和网膜支，分布于胃和大网膜。又称 *arteria gastroomentalis sinistra*；**gastro-omental a., right,** *origin*, gastroduodenal artery; *branches*, gastric, omental branches; *distribution*, stomach, greater omentum 胃网膜右动脉，起源于胃十二指肠动脉，分支包括胃支和网膜支，分布于胃和大网膜。又称 *arteria gastroomentalis dextra*；**genicular a., descending,** *origin*, femoral artery; *branches*, saphenous, articular; *distribution*, knee joint, upper and medial leg 膝降动脉，起源于股动脉，分支包括隐支和关节支，分布于膝关节和下肢中上段。又称 *arteria descendens genus*；**genicular a., lateral inferior,** *origin*, popliteal artery; *branches*, none; *distribution*, knee joint. 膝下外侧动脉，起源于胭动脉，无分支，分布于膝关节。又称 *arteria inferior lateralis genus*；**genicular a., lateral superior,** *origin*, popliteal artery; *branches*, none; *distribution*, knee joint, femur, patella, contiguous muscles 膝上外侧动脉，起源于胭动脉，无分支，分布于膝关节、股骨、髌骨及邻近肌肉。又称 *arteria superior lateralis genus*；**genicular a., medial inferior,** *origin*, popliteal artery; *branches*, none; *distribution*, knee joint 膝下内侧动脉，起源于胭动脉，无分支，分布于膝关节。又称 *arteria inferior medialis genus*；**genicular a., medial superior,** *origin*, popliteal artery; *branches*, none; *distribution*, knee joint, femur, patella, contiguous muscles 膝上内侧动脉，起源于胭动脉，无分支，分布于膝关节、股骨、髌骨及其邻近肌肉。又称

arteria superior medialis genus; **genicular a.,** *middle, origin,* popliteal artery; *branches,* none; *distribution,* knee joint, cruciate ligaments, patellar synovial and alar folds 膝中动脉，起源于腘动脉，无分支，分布于膝关节、交叉韧带、髌骨滑膜和翼状襞。又称 *arteria media genus*; **gluteal a.,** *inferior, origin,* internal iliac artery; *branches,* sciatic artery; *distribution,* buttock, back of thigh 臀下动脉，起源于髂内动脉，分支包括左股动脉，分布于臀部和大腿后部。又称 *arteria glutea inferior*; **gluteal a.,** *superior, origin,* internal iliac artery; *branches,* superficial and deep branches; *distribution,* buttocks 臀上动脉，起源于髂内动脉，分支包括浅支和深支，分布于臀部。又称 *arteria glutea superior*; **gonadal a's,** the ovarian arteries or the testicular arteries 性腺动脉，女性卵巢动脉或男性睾丸动脉; **great radicular a.,** 见 l. of Adamkiewicz; **helicine a's,** small arteries that for their entire length have a band of thickened intima on one side, in which longitudinal muscle fibers are embedded. They follow a convoluted or curled course and open directly into cavernous sinuses instead of capillaries; they play a dominant role in erection of erectile tissue 螺旋动脉，一种小动脉，其全长皆有一侧有一条增厚的内膜带，纵向肌纤维嵌入其中。螺旋动脉沿着旋绕或弯曲的路线走行，直接汇入海绵窦而非毛细血管；该动脉在组织勃起中起主导作用; **helicine a's of penis,** helicine arteries arising from the vessels of the penis, whose engorgement causes erection of the organ 阴茎螺旋动脉，从阴茎血管中发出的螺旋动脉，其充血可导致阴茎勃起。又称 *arteriae helicinae penis*; **hemorrhoidal a's,** the rectal arteries (inferior, middle, and superior) 痔动脉，直肠动脉（直肠下、中、上动脉）; **hepatic a., common,** *origin,* celiac trunk; *branches,* right gastric and gastroduodenal arteries and hepatic artery proper; *distribution,* stomach, pancreas, duodenum, liver, gallbladder, greater omentum 肝总动脉，起源于腹腔干，分支包括胃右动脉、胃十二指肠动脉和肝固有动脉，分布于胃、胰腺、十二指肠、肝、胆囊和大网膜。又称 *arteria hepatica communis*; **hepatic a., proper,** *origin,* common hepatic artery; *branches,* right and left branches; *distribution,* liver, gallbladder 肝固有动脉，起源于肝总动脉，分支包括左右两支，分布于肝和胆囊。又称 *arteria hepatica propria*; **humeral nutrient a's,** *origin,* brachial and profunda brachii arteries; *branches,* none; *distribution,* humerus 肱骨滋养动脉，起源于肱动脉和股深动脉，无分支，分布于肱骨。又称 *arteriae nutriciae humeri*; **hyaloid a.,** a fetal vessel that continues forward from the central artery of retina through the vitreous body to supply the lens; it normally is not present after birth 玻璃体动脉，一种胎儿血管，由视网膜中央动脉发出，向前穿过玻璃体，供应晶状体血供；该动脉正常情况下在出生后即不存在; **hypogastric a.,** internal iliac a. 髂内动脉; **hypophysial a., inferior,** a small branch from the cavernous part of the internal carotid artery that supplies the pituitary gland 垂体下动脉，颈内动脉海绵窦段的一个小分支，供应垂体。又称 *arteria hypophysialis inferior*; **hypophysial a., superior,** a small branch from the cerebral part of the internal carotid artery that supplies the pituitary gland 垂体上动脉，颈内动脉颅内段的一个小分支，供应垂体。又称 *arteria hypophysialis superior*; **ileal a's,** *origin,* superior mesenteric artery; *branches,* none; *distribution,* ileum. 回肠动脉，起源于肠系膜上动脉，无分支，分布于回肠。又称 *arteriae ileales*; **ileocolic a.,** *origin,* superior mesenteric artery; *branches,* anterior and posterior cecal and appendicular arteries and colic (ascending) and ileal branches; *distribution,* ileum, cecum, vermiform appendix, ascending colon. 回结肠动脉，起源于肠系膜上动脉，分支包括盲肠前动脉、盲肠后动脉、阑尾动脉，以及升结肠支、回肠支，分布于回肠、盲肠、阑尾和升结肠。又称 *arteria ileocolica*; **iliac a., common,** *origin,* abdominal aorta; *branches,* internal and external iliac arteries; *distribution,* pelvis, abdominal wall, lower limb 髂总动脉，起源于腹主动脉，分支包括髂内动脉和髂外动脉，分布于骨盆、腹壁和下肢。又称 *arteria iliaca communis*; **iliac a., external,** *origin,* common iliac; *branches,* inferior epigastric, deep circumflex iliac arteries; *distribution,* abdominal wall, external genitalia, lower limb 髂外动脉，起源于髂总动脉，分支包括腹壁下动脉和旋髂深动脉，分布于腹壁、外生殖器和下肢。又称 *arteria iliaca externa*; **iliac a., internal,** *origin,* continuation of common iliac artery; *branches,* iliolumbar, obturator, superior gluteal, inferior gluteal, umbilical, inferior vesical, uterine, middle rectal, and internal pudendal arteries; *distribution,* wall and viscera of pelvis, buttock, reproductive organs, medial aspect of thigh 髂内动脉，是髂总动脉的直接延续，分支包括髂腰动脉、闭孔动脉、臀上动脉、臀下动脉、脐动脉、膀胱下动脉、子宫动脉、直肠中动脉和阴部内动脉，分布于骨盆壁及其内部脏器、臀部、生殖器官和大腿内侧。又称 *arteria iliaca interna*; **iliolumbar a.,** *origin,* internal iliac artery; *branches,* iliac, spinal, and lumbar branches; *distribution,* pelvic muscles and bones, fifth lumbar segment, sacrum 髂腰动脉，起源于髂内动脉，分支包括髂支、脊椎支和腰支，分布于骨盆肌肉和骨骼，第五腰椎节段和骶骨。又称 *arteria iliolumbalis*; **infraorbital a.,** *origin,* maxillary artery; *branches,* anterior superior alveolar arteries; *distribution*, maxilla, maxillary sinus, upper teeth, lower eyelid, cheek, nose 眶下动脉，起源于上颌动脉，分支包括上牙槽前动脉，分布于上颌、上颌窦、上颌牙、下眼睑、颊部和鼻部。又 称 *arteria infraorbitalis*; **innominate a.,** brachiocephalic trunk 无名动脉，头臂干；**insular a's,** *origin*, insular part of middle cerebral artery; *branches*, none; *distribution*, cortex of insula 内囊动脉，起源于大脑中动脉内囊段，无分支，分布于内囊皮质。又称 *arteriae insulares*; **intercostal a's, anterior,** the twelve anterior intercostal branches of the internal thoracic artery, two in each of the upper six intercostal spaces, supplying the intercostal spaces and the pectoralis major muscle. Within each space both branches run laterally, the upper anastomosing with the posterior intercostal artery, the lower with the collateral branch of that artery 肋间前动脉，胸廓内动脉的 12 个肋间前支，1~6 肋间为每个肋间隙 2 支，供应肋间隙和胸大肌。在每个肋间隙内两个分支都向两侧走行，上 6 个肋间隙的肋间前动脉与对应的肋间后动脉吻合，下 6 个肋间隙的肋间前动脉与其侧支吻合；**intercostal a., first posterior,** *origin*, supreme intercostal artery; *branches*, dorsal and spinal branches; *distribution*, upper thoracic wall 第一肋间后动脉，起源于最上肋间动脉，分支包括背侧支和脊支，分布于上胸壁。又称 *arteria intercostalis posterior prima*; **intercostal a., highest,** supreme intercostal a. 最上肋间动脉；**intercostal a's, posterior,** for the first two, see *first posterior intercostal a.* and *second posterior intercostal a.*; there are nine other pairs (Ⅲ–Ⅺ): *origin*, descending thoracic aorta; *branches*, dorsal, collateral, muscular, and lateral cutaneous branches; *distribution*, thoracic wall 肋间后动脉，前 2 对肋间后动脉见 first posterior intercostal a. 和 second posterior intercostal a.；其余 9 对（Ⅲ – Ⅺ）：起源于胸主动脉，分支包括背侧支、侧副支、肌支和皮侧支，分布于胸壁。又称 *arteriae intercostales posteriores*; **intercostal a., second posterior,** *origin*, supreme intercostal artery; *branches*, dorsal and spinal branches; *distribution*, upper thoracic wall 第二肋间后动脉，起源于最上肋间动脉，分支包括背侧支和脊支，分布于上胸壁。又称 *arteria intercostalis posterior secunda*; **intercostal a., superior, intercostal a., supreme,** *origin*, costocervical trunk; *branches*, first and second posterior intercostal arteries; *distribution*, upper thoracic wall 最上肋间动脉，起源于肋颈干，分支包括第一和第二肋间后动脉，分布于上胸壁。又 称 *arteria intercostalis suprema*; **interlobar a's of kidney,** *origin*, lobar branches of segmental arteries; *branches*, arcuate arteries; *distribution*, parenchyma of kidney 肾叶间动脉，起源于肾段动脉的

大叶分支，分支包括弓状动脉，分布于肾实质。又 称 *arteriae interlobares renis*; **interlobular a's of kidney,** arteries originating from the arcuate arteries of the kidney and distributed to the renal glomeruli 肾小叶间动脉，起源于肾弓状动脉，分布于肾小球。又称 *arteriae corticales radiatae renis*; **interlobular a's of liver,** arteries originating from the right or left branch of the hepatic artery proper, forming a plexus outside each hepatic lobule and supplying the walls of the interlobular veins and the accompanying bile ducts 肝小叶间动脉，起源于肝固有动脉的左支或右支，在每个肝小叶外侧形成血管丛，供应小叶间静脉的血管壁，与胆管伴行。又称 *arteriae interlobulares hepatis*; **internal auditory a.,** 见 labyrinthine a.; **interosseous a., anterior,** *origin*, posterior or common interosseous artery; *branches*, median artery; *distribution*, deep parts of front of forearm 骨间前动脉，起源于骨间后动脉或骨间总动脉，分支包括正中动脉，分布于前臂深部。又称 *arteria interossea anterior*; **interosseous a., common,** *origin*, ulnar artery; *branches*, anterior and posterior interosseous arteries; *distribution*, antecubital fossa 骨间总动脉，起源于尺动脉，分支包括骨间前、后动脉，分布于肘窝。又称 *arteria interossea communis*; **interosseous a., posterior,** *origin*, common interosseous artery; *branches*, recurrent interosseous artery; *distribution*, deep parts of back of forearm 骨间后动脉，起源于骨间总动脉，分支包括骨间返动脉，分布于前臂后侧深部。又称 *arteria interossea posterior*; **interosseous a., recurrent,** *origin*, posterior interosseous or common interosseous artery; *branches*, none; *distribution*, back of elbow joint 骨间返动脉，起源于骨间后动脉或骨间总动脉，无分支，分布于肘关节后侧。又称 *arteria interossea recurrens*; **interventricular septal a's, anterior,** anterior septal a's 前室间隔动脉；**interventricular septal a's, posterior,** posterior septal a's 后室间隔动脉；**intestinal a's,** the arteries arising from the superior mesenteric, and supplying the intestines, including the pancreaticoduodenal, jejunal, ileal, ileocolic, and colic arteries 小肠动脉，起源于肠系膜上动脉，供应小肠，包括胰十二指肠动脉、空肠动脉、回肠动脉、回结肠动脉和结肠动脉；**intrarenal a's,** the arteries within the kidney, including the interlobar, arcuate, and cortical radiate (interlobular) arteries, and the straight arterioles 肾内动脉，肾内部的动脉，包括叶间动脉、弓状动脉、皮质放射动脉（小叶间动脉）和直小动脉。又称 *arteriae intrarenales*; **jejunal a's,** *origin*, superior mesenteric; *branches*, none; *distribution*, jejunum 空肠动脉，起源于肠系膜上动脉，无分支，分布于空肠。又称 *arteriae jejunales*; **a's of kid-**

ney, intrarenal a's 肾内动脉; **labial a., inferior,** *origin,* facial artery; *branches,* none; *distribution,* lower lip 下唇动脉，起源于面动脉，无分支，分布于下唇。又称 *arteria labialis inferior*; **labial a., superior,** *origin,* facial artery; *branches,* septal and alar; *distribution,* upper lip, nose 上唇动脉，起源于面动脉，分支包括鼻中隔支和翼支，分布于上唇和鼻部。又称 *arteria labialis superior*; **labyrinthine a.,** *origin,* anterior inferior cerebellar or basilar artery; *branches,* anterior vestibular and common cochlear arteries; *distribution,* through the internal acoustic meatus to the internal ear 迷路动脉，起源于小脑前下动脉或基底动脉，分支包括前庭前动脉和耳蜗总动脉，沿内耳道走行至内耳。又称 *arteria labyrinthi*; **lacrimal a.,** *origin,* ophthalmic artery; *branches,* lateral palpebral arteries and anastomotic branch with middle meningeal artery; *distribution,* lacrimal gland, upper and lower eyelids, conjunctiva 泪腺动脉，起源于眼动脉，分支包括睑外侧动脉以及与脑膜中动脉的吻合支，分布于泪腺、上下眼睑和结膜。又称 *arteria lacrimalis*; **laryngeal a., inferior,** *origin,* inferior thyroid artery; *branches,* none; *distribution,* larynx, trachea, esophagus 喉下动脉，起源于甲状腺下动脉，无分支，分布于喉部、气管和食管。又称 *arteria laryngea inferior*; **laryngeal a., superior,** *origin,* superior thyroid artery; *branches,* none; *distribution,* larynx 喉上动脉，起源于甲状腺上动脉，无分支，分布于喉部。又称 *arteria laryngea superior*; **lenticulostriate a's,** anterolateral central a's 豆状核纹状体动脉，前外侧中央动脉; **lingual a.,** *origin,* external carotid artery; *branches,* suprahyoid, sublingual, dorsal lingual, deep lingual; *distribution,* tongue, sublingual gland, tonsil, epiglottis 舌动脉，起源于颈外动脉，分支包括舌骨上动脉、舌下动脉、舌背动脉和舌深动脉，分布于舌部、舌下腺、扁桃体和会厌。又称 *arteria lingualis*; **lingular a.,** a branch of the left pulmonary artery to the superior lobe of the left lung, consisting almost entirely of the superior and inferior lingular arteries and supplying the lingular segments 舌动脉，左肺动脉舌支，在肺动脉发至左肺上叶的一个分支，几乎包含舌上、下动脉全长，供应左肺上叶舌段。又称 *arteria lingularis*; **lingular a., inferior,** a branch of the lingular artery, supplying the inferior lingular segment of the superior lobe of the left lung 舌下动脉，左肺动脉舌支的分支，供应左肺上叶舌段下部。又称 *arteria lingularis inferior*; **lingular a., superior,** a branch of the lingular artery, supplying the superior lingular segment of the superior lobe of the left lung 舌上动脉，左肺动脉舌支的分支，供应左肺上叶舌段上部。又称 *arteria lingularis superior*; **lobar a's, inferior,** the branches of each pulmonary artery that supply the inferior lobe of the corresponding lung, consisting of the superior, anterior basal, lateral basal, medial basal, and posterior basal segmental arteries 肺下叶动脉，供应肺下叶的肺动脉分支，包含上、前基底、外侧基底、内侧基底和后基底肺段动脉。又称 *arteriae lobares inferiores*; **lobar a., middle,** the branch of the right pulmonary artery that carries blood to the middle lobe of the right lung, giving rise to the lateral and medial segmental arteries 肺中叶动脉，供应右肺中叶的右肺动脉分支，分出外侧和内侧肺段动脉。又称 *arteria lobaris media pulmonis dextri*; **lobar a's, superior,** the branches of each pulmonary artery that supply the superior lobe of the corresponding lung, consisting of the apical, anterior, and posterior segmental arteries 肺上叶动脉，供应肺上叶的肺动脉分支，包含肺尖和前、后肺段动脉。又称 *arteriae lobares superiores*; **lumbar a's,** *origin,* abdominal aorta; *branches,* dorsal and spinal branches; *distribution,* posterior abdominal wall, renal capsule 腰动脉，起源于腹主动脉，分支包括背侧支和脊支，分布于后腹壁和肾包膜。又称 *arteriae lumbales*; **lumbar a's, lowest,** *origin,* median sacral artery; *branches,* none; *distribution,* sacrum, gluteus maximus muscle 腰最下动脉，起源于骶正中动脉，无分支，分布于骶骨和臀大肌。又称 *arteria malleolaris anterior lateralis*; **malleolar a., anterior lateral,** *origin,* anterior tibial artery; *branches,* none; *distribution,* ankle joint 踝动脉，起源于胫前动脉，无分支，分布于踝关节。又称 *arteria malleolaris anterior lateralis*; **malleolar a., anterior medial,** *origin,* anterior tibial artery; *branches,* none; *distribution,* ankle joint 内踝前动脉，起源于胫前动脉，无分支，分布于踝关节。又称 *arteria malleolaris anterior medialis*; **mammary a., external,** lateral thoracic. 乳外动脉，胸廓外动脉; **mammary a., internal,** internal thoracic a. 乳内动脉，胸廓内动脉; **mammillary a's,** *origin,* posterior communicating artery; *branches,* none; *distribution,* mammillary bodies 乳头外动脉，起源于后交通动脉，无分支，分布于乳头体。又称 *arteriae mammillares*; **mandibular a.,** inferior alveolar a. 下颌动脉，下牙槽动脉; **marginal a., left,** a branch of the circumflex branch of the left coronary artery, which follows the left margin of the heart and supplies the left ventricle 左缘动脉，左冠状动脉回旋支的分支，沿心脏左缘走行，供应左心室; **marginal a., right,** a branch of the right coronary artery passing toward the apex of the heart along the acute margin of the heart and ramifying over the right ventricle 右缘动脉，右冠状动脉的分支，沿心脏锐缘行经心尖部，在右心室发出分支; **marginal a. of colon,** a continuous vessel running along the inner perimeter of the large intestine from the ileocolic junction to the rectum, formed by branches from the superior and inferior mesenteric arteries and giving rise to straight arteries that supply the intestinal wall. 结肠缘动脉，一个沿大肠内周自回结肠交界处走行至直肠的连续血管，由肠系膜上、下动脉的分支共同形成，发出供应肠壁的直动脉。又称 *arteria marginalis coli*；**masseteric a., origin**, maxillary artery; *branches*, none; *distribution*, masseter muscle 咬肌动脉，起源于上颌动脉，无分支，分布于咬肌。又称 *arteria masseterica*；**maxillary a., origin**, external carotid artery; *branches*, deep auricular, anterior tympanic, inferior alveolar, middle meningeal, pterygomeningeal, masseteric, anterior and posterior deep temporal, buccal, posterior superior alveolar, infraorbital, descending palatine, and sphenopalatine arteries, and artery of pterygoid canal; *distribution*, both jaws, teeth, muscles of mastication, ear, meninges, nose, paranasal sinuses, palate 上颌动脉，起源于颈外动脉，分支包括耳深动脉、鼓室前动脉、下牙槽动脉、脑膜中动脉、翼突脑膜动脉、咬肌动脉、颞深前、后动脉、颊动脉、上牙槽后动脉、眶下动脉、腭降动脉、蝶腭动脉和翼状动脉，分布于两侧下颌、牙齿、咀嚼肌、耳、脑膜、鼻、鼻旁窦和腭部。又称 *arteria maxillaris*；**maxillary a., external,** 见 facial a.；**maxillary a., internal,** 见 maxillary a.；**median a., origin**, anterior interosseous artery; *branches*, none; *distribution*, median nerve, muscles of front of forearm 正中动脉，起源于骨间前动脉，无分支，分布于正中神经和前臂肌肉。又称 *arteria comitans nervi mediani*；**median callosal a., origin**, anterior communicating artery; *distribution*, runs above the lamina terminalis to supply anterior hypothalamic and subcallosal areas and corpus callosum 胼胝体正中动脉，起源于前交通动脉，走行于下丘脑终板上方，供应下丘脑前部、胼胝体下部区域和胼胝体。又称 *arteria callosa mediana*；**median commissural a., origin**, anterior communicating artery; *branches*, none; *distribution*, supraoptic commissures and optic chiasm 连合中动脉，起源于前交通动脉，无分支，分布于眶上连合纤维和视交叉。又称 *arteria commissuralis mediana*；**medullary a.,** 见 nutrient a.；**meningeal a., accessory,** 见 pterygomeningeal a.；**meningeal a., anterior,** the anterior meningeal branch of the anterior ethmoidal artery, supplying the dura mater 脑膜前动脉，筛前动脉的脑膜前支，供应硬脑膜；**meningeal a., middle, origin**, maxillary artery; *branches*, frontal, parietal, and lacrimal anastomotic, accessory meningeal, and petrosal branches, and superior tympanic artery; *distribution*, cranial bones, dura mater 脑膜中动脉，

起源于上颌动脉，分支包括额叶支、顶叶支、泪腺吻合支、脑膜副支、颞骨岩支和鼓室上支，分布于颅骨和硬脑膜。又称 *arteria meningea media*；**meningeal a., posterior, origin**, ascending pharyngeal artery; *branches*, none; *distribution*, bones and dura mater of posterior cranial fossa 脑膜后动脉，起源于咽升动脉，无分支，分布于颅后窝的骨骼和硬脑膜。又称 *arteria meningea posterior*；**mental a.,** the mental branch of the inferior alveolar artery, arising from the inferior alveolar artery in the mandibular canal, leaving the canal at the mental foramen, supplying the chin, and anastomosing with its fellow of the opposite side and with the submental and inferior labial arteries 颏动脉，下牙槽动脉颏支，起自下颌管内的下牙槽动脉，从颏孔处离开下颌管，供应颏部，与其对侧颏动脉、颏下动脉和下唇动脉相吻合；**mesencephalic a's, origin**, basilar artery; *branches*, none; *distribution*, cerebral peduncle 中脑动脉，起源于基底动脉，无分支，分布于大脑脚。又称 *arteriae mesencephalicae*；**mesenteric a., inferior, origin**, abdominal aorta; *branches*, left colic, sigmoid, and superior rectal arteries; *distribution*, descending colon, rectum 肠系膜下动脉，起源于腹主动脉，分支包括左结肠动脉、乙状结肠动脉和直肠上动脉，分布于降结肠和直肠。又称 *arteria mesenterica inferior*；**mesenteric a., superior, origin**, abdominal aorta; *branches*, inferior pancreaticoduodenal, jejunal, ileal, ileocolic, right colic, and middle colic arteries; *distribution*, small intestine, proximal half of colon 肠系膜上动脉，起源于腹主动脉，分支包括胰十二指肠下动脉、空肠动脉、回肠动脉、回结肠动脉、右结肠动脉和结肠中动脉，分布于小肠和结肠近半部分。又称 *arteria mesenterica superior*；**metacarpal a's, dorsal, origin**, dorsal carpal rete and radial artery; *branches*, dorsal digital arteries; *distribution*, dorsum of fingers 掌背动脉，起源于腕背侧动脉网和桡动脉，分支包括指背动脉，分布于手指背侧。又称 *arteriae metacarpales dorsales*；**metacarpal a's, palmar, origin**, deep palmar arch; *branches*, none; *distribution*, deep parts of metacarpus 掌骨掌侧动脉，起源于掌深弓，无分支，分布于掌深部。又称 *arteriae metacarpales palmares*；**metatarsal a's, dorsal, origin**, arcuate artery of foot; *branches*, dorsal digital arteries; *distribution*, dorsal region of foot, including toes 跖背动脉，起源于足弓状动脉，分支包括趾背动脉，分布于足背侧区域包括足趾。又称 *arteriae metatarsales dorsales*；**metatarsal a's, plantar, origin**, plantar arch; *branches*, perforating branches, common and proper plantar digital arteries; *distribution*, toes 跖底动脉，起源于足底弓，分支包括穿通支、趾足底总动脉和趾足底固有动脉，分布于足趾。

又称 *arteriae metatarsales plantares*; **muscular a's,**
1. branches of the ophthalmic artery consisting of a
superior group and an inferior group; the inferior
group gives origin to the anterior ciliary arteries 肌
性动脉，眼动脉的分支，包括上、下两组血管，
下组发出睫状前动脉。又称 *arteriae muscu-
lares*; 2. distributing a's 分配动脉，即中动脉；
musculophrenic a., *origin*, internal thoracic artery;
branches, none; *distribution*, respiratory diaphragm,
abdominal and thoracic walls. 肌膈动脉，起源于
胸廓内动脉，无分支，分布于横膈、腹壁和胸壁。
又 称 *arteria musculophrenica*; **mylohyoid a.,** a
branch of the inferior alveolar artery that descends
with the mylohyoid nerve in the mylohyoid sulcus
to supply the floor of the mouth 下颌舌骨动脉，下
牙槽动脉的分支，沿下颌舌骨沟走行，伴行下颌
舌骨肌神经，供应口底; **nasal a., dorsal, nasal a.,
external,** *origin*, ophthalmic artery; *branches*,
branch to nasolacrimal sac and branch anastomosing
with terminal part of facial artery; *distribution*, skin
of nose 鼻背动脉，鼻外侧动脉，起源于眼动脉，
分支包括鼻泪囊分支及与面动脉终末段吻合的分
支，分布于鼻部皮肤。又称 *arteria dorsalis
nasi*; **nasal a's, posterior lateral,** *origin*, sphenopalatine artery; *branches*, none; *distribution*, frontal,
maxillary, ethmoidal, and sphenoidal sinuses 鼻后
外侧动脉，起源于蝶腭动脉，无分支，分布于额
叶、上颌、筛骨和蝶窦。又称 *arteriae nasales
posteriores laterales*; **nutrient a.,** any artery that
supplies the marrow of a long bone 滋养动脉，供
应长骨骨髓的动脉血管; **obturator a.,** *origin*, internal iliac artery; *branches*, pubic, acetabular, anterior, and posterior branches; *distribution*, pelvic
muscles, hip joint 闭孔动脉，起源于髂内动脉，
分支包括耻骨支、髋臼支、前支和后支，分布于
骨盆肌肉和髋关节。又称 *arteria obturatoria*;
occipital a., *origin*, external carotid artery; *branches*, auricular, meningeal, mastoid, descending, occipital, and sternocleidomastoid branches; *distribution*, muscles of neck and scalp, meninges, mastoid
cells 枕动脉，起源于颈外动脉，分支包括耳支、
脑膜支、乳突支、降支、枕支和胸锁乳突支，分
布于颈部肌肉、头皮、脑膜和乳突细胞。又称
arteria occipitalis; **occipital a., lateral,** *origin*,
third segment of posterior cerebral artery; *branches*,
anterior temporal, intermediate temporal, and posterior temporal arteries; *distribution*, cortex of anteri-
or, middle, and posterior parts of temporal lobe 枕
叶外侧动脉，起源于大脑后动脉的第三节段，分
支包括颞叶前、中、后动脉，分布于颞叶前、中、
后部皮质。又称 *arteria occipitalis lateralis*; **occipital a., medial,** *origin*, fourth segment of posteri-
or cerebral artery; *branches*, parietal, parietoocci-

tal, calcarine, and occipitotemporal branches, and
branch to dorsal corpus callosum; *distribution*, dorsum of corpus callosum, precuneus, cuneus, lingual
gyrus, and posterior part of lateral surface of occipital lobe 枕叶内侧动脉，起源于大脑后动脉的第
四节段，分支包括顶叶支、顶枕叶支、距状皮层
支、枕颞叶支和胼胝体背侧支，分布于胼胝体背
侧、楔前叶、楔状叶、舌回和枕叶外侧面后部。
又 称 *arteria occipitalis medialis*; **ophthalmic a.,**
origin, internal carotid artery; *branches*, lacrimal
and supraorbital arteries, central artery of retina, ciliary, muscular, posterior and anterior ethmoidal, palpebral, supratrochlear, and dorsal nasal arteries, and
recurrent meningeal branch; *distribution*, eye, orbit,
adjacent facial structures 眼动脉，起源于颈内动脉，
分支包括泪腺动脉、眶上动脉、视网膜中央动脉、
睫状动脉、肌性动脉、筛前动脉、筛后动脉、眼
睑动脉、滑车上动脉、鼻背动脉和脑膜返支等，
分布于眼、眶及邻近面部结构。又称 *arteria
ophthalmica*; **ovarian a.,** *origin*, abdominal aorta;
branches, ureteral, tubal; *distribution*, ureter, ovary,
uterine tube 卵巢动脉，起源于腹主动脉，分支包
括输尿管动脉和输卵管动脉，分布于输尿管、卵
巢和输卵管。又称 *arteria ovarica*; **palatine a.,
ascending,** *origin*, facial artery; *branches*, none;
distribution, soft palate, wall of pharynx, tonsil, auditory tube 腭升动脉，起源于面动脉，无分支，
分布于软腭、咽壁、扁桃体和咽鼓管。又称 *ar-
teria palatina ascendens*; **palatine a., descending,**
origin, maxillary artery; *branches*, greater and lesser
palatine arteries; *distribution*, soft palate, hard palate, tonsil 腭降动脉，起源于上颌动脉，分支包
括腭大动脉和腭小动脉，分布于软腭、硬腭和扁
桃体。又称 *arteria palatina descendens*; **palatine
a., greater,** *origin*, descending palatine artery;
branches, none; *distribution*, hard palate 腭大动脉，
起源于腭降动脉，无分支，分布于硬腭。又称
arteria palatine major; **palatine a's, lesser,** *origin*,
descending palatine artery; *branches*, none; *distribution*, soft palate, tonsil 腭小动脉，起源于腭降
动脉，无分支，分布于软腭和扁桃体。又称 *ar-
teriae palatinae minores*; **palmar digital a's, common,** *origin*, superficial palmar arch; *branches*,
proper palmar digital arteries; *distribution*, fingers
指掌侧总动脉，起源于掌浅弓，分支有指掌侧固
有动脉，分布于手指。又称 *arteriae digitales pal-
mares communes*; **palmar digital a's, proper,** *origin*, common palmar digital arteries; *branches*,
none; *distribution*, fingers 指掌侧固有动脉，起源
于指掌侧总动脉，无分支，分布于手指。又称
arteriae digitales palmares propriae; **palpebral a's,
lateral,** *origin*, lacrimal artery; *branches*, none; *distribution*, eyelids, conjunctiva 睑外侧动脉，起源

于泪腺动脉，无分支，分布于眼睑和结膜。又称 *arteriae palpebrales laterales*；palpebral a's, medial, *origin*, ophthalmic artery; *branches*, posterior conjunctival arteries and superior and inferior palpebral arches; *distribution*, eyelids. There are two (superior and inferior) 睑内侧动脉，起源于眼动脉，分支包括结膜后动脉和睑上、下动脉，分布于眼睑。睑内侧动脉有两支（上支和下支）。又称 *arteriae palpebrales mediales*；pancreatic a., caudal, *origin*, splenic artery; *branches and distribution*, supplies branches to tail of pancreas, and accessory spleen (if present) 胰尾动脉，起源于脾动脉，其分支供应胰尾部和副脾（若存在副脾的话）。又 称 *arteria caudae pancreatis*；pancreatic a., dorsal, *origin*, splenic artery; *branches*, inferior pancreatic artery; *distribution*, neck and body of pancreas 胰背动脉，起源于脾动脉，分支包括胰下动脉，分布于胰腺颈部和体部。又称 *arteria pancreatica dorsalis*；pancreatic a., greater, *origin*, splenic artery; *branches and distribution*, right and left branches anastomose with other pancreatic arteries 胰大动脉，起源于脾动脉，其左、右支与其他胰腺动脉相吻合。又称 *arteria pancreatica magna*；pancreatic a., inferior, *origin*, dorsal pancreatic artery; *branches*, none; *distribution*, body and tail of pancreas 胰下动脉，起源于胰背动脉，无分支，分布于胰腺体部和尾部。又称 *arteria pancreatica inferior*；pancreaticoduodenal a., anterior superior, *origin*, gastroduodenal artery; *branches*, pancreatic and duodenal; *distribution*, pancreas and duodenum 胰十二指肠前上动脉，起源于胃十二指肠动脉，分支包括胰支和十二指肠支，分布于胰腺和十二指肠。又称 *arteria pancreaticoduodenalis superior anterior*；pancreaticoduodenal a., inferior, *origin*, superior mesenteric artery; *branches*, anterior, posterior; *distribution*, pancreas, duodenum 胰十二指肠下动脉，起源于肠系膜上动脉，分支包括前支和后支，分布于胰腺和十二指肠。又称 *arteria pancreaticoduodenalis inferior*；pancreaticoduodenal a., posterior superior, *origin*, gastroduodenal artery; *branches*, pancreatic and duodenal; *distribution*, pancreas, duodenum 胰十二指肠前下动脉，起源于胃十二指肠动脉，分支包括胰支和十二指肠支，分布于胰腺和十二指肠。又称 *arteria pancreaticoduodenalis posterior superior*；paracentral a., the paracentral branches of the callosomarginal artery, which arise from the anterior cerebral artery and supply the cerebral cortex and medial central sulcus 旁中央动脉，胼胝体缘动脉的旁中央支，发自大脑前动脉，供应大脑皮质和内中央沟；paramedian a's, posteromedial central a's of posterior communicating artery 旁正中动脉，后交通动脉的后内侧中央动

脉；parietal a., anterior, *origin*, superior terminal branch of middle cerebral artery; *branches*, none; *distribution*, anterior parietal lobe 顶叶前动脉，起源于大脑中动脉的终末上支，无分支，分布于顶叶前部。又称 *arteria parietalis anterior*；parietal a., posterior, *origin*, superior terminal branch of middle cerebral artery; *branches*, none; *distribution*, posterior parietal lobe 顶叶后动脉，起源于大脑中动脉的终末上支，无分支，分布于顶叶后部。又称 *arteria parietalis posterior*；perforating a's, *origin*, branches (usually three) of the deep femoral artery that perforate the insertion of the adductor magnus to reach the back of the thigh; *branches*, nutrient arteries; *distribution*, adductor, hamstring, and gluteal muscles, and femur. 穿通动脉，股深动脉的分支（通常有三支），穿过大收肌附着点到达大腿后侧，分支包括滋养动脉，分布于内收肌、腘绳肌腱、臀肌和股骨。又称 *arteriae perforantes*；perforating a's, anterior, *origin*, anterior cerebral artery; *branches*, none; *distribution*, enter anterior perforated substance 前穿通动脉，起源于大脑前动脉，无分支，分布于前穿质。又称 *arteriae perforantes anteriores*；perforating radiate a's of kidney, small arteries that are continuations of the interlobular arteries and perforate the renal capsule 肾穿通放射状动脉，小叶间动脉的直接延续，穿过肾包膜。又称 *arteriae perforantes radiatae renis*；pericallosal a., *origin*, anterior cerebral artery, distal to the origin of the callosomarginal artery; *branches*, precuneal and parietooccipital branches; *distribution*, runs along corpus callosum, supplying cerebral cortex 胼胝体周围动脉，起源于大脑前动脉，位于胼胝体缘动脉起点远端，分支包括楔叶前支和顶枕叶支，沿胼胝体走行，供应大脑皮质。又称 *arteria pericallosa*；pericardiacophrenic a., *origin*, internal thoracic artery; *branches*, none; *distribution*, pericardium, respiratory diaphragm, pleura 心包膈动脉，起源于胸廓内动脉，无分支，分布于心包、横膈和胸膜。又称 *arteria pericardiacophrenica*；perineal a., *origin*, internal pudendal artery; *branches*, none; *distribution*, perineum, skin of external genitalia 会阴动脉，起源于阴部内动脉，无分支，分布于回阴、外生殖器皮肤。又称 *arteria perinealis*；perirenal a's, 见 capsular a's.；peroneal a., *origin*, posterior tibial artery; *branches*, perforating, communicating, calcaneal, and lateral and medial malleolar branches, and calcaneal rete; *distribution*, outside and back of ankle, deep calf muscles 腓动脉，起源于胫后动脉，分支包括穿通支、交通支、跟骨支、外踝支、内踝支和跟骨动脉网，分布于踝关节外侧和后侧以及小腿深部肌肉。又称 *arteria fibularis*；phrenic a., great, phrenic a., inferior, *origin*, abdominal aorta; *branches*, superior suprarenal arteries; *distribution*, respiratory diaphragm, suprarenal gland 膈下动脉，起源于腹主动脉，分支包括肾上腺上动脉，分布于横膈和肾上腺。又称 *arteria phrenica inferior*；**phrenic a's, superior, *origin***, descending thoracic aorta; *branches*, none; *distribution*, upper surface of vertebral portion of respiratory diaphragm 膈上动脉，起源于胸主动脉，无分支，分布于横膈椎体部分的上表面。又称 *arteriae phrenicae superiores*；**plantar a., deep, *origin***, dorsalis pedis artery; *branches*, none; *distribution*, sole of foot to help form plantar arch 足底深动脉，起源于足背动脉，无分支，分布于足底，参与构成足底动脉弓。又称 *arteria plantaris profunda*；**plantar a., lateral, *origin***, posterior tibial artery; *branches*, plantar arch and plantar metatarsal arteries; *distribution*, sole of foot and toes 足底外侧动脉，起源于胫后动脉，分支包括足底弓和跖底动脉，分布于足底和足趾。又称 *arteria plantaris lateralis*；**plantar a., medial, *origin***, posterior tibial artery; *branches*, deep and superficial branches; *distribution*, sole of the foot and toes 足底内侧动脉，起源于胫后动脉，分支包括深支和浅支，分布于足底和足趾。又称 *arteria plantaris medialis*；**plantar digital a's, common, *origin***, plantar metatarsal arteries; *branches*, proper plantar digital arteries; *distribution*, toes 趾足底总动脉，起源于跖底动脉，分支包括趾足底固有动脉，分布于足趾。又称 *arteriae digitales plantares communes*；**plantar digital a's, proper, *origin***, common plantar digital arteries; *branches*, none; *distribution*, toes 趾足底固有动脉，起源于趾足底总动脉，无分支，分布于足趾。又称 *arteriae digitales plantares propriae*；**polar frontal a., *origin***, anterior cerebral artery; *branches*, none; *distribution*, frontal pole of cerebral hemisphere 额极动脉，起源于大脑前动脉，无分支，分布于大脑半球额极。又称 *arteria polaris frontalis*；**polar temporal a., *origin***, middle cerebral artery; *branches*, none; *distribution*, temporal pole of cerebral hemisphere 颞极动脉，起源于大脑中动脉，无分支，分布于大脑半球颞极。又称 *arteria polaris temporalis*；**pontine a's, *origin***, basilar artery; *branches*, none; *distribution*, pons and adjacent areas of brain 脑桥动脉，起源于基底动脉，无分支，分布于脑桥及邻近区域。又称 *arteriae pontis*；**popliteal a., *origin***, continuation of femoral artery; *branches*, lateral and medial superior genicular, middle genicular, sural, lateral and medial inferior genicular, anterior and posterior tibial arteries, and the genicular articular and the patellar retes; *distribution*, knee, calf 腘动脉，是股动脉的直接延续，分支包括膝关节上外侧和上内侧动脉、膝关节中动脉、腓肠肌动脉、膝关节外下侧和内下侧动脉、膝关节及髌骨动脉网，分布于膝关节和小腿。又称 *arteria poplitea*；**a. of postcentral sulcus, *origin***, middle cerebral artery; *branches*, none; *distribution*, cortex on either side of postcentral sulcus 后中央沟动脉，起源于大脑中动脉，无分支，分布于后中央沟两侧皮质。又称 *arteria sulci postcentralis*；**a. of precentral sulcus, *origin***, middle cerebral artery; *branches*, none; *distribution*, cortex on either side of precentral sulcus 前中央沟动脉，起源于大脑中动脉，无分支，分布于前中央沟两侧皮质。又称 *arteria sulci precentralis*；**precuneal a's**, branches of the pericallosal artery originating in the anterior cerebral artery and supplying the inferior precuneus 楔前动脉，胼胝体周围动脉的分支，发自大脑前动脉，供应楔叶前沟；**prefrontal a., *origin***, superior terminal branch of middle cerebral artery; *branches*, none; *distribution*, prefrontal area of cerebrum 额前动脉，起源于大脑中动脉的终末上支，无分支，分布于大脑额叶前区。又称 *arteria prefrontalis*；**preoptic a's, *origin***, anterior cerebral artery; *branches*, none; *distribution*, preoptic region 视前动脉，起源于大脑前动脉，无分支，分布于视叶前区。又称 *arteriae preopticae*；**prepancreatic a.**, an arterial arch between the neck and uncinate process of the pancreas, formed by branches from the splenic artery and the anterior superior pancreaticoduodenal artery 胰前动脉，胰腺颈部和钩突之间的动脉弓，由脾动脉和胰十二指肠前上动脉的分支构成。又称 *arteria prepancreatica*；**princeps pollicis a., *origin***, radial artery; *branches*, radialis indicis artery of index finger; *distribution*, each side and palmar aspect of thumb 拇主要动脉，起源于桡动脉，分支包括示指桡侧动脉，分布于拇指的左右两侧和掌侧。又称 *arteria princeps pollicis*；**profunda brachii a., *origin***, brachial artery; *branches*, deltoid branch, nutrient of humerus and middle and radial collateral arteries; *distribution*, humerus, muscles and skin of arm 肱深动脉，起源于肱动脉，分支包括三角肌支、肱骨滋养动脉、中副动脉和桡侧副动脉，分布于肱骨、上肢肌肉和皮肤。又称 *arteria profunda brachii*；**profunda femoris a.**, deep femoral a. 股深动脉；**a. of pterygoid canal, 翼管动脉，**1. *origin*, maxillary artery; *branches*, pterygoid; *distribution*, roof of pharynx, auditory tube 起源于上颌动脉，分支包括翼支，分布于咽顶和咽鼓管；2. *origin*, internal carotid artery; *branches*, none; *distribution*, pterygoid canal, anastomosing with the artery of the pterygoid canal that branches from the maxillary artery 起源于颈内动脉，无分支，分布于翼管，与自上颌动脉发出的翼管动脉相吻合。又称 *arteria canalis pterygoidei*；**pterygomeningeal a.**, a branch arising from the middle meningeal artery, or directly from the maxillary artery, and entering the middle cranial fossa through the foramen ovale to supply the trigeminal ganglion, walls of the cavernous sinus, and neighboring dura mater 翼突脑膜动脉、脑膜中动脉的分支，或直接发自上颌动脉，经卵圆孔进入颅中窝，供应三叉神经节、海绵窦壁和邻近硬脑膜；**pudendal a., deep external**, *origin*, femoral artery; *branches*, anterior scrotal or anterior labial branches, inguinal branches; *distribution*, external genitalia, upper medial thigh 阴部外深动脉，起源于股动脉，分布包括阴囊前支或阴唇前支，以及腹股沟支，分布于外生殖器和大腿上内侧。又称 *arteria pudenda externa profunda*；**pudendal a., internal**, *origin*, internal iliac artery; *branches*, posterior scrotal or posterior labial branches and inferior rectal, perineal, urethral arteries, artery of bulb of penis or vestibule, deep artery of penis or clitoris, dorsal artery of penis or clitoris; *distribution*, external genitalia, anal canal, perineum 阴部内动脉，起源于髂内动脉，分支包括阴囊后支或阴唇后支、直肠下动脉、会阴动脉、尿道动脉、阴茎球动脉或前庭球动脉、阴茎深动脉或阴蒂深动脉，以及阴茎或阴蒂背侧动脉，分布于外生殖器、肛管和会阴。又称 *arteria pudenda interna*；**pudendal a., superficial external**, *origin*, femoral artery; *branches*, none; *distribution*, external genitalia 阴部外浅动脉，起源于股动脉，无分支，分布于外生殖器。又称 *arteria pudenda externa superficialis*；**pulmonary a., left**, *origin*, pulmonary trunk; *branches*, numerous, named according to the segments of the lung to which they distribute unaerated blood; *distribution*, left lung 左肺动脉，起源于肺动脉干，分支众多，根据其输送未氧合血液的肺段进行命名，分布于左肺。又称 *arteria pulmonalis sinistra*；**pulmonary a., right**, *origin*, pulmonary trunk; *branches*, numerous, named according to the segments of the lung to which they distribute unaerated blood; *distribution*, right lung 右肺动脉，起源于肺动脉干，分支众多，根据其输送未氧合血液的肺段进行命名，分布于右肺。又称 *arteria pulmonalis dextra*；**quadrigeminal a.**，见 collicular a.；**radial a.**, *origin*, brachial artery; *branches*, palmar carpal, superficial palmar, and dorsal carpal branches, recurrent radial artery, princeps pollicis artery, deep palmar arch; *distribution*, forearm, wrist, hand 桡动脉，起源于肱动脉，分支包括腕掌支、掌浅支、腕背支、桡侧返动脉、拇主要动脉和掌深弓，分布于前臂、腕部和手。又称 *arteria radialis*；**radial recurrent a.**, *origin*, radial artery; *branches*, none; *distribution*, brachioradialis, brachialis, elbow region 桡侧返动脉，起源于桡动脉，无分支，分布于肱桡肌、肱肌和肘关节区域。又称 *arteria*

recurrens radialis；**radial a's of uterus**, branches of the uterine arcuate arteries that supply the deeper layers of the myometrium and penetrate the endometrium, giving rise to the spiral arteries 子宫放射动脉，子宫弓状动脉分支，供应子宫肌层深层组织，并且穿过子宫内膜，发出螺旋动脉；**radialis indicis a.**, *origin*, princeps pollicis artery; *branches*, none; *distribution*, index finger 示指桡侧动脉，起源于拇主要动脉，无分支，分布于示指。又称 *arteria radialis indicis*；**radiate a's of kidney**，见 interlobular a's of kidney；**radicular a., anterior**, one of the spinal branches of the dorsal branch of a posterior intercostal artery; it is the branch supplying the anterior root of a particular spinal nerve 前根动脉，肋间后动脉背侧支的脊髓支，该分支供应某个特定脊神经的前根。又称 *arteria radicularis anterior*；**radicular a., posterior**, one of the spinal branches of the dorsal branch of a posterior intercostal artery; it is the branch supplying the posterior root of a particular spinal nerve 后根动脉，肋间后动脉背侧支的脊髓支，该分支供应某个特定脊神经的后根。又称 *arteria radicularis posterior*；**ranine a.**，见 deep lingual a.；**rectal a., inferior**, *origin*, internal pudendal artery; *branches*, none; *distribution*, rectum, anal canal 直肠下动脉，起源于阴部内动脉，无分支，分布于直肠和肛管。又称 *arteria rectalis inferior*；**rectal a., middle**, *origin*, internal iliac artery; *branches*, vaginal; *distribution*, rectum, prostate, seminal vesicles, vagina 直肠中动脉，起源于髂内动脉，分支包括阴道支，分布于直肠、前列腺、精囊和阴道。又称 *arteria rectalis media*；**rectal a., superior**, *origin*, inferior mesenteric artery; *branches*, none; *distribution*, rectum 直肠上动脉，起源于肠系膜下动脉，无分支，分布于直肠。又称 *arteria rectalis superior*；**renal a.**, *origin*, abdominal aorta; *branches*, ureteral branches, inferior suprarenal artery; *distribution*, kidney, suprarenal gland, ureter 肾动脉，起源于腹主动脉，分支包括输尿管支、肾上腺下动脉，分布于深、肾上腺和输尿管。又称 *arteria renalis*；**retroduodenal a's**, *origin*, first branch of gastroduodenal artery; *branches*, none; *distribution*, bile duct, duodenum, head of pancreas 十二指肠后动脉，起源于胃十二指肠动脉的第一个分支，无分支，分布于胆管、十二指肠和胰头。又称 *arteriae retroduodenales*；**a. of round ligament of uterus**, *origin*, inferior epigastric artery; *branches*, none; *distribution*, round ligament of uterus 子宫圆韧带动脉，起源于腹壁下动脉，无分支，分布于子宫圆韧带。又称 *arteria ligamenti teretis uteri*；**sacral a's, lateral**, *origin*, posterior trunk of internal iliac artery; *branches*, spinal branches; *distribution*, structures about coccyx and sacrum. There are usually two on each side (superior and inferior) 骶外侧动脉, 起源于髂内动脉后干, 分支包括骶支, 分布于骶尾骨的相关结构。通常每侧有两支骶外侧动脉（上支和下支）。又称 *arteriae sacrales laterales*；**sacral a., median**, *origin*, continuation of abdominal aorta；*branches*, lowest lumbar artery；*distribution*, sacrum, coccyx, rectum 骶正中动脉, 是腹主动脉的直接延续, 分支包括腰最下动脉, 分布于骶骨、尾骨和直肠。又称 *arteria sacralis mediana*；**scapular a., dorsal**, *origin*, second or third part of subclavian artery (or may be deep branch of transverse cervical artery)；*branches*, none；*distribution*, rhomboid, latissimus dorsi, and trapezius muscles 肩胛背动脉, 起源于肩胛下动脉的第二或第三部分（亦可能是起自颈横动脉深支）, 无分支, 分布于菱形肌、背阔肌和斜方肌。又称 *arteria dorsalis scapulae*；**scapular a., transverse**, 见 suprascapular a.；**sciatic a., a. to sciatic nerve**, *origin*, inferior gluteal artery；*branches*, none；*distribution*, accompanies sciatic nerve 坐骨动脉, 起源于臀下动脉, 无分支, 与坐骨神经伴行。又称 *arteria comitans nervi ischiadici*；**segmental a's of kidney**, a group of arteries originating from the anterior or posterior branch of the renal artery, consisting of anterior inferior, anterior superior, inferior, posterior, and superior segmental arteries；each supplies the corresponding renal segment 肾段动脉, 一组起自肾动脉前支或后支的动脉, 包括前下、前上、下、后和上段动脉, 每一支供应其相应的肾段；**segmental a's of left lung**, branches of the left pulmonary artery that supply segments of the left lung；variable but often including lingular arteries and anterior, apical, posterior, superior, anterior basal, lateral basal, medial basal, and posterior basal segmental arteries, named for the segment supplied 左肺段动脉, 左肺动脉分支, 供应左肺肺段, 其分支具有一定差异, 但通常包括舌动脉和前、顶端、后、上、前基底动脉, 外侧基底、内侧基底和后基底肺段动脉, 根据其供应的肺段进行命名；**segmental a's of liver**, a group of arteries originating from the right or left branch of the hepatic artery proper, consisting of anterior, posterior, medial, and lateral segmental arteries；each supplies the corresponding region of the liver 肝段动脉, 一组起自肝固有动脉左支或右支的动脉, 包括前、后、内侧和外侧肝段动脉, 每一支供应其相应的肝的区域；**segmental medullary a.**, one of the spinal branches of the vertebral artery, of the dorsal branch of a posterior intercostal artery, or of a lumbar artery；it supplies the root of a particular spinal nerve and extends to anastomose with the anterior and posterior spinal arteries 脊髓段动脉, 脊椎动脉的脊髓支、肋间后动脉的背侧支或腰动脉的背侧支, 该血管供应某个特定脊神经的神经根, 并延伸至于脊髓前、后动脉相吻合。又称 *arteria medullaris segmentalis*；**segmental medullary a., great anterior**, 见 a. of Adamkiewicz；**segmental a's of right lung**, branches of the right pulmonary artery that supply segments of the right lung；variable but often including anterior, apical, medial, lateral, posterior, superior, anterior basal, lateral basal, medial basal, and posterior basal segmental arteries, named for the segment supplied 右肺段动脉, 右肺动脉的分支, 供应右肺肺段, 分支有一定差异, 但通常包括前、肺尖、内侧、外侧、后、上、前基底、外侧基底、内侧基底和后极低肺段动脉, 根据其供应的相应肺段命名；**segmental spinal a.**, any artery that supplies, or that provides a branch supplying, one or more segments of the spinal cord, including the vertebral, ascending cervical, posterior intercostal, subcostal, iliolumbar, lumbar, and lateral sacral arteries 脊髓段动脉, 供应或发出分支供应脊髓的一个或多个节段的动脉, 此类动脉包括椎动脉、颈升动脉、肋间后动脉、肋下动脉、髂腰动脉、腰动脉和骶外侧动脉；**septal a's, anterior**, interventricular septal branches of left coronary artery: branches of the anterior interventricular branch of the left coronary artery that supply approximately the anterior two-thirds of the interventricular septum 前室间隔动脉, 左冠状动脉的室间隔支, 大约供应室间隔的前 2/3 部分；**septal a's, posterior**, interventricular septal branches of right coronary artery: numerous relatively small branches of the inferior interventricular branch of the right coronary artery that supply the posterior one-third of the interventricular septum 后室间隔动脉, 右冠状动脉的室间隔支的众多相对细小的分支, 供应室间隔的后 1/3 部分；**short circumferential a's**, *origin*, basilar artery and posterior cerebral artery；*branches*, none；*distribution*, part of the ventrolateral surface of the pons 短旋动脉, 起源于基底动脉和大脑后动脉, 无分支, 分布于脑桥腹外侧面。又称 *arteriae circumferentiales breves*；**sigmoid a's**, *origin*, inferior mesenteric artery；*branches*, none；*distribution*, sigmoid colon 乙状结肠动脉, 起源肠系膜下动脉, 无分支, 分布于乙状结肠。又称 *arteriae sigmoideae*；**sinoatrial nodal a.**, a branch of the right coronary artery that supplies the right atrium, encircles the base of the superior vena cava, and inserts into the sinoatrial node 窦房结动脉, 右冠状动脉的分支, 供应右心房, 环绕上腔静脉的基底部, 插入并供应窦房结；**spermatic a., external**, 见 cremasteric a.；**spermatic a., internal**, 精索内动脉, 见 testicular a.；**sphenopalatine a.**, *origin*, maxillary artery；*branches*, posterior lateral nasal artery and posterior septal branches; *distribution*, structures adjoining nasal cavity, the nasopharynx 蝶腭动脉，起源于上颌动脉，分支包括鼻后外侧动脉和鼻中隔后动脉，分布于鼻腔附近的结构和鼻咽。又称 *arteria sphenopalatina*；**spinal a.**, any artery supplying the spinal cord, including the segmental spinal arteries and the anterior and posterior spinal arteries 脊髓动脉，供应脊髓的动脉，包括脊髓段动脉和脊髓前后动脉；**spinal a., anterior**, *origin*, vertebral artery; *branches*, none; *distribution*, the two branches, one from each vertebral artery, unite to form a single vessel, which descends on the anterior midline of the spinal cord, supplying the anterior region of the cord 脊髓前动脉，起源于椎动脉，无分支，两侧椎动脉发出的两个分支相汇合、形成一个单一血管，沿脊髓前正中线下行，供应脊髓前部。又称 *arteria spinalis anterior*；**spinal a., posterior**, *origin*, posterior inferior cerebellar artery (usually) or vertebral artery; *branches*, none; *distribution*, posterior column nuclei and posterior region of spinal cord 脊髓后动脉，起源于小脑后下动脉（通常）或椎动脉，无分支，分布于脊髓后部核团和后部区域。又称 *arteria spinalis posterior*；**spiral a's, spiral endometrial a's**, tightly coiled branches of the uterine radial arteries, which supply the endometrium and in pregnancy supply blood to the intervillous space 螺旋动脉，子宫内膜螺旋动脉，子宫放射动脉的紧密螺旋状分支，供应子宫内膜，妊娠期可向绒毛间隙供血；**spiral modiolar a.**, *origin*, common cochlear artery; *branches*, none; *distribution*, internal auditory meatus, running a spiral course around the auditory nerve 耳蜗螺旋动脉，起源于耳蜗总动脉，无分支，分布于内耳道，围绕听神经螺旋状走行。又称 *arteria spiralis modioli*；**splenic a.**, *origin*, celiac trunk; *branches*, pancreatic and splenic branches, prepancreatic, left gastro-omental, and short gastric arteries; *distribution*, spleen, pancreas, stomach, greater omentum 脾动脉，起源于腹腔干，分支包括胰支、脾支、胰前动脉、胃网膜左动脉和胃短动脉，分布于脾、胰腺、胃和大网膜。又称 *arteria splenica*；**straight a's of kidney**, 肾直动脉，见 *arteriole*. 下词条；**striate a., distal medial**, *origin*, anterior cerebral artery; *branches*, none; *distribution*, anterior part of head of caudate nucleus and adjacent regions of putamen and internal capsule. 远端内侧纹状动脉，起源于大脑前动脉，无分支，分布于尾状核头前部及壳核、内囊邻近区域。又称 *arteria striata medialis distalis*；**striate a's, proximal medial**, *origin*, anterior cerebral artery; *branches*, none; *distribution*, anterior part of head of caudate nucleus and adjacent regions of putamen and internal capsule 近端内侧纹状动脉，起源于

大脑前动脉，无分支，分布于尾状核头前部和壳核、内囊邻近区域。又称 *arteriae striatae mediales proximales*；**stylomastoid a.**, *origin*, posterior auricular artery; *branches*, mastoid and stapedial branches, posterior tympanic artery; *distribution*, tympanic cavity walls, mastoid cells, stapedius muscle 茎乳突动脉，起源于耳后动脉，分支包括乳头支、茎突支和鼓室后动脉，分布于鼓室壁、乳突细胞和镫骨肌。又称 *arteria stylomastoidea*；**subclavian a.**, *origin*, brachiocephalic trunk (right), arch of aorta (left); *branches*, vertebral, internal thoracic arteries, thyrocervical and costocervical trunks; *distribution*, neck, thoracic wall, spinal cord, brain, meninges, upper limb 锁骨下动脉，起源于头臂干（右侧）或主动脉弓（左侧），分支包括椎动脉、胸廓内动脉、甲状颈干和肋颈干，分布于颈部、胸壁、脊髓、大脑、脑膜和上肢。又称 *arteria subclavia*；**subcostal a.**, *origin*, descending thoracic aorta; *branches*, dorsal and spinal branches; *distribution*, upper posterior abdominal wall 肋下动脉，起源于胸主动脉，分支包括背侧支和脊支，分布于后腹壁上部。又称 *arteria subcostalis*；**sublingual a.**, *origin*, lingual artery; *branches*, none; *distribution*, sublingual gland 舌下动脉，起源于舌动脉，无分支，分布于舌下腺。又称 *arteria sublingualis*；**submental a.**, *origin*, facial artery; *branches*, none; *distribution*, tissues under chin 颏下动脉，起源于面动脉，无分支，分布于颏下组织。又称 *arteria submentalis*；**subscapular a.**, *origin*, axillary artery; *branches*, thoracodorsal and circumflex scapular arteries; *distribution*, scapular and shoulder region 肩胛下动脉，起源于腋动脉，分支包括胸背动脉和旋肩胛动脉，分布于肩胛骨和肩部区域。又称 *arteria subscapularis*；**suprachiasmatic a.**, *origin*, anterior communicating artery; *branches*, none; *distribution*, optic chiasm 视交叉上动脉，起源于前交通动脉，无分支，分布于视交叉。又称 *arteria suprachiasmatica*；**supraduodenal a.**, *origin*, gastroduodenal artery; *branches*, duodenal branch; *distribution*, descending part of duodenum 十二指肠上动脉，起源于胃十二指肠动脉，分支包括十二指肠支，分布于十二指肠降段。又称 *arteria supraduodenalis*；**supraoptic a.**, *origin*, anterior cerebral artery; *branches*, none; *distribution*, superior surface of optic nerve and optic chiasm 视上动脉，起源于大脑前动脉，无分支，分布于视神经上表面和视交叉。又称 *arteria supraoptica*；**supraorbital a.**, *origin*, ophthalmic artery; *branches*, superficial, deep, diploic; *distribution*, forehead, upper muscles of orbit, upper eyelid, frontal sinus 眶上动脉，起源于眼动脉，分支包括浅支、深支和板障支，分布于前额、眶上肌、上眼睑和额窦。又称 *arteria supraorbit-*

alis；**suprarenal a., inferior,** *origin*, renal artery; *branches*, none; *distribution*, suprarenal gland 肾上腺下动脉，起源于肾动脉，无分支，分布于肾上腺。又称 *arteria suprarenalis inferior*；**suprarenal a., middle,** *origin*, abdominal aorta; *branches*, none; *distribution*, suprarenal gland 肾上腺中动脉，起源于腹主动脉，无分支，分布于肾上腺。又称 *arteria suprarenalis media*；**suprarenal a's, superior,** *origin*, inferior phrenic artery; *branches*, none; *distribution*, suprarenal gland 肾上腺上动脉，起源于膈下动脉，无分支，分布于肾上腺。又称 *arteriae suprarenales superiores*；**suprascapular a.,** *origin*, thyrocervical trunk; *branches*, acromial branch; *distribution*, clavicular, deltoid, and scapular regions 肩胛上动脉，起源于甲状颈干，分支包括肩峰支，分布于锁骨、三角肌和肩胛骨区域。又称 *arteria suprascapularis*；**supratrochlear a.,** *origin*, ophthalmic artery; *branches*, none; *distribution*, anterior scalp 滑车上动脉，起源于眼动脉，无分支，分布于头皮前部。又称 *arteria supratrochlearis*；**sural a's,** *origin*, popliteal artery; *branches*, none; *distribution*, popliteal space, calf 腓肠动脉，起源于腘动脉，无分支，分布于腘窝和小腿。又称 *arteriae surales*；**sylvian a.,** middle cerebral a. 大脑中动脉；**a. to tail of pancreas,** caudal pancreatic a. 胰尾动脉；**tarsal a., lateral,** *origin*, dorsalis pedis artery; *branches*, none; *distribution*, tarsus 跗外侧动脉，起源于足背动脉，无分支，分布于跗骨。又称 *arteria tarsalis lateralis*；**tarsal a's, medial,** *origin*, dorsalis pedis artery; *branches*, none; *distribution*, side of foot 跗内侧动脉，起源于足背动脉，无分支，分布于足侧面。又称 *arteriae tarsales mediales*；**temporal a., anterior,** 颞前动脉 1. *origin*, sphenoid part of middle cerebral artery; *branches*, none; *distribution*, cortex of anterior temporal lobe 起源于大脑中动脉蝶骨段，无分支，分布于颞叶前部皮质，又称 *arteria temporalis anterior*；2. anterior temporal branch of middle cerebral artery, arising from the inferior terminal branch of the middle cerebral artery and supplying the lateral surface of the anterior temporal lobe 大脑中动脉的颞前分支，起自大脑中动脉的终末下支，供应颞叶前部的外侧面；**temporal a., anterior deep,** *origin*, maxillary artery; *branches*, to zygomatic bone and greater wing of sphenoid bone; *distribution*, temporalis muscle, and anastomoses with middle temporal artery 颞深前动脉，起源于上颌动脉，分支发至颧骨和蝶骨大翼，分布于颞肌，与颞中动脉相吻合。又称 *arteria temporalis profunda anterior*；**temporal a., middle,** 颞中动脉 1. *origin*, superficial temporal artery; *branches*, none; *distribution* temporal region 起源于颞浅动脉，无分支，分布于颞叶区域，又称 *arteria tem-*

poralis media；2. middle temporal branch of middle cerebral artery, arising from the inferior terminal branch of the middle cerebral artery and supplying the lateral surface of the temporal lobe between the anterior and posterior branches 大脑中动脉的颞中支，起自大脑中动脉的终末下支，供应颞前支和颞后支之间的颞叶外侧面；**temporal a., posterior,** posterior temporal branch of middle cerebral artery, arising from the inferior terminal branch of the middle cerebral artery and supplying the lateral surface of the posterior temporal lobe 颞后动脉，大脑中动脉的颞后支，起自大脑中动脉的终末下支，供应颞叶后部的外侧面；**temporal a., posterior deep,** *origin*, maxillary artery; *branches*, none; *distribution*, temporalis muscle, and anastomoses with middle temporal artery 颞后深动脉，起源于上颌动脉，无分支，分布于颞肌，与颞中动脉相吻合。又称 *arteria temporalis profunda posterior*；**temporal a., superficial,** *origin*, external carotid artery; *branches*, parotid, auricular, and occipital branches, transverse facial, zygomaticoorbital, and middle temporal arteries 颞浅动脉，起源于颈外动脉，分支包括腮腺支、耳支、枕叶支、面横动脉、颧眶动脉和颞中动脉，分布于腮腺和颞叶区域。又称 *arteria temporalis superficialis*；**terminal a.,** 1. end a. 末梢动脉，终动脉；2. an artery that does not divide into branches but is directly continuous with capillaries 不发出分支而直接延续为毛细血管的动脉；**testicular a.,** *origin*, abdominal aorta; *branches*, ureteral, epididymal; *distribution*, ureter, epididymis, testis 睾丸动脉，起源于腹主动脉，分支包括输尿管支和附睾支，分布于输尿管、附睾和睾丸。又称 *arteria testicularis*；**thalamogeniculate a.,** *origin*, posterior cerebral artery; *branches*, none; *distribution*, caudal thalamus 丘脑膝状体动脉，起源于大脑后动脉，无分支，分布于丘脑尾部。又称 *arteria thalamogeniculata*；**thalamoperforating a.,** *origin*, posterior cerebral artery; *branches*, none; *distribution*, penetrates posterior perforating substance to supply the thalamus and midbrain 丘脑穿通动脉，起源于大脑后动脉，无分支，穿过后穿质，供应丘脑和中脑。又称 *arteria thalami perforans*；**thalamotuberal a.,** *origin*, posterior communicating artery; *branches*, none; *distribution*, premammillary area 丘脑结节动脉，起源于后交通动脉，无分支，分布于乳头体前区。又称 *arteria thalamotuberalis*；**thoracic a., internal,** *origin*, subclavian artery; *branches*, mediastinal, thymic, bronchial, tracheal, sternal, perforating, medial mammary, lateral costal, and anterior intercostal branches, pericardiacophrenic, musculophrenic, and superior epigastric arteries; *distribution*, anterior thoracic wall, mediastinal structures, respiratory diaphragm 胸廓内动脉，起源于锁骨下动脉，分支包括横膈支、胸腺支、支气管支、气管支、胸骨支、穿通支、乳内支、肋外侧支、肋间前支、心包膈动脉、肌膈动脉和腹壁上动脉，分布于前胸壁、纵隔结构和横膈。又称 *arteria thoracica interna*；**thoracic a., lateral,** *origin,* axillary artery; *branches,* mammary branches; *distribution,* pectoral muscles, mammary gland 胸外侧动脉，起源于腋动脉，分支包括乳腺支，分布于胸大肌和乳腺。又称 *arteria thoracica lateralis*；**thoracic a., superior,** *origin,* axillary artery; *branches,* none; *distribution,* axillary aspect of chest wall 胸上动脉，起源于腋动脉，无分支，分布于胸壁腋窝侧。又称 *arteria thoracica superior*；**thoracoacromial a.,** *origin,* axillary artery; *branches,* clavicular, pectoral, deltoid, acromial branches; *distribution,* deltoid, clavicular, and thoracic regions 胸肩峰动脉，起源于腋动脉，分支包括锁骨支、胸肌支、三角肌支和肩峰支，分布于三角肌、锁骨和胸骨区域。又称 *arteria thoracoacromialis*；**thoracodorsal a.,** *origin,* subscapular artery; *branches,* none; *distribution,* subscapularis and teres muscles 胸背动脉，起源于肩胛下动脉，无分支，分布于肩胛下肌和圆肌。又称 *arteria thoracodorsalis*；**thyroid a., inferior,** *origin,* thyrocervical trunk; *branches,* pharyngeal, esophageal, and tracheal branches, inferior laryngeal and ascending cervical arteries; *distribution,* thyroid gland and adjacent structures 甲状腺下动脉，起源于甲状颈干，分支包括咽支、食管支、气管支、咽下动脉和颈升动脉，分布于甲状腺及邻近结构。又称 *arteria thyroidea inferior*；**thyroid a., lowest,** thyroid ima a. 甲状腺最下动脉；**thyroid a., superior,** *origin,* external carotid artery; *branches,* hyoid, sternocleidomastoid, superior laryngeal, cricothyroid, muscular, and anterior, posterior, and lateral glandular branches; *distribution,* thyroid gland and adjacent structures 甲状腺上动脉，起源于颈外动脉，分支包括舌骨支、胸锁乳突肌支、喉上支、环甲肌支、肌支、前支、后支和腺体侧支，分布于甲状腺及邻近结构。又称 *arteria thyroidea superior*；**thyroid ima a.,** *origin,* arch of aorta, brachiocephalic trunk, or right common carotid, internal mammary, subclavian, or inferior thyroid arteries; *branches,* none; *distribution,* thyroid gland 甲状腺最下动脉，起源于主动脉弓、头臂干或右颈总动脉、乳内动脉、锁骨下动脉或甲状腺下动脉，无分支，分布于甲状腺。又称 *arteria thyroidea ima*；**tibial a., anterior,** *origin,* popliteal artery; *branches,* posterior and anterior tibial recurrent, and lateral and medial anterior malleolar arteries; lateral and medial malleolar retes; *distribution,* leg, ankle, foot 胫前动脉，起源于腘动脉，

分支包括胫前返动脉和胫后返动脉、前外侧和前内侧踝动脉、内外侧踝动脉网，分布于下肢、踝关节和足。又称 *arteria tibialis anterior*；**tibial a., posterior,** *origin,* popliteal artery; *branches,* fibular circumflex branch, fibular, medial plantar, and lateral plantar arteries; *distribution,* leg, foot 胫后动脉，起源于腘动脉，分支包括旋腓骨支、腓动脉、足底内侧动脉和足底外侧动脉，分布于小腿和足部。又称 *arteria tibialis posterior*；**tibial nutrient a.,** *origin,* posterior tibial artery; *branches,* none; *distribution,* tibia 胫骨滋养动脉，起源于胫后动脉，无分支，分布于胫骨。又称 *arteria nutricia tibiae*；**tibial recurrent a., anterior,** *origin,* anterior tibial artery; *branches,* none; *distribution,* tibialis anterior, extensor digitorum longus, knee joint, contiguous fascia and skin 胫骨前返动脉，起源于胫前动脉，无分支，分布于胫骨前肌、趾长伸肌、膝关节及其邻近筋膜和皮肤。又称 *arteria recurrens tibialis anterior*；**tibial recurrent a., posterior,** *origin,* anterior tibial artery; *branches,* none; *distribution,* knee 胫骨后返动脉，起源于胫前动脉，无分支，分布于膝关节。又称 *arteria recurrens tibialis posterior*；**transverse cervical a.,** *origin,* subclavian artery; *branches,* deep and superficial branches; *distribution,* root of neck, muscles of scapula 颈横动脉，起源于锁骨下动脉，分支包括深支和浅支，分布于颈根部和肩胛肌。又称 *arteria transversa colli*；**transverse facial a.,** *origin,* superficial temporal artery; *branches,* none; *distribution,* parotideomasseteric region 面横动脉，起源于颞浅动脉，无分支，分布于腮腺咬肌区域。又称 *arteria transversa faciei*；**a. of tuber cinereum,** *origin,* posterior communicating artery; *branches,* medial and diagonal branches; *distribution,* tuber cinereum 灰结节动脉，起源于后交通动脉，分支包括内侧支和对角支，分布于灰结节。又称 *arteria tuberis cinerei*；**tympanic a., anterior,** *origin,* maxillary artery; *branches,* none; *distribution,* tympanic cavity 鼓室前动脉，起源于上颌动脉，无分支，分布于鼓室。又称 *arteria tympanica anterior*；**tympanic a., inferior,** *origin,* ascending pharyngeal artery; *branches,* none; *distribution,* tympanic cavity 鼓室下动脉，起源于咽升动脉，无分支，分布于鼓室。又称 *arteria tympanica inferior*；**tympanic a., posterior,** *origin,* stylomastoid artery; *branches,* none; *distribution,* tympanic cavity 鼓室后动脉，起源于茎乳突动脉，无分支，分布于鼓室。又称 *arteria tympanica posterior*；**tympanic a., superior,** *origin,* middle meningeal artery; *branches,* none; *distribution,* tympanic cavity 鼓室上动脉，起源于脑膜中动脉，无分支，分布于鼓室。又称 *arteria tympanica superior*；**ulnar a.,** *origin,* brachial artery; *branches,* palmar carpal, dorsal carpal, and deep palmar branches, ulnar recurrent and common interosseous arteries, superficial palmar arch; *distribution*, forearm, wrist, hand 尺动脉，起源于肱动脉，分支包括腕掌支、腕背支、掌深支、尺侧返动脉、骨间总动脉和掌浅弓，分布于前臂、腕部和手部。又称 *arteria ulnaris*；**ulnar collateral a., inferior**, *origin*, brachial artery; *branches*, none; *distribution*, arm muscles at back of elbow 尺侧下副动脉，起源于肱动脉，无分支，分布于肘关节背侧的前臂肌肉。又称 *arteria collateralis ulnaris inferior*；**ulnar collateral a., superior**, *origin*, brachial artery; *branches*, none; *distribution*, elbow joint, triceps muscle 尺侧上副动脉，起源于肱动脉，无分支，分布于肘关节和肱三头肌。又称 *arteria collateralis ulnaris superior*；**ulnar recurrent a.**, *origin*, ulnar artery; *branches*, anterior and posterior; *distribution*, elbow joint region 尺侧返动脉，起源于尺动脉，分支包括前支和后支，分布于肘关节区域。又称 *arteria recurrens ulnaris*；**umbilical a.**, *origin*, internal iliac artery; *branches*, artery of ductus deferens and superior vesical arteries; *distribution*, ductus deferens, seminal vesicles, testes, urinary bladder, ureter 脐动脉，起源于髂内动脉，分支包括输精管动脉和膀囊上动脉，分布于输精管、精囊、睾丸、膀胱和输尿管。又称 *arteria umbilicalis*；**uncal a.**, a branch of the internal carotid, or rarely the middle cerebral, artery; it supplies the uncus 钩动脉，颈内动脉分支，偶尔可为大脑中动脉分支，供应钩回。又称 *arteria uncalis*；**urethral a.**, *origin*, internal pudendal artery; *branches*, none; *distribution*, urethra 尿道动脉，起源于阴部内动脉，无分支，分布于尿道。又称 *arteria urethralis*；**uterine a.**, *origin*, internal iliac artery; *branches*, ovarian and tubal branches, vaginal artery; *distribution*, uterus, vagina, round ligament of uterus, uterine tube, ovary 子宫动脉，起源于髂内动脉，分支包括卵巢支、输卵管支和阴道支，分布于子宫、阴道、子宫圆韧带、输卵管和卵巢。又称 *arteria uterina*；**vaginal a.**, *origin*, uterine artery; *branches*, none; *distribution*, vagina, fundus of bladder 阴道动脉，起源于子宫动脉，无分支，分布于阴道和膀胱底部。又称 *arteria vaginalis*；**vertebral a.**, *origin*, subclavian artery; it is divided into four parts: *first* or *prevertebral part*, *second* or *cervical part*, *third* or *atlantal part*, and *fourth* or *intracranial part*; *branches*, (cervical part) spinal and muscular branches; (intracranial part) anterior spinal artery and posterior inferior cerebellar artery and its branches, meningeal branches, and lateral and medial medullary branches; *distribution*, muscles of neck, vertebrae, spinal cord, cerebellum, medulla oblongata 椎动脉，起源于锁骨下动脉，分为四部分：第一部分或椎前段、第二部

分或颈段、第三部分或寰椎段，以及第四部分或颅内段；分支包括（颈段）脊支和肌支、（颅内段）脊髓前支。又称 *arteria vertebralis*；**vesical a., inferior**, *origin*, internal iliac artery; *branches*, prostatic branches; *distribution*, bladder, prostate, seminal vesicles, lower ureter 膀胱下动脉。又称 *arteria vesicalis inferior*；**vesical a's, superior**, *origin*, umbilical artery; *branches*, none; *distribution*, bladder, urachus, ureter 膀胱上动脉。又称 *arteriae vesicales superiores*；**vestibular a., anterior**, *origin*, labyrinthine artery; *branches*, none; *distribution*, vestibular nerves, utricle, part of the cristae and semicircular canals 前庭动脉。又称 *arteria vestibularis anterior*；**vestibulocochlear a.**, *origin*, common cochlear artery; *branches*, cochlear and posterior vestibular branches; *distribution*, cochlea, saccule, semicircular canals 前庭耳蜗动脉。又称 *arteria vestibulocochlearis*；**zygomatico-orbital a.**, *origin*, superficial temporal artery; *branches*, none; *distribution*, lateral side of orbit 颧眶动脉。又称 *arteria zygomaticoorbitalis*

ar·thral·gia (ahr-thral′jə) pain in a joint 关节疼痛

ar·thres·the·sia (ahr″thres-the′zhə) joint sensibility 关节感觉；the perception of joint motions 关节运动觉

ar·thrit·ic (ahr-thrit′ik) pertaining to or affected with arthritis 关节炎相关的；由关节炎引起的

ar·thri·tis (ahr-thri′tis) pl. *arthri′tides*. Inflammation of a joint 关节炎；**acute a.**, arthritis marked by pain, heat, redness, and swelling 急性关节炎；**chronic inflammatory a.**, inflammation of joints in chronic disorders such as rheumatoid arthritis 慢性关节炎病；**a. defor′mans**, severe destruction of joints, seen in disorders such as rheumatoid arthritis 关节炎畸形；**degenerative a.**, osteoarthritis 退变性关节炎，骨关节炎；**enteropathic a.**, arthritis associated with inflammatory bowel disease or following bacterial infection of the bowel 炎性肠病性关节炎；**hypertrophic a.**, osteoarthritis 增生性关节炎；**infectious a.**, arthritis caused by bacteria, rickettsiae, mycoplasmas, viruses, fungi, or parasites 感染性关节炎；**juvenile rheumatoid a.**, rheumatoid arthritis in children, with swelling, tenderness, and pain involving one or more joints, sometimes leading to impaired growth and development, limitation of movement, and ankylosis and flexion contractures of the joints 幼年型类风湿关节炎；**Lyme a.**, 莱姆关节炎，见 *disease* 下词条；**menopausal a.**, that seen in some menopausal women, due to ovarian hormonal deficiency, and marked by pain in the small joints, shoulders, elbows, or knees 绝经期关节炎；**a. mu′tilans**, severe deforming polyarthritis with gross bone and cartilage destruction, an atypical variant of rheumatoid arthritis 毁形性关节炎；**reactive a.**, acute aseptic arthritis associated with infection in the gastrointestinal or genital tracts or other distant site 反应性关节炎；**rheumatoid a.**, a chronic systemic disease primarily of the joints, usually polyarticular, marked by inflammatory changes in the synovial membranes and articular structures and by atrophy and rarefaction of the bones. In late stages, deformity and ankylosis develop 类风湿关节炎；**septic a.**, **suppurative a.**, a form marked by purulent joint infiltration, chiefly due to bacterial infection but also seen in Reiter disease 化脓性关节炎；**systemic onset juvenile rheumatoid a.**, a form of juvenile rheumatoid arthritis with fever, rash, and other systemic manifestations 全身型幼年型类风湿关节炎；**tuberculous a.**, that secondary to tuberculosis, usually affecting a single joint, marked by chronic inflammation with effusion and destruction of contiguous bone 结核性关节炎

Ar·thro·bac·ter (ahr'thro-bak″tər) a genus of bacteria of the family Micrococcaceae; several species cause septicemia in immunocompromised persons 节杆菌属

ar·thro·cen·te·sis (ahr″thro-sen-te'sis) puncture of a joint cavity with aspiration of fluid 关节穿刺术

ar·thro·cha·la·sis (ahr″thro-kal'ə-sis) abnormal relaxation or flaccidity of a joint 关节松弛症

ar·thro·chon·dri·tis (ahr″thro-kon-dri'tis) [*arthro-* + *chondritis*] inflammation of the cartilage of a joint 关节软骨炎

ar·thro·cla·sia (ahr″thro-kla'zhə) surgical breaking of an ankylosis to permit a joint to move 关节松动术

Ar·thro·der·ma (ahr″thro-dur'mə) a genus of fungi containing the known teleomorphs of the dermatophytes; corresponding anamorphs are classified in *Microsporum* and *Trichophyton* 节皮菌属

ar·thro·de·sis (ahr″thro-de'sis) the surgical fixation of a joint by a procedure designed to accomplish fusion of the joint surfaces by promoting the proliferation of bone cells 关节融合术；又称 *artificial ankylosis*

ar·thro·dia (ahr-thro'de-ə) a synovial joint that allows a gliding motion 滑动关节；**arthro'dial** *adj.*

ar·thro·dys·pla·sia (ahr″thro-dis-pla'zhə) hereditary deformity of various joints 关节发育不良

ar·thro·em·py·e·sis (ahr″thro-em″pi-e'sis) suppuration within a joint 关节积脓

Ar·thro·graph·is (ahr″thro-graf'is) a genus of anamorphic fungi; *A. kal'rae* and other species have been occasional causes of opportunistic hyalohyphomycosis 爪甲白癣菌属

ar·throg·ra·phy (ahr-throg'rə-fe) radiography of a joint after injection of opaque contrast material 关节腔造影术；**air a.**, pneumarthrography 关节空气造影术

ar·thro·gry·po·sis (ahr″thro-grə-po'sis) persistent flexure of a joint 关节挛缩症；**distal a.**, an autosomal dominant condition, occurring alone or in combination with other anomalies, characterized by contractures of the hands and feet, causing severe deformity, with variable involvement of more proximal joints 远端关节挛缩症

ar·thro·lith (ahr'thro-lith) calculus deposit within a joint 关节石

ar·throl·o·gy (ahr-throl'ə-je) the study of or the sum of knowledge regarding the joints and ligaments 关节学

ar·thro·neu·ral·gia (ahr″thro-noo-ral'jə) pain in or around a joint 关节神经痛

ar·thro·oph·thal·mop·a·thy (ahr″thro-ofthəl-mop′ə-the) an association of degenerative joint disease and eye disease 关节—眼病

ar·throp·a·thy (ahr-throp'ə-the) any joint disease 关节病；**arthropath'ic** *adj.*；**Charcot a.**, 见 neuropathic a.；**chondrocalcific a.**, progressive polyarthritis with joint swelling and bony enlargement, most commonly in the small joints of the hand but also affecting other joints, characterized radiographically by narrowing of the joint space with subchondral erosions and sclerosis and frequently chondrocalcinosis 软骨钙化性关节病；**neuropathic a.**, chronic progressive degeneration of the stress-bearing portion of a joint, with hypertrophic changes at the periphery; it is associated with neurologic disorders involving loss of sensation in the joint 夏科氏关节病；**osteopulmonary a.**, clubbing of fingers and toes and enlargement of ends of the long bones, in cardiac or pulmonary disease 肺性骨关节病

ar·thro·plas·ty (ahr'thro-plas″te) joint replacement; plastic repair of a joint 关节置换术

Ar·throp·o·da (ahr-throp'ə-də) the largest phylum of animals, composed of bilaterally symmetrical organisms with hard, segmented bodies bearing jointed legs, including, among other related forms, arachnids, crustaceans, and insects, many species of which are parasites or are vectors of diseasecausing organisms 节肢动物（门）

ar·thro·py·o·sis (ahr″thro-pi-o'sis) formation of pus in a joint cavity 关节化脓

ar·thro·scle·ro·sis (ahr″thro-sklə-ro'sis) stiffening or hardening of the joints 关节硬化

ar·thro·scope (ahr'thro-skōp) an endoscope for examining the interior of a joint and for performing diagnostic and therapeutic procedures within the joint 关节镜

ar·thros·copy (ahr-thros′kə-pe) examination of the interior of a joint with an arthroscope 关节镜检查

ar·thro·sis (ahr-thro′sis) 1. joint 关节; 2. arthropathy 关节病

ar·thros·to·my (ahr-thros′tə-me) surgical creation of an opening into a joint, as for drainage 关节腔引流

ar·tic·u·lar (ahr-tik′u-lər) pertaining to a joint 关节的

ar·tic·u·la·re (ahr-tik″u-lar′e) the point of intersection of the dorsal contours of the articular process of the mandible and the temporal bone 下颌关节突

ar·tic·u·late[1] (ahr-tik′u-lāt) 1. to pronounce clearly and distinctly 清楚明白地发音; 2. to make speech sounds by manipulation of the vocal organs 通过操纵发声器官发出声音; 3. to express in coherent verbal form 用连贯的语言表达; 4. to divide into or unite so as to form a joint 分离或相桥接以形成关节; 5. in dentistry, to adjust or place the teeth in their proper relation to each other in making an artificial denture 牙科学中, 制作义齿时, 将义齿调至适当位置

ar·tic·u·late[2] (ahr-tik′u-lət) 1. divided into distinct, meaningful syllables or words 吐字清楚的; 2. endowed with the power of speech 善于表达的; 3. characterized by the use of clear, meaningful language 言简意赅的; 4. divided into or united by joints 关节的, 关节连接的

ar·tic·u·la·tio (ahr-tik″u-la′she-o) pl. *articulatio′nes* [L.] 1. joint 关节; 2. synovial joint 滑膜关节

ar·tic·u·la·tion (ahr-tik″u-la′shən) 1. a joint or place of junction between two different parts or objects 两个物体或同一物体两个部分之间的接合部或接头; 2. the forming of speech sounds 声音的形成; 3. in dentistry 在牙科学中: (*a*) the contact relationship of the occlusal surfaces of the teeth while in action 牙齿活动时咬合面的接触关系; (*b*) the arrangement of artificial teeth so as to accommodate the various positions of the mouth and to serve the purpose of the natural teeth that they are to replace 假牙的排列方式, 以适应口腔的各种位置并达到替换天然牙齿的目的

ar·tic·u·lo (ahr-tik′u-lo) [L.] at the moment, or crisis 时刻, 危象; **a. mor′tis,** at the point or moment of death 濒死

ar·ti·fact (ahr′tĭ-fakt″) any artificial (manmade) product; anything not naturally present, but introduced by some external source 手工制品。Spelled also *artefact*

ARVO Association for Research in Vision and

Ophthalmology 视觉与眼科研究协会

ary·ep·i·glot·tic (ar″e-ep″ĭ-glot′ik) arytenoepiglottic 会厌软骨

aryl (ar′əl) a radical derived from an aromatic compound by removal of a hydrogen atom from the ring; also used as a prefix 芳基

ar·yl·for·mam·i·dase (ar″əl-for-mam′ĭdās) an enzyme that catalyzes the hydrolytic cleavage of formylkynurenine in the catabolism of tryptophan; it also acts on other formyl aromatic amines 芳基甲酰胺酶

ar·y·te·no·ep·i·glot·tic (ar-it″ə-no-ep″ĭglot′ik) pertaining to the arytenoid cartilage and to the epiglottis 会厌软骨

ar·y·te·noid (ar″ə-te′noid) shaped like a jug or pitcher, as arytenoid cartilage 杓状软骨

ar·y·te·noi·do·pexy (ar″ə-te-noi′dopek″se) surgical fixation of arytenoid cartilage or muscle 杓状软骨固定术

AS [L.] au′ris sinis′tra (left ear) 左耳

AS aortic stenosis 主动脉狭窄; arteriosclerosis 动脉硬化

As arsenic 砷

ASA acetylsalicylic acid 乙酰水杨酸; American Society on Aging 美国衰老学会; American Society of Anesthesiologists 美国麻醉师学会; American Standards Association 美国标准协会; American Surgical Association 美国外科学会; antisperm antibody 抗精子抗体; argininosuccinic acid 精氨酸丁二酸

5-ASA mesalamine (5-aminosalicylic acid) 5-氨基水杨酸

ASAHP Association of Schools of Allied Health Professions 卫生职业学院联盟协会

asa·na (ə-sah′nə) [Sanskrit] any of the postures used in hatha yoga for the purpose of achieving balance, promoting physical health, and attaining mental relaxation 梵语, 泛指所有能保持平衡, 促进身体健康, 放松精神的 hatha 瑜伽姿势

as·bes·tos (as-bes′təs) a fibrous incombustible magnesium and calcium silicate used in thermal insulation; its dust causes asbestosis and acts as an epigenetic carcinogen for pleural mesothelioma. It is divided into two main classes: *amphibole a.,* less widely used and more highly carcinogenic and including amosite and crocidolite, and *serpentine a.,* including chrysotile 石棉

as·bes·to·sis (as″bes-to′sis) pneumoconiosis caused by inhaled asbestos fibers, characterized by interstitial fibrosis, sometimes followed by pleural mesothelioma and bronchogenic carcinoma 石棉肺

as·ca·ri·a·sis (as″kə-ri′ə-sis) infection with the roundworm *Ascaris lumbricoides.* After ingestion, the larvae migrate first to the lungs then to the intestine 蛔虫病

as·car·i·cide (as-kar′ĭ-sīd″) an agent that destroys ascarids 驱蛔虫药；**ascarici′dal** *adj.* 杀蛔虫的

as·ca·rid (as′kə-rid) any of the phasmid nematodes of the Ascaridoidea, which includes the genera *Ascaridia*, *Ascaris*, and *Toxocara* 蛔虫。包括禽蛔虫属，蛔线虫属，弓蛔虫属

As·ca·ris (as′kə-ris) a genus of nematode parasites of the large intestine. *A. lumbricoi′des* causes ascariasis 蛔虫属

as·cend·ing (ə-send′ing) having an upward course 上升

as·cer·tain·ment (ă″sər-tān′mənt) in genetic studies, the method by which persons with a trait or disease are selected or found by an investigator 查明，确定

ASCH American Society of Clinical Hypnosis 美国临床催眠学会

Asc·hel·min·thes (ask″həl-minth′ēz) a phylum of unsegmented, bilaterally symmetrical, pseudocoelomate, mostly vermiform animals whose bodies are almost entirely covered with a cuticle, and that possess a complete digestive tract lacking definite muscular walls 袋形动物（门）

ASCI American Society for Clinical Investigation 美国临床调查学会

as·ci·tes (ə-si′tēz) effusion and accumulation of serous fluid in the abdominal cavity 腹腔积液；**ascit′ic** *adj* 腹水的；**chylous a.,** the presence of chyle in the peritoneal cavity as a result of anomalies, injuries, or obstruction of the thoracic duct 乳糜性腹水。又称 *chyloperitoneum*

ASCLS American Society for Clinical Laboratory Science 美国临床实验室科学学会

ASCO American Society of Clinical Oncology 美国临床肿瘤学会；American Society of Contemporary Ophthalmology 美国当代眼科学会

as·co·my·cete (as″ko-mi′sēt) an individual fungus of the Ascomycota 子囊菌纲；**ascomyce′tous** *adj.* 子囊菌类的

As·co·my·co·ta (as″ko-mi-ko′tə) the sac fungi, a large phylum of fungi originally defined by the formation of an ascus in which sexual spores (ascospores) are produced; some asexual species are now included 子囊菌（门）

ascor·bic ac·id (ə-skor′bik) vitamin C, a water-soluble vitamin found in many vegetables and fruits, and an essential element in the diet of humans and many other animals; deficiency produces scurvy and poor wound repair. It is used as an antiscorbutic and nutritional supplement, in the treatment of iron-deficiency anemia and chronic iron toxicity,

and in the labeling of red blood cells with sodium chromate Cr 51 维生素 C

ASCP American Society of Clinical Pathologists 美国临床病理学会

ASCT American Society for Cytotechnology 美国细胞技术学会

ASCVD arteriosclerotic cardiovascular disease 动脉硬化性心血管疾病

ASDP American Society of Dermatopathology 美国皮肤病学会

ASE American Society of Electrocardiography 美国心电图学会

ase suffix used in enzyme names, affixed to a stem indicating the substrate (luciferase), the general nature of the substrate (proteinase), the reaction catalyzed (hydrolase), or a combination of these (transaminase)（后缀）表示酶

ase·mia (a-se′me-ə) aphasia with inability to employ or to understand either speech or signs 失语症。又称 *asemasia*

asep·sis (a-sep′sis) 1. freedom from infection 抗感染；2. the prevention of contact with microorganisms 防菌

asep·tic (a-sep′tik) free from infection or septic material 无菌的

ASET American Society of Electroneurodiagnostic Technologists 美国神经诊断技术专家学会

asex·u·al (a-sek′shoo-əl) having no sex; not sexual; not pertaining to sex 无性行为的

ASGE American Society for Gastrointestinal Endoscopy 美国胃肠内镜学会

ASH American Society of Hematology 美国血液病学会；asymmetrical septal hypertrophy 非对称性室间隔肥大

ASHA American School Health Association 美国学校健康协会；American Speech and Hearing Associaton 美国演讲和倾听协会

ASHD arteriosclerotic heart disease 动脉硬化性心脏病；见 *disease* 下词条 *ischemic heart disease*

ASHG American Society for Human Genetics 美国人类遗传学学会

ASHNR American Society of Head and Neck Radiology 美国头颈放射学学会

ASHP American Society of Health-System Pharmacists 美国卫生系统药剂师协会

ASHT American Society of Hand Therapists 美国手理疗协会

asi·a·lia (a″si-a′le-ə) aptyalism 唾液缺乏

asid·er·o·sis (a″sid-ər-o′sis) deficiency of iron reserve of the body 铁缺乏

ASII American Science Information Institute 美国科学信息研究院

ASIM American Society of Internal Medicine 美

国内科学会

ASMBS American Society for Metabolic and Bariatric Surgery 美国代谢与肥胖外科学会

ASN American Society of Nephrology 美国肾病学会

Asn asparagine 天冬酰胺

ASO arteriosclerosis obliterans 动脉硬化闭塞

aso·ma·tog·no·sia (ə-so″mə-tog-no′zhə) lack of awareness of the condition of all or part of one's body 躯体失认，本体感觉缺乏

ASP American Society of Parasitologists 美国寄生虫学家协会

Asp aspartic acid 天冬氨酸

ASPAN American Society of PeriAnesthesia Nurses 美国麻醉护士协会

as·par·a·gin·ase (as-par′ə-jin-ās″) an enzyme that catalyzes the deamination of asparagine; a preparation is used as an antineoplastic agent in acute lymphoblastic leukemia to reduce availability of asparagine to tumor cells 天冬酰胺酶

as·par·a·gine (**Asn, N**) (ə-spar′ə-jēn) (ə-spar′ə-jin) the β-amide of aspartic acid, a nonessential amino acid occurring in proteins; used in bacterial culture media 天冬酰胺

as·par·tame (ə-spahr′tām) (as′pahr-tām″) an artificial sweetener about 200 times as sweet as sucrose and used as a low-calorie sweetener 阿斯巴甜（甜味剂）

as·par·tate (ə-spahr′tāt) a salt of aspartic acid, or aspartic acid in dissociated form 天冬氨酸

as·par·tate trans·am·i·nase (**AST, ASAT**) (ə-spahr′tāt trans-am′ĭ-nās) an enzyme normally present in body tissues, especially in the heart and liver; it is released into the serum as the result of tissue injury; hence the concentration in the serum (SGOT) may be increased in disorders such as myocardial infarction or acute damage to hepatic cells 天冬氨酸转氨酶

as·par·tic ac·id (**Asp**) (**D**) (ə-spahr′tik) a nonessential, natural dibasic amino acid occurring in proteins and also an excitatory neurotransmitter in the central nervous system 天冬氨酸

ASPE Association of Standardized Patient Educators 标准患者宣教者协会

as·pect (as′pekt) that part of a surface facing in some designated direction 方面; **dorsal a.,** that surface of a body viewed from the back (human anatomy) or from above (veterinary anatomy) 背侧面; **ventral a.,** that surface of a body viewed from the front (human anatomy) or from below (veterinary anatomy) 腹侧面

ASPEN American Society for Parenteral and Enteral Nutrition 美国肠外营养与肠内营养学会

as·per·gil·lo·ma (as″pər-jil-o′mə) the most common kind of fungus ball, caused by *Aspergillus* in a bronchus or lung cavity 曲霉球

as·per·gil·lo·sis (as″pər-jil-o′sis) infection by species of *Aspergillus*, marked by inflammatory granulomatous lesions in the skin, ear, orbit, nasal sinuses, lungs, bones, and meninges 曲霉病

as·per·gil·lo·tox·i·co·sis (as″pər-jil″o-tok″sīko′sis) mycotoxicosis caused by *Aspergillus* 曲霉菌感染

Asper·gil·lus (as″pər-jil′əs) a genus of anamorphic fungi, including various species that are opportunistic pathogens causing invasive disease, most notably *A fumiga'tus, A. fla'vus, A. ter'reus,* and *A. ni'ger.* It also includes several species that produce aflatoxin, and others that produce various antibiotics 曲霉菌属

asper·ma·to·gen·e·sis (a-spur″mə-to-jen′ə-sis) failure in a male of production of spermatozoa 精子生成缺乏

asper·mia (ə-spur′me-ə) 1. aspermatogenesis 无精症; 2. anejaculation 射精不能

as·phyx·ia (as-fik′se-ə) pathological changes caused by lack of oxygen in respired air, resulting in hypoxia and hypercapnia 窒息; **asphyx′ial** adj. 窒息的; **fetal a.,** asphyxia in utero due to hypoxia 胎儿窘迫; **a. neonato′rum,** respiratory failure in the newborn, as with neonatal respiratory distress syndrome 新生儿窒息; **traumatic a.,** that due to sudden or severe compression of the thorax or upper abdomen, or both 创伤性窒息

as·phyx·i·a·tion (as-fik″se-a′shən) suffocation; the stoppage of respiration 窒息

as·pi·ra·tion (as″pī-ra′shən) 1. the drawing of a foreign substance into the respiratory tract during inhalation 吸入; 2. removal by suction, as the removal of fluid or gas from a body cavity or the procurement of biopsy specimens 抽吸; **meconium a.,** aspiration of meconium by the fetus or newborn, which may result in atelectasis, emphysema, pneumothorax, or pneumonia 胎粪吸入; **microsurgical epididymal sperm a. (MESA),** retrieval of sperm from the epididymis using microsurgical techniques, done in men with obstructive azoospermia 微创附睾穿刺采精术 **vacuum a.,** 见 *curettage* 下词条

as·pi·rin (as′pī-rin) acetylsalicylic acid, a nonsteroidal antiinflammatory drug having analgesic, antipyretic, antiinflammatory, and antirheumatic activity; also an inhibitor of platelet aggregation 乙酰水杨酸（阿司匹林）

asple·nia (a-sple′ne-ə) absence of the spleen 无脾综合征; **functional a.,** impaired reticuloendothelial function of the spleen, as seen in children with sickle cell anemia 功能性无脾

ASPMN American Society of Pain Management Nurses 美国疼痛管理护士协会

ASPS alveolar soft part sarcoma 腺泡状软组织肉瘤

ASRT American Society of Radiologic Technologists 美国放射学专家协会

as·say (as′a) determination of the amount of a particular constituent of a mixture, or of the potency of a drug 测定，化验；**biological a.,** bioassay 生物测定；**CH50 a.,** a test of total complement activity as the capacity of serum to lyse a standard preparation of sheep red blood cells coated with antisheep erythrocyte antibody. The reciprocal of the dilution of serum that lyses 50 percent of the erythrocytes is the whole complement titer in CH50 units per milliliter of serum CH50 溶血试验；**enzyme-linked immunosorbent a.,** 酶联免疫吸附试验，见 *ELISA*；. **microbiological a.,** assay by the use of microorganisms 微生物测定；**microcytotoxicity a.,** one using the pattern of lysis of peripheral blood lymphocytes in the presence of complement and typing sera to type serologically defined HLA antigens (HLA-A, -B, and -C antigens) 微量细胞毒实验；**radioimmunoprecipitation a. (RIPA),** immunoprecipitation conducted with radiolabeled antibody or antigen 放射免疫沉淀法；**radioligand a.,** any assay procedure that uses radioisotopic labeling and biologically specific binding of reagents 放射性配体试验；**stem cell a.,** a measurement of the potency of antineoplastic drugs, based on their ability to retard the growth of cultures of human tumor cells 干细胞测定

as·ser·tive·ness (ə-sur′tiv-nes) the quality or state of bold or confident self-expression, neither aggressive nor submissive 自信，魄力

ASSH American Society for Surgery of the Hand 美国手外科协会

as·sim·i·la·tion (ə-sim″ĭ-la′shən) 1. psychologically, absorption of new experiences into existing psychologic make-up 接受，理解；2. anabolism 同化，吸收

as·so·ci·at·ed (ə-so′she-āt″əd) connected; accompanying; joined with another or others 相关联

as·so·ci·a·tion (ə-so″se-a′shən) 1. a state in which two attributes occur together either more or less often than expected by chance 相关，概率上存在相关性；2. a term applied to those regions of the brain that link the primary motor and sensory cortices 大脑中连接初级运动皮质和感觉皮质的区域；见 *area* 下 *association areas*；3. the occurrence together of two or more phenotypic characteristics more often than would be expected by chance(基因) 连锁；4. a connection between ideas or feelings, especially between conscious thoughts and elements of the unconscious, or the formation of such a connection 思想或感觉之间的联系，尤指有意识的思想和无意识的要素之间的联系，或这种联系的形成；**CHARGE a.,** 见 *syndrome* 下词条；**free a.,** verbal expression of one's ideas as they arrive spontaneously; a method used in psychoanalysis 自由联想

as·sor·ta·tive (ə-sor′tə-tiv) characterized by or pertaining to selection on the basis of likeness or kind 相配的

as·sor·tive (ə-sor′tiv) assortative 相配的

as·sort·ment (ə-sort′mənt) the random distribution of different combinations of the parental chromosomes to the gametes, each gamete thus containing one chromosome of each homologous pair, but randomly receiving the maternal versus paternal homologue for any pair 多样性 **independent a.,** 1. the independent behavior of alleles of different, unlinked genes in gametogenesis, a consequence of the random distribution of the chromosomal homologues 自由组合；2. assortment 多样性

AST aspartate transaminase 天冬氨酸转氨酶；Association of Surgical Technologists 外科技术专家协会

asta·sia (as-ta′zhə) motor incoordination with inability to stand 站立不能；**astat′ic** *adj.* 不稳定的 **a.-aba′sia,** inability to stand or walk although the legs are otherwise under control 站立不能

as·ta·tine (At) (as′tə-tēn) a rare radioactive element, the heaviest known halogen; at. no. 85, at. wt. 210 砹

aste·a·to·sis (as″te-ə-to′sis) any disease in which persistent dry scaling of the skin suggests scantiness or absence of sebum 皮脂缺乏症；**asteatot′ic** *adj.* 皮脂缺乏的

as·ter (as′tər) [L.] a system of microtubules arranged in starlike rays around each pair of centrioles during mitosis 星体

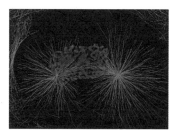

▲ 有丝分裂前体阶段免疫荧光图像中的星体（**aster**），显示纺锤丝微管（绿色）和染色体（蓝色）

as·te·ri·on (as-te′re-on) pl. *aste′ria* [Gr.] the point on the skull at the junction of occipital, parietal, and temporal bones 星点

as·ter·ix·is (as″tər-ik′sis) a motor disturbance marked by intermittent lapses of an assumed posture as a result of intermittency of sustained contraction of groups of muscles; called *liver flap* because of its occurrence in hepatic coma, but observed also in other conditions 扑翼样震颤

aster·nal (a-stur′nəl) 1. not joined to the sternum 未连接至胸骨; 2. lacking a sternum 无胸骨畸形

as·ter·oid (as″tər-oid) star-shaped 星形的

as·the·nia (as-the′ne-ə) lack or loss of strength and energy; weakness 虚弱; **neurocirculatory a.**, a syndrome of breathlessness, fear of effort, a sense of fatigue, precordial pain, and palpitation, generally considered to be a particular presentation of an anxiety disorder 神经循环性衰弱; **tropical anhidrotic a.**, a condition due to generalized anhidrosis in conditions of high temperature, characterized by a tendency to overfatigability, irritability, anorexia, inability to concentrate, and drowsiness, with headache and vertigo 热带性汗闭性衰弱

as·the·no·co·ria (as″thə-no-kor′e-ə) sluggishness of the pupillary light reflex; seen in hypoadrenalism 瞳孔反应迟钝

as·the·no·pia (as″thə-no′pe-ə) weakness or easy fatigue of the eye, with pain in the eyes, headache, dimness of vision, etc. 视疲劳; **asthenop′ic** *adj.* 视疲劳的; **accommodative a.**, asthenopia due to strain of the ciliary muscle 调节性视疲劳; **muscular a.**, asthenopia due to weakness of external ocular muscles 肌性视疲劳

as·the·no·sper·mia (as″thə-no-spur′me-ə) asthenozoospermia 弱精子症

as·the·no·zo·o·sper·mia (as″thə-no-zo″ospur′me-ə) reduced motility or vitality of spermatozoa 弱精子症

as·thma (az′mə) recurrent attacks of paroxysmal dyspnea, with wheezing due to spasmodic contraction of the bronchi. It is usually either an allergic manifestation (*allergic* or *extrinsic a.*) or secondary to a chronic or recurrent condition (*intrinsic a.*) 哮喘; **asthmat′ic** *adj.* 哮喘的; **bronchial a.**, asthma 支气管哮喘

astig·ma·tism (ə-stig′mə-tiz-əm) ametropia caused by differences in curvature in different meridians of the refractive surfaces of the eye so that light rays are not sharply focused on the retina 屈光不正; **astigmat′ic, astigmic** *adj.* 散光的; **compound a.**, that complicated with hypermetropia or myopia in all meridians 复性散光; **corneal a.**, astigmatism due to irregularity in the curvature or refracting power of the cornea 角膜性散光; **irreg-**

ular a., that in which the curvature varies in different parts of the same meridian or in which refraction in successive meridians differs irregularly 不规则散光; **mixed a.**, astigmatism in which one principal meridian is myopic and the other hyperopic 混合性散光; **myopic a.**, that in which the light rays are brought to a focus in front of the retina 近视散光; **regular a.**, that in which the refractive power of the eye shows a uniform increase or decrease from one meridian to another 规则散光

as·trag·a·lus (as-trag′ə-ləs) talus 距骨; **as-trag′alar** *adj.* 距骨的

as·tral (as′trəl) of or relating to an aster 星状体的

as·tra·pho·bia (as″trə-fo′be-ə) irrational fear of thunder and lightning 雷电恐惧症

astrin·gen·cy (ə-strin′jən-se) the quality of being astringent 收敛性

astrin·gent (ə-strin′jənt) 1. causing contraction, usually locally after topical application 局部应用后产生收缩效应的收敛剂; 2. an agent that so acts 产生收敛效应

ASTRO American Society for Therapeutic Radiology and Oncology 美国放射治疗和肿瘤学会

as·tro·blast (as′tro-blast) an embryonic cell that develops into an astrocyte 成星形胶质细胞

as·tro·blas·to·ma (as″tro-blas-to′mə) an astrocytoma of Grade Ⅱ; its cells resemble astroblasts, with abundant cytoplasm and two or three nuclei 星形母细胞瘤

as·tro·cyte (as′tro-sīt) a neuroglial cell of ectodermal origin, characterized by fibrous, protoplasmic, or plasmatofibrous processes 星形胶质细胞。统称 *astroglia*

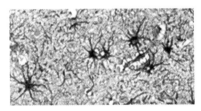

▲ 胶质纤维酸性蛋白（棕色）免疫组化染色显示星形胶质细胞（**astrocyte**) 发育良好

as·tro·cy·to·ma (as″tro-si-to′mə) a tumor composed of astrocytes; the most common type of primary brain tumor and also found throughout the central nervous system, classified on the basis of histology or in order of malignancy (Grades Ⅰ–Ⅳ) 星形细胞瘤; **glioblastoma a.**, an astrocytoma of GradeⅣ 胶质母细胞瘤; **malignant a.**, an astrocytoma of Grade Ⅲ 恶性星形细胞瘤；**protoplasmic a.**, a tumor composed of protoplasmic astrocytes 原生质星形胞瘤；**subependymal giant cell a.**, a rare, usually slow-growing astrocytoma found in the wall of the lateral ventricle; it is sometimes associated with tuberous sclerosis complex 室管膜下巨细胞星形细胞瘤

as·trog·lia (as-trog′le-ə) 1. astrocytes 星形胶质细胞；2. the astrocytes considered as tissue；被认为是组织的星形胶质细胞

As·tro·vi·ri·dae (as″tro-vi′rĭ-de) a family of RNA viruses that cause gastroenteritis in humans and other animals; the single genus is *Astrovirus* 星状病毒科

As·tro·vi·rus (as′tro-vi″rəs) the sole genus in the family Astroviridae, RNA viruses that cause gastroenteritis in humans and other animals 星状病毒属

as·tro·vi·rus (as′tro-vi″rəs) any virus belonging to the family *Astroviridae* 星状病毒

a·su·na·pre·vir (ə-soo′nă-prə-veer) inhibitor of NS3 protease, approved in Japan for the treatment of hepatitis C virus; administered orally in tablet formulation 阿那匹韦，NS3 蛋白酶抑制剂

asym·me·try (a-sim′ə-tre) 1. lack or absence of symmetry; dissimilarity in corresponding parts or organs on opposite sides of the body which are normally alike 不对称的；2. in chemistry, lack of symmetry in the special arrangements of the atoms and radicals within the molecule or crystal（分子）非对称性；**asymmet′ric, asymmet′rical adj.** 不对称的

asyn·chro·nism (a-sing′krə-niz-əm) asynchrony 不同步的

asyn·chro·ny (a-sing′krə-ne) 1. lack of synchronism; disturbance of coordination 缺乏同步性，协调受阻；2. occurrence at distinct times of events normally synchronous; disturbance of coordination 通常同步的事件不同步发生；**asyn′chronous adj.** 不同步的

asyn·cli·tism (ə-sin′klī-tiz-əm) 1. oblique presentation of the fetal head in labor, called *anterior a.* when the anterior parietal bone is designated the point of presentation, and *posterior a.* when the posterior parietal bone is so designated 前不均倾位；2. maturation at different times of the nucleus and cytoplasm of blood cells 血细胞胞核与胞质成熟的不同时期

asyn·de·sis (ə-sin′də-sis) a language disorder in which related elements of a sentence cannot be welded together as a whole 言语不连贯

asyn·ech·ia (a″sin-ek′e-ə) absence of continuity of structure 不连续（结构）

asyn·er·gy (a-sin′ər-je) lack of coordination among parts or organs normally acting in unison 共济失调

asys·to·le (a-sis′to-le) cardiac standstill or arrest; absence of heartbeat 心脏停搏；**asystol′ic adj.** 心搏停止的

AT atrial tachycardia 房性心动过速

At astatine 砹

ATA American Telemedicine Association 美国远程医疗协会；American Thyroid Association 美国甲状腺协会

atac·ti·form (ə-tak′tĭ-form) resembling ataxia 共济失调样

at·a·vism (at′ə-viz-əm) apparent inheritance of a characteristic from remote rather than immediate ancestors 隔代遗传；**atavis′tic adj.** 隔代遗传的，返祖的

atax·ia (ə-tak′se-ə) failure of muscular coordination; irregularity of muscular action 共济失调；**atac′tic, atax′ic adj.** 共济失调的；**Bruns frontal a.**, gait apraxia 步态失调；**Friedreich a.**, an autosomal recessive inherited disorder that causes progressive damage to the nervous system resulting in symptoms ranging from gait disturbance and speech problems to heart disease; it is a triplet repeat disorder in which the repeat expansion intereferes with expression of a mitochondrial protein important in iron metabolism 遗传性共济失调；**locomotor a.**, tabes dorsalis 脊髓痨；**motor a.**, inability to control the coordinate movements of the muscles 运动性共济失调；**sensory a.**, ataxia due to loss of joint position sense, resulting in poorly judged movements, the incoordination becoming aggravated when the eyes are closed 感觉性共济失调；**spinocerebellar a.**, any of a group of hereditary disorders characterized by progressive degeneration of the cerebellum and other regions of the brain, with neuronal loss and secondary degeneration of white matter tracts. Those of autosomal dominant inheritance are triplet repeat disorders 脊髓小脑性共济失调；**a.-telangiectasia**, a severe autosomal recessive progressive cerebellar ataxia, associated with oculocutaneous telangiectasia, abnormal eye movements, sinopulmonary disease, and immunodeficiency 共济失调微血管扩张综合征

at·a·za·na·vir (at″ə-zan′ə-vir) an inhibitor of human immunodeficiency virus-1 (HIV-1) protease, used as the sulfate salt in the treatment of HIV-1 infection 阿扎那韦

at·e·lec·ta·sis (at″ə-lek′tə-sis) incomplete expansion of the lungs at birth, or collapse of the adult lung 肺不张；**atelectat′ic adj.** 肺不张的；**absorption a., acquired a.**, obstructive a.; that caused by an obstruction of the airway that prevents intake of air 吸收性肺不张；**lobar a.**, that affecting only one lobe of the lung 肺叶性肺不张；**lobular a.**, that affecting only a lobule of the lung 肺小叶性肺不张；**obstructive a.**, acquired a. 阻塞性肺不张；**segmental a.**, that affecting one segment of a lung 肺段性肺不张；**tympanic membrane a.**, a complication of chronic serous otitis media, with viscous fluid in the middle ear and thinning of the tympanic membrane, which adheres to middle ear structures; there is usually conductive hearing loss 鼓膜不张

ate·lia (ə-te′le-ə) imperfect or incomplete development 发育不全；**ateliot′ic adj.** 发育不全的

at·e·lo·car·dia (at″ə-lo-kahr′de-ə) imperfect development of the heart 心脏发育不全

aten·o·lol (ə-ten′ə-lol) a cardioselective β₁-adrenergic blocking agent used in the treatment of hypertension and chronic angina pectoris and the prophylaxis and treatment of myocardial infarction and cardiac arrhythmias 阿替洛尔

ATG antithymocyte globulin 抗胸腺细胞球蛋白

athe·lia (ə-the′le-ə) congenital absence of the nipples 先天乳头缺如

ath·er·ec·to·my (ath″ər-ek′tə-me) the removal of atherosclerotic plaque from an artery using a rotary cutter inside a special catheter guided radiographically; it does not extend to the tunica intima as endarterectomy does 动脉粥样斑块旋切术

ather·mic (a-thur′mik) without rise of temperature; afebrile; apyretic 不发热的

ather·mo·sys·tal·tic (ə-thur″mo-sistal′tik) not contracting under the action of cold or heat; said of skeletal muscle 骨骼肌无温觉收缩

ath·ero·em·bo·lus (ath″ər-o-em′bo-ləs) pl. *atheroem′boli.* An embolus composed of cholesterol or its esters or of fragments of atheromatous plaques, typically lodging in small arteries 粥样硬化栓子

ath·ero·gen·e·sis (ath″ər-o-jen′ə-sis) formation of atheromatous lesions in arterial walls 动脉粥样硬化形成；**atherogen′ic adj.** 致粥样硬化的

ath·er·o·ma (ath″ər-o′mə) a mass or plaque of degenerated thickened arterial intima, occurring in atherosclerosis 动脉粥样硬化

ath·er·o·ma·to·sis (ath″ər-o″mə-to′sis) diffuse atheromatous arterial disease 弥漫性动脉粥样化病

ath·ero·scle·ro·sis (ath″ər-o-sklə-ro′sis) a form of arteriosclerosis in which atheromas containing cholesterol, lipoid material, and lipophages are formed within the intima and inner media of large and medium-sized arteries 动脉粥样硬化；**atherosclerot′ic adj.** 动脉粥样硬化的

ath·e·to·sis (ath″ə-to′sis) repetitive involuntary, slow, sinuous, writhing movements, especially severe in the hands 手足徐动症

athym·ia (ə-thīm′e-ə) absence of the thymus or

the condition resulting from such absence 无胸腺

athy·ria (ə-thi′re-ə) 1. hypothyroidism 甲状腺功能减退；2. complete absence of thyroid function 无甲状腺功能；**athyrot′ic adj.** 无甲状腺的

ATL adult T-cell leukemia/lymphoma 成人 T 细胞白血病 / 淋巴瘤

at·lan·tad (at-lan′tad) toward the atlas 向寰椎的

at·lan·tal (at-lan′təl) pertaining to the atlas 寰椎的

at·lan·to·ax·i·al (at-lan″to-ak′se-əl) pertaining to the atlas and the axis 寰枢椎的

at·lan·to·oc·cip·i·tal (at-lan″to-ok-sip′ĭ-təl) pertaining to the atlas and the occiput 寰枕的

at·las (at′ləs) the first cervical vertebra, which articulates above with the occipital bone and below with the axis 寰椎

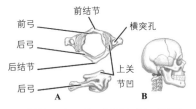

前结节

前弓 横突孔

后弓

后结节 上关节凹

后弓

A B

▲ 寰椎（**atlas**）。A.上一俯视图；下一侧视图。**B. 位置**

at·lo·ax·oid (at″lo-ak′soid) atlantoaxial 寰枢的

atm 见 atmosphere (3)

at·mos·pher·ic (at″məs-fer′ik) of or pertaining to the atmosphere 大气的

at no atomic number 原子序数

ato·cia (a-to′shə) sterility in the female 女性不育

at·om (at′əm) the smallest particle of an element with all the properties of the element; it consists of a positively charged nucleus (made up of protons and neutrons) and negatively charged electrons, which move in orbits about the nucleus 原子 **atom′ic adj.** 原子的

at·om·i·za·tion (at″əm-ĭ-za′shən) nebulization 雾化

at·om·iz·er (at′əm-i″zər) nebulizer 雾化器

at·om·ox·e·tine (at″ə-mok′sə-tēn) a selective norepinephrine reuptake inhibitor used as the hydrochloride salt in the treatment of attentiondeficit/hyperactivity disorder 托莫西汀

at·o·ny (at′ə-ne) lack of normal tone or strength; flaccidity 失张力；松弛；**aton′ic adj.** 失张力的，平音

atop·ic (a-top′ik) (a-top′ik) 1. ectopic 异位的；2. pertaining to atopy; allergic 过敏的

Ato·po·bi·um (at″ə-po′be-əm) a genus of grampositive, anaerobic bacteria that cause soft tissue infections; *A. vagi'nae* causes vaginal disease 奇异菌属

atop·og·no·sia (ə-top″og-no′zhə) loss of the power of topognosia (ability to correctly locate a sensation) 位置觉缺失

at·o·py (at′ə-pe) a genetic predisposition toward the development of immediate hypersensitivity reactions against common environmental antigens (atopic allergy), most commonly manifested as allergic rhinitis but also as bronchial asthma, atopic dermatitis, or food allergy 特异反应性

ator·va·stat·in (ə-tor′və-stat″in) an antihyperlipidemic agent that acts by inhibiting cholesterol synthesis, used as the calcium salt in the treatment of hypercholesterolemia and other forms of dyslipidemia 阿托伐他汀

ato·va·quone (ə-to′və-kwōn″) an antibiotic used in treatment of mild to moderate pneumocystis pneumonia and the prophylaxis and treatment of falciparum malaria 阿托伐醌

atox·ic (a-tok′sik) not poisonous; not due to a poison 无毒

ATP adenosine triphosphate 三磷酸腺苷

ATP·ase (a-te-pe′ās) adenosinetriphosphatase 三磷酸腺苷酶

atra·cu·rium (at″rŏ-kūr′e-əm) a nondepolarizing neuromuscular blocking agent of intermediate duration, used as the besylate salt as an adjunct to general anesthesia 阿曲库铵

atrans·fer·ri·ne·mia (a-trans″fer-ĭ-ne′me-ə) absence of circulating iron-binding protein (transferrin) 血转铁蛋白缺乏

atrau·mat·ic (a″traw-mat′ik) not producing injury or damage 无创的

atre·sia (ə-tre′zhə) congenital absence or closure of a normal body opening or tubular structure 闭锁; **atret′ic** *adj.* 闭锁的; **anal a.**, **a. a′ni**, imperforate anus 肛门闭锁; **aortic a.**, congenital absence of the aortic orifice of the heart 先天性主动脉闭锁; **biliary a.**, obliteration or hypoplasia of part of the bile ducts due to arrested fetal development, causing persistent jaundice and liver damage ranging from biliary stasis to biliary cirrhosis, with splenomegaly as portal hypertension progresses 胆道闭锁; **follicular a.**, degeneration and resorption of an ovarian follicle before it reaches maturity and ruptures 卵泡闭锁; **laryngeal a.**, congenital lack of the normal opening into the larynx 喉闭锁; **mitral a.**, congenital obliteration of the mitral orifice of the heart, often associated with hypoplastic left heart syndrome or transposition of great vessels 二尖瓣闭锁; **prepyloric a.**, pyloric atresia; congenital membranous obstruction of the gastric outlet, with vomiting

of gastric contents only 幽门闭锁; **pulmonary a.**, congenital severe narrowing or obstruction of the pulmonary orifice of the heart, with cardiomegaly, reduced pulmonary vascularity, and right ventricular atrophy. It is usually associated with tetralogy of Fallot, transposition of great vessels, or other cardiovascular anomalies 肺动脉闭锁; **pyloric a.**, 见 prepyloric a.; **tricuspid a.**, congenital absence of the tricuspid orifice of the heart; circulation is made possible by the presence of an atrial septal defect 三尖瓣闭锁; **urethral a.**, congenital imperforation of the urethra 尿道闭锁

atri·al (a′tre-əl) pertaining to an atrium 心房的

atrio·his·i·an (a″tre-o-his′e-ən) connecting the atrium and the bundle of His 心房希氏束的

atrio·meg·a·ly (a″tre-o-meg′ə-le) abnormal enlargement of an atrium of the heart 心房肥大

atrio·sep·tal (a″-tre-o-sep′təl) pertaining to or occurring in the interatrial septum 房间隔的

atrio·sep·to·pexy (a″tre-o-sep′to-pek″se) surgical correction of a defect in the interatrial septum 房间隔修补术

atrio·sep·to·plas·ty (a″tre-o-sep′to-plas″te) plastic repair of the interatrial septum 房间隔修补术

atrio·ven·tric·u·lar (a″tre-o-ven-trik′ulər) pertaining to both an atrium and a ventricle of the heart (心)房室的

atri·o·ven·tric·u·la·ris com·mu·nis (a″tre-oven-trik″u-la′ris kə-mu′nis) a congenital cardiac anomaly in which the endocardial cushions fail to fuse, the ostium primum persists, the atrioventricular canal is undivided, a single atrioventricular valve has anterior and posterior leaflets, and there is a defect of the membranous interventricular septum 房室共道

atri·um (a′tre-əm) pl. *a′tria* [L.] a chamber; in anatomy, a chamber affording entrance to another structure or organ, especially the upper, smaller cavity (*a. cordis*) on either side of the heart, which receives blood from the pulmonary veins (*left a.*) or venae cavae (*right a.*) and delivers it to the ventricle on the same side 心房; **a′trial** *adj.* 心房的; **common a.**, the single atrium found in a form of three-chambered heart 单心房

atro·phic (a-tro′fik) pertaining to or characterized by atrophy 萎缩的

at·ro·pho·der·ma (at″ro-fo-dur′mə) atrophy of the skin 皮萎缩

at·ro·phy (at′rŏ-fe) 1. a wasting away; a diminution in the size of a cell, tissue, organ, or part 萎缩; 2. to undergo or cause atrophy 萎缩的或在萎缩的; **Aran-Duchenne muscular a.**, 见 spinal muscular a.; **bone a.**, resorption of bone evident in both external form and internal density 骨萎缩；**Duchenne-Aran muscular a.**, 见 spinal muscular a.；**fibular a., fibular muscular a.**, Charcot-Marie-Tooth disease 腓骨萎缩，又称 *peroneal atrophy*；**healed yellow a.**, macronodular cirrhosis 大结节性肝硬化；**Leber hereditary optic a.**, 见 *neuropathy* 下词条；**lobar a.**, 见 Pick disease (1)；**multiple system a. (MSA)**, a progressive disorder characterized by striatonigral and olivopontocerebellar degeneration, formation of Papp-Lantos bodies, and varying combinations of parkinsonism, cerebellar ataxia, autonomic failure, urogenital dysfunction, and corticospinal disorders. It is divided into two categories, MSA with predominant parkinsonism (MSA-P) and MSA with predominant cerebellar ataxia (MSA-C) 多系统萎缩；**myelopathic muscular a.**, muscular atrophy due to lesion of the spinal cord, as in spinal muscular atrophy 脊髓型肌萎缩；**olivopontocerebellar a.**, any of a group of progressive hereditary disorders involving degeneration of the cerebellar cortex, middle peduncles, ventral pontine surface, and olivary nuclei in the young to middle-aged, characterized by ataxia, dysarthria, and tremors similar to those of parkinsonism 橄榄体脑桥小脑萎缩；**optic a.**, atrophy of the optic disk due to degeneration of the nerve fibers of the optic nerve and optic tract 视神经萎缩；**physiologic a.**, that affecting certain organs in all individuals as part of the normal aging process 生理性萎缩；**senile a.**, the natural atrophy of tissues and organs occurring with advancing age 老年性萎缩；**senile a. of skin**, the mild atrophic changes in the dermis and epidermis that occur naturally with aging 老年性皮肤萎缩；**spinal muscular a.**, a group of hereditary progressive degenerative disorders affecting the motor cells of the spinal cord, beginning usually in the small muscles of the hands, but in some cases (scapulohumeral type) in the upper arm and shoulder muscles, and progressing slowly to the leg muscles 脊髓型肌萎缩；**spinobulbar muscular a. (SBMA)**, an X-linked, adult-onset disorder with degeneration of the lower motor neurons in the brainstem and spinal cord; characterized by distal limb amyotrophy, bulbar signs, and androgen insensitivity. It is a triplet repeat disorder caused by mutation in the androgen receptor gene 脊髓延髓肌萎缩症；**Sudeck a.**, posttraumatic osteoporosis 创伤后骨质疏松

at·ro·pine (at′ro-pēn) an anticholinergic and antispasmodic alkaloid used as the sulfate salt to relax smooth muscles and increase and regulate the heart rate by blocking the vagus nerve, and to act as a preanesthetic antisialagogue, an antidote for various toxic and anticholinesterase agents, and as an antisecretory, mydriatic, and cycloplegic 阿托品

ATS American Thoracic Society 美国胸外科学会；American Trauma Society 美国创伤学会

at·tack (ə-tak′) an episode or onset of illness. 发作；**Adams-Stokes a.**, an episode of syncope in Adams-Stokes syndrome 阿‑斯综合征发作；**drop a.**, sudden loss of balance without loss of consciousness, usually seen in elderly women 跌倒发作；**panic a.**, an episode of acute intense anxiety, the essential feature of panic disorder 惊恐发作；**transient ischemic a. (TIA)**, a brief attack (an hour or less) of cerebral dysfunction of vascular origin, without lasting neurological effect 短暂性脑缺血发作

at·ta·pul·gite (at″ə-pul′jīt) a hydrated silicate of aluminum and magnesium, a clay mineral that is the main ingredient of fuller's earth; *activated a.* is a heat-treated form that is used in the treatment of diarrhea 硅镁土

at·tend·ing (ə-ten′ding) 1. attending physician 主治医师；2. being or pertaining to such a physician 主治医师的

at·ten·u·ate (ə-ten′u-āt) 1. to render thin 变薄；2. to render less virulent 解毒

at·ten·u·a·tion (ə-ten″u-a′shən) the act of thinning or weakening, as 衰减 (*a*) the alteration of virulence of a pathogenic microorganism by passage through another host species, decreasing the virulence of the organism for the native host and increasing it for the new host, 通过寄主的更替以致改变病微生物自身的毒力，削弱原寄主的生物体毒力，增加新寄主的毒力 or (*b*) the process by which a beam of radiation is reduced in energy when passed through tissue or other material. 当辐射通过组织或其他材料时能量减少的过程

at·tic (at′ik) epitympanic recess 鼓室上隐窝

at·ti·co·an·trot·o·my (at″ĭ-ko-an-trot′ə-me) surgical exposure of the attic and mastoid antrum 上鼓室、鼓窦凿开术

at·ti·tude (at′ĭ-tood) 1. a position of the body 姿势；in obstetrics, the relation of the various parts of the fetal body 胎儿姿态；2. a pattern of mental views established by cumulative prior experience 态度

atto- word element [Danish], *eighteen* 丹麦语词素，18; used in naming units of measurement to designate an amount one quintillionth (10^{-18}) the size of the unit to which it is joined 计量单位 (10^{-18}); symbol a 符号 a

at·trac·tion (ə-trak′shən) 1. the force, act, or process that draws one body toward another 吸引；2. malocclusion in which the occlusal plane is closer than normal to the eye-ear plane, causing shortening of the face; cf. *abstraction* (3) 咬合平面比正常情

况下更靠近眼耳平面的错位咬合，导致面部缩短；参见 abstra ction (3)；**capillary a.**, the force which causes a liquid to rise in a fine-caliber tube 毛细现象（毛细血管作用）

at wt atomic weight 原子量

atyp·ia (a-tip′e-ə) deviation from the normal 异型性；**koilocytotic a.**, vacuolization and nuclear abnormalities of cells of the stratified squamous epithelium of the uterine cervix; it may be premalignant 空泡变性

atyp·i·cal (a-tip′ĭ-kəl) irregular; not conforming to type; in microbiology, applied specifically to strains of unusual type 非典型

AU [L.] aures unitas, both ears together 双耳；auris uterque, each ear 每只耳

Au gold (L. *au′rum*) 金

AUA American Urological Association 美国泌尿外科学会

Au·bag·i·o (ō-bah-zhē′ō) trademark for a preparation of teriflunomide 特立氟胺制剂的商品名

au·dio·gen·ic (aw″de-o-jen′ik) produced by sound 听觉的

au·di·ol·o·gy (aw″de-ol′ə-je) the study of impaired hearing that cannot be improved by medication or surgical therapy 听力学

au·di·om·e·try (aw″de-om′ə-tre) measurement of the acuity of hearing for the various frequencies of sound waves 听力测试；**audiomet′ric adj.** 听力测试的；**Békésy a.**, that in which the patient, by pressing a signal button, traces monaural thresholds for pure tones: the intensity of the tone decreases as long as the button is depressed and increases when it is released; both continuous and interrupted tones are used 贝克赛测听法；**cortical a.**, an objective method of determining auditory acuity by recording and averaging electric potentials evoked from the cortex of the brain in response to stimulation by pure tones 皮质测听法；**electrocochleographic a.**, measurement of electrical potentials from the middle ear or external auditory canal (cochlear microphonics and eighth nerve action potentials) in response to acoustic stimuli 耳蜗电图测听法；**electrodermal a.**, audiometry in which the subject is conditioned by harmless electric shock to pure tones, thereafter anticipating a shock when hearing a pure tone; the anticipation results in a brief electrodermal response, which is recorded; the lowest intensity at which the response is elicited is taken to be the hearing threshold 皮电（阻）测听法；**localization a.**, a technique for measuring the capacity to locate the source of a pure tone received binaurally in a sound field 声源定位测听法；**pure tone a.**, audiometry utilizing pure tones that are relatively free of noise and overtones 纯音听阈测试

au·di·tion (aw-dish′ən) hearing 听力；**chromatic a.**, color hearing 色听

au·di·to·ry (aw′dĭ-tor″e)1. aural or otic; pertaining to the ear 听觉的；耳科或耳朵的；2. pertaining to hearing 听力的

aug·men·ta·tion (awg″men-ta′shən) an adding on, or the resulting condition 增大

AUL acute undifferentiated leukemia 急性未分化白血病

au·la (aw′lə) the red areola formed around a vaccination vesicle 红晕

AUR Association of University Radiologists 大学放射科医师协会

au·ra (aw′rə) pl. **auras** or **au′rae** [L.] a subjective sensation or motor phenomenon that precedes and marks the onset of a neurological condition, particularly an epileptic seizure (*epileptic a.*) or migraine (*migraine a.*) 先兆；**epileptic a.**, a type of simple partial seizure, experienced as a subjective sensation or motor phenomenon, that sometimes signals an approaching generalized or complex partial seizure 癫痫先兆；**vertiginous a.**, a sensory seizure affecting the vestibular sense, causing a feeling of vertigo 眩晕先兆

au·ral (aw′rəl) 1. 见 auditory (1)；2. pertaining to an aura 先兆的

au·ran·o·fin (aw-ran′ə-fin) a gold-containing compound used in the treatment of active rheumatoid arthritis 金诺芬

au·ric (aw′rik) pertaining to or containing gold 金的或含金的

au·ri·cle (aw′rĭ-kəl) [*aur′icula* L.] 1. pinna; the flap of the ear 耳廓；2. the ear-shaped appendage of either atrium of the heart 心耳；3. formerly, either atrium of the heart 心房

au·ric·u·lar (aw-rik′u-lər) 1. pertaining to an auricle 耳廓的；2. pertaining to the ear 耳朵的

au·ric·u·la·re (aw-rik″u-lar′e) a point at the top of the opening of the external auditory meatus 耳点

au·ric·u·la·ris (aw-rik″u-lar′is) [L.] pertaining to the ear 耳朵的；auricular 耳廓的

au·ris (aw′ris) [L.] ear 耳

au·ri·scope (aw′rĭ-skōp) otoscope 耳镜

au·ro·thio·glu·cose (aw″ro-thi″o-gloo′kōs) a monovalent gold salt used in treating rheumatoid arthritis 葡糖硫金

aus·cul·ta·tion (aws″kəl-ta′shən) listening for sounds within the body, chiefly to ascertain the condition of the thoracic or abdominal viscera and to detect pregnancy; it may be performed with the unaided ear (*direct* or *immediate a.*) or with a stethoscope (*mediate a.*) 听 诊；**auscul′tatory** *adj.* 听诊的

au·te·cic (aw-te′sik) autoecious 单寄生

au·te·cious (aw-te′shəs) characterized by a life cycle spent on the same host; said of parasitic fungi. Spelled also autoecious 单寄生；**aute′cic** *adj.* 单寄生的

au·tism (aw′tiz-əm) 1. autistic disorder 自闭症；2. autistic thinking 自闭思维；**infantile a.**, autistic disorder 自闭症

au·tis·tic (aw-tis′tik) characterized by selfabsorption, impairment in social interaction and communication, and a restricted range of activities and interests 自闭症的

au·to·ag·glu·ti·na·tion (aw″to-ə-gloo″tĭna′shən) 1. clumping or agglutination of an individual's cells by his or her own serum, as in autohemagglutination 自体凝集；2. agglutination of particulate antigens, e.g., bacteria, that does not involve antibody 抗原自凝

au·to·ag·glu·ti·nin (aw″to-ə-gloo′tĭ-nin) a factor in serum capable of causing clumping together of the subject's own cellular elements 自体凝集素

au·to·am·pu·ta·tion (aw″to-am″pu-ta′shən) spontaneous detachment from the body and elimination of an appendage or an abnormal growth, such as a polyp 自体截肢

au·to·an·ti·body (aw″to-an′tĭ-bod″e) an antibody formed in response to, and reacting against, an antigenic constituent of one's own tissues 自身抗体

au·to·an·ti·gen (aw″to-an′tĭ-jen) an antigen that despite being a normal tissue constituent is the target of a humoral or cell-mediated immune response, as in autoimmune disease 自身抗原

au·to·ca·tal·y·sis (aw″to-kə-tal′ə-sis) catalysis in which a product of the reaction hastens the catalysis 自催化作用

au·toch·tho·nous (aw-tok′thə-nəs) 1. originating in the same area in which it is found 土著的；2. denoting a tissue graft to a new site on the same individual 自体移植

au·toc·la·sis (aw-tok′lə-sis) destruction of a part by influences within itself, as by autoimmune processes 自裂

au·to·clave (aw′to-klāv) a self-locking apparatus for the sterilization of materials by steam under pressure 高压灭菌器，高压釜

au·to·coid (aw′to-koid) local hormone 内分泌物

au·to·crine (aw′to-krin) denoting a mode of hormone action in which a hormone binds to receptors on and affects the function of the cell type that produced it 自分泌

au·to·di·ges·tion (aw″to-di-jes′chən) autolysis 自

身溶解

au·toe·cious (aw-te′shəs) characterized by a life cycle spent on the same host; said of parasitic fungi 单寄生。Spelled also *autecious*

au·to·ec·zem·a·ti·za·tion (aw″to-ek-zem″ə-tī-za′shən) the spread, at first locally and later more generally, of lesions from an originally circumscribed focus of eczema 自身湿疹化

au·to·erot·i·cism (aw″to-ə-rot′ĭ-siz-əm) sexual self-gratification or arousal without the participation of another person 自慰；**autoerot′ic** *adj.* 自慰的

au·to·gen·e·sis (aw″to-jen′ə-sis) selfgeneration；origination within the organism 单性生殖；**autogenet′ic** *adj.* 单性生殖的

au·tog·e·nous (aw-toj′ə-nəs) autologous 自体的

au·to·graft (aw′to-graft) a tissue graft transferred from one part of the patient's body to another part 自体移植

au·to·he·mag·glu·ti·na·tion (aw″to-he″mə-gloo″tī-na′shən) hemagglutination caused by a factor produced in the subject's own body 自身凝集反应

au·to·he·mag·glu·ti·nin (aw″to-he″mə-gloo′tĭ-nin) a hemagglutinin produced in the subject's own body 自体凝血素

au·to·he·mol·y·sin (aw″to-he-mol′ĭ-sin) a hemolysin that causes complement-dependent hemolysis of the patient's own erythrocytes 自身溶血素

au·to·he·mol·y·sis (aw″to-he-mol′ĭ-sis) hemolysis of an individual's blood cells by his or her own serum 自体溶血；**autohemolyt′ic** *adj.* 自体溶血的

au·to·he·mo·ther·a·py (aw″to-he″mother′ ə-pe) treatment using an autotransfusion 自体输血

au·to·hyp·no·sis (aw″to-hip-no′sis) the act or process of hypnotizing oneself 自 我 催 眠；**autohypnot′ic** *adj.* 自我催眠的

au·to·im·mune (aw″to-ĭ-mūn′) directed against the body's own tissue 自 身 免 疫；见 *disease* 和 *response* 下词条

au·to·im·mu·ni·ty (aw″to-ĭ-mu′nĭ-te) a condition characterized by a specific humoral or cell-mediated immune response against the constituents of the body's own tissues (autoantigens); it may result in hypersensitivity reactions or, if severe, in autoimmune disease 自身免疫反应

au·to·im·mu·ni·za·tion (aw″to-im″u-nīza′shən) induction in an organism of an immune response to its own tissue constituents 自身免疫

au·to·in·oc·u·la·tion (aw″to-in-ok′u-la″shən) inoculation with microorganisms from one's own body 自体接种

au·to·isol·y·sin (aw″to-i-sol′ĭ-sin) a substance that lyses cells (e.g., blood cells) of the individual in which it is formed, as well as those of other members of the same species 自体同族溶素

au·to·ker·a·to·plas·ty (aw″to-ker′ə-toplas″te) grafting of corneal tissue from one eye to the other 自体角膜移植术

au·to·le·sion (aw″to-le′zhən) a self-inflicted injury 自损

au·tol·o·gous (aw-tol′ə-gəs) related to self; belonging to the same organism 自体的

au·tol·y·sin (aw-tol′ĭ-sin) a lysin originating in an organism and capable of destroying its own cells and tissues 自溶素

au·tol·y·sis (aw-tol′ĭ-sis) 1. spontaneous disintegration of cells or tissues by autologous enzymes, as occurs after death and in some pathologic conditions 生理性的自身溶解; 2. destruction of cells of the body by its own serum 血清性自身溶解; **autolyt′ic** adj. 自溶的

au·to·ly·so·some (aw″to-li′so-sōm) an organelle, formed by the fusion of an autophagosome with a lysosome, in which digestion of intracellular elements occurs in autophagy 自身溶酶体

au·to·ma·tic·i·ty (aw″to-mə-tis′ĭ-te) 1. the state or quality of being spontaneous, involuntary, or self-regulating 自动化; 2. the capacity of a cell to initiate an impulse without an external stimulus 自律性; **triggered a.**, pacemaker activity occurring as a result of a propagated or stimulated action potential, such as an afterpotential, in cells or tissues not normally displaying spontaneous automaticity 触发活动

au·tom·a·tism (aw-tom′ə-tiz-əm) performance of nonreflex acts without conscious volition 自动性; **command a.**, abnormal responsiveness to commands, as in hypnosis 服从自动症

au·to·nom·ic (aw″tə-nom′ik) not subject to voluntary control 自主的。见 *system* 下词条

au·to·nomo·tro·pic (aw″to-nom-o-tro′pik) having an affinity for the autonomic nervous system 亲自主神经系统的

au·ton·o·my (aw-ton′ə-me) the state of functioning independently, without extraneous influence 自治; **auton′omous** adj. 自治的

au·to-ox·i·da·tion (aw″to-ok′sĭ-da′shən) spontaneous direct combination, at normal temperatures, with molecular oxygen 自发氧化

au·to·pha·gia (aw″to-fa′jə) 1. eating one's own flesh 自噬; 2. nutrition of the body by consumption of its own tissues 自身消耗; **autopha′gic** adj. 自噬的

au·to·phago·some (aw″to-fag′ə-sōm) an intracytoplasmic vacuole containing elements of a cell's own cytoplasm; it fuses with a lysosome and the

contents are subjected to enzymatic digestion 自噬小体

au·toph·a·gy (aw-tof′ə-je) 1. lysosomal digestion of a cell's own cytoplasmic material 溶酶体吞噬自身胞质; 2. autophagia 自噬

au·toph·o·ny (aw-tof′ə-ne) abnormal hearing of one's own voice and respiratory sounds, usually as a result of a patulous eustachian tube 自听增强

au·to·plas·ty (aw′to-plas″te) 1. autotransplantation 自体移植术; 2. in psychoanalytic theory, adaptation by changing one's self rather than the external environment 自适应; **autoplas′tic** adj. 自身移植的

au·top·sy (aw′top-se) postmortem examination of a body to determine the cause of death or the nature of pathological changes 验尸; necropsy 尸检

au·to·ra·di·og·ra·phy (aw″to-ra″de-og′rə-fe) the making of a radiograph of an object or tissue by recording on a photographic plate the radiation emitted by radioactive material within the object 放射自显影术

au·to·reg·u·la·tion (aw″to-reg″u-la′shən) 1. the process occurring when some mechanism within a biological system detects and adjusts for changes within the system 自体调节; 2. in circulatory physiology, the intrinsic tendency of an organ or tissue to maintain constant blood flow despite changes in arterial pressure, or the adjustment of blood flow through an organ in accordance with its metabolic needs 自身调节; **heterometric a.**, intrinsic mechanisms controlling the strength of ventricular contractions that depend on the length of myocardial fibers at the end of diastole 异长调节; **homeometric a.**, 1. intrinsic mechanisms controlling the strength of ventricular contractions that are independent of the length of myocardial fibers at the end of diastole 等长调节; 2. Anrep effect Anrep 效应

au·to·sen·si·ti·za·tion (aw″to-sen″sĭ-tĭ-za′-shən) autoimmunization 自身免疫

au·to·sep·ti·ce·mia (aw″to-sep″tĭ-se′me-ə) septicemia from poisons developed within the body 自体败血症

au·to·site (aw′to-sīt) the larger, more normal member of asymmetrical conjoined twin fetuses, to which the parasite is attached 优势定植

au·to·some (aw′to-sōm) any non-sex-determining chromosome; in humans there are 22 pairs 常染色体; **autoso′mal** adj. 常染色体的

au·to·sple·nec·to·my (aw″to-sple-nek′tə-me) almost complete disappearance of the spleen through progressive fibrosis and shrinkage 自体脾切除

au·to·sug·ges·tion (aw″to-səg-jes′chən) the process of inducing in oneself the uncritical acceptance of an idea, belief, or opinion 自我暗示

au·to·to·mog·ra·phy (aw″to-to-mog′rə-fe) a method of body section radiography involving movement of the patient instead of the x-ray tube 自体断层摄影；**autotomograph′ic** adj. 自体断层摄影的

au·to·trans·fu·sion (aw″to-trans-fu′zhən) reinfusion of a patient's own blood 自体输血

au·to·trans·plan·ta·tion (aw″to-trans″planta′shən) transfer of tissue from one part of the body to another part 自体移植

au·to·troph (aw′to-trōf) an autotrophic organism 自养生物

au·to·tro·phic (aw″to-tro′fik) self-nourishing 自养的；able to build organic constituents from carbon dioxide and inorganic salts 能利用二氧化碳和无机盐生成有机成分的

au·to·vac·cine (aw″to-vak-sēn′) a vaccine prepared from cultures of organisms isolated from the patient's own tissues or secretions 自体疫苗

au·tox·i·da·tion (aw″tok-sī-da′shən) auto-oxidation 自氧化

aux·an·og·ra·phy (awk″san-og′rə-fe) a method used for determining the most suitable medium for the cultivation of microorganisms 生长谱法；**auxanograph′ic** adj. 生长谱法的

aux·e·sis (awk-se′sis) increase in size of an organism, especially that due to growth of its individual cells rather than an increase in their number 无分裂生长；**auxet′ic** adj. 无分裂生长的

aux·i·lyt·ic (awk-sī-lit′ik) increasing the lytic or destructive power 促溶

auxo·tro·phic (awk″so-tro′fik) 1. requiring a growth factor not required by the parental or prototype strain; said of microbial mutants（微生物突变型）营养缺陷型；2. requiring specific organic growth factors in addition to the carbon source present in a minimal medium 除基本碳源外仍需其他特定有机生长因子的

AV, A-V atrioventricular 房室的；arteriovenous 动静脉的

av avoirdupois 常衡；见 *weight* 下 *avoirdupois weight*

avas·cu·lar (a-vas′ku-lər) not vascular 无血管的；bloodless 少血的

avas·cu·lar·i·za·tion (a-vas″ku-lər-ī-za′shən) diversion of blood from tissues, as by ligation of vessels or tight bandaging 驱血法

aver·sive (ə-vur′siv) characterized by or giving rise to avoidance 厌恶；noxious 有害的

avi·an (a′ve-ən) of or pertaining to birds 禽类的

avid·i·ty (ə-vid′ĭ-te) 1. the strength of an acid or base 酸碱度；2. in immunology, an imprecise measure of the strength of antigen-antibody binding based on the rate at which the complex is formed 亲

和力。Cf. *affinity* (3)

avir·u·lence (a-vir′u-ləns) lack of virulence of an infectious agent 无毒力；**avir′ulent** adj. 无毒力的

AVMA American Veterinary Medical Association 美国兽医学协会

av·o·ben·zone (av″o-ben′zōn) a sunscreen that absorbs light in the UVA range 亚佛苯酮

avoid·ance (ə-void′əns) a conscious or unconscious defense mechanism consisting of refusal to encounter situations, activities, or objects that would produce anxiety or conflict 避免

avoid·ant (ə-void′ənt) moving away from; negatively oriented 驱避

av·oir·du·pois (av″ər-də-poiz′) (av-wahr″doopwah′) 见 *weight* 下词条

AVRT atrioventricular reciprocating tachycardia 房室折返性心动过速

AVTE Association of Veterinary Technician Educators 兽医技术教育工作者协会

Avu·la·vi·rus (a′vu-lə-vi″rəs) a genus of viruses of the family Paramyxoviridae, subfamily Paramyxovirinae; it includes Newcastle disease virus 腮腺炎病毒属，包括新城疫病毒

avul·sion (ə-vul′shən) the tearing away of a structure or part 撕脱

AWHONN Association of Women's Health, Obstetric, and Neonatal Nurses 女性健康、产科和新生儿护士协会

ax. axis 轴

axen·ic (a-zen′ik) not contaminated by or associated with any foreign organisms; used in reference to pure cultures of microorganisms or to germ-free animals 未感染的；无菌的。Cf. *gnotobiotic*

ax·e·til (ak′sə-til″) USAN contraction for 1-acetoxyethyl 醋氧乙（基）

ax·i·al (ak′se-əl) *axialis* [L.] of or pertaining to the axis of a part or body 轴的

ax·i·a·tion (ak″se-a′shən) establishment of an axis; development of polarity in an oocyte, embryo, organ, or other body structure 轴性发展

ax·il·la (ak-sil′ə) pl. *axil′lae* [L.] the pyramidal region between the upper thoracic wall and the upper limb, containing adipose tissue, vessels, nerves, and lymphatics 腋窝；**ax′illary** adj. 腋窝的

ax·ip·e·tal (ak-sip′ə-təl) directed toward an axis or axon 轴向的

ax·is (ak′sis) pl. *ax′es* [L.] 1. a line through the center of a body, or about which a structure revolves 体轴；a line around which body parts are arranged 轴线；2. the second cervical vertebra, which articulates with the atlas above and the third cervical vertebra below 枢椎；**ax′ial** adj. 枢椎的；**basibregmatic a.**, the vertical line from the basion to the bregma 颅顶轴；**basicranial**

a., a line from basion to gonion 颅底轴；**basifacial a.**, a line from gonion to subnasal point 面基轴；**binauricular a.**, a line joining the two auricular points 双耳轴；**celiac a.**, 见 *trunk* 下词条；**dorsoventral a.**, one passing from the back to the belly surface of the body 背腹轴；**electrical a. of heart**, the resultant of the electromotive forces within the heart at any instant 额面心电轴；**frontal a.**, an imaginary line running from right to left through the center of the eyeball 冠状轴；**a. of heart**, a line passing through the center of the base of the heart and the apex 心轴；**optic a.**, 1. a line connecting the center of the anterior curvature of the cornea (anterior pole) with that of the posterior curvature of the sclera (posterior pole) 眼轴；2. the straight line that passes through the centers of the surfaces and the centers of curvature of a lens system 光轴；**visual a.**, the line between the central fovea of the retina and the point of fixation, intersecting the optic axis as it passes through the nodal point 视轴

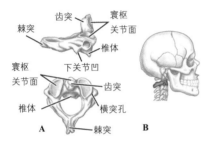

▲ 枢椎（**axis**）。A. 上一侧视图；下一俯视图。B. 位置

ax·it·i·nib (ak-sit′ĭ-nib) a tyrosine kinase inhibitor selective for vascular endothelial growth factor (VEGF) receptors 1, 2, and 3, used in the treatment of advanced renal cell carcinoma 阿西替尼

axo·ax·on·ic (ak″so-ak-son′ik) referring to a synapse between the axon of one neuron and the axon of another 轴突突触

axo·den·drit·ic (ak″so-den-drit′ik) referring to a synapse between the axon of one neuron and the dendrites of another 树突突触

axo·lem·ma (ak-so-lem′ə) the plasma membrane of an axon 轴膜

ax·ol·ysis (ak-sol′ĭ-sis) degeneration of an axon 神经轴分解

ax·on (ak′son) 1. that process of a neuron by which impulses travel away from the cell body 轴突传导；at the terminal arborization of the axon, the impulses are transmitted to other nerve cells or to effector organs. Larger axons are covered by a myelin sheath 轴索；2. vertebral column 脊柱；**ax′onal**

adj. 脊柱的

ax·o·neme (ak′so-nēm) the central core of a cilium or flagellum, consisting of a central pair of microtubules surrounded by nine other pairs 中轴丝

axo·nop·a·thy (ak″sə-nop′ə-the) a disorder disrupting the normal functioning of the axons; in *distal a.* the disease progresses from the center toward the periphery and in *proximal a.* the disease progresses from the periphery toward the center 轴突病变

ax·on·ot·me·sis (ak″son-ot-me′sis) nerve injury characterized by disruption of the axon and myelin sheath but with preservation of the connective tissue fragments, resulting in degeneration of the axon distal to the injury site; regeneration of the axon is spontaneous and of good quality 轴突裂伤. Cf. *neurapraxia* and *neurotmesis*

axo·phage (ak′so-fāj) a glial cell occurring in excavations in the myelin in myelitis 噬髓鞘细胞

axo·plasm (ak′so-plaz″əm) cytoplasm of an axon 轴浆；**axoplas′mic** *adj.* 轴浆的

axo·po·di·um (ak″so-po′de-əm) pl. *axopo′dia*. A long and slender, semipermanent type of locomotor pseudopodium with a central axial filament composed of a bundle of microtubules 轴足

axo·so·mat·ic (ak″so-so-mat′ik) referring to a synapse between the axon of one neuron and the cell body of another 轴-体的

axo·style (ak′so-stīl) 1. the central supporting structure of an axopodium 轴柱；2. a supporting rod running through the body of a trichomonad and protruding posteriorly 轴杆

ax·ot·o·my (ak-sot′ə-me) transection or severing of an axon 轴突横断术

ayur·ve·da (i-yur′ved-ə) (i″yər-va′də) [Sanskrit] a classical system of medicine founded 5000 years ago and currently practiced in India. Its emphasis is on balance with the environment and interpersonal communication and is based on the principles that humans are microcosmic representations of the entire universe and that health is the natural end of living in harmony with the environment. Disease results from disharmony between the person and the environment, and each case of disease is a manifestation of a unique state in a unique individual, therefore requiring a unique cure. The practitioner attempts to maintain or restore the balance of the doshas, with therapies including diet; herbal, color, and sound therapies; aromatherapy; application of medicated oils to the skin and massage; and meditation. 印度阿育吠陀医疗体系. Written also *Ayurveda*；**ayurve′dic** *adj.* 阿育吠陀的

azat·a·dine (ə-zat′ə-dēn) an antihistamine with

anticholinergic and sedative effects, used as the maleate salt 阿扎他定

aza·thio·prine (az′ə-thi′o-prēn) a 6-mercaptopurine derivative used as the base or the sodium salt as an immunosuppressant for prevention of transplant rejection and for treatment of rheumatoid arthritis and various autoimmune diseases 硫唑嘌呤

az·e·la·ic ac·id (az″ə-la′ik) a topical antibacterial used in the treatment of acne vulgaris 壬二酸

azel·as·tine (ə-zel′ə-stēn) a topical antihistamine used as the hydrochloride salt in the treatment of seasonal allergic rhinitis and allergic conjunctivitis 氮卓斯汀

azeo·trope (a′ze-o-trōp″) a mixture of two substances that has a constant boiling point and cannot be separated by fractional distillation 共 沸 物； **azeotrop′ic** adj. 共沸的

azil·sar·tan me·dox·o·mil (a″zil-sahr′tan mə-dok′sə-mil) an angiotensin Ⅱ receptor antagonist, used in the treatment of hypertension 阿齐沙坦酯

az·ith·ro·my·cin (az-ith″ro-mi′sin) a macrolide antibiotic derived from erythromycin, effective against a wide range of gram-positive, gram-negative, and anaerobic bacteria 阿奇霉素

azoo·sper·mia (a-zo″ə-spur′me-ə) lack of live spermatozoa in the semen; classified as obstructive or nonobstructive depending on whether or not the cause is blockage of the tubules or ducts 无精症

az·ote (az′ōt) nitrogen (in France) 氮（法语）

az·o·te·mia (az″o-te′me-ə) uremia; an excess of urea or other nitrogenous compounds in the blood 氮质血症

az·o·tu·ria (az″o-tu′re-ə) excess of urea or other nitrogenous compounds in the urine 氮尿症； **azo-tu′ric** adj. 氮尿症的

az·oxy·gly·co·side (ə-zok″se-gli′co-sīd) any of a group of related compounds in which an azoxy group is linked to a carbohydrate moiety 氧化偶氮基糖苷

AZQ diaziquone 地吖醌

AZT zidovudine 齐多夫定

az·tre·o·nam (az′tre-o-nam″) a narrow-range monobactam antibiotic effective against aerobic gram-negative bacteria 氨曲南

az·ure (azh′ər) one of three metachromatic basic dyes (A, B, and C) 天蓝

az·u·res·in (azh″u-rez′in) a complex combination of azure A dye and carbacrylic cationic exchange resin used as a diagnostic aid in detection of gastric secretion 天青树脂

az·u·ro·phil (azh′u-ro-fil) a tissue constituent staining with azure or a similar metachromatic thiazin dye 嗜天青的

az·u·ro·phil·ia (azh″u-ro-fil′e-ə) a condition in which the blood contains cells having azurophilic granules 嗜天青性

az·y·gog·ra·phy (az″ī-gog′rə-fe) radiography of the azygous venous system 奇静脉造影； **azygo-graph′ic** adj. 奇静脉造影的

az·y·gos (az′ī-gəs) (ə-zi′gəs) 1. unpaired 奇数的； 2. any unpaired part, as the azygos vein 不成对的器官

B bel 贝尔；boron 硼

b base (in nucleic acid sequences) 碱基；born 出生

β (beta, the second letter of the Greek alphabet) β chain of hemoglobin（希腊字母表中的第二个字母）血红蛋白的 β 链

β- a prefix designating 指定前缀 (1) the position of a substituting atom or group in a chemical compound 亚原子或基团在化合物中的位置；(2) the specific rotation of an optically active compound 光学活性化合物的旋光率；(3) the orientation of an exocyclic atom or group 异环原子或基团的方向；(4) a plasma protein migrating with the β band in electrophoresis 电泳时血浆蛋白随 β 带迁移；(5) second in a series of two or more related entities or chemical compounds 在两个或两个以上相关实体或化合物序列中的第二个

BA Bachelor of Arts 文学学士学位

Ba barium 钡

BAA bone age assessment 骨龄测定

Ba·be·sia (bə-be′ze-ə) a genus of protozoa found as parasites in red blood cells and transmitted by ticks; its numerous species include *B. bige′mina, B. bo′vis, B. ma′jor,* and *B. micro′ti,* and cause babesiosis in wild and domestic animals and sometimes humans 巴贝斯原虫属

ba·be·si·a·sis (bă″be-zi′ə-sis) 1. chronic, asymptomatic infection with protozoa of the genus *Babesia* 巴贝斯虫无症状性慢性感染；2. babesiosis 巴贝斯虫病

ba·be·si·o·sis (bə-be″ze-o′sis) a group of tick-borne diseases due to infection with species of *Babesia,* seen in wild and domestic animals associated with anemia, hemoglobinuria, and hemoglobinemia;

124

it may spread to humans as a zoonosis that resembles malaria 巴贝斯虫病

ba·by (ba′be) infant 婴 儿; **blue b.**, an infant born with cyanosis due to a congenital heart lesion or atelectasis 青紫婴儿; **collodion b.**, an infant born encased in a collodion- or parchment-like membrane, which usually leaves fissures in the skin when it is shed so that the infant has lamellar ichthyosis. Occasionally it is shed without major problems *(lamellar exfoliation of the newborn)* 火棉胶样婴儿

ba·cam·pi·cil·lin (bə-kam″pī-sil′in) a semisynthetic penicillin of the ampicillin class; its hydrochloride salt has the same actions and uses as ampicillin 巴氨西林

bac·cate (bak′āt) resembling a berry 浆果状的

Ba·cil·la·ceae (bas″ī-la′se-e) a family of mostly saprophytic bacteria of the order Bacillales, commonly found in soil and as animal parasites; members of genus *Bacillus* cause disease in humans 芽孢菌科

Ba·cil·la·les (bas″ī-la′lēz) an order of grampositive, endospore-forming bacteria of the class Bacilli 芽孢杆菌目

bac·il·lary (bas′ ī-lar″e) pertaining to bacilli or to rodlike structures 杆菌的

ba·cille (bah-sēl′) [Fr.] bacillus 芽 孢 杆 菌; **b. Calmette-Guérin (BCG)**, *Mycobacterium bovis* rendered completely avirulent by cultivation over a long period on bile-glycerol-potato medium 卡介苗; 见 *BCG vaccine*

Ba·cil·li (bə-sil′i) a class of bacteria of the phylum Firmicutes 芽孢杆菌

ba·cil·li (bə-sil′i) 杆菌属。*bacillus* 的复数形式

ba·cil·lin (bə-sil′in) an antibiotic substance isolated from strains of *Bacillus subtilis*, highly active on both gram-positive and gram-negative bacteria 杆菌素

ba·cil·lu·ria (bas″ī-lu′re-ə) bacilli in the urine 尿杆菌

Ba·cil·lus (bə-sil′əs) a genus of bacteria, including gram-positive, spore-forming bacteria of the family Bacillaceae. Most species are soil saprophytes, but three are potentially pathogenic 芽 孢 杆 菌; **B. an′thracis**, the species that causes anthrax 炭疽芽孢杆菌; **B. ce′reus,** a common soil saprophyte that causes food poisoning by the formation of an enterotoxin in contaminated foods 蜡状芽孢杆菌; **B. sub′tilis,** a common saprophytic soil and water form, often occurring as a laboratory contaminant and occasionally causing conjunctivitis 枯草芽孢杆菌

ba·cil·lus (bə-sil′əs) pl. *bacil′li* [L.] 芽 孢 杆 菌 1. an organism of the genus *Bacillus* 隶属于芽孢杆

菌属的有机体; 2. any rod-shaped bacterium 任何杆状的细菌; **Calmette-Guérin b.**, bacille Calmette-Guérin 卡介苗; **coliform bacilli,** gram-negative bacilli resembling *Escherichia coli* that are found in the intestinal tract; the term generally refers to the genera *Citrobacter, Edwardsiella, Enterobacter, Escherichia, Klebsiella,* and *Serratia* 大肠杆菌; **dysentery bacilli,** gram-negative non–spore-forming rods causing dysentery in humans 痢疾杆菌; 见 *Shigella*; **enteric b.,** a bacillus belonging to the family Enterobacteriaceae 肠杆菌; **tubercle b.,** *Mycobacterium tuberculosis* 结核分枝杆菌

bac·i·tra·cin (bas″ī-tra′sin) an antibacterial produced by the licheniformis group of *Bacillus subtilis* that acts by interfering with bacterial cell wall synthesis; it is effective against a wide range of gram-positive and a few gram-negative bacteria; also used as the zinc salt 杆菌肽

back (bak) the posterior part of the trunk from the neck to the pelvis 背例; **angry b.**, excited skin syndrome 愤怒背, 兴奋性皮肤综合征

back blow (bak blo) sharp blows given with the heel of the hand between a person's shoulder blades; an action taken to dislodge an airway blockage in a person who is choking; part of the "five-and-five" approach recommended by the Red Cross 背部扣击

back·cross (bak′kros) a cross between an offspring and one of its parents, or an organism genetically identical to one of its parents 回交

back·flow (bak′flo) reflux or regurgitation (1) 回流; **pyelovenous b.**, drainage from the renal pelvis into the venous system occurring under certain conditions of back pressure 肾盂静脉回流

back·scat·ter (bak′skat-ər) in radiology, radiation deflected by scattering processes at angles greater than 90 degrees to the original direction of the beam of radiation 反向散射

bac·lo·fen (bak′lo-fen″) an analogue of γ- aminobutyric acid used to treat severe spasticity 巴氯芬

bac·ter·as·ci·tes (bak″tər-ə-si′tēz) bacterial infection of ascitic fluid 细菌性腹水; **monomicrobial non-neutrocytic b.**, bacterial infection of ascitic fluid with no intra-abdominal source of infection and a neutrophil count less than 250 cells/mm³ 单菌型非中性粒细胞性细菌性腹水; **polymicrobial b.,** bacterial infection of ascitic fluid caused by several species and resulting from bowel puncture during paracentesis 多菌型细菌性腹水

bac·ter·e·mia (bak″tər-e′me-ə) the presence of bacteria in the blood 菌血症

Bac·te·ria (bak-tēr′e-ə) one of the two large divisions into which prokaryotes are usually grouped, comprising unicellular microorganisms that commonly multiply by cell division and whose cell is typically contained within a cell wall 细 菌。Cf. *Archaea*；见 *bacterium*

bac·te·ria (bak-tēr′e-ə) 细菌。*bacterium* 的复数形式

bac·te·ri·al (bak-tēr′e-əl) pertaining to or caused by bacteria 细菌的或由细菌引起的

bac·te·ri·ci·dal (bak-tēr″ĭ-si′dəl) destructive to bacteria 灭菌剂，杀菌的

bac·te·ri·ci·din (bak-tēr″ĭ-si′din) bactericidal antibody 杀菌素

bac·ter·id (bak′tər-id) a skin eruption caused by bacterial infection elsewhere in the body 细菌疹

bac·te·rio·chlo·ro·phyll (bak-tēr″e-o-klor′ə-fĭl) a form of chlorophyll produced by certain bacteria and capable of carrying out photosynthesis 菌绿素

bac·te·rio·ci·din (bak-tēr″e-o-si′din) a bactericidal antibody 抗菌素

bac·te·rio·cin (bak-tēr″e-o″sin) any of a group of substances, e.g., colicin, released by certain bacteria that kill other strains of bacteria by inducing metabolic block 细菌素

bac·te·ri·o·cin·o·gen·ic (bak-tēr″e-o-sin″ə-jen′ik) giving rise to bacteriocin; denoting bacterial plasmids that synthesize bacteriocin 产菌素的

bac·te·ri·ol·o·gy (bak-tēr″e-ol′ə-je) the scientific study of bacteria 细菌学；**bacteriolog′ic, bacteriolog′ical** *adj.*

bac·te·ri·ol·y·sin (bak-tēr″e-ol′ĭ-sin) an antibacterial antibody that lyses bacterial cells 溶菌素

bac·te·rio·phage (bak-tēr′e-o-fāj″) a virus that lyses bacteria 噬菌体；**bacteriopha′gic** *adj.* 噬菌的；**temperate b.,** one whose genetic material (prophage) becomes an intimate part of the bacterial genome, persisting and being reproduced through many cell division cycles; the affected bacterial cell is known as a *lysogenic bacterium* (q.v.) 温和噬菌体

bac·te·ri·op·so·nin (bak-tēr″e-op′so-nin) an antibody that acts on bacteria 噬菌调理素

bac·te·rio·stat·ic (bak-tēr″e-o-stat′ik) 1. inhibiting growth or multiplication of bacteria 抑菌剂；2. an agent that so acts 抑菌的

bac·te·ri·um (bak-tēr′e-əm) pl. *bacte·ria* [L.] any of the unicellular prokaryotic microorganisms that commonly multiply by cell division, lack a nucleus or membrane-bound organelles, and possess a cell wall; they may be aerobic or anaerobic, motile or nonmotile, free-living, saprophytic, parasitic, or pathogenic 细 菌；**bacter′ial** *adj.* 细 菌 的；**acid-fast b.,** one not readily decolorized by acids after staining 耐 酸 菌；**coliform b.,** one of the facultative, gram-negative, rod-shaped bacteria

that are normal inhabitants of the intestinal tract 大肠杆菌；见 *Escherichia, Klebsiella* 和 *Serratia*；**coryneform bacteria,** a group of bacteria that are morphologically similar to organisms of the genus *Corynebacterium* 棒 状 杆 菌；**gram-negative b.,** 见 G. 下 *gram-negative*；**gram-positive b.,** 见 G. 下 *gram-positive*；**hemophilic b.,** one that has a nutritional affinity for constituents of fresh blood or whose growth is stimulated by bloodenriched media 嗜 血 菌；**lysogenic b.,** a bacterial cell that harbors in its genome the genetic material (prophage) of a temperate bacteriophage and thus reproduces the bacteriophage in cell division; occasionally the prophage develops into the mature form, replicates, lyses the bacterial cell, and is free to infect other cells 溶原细菌

bac·te·ri·uria (bak-tēr″e-u′re-ə) the presence of bacteria in the urine 细菌尿

Bac·te·roi·da·ceae (bak″tər-oi-da′se-e) a family of gram-negative, rod-shaped bacteria of the phylum Bacteroidetes, occurring naturally in body cavities and isolated from infections 拟杆菌科

Bac·te·roi·des (bak″tər-oi′dēz) a genus of gram-negative, anaerobic, rod-shaped bacteria of the family Bacteroidaceae, which are normal inhabitants of the oral, respiratory, intestinal, and urogenital cavities; some species can cause potentially fatal abscesses and bacteremias. The most important such organisms belong to the *B. fra′gilis* group 拟杆菌属

bac·te·roi·des (bak″tər-oi′dēz) 1. any highly pleomorphic rod-shaped bacteria 拟杆菌属；2. an organism of the genus *Bacteroides* 隶属拟杆菌属的有机体

Bac·te·roi·de·tes (bak″tər-oid′ə-tēz) a phenotypically diverse phylum of bacteria that includes a number of human and animal pathogens; with Firmicutes it is one of the two major constituents of the intestinal flora 拟杆菌门

BAE bounded area elimination 界域消除

bag (bag) sac 袋；a flexible container 灵活的容器；**colostomy b.,** a bag worn over the stoma to receive fecal discharge after colostomy 结肠造口袋；**ileostomy b.,** a plastic or latex bag attached to the body for collection of urine or fecal material after ileostomy or cystoplasty 回肠造口袋；**Politzer b.,** a soft bag of rubber for inflating the auditory tube 波氏球；**b. of waters,** popular name for the amniotic sac 羊膜囊

bag·as·so·sis (bag″ə-so′sis) hypersensitivity pneumonitis due to inhalation of dust from bagasse (the residue of cane after extraction of sugar) 蔗尘肺

BAL dimercaprol (British antilewisite) 二巯基丙醇

bal·ance (bal′əns) 1. an instrument for weighing

天平；2. equilibrium 平衡；**acid-base b.**, a normal balance between production and excretion of acid or alkali by the body, resulting in a stable concentration of H$^+$ in body fluids 酸碱平衡；**analytical b.**, a balance used in the laboratory, sensitive to variations of the order of 0.05 to 0.1 mg 分析天平；**fluid b.**, the state of the body in relation to ingestion and excretion of water and electrolytes 体液平衡；**nitrogen b.**, the state of the body in regard to ingestion and excretion of nitrogen. In *negative nitrogen b.* the amount excreted is greater than the quantity ingested; in *positive nitrogen b.* the amount excreted is smaller than the quantity ingested 氮平衡；**water b.**, 体液平衡，见 fluid b.

bal·anced (bal′ənst) existing in or maintaining an equilibrium 平衡的

ba·lan·ic (bə-lan′ik) pertaining to the glans penis or glans clitoridis 阴茎头的

bal·a·ni·tis (bal″ə-ni′tis) inflammation of the glans penis 阴茎头炎；**gangrenous b.**, a rapidly destructive infection producing erosion of the glans penis and often destruction of the entire external genitals; believed to be due to a spirochete 坏疽性阴茎头炎；**plasma cell b., Zoon b.**, a benign erythroplasia of the inner surface of the prepuce or the glans penis, characterized histologically by plasma cell infiltration of the dermis, and clinically by a single erythematous, moist, shiny lesion 浆细胞性阴茎头炎

bal·a·no·pos·thi·tis (bal″ə-no-pos-thi′tis) inflammation of the glans penis and prepuce 阴茎头包皮炎

bal·an·ti·di·a·sis (bal″an-tī-di′ə-sis) infection by protozoa of the genus *Balantidium*; in humans, *B. coli* may cause diarrhea and dysentery with ulceration of the colonic mucosa 结肠小袋纤毛虫病

Bal·an·tid·i·um (bal″an-tid′e-əm) a genus of ciliated protozoa, including many species found in the intestine in vertebrates and invertebrates, including *B. co'li*, a common parasite of swine, rarely in humans, in whom it may cause dysentery 纤毛虫属

bald·ness (bawld′nis) alopecia, especially of the scalp 秃头；**female pattern b.**, 见 *alopecia* 下 *androgenetic alopecia*；**male pattern b.**, 见 *alopecia* 下 *androgenetic alopecia*

ball (bawl) a more or less spherical mass 球。另见 *globus* 和 *sphere*；**fungus b.**, a tumorlike granulomatous mass formed by colonization of a fungus, usually *Aspergillus*, in a body cavity 真菌球

bal·lis·mus (bə-liz′məs) violent movements of the limbs, as in chorea, sometimes affecting only one side of the body (hemiballismus) 舞蹈病

balm (bahm) a soothing or healing medicine 镇痛药膏；**lemon b., sweet b.**, a preparation of the fresh or dried herb of *Melissa officinalis*, or the volatile oil; used for nervousness and insomnia, as a homeopathic preparation for menstrual irregularities, and in folk medicine 香蜂叶

bal·sal·a·zide (bal-sal′ə-zīd) a prodrug of the antiinflammatory mesalamine, to which it is converted in the colon; administered orally as the sodium salt in the treatment of ulcerative colitis 巴柳氮

bal·sam (bawl′səm) a semifluid, resinous, and fragrant liquid of vegetable origin, usually trees; often composed chiefly of resins, volatile oils, and various esters 香脂；**balsam′ic** *adj.* 香膏质的；**Canada b.**, an oleoresin from the balsam fir, used as a microscopic mounting medium 加拿大香脂；**b. of Peru, peruvian b.**, a thick brown liquid from the tree *Myroxylon pereirae*, used as a local protectant and rubefacient 秘鲁香脂；**tolu b.**, a balsam obtained from the tree *Myroxylon balsamum*, used as an expectorant and pharmaceutical aid 吐鲁香胶；

band (band) 1. a strip that holds together or binds separate objects or parts; for anatomical structures 带子，见 *frenulum, taenia, trabecula*, and *vinculum*；2. an object or appliance that confines or restricts while allowing a limited range of movement 箍；3. an elongated area with parallel or roughly parallel borders that is distinct from the surrounding surface, as by color or texture 条纹。另见 *layer* 和 *stria*；4. chromosome band; a segment of a chromosome stained brighter or darker than the adjacent bands; used in identifying the chromosomes and in examining chromosomal abnormalities. Called *Q b's, G b's, C b's, T b's*, etc., according to the staining method used 染色体带；5. in dentistry, a thin metal hoop that horizontally encircles the crown or root of a natural tooth 牙套；**A b.**, the dark-staining zone of a sarcomere, whose center is traversed by the H band 暗带；**b. of Broca**, a band of nerve fibers that forms the caudal zone of the anterior perforated substance where it adjoins the optic tract 布罗卡带；**H b.**, a pale zone sometimes seen traversing the center of the A band of a striated myofibril H带；**I b.**, the band within a striated myofibril, seen as a light region under the light microscope and as a dark region under polarized light 明带；**iliotibial b.**, 见 *tract* 下词条；**M b.**, the narrow dark band in the center of the H band M带；**matrix b.**, a thin piece of metal or plastic fitted around a tooth to serve as a mold or form for impression or restorative materials 牙套模片；**oligoclonal b's**, discrete bands of immunoglobulins with decreased electrophoretic mobility whose presence in the cerebrospinal fluid when absent from the serum may be indicative of multiple sclerosis or other disease of the central nervous system 寡克隆

区 带；Z b., a thin membrane in a myofibril, seen on longitudinal section as a dark line in the center of the I band; the distance between Z bands delimits the sarcomeres of striated muscle Z 线

ban·dage (ban′dəj) 1. a strip or roll of gauze or other material for wrapping or binding a body part 绷 带；2. to cover by wrapping with such material 包 扎；**Ace b.,** trademark for a bandage of woven elastic material Ace 牌弹性绷带；**Barton b.,** a double figure-of-8 bandage for fracture of the lower jaw 巴 尔 通 氏 绷 带；**demigauntlet b.,** one that covers the hand but leaves the fingers exposed 半 手套式绷带；**Desault b.,** one binding the elbow to the side, with a pad in the axilla, for fractured clavicle 德佐氏绷带；**Esmarch b.,** a rubber bandage applied upward around a limb from distal to proximal in order to expel blood from it; the limb is often elevated as the elastic pressure is applied 驱 血绷带；**gauntlet b.,** one that covers the hand and fingers like a glove 手套式绷带；**Gibney b.,** strips of adhesive 1.2 cm wide, overlapped along the sides and back of the foot and leg to hold the foot in the slight varus position and leave the dorsal region of the foot and anterior aspect of the leg exposed 吉 布 尼 氏 绷 带；**plaster b.,** one stiffened with a paste of plaster of Paris 石膏绷带；**pressure b.,** one for applying pressure 加压包扎；**roller b.,** a tightly rolled, circular bandage of varying width and materials, often commercially prepared 绷 带 卷；**Scultetus b.,** a many-tailed bandage applied with the tails overlapping each other and held in position by safety pins 多 头 绷 带；**spica b.,** a figure-of-8 bandage with turns that cross one another regularly like the letter V, usually applied to anatomical areas whose dimensions vary, such as the pelvis and thigh 人字形绷带；**Velpeau b.,** one used in immobilization of certain fractures involving the upper end of the humerus and glenohumeral joint, binding the arm and shoulder to the chest 韦尔波绷带

band·ing (band′ing) 1. the act of encircling and binding with a thin strip of material 捆绑；2. any of several techniques of staining chromosomes so that a characteristic pattern of transverse dark and light bands becomes visible, permitting identification of individual chromosome pairs 染色体分带；又称 *chromosome b.*

ban·dy (band′e) bowed or bent in an outward curve 向外弯曲

bank (bangk) a stored supply of human material or tissues for future use by other individuals, such as a *blood b., bone b., eye b., human-milk b.,* or *skin b.* 库存

bar (bahr) 1. a structure having greater length than width, and often some degree of rigidity 棒；2. a heavy wire or wrought or cast metal segment, longer than its width, used to connect parts of a removable partial denture 牙 基；**median b.,** a fibrotic formation across the neck of the prostate gland, producing obstruction of the urethra 前列腺正中嵴；**Mercier b.,** interureteric ridge 输尿管间嵴；**terminal b's,** zones of epithelial cell contact, once thought to represent an accumulation of dense cementing substance, but with the electron microscope shown to be a junctional complex 上皮细胞接触区

bar·ag·no·sis (bar″ag-no′sis) lack or loss of the faculty of barognosis, the conscious perception of weight 重力、压力感受缺失

bar·bi·tur·ate (bahr-bich′ər-ət) any of a class of compounds derived from barbituric acid; used for their hypnotic and sedative effects 巴比妥酸盐

bar·bi·tur·ic ac·id (bahr-bĭ-tūr′ik) the parent substance of the barbiturates, not itself a central nervous system depressant 巴比妥酸

bar·bo·tage (bahr″bo-tahzh′) [Fr.] repeated alternate injection and withdrawal of fluid with a syringe, as in gastric lavage or administration of an anesthetic agent into the subarachnoid space by alternate injection of part of the anesthetic and withdrawal of cerebrospinal fluid into the syringe 往返吸注麻醉法

bar·es·the·si·om·e·ter (bar″əs-the″ze-om′ə-tər) instrument for estimating sense of weight or pressure 压力计

bar·i·at·rics (bar″e-at′riks) the study of obesity and its causes, prevention, and treatment 肥胖病学

bar·ium (Ba) (bar′e-əm) a soft, silvery, alkaline earth metallic element; at. no. 56, at. wt. 137.327. Its acid-soluble salts are poisonous, causing gastrointestinal symptoms followed by severe, sometimes fatal hypokalemia with paralysis 钡；**b. sulfate,** a water-insoluble salt, $BaSO_4$, used as an opaque contrast medium in radiography of the digestive tract 硫酸钡

bark (bahrk) the rind or outer cortical cover of the woody parts of a plant, tree, or shrub 树皮；**cramp b.,** the dried bark of *Viburnum opulus,* the high bush or cranberry tree; it has been used as an antispasmodic, uterine sedative, and antiscorbutic 黄杨的干燥树皮，一种高大的灌木或蔓越莓树；它被用作解痉药、子宫镇静剂和抗坏血病药；**elm b., slippery elm b.,** the dried inner bark of the slippery elm, *Ulmus rubra,* which is mucilaginous and demulcent 赤榆皮；**white willow b.,** a preparation of the bark of various *Salix* species collectively known as white willow, containing salicin, a precursor of salicylic acid; used as an antiinflammatory and antipyretic 白

柳树皮；**yohimbe b.**, a preparation of the bark of *Pausinystalia yohimbe*, used for the same indications as yohimbine hydrochloride; it has also been used traditionally as an aphrodisiac and for skin diseases and obesity 育亨宾树皮

bar·o·don·tal·gia (bar″o-don-tal′jə) pain in an otherwise asymptomatic tooth caused by a change in barometric pressure 气压性牙痛。又称 *aerodontalgia*

bar·og·no·sis (bar″og-no′sis) conscious perception of weight 重力觉

baro·phil·ic (bar″o-fil′ik) growing best under high atmospheric pressure; said of bacteria 嗜压的

baro·re·cep·tor (bar″o-re-sep′tər) a type of interoceptor that is stimulated by pressure changes, such as those in blood vessel walls 压力感受器。又称 *baroceptor*

baro·re·flex (bar′o-re″fleks) baroreceptor reflex 感压反射

baro·si·nus·itis (bar″o-si″nəs-i′tis) a symptom complex due to differences in environmental atmospheric pressure and the air pressure in the paranasal sinuses 气压性鼻窦炎

baro·tax·is (bar″o-tak′sis) stimulation of living matter by change of atmospheric pressure 趋压性

bar·oti·tis (bar″o-ti′tis) a morbid condition of the ear due to exposure to differing atmospheric pressures 气压损伤性中耳炎；**b. me′dia**, a symptom complex due to the difference between atmospheric pressure of the environment and air pressure in the middle ear 航空性中耳炎

baro·trau·ma (bar″o-traw′mə) injury due to pressure, as to structures of the ear, in highaltitude flyers, owing to differences between atmospheric and intratympanic pressures 气压损伤。见 *barosinusitis* 和 *barotitis*；**bar·ri·er** (bar′e-ər) an obstruction 障碍；**alveolarcapillary b., alveolocapillary b.**, 见 *membrane* 下 词 条；**blood-air b.**, alveolocapillary membrane 血气屏障；**blood-aqueous b.**, the physiologic mechanism that prevents exchange of materials between the chambers of the eye and the blood 血 - 房水屏障；**blood-brain b. (BBB)**, **blood-cerebral b.**, the selective barrier separating the blood from the parenchyma of the central nervous system 血脑屏障；**blood-gas b.**, alveolocapillary membrane 血气屏障；**blood-testis b.**, a barrier separating the blood from the convoluted seminiferous tubules, consisting of special junctional complexes between adjacent Sertoli cells near the base of the seminiferous epithelium 血 - 睾屏障；**placental b.**, term sometimes used for the placental membrane, because it prevents the passage of some materials between the maternal and fetal blood 胎盘

屏障

Bar·to·nel·la (bahr″tə-nel′ə) a genus of the family Bartonellaceae, including *B. bacillifor′mis*, the etiologic agent of Carrión disease, and *B. hen′selae*, the agent of cat-scratch disease 巴尔通体属

Bar·to·nel·la·ceae (bahr″tə-nel-a′se-e) a family of the order Rhizobiales, transmitted as arthropods and occurring as pathogenic parasites in the erythrocytes of humans and other animals. 巴尔通体科

bar·to·nel·lo·sis (bahr-tə-nel-o′sis) 1. any infection with a species of *Bartonella* 巴尔通体感染；2. an infectious disease in South America due to *Bartonella bacilliformis*, transmitted by a sandfly; the first stage, Oroya fever, is often fatal; the second stage is a skin eruption, verruga peruana 巴尔通体病

ba·sad (ba′sad) toward a base or basal aspect 向基底的

ba·sal (ba′səl) ba′salis [L.] pertaining to or situated near a base 基底的

bas·cule (bas′kūl) [Fr.] a device working on the principle of the seesaw, so that when one end is raised the other is lowered 开 启 桥，**cecal b.**, a form of cecal volvulus in which the cecum becomes folded across bands or adhesions that run across the ascending colon 开启式盲肠扭转

base (bās) 1. the lowest part or foundation of anything 基础，另见 *basis*；2. the main ingredient of a compound 化合物基本成分；3. in chemistry, a substance that combines with acids to form salts; a substance that dissociates to give hydroxide ions in aqueous solutions; a substance whose molecule or ion can combine with a proton (hydrogen ion); a substance capable of donating a pair of electrons (to an acid) for the formation of a coordinate covalent bond 碱；4. a unit of a removable dental prosthesis 假牙的一种；5. in genetics, a nucleotide, particularly one in a nucleic acid sequence 碱 基；**buffer b.**, the sum of all the buffer anions in the blood, used as an index of the degree of metabolic disturbance in the acid-base balance 缓 冲 碱；**denture b.**, the material in which the teeth of a denture are set and which rests on the supporting tissues when the denture is in place in the mouth 义 齿 基 托；**nitrogenous b.**, an aromatic, nitrogen-containing molecule that serves as a proton acceptor, e.g., purine or pyrimidine 含氮碱基；**ointment b.**, a vehicle for the medicinal substances carried in an ointment 软膏基质；**purine b's**, a group of chemical compounds of which purine is the base, including adenine, guanine, hypoxanthine, theobromine, uric acid, and xanthine 嘌 呤 碱 基；**pyrimidine b's**, a group of chemical compounds of which pyrimidine is the base, including uracil, thymine, and cytosine 嘧啶碱基；**record b.**, baseplate 记录基底；**b. of stapes**, footplate 镫骨足板；**temporary b., trial b.**, baseplate 义齿托

base·line (bās′līn) a value representing a normal background level or an initial level of a measurable quantity and used for comparison with values representing the response to an environmental stimulus or intervention 基线

base·plate (bās′plāt) a sheet of plastic material used in making trial plates for artificial dentures 义齿托

ba·si·al (ba′se-əl) pertaining to the basion 颅底点的

ba·sic (ba′sik) 1. pertaining to or having properties of a base 碱性的；2. capable of neutralizing acids 碱化

ba·sic·i·ty (bə-sis′ĭ-te) 1. the quality of being a base, or basic 基性度；2. the combining power of an acid 碱度

ba·sid·i·ob·o·lo·my·co·sis (bə-sid″e-ob″ə-lomi-ko′sis) chronic localized fungal infection by *Basidiobolus ranarum*, with formation of gradually enlarging granulomas in the subcutaneous tissues of the upper limbs, chest, and trunk; it occurs in tropical areas, mainly affecting children and adolescents, particularly males, who are otherwise healthy 蛙粪霉病

Ba·sid·i·ob·o·lus (bə-sid″e-ob′ə-ləs) a mainly saprobic genus of fungi of the family Basidiobolaceae (phylum Zygomycota), including *B. rana′rum*, which causes basidiobolomycosis 蛙粪霉属

ba·sid·io·my·cete (bə-sid″e-o-mi′sēt) an individual fungus of the Basidiomycota 担子菌亚门；**basidiomyce′tous** *adj.* 担子菌的

Ba·sid·i·o·my·co·ta (bə-sid″e-o-mi-ko′tə) the club fungi; a phylum of fungi reproducing sexually via basidiospores borne on clubshaped basidia; the group includes mushrooms, puffballs, stinkhorns, bracket fungi, jelly fungi, boletes, chanterelles, earth stars, smuts, bunts, and rusts 担子菌门

ba·sid·i·um (bə-sid′e-əm) pl. *basi′dia* [L.] the clublike organ of the basidiomycetes that bears the basidiospores 担子

ba·si·hy·oid (ba″sī-hi′oid) the body of the hyoid bone；in certain animals other than humans, either of two lateral bones that are its homologues 舌骨体；某些动物中成对骨中的任意一个

bas·i·lad (bas′ĭ-lad) toward the base 向底的

bas·i·lar (bas′ĭ-lər) ba′silaris [L.] pertaining to a base or basal part 基底的

ba·si·lem·ma (ba″sī-lem′ə) basement membrane 基底膜

bas·i·lix·i·mab (bas″ĭ-liks′ĭ-mab) a chimeric monoclonal antibody that is an interleukin-2 receptor antagonist; used in the prophylaxis of acute organ rejection after renal transplantation 巴利昔单抗

ba·si·on (ba′se-on) the midpoint of the anterior border of the foramen magnum 颅底点

ba·sis (ba′sis) pl. *ba′ses* [L.] the lower, basic, or fundamental part of an object, organ, or substance 基础；**b. pedun′culi ce′rebri**, the part of the midbrain consisting of the crus cerebri and the substantia nigra; sometimes excluding the latter 大脑脚底

ba·si·sphe·noid (ba″sī-sfe′noid) 1. postsphenoid 后蝶骨；2. an embryonic bone that becomes the back part of the body of the sphenoid bone 基蝶骨

bas·ket (bas′kət) 1. a container made of material woven together, or something resembling it 篮子；2. basket cell 篮状细胞；**stone b.**, a tiny apparatus of several wires that can be advanced through an endoscope into a body cavity or tube, manipulated to trap a calculus or other object, and withdrawn 结石网篮

ba·so·phil (ba′so-fil) 1. any structure, cell, or histologic element staining readily with basic dyes 嗜碱性的；2. a granular leukocyte with an irregularly shaped, relatively pale-staining nucleus that is partially constricted into two lobes, and with cytoplasm containing coarse bluish-black granules of variable size 嗜碱粒细胞；3. one of the hormoneproducing basophilic cells of the anterior lobe of the pituitary; types include *gonadotrophs* and *thyrotrophs* 腺垂体β细胞；4. basophilic 嗜碱性

ba·so·phil·ia (ba″so-fil′e-ə) 1. abnormal increase of basophils in the blood 嗜碱细胞增多症；2. reaction of immature erythrocytes to basic dyes, becoming blue to gray in color; stippling is seen in lead poisoning 点彩红细胞碱染

ba·so·phil·ic (ba-so-fil′ik) 1. pertaining to basophils 嗜碱性粒细胞；2. staining readily with basic dyes 嗜碱

ba·soph·i·lism (ba-sof′ĭ-liz-əm) abnormal increase of basophilic cells 嗜碱性细胞异常增多

ba·so·phil·o·pe·nia (ba″so-fil″o-pe′ne-ə) abnormal reduction in the number of basophils in the blood 嗜碱性粒细胞减少

bath (bath) 1. a medium, e.g., water, vapor, sand, or mud, with which the body is washed or in which the body is wholly or partially immersed for therapeutic or cleansing purposes; application of such a medium to the body 洗浴；2. the equipment or apparatus in which a body or object may be immersed 浴缸；**colloid b.**, one containing gelatin, starch, bran, or similar substances 胶体浴；**contrast b.**, alternate immersion of a body part in hot and cold water 冷热交替浴法；**emollient b.**, one in an emollient liquid, e.g., a decoction of bran 润肤浴；**hip b.**, sitz b 坐浴；**sitz b.**, immersion of only the hips and buttocks 坐浴；**sponge b.**, one in which the body is not immersed but is rubbed with a wet cloth or sponge 擦浴；**whirlpool b.**, one in which the water is kept in constant motion by mechanical means 涡流浴

batho·rho·dop·sin (bath″o-ro-dop′sin) a transient intermediate produced upon irradiation of rhodopsin in the visual cycle 红光视紫红质

bath·ro·ceph·a·ly (bath″ro-sef′ə-le) a developmental anomaly marked by a steplike posterior projection of the skull, caused by excessive growth of the lambdoid suture 梯形头

bathyp·nea (bath″ip-ne′ə) deep breathing 深呼吸

bat·te·ry (bat′ər-e) 1. a set or series of cells that yield an electric current 电池；2. any set, series, or grouping of similar things, as a battery of tests 系列

Bay·lis·as·car·is (ba″lis-as′kə-ris) a genus of nematodes of the family Ascaridae; human infection via contaminated animal feces results in larval migration through tissues, causing mechanical trauma; migration through brain tissue can cause lethal eosinophilic meningitis 贝蛔属

BBBB bilateral bundle branch block 双侧束支传导阻滞

BBT basal body temperature 基础体温

BCDF B cell differentiation factors B 细胞分化因子

BCG bacille Calmette-Guérin 卡介苗

BCNU carmustine 卡莫司汀。Spelled also BiCNU

B-E BE below-elbow 腋下；见 *amputation* 下词条

Be beryllium 铍

bead (bēd) a small spherical structure or mass 珠子；**rachitic b's**, a series of prominences at the points where the ribs join their cartilages; seen in certain cases of rickets 佝偻病串珠

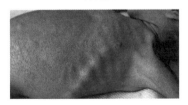

▲ 佝偻病串珠（**rachitic beads**）

bead·ed (bēd′əd) having the appearance of beads or a string of beads 珠状的

bear·ber·ry (ber′ber-e) 1. uva ursi 熊果；2. *Rhamnus purshiana* 鼠李

beat (bēt) a throb or pulsation, as of the heart or of an artery 搏动；**apex b.**, the beat felt over the apex of the heart, normally in or near the fifth left intercostal space 心尖搏动；**atrioventricular (AV) junctional escape b.**, a depolarization initiated in the atrioventricular junction when one or more impulses from the sinus node are ineffective or nonexistent 房室交界性逸搏；**atrioventricular (AV) junctional premature b.**, 见 *complex* 下词条；**capture b's**, in atrioventricular dissociation, occasional ventricular responses to a sinus impulse that reaches the atrioventricular node in a nonrefractory phase 心室夺获；**ectopic b.**, a heart beat originating at some point other than the sinus node 异位搏动；**escape b., escaped b.**, heart beats that follow an abnormally long pause 逸搏；**forced b.**, an extrasystole produced by artificial stimulation of the heart 刺激性期外收缩；**fusion b.**, in electrocardiography, the complex resulting when an ectopic ventricular beat coincides with normal conduction to the ventricle 融合波；**heart b.**, heartbeat 心跳；**interpolated b.**, a contraction occurring exactly between two normal beats without altering the sinus rhythm 间位性搏动；**junctional escape b.**, atrioventricular junctional escape b. 交界性逸搏；**junctional premature b.**, atrioventricular junctional premature complex 交界性早搏；**postectopic b.**, the normal beat following an ectopic beat 异搏后搏动；**premature b.**, extrasystole 早搏；**pseudofusion b.**, an ineffective pacing stimulus delivered during the absolute refractory period following a spontaneous discharge but before sufficient charge accumulates to prevent pacemaker discharge 假性融合波；**reciprocal b.**, a cardiac impulse that in one cycle causes ventricular contraction, travels backward toward the atria, then reexcites the ventricles 反复搏动；**reentrant b.**, any of the characteristic beats of a reentrant circuit 折返搏动；**retrograde b.**, a beat resulting from impulse conduction that is backward relative to the normal atrioventricular direction 逆行搏动；**ventricular escape b.**, an ectopic beat of ventricular origin occurring in the absence of supraventricular impulse generation or conduction 室性逸搏；**ventricular premature b. (VPB)**, 见 *complex* 下词条

be·cap·ler·min (bə-kap′lər-min) a recombinant platelet-derived growth factor used in the treatment of chronic severe dermal ulcers of the lower limbs in diabetes mellitus 贝卡普明

bec·lo·meth·a·sone (bek″lo-meth′ə-sōn) a glucocorticoid used in the dipropionate form in the treatment of bronchial asthma, seasonal and nonseasonal allergic rhinitis or other allergic or inflammatory nasal conditions, and some dermatoses, and to prevent

recurrence of nasal polyps 倍氯米松

bec·que·rel (Bq) (bek″ə-rel′) a unit of radioactivity, defined as the quantity of a radionuclide that undergoes one decay per second (s^{-1}). One curie equals 3.7×10^{10} becquerels 贝可

bed (bed) 1. a supporting structure or tissue 支撑结构; 2. a couch or support for the body during sleep 床; **capillary b.**, the capillaries, collectively, and their volume capacity 毛细血管床; 见图 22; **nail b.**, matrix unguis; the area of modified epithelium beneath the nail, over which the nail plate slides forward as it grows 甲床; **vascular b.**, the sum of the blood vessels supplying an organ or region 血管床

bed·aq·ui·line (bĕd-ak′wi-leen) antibiotic inhibitor of ATP synthase in mycobacteria, used in combination therapy to treat pulmonary multidrug-resistant tuberculosis 贝达喹啉

bed·bug (bed′bug) a bug of the genus *Cimex* 臭虫

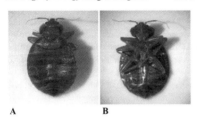

▲ 温带地区常见的臭虫 (bedbug)，温带臭虫。A. 背视图；B. 腹视图

bed·sore (bed′sor″) decubitus ulcer 褥疮

bees·wax (bēz′waks) wax derived from the honeycomb of the bee *Apis mellifera* 蜂蜡; 见 *wax* 下 *yellow wax* (unbleached b.) 和 *white wax* (bleached b.)

be·hav·ior (be-hāv′yər) deportment or conduct; any or all of a person's total activity, especially that which is externally observable 行 为; **behav′ioral** *adj.* 行为的

be·hav·ior·ism (be-hāv′yər-iz-əm) the psychologic theory based upon objectively observable, tangible, and measurable data, rather than subjective phenomena, such as ideas and emotions 行为主义

bel (B) (bel) a unit used to express the ratio of two powers, usually electric or acoustic powers; an increase of 1 bel in intensity approximately doubles the loudness of most sounds 贝 尔。另 见 *decibel*

bel·at·a·cept (bel-at′a-sept) immunosuppressant that blocks T-cell stimulation to prevent organ rejection after transplantation; administered by intravenous injection 贝拉西普

bel·la·don·na (bel′ə-don′ə) the deadly nightshade, *Atropa belladonna*, a perennial plant containing various anticholinergic alkaloids, including atropine, hyoscyamine, and scopolamine, which are used medicinally; however, the plant or its alkaloids can cause poisoning 颠茄

bel·ly (bel′e) 1. abdomen 腹部; 2. venter (1) 下腹

bel·o·noid (bel′o-noid) needle-shaped 针 形 的; styloid 茎突的

Bel·viq (bel-vēk) trademark for a preparation of lorcaserin 盐酸氯卡色林

ben·a·ze·pril (ben-a′zə-pril) an angiotensinconverting enzyme inhibitor used as the hydrochloride salt in the treatment of hypertension 贝那普利

bend (bend) a flexure or curve 弯 曲; a flexed or curved part 弯曲的部分; **varolian b.**, the third cerebral flexure in the developing fetus 发育中胎儿的第三脑曲

ben·dro·flu·me·thi·a·zide (ben″dro-floo″mə-thi′ə-zīd) a thiazide diuretic used to treat hypertension and edema 苄氟噻嗪

bends (bendz) pain in the limbs and abdomen due to rapid reduction of air pressure 减压病; 见 *sickness* 下 *decompression sickness*

be·nign (bə-nīn′) not malignant 良 性; not recurrent 不复发的; favorable for recovery 预后好的

ben·ox·i·nate (ben-ok′sĭ-nāt) a topical anesthetic for the eye, used as the hydrochloride salt 丁氧普鲁卡因

ben·ser·a·zide (ben-ser′ə-zīd) an inhibitor of decarboxylation of levodopa in extracerebral tissues, used in combination with levodopa as an antiparkinsonian agent 苄丝肼

ben·to·qua·tam (ben′to-kwah″tam) a topical skin protectant used to prevent or reduce allergic contact dermatitis resulting from contact with urushiol (poison ivy, poison oak, poison sumac) 本托奎坦

ben·zal·de·hyde (ben-zal′də-hīd) an aldehyde derivative of benzene, occurring in the kernels of bitter almonds or produced synthetically; used as a pharmaceutical flavoring agent 苯甲醛

ben·zal·ko·ni·um chlo·ride (ben″zal-ko′ne-əm) a quaternary ammonium compound used as a surface disinfectant and detergent, topical antiseptic, and antimicrobial preservative 苯扎氯铵

ben·zene (ben′zēn) a liquid hydrocarbon, C_6H_6, from coal tar; used as a solvent. It is toxic by transdermal absorption, ingestion, or inhalation; chronic exposure may cause bone marrow depression and aplasia and leukemia 苯; **b. hexachloride** (BHC), a chlorinated hydrocarbon, $C_6H_6Cl_6$, having numerous isomers; the gamma isomer is *lindane* 六氯化苯

ben·ze·tho·ni·um chlo·ride (ben″zə-tho′ne-əm)

a quaternary ammonium compound used as a local antiseptic, pharmaceutical preservative, and detergent and disinfectant 氯化苄乙氧铵

ben·zi·dine (ben′zĭ-dēn) a carcinogen and toxin once widely used as a test for occult blood 联苯胺

ben·zo·ate (ben′zo-āt) a salt of benzoic acid 苯甲酸盐

ben·zo·caine (ben′zo-kān) a local anesthetic applied topically to the skin and mucous membranes; also used to suppress the gag reflex in various procedures 苯佐卡因

ben·zo·di·az·e·pine (ben″zo-di-az′ə-pēn) any of a group of compounds having a common molecular structure and similar pharmacological activities, including antianxiety, muscle relaxing, and sedative and hypnotic effects 苯二氮䓬类

ben·zo·ic ac·id (ben-zo′ik) a fungistatic compound used as a pharmaceutical and food preservative and, with salicylic acid, as a topical antifungal agent 苯甲酸

ben·zo·na·tate (ben-zo′nə-tāt) an antitussive that reduces the cough reflex by anesthetizing the stretch receptors in the respiratory passages, lungs, and pleura 苯甲酸钠

ben·zo·pur·pu·rine (ben′zo-pur′pu-rin) any one of a series of azo dyes of a scarlet color 苯并红紫

ben·zo·qui·none (ben″zo-kwin′ōn) 1. a substituted benzene ring containing two carbonyl groups, usually in the *para* (1,4) position; pbenzoquinone is used in manufacturing and in fungicides and is toxic by inhalation and an irritant to skin and mucous membranes 苯醌; 2. any of a subclass of quinones derived from or containing this structure 醌的一个亚类

ben·zo·thi·a·di·a·zine (ben″zo-thi″ə-di′ə-zēn) thiazide 苯并噻二嗪

ben·zo·yl (ben′zo-əl) the acyl radical formed from benzoic acid, C_6H_5CO— 苯甲酰; **b. peroxide,** a topical keratolytic and antibacterial used in the treatment of acne vulgaris 过氧化苯甲酰

ben·zo·yl·ec·go·nine (ben″zo-əl-ek′go-nēn) the major metabolite of cocaine; detectable in the blood by laboratory testing 苯甲酰芽子碱

benz·phet·amine (benz-fet′ə-mēn) a sympathomimetic amine used as an anorectic in the form of the hydrochloride salt 甲苯异丙胺

benz·tro·pine (benz′tro-pēn) an antidyskinetic used as the mesylate salt in the treatment of parkinsonism and for the control of druginduced extrapyramidal reactions 苯托品

ben·zyl (ben′zəl) the hydrocarbon radical, C_7H_7 苄基; **b. benzoate,** one of the active substances in peruvian and tolu balsams, and produced synthetically;

applied topically as a scabicide 苯甲酸苄酯

ben·zyl·pen·i·cil·lin (ben″zəl-pen″ĭ-sil′in) penicillin G 青霉素 G

ben·zyl·pen·i·cil·lo·yl poly·ly·sine (ben″zəl-pen″ĭ-sil′o-əl) a skin test antigen composed of a benzylpenicilloyl moiety and a polylysine carrier, used in assessing hypersensitivity to penicillin by scratch test or intradermal test 青霉噻唑酰多聚赖氨酸

bep·ri·dil (bep′rĭ-dil) a calcium channel blocking agent used as the hydrochloride salt in the treatment of chronic angina pectoris 苄普地尔

ber·ac·tant (bər-ak′tənt) a modified bovine lung extract that mimics the action of pulmonary surfactant, used in the prevention and treatment of neonatal respiratory distress syndrome 贝雷克坦

ber·ber·ine (bur′bər-ēn) an alkaloid from species of *Berberis* and related plants, and from *Hydrastis canadensis*; it has antimicrobial activity and has been used in treatment of various infections and in ulcer dressings 黄连素

beri·beri (ber″e-ber′e) a disease due to thiamine (vitamin B1) deficiency, marked by polyneuritis, cardiac pathology, and edema; the epidemic form occurs primarily in areas in which white (polished) rice is the staple food 脚气病

ber·ry (ber′e) a small fruit with a succulent pericarp 浆果; **bear b.,** bearberry 熊果

be·ryl·li·o·sis (bə-ril″e-o′sis) a morbid condition caused by exposure to fumes or fine dust of beryllium salts, with formation of granulomas, usually in the lungs and less often the skin, superficial fascia, lymph nodes, liver, or other organs 铍中毒

be·ryl·li·um (Be) (bə-ril′e-əm) a rare, steel gray, brittle, alkaline earth metallic element; at. no. 4, at. wt. 9.012; inhalation of its fumes causes berylliosis 铍

bes·ti·al·i·ty (bes-te-al′ĭ-te) 兽奸, 见 zoophilia (2)

bes·y·late (bes′ə-lāt) USAN contraction for benzenesulfonate 苯磺酸盐

be·ta (ba′tə) β, the second letter of the Greek alphabet 希腊字母表的第二个字母; 另见 β-

be·ta·car·o·tene (ba″tə-kar′ə-tēn) 见 *carotene* 下词条

be·ta·his·tine (ba″tə-his′tēn) a histamine analogue used as the hydrochloride salt to reduce the frequency of attacks of vertigo in Meniere disease 倍他司汀

be·ta·ine (be′tə-ēn) the carboxylic acid derived by oxidation of choline; it acts as a transmethylating metabolic intermediate and is used in the treatment of homocystinuria. The hydrochloride salt is used as a gastric acidifier 甜菜碱

be·ta·meth·a·sone (ba″tə-meth′ə-sōn) a synthetic

glucocorticoid, the most active of the antiinflammatory steroids; used topically as the benzoate, dipropionate, or valerate salts as an antiinflammatory, topically or rectally as the sodium phosphate salt as an antiinflammatory, and systemically as the base or the combination of sodium phosphate and acetate salts as an antiinflammatory, as a replacement for adrenal insufficiency, and as an immunosuppressant 倍他米松

Be·ta·pap·il·lo·ma·vi·rus (ba″tə-pap″ĭ-lo′mə-vi″rəs) a genus of viruses of the family Papillomaviridae that contains several of the human papillomaviruses β 乳头状瘤病毒属

Be·ta·pro·teo·bac·te·ria (ba″tə-pro″te-obak-tēr′e-ə) a class of bacteria of the Proteobacteria β 变形菌门

be·tax·o·lol (ba-tak′sə-lol) a cardioselective β-adrenergic blocking agent, used in the form of the hydrochloride salt as an antihypertensive and in the treatment of glaucoma and ocular hypertension 倍他洛尔

be·than·e·chol (bə-than′ə-kol) a cholinergic agonist, used as the chloride salt to stimulate smooth muscle contraction of the urinary bladder in cases of postoperative, postpartum, or neurogenic atony and retention 氯贝胆碱

bev·a·ciz·u·mab (bev″ə-siz′u-mab) a monoclonal antibody that interferes with tumor blood supply by inhibiting vascular endothelial growth factor, used for the treatment of metastatic colorectal cancer 贝伐单抗

bex·ar·o·tene (bek-sar′ə-tēn) a retinoid used as an antineoplastic in the treatment of cutaneous T-cell lymphoma and the cutaneous lesions of T-cell lymphomas and Kaposi sarcoma 蓓萨罗丁

be·zoar (be′zor) a concretion of foreign material found in the gastrointestinal or urinary tract 牛黄

BFRB body-focused repetitive behavior 以身体为中心的重复性行为

BH4, BH4 tetrahydrobiopterin 四氢生物蝶呤

BHA butylated hydroxyanisole, an antioxidant used in foods, cosmetics, and pharmaceuticals that contain fats or oils 丁基羟基茴香醚

BHC benzene hexachloride 六氯化苯

BHPr Bureau of Health Professions 卫生专业处

BHT butylated hydroxytoluene, an antioxidant used in foods, cosmetics, pharmaceuticals, and petroleum products 丁基羟基甲苯

Bi bismuth 铋

bi·acro·mi·al (bi-ə-kro′me-əl) between the two acromia 肩峰间的

bi·au·ric·u·lar (bi″aw-rik′u-lər) pertaining to the auricles of both ears 双耳的

bi·ax·i·al (bi-ak′se-əl) having, pertaining to, or occurring in two axes 双轴的

bib·lio·ther·a·py (bib″le-o-ther′ə-pe) the reading of selected books as part of the treatment of mental disorders or for mental health 阅读疗法

bi·ca·lu·ta·mide (bi″kə-loo′tə-mīd) an antiandrogen used in the treatment of prostatic carcinoma 比卡鲁胺

bi·cam·er·al (bi-kam′ər-əl) having two chambers or cavities 双腔的

bi·car·bo·nate (bi-kahr′bə-nāt) any salt containing the HCO_3^- anion 碳酸氢盐; **blood b., plasma b.,** the bicarbonate of the blood plasma, an index of alkali reserve 血碳酸氢盐; **b. of soda,** sodium bicarbonate 碳酸氢钠; **standard b.,** the plasma bicarbonate concentration in blood equilibrated with a specific gas mixture under specific conditions 标准碳酸氢盐

bi·ceps (bi′seps) a muscle having two heads 肱二头肌

bi·cip·i·tal (bi-sip′ĭ-təl) having two heads 双头的; pertaining to a biceps muscle 肱二头肌的

bi·col·lis (bi-kol′is) having a double cervix 双子宫颈

bi·con·cave (bi″kon-kāv′) having two concave surfaces 双凹的

bi·con·vex (bi″kon-veks′) having two convex surfaces 双凸形的

bi·cor·nate (bi-kor′nāt) bicornuate 两角的

bi·cor·nu·ate (bi-kor′nu-āt) having two horns or cornua 双角的

bi·cus·pid (bi-kus′pid) 1. having two cusps 双尖的; 2. pertaining to a mitral (bicuspid) valve 二尖瓣; 3. (pl.) premolar teeth 前磨牙

b.i.d. [L.] bis in die (twice a day) 每日两次

bi·der·mo·ma (bi″dər-mo′mə) didermoma 双胚叶瘤

bi·fas·cic·u·lar (bi″fə-sik′u-lər) pertaining to two bundles, or fasciculi 双束支的

bi·fid (bi′fid) cleft into two parts or branches 二裂的

Bi·fi·do·bac·te·ri·a·ceae (bi″fid-o-bak-tēr″ea′se-e) a family of bacteria of the order Bifidobacteriales 双歧杆菌科

Bi·fi·do·bac·te·ri·a·les (bi″fid-o-bak-tēr″ea′lēz) an order of bacteria of the subclass Actinobacteridae 双歧杆菌目

Bi·fid·o·bac·te·ri·um (bi″fid-o-bak-tēr′e-əm) a genus of gram-positive, anaerobic bacteria of the family Bifidobacteriaceae, commonly occurring in the feces 双歧杆菌属

bi·fo·cal (bi-fo′-) (bi′fo-kəl) 1. having two foci 双焦点的; 2. containing one part for near vision and another part for distant vision, as in a bifocal lens 双

焦透镜

bi·fo·cals (bi'fo-kəlz) bifocal glasses 双焦眼镜

bi·fo·rate (bi-for'āt) having two perforations or foramina 双孔的

bi·fur·ca·tion (bi″fər-ka'shən) 1. a division into two branches 分叉；2. the point at which division into two branches occurs 分支点

bi·gem·i·ny (bi-jem'ĭ-ne) 1. occurring in pairs 成对发生的；2. the occurrence of two beats of the pulse in rapid succession 二联律；**bigem'inal** *adj.* 二重的；**atrial b.**, an arrhythmia consisting of the repetitive sequence of one atrial premature complex followed by one normal sinus impulse 房性二联律；**atrioventricular nodal b.**, an arrhythmia in which an atrioventricular extrasystole is followed by a normal sinus impulse in repetitive sequence 房室结二联律；**ventricular b.**, an arrhythmia consisting of the repeated sequence of one ventricular premature complex followed by one normal beat 室性二联律；

bi·lat·er·al (bi-lat'ər-əl) having two sides, or pertaining to both sides 双边的

bi·lay·er (bi'la-ər) a membrane consisting of two molecular layers 双层的；**lipid b., phospholipid b.**, the structure common to all biological membranes, consisting of two layers of phospholipids with their hydrophilic head groups exposed to the aqueous medium and hydrophobic tails directed inward 磷脂双分子层

bil·ber·ry (bil'ber-e) the leaves and fruit of *Vaccinium myrtillus*, having astringent and antidiarrheal effects, used topically for inflammation, burns, and skin diseases, and orally for gout, arthritis, dermatitis, diabetes mellitus, and gastrointestinal, urinary tract, and kidney disorders 欧洲越橘

bile (bīl) a fluid secreted by the liver, concentrated in the gallbladder, and poured into the small intestine via the bile ducts, which helps in alkalinizing the intestinal contents and plays a role in emulsification, absorption, and digestion of fat; its chief constituents are conjugated bile salts, cholesterol, phospholipid, bilirubin, and electrolytes 胆汁

bile ac·id (bīl) any of the steroid acids derived from cholesterol; classified as *primary*, thus synthesized in the liver, e.g., cholic and chenodeoxycholic acids, or *secondary*, those produced from primary bile acids by intestinal bacteria, e.g., deoxycholic and lithocholic acids. Most of the bile acids are reabsorbed and returned to the liver via the enterohepatic circulation 胆汁酸。Cf. *bile salt* under *salt*

Bil·har·zia (bil-hahr'ze-ə) *Schistosoma* 血吸虫

bil·har·zi·a·sis (bil″hahr-zi'ə-sis) schistosomiasis 血吸虫病

bil·i·ary (bil'e-ar-e) pertaining to the bile, to the bile ducts, or to the gallbladder 胆的

bil·i·blank·et (bil″ĭ-blank'-ət) a portable phototherapy device used to treat hyperbilirubinemia and jaundice in infants 毛毯。Spelled also *bili blanket*

bil·i·ra·chia (bil″ĭ-ra'ke-ə) presence of bile pigments in spinal fluid 胆汁脊液

bil·i·ru·bin (bil″ĭ-roo'bin) a bile pigment produced by breakdown of heme and reduction of biliverdin; it normally circulates in plasma and is taken up by liver cells and conjugated to form bilirubin diglucuronide, the water-soluble pigment excreted in bile. High concentrations of bilirubin may result in jaundice 胆红素；**conjugated b., direct b.**, bilirubin that has been taken up by the liver cells and conjugated to form the water-soluble bilirubin diglucuronide 直接胆红素；**indirect b., unconjugated b.**, the lipid-soluble form of bilirubin that circulates in loose association with the plasma proteins 间接胆红素

bil·i·uria (bil″ĭ-u're-ə) choluria 胆汁尿

bil·i·ver·din (bil″ĭ-vur'din) a green bile pigment formed by catabolism of hemoglobin and converted to bilirubin in the liver; it may also arise from oxidation of bilirubin 胆绿素

bi·loc·u·lar (bi-lok'u-lər) having two compartments. 双房的

bi·lo·ma (bi-lo'mə) an encapsulated collection of bile in the peritoneal cavity 胆汁积聚

Bi·lo·phi·la (bi-lof'ĭ-lə) a genus of gramnegative, anaerobic bacteria, including *B. wadswor'thia*, which causes intra-abdominal and other infections 嗜胆菌属

bi·man·u·al (bi-man'u-əl) with both hands 双手的；performed by both hands 双手执行的

bi·mat·o·prost (bī-mat'o-prost) a synthetic prostaglandin analogue used topically in the treatment of open-angle glaucoma and ocular hypertension 比马前列素

bi·na·ry (bi'nə-re) 1. made up of two elements or of two equal parts 二元的；2. denoting a number system with a base of two 二进制的

bi·nau·ral (bi-naw'rəl) pertaining to both ears 两耳的

bi·nau·ric·u·lar (bi″naw-rik'u-lər) biauricular 双耳的

bind·er (bīnd'ər) a girdle or large bandage for support of the abdomen or breasts, particularly one applied to the abdomen after childbirth to support the relaxed abdominal walls 产后束腹带

binge (binj) 1. a period of uncontrolled or excessive self-indulgent activity, particularly of eating or drinking 暴饮暴食；2. to indulge in such activity 沉迷于暴饮暴食中

bin·oc·u·lar (bǐ-nok′u-lər) 1. pertaining to both eyes 双眼的；2. having two eyepieces, as in a microscope 双目镜

bi·no·mi·al (bi-no′me-əl) composed of two terms, e.g., names of organisms formed by the combination of genus and species names 二项式

bin·ov·u·lar (bin-ov′u-lər) pertaining to or derived from two distinct oocytes or ova 双卵性的

bi·nu·cle·a·tion (bi″noo-kle-a′shən) formation of two nuclei within a cell through division of the nucleus without division of the cytoplasm 双核化

bio·ac·tive (bi″o-ak′tiv) having an effect on or eliciting a response from living tissue 生物活性的

bio·am·in·er·gic (bi″o-am″in-ur′jik) of or pertaining to neurons that secrete biogenic amines 生物胺能的

bio·as·say (bi″o-as′a) determination of the active power of a drug sample by comparing its effects on a live animal or an isolated organ preparation with those of a reference standard 生物测定

bio·avail·a·bil·i·ty (bi″o-ə-vāl″ə-bil′ ĭ-te) the degree to which a drug or other substance becomes available to the target tissue after administration 生物利用率

bio·chem·is·try (bi″o-kem′is-tre) the chemistry of living organisms and of vital processes 生物化学；**biochem′ical** *adj.* 生物化学的

bio·com·pat·i·ble (bi″o-kom-pat′ĭ-bəl) being harmonious with life; not having toxic or injurious effects on biological function 生物相容性

bio·de·grad·a·ble (bi″o-de-grād′ə-bəl) susceptible of degradation by biological processes, as by bacterial or other enzymatic action 可生物降解的

bio·deg·ra·da·tion (bi″o-deg″rə-da′shən) the series of processes by which living systems render chemicals less noxious to the environment 生物降解

bio·equiv·a·lent (bi″o-e-kwiv′ə-lənt) having the same strength and similar bioavailability in the same dosage form as another specimen of a given drug substance 生物等效性；**bioequiv′alence** *n.* 生物等效

bio·eth·ics (bi″o-eth′iks) obligations of a moral nature relating to biological research and its applications 生命伦理学

bio·feed·back (bi″o-fēd′bak) the process of furnishing someone with information on one or more physiologic variables, such as heart rate, blood pressure, or skin temperature; this may help the person gain some voluntary control over them 生物反馈；**alpha b.,** presentation of continuous information on the state of the brain-wave pattern, to assist in purposeful increase in the percentage of alpha activity and thus a state of relaxation and peaceful wakefulness α 生物反馈

bio·fla·vo·noid (bi″o-fla′və-noid) any of the flavonoids with biological activity in mammals 生物类黄酮

bio·gen·e·sis (bi″o-jen′ə-sis) biosynthesis 生物合成

bi·o·gen·ic (bi″o-jen′ik) having origins in biological processes 生物源的

bio·im·plant (bi″o-im′plant) a prosthesis made of biosynthetic material 生物植入物

bio·in·com·pat·i·ble (bi″o-in″kəm-pat′ə-bəl) inharmonious with life; having toxic or injurious effects on life functions 生物不相容

bio·in·for·mat·ics (bi″o-in″for-mat′iks) the organization and use of biological information, particularly computer-driven storage, processing, and analysis of data and databases in the fields of molecular biology and genetics 生物信息学

bio·ki·net·ics (bi″o-kǐ-net′iks) 1. the science of the movements within organisms 生物动力学；2. the application of therapeutic exercise in rehabilitative treatment or performance enhancement 运动疗法的运用

bi·o·log·i·cal (bi-o-loj′ ĭ-kəl) 1. pertaining to biology 生物学的；2. a medicinal preparation made from living organisms and their products, including serums, vaccines, antigens, antitoxins, etc. 生物学

bi·ol·o·gy (bi-ol′ə-je) scientific study of living organisms 生理；**biolog′ic** *adj.* 生物学；**cell b.,** the study of the origin, structure, function, behavior, growth, and reproduction of cells and their components 细胞生物学。又称 *cytology*；**molecular b.,** study of molecular structures and events underlying biological processes, including relationships between genes and the functional characteristics they determine 分子生物学；**radiation b.,** scientific study of effects of ionizing radiation on living organisms 核生物学

bio·mark·er (bi″o-mahr″kər) 1. a biological molecule used as a marker for a substance or process of interest 生物标记物；2. a tumor marker 肿瘤标记物

bio·mass (bi′o-mas″) the entire assemblage of living organisms of a particular region, considered collectively 生物量

bio·ma·te·ri·al (bi″o-mə-tēr-e-əl) a synthetic dressing with selective barrier properties, used in the treatment of burns; it consists of a liquid solvent (polyethylene glycol-400) and a powdered polymer 生物材料

bio·med·i·cine (bi″o-med′ĭ-sin) medicine based on the principles of the natural sciences (biology, biochemistry, etc.) 生物医学；**biomed′ical** *adj.* 生物医学的

bio·mem·brane (bi″o-mem′brān) the lipid bilayer, with associated proteins, that surrounds cells and organelles 生物膜；**biomem′ branous** *adj.* 生物膜的

bi·om·e·try (bi-om′ə-tre) the application of statistical methods to biological phenomena 生物统计学

bio·mi·cro·scope (bi″o-mi′krə-skōp) a microscope for examining living tissue in the body 生物显微镜

bio·mi·met·ic (bi″o-mī-met′ik) imitating something that exists in nature; said of a synthetic product or process 仿生的

bio·mod·u·la·tion (bi″o-mod″u-la′shən) reactive or associative adjustment of the biochemical or cellular status of an organism 生物调控

bio·mod·u·la·tor (bi″o-mod″u-la″tər) biologic reponse modifier 生物调节剂

bio·mol·e·cule (bi″o-mol′ə-kūl) a molecule produced by living cells, e.g., a protein, carbohydrate, lipid, or nucleic acid 生物分子

bi·on·ics (bi-on′iks) scientific study of functions, characteristics, and phenomena observed in the living world, and the application of knowledge gained therefrom to nonliving systems 仿生学

bio·phys·ics (bi-o-fiz′iks) the science dealing with the application of physical methods and theories to biological problems 生物物理学；**biophys′ical** *adj.* 生物物理学的

bio·phys·i·ol·o·gy (bi″o-fiz-e-ol′ə-je) that portion of biology including organogeny, morphology, and physiology 生物生理学

bio·pros·the·sis (bi″o-pros-the′sis) a prosthesis that contains biological material 生物假体；**bioprosthet′ic** *adj.* 生物假体的

bi·op·sy (bi′op-se) removal and examination, usually microscopic, of tissue from the living body, performed to establish a precise diagnosis 活检；**aspiration b.**, biopsy in which tissue is obtained by application of suction through a needle attached to a syringe 抽吸活检；**brush b.**, biopsy in which cells or tissue are obtained by manipulating tiny brushes against the tissue or lesion in question (e.g., through a bronchoscope) at the desired site 刷试活检；**cone b.**, conization 锥切活检；**core b., core needle b.**, needle biopsy with a large hollow needle that extracts a core of tissue 粗针穿刺活检；**endoscopic b.**, removal of tissue by appropriate instruments through an endoscope 内镜活检；**excisional b.**, biopsy of tissue removed by surgical cutting 切除活检；**incisional b.**, biopsy of a selected portion of a lesion 切取活检；**needle b.**, biopsy in which tissue is obtained by puncture of a tumor, the tissue within

the lumen of the needle being detached by rotation, and the needle withdrawn 穿刺活检。又称 *percutaneous b.*；**percutaneous b.**, 见 needle b.；**punch b.**, biopsy in which tissue is obtained by a punch 钻取活检；**shave b.**, biopsy of a skin lesion in which the sample is excised using a cut parallel to the surface of the surrounding skin 刮取活检；**stereotactic b.**, biopsy of the brain using stereotactic surgery to locate the biopsy site 立体定位切片活检；**sternal b.**, biopsy of bone marrow of the sternum removed by puncture or trephining 胸骨骨髓活检

bio·psy·chol·o·gy (bi″o-si-kol′ə-je) 生物心理学，见 psychobiology (1)

bi·op·tome (bi′op-tōm″) a cutting instrument for taking biopsy specimens 活检钳

bio·re·ver·si·ble (bi″o-re-vur′sī-bəl) capable of being changed back to the original biologically active chemical form by processes within the organism; said of drugs 生物可逆的

bio·sci·ence (bi″o-si′ens) the study of biology wherein all the applicable sciences (physics, chemistry, etc.) are applied. 生物科学

bio·sta·tis·tics (bi″o-stə-tis′tiks) biometry 生物统计学

bio·syn·the·sis (bi″o-sin′thə-sis) creation of a compound by physiologic processes in a living organism 生物合成；**biosynthet′ic** *adj.* 生物合成的；

bi·o·ta (bi-o′tə) all the living organisms of a particular area; the combined flora and fauna of a region 生物群

bio·tech·nol·o·gy (bi″o-tek-nol′ə-je) any application of technology that uses biological systems, organisms, or their derivatives to create new products or processes or modify existing ones 生物技术

bio·te·lem·e·try (bi″o-tə-lem′ə-tre) the recording and measuring of certain vital phenomena of living organisms that are situated at a distance from the measuring device 生物遥测学

bio·ther·a·py (bi″o-ther′ə-pe) biological therapy 生物疗法

bi·ot·ic (bi-ot′ik) 1. pertaining to life or living matter 生命的；2. pertaining to the biota 生物的

bio·tin (bi′o-tin) a member of the vitamin B complex; it is a cofactor for several enzymes, plays a role in fatty acid and amino acid metabolism, and is used in vitro in some biochemical assays 生物素

bio·tox·i·col·o·gy (bi″o-tok″sī-kol′ə-je) scientific study of poisons produced by living organisms, and treatment of conditions produced by them 生物毒物学

bio·trans·for·ma·tion (bi″o-trans″for-ma′shən) the series of chemical alterations of a compound (e.g., a drug) occurring within the body, as by enzymatic activity 生物转化

bio·type (bi′o-tīp) 1. a group of individuals having the same genotype 生物型；2. biovar 生化变种

bio·var (bi′o-vahr) (bi′o-var) in bacteriology, a variant strain of a species having differentiable physiological or biochemical characteristics 生化变种；又称 *biotype*

bi·ov·u·lar (bi-ov′u-lər) binovular 双卵性的

bip·a·rous (bip′ə-rəs) producing two offspring or eggs at one time 双胎的

bi·pen·ni·form (bi-pen′ĭ-form) doubly feather-shaped; said of muscles whose fibers are arranged on each side of a tendon like barbs on a feather shaft 双羽状

bi·per·i·den (bi-per′ĭ-den) an antidyskinetic used as the hydrochloride and lactate salts in the treatment of parkinsonism and drug-induced extrapyramidal reactions 安克痉

bi·phen·yl (bi-fen′əl) diphenyl 联苯；**polybrominated b.,** any of various brominated derivatives of biphenyl; uses and toxic hazards are similar to those of polychlorinated biphenyls 多溴联苯；**polychlorinated b. (PCB),** any of a group of chlorinated derivatives of biphenyl, used as heattransfer agents and electrical insulators; they are toxic, carcinogenic, and non-biodegradable 多氯联苯

bi·po·lar (bi-po′lər) 1. having two poles or pertaining to both poles 双极的；2. describing neurons that have processes at both ends 双极神经元；3. pertaining to mood disorders in which both depressive episodes and manic or hypomanic episodes occur 躁狂抑郁性精神病的

Bi·po·la·ris (bi-po-lar′is) a genus of dematiaceous anamorphic fungi including opportunistic pathogens that are common causes of phaeohyphomycosis, particularly fungal sinusitis and cutaneous infections 孢菌属

bi·po·ten·ti·al·i·ty (bi″po-ten″she-al′ĭ-te) ability to develop or act in either of two possible ways 双性潜能；**bipoten′tial** *adj.* 双电位的

bi·ra·mous (bi-ra′məs) having two branches 双支的

bi·re·frin·gence (bi″re-frin′jəns) the quality of transmitting light unequally in different directions 双折射；**birefrin′gent** *adj.* 双折射的

birth (burth) a coming into being; act or process of being born 出生；**multiple b.,** the birth of two or more offspring produced in the same gestation period 多胎妊娠；**postterm b.,** birth of an infant at or after 42 completed weeks (294 days) of gestation 延迟分娩；**premature b., preterm b.,** birth of an infant before 37 completed weeks (259 days) of gestation 早产

birth·mark (burth′mahrk) a congenital circumscribed blemish or spot on the skin 胎记；见 *nevus*

bis·ac·o·dyl (bis-ak′o-dəl) (bis″ə-ko′dəl) a contact laxative, used as the base or as a complex with tannic acid (*b. tannex*) 双醋苯啶

bis·acro·mi·al (bis-ə-kro′me-əl) pertaining to the two acromial processes 双肩峰的

bi·sec·tion (bi-sek′shən) division into two parts by cutting 平分点

bi·sex·u·al (bi-sek′shoo-əl) 1. pertaining to or characterized by bisexuality 双性的；2. an individual exhibiting bisexuality 双性恋者；3. hermaphroditic 雌雄同体的

bi·sex·u·al·i·ty (bi-sek″shoo-al′ĭ-te) 1. sexual attraction to both sexes; exhibition of or interest in both homosexual and heterosexual behavior 双性恋；2. hermaphroditism 两性现象

bis·fe·ri·ens (bis-fe′re-ənz) [L.] bisferious. 二联律的

bis·fe·ri·ous (bis-fe′re-əs) having two beats 二联律的

bis·il·i·ac (bis-il′e-ak) pertaining to the two iliac bones or to any two corresponding points on them 双髂嵴的

bis·muth (Bi) (biz′məth) a silver-white to pinkish, brittle, heavy metal element; at. no. 83, at. wt. 208.980. Its salts are used to treat diarrhea, nausea, and other gastrointestinal conditions 铋；**b. subsalicylate,** a bismuth salt of salicylic acid, used in the treatment of diarrhea and gastric distress, including nausea, indigestion, and heartburn 碱式水杨酸铋

bis·mu·tho·sis (biz″mə-tho′sis) bismuth poisoning, with anuria, stomatitis, dermatitis, and diarrhea 铋中毒

bis·o·pro·lol (bis″o-pro′lol) a cardioselective beta-adrenergic blocking agent, used as the fumarate salt in the treatment of hypertension 比索洛尔

2,3-bis·phos·pho·glyc·er·ate (bis-fos″foglis′ər-āt) an intermediate in the conversion of 3-phosphoglycerate to 2-phosphoglycerate; it also acts as an allosteric effector in the regulation of oxygen binding by hemoglobin 2,3-二磷酸甘油酯

bis·phos·pho·nate (bis-fos″fə-nāt) diphosphonate 二磷酸盐

bis·tou·ry (bis′too-re) a long, narrow, straight or curved surgical knife 柳叶刀

bi·sul·fate (bi-sul′fāt) an acid sulfate 酸性硫酸盐

bi·tar·trate (bi-tahr′trāt) any salt containing the anion $C_4H_5O_6$- derived from tartaric acid ($C_4H_6O_6$) 酒石酸氢盐

bite (bīt) 1. seizure with the teeth 咬；2. a wound or puncture made by a living organism 咬伤；3. an impression made by closure of the teeth upon some plastic material, e.g., wax 咬痕；4. occlusion (2) 咬合；**closed b.**, malocclusion in which the incisal edges of the mandibular anterior teeth protrude past those of the maxillary teeth 闭锁𬌗；**cross b.**, crossbite 反𬌗；**edge-to-edge b., end-to-end b.**, occlusion in which the incisors of both jaws are closed 对刃𬌗；**open b.**, occlusion in which certain opposing teeth fail to come together when the jaws are closed; usually confined to anterior teeth 开𬌗 **over b.**, overbite 深覆𬌗

bite-block (bīt'blok) occlusion rim 牙垫

bite·lock (bīt'lok) a dental device for retaining occlusion rims in the same relation outside the mouth which they occupied in the mouth 咬锁

bi·tem·po·ral (bi-tem'pə-rəl) pertaining to both temples or temporal bones 双颞的

bite·plate (bīt'plāt) an appliance, usually plastic and wire, worn in the palate as a diagnostic or therapeutic adjunct in orthodontics or prosthodontics 咬合板

bite-wing (bīt'wing) a wing or fin attached along the center of the tooth side of a dental x-ray film and bitten on by the patient, permitting production of images of the corona of the teeth in both dental arches and their contiguous periodontal tissues 咬翼片

Bi·tis (bi'tis) a genus of venomous, brightly colored, thick-bodied, viperine snakes, possessing heart-shaped heads; it includes the puff adder (*B. arie'tans*), Gaboon viper (*B. gabo'nica*), and rhinoceros viper (*B. nasicor'nis*) 咝蝰属

bi·tol·ter·ol (bi-tol'tər-ol) a β 2-adrenergic receptor agonist, administered by inhalation in the form of the mesylate salt as a bronchodilator 比托特罗

bi·tro·chan·ter·ic (bi″tro-kan-ter'ik) pertaining to both trochanters on one femur or to both greater trochanters 转子间的

bi·tu·mi·no·sis (bi-too″mĭ-no'sis) a mild form of pneumoconiosis due to inhalation of dust from soft coal 沥青末沉着病

bi·u·ret (bi'u-rət) a urea derivative 双缩脲；见 *reaction* 下词条

bi·va·lent (bi-va'lənt) 1. having a valence of two; divalent 二价的；2. the structure formed by a pair of homologous chromosomes by synapsis along their length during the zygotene and pachytene stages of the first meiotic prophase 二价染色体；3. effective against two different entities, as diseases or strains of a pathogen 二价体

bi·val·i·ru·din (bi-val'ĭ-roo-din) an anticoagulant used with aspirin in patients with unstable angina pectoris who are undergoing percutaneous transluminal coronary angioplasty 比伐卢定

bi·ven·tric·u·lar (bi″ven-trik'u-lər) pertaining to or affecting both ventricles of the heart 双心室

bi·zy·go·mat·ic (bi″zi-go-mat'ik) pertaining to the two most prominent points on the two zygomatic arches 两颧的

B-K, BK below-knee 膝下；见 *amputation* 下 *transtibial amputation*

BKV BK virus BK 病毒；见 *polyomavirus*

black (blak) reflecting no light or true color 不反射光线的；of the darkest hue 黑色

black·head (blak'hed) open comedo 黑头粉刺

black·out (blak'out) loss of vision and momentary lapse of consciousness due to diminished circulation to the brain and retina 黑视；脑或视网膜缺血导致暂时性意识丧失；**alcoholic b.**, anterograde amnesia experienced by alcoholics during episodes of drinking, even when not fully intoxicated; indicative of early, reversible brain damage 饮酒期间（即使没有完全喝醉）酗酒者经历的顺行性遗忘；表明早期可逆性脑损伤

black·snake (blak'snāk) 1. *Pseudechis porphyriacus*, a large venomous semiaquatic Australian snake whose body is black on top and red underneath 红腹伊澳蛇：体型大，剧毒，半水栖的澳大利亚蛇，因背部呈黑色而腹部为红色得名；2. *Coluber constrictor*, a nonvenomous snake found in North America 黑索游蛇：分布于北美，无毒

blad·der (blad'ər) 1. a membranous sac, such as one serving as a receptacle for a secretion 膜囊，例如作为分泌物容器的膜囊；2. urinary bladder 膀胱；**atonic neurogenic b.**, neurogenic bladder due to destruction of sensory nerve fibers from the bladder to the spinal cord, with absence of control of bladder functions and of desire to urinate, bladder overdistention, and an abnormal amount of residual urine; usually associated with tabes dorsalis or pernicious anemia 弛缓性神经源性膀胱，由于从膀胱到脊髓的感觉神经纤维的破坏，失去对膀胱功能和排尿欲望的控制，膀胱过度膨胀和异常尿量残留；通常与脊髓痨或恶性贫血有关；**automatic b.**, neurogenic bladder due to complete transection of the spinal cord above the sacral segments, with loss of micturition reflexes and bladder sensation, involuntary urination, and an abnormal amount of residual urine 神经源性膀胱，由于骶骨段以上脊髓完全横断，排尿反射和膀胱感觉丧失，无意识排尿，残余尿量异常；**autonomic b., autonomous b.**, neurogenic bladder due to a lesion in the sacral spinal cord, interrupting the reflex arc controlling the bladder, with loss of normal bladder sensation and reflexes, inability to initiate urination normally, and incontinence 脊髓损伤引起的神经源性膀胱，控制膀胱的反射弧中断，丧失正常的

膀胱感觉和反射，无法引发正常排尿，引起尿失禁及异常尿量潴留；**gall b.,** gallbladder 胆囊；**ileal b.,** a neobladder made from a section of ileum 回肠膀胱，由一段回肠制成的新膀胱；**irritable b.,** a condition of the bladder marked by increased frequency of contraction with associated desire to urinate 易激性膀胱，膀胱收缩频率增加并伴有排尿欲望；**motor paralytic b.,** neurogenic bladder due to impairment of motor neurons or nerves controlling the bladder; the *acute* form is marked by painful distention and inability to initiate urination, and the *chronic* form by difficulty initiating urination, straining, decreased size and force of stream, interrupted stream, and recurrent urinary tract infection 运动麻痹性膀胱，由运动神经元或控制膀胱的神经受损引起的神经源性膀胱；急性型以疼痛性扩张和排尿困难为特征，慢性型以排尿困难、尿急、尿流减小、尿力减弱、尿流中段、反复尿路感染为特征；**neurogenic b.,** dysfunction of the urinary bladder caused by a lesion of the central or peripheral nervous system 神经源性膀胱，中枢或外周神经系统受损导致的膀胱功能障碍；**uninhibited neurogenic b.,** neurogenic bladder due to a lesion in upper motor neurons with subtotal interruption of corticospinal pathways, with urgency, frequent involuntary urination, and small-volume threshold of activity 非抑制性神经源性膀胱，上运动神经元损伤导致的神经源性膀胱，皮质脊髓通路中断，造成尿急，频繁不自主排尿和引起膀胱活动的体积阈值减小；**urinary b.,** the musculomembranous sac in the anterior part of the pelvic cavity that serves as a reservoir for urine, which it receives through the ureters and discharges through the urethra 膀胱

blast[1] (blast) 1. an immature stage in cellular development before appearance of the definitive characteristics of the cell; used also as a word termination (see *-blast*) 具有细胞特性之前的不成熟阶段；也用作词尾（见 -blast）；2. 母细胞，见 blast cell (2)

blast[2] (blast) the wave of air pressure produced by the detonation of high-explosive bombs or shells or by other explosions; it causes pulmonary concussion and hemorrhage (*lung blast, blast chest*), laceration of other thoracic and abdominal viscera, ruptured eardrums, and minor effects in the central nervous system 高爆炸弹或炮弹爆炸或其他爆炸产生的气压波；引起肺部震荡和出血（肺部爆炸，爆炸胸部）其他胸腹部内脏撕裂，耳膜破裂，中枢神经系统轻微影响

blas·te·ma (blas-te′mə) a group of cells giving rise to a new individual (in asexual reproduction) or to an organ or part (in either normal development or in regeneration) 胚基；芽基；原基；胚茎，一组细胞可产生一个新的个体（在无性繁殖中）或一个或部分器官（在正常发育或再生中）**blaste′mic** *adj.*

blas·to·coele (blas′to-sēl) the fluid-filled central segmentation cavity of the blastula 囊胚腔；卵裂腔；胚泡腔；**blastocoe′lic, blastocoe′lic** *adj.*

blas·to·cyst (blas′to-sist) the mammalian conceptus in the postmorula stage, consisting of an embryoblast (inner cell mass) and a thin trophoblast layer enclosing a blastocyst cavity 胚泡；囊胚，由胚细胞（内细胞团）和包围胚泡腔的薄滋养层组成

blas·to·cyte (blas′to-sīt) an undifferentiated embryonic cell 胚细胞

blas·to·derm (blas′to-dərm) the single layer of cells forming the wall of the blastula, or the cellular cap above the floor of segmented yolk in the discoblastula of telolecithal eggs. 胚盘；**blastoder′mal, blastoder′mic** *adj.*

blas·to·gen·e·sis (blas″to-jen′ə-sis) 1. development of an individual from a blastema, i.e., by asexual reproduction 芽基发育，如无性繁殖；2. transmission of inherited characters by the germ plasm 细胞质遗传；3. morphological transformation of small lymphocytes into larger cells resembling blast cells on exposure to phytohemagglutinin or to antigens to which the donor is immunized 小淋巴细胞在接触植物血凝素或免疫供体的抗原时形成类似于母细胞的较大细胞的形态转化；**blastogenet′ic, blastogen′ic** *adj.*

blas·to·ma (blas-to′mə) pl. *blastomas, blasto′mata*. A neoplasm composed of embryonic cells derived from the blastema of an organ or tissue 母细胞瘤；**blasto′matous** *adj.*

blas·to·mere (blas′to-mēr) one of the cells produced by cleavage of a zygote 卵裂球

Blas·to·my·ces (blas″to-mi′sēz) a genus of anamorphic fungi comprising the single species *B. dermati′tidis*, a thermally dimorphic organism growing as a mold at 37℃ and a yeast at 25℃ and causing North American blastomycosis 芽生菌属，变形真菌的一个属，由单种皮炎芽生菌——一种在37℃以霉菌形式生长的热双形生物和一种在25℃以酵母形式生长并引起北美芽生菌病

Blas·to·my·ce·tes (blas″to-mi-se′tēz) formerly, a class of fungi comprising the anamorphic yeasts; still used informally to describe the group 芽孢菌纲，既往用于表示一类包含变形酵母的真菌；目前仍非正式地用来形容这个群体

blas·to·my·co·sis (blas″to-mi-ko′sis) 1. infection due to *Blastomyces dermatitidis*, usually acquired by inhalation and predominantly involving the skin, lungs, and bones 皮肤芽孢杆菌引起的感染，通常经吸入感染，主要涉及皮肤，肺和骨骼; 2. any infection caused by a yeastlike organism 任何由酵母样生物引起的感染; **North American b.**, blastomycosis (1) 北美芽生菌病; **South American b.**, paracoccidioidomycosis 副球孢子菌病

blas·to·pore (blas′to-por) the opening of the archenteron to the exterior of the embryo at the gastrula stage 胚孔

Blas·to·schizo·my·ces (blas″to-skiz″omi′sēz) a genus of anamorphic fungi whose sole species, *B. capita′tus*, has been reclassified as *Saprochaete capitata* 芽生裂殖菌属，一种变形真菌，其唯一的物种，头状芽生裂殖酵母，被重新分类为 Saprochaete capitata

blas·tu·la (blas′tu-lə) pl. *blas′tulae* [L.] the usually spherical structure produced by cleavage of a zygote, consisting of a single layer of cells (blastoderm) surrounding a fluid-filled cavity (blastocoele) 囊胚，受精卵分裂产生的球形结构，由单层细胞的胚盘及其周围充满液体的腔组成

bleb (bleb) bulla (1) 疱疹

bleed·er (blēd′ər) 1. one who bleeds freely 易出血者; 2. any blood vessel cut during surgery that requires clamping, ligature, or cautery 手术过程中需要夹紧，结扎或烧灼的血管损伤

bleed·ing (blēd′ing) 1. the escape of blood, as from an injured vessel 出血; 2. phlebotomy 放血; **dysfunctional uterine b. (DUB)**, bleeding from the uterus when no organic lesions are present 功能失调性子宫出血，没有器质性病变时的子宫出血; **implantation b.**, bleeding in the uterus at the time of implantation of the blastocyst in the decidua 胚泡植入蜕膜时子宫内出血; **obscure gastrointestinal b.**, persistent or recurrent gastrointestinal bleeding when a standard endoscopic evaluation is negative; it may be either overt, with melena or hematochezia, or occult, with anemia or a positive test for occult blood 不明原因消化道出血，内镜检查为阴性的持续性或复发性胃肠道出血，可能为明显的呕血或黑粪，或者隐匿性的，伴有贫血或潜血检测阳性; **occult b.**, escape of blood in such small quantity that it can be detected only by chemical test or by microscopic or spectroscopic examination 潜血，出血量很小，只能通过化学试验、显微镜和光谱检查来检测

blen·nad·e·ni·tis (blen″ad-ə-ni′tis) myxadenitis 黏液腺炎

blen·noid (blen′oid) mucoid (1) 黏液

blen·nor·rhea (blen″o-re′ə) any free discharge of mucus, especially a gonorrheal discharge from the urethra or vagina 任何自由排出的黏液，特别是从尿道或阴道排出的淋病（溢脓）; **blennorrhagic,**

blennorrhe′al *adj.*

blen·no·tho·rax (blen″o-thor′aks) a pleural effusion with mucus 脓胸

ble·o·my·cin (ble″o-mi′sin) a polypeptide antibiotic mixture obtained from cultures of *Streptomyces verticellus*; used as the sulfate salt as an antineoplastic 博来霉素，从链霉菌培养物中获得的多肽抗生素混合物; 以硫酸盐作为抗肿瘤药

bleph·a·rad·e·ni·tis (blef″ə-rad″ə-ni′tis) inflammation of the meibomian glands 睑板腺炎

bleph·a·ri·tis (blef″ə-ri′tis) inflammation of the eyelids 眼睑炎; **angular b., b. angula′ris**, inflammation involving the angles of the eyelids 眦角性睑缘炎; **b. cilia′ris, marginal b.**, a chronic inflammation of the hair follicles and sebaceous gland openings of the margins of the eyelids 睑缘炎，眼睑边缘的毛囊和皮脂腺开口的慢性炎症; **nonulcerative b., seborrheic b.**, blepharitis with seborrhea of the scalp, brows, and skin behind the ears, marked by greasy scaling, hyperemia, and thickening 脂溢性睑炎，睑缘炎伴头皮、眉毛和耳后皮肤的皮脂溢出，以油腻的皮屑、充血和增厚为特征; **ulcerative b.**, that marked by small ulcerated areas along the eyelid margin, multiple suppurative lesions, and loss of lashes 疡性睑缘炎，以沿着眼睑边缘的小溃疡区域，多个化脓性病变和睫毛丢失为特征

bleph·a·ro·ath·er·o·ma (blef″ə-ro-ath″əro′mə) an encysted tumor or sebaceous cyst of an eyelid 眼睑肿瘤或眼睑皮脂腺囊肿

bleph·a·ro·chal·a·sis (blef″ə-ro-kal′ə-sis) hypertrophy and loss of elasticity of the skin of the upper eyelid 眼睑松弛症，上睑皮肤肥大和失去弹性

bleph·a·ron·cus (blef″ə-rong′kəs) a tumor on the eyelid 眼睑肿瘤

bleph·a·ro·phi·mo·sis (blef″ə-ro-fī-mo′sis) abnormal narrowness of the palpebral fissures 睑裂狭小，睑板的异常狭窄

bleph·a·ro·plas·ty (blef′ə-ro-plas″te) plastic surgery of the eyelids 眼睑成形术

bleph·a·ro·ple·gia (blef″ə-ro-ple′jə) paralysis of an eyelid 眼睑麻痹

bleph·a·rop·to·sis (blef″ə-rop-to′sis) ptosis (2) 上睑下垂

bleph·a·ro·py·or·rhea (blef″ə-ro-pi″ə-re′ə) purulent ophthalmia 化脓性眼炎

bleph·a·ror·rha·phy (blef″ə-ror′ə-fe) 1. suture of an eyelid 眼睑缝合; 2. tarsorrhaphy 睑裂缝合术; 眦缝合术; 睑缝合术

bleph·a·ro·ste·no·sis (blef″ə-ro-stə-no′sis) blepharophimosis 睑裂

bleph·a·ro·syn·ech·ia (blef″ə-ro-sī-nek′e-ə) a growing together or adhesion of the eyelids 眼睑黏连

bleph·a·rot·o·my (blef″ə-rot′ə-me) surgical incision of an eyelid 眼睑切开术

blind (blīnd) [A.S.] 1. not having the sense of sight 盲的，视力缺失的；2. pertaining to a clinical trial or other experiment in which one or more of the groups receiving, administering, and evaluating the treatment are unaware of which treatment any particular subject is receiving 盲法

blind·ness (blīnd′nis) lack or loss of ability to see 缺乏或丧失视物的能力；lack of perception of visual stimuli 缺乏对视觉刺激的感知；**blue b.**, **blue-yellow b.**, popular names for imperfect perception of blue and yellow tints 青盲，蓝黄色盲；见 *tritanopia* 和 *tetartanopia*；**color b.**, 1. popular name for *color vision deficiency* 色盲；2. 见 *monochromatic vision*；**complete color b.**, monochromatic vision 单色视；**day b.**, hemeralopia 黑夜睛明；**flight b.**, amaurosis fugax due to high centrifugal forces encountered in aviation 飞行盲，由于飞行中遇到的高离心力导致的黑矇；**green b.**, imperfect perception of green tints 绿色盲，对绿色感知不全；见 *deuteranopia* 和 *protanopia*；**legal b.**, that defined by law; usually, maximal visual acuity in the better eye after correction of 20/200 with a total diameter of the visual field in that eye of 20 degrees 法定盲，法律规定的盲症；**letter b.**, alexia characterized by inability to recognize individual letters 文盲；**music b.**, musical alexia 乐盲；**night b.**, failure or imperfection of vision at night or in dim light 夜盲；**object b.**, **psychic b.**, visual agnosia 视觉失认症；**red b.**, popular name for *protanopia* 红色盲；第一原色盲；**red-green b.**, popular name for any imperfect perception of red and green tints, including all the most common types of color vision deficiency 红绿色盲。见 *deuteranomaly, deuteranopia, protanomaly* 和 *protanopia*；**snow b.**, dimness of vision, usually temporary, due to glare of sun upon snow 雪盲；**text b.**, alexia 失读；**total color b.**, monochromatic vision 单色视；**word b.**, alexia 失读

blis·ter (blis′tər) a vesicle, especially a bulla 水泡，特别是大疱；**blood b.**, a vesicle having bloody contents, as may be caused by a pinch or bruise 由捏或瘀伤引起的血泡；**fever b.**, herpes febrilis 唇疱疹；**water b.**, a blister with clear watery contents 水疱

block (blok) 1. obstruction 阻塞；2. to obstruct 使阻塞；3. regional anesthesia 区域麻醉；**ankle b.**, regional anesthesia of the foot by injection of anesthetic around the tibial nerves at the ankle 踝部阻滞麻醉，通过在踝关节周围的胫神经周围注射麻醉剂进行足部局部麻醉；**atrioventricular b.**, **AV b.**, impairment of conduction of cardiac impulses from the atria to the ventricles, usually due to a block in the atrioventricular junctional tissue, and generally subclassified on the basis of severity as first, second, or third degree 房室传导阻滞，心房冲动从心房到心室的传导受损，通常是由于房室交界处组织阻塞，并且通常根据严重程度分为一度、二度或三度；**Bier b.**, regional anesthesia by intravenous injection; used for surgical procedures on the arm below the elbow or leg below the knee that are done in a bloodless field maintained by a pneumatic tourniquet 静脉注射局部麻醉；用于在肘部以下的手臂或膝盖下方的小腿上进行的外科手术，此手术是在流动气场维持的无血区域中进行的；**bifascicular b.**, impairment of conduction in two of the three fascicles of the bundle branches 双束支传导阻滞，心室传导三个束支中的两个发生传导阻滞；**bilateral bundle branch b. (BBBB)**, interruption of cardiac impulses through both bundle branches, clinically indistinguishable from third-degree (complete) heart block 双侧束支传导阻滞，三束支传导阻滞，通过两个束分支中断心脏冲动，临床上与三度（完全）心脏阻滞无法区分；**brachial plexus b.**, regional anesthesia of the shoulder, arm, and hand by injection of anesthetic into the brachial plexus 臂丛阻滞麻醉；**bundle branch b. (BBB)**, interruption of conduction in one of the main bundle branches, so that the impulse first reaches one ventricle, then travels to the other 束支传导阻滞，其中一个主束分支的传导中断，使脉冲首先到达一个心室，然后传播到另一个心室；**caudal b.**, regional anesthesia by injection of local anesthetic into the caudal or sacral canal 骶管阻滞；**cervical plexus b.**, regional anesthesia of the neck by injection of a local anesthetic into the cervical plexus 颈丛阻滞麻醉；**complete heart b.**, 见 *heart b.*；**conduction b.**, a blockage in a nerve that prevents impulses from being conducted across a given segment although the nerve beyond is viable 传导阻滞；**elbow b.**, regional anesthesia of the forearm and hand by injection of local anesthetic around the median, radial, and ulnar nerves at the elbow 肘部阻滞麻醉，通过在肘部的正中神经、桡神经和尺神经周围注射局部麻醉剂对前臂和手进行局部麻醉；**entrance b.**, in cardiology, a unidirectional impasse to conduction that prevents an impulse from entering a specific region of excitable tissue; part of the mechanism underlying parasystole 传入阻滞，在心脏病学中，不可逆传的传导通路可防止冲动进入可兴奋组织的特定区域；**epidural b.**, that produced by injection of the anesthetic into the epidural space, either between the vertebral spines or into the sacral hiatus (*caudal block*) 硬膜外阻滞；**exit b.**, in cardiology, delay or failure of an impulse to be conducted from a specific region to surrounding tissues 传出阻滞；**fascicular b.**, any of a group of disorders of conduction localized within any combination of the three fascicles of the bundle branches or their ramifications 分支传递阻滞；**femoral b.**, regional anesthesia of the posterior thigh and the leg below the knee by injection of a local anesthetic around the femoral nerve just below the inguinal ligament at the lateral border of the fossa ovalis 股部阻滞，通过在卵圆窝外侧边缘的腹股沟韧带正下方的股神经周围注射局部麻醉剂，对大腿后部和膝盖以下的腿进行局部麻醉；**field b.**, regional anesthesia by encircling the operative field with injections of a local anesthetic 局部麻醉，通过注射局部麻醉剂包围手术区域；**first-degree heart b.**, 见 *heart b.*；另见 *atrioventricular b.*；**heart b.**, impairment of conduction of an impulse in heart excitation; it is subclassified as *first degree* when conduction time is prolonged, *second degree* (*partial heart b.*) when some atrial impulses are not conducted, and *third degree* (*complete heart b.*) when no atrial impulses are conducted; the term and its subcategories are often used specifically for atrioventricular block 心脏传导阻滞，心脏激发中脉冲传导受损；当传导时间延长时，为一度，部分传导受损，为二度（部分心脏传导阻滞），当心房冲动完全受损时，为三度（完全性心脏传导阻滞）；该术语及其子类别通常专指房室传导阻滞；**high grade atrioventricular b.**, second- or third-degree atrioventricular block 第二或第三级房室传导阻滞；**incomplete heart b.**, first- or second-degree heart block 不完全性传导阻滞，第一或第二级心脏传导阻滞；**intraspinal b.**, spinal anesthesia (1) 椎管内麻醉；**intravenous b.**, Bier b. 静脉内麻醉；**lumbar plexus b.**, regional anesthesia of the anterior and medial aspects of the leg by injection of a local anesthetic into the lumbar plexus 腰麻，通过局部麻醉剂注入腰从，麻醉腿的前部和内侧；**mental b.**, 见 *blocking* (2)；**metabolic b.**, the blocking of a biosynthetic pathway due to a genetic enzyme defect or to inhibition of an enzyme by a drug or other substance 代谢阻断，由于遗传酶缺陷或通过药物或其他物质抑制酶而阻断生物合成途径；**Mobitz type I b.**, Wenckebach b. 莫氏Ⅰ型阻滞，文氏阻滞；**Mobitz type Ⅱ b.**, a type of second-degree atrioventricular block in which dropped beats occur periodically without previous lengthening of the P–R interval, due to a block within or below the bundle of His 莫氏Ⅱ型阻滞，一种二度房室传导阻滞，由于 His 束内或下的阻滞，其前 P–R 期不延长情况下发生周期性心脏停搏；**motor point b.**, interruption of impulses, by anesthesia or destruction of the nerve, at a motor point in order to relieve spasticity 运动点阻滞，在运动点通过麻醉或神经破坏来中断冲动以减

轻痉挛；**nerve b.**, regional anesthesia by injection of anesthetics close to the appropriate nerve 神经阻滞；**paracervical b.**, regional anesthesia of the inferior hypogastric plexus and ganglia produced by injection of the local anesthetic into the lateral fornices of the vagina 宫颈旁阻滞，将局部麻醉药注射到阴道外侧穹窿以麻醉下腹下神经丛和神经节；**parasacral b.**, regional anesthesia produced by injection of a local anesthetic around the sacral nerves as they emerge from the sacral foramina 骶旁阻滞，在骶神经（骶孔）周围注射局部麻醉剂产生局部麻醉；**paravertebral b.**, infiltration of anesthetic into an area near the vertebrae 椎旁阻滞；**partial heart b.**, 见 *heart b.*；**periinfarction b.**, disturbance of intraventricular conduction after a myocardial infarction, due to delayed conduction in the infarct region 梗死周围传导阻滞；**presacral b.**, anesthesia produced by injection of the local anesthetic into the sacral nerves on the anterior aspect of the sacrum 骶前阻滞，将局部麻醉药注射到骶骨前部的骶神经中产生麻醉；**pudendal b.**, anesthesia produced by blocking the pudendal nerves, accomplished by injection of the local anesthetic into the tuber of the ischium 阴部阻滞；**retrobulbar b.**, anesthetization and immobilization of the eye achieved by injection of a local anesthetic into the retrobulbar space 眼部后阻滞；**sacral b.**, 参见 anesthesia；**saddle b.**, regional anesthesia in an area of the buttocks, perineum, and inner aspects of the thighs, by introducing the anesthetic agent low in the dural sac 鞍区阻滞；**second-degree heart b.**, 见 *heart b.*；另见 *atrioventricular b.*；**sinoatrial b.**, delay or absence of the atrial beat due to partial or complete interference with the propagation of impulses from the sinoatrial node to the atria 窦房传导阻滞；**spinal b.**, 参见 anesthesia；**subarachnoid b.**, spinal anesthesia (1) 蛛网膜下腔阻滞；**third-degree heart b.**, 见 *heart b.*；另见 *atrioventricular b.*；**trifascicular b.**, impairment of conduction in all three fascicles of the bundle branches, a form of complete heart block 三束支传导阻滞；**unifascicular b.**, impairment of conduction in only one fascicle of the bundle branches 单束支传导阻滞；**vagal b., vagus nerve b.**, blocking of vagal impulses by injection of a solution of local anesthetic into the vagus nerve at its exit from the skull 迷走神经阻滞；**Wenckebach b.**, a type of second-degree atrioventricular block in which one or more dropped beats occur periodically after a series of steadily increasing P–R intervals 文氏阻滞；**wrist b.**, regional anesthesia of the hand by injection of a local anesthetic around the median, radial, and ulnar nerves of the wrist 腕阻滞

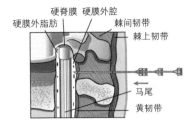

硬膜外脂肪　硬脊膜　硬膜外腔
棘间韧带
棘上韧带
马尾
黄韧带

▲　**硬膜外阻滞（epidural block）**。通过黄韧带注射麻醉药进入硬膜外腔，针头刚好停在硬脊膜外

block·ade　(blok-ād′) 1. the blocking of the effect of a hormone or neurotransmitter at a cell-surface receptor by a pharmacologic antagonist bound to the receptor 拮抗剂与细胞表面受体结合后，阻断相应激素或神经递质的作用；2. in histochemistry, a chemical reaction that modifies certain chemical groups and blocks a specific staining method（组织化学中）封闭；3. regional anesthesia 局部麻醉；**adrenergic b.,** selective inhibition of the response to sympathetic impulses transmitted by epinephrine or norepinephrine at alpha or beta receptor sites of an effector organ or postganglionic adrenergic neuron 肾上腺素能阻滞；**cholinergic b.,** selective inhibition of cholinergic nerve impulses at autonomic ganglial synapses, postganglionic parasympathetic effectors, or the neuromuscular junction 胆碱能阻断；**ganglionic b.,** inhibition by drugs of nerve impulse transmission at autonomic ganglial synapses 神经节阻滞，神经冲动传递药物对自主神经神经节突触的抑制作用；**narcotic b.,** inhibition of the euphoric effects of narcotic drugs by the use of other drugs, such as methadone, in the treatment of addiction 通过使用其他药物（例如美沙酮）来治疗成瘾，从而抑制麻醉药品的欣快效应；**neuromuscular b.,** a failure in neuromuscular transmission that can be induced pharmacologically or may result from pathological disturbances at the myoneural junction 神经肌肉传导阻断

block·er　(blok′ər) something that blocks or obstructs passage, activity, etc. 阻断剂，拮抗剂，阻断或阻碍活性的事物；**α-b.,** alphaadrenergic blocking agent α受体拮抗药；见 *adrenergic blocking agent*；**β-b.,** beta-adrenergic blocking agent β受体拮抗药；见 *adrenergic blocking agent*；**calcium channel b.,** calcium channel blocking agent 钙通道阻滞药；**potassium channel b.,** potassium channel blocking agent 钾通道阻滞药；**sodium channel b.,** sodium channel blocking agent 钠通道阻滞药

block·ing　(blok′ing) 1. interruption of an afferent nerve pathway 传入神经通路中断；见 *block.*；2. difficulty in recollection, or interruption of a train of thought or speech, due to emotional factors, usually unconscious 由于情绪因素，通常是无意识的，在思维或言语的回忆或中断方面存在困难

blood　(blud) the fluid circulating through the heart, arteries, capillaries, and veins, carrying nutriment and oxygen to body cells, and removing waste products and carbon dioxide. It consists of the liquid portion (the plasma) and the formed elements (erythrocytes, leukocytes, and platelets) 血液；循环于心脏，动脉，毛细血管和静脉中，将营养物质和氧气传播到体细胞，去除废物和二氧化碳。它由液体部分（血浆）和有形成分（红细胞，白细胞和血小板）组成；**arterial b.,** oxygenated blood, found in the pulmonary veins, the left chambers of the heart, and the systemic arteries 动脉血；**citrated b.,** blood treated with sodium citrate or citric acid to prevent its coagulation 用柠檬酸钠或柠檬酸处理的血液以防止其凝结；**cord b.,** that contained in umbilical vessels at time of delivery of the infant 脐带血；**occult b.,** that present in such small quantities that it is detectible only by chemical tests or by spectroscopic or microscopic examination 潜血；**predonated autologous b.,** blood donated prior to surgery or other invasive procedure for use in a possible autotransfusion 在手术或其他侵入性手术之前捐献的血液用于可能的自体输血；**venous b.,** blood that has given up its oxygen to the tissues and is carrying carbon dioxide back through the systemic veins for gas exchange in the lungs 静脉血；**whole b.,** that from which none of the elements has been removed, sometimes specifically that drawn from a selected donor under aseptic conditions, containing citrate ion or heparin, and used as a blood replenisher 全血

blood group　(blud groop) 1. an erythrocytic allotype (or phenotype) defined by one or more cellular antigenic groupings controlled by allelic genes. Numerous blood group systems are now known, the most widely used in matching blood for transfusion being the ABO and Rh groups 由等位基因控制的一个或多个细胞抗原决定簇定义的红细胞同种异型（或表型）。现在已知许多血型系统，最广泛用于匹配输血的血液是 ABO 和 Rh 血型；2. any of various other characteristics or traits of cellular or fluid components of blood, considered as the expression (phenotype or allotype) of the actions and interactions of dominant genes, and useful in medicolegal and other studies of human inheritance 血液的细胞或流体组分的任何其他特征或性状，被认为是显性基因的作用和相互作用的表达（表型或同种异型），并且可用于法医学和人类遗传的其他研究

blood·stream　(blud′strēm) the blood flowing

B

through the circulatory system in the living body 血流。Written also *blood stream*

blot (blot) 1. to transfer ionic solutes onto a membrane or other immobilizing matrix for analysis 印迹；2. the substrate containing the transferred material in such a process 印迹物；**dot b.**, a technique used to detect and analyze nucleic acids or proteins, in which samples are spotted directly onto the substrate, without first being separated electrophoretically, then hybridized to the probe of interest 斑点印迹；**Northern b.**, a technique analogous to a Southern blot but performed on fragments of RNA 一种类似于 Southern 印迹但用于 RNA 片段分析的技术；**Southern b.**, a blot obtained by transferring electrophoretically separated DNA fragments onto an immobilizing membrane, then detecting specific fragments by their hybridization to defined DNA or RNA probes 通过电泳分离的 DNA 片段转移到固定膜上获得的印迹，然后通过它们与标记的 DNA 或 RNA 探针杂交来检测特异性片段；**Western b.**, a blot obtained by separating proteins electrophoretically, transferring them in place to a filter or membrane, and probing with specific antibodies 通过电泳分离蛋白质，将它们转移到过滤器或膜上，并用特异性抗体探测获得的印迹
blot·ting (blot′ing) soaking up with or transferring to absorbent material 印迹

blue (bloo) 1. a color between green and indigo, produced by energy with wavelengths between 420 and 490 nm 蓝色；2. a dye or stain with this color 蓝色染料或染色剂；**aniline b., aniline b. WS**, a mixture of methyl blue and water blue, or either one individually; used as a counterstain, as a stain for collagen and for connective tissue, and as a component of bacteriological media 苯胺蓝，甲基蓝和水蓝的混合物，或单独一个；用作复染剂，用作胶原蛋白和结缔组织的染色剂，以及作为细菌培养基的组分；**brilliant cresyl b.**, an oxazin dye used in staining blood cells; also used as a less toxic alternative to ethidium bromide in staining nucleic acids 亮甲酚蓝，一种用于染色血细胞的恶嗪染料；在核酸染色中也用作溴化乙锭的毒性较小的替代品；**isosulfan b.**, a dye injected subcutaneously to delineate lymphatic vessels draining the region injected 异硫蓝，皮下注射染料以描绘引流注射区域的淋巴管；**methyl b.**, a blue dye of the triarylmethane class; used, alone or in combination with water blue, as a biological stain 三芳基甲烷类的蓝色染料；单独使用或与水蓝组合使用作为生物染色剂；见 *aniline b. WS.*；**methylene b.**, dark green crystals or crystalline powder with a bronzelike luster; used in the treatment of congenital or toxic methemoglobinemia, as a bacteriologic, biologic, and

pathologic stain, as a colorimetric indicator, and as a dye to stain tissues prior to surgery 亚甲基蓝，深绿色晶体或结晶粉末，具有青铜色光泽；用于治疗先天性或毒性甲状腺球蛋白血症，作为细菌学、生物学和病理学染色剂，作为比色指示剂，以及作为染色在手术前染色组织的染料；**Prussian b.**, an amorphous blue powder used as a dye; it is also used in the treatment of internal contamination with radioactive cesium and radioactive or nonradioactive thallium, to speed their elimination 普鲁士蓝，用作染料的无定形蓝色粉末；它还用于处理放射性铯和放射性或非放射性铊的内部污染，以加速其消除；**toluidine b. O**, a basic blue dye related to methylene blue; used for both orthochromatic and metachromatic staining 甲苯胺蓝，与亚甲基有关的碱性蓝染料；用于正色染色和异染色；**water b.**, a blue dye of the triarylmethane class; used, alone or in combination with methyl blue, as a biological stain 水蓝；见 *aniline b. WS*

blunt (blunt) having a thick or dull edge or point; not sharp 钝的
blur (blər) indistinctness, clouding, or fogging 模糊不清，混浊或迷雾；**spectacle b.**, the indistinct vision with spectacles occurring after removal of contact lenses, especially non–gas-permeable lenses 去除隐形眼镜后出现的眼镜模糊不清，尤其是非透气性镜片；it is believed to result from chronic corneal hypoxia and edema 据报道是由慢性角膜缺氧和水肿引起的
BMA British Medical Association 英国医学会
BMI body mass index 体质量指数，体重指数
BMIS Bioresearch Monitoring Information System 生物研究监测信息系统
BMP bone morphogenetic protein 骨形态发生蛋白
BMR basal metabolic rate 基础代谢率
BMT bone marrow transplantation 骨髓移植
BOA British Orthopaedic Association 英国矫形外科协会
bob·bing (bob′ing) a quick, jerky, up-and-down movement 快速、抽动性的上下运动；**ocular b.**, a jerky downward deviation of the eyes with slow return, seen in comatose patients and believed to be due to a pontine lesion 在昏迷的患者中看到眼睛的急剧向下偏离和缓慢的返回，认为是由于脑桥病变
bo·cep·re·vir (bō-sep′rə-vir) a first-generation protease inhibitor previously used in combination therapy to treat chronic hepatitis C virus 波西普韦，用于联合治疗的第一代蛋白酶抑制剂，用于治疗慢性丙型肝炎病毒
body (bod′e) 1. the entire physical substance of an organism 身体；2. the largest and most important part

of any organ 器官的主体部分；3. any mass or collection of material 实体；4. a cadaver or corpse 尸体；**acetone b's,** ketone bodies 酮体；**amygdaloid b.,** corpus amygdaloideum 杏仁核；**anococcygeal b.,** 见 *ligament* 下条；**aortic b's,** small neurovascular structures on either side of the aorta in the region of the aortic arch, containing chemoreceptors that play a role in reflex regulation of respiration 主动脉体，在主动脉弓区域的主动脉两侧的小神经血管结构，含有化学感受器，其在呼吸调节中发挥作用；**b's of Arantius,** small tubercles, one at the center of the free margin of each of the three leaflets of the aortic and pulmonary valves 小结节状，位于主动脉瓣、肺动脉瓣各瓣叶的游离缘中心；**asbestos b's,** ferruginous bodies whose center is asbestos 石棉小体；**Aschoff b's,** perivascular foci of inflammation in the interstitial tissues of the heart in rheumatic fever 阿绍夫小体；**asteroid b.,** an irregularly star-shaped inclusion body found in the giant cells in sarcoidosis and other diseases 在结节病和其他疾病的巨细胞中发现的不规则星形包涵体；**Auer b's,** finely granular, lamellar bodies having acid-phosphatase activity, found in the cytoplasm of myeloblasts, myelocytes, monoblasts, and granular histiocytes, rarely in plasma cells, and virtually pathognomonic of leukemia 棒状小体，具有酸性磷酸酶活性的细小的层状体，存在于成髓细胞、骨髓细胞、原始单核细胞和颗粒状组织细胞的细胞质中，很少存在于浆细胞中，并且几乎是白血病的病理学特征；**Barr b.,** a chromatin mass in the nucleus of somatic cells of females of most mammalian species, including humans. It represents a single, inactive, condensed X chromosome 巴氏小体，大多数哺乳动物物种（包括人类）雌性体细胞核内的染色质团。它代表一个单一的，无活性的，浓缩的X染色体；**basal b.,** a modified centriole that occurs at the base of a flagellum or cilium 基体，特化的中心粒，发生在鞭毛或纤毛的基部；**Cabot ring b's,** lines in the form of loops or figures-of-8, seen in stained erythrocytes in severe anemias Cabot 环，见于严重贫血患者的红细胞；**carotid b.,** a small neurovascular structure lying in the bifurcation of the right and left carotid arteries, containing chemoreceptors that monitor oxygen content in blood and help to regulate respiration 颈动脉体，一种小的神经血管结构，位于右颈动脉和左颈动脉的分叉处，含有可以监测血液中氧含量并有助于调节呼吸的化学感受器；**cavernous b. of penis,** corpus cavernosum penis 阴茎海绵体；**cell b.,** the portion of a cell that contains the nucleus, independent of projections such as an axon or dendrites 细胞体，包含细胞核的细胞主体部分；**ciliary b.,** the thickened part of the vascular tunic of the eye, connecting the choroid and iris 睫状体，眼球血管膜的增厚部分，连接脉

络膜和虹膜；**Döhle inclusion b's,** small bodies seen in the cytoplasm of neutrophils in many infectious diseases, burns, aplastic anemia, and other disorders, and after the administration of toxic agents Döhle 包涵体 在许多传染病、烧伤、再生障碍性贫血、其他疾病以及毒性剂给药后，中性粒细胞的细胞质中看到的小体；**Donovan b.,** *Klebsiella granulomatis* Donovan 小体；**embryoid b's,** structures resembling embryos, seen in several types of germ cell tumors 胚状体，类似于胚胎的结构，见于几种生殖细胞肿瘤；**ferruginous b's,** small masses of mineral matter in the lungs resulting from deposition of calcium salts, iron salts, and protein around a central core of foreign matter 含铁小体，由于钙盐、铁盐和蛋白质在外来物质核心周围沉积而导致的肺部少量矿物质；**foreign b.,** a mass or particle of material that is not normal to the place where it is found 异物；**fruiting b.,** a specialized structure, as an apothecium, which produces spores 子实体一种专门的结构，作为产生孢子的子囊盘；**Gamna-Gandy b's,** brown or yellow pigmented nodules seen in some types of splenomegaly 在某些类型的脾肿大中可见褐色或黄色色素性结节；**geniculate b., lateral,** an eminence of the metathalamus, just lateral to the medial geniculate body, marking the end of the optic tract 外侧膝状体，在内侧膝状体外侧的后丘脑的隆起，标志着视神经束的末端；**geniculate b., medial,** an eminence of the metathalamus, just lateral to the superior colliculi, concerned with hearing 在上丘的侧面，与听觉有关的后丘脑的隆起；**glomus b.,** a specialized arteriovenous shunt occurring predominantly in the skin of the hands and feet, regulating blood flow and temperature 血管球体，一种专门的动静脉分流，主要发生在手脚皮肤，调节血液流量和温度；**Golgi b.,** 高尔基体；见 *complex* 下词条；**Hassall b's,** one of the formed elements of the blood; a leukocyte, erythrocyte, or platelet 胸腺小体，血液中有形成分；白细胞、红细胞或血小板；**Heinz b's, Heinz-Ehrlich b's,** inclusion bodies resulting from oxidative injury to and precipitation of hemoglobin; seen in the presence of certain abnormal hemoglobins and erythrocytes with enzyme deficiencies 由氧化损伤和血红蛋白沉淀引起的包涵体；存在于某些异常血红蛋白病和酶缺陷红细胞；**hematoxylin b.,** a dense, homogeneous particle consisting of the denatured nuclear material of an injured cell, occurring in systemic lupus erythematosus; lymphocytes that ingest such particles are known as LE cells 苏木精体，一种致密的、均匀的颗粒，由受损细胞的变性核物质组成，存在于系统性红斑狼疮中；摄取这种颗粒的淋巴细胞称为 LE 细胞。又称 *LE b.*；**Howell-Jolly b's,** smooth, round remnants of nuclear chromatin seen in erythrocytes in megaloblastic anemia, hemolytic anemia, and after splenec-

B

tomy 染色质小体，在巨幼红细胞性贫血，溶血性贫血和脾切除术后的红细胞中见到的光滑的圆形核染色质残留物；**hyaloid b.**，见 vitreous b.；**immune b.**, antibody 抗体；**inclusion b's**, round, oval, or irregular-shaped bodies in the cytoplasm and nuclei of cells, as in disease due to viral infection, such as rabies or smallpox 包涵体，细胞质和细胞核中的圆形、椭圆形或不规则形状的小体，如病毒感染引起的疾病，如狂犬病或天花；**ketone b's**, the substances acetone, acetoacetic acid, and β-hydroxybutyric acid; except for acetone (which may arise spontaneously from acetoacetic acid), they are normal metabolic products of lipid within the liver, and are oxidized by muscles; excessive production leads to urinary secretion of these bodies, as in diabetes mellitus 酮体，物质丙酮，乙酰乙酸和 β- 羟丁酸；除丙酮（可能由乙酰乙酸自发产生）外，它们是肝脏内脂质的正常代谢产物，被肌肉氧化；过量生产导致其从尿液分泌，如糖尿病；**Lafora b's**, intracytoplasmic inclusions consisting of a complex of glycoprotein and acid mucopolysaccharide; found in Lafora disease 拉福拉小体，胞浆内包涵体由糖蛋白和酸性黏多糖组成的复合物组成；发现于拉福拉病；**lamellar b.**, keratinosome; a type of spherical granule in cells of the skin that migrates to the cytoplasm and discharges its contents into the intercellular space, where the granules are believed to function as a barrier against foreign substances 皮肤细胞中的一种球形颗粒，它迁移到细胞质中并将其内容物排放到细胞间隙中，该颗粒被认为是对抗外来物质的屏障；**LE b.**，见 hematoxylin b.；**Leishman-Donovan b.**, amastigote 利杜体，无鞭毛体；**Lewy b's**, concentrically laminated inclusion bodies consisting of α -synuclein, seen in neurodegenerative conditions such as Parkinson disease and multiple system atrophy 路易体，同心层叠的包涵体由 α- 突触核蛋白组成，见于神经退行性疾病如帕金森病和多系统萎缩；**mammillary b.**, either of the pair of small spherical masses in the interpeduncular fossa of the midbrain, forming part of the hypothalamus 乳头体，在大脑中间的间隙窝中的一对小球形块中的任何一个，形成下丘脑的一部分；**Masson b's**, cellular tissue that fills the pulmonary alveoli and alveolar ducts in rheumatic pneumonia; they may be modified Aschoff bodies 在风湿性肺炎中填充肺泡和肺泡管的细胞组织；可能特化为 Aschoff 小体；**metachromatic b's**, 异染小体，见 granule 下词条；**Negri b's**, round or oval inclusion bodies seen in the cytoplasm and sometimes in the processes of certain nerve cells in rabies; pathognomonic for the disease 内氏小体，在细胞质中看到的圆形或椭圆形包涵体，有时见于狂犬病的某些神经细胞中；为这种疾病的特征；**Nissl b's**, large granular basophilic bodies found in the cytoplasm of neurons, composed of rough endoplasmic reticulum and free polyribosomes 尼氏体，在神经元的细胞质中发现的大颗粒嗜碱性体，由粗面内质网和游离多聚体组成；**olivary b.**, olive (2) 橄榄体；**pacchionian b.**, arachnoidal granulations 蛛网膜颗粒；**Papp-Lantos b's**, inclusion bodies composed of α-synuclein, found chiefly in the cytoplasm of oligodendrocytes, that are characteristic of multiple system atrophy 由 α- 突触蛋白组成的包涵体，见于少突胶质细胞的细胞质，是多系统萎缩的特征；**para-aortic b's**, enclaves of chromaffin cells near the sympathetic ganglia along the abdominal aorta, serving as chemoreceptors responsive to oxygen, carbon dioxide, and hydrogen ion concentration and which help control respiration 主动脉旁体，沿着腹主动脉的交感神经节附近的嗜铬细胞区，作为对氧气、二氧化碳和氢离子浓度有响应的化学感受器，有助于控制呼吸；**pineal b.**，见 gland 下词条；**pituitary b.**, hypophysis 垂体；**polar b's**, 1. small nonfunctional cells consisting of a tiny bit of cytoplasm and a nucleus, resulting from unequal division of the primary oocyte (first polar b.) and, if fertilization occurs, of the secondary oocyte (second polar b.) 极体，小的非功能性细胞，由一小部分细胞质和细胞核组成，由初级卵母细胞（第一极体）的不均等分裂产生，如果受精，则由次级卵母细胞(第二极体) 产生；2. metachromatic granules located at the ends of bacteria 位于细菌的末端的异染色颗粒端；**psammoma b.**, a spherical, concentrically laminated mass of calcareous material, usually of microscopic size; such bodies occur in both benign and malignant epithelial and connective tissue tumors, and are sometimes associated with chronic inflammation 砂粒体，球形，同心层叠的钙质材料，通常具有微观尺寸；这些小体发生在良性和恶性上皮和结缔组织肿瘤中，并且有时与慢性炎症有关；**quadrigeminal b's**, corpora quadrigemina 四叠体；**restiform b.**, the larger part of the inferior cerebellar peduncle (and formerly equated with it), located on the dorsolateral aspect of the medulla oblongata and containing various cerebellar afferent fibers 绳状体，较低部分的小脑下脚，位于延髓的背外侧，包含各种小脑传入纤维；**Russell b's**, globular plasma cell inclusions, representing aggregates of immunoglobulins synthesized by the cell 球状类细胞包涵体，代表由细胞合成的免疫球蛋白的聚集体；**b. of sternum**, the principal portion of the sternum, located between the manubrium above and the xiphoid process below 胸骨体；**trachoma b's**, inclusion bodies found in clusters in the cytoplasm of the epithelial cells of the conjunctiva in trachoma 包涵体在沙眼结膜上皮细胞的细胞质中聚集；**trapezoid b.**, a mass of transverse fibers extending through the central part of the caudal pons and forming a part of the path of the cochlear nerve 斜方体，延伸于脑桥尾部并构成部分耳蜗神经的一群横行纤维斜方体，延伸于脑桥尾部并构成部分耳蜗神经的一群横行纤维；**tympanic b.,** an ovoid body in the upper part of the superior bulb of the internal jugular vein, believed similar to the carotid body in structure and function 颈静脉球体，颈内静脉上部球茎上部的卵圆形体，在结构和功能上与颈动脉体相似；**vermiform b's,** peculiar sinuous invaginations of the plasma membrane of Kupffer cells of the liver 肝脏库普弗细胞质膜的特殊蜿蜒内陷；**vitreous b.,** the loose fibrillar mesh and transparent gel filling the inner portion of the eyeball between the lens, ciliary body, and retina; sometimes incorrectly equated with *vitreous humor* 玻璃体；**Weibel-Palade b's,** rod-shaped intracytoplasmic bundles of microtubules specific for vascular endothelial cells and used as markers for endothelial cell neoplasms W-P 小体，血管内皮细胞特有的杆状胞质内微管束，用作内皮细胞肿瘤的标记物

body·work (bod′e-wurk″) a general term for therapeutic methods that center on the body for the promotion of physical health and emotional and spiritual well-being, including massage, various systems of touch and manipulation, relaxation techniques, and practices designed to affect the body's energy flow 治疗方法的一般术语，以身体为中心，促进身体，情感和精神健康，包括按摩，各种触觉和操作系统，放松技术，以及旨在影响身体能量流动的实践

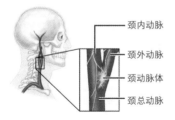

▲ 颈动脉体（**carotid body**），位于颈动脉分叉深处，由舌咽、迷走神经和交感神经支配

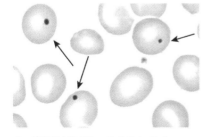

▲ 染色质小体（**Howell−Jolly bodies**）

boil (boil) furuncle 疖

Bo·le·tus (bo-le′təs) a genus of fungi containing both edible and poisonous species; several species produce the toxin muscarine 牛肝菌属，含有食用和有毒物种的真菌；几物种产生毒素毒蕈碱

bo·lus (bo′ləs) 1. a rounded mass of food or pharmaceutical preparation ready to swallow, or such a mass passing through the gastrointestinal tract 丸；2. a concentrated mass of pharmaceutical preparation, e.g., an opaque contrast medium, given intravenously 浓缩的药物制剂，例如不透明的造影剂，静脉内给药；3. a mass of scattering material, such as wax or paraffin, placed between the radiation source and the skin to achieve a precalculated isodose pattern in the tissue irradiated 放置在辐射源和皮肤之间的大量散射材料，例如蜡或石蜡，以在被照射的组织中实现预先精制的等剂量图案

bom·be·sin (bom′bə-sin) a tetradecapeptide neurotransmitter and hormone found in the brain and gut 蛙皮素，一种十四肽神经递质和激素大脑和肠道

bond (bond) the linkage between atoms or radicals of a chemical compound, or the mark indicating the number and attachment of the valences of an atom in constitutional formulas, represented by a pair of dots or a line between atoms, e.g., H—O—H, H—C ≡ C—H or H:O:H, H:C:::C:H 化学键；**coordinate covalent b.,** a covalent bond in which one of the bonded atoms furnishes both of the shared electrons 配位共价键；**covalent b.,** a chemical bond between two atoms or radicals formed by the sharing of a pair (single bond), two pairs (double bond), or three pairs of electrons (triple bond) 共价键；**disulfide b.,** a strong covalent bond, —S—S—, important in linking polypeptide chains in proteins, the linkage arising as a result of the oxidation of the sulfhydryl (SH) groups of two molecules of cysteine 二硫键；**high energy b.,** a chemical bond the hydrolysis of which yields high levels of free energy; it may involve phosphate (*high energy phosphate b.*) or sulfur (*high energy sulfur b.*) or other mixed anhydride types of chemical structure 高能键；**hydrogen b.,** a weak, primarily electrostatic, bond between a hydrogen atom bound to a highly electronegative element in a given molecule and a second highly electronegative atom in another molecule or elsewhere in the same molecule; it is usually represented by three dots, e.g., X—H···Y 氢键；**ionic b.,** a chemical bond in which electrons are transferred from one atom to another so that one bears a negative and the other a positive charge, the attraction between these opposite charges forming the bond 离子键；**peptide b.,** a—CO—NH— linkage formed between the carboxyl group of one amino acid and the amino group of another; it is an amide linkage joining amino acids to form peptides 肽键

bone (bōn) 1. the hard, rigid form of connective tissue constituting most of the skeleton of vertebrates, composed chiefly of calcium salts 骨; 2. any distinct piece of the skeleton of the body 人体骨骼系统的任何独立部分。见附表和 Plate1，Plate2；**acetabular b.**, acetabulum 髋臼；**alveolar b.**, the thin layer of bone making up the bony processes of the maxilla and mandible, and surrounding and containing the teeth; it is pierced by many small openings through which blood vessels, lymphatics, and nerve fibers pass 牙槽骨；**ankle b.**, talus 踝骨；**back b.**, vertebral column 脊柱；**breast b.**, sternum 胸骨；**brittle b's**, osteogenesis imperfecta 成骨不全；**cancellous b.**, 松质骨，见 *lamellar b.*；**capitate b.**, the bone in the distal row of carpal bones lying between the trapezoid and hamate bones 头状骨；又称 *os capitatum*；**carpal b's**, the eight bones of the wrist (carpus), including the capitate, hamate, lunate, pisiform, scaphoid, trapezoid, and triquetral bones and the trapezium bone 腕骨，包括与桡骨相连的近侧列的手舟骨、月骨、三角骨、豌豆骨，以及与掌骨相连的远侧列的大多角骨、小多角骨、头状骨、钩骨。又称 *ossa carpi*；**cartilage b.**, bone developing within cartilage, ossification taking place within a cartilage model 软骨；**cheek b.**, 见 zygomatic b.；**collar b.**, clavicle 锁骨；**compact b.**, 见 *lamellar b.*；**cortical b.**, the compact outer surface of the shaft of a bone that surrounds the medullary cavity 骨皮质；**coxal b.**, hip bone; pelvic bone 髋骨；**cuboid b.**, a bone on the lateral side of the tarsus between the calcaneus and the fourth and fifth metatarsal bones 骰骨；又称 *os cuboideum*；**cuneiform b., intermediate,** the intermediate and smallest of the three wedge-shaped tarsal bones located medial to the cuboid and between the navicular and the first three metatarsal bones 中间楔骨；又称 *os cuneiforme intermedium*；**cuneiform b., lateral,** the most lateral of the three wedgeshaped tarsal bones located medial to the cuboid and between the navicular and the first three metatarsal bones 外侧楔骨；又称 *os cuneiforme laterale*；**cuneiform b., medial,** the medial and largest of the three wedge-shaped tarsal bones located medial to the cuboid and between the navicular and the first three metatarsal bones 内侧楔骨；又称 *os cuneiforme mediale*；**ethmoid b.**, the cubical bone located between the orbits and consisting of the lamina cribrosa, the lamina perpendicularis, and the paired lateral masses 筛骨；又称 *os ethmoidale*；**flat b.**, one whose thickness is slight, sometimes consisting of only a thin layer of compact bone, or of two layers with intervening cancellous bone and marrow; usually curved rather than flat 扁骨；**frontal b.**, a single bone that closes the anterior part of the cranial cavity and forms the skeleton of the forehead; it is developed from two halves, the line of separation (the metopic suture) sometimes persisting in adult life 额骨。又称 *os frontale*；**funny b.**, the region of the medial epicondyle of the humerus where it is crossed by the ulnar nerve 鹰嘴突，肱骨内侧上髁区域，与尺神经交叉；**hamate b.**, the medial bone in the distal row of carpal bones 钩骨；又称 *os hamatum*；**heel b.**, calcaneus 跟骨；**hip b.**, the large bone in the hip, consisting of the ilium, ischium, and pubic bone 髋骨，由髂骨、坐骨和耻骨组成。又称 *os coxae*；**hyoid b.**, a horseshoe-shaped bone situated at the base of the tongue, just superior to the thyroid cartilage 舌骨；又称 *os hyoideum*；**incisive b.**, the portion of the maxilla bearing the incisors; developmentally, it is the premaxilla, which in humans later fuses with the maxilla, but in most other vertebrates persists as a separate bone 切牙骨，带有门牙的上颌骨部分；在发育上，它是前颌骨，在人类中，它后来与上颌骨融合，但在大多数其他脊椎动物中仍作为单独的骨骼；**innominate b.**, 见 hip b. 髋骨；**jaw b.**, the mandible or maxilla, especially the mandible 颌骨；**jugal b.**, 见 zygomatic b.；**lacrimal b.**, a thin scalelike bone at the anterior part of the labyrinthine wall of the orbit, articulating with the frontal and ethmoid bones and the maxilla and inferior nasal concha 泪骨。又称 *os lacrimale*；**lamellar b.**, the normal type of adult bone, organized in layers (lamellae), which may be parallel (*cancellous b.*) or concentrically arranged (*compact b.*) 板层骨；**lingual b.**, 见 hyoid b.；**long b.**, a bone that has a longitudinal axis of considerable length, consisting of a body or shaft (diaphysis) and an expanded portion (epiphysis) at each end that is usually articular; typically found in the limbs 长骨。又称 *os longum*；**lunate b.**, the bone in the proximal row of carpal bones lying between the scaphoid and triquetral bones 月骨；又称 *os lunatum*；**malar b.**, 见 zygomatic b.；**marble b's**, osteopetrosis 硬骨症；**mastoid b.**, mastoid part of temporal bone 乳突骨；见 *part* 下词条；**metacarpal b's**, metacarpals; the five cylindrical bones of the hand, which articulate proximally with the bones of the carpus and distally with the proximal phalanges of the fingers; numbered from that articulating with the phalanx of the thumb to that articulating with the phalanx of the little finger 掌骨。又称 *ossa metacarpi*；**metatarsal b's**, metatarsals; the five bones extending from the tarsus to the phalanges of the toes, being numbered in the same sequence from the most medial to the most lateral 跖骨；又称 *ossa metatarsi*；**nasal b.**, either of the two small, oblong bones that together form the bridge of the nose 鼻骨；又称 *os nasale*；**navicular b.**, the ovoid-shaped tarsal bone found between the talus and the three cuneiform bones 足舟骨；又称 *os naviculare*；**occipital b.,** a single trapezoid-shaped bone situated at the lower posterior part of the cranium, articulating with the two parietal and two temporal bones, the sphenoid bone, and the atlas; it contains a large opening, the foramen magnum 枕骨。又称 *os occipitale*；**palatine b.,** the irregularly shaped bone forming the posterior part of the hard palate, the lateral wall of the nasal fossa between the medial pterygoid plate and the maxilla, and the posterior part of the floor of the orbit 腭骨。又称 *os palatinum*；**parietal b.,** either of the two quadrilateral bones forming part of the superior and lateral surfaces of the skull, and joining each other in the midline at the sagittal suture 顶骨。又称 *os parietale*；**pelvic b.,** hip b. 骨盆；**petrous b.,** petrous part of temporal bone 颞骨岩部；见 *part* 下词条；**pisiform b.,** the medial bone of the proximal row of carpal bones 豌豆骨；又称 *os pisiforme*；**pneumatic b.,** bone that contains air-filled spaces 含气骨；**premaxillary b.,** premaxilla 前颌骨；**pterygoid b.,** 翼骨，见 *process* 下词条；**pubic b.,** pubis; the lower anterior part of the coxal bone on either side, articulating with its fellow in the anterior midline at the pubic symphysis 耻骨。又称 *os pubis*；**rider's b.,** localized ossification of the inner aspect of the lower end of the tendon of the adductor muscle of the thigh; sometimes seen in horseback riders 大腿内收肌腱下端内侧的局部骨化；有时在骑马者身上看到过；**scaphoid b.,** the most lateral bone of the proximal row of carpal bones 舟骨；又称 *os scaphoideum*；**semilunar b.,** 见 lunate b.；**sesamoid b's,** numerous ovoid nodular bones, often small, usually found embedded within a tendon or joint capsule, principally in the hands and feet (where they are called also *ossa sesamoidea*); two sesamoid bones, the fabella and patella, are associated with the knee 籽骨；**shin b.,** tibia 胫骨；**sphenoid b.,** a single irregular, wedge-shaped bone at the base of the skull, forming a part of the floor of the anterior, middle, and posterior cranial fossae 蝶骨；又称 *os sphenoidale*；**spongy b.,** cancellous b. 松质骨；见 *lamellar b.*；**squamous b.,** squamous part of temporal bone 鳞状骨；见 *part* 下词条；**sutural b.,** variable and irregularly shaped bones in the sutures between the bones of the skull 缝间骨；**tail b.,** coccyx 尾骨；**tarsal b's,** the seven bones of the ankle (tarsus), including the calcaneus, talus, cuboid and navicular bones, and intermediate, lateral, and medial cuneiform bones 足骨中的跗骨，共7块，包括跟骨、距骨、足舟骨、骰骨、中间楔骨、内侧楔骨、外侧楔骨。又称 *ossa tarsi*；**temporal b.,** one of the two irregular bones forming part of the lateral surfaces and base of the skull, and containing the organs of hearing. It is divided anatomically into pe-

trous, mastoid, squamous, and tympanic parts 颞骨。又称 *os temporale*；**thigh b.,** femur 股骨；**trabecular b.,** cancellous b. 小梁骨；见 *lamellar b.*；**trapezoid b.,** the bone in the distal row of carpal bones lying between the trapezium and capitate bones; called also *os trapezoideum* 小多角骨；**triquetral b.,** the bone in the proximal row of carpal bones lying between the lunate and pisiform bones 三角骨；又称 *os triquetrum*；**turbinate b.,** any of the nasal conchae 鼻甲骨；**tympanic b.,** tympanic ring of temporal bone 鼓骨；见 *part* 下词条；**unciform b., uncinate b.,** 见 hamate b.；**wormian b.,** sutural b. 缝间骨；**zygomatic b.,** the quadrangular bone of the cheek, articulating with the frontal bone, maxilla, temporal bone, and greater wing of sphenoid bone 颧骨。又称 *os zygomaticum*

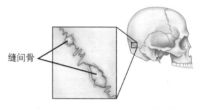

缝间骨

bony (bo′ne) 1. pertaining to, characterized by, resembling, or consisting of bone 骨的；2. having an internal skeleton made of bones 具有由骨头制成的内部骨架；3. having prominent bones or being lean or scrawny 瘦骨嶙峋

Bo·oph·i·lus (bo-of′ĭ-ləs) a genus of hardbodied ticks that are vectors of babesiosis, including *B. annula′tus,* the vector of *Babesia bigemina*；*B. mi′croplus,* the vector of *Babesia bovis*；and *B. cal-cara′tus,* the vector of *Babesia major* 牛蜱属，一种硬体蜱，是巴贝虫病的载体

boost·er (boost′ər) 见 *dose* 下词条

boot (boot) an encasement for the foot; a protective casing or sheath 靴子；**Gibney b.,** an adhesive tape support used in treatment of sprains and other painful conditions of the ankle, the tape being applied in a basketweave fashion with strips placed alternately under the sole of the foot and around the back of the leg 一种用于治疗扭伤和脚踝其他疼痛胶带支撑物，该胶带以篮网方式施加，条带交替地放置在脚底和脚后部周围

bor·age (bor′ij) *Borago officinalis* or preparations of its flowers, stems, and seeds, which are used in folk medicine for a wide variety of disorders 玻璃苣或其花、茎、种子的制品，在民间用于治疗各种疾病；见 *oil*

bo·rate (bor′āt) a salt of boric acid 硼酸盐

bo·rax (bor′aks) sodium borate 硼砂

150

Skeleton (Total = 80) 骨骼 (总数 =80)

Region 部位	Total Number 总数	Name 名称
Skull 头骨	21	(eight paired-16)（8 对 -16） Nasal concha 鼻甲 Lacrimal 泪骨 Maxilla 上颌骨 Nasal 鼻骨 Palatine 腭骨 Parietal 顶骨 Temporal 颞骨 Zygomatic 颧骨 (five unpaired-5)（5 个不成对的 -5） Ethmoid 筛骨 Frontal 额骨 Occipital 枕骨 Sphenoid 蝶骨 Vomer 犁骨
Auditory ossicles (×2) 听觉鼓膜处(x2)	6	Incus 砧骨 Malleus 锤骨 Stapes 镫骨
Lower jaw 下颌	1	Mandible 下颌骨
Neck 颈部	1	Hyoid 舌骨
Vertebral column 脊柱	26	Cervical vertebrae (C1–C7) 颈椎 (C1–C7) Atlas (C1) 寰椎 (C1) Axis (C2) 枢椎 (C2) Thoracic vertebrae (T1–T12) 胸椎 (T1–T12) Lumbar vertebrae (L1–L5) 腰椎 (L1–L5) Sacrum (S1–S5, fused) 骶骨 (S1–S5, 融合) Coccyx (4, fused) 尾骨 (融合)
Chest 胸部	25	Sternum 胸骨 Ribs (12 pairs) 肋骨 (12 对)

Upper Limb (× 2) (Total = 64) 上肢（x2）（总数 =64）

Region 部位	Total Number 总数	Name 名称
Shoulder 肩部	2	Scapula 肩胛骨 Clavicle 锁骨
Upper arm 上臂	1	Humerus 肱骨
Lower arm Ulna 下臂 尺骨	2	Radius 桡骨
Carpus 腕部	8	Capitate 头状骨 Hamate 钩骨 Lunate 月骨 Pisiform 豌豆骨 Scaphoid 手舟骨 Trapezium 大多角骨 Trapezoid 小多角骨 Triquetral 三角骨
Hand 手	5	Metacarpal 掌骨
Fingers 手指	14	Phalanges 指骨

Lower Limb (× 2) (Total = 62) 下肢（x2）（总数 =62）

Region 部位	Total Number 总数	Name 名称
Pelvis 骨盆	1	Coxal bone 髋骨 (Ilium) (髂骨) (Ischium) (坐骨) (Pubis) (耻骨)
Thigh 大腿	1	Femur 股骨
Knee 膝	1	Patella 髌骨
Leg 小腿	2	Tibia 胫骨 Fibula 腓骨
Tarsus 跗骨	7	Calcaneus 跟骨 Cuboid 骰骨 Intermediate cuneiform 内侧楔状骨 Lateral cuneiform 外侧楔状骨 Medial cuneiform 中间楔状骨 Navicular 足舟骨 Talus 距骨
Foot 脚	5	Metatarsal 跖骨
Toes 脚趾	14	Phalanges 趾骨

bor·bo·ryg·mus (bor"bə-rig'məs) pl. *borboryg'mi* [L.] a rumbling noise caused by propulsion of gas through the intestines 肠鸣

bor·der (bor'dər) a bounding line, edge, or surface 边界; brush b., a specialization of the free surface of a cell, consisting of minute cylindrical processes (microvilli) that greatly increase the surface area 刷状缘; vermilion b., the exposed red portion of the upper and lower lips 上唇和下唇的外露红色部分

bor·der·line (bor'dər-līn) of a phenomenon, straddling the dividing line between two categories 分界线

Bor·de·tel·la (bor"də-tel'ə) a genus of gramnegative, aerobic bacteria of the family Alcaligenaceae, made up of organisms that are parasites and pathogens of the respiratory tract 鲍特菌，产碱杆菌科的革兰阳性需氧菌; *B. parapertus'sis*, a species that is immunologically related to *B. pertussis* and causes parapertussis and occasionally classic pertussis 副百日咳鲍特菌，与百日咳鲍特菌免疫相关并引起副百日咳和偶尔经典百日咳的物种; *B. pertus'sis*, the usual cause of pertussis (whooping cough) 副博德特氏菌

bo·ric ac·id (bor'ik) H_3BO_3; used as a buffer and weak antimicrobial, and as a pesticide to kill ants and cockroaches 硼酸，用作缓冲剂和弱抗菌剂，以及用作杀灭蚂蚁和蟑螂的杀虫剂。另见 *sodium borate*

bo·ron (B) (bor'on) a metalloid element occurring as amorphous brown powder and gray-black crystals; at. no. 5, at. wt. 10.81 硼，非金属元素，呈无定形棕色粉末和灰黑色晶体

Bor·rel·ia (bə-rel'e-ə) a genus of bacteria of the family Spirochaetaceae, parasitic in many animals. *B. burgdor'feri* causes Lyme disease and skin disease, and numerous species cause relapsing fever 包柔氏螺旋体科的一种细菌，寄生在许多动物身上。包柔氏螺旋体引起莱姆病和皮肤病，许多物种引起复发性发热

bor·rel·i·o·sis (bə-rel"e-o'sis) infection with spirochetes of the genus *Borrelia* 疏螺旋体属病; Lyme b., any of several diseases caused by *Borrelia burgdorferi* and having similar manifestations, including Lyme disease, acrodermatitis chronica atrophicans, and erythema chronicum migrans 由伯氏疏螺旋体引起并具有相似表现的几种疾病中的任何一种，包括莱姆病、慢性萎缩性皮炎和慢性迁移性红斑病

boss (bos) a rounded eminence 疣突

bot (bot) the larva of botflies, which may be

parasitic in the stomach of animals and sometimes humans 马蝇的幼虫，可能寄生在动物的胃中，有时也会寄生在人体内

Both·rio·ceph·a·lus (both″re-o-sef′ə-ləs) *Diphyllobothrium* 阔节裂头绦虫

bot·ry·oid (bot′re-oid) shaped like a bunch of grapes 葡萄状

bot·u·li·form (boch′u-lĭ-form) sausageshaped 香肠状的

bot·u·li·nal (boch″u-lī′nəl) 1. pertaining to *Clostridium botulinum* 与肉毒梭菌有关；2. pertaining to botulinum toxin 与肉毒梭菌毒素有关

bot·u·lism (boch′ə-liz-əm) an extremely severe type of food poisoning due to a neurotoxin (botulin) produced by *Clostridium botulinum* in improperly canned or preserved foods 肉毒梭菌中毒，由于肉毒梭菌在罐装或保存不当的食品中产生的神经毒素（肉毒梭菌）引起的极其严重的食物中毒；**infant b.,** that affecting infants, thought to result from toxin produced in the gut by ingested organisms, rather than from preformed toxins 影响婴儿的，被认为是由摄入肠道有机体产生的毒素，而不是来自预先形成的毒素；**wound b.,** a form resulting from infection of a wound with *Clostridium botulinum* 肉毒梭菌感染伤口

bou·gie (boo-zhe′) a slender, flexible, hollow or solid, cylindrical instrument for introduction into the urethra or other tubular organ, usually for calibrating or dilating constricted areas 探条，细长的，柔软的，中空的或实心的圆柱形器械，用于引入尿道或其他管状器官，通常用于校准或扩张狭窄区域；**bulbous b.,** one with a bulb-shaped tip 球头探条；**filiform b.,** one of very slender caliber 丝状探头

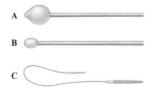

▲ 探条（bougie）。A 和 B. 球头探头。C. 丝状探头

bound (bound) 1. restrained or confined 被克制的；not free 被限制的；2. held in chemical combination 被化学结合的

bou·ton (boo-tahn′) [Fr.] a buttonlike swelling on an axon where it has a synapse with another neuron 轴突上的膨大，位于其通过突触与其他神经连接处；**synaptic b.,** 见 b. terminal；**b. terminal,** (ter-mĭ-nahl′) a buttonlike terminal enlargement of an axon that ends in relation to another neuron at a

synapse 突触结

bo·vine (bo′vīn) pertaining to, characteristic of, or derived from cattle 与牛有关的

bow (bo) an arched or curved appliance or device 拱形或弯曲的器具或装置

bow·el (bou′əl) the intestine 肠

bow·en·oid (bo′ə-noid) pertaining to or resembling the lesions of Bowen disease 属于或类似鲍恩病的病变

bowl (bōl) a rounded, more or less hemispherical open container 碗；**mastoid b., mastoidectomy b.,** the hollow bony defect in the temporal bone created by open mastoidectomy 开放性乳突切除术产生的颞骨中空骨缺损

bow·leg (bo′leg) genu varum; an outward curvature of one or both legs near the knee O 型腿

box (boks) a rectangular structure 盒，箱；**anatomical snuff-b.,** a triangular depression on the dorsum of the wrist at its lateral border when the thumb is abducted and extended; between the tendon of the extensor pollicis longus medially and the tendons of the extensor pollicis brevis and abductor pollicis longus laterally 鼻烟窝

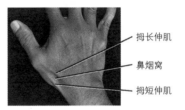

拇长伸肌

鼻烟窝

拇短伸肌

▲ 鼻烟窝 (anatomical snuff-box)

BP blood pressure 血压；*British Pharmacopoeia,* a publication of the General Medical Council, describing and establishing standards for medicines, preparations, materials, and articles used in the practice of medicine, surgery, or midwifery 英国药典

bp base pair 碱基对

BPA British Paediatric Association 英国儿科协会

BPH benign prostatic hyperplasia 良性前列腺增生症

BPIG bacterial polysaccharide immune globulin 细菌多糖免疫球蛋白

Bq becquerel 贝可，放射性活度的国际单位制单位

Br bromine 溴

brace (brās) 1. an orthosis used to support, align, or hold parts of the body in correct position 矫形器，用于支撑，对齐或保持身体各部位的正确位置；2. (*in the pl.*) orthodontic appliance 正畸矫

治器

bra·chi·al (bra′ke-əl) pertaining to the upper limb.

腕板

bra·chi·al·gia (bra″ke-al′jə) pain in the arm 臂痛

bra·chio·ce·phal·ic (bra″ke-o-sə-fal′ik) pertaining to the arm and head 与手臂和头相关的

bra·chio·cu·bi·tal (bra″ke-o-ku′bĭ-təl) pertaining to the arm and elbow or forearm 与手臂、肘部及前臂有关的

bra·chi·um (bra′ke-əm) pl. *bra′chia* [L.] 见 arm (1, 3).; **b. colli′culi inferio′ris,** fibers of the auditory pathway connecting the inferior quadrigeminal body to the medial geniculate body 下 丘 臂; **b. colli′culi superio′ris,** fibers connecting the optic tract and lateral geniculate body with the superior quadrigeminal body 上 丘 臂; **b. conjunc′tivum,** usually, the superior cerebellar peduncle, although it can specifically denote the large mass of cerebellar efferents of the peduncle 小脑上脚

brachy·ba·sia (brak″e-ba′zhə) a slow, shuffling, short-stepped gait 缓慢步态

brachy·ceph·a·ly (brak″e-sef′ə-le) the condition of having a comparatively short head 短头畸形

brachy·dac·ty·ly (brak″e-dak′tə-le) abnormal shortness of fingers and toes 短指（趾）

brach·yg·na·thia (brak″ig-na′the-ə) abnormal shortness of the lower jaw 短颌

brachy·pha·lan·gia (brak″e-fə-lan′jə) abnormal shortness of one or more of the phalanges 短指节畸形

brachy·ther·a·py (brak″e-ther′ə-pe) treatment with ionizing radiation whose source is applied to the surface of the body or within the body a short distance from the area being treated 近程放射治疗

brady·ar·rhyth·mia (brad″e-ə-rith′me-ə) any disturbance in the heart rhythm in which the heart rate is abnormally slowed 心动过缓

brady·car·dia (brad″e-kahr′de-ə) slowness of the heartbeat, as evidenced by slowing of the pulse rate to less than 60 心动过缓; **bradycar′diac** *adj.*

brady·dys·rhyth·mia (brad″e-dis-rith′me-ə) an abnormal heart rhythm with rate less than 60 beats per minute in an adult; *bradyarrhythmia* is usually used instead 缓慢性心律失常

brady·es·the·sia (brad″e-es-the′zhə) slowness or dullness of perception 感觉迟钝

brady·ki·ne·sia (brad″e-kĭ-ne′zhə) abnormal slowness of movement 行动迟缓; **bradykinet′ic** *adj.*

brady·ki·nin (brad″e-ki′nin) a nonapeptide kinin formed from HMW kininogen by the action of kallikrein; it is a very powerful vasodilator and increases capillary permeability; in addition, it constricts smooth muscle and stimulates pain receptors 缓激肽

brady·pnea (brad-ip′ne-ə) abnormal slowness of breathing 呼吸缓慢

brady·sphyg·mia (brad″e-sfig′me-ə) abnormal slowness of the pulse, usually linked to bradycardia 脉搏徐缓

brady·tachy·car·dia (brad″e-tak″ĭ-kahr′de-ə) alternating attacks of bradycardia and tachycardia 心动过缓和心动过速的交替发作

brain (brān) encephalon; that part of the central nervous system contained within the cranium, comprising the forebrain (prosencephalon), midbrain (mesencephalon), and hindbrain (rhombencephalon); it develops from the anterior part of the embryonic neural tube 脑。另见 *cerebrum*; **eloquent b.,** regions of the brain directly involved in speech, motor functions, sensory reception, and cranial nerve function (motor and sensory); such regions are essential to localize in treating brain lesions 大脑功能区; **split b.,** one in which the connections between the hemispheres have been disrupted or severed; used to provide access to the third ventricle or to control epilepsy 半球之间的连接被破坏或切断一个，以便进入第三脑室或控制癫痫

brain·stem (brān′stem) the stemlike portion of the brain connecting the cerebral hemispheres with the spinal cord, and comprising the pons, medulla oblongata, and midbrain; considered by some to include the diencephalon 脑干

brain·wash·ing (brān′wahsh″ing) any systematic effort aimed at instilling certain attitudes and beliefs against a person's will, usually beliefs in conflict with prior beliefs and knowledge 洗脑

bran (bran) the meal derived from the outer covering of a cereal grain; a source of dietary fiber 糠，麸皮

branch (branch) ramus; a division or offshoot from a main stem, especially of blood vessels, nerves, or lymphatics 主干的分裂或分支，特别是血管、神经或淋巴管; **bundle b.,** a branch of the bundle of His 希氏束的分支

branch·er en·zyme (branch′ər en′zīm) 见 *enzyme* 下词条

bran·chi·al (brang′ke-əl) pertaining to or resembling gills of a fish or derivatives of homologous parts in higher forms 属于或类似于鳃或更高形式的同源部分的衍生物

Bran·ha·mel·la (bran″hə-mel′ə) *Moraxella* (*Branhamella*) 布拉汉氏菌属

brash (brash) heartburn 胃灼热; **water b.,** heartburn with regurgitation of sour fluid or almost tasteless saliva into the mouth 反酸

BRB   bright red blood 鲜红血液

BRBNS   blue rubber bleb nevus syndrome 蓝色橡皮疱疹痣综合征

break·down   (brāk′doun) 1. the act or process of ceasing to function 停止运作的行为或过程；2. an often sudden collapse in health 身体状况突然变坏；3. loss of self-control 失去自制力；**nervous b.,** a nonspecific, popular name for any type of mental disorder that interferes with the affected individual's normal activities, often implying a severe episode with sudden onset 非特异性，任何类型的精神障碍的流行名称，干扰受影响的个体的正常活动，通常暗示严重、突然发作

breast   (brest) the front of the chest, especially its modified glandular structure, the mamma 乳腺；另见 *gland* 下 *mammary gland*；**chicken b.,** pectus carinatum 鸡胸；**funnel b.,** pectus excavatum 漏斗胸；**pigeon b.,** pectus carinatum 鸡胸

breast·feed·ing   (brest′ fēd′ing) nursing; the feeding of an infant at the mother's breast 母乳喂养

breath   (breth) the air inhaled and exhaled during ventilation 呼吸

breath·ing   (brēth′ing) ventilation (1) 呼吸；**frog b., glossopharyngeal b.,** breathing in which air is "swallowed" into the lungs by the tongue and muscles of the pharynx, unaided by primary or ordinary accessory muscles of respiration; used by those with chronic muscle paralysis to augment their breathing 舌咽呼吸，在呼吸的主要或普通辅助肌肉的帮助下，通过咽部的舌头和肌肉将空气"吞入"肺部的呼吸；慢性肌肉麻痹患者使用它来增加呼吸；**intermittent positive pressure b.,** the active inflation of the lungs during inhalation under positive pressure from a cycling valve 间断正压通气；**rescue b.,** any artificial respiration technique in which ventilation is supplied by exhaling into the patient's nose or throat, or into a laryngectomy site, airway, or special mask made for the purpose 人工呼吸

breech   (brēch) the buttocks 臀部

breg·ma   (breg′mə) the point on the surface of the skull at the junction of the coronal and sagittal sutures 前囟；**bregmat′ic** *adj.*

bren·tux·i·mab   (bren-tux′i-mab) an antibodydrug conjugate that targets CD30 with cytotoxic activity against lymphomas; administered by injection 维布妥昔单抗，一种抗 CD30 抗体，具有针对淋巴瘤的细胞毒活性，通过注射给药

bre·tyl·i·um   (brə-til′e-əm) an adrenergic blocking agent used as the tosylate salt as an antiarrhythmic in certain cases of ventricular tachycardia or fibrillation 溴苄胺，抗心律失常的药物

brevi·col·lis   (brev″ĭ-kol′ĭs) shortness of the neck 短颈畸形

Bre·vun·di·mo·nas   (brev-un″dĭ-mo′nəs) a genus of aerobic, gram-negative bacteria; *B. vesicula'ris* (formerly *Pseudomonas vesicularis*) causes urinary tract infections and is a rare nosocomial pathogen 短波单胞菌属，一种需氧，革兰阴性细菌；引起尿路感染，是一种罕见的院内感染病原体

bridge   (brij) 1. a structure connecting two separate points, including parts of an organ 桥；2. a fixed partial denture 齿桥；3. tarsal coalition 跗骨联合；**cantilever b.,** a bridge having an artificial tooth attached beyond the point of anchorage of the bridge (口腔医学) 单端固定桥；**cytoplasmic b.,** 1. protoplasmic b. 细胞质桥；2. 见 *intercellular b.*;**disulfide b.,** 二硫键，见 *bond.* 下词条；**extension b.,** cantilever b. 延伸式牙桥；**intercellular b.,** a misnomer for the appearance of the junction of epithelial cells at a desmosome as a result of dehydration during fixation; it was formerly thought to constitute a bridge for cytoplasmic continuity (cytoplasmic bridge) 细胞间桥；**protoplasmic b.,** a strand of protoplasm connecting two secondary spermatocytes, occurring as a result of incomplete cytokinesis 连接两个次级精母细胞的原生质链，由于不完全胞质分裂而发生

bridge·work   (brij′wərk) a partial denture retained by attachments other than clasps 假牙的齿桥；**fixed b.,** one retained with crowns or inlays cemented to the natural teeth 固定齿桥；**removable b.,** one retained by attachments allowing removal 移动性齿桥

brim   (brim) the upper edge of a basin 边缘；**pelvic b.,** the upper edge of the superior strait of the pelvis 骨盆边缘

bri·mo·ni·dine   (brĭ-mo′nə-dēn) an α-adrenergic receptor agonist used as the tartrate salt in the treatment of open-angle glaucoma and ocular hypertension 溴莫尼定，一种 α-肾上腺素能受体激动药，用于用酒石酸盐治疗开角型青光眼和高眼压症

brin·zo·la·mide   (brin-zo′lə-mīd) a carbonic anhydrase inhibitor used in the treatment of open-angle glaucoma and ocular hypertension 布林佐胺，碳酸酐酶抑制剂，用于治疗开角型青光眼和高眼压症

brise·ment   (brēz-maw′) [Fr.] the breaking up or tearing of anything 打碎，撕碎；**b. forcé,** (for-sa′) the breaking up or tearing of a bony ankylosis 关节强直的破裂或撕裂

brit·tle   (brit′əl) 1. easily broken, snapped, or cracked, especially under slight pressure 易碎的；2. easily disrupted 易被打碎的

BRM biologic response modifier 生物反应修饰剂

broach (brōch) a fine barbed instrument for dressing a tooth canal or extracting the pulp 拉刀，一种用于修整牙齿管或拔除牙髓的尖刺器械

bro·me·lain (bro′mə-lān) any of several endopeptidases that catalyze the cleavage of specific bonds in proteins. Different forms are derived from the fruit (*fruit b.*) and stem (*stem b.*) of the pineapple plant, *Ananas comosus*. As the concentrate *bromelains*, it is used as an antiinflammatory agent 菠萝蛋白酶；催化蛋白质特异性键断裂的几种内肽酶中的任何一种

brom·hi·dro·sis (bro″mī-dro′sis) axillary (apocrine) sweat that has become foul smelling as a result of its bacterial decomposition 腋臭

bro·mide (bro′mīd) any binary compound of bromine in which the bromine carries a negative charge (Br⁻); specifically a salt (or organic ester) of hydrobromic acid (H⁺Br⁻) 溴化物

bro·mine (**Br**) (bro′mēn) (bro′min) a fuming reddish-brown liquid element of the halogen group; at. no. 35, at. wt. 79.904 溴

bro·mo·crip·tine (bro″mo-krip′tēn) an ergot alkaloid dopamine agonist, used as the mesylate salt to suppress prolactin secretion and thereby treat prolactinomas and endocrine disorders secondary to hyperprolactinemia; also used as an antidyskinetic in parkinsonism and a growth hormone suppressant in acromegaly 溴隐亭；一种麦角生物碱多巴胺激动剂，用作甲磺酸盐抑制催乳素分泌，从而治疗继发于高催乳素血症的催乳素瘤和内分泌疾病；也用作帕金森病的抗运动障碍和肢端肥大症的生长激素抑制剂

bro·mo·di·phen·hy·dra·mine (bro″modi′fen-hi′drə-mēn) a derivative of monoethanolamine used as the hydrochloride salt as an antihistamine 溴苯海拉明，单乙醇胺的衍生物，用作盐酸盐，作为抗组胺药

bro·mo·men·or·rhea (bro″mo-men-o-re′ə) menstruation characterized by an offensive odor 臭经

brom·phen·ir·amine (brōm″fən-ir′ə-mēn) an antihistamine with anticholinergic and sedative effects, used as the maleate salt 溴苯那敏，具有抗胆碱能和镇静作用的抗组胺药，用作马来酸盐

bronch·ad·e·ni·tis (brongk″ad-ə-ni′tis) inflammation of the bronchial glands 在支气管腺体的炎症

bron·chi (brong′ki) *bronchus* 的复数形式

bron·chi·al (brong′ke-əl) pertaining to or affecting one or more bronchi 支气管的

bron·chi·ec·ta·sis (brong″ke-ek′tə-sis) chronic dilatation of one or more bronchi 支气管扩张

bron·chil·o·quy (brong-kil′ə-kwe) bronchophony

(2) 支气管语音

bron·chio·cele (brong′ke-o-sēl) bronchocele 细支气管扩大

bron·chi·ole (brong′ke-ōl) a subdivision of a bronchus, itself subdividing into terminal bronchioles 细支气管；**respiratory b.**, a branch of a terminal bronchiole, dividing further and terminating as several alveolar ducts; it is the first part of the bronchiole that contains alveoli and in which gas exchange occurs 呼吸性细支气管；**terminal b.**, a subdivision of a bronchiole; it is the last part of the bronchiole that does not contain alveoli, and it subdivides into respiratory bronchioles 终末细支气管

bron·chio·lec·ta·sis (brong″ke-o-lek′tə-sis) dilatation of the bronchioles 细支气管扩张

bron·chi·o·li·tis (brong″ke-o-li′tis) inflammation of the bronchioles 细支气管炎

bron·chi·o·lus (brong-ki′o-ləs) pl. *bronchi′oli* [L.] bronchiole 细支气管

bron·chio·spasm (brong′ke-o-spaz″əm) bronchospasm 支气管痉挛

bron·chi·tis (brong-ki′tis) inflammation of one or more bronchi 支气管炎；**bronchit′ic** *adj.*；**acute b.**, a short, severe attack of bronchitis, with fever and a productive cough 急性支气管炎；**chronic b.**, a type of chronic obstructive pulmonary disease with bronchial irritation, increased secretions, and a productive cough lasting at least 3 months, 2 years in a row 慢性支气管炎；**fibrinous b.**, bronchitis with violent cough, paroxysmal dyspnea, and expectoration of bronchial casts containing Charcot-Leyden crystals 纤维素性支气管炎，支气管炎，伴有剧烈咳嗽，阵发性呼吸困难，以及含有 Charcot-Leyden 结晶支气管管型的咳痰；**b. obli′terans**, that in which the smaller bronchi become filled with nodules composed of fibrinous exudate 闭塞性支气管炎；**pseudomembranous b.**, fibrinous b. 假膜性支气管炎

bron·cho·al·ve·o·lar (brong″ko-al-ve′ə-lər) pertaining to a bronchus and alveoli 支气管肺泡

bron·cho·can·di·di·a·sis (brong″ko-kan-di-di′ə-sis) bronchopulmonary candidiasis 支气管肺念珠菌病

bron·cho·cele (brong′ko-sēl) localized dilatation of a bronchus 局部支气管扩张

bron·cho·con·stric·tion (brong″ko-kənstrik′shən) narrowing of air passages of the lungs from smooth muscle contraction, as in asthma 支气管收缩，平滑肌收缩导致肺部空气通道变窄，如哮喘

bron·cho·con·stric·tor (brong″ko-kənstrik′tər) 1. narrowing the lumina of the air passages of the lungs 缩小肺部空气通道的腔；2. an agent that causes such constriction 支气管收缩药

bron·cho·di·la·tor (brong″ko-di′la-tər) (-dila′tər) 1. expanding the lumina of the air passages of the lungs 扩张肺部空气通道的腔；2. an agent that causes dilatation of the bronchi 支气管扩张药

bron·cho·esoph·a·ge·al (brong″ko-ə-sof″ə-je′əl) pertaining to or communicating with a bronchus and the esophagus 支气管食管的

bron·cho·esoph·a·gos·co·py (brong″ko-ə-sof″ə-gos′kə-pe) instrumental examination of the bronchi and esophagus 支气管食管镜

bron·cho·fi·ber·scope (brong″ko-fi′bər-skōp) fiberoptic bronchoscope; a flexible bronchoscope using fiberoptics 纤维支气管镜

bron·cho·fi·bros·co·py (brong″ko-fi-bros′kə-pe) examination of bronchi through a bronchofiberscope 纤维支气管镜检查

bron·cho·gen·ic (brong-ko-jen′ik) originating in bronchi 支气管原的

bron·chog·ra·phy (brong-kog′rə-fe) radiography of the lungs after instillation of an opaque medium in the bronchi 支气管造影；**bronchograph′ic** adj.

bron·cho·li·thi·a·sis (brong″ko-lĭ-thi′ə-sis) the presence of calculi in the lumen of the tracheobronchial tree 支气管结石症

bron·chol·o·gy (brong-kol′ə-je) the study and treatment of diseases of the tracheobronchial tree 支气管病学；**bronchologic′ic** adj.

bron·cho·ma·la·cia (brong″ko-mə-la′shə) a deficiency in the cartilaginous wall of the trachea or a bronchus that may lead to atelectasis or obstructive emphysema 支气管软化，气管或支气管软骨壁的缺陷可能导致肺不张或阻塞性肺气肿

bron·cho·mo·tor (brong″ko-mo′tər) affecting the caliber of the bronchi 支气管舒缩的

bron·cho·mu·co·tro·pic (brong″ko-mu″kotro′pik) augmenting secretion by the respiratory mucosa 促支气管分泌的

bron·cho·pan·cre·at·ic (brong″ko-pan″kreat′ik) communicating with a bronchus and the pancreas, such as a fistula 支气管胰腺的，如支气管胰腺瘘

bron·choph·o·ny (brong-kof′ə-ne) 1. normal voice sounds heard over a large bronchus 支气管语音；2. abnormal voice sounds heard over the lung, with the voice too clear and high-pitched, indicating solidification 在肺部听到异常的声音，声音清晰、高调，指示实变

bron·cho·plas·ty (brong′ko-plas″te) plastic surgery of a bronchus; surgical closure of a bronchial fistula 支气管成形术

bron·cho·ple·gia (brong″ko-ple′jə) paralysis of bronchial tube muscles 支气管麻痹

bron·cho·pleu·ral (brong″ko-ploor′əl) pertaining to or communicating between a bronchus and the pleura or pleural cavity 支气管胸膜的

bron·cho·pneu·mo·nia (brong″ko-noomo′nyə) bronchial pneumonia 支气管肺炎；inflammation of the lungs beginning in the terminal bronchioles 从末端细支气管开始的肺部炎症

bron·cho·pul·mo·nary (brong″ko-pool′mə-nar″e) pertaining to the bronchi and the lungs 支气管肺

bron·chor·rha·phy (brong-kor′ə-fe) suture of a bronchus 支气管缝合术

bron·cho·scope (brong′ko-skōp) an instrument for inspecting the interior of the tracheobronchial tree and doing diagnostic and therapeutic maneuvers such as removing specimens or foreign bodies 支气管镜；**bronchoscop′ic** adj.；fiberoptic b., bronchofiberscope 纤维支气管镜

bron·chos·co·py (brong-kos′kə-pe) examination of the bronchi through a bronchoscope 支气管镜检查；fiberoptic b., bronchofibroscopy 纤维支气管镜检查

bron·cho·spasm (brong′ko-spaz″əm) bronchial spasm; spasmodic contraction of the smooth muscle of the bronchi, as in asthma 支气管痉挛；支气管平滑肌的痉挛性收缩，如哮喘

bron·cho·spi·rom·e·try (brong″ko-spirom′ə-tre) determination of vital capacity, oxygen intake, and carbon dioxide excretion of a lung, or simultaneous measurements of the function of each lung separately 支气管肺量测量法；differential b., measurement of the function of each lung separately 对比支气管肺量测定法

bron·cho·ste·no·sis (brong″ko-stə-no′sis) narrowing of a bronchial tube by scarring or other stricture 支气管狭窄

bron·chos·to·my (brong-kos′tə-me) the surgical creation of an opening through the chest wall into a bronchus 支气管造口术

bron′cho·tra·che·al (brong″ko-tra′ke-əl) tracheobronchial 气管支气管的

bron·cho·ve·sic·u·lar (brong″ko-vĕ-sik′u-lər) bronchoalveolar 支气管肺泡的

bron·chus (brong′kəs) pl. bron′chi [L.] one of the larger passages conveying air to a lung (right or left primary bronchus) and within the lungs (lobar and segmental bronchi) 支气管

brow (brou) forehead 前额

BRS British Roentgen Society 英国放射线学会

Bru·cel·la (broo-sel′ə) a genus of gramnegative, aerobic coccobacilli of the family Brucellaceae. Several species cause human infection; the most important are *B. abor′tus*, which causes infectious abortion in cattle and is the most common cause of brucellosis in humans, and *B. su′is*, which usually infects swine 布鲁氏菌，布鲁氏菌科的一种革兰阴性好氧球菌。几种物种引起人类感染；最重要的是流产布鲁氏菌，

它导致牛的传染性流产，是人类布鲁氏菌病的最常见原因，而猪布鲁氏菌通常感染猪

bru·cel·la (broo-sel′ə) any member of the genus *Brucella* 布鲁氏菌属；**brucel′lar** *adj.*

Bru·cel·la·ceae (broo″sə-la′se-e) a family bacteria of the order Rhizobiales, consisting of gram-negative, aerobic cocci and rod-shaped bacteria 布鲁氏菌科

bru·cel·lo·sis (broo″sə-lo′sis) a generalized infection involving primarily the reticuloendothelial system, caused by species of *Brucella*. 布鲁氏菌病

Brug·ia (broo′je-ə) a genus of filarial worms, including *B. mala′yi*, a species similar to, and often found in association with, *Wuchereria bancrofti*, which causes human filariasis and elephantiasis throughout Southeast Asia, the China Sea, and eastern India 布鲁丝虫属，一种野生蠕虫属，包括马来丝虫，一种与班氏丝虫相似并与之相关的物种，在整个东南亚、中国沿海和印度东部引起人类丝虫病和象皮病

bruise (brooz) contusion 挫伤

bruit (brwe) (broot) [Fr.] sound (3) 杂音；**aneurysmal b.**, a blowing sound heard over an aneurysm 动脉瘤杂音；**placental b.**, 胎盘杂音，见 *souffle* 下词条

brux·ism (bruk′siz-əm) grinding of the teeth, especially during sleep 磨牙

BS Bachelor of Science 理学学士；Bachelor of Surgery 外科学士；breath sounds 呼吸音；blood sugar 血糖

BSF B lymphocyte stimulatory factor B 淋巴细胞刺激因子

BTU British thermal unit 英国热量单位

bu·bo (bu′bo) an enlarged and inflamed lymph node, particularly in the axilla or inguinal region, due to such infections as plague, syphilis, gonorrhea, lymphogranuloma venereum, and tuberculosis(腋下或腹股沟的) 淋巴结炎；**bubon′ic** *adj.*

buc·ca (buk′ə) [L.] cheek (1) 脸颊；**buc′cal** *adj.*

buc·co·clu·sion (buk″o-kloo′zhən) malocclusion in which the dental arch or a quadrant or group of teeth is buccal to the normal 颊咬合

buc·co·ver·sion (buk″o-vur′zhən) position of a tooth lying buccally to the line of occlusion 颊向错位，牙齿位于咬合线的位置

buck·ling (buk′ling) the process or an instance of becoming crumpled or warped 屈曲，波状变形；**scleral b.**, a technique for repair of a detached retina, in which indentations or infoldings of the sclera are made over the tears in the retina to promote adherence of the retina to the choroid 巩膜扣带术，一种用于修复分离的视网膜的技术

bu·cli·zine (bu′kli-zēn) an antihistamine, used as the hydrochloride salt as an antinauseant in the man-agement of motion sickness 氯苯丁嗪，一种抗组胺药，用作盐酸盐治疗晕动病

bud (bud) 1. a structure on a plant, often round, that encloses an undeveloped flower or leaf 芽；2. any small part of the embryo or adult metazoon more or less resembling such a plant structure and presumed to have potential for growth and differentiation 胚胎或成虫变种的任何一小部分或多或少类似于这种植物结构，并被认为具有生长和分化的潜力；**end b.**, caudal eminence 尾芽；**limb b.**, a swelling on the trunk of an embryo that becomes a limb 肢芽；**periosteal b.**, vascular connective tissue from the periosteum growing through apertures in the periosteal bone collar into the cartilage matrix of the primary center of ossification 骨膜芽；**tail b.**, 1. in animals having a tail, the primordium that forms it 尾芽，在有尾动物中，形成尾部的原基；2. caudal eminence 尾部隆起；**taste b.**, one of the end organs of the gustatory nerve containing the receptor surfaces for the sense of taste 味蕾；**ureteric b.**, an outgrowth of the mesonephric duct giving rise to all but the nephrons of the permanent kidney 输尿管芽

bu·des·o·nide (bu-des′ə-nīd) an antiinflammatory glucocorticoid used to treat allergic rhinitis, bronchial asthma, nasal inflammation, ulcerative colitis, and Crohn disease 布地奈德，一种糖皮质激素抗炎药物，用于治疗过敏性鼻炎、支气管哮喘、鼻炎、溃疡性结肠炎和克罗恩病

buf·fer (buf′ər) 1. a chemical system that prevents changes in hydrogen ion concentration 缓冲液；2. a physical or physiological system that tends to maintain constancy 保持恒定的物理或生理系统

bulb (bulb) a rounded mass or enlargement 鳞茎，灯泡体，球状物；**bul′bar** *adj.*；**b. of aorta**, the enlargement of the aorta at its point of origin from the heart 动脉球；**hair b.**, **b. of hair**, the bulbous expansion at the proximal end of a hair in which the hair shaft is generated 毛球；**olfactory b.**, the bulb-like expansion of the olfactory tract on the undersur-face of the frontal lobe of each cerebral hemisphere; the olfactory nerves enter it 嗅球；**onion b.**, in neuropathology, a collection of overlapping Schwann cells resembling the bulb of an onion, encircling an axon that has become demyelinated; seen when an axon has repeatedly become demyelinated and remyelinated 在神经病理学中，一组重叠的施万细胞，类似于洋葱的鳞茎，环绕着一个已脱髓鞘的轴突，当轴突反复变为脱髓鞘和髓鞘再生时出现；**b. of penis**, the enlarged proximal part of the corpus spongiosum. 阴茎球，尿道海绵体的近端膨大部分；**b. of vestibule of vagina**, a body consisting of paired masses of erectile tissue, one on either side of the vaginal opening 阴道前庭球

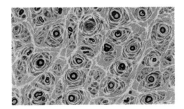

▲ 腓肠肌萎缩症中腓肠神经横截面洋葱鳞茎（onion bulb）样改变

bul·bar (bul′bər) 1. pertaining to a bulb 球状的；2. pertaining to or involving the medulla oblongata 与延髓相关的

bul·bi·tis (bul-bi′tis) inflammation of the bulb of the penis 尿道球炎

bul·bo·cav·er·no·sus (bul″bo-kav″ər-no′səs) bulbocavernous muscle 球海绵体肌

bul·bo·cav·er·nous (bul″bo-kav′ər-nəs) pertaining to the bulb of the penis or to the bulbocavernous muscle 阴茎球的或球海绵体肌的

bul·bo·spi·ral (bul″bo-spi′rəl) pertaining to the root of the aorta (bulbus aortae) and having a spiral course; said of certain bundles of cardiac muscle fibers 延髓

bul·bo·spon·gi·o·sus (bul″bo-spon″je-o′səs) bulbocavernous muscle 球海绵体肌

bul·bo·ure·thral (bul″bo-u-re′thrəl) pertaining to the bulb of the penis 尿道球部的

bul·bous (bul′bəs) 1. bulbar 球状的；2. shaped like, bearing, or arising from a bulb 茎状的，有球茎的，或由球茎产生的

bul·bus (bul′bəs) pl. *bul′bi* [L.] 见 bulb

bu·lim·ia (boo-le′me-ə) [Gr.] episodic binge eating usually followed by behavior designed to negate the caloric intake of the ingested food, most commonly purging behaviors such as selfinduced vomiting or laxative abuse but sometimes other methods such as excessive exercise or fasting 贪食症，偶发性暴食通常伴随着旨在消除摄入食物热量的行为，最常见的是清除行为，如自我诱发的呕吐或泻药滥用，但有时采用其他方法，如过度运动或禁食；**bulim′ic** *adj.*；**b. nervo′sa,** an eating disorder occurring mainly in girls and young women, characterized by episodic binge eating followed by purging or other behaviors designed to prevent weight gain and by excessive influence of body shape and size on the patient's sense of self-worth. Bingeing episodes involve intake of quantifiably excessive quantities of food within a short, discrete period and a sense of loss of control over food intake during these periods. Unlike anorexia nervosa, no extreme weight loss occurs 神经性贪食症

bul·la (bul′ə) pl. *bul′lae* [L.] 1. a large blister 大疱；2. a rounded, projecting anatomical structure 圆形、突出的解剖结构；**bul′late, bul′lous** *adj.*

bul·lec·to·my (bə-lek′tə-me) excision of giant bullae from the lung in emphysema to improve pulmonary function 肺大疱切除术

bul·lo·sis (bul-o′sis) the production of, or a condition characterized by, bullous lesions 大疱性病变的产生或病症

bul·lous (bul′əs) pertaining to or characterized by bullae 大泡的，大疱的

bu·met·a·nide (bu-met′ə-nīd) a loop diuretic used in the treatment of edema, including that associated with congestive heart failure or hepatic or renal disease, and hypertension 布美他尼，用于治疗水肿的襻利尿剂，包括与充血性心力衰竭或肝脏或肾脏疾病和高血压相关的利尿剂

BUN blood urea nitrogen 血尿素氮；见 *urea nitrogen*

bun·dle (bun′dəl) a collection of fibers or strands, as of muscle fibers, or a fasciculus or band of nerve fibers 束；**atrioventricular b., AV b.,** bundle of His 房室束；**common b.,** the undivided portion of the bundle of His, from its origin at the atrioventricular node to the point of division into the right and left bundle branches 总支，希氏束尚未分支的部分；**b. of His,** a band of atypical cardiac muscle fibers connecting the atria with the ventricles of the heart, occurring as a trunk and two bundle branches; it propagates the atrial contraction rhythm to the ventricles, and its interruption produces heart block. The term is sometimes used specifically to denote only the trunk of the bundle 希氏束；**medial forebrain b.,** a group of nerve fibers containing the midbrain tegmentum and elements of the limbic system 内侧前脑束；**Thorel b.,** a bundle of muscle fibers in the human heart connecting the sinoatrial and atrioventricular nodes 连接窦房结和房室结的人类心脏中的一束肌肉

bun·dle branch (bun′dəl branch) 见 *branch* 下词条

bun·ion (bun′yən) abnormal prominence of the medial eminence of the first metatarsal head, with bursal hypertrophy and associated with valgus displacement of the great toe 踇趾滑囊炎，第一跖骨头内侧隆突异常突出，滑膜囊肥大并伴有大脚趾外翻；**tailor's b.,** bunionette 小趾囊肿

bun·ion·ette (bun″yən-et′) enlargement of the lateral aspect of the fifth metatarsal head 小趾囊肿

Bun·ya·vi·ri·dae (bun″yə-vir′ĭ-de) the bunyaviruses, a family of RNA viruses that includes the genera *Orthobunyavirus*, *Hantavirus*, *Nairovirus*, and *Phlebovirus* 布尼亚病毒科，布尼亚病毒是一类 RNA 病毒，包括布尼亚病毒属，汉坦病毒属，

B

内罗病毒属以及白蛉病毒属

Bun·ya·vi·rus (bun'yə-vi″rəs) *Orthobunyavirus* 的旧称

bun·ya·vi·rus (bun'yə-vi″rəs) any virus of the family Bunyaviridae 布尼亚病毒科病毒

bu·piv·a·caine (bu-piv'ə-kān) a local anesthetic, used as the hydrochloride salt for local infiltration, peripheral nerve block, and retrobulbar, subarachnoid, sympathetic, caudal, or epidural block. 布比卡因，局部麻醉剂，其盐酸盐用于局部浸润、周围神经阻滞和眼球后、蛛网膜下腔、交感神经、尾侧或硬膜外阻滞

bu·pre·nor·phine (bu″prə-nor'fēn) an opioid partial agonist; used as the base or as the hydrochloride salt in the treatment of opioid addiction, as an analgesic, and as an anesthesia adjunct 丁丙诺啡，阿片类药物部分激动剂；用作碱或盐酸盐治疗阿片类药物成瘾，作为镇痛药，以及作为麻醉剂的辅助剂

bu·pro·pi·on (bu-pro'pe-on) a monocyclic compound structurally similar to amphetamine, used as the hydrochloride salt as an antidepressant and as an aid in smoking cessation 安非他酮，使用结构上类似于苯丙胺的单环化合物，其盐酸盐作为抗抑郁药和帮助戒烟

bur (bur) a rotary instrument for creating openings in teeth, bones, or similar hard material 钻，用于牙齿、骨骼或类似硬质材料中形成开口的旋转器械

bur·bu·lence (bur'bu-ləns″) gaseousness; a group of intestinal symptoms including fullness, bloating or distention, borborygmus, and flatulence 胃肠气症，一组肠道症状，包括饱胀，腹胀或腹胀，腹胀和痉挛

bu·ret (bu-ret') a graduated glass tube with a stopcock at its bottom end, used to deliver a measured amount of liquid 滴定管

Burk·hol·de·ria (burk″hol-dēr'e-ə) a genus of gram-negative, rod-shaped bacteria of the family Burkholderiaceae, formerly included in the genus *Pseudomonas. B. cepa'cia* is an opportunistic pathogen causing nosocomial infections, and *B. pseudomal'lei* causes melioidosis 伯克霍尔德氏菌属，伯克霍尔德氏科的一种革兰阴性棒状细菌，曾属于假单胞菌属。洋葱伯克霍尔德菌是引起医院感染的机会致病菌，类鼻疽伯克霍尔德菌导致类鼻疽

Burk·hol·de·ri·a·ceae (burk″hol-dēr″e-a'se-e) a family of phenotypically, metabolically, and ecologically diverse bacteria of the order Burkholderiales 伯克氏菌科一种表型，代谢和生态多样的细菌

Burk·hol·de·ri·a·les (burk″hol-dēr″e-a'les) an order of phenotypically, metabolically, and ecologically diverse bacteria of the class Betaproteobacteria 伯克氏菌目

burn (burn) injury to tissues caused by the contact with heat, flame, chemicals, electricity, or radiation. First-degree burns show redness; second-degree burns show vesication; thirddegree burns show necrosis through the entire skin. Burns of the *first* and *second degree* are partial-thickness burns; those of the *third degree* are full-thickness burns 烧伤；**first-degree b.**, a burn that affects the epidermis only, causing erythema without blistering 一度烧伤，只影响表皮的灼伤，导致红斑，不起水疱；**fourth-degree b.**, a burn that extends deeply into the subcutaneous tissue; it may involve muscle, fascia, or bone 四度烧伤，烧伤深深地延伸到皮下组织中，可能涉及肌肉，筋膜或骨骼；**full-thickness b.**, 见 third-degree b.; **partial-thickness b.**, 见 second-degree b.; **second-degree b.**, a burn that affects the epidermis and the dermis, classified as *superficial* (involving the epidermis and the papillary dermis) or *deep* (extending into the reticular dermis) 二度烧伤，影响表皮和真皮的烧伤，表现为浅层（涉及表皮和乳头状真皮）或深部（延伸到网状真皮中）。又称 *partial-thickness b*; **third-degree b.**, a burn that destroys both the epidermis and the dermis, often also involving the superficial fascia 烧伤会破坏表皮和真皮，通常还会涉及浅层筋膜。又称 *full-thickness b*

bur·nish·ing (bur'nish-ing) a dental procedure somewhat related to polishing and abrading 与抛光和磨蚀有关的牙科手术

burr (bur) bur 毛刺，角环

bur·sa (bur'sə) pl. *bur'sae* [L.] a fluid-filled sac or saclike cavity situated in places in tissues where friction would otherwise occur 囊；黏液囊；**bur'sal** *adj.*; **b. of Achilles tendon**, a bursa between the calcaneal tendon and the back of the calcaneus 跟腱囊; **anserine b.**, a bursa between the tendons of the sartorius, gracilis, and semitendinosus muscles, and the tibial collateral ligaments 缝匠肌、股薄肌和半腱肌腱与胫骨侧副韧带之间的囊; **His b.**, the dilatation at the end of the archenteron 原肠末端的扩张; **omental b.**, the lesser sac of the peritoneum 网膜囊; **pharyngeal b.**, an inconstant blind sac located above the pharyngeal tonsil in the midline of the mastoid wall of the nasopharynx; it represents persistence of an embryonic communication between the anterior tip of the notochord and the roof of the pharynx 咽囊; **popliteal b.**, a prolongation of the synovial tendon sheath of the popliteus muscle outside knee joint into the popliteal space 腘囊，腘肌囊，腘下隐窝; **prepatellar b.**, one of the bursae in front of the patella; it may be subcutaneous, subfascial, or subtendinous in location 髌前滑囊；**subacromial b.**, one between the acromion and the insertion of the supraspinatus muscle, extending between the deltoid and greater tubercle of the humerus 肩峰下滑囊；**subdeltoid b.**, one between the deltoid and the glenohumeral joint capsule, usually connected to the subacromial bursa 三角肌下滑液囊；**subtendinous b. of iliacus**, one at the point of insertion of the iliopsoas muscle into the lesser trochanter 髂肌腱下囊；**synovial b.**, a closed synovial sac interposed between surfaces that glide upon each other; it may be subcutaneous, submuscular, subfascial, or subtendinous in nature 滑膜囊

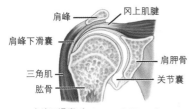

▲ 肩峰下滑囊（**subacromial bursa**）

bur·si·tis (bər-si′tis) inflammation of a bursa; specific types of bursitis are named according to the bursa affected, e.g., prepatellar bursitis, subacromial bursitis 滑囊炎；**Achilles b.**, 见 retrocalcaneal b.；**calcific b.**, 见 *tendinitis* 下词条；**ischiogluteal b.**, inflammation of the bursa over the ischial tuber, characterized by sudden onset of excruciating pain over the center of the buttock and down the back of the leg 臀大肌坐骨囊炎；**retrocalcaneal b.**, inflammation and thickening of the bursae in front of the Achilles tendon 跟骨后滑囊炎；**subacromial b.**, calcific tendinitis of the subacromial bursa 肩峰下滑囊炎；**subdeltoid b.**, calcific tendinitis of the subdeltoid bursa 三角肌下滑囊炎；**Tornwaldt b.**, chronic inflammation of the pharyngeal bursa 慢性咽囊炎

bur·sot·o·my (bər-sot′ə-me) incision of a bursa 滑液囊切开术

bu·spi·rone (bu-spi′rōn) an antianxiety agent used as the hydrochloride salt in the treatment of anxiety disorders and the short-term relief of anxiety symptoms 丁螺环酮，一种抗焦虑药，用其盐酸盐治疗焦虑症和短期缓解焦虑症状

bu·sul·fan (bu-sul′fan) an antineoplastic used in treating chronic myelogenous leukemia, polycythemia vera, myeloid metaplasia, and myeloproliferative syndrome; also used in lieu of whole body irradiation in stem cell transplantation 白消安，用于治疗慢性粒细胞白血病，真性红细胞增多症，骨髓增生和骨髓增生综合征的抗肿瘤药，也用于代替干细胞移植中的全身照射

bu·ta·bar·bi·tal (bu-tə-bahr′bĭ-təl) an intermediate-acting barbiturate used for preoperative sedation; used also as the sodium salt 另丁巴比妥，用于术前镇静的中效作用的巴比妥酸盐；也用作钠盐

bu·tal·bi·tal (bu-tal′bĭ-təl) a short- to intermediate-acting barbiturate used as a sedative in combination with an analgesic in the treatment of headache 布他比妥，短效至中效巴比妥酸盐，用作镇痛剂，配合镇痛药治疗头痛

bu·tam·ben (bu-tam′bən) a topical anesthetic, used as the base or picrate salt 氨苯丁酯，局部麻醉药，用作碱或苦味酸盐

bu·tane (bu′tān) an aliphatic hydrocarbon from petroleum, occurring as a colorless flammable gas; used in pharmacy as an aerosol propellant 丁烷，来自石油的脂肪烃，以无色可燃气体形式存在；在药房中用作气溶胶推进剂

butch·er's broom (booch′ərz) the European evergreen *Ruscus aculeatus* or preparations of its rhizome, which are used in the treatment of hemorrhoids and venous insufficiency 假叶树或根茎制剂，用于治疗痔疮和静脉功能不全

bu·ten·a·fine (bu-ten′ə-fēn) a topical antifungal used as the hydrochloride salt in the treatment of tinea pedis, tinea corporis, and tinea cruris 布替萘芬，局部抗真菌药，用其盐酸盐治疗足癣、体癣和股癣

bu·to·con·a·zole (bu″to-kon′ə-zōl) an imidazole antifungal used as the nitrate salt in the treatment of vulvovaginal candidiasis 布康唑，咪唑类抗真菌药，用其硝酸盐治疗外阴阴道念珠菌病

bu·tor·pha·nol (bu-tor′fə-nol) a synthetic opioid used as the tartrate salt as an analgesic and anesthesia adjunct 布托啡诺，一种合成阿片类药物，用其酒石酸盐作为镇痛和麻醉辅助剂

but·tocks (but′əks) the two fleshy prominences formed by the gluteal muscles on the lower part of the back 臀部

but·ton (but′ən) 1. a knoblike elevation or structure 山丘状的隆起或结构；2. a spool- or disk-shaped device used in surgery for construction of intestinal anastomosis 肠吻合器；**mescal b's**, transverse slices of the flowering heads of a Mexican cactus, *Lophophora williamsii*, whose major active principle is mescaline 墨西哥仙人掌花香头的横切面，主要活性成分是美斯卡林；**skin b.**, a connector or stretch of tubing covered with a velour fabric, designed to encourage tissue ingrowth where it passes through the skin 一种覆盖有丝绒织物的连接件或延伸管，其设计目的是促进组织进入皮肤

bu·tyl (bu′təl) a hydrocarbon radical, C_4H_9 丁基

bu·ty·rate (bu′tə-rāt) a salt, ester, or anionic form

of butyric acid 丁酸的盐、酯或阴离子形式

bu·tyr·ic ac·id (bu-tēr'ik) 1. any four-carbon carboxylic acid, either n-butyric acid or isobutyric acid 四碳羧酸, 正丁酸或异丁酸; 2. *n*-butyric acid, occurring in butter, particularly rancid butter, and in much animal fat 正丁酸, 存在于黄油中, 特别是腐臭的黄油, 以及大量的动物脂肪中

bu·ty·ro·phe·none (bu″tə-ro-fe′nōn) any of a class of structurally related antipsychotic agents, including haloperidol 丁酰苯类, 任何一种结构相关的抗精神病药物, 包括氟哌啶醇

BVAD biventricular assist device 双心室辅助装置

by·pass (bi′pas) an auxiliary flow 辅助流动; a shunt 分流; a surgically created pathway circumventing the normal anatomical pathway, as in an artery or the intestine 手术创建的通路, 绕过正常的解剖路径, 如动脉或肠道; **cardiopulmonary b.,** diversion of the flow of blood to the heart directly to the aorta, via a pump oxygenator, avoiding both the heart and the lungs; a form of extracorporeal circulation used in heart surgery 心肺转流术; **coronary artery b.,** a section of vein or other conduit grafted between the aorta and a coronary artery distal to an obstructive lesion in the latter 冠状动脉旁路术; **gastric b.,** surgical treatment of morbid obesity by transecting the stomach high on its body, and joining the proximal remnant to a loop of jejunum in end-to-side anastomosis 胃旁路术

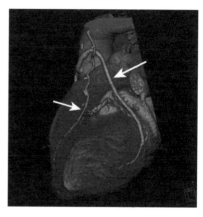

▲ 冠状动脉旁路 (**coronary artery bypass**) 移植到左冠状动脉的前室间支 (左箭) 和静脉移植到左回旋支 (右箭)

bys·si·no·sis (bis″ĭ-no′sis) brown lung; pulmonary disease due to inhalation of the dust of cotton or other textiles 棉屑沉着病, 由于吸入棉花或其他纺织品的粉尘引起的肺部疾病; **byssinot′ic** *adj.*

C canine (tooth) 犬 (齿); carbon 元素碳的符号; cathode 阴极; Celsius (scale) 摄氏度; clonus 克隆; complement 补体; compliance 顺应性; contraction 收缩; coulomb 库仑 (电量单位); cytosine or cytidine 胞嘧啶或胞苷; cylindrical lens 柱面透镜; color sense 色感; cervical vertebrae ($C_1 \sim C_7$) 颈椎 ($C_1 \sim C_7$); large calorie 千卡 (热量单位)

C capacitance 电容的符号; heat capacity 热容量; clearance (subscripts denote the substance, e.g., C_1 or C_{In}, inulin clearance) 清除率 (下标表示物质, 例如 C_1 或 C_{In}, 菊粉清除率)

°C degree Celsius 摄氏度; 见 *scale* 下 *Celsius scale*

c small calorie 小卡 (热量单位); centi- 厘, 百分之一

c molar concentration 摩尔浓度; the velocity of light in a vacuum. 真空中光速的符号

χ^2 (chi, the twenty-second letter of the Greek alphabet) chi-squared 卡方; 见 *distribution* 下 *chi-square distribution* 和 *test* 下 *chi-square test*

CA cardiac arrest 心脏停搏; coronary artery 冠状动脉

CA 125 cancer antigen 125 癌抗原 125

Ca calcium 元素钙的符号

Ca^{2+}-ATP·ase (a-te-pe′ās) a membrane-bound enzyme that hydrolyzes ATP to provide energy to drive the cellular calcium pump 钙腺苷三磷酸酶, 膜结合酶, 水解 ATP, 提供能量驱动细胞钙泵

ca·ber·go·line (kə-bur′go-lēn) a dopamine receptor agonist used in the treatment of hyperprolactinemia 卡麦角林, 多巴胺受体激动剂, 用于治疗高催乳素血症

CABG coronary artery bypass graft 冠状动脉搭桥术

CACCN Canadian Association of Critical Care Nurses 加拿大重症监护护士协会

ca·chec·tin (kə-kek′tin) former name for tumor necrosis factor α 恶病质素, 肿瘤坏死因子 α 的旧称

ca·chet (kā-sha′) a disk-shaped wafer or capsule enclosing a dose of medicine 圆盘形晶片或胶囊, 里面含有药物

ca·chex·ia (kə-kek′se-ə) a profound and marked state of constitutional disorder; general ill health and malnutrition 恶病质；**cachec′tic** adj.；**cancer c.**, anorexia-cachexia syndrome in cancer patients 癌症恶病质；c. hypophysiopri′va, the train of symptoms resulting from total deprivation of pituitary function, including loss of sexual function, bradycardia, hypothermia, and coma 垂体缺失性恶病质，完全剥夺垂体功能导致的一系列症状，包括丧失性功能、心动过缓、体温过低和昏迷；**malarial c.**, the physical signs resulting from antecedent attacks of severe malaria, including anemia, sallow skin, yellow sclera, splenomegaly, hepatomegaly, and, in children, retardation of growth and puberty 疟疾恶病质，由严重疟疾的发作前期引起的体征，包括贫血、皮肤灰黄、巩膜黄化、脾肿大、肝肿大、以及儿童生长和青春期发育迟缓；**pituitary c.**, 垂体性恶病质，见 *panhypopituitarism*

cach·in·na·tion (kak″ĭ-na′shən) excessive, hysterical laughter 大笑，哄笑，放纵地笑

cac·o·dyl·ic ac·id (kak″o-dil′ik) dimethyl arsinic acid, a highly toxic herbicide 二甲胂酸，一种剧毒的除草剂

caco·geu·sia (kak″o-goo′zhə) a parageusia consisting of a bad taste not related to ingestion of specific substances, or associated with gustatory stimuli usually considered to be pleasant 劣味，恶味，属于味觉倒错或味觉异常

caco·me·lia (kak″o-me′le-ə) dysmelia 肢体畸形，肢体发育异常

CAD chronic actinic dermatitis; coronary artery disease 慢性光化性皮炎，冠状动脉疾病

ca·dav·er (kə-dav′ər) a dead body; generally applied to a human body preserved for anatomic study 尸体。Cf. *corpse*；**cadav′eric** adj. 尸体的

ca·dav·er·ine (kə-dav′ər-in) a foul-smelling polyamine produced by decarboxylation of lysine and contributing to the odor of decaying meat and feces 尸胺，一种恶臭的多胺，由赖氨酸脱羧产生，是腐烂肉和粪便的气味的原因

ca·dav·er·ous (kə-dav′ər-əs) resembling a cadaver 像尸体一样

cad·he·rin (kad-hēr′in) any of a family of over 80 calcium-dependent cell adhesion molecules, having in common a structure called the CAD domain 钙黏着蛋白，任何超过 80 个钙依赖性细胞黏附分子的家族，具有共同的称为 CAD 结构域的结构

cad·mi·um (Cd) (kad′me-əm) a blue-white heavy metal element; at. no. 48, at. wt. 112.411. Cadmium and its salts are poisonous on ingestion or inhalation and can cause pneumoconiosis, severe gastrointestinal symptoms, and damage to the liver and kidneys 镉

ca·du·ce·us (kə-doo′shəs) [L.] the wand of Hermes or Mercury 使者杖（希腊神话中 Hermes 或 Mercury 所持的带有两条互相缠绕的蛇的带翼权杖）；used as a symbol of the medical profession and as the emblem of the Medical Corps of the U.S. Army. 另见 *staff of Aesculapius* 作为医学的标志，也是美国陆军卫生队的队徽。

caf·feine (kă-fēn′) (kaf′ēn) a xanthine found in coffee, tea, chocolate, and colas; it is a central nervous system stimulant, diuretic, and striated muscle stimulant, and it acts on the cardiovascular system. As the base or the citrate salt, it is used as a central nervous system stimulant and as an adjunct in treating neonatal apnea; as the base it is also used in the treatment of vascular headaches and as an adjunct to analgesics 咖啡因，在咖啡、茶、巧克力和可乐中发现的黄嘌呤；一种中枢兴奋药，利尿药和横纹肌刺激药，作用于心血管系统。作为碱或柠檬酸盐，被用作中枢兴奋药和治疗新生儿呼吸暂停的辅助手段；还用于治疗血管性头痛和作为镇痛药的辅助剂

caf·fein·ism (kaf′ēn-iz-əm) a morbid condition resulting from ingestion of excessive amounts of caffeine; characteristics include insomnia, restlessness, excitement, tachycardia, tremors, and diuresis 咖啡因中毒，摄入过量咖啡因导致的病态情况；特征包括失眠、烦躁不安、兴奋、心动过速、震颤和利尿

cage (kāj) a box or enclosure 罐笼，保持架；**rib c., thoracic c.**, the bony structure enclosing the thorax, consisting of the ribs, vertebral column, and sternum 胸廓

CAH congenital adrenal hyperplasia 先天性肾上腺皮质增生症

caj·e·put (kaj′ə-poot) the tree *Melaleuca leucaden′dron*, whose fresh leaves and twigs yield cajeput oil 白千层（一种花叶可提香油之月桂树）

cal calorie 卡路里

cal·a·mine (kal′ə-mīn) a preparation of zinc oxide and the coloring agent ferric oxide; used topically as a protectant 炉甘石

cal·a·mus (kal′ə-məs) a reed or reedlike structure 芦苇或芦苇样结构；**c. scripto′rius**, the lowest portion of the floor of the fourth ventricle, situated between the restiform bodies 第四脑室底的最下部分，位于绳状体之间

cal·ca·ne·al (kal-ka′ne-əl) pertaining to the calcaneus 与跟骨相关的

cal·ca·neo·as·trag·a·loid (kal-ka″ne-o-ə-strag′ə-loid) pertaining to the calcaneus and astrag-a-lus 跟距的

cal·ca·ne·odyn·ia (kal-ka″ne-o-din′e-ə) pain in the heel 跟痛症

cal·ca·ne·us (kal-ka′ne-əs) pl. *calca′nei* [L.] heel bone; the irregular quadrangular bone at the back of the tarsus 见图 1。**calca′neal** adj. 跟骨；跗骨；

后面不规则的四边形骨。

cal·car (kal'kər) a spur or spur-shaped structure. 距或距样的；c. a′vis, the lower of the two medial elevations in the posterior horn of the lateral cerebral ventricle, produced by the impression of the calcarine sulcus on the ventricular wall 禽距，侧脑室后角两个内侧隆起的下部，由脑室壁上的距状沟形成

cal·car·e·ous (kal-kar′e-əs) pertaining to or containing lime 石灰质的；chalky 碳酸钙的

cal·ca·rine (kal′kə-rīn) 1. 距状的；2. pertaining to a calcar 距的

cal·ce·mia (kal-se′me-ə) hypercalcemia 高钙血症

cal·ci·bil·ia (kal″sī-bil′e-ə) presence of calcium in the bile 钙胆汁

cal·cif·e·di·ol (kal″sif-ə-di′ol) 见 *25-hydroxycholecalciferol*

cal·cif·er·ol (kal-sif′ər-ol) 1. a compound having vitamin D activity, e.g., cholecalciferol or ergocalciferol 醇；2. ergocalciferol 钙化醇

cal·cif·ic (kal-sif′ik) forming lime 钙化

cal·ci·fi·ca·tion (kal″sī-fī-ka′shən) the deposit of calcium salts in a tissue 钙 化；**dystrophic c.**, the deposition of calcium in abnormal tissue, such as scar tissue or atherosclerotic plaques, without abnormalities of blood calcium 营养不良性钙化；**eggshell c.**, deposition of a thin layer of calcium around a thoracic lymph node, often seen in silicosis 蛋壳样钙化；**Mönckeberg c.**, 见 *arteriosclerosis* 下词条

cal·ci·no·sis (kal″sī-no′sis) a condition marked by dystrophic calcifications 钙质沉着；**c. circumscrip′ta**, localized dystrophic calcifications in superficial fascia or muscle. 限 界 性 钙 化；**c. universa′lis**, widespread dystrophic calcifications in the dermis, panniculus, and muscles 普遍性钙化

cal·ci·pex·is (kal″sī-pek′sis) calcipexy 钙固定

cal·ci·pexy (kal′sī-pek″se) fixation of calcium in the tissues 钙固定；**calcipec′tic, calcipex′ic** *adj.*

cal·ci·phy·lax·is (kal″sī-fə-lak′sis) a condition of induced hypersensitivity characterized by formation of calcified tissue in response to administration of a challenging agent 钙过敏

cal·ci·po·tri·ene (kal″sī-po-tri′ēn) a synthetic derivative of vitamin D_3 (cholecalciferol), applied topically in the treatment of psoriasis 卡泊三醇

cal·ci·priv·ia (kal″sī-priv′e-ə) deprivation or loss of calcium 缺钙；**calcipri′vic** *adj.*

cal·ci·to·nin (kal″sī-to′nin) a polypeptide hormone secreted by C cells of the thyroid gland, and sometimes of the thymus and parathyroids, which lowers calcium and phosphate concentrations in plasma and inhibits bone resorption. Preparations (*c.-human, c.-salmon*) are used in the treatment of osteitis deformans, postmenopausal osteoporosis, and hypercalcemia 降钙素

cal·ci·tri·ol (kal″sī-tri′ol) 1. 见 *dihydroxycholecalciferol*；2. a preparation of this compound, used in the treatment of hypocalcemia, hypophosphatemia, rickets, and osteodystrophy associated with a variety of disorders 钙三醇

cal·ci·um (Ca) (kal′se-əm) a light, silvery white, alkaline earth metal element; at. no. 20, at. wt. 40.078. Calcium phosphate salts form the dense hard material of teeth and bones. It is an essential dietary element, a constant blood calcium level being essential for normal function of the heart, nerves, and muscles. It is involved in blood coagulation (in which it is called *coagulation factor IV*) and in many enzymatic processes 钙；**c. acetate**, the calcium salt of acetic acid, used as a source of calcium and as a phosphate binder 醋酸 钙；**c. carbonate**, an insoluble salt, $CaCO_3$, occurring naturally in shells, limestone, and chalk and also used in more purified forms; used as an antacid and calcium replenisher and in the treatment of osteoporosis 碳酸钙；**c. chloride**, a salt, $CaCl_2$, used in the treatment of hypocalcemia, electrolyte depletion, and hyperkalemia, and as a treatment adjunct in cardiac arrest and in magnesium poisoning 氯化钙；**c. citrate**, a calcium replenisher also used in the treatment of hyperphosphatemia in renal osteodystrophy 柠 檬 酸 钙；**c. glubionate**, a calcium replenisher, used as a nutritional supplement and for the treatment of hypocalcemia 葡乳醛酸钙；**c. gluceptate**, a calcium salt used in the treatment and prophylaxis of hypocalcemia and as an electrolyte replenisher 葡庚糖酸钙；**c. gluconate**, a calcium salt used to treat or prevent hypercalcemia, nutritional deficiency, and hyperkalemia; also used as a treatment adjunct in cardiac arrest 葡萄糖酸钙；**c. hydroxide**, a salt, $Ca(OH)_2$, used in solution as a topical astringent 氢氧化钙；**c. lactate**, a calcium replenisher, used as a nutritional supplement and for the treatment of hypocalcemia 乳酸钙；**c. oxalate**, a salt of oxalic acid, which in excess in the urine may lead to formation of oxalate calculi 草酸钙；**c. oxide**, lime (1) 氧化钙；**c. phosphate**, a salt containing calcium and the phosphate radical; *dibasic* and *tribasic c. phosphate* are used as sources of calcium 磷酸钙；**c. polycarbophil**, a calcium salt of a hydrophilic resin of the polycarboxylic type; a bulk laxative 聚卡波非钙，导泻药；**c. pyrophosphate**, the pyrophosphate salt of calcium, used as a polishing agent in dentifrices. Crystals of the dihydrate form occur in the joints in calcium pyrophosphate deposition disease 焦磷酸钙。钙的焦磷酸盐，用作洁齿剂中的抛光剂。二水合物形式的晶体出现在焦磷酸钙沉积疾病的关节；c. sulfate, the sulfate salt of calcium, CaSO$_4$, occurring in the anhydrous form and in a hydrated form (*gypsum*, q.v.), which upon being calcined forms *plaster of Paris* 硫酸钙

cal·co·spher·ite (kal″ko-sfĕr′ĭt) one of the tiny round bodies formed during calcification by chemical union of calcium particles and albuminous matter of cells 钙球体，在钙化过程中钙颗粒和细胞的白蛋白化学结合形成的一个小圆体

cal·cu·lo·sis (kal″ku-lo′sis) lithiasis 结石

cal·cu·lus (kal′ku-ləs) pl. *cal'culi* [L.] an abnormal concretion, usually composed of mineral salts, occurring within the animal body 结石，在动物体内发生的异常结石，通常由矿物盐组成；**cal'culous** adj. **biliary c.**, gallstone 胆结石；**dental c.**, calcium phosphate and carbonate, with organic matter, deposited on tooth surfaces 牙结石；**lung c.**, one formed in the bronchi by accretion about an inorganic nucleus, or from calcified portions of lung tissue or adjacent lymph nodes 肺结石；**oxalate c.**, a urinary calculus made of calcium oxalate; some have tiny sharp spines and others are smooth 草酸盐结石；**renal c.**, one in the kidney 肾结石；**salivary c.**, 1. sialolith 涎石；2. supragingival c. 牙龈结石；**struvite c.**, a urinary calculus of crystals of struvite (magnesium ammonium phosphate) 鸟粪石（磷酸铵镁）结晶尿路；**supragingival c.**, that covering the coronal surface of the tooth to the crest of the gingival margin 牙龈结石；**urinary c.**, one in any part of the urinary tract 尿结石；**uterine c.**, uterolith; a concretion in the uterus 子宫结石；**vesical c.**, one in the urinary bladder 膀胱结石

cal·e·fa·cient (kal″ə-fa′shənt) causing a sensation of warmth 变暖；an agent that so acts 发暖剂

Ca·len·du·la (kə-len′du-lə) [L.] a genus of composite-flowered plants. The dried florets of *C. offici·na'lis*, the pot marigold, have antimicrobial and antiinflammatory properties; they are used topically for inflammatory lesions and to promote healing and are used in homeopathy and folk medicine 金盏草，干燥的金盏花，具有抗微生物和抗炎作用；局部用于炎症性病变并促进愈合，用于顺势疗法和民间医学

calf (kaf) sura（可兰经的）章、节；the fleshy back part of the leg below the knee 膝盖以下腿的后部肌肉

cal·fac·tant (kal-fak′tənt) a pulmonary surfactant from calf lung, used in the prophylaxis and treatment of neonatal respiratory distress syndrome 来自小牛肺的肺表面活性物质，用于预防和治疗新生儿呼吸窘迫综合征

cal·i·ber (kal′ĭ-bər) the diameter of the opening of a canal or tube 管道或管道开口的直径

cal·i·bra·tion (kal″ĭ-bra′shən) determination of the accuracy of an instrument, usually by measurement of its variation from a standard, to ascertain necessary correction factors 校准

cal·i·cec·ta·sis (kal″ĭ-sek′tə-sis) caliectasis 肾盏扩张

Ca·li·ci·vi·ri·dae (kə-lis″ĭ-vir′ĭ-de) the caliciviruses, a family of RNA viruses that cause disease in humans and other animals; genera that cause human disease are *Norovirus* and *Sapovirus*；杯状病毒，一种在人类和其他动物身上引起疾病的 RNA 病毒家族；引起人类疾病的属是诺如病毒和沙波病毒

ca·li·ci·vi·rus (kə-lis′ĭ-vi′rəs) any virus of the family Caliciviridae 萼状病毒

ca·lic·u·lus (kə-lik′u-ləs) pl. *cali'culi* [L.] a budshaped or cup-shaped structure 小杯；杯状物

ca·li·ec·ta·sis (ka″le-ek′tə-sis) dilatation of a renal calyx 肾盏扩张

cal·i·for·ni·um (Cf) (kal″ĭ-for′ne-əm) a synthetic metallic transuranium element; at. no. 98, at. wt. 251 锎

cal·i·pers (kal′ĭ-pərz) an instrument with two bent or curved legs used for measuring thickness or diameter of a solid 游标卡尺

Cal'liph·o·ra (kə-lif′o-rə) a genus of flies, including the blowflies and bluebottle flies, which deposit their eggs in decaying matter, on wounds, or in body openings; the maggots are a cause of myiasis 丽蝇属

cal·los·i·ty (kə-los′ĭ-te) a callus (1) 胼胝

cal·lo·sum (kə-lo′səm) corpus callosum 胼胝体；**callo'sal** adj.

cal·lo·ta·sis (kal″ō-tā′sis) a method of limb lengthening using a telescoping device to slowly distract and hold in place the callus that forms after corticotomy. Used to treat such bone defects as congenital or traumatic amputation, phocomelia, radial agenesis, and infected fracture with bone loss 一种使用伸缩装置延长肢体的方法，以缓慢地分散和保持截骨后形成的愈伤组织。用于治疗先天性或创伤性截肢，海豹肢畸形，桡骨发育不全和骨质流失的感染性骨折等骨缺损

cal·lous (kal′əs) 1. hardened 硬化；2. pertaining to or characterized by callus 与愈伤组织有关或以愈伤组织为特征的

cal·lus (kal′əs) [L.] 1. localized hyperplasia of the stratum corneum of the epidermis due to pressure or friction 由于压力或摩擦，表皮角质层局部增生；2. an unorganized network of woven bone formed about the ends of a broken bone, which is absorbed as repair is completed (*provisional c.*), and ultimately replaced by true bone (*definitive c.*) 一个无组织的编织骨网络，围绕骨折的末端形成，当修复完成时被吸收 (provisional c.)，最终被真骨取代 (definitive c.)

cal·mod·u·lin (kal-mod′u-lin) a calcium-binding protein, present in all nucleated cells, that mediates a wide variety of calcium-dependent cellular processes 钙调蛋白，钙结合蛋白，存在于所有有核细胞中，介导多种钙依赖性细胞过程

ca·lor (kal′or) [L.] heat 热；one of the cardinal signs of inflammation 炎症的一个主要迹象

ca·lor·ic (kə-lor′ik) pertaining to heat or to calories 与热量或卡路里有关

cal·o·rie (cal) (kal′ə-re) any of several units of heat defined as the amount of heat required to raise 1 g of water 1℃ at a specified temperature; the calorie used in chemistry and biochemistry is equal to 4.184 joules 卡路里，一种热量单位，定义为在特定温度下将 1 克水升至 1℃ 所需的热量；化学和生物化学中使用的卡路里等于 4.184 焦耳 **large c. (C)**, the calorie now used only in metabolic studies; also used to express the fuel or energy value of food. It is equivalent to the kilocalorie 卡路里现在只用于代谢研究，也用于表示食物的燃料或能量值。它相当于千卡；**small c.**, calorie, when the term large calorie had broader meaning 小卡（热量单位）

ca·lor·i·gen·ic (kə-lor″ĭ-jen′ik) producing or increasing production of heat or energy; increasing oxygen consumption 增加热量或能量的产生；增加氧气消耗

cal·o·rim·e·ter (kal″ə-rim′ə-tər) an instrument for measuring the amount of heat produced in any system or organism 量热仪

cal·re·tic·u·lin (kal″rə-tik′u-lin) a calciumbinding protein in the sarcoplasmic reticulum and in the endoplasmic reticulum of nonmuscle cells; its roles include calcium homeostasis, control of viral RNA replication, lymphocyte activation, and cytotoxicity 钙网蛋白，肌浆网和非肌肉细胞内质网中的钙结合蛋白；其作用包括钙稳态，病毒 RNA 复制的控制，淋巴细胞活化和细胞毒性

cal·se·ques·trin (kal″sə-kwes′trin) a calciumbinding protein rich in carboxylate side chains, occurring on the inner membrane surface of the sarcoplasmic reticulum 隐钙素，富含羧酸盐侧链的钙结合蛋白，存在于肌浆网的内膜表面

cal·va·ria (kal-var′e-ə) [L.] the domelike superior portion of the cranium, comprising the superior portions of the frontal, parietal, and occipital bones 颅盖，颅骨的穹顶状上部，包括额骨、顶骨和枕骨的上部

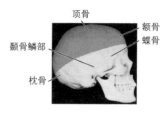

▲ **颅盖（calvaria）**

calx (kalks) 1. lime or chalk 石灰；2. heel 脚跟

ca·lyx (ka′liks) pl. *ca′lyces, ca′lices* [Gr.] a cup-shaped organ or cavity, e.g., one of the recesses of the pelvis of the kidney that encloses the pyramids 花萼；杯状结构。Spelled also *calix*. **calice′al, calyce′al** *adj.*

CAM complementary and alternative medicine 补充和替代医学

cam·era (kam′ə-rə) pl. *ca′merae, cameras* [L.] 1. chamber; an enclosed space or ventricle 室；封闭的空间或心室；2. a device for converting light or other energy from an object into a visible image 相机；**Anger c.**, the original, and by far the most commonly used, form of scintillation (or gamma) camera, so that the terms are often used interchangeably 闪烁照相机；**ca′merae bul′bi o′culi**, the anterior, posterior, and vitreous chambers of the eye 眼的前部、后部和玻璃体室；见 *chamber*. 下词条；**gamma c.**, scintillation c. 射线照相机；**scintillation c.**, an electronic instrument that produces photographs or cathode-ray tube images of the gamma ray emissions from organs containing tracer compounds; the term is often equated with *Anger camera*, the original and most used version 闪烁照相机

cAMP cyclic adenosine monophosphate 环磷腺苷

cam·phor (kam′for) (kam′fər) a ketone derived from the Asian tree *Cinnamomum camphora* or produced synthetically 樟脑；来自亚洲樟树的酮或合成产生的酮；used topically as an antipruritic and antiinfective and inhaled as a nasal decongestant 局部用作抗瘙痒症和抗感染药，并作为鼻腔减充血剂吸入；also used in folk medicine and in Indian medicine 也用于民间医学和印度医学

cam·pim·e·ter (kam-pim′ə-tər) an apparatus for mapping the central portion of the visual field on a flat surface 平面视野计，一种用于将视野的中心部分映射到表面上的装置

cam·pot·o·my (kam-pot′ə-me) the stereotaxic surgical technique of producing a lesion in the Forel fields, beneath the thalamus, for correction of tremor in Parkinson disease 切开术，在丘脑下方前路产生病变部位的立体定向手术技术，用于治疗帕金

森病的震颤

camp·to·cor·mia (kamp″to-kor′me-ə) a static deformity consisting of forward flexion of the trunk 躯干前曲症，驼背

camp·to·dac·ty·ly (kamp″to-dak′tə-le) permanent flexion of one or more fingers 先天性指屈曲

camp·to·me·lia (kamp″to-me′le-ə) bending of the limbs, producing permanent bowing or curving of the affected part 弯肢，四肢弯曲，造成受影响部分永久弯曲或弯曲，**camptomel′ic** *adj.*

Cam·py·lo·bac·ter (kamp″pə-lo-bak′tər) a genus of gram-negative bacteria of the family Campylobacteraceae, made up of motile, spirally curved rods. *C. co′li, C. jeju′ni,* and certain subspecies of *C. fe′tus* can cause gastroenteritis; *C. rec′tus* is associated with periodontal disease 弯曲杆菌属

Cam·py·lo·bac·ter·a·ceae (kam″pə-lobak″tər-a′se-e) a family of gram-negative, rodshaped bacteria of the order Campylobacterales 弯曲杆菌科，一种革兰阴性杆状细菌，弯曲杆菌属，具有特征性的螺旋状运动

Cam·py·lo·bac·ter·a·les (kam″pə-lo-bak″təra′lēz) a metabolically and ecologically diverse order of bacteria of the class Epsilonproteobacteria; many are human and animal pathogens 弯曲杆菌属

cam·sy·late (kam′sə-lāt) USAN contraction for camphorsulfonate 右旋樟脑磺酸

can·a·gli·flo·zin (kan′a-gli-flo′zin) sodiumglucose cotransporter 2 (SGLT2) inhibitor for the treatment of type 2 diabetes mellitus in adults; administered orally in tablet formulation 卡格列净，钠 - 葡萄糖协同转运蛋白 2（SGLT2）抑制剂，用于治疗成人 2 型糖尿病，以片剂形式口服给药

ca·nal (kə-nal′) a relatively narrow tubular passage or channel 相对狭窄的管状通道或通道；**adductor c.,** a fascial tunnel in the middle third of the medial part of the thigh, containing the femoral vessels and saphenous nerve 收肌管，大腿内侧中间 1/3 的筋膜隧道，包含股骨血管和隐神经 **Alcock c.,** pudendal c.; **alimentary c.,** the musculomembranous digestive tube extending from the mouth to the anus 消 化 道；**anal c.,** the terminal portion of the alimentary canal, from the rectum to the anus 肛管，消化道的末端部分，从直肠到肛门；**Arnold c.,** a channel in the petrous portion of the temporal bone for passage of the vagus nerve 乳突小管，颞骨岩部中的通道，用于迷走神经的 通 过；**atrioventricular c.,** the common canal connecting the primordial atrium and ventricle; it sometimes persists as a congenital anomaly 房室管；**birth c.,** the canal through which the fetus passes in birth 产 道；**caroticotympanic c's,** tiny passages in the temporal bone connecting the carotid canal and the tympanic cavity, carrying communicating twigs between the internal carotid and tympanic plexuses 颈鼓小管；**carotid c.,** a tunnel in the petrous portion of the temporal bone that transmits the internal carotid artery to the cranial cavity 颈 动 脉 管；**cochlear c.,** 见 duct 下词条，耳蜗管；**condylar c., condyloid c.,** an occasional opening in the condylar fossa for transmission of the transverse sinus 髁管；**Dorello c.,** an occasional opening in the temporal bone through which the abducens nerve and inferior petrosal sinus enter the cavernous sinus Dorello 管，颞骨中的一个开口，通过它外展神经和岩下窦进入海绵窦；**facial c.,** a canal for the facial nerve in the petrous portion of the temporal bone 面神经管；**femoral c.,** the medial part of the femoral sheath lateral to the base of the lacunar ligament 股 管；**Gartner c.,** a closed rudimentary duct, lying parallel to the uterine tube, into which the transverse ducts of the epoöphoron open; it is the remains of the part of the mesonephros that participates in formation of the reproductive organs 加 特 纳 氏 管；**genital c.,** any canal for the passage of ova or for copulatory use 生殖管；**haversian c.,** any of the anastomosing channels of the haversian system in compact bone, containing blood and lymph vessels and nerves 哈弗斯管；**Huguier c.,** a small canal opening into the facial canal just before its termination, transmitting the chorda tympani nerve Huguier 管，鼓 索 出 口小管，传输鼓膜脊索神经；**Huschke c.,** a canal formed by the tubercles of the tympanic ring, usually disappearing during childhood Huschke 管，鼓膜管由鼓膜环结节形成的管，通常在儿童时期消失；**hyaloid c.,** a passage running from in front of the optic disk to the lens of the eye; in the fetus, it transmits the hyaloid artery 透明管，玻璃体管，玻璃体动脉导管；**hypoglossal c.,** an opening in the occipital bone, transmitting the hypoglossal nerve and a branch of the posterior meningeal artery 舌下神经管；**incisive c's,** the small canals opening into the incisive fossa of the hard palate, transmitting the nasopalatine nerves 切管；**infraorbital c.,** a small canal running obliquely through the floor of the orbit, transmitting the infraorbital vessels and nerve 眶下管；**inguinal c.,** the oblique passage in the lower anterior abdominal wall, through which passes the round ligament of the uterus in the female, and the spermatic cord in the male 腹股沟管；**interdental c's,** channels in the alveolar process of the mandible between the roots of the central and lateral incisors, for passage of anastomosing blood vessels between the sublingual and inferior dental arteries 牙间管；

medullary c., 1. vertebral c.; 2. 见 *cavity*. 下词条，髓管；**nasal c.**, **nasolacrimal c.**, a canal formed by the maxilla laterally and the lacrimal bone and inferior nasal concha medially, transmitting the nasolacrimal duct 鼻管；**neurenteric c.**, a temporary communication in the embryo between the posterior part of the neural tube and the archenteron 神经肠管；**c. of Nuck**, a pouch of peritoneum extending into the inguinal canal, accompanying the round ligament, in the female; usually obliterated after birth Nuck 管 女性的腹膜囊，伴随圆韧带延伸至腹股沟管，通常在出生后消失；**nutrient c.**, 见 haversian c.；**optic c.**, one of the paired openings in the sphenoid bone that transmits an optic nerve and its associated ophthalmic artery 视神经管；**perivascular c.**, a lymph space about a blood vessel 血管周隙；**Petit c.**, zonular spaces Petit 管，小带间隙（存在于睫状小带间的淋巴间隙）；**portal c.**, a space within the capsule of Glisson and liver substance, containing branches of the portal vein, of the hepatic artery, and of the hepatic duct 门脉管；**pterygoid c.**, a canal in the sphenoid bone transmitting the pterygoid vessels and nerves 翼管；**pterygopalatine c.**, a passage in the sphenoid and palatine bones for the greater palatine vessels and nerve 翼腭管；**pudendal c.**, a tunnel formed by a splitting of the obturator fascia, which encloses the pudendal vessels and nerve 阴部管；**pyloric c.**, the short narrow part of the stomach extending from the gastroduodenal junction to the pyloric antrum 幽门管；**root c.**, that part of the pulp cavity extending from the pulp chamber to the apical foramen 牙根管；牙根管填充手术；**saccu-locochlear c.**, the canal connecting the saccule and cochlea 连合管（耳蜗）；**sacral c.**, the continuation of the vertebral canal through the sacrum 骶管；**semicircular c's**, three long canals (anterior, lateral, and posterior) of the bony labyrinth, important in the sense of equilibrium（内耳的）半规管；**spermatic c.**, the inguinal canal in the male 腹股沟管（男）；**spiral c. of cochlea**, cochlear duct（耳）蜗螺旋管；**spiral c. of modiolus**, a canal following the course of the bony spiral lamina of the cochlea and containing the spiral ganglion 蜗轴螺旋管；**tarsal c.**, 见 *sinus* 下词条，跗骨窦；**tympanic c. of cochlea**, scala tympani 耳蜗鼓室管，鼓阶；**uterine c.**, the cavity of the uterus 子宫腔；**vertebral c.**, the canal formed by the series of vertebral foramina together, enclosing the spinal cord and meninges 椎管；**Volkmann c's**, canals communicating with the haversian canals, for passage of blood vessels through bone Volkmann 管，哈弗森管相通的管道，用于血管通过骨骼；**zygomaticotemporal c.**, 见 *foramen* 下词条，颧颞管

can·a·lic·u·lus (kan″ə-lik′u-ləs) pl. *canali′culi* [L.] an extremely narrow tubular passage or channel 小管；**canalic′ular** *adj.*；**apical c.**, one of the numerous tubular invaginations arising from the clefts between the microvilli of the proximal convoluted tubule of the kidney and extending downward into the apical cytoplasm 顶小管；**bone canaliculi**, branching tubular passages radiating like wheel spokes from each bone lacuna to connect with the canaliculi of adjacent lacunae, and with the haversian canal 骨小管；**cochlear c.**, a small canal in the petrous part of the temporal bone that interconnects the scala tympani with the subarachnoid space; it houses the perilymphatic duct and a small vein 耳蜗小管；**dental canaliculi**, minute channels in dentin, extending from the pulp cavity to the overlying cement and enamel 牙小管；**intercellular c.**, one located between adjacent cells, such as one of the secretory capillaries, or canaliculi, of the gastric parietal cells 细胞间小管；**intracellular canaliculi of parietal cells**, a system of canaliculi that seem to be intracellular but are formed by deep invaginations of the surface of the gastric parietal cells rather than extending into the cytoplasm of the cell 壁细胞细胞内分泌小管；**lacrimal c.**, the short passage in the eyelid, beginning at the lacrimal point and draining tears from the lacrimal lake to the lacrimal sac 泪小管；**mastoid c.**, a small channel in the temporal bone transmitting the auricular branch of the vagus nerve 乳突小管；**tympanic c.**, a small opening on the inferior surface of the petrous portion of the temporal bone, transmitting the tympanic branch of the glossopharyngeal nerve and a small artery 鼓室小管

ca·na·lis (kə-na′lis) pl. *cana′les* [L.] canal 沟；管；道

can·a·li·za·tion (kan″ə-lĭ-za′shən) 1. formation of canals, natural or pathologic 自然或病理性形成的通道；2. surgical creation of canals for drainage 外科引流管路；3. recanalization 再通；4. in psychology, formation in the central nervous system of new pathways by repeated passage of nerve impulses 心理学中，通过反复传递神经冲动在中枢神经系统中形成新的通路

can·cel·lous (kan-səl′əs) of a reticular, spongy, or lattice-like structure 网状、海绵状或格子状结构

can·cel·lus (kan-səl′əs) pl. *cancel′li* [L.] the lattice-like structure in bone; any structure arranged like a lattice 骨骼中的格子状结构；任何排列成格子的结构

can·cer (kan′sər) a neoplastic disease the natural course of which is fatal. Cancer cells, unlike benign tumor cells, exhibit the properties of invasion and

C

metastasis and are highly anaplastic. The term includes the two broad categories of carcinoma and sarcoma, but is often used synonymously with the former 癌症；**can′cerous** *adj.*；**bladder c.**, malignancy of the urinary bladder 膀胱癌；**epithelial c.**, carcinoma 上皮癌；**hereditary nonpolyposis colorectal c. (HNPCC)**, a group of autosomal dominant cancers characterized by adenomas of the colon and rectum without polyposis; caused by mutations in genes involved in repair of mismatch errors introduced during DNA replication 遗传性非息肉病结直肠癌；**ovarian c.**, cancer of the ovary; most often indicated by a pelvic mass 卵巢癌

can·cer·emia (kan″sər-e′me-ə) the presence of cancer cells in the blood 癌细胞血症

can·cer·i·gen·ic (kan″sər-ĭ-jen′ik) giving rise to a malignant tumor 致癌的

can·cer·pho·bia (kan″sər-fo′be-ə) irrational fear of cancer 恐癌症

can·croid (kang′kroid) resembling cancer 软下疳

can·crum (kang′krəm) [L.] canker 溃疡；**c. o′ris**, 见 *noma*；**c. puden′di**, 见 *noma*

can·dela (cd) (kan-del′ə) the base SI unit of luminous intensity 坎德拉发光强度的国际单位制基本单位

can·de·sar·tan (kan″də-sahr′tan) an angiotensin II receptor antagonist, used in the treatment of hypertension; administered orally as *c. cilexetil* 坎地沙坦

Can·di·da (kan′dĭ-də) a genus of anamorphic fungi that grow as yeast cells; most also produce a filamentous form. Some species are part of the normal flora of the skin and mucous membranes but can cause a variety of localized and systemic infections; common pathogens include *C. al′bicans, C. glabra′ta,* and *C. tropica′lis* 念珠菌属，变形真菌的一个属，以酵母细胞的形式生长；大多数也产生丝状体。有些物种是皮肤和黏膜正常菌群的一部分，但可引起多种局部和全身感染。包括白色念珠菌、光滑念珠菌和热带念珠菌

can·di·dal (kan′dĭ-dəl) pertaining to or caused by *Candida* 与念珠菌有关或由其引起的

can·di·di·a·sis (kan″dĭ-di′ə-sis) infection by fungi of the genus *Candida*, generally *C. albicans*, most commonly involving the skin, oral mucosa, respiratory tract, or vagina; rarely there is a systemic infection or endocarditis 念球菌病，念珠菌属真菌感染，通常是白色念珠菌，最常见的是皮肤、口腔黏膜（鹅口疮）、呼吸道或阴道；很少有全身性感染或心内膜炎；**acute pseudomembranous c.**, thrush 急性假膜性念珠菌病；**atrophic c.**, a type of oral candidiasis marked by erythematous pebbled patches on the hard or soft palate, buccal mucosa, and dorsal surface of the tongue 萎缩性念珠菌病；**bronchopulmonary c.**, bronchocandidiasis; that found in the respiratory tract 支气管肺念珠菌病；**chronic mucocutaneous c.**, any of various forms characterized by chronic candidiasis of oral and vaginal mucosa, skin, and nails, resistant to treatment, and sometimes familial 慢性黏膜皮肤念珠菌病；**oral c.**, thrush. 口腔念珠菌病 **vaginal c., vulvovaginal c.**, candidal infection of the vagina, and usually also the vulva, commonly characterized by pruritus, creamy white discharge, vulvar erythema and swelling, and dyspareunia 外阴阴道念珠菌病

can·di·din (kan′dĭ-din) a skin test antigen derived from *Candida albicans*, used in testing for the development of delayed-type hypersensitivity to the microorganism 白色念珠菌的皮肤试验抗原，用于测试对微生物的迟发型超敏反应的发展

ca·nine (ka′nīn) 1. of, pertaining to, or characteristic of a dog 犬齿；2. cuspid tooth 尖牙

ca·ni·ti·es (kə-nish′e-ēz) grayness or whiteness of the scalp hair 白发病

can·ker (kang′kər) an ulceration, especially of the oral mucosa 溃疡，尤指口腔溃疡

can·nab·i·noid (kə-nab′ĭ-noid) any of the principles of *Cannabis*, including tetrahydrocannabinol, cannabinol, and cannabidiol 大麻素

can·na·bis (kan′ə-bis) the dried flowering tops of hemp plants (*Cannabis sativa*), which have euphoric principles (tetrahydrocannabinols); classified as a hallucinogen and prepared as bhang, ganja, hashish, and marihuana 大麻制品

can·nu·la (kan′u-lə) a tube for insertion into a vessel, duct, or cavity; during insertion its lumen is usually occupied by a trocar 插管

can·thi·tis (kan-thi′tis) inflammation of the canthus 眼角炎

can·tho·plas·ty (kan′tho-plas″te) plastic surgery of a canthus 眼角膜整形手术

can·thot·o·my (kan-thot′ə-me) incision of a canthus 切开眼角术

can·thus (kan′thəs) pl. *can′thi* [L.] the angle at either end of the fissure between the eyelids, lateral or medial 眼角

can·ti·le·ver (kan″tĭ-le′vər) a projecting structure supported on only one end and carrying a load at the other end or along its length 悬臂

CAOS computer-assisted orthopedic surgery 计算机辅助整形外科

CAP College of American Pathologists 美国病理学家学院；community-acquired pneumonia 社区获得性肺炎

cap (kap) a protective covering for the head or for a similar structure; a structure resembling such a

covering 帽子；**acrosomal c.**, acrosome 顶体帽；
cradle c., crusta lactea 乳痂；**duodenal c.**, the part
of the duodenum adjacent to the pylorus, forming
the superior flexure 十二指肠球部；**enamel c.**, the
enamel organ after it covers the top of the growing
tooth papilla 釉质；**head c.**, the double-layered caplike structure over the upper two-thirds of the acrosome of a spermatozoon, consisting of the collapsed
acrosomal vesicle 帽（精子），双层帽状结构，
位于精子顶体的上 2/3 处，由顶体塌陷的囊泡组
成；**knee c.**, patella 髌骨

ca·pac·i·tance (C) (kə-pas′ ĭ-təns) 1. the property
of being able to store an electric charge 电容；
2. the ratio of the charge stored by a capacitor to the
voltage across the capacitor 电流容量

ca·pac·i·ta·tion (kə-pas″ĭ-ta′shən) the process by
which spermatozoa in the ampullary portion of a
uterine tube become capable of going through the
acrosome reaction and fertilizing an oocyte（精子）
获能

ca·pac·i·ty (kə-pas′ ĭ-te) the power to hold,
retain, or contain, or the ability to absorb; usually
expressed numerically as the measure of such ability
容量，容纳能力；**forced vital c. (FVC)**, vital
capacity measured when the patient is exhaling with
maximal speed and effort 用力肺活量；**functional
residual c.**, the amount of air remaining at the end
of normal quiet respiration 功能残气量；**heat c. (C.)**,
the amount of heat required to raise the temperature
of a specific quantity of a substance by one degree
Celsius 热容，将特定物质的温度升高 1℃所需
的热量；**inspiratory c.**, the volume of gas that can
be taken into the lungs in a full inhalation, starting
from the resting inspiratory position; equal to the
tidal volume plus the inspiratory reserve volume 吸
气量；**maximal breathing c.**, maximum voluntary
ventilation 最大呼吸容量；**thermal c.**, heat c.；**total lung c.**, the amount of gas contained in the lung
at the end of a maximal inhalation 肺总量；**virus
neutralizing c.**, the ability of a serum to inhibit
the infectivity of a virus 中和病毒能力；**vital c.
(VC)**, the volume of gas that can be expelled from
the lungs from a position of full inspiration, with no
limit to duration of inspiration; equal to inspiratory
capacity plus expiratory reserve volume 肺活量

cap·e·ci·ta·bine (kap″ə-si′tə-bēn) an antineoplastic used in the treatment of metastatic breast or
colorectal carcinoma 卡培他滨，一种用于治疗转
移性乳腺癌或结直肠癌的抗肿瘤药

cap·il·lar·ec·ta·sia (kap″ĭ-lar″ək-ta′zhə) dilatation
of capillaries 毛细血管扩张

Ca·pil·la·ria (kap″ĭ-lar′e-ə) a genus of parasitic
nematodes, including *C. hepat′ica*, found in the liver
of rats and other mammals, including humans; and *C.
philippinen′sis*, found in the human intestine in the
Philippines, causing severe diarrhea, malabsorption,
and high rates of mortality 毛细线虫属，一种寄生
线虫，包括肝毛细线虫，存在于大鼠和其他哺乳
动物（包括人类）的肝脏中；在菲律宾的人体肠
道中发现的菲律宾毛细线虫导致严重的腹泻，吸
收不良和高死亡率

cap·il·la·ri·a·sis (kap″ĭ-lə-ri′ə-sis) infection with
nematodes of the genus *Capillaria*, especially *C.
philippinensis* 毛细线虫病，感染了毛细线虫属的
线虫，特别是菲律宾毛细线虫

cap·il·lar·i·ty (kap″ĭ-lar′ ĭ-te) the action by which
the surface of a liquid in contact with a solid, as in a
capillary tube, is elevated or depressed 毛细现象，
液体表面与固体接触的作用，如在毛细管中，升
高或降低的作用

cap·il·lary (kap″ĭ-lar″e) 1. pertaining to or resembling a hair 毛细管；2. one of the minute vessels
connecting the arterioles and venules, the walls of
which act as a semipermeable membrane for inter-
change of various substances between the blood and
tissue fluid 毛细血管；见图 22；**arterial c.**, precapillary; a type of minute vessel lacking a continuous
muscular coat, intermediate in structure and location
between an arteriole and a capillary 动脉毛细血
管；**continuous c's**, one of the two major types
of capillaries, found in muscle, skin, lung, central
nervous system, and other tissues, characterized by
the presence of an uninterrupted endothelium and a
continuous basal lamina, and by fine filaments and
numerous pinocytotic vesicles 在肌肉、皮肤、
肺、中枢神经系统和其他组织中发现的两种主要
类型的毛细血管之一，其特征在于存在不间断
的内皮和连续的基底层，以及细胞和许多胞饮
囊泡；**fenestrated c's**, one of the two major types
of capillaries, found in the intestinal mucosa, renal
glomeruli, pancreas, endocrine glands, and other
tissues, and characterized by the presence of circular
fenestrae or pores that penetrate the endothelium;
these pores may be closed by a very thin diaphragm
有孔毛细管；两种主要类型的毛细血管中的一
种，存在于肠黏膜、肾小球、胰腺、内分泌腺和
其他组织中，其特征在于存在穿透内皮的圆形
窗孔或孔；这些孔可以被非常薄的隔膜封闭；
lymph c., **lymphatic c.**, one of the minute vessels
of the lymphatic system 毛细淋巴管，见图 22.；
secretory c., any of the extremely fine intercellular
canaliculi situated between adjacent gland cells,
being formed by the apposition of grooves in the parietal cells and opening into the gland's lumen. 分泌
毛细血管；**venous c.**, postcapillary venule; a type
of minute vessel lacking a muscular coat, intermedi-

ate in structure and location between a venule and a capillary 静脉毛细血管，毛细血管后小静脉；一种缺乏肌肉外层的微小血管，结构和位置介于小静脉和毛细血管之间

cap·il·lus (kə-pil′əs) pl. *capil′li* [L.] a hair of the scalp; in the plural, denoting the aggregate of scalp hair 头发

cap·i·tate (kap′ĭ-tāt) head-shaped 头形的

cap·i·ta·tion (kap″ĭ-ta′shən) the annual fee paid to a physician or group of physicians by each participant in a health plan 按人头付费，由健康计划中的每个参与者支付给医生或医生组的年费

cap·i·ta·tum (kap″ĭ-ta′təm) [L.] capitate bone 头骨

cap·i·tel·lum (kap″ĭ-tel′əm) capitulum 肱骨小头

cap·i·ton·nage (kap″ĭ-to-nahzh′) [Fr.] closure of a cyst by applying sutures to approximate the opposing surfaces of the cavity 缝合

ca·pit·u·lum (kə-pit′u-ləm) pl. *capi′tula* [L.] a small eminence on a bone, as on the distal end of the humerus, by which it articulates with another bone; **capit′ular** *adj.*

Cap·no·cy·toph·a·ga (kap″no-si-tof′ə-gə) a genus of anaerobic, gram-negative, rod-shaped bacteria of the family Flavobacteriaceae; it has been implicated in the pathogenesis of periodontal disease and is associated with systemic disease in debilitated persons 二氧化碳噬纤维菌属，黄杆菌科一种厌氧、革兰阴性、杆状细菌；它与牙周病的发病机制有关，并且与衰弱的人的全身性疾病有关；*C. canimor′sus*, a species that is part of the normal oral flora of dogs and cats; following a bite it may cause serious local or systemic infection or death 犬咬二氧化碳嗜纤维菌，一种属于狗和猫正常口腔的物种；被咬后，可能会导致严重的局部或全身性感染或死亡

cap·no·gram (kap′no-gram″) a real-time waveform record of the concentration of carbon dioxide in the respiratory gases 二氧化碳描记图，实时波形记录呼吸气体中二氧化碳的浓度

cap·no·graph (kap′no-graf″) a system for monitoring the concentration of exhaled carbon dioxide 二氧化碳分析仪

cap·nog·ra·phy (kap-nog′rə-fe) monitoring of the concentration of exhaled carbon dioxide in order to assess the physiologic status or determine the adequacy of ventilation during anesthesia 二氧化碳监测仪

cap·nom·e·ter (kap-nom′ə-tər) a device for monitoring the end-tidal partial pressure of carbon dioxide 二氧化碳监测仪

cap·nom·e·try (kap-nom′ə-tre) the determination of the end-tidal partial pressure of carbon dioxide 二氧化碳测定术

cap·ping (kap′ing) 1. the provision of a protective or obstructive covering 封盖；2. the formation of a polar cap on the surface of a cell concerned with immunologic responses, occurring as a result of movement of components on the cell surface into clusters or patches that coalesce to form the cap. The process is produced by reaction of antibody with the cell membrane and appears to involve cross-linking of antigenic determinants 因免疫反应在细胞表面形成极帽，主要是由于细胞表面成分移动聚集成簇或堆，该过程通过抗体与细胞膜的反应产生，且涉及抗原决定簇的交联；**pulp c.**, the covering of an exposed or nearly exposed dental pulp with some material to provide protection against external influences and to encourage healing 盖髓术；用一些材料覆盖暴露或接近暴露的牙髓，以防止外部影响并促进愈合

cap·reo·my·cin (kap″re-o-mi′sin) a polypeptide antibiotic produced by *Streptomyces capreolus*, which is active against human strains of *Mycobacterium tuberculosis*; used as the disulfate salt 卷曲霉素

cap·ric ac·id (kap′rik) a saturated ten-carbon fatty acid, occurring as a minor constituent in many fats and oils 癸酸，饱和的十碳脂肪酸，在许多脂肪和油中作为次要成分出现

cap·ro·ate (kap′ro-āt) 1. any salt or ester of caproic acid (hexanoic acid) 盐或己酸的酯；2. USAN contraction for hexanoate USAN 收缩己酸盐

ca·pro·ic ac·id (kə-pro′ik) a saturated sixcarbon fatty acid occurring in butterfat and coconut and palm oils 饱和的六碳脂肪酸，存在于乳脂、椰子油和棕榈油中

cap·ry·late (kap′rə-lāt) any salt, ester, or anionic form of caprylic acid 盐、酯或阴离子形式的辛酸

ca·pryl·ic ac·id (kə-pril′ik) an eight-carbon saturated fatty acid occurring in butterfat and palm and coconut oils 辛酸，一种八碳饱和脂肪酸，存在于乳脂、棕榈和椰子油中

cap·sa·i·cin (kap-sa′ĭ-sin) an alkaloid irritating to the skin and mucous membranes, the active ingredient of capsicum; used as a topical counterirritant and analgesic 辣椒素，生物碱刺激皮肤和黏膜，辣椒的有效成分；用作局部抗刺激剂和止痛剂

cap·si·cum (kap′sĭ-kəm) a plant of the genus *Capsicum*, the hot peppers, or the dried fruit derived from certain of its species (cayenne or red pepper), containing the active principle capsaicin; used as a counterirritant and analgesic and also in pepper spray 辣椒

cap·sid (kap′sid) the shell of protein that protects the nucleic acid of a virus; it is composed of structural units, or capsomers 衣壳

cap·so·mer (kap′so-mər) the morphologic unit of the capsid of a virus 壳粒

cap·su·la (kap′su-lə) pl. *cap′sulae* [L.] capsule 囊

cap·sule (kap′səl) 1. an enclosing structure, as a soluble container enclosing a dose of medicine 胶囊; 2. a cartilaginous, fatty, fibrous, membranous structure enveloping another structure, organ, or part 软骨、脂肪、纤维、膜状结构，包裹着另一结构，器官或部分; **cap′sular** *adj.*; **adipose c. of kidney,** the investment of fat surrounding the fibrous capsule of the kidney, continuous at the hilum with the fat in the renal sinus 肾脏脂肪囊; **articular c.,** joint c.; **auditory c.,** the cartilaginous capsule of the embryo that develops into the bony labyrinth of the internal ear 听囊，胚胎的软骨囊发展成内耳的骨迷路; **bacterial c.,** an envelope of gel surrounding a bacterial cell, usually polysaccharide but sometimes polypeptide in nature; it is associated with the virulence of pathogenic bacteria 荚膜; **cartilage c.,** a basophilic zone of cartilage matrix bordering on a lacuna and its enclosed cartilage cells 软骨囊; **external c.,** the layer of white fibers between the putamen and claustrum 外囊; **fibrous c. of kidney,** the connective tissue investment of the kidney, continuous through the hilum to line the renal sinus 肾脏纤维囊; **Glisson c.,** the connective tissue sheath accompanying the hepatic ducts and vessels through the hepatic portal Glisson 囊实际是一种纤维囊。它包绕肝门静脉、肝管、肝固有动脉三部分。由于肝门静脉、肝管、肝固有动脉在肝内的分布与分支情况基本一致，因此就将 Glisoon 囊包绕的这部分统称为门脉系统，并以此进行肝叶及肝段的划分; **glomerular c., c. of glomerulus,** the globular dilatation forming the beginning of a uriniferous tubule within the kidney and surrounding the glomerulus 肾小囊; **internal c.,** a fanlike mass of white fibers separating the lentiform nucleus laterally from the head of the caudate nucleus, the dorsal thalamus, and the tail of the caudate nucleus medially 内囊，一种扇形的白色纤维，从尾状核的头部、背侧丘脑和尾状核的尾部向内侧分离豆状核; **joint c.,** articular c.; the saclike envelope enclosing the cavity of a synovial joint 关节囊; **lens c., c. of lens,** the elastic envelope covering the lens of the eye 晶状体囊; **optic c.,** the embryonic structure from which the sclera develops 视神经囊，巩膜发育的胚胎结构; **otic c.,** the skeletal element enclosing the inner ear mechanism. In the human embryo, it develops as cartilage at various ossification centers and becomes completely bony and unified at about the 23rd week of fetal life 耳囊，包绕内耳的骨骼结构。在人类胚胎中，它在不同的骨化中心形成软骨，在胎儿 23 周左右完

全成骨; **renal c's,** the investing tissue around the kidney, divided into the *fibrous renal capsule* and the *adipose renal capsule* 肾包膜; **Tenon c.,** the connective tissue enveloping the posterior eyeball 后部眼球筋膜

cap·su·lec·to·my (kap″su-lek′tə-me) excision of a capsule, especially a joint capsule or lens capsule 囊切除术，特别是关节囊或晶状体囊

cap·su·li·tis (kap″su-li′tis) inflammation of a capsule, such as the lens capsule 囊炎，例如晶状体囊炎; **adhesive c.,** adhesive inflammation between the joint capsule and the peripheral articular cartilage of the shoulder, with obliteration of the subdeltoid bursa, characterized by increasing pain, stiffness, and limitation of motion 黏连性囊炎

cap·su·lo·plas·ty (kap″su-lo-plas″te) plastic repair of a joint capsule 关节囊修复

cap·su·lor·rhex·is (kap″su-lo-rek′sis) the making of a continuous circular tear in the anterior capsule during cataract surgery in order to allow expression or phacoemulsification of the nucleus of the lens 撕囊术

cap·su·lot·o·my (kap″su-lot′ə-me) incision of a capsule, as that of the lens, the kidney, or a joint 囊切开术，如晶状体、肾脏或关节囊的切除术

cap·to·pril (kap′to-pril) an angiotensin-converting enzyme inhibitor used in the treatment of hypertension, congestive heart failure, and post–myocardial infarction left ventricular dysfunction 卡托普利，一种血管紧张素转换酶抑制剂，用于治疗高血压、充血性心力衰竭和心肌梗死后左心室功能障碍

cap·ture (kap′chər) 1. to seize or catch 抓住; 2. the coalescence of an atomic nucleus and a subatomic particle, usually resulting in an unstable mass 原子核和亚原子粒子的结合，通常导致质量不稳定; **atrial c.,** depolarization of the atria in response to a stimulus originating elsewhere in the heart or induced by a pacemaker 心房捕获; **ventricular c.,** depolarization of the ventricles in response to an impulse originating either in the supraventricular region or in an artificial pacemaker 心室捕获

cap·ut (kap′ət) pl. *cap′ita* [L.] 1. head 头; 2. the expanded or chief extremity of an organ or part 器官或部分器官的扩张或主要末端; **c. medu′sae,** dilated cutaneous veins around the umbilicus, seen mainly in the newborn and in patients with cirrhosis 水母头样扩张的静脉，脐周围皮肤静脉扩张，主要见于新生儿和肝硬化患者; **c. succeda′neum,** edema occurring in and under the fetal scalp during labor 产瘤，在分娩期间发生在胎儿头皮内和头皮下的水肿

CAR Canadian Association of Radiologists 加拿

大放射学家协会

car·ba·ceph·em (kahr″bə-sef′əm) any of a class of antibiotics closely related to the cephalosporins in structure and use, but chemically more stable 碳头孢烯，在结构和用途上与头孢菌素密切相关的一类抗生素，但化学性质更稳定

car·ba·chol (kahr′bə-kol) a cholinergic agonist used as a miotic and to lower intraocular pressure in the treatment of glaucoma and following cataract surgery 卡巴可，氯化氨甲酰胆碱，碳酰胆碱，一种胆碱能激动剂，作为缩瞳剂用于降低眼压，治疗青光眼和白内障手术

car·ba·mate (kahr′bə-māt) any ester of carbamic acid 氨基甲酸酯

car·ba·maz·e·pine (kahr″bə-maz′ə-pēn) an anticonvulsant and analgesic used in the treatment of pain associated with trigeminal neuralgia and in epilepsy manifested by certain types of seizures 卡马西平，一种抗惊厥药和止痛药，用于治疗与三叉神经痛以及表现为某些类型癫痫发作的疼痛

car·bam·ic ac·id (kahr-bam′ik) NH_2COOH, a compound existing only in the form of salts or esters (carbamates), amides (carbamides), and other derivatives 氨基甲酸

car·bam·ide (kahr′bə-mīd) urea 尿素；**c. peroxide,** a compound of urea and hydrogen peroxide used as a cerumen-softening agent, dental cleanser, bleaching agent, and antiinflammatory 过氧化脲

car·bam·i·no·he·mo·glo·bin (kahr-bam″ĭno-he′mo-glo″bin) a combination of carbon dioxide and hemoglobin, CO_2HHb, being one of the forms in which carbon dioxide exists in the blood 氨基甲酸血红蛋白，二氧化碳和血红蛋白的结合物，CO_2HHb，是二氧化碳存在于血液中的一种形式

car·bam·o·yl (kahr-bam′o-əl) the radical NH_2CO-氨甲酰基，见 *carbamoyltransferase*

car·bam·o·yl·trans·fer·ase (kahr-bam″o-əl-trans′fər-ās) an enzyme that catalyzes the transfer of a carbamoyl group, as from carbamoylphosphate to l-ornithine to form orthophosphate and citrulline in the synthesis of urea 氨基甲酰转移酶

car·ben·i·cil·lin (kahr″bən-ĭ-sil′in) a semisynthetic penicillin, with activity against *Pseudomonas aeruginosa* and some other gram-negative bacteria; used as the disodium salt. It is also used as *c. indanyl sodium* in the treatment of urinary tract infections and prostatitis 羧苄青霉素

car·bi·do·pa (kahr″bĭ-do′pə) an inhibitor of decarboxylation of levodopa in extracerebral tissues, used in combination with levodopa as an antiparkinsonian agent 卡比多巴

car·bi·nol (kahr′bĭ-nol) 1. methyl alcohol 甲醇；2. any aromatic or fatty alcohol formed by substituting one, two, or three hydrocarbon groups for hydrogen in methanol 甲醇中以一个、两个或三个烃基取代氢而形成的芳香醇或脂肪醇

car·bi·nox·amine (kahr″bin-ok′sə-mēn) an antihistamine with anticholinergic and sedative effects, used as the maleate salt 卡比沙明，具有抗胆碱能和镇静作用的抗组胺药，用作马来酸盐

car·bo·hy·drate (kahr″bo-hi′drāt) any of a class of aldehyde or ketone derivatives of polyhydric alcohols, so named because the hydrogen and oxygen are usually in the proportion of water, $C_n(H_2O)$; the most important comprise the starches, sugars, glycogens, celluloses, and gums 碳水化合物，糖类

car·bol·fuch·sin (kahr″bol-fūk′sin) a solution containing basic fuchsin and dilute phenol; used in various stains for demonstrating acid-fast bacteria 石炭酸品红，含有碱性品红和稀释酚；用于各种污渍，用于证明耐酸细菌

car·bol·ic ac·id (kahr-bol′ik) phenol (1) 苯酚

car·bol·ism (kahr′bəl-iz-əm) phenol poisoning 石炭酸中毒；见 *phenol* (1)

car·bon (C) (kahr′bən) a nonmetallic tetrad element occurring in several forms, including diamond, graphite, and amorphous carbon; at. no. 6, at. wt. 12.011. There are three naturally occurring isotopes; two are stable (^{12}C and ^{13}C) and one is unstable (^{14}C, half-life 5730 years) 碳（C）；**c. dioxide,** an odorless, colorless gas, CO_2, resulting from oxidation of carbon, and formed in the tissues and eliminated by the lungs; used in some pump oxygenators to maintain blood carbon dioxide tension. In solid form it is *carbon dioxide snow* (see under *snow*) 二氧化碳；**c. monoxide,** an odorless gas, CO, formed by burning carbon or organic fuels with a scanty supply of oxygen; inhalation causes central nervous system damage and asphyxiation by combining irreversibly with blood hemoglobin 一氧化碳；**c. tetrachloride,** a clear, colorless, volatile liquid; inhalation of its vapors can depress central nervous system activity and cause degeneration of the liver and kidneys 四氯化碳

car·bon·ate (kahr′bə-nāt) a salt of carbonic acid 碳酸盐

car·bon·ic ac·id (kahr-bon′ik) an aqueous solution of carbon dioxide, H_2CO_3 碳酸

car·bon·ic an·hy·drase (kahr-bon′ik anhi′drās) an enzyme that catalyzes the decomposition of carbonic acid into carbon dioxide and water, facilitating the transfer of carbon dioxide from tissues to blood and from blood to alveolar air 碳酸酐酶

car·bon·yl (kahr′bə-nəl) the bivalent organic radical, C:O, characteristic of aldehydes, ketones, carboxylic acid, and esters 羰基

car·bo·pla·tin (kahr″bo-plat″in) an antineoplastic used in the treatment of carcinomas of the ovary and numerous other organs 卡铂, 用于治疗卵巢癌和许多其他器官的抗肿瘤药

car·bo·prost (kahr″bo-prost) a synthetic analogue of dinoprost, a prostaglandin of the F type; used as the tromethamine salt as an oxytocic for termination of pregnancy and missed abortion 卡前列素, 地诺前列素合成类似物, 是一种 F 型前列腺素；作为催产药用于终止妊娠和流产

γ-car·boxy·glu·ta·mic ac·id (kahr-bok″segloo-tam′ik) an amino acid occurring in biologically active prothrombin, and formed in the liver in the presence of vitamin K by carboxylation of glutamic acid residues in prothrombin precursor molecules γ-羧基谷氨酸

car·boxy·he·mo·glo·bin (kahr-bok″se-he′moglo″bin) hemoglobin combined with carbon monoxide, which occupies the sites on the hemoglobin molecule that normally bind with oxygen and which is not readily displaced from the molecule 碳氧血红蛋白

car·box·yl (kahr-bok″səl) the monovalent radical −COOH, occurring in those organic acids termed carboxylic acids 羧基

car·box·y·lase (kahr-bok′sə-lās) an enzyme that catalyzes the removal of carbon dioxide from the carboxyl group of alpha amino keto acids 羧化酶

car·box·y·la·tion (kahr-bok″sə-la′shən) the addition of carbon dioxide or bicarbonate to form a carboxyl group, as to pyruvate to form oxaloacetate 羧化

car·box·yl·es·ter·ase (kahr-bok″səl-es′tər-ās) an enzyme of wide specificity that catalyzes the hydrolytic cleavage of the ester bond in a carboxylic ester to form an alcohol and a carboxylic acid, including acting on esters of vitamin A 羧酸酯酶

car·box·yl·trans·fer·ase (kahr-bok″səl-trans′fər-ās) any of a group of enzymes that catalyze the transfer of a carboxyl group from a donor to an acceptor compound 羧基转移酶

car·boxy·ly·ase (kahr-bok″səl-li′ās) any of a group of lyases that catalyze the removal of a carboxyl group; it includes the carboxylases and decarboxylases 羧基裂解酶

car·boxy·meth·yl·cel·lu·lose (kahr-bok″se-meth″əl-sel′u-lōs) a substituted cellulose polymer of variable size, used as the sodium or calcium salt as a pharmaceutical suspending agent, tablet excipient, and viscosity-increasing agent; the former is also used as a laxative 羧甲基纤维素

car·boxy·myo·glo·bin (kahr-bok″se-mi″oglo′bin) a compound formed from myoglobin on exposure to carbon monoxide 碳氧肌红蛋白

car·boxy·pep·ti·dase (kahr-bok″se-pep′tīdās) any exopeptidase that catalyzes the hydrolytic cleavage of the terminal or penultimate bond at the end of a peptide or polypeptide where the free carboxyl group occurs 羧肽酶

car·bun·cle (kahr′bəng-kəl) a necrotizing infection of skin and superficial fascia composed of a cluster of furuncles, usually due to *Staphylococcus aureus*, with multiple drainage sinuses 痈, 有头疽；**carbunc′ular** adj.; **malignant c.**, anthrax 恶性痈, 炭疽

car·ci·no·em·bry·on·ic (kahr″sĭ-no-em″breon′ik) occurring both in carcinoma and in embryonic tissue; see under *antigen* 癌胚的, 发生于癌和胚胎的

car·cin·o·gen (kahr-sin′ə-jen) any substance which causes cancer 致癌物质；**carcinogen′ic** adj. **epigenetic c.**, one that does not itself damage DNA but causes alterations that predispose to cancer 表观遗传毒性致癌物；**genotoxic c.**, one that reacts directly with DNA or with macromolecules that then react with DNA 基因毒性致癌物

car·ci·no·gen·e·sis (kahr″sĭ-no-jen′ə-sis) the production of carcinoma 致癌作用

car·ci·no·ge·nic·i·ty (kahr″sĭ-no-jə-nis′ ĭ-te) the ability or tendency to produce cancer 致癌性

car·ci·noid (kahr′sĭ-noid) carcinoid tumor 良性肿瘤；**ECL cell c.**, enterochromaffin-like cell c., a carcinoid tumor of the gastric fundus consisting of enterochromaffin-like (ECL) cells; multiple tumors are usually present 肠嗜铬细胞样癌

car·ci·nol·y·sis (kahr″sĭ-nol′ə-sis) destruction of cancer cells 癌细胞溶解；**carcinolyt′ic** adj.

car·ci·no·ma (kahr″sĭ-no′mə) pl. *carcinomas, carcino′mata*. A malignant new growth made up of epithelial cells tending to infiltrate surrounding tissues and to give rise to metastases 癌；**acinar c., acinic cell c., acinous c.**, a slow-growing malignant tumor with acinic cells in small glandlike structures, usually in the pancreas or salivary glands 腺泡癌；**adenocystic c., adenoid cystic c.**, cylindroma; carcinoma marked by cylinders or bands of hyaline or mucinous stroma separating or surrounded by nests or cords of small epithelial cells, occurring particularly in the salivary glands 腺样囊性癌；**adenosquamous c.**, 1. adenoacanthoma 腺棘皮癌；2. a diverse category of bronchogenic carcinoma, with areas of glandular, squamous, and large-cell differentiation 腺鳞癌；**adnexal c's**, a large group of carcinomas arising from, or forming structures resembling, the skin appendages, particularly the sweat or sebaceous glands 附件癌；**adrenocortical c.,** a malignant adrenal cortical tumor that can cause endocrine disorders such as Cushing syndrome or adrenogenital syndrome 肾上腺皮质癌；**alveolar c.,** bronchioloalveolar c. 肺泡细胞癌；**ameloblastic c.,** a type of ameloblastoma in which there has been malignant epithelial transformation, with metastases usually resembling squamous cell c. 成釉细胞癌；**apocrine c.,** 1. adnexal carcinoma in an apocrine gland（皮肤）大汗腺癌；2. a rare breast malignancy with a ductal or acinar growth pattern and apocrine secretions 乳腺大汗腺癌；**basal cell c.,** an epithelial tumor of the skin that seldom metastasizes but has the potential for local invasion and destruction; the most common is the *nodular* type, characterized by small pearly nodules with central depressions on the sunexposed skin of fair-skinned older adults 基底细胞癌；**basosquamous cell c.,** a type of carcinoma of the skin that has elements of both basal cell and squamous cell types 基底鳞状细胞癌；**bronchioloalveolar c.,** a variant type of adenocarcinoma of the lung, with columnar to cuboidal cells lining the alveolar septa and projecting into alveolar spaces 细支气管肺泡癌；**bronchogenic c.,** any of a group of carcinomas of the lung, so called because it arises from the epithelium of the bronchial tree 支气管肺癌；**cholangiocellular c.,** a rare primary carcinoma of the liver originating in bile duct cells 胆管细胞癌；**chorionic c.,** choriocarcinoma 绒毛膜癌；**clear cell c.,** 1. 见 *adenocarcinoma* 下词条，透明细胞癌；2. renal cell c. 肾透明细胞癌；**colloid c.,** mucinous c. 胶质瘤；**cribriform c.,** 1. adenoid cystic c. 腺样囊性癌；2. an adenoid cystic carcinoma of the lactiferous ducts, one of the subtypes of ductal carcinoma in situ 筛状癌；**cylindrical cell c.,** carcinoma in which the cells are cylindrical or nearly so 柱状细胞癌；**ductal c. in situ (DCIS),** any of a large group of in situ carcinomas of the lactiferous ducts 导管原位癌；**eccrine c.,** an adnexal carcinoma that originates in eccrine sweat glands 小汗腺癌；**embryonal c.,** a highly malignant, primitive form of carcinoma, probably of germinal cell or teratomatous derivation, usually arising in a gonad 胚胎癌；**c. en cuirasse,** carcinoma of the skin manifest as areas of thickening and induration over large areas of the thorax, frequently as a result of metastasis from a primary breast lesion 铠甲状癌；**endometrioid c.,** that characterized by glandular patterns resembling those of the endometrium, occurring in the uterine fundus and ovaries 子宫内膜癌；**epidermoid c.,** squamous cell c. (2) 表皮样癌；**c. ex mixed tumor,**

c. ex pleomorphic adenoma, a type of malignant pleomorphic adenoma usually occurring in the salivary glands of older adults; an epithelial malignancy arises in a preexisting mixed tumor 多形性腺瘤癌；**follicular c. of thyroid gland,** a type of thyroid gland carcinoma with many follicles 甲状腺滤泡癌；**giant cell c.,** a poorly differentiated, highly malignant, epithelial neoplasm containing many giant cells, such as occurs in the lungs or thyroid gland 巨细胞癌；**hepatocellular c.,** primary carcinoma of the liver cells; it has been associated with chronic hepatitis B virus infection, some types of cirrhosis, and hepatitis C virus infection 肝细胞癌；**Hürthle cell c.,** a malignant Hürthle cell tumor Hürthle 细胞癌；**inflammatory c. of breast,** a highly malignant carcinoma of the breast, with pink to red skin discoloration, tenderness, edema, and rapid enlargement 炎性乳腺癌；**c. in si'tu,** a type whose tumor cells are still confined to the epithelium of origin, without invasion of the basement membrane; the likelihood of subsequent invasive growth is presumed to be high 原位癌；**intraductal c.,** 1. any carcinoma of the epithelium of a duct 导管上皮细胞癌；2. ductal carcinoma in situ 导管内原位癌；**invasive lobular c.,** an invasive type of carcinoma of the breast characterized by linear growth into desmoplastic stroma around the terminal part of the lobules of the mammary glands; usually developing from lobular carcinoma in situ 乳腺浸润性小叶癌；**large cell c.,** a bronchogenic tumor of undifferentiated (anaplastic) cells of large size 大细胞癌；**lobular c.,** 1. terminal duct c. 终末导管癌；2. 见 *lobular c. in situ*; **lobular c. in situ (LCIS),** a type of precancerous neoplasia found in the lobules of mammary glands, progressing slowly, sometimes to invasive lobular carcinoma, after many years 小叶原位癌；**medullary c.,** that composed mainly of epithelial elements with little or no stroma; commonly occurring in the breast and thyroid gland 髓样癌；**meningeal c.,** primary or secondary carcinomatous infiltration of the meninges, particularly the pia and arachnoid 脑膜癌；**Merkel cell c.,** a rapidly growing malignant dermal or subcutaneous tumor occurring on sun-exposed areas in middled-aged or older adults and containing irregular anastomosing trabeculae and small dense granules typical of Merkel cells 梅克尔细胞癌；**mucinous c.,** adenocarcinoma producing significant amounts of mucin 黏液癌；**mucoepidermoid c.,** a malignant epithelial tumor of glandular tissue, particularly the salivary glands, characterized by acini with mucus-producing cells and by malignant squamous elements 黏液表皮样癌；**nasopharyngeal c.,** a malignant tumor arising in the epithelial lining of the nasopharynx, seen most often in people of Chinese ancestry. Human herpesvirus 4 (Epstein-Barr virus) has been implicated as a cause 鼻咽癌；**non-small cell c., nonsmall cell lung c. (NSCLC)**, a general term comprising all lung carcinomas except small cell c. 非小细胞肺癌；**oat cell c.**, a form of small cell carcinoma in which the cells are round or elongated, have scanty cytoplasm, and clump poorly 燕麦细胞癌；**papillary c.**, carcinoma in which there are papillary excrescences. 乳头状癌；**renal cell c.**, clear cell carcinoma; carcinoma of the renal parenchyma, composed of tubular cells in varying arrangements 肾细胞癌；**scirrhous c.**, carcinoma with a hard structure due to the formation of dense connective tissue in the stroma 硬癌；**sebaceous c.**, adnexal carcinoma of the sebaceous glands, usually occurring as a hard yellow nodule on the eyelid 皮脂腺癌；**signet ring cell c.**, a highly malignant mucus-secreting tumor in which the cells are anaplastic, with nuclei displaced to one side by a globule of mucus 印戒细胞癌；**c. sim′plex**, an undifferentiated carcinoma 单纯癌；**small cell c., small cell lung c. (SCLC)**, a common, highly malignant form of bronchogenic carcinoma in the wall of a major bronchus, usually in middle-aged smokers, composed of small, oval, undifferentiated hematoxyphilic cells 小细胞肺癌；**spindle cell c.**, carcinoma, usually of the squamous cell type, marked by fusiform development of rapidly proliferating cells 梭形细胞癌；**squamous c., squamous cell c.**, 1. an initially local carcinoma developed from squamous epithelium, including sun-damaged skin, characterized by cuboid cells and keratinization 鳞状上皮细胞癌；2. a form of bronchogenic carcinoma, usually in middle-aged smokers, generally forming polypoid or sessile masses obstructing the bronchial airways 支气管鳞癌；**terminal duct c.**, a slow-growing, locally invasive, malignant neoplasm composed of myoepithelial and ductal elements, occurring in the minor salivary glands 终末导管癌；**transitional cell c.**, a malignant tumor arising from a transitional type of stratified epithelium, usually affecting the urinary bladder 移行细胞癌；**tubular c.**, 1. an adenocarcinoma in which the cells are arranged in tubules 管状腺癌；2. a type of breast cancer in which small glandlike structures are formed and infiltrate the stroma, usually developing from a ductal carcinoma in situ 乳腺小管癌；**verrucous c.**, a variety of locally invasive squamous cell carcinoma with a predilection for the buccal mucosa but also affecting other oral soft tissues and the larynx; sometimes used for the similar Buschke-Löwenstein tumor on the genitals 疣状癌

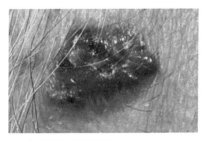

▲　色素性基底细胞癌（**Pigmented basal cell carcinoma**）

car·ci·no·ma·to·sis (kahr″sĭ-no-mə-to′sis) the condition of widespread dissemination of cancer throughout the body 癌扩散

car·ci·nom·a·tous (kahr″sĭ-nom′ə-təs) pertaining to or of the nature of cancer 癌性的

car·ci·no·sar·co·ma (kahr″sĭ-no-sahr-ko′mə) a malignant tumor composed of carcinomatous and sarcomatous tissues 癌肉瘤；**embryonal c.**, Wilms tumor 胚胎学癌肉瘤

car·da·mom (kahr′də-məm) 1. a plant of the species *Elettaria cardamomum* or any of various closely related plants having similar seeds 小豆蔻属的植物或具有类似种子、亲缘关系密切的植物；2. a preparation of the seeds of *E. cardamomum*, used for respiratory and gastrointestinal tract disorders, as well as in traditional Chinese medicine and ayurveda 中医和阿育吠陀中，使用小豆蔻种子的处方，用作治疗呼吸道和胃肠道疾病

car·dia (kahr′de-ə) the cardiac part of the stomach, surrounding the esophagogastric junction and distinguished by the presence of cardiac glands 贲门

car·di·ac (kahr′de-ak) 1. pertaining to the heart 心脏的；2. pertaining to the cardia 贲门的

car·di·ac rhy·thm (car′dē-ack rithm) heart rhythm 心律

car·di·al·gia (kahr″de-al′jə) cardiodynia 心痛

car·di·ec·ta·sis (kahr″de-ek′tə-sis) dilatation of the heart 心脏扩张

car·di·nal (kahr′dĭ-nəl) 1. of primary or preeminent importance 主要的；2. in embryology, pertaining to the main venous drainage 胚胎主要静脉回流的

car·dio·ac·cel·er·a·tor (kahr″de-o-ak-sel′ərə-tər) quickening the heart action; an agent that so acts 心动加速药

car·dio·an·gi·ol·o·gy (kahr″de-o-an″je-ol′ə-je) the medical specialty dealing with the heart and blood vessels 心血管学

car·dio·ar·te·ri·al (kahr″de-o-ahr-tēr′e-əl) pertaining to the heart and the arteries 心动脉的

Car·dio·bac·te·ri·a·ceae (kahr″de-o-bak-tēr″ea′se-e) a family of gram-negative, rod-shaped bacteria of the order Cardiobacteriales 心杆菌科

Car·dio·bac·ter·i·a·les (kahr″de-o-bak-tēr″ea′lēz) an order of gram-negative, mainly aerobic bacteria of the class Gammaproteobacteria 心杆菌目

Car·dio·bac·te·ri·um (kahr″de-o-bak-tēr′e-əm) a genus of gram-negative, rod-shaped bacteria of the family Cardiobacteriaceae, which are part of the normal flora of the nose and throat and are also isolated from the blood. *C. ho′minis* is a cause of endocarditis 心杆菌属

car·dio·cele (kahr′de-o-sēl″) hernial protrusion of the heart through a fissure of the respiratory diaphragm or through a wound 通过呼吸隔膜的裂口或伤口引发的心脏突出

car·dio·cen·te·sis (kahr″de-o-sen-te′sis) surgical puncture of the heart 心脏穿刺术

car·dio·cir·rho·sis (kahr″de-o-sĭ-ro′sis) cardiac cirrhosis 心性肝硬变

car·dio·cyte (kahr′de-o-sīt″) myocyte 心肌细胞

car·dio·di·a·phrag·mat·ic (kahr″de-o-di″ə-frag-mat′ik) pertaining to the heart and the respiratory diaphragm 心膈的

car·dio·dy·nam·ics (kahr″de-o-di-nam′iks) study of the forces involved in the heart's action 心脏动力学

car·di·odyn·ia (kahr″de-o-din′e-ə) pain in the heart 心痛

car·dio·esoph·a·ge·al (kahr″de-o-ə-sof″ə-je′əl) pertaining to the cardia of the stomach and the esophagus, as the cardioesophageal junction or sphincter 贲门食管的

car·dio·gen·e·sis (kahr″de-o-jen′ə-sis) the development of the heart in the embryo 心脏发育

car·dio·gen·ic (kahr″de-o-jen′ik) 1. originating in the heart; caused by normal or abnormal function of the heart 源于心的; 2. pertaining to cardiogenesis 心脏发育的

car·dio·gram (kahr′de-o-gram″) a tracing of a cardiac event made by cardiography 心电图; **apex c.**, apexcardiogram 心尖心动图; **precordial c.**, kinetocardiogram 心振动图

car·di·og·ra·phy (kahr″de-og′rə-fe) the graphic recording of a physical or functional aspect of the heart, e.g., apexcardiography, echocardiography, electrocardiography, kinetocardiography, phonocardiography, telecardiography, and vectorcardiography 心动描记法; **ultrasonic c.**, echocardiography 超声心动描记法

car·dio·in·hib·i·tor (kahr″de-o-in-hib′ ĭ-tər) an agent that restrains the heart's action 心动抑制药

car·dio·in·hib·i·to·ry (kahr″de-o-in-hib′ ĭ-tore) restraining or inhibiting the movements of the heart 心动抑制的

car·dio·ki·net·ic (kahr″de-o-kĭ-net′ik) 1. exciting or stimulating the heart 兴奋心脏的; 2. an agent that so acts 兴奋心脏的药物

car·dio·ky·mog·ra·phy (kahr″de-o-ki-mog′rə-fe) the recording of the motion of the heart by means of the electrokymograph 心动记波法; **cardiokymograph′ic** *adj.*

car·dio·lip·in (kahr″de-o-lip′in) a phospholipid occurring primarily in mitochondrial inner membranes and in bacterial plasma membranes; used in certain tests for syphilis 心磷脂

car·di·ol·o·gy (kahr″de-ol′ə-je) the study of the heart and its functions 心脏病学

car·di·ol·y·sis (kahr″de-ol′ə-sis) the operation of freeing the heart from its adhesions to the sternal periosteum in adhesive mediastinopericarditis 心松解术

car·dio·ma·la·cia (kahr″de-o-mə-la′shə) morbid softening of the muscular substance of the heart 心肌软化

car·dio·meg·a·ly (kahr″de-o-meg′ə-le) abnormal enlargement of the heart 心肌肥大症

car·dio·mel·a·no·sis (kahr″de-o-mel″ə-no′sis) melanosis of the heart 心脏黑变

car·dio·mo·til·i·ty (kahr″de-o-mo-til′ ĭ-te) the movements of the heart; motility of the heart 心脏活动

car·dio·myo·li·po·sis (kahr″de-o-mi″o-lĭpo′sis) fatty degeneration of the heart muscle 心肌脂肪变性

car·dio·my·op·a·thy (kahr″de-o-mi-op′ə-the) 1. a general diagnostic term designating primary noninflammatory disease of the heart 心脏原发性非炎症性疾病的一般诊断术语; 2. more restrictively, only those disorders in which the myocardium alone is involved and in which the cause is unknown and not part of a disease affecting other organs 仅与心肌有关、病因不明且不影响其他器官造成疾病的一部分心脏疾病; **cardiomyopath′ic** *adj.*; **alcoholic c.**, dilated cardiomyopathy in patients chronically abusing alcohol 酒精性心肌病; **beer-drinkers' c.**, cardiac dilatation and hypertrophy due to excessive beer consumption; in at least some cases it has been due to the addition of cobalt to the beer during the manufacturing process 啤酒心; **dilated c.**, ventricular dilatation, systolic contractile dysfunction, and often congestive heart failure, usually progressive; it may be inherited or acquired. Inherited forms have been associated with numerous autosomal dominant mutations, most encoding proteins involved in muscle structure and assembly; causes of acquired cases include myocarditis, coronary artery disease, systemic diseases, and myocardial toxins 扩张性心肌病；**hypertrophic c. (HCM)**, a form marked by ventricular hypertrophy, particularly of the left ventricle, with impaired ventricular filling due to diastolic dysfunction 肥厚性心肌病；**hypertrophic obstructive c. (HOCM)**, a form of hypertrophic cardiomyopathy in which the location of the septal hypertrophy causes obstructive interference to left ventricular outflow 肥厚型梗阻性心肌病；**infiltrative c.**, restrictive cardiomyopathy characterized by deposition in the heart tissue of abnormal substances, as may occur in amyloidosis, hemochromatosis, etc 浸润性心肌病；**ischemic c.**, heart failure with left ventricular dilatation resulting from ischemic heart disease 缺血性心肌病；**restrictive c.**, a form in which the ventricular walls are excessively rigid, impeding ventricular filling 限制性心肌病；**right ventricular c.**, a right-sided cardiomyopathy occurring particularly in young males, with dilatation of the right ventricle with partial to total replacement of its muscle by fibrous or adipose tissue, palpitations, syncope, and sometimes sudden death 右室心肌病；**takotsubo c., tako-tsubo c.**, a reversible, stress-related syndrome mimicking acute coronary syndrome, with apical ballooning of the left ventricle but without angiographically significant coronary artery stenosis 应激性心肌病

car·di·op·a·thy (kahr″de-op′ə-the) any disorder or disease of the heart 心脏病

car·dio·pho·bia (kahr″de-o-fo′be-ə) irrational dread of heart disease 心脏病恐惧症

car·dio·plas·ty (kahr′de-o-plas″te) esophagogastroplasty 贲门成形术

car·dio·ple·gia (kahr″de-o-ple′jə) arrest of myocardial contractions, as by use of chemical compounds or cold in cardiac surgery 心脏停搏；**cardiople′gic adj.**

car·dio·pneu·mat·ic (kahr″de-o-noo-mat′ik) of or pertaining to the heart and respiration 心肺的

car·dio·pro·tec·tant (kahr″de-o-pro-tek′tənt) counteracting cardiotoxicity, or an agent that so acts 抗心脏毒性的药物

car·di·op·to·sis (kahr″de-op-to′sis) downward displacement of the heart 心脏下垂

car·dio·pul·mo·nary (kahr″de-o-pool′mə-nar-e) pertaining to the heart and lungs 心肺的

car·di·or·rha·phy (kahr″de-or′ə-fe) suture of the heart muscle 心脏修补术

car·di·or·rhex·is (kahr″de-o-rek′sis) rupture of the heart 心脏破裂

car·dio·scle·ro·sis (kahr″de-o-sklə-ro′sis) fibrous induration of the heart 心硬化

car·dio·se·lec·tive (kahr″de-o-sə-lek′tiv) having greater activity on heart tissue than on other tissue 心选择性的

car·dio·spasm (kahr′de-o-spaz″əm) achalasia of the esophagus 贲门痉挛

car·dio·ta·chom·e·ter (kahr″de-o-tə-kom′ə-tər) an instrument for continuously portraying or recording the heart rate 心率计

car·dio·ther·a·py (kahr″de-o-ther′ə-pe) the treatment of diseases of the heart 心脏病的治疗

car·dio·tho·rac·ic (kahr″de-o-thə-ras′ik) pertaining to the heart and the thorax 心和胸部的

car·dio·to·cog·ra·phy (kahr″de-o-to-kog′rə-fe) the monitoring of the fetal heart rate and uterine contractions, as during delivery 心分娩力描记法

car·di·ot·o·my (kahr″de-ot′ə-me) 1. surgical incision of the heart 心切开术；2. surgical incision into the cardia 贲门切开术

car·dio·ton·ic (kahr″de-o-ton′ik) having a tonic effect on the heart; an agent that so acts 强心的，强心药

car·dio·to·pom·e·try (kahr″de-o-tə-pom′ə-tre) measurement of the area of superficial cardiac dullness observed in percussion of the chest 心浊音区测定法

car·dio·tox·ic (kahr′de-o-tok″sik) having a poisonous or deleterious effect upon the heart 心脏毒性的

car·dio·tox·ic·i·ty (kahr″de-o-tok-sis′ ĭ-te) the quality of being cardiotoxic 心脏毒性

car·dio·val·vu·li·tis (kahr″de-o-val′vu-li′tis) inflammation of the heart valves 心瓣膜炎

car·dio·val·vu·lo·tome (kahr″de-o-val′vu-lə-tōm″) an instrument for incising a heart valve 心瓣膜刀

car·dio·vas·cu·lar (kahr″de-o-vas′ku-lər) pertaining to the heart and blood vessels 心血管的

car·dio·ver·sion (kahr′de-o-vur″zhən) the restoration of normal rhythm of the heart by electrical shock 心脏复律

car·dio·ver·ter (kahr′de-o-vur″tər) an energystorage capacitor-discharge type of condenser that is discharged with an inductance; it delivers a direct-current shock that restores the normal rhythm of the heart 心脏复律器；**automatic implantable c.-defibrillator,** an implantable device that detects sustained ventricular tachycardia or fibrillation and terminates it by a shock or shocks delivered directly to the atrium 植入型自动心律转复除颤器

Car·dio·vi·rus (kahr′de-o-vi″rəs) EMC-like viruses; a genus of viruses of the family Picornaviridae that cause encephalomyelitis and myocarditis. The one species that causes disease in humans is encephalomyocarditis virus 心病毒属

car·di·tis (kahr-di′tis) inflammation of the heart; myocarditis 心肌炎

care (kār) the services rendered by members of the health professions for the benefit of a patient 医疗服务; coronary c., 见 *unit*. 下词条, 心脏监护; **critical c.,** 见 unit 下 *intensive care unit*, 重症照顾; **intensive c.,** 见 *unit*. 加强临护; **primary c.,** the care a patient receives at first contact with the health care system, usually involving coordination of care and continuity over time 初级医疗; **respiratory c.,** 1. the health care profession providing, under a physician's supervision, diagnostic evaluation, therapy, monitoring, and rehabilitation of patients with cardiopulmonary disorders 心肺疾病保健; 2. respiratory therapy; the diagnostic and therapeutic use of medical gases and their apparatuses, and other forms of ventilatory support, including cardiopulmonary resuscitation 呼吸治疗; **secondary c.,** treatment by specialists to whom a patient has been referred by primary care providers 二级医疗; **tertiary c.,** treatment given in a health care center that includes highly trained specialists and often advanced technology 三级医疗

car·filz·o·mib (kar-filz′oh-mib) an irreversible proteasome inhibitor used as an antineoplastic, alone or in combination, to treat refractory multiple myeloma 卡非佐米, 一种不可逆的蛋白酶体抑制剂, 用作抗肿瘤药物, 单独或联合使用时可治疗难治性多发性骨髓瘤

car·ies (kar′ēz) (kar′e-ēz) decay, as of bone or teeth 骨头或牙齿的腐烂; **ca′rious** *adj.*; **dental c.,** a destructive process causing decalcification of the tooth enamel and leading to continued destruction of enamel and dentin, and cavitation of the tooth 龋齿

ca·ri·na (kə-ri′nə) pl. *cari′nae* [L.] a ridgelike structure 脊; **c. tra′cheae,** a downward and backward projection of the lowest tracheal cartilage, forming a ridge between the openings of the right and left principal bronchi 气管隆嵴; **c. urethra′lis vagi′nae,** the column of rugae in the lower anterior wall of the vagina, immediately below the urethra 阴道尿道隆嵴

car·i·nate (kar′ĭ-nāt) keel-shaped; having a keel-like process 龙骨状的, 隆突的

car·io·gen·e·sis (kar″e-o-jen′ə-sis) development of caries 龋发生

car·iso·pro·dol (kar″i-so-pro′dol) an analgesic and skeletal muscle relaxant used to relieve symptoms of acute painful skeletomuscular disorders 异

丙基甲丁双脲; 肌安宁, 一种肛门和骨骼肌松弛药, 用于缓解急性疼痛性骨骼肌疾病的症状

car·min·a·tive (kahr-min′ə-tiv) 1. relieving flatulence 排气的; 2. an agent that relieves flatulence 排气药

car·mine (kahr′min) a red coloring matter used as a histologic stain 用作组织学染色的红色物质; **indigo c.,** indigotindisulfonate sodium 靛胭脂

car·min·ic ac·id (kahr-min′ik) the active principle of carmine and cochineal, $C_{22}H_{20}O_{13}$ 胭脂红酸

car·min·o·phil (kahr-min′ə-fil) 1. easily stainable with carmine 嗜胭脂红的; 2. a cell or element readily taking a stain from carmine 易被胭脂红染色的细胞或成分

car·mus·tine (kahr-mus′tēn) a cytotoxic alkylating agent of the nitrosourea group, used as an antineoplastic agent 卡莫司汀, 一种细胞毒性的亚硝基烷基化剂, 用作抗肿瘤药

car·ni·tine (kahr′nĭ-tēn) a betaine derivative involved in the transport of fatty acids into mitochondria, where they are metabolized 肉毒碱, 一种甜菜碱衍生物, 参与脂肪酸进入线粒体的运输, 并在线粒体中进行代谢

car·no·sin·ase (kahr′no-sĭ-nās″) an enzyme that hydrolyzes carnosine and related dipeptides into component amino acids. There are two: a nonspecific cytosolic form and a highly specific, metal-dependent form found in serum, brain, and cerebrospinal fluid 肌肽酶

car·no·sine (kahr′no-sēn) a dipeptide composed of β-alanine and histidine, found in skeletal muscle and the brain 肌肽

car·no·si·ne·mia (kahr″no-sĭ-ne′me-ə) accumulation of carnosine in the blood 肌肽血症

car·no·sin·u·ria (kahr″no-sĭ-nu′re-ə) urinary excretion of high levels of carnosine, as after ingestion of meat or in serum carnosinase deficiency 肌肽尿

car·o·tene (kar′ə-tēn) one of four isomeric pigments (α-, β-, γ-, and δ-carotene), having colors from violet to red-yellow to yellow and occurring in many dark green, leafy, and yellow vegetables and yellow fruits. They are fatsoluble, unsaturated hydrocarbons that can be converted into vitamin A in the body; in humans the β- isomer (β- or beta carotene) is the major precursor of this vitamin 胡萝卜素; **beta c.,** the β- isomer of carotene; a preparation is used to prevent vitamin A deficiency and to reduce the severity of photosensitivity in patients with erythropoietic protoporphyria β- 胡萝卜素

car·o·ten·emia (kar″ə-tə-ne′me-ə) hypercarotenemia 胡萝卜素血症

ca·rot·e·noid (kə-rot′ə-noid) 1. any of a group of red, orange, or yellow pigmented polyisoprenoid hydrocarbons synthesized by prokaryotes and higher plants and concentrating in animal fat when eaten; examples are β-carotene, lycopene, and xanthophyll 类胡萝卜素； 2. marked by yellow color 用黄色标记的； **provitamin A c's,** carotenoids, particularly the carotenes, that can be converted to vitamin A in the body 类胡萝卜素的一种，主要是胡萝卜素，可在体内转化为维生素 A

car·o·te·no·sis (kar″o-tə-no′sis) the yellowish discoloration of the skin occurring in hypercarotenemia 胡萝卜素沉着，胡萝卜素过多引起皮肤发黄的现象

ca·rot·i·co·tym·pan·ic (kə-rot″ĭ-ko-tim-pan′ik) pertaining to the carotid canal and the tympanum 颈动脉管和鼓室的

ca·rot·id (kə-rot′id) pertaining to the carotid artery, the principal artery of the neck 颈动脉的

ca·rot·i·dyn·ia (kə-rot″ĭ-din′e-ə) episodic, usually unilateral neck pain with tenderness along the course of the common carotid artery 颈动脉痛

car·pal (kahr′pəl) pertaining to the carpus 腕骨的

car·pec·to·my (kahr-pek′tə-me) excision of a carpal bone 腕骨切除术

car·phol·o·gy (kahr-fol′ə-je) floccillation 摸空症

car·pi·tis (kahr-pi′tis) inflammation of the synovial membranes of the bones of the carpal joint in domestic animals, producing swelling, pain, and lameness 腕关节炎

car·po·ped·al (kahr″po-ped′əl) pertaining to or affecting the wrist (or the hand) and the foot 腕足的

car·pop·to·sis (kahr″pop-to′sis) wristdrop 腕下垂

car·pus (kahr′pəs) the joint between the arm and hand, made up of eight bones; the wrist 腕骨

car·ri·er (kar′e-ər) 1. an instrument or apparatus for carrying something 携带某物的仪器或装置； 2. one who harbors disease organisms in their body without manifest symptoms, thus acting as a distributor of infection 病原携带者，有疾病但无明显机体症状，是感染的传播者； 3. a chemical substance that can accept electrons and then donate them to another substance (being reduced and then reoxidized) 一种化学物质，它能接收电子，然后将电子传递给另一种物质 (还原后再氧化)； 4. an individual who is heterozygous for a recessive gene and thus does not express the recessive phenotype but can transmit it to offspring 隐性基因的杂合个体，不表达隐性表现型，但能将其遗传给后代； 5. a substance that carries a radioisotopic or other label; also used for a second isotope mixed with a particular isotope 带有放射性同位素或其他标记的物质；与特定同位素混合的第二同位素 (见 *carrier-free*)； 6. transport protein 载体蛋白； 7. in immunology, a macromolecular substance to which a hapten is coupled in order to produce an immune response against the hapten 免疫学中，为产生对半抗原的免疫反应而与半抗原结合的一种大分子物质

car·ri·er-free (kar′e-ər-fre′) denoting or pertaining to a radioisotope of an element in pure form, i.e., undiluted with a stable isotope carrier 纯元素放射性同位素的，未使用稳定同位素载体稀释

car·sick·ness (kahr′sik-nis) motion sickness due to automobile or other vehicular travel 晕车

cart (kahrt) a vehicle for conveying patients or equipment and supplies in a hospital 运送病人或医院设备用品的车辆； **crash c.,** resuscitation c. 急救车； **dressing c.,** one containing all supplies necessary for changing dressings of surgical or injured patients 敷料车； **resuscitation c.,** one containing all equipment for initiating emergency resuscitation 抢救车

car·te·o·lol (kahr′te-ə-lol) a beta-adrenergic blocking agent used as the hydrochloride salt in the treatment of hypertension and of glaucoma and ocular hypertension 卡替洛尔，一种 β 肾上腺素阻断剂，盐酸盐用作治疗高血压、青光眼和眼压升高

car·ti·lage (kahr′tĭ-ləj) a specialized, fibrous connective tissue present in adults, and forming the temporary skeleton in the embryo, providing a model in which the bones develop, and constituting a part of the organism's growth mechanism 软骨 **alar c's,** the cartilages of the wings of the nose 鼻翼软骨； **aortic c.,** the second costal cartilage on the right side 主动脉软骨，右侧第二肋软骨； **arthrodial c., articular c.,** that lining the articular surface of synovial joints 关节软骨； **arytenoid c.,** one of the two pyramidshaped cartilages of the larynx 杓状软骨； **connecting c.,** that connecting the surfaces of an immovable joint 连接软骨； **corniculate c.,** a nodule of cartilage at the apex of each arytenoid cartilage 小角状软骨； **costal c.,** a bar of hyaline cartilage that attaches a rib to the sternum in the case of true ribs, or to the rib immediately above in the case of the upper false ribs 肋软骨； **cricoid c.,** a ringlike cartilage forming the lower and back part of the larynx 环状软骨； **cuneiform c.,** either of a pair of cartilages, one on either side in the aryepiglottic fold 楔状软骨； **dentinal c.,** the substance remaining after the lime salts of dentin have been dissolved in an acid 牙质架； **diarthrodial c.,** articular c. 关节软骨； **elastic c.,** cartilage whose matrix contains yellow elastic fibers 弹性软骨； **ensiform c.,** xiphoid process 剑状软骨； **epiphyseal c.,** the cartilage composing the epiphysis prior to ossification 骺软骨； **floating c.,** a detached portion of semilunar cartilage in the knee joint 膝关节中半月板软骨脱

落 的 部 分；**hyaline c.,** a flexible semitransparent substance with an opalescent tint, composed of a basophilic, fibril-containing substance with cavities in which the chondrocytes occur 透明软骨；**interosseous c.,** connecting c.; **Jacobson c.,** vomeronasal c. Jacobson 软骨；**permanent c.,** cartilage that does not normally become ossified 永久性软骨；**precursory c.,** temporary c. 骨化软骨；**Santorini c.,** corniculate c. Santorini 软骨；**semilunar c.,** either of the two interarticular cartilages of the knee joint 半 月 软 骨；**sesamoid c's,** small cartilages found in the thyrohyoid ligament (*sesamoid c. of larynx*), on either side of the nose (*sesamoid c. of nose*), and occasionally in the vocal ligaments (*sesamoid c. of vocal ligament*) 籽状软骨；**slipping rib c.,** a loosened or deformed cartilage whose slipping over an adjacent rib cartilage may produce discomfort or pain 滑动肋软骨；**temporary c.,** cartilage that is being replaced by bone or that is destined to be replaced by bone 暂时性软骨；**thyroid c.,** the shield-shaped cartilage of the larynx 甲状软骨；**tracheal c's,** 见 *ring* 下词条，气管软骨；**triticeous c.,** a small cartilage in the thyrohyoid ligament 麦 粒 软 骨；**vomeronasal c.,** either of the two strips of cartilage of the nasal septum supporting the vomeronasal organ 犁鼻软骨；**Weitbrecht c.,** a pad of fibrocartilage sometimes present within the articular cavity of the acromioclavicular joint Weitbrecht 软 骨，一种纤维软骨垫，有时存在于肩锁关节的关节腔内；**Wrisberg c.,** cuneiform c. Wrisberg 软 骨；**xiphoid c.,** 见 *process* 下词条，胸骨剑突；**Y c.,** Y-shaped cartilage within the acetabulum, joining the ilium, ischium, and pubes Y 形软骨，存在于髋臼内，连接髂骨、坐骨和耻骨；**yellow c.,** elastic c. 黄色软骨

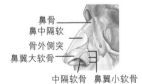

鼻骨
鼻中隔软
骨外侧突
鼻翼大软骨
中隔软骨　鼻翼小软骨

▲ **鼻软骨（nasal cartilages）**

car·ti·lag·i·nous (kahr″tĭ-laj′ ĭ-nəs) consisting of or of the nature of cartilage 软骨的

car·ti·la·go (kahr″tĭ-lah′go) pl. *cartila'gines* [L.] cartilage 软骨

car·un·cle (kar′ŏng-kəl) [*caruncula* L.] a small fleshy eminence, often abnormal 肉 阜；**hymenal c's,** small elevations of the mucous membrane around the vaginal opening, being relics of the torn hymen 处 女 膜 痕；**lacrimal c.,** the red eminence at the medial angle of the eye 泪阜；**sublingual c.,** an eminence on either side of the frenulum of the tongue, on which the major sublingual duct and the submandibular duct open 舌 下 阜；**urethral c.,** a polypoid, deep red growth on the mucous membrane of the urinary meatus in women 尿道肉阜

car·ve·dil·ol (kahr′və-dil″ol) a beta-adrenergic blocking agent used in the treatment of hypertension and as an adjunct in the treatment of congestive heart failure 卡维地洛，一种 β 肾上腺素阻断剂，用于治疗高血压和充血性心力衰竭

car·ver (kahr′vər) a tool for producing anatomic form in artificial teeth and dental restorations 牙科雕刻刀，在假牙和牙体修复中产生解剖形状的工具

ca·san·thra·nol (kə-san′thrə-nol) a purified mixture of glycosides derived from cascara sagrada; used as a laxative 鼠李蒽酚，从鼠李中提取的纯化的糖苷混合物，用作泻药

cas·cade (kas-kād′) a series that once initiated continues to the end, each step being triggered by the preceding one, sometimes with cumulative effect 级联反应；**coagulation c.,** the series of steps beginning with activation of the intrinsic or extrinsic pathways of coagulation, or of one of the related alternative pathways, and proceeding through the common pathway of coagulation to the formation of the fibrin clot 凝血级联反应

cas·ca·ra (kas-kah′rə) [Sp.] bark 树皮；**c. sagra′da,** dried bark of the shrub *Rhamnus purshiana*, used as a cathartic 鼠李皮，一种灌木的干树皮，用作泻药

case (kās) an instance of a disease 病例；**index c.,** 1. the first case observed in a family or other defined group, which provides the stimulus for a genetic study; the affected individual is called the propositus 先证者，在一个家庭或其他特定群体中观察到的第一个病例，它为遗传研究提供了信息；2. the first case of a contagious disease, as opposed to subsequent cases 首发病例，传染病的第一个病例而不是后续病例

ca·se·a·tion (ka″se-a′shən) 1. the precipitation of casein 酪蛋白沉淀；2. necrosis in which tissue is changed into a dry mass resembling cheese 干酪样变

case his·to·ry (kās′ his′tə-re) the data concerning an individual, their family, and their environment, including medical history that may be useful in analyzing and diagnosing the case or for instructional purposes 病历

ca·sein (ka′sēn) a phosphoprotein, the principal protein of milk, the basis of curd and of cheese. note: In British nomenclature casein is called *ca-*

seinogen, and paracasein is called *casein* 酪蛋白

ca·sein·o·gen (ka-sēn′o-jen) the British term for casein 酪蛋白的英国表述

ca·se·ous (ka′se-əs) resembling cheese or curd; cheesy 干酪样的

case·worm (kās′wərm) echinococcus 棘球绦虫

cas·po·fun·gin (kas″po-fun′jin) an antifungal used as the acetate salt in the treatment of invasive aspergillosis 卡泊芬净，用于治疗侵袭性曲霉菌病的一种醋酸盐抗真菌剂

cas·sette (kə-set′) [Fr.] 1. a flat case for film or magnetic tape 盒式磁带；2. X-ray c. X 射线暗盒；**X-ray c.**, a lightproof housing for x-ray film, containing front and back intensifying screens, between which the film is placed; a magazine for film or magnetic tape X射线暗盒，一种用于 X 射线胶片的防光外壳，包括用于放置胶片的前后增强遮挡；电影或磁带胶卷盒

cast (kast) 1. a positive copy of an object, e.g., a mold of a tube or hollow organ, formed of effused matter such as fat or cellular debris and later extruded from the organ, such as a urinary cast 一种物体的阳性拷贝，如由渗出物（如脂肪或细胞碎片）构成的管状或中空器官模子，之后从器官挤压出，如肾铸；2. a positive copy of the tissues of the jaws, made in an impression, and over which denture bases or other restorations may be fabricated 假牙模，印在印模上的下颌组织正片复制品，可在其上制作义齿基托或其他修复体；3. to form an object in a mold 铸型；4. a rigid dressing, molded to the body while pliable, and hardening as it dries, to give firm support 一种坚硬的敷料，在身体柔韧时模压成型，在干燥时硬化，以提供牢固的支撑；5. strabismus 斜视；**dental c.**, 见 *cast* (2), 牙模；**hanging c.**, one applied to the arm in a fracture of the shaft of the humerus, suspended by a sling looped around the neck 一种环绕在脖子上的吊索，悬挂肱骨干骨折时的手臂；**renal c.**, **urinary c.**, one formed from gelled protein in the renal tubules, molded to the shape of the tubular lumen 尿液管型，肾铸

cas·trate (kas′trāt) 1. to deprive of the gonads, rendering the individual incapable of reproduction 阉割；2. a castrated individual 阉割个体

cas·tra·tion (kas-tra′shən) excision of the gonads, or their destruction as by radiation or parasites 去势；**female c.**, bilateral oophorectomy 女性去势术，双侧卵巢切除术；**male c.**, bilateral orchiectomy 男性去势术，双侧睾丸切除术

ca·su·al·ty (kazh′oo-əl-te) 1. an accident; an accidental wound; death or disablement from an accident; also the person so injured 意外事故，也指伤员；2. in the armed forces, one missing from a unit as a result of death, injury, illness, or capture; because the person's whereabouts are unknown; or for other reasons 伤亡人数

cas·u·is·tics (kazh″u-is′tiks) the recording and study of cases of disease 病例讨论

CAT computerized axial tomography 计算机 X 线断层造影

ca·tab·o·lism (kə-tab′o-liz-əm) any destructive process by which complex substances are converted by living cells into more simple compounds, with release of energy 分解代谢；**catabol′ic** *adj.*

ca·tab·o·lize (kə-tab′o-līz) to subject to catabolism; to undergo catabolism 进行分解代谢

ca·tac·ro·tism (kə-tak′ro-tiz-əm) a pulse anomaly in which a small additional wave or notch appears in the descending limb of the pulse tracing 降线一波脉现象，一种脉搏波异常，在脉搏传导的下行分支上出现一个小的附加波或缺口；**catacrot′ic** *adj.*

cata·di·cro·tism (kat″ə-di′kro-tiz-əm) a pulse anomaly in which two small additional waves or notches appear in the descending limb of the pulse tracing 降线二波脉现象，一种脉搏波异常，在脉搏传导的下行分支上出现两个小的附加波或缺口；**catadicrot′ic** *adj.*

cat·a·gen (kat′ə-jən) the brief portion in the hair cycle in which growth (anagen) stops and resting (telogen) starts 毛发生长中期

cat·a·lase (kat′ə-lās) a hemoprotein enzyme that catalyzes the decomposition of hydrogen peroxide to water and oxygen, protecting cells. It is found in almost all animal cells except certain anaerobic bacteria; genetic deficiency of the enzyme results in acatalasia 过氧化氢酶；**catalat′ic** *adj.*

cat·a·lep·sy (kat′ə-lep″se) indefinitely prolonged maintenance of a fixed body posture; seen in severe cases of catatonic schizophrenia. The term is sometimes used to denote *cerea flexibilitas* 僵住

ca·tal·y·sis (kə-tal′ə-sis) increase in the velocity of a chemical reaction or process produced by the presence of a substance that is not consumed in the net chemical reaction or process; *negative c.* denotes the slowing down or inhibition of a reaction or process by the presence of such a substance 催化作用；**catalyt′ic** *adj.*

cat·am·ne·sis (kat″am-ne′sis) 1. the followup history of a patient after discharge from treatment or a hospital 病人出院或出院后的随访史；2. the history of a patient after onset of a medical or psychiatric illness 病人发病后的病史；**catamnes′tic** *adj.*

cata·pha·sia (kat″ə-fa′zhə) verbigeration 言语重复

cata·pho·ria (kat″ə-for′e-ə) a permanent downward turning of the visual axis of both eyes after visual functional stimuli have been removed 下隐斜视; **cataphor′ic** *adj.*

cata·phy·lax·is (kat″ə-fə-lak′sis) breaking down of the body's natural defense to infection 自然防御系统崩解; **cataphylac′tic** *adj.*

cat·a·plexy (kat′ə-plek″se) a condition marked by abrupt attacks of muscular weakness and hypotonia triggered by such emotional stimuli as mirth, anger, fear, etc., often associated with narcolepsy 猝倒症; **cataplec′tic** *adj.*

cat·a·ract (kat′ə-rakt) an opacity of the crystalline lens of the eye or its capsule 白内障; **catarac′tous** *adj.*; **after-c.**, a recurrent capsular cataract 后发性白内障; **atopic c.**, cataract in those with long-standing atopic dermatitis 特应性白内障; **black c.**, 见 *senile nuclear sclerotic c.*,黑色内障; **blue c., blue dot c.**, blue punctate opacities scattered throughout the nucleus and cortex of the lens 蓝点状内障; **brown c., brunescent c.,** 见 senile *nuclear sclerotic c.*; 棕色内障; **capsular c.**, one consisting of an opacity in the lens capsule 囊膜性白内障; **complicated c.**, secondary c. 并发性白内障; **congenital c.,** 1. cataract present at birth, usually bilaterally; it may be mild or severe and may or may not impair vision depending on size, density, and location 先天性白内障; 2. developmental c. 发育性白内障; **coronary c.**, cataract in which tiny white opacities are present in a ring around the lens, the center and periphery of the lens remaining clear 冠状白内障; **cortical c.,** 皮质性白内障 1. developmental punctate opacity common in the cortex and present in most lenses. The cataract is white or cerulean, increases in number with age, but rarely affects vision 常见于皮质，多见于晶状体的发育性点状混浊。白内障呈白色或天蓝色，随年龄增长而增多，但很少影响视力; 2. the most common senile cataract; white, wedge-like opacities are like spokes around the periphery of the cortex 最常见的老年性白内障; 白色的楔状混浊物像辐条一样环绕在皮质的边缘; **cupuliform c.**, a senile cataract in the posterior cortex of the lens just under the capsule 杯状白内障; **developmental c.**, a type of small cataract in youth, resulting from heredity, malnutrition, toxicity, or inflammation; it seldom affects vision 发育性白内障; **electric c.**, one occurring after an electric shock, especially to the head. Anterior subcapsular cataracts may form and develop within days; slowly developing or stationary opacities may follow a shock not to the head 电击性白内障; **glassblowers' c., heat c.**, posterior subcapsular opacities caused by chronic exposure to infrared (heat) radiation 热性白内障; **hypermature c.**, one with a swollen, milky cortex,

the result of autolysis of the lens fibers of a mature cataract 过熟期白内障; **lamellar c.**, one affecting only certain layers between the cortex and nucleus of the lens 板层白内障; **mature c.**, one producing swelling and opacity of the entire lens 成熟期白内障; **membranous c.**, a condition in which the lens substance has shrunk, leaving remnants of the capsule and fibrous tissue formation 膜性白内障; **morgagnian c.**, a mature cataract in which the cortex has liquefied and the nucleus moves freely within the lens 硬核液化白内障; **nuclear c.**, one in which the opacity is in the central nucleus of the eye 核性白内障; **overripe c.**, hypermature c.; **polar c.**, one at the center of the anterior (*anterior polar c.*) or posterior (*posterior polar c.*) pole of the lens 极性白内障; **pyramidal c.**, a conoid anterior cataract with its apex projecting forward into the aqueous humor 锥体白内障; **radiation c.**, one caused by ionizing radiation, e.g., x-rays, or by nonionizing radiation, e.g., infrared (heat) rays, ultraviolet rays, microwaves 放射性白内障; **ripe c.**, mature c.; **secondary c.**, one resulting from disease, e.g., iridocyclitis; degeneration, e.g., chronic glaucoma, retinal detachment; or from surgery, e.g., glaucoma filtering, retinal reattachment 继发性白内障; **senile c.**, cataract in the elderly 老年性白内障; **senile nuclear sclerotic c.**, slowly increasing hardening of the nucleus, usually bilateral and brown or black, with the lens becoming inelastic and unable to accommodate 老年性核硬化性白内障; **snow-flake c., snowstorm c.**, one marked by gray or blue to white flaky opacities, seen in young diabetics 雪花状白内障; **total c.**, an opacity of all the fibers of a lens 全内障; **toxic c.**, that due to exposure to a toxic drug, e.g., naphthalene 中毒性白内障; **traumatic c.**, one due to injury to the eye 外伤性白内障; **zonular c.**, lamellar c.

cat·a·rac·ta (kat″ə-rak′tə) cataract 白内障; **c. brunes′cens**, brown cataract 棕色内障; 见 *senile nuclear sclerotic cataract*; **c. caeru′lea**, blue dot cataract 蓝点状内障

ca·tarrh (kə-tahr′) inflammation of a mucous membrane, particularly of the head and throat, with free discharge of mucus 黏膜炎, 卡他; **catar′rhal** *adj.*

cat·a·to·nia (kat″ə-to′ne-ə) a wide group of motor abnormalities, most involving extreme under- or overactivity, associated primarily with catatonic schizophrenia. It may also be diagnosed as a specifier for depressive, bipolar, and psychotic disorders; as a separate diagnosis in the context of another medical condition; or as an other-specified diagnosis 畸张症; **cataton′ic** *adj.*

ca·ta·tri·cro·tism (kat″ə-tri′kro-tiz-əm) a pulse anomaly in which three small additional waves or notches appear in the descending limb of the pulse tracing 降线三波脉，一种脉搏波异常，在脉搏传导的下行分支中出现三个小的附加波或缺口；**catatricrot′ic** *adj.*

cat·e·chin (kat′ə-kin) an astringent principle from the heartwood of *Acacia catechu* (catechu) and *Uncaria gambier* (gambir) 儿茶素

cat·e·chol (kat′ə-kol) 1. catechin 儿茶素；2. pyrocatechol 邻苯二酚

cat·e·chol·amine (kat″ə-kol′ə-mēn) any of a group of sympathomimetic amines (including dopamine, epinephrine, and norepinephrine), the aromatic portion of whose molecule is catechol 阴茎套导尿管；儿茶酚胺

cat·e·chol·am·in·er·gic (kat″ə-kol″ə-mĭnur′jik) activated by or secreting catecholamines 含儿茶酚胺的

cat·gut (kat′gut) surgical gut 肠线

ca·thar·sis (kə-thahr′sis) 1. purgation; a cleansing or emptying 导泻 2. in psychiatry, the expression and discharge of repressed emotions and ideas 情感宣泄

ca·thar·tic (kə-thahr′tik) 1. causing emptying of the bowels 导泻 的；2. an agent that empties the bowels. 泻药；3. producing emotional catharsis 情感宣泄 的；**bulk c.**, one stimulating bowel evacuation by increasing fecal volume 容积性泻药；**lubricant c.**, one that acts by softening the feces and reducing friction between them and the intestinal wall 滑润性泻药；**saline c.**, one that increases fluidity of intestinal contents by retention of water by osmotic forces and indirectly increases motor activity 盐类泻药；**stimulant c.**, one that directly increases motor activity of the intestinal tract 刺激性泻剂

ca·the·li·ci·din (kə-the″lĭ-si′din) a peptide expressed by leukocytes and epithelial cells and having a wide spectrum of antimicrobial activity; overexpression results in rosacea 抗菌肽

ca·thep·sin (kə-thep′sin) one of a number of enzymes each of which catalyzes the hydrolytic cleavage of specific peptide bonds 组织蛋白酶

cath·e·ter (kath′ə-tər) 1. a tubular, flexible surgical instrument that is inserted into a cavity of the body to withdraw or introduce fluid 导管；2. urethral c. 导尿管；**angiographic c.**, one through which a contrast medium is injected for visualization of the vascular system of an organ 血管造影导管；**atherectomy c.**, one with a rotating cutter and a collecting chamber for debris, used for atherectomy and endarterectomy and inserted under radiographic

guidance 粥样硬化切除导管；**balloon c.**, one whose tip has an inflatable balloon that holds the catheter in place or can dilate the lumen of a vessel, as in angioplastic procedures 气囊导管；**cardiac c.**, a long, fine catheter designed for passage, usually through a peripheral blood vessel, into the chambers of the heart under radiographic control 心导管；**cardiac c.-microphone**, phonocatheter 心音导管；**central venous c.**, a long, fine catheter introduced via a large vein into the superior vena cava or right atrium for administration of parenteral fluids or medications or for measurement of central venous pressure 中心静脉导管；**condom c.**, an external urinary collection device that fits over the penis like a condom; used in the management of urinary incontinence; **DeLee c.**, one used to suction meconium and amniotic debris from the nasopharynx and oropharynx of neonates Delee 吸管，一种用于从新生儿的鼻咽和口咽吸胎粪和羊膜碎片的装置；**double-channel c., double-lumen c.**, one with two channels, one for injection and the other for fluid removal 双腔导管；**elbowed c.**, a urethral catheter with a sharp bend near the beak, used to get around an enlarged prostate 弯头导管；**electrode c.**, a cardiac catheter containing electrodes; it may be used to pace the heart or to deliver high-energy shocks 电极导管；**female c.**, a short urethral catheter for passage through the female urethra 女用导尿管；**fluid-filled c.**, an intravascular catheter connected by a saline-filled tube to an external pressure transducer; used to measure intravascular pressure 一种血管内导管，由一盐水充注的导管连接到外部压力传感器；用于测量血管内压力；**Foley c.**, an indwelling catheter retained in the bladder by a balloon inflated with air or liquid Foley 导尿管，一种通过充气或充液的气球留在膀胱内的留置导管；**Gouley c.**, a solid, curved steel urethral catheter grooved on its inferior surface so that it can pass over a guide through a urethral stricture Gouley 导管，一种坚固的弯曲钢制导尿管，在其下表面开槽，以便导尿管穿过尿道狭窄；**Gruentzig balloon c.**, a flexible balloon catheter with a short guidewire fixed to the tip, used for dilation of arterial stenoses 球囊导管，一种有短导丝固定在顶端的柔性球囊导管，用于扩张动脉狭窄；**indwelling c.**, one held in position in the urethra 留置导管；**pacing c.**, a cardiac catheter containing one or more electrodes on pacing wires; used as a temporary cardiac pacing lead 起搏导管；**prostatic c.**, elbowed c. 前列腺导管；**self-retaining c.**, indwelling c. 自流导尿管；**snare c.**, a catheter designed to remove catheter fragments introduced into the heart iatrogenically 勒除器导管，一种医学上用于移除插入心脏导管的碎片的

导管；**Swan-Ganz c.**, a soft, flow-directed catheter with a balloon at the tip for measuring pulmonary arterial pressures 斯旺－甘兹导管（又称血流导向气囊导管），一种软的、有流向的导管，顶端有一个气囊，用于测量肺动脉压力；**Tenckhoff c.**, any of several types commonly used in peritoneal dialysis, having end and side holes and one or more extraperitoneal felt cuffs making a bacteriatight seal Tenckhoff 导管，腹膜透析中常用的一种导管，有端孔和侧孔以及一个或多个腹膜外毛毡袖口，使之具有无菌密封的特性；**toposcopic c.**, a miniature catheter that can pass through narrow, tortuous vessels to convey chemotherapy directly to specific sites 局部介入放射导管；**two-way c.**, double-lumen c.; **ureteral c.**, one inserted into the ureter, either through the urethra and bladder or posteriorly via the kidney 输尿管导管；**urethral c.**, one inserted through the urethra into the urinary bladder 尿道导管；**winged c.**, a urethral catheter with two projections on the end to retain it in place 翼状导管，于尿管末端有两个突出物，以保持导尿管的位置

cath·e·ter·iza·tion (kath″ə-tur″ĭ-za′shən) passage of a catheter into a body channel or cavity 导管插入；**cardiac c.**, passage of a small catheter through a vein in an arm or leg or the neck and into the heart, permitting the securing of blood samples, determination of intracardiac pressure, detection of cardiac anomalies, planning of operative approaches, and determination, implementation, or evaluation of appropriate therapy 心导管插入术；**retrograde c.**, passage of a cardiac catheter against the direction of blood flow and into the heart 逆行性导管插入术；**transseptal c.**, passage of a cardiac catheter through the right atrium into the left atrium, performed to relieve valve obstruction and in techniques such as balloon mitral valvuloplasty 经房间导管插入术

ca·thex·is (kə-thek′sis) conscious or unconscious investment of psychic energy in a person, idea, or any other object 全神贯注的；**cathec′tic** adj.

cath·ode (kath′ōd) the electrode at which reduction occurs and to which cations are attracted 阴极；**cathod′ic** adj.

cat·ion (kat′i-on) a positively charged ion 阳离子；**cation′ic** adj.

cau·da (kaw′də) pl. **cau′dae** [L.] a tail or taillike appendage 尾或尾状物；**c. equi′na**, the collection of spinal roots descending from the lower spinal cord and occupying the lumbar cistern of the caudal dural sac; resembling a horse's tail 马尾

cau·dad (kaw′dad) directed toward the tail or distal end; opposite to cephalad 近尾部

cau·dal (kaw′dəl) [caudalis L.] 1. pertaining to a

cauda or tail 尾部的；2. situated more toward the cauda, or tail; in human anatomy, synonymous with *inferior* 近尾部的

cau·date (kaw′dāt) having a tail 有尾的

caul (kawl) a piece of amnion sometimes enveloping a child's head at birth 胎膜

cau·sal (kaw′zəl) pertaining to, involving, or indicating a cause 有原因的

cau·sal·gia (kaw-zal′jə) complex regional pain syndrome type 2 灼性神经痛，2 型复杂性区域疼痛综合征

caus·tic (kaws′tik) 1. burning or corrosive; destructive to living tissues 燃烧，腐蚀，对活组织有破坏性；2. having a burning taste 烧灼气味的；3. an escharotic or corrosive agent 腐蚀剂

cau·ter·ant (kaw′tər-ənt) an agent that cauterizes 腐蚀剂

cau·ter·ize (kaw′tər-īz) 1. to apply a cautery; to destroy tissue by the application of heat, cold, or a caustic agent 烧灼；用热、冷或腐蚀性物质破坏组织；2. cauterization 腐蚀

cau·tery (kaw′tər-e) 1. an agent used for cauterization 腐蚀剂；2. cauterization. 腐蚀，烧灼 **actual c.**, 1. an instrument that destroys tissue by burning 火烙；2. the application of such an instrument 火烙；**cold c.**, cryocautery 冻烙；**electric c., galvanic c.**, electrocautery 电烙；**potential c., virtual c.**, cauterization by an escharotic, without applying heat 腐蚀剂烙

ca·va (ka′və) [L.] 1. *cavum* 的复数；2. vena cava 腔静脉

ca·ve·o·la (ka-ve-o′lə) pl. *caveo′lae* [L.] one of the minute pits or incuppings of the cell membrane formed during pinocytosis 陷窝，小凹，胞膜窖

ca·ver·na (ka-vur′nə) pl. *caver′nae* [L.] cavity (1) 洞

cav·er·nil·o·quy (kav″ər-nil′ə-kwe) lowpitched pectoriloquy indicative of a pulmonary cavity 空洞语音

cav·er·ni·tis (kav″ər-ni′tis) inflammation of the corpora cavernosa or corpus spongiosum of the penis 海绵体炎

cav·er·no·sal (kav″ər-no′səl) 1. pertaining to a corpus cavernosum 海绵体的；2. cavernous 海绵状的

cav·er·no·sog·ra·phy (kav″ər-no-sog′rə-fe) radiographic visualization of the corpus cavernosum of the penis 阴茎海绵体造影术

cav·er·no·som·e·try (kav″ər-no-som′ə-tre) measurement of the vascular pressure in the corpus cavernosum 阴茎海绵体测压法

cav·er·nous (kav′ər-nəs) 1. pertaining to a hollow, or containing hollow spaces 海绵状的；2. having a hollow sound, such as certain abnormal breath sounds 空洞声音的

cav·i·tary (kav′ĭ-tar″e) characterized by a cavity or cavities 空洞的

ca·vi·tis (ka-vi′tis) inflammation of a vena cava 腔静脉炎

cav·i·ty (kav′ĭ-te) [*cavitas* L.] 1. a hollow place or space, or a potential space, within the body or one of its organs 腔，洞；2. in dentistry, the lesion produced by caries 龋洞；**abdominal c.,** the cavity of the body between the respiratory diaphragm and pelvis, containing the abdominal organs 腹腔；**absorption c's,** cavities in developing compact bone due to osteoclastic erosion, usually occurring in the areas laid down first 吸收腔；**amniotic c.,** the closed sac between the embryo and the amnion, containing the amniotic fluid 羊膜腔；**cleavage c.,** blastocoele 卵裂腔；**complex c.,** a carious lesion involving three or more surfaces of a tooth in its prepared state 复杂洞；**compound c.,** a carious lesion involving two surfaces of a tooth in its prepared state 复面洞；**cotyloid c.,** acetabulum 髋臼；**cranial c.,** the space enclosed by the bones of the cranium 颅腔；**dental c.,** the carious defect (lesion) produced by destruction of enamel and dentin in a tooth 牙腔；**glenoid c.,** a depression in the lateral angle of the scapula for articulation with the humerus 关节盂；**marrow c., medullary c.,** the cavity in the diaphysis of a long bone containing the marrow 骨髓腔；**nasal c.,** the proximal part of the respiratory tract, separated by the nasal septum and extending from the nares to the pharynx 鼻腔；**oral c.,** the mouth; the anterior opening of the alimentary canal, bounded externally by the lips and cheeks and extending to the oropharynx, and which also includes the palate, oral mucosa, teeth, tongue, and various glands 口腔；**pelvic c.,** the space within the walls of the pelvis 盆腔；**pericardial c.,** the potential space between the epicardium and the parietal layer of the serous pericardium 心包腔；**peritoneal c.,** the potential space between the parietal and the visceral peritoneum 腹膜腔；**pleural c.,** the potential space between the parietal and visceral pleurae 胸膜腔；**pleuroperitoneal c.,** the temporarily continuous coelomic cavity in the embryo that is later partitioned by the developing respiratory diaphragm 胸膜腹腔的；**prepared c.,** a lesion from which all carious tissue has been removed, preparatory to filling of the tooth 备填腔，清除所有的龋病组织，准备补牙的创口；**pulp c.,** the pulp-filled central chamber in the crown of a tooth 牙髓腔；**Rosenmüller c.,** pharyngeal recess Rosenmüller 窝，咽隐窝；**serous c.,** a coelomic cavity, like that enclosed

by the pericardium, peritoneum, or pleura, not communicating with the outside body, and whose lining membrane secretes a serous fluid 浆膜腔；**sigmoid c.,** 1. either of two depressions in the head of the ulna for articulation with the humerus. 尺骨大、小乙状窝；2. a depression on the distal end of the medial side of the radius for articulation with the ulna 桡骨乙状窝；**simple c.,** a carious lesion whose preparation involves only one tooth surface 单面洞；**somatic c.,** the intraembryonic portion of the coelom 体腔；**tension c's,** cavities of the lung in which the air pressure is greater than that of the atmosphere 肺腔肺中气压大于大气压力的空洞；**thoracic c.,** the part of the ventral body cavity between the neck and the respiratory diaphragm 胸腔；**tympanic c.,** the major portion of the middle ear, consisting of a narrow air-filled cavity in the temporal bone that contains the auditory ossicles 鼓；**uterine c.,** the flattened space within the uterus communicating proximally on either side with the uterine tubes and below with the vagina 子宫腔；**yolk c.,** the space between the embryonic disk and the yolk of the developing ovum of some animals 卵黄囊

ca·vum (ka′vəm) pl. *ca′va* [L.] cavity (1) 空洞；**ca′val** *adj.* **c. sep′ti pellu′cidi,** fifth ventricle 第五脑室

ca·vus (ka′vəs) [L.] hollow 洞

CBC complete blood (cell) count 全血细胞计数

Cbl cobalamin 钴胺素，维生素 B_{12}

cc cubic centimeter (*on The Joint Commission "Do Not Use" List*) 立方厘米

CCK cholecystokinin 缩胆囊素

CCNU lomustine 环己亚硝脲

CD cadaveric donor 尸体供体；cluster designation (见 *antigen* 下 CD antigen) 胞表面标志；curative dose 治愈剂量

CD₅₀ median curative dose 半数治愈量

Cd cadmium 元素镉的符号；caudal or coccygeal 尾或尾骨的

cd candela 坎德拉，发光强度单位

CDC Centers for Disease Control and Prevention 疾病预防控制中心

CDI *Clostridium difficile* infection 艰难梭菌感染

cDNA complementary (or copy) DNA 互补（或复制）DNA

Ce cerium 铈

CEA carcinoembryonic antigen 癌胚抗原

ce·as·mic (se-as′mik) characterized by persistence of embryonic fissures after birth 出生后胚胎裂隙持续存在的

ce·cal (se′kəl) 1. ending in a blind passage 盲端的；2. pertaining to the cecum 盲肠的

ce·cec·to·my (se-sek′tə-me) excision of the cecum 盲肠切除术

ce·ci·tis (se-si′tis) inflammation of the cecum 盲肠炎

ce·co·co·los·to·my (se″ko-kə-los′tə-me) surgical anastomosis of the cecum and colon 盲肠结肠吻合术

ce·co·cys·to·plas·ty (se″ko-sis′to-plas″te) augmentation cystoplasty using an isolated part of the cecum for the added segment 利用盲肠独立的部分来增加节段的膀胱扩大成形术

ce·co·pli·ca·tion (se″ko-plĭ-ka′shən) plication of the cecal wall to correct ptosis or dilatation 折叠盲肠壁以矫正盲肠下垂或扩张

ce·cor·rha·phy (se-kor′ə-fe) suture or repair of the cecum 盲肠缝合术

ce·co·sig·moid·os·to·my (se″ko-sig″moidos′tə-me) formation, usually by surgery, of an opening between the cecum and sigmoid 盲肠乙状结肠吻合术

ce·cos·to·my (se-kos′tə-me) surgical creation of an artificial opening or fistula into the cecum 盲肠造瘘术

ce·cot·o·my (se-kot′ə-me) typhlotomy; incision of the cecum 盲肠切开术

ce·co·ure·ter·o·cele (se″ko-u-re′tər-o-sēl) a ureterocele in which a blind pouch or cecum extends into the submucosa of the bladder or urethra 盲囊或盲肠伸入膀胱或尿道黏膜下层的输尿管疝

ce·cum (se′kəm) 1. the first part of the large intestine, forming a dilated pouch distal to the ileum and proximal to the colon, and giving off the vermiform appendix 盲肠; 2. cul-de-sac 盲管

cef·a·clor (sef′ə-klor) a semisynthetic, secondgeneration cephalosporin effective against a wide range of gram-positive and gram-negative bacteria 头孢克洛, 对多种革兰阳性菌和革兰阴性菌有效的半合成第二代头孢菌素

cef·a·drox·il (sef″ə-droks′il) a semisynthetic first-generation cephalosporin antibiotic effective against a wide range of gram-positive bacteria and a very limited number of gramnegative bacteria 头孢羟氨苄, 半合成第一代头孢菌素类抗生素, 对多种革兰阳性菌和小部分革兰阴性菌有效

cef·a·man·dole (sef″ə-man′dōl) a semisynthetic second-generation cephalosporin antibiotic; used primarily as c. nafate, the sodium salt of the cefamandole formyl ester 头孢孟多, 半合成第二代头孢菌素类抗生素; 主要使用头孢孟多钠, 一种头孢孟多甲酰酯钠盐

cef·az·o·lin (sə-faz′o-lin) a first-generation cephalosporin effective against a wide range of gram-positive bacteria and a limited range of gram-negative

bacteria; used as the sodium salt 头孢唑啉, 第一代头孢菌素, 对多种革兰阳性菌和少量革兰阴性菌有效; 以其钠盐形式使用

cef·din·ir (sef′dĭ-nir) a third-generation cephalosporin effective against a wide range of bacteria 头孢地尼, 对多种细菌有效的第三代头孢菌素

cef·e·pime (sef′ə-pēm) a fourth-generation cephalosporin antibiotic; used as the hydrochloride salt 头孢吡肟, 第四代头孢菌素类抗生素; 以其盐酸盐形式使用

ce·fix·ime (sə-fik′sēm) a third-generation cephalosporin effective against a wide range of bacteria, used in the treatment of otitis media, bronchitis, pharyngitis, tonsillitis, gonorrhea, and urinary tract infections 头孢克肟, 对多种细菌有效的第三代头孢菌素, 用于治疗中耳炎、支气管炎、咽炎、扁桃体炎、淋病和尿路感染

ce·fon·i·cid (sĕ-fon′ĭ-sid) a semisynthetic, second-generation, β-lactamase–resistant cephalosporin effective against a wide range of grampositive and gram-negative bacteria; used as the sodium salt 头孢尼西, 半合成抗β-内酰胺酶第二代头孢菌素, 对多种革兰阴性菌有效; 以其盐酸盐形式使用

cef·o·per·a·zone (sef″o-per′ə-zōn) a β-lactamase–resistant, third-generation cephalosporin effective against a wide range of aerobic and anaerobic gram-positive and gram-negative bacteria; used as the sodium salt 头孢哌酮, 抗β-内酰胺酶第三代头孢菌素, 对各种需氧和厌氧革兰阳性和革兰阴性细菌有效; 以其盐酸盐形式使用

cef·o·tax·ime (sef″o-tak′sēm) a semisynthetic, broad-spectrum, β-lactamase–resistant, thirdgeneration cephalosporin effective against a wide variety of gram-negative bacteria but less active against gram-positive cocci than are the firstand second-generation cephalosporins; used as the sodium salt 头孢噻肟, 半合成广谱抗β-内酰胺酶第三代头孢菌素, 对多种革兰阴性细菌有效, 但对革兰阳性球菌的有效性低于第一代和第二代头孢菌素; 以盐酸盐形式使用

cef·o·te·tan (sef′o-te″tən) a β-lactamase–resistant second-generation cephalosporin effective against a wide range of gram-positive and gramnegative bacteria; used as the disodium salt 头孢替坦, 抗β-内酰胺酶第二代头孢菌素, 对多种革兰阳性菌和革兰阴性菌有效; 以其盐酸盐形式使用

ce·fox·i·tin (sə-fok′sĭ-tin) a strongly β-lactamase–resistant cephamycin antibiotic, classified as a second-generation cephalosporin and especially effective against gram-negative organisms; used as the sodium salt 头孢西丁, 强抗β-内酰胺酶头孢菌素类抗生素, 被归类为第二代头孢菌素, 对革兰阴性菌特别有效; 以其盐酸盐形式

使用

cef·po·dox·ime (sef″po-dok′sēm) a β-lactamase–resistant third-generation cephalosporin effective against a wide range of gram-positive and gram-negative bacteria; used as c. *proxetil* 头孢泊肟，抗 β- 内酰胺酶第三代头孢菌素，对多种革兰阳性和革兰阴性菌有效；用作头孢泊肟酯

cef·pro·zil (sef-pro′zil) a broad-spectrum, second-generation cephalosporin effective against a wide range of gram-positive and gramnegative bacteria 头孢丙烯，广谱的第二代头孢菌素，对多种革兰阳性菌和革兰阴性菌有效

cef·ta·ro·line (sef″tə-ro′lēn fos′ə-mil) a broad-spectrum, β-lactamase–resistant cephalosporin effective against a wide range of gram-negative and gram-positive organisms; used as c. *fosamil* 头孢洛林，广谱抗 β- 内酰胺酶头孢菌素，对各种革兰阴性菌和革兰阳性微生物有效；用作头孢洛林酯

cef·ta·zi·dime (sef-taz′ĭ-dēm″) a third-generation cephalosporin effective against gram-positive and gram-negative bacteria 头孢他啶，第三代头孢菌素，对革兰阳性和革兰阴性细菌有效

cef·ti·bu·ten (sef-ti′bu-tən) a third-generation cephalosporin used in treatment of bronchitis, pharyngitis, tonsillitis, and otitis media 头孢布坦，用于治疗支气管炎、咽炎、扁桃体炎和中耳炎的第三代头孢菌素

cef·ti·zox·ime (sef″tĭ-zok′sēm) a semisynthetic, β-lactamase–resistant, third-generation cephalosporin effective against a wide range of grampositive and gram-negative bacteria; used as the sodium salt 头孢噻肟，半合成抗 β- 内酰胺酶第三代头孢菌素，对多种革兰阴性菌有效；以其盐铵盐形式使用

cef·tri·ax·one (sef″tri-ak′sōn) a semisynthetic, β-lactamase–resistant, third-generation cephalosporin effective against a wide range of grampositive and gram-negative bacteria; used as the sodium salt 头孢曲松，半合成抗 β- 内酰胺酶第三代头孢菌素，对多种革兰阴性菌有效，以盐酸盐形式使用

cef·u·rox·ime (sef″u-rok′sēm) a semisynthetic, β -lactamase–resistant, second-generation cephalosporin effective against a wide range of gram-positive and gram-negative bacteria; used as the sodium salt and the axetil ester 头孢呋辛，半合成抗 β- 内酰胺酶第二代头孢菌素，对各种革兰阳性和革兰阴性菌有效；以盐酸盐形式使用

cel·e·cox·ib (sel″ə-kok′sib) a nonsteroidal antiinflammatory drug that inhibits cyclooxygenase-1 activity, used for the treatment of osteoarthritis and rheumatoid arthritis 塞来昔布，抑制环氧合酶 -1 活性的非甾体抗炎药，用于治疗骨关节炎和类风湿关节炎

ce·li·ac (se′le-ak) abdominal 腹部

ce·li·o·ma (se″le-o′mə) a tumor of the abdomen 腹部肿瘤

ce·li·op·a·thy (se″le-op′ah-the) any abdominal disease 腹部疾病

ce·li·os·co·py (se″le-os′kə-pe) laparoscopy 腹腔镜检查

ce·li·ot·o·my (se″le-ot′ə-me) laparotomy 剖腹术

ce·li·tis (se-li′tis) any abdominal inflammation 腹腔炎

cell (sel) 1. the smallest living unit capable of independent function, consisting of cytoplasm containing various subcellular compartments and separated from the external environment by the plasma membrane. Eukaryotic cells also include a nucleus containing the genome and nucleolus; prokaryotic cells contain DNA but lack a nucleus 细胞，能够独立工作的最小的生物单位，由含有各种亚细胞结构的细胞质组成，并通过质膜与外界环境分离。真核细胞还包括包含基因组和核仁的细胞核；原核细胞包含 DNA，但缺少细胞核；2. a small, more or less closed space 几乎封闭的空间 **accessory c.,** a type of macrophage involved in processing and presentation of antigens, making them more immunogenic 辅助细胞，一种巨噬细胞，参与抗原的加工和表达，使其更具免疫原性；**acid c's,** parietal c's. 酸细胞，胃壁细胞；**acinar c., acinic c., acinous c.,** any of the cells lining an acinus, especially the zymogen-secreting cells of the pancreatic acini 腺泡细胞，腺泡内的任何一种细胞，尤其是胰腺腺泡内分泌酶的细胞；**adventitial c.,** pericyte 周细胞；**air c.,** 1. any minute bodily chamber filled with air, such as an alveolus of the lung 身体内充满空气的微小腔，如肺泡；2. a cavity containing air and surrounded by a bodily structure, usually one of the bones of the head, such as the ethmoid or mastoid 由身体结构包围的含有空气的空腔，通常是头部的骨头之一，如筛骨或乳突；**alpha c.,** 1. a type of cell found in the periphery of the islets of Langerhans that secretes glucagon α 细胞，一种存在于胰岛周围分泌胰高血糖素的细胞；2. acidophil (2); **alveolar c.,** pneumonocyte; any cell of the walls of the pulmonary alveoli; often restricted to the cells of the alveolar epithelium (squamous alveolar cells and great alveolar cells) and alveolar phagocytes 肺泡上皮细胞；肺泡壁上的任何细胞；通常仅指肺泡上皮细胞（鳞状肺泡细胞和大肺泡细胞）和肺泡吞噬细胞；**Alzheimer c.,** 1. a type of giant astrocyte with a large prominent nucleus, found in the brain in hepatolenticular degeneration and hepatic coma 具有大而突出的细胞核的巨大星形胶质细胞，见于肝豆状核变性和肝昏迷的大脑中；2. degenerated astrocytes 变形星形胶质细胞；**amacrine c.,** any of five types of retinal neurons that seem to lack large axons, having only processes that resemble dendrites 无轴突细胞，缺少大轴突的视网膜神经元，只有类似树突的突起；**ameboid c.,** a cell that shows ameboid movement 变形细胞，表现为阿米巴运动的细胞；**Anichkov c.,** a plump modified histiocyte in the inflammatory lesions of the heart (Aschoff bodies) characteristic of rheumatic fever Anichkov 细胞，风湿性心脏病炎性病变中的肥大组织细胞（阿绍夫小体）；**APUD c's,** a group of cells that manufacture polypeptides and biogenic amines serving as hormones or neurotransmitters. The polypeptide production is linked to the uptake of a precursor amino acid and its decarboxylation to an amine 胺前体摄取及脱羧细胞，一组其产生的多肽和生物胺被用作激素或神经递质的细胞，多肽的产生与前体氨基酸的吸收及其对胺的脱羧作用有关；**argentaffin c's,** enterochromaffin cells whose granules stain readily with chromium and silver salts; located in the basilar portions of the glands of the gastrointestinal tract 亲银细胞，其颗粒易被铬和银盐染色；位于胃肠道腺体的基底部；**argyrophilic c's,** enterochromaffin cells that require exposure to a reducing substance before their granules will react with silver; located in the fundic and pyloric glands 嗜银细胞，肠嗜铬细胞需在颗粒与银反应之前接触还原物质；位于胃底腺和幽门腺；**Arias-Stella c's,** columnar cells in the endometrial epithelium that have a hyperchromatic enlarged nucleus; they appear to be associated with chorionic tissue in an intrauterine or extrauterine site Arias-Stella 细胞，子宫内膜上皮中的柱状细胞，细胞核呈深染增大；可能与子宫内或异位的绒毛膜组织有关；**Askanazy c's,** large eosinophilic cells found in the thyroid gland in autoimmune thyroiditis and Hürthle cell tumors Askanazy 细胞，自身免疫性甲状腺炎的甲状腺和 Hürthle 细胞腺瘤中发现的大嗜酸性细胞；**automatic c.,** pacemaker c.; **B c.,** B 细胞 1. beta c. (1); 2. basophil (3); 3.（复数形式）见 *lymphocyte* 下词条；**balloon c.,** a type of swollen, degenerated cell with pale, almost clear, abundant cytoplasm; one variety is seen in the vesicles of herpes zoster and varicella and another is seen in a balloon cell nevus 气球状细胞，肿胀、退化的细胞，胞质丰富、色淡、几乎透明；见于带状疱疹和水痘的囊泡，或见于气球细胞痣；**band c.,** a late metamyelocyte in which the nucleus is in the form of a curved or coiled band 杆状核细胞，晚期晚幼粒细胞，其核呈弯曲或盘绕杆状；**basal c.,** a type of keratinocyte found in the stratum basale of the epidermis 基底细胞，表皮基底层中的角蛋白形成细胞；**basal granular c's,** enteroendocrine c's. 基底颗粒细胞；**basket c.,** a neuron of the cerebral cortex whose fibers form a basket-like nest in which a Purkinje cell rests 篮状细胞，大脑皮层的神经元，处于浦肯野细胞纤维形成的篮

状巢中；**beaker c.,** goblet c.; **beta c.,** β 细胞；1. one of the cells that compose the bulk of the islets of Langerhans and secrete insulin 组成胰岛大部分并分泌胰岛素的细胞之一；2. basophil (3); **Betz c's,** large pyramidal ganglion cells forming a layer of the gray matter of the brain 贝兹细胞，大脑灰质层的大锥体神经节细胞；**bipolar c.,** a neuron with two processes 双极细胞，双极的神经元；**blast c.,** 母细胞 1. blast1 (1).; 2. the least differentiated blood cell without commitment as to its particular series; it precedes a stem cell 无特定分化倾向的分化程度最低的血细胞，它先于干细胞出现；**blood c.,** one of the formed elements of the blood; a leukocyte, erythrocyte, or platelet 血细胞，血液的组成成分之一；白细胞、红细胞或血小板；**bone c.,** osteocyte 骨细胞；**burr c.,** echinocyte: a spiculed erythrocyte with multiple small projections evenly spaced over its circumference 棘细胞：一种棘刺状红细胞，周围有多个均匀分布的小突起；**cartilage c.,** chondrocyte 软骨细胞；**CD4 c's,** a major classification of T lymphocytes; most are helper cells CD4 细胞，是 T 淋巴细胞的主要类型之一，指携带 CD4 抗原的细胞；大多数是辅助细胞；**CD8 c's,** a major classification of T lymphocytes, referring to those that carry the CD8 antigen, including cytotoxic T lymphocytes and suppressor cells CD8 细胞，是 T 淋巴细胞的主要类型之一，指携带 CD8 抗原的细胞，包括细胞毒性 T 淋巴细胞和抑制细胞；**chief c's,** 主细胞 1. columnar or cuboidal epithelial cells that line the lower portions of the gastric glands and secrete pepsin 排列在胃腺底部并分泌胃蛋白酶的柱状或立方状上皮细胞；2. pinealocytes. 松果体细胞；3. the most abundant parenchymal cells of the parathyroid, being polygonal epithelial cells rich in glycogen, having granular cytoplasm and vesicular nuclei, and being arranged in plates or cords; cf. *oxyphil c's* 甲状腺中最多的实质细胞，富含糖原的多边形上皮细胞，有颗粒状胞浆和泡状核，排列成板状或索状；4. the principal chromaffin cells of the paraganglia, each of which is surrounded by supporting cells 副神经节的主要嗜铬细胞，每一个都被支持细胞包围；5. chromophobe c's 嫌色细胞；

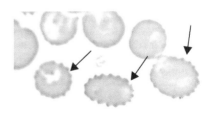

▲　棘细胞（**burr cell**）（箭）

C

chromaffin c's, cells staining readily with chromium salts, especially those of the adrenal medulla and similar cells occurring in widespread accumulations throughout the body in various organs, whose cytoplasm shows fine brown granules when stained with potassium bichromate 嗜铬细胞，易被铬盐染色的细胞，尤其是肾上腺髓质细胞和类似的细胞，在全身各器官广泛聚集，重铬酸钾染色时胞浆呈棕色颗粒；**chromophobe c's,** faintly staining cells in the anterior lobe of the pituitary; some are nongranular (either nonsecretory, immature presecretory, or degenerating cells), while others have extremely small granules; they are increased in chromophobe adenomas 嫌色细胞，垂体前叶淡染细胞；一些是非颗粒细胞（非分泌性、未成熟的前体或退化细胞），另一些则有非常小的颗粒；嫌色细胞瘤中其数目增加；**Claudius c's,** cuboidal cells, which along with Böttcher cells form the floor of the external spiral sulcus, external to the organ of Corti 克劳迪与斯细胞，立方细胞，与 Böttcher 细胞一起形成外螺旋沟的底部，位于螺旋器的外部；**clear c's,** cells with empty-appearing cytoplasm, seen normally in the sweat glands, parathyroid glands, renal collecting tubules, and epididymis, and pathologically in some neoplastic conditions 透明细胞，细胞质为空的细胞，通常见于汗腺、甲状旁腺、肾集合管和附睾，某些肿瘤病理上可见；**columnar c.,** an elongated epithelial cell 柱状细胞，细长的上皮细胞；**committed c.,** a lymphocyte that, after contact with antigen, is obligated to follow an individual course of development leading to antibody synthesis or immunologic memory 定型细胞，一种淋巴细胞，与抗原接触后经由独立的发育过程，导致抗体合成或免疫记忆形成；**cuboidal c.,** an epithelial cell whose transverse and vertical diameters are approximately equal 立方细胞，横径和竖径大致相等的上皮细胞；**daughter c.,** one of the two or more cells formed by the division of a mother cell 子细胞，母细胞分裂形成的两个或多个细胞之一；**decidual c's,** connective tissue cells of the uterine mucous membrane, enlarged and specialized during pregnancy 蜕膜细胞，子宫黏膜的结缔组织细胞，在怀孕期间增大并特化；**Deiters c's,** the outer phalangeal cells of the organ of Corti; they support the outer hair cells 戴特斯细胞，螺旋器的外指细胞；起支持外毛细胞的作用；**delta c's,** cells in the pancreatic islets that secrete somatostatin D 细胞，胰岛中分泌生长抑素的细胞；**dendritic c's,** cells with long cytoplasmic processes in the lymph nodes and germinal centers of the spleen; such processes, which extend along lymphoid cells, retain antigen molecules for extended periods of time 树突状细胞，即在淋巴结和脾脏生发中心具有长胞质突起的细胞；这种沿着淋巴细胞延伸的突起可将抗原分子

保留较长时间；**ECL c.,** enterochromaffin-like c.; **effector c.,** any cell, such as an activated lymphocyte or plasma cell, which is instrumental in causing antigen disposal accomplished by either a cell-mediated or a humoral immunologic response 效应细胞，如激活的淋巴细胞或浆细胞，可通过细胞介导或体液免疫反应来实现抗原清除；**embryonic stem c's,** totipotent stem cells derived from the embryoblast or inner cell mass of the blastocyst 胚胎干细胞，来自胚泡母细胞或胚泡内细胞团的全能性干细胞；**enamel c.,** ameloblast 釉质细胞；**enterochromaffin c's,** endocrine cells that stain with chromium salts and are impregnable with silver; they occur throughout the body but are seen most frequently in the intestinal and bronchial submucosa and are sites of synthesis and storage of serotonin 肠嗜铬细胞，可被铬盐染色并能被银染的内分泌细胞，分布于全身，但最常见于肠和支气管黏膜下层，是血清素合成和储存的场所；**enterochromaffin-like c.,** a paracrine cell of the fundic glands that controls the secretion of acid by releasing histamine in response to stimulation by gastrin 肠嗜铬样细胞，在胃泌素刺激下通过释放组胺来控制胃酸分泌的旁分泌细胞。称 *ECL c.* **enteroendocrine c's,** a group of APUD cells, divisible into a number of populations on the basis of polypeptide hormone and biogenic amine production; found scattered throughout the gastrointestinal epithelium, mainly at the base of the epithelium 肠内分泌细胞，一组 APUD 细胞，根据多肽激素和生物胺的产生类型可分成许多群体；分布在整个胃肠道上皮，主要分布在上皮的底部；**epithelial c.,** any of the cells that cover the surface of the body and line its cavities 上皮细胞，覆盖身体及空腔表面的细胞；**epithelioid c.,** 上皮样细胞 1. large polyhedral cells of connective tissue origin 结缔组织起源的大、多面体细胞；2. highly phagocytic, modified macrophages, resembling epithelial cells, which are characteristic of granulomatous inflammation 高吞噬性、修饰性巨噬细胞，类似上皮细胞，具有肉芽肿性炎症特征；3. pinealocytes 松果体细胞；**erythroid c's,** blood cells of the erythrocytic series 类红细胞；**ethmoid c's, ethmoidal c's, ethmoidal air c's,** ethmoidal sinuses; paranasal sinuses found in spaces within the ethmoid bone and communicating with the ethmoidal infundibulum and bulla and the superior and highest meatuses; often subdivided into *anterior, middle,* and *posterior* 筛窦；筛骨中的成组的副鼻窦通过筛窦漏斗、筛窦泡及最上、最高的管道相通。通常分为前、中、后三部分；**eukaryotic c.,** a cell with a true nucleus 真核细胞，见 *eukaryote*；**excitable c.,** a cell that can generate an action potential at its membrane in response to depolarization and may transmit an impulse along the membrane 可兴奋细胞，对去极化反应产生动作电

位的细胞，可以沿着细胞膜传递脉冲；**fat c.**, adipocyte; a connective tissue cell specialized for synthesis and storage of fat; these are bloated with globules of triglycerides surrounded by a thin line of cytoplasm and have the nucleus displaced to one side 脂肪细胞；专门用于合成和储存脂肪的结缔组织细胞；细胞内充满了甘油三酯，周围有一条薄薄的细胞质线，细胞核移向一边；**fat-storing c. of liver**, lipid-accumulating, stellate cells located in the perisinusoidal space of the liver 肝脂肪储存细胞，位于肝窦周围的脂肪聚集、星状细胞；**foam c.**, a cell with a fluid-filled appearance due to the presence of complex lipoids, such as a type of macrophage seen in xanthoma 泡沫细胞，由于存在复杂的类脂物质而具有液体填充外观的细胞，例如黄体瘤中的巨噬细胞；**follicle c's, follicular c's**, cells located in the epithelium of follicles, such as those of the thyroid or ovarian follicles 滤泡细胞，位于滤泡上皮的细胞，如甲状腺或卵巢滤泡；**follicular center c.**, any of a series of B lymphocytes occurring normally in the germinal center and pathologically in the neoplastic nodules of follicular center cell lymphoma; believed to be intermediate stages in the development of lymphoblasts and plasma cells and are distinguished according to size (large or small) and the presence or absence of nuclear folds or clefts (cleaved or noncleaved) 滤泡中心细胞，正常生发中心和淋巴瘤新生结节病理性滤泡中心的一系列 B 淋巴细胞；被认为是淋巴母细胞和浆细胞发育的中间阶段，根据大小和是否有核皱褶或裂隙（有裂隙或无裂隙）来区分；**G c's**, granular enterochromaffin cells in the mucosa of the pyloric part of the stomach, a source of gastrin G 细胞，胃幽门部黏膜中的颗粒状肠嗜铬细胞，分泌胃泌素；**ganglion c.**, a large nerve cell, especially one of those of the spinal ganglia 神经节细胞，一种大神经细胞，尤指脊髓神经节中的细胞；**Gaucher c.**, a large cell characteristic of Gaucher disease, with eccentrically placed nuclei and fine wavy fibrils parallel to the long axis of the cell 戈谢细胞，戈谢病的特征性大细胞，具有偏心排列的细胞核和平行于细胞长轴的细小波浪状纤维；**germ c's**, the cells of an organism whose function is to reproduce its kind, i.e., oocytes and spermatozoa and their immature stages 生殖细胞，生命体中用于繁殖的一类细胞，即卵母细胞和精子及其未成熟阶段；**ghost c.**, 血影细胞 1. a keratinized denucleated cell with an unstained, shadowy center where the nucleus has been 一种角质化的无核细胞，其中心不着色，有阴影；2. a degenerating or fragmented erythrocyte with no hemoglobin 没有血红蛋白的退化或分裂的红细胞；**giant c.**, a very large cell, often specifically a large, multinucleate, modified macrophage formed by coalescence of epithelioid cells or by nuclear division without cytoplas-

mic division of monocytes 巨细胞，由上皮样细胞聚集形成的多核巨噬细胞，核分裂而胞质不分裂的单核细胞；**glial c's**, neuroglial c's.; **globoid c.**, an abnormal large histiocyte found in large numbers in intracranial tissues in Krabbe disease 球样细胞，异常大的组织细胞，在克拉伯病的颅内组织中大量存在；**glomus c.**, 球细胞 1. any of the specific cells of the carotid body that contain many dense-cored vesicles and occur in clusters surrounded by other cells not having cytoplasmic granules 颈动脉体的一种特殊细胞，含有许多致密的有核小泡，呈簇状分布，周围有其他细胞，无细胞质颗粒；2. any of the modified smooth muscle cells surrounding the arterial segment of a glomeriform arteriovenous anastomosis 环绕在球形动静脉吻合术动脉段周围的经修饰的平滑肌细胞；**goblet c.**, a unicellular mucous gland found in the epithelium of various mucous membranes, especially that of the respiratory passages and intestines 杯状细胞，单细胞黏液腺，见于各种黏膜的上皮细胞，特别是呼吸道和肠道的上皮细胞；**Golgi c's**, 见 *neuron* 下词条，高尔基细胞；**granular c.**, a type of keratinocyte in the stratum granulosum of the epidermis, containing keratohyalin granules 颗粒细胞，表皮颗粒层中的一角质形成细胞，含有角蛋白颗粒；**granule c's**, 颗粒细胞 1. tiny cells found in the granular layers of the cerebellar and cerebral cortices 小脑和大脑皮质颗粒层中发现的微小细胞；2. small nerve cells without axons, found in the granular layer of the olfactory bulb 无轴突的小神经细胞，见于嗅球的颗粒层；**granulosa c's**, cells surrounding the graafian follicle and forming the stratum granulosum and cumulus oophorus, after ovulation becoming lutein cells 卵泡颗粒细胞，成熟卵泡（格拉夫卵泡）周围的细胞，在排卵后形成颗粒层和卵丘，成为黄体细胞；**granulosa-lutein c's**, lutein cells of the corpus luteum derived from granulosa cells 黄体颗粒细胞，含有黄体素的黄体细胞，来源于颗粒细胞；**gustatory c's**, taste c's.; **hair c's**, sensory epithelial cells with long hairlike processes (kinocilia or stereocilia); *auditory hair cells* are found in the organ of Corti and regulate hearing, and *vestibular hair cells* are found in the vestibular labyrinth and regulate the sense of equilibrium 毛细胞，长毛状突起的感觉上皮细胞（动纤毛或静纤毛）；听觉毛细胞存在于柯蒂氏器中调节听觉，前庭毛细胞存在于前庭迷路中调节平衡感；**hairy c.**, one of the abnormal large leukocytes found in the blood in hairy cell leukemia, having numerous irregular cytoplasmic villi that give the cell a flagellated or hairy appearance 毛细胞，白血病患者血液中发现的异常大白细胞，有许多不规则的胞质绒毛，使细胞呈现毛状外观；**heart disease c's, heart failure c's**, macrophages containing granules of iron, found in the pulmonary alveoli and sputum in congestive heart failure 心脏病细胞，心衰细胞，含铁颗粒的巨噬细胞，见于充血性心力衰竭的肺泡和痰中；**HeLa c's,** cells of the first continuously cultured carcinoma strain, descended from a human cervical carcinoma 海拉细胞，第一个连续培养的癌细胞株，源于人宫颈癌；**helmet c.,** schistocyte 盔形红细胞，裂红细胞；**helper c's, helper T c's,** differentiated T lymphocytes that cooperate with B lymphocytes in the synthesis of antibody to many antigens; they play an integral role in immunoregulation 辅助细胞、辅助 T 细胞，与 B 淋巴细胞协同合成多种抗原抗体的分化 T 淋巴细胞，在免疫调节中起着不可分割的作用；**hematopoietic stem c.,** a type of blood cell precursor that is a slightly later stage than a blast cell 造血干细胞，血细胞前体，比母细胞分化稍晚；**Hensen c's,** tall supporting cells constituting the outer border of the organ of Corti 汉森细胞，位于螺旋器外侧缘的几行高柱状细胞；**hepatic c.,** one of the polyhedral epithelial cells that constitute the substance of an acinus of the liver 肝细胞，构成肝腺泡的多形上皮细胞之一；**horizontal c.,** a retinal neuron, occurring in two types, each with one long neural process and several short ones 水平细胞，一种视网膜神经元，有两种类型，每种类型均有一长时神经传到过程和几个短时神经传到过程；**Hürthle c's, Askanazy c's; interdental c's,** cells found in the spiral limbus between the dens acustici which secrete the tectorial membrane of the cochlear duct 齿间细胞，位于听齿间的螺旋缘上细胞，分泌耳蜗管覆膜；**interstitial c's,** 间质细胞 1. Leydig c's (1); 2. large epithelioid cells in the ovarian stroma, believed to have a secretory function, derived from the theca interna of atretic ovarian follicles 卵巢基质中的大上皮样细胞，被认为具有分泌功能，来源于闭锁性卵巢滤泡的卵巢膜细胞；3. cells found in the perivascular areas and between the cords of pinealocytes in the pineal body 松果体血管周围和松果体细胞索之间的细胞；4. fat-storing c's of liver 肝脏脂肪储存细胞；**interstitial c's of Cajal,** pleomorphic cells having an oval nucleus and long, branching cytoplasmic processes that interlace with processes of adjacent cells, found in the gastrointestinal tract and esophagus and thought to act as pacemakers 间质卡哈尔细胞，多形性细胞，有椭圆形核和长的、分支状突起，与邻近细胞突起相互交错，见于胃肠道和食道，被认为是起搏细胞；**islet c's,** the alpha and beta cells of the islets of Langerhans 胰岛细胞；**juxtaglomerular c's,** specialized cells containing secretory granules, located in the tunica media of the afferent glomerular arterioles, thought to stimulate aldosterone secretion and to play a role in renal autoregulation. These cells secrete the enzyme renin 肾小球球旁细胞，含有分泌颗粒的特殊细胞，位于肾小球入球

小动脉的中膜，能刺激醛固酮的分泌，并在肾脏自动调节中起到作用。这些细胞分泌肾素；**K c's,** K 细胞 1. killer cells; cells mediating antibody-dependent cell-mediated cytotoxicity; they are small lymphocytes without T- or B-cell surface markers, having cytotoxic activity against target cells coated with specific IgG antibody 杀伤细胞；介导抗体依赖细胞介导的细胞毒性作用的细胞；为没有 T 细胞或 B 细胞表面标记物的小淋巴细胞，对特异性 IgG 抗体的靶细胞具有细胞毒活性；2. cells in the duodenal and jejunal mucosa that synthesize gastric inhibitory polypeptide 十二指肠和空肠黏膜中合成抑胃肽的细胞；**killer c's,** 杀伤细胞 1. K c's (1); 2. cytotoxic T lymphocytes 细胞毒性 T 淋巴细胞；**killer T c's,** cytotoxic T lymphocytes 杀伤 T 细胞，细胞毒性 T 淋巴细胞；**Kupffer c's,** large, stellate or pyramidal, intensely phagocytic cells lining the walls of the hepatic sinusoids and forming part of the reticuloendothelial system 库普弗细胞，大的星状或锥形吞噬细胞，排列在肝窦壁上，形成网状内皮系统的一部分；**L c's,** endocrine cells of the gut, resembling the alpha cells of the islets of Langerhans, they secrete glucagon-like peptides 1 and 2 L 细胞，肠道的内分泌细胞，类似于胰岛的 α 细胞，分泌胰高血糖素样肽 1 和肽 2；**lacunar c.,** a variant of the Reed-Sternberg cell, primarily associated with the nodular sclerosis type of Hodgkin disease 腔隙细胞，是里－施细胞的变异细胞，主要与结节硬化型霍奇金病有关；**LAK c's,** lymphokine-activated killer c's LAK 细胞；**Langerhans c's,** stellate dendritic cells, derived from precursors in the bone marrow, containing characteristic inclusions (*Birbeck granules*) in the cytoplasm and found principally in the epidermis; they are antigenpresenting cells involved in cell-mediated immune reactions in the skin 朗格汉斯细胞，星状树突状细胞，来源于骨髓前体，细胞质中含有特征性包涵体（伯贝克颗粒），主要发现于表皮；为参与皮肤细胞介导的免疫反应的抗原呈递细胞；**large cleaved c.,** 见 *follicular center c.* 大裂细胞；**large noncleaved c., large uncleaved c.,** 见 *follicular center c.* 大无裂细胞；见 follicular center c. **LE c.,** a neutrophil or macrophage that has phagocytized the denatured nuclear material of an injured cell (hematoxylin body); a characteristic of lupus erythematosus, but also found in analogous connective tissue disorders LE 细胞，吞噬受损细胞变性核（苏木精体）的中性粒细胞或巨噬细胞；红斑狼疮的特征细胞，但也存在于类似的结缔组织疾病中；**Leydig c's,** 睾丸间质细胞 1. clusters of epithelioid cells constituting the endocrine tissue of the testis, which elaborate androgens, chiefly testosterone 构成睾丸内分泌组织的上皮样细胞群，产生雄激素，主要是睾酮；2. mucous cells that do not pour their secretion out over the epithelial surface 分泌物不排出上皮表面的黏液细胞；**littoral c's,** flattened cells lining the walls of lymph or blood sinuses 衬细胞，淋巴或血窦壁上的扁平细胞；**luteal c's, lutein c's,** the plump, pale-staining, polyhedral cells of the corpus luteum 黄体细胞，丰满、淡染色的多形黄体细胞；**lymph c.,** lymphocyte 淋巴细胞；**lymphoid c's,** lymphocytes and plasma cells; cells of the immune system that react specifically with antigen and elaborate specific cell products 淋巴细胞和浆细胞；免疫系统中与抗原特异性反应的细胞，并产生特异性细胞产物；**lymphokine-activated killer c's,** killer cells activated by interleukin-2 and having specificity for tumors refractory to NK cells 淋巴因子激活的杀伤细胞，白细胞介素 -2 激活的杀伤细胞，对 NK 细胞不敏感的肿瘤细胞有特异性杀伤作用；**mast c.,** a connective tissue cell capable of elaborating basophilic, metachromatic cytoplasmic granules that contain histamine, heparin, hyaluronan, slowreacting substance of anaphylaxis, and, in some species, serotonin 肥大细胞，结缔组织细胞，具有嗜碱性、异染胞质颗粒，其中含有组胺、肝素、透明质酸、过敏性慢反应物质，在某些颗粒中还含有血清素；**mastoid c's,** air cells of various sizes and shapes in the mastoid process of the temporal bone 颞骨乳突中大小和形状不等的气腔；**memory c's,** T and B lymphocytes that mediate immunologic memory; believed to retain information that permits a subsequent antigenic challenge to be followed by a more rapid, efficient immunologic reaction than that seen with the first exposure 记忆细胞，介导免疫记忆的 T 淋巴细胞和 B 淋巴细胞；可记忆免疫信息，在次接触抗原刺激时比第一次更迅速、更有效地发生免疫反应；**Merkel c.,** a specialized cell at or near the epithelial-dermal junction and believed to act as a touch receptor by association with the flat, disklike ending of a nerve fiber (tactile meniscus) 梅克尔细胞，位于或接近上皮 - 真皮连接处的一种特殊细胞，与神经纤维的扁平、盘状末端（触盘）有关，起触感受器的作用；**Mexican hat c.,** target c. (1) 墨西哥帽形细胞；**microglial c.,** a cell of the microglia 小胶质细胞；**mother c.,** one that divides to form new, or daughter, cells 母细胞，分裂形成新细胞或子细胞；**mucous c's,** cells that secrete mucus or mucin. 黏液细胞，分泌黏液或黏蛋白的细胞；**muscle c.,** 肌细胞，见下 fiber。**myoid c's,** cells in the convoluted seminiferous tubules that seem to be contractile and that are probably responsible for the rhythmic shallow contractions of the tubules 肌样细胞，迂回的生精小管中的细胞是可收缩的，这可能是生精小管有节奏的浅收缩的原因；**natural killer c's,** NK c's.；**nerve c.,** neuron 神经细胞，神经元；**neuroendocrine c's,** the specialized neurons that secrete neurohormones 神经内分泌细胞，分泌神经激素的特殊神经元；**neuroglia c's, neuroglial c's,** the branching, non-neural cells of the neuroglia; they are of three types: astroglia, oligodendroglia (collectively termed macroglia), and microglia 神经胶质细胞，分支状、非神经细胞的神经胶质细胞；它们有三种类型：星形胶质型、少突胶质型（统称为大胶质）和小胶质型；**neurosecretory c.,** any cell with neuronlike properties that secretes a biologically active substance acting on another structure, often at a distant site 神经分泌细胞，任何具有神经活性，并分泌生物活性物质作用于另一结构的细胞，通常为远距分泌；**nevus c.,** a small cell with a deeply staining nucleus, pale cytoplasm, and sometimes melanin granules, found in clusters in the epidermis, and reaching the dermis by a kind of extrusion 痣细胞，胞核深染、胞质苍白的小细胞，有时为黑色素颗粒，在表皮呈簇状，通过挤压到达真皮；**Niemann-Pick c's, Pick c's; NK c's,** natural killer cells; cells capable of mediating cytotoxic reactions without themselves being specifically sensitized against the target NK 细胞，自然杀伤细胞，能够介导细胞毒性反应而对自身靶点不敏感的细胞；**nonpacemaker c.,** a cardiac cell that is incapable of self-excitation and must wait in a state of equilibrium for an outside stimulus. 非起搏器细胞，须在平衡状态下等待外界刺激，而无自主兴奋性的心脏细胞；**null c's,** lymphocytes that lack the surface antigens characteristic of B and T lymphocytes; seen in active systemic lupus erythematosus and other disease states 裸细胞，缺乏 B 和 T 淋巴细胞表面抗原的淋巴细胞；见于活动期的系统性红斑狼疮和其他疾病；**olfactory c's,** a set of specialized cells of the mucous membranes of the nose, which are receptors of smell 嗅细胞，鼻黏膜的一组特殊细胞，是嗅觉的受体；**osteoprogenitor c's,** relatively undifferentiated cells found on or near the free surfaces of bone; under certain circumstances they either undergo division and transform into osteoblasts or coalesce to give rise to osteoclasts 骨祖细胞，在骨表面游离或其附近发现的相对未分化细胞；在某些情况下，它们或被分裂并转化为成骨细胞，或融合成破骨细胞；**oxyphil c's, oxyphilic c's,** 嗜酸性细胞 1. acidophilic cells found, along with the more numerous chief cells, in the parathyroid glands 甲状旁腺中发现的伴随着大量主细胞的嗜酸性细胞；2. Askanazy c's. Askanazy 细胞；**P c's,** poorly staining, pale, small cells almost devoid of myofibrils, mitochondria, or other organelles; they are clustered in the sinoatrial node (where they are thought to be the center of impulse generation), as well as in the atrioventricular node P 细胞，染色不良，苍白，几乎没有肌原纤维、线粒体或其他细胞器的小细胞；聚集在窦房结（被认为是冲动产生的中心）以及房室结；**pacemaker c.,** a myocardial cell displaying automaticity 起搏细胞，具有自律性的 心 肌 细 胞；**packed red blood c's**, whole blood from which plasma has been removed; used therapeutically in blood transfusions 浓缩红细胞，无血浆的全血；用于输血治疗；**Paget c., pagetoid c.**, a large, irregularly shaped, pale anaplastic tumor cell found in the epidermis in Paget disease of the nipple and in extramammary Paget disease 佩吉特细胞，乳房佩吉特病和乳房外佩吉特病的表皮中发现大的、不规则形状的、苍白的间变性肿瘤细胞；**Paneth c's**, narrow, pyramidal, or columnar epithelial cells with a round or oval nucleus near the base, found in the fundus of the crypts of Lieberkühn; they contain large secretory granules that may contain peptidase 帕内特细胞，狭长的、锥形或柱状上皮细胞，基部附近有圆形或椭圆形的细胞核，见于肠腺的基底部；含有分泌肽酶的大分泌颗；**parafollicular c's**, ovoid epithelial cells located in the thyroid follicles; they secrete calcitonin 滤泡旁细胞，位于甲状腺滤泡内的卵球形上皮细胞，分泌降钙素；**parietal c's**, large spheroidal or pyramidal cells that are the source of gastric hydrochloric acid and are the site of intrinsic factor production 壁细胞，大的球状或锥形细胞，分泌胃酸及内因子；**peptic c's**, chief c's (1) 胃酶细胞；**pessary c.**, an erythrocyte that has lost its color because its hemoglobin is present only as a circumferential rim 子宫托形红细胞，一种红细胞，其血红蛋白存在于周缘而中心失去颜色；**phalangeal c's**, elongated supporting cells of the organ of Corti with bases that rest on the basilar membrane adjacent to the pillar cells; the *inner* ones are arranged in a row on the inner surface of the inner pillar cells and surround the inner hair cells; the *outer* ones (*Deiters c's*) support the outer hair cells 指细胞，螺旋器上细长的支持细胞，其基部位于邻近柱状细胞的基底膜上；内柱细胞排列在内表面上，并包围内毛细胞；外指细胞（戴特斯细胞）支持外毛细胞；**pheochrome c's**, chromaffin c's.; **Pick c's**, round, oval, or polyhedral cells with foamy, lipid-containing cytoplasm, found in the bone marrow and spleen in Niemann-Pick disease 皮克细胞，在尼曼 - 皮克病的骨髓和脾脏中发现的圆形、卵圆形或多形性细胞，胞浆呈泡沫状，含脂质；**pigment c.**, any cell containing pigment granules 色素细胞，任何含有色素颗粒的细胞；**pillar c's**, elongated supporting cells in a double row (*inner* and *outer pillar c's*) in the organ of Corti, arranged to form the inner tunnel 柱细胞，螺旋器中呈双列（内柱细胞和外柱细胞）的细长支持细胞，排列成内部管道；**plasma c.**, spherical or ellipsoidal cells with a single nucleus containing chromatin, an area of perinuclear clearing, and generally abundant, sometimes vacuolated, cytoplasm; they are involved in the synthesis, stor-

age, and release of antibody 浆细胞，球形或椭圆形细胞，单核含染色质及核周淡染区，胞质丰富，有时呈空泡状，参与抗体的合成、储存和释放；**polychromatic c's, polychromatophil c's**, immature erythrocytes that stain with both acid and basic stains in a diffuse mixture of blue-gray and pink 多色素性红细胞，嗜多色性红细胞，同时有酸性和碱性染色的灰蓝色和灰红色未成熟红细胞；**pre-B c's**, lymphoid cells that are immature and contain cytoplasmic IgM; they develop into B lymphocytes 前 B 细胞，不成熟的含 IgM 的淋巴细胞；发育成 B 淋巴细胞；**pre-T c's**, a T-lymphocyte precursor before undergoing induction of the maturation process in the thymus; it lacks the characteristics of a mature T lymphocyte 前 T（淋巴）细胞，胸腺诱导成熟前的 T 淋巴细胞前体，缺乏成熟 T 淋巴细胞的特征；**prickle c.**, a keratinocyte with delicate radiating processes connecting with similar cells, found in the stratum spinosum (prickle cell layer) of the epidermis 棘细胞，角蛋白形成细胞纤细突起辐射交联，见于表皮的刺细胞层；**primordial germ c.**, the earliest recognizable precursor in the embryo of a germ cell; these originate extragonadally but migrate early in embryonic development to the gonads 原始生殖细胞，胚胎中最先可识别的生殖细胞前体；起源于性腺外，但在胚胎发育早期迁移至性腺；**prokaryotic c.**, a cell without a true nucleus 原核细胞，没有真核的细胞；见 *prokaryote*；**pulmonary epithelial c's**, extremely thin nonphagocytic squamous cells with flattened nuclei, constituting the outer layer of the alveolar wall in the lungs 肺泡上皮细胞，极薄的非吞噬性鳞状细胞，细胞核扁平，构成肺泡壁的外层；**Purkinje c's**, 浦肯野细胞 1. large branching neurons in the middle layer of the cerebellar cortex. 小脑皮质中层的大分支神经元；2. large, clear, tightly packed, impulseconducting cells of the cardiac Purkinje fibers 心脏浦肯野纤维中的大的、透明的、紧密的、冲动传导细胞；**pyramidal c.**, a type of large multipolar pyramid-shaped cell found in the cerebral cortex, having one apical dendrite extending outward toward the surface and several dendrites; a few are inverted and have apical dendrites extending inward 锥体细胞，大脑皮层中的大多极锥体状细胞，有一向外延伸到表面的顶端树突和几个树突；少数是顶端树突向内延伸；**red c.**, **red blood c.**, erythrocyte 红 细 胞；**red blood c's**, official terminology for *packed red blood c's* 红 细 胞的专业术语；**Reed c's, Reed-Sternberg c's**, the giant histiocytic cells, typically multinucleate, that are the common histologic characteristic of Hodgkin disease 里 - 施细胞巨大的组织细胞，典型的多核细胞，是霍奇金病的常见组织学特征；**reticu-**

lar c's, the cells forming the reticular fibers of connective tissue; those forming the framework of lymph nodes, bone marrow, and spleen form part of the reticuloendothelial system and may differentiate into macrophages 网状细胞，形成结缔组织网状纤维的细胞；形成淋巴结、骨髓和脾脏框架的细胞，构成网状内皮系统的一部分，并可分化为巨噬细胞；**reticuloendothelial c.**, 网状内皮细胞，见 *system* 下 词 条；Sala **c's**, star-shaped cells of connective tissue in the fibers that form the sensory nerve endings in the pericardium Sala 细胞，纤维结缔组织中的星形细胞，在心包中形成感觉神经末梢；**Schwann c.**, any of the large nucleated cells whose cell membrane spirally enwraps the axons of myelinated peripheral neurons supplying the myelin sheath between two nodes of Ranvier 施万细胞，神经膜细胞有核大细胞，其细胞膜膜螺旋地包裹在外周有髓神经元的轴突，在两个郎飞氏结之间形成髓鞘；**segmented c.**, a mature granulocyte whose nucleus is divided into distinct lobes joined by a filamentous connection 分叶核粒细胞，成熟的粒细胞，其核分裂成由细丝连接的不同叶；**sensitized c.**, 致 敏 细 胞 1. a cell that has been immunologically activated (primed) by an antigen 被抗原免疫激活（启动）的细胞；2. an antibodycoated cell used in complement fixation tests 补体结合试验中的一种抗体细胞；**Sertoli c's**, cells in the seminiferous tubules to which the spermatids become attached and which support, protect, and apparently nourish the spermatids until they develop into mature spermatozoa 支持细胞，附着在生精小管中，支持、保护和滋养精母细胞，直到其发育为成熟精子；**sex c's**, **sexual c's**, germ c's 性细胞，生殖细胞；**Sézary c.**, an abnormal mononuclear T lymphocyte seen in mycosis fungoides and Sézary syndrome Sézary 细胞，蕈样真菌病和 Sézary 综合征中异常的单核 T 淋巴细胞；**sickle c.**, a crescentic or sickleshaped erythrocyte, characteristic of sickle cell anemia 镰状细胞，新月形或镰状红细胞，镰状细胞贫血的特征性细胞；**signet ring c.**, a cell whose nucleus has been pressed to one side by an accumulation of intracytoplasmic mucin, as in a Krukenberg tumor or signet ring cell carcinoma 印戒细胞，核被细胞质内的黏蛋白挤向一侧的细胞，如 Krukenberg 瘤或印戒细胞癌；**small cleaved c.**, 小 裂 细 胞，见 *follicular center c.*；**small noncleaved c.**, **small uncleaved c.**, 小无裂细胞，见 *follicular center c.*；**somatic c's**, any of the cells of an organism other than the germ cells 体细胞，有机体内除生殖细胞以外的任何细胞；**somatostatin c's**, endocrine cells of the oxyntic and pyloric glands that secrete somatostatin 生长抑素细胞，泌酸腺和幽门腺内分泌生长抑素的内分泌细胞；**sperm c.**, spermatozoon 精子；**spindle c.**, any of various cells that are shaped like spindles, being more or less round in the middle with two ends that are pointed 梭形细胞，形状似纺锤的细胞，中间为圆形，两端呈尖状；**spur c.**, acanthocyte 棘细胞；**squamous c.**, a flat, scalelike type of epithelial cell 鳞状细胞，扁平的鳞状上皮细胞；**stab c.**, **staff c.**, band c. 杆状细胞；**stellate c.**, any star-shaped cell, such as a Kupffer cell or astrocyte, having many filaments extending in all directions 星形细胞，如库普弗细胞或星形细胞，有许多细丝向各个方向延伸；**stem c's**, undifferentiated cells with the ability to divide and proliferate to provide precursor cells that can differentiate into specialized cells 干细胞，具有分裂和增殖能力的未分化细胞，可分化成特异性细胞的前体细胞；**stippled c.**, an erythrocyte whose granules take a basic or bluish stain with Wright stain 点彩细胞，瑞特染色红细胞颗粒呈碱性或蓝色，见 basophilia；**suppressor c's**, lymphoid cells, especially T lymphocytes, that inhibit humoral and cell-mediated immune responses. They play an integral role in mmunoregulation, and are believed to be operative in various autoimmune and other immunologic disease states 抑制细胞，尤其是 T 淋巴细胞，抑制体液和细胞介导的免疫反应。它们在免疫接种中起着不可分割的作用，在各种自身免疫和其他免疫疾病中起作用；**synovial c's**, fibroblasts found between the cartilaginous fibers in the synovial membrane of a joint 滑膜细胞，在关节滑膜软骨纤维之间的成纤维细胞；**T c.**, T lymphocyte T 细胞，T 淋巴细胞；**target c.**, 1. an abnormally thin erythrocyte that when stained shows a dark center surrounded by a pale unstained ring and a peripheral ring of hemoglobin 靶细胞，异常稀疏的红细胞，染色时中心暗，周围有苍白的未着色环和血红蛋白外周环；2. any cell selectively affected by a particular agent, such as a hormone or drug 靶细胞，任何受特定因子选择性影响的细胞，如激素或药物；**taste c's**, cells in the taste buds that have gustatory receptors 味觉细胞，味蕾中有味觉感受器的细胞；**tendon c's**, flattened cells of connective tissue occurring in rows between the pri-

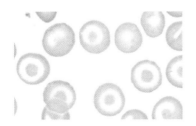

▲ 靶细胞（starget cell）

C

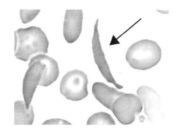

▲ 镰状细胞（sickle cell）（箭）

mary bundles of the tendons 肌腱细胞，扁平的结缔组织细胞，出现在肌腱原始束之间；**theca c's, theca-lutein c's,** lutein cells derived from the theca interna of the graafian follicle 膜细胞，膜黄体细胞，来源于成熟卵泡膜间隙的黄体细胞；**totipotential c.,** an embryonic cell that is capable of developing into any type of body cell 全能细胞，能够发育成任何类型细胞的胚胎细胞；**transitional c's,** 1. cells in the process of changing from one type to another 从一种类型转化为另一种类型的细胞；2. in the sinoatrial and atrioventricular nodes, small, slow-conducting, heterogeneous cells interposed between the P cells and Purkinje cells 移行细胞，在窦房结和房室结中，位于 P 细胞与浦肯野细胞之间小的、传导缓慢的异质性细胞；**tubal air c's,** air cells on the floor of the eustachian tube close to the carotid canal 咽鼓管含气小房，位于咽鼓管底部靠近颈动脉管的含气腔；**tympanic c's, tympanic air c's,** spaces in the tympanic cavity between the bony projections of the floor or jugular wall; they sometimes communicate with the tubal air cells 鼓室小房，鼓室底部或颈静脉壁的骨状突起之间的空间；它们有时与咽鼓管含气小房相通；**visual c's,** the neuroepithelial elements of the retina 视觉细胞，视网膜的神经上皮成分；**white c., white blood c.,** leukocyte 白细胞

cel·loi·din (sə-loi′din) a concentrated preparation of pyroxylin, used in microscopy for embedding specimens for section cutting 火棉胶，聚焦木素的浓缩制剂，用于显微镜下嵌入切片标本

cel·lu·lar (sel′u-lər) pertaining to or composed of cells 细胞的

cel·lu·lar·i·ty (sel″u-lar′ ĭ-te) the state of a tissue or other mass as regards the number of constituent cells 细胞性，由细胞数量决定的组织或其他物质状态

cel·lu·lif·u·gal (sel″u-lif′ə-gəl) directed away from a cell body 离细胞性，背离细胞

cel·lu·lip·e·tal (cel″u-lip′ə-təl) directed toward a cell body 向细胞性，向着细胞

cel·lu·li·tis (sel″u-li′tis) inflammation of the soft or connective tissue, in which a thin, watery exudate spreads through the cleavage planes of interstitial and tissue spaces; it may lead to ulceration and abscess 蜂窝织炎，软组织或结缔组织的炎症，其稀薄而湿润的渗出物通过间质和组织间扩散，导致溃疡和脓肿；**anaerobic c.,** that due to a necrotizing infection with anaerobic bacteria, including *Clostridium perfringens* and others, in a contaminated wound or otherwise compromised tissue 厌氧性蜂窝织炎，受污染伤口或其他受损组织中的厌氧细菌（包括产气荚膜梭菌和其他细菌）引起的坏死性感染；**gangrenous c.,** that leading to death of the tissue followed by bacterial invasion and putrefaction 坏疽性蜂窝织炎，随着细菌入侵和腐败，而出现组织坏死；**pelvic c.,** parametritis 盆腔蜂窝织炎子宫旁（组织）炎

Cel·lu·lo·mo·na·da·ceae (sel″u-lo-mo″nə-da′se-e) a family of bacteria of the suborder Micrococcineae, order Actinomycetales, consisting of gram-positive, branching rods 微杆菌亚目，革兰阳性分枝杆菌组成的微球菌亚目放线菌属细菌

cel·lu·lose (sel′u-lōs) a rigid, colorless, unbranched, insoluble, long-chain polysaccharide, consisting of 3000 to 5000 glucose residues and forming the structure of most plant structures and of plant cells 纤维素，一种坚硬、无色、无分枝、不溶性长链多糖，由 3000 到 5000 个葡萄糖残基组成，形成大多数植物结构和植物细胞的结构；**absorbable c.,** oxidized c. 可吸收纤维素；**c. acetate,** an acetylated cellulose used in membrane filters 纤维素乙酸酯，用于膜过滤器的乙酰化纤维素；**oxidized c.,** an absorbable oxidation product of cellulose, used as a local hemostatic 氧化纤维素，纤维素的可氧化吸收产物，用作局部止血剂；**c. sodium phosphate,** an insoluble, nonabsorbable cation exchange resin prepared from cellulose; it binds calcium and is used to prevent formation of calcium-containing renal calculi 纤维素磷酸钠，由纤维素制备的不溶性、不可吸收的阳离子交换树脂，能结合钙，用于防止含钙肾结石的形成

ce·lom (se′ləm) coelom 体腔

ce·los·chi·sis (se-los′kĭ-sis) abdominal fissure 腹裂

ce·lo·so·mia (se″lo-so′me-ə) congenital fissure or absence of the sternum, with hernial protrusion of the viscera 露脏畸形，先天性胸骨裂或缺失，内脏突出

ce·ment (sə-ment′) 1. a substance that produces a solid union between two surfaces 黏固剂，两个表面之间产生固体结合的物质；2. dental c.; 3. cementum 牙骨质；**cemen′tal** *adj.*; **dental c.,** any of various bonding substances that are placed in the mouth as a viscous liquid and set to a hard mass; used in restorative and orthodontic dental procedures as luting (cementing) agents, as protective, insulating, or sedative bases, and as restorative materials 牙科水门汀，黏性液体放入口中并固定成硬块的黏接剂；用于牙科修复和正畸手术中的黏合剂，保护、隔热或止痛的修复性材料

ce·men·ti·cle (sə-men′tĭ-kəl) a small, discrete globular mass of cementum in the region of a tooth root 牙骨质小体，牙根区牙骨质小的、不连续的球状团块

ce·men·ti·fi·ca·tion (sə-men″tĭ-fĭ-ka′shən) cementogenesis 牙骨质形成

ce·men·to·blast (sə-men′to-blast) a large cuboidal cell, found between the fibers on the surface of the cementum, which is active in cementum formation 成牙骨质细胞，在牙骨质表面纤维之间的大立方形细胞，在牙骨质形成中起作用

ce·men·to·blas·to·ma (sə-men″to-blas-to′mə) a rare, benign odontogenic tumor arising from the cementum and presenting as a proliferating mass contiguous with a tooth root 成牙骨质细胞瘤，起源于牙骨质的罕见良性牙源性肿瘤，与牙根相邻的增生肿块

ce·men·to·cyte (sə-men′to-sīt) a cell in the lacunae of cellular cementum, frequently having long processes radiating from the cell body toward the periodontal surface of the cement 牙骨质细胞，牙骨质间隙中的细胞，通常从细胞体向牙骨质牙周表面辐射性生长

ce·men·to·enam·el (sə-men″to-ə-nam′əl) pertaining to the cementum and the dental enamel 牙骨质釉质的，牙骨质和牙釉质

ce·men·to·gen·e·sis (sə-men″to-jen′ə-sis) development of cementum on the root dentin of a tooth 牙骨质形成

ce·men·to·ma (se″mən-to′mə) any of a variety of benign cement-producing tumors, including cementoblastoma, cementifying fibroma, florid osseous dysplasia, and periapical cemental dysplasia, particularly the last 牙骨质瘤，良性牙骨质瘤，包括成骨细胞瘤、牙骨质纤维瘤、繁茂性牙骨质结构不良和根尖周牙骨质结构不良，尤其是最后一种；**gigantiform c.,** florid osseous dysplasia 巨大牙骨质瘤，繁茂性牙骨质结构不良

ce·men·tum (sə-men′təm) the bonelike connective tissue covering the root of a tooth and assisting in tooth support 牙骨质，覆盖牙齿根部并协助牙齿支撑的骨状结缔组织，又称 *cement*

ce·nes·the·sia (se″nes-the′zhə) somatognosis. **cenesthe′sic, cenesthe′tic** *adj.*

ce·no·site (se′no-sīt) coinosite 半自由寄生物

cen·te·nar·ian (sen-ten″ə-rēən) a person who lives to be at least 100 years of age 百岁老人

cen·ter (sen′tər) 1. the middle point of a body 身

体的中点；2. a collection of neurons in the central nervous system that are concerned with performance of a particular function 中枢神经系统中与特定功能表现有关的神经元集合；**accelerating c.,** the part of the vasomotor center involved in acceleration of the heart 加速中枢，参与心动过速的血管运动中枢；**apneustic c.,** the neurons in the brainstem controlling normal respiration 长吸中枢，控制正常呼吸的脑干神经元；**Broca c.,** Broca motor speech area 布罗卡中枢；**cardioinhibitory c.,** the part of the vasomotor center that exerts an inhibitory influence on the heart 心脏抑制中枢，血管运动中枢对心脏产生抑制作用的部分；**c's of chondrification,** dense aggregations of embryonic mesenchymal cells at sites of future cartilage formation 软骨化中心，胚胎间充质细胞在未来软骨形成部位的聚集；**ciliospinal c.,** one in the lower cervical and upper thoracic portions of the spinal cord, involved in dilatation of the pupil 睫脊中枢，位于脊髓的下颈部和上胸部，参与瞳孔的扩张；**community mental health c. (CMHC),** a mental health facility or group of affiliated agencies that provide various psychotherapeutic services to a designated geographic area 社区心理卫生中心（CMHC），心理健康机构及其附属机构，为指定的区域提供各种心理治疗服务；**coughing c.,** one in the medulla oblongata above the respiratory center, which controls the act of coughing 咳嗽中枢，位于呼吸中枢上方的延髓，控制咳嗽行为；**deglutition c.,** a nerve center in the medulla oblongata that controls the function of swallowing 吞咽中枢，延髓中控制吞咽功能的神经中枢；**C's for Disease Control and Prevention (CDC),** an agency of the U.S. Department of Health and Human Services, serving as a center for the control, prevention, and investigation of diseases 疾病防治中心（CDC），美国卫生和公众服务机构，是疾病控制、预防和调查的中心；**ejaculation c.,** the reflex center in the lumbar spinal cord that regulates ejaculation of semen during sexual stimulation 射精中枢，在性刺激过程中调节精液射精的腰脊髓反射中枢；**epiotic c.,** the center of ossification that forms the mastoid process 乳突骨化中心；**erection c.,** a reflex center in the sacral spinal cord that regulates erection of the penis or clitoris 勃起中枢，骶脊髓中调节阴茎或阴蒂勃起的反射中枢；**feeding c.,** a center formed by a group of cells in the lateral hypothalamus; when stimulated, it causes a sensation of hunger 摄食中枢，下丘脑外侧的一组细胞形成的中枢；当受到刺激时，会引起饥饿感；**germinal c.,** the spherical area in the center of a lymphoid nodule that has been exposed to antigen, containing aggregations of actively proliferating B lymphocytes 生发中心，淋巴结中心暴露于抗原的球形区域，活跃增殖的 B 淋巴细胞聚集；**health c.,** 健康中心 1. a community health organization for creating health work and coordinating the efforts of all health agencies 创建卫生工作并协调所有卫生机构工作的社区卫生组织；2. an educational complex consisting of a medical school and various allied health professional schools 由一所医学院和多所联合的健康专业学校组成的教育机构；**medullary respiratory c.,** the part of the respiratory centers that is in the medulla oblongata 延髓呼吸中枢，呼吸中枢位于延髓的部分；**micturition c's,** centers in the pons and sacral spinal cord that control bladder and urethral function in micturition 排尿中枢，位于脑桥和骶脊髓，控制排尿时膀胱和尿道的功能；**nerve c.,** center (2)；**ossification c.,** any point at which the process of ossification begins in a bone; in a long bone there is a *primary center* for the diaphysis and one *secondary center* for each epiphysis 骨化中心；在长骨中，骨干有一主骨化中心，每个骨骺有一个次级骨化中心；**pneumotaxic c.,** one in the upper pons that rhythmically inhibits inspiration 呼吸调整中枢，位于脑桥上部，有节奏地抑制呼吸；**reflex c.,** any center in the brain or spinal cord in which a sensory impression is changed into a motor impulse 反射中枢，大脑或脊髓中的中枢，在中枢中感觉被转变为运动冲动；**respiratory c's,** a series of centers (apneustic and pneumotaxic respiratory centers and dorsal and ventral respiratory groups) in the medulla and pons that coordinate respiratory movements 呼吸中枢，延髓和脑桥内协调呼吸运动的一系列中枢（长吸中枢和呼吸暂停中枢以及背侧和腹侧呼吸群）；**satiety c.,** a group of cells in the ventromedial hypothalamus that when stimulated suppress a desire for food 饱食中枢，下丘脑腹内侧的一组细胞，当受到刺激时抑制对食物的欲望；**sudorific c.,** sweat cell 发汗中枢；**swallowing c.,** deglutition c.；**sweat c.,** 发汗中枢 1. a center in the anterior hypothalamus controlling diaphoresis 下丘脑前部控制发汗的中枢；2. any of several centers in the medulla oblongata or spinal cord that exercise parasympathetic control over diaphoresis 延髓或脊髓中的任何一个对发汗进行副交感神经控制的中枢；**thermoregulatory c's,** hypothalamic centers regulating the conservation and dissipation of heat 体温调节中枢，下丘脑中枢调节保温和散热；**thirst c.,** a group of cells in the lateral hypothalamus that when stimulated cause a sensation of thirst 渴觉中枢，位于下丘脑外侧的一组细胞，当受到刺激时会引起口渴感；**vasomotor c's,** centers in the medulla oblongata and lower pons that regulate the caliber of blood vessels and the heart rate and contractility 血管运动中枢，位于延髓和下脑桥的中枢，调节血管的直径、心率和收缩力

cen·tes·i·mal (sen-tes′ĭ-məl) divided into hundredths 百分之一的

cen·te·sis (sen-te′sis) [Gr.] perforation or tapping, as with a trocar or needle 穿刺术，如用套管针或针

cen·ti·grade (sen′tĭ-grād) having 100 gradations (steps or degrees) 百分度，见 scale 下词条

cen·ti·gray (cGy) (sen′tĭ-gra″) a unit of absorbed radiation dose equal to one-hundredth (10^{-2}) of a gray, or 1 rad 厘戈瑞（cGy），吸收剂量单位，等于百分之一（10^{-2}）戈瑞或 1 拉德

cen·ti·me·ter (cm) (sen′tĭ-me″tər) one-hundredth (10^{-2}) of a meter 厘米（cm）；**cubic c. (cm³, cc),** a unit of capacity, being that of a cube each side of which measures 1 cm; equal to 1 mL 立方厘米（cm³, ml），容量单位

cen·trad (sen′trad) toward a center 向心，朝向中心

cen·tral (sen′trəl) situated at or pertaining to a center; not peripheral 中心

cen·tren·ce·phal·ic (sen″trən-sə-fal′ik) pertaining to the center of the encephalon 中脑

cen·tri·ac·i·nar (sen″trī-as′ĭ-nər) pertaining to the central portion of one or more acini 一个或多个腺泡的中心部分

cen·tric (sen′trik) 1. central 中央；2. having a center 有中心的

cen·tric·i·put (sən-tris′ĭ-pət) the central part of the upper surface of the head, located between the occiput and sinciput 头中部

cen·trif·u·gal (sen-trif′ə-gəl) efferent (1) 离心的

cen·trif·u·gate (sən-trif′u-gāt) material subjected to centrifugation 离心液

cen·trif·u·ga·tion (sen-trif″u-ga′shən) the process of separating lighter portions of a solution, mixture, or suspension from the heavier portions by centrifugal force 离心，用离心力将溶液、混合物或悬浮液的较轻部分与较重部分分离的过程

cen·tri·fuge (sen′trĭ-fūj) 1. a machine by which centrifugation is effected 离心机；2. to subject to centrifugation 离心分离

cen·tri·lob·u·lar (sen″trī-lob′u-lər) pertaining to the central portion of a lobule 小叶中心的

cen·tri·ole (sen′tre-ōl) either of the two cylindrical organelles located in the centrosome; during cell division they are duplicated and migrate to opposite poles of the cell, where they organize the spindles. They are capable of independent replication and of migrating to form basal bodies 中心粒，中心体中两个圆柱形细胞器的任意一个；在细胞分裂过程中，它们被复制并迁移到细胞的两极，组织形成

纺锤；其能独立复制和迁移形成基粒

cen·trip·e·tal (sən-trip′ə-təl) 1. afferent (1) 向 心 的；2. corticipetal 向皮质的

cen·tro·blast (sen′tro-blast″) a general term encompassing both large and small noncleaved follicular center cells 生发中心母细胞，大小无裂滤泡中心细胞的总称

cen·tro·ce·cal (sen″tro-se′kəl) pertaining to the central macular area and the blind spot 中心盲点的

cen·tro·cyte (sen′tro-sīt″) a general term encompassing both large and small cleaved follicular center cells 中心细胞，大小有裂滤泡中心细胞的总称；**centrocyt′ic** *adj.*

cen·tro·mere (sen′tro-mēr) the region of the chromosome at which the chromatids are joined and by which the chromosome is attached to the spindle during cell division 着丝粒，染色单体结合及细胞分裂时纺锤体附着的区域；**centromer′ic** *adj.*

cen·tro·nu·cle·ar (sen″tro-noo′kle-ər) having or pertaining to a centrally located nucleus 中央核

cen·tro·scle·ro·sis (sen″tro-sklə-ro′sis) osteosclerosis of the medullary cavity of a bone 骨髓腔骨化

cen·tro·some (sen′tro-sōm) an organelle, located near the nucleus of animal cells, that contains the centrioles and directs the assembly of the spindle in mitosis 中心体，动物细胞核附近的细胞器，包含中心粒并在有丝分裂中引导纺锤体的形成

cen·trum (sen′trəm) pl. **cen′tra** [L.] 1. a center 中心；2. the body of a vertebra 椎体

CEP congenital erythropoietic porphyria 先天性红细胞生成性卟啉病

ceph·a·lad (sef′ə-lad) toward the head 向头部地，朝向头部

ceph·a·lal·gia (sef″ə-lal′jə) [Gr.] headache 头痛；**trigeminal autonomic c.**, any of a group of primary headaches characterized by unilateral head pain accompanied by ipsilateral autonomic manifestations such as conjunctival injection, lacrimation, and Horner syndrome. It includes cluster headache 三叉神经自主神经性头痛，一种原发性头痛，以单侧头痛为特征，伴有同侧自主神经症状，如结膜充血、流泪和霍纳综合征；包括丛集性头痛

ceph·al·ede·ma (sef″əl-ə-de′mə) edema of the head 脑水肿

ceph·a·lex·in (sef″ə-lek′sin) a semisynthetic first-generation cephalosporin, effective against a wide range of gram-positive and a limited range of gram-negative bacteria; used as the base or the hydrochloride salt 头孢氨苄，半合成第一代头孢菌素，对多种革兰阳性和少量革兰阴性细菌有效；用作碱或盐酸盐

ceph·al·he·mat·o·cele (sef″əl-he-mat′o-sēl) a hematocele under the pericranium, communicating with one or more dural sinuses 头血囊肿颅骨外膜下的血肿，与一个或多个硬脑膜窦相通

ceph·al·he·ma·to·ma (sef″əl-he″mə-to′mə) a subperiosteal hemorrhage limited to the surface of one cranial bone; a usually benign condition seen in the newborn as a result of bone trauma 头颅血肿，局限于头骨表面的骨膜下出血；一种常见于新生儿的良性疾病，由骨外伤引起

ceph·al·hy·dro·cele (sef″əl-hi′dro-sēl) a serous or watery accumulation under the pericranium 脑积水

ce·phal·ic (sə-fal′ik) pertaining to the head, or to the head end of the body 头部的

ceph·a·lo·cele (sef′ə-lo-sēl″) encephalocele. 脑膨出

ceph·a·lo·cen·te·sis (sef″ə-lo-sen-te′sis) surgical puncture of the skull 头颅穿刺术

ceph·a·lo·dac·ty·ly (sef″ə-lo-dak′tə-le) malformation of the head and digits 头指（趾）畸形，头部和手指的畸形

ceph·a·lo·gram (sef′ə-lo-gram) an x-ray image of the structures of the head; cephalometric radiograph 测颅 X 射线片

ceph·a·log·ra·phy (sef″ə-log′rə-fe) radiography of the head 头部射线照相

ceph·a·lo·gy·ric (sef″ə-lo-ji′rik) pertaining to turning motions of the head 头部转动

ceph·a·lom·e·ter (sef″ə-lom′ə-tər) an instrument for measuring the head; an orienting device for positioning the head for radiographic examination and measurement 头颅定位仪，测量头部的仪器；用于定位头部以进行射线照相检查和测量的定向装置

ceph·a·lom·e·try (sef″ə-lom′ə-tre) scientific measurement of the dimensions of the head 头影测量学

ceph·a·lo·mo·tor (sef″ə-lo-mo′tər) moving the head; pertaining to motions of the head 头颅运动

ceph·a·lo·nia (sef″ə-lo′ne-ə) a condition in which the head is abnormally enlarged, with sclerotic hyperplasia of the brain 巨头症，头部异常增大，伴有大脑硬化性增生

ceph·a·lop·a·thy (sef″ə-lop′ə-the) any disease of the head 头部病

ceph·a·lo·pel·vic (sef″ə-lo-pel′vik) pertaining to the relationship of the fetal head to the maternal pelvis 胎头骨盆的，胎头与母体骨盆的位置关系

ceph·a·lo·spo·rin (sef″ə-lo-spor′in) any of a group of broad-spectrum, penicillinase-resistant antibiotics from *Acremonium*, related to the penicillins in both structure and mode of action. Those used medicinally are semisynthetic derivatives of the natural antibiotic cephalosporin C. First-generation cephalosporins have a broad range of activity against gram-positive organisms and a narrow

C

range of activity against gram-negative organisms; second-, third-, and fourth-generation agents are progressively more active against gram-negative organisms and less active against gram-positive organisms 头孢菌素，抗青霉素酶的广谱抗生素，从顶孢霉中提取，在结构和作用方式上与青霉素相似；医学上使用的是天然抗生素头孢菌素 C 的半合成衍生物；第一代头孢菌素对革兰阳性微生物有广泛的杀菌活性，对革兰阴性微生物的杀菌范围很窄；第二代、第三代和第四代药剂对革兰阴性微生物的杀菌性逐渐增强，而对革兰阳性微生物则逐渐减弱

ceph·a·lo·spo·rin·ase (sef″ə-lo-spor′in-ās) a β-lactamase preferentially acting on cephalosporins 头孢菌素酶，优先作用于头孢菌素类的β-内酰胺酶

Ceph·a·lo·spo·ri·um (sef″ə-lo-spor′e-əm) former name for *Acremonium* 头孢菌属，支顶孢属的曾用名

ceph·a·lo·stat (sef′ə-lo-stat″) a head-positioning device that ensures reproducibility of the relations between an x-ray beam, a patient's head, and an x-ray film 头颅固定架，头部定位装置，确保 X 射线束、患者头部和 X 射线胶片之间关系的一致性

ceph·a·lot·o·my (sef″ə-lot′ə-me) 1. the cutting up of the fetal head to facilitate delivery 胎头切开术，切开胎儿头部以便于分娩；2. dissection of the fetal head 胎头解剖

ceph·a·my·cin (sef″ə-mi′sin) any of a family of natural and semisynthetic, β-lactamase–resistant antibiotics derived from various species of *Streptomyces*, generally classed as second-generation cephalosporins but more active against anaerobes 头霉素，天然及半合成β-内酰胺酶抗生素，由链霉菌属的不同种类衍生而来，通常被归类为第二代头孢菌素类，对厌氧菌更为有效

ceph·a·pi·rin (sef-ə-pi′rin) a semisynthetic analogue of the natural antibiotic cephalosporin C, effective against a wide range of gram-negative and gram-positive bacteria; used as the sodium salt 头孢匹林，天然抗生素，头孢菌素 C 的半合成类似物，对多种革兰阴性和革兰阳性细菌有效；用作钠盐

ceph·ra·dine (sef′rə-dēn) a semisynthetic first-generation cephalosporin, effective against a wide range of gram-positive bacteria and a limited range of gram-negative bacteria 头孢拉定，半合成第一代头孢菌素，对多种革兰阳性菌和少量的革兰阴性菌有效

cer·am·i·dase (sə-ram′ ĭ-dās) an enzyme occurring in most mammalian tissue that catalyzes the reversible acylation-deacylation of ceramides 神经酰胺酶，存在于大多数哺乳动物组织中的酶，对神经酰胺的可逆酰化 - 脱酰化作用进行催化

cer·a·mide (ser′ə-mīd) the basic unit of the sphingolipids; it is sphingosine, or a related base, attached to a long chain fatty acyl group. Ceramides are accumulated abnormally in Farber disease 神经酰胺 鞘脂的基本单位；由鞘氨醇或相关的碱与长链脂肪酰基相连；神经酰胺在法布里病中异常积累；

c. trihexoside, any of a specific family of glyco-sphingolipids; due to a deficiency of α-galactosidase A, they accumulate in Fabry disease 神经酰胺三己糖苷，特殊的糖脂类家族；由于α- 半乳糖苷酶 A 的缺乏，使其累积在法布里病中

Cer·a·to·phyl·lus (ser″ə-to-fil′əs) a genus of fleas 角叶蚤属

cer·ca·ria (sər-kar′e-ə) pl. *cerca′riae*. The final, free-swimming larval stage of a trematode parasite 尾蚴，吸虫可自由游动的末期幼虫； **cercar′ial** *adj.* **cer·clage** (ser-klahzh′) [Fr.] encircling of a part with a ring or loop, as for correction of an incompetent cervix uteri or fixation of adjacent ends of a fractured bone 环扎术，如用于矫正子宫颈功能不全或固定骨折的邻近端

cer·e·bel·lar (ser″ə-bel′ər) pertaining to the cerebellum 小脑的

cer·e·bel·lif·u·gal (ser″ə-bel-if′ə-gəl) conducting away from the cerebellum 离小脑的，小脑传出的

cer·e·bel·lip·e·tal (ser″ə-bel-ip′ə-təl) conducting toward the cerebellum 向小脑的，传入小脑的

cer·e·bel·lo·spi·nal (ser″ə-bel′o-spi′nəl) proceeding from the cerebellum to the spinal cord 小脑脊髓的

cer·e·bel·lum (ser″ə-bel′əm) the part of the metencephalon situated on the back of the brainstem, to which it is attached by three cerebellar peduncles on each side; it consists of a median lobe (vermis) and two lateral lobes (the hemispheres) 小脑，位于脑干后部的一部分，每侧由三个小脑足连在脑干上；由中叶（蚓部）和两个侧叶（半球）组成

cer·e·bral (sə-re′brəl) (ser′ə-brəl) pertaining to the cerebrum 大脑的

cer·e·bra·tion (ser″ə-bra′shən) functional activity of the brain 大脑，脑的功能活动

cer·e·brif·u·gal (ser″ə-brif′u-gəl) conducting or proceeding away from the cerebrum 离大脑的，大脑传出的

cer·e·brip·e·tal (ser″ə-brip′ə-təl) conducting or proceeding toward the cerebrum 向大脑的，传入大脑的

cer·e·bro·mac·u·lar (ser″ə-bro-mak′u-lər) maculocerebral; pertaining to or affecting the brain and the macula retinae 脑黄斑的，累及或侵犯脑和视网膜的黄斑

cer·e·bro·ma·la·cia (ser″ə-bro-mə-la′shə) abnormal softening of the substance of the cerebrum 脑软化，大脑实质异常软化

cer·e·bro·men·in·gi·tis (ser″ə-bro-men″inji′tis) meningoencephalitis 脑膜脑炎

cer·e·bron·ic ac·id (ser″ə-bron′ik) a fatty acid found in cerebrosides such as phrenosine 脑羟脂酸，存在于脑中的脂肪酸，如羟脑苷脂

cer·e·bro·path·ia (ser″ə-bro-path′e-ə) [L.] cerebropathy 脑病；**c. psy′chica toxe′mica,** Korsakoff psychosis 精神病

cer·e·brop·a·thy (ser″ə-brop′ə-the) any disorder of the cerebrum 脑病，大脑的任何疾病；另见 *encephalopathy*。又称 *cerebrosis*

cer·e·bro·phys·i·ol·o·gy (ser″ə-bro-fiz″e-ol′ə-je) the physiology of the cerebrum 脑生理学

cer·e·bro·pon·tile (ser″ə-bro-pon′tīl) pertaining to the cerebrum and pons 脑桥

cer·e·bro·side (sə-re′bro-sīd) a general designation for sphingolipids in which sphingosine is combined with galactose or glucose; found chiefly in nervous tissue 脑苷脂，神经鞘脂的总称，其中鞘脂与半乳糖或葡萄糖结合；主要存在于神经组织中

cer·e·bro·spi·nal (ser″ə-bro-spi′nəl) pertaining to the brain and spinal cord 脑脊髓的

cer·e·bro·spi·nant (ser″ə-bro-spi′nənt) an agent that affects the brain and spinal cord 影响大脑和脊髓的药物

cer·e·brot·o·my (ser″ə-brot′ə-me) encephalotomy 脑切除术

cer·e·brum (sə-re′brəm) (ser″ə-brəm) the main portion of the brain, occupying the upper part of the cranial cavity; its two hemispheres, united by the corpus callosum, form the largest part of the central nervous system in humans. The term is sometimes applied to the postembryonic forebrain and midbrain together or to the entire brain 大脑的主要部分，位于颅腔的上部，两半球，由胼胝体连接，构成人类中枢神经系统的最大部分。这个术语有时用于胚胎后的前脑和中脑，或者用于整个大脑

ce·ri·um (Ce) (sēr′e-əm) a soft, silvery, ductile, rare earth element; at. no. 58, at. wt. 140.116 铈，一种软的、银色的、可延展的稀土元素；原子序数 58，原子质量 140.116

ce·ru·lo·plas·min (sə-roo″lo-plaz′min) an α₂-globulin of plasma that functions in copper transport and its maintenance at appropriate levels in tissue; absent in Wilson disease 铜蓝蛋白，血浆中的 α_2 球蛋白，在组织中起铜转运和维持铜正常水平的作用；在威尔逊氏症中缺失

ce·ru·men (sə-roo′mən) earwax; the waxlike substance found within the external meatus of the ear 耵聍，耳垢；在外耳道内发现的蜡状物质；**ceru′minal, ceru′minous** *adj.*

ce·ru·min·ol·y·sis (sə-roo″mĭ-nol′ə-sis) dissolution or disintegration of cerumen in the external auditory meatus 耵聍溶解；**ceruminolyt′ic** *adj.*

cer·vi·cal (sur′vĭ-kəl) 1. pertaining to the neck 颈部；2. pertaining to the neck or cervix of any organ or structure 任何器官或结构的颈部

cer·vi·cec·to·my (sur″vĭ-sek′tə-me) excision of the cervix uteri 宫颈切除术

cer·vi·ci·tis (sur″vĭ-si′tis) inflammation of the cervix uteri 宫颈炎

cer·vi·co·bra·chi·al·gia (sur″vĭ-ko-bra″keal′jə) pain in the neck radiating to the arm, due to compression of nerve roots of the cervical spinal cord 颈肩痛，由于颈脊髓神经根压迫而放射到手臂的疼痛

cer·vi·co·col·pi·tis (sur″vĭ-ko-kol-pi′tis) inflammation of the cervix uteri and vagina 子宫颈阴道炎

cer·vi·co·med·ul·lary (sur″vĭ-ko-med′ə-lar″e) pertaining to or connecting the cervical spinal cord and the medulla oblongata 颈脊髓延髓的

cer·vi·co·tho·rac·ic (sur″vĭ-ko-thə-ras′ik) pertaining to the neck and thorax 颈胸的

cer·vi·co·uter·ine (sur″vĭ-ko-u′tər-in) of or pertaining to the uterine cervix 子宫颈

cer·vi·co·ves·i·cal (sur″vĭ-ko-ves′ ĭ-kəl) vesicocervical 子宫颈膀胱的

cer·vix (sur′viks) pl. *cer′vices* [L.] 1. neck 脖子；2. the front portion of the neck 颈部的前部；3. cervix uteri 子宫颈；**incompetent c.,** a uterine cervix that is abnormally prone to dilate in the second trimester of pregnancy, resulting in premature expulsion of the fetus 子宫颈内口松弛症，子宫颈在妊娠中期异常扩张，导致胎儿过早娩出；**c. u′teri, uterine c.,** the narrow lower end of the uterus, between the isthmus and the opening of the uterus into the vagina 子宫颈，子宫下端狭窄部位，在峡部和子宫开口之间进入阴道；**c. vesi′cae urina′riae,** the lower, constricted part of the urinary bladder, proximal to the opening of the urethra 膀胱颈，膀胱下部狭窄的部分，靠近尿道开口

ce·sar·e·an (sə-zar′e-ən) 剖腹产，见 *section* 下词条

CESD cholesteryl ester storage disease 胆固醇酯贮积病

ce·si·um (Cs) (se′ze-əm) a rare, soft, silverygold alkali metal element; at. no. 55, at. wt. 132.905 铯（Cs），稀有、柔软、银色的碱性金属元素；原子序数 55，原子质量 132.905

ces·ti·ci·dal (ses″tĭ-si′dəl) destructive to cestodes (tapeworms) 杀绦虫的

Ces·to·da (səs-to′də) a subclass of Cestoidea

comprising the true tapeworms, which have a head (scolex) and segments (proglottides). The adults are endoparasitic in the alimentary tract and associated ducts of various vertebrate hosts; their larvae may be found in various organs and tissues 真绦虫亚纲，由真绦虫组成的绦虫亚纲，有头（头节）和节（前驱体），成虫在各种脊椎动物宿主的消化道和相关管道内寄生；其幼虫可存活于各种器官和组织中

Ces·to·da·ria (ses″to-dar′e-ə) a subclass of tapeworms, the unsegmented tapeworms of the class Cestoidea, which are endoparasitic in the intestines and coelom of various primitive fishes and rarely in reptiles 单节绦虫亚纲，绦虫纲中的一个亚纲，属于绦虫纲的未分类绦虫，在各种原始鱼类的睾丸和体腔内寄生，很少在爬行动物中寄生

ces·tode (ses′tōd) 1. tapeworm 绦虫；2. resembling a tapeworm 绦虫状的。又称 *cestoid*

Ces·toi·dea (ses-toi′de-ə) a class of tapeworms (phylum Platyhelminthes), characterized by the absence of a mouth or digestive tract, and by a noncuticular layer covering their bodies 绦虫纲（扁形动物门），特征是没有嘴或消化道，表皮覆盖着一层非角质膜

cet·al·ko·ni·um chlo·ride (set″al-ko′ne-əm) a cationic quaternary ammonium surfactant used as a topical anti-infective and disinfectant 西他氯铵，阳离子季铵表面活性剂，用作局部抗感染和消毒剂

ce·ti·ri·zine (sə-tir′ ĭ-zēn) a nonsedating antihistamine used as the hydrochloride salt in the treatment of allergic rhinitis, chronic idiopathic urticaria, and asthma 西替利嗪，非镇静抗组胺药，用作治疗变应性鼻炎、慢性特发性荨麻疹和哮喘的盐酸盐

cet·ro·rel·ix (set″ro-rel′iks) a gonadotropinreleasing hormone antagonist, used as the acetate salt to inhibit premature surges of luteinizing hormone in women undergoing controlled ovarian stimulation during infertility treatment 西曲瑞克，促性腺激素拮抗剂，用作醋酸盐，不孕症妇女接受控制性卵巢刺激治疗期间抑制黄体生成素的过早释放

ce·tux·i·mab (sə-tuk′sĭ-mab) a monoclonal antibody that binds to the epidermal growth factor (EGF) receptor and inhibits the growth and survival of cells that overexpress the EGF receptor; used in the treatment of metastatic colorectal carcinoma 西妥昔单抗，能结合表皮生长因子（EGF）受体并抑制过度表达 EGF 受体的细胞生长和存活的单克隆抗体；用于治疗转移性大肠癌

ce·tyl·pyr·i·din·i·um chlo·ride (se″təl-pir″ĭ-din′e-əm) a cationic disinfectant; used as a local antiinfective administered sublingually or applied topically to intact skin and mucous membranes, and as a preservative in pharmaceutical preparations 西吡氯铵（氯化十六烷基吡啶），阳离子消毒剂；作为局部抗感染剂，舌下给药或局部应用于完整的皮肤和黏膜，并作为药物制剂中的防腐剂

cev·i·mel·ine (sə-vim′ə-lēn) a cholinergic agonist used as the hydrochloride salt in the treatment of xerostomia associated with Sjögren syndrome 西维美林，胆碱能激动药，用作盐酸盐，治疗与干燥综合征相关的口腔干燥

CF carbolfuchsin 卡硫菌素；cardiac failure 心力衰竭（见 *failure* 下的 *heart failure*）；Christmas factor. 血友病因子

Cf californium 锎

CFT complement fixation test; 补体结合试验；见 *fixation* 下词条

CFTR cystic fibrosis transmembrane regulator 囊性纤维化穿膜传导调节蛋白

CGNA Canadian Gerontological Nursing Association 加拿大老年护理协会

CGS centimeter-gram-second system 厘 - 克 - 秒制

cGy centigray 厘戈瑞

CH50 见 *assay* 和 *unit* 下词条

CHA Canadian Healthcare Association 加拿大医疗协会

chafe (chāf) to irritate the skin, as by rubbing together of opposing skin folds 刺激皮肤，如相对的皮肤褶襞共同摩擦

cha·gas·ic (chə-gās′ik) pertaining to or due to Chagas disease Chagas 病（美洲锥虫病）的

cha·go·ma (chə-go′mə) a skin tumor occurring in Chagas disease 南美锥虫病的

chain (chān) a collection of objects linked end to end 链；**branched c.**, an open chain of atoms, usually carbon, with one or more side chains attached to it 支链，通常是碳原子的开放链，有一个或多个侧链连接；**electron transport c.**, the final common pathway of biologic oxidation, the series of electron carriers in the inner mitochondrial membrane that pass electrons from reduced coenzymes to molecular oxygen via sequential redox reactions coupled to proton transport, generating energy for biologic processes 电子传递链，生物氧化的最终共同途径，线粒体内膜中的一系列电子载体，通过连续的氧化还原反应将电子从还原的辅酶传递到分子氧，再结合质子传递，为生物过程提供能量；**H c., heavy c.**, any of the large polypeptide chains of five classes that, paired with the light chains, make up the antibody molecule. Heavy chains bear the antigenic determinants that differentiate the immunoglobulin classes H 链、重链，大多肽链中的一种，与轻链配对构成抗体分子；重链具有区分免疫球蛋白种类的抗原决定簇；**J c.**, a polypeptide occurring in polymeric IgM and IgA molecules J 链，

聚合 IgM 和 IgA 分子中的多肽链; **L c., light c.,** either of the two small polypeptide chains (molecular weight 22,000) that, when linked to heavy chains by disulfide bonds, make up the antibody molecule; they are of two types, kappa and lambda, which are unrelated to immunoglobulin class differences L 链, 轻链, 两条小多肽链（分子量 22 000）中的任意一条, 通过二硫键与重链连接, 构成抗体分子; 有两种类型, kappa 和 lambda, 与免疫球蛋白分类无关; **open c.,** a series of atoms united in a straight line; compounds of this series are related to methane 开链化合物, 一系列结合成线性的原子; 这类化合物与甲烷有关; **polypeptide c.,** the structural element of protein, consisting of a series of amino acid residues (peptides) joined together by peptide bonds 多肽链, 蛋白质的结构元素, 由肽键连接在一起的氨基酸残基（肽）组成; **respiratory c.,** electron transport c. 呼吸链, 电子传递链; **side c.,** a group of atoms attached to a larger chain or to a ring 侧链, 一组原子连接到较大的链或环上

chak·ra (chuk′rə) (shah′krə) any of the seven energy centers, located from the perineum to the crown of the head, of yoga philosophy; also used in some energy-based complementary medicine systems 脉轮, 瑜伽哲学中从会阴到头顶的七个能量中心中的任何一个; 也用于一些基于能量的补充医学系统中

cha·la·sia (kə-la′zhə) relaxation of a bodily opening, such as the cardiac sphincter (a cause of vomiting in infants) 松弛, 如贲门括约肌松弛（婴儿呕吐的原因之一）

cha·la·zi·on (kə-la′ze-on) pl. *chala′zia, chalazions* [Gr.] a small eyelid mass due to inflammation of a meibomian gland 麦粒肿, 眼睑腺发炎而形成的小眼睑肿块

chal·co·sis (kal-ko′sis) copper deposits in tissue 铜质沉着症

chal·i·co·sis (kal-ĭ-ko′sis) pneumoconiosis due to inhalation of fine particles of stone 石末沉着病, 吸入石末引起的尘肺

chal·lenge (chal′enj) 激 发 1. to administer a substance to monitor for the normal physiologic response 给药以监测正常生理反应; 2. in immunology, to administer an antigen to monitor the response in a sensitized person 在免疫学中, 给予抗原以监测致敏者的反应

chal·one (kal′ōn) a group of tissue-specific water-soluble substances that are produced within a tissue and that inhibit mitosis of cells of that tissue and the action of which is reversible 抑素, 组织内产生的一组组织特异性水溶性物质, 抑制该组织细胞的有丝分裂, 其作用是可逆的

cham·ae·ceph·a·ly (kam″e-sef′ə-le) the condition of having a low flat head, i.e., a cephalic index of 70 or less 扁头畸形, 头部低平的状态, 即头颅指数为 70 或更低; **chamaecephal′ic** adj.

cham·ber (chām′bər) an enclosed space 室, 封 闭 的 空 间; **anterior c. of eye,** the part of the aqueouscontaining space of the eyeball between the cornea and the iris 眼球前房, 眼角膜与虹膜之间的间隙部分; **aqueous c.,** the part of the eyeball filled with aqueous humor 眼房, 眼球充满房水的部 分; 见 *anterior c.* 和 *posterior c*; **counting c.,** the part of a hemacytometer consisting of a microscopic slide with a depression whose base is marked in grids, and into which a measured volume of a sample of blood or bacterial culture is placed and covered with a cover glass. Cells and formed blood elements in any given square can then be counted under a microscope 计数板, 血细胞计数器, 由一个带有凹陷的载玻片组成, 该载玻片的基部以网格标记, 将测得体积的血液或细菌培养样品放入其中, 并用盖玻片覆盖, 在显微镜下, 对任何一个指定的正方形, 计数细胞和血液成分; **diffusion c.,** an apparatus for separating a substance by means of a semipermeable membrane 扩散室, 通过半透膜分离物质的装置; **hyperbaric c.,** an enclosed space in which gas (oxygen) can be raised to greater than atmospheric pressure 高压舱, 封闭的空间, 其气体（氧气）可以升高到一个大气压以上; **ionization c.,** an enclosure containing two or more electrodes between which an electric current may be passed when the enclosed gas is ionized by radiation; used for determining the intensity of x-rays and other rays 电离室, 含有两个或多个电极外壳, 当封闭的气体被辐射电离时, 电流可在两个或多个电极之间通过; 用于确定 X 射线和其他射线的强度; **posterior c. of eye,** the part of the aqueous-containing space of the eyeball between the iris and the lens 眼后房, 眼球中位于虹膜和晶状体之间的含水空间; **pulp c.,** the natural cavity in the central portion of the tooth crown that is occupied by the dental pulp 牙髓腔, 牙冠中央被牙髓占据的自然腔; **relief c.,** the recess in a denture surface that rests on the oral structures, to reduce or eliminate pressure 减压腔, 口腔义齿表面的凹处, 用于降低或消除压力; **vitreous c.,** the vitreous-containing space in the eyeball, bounded anteriorly by the lens and ciliary body and posteriorly by the posterior wall of the eyeball 玻璃体腔, 眼球内含有玻璃体的空间, 晶状体和纤毛体为前界, 眼球后壁为后界

cham·o·mile (kam′ə-mēl) (-mīl) German chamomile; the dried flower heads of the herb *Matricaria recutita*, used for inflammatory diseases of the

C

gastrointestinal tract and as a topical counterirritant and antiinflammatory 德国洋甘菊；苦参的干燥花头，用于胃肠道炎性疾病以及局部抗刺激和消炎；**English c., Roman c.,** the dried flowers of the perennial herb *Chamaemelum nobile*, used as a homeopathic preparation and in folk medicine as a carminative and counterirritant 英国洋甘菊，罗马洋甘菊，多年生草本果香菊的干花，用作顺势疗法制剂，在民间医学中用作驱虫剂和抗刺激剂

chan·cre (shang′kər) [Fr.] 1. the primary sore of syphilis, occurring at the site of entry of the infection 下疳，梅毒感染部位的原发性疼痛；2. the primary cutaneous lesion of such diseases as sporotrichosis and tuberculosis 孢子菌病、肺结核等疾病的原发性皮肤病变；**hard c., hunterian c.,** chancre (1) 硬下疳；**soft c.,** chancroid 软下疳，Hunter 下疳；**tuberculous c.,** a brownish red papule that develops into an indurated nodule or plaque, representing the initial cutaneous infection of the tubercle bacillus into the skin or mucosa 结核性下疳，棕红色丘疹发展成硬结节或斑块，皮肤或黏膜结核杆菌感染的最初皮肤表现

chan·croid (shang′kroid) a sexually transmitted disease caused by *Haemophilus ducreyi*, characterized by a painful primary ulcer at the site of inoculation, usually on the external genitalia, associated with regional lymphadenitis 软下疳，由杜克雷嗜血杆菌引起的性传播疾病，其特征是在接触部位（通常在外生殖器）出现疼痛性原发性溃疡，与局部淋巴结炎有关；**chancroi′dal** adj. **phageden-lc c.,** chancroid with a tendency to slough 崩蚀性软下疳，有蚀皮倾向的下疳；**serpiginous c.,** a variety tending to spread in curved lines 匍行性软下疳，倾向于伸展成线性溃疡的下疳

change (chānj) an alteration 改变；**fatty c.,** abnormal accumulation of fat within parenchymal cells 脂肪变，实质细胞内脂肪异常积累；**hyaline c.,** a pale, eosinophilic, homogeneous glassy appearance seen in histologic specimens; it is a purely descriptive term and has a variety of causes 玻璃样变，组织标本中出现的苍白、嗜酸性、均匀玻璃状外观；为描述性术语，有多种原因可导致

chan·nel (chan′əl) that through which anything flows; a cut or groove 通 道；**calcium c., calcium-sodium c.,** a voltage-gated channel that is very permeable to calcium ions and slightly permeable to sodium ions 钙通道（钙钠通道），电压门控通道，对钙离子具有很强的通透性，对钠离子具有轻微的通透性；**gated c.,** a protein channel that opens and closes in response to signals, such as binding of a ligand (*ligand-gated c.*) or changes in the electric potential across the cell membrane (*voltage-gated c.*) 门通道，根据信号打开和关闭的蛋白质通道，如配体（配体门控通道）的结合或细胞膜电位的变化（电压门控通道）；**ion c.,** a cell membrane protein with an ion-specific transmembrane pore, through which ions and small molecules pass into or out of a cell by diffusion downward along their electrochemical gradient 离子通道，具有离子特异性跨膜孔的细胞膜蛋白，离子和小分子通过电化学梯度扩散进入或流出细胞，又称 protein c.；**potassium c.,** a voltage-gated protein channel selective for the passage of potassium ions 钾通道，选择钾离子通过的电压门控蛋白通道；**protein c.,** ion c. 蛋白质通道，离子通道；**sodium c.,** a voltage-gated protein channel selective for the passage of sodium ions 钠通道，选择钠离子通过的电压门控蛋白通道；**water c.,** aquaporin 水通道

chap·er·one (shap′ər-ōn) someone or something that accompanies and oversees another 伴 侣；**molecular c.,** any of a diverse group of proteins that oversee the correct intracellular folding and assembly of polypeptides without being components of the final structure 分子伴侣，不作为最终结构的组成部分而是监督多肽正确细胞内折叠和组装的蛋白质

chap·er·o·nin (shap″ər-o′nin) any of various heat shock proteins that act as molecular chaperones in bacteria, plasmids, mitochondria, and eukaryotic cytosol 伴侣蛋白，热休克蛋白，在细菌、质粒、线粒体和真核细胞质中作为分子伴侣

char·ac·ter (kar′ak-tər) 1. a quality indicative of the nature of an object or an organism 特征，指一个物体或有机体性质的品质；2. in genetics, the expression in the phenotype of a gene or group of genes 性状，遗传学中，一个基因或一组基因表型的表达；3. in psychiatry, a term used in much the same way as personality, particularly for those personality traits shaped by life experiences 精神病学中的一个术语，与人格的用法大致相同，特别是对那些由生活经历形成的人格特征；**acquired c.,** a noninheritable modification produced in an animal as a result of its own activities or of environmental influences 获得性状，动物因自身活动或环境影响而产生的不可遗传的改变；**primary sex c's,** those characters in the male or female that are directly involved in reproduction; the gonads and their accessory structures 第一性征，与生殖直接相关的男性或女性的特征；性腺及其附属结构；**secondary sex c's,** those characters specific to the male or female but not directly involved in reproduction 第二性征，特定于男性或女性，但不直接参与生殖的特征，另见 *masculinization* 和 *feminization*

char·ac·ter·is·tic (kar″ak-tər-is′tik) 1. character. 特点；2. typical of an individual or other entity 个

人或其他实体的典型特征；**demand c's,** behavior exhibited by the subject of an experiment in an attempt to accomplish certain goals as a result of cues communicated by the experimenter (expectations or hypothesis) 需求特征，实验对象为了达到某一目标而表现出的行为，由实验者传达的线索（期望或假设）所致

char·coal (chahr'kōl) carbon prepared by charring wood or other organic material 木炭，炭化木材或其他有机材料制备的碳；**activated c.,** residue of destructive distillation of various organic materials, treated to increase its adsorptive power; used as a general-purpose antidote 活性炭，各种有机物破坏性蒸馏残渣，经过处理以增加其吸附能力；为通用解毒剂；**animal c.,** charcoal prepared from bone; it may be purified (*purified animal c.*) by removal of materials dissolved by hot hydrochloric acid and water; adsorbent and decolorizer 骨炭，由骨制备的木炭；通过热盐酸和水溶解、吸附剂和脱色剂来提纯（纯化动物木炭）

char·ley horse (chahr'le hors) soreness and stiffness in a muscle, especially the quadriceps, due to overstrain or contusion 抽筋，肌肉酸痛和僵硬，尤指过度拉伸或挫伤股四头肌

chart (chahrt) a record of data in graphic or tabular form 图表，以图形或表格形式记录的数据；**reading c.,** a chart printed in gradually increasing type sizes, used in testing acuity of near vision 阅读视力表，逐渐增大字体尺寸的图表，用于测试近视力；**Snellen c.,** a chart with block letters in gradually decreasing sizes, used in testing visual acuity 斯内伦视力表，印刷体字母逐渐缩小的图表，用于测试视力

chaste tree (chāst' tre″) the shrub *Vitex agnuscastus* or an extract prepared from its berries and root bark, which is used for the treatment of premenstrual syndrome and menopause; also used in homeopathy 牡荆，灌木黄荆或从其浆果和根皮中的提取物，用于治疗经前综合征和更年期；也用于顺势疗法

CHAT Checklist for Autism in Toddlers 婴幼儿孤独症筛查量表

ChB [L.] Chirur'giae Baccalau'reus (Bachelor of Surgery) 外科学士

CHD coronary heart disease 冠状动脉粥样硬化性心脏

ChE cholinesterase 胆碱酯酶

check-bite (chek'bīt) a sheet of hard wax or modeling compound placed between the teeth, used to check occlusion of the teeth 殆校正，置于牙齿之间的一层硬蜡或模型化合物，用于检查牙齿的咬合情况

cheek (chēk) 1. the fleshy portion of either side of the face, or the fleshy mucous membrane-covered side of the oral cavity 面颊；2. any fleshy protuberance resembling the cheek of the face 颊状突起；**cleft c.,** facial cleft caused by developmental failure of union between the maxillary and frontonasal processes 颊裂，由上颌和额突结合发育失败引起的面部裂口

chei·lec·tro·pi·on (ki″lek-tro'pe-on) eversion of the lip 唇外翻

chei·li·tis (ki-li'tis) inflammation of the lips 唇炎；**actinic c.,** pain and swelling of the lips and development of a scaly crust on the vermilion border after exposure to actinic rays; it may be acute or chronic 日光性唇炎，嘴唇暴露于光线后，出现疼痛和肿胀及红唇部边缘形成鳞状痂；急性或慢性病程；**angular c.,** perlèche 口角炎，传染性口角炎；**solar c.,** actinic c

chei·lo·gnatho·pros·o·pos·chi·sis (ki″lona″thopros″o-pos'kĭ-sis) congenital oblique facial cleft continuing into the upper jaw and lip 唇腭裂，先天性面部斜裂，一直延伸到上腭及嘴唇

chei·lo·plas·ty (ki'lo-plas″te) surgical repair of a defect of the lip 唇成形术

chei·lor·rha·phy (ki-lor'ə-fe) suture of the lip; surgical repair of harelip 唇裂修复术

chei·los·chi·sis (ki-los'kĭ-sis) harelip 唇裂，兔唇

chei·lo·sis (ki-lo'sis) fissuring and dry scaling of the vermilion surface of the lips and angles of the mouth, a characteristic of riboflavin deficiency 口角炎，嘴唇和嘴角红唇部的裂痕和干裂，是核黄素缺乏的特征；**angular c.,** perlèche 口角干裂

chei·lo·sto·ma·to·plas·ty (ki″lo-sto-mat'oplas″te) surgical restoration of the lips and mouth 口唇成形术

chei·ro·kin·es·the·sia (ki″ro-kin″es-the'zhə) the subjective perception of movements of the hand, especially in writing 手运动觉，对手运动的主观感觉，尤指在书写中

chei·ro·meg·a·ly (ki-ro-meg'ə-le) megalocheiria 巨手

chei·ro·plas·ty (ki'ro-plas″te) plastic surgery on the hand 手整形术

chei·ro·pom·pho·lyx (ki″ro-pom'fo-liks) pompholyx 掌跖汗疱

chei·ro·spasm (ki'ro-spaz″əm) spasm of the muscles of the hand 手痉挛

che·late (ke'lāt) 1. to combine with a metal in complexes in which the metal is part of a ring 螯合作用；2. by extension, a chemical compound in which a metallic ion is sequestered and firmly bound into a ring within the chelating molecules. Chelates are used in chemotherapy of metal poisoning 螯合物，一种化合物，金属离子被隔离并牢固地结合成螯合分子中的一个环；螯合物用于金属中毒的

化学治疗

chem·abra·sion (kēm″ə-bra′zhən) superficial destruction of the epidermis and the dermis by application of a cauterant to the skin; done to remove lesions such as scars or tattoos 化学脱皮法，在皮肤上施加烧灼物，破坏表皮和真皮的表面；用来去除疤痕或纹身等损伤

chem·ex·fo·li·a·tion (kēm″eks-fo″le-a′shən) chemabrasion 化学剥脱术，化学脱皮法

chem·i·cal (kem′ĭ-kəl) 1. pertaining to chemistry 化学的；2. a substance composed of chemical elements, or obtained by chemical processes 由化学元素组成的物质，或通过化学反应获得的物质

chemi·lu·mi·nes·cence (kem″ĭ-loo″mīnes′əns) luminescence produced by direct transformation of chemical energy into light energy 化学发光，化学反应直接转化为光能而产生的光

chem·ist (kem′ist) 1. a specialist in chemistry 化学家；2. (*British*) pharmacist（英国）药剂师

chem·is·try (kem′is-tre) the science dealing with the elements and atomic relations of matter, and of various compounds of the elements 化学; **colloid c.,** chemistry dealing with the nature and composition of colloids 胶体化学; **inorganic c.,** that branch of chemistry dealing with compounds not occurring in the plant or animal worlds 无机化学，化学中的一个分支，涉及植物或动物界以外的化合物; **organic c.,** that branch of chemistry dealing with carbon-containing compounds 有机化学，研究含碳化合物的化学分支

che·mo·at·trac·tant (ke″mo-ə-trak′tənt) a substance that induces positive chemotaxis 化学引诱物，诱导阳性趋化性的物质

che·mo·au·to·troph (ke″mo-aw′to-trōf) a chemoautotrophic microorganism 化能自养生物

che·mo·au·to·tro·phic (ke″mo-aw″to-tro′fik) capable of synthesizing cell constituents from carbon dioxide with energy from inorganic reactions 化能自养的，利用二氧化碳和无机反应产生的能量合成细胞成分

che·mo·cau·tery (ke″mo-kaw′tər-e) cauterization by application of a caustic substance 化学烧灼，用腐蚀性物质烧灼

che·mo·dec·to·ma (ke″mo-dek-to′mə) any benign, chromaffin-negative tumor of the chemoreceptor system, e.g., a carotid body tumor or glomus jugulare tumor 化学感受器瘤，化学感受器系统任何良性、嗜铬阴性肿瘤，例如颈动脉体肿瘤或颈静脉球肿瘤

che·mo·en·do·crine (ke″mo-en′do-krin) chemohormonal 化学内分泌，化学激素

che·mo·hor·mo·nal (ke″mo-hor-mo′nəl) chemoendocrine; pertaining to drugs that have hormonal activity 化学激素，化学内分泌；具有激素活性的药物

che·mo·kine (ke′mo-kīn) any of a group of low-molecular-weight cytokines identified that induce chemotaxis or chemokinesis in leukocytes (or in particular populations of leukocytes) in inflammation 趋化因子，低分子量细胞因子中的任何一种，在炎症中诱导白细胞趋化

che·mo·ki·ne·sis (ke″mo-kĭ-ne′sis) increased nondirectional activity of cells due to the presence of a chemical substance 化学增活现象，化学激动作用，由于化学物质的存在而增加了细胞的非定向活性

che·mo·litho·tro·phic (ke″mo-lith″o-tro′fik) deriving energy from the oxidation of inorganic compounds of iron, nitrogen, sulfur, or hydrogen; said of bacteria 化能无机营养生物，细菌从铁、氮、硫或氢的无机化合物的氧化中获得能量

che·mo·nu·cle·ol·y·sis (ke″mo-noo″kle-ol′ə-sis) dissolution of a portion of the nucleus pulposus of an intervertebral disk by injection of a proteolytic agent such as chymopapain, particularly used for treatment of a herniated intervertebral disk 化学髓核溶解术，通过注射蛋白水解剂（如凝乳蛋白酶）溶解椎间盘髓核的一部分，特别用于治疗椎间盘突出

che·mo·or·gano·troph (ke″mo-or′gə-notrōf″) an organism that derives its energy and carbon from organic compounds 化能有机营养生物，从有机化合物中获取能量和碳的微生物; **chemoorganotro′phic** adj.

che·mo·pal·li·dec·tomy (ke″mo-pal″ĭ-dek′tə-me) chemical destruction of tissue of the globus pallidus 苍白球化学破坏术

che·mo·pro·phy·lax·is (ke″mo-pro″fə-lak′sis) prevention of disease by means of a chemotherapeutic agent 化学预防

che·mo·pro·tec·tant (ke″mo-pro-tek′tənt) providing protection, or an agent providing protection, against the toxic effects of chemotherapeutic agents 化学保护药，对化疗药物的毒性作用提供保护的药物

che·mo·ra·dio·ther·a·py (ke″mo-ra″de-other′ə-pe) combined modality therapy using chemotherapy and radiotherapy, maximizing their interaction 放化疗，采用化疗和放疗的综合疗法，最大限度地发挥相互作用

che·mo·re·cep·tor (ke″mo-re-sep′tər) a receptor sensitive to stimulation by chemical substances 化学受体，对化学物质刺激敏感的受体

che·mo·re·pel·lent (ke″mo-re-pel′ənt) a substance that induces negative chemotaxis 化学驱避剂，引起负趋化性的物质

che·mo·re·sis·tance (ke″mo-re-zis′təns) specific resistance acquired by cells to the action of certain chemicals 化学抗性，细胞获得对某些化学物质的特异性抵抗

che·mo·sen·si·tive (ke″mo-sen′sĭ-tiv) sensitive to changes in chemical composition 化学敏感性，对化学成分的变化敏感

che·mo·sen·sory (ke″mo-sen′sər-e) relating to the perception of chemicals, as in odor detection 化学感应，与感觉化学物质有关，如检测气味

che·mo·sis (ke-mo′sis) edema of the conjunctiva of the eye 球结膜水肿；**chemot′ic** adj.

che·mo·sur·gery (ke″mo-sur′jər-e) destruction of tissue by chemical means for therapeutic purposes 化学外科，为达到治疗目的，使用化学方法破坏组织

che·mo·syn·the·sis (ke″mo-sin′thə-sis) the building up of chemical compounds under the influence of chemical stimulation, specifically the formation of carbohydrates from carbon dioxide and water as a result of energy derived from chemical reactions 化学合成，在化学反应的作用下形成化合物，特别是利用化学反应产生的能量使二氧化碳和水形成碳水化合物；**chemosynthet′ic** adj.

che·mo·tax·in (ke″mo-tak′sin) a substance, e.g., a complement component, that induces chemotaxis 化学吸引（趋向）素，诱导趋化作用的物质，如补体成分

che·mo·tax·is (ke″mo-tak′sis) movement of a cell or organism in response to differences in concentration of a dissolved substance, either in the direction of increasing concentration (*positive*) or in the direction of decreasing concentration (*negative*) 趋化作用，因溶解物浓度的差异使细胞或微生物运动，或向浓度增加（正）或向浓度降低（负）方向运动；**chemotac′tic** adj.

che·mo·ther·a·py (ke″mo-ther′ə-pe) treatment of disease by chemical agents 化疗；**adjuvant c.**, cancer chemotherapy employed after the primary tumor has been removed by some other method 辅助化疗，原发肿瘤切除后对肿瘤进行化疗；**combination c.**, that combining several different agents simultaneously in order to enhance their effectiveness 联合化疗，同时将几种不同的药物组合在一起进行化疗，以提高治疗有效性；**induction c.**, the use of drug therapy as the initial treatment for patients presenting with advanced cancer that cannot be treated by other means 诱导化疗，对无其他治疗方法的晚期癌症患者，使用药物治疗作为初始治疗；**neoadjuvant c.**, initial use of chemotherapy in patients with localized cancer in order to decrease the tumor burden prior to treatment by other modalities 新辅助化疗，为减轻治疗癌症前的肿瘤负担，

在局限性肿瘤患者中先使用化疗；**regional c.**, chemotherapy, especially for cancer, administered as a regional perfusion 局部化疗，局部灌注进行化疗，尤其针对癌症

che·mot·ic (ke-mot′ik) pertaining to or affected with chemosis 球结膜水肿的

che·mo·tro·phic (ke″mo-tro′fik) deriving energy from the oxidation of organic (chemoorganotrophic) or inorganic (chemolithotrophic) compounds; said of bacteria 化能自养的，细菌从有机（化能有机营养）或无机（化能无机营养）化合物的氧化中获得能量

che·mot·rop·ism (ke-mot′ro-piz-əm) tropism due to chemical stimulation 趋化性，化学刺激引起的趋向性；**chemotrop′ic** adj.

che·no·de·oxy·cho·lic ac·id (ke″no-de-ok″se-kol′ik) a primary bile acid, usually conjugated with glycine or taurine; it facilitates fat absorption and cholesterol excretion 鹅去氧胆酸，一种胆汁酸，通常与甘氨酸或牛磺酸结合；促进脂肪吸收和胆固醇排泄

che·no·di·ol (ke″no-di′ol) chenodeoxycholic acid used as an anticholelithogenic agent to dissolve radiolucent, noncalcified gallstones 鹅去氧胆酸，抗胆结石药，用来溶解射线可透过的、未钙化的胆结石

cher·ub·ism (cher′əb-iz-əm) hereditary progressive bilateral swelling at the angle of the mandible, and sometimes the entire jaw, giving a cherubic look to the face, in some cases enhanced by upturning of the eyes 家族性巨颌症，遗传性进行性双侧下颌角肿胀，有时是整个下颌，看起来像天使面容，在某些情况下，眼球上翻增强

chest (chest) thorax 胸部；**flail c.**, paradoxical movement of the chest wall with respiration, owing to multiple fractures of the ribs 连枷胸，由于肋骨多处骨折，胸壁在呼吸时出现反常运动；**funnel c.**, pectus excavatum 漏斗胸；**pigeon c.**, pectus carinatum 鸡胸

chest·nut (chest′nət) a tree of the genus *Castanea* or a nut of various species; the wood and leaves of *C. dentata* (American chestnut) contain tannin and it has been used as an astringent and in pertussis 板栗属树木或多种坚果树；板栗的木材和叶子含有单宁，用作收敛剂和治疗百日咳；**horse c.**, the tree *Aesculus hippocastanum* or a preparation of the medicinal parts of its seeds, having antiexudative, antiinflammatory, and immunomodulatory activity and used in the treatment of chronic venous insufficiency, in homeopathy and in folk medicine 七叶树或其种子制备的药物，具有抗渗出、抗炎和免疫调节活性，用于慢性静脉功能不全治疗、顺势疗法和民间医学

C

CHF congestive heart failure 充血性心力衰竭

chi ch'i (che) qi 气

chi·asm (ki′az-əm) a decussation or X-shaped crossing 交叉或 X 形交叉; **optic c.**, the structure in the forebrain formed by the decussation of the fibers of the optic nerve from each half of each retina 视交叉, 位于前脑, 双侧视网膜的视神经纤维交叉形成

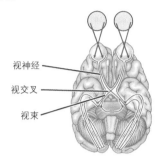

视神经
视交叉
视束

chi·as·ma (ki-az′mə) pl. *chias′mata* [L.] 1. chiasm 交叉; 2. in genetics, a point where pairs of homologous chromatids remain in contact during meiosis, indicating recombination between nonsister chromatids 遗传学中, 一对同源染色单体在减数分裂期间保持接触的点, 预示非同源染色单体之间的重组

chick·en·pox (chik′ən-poks) varicella; a highly contagious disease caused by human herpesvirus 3, characterized by vesicular eruptions appearing over a period of several days after an incubation period of 17 to 21 days; usually benign in children, but in infants, some adults, and immunocompromised patients there may be severe symptoms 水痘, 人类疱疹病毒 3 引起的高度传染性疾病, 特征是在潜伏期 17～21 天后的几天内出现水疱疹; 通常是儿童中的良性疾病, 但在婴儿、某些成人和免疫功能受损的患者中可有严重症状

chig·ger (chig′ər) the red larva of a mite of the family Trombiculidae; it attaches to a host's skin, and its bite produces a wheal with severe itching and dermatitis. Some species are vectors of the rickettsiae of scrub typhus 恙螨科螨虫的红色幼虫; 附着在宿主皮肤上, 被咬后会产生严重瘙痒和皮炎, 某些为斑疹伤寒立克次体的载体

chig·oe (chig′o) the flea, *Tunga penetrans*, of subtropical and tropical America and Africa; the pregnant female burrows into the skin of the feet, legs, or other part of the body, causing intense irritation and ulceration, sometimes leading to spontaneous amputation of a digit 跳蚤, 产于亚热带和热带美洲和非洲; 怀孕的雌性跳蚤钻入脚、腿或身体其

他部位的皮肤, 引起强烈的瘙痒和溃疡, 有时会导致手指的自发截断

chil·blain (chil′blān) a recurrent localized itching, swelling, and painful erythema of the fingers, toes, or ears, caused by mild frostbite and dampness 冻疮, 因轻度冻伤和潮湿而引起的手指、脚趾或耳朵的复发性局部瘙痒、肿胀和疼痛性红斑, 又称 *chilblains*

child·birth (chīld′bərth) parturition; the process of giving birth to a child 分娩

chill (chil) a sensation of cold, with convulsive shaking of the body 寒战

Chi·lo·mas·tix (ki″lo-mas′tiks) a genus of parasitic protozoa found in the intestines of vertebrates, including *C. mesni'li*, a common species found as a commensal in the human cecum and colon 唇鞭虫属, 在脊椎动物肠道中发现的一个寄生原生动物属, 在人类盲肠和结肠中作为共生体存在的一种常见物种

chi·me·ra (ki-mēr′ə) 1. an organism with different cell populations derived from different zygotes of the same or different species, occurring spontaneously or produced artificially 嵌合体, 自发发生或人工产生的由同种或不同种的不同合子结合产生的具有不同细胞群的有机体; 2. a substance created from proteins or genes of two species, as by genetic engineering 两种物种的蛋白质或基因通过基因工程, 产生的物质; **chimer′ic** *adj.*

chin (chin) the anterior prominence of the lower jaw; the mentum 颏

chi·rop·o·dy (ki-rop′ə-de) podiatry 足病学

chi·ro·prac·tic (ki″ro-prak′tik) a nonpharmaceutical, nonsurgical system of health care based on the self-healing capacity of the body and the primary importance of the proper function of the nervous system in the maintenance of health; therapy is aimed at removing irritants to the nervous system and restoring proper function. The most common method of treatment is by spinal manipulation and is primarily done for musculoskeletal complaints; other methods include lifestyle modification, nutritional therapy, and physiotherapy 脊柱推拿疗法, 基于身体自愈能力和神经系统在维持健康中的重要作用的非药物、非手术保健系统; 治疗的目的是消除对神经系统的刺激并恢复正常功能; 最常见的治疗方法是脊柱推拿, 主要用于肌肉骨骼疾病; 其他方法包括生活方式调整、营养疗法和物理疗法

chi-square (ki′skwār) 卡方, 见 *distribution* 和 *test* 下词条

chi·tin (ki′tin) an insoluble, linear polysaccharide forming the principal constituent of arthropod exoskeletons and found in some plants, particularly fungi 壳多糖, 一种不溶的线状多糖, 形成节肢

动物外骨骼的主要成分,在一些植物中也有发现,特别是真菌

CHL crown-heel length 顶踵长度

Chla·my·dia (klə-mid'e-ə) a genus of bacteria of the family Chlamydiaceae; some species are now classified in the genus *Chlamydophila. C. tracho'matis* causes trachoma, inclusion conjunctivitis, urethritis, proctitis, and lymphogranuloma venereum 衣原体,衣原体科的一个菌属;有些种类现在被归入衣原体属;沙眼衣原体引起沙眼、包涵体结膜炎、尿道炎、直肠炎和性病淋巴肉芽肿

Chla·myd·i·a·ceae (klə-mid"e-a'se-e) a family of bacteria of the order Chlamydiales consisting of small coccoid microorganisms that have a unique, obligately intracellular developmental cycle and are incapable of synthesizing ATP. They induce their own phagocytosis by host cells, in which they then form intracytoplasmic colonies. They are parasites of birds and mammals (including humans) 衣原体科,衣原体目的一个家族,由小的球形微生物组成,具有独特的细胞内发育周期,不能合成ATP;它们通过诱导宿主细胞的吞噬作用,在宿主胞质内进行克隆;是鸟类和哺乳动物(包括人类)的寄生虫

Chla·my·diae (klə-mid'e-e) 衣原体 1. a phylum of gram-positive or gram-variable, nonmotile, obligately parasitic bacteria that multiply by means of a complex life cycle within cytoplasmic vacuoles of mammalian and avian host cells 革兰阳性或革兰染色不定的、不动的、专性寄生菌的门,借助哺乳动物和鸟类宿主细胞的胞浆的复杂生命周期进行繁殖;2. the sole class of this phylum 衣原体门的唯一一类

Chla·myd·i·al·es (klə-mid'e-a"lēz) an order of coccoid, gram-negative bacteria of the class Chlamydiae 衣原体目,衣原体类的球形革兰阳性菌

chla·myd·i·o·sis (klə-mid"e-o'sis) any infection or disease caused by members of the Chlamydiales 衣原体病,由衣原体成员引起的任何感染或疾病

Chla·my·do·phi·la (klam"ĭ-dof'ĭ-lə) a genus of bacteria of the family Chlamydiaceae, including several species formerly classified in the genus *Chlamydia. C. pneumo'niae* is an important cause of pneumonia, bronchitis, and sinusitis, and *C. psit'taci* causes psittacosis 衣原体属,衣原体科衣原体科的一个菌属,包括以前归入衣原体属的几种细菌;肺炎衣原体是引起肺炎、支气管炎和鼻窦炎的重要原因,而鹦鹉体衣原体引起鹦鹉热

chlam·y·do·spore (klam'ĭ-do-spor") a thick-walled intercalary or terminal asexual spore formed by the rounding-up of a cell; it is not shed 厚垣孢子,厚壁有抵抗能力的无性孢子,不会脱落

chlo·as·ma (klo-az'mə) melasma 黄褐斑

chlor·ac·ne (klor-ak'ne) an acneiform eruption due to exposure to chlorine compounds 氯痤疮,由于暴露在氯化合物中而引起的痤疮

chlo·ral (klor'əl) 1. an oily liquid with a pungent, irritating odor; used in the manufacture of chloral hydrate and DDT 氯醛,一种有刺激性气味的油状液体;用于制造水合氯醛和DDT;水合氯醛;2. c. hydrate **c. hydrate**, a hypnotic and sedative, now used mainly as an adjunct to anesthesia and as a sedative for children undergoing medical and dental procedures 水合氯醛,催眠药和镇静药,目前主要用作麻醉的辅助药物,也用于正在接受治疗和牙科手术的儿童镇静药

chlor·am·bu·cil (klor-am'bu-sil) an alkylating agent from the nitrogen mustard group, used as an antineoplastic 苯丁酸氮芥,氮芥基烷基化剂,用作抗肿瘤药

chlor·am·phen·i·col (klor"əm-fen'ĭ-kol) a broad-spectrum antibiotic effective against rickettsiae, gram-positive and gram-negative bacteria, and certain spirochetes; used also as the palmitate ester and as the sodium succinate derivative 氯霉素,广谱抗生素,对立克次体、革兰阳性菌和革兰阴性菌以及某些螺旋体有效;也用作棕榈酸酯和琥珀酸钠衍生物

chlor·cy·cli·zine (klor-si'klī-zēn) an H₁ histamine receptor antagonist with anticholinergic, antiemetic, and local anesthetic properties, used as the hydrochloride salt as an antihistaminic and antipruritic 氯环力嗪,具有抗胆碱、止吐和局部麻醉特性的H₁组胺受体拮抗药,盐酸盐用作抗组胺和止痒药

chlor·dane (klor'dān) a poisonous substance of the chlorinated hydrocarbon group, used as an insecticide 氯丹,有毒的氯化烃类物质,用作杀虫剂

chlor·di·az·ep·ox·ide (klor"di-az"ə-pok'sīd) a benzodiazepine used as the base or hydrochloride salt in the treatment of anxiety disorders and short-term or preoperative anxiety, for alcohol withdrawal, and as an antitremor agent 氯氮草,苯二氮草类药物,其碱或盐酸盐用作治疗焦虑症和短期或术前焦虑症,可用于戒酒和作为抗肿瘤药

chlor·emia (klor-e'me-ə) hyperchloremia 高氯血症

chlor·hex·i·dine (klor-heks'ĭ-dēn) an antibacterial effective against a wide variety of gramnegative and gram-positive organisms; used also as the acetate ester, as a preservative for eyedrops, and as the gluconate or hydrochloride salt, as a topical anti-infective 氯己定,对多种革兰阴性和革兰阳性微生物有效的抗菌剂;其醋酸酯用作眼药水防腐剂,其葡萄糖酸盐或盐酸盐用作局部抗感染剂

chlor·hy·dria (klor-hi'dre-ə) hyperchlorhydria 胃

酸过多症

chlo·ride (klor′īd) a salt of hydrochloric acid; any binary compound of chlorine in which the latter is the negative element 氯化物

chlor·id·or·rhea (klor″ĭ-də-re′ə) diarrhea with an excess of chlorides in the stool 高氯性腹泻

chlo·ri·nat·ed (klor′ ĭ-nāt″əd) treated or charged with chlorine 氯化处理

chlo·rine (Cl) (klor′ēn) a yellowish green, gaseous element of the halogen group, with a suffocating odor; at. no. 17, at. wt. 35.45. It is a disinfectant, decolorant, and irritant poison, used for disinfecting, fumigating, and bleaching 氯（Cl），一种黄绿色的卤素族气体元素，有令人窒息的气味；原子序数17，原子质量35.45；是消毒剂、脱色剂和刺激性毒物，用于消毒、熏蒸和漂白

chlo·rite (klor′īt) a salt of chlorous acid; disinfectant and bleaching agent 亚氯酸盐，一种氯酸盐；用作消毒剂和漂白剂

chlo·ro·form (klor′ə-form) a colorless, mobile liquid, CHCl₃, with an ethereal odor and sweet taste, used as a solvent; once widely used as an inhalation anesthetic and analgesic, and as an antitussive, carminative, and counterirritant. It is hepatotoxic and nephrotoxic by ingestion 氯仿，无色的液体，CHCl₃，具有特殊气味和甜味，用作溶剂；曾被广泛用作吸入麻醉药和镇痛药，以及镇咳、驱风和抗刺激剂；口服有肝毒性和肾毒性

chlo·ro·ma (klor-o′mə) a malignant, greencolored tumor arising from myeloid tissue, associated with myelogenous leukemia. 绿色瘤，骨髓组织产生的恶性绿色肿瘤，与髓性白血病有关，又称chloroleukemia

chlo·ro·phyll (klor′o-fil) any of a group of green magnesium-containing porphyrin derivatives occurring in all photosynthetic organisms; they convert light energy to reducing potential for the reduction of CO₂. Preparations of watersoluble chlorophyll salts are used as deodorizers 叶绿素，含镁的绿色卟啉衍生物，存在于有光合作用的有机体中；将光能转化，二氧化碳的产生；水溶性叶绿素盐被用作除臭剂；见 *chlorophyllin*

chlo·ro·phyl·lin (klor′o-fil-in) any of the water-soluble salts from chlorophyll; used topically and orally for deodorizing skin lesions and orally for deodorizing the urine and feces in colostomy, ileostomy, and incontinence; used particularly in the form of the copper complex 水溶性叶绿素盐；局部和口服用于皮肤病变的除臭，口服用于结肠造口术、回肠造口术和尿失禁中的尿液和粪便的除臭；以铜络合物的形式使用

Chlo·ro·phyl·lum (klo-rof′ ĭ-ləm) a genus of mushrooms including the species *C. molyb′dites*, easily confused with the common cultivated mushroom but causing gastrointestinal irritation 绿褶菇，蘑菇属，包括青褶伞属，易与普通栽培蘑菇混淆，其可引起胃肠道刺激

chlo·ro·plast (klor′o-plast) any of the chlorophyll-bearing bodies of plant cells 叶绿体，含叶绿素的植物细胞体

chlo·ro·priv·ic (klor″o-priv′ik) deprived of chlorides; due to loss of chlorides 氯化物缺失的

chlo·ro·pro·caine (klor″o-pro′kān) a local anesthetic, used as the hydrochloride salt 普鲁卡因，局部麻醉药，常用其盐酸盐

chlo·rop·sia (klor-op′se-ə) defect of vision in which objects appear to have a greenish tinge 绿视症，视物呈绿色的视觉缺陷

chlo·ro·quine (klor′o-kwin) an antiamebic and anti-inflammatory used in the treatment of malaria, giardiasis, extraintestinal amebiasis, lupus erythematosus, and rheumatoid arthritis; used also as the hydrochloride and phosphate salts 氯喹，用于治疗疟疾、贾第虫病、肠外阿米巴病、红斑狼疮和类风湿关节炎的抗阿米巴和抗炎药；常用其盐酸盐和磷酸盐

chlo·ro·thi·a·zide (klor″o-thi′ə-zīd) a thiazide diuretic used in the form of the base or the sodium salt to treat hypertension and edema. 氯噻嗪，噻嗪类利尿药，其碱或钠盐用于治疗高血压和水肿

chlo·rox·ine (klor-ok′sēn) a synthetic antibacterial used in the topical treatment of dandruff and seborrheic dermatitis of the scalp 二氯羟喹，合成抗菌剂，用于头皮屑和脂溢性皮炎的局部治疗

chlor·phen·ir·amine (klor″fən-ir′ə-mēn) an antihistamine with sedative and anticholinergic effects; used as *c. maleate*, *c. polistirex*, and *c. tannate*. 氯苯吡胺，具有镇静和抗胆碱作用的抗组胺药

chlor·pro·ma·zine (klor-pro′mə-zēn) a phenothiazine used in the form of the base or the hydrochloride salt as an antipsychotic, antiemetic, and presurgical sedative, and in the treatment of intractable hiccups, acute intermittent porphyria, tetanus, the manic phase of bipolar disorder, and severe behavioral problems in children 氯丙嗪，吩噻嗪，其碱或盐酸盐用作抗精神病药、止吐药和术前镇静药，用于治疗顽固性打嗝、急性间歇性卟啉症、破伤风、双相情感障碍的躁狂期及儿童严重的行为问题

chlor·pro·pa·mide (klor-pro′pə-mīd) a sulfonylurea used as a hypoglycemic in the treatment of type 2 diabetes mellitus 氯磺丙脲，磺酰脲类药物，用于治疗2型糖尿病

chlor·tet·ra·cy·cline (klor″tet-rə-si′klēn) a broad-spectrum antibiotic obtained from *Streptomyces aureofaciens*; used as the hydrochloride salt 氯

四环素，金色链霉菌中提取的广谱抗生素；用作盐酸盐

chlor·thal·i·done (klor-thal′ĭ-dōn) a sulfonamide with similar actions to the thiazide diuretics; used in the treament of hypertension and edema 氯噻酮，具有类似噻嗪类利尿药作用的磺胺类药物；用于治疗高血压和水肿

chlor·ure·sis (klor″u-re′sis) excretion of excessive chlorides in the urine 尿氯排泄，尿液中氯化物过量

chlor·uret·ic (klor″u-ret′ik) 1. promoting chloruresis 促尿氯排泄；2. an agent that promotes the excretion of chlorides in the urine 促进尿液中氯化物排泄的药物

chlor·zox·a·zone (klor-zok′sə-zōn) a skeletal muscle relaxant used to relieve discomfort of painful musculoskeletal disorders 氯唑沙宗，骨骼肌松弛药，用于缓解疼痛性骨骼肌肉疾病的不适

ChM [L.] Chirur′giae Magis′ter (Master of Surgery) 外科学硕士

cho·a·na (ko′ə-nə) pl. *cho′anae* [L.] 1. infundibulum 漏斗；2. one of the pair of openings between the nasal cavity and the nasopharynx 鼻腔和鼻咽之间的一对开口，后鼻孔

cho·a·no·mas·ti·gote (ko″ə-no-mas′tĭ-gōt) a morphologic stage in the life cycle of some trypanosomatid protozoa; the kinetoplast and basal body are anterior to the nucleus and the flagellum emerges through a collarlike extension at the anterior end of the cell 领鞭毛体期，某些锥虫原生动物生命周期中的一个形态阶段；动基体和基体位于细胞核前，鞭毛通过细胞前端的一个锁状环延伸而出

choke (chōk) 1. strangle; to interrupt respiration by obstruction or compression. 使窒息；2. strangulation; the condition resulting from such an interruption 窒息，由此种阻断引起的窒息状态

chol·a·gogue (ko′lə-gog) an agent that stimulates gallbladder contraction to promote bile flow 利胆药，刺激胆囊收缩以促进胆汁流动的药物；**cholagog′ic** *adj.*

cho·lan·gi·ec·ta·sis (ko-lan″je-ek′tə-sis) dilatation of a bile duct 胆管扩张

cho·lan·gio·car·ci·no·ma (ko-lan″je-o-kahr″sīno′mə) 1. an adenocarcinoma arising from the epithelium of bile ducts and composed of epithelial cells in tubules or acini with fibrous stroma. There are both *intrahepatic* and *extrahepatic* varieties 胆管癌，胆管上皮的腺癌，由胆管或腺泡中的上皮细胞和纤维间质组成，有肝内和肝外两种类型；2. cholangiocellular carcinoma 胆管细胞癌

cho·lan·gio·cel·lu·lar (ko-lan″je-o-sel′u-lər) of, resembling, or pertaining to cells of the cholangioles 胆管细胞的

cho·lan·gio·en·ter·os·to·my (ko-lan″je-oen″tər-os′tə-me) surgical anastomosis of a bile duct to the intestine 胆管小吻合术

cho·lan·gio·gas·tros·to·my (ko-lan″je-ogas-tros′tə-me) anastomosis of a bile duct to the stomach 胆管胃吻合术

cho·lan·gi·og·ra·phy (ko-lan″je-og′rə-fe) radiography of the bile ducts 胆管造影术

cho·lan·gio·hep·a·to·ma (ko-lan″je-o-hep″ə-to′mə) hepatocellular carcinoma of mixed liver cell and bile duct cell origin 胆管肝细胞癌，肝细胞癌起源于混合肝细胞和胆管细胞

cho·lan·gi·ole (ko-lan′je-ōl) one of the fine terminal elements of the bile duct system 毛细胆管，胆管系统的终端；**cholangi′olar** *adj.*

cho·lan·gi·o·li·tis (ko-lan″je-o-li′tis) inflammation of the cholangioles 胆管炎；**cholangiolit′ic** *adj.*

cho·lan·gi·o·ma (ko-lan″je-o′mə) cholangiocellular carcinoma 胆管细胞癌

cho·lan·gio·sar·co·ma (ko-lan″je-o-sahr-ko′mah) sarcoma of bile duct origin 胆管肉瘤

cho·lan·gi·os·to·my (ko-lan″je-os′tə-me) fistulization of a bile duct 胆管造口术

cho·lan·gi·ot·o·my (ko-lan″je-ot′ə-me) incision into a bile duct 胆管切开术

cho·lan·gi·tis (ko″lan-ji′tis) inflammation of a bile duct 胆管炎。Spelled also *cholangeitis.* **cholangit′ic** *adj.*

cho·lano·poi·e·sis (ko″lə-no-poi-e′sis) the synthesis of bile acids or of their conjugates and salts by the liver 胆酸盐生成，肝脏合成胆汁酸或其结合物和盐

cho·lano·poi·et·ic (ko″lə-no-poi-et′ik) 1. promoting cholanopoiesis 促进胆汁生成；2. an agent that promotes cholanopoiesis 促进胆汁生成的药物

cho·late (ko′lāt) a salt, anion, or ester of cholic acid 胆酸盐

chole·cal·ci·fer·ol (ko″lə-kal-sif′ər-ol) vitamin D₃; a hormone synthesized in the skin on irradiation of 7-dehydrocholesterol or obtained from the diet; it is activated when metabolized to 1,25-dihydroxy-cholecalciferol. It is used as an antirachitic and in the treatment of hypocalcemic tetany and hypoparathyroidism 维生素 D₃；在紫外线照射下，7-脱氢胆固醇在皮肤中合成的激素或从饮食中获得的激素；代谢物 1,25- 二羟维生素 D₃ 为活化状态；被用作抗风湿药，用于治疗低血钙性手足强直和甲状旁腺功能减退

cho·le·cyst (ko′lə-sist) gallbladder 胆囊

cho·le·cyst·a·gogue (ko″lə-sis′tə-gog) an agent that promotes evacuation of the gallbladder 利胆药，促进胆囊排空的药物

cho·le·cys·tal·gia (ko″lə-sis-tal′jə) 1. biliary colic

胆绞痛；2. pain due to inflammation of the gall-bladder 胆囊炎引起的疼痛

cho·le·cys·tec·ta·sia (ko″lə-sis″tek-ta′zhə) distention of the gallbladder 胆囊扩张症

cho·le·cys·tec·to·my (ko″lə-sis-tek′tə-me) excision of the gallbladder 胆囊切除术

cho·le·cyst·en·ter·os·to·my (ko″lə-sis″tentər-os-′tə-me) formation of a new communication between the gallbladder and the intestine 胆囊小肠吻合术

cho·le·cys·ti·tis (ko″lə-sis-ti′tis) inflammation of the gallbladder 胆囊炎；emphysematous c., that due to gas-producing organisms, marked by gas in the gallbladder lumen, often infiltrating into the gallbladder wall and surrounding tissues 气肿性胆囊炎，胆囊腔中有以产气为特征的微生物，胆囊腔中存在气体，常常渗入胆囊壁和周围组织

cho·le·cys·to·co·los·to·my (ko″lə-sis″to-kə-los′tə-me) anastomosis of the gallbladder and colon 胆囊结肠吻合术

cho·le·cys·to·du·o·de·nos·to·my (ko″lə-sis″to-doo″o-də-nos′tə-me) anastomosis of the gallbladder and duodenum 胆囊十二指肠吻合术

cho·le·cys·to·gas·tros·to·my (ko″lə-sis″togas-tros′tə-me) anastomosis between the gallbladder and stomach 胆囊胃吻合术

cho·le·cys·to·gram (ko″lə-sis′to-gram) a radiograph of the gallbladder 胆囊照片

cho·le·cys·tog·ra·phy (ko″lə-sis-tog′rə-fe) radiography of the gallbladder 胆囊造影术；**cholecystograph′ic** adj.

cho·le·cys·to·je·ju·nos·to·my (ko″lə-sis″tojə-joo-nos′tə-me) anastomosis of the gallbladder and jejunum 胆囊空肠吻合术

cho·le·cys·to·ki·net·ic (ko″lə-sis″to-kīnet′ik) stimulating contraction of the gallbladder 胆囊收缩素

cho·le·cys·to·ki·nin (CCK) (ko″lə-sis″to-ki′nin) a polypeptide hormone secreted in the small intestine that stimulates gallbladder contraction and secretion of pancreatic enzymes 胆囊收缩素（CCK），小肠分泌的多肽激素，刺激胆囊收缩和胰腺酶的分泌

cho·le·cys·to·li·thi·a·sis (ko″lə-sis″to-līthi′ə-sis) the occurrence of gallstones (see cholelithiasis) within the gallbladder 胆结石

cho·le·cys·to·li·thot·o·my (ko″lə-sis″tolī-thot′ə-me) incision of the gallbladder for removal of gall-stones 胆结石切除术

cho·le·cys·to·pexy (ko″lə-sis′to-pek″se) surgical suspension or fixation of the gallbladder 胆囊固定术，胆囊的外科悬吊或固定

cho·le·cys·tor·rha·phy (ko″lə-sis-tor′ə-fe) suture or repair of the gallbladder 胆囊缝合术

cho·le·cys·tot·o·my (ko″lə-sis-tot′ə-me) incision of the gallbladder 胆囊切开术

cho·led·o·chal (ko-led′o-kəl) pertaining to the common bile duct 胆总管的

cho·le·do·chec·to·my (ko″lə-do-kek′tə-me) excision of part of the common bile duct 胆总管部分切除术

cho·le·do·chi·tis (ko″lə-do-ki′tis) inflammation of the common bile duct 胆总管炎

cho·led·o·cho·du·o·de·nos·to·my (ko-led″o-ko-doo″o-də-nos′tə-me) anastomosis of the common bile duct to the duodenum 胆总管 - 十二指肠吻合术

cho·led·o·cho·en·ter·os·to·my (ko-led″ə-ko-en″tər-os′ə-me) anastomosis of the bile duct to the intestine 胆总管 - 小肠吻合术

cho·led·o·cho·gas·tros·to·my (ko-led″ə-kogas-tros′ə-me) anastomosis of the bile duct to the stomach 胆总管 - 胃吻合术

cho·led·o·cho·je·ju·nos·to·my (ko-led″ə-ko-jə-joo-nos′ə-me) anastomosis of the bile duct to the jejunum 胆总管 - 空肠吻合术

cho·led·o·cho·li·thi·a·sis (ko-led″ə-ko-līthi′ə-sis) the occurrence of calculi (see cholelithiasis) in the common bile duct 胆总管结石

cho·led·o·cho·li·thot·o·my (ko-led″ə-ko-līthot′ə-me) incision into the common bile duct for stone removal 胆总管切开取石术

cho·led·o·cho·plas·ty (ko-led′ə-ko-plas″te) plastic repair of the common bile duct 胆管成形术

cho·led·o·chor·rha·phy (ko-led″ə-kor′ə-fe) suture or repair of the common bile duct 胆总管缝合术

cho·led·o·chos·to·my (ko-led″ə-kos′ə-me) creation of an opening into the common bile duct for drainage 胆总管造口术

cho·led·o·chot·o·my (ko-led″ə-kot′ə-me) incision into the common bile duct 胆总管切开术

cho·led·o·chus (ko-led′ə-kəs) common bile duct 胆总管

cho·le·ic (ko-le′ik) biliary 胆管的

cho·le·ic ac·id (ko-le′ik) any of the complexes formed between deoxycholic acid and a fatty acid or other lipid 胆汁酸，脱氧胆酸与脂肪酸或其他脂类形成的复合物

cho·le·lith (ko″lə-lith) gallstone 胆结石

cho·le·li·thi·a·sis (ko″lə-lī-thi′ə-sis) the presence or formation of gallstones 胆石症

cho·le·li·thot·o·my (ko″lə-lī-thot′ə-me) incision of the biliary tract for removal of gallstones 胆石切除术

cho·le·litho·trip·sy (ko″lə-lith′o-trip-se) crushing of a gallstone 碎胆石术

cho·lem·e·sis (ko-lem′ə-sis) vomiting of bile 呕胆
cho·le·mia (ko-le′me-ə) bile or bile pigment in the blood 胆血症，血液中有胆汁或胆色素；**chole′mic** adj.

cho·le·peri·to·ne·um (ko″lə-per″ĭ-to-ne′əm) the presence of bile in the peritoneum 胆汁性腹膜炎
cho·le·poi·e·sis (ko″lə-poi-e′sis) the formation of bile in the liver 胆汁生成；**cholepoiet′ic** adj.

chol·era (kol′ər-ə) an acute infectious disease endemic and epidemic in Asia, caused by *Vibrio cholerae*, marked by severe diarrhea with extreme fluid and electrolyte depletion, and by vomiting, muscle cramps, and prostration 霍乱，亚洲流行的急性传染病，由霍乱弧菌引起，以严重腹泻、体液和电解质极度紊乱、呕吐、肌肉痉挛和虚脱为特征；**Asiatic c.**, cholera 亚洲霍乱；**pancreatic c.**, a condition usually due to an islet-cell tumor (other than beta cell), with profuse watery diarrhea, hypokalemia, and usually achlorhydria 胰腺霍乱，通常由胰岛细胞瘤（β细胞除外）引起的疾病，伴有大量的水样腹泻、低钾血症且常有胃酸缺乏

chol·er·a·gen (kol′ər-ə-jen) cholera toxin 霍乱肠毒素

chol·e·ra·ic (kol″ə-ra′ik) pertaining to or characterized by cholera 霍乱的，与霍乱有关或以霍乱为特征

cho·ler·e·sis (ko-ler′ə-sis) the secretion of bile by the liver 胆汁分泌，由肝脏分泌的胆汁

cho·ler·et·ic (ko″lər-et′ik) stimulating bile production by the liver; an agent that so acts 利胆药，刺激肝脏胆汁产生的药物

cho·ler·i·form (ko-ler′ ĭ-form) resembling cholera 霍乱样的

cho·le·sta·sis (ko″lə-sta′sis) stoppage or suppression of bile flow, having intrahepatic or extrahepatic causes 胆汁淤积，肝内或肝外胆汁分泌停止或受抑，有肝内或肝外原因；**cholestat′ic** adj.

cho·le·ste·a·to·ma (ko″lə-ste″ə-to′mə) a cystlike mass lined with stratified squamous epithelium filled with desquamating debris, often including cholesterol, usually in the middle ear and mastoid region 胆脂瘤，囊状肿块，内衬复层鳞状上皮，其内充满脱皮碎屑、通常发生于中耳和乳突区

cho·les·te·a·to·sis (ko″lə-ste″ə-to′sis) fatty degeneration due to cholesterol esters 胆固醇沉着病性变性

cho·les·ter·ol (kə-les′tər-ol″) a eukaryotic sterol that in higher animals is the precursor of bile acids and steroid hormones and a key constituent of cell membranes. Most is synthesized by the liver and other tissues, but some is absorbed from dietary sources, with each kind transported in the plasma by specific lipoproteins. It can accumulate or deposit abnormally, as in some gallstones and in atheromas.

Preparations are used as emulsifiers in pharmaceuticals 胆固醇，真核生物甾醇，高等动物中是胆汁酸和类固醇激素的前体，且为细胞膜的关键成分，大多数是由肝脏和其他组织合成，但有些是从饮食中吸收的，每一种都通过特定的脂蛋白在血浆中运输；可不正常地积聚或沉积，如胆结石和动脉粥样硬化；制剂在药物中用作乳化剂；**HDL c.**, high-density–lipoprotein c. (HDL-C), the serum cholesterol carried on high-density lipoproteins, approximately 20 to 30 percent of the total 高密度脂蛋白胆固醇（HDL-C），高密度脂蛋白携带的血清胆固醇，占总胆固醇的20%～30%；**LDL c.**, low-density–lipoprotein c. (LDL-C), the serum cholesterol carried on low-density lipoproteins, approximately 60 to 70 percent of the total 低密度脂蛋白胆固醇（LDL-C），低密度脂蛋白携带的血清胆固醇，占总胆固醇的60%—70%

cho·les·ter·ol·emia (kə-les′tər-ol-e′me-ə) hypercholesterolemia 高胆固醇血症

cho·les·ter·ol es·ter·ase (kə-les′tər-ol es′tərās) acid lipase; an enzyme that catalyzes the hydrolytic cleavage of cholesterol and other sterol esters and triglycerides. Deficiency of the lysosomal enzyme causes the allelic disorders Wolman disease and cholesteryl ester storage disease 胆固醇酯酶，酸性脂肪酶；催化胆固醇和其他甾醇酯和甘油三酯水解的酶；溶酶体酶缺乏可引起等位基因紊乱、酸性脂肪酶缺乏症和胆固醇酯贮积病

cho·les·ter·ol·o·sis (kə-les″tər-ol-o′sis) cholesterosis 胆固醇贮积病

cho·les·ter·ol·uria (kə-les″tər-ol-u′re-ə) cholesterol in the urine 胆固醇尿症

cho·les·ter·o·sis (kə-les″tər-o′sis) abnormal deposition of cholesterol in tissues 胆固醇贮积病，组织中胆固醇异常沉积

cho·les·ter·yl (kə-les′tə-rəl″) the radical of cholesterol, formed by removal of the hydroxyl group 胆固醇基，胆固醇除去羟基形成的自由基

cho·le·sty·ra·mine (ko″lə-sti′rə-mēn) 考来烯胺 见 resin 下 *cholestyramine resin*

cho·lic ac·id (ko′lik) 1. one of the primary bile acids, usually occurring conjugated with glycine or taurine; it facilitates fat absorption and cholesterol excretion 胆酸，胆汁酸的一种，通常与甘氨酸或牛磺酸结合；促进脂肪吸收和胆固醇排泄；2. any of the substituted derivatives of cholic acid collectively constituting the bile acids 胆酸的任何取代衍生物，共同构成胆汁酸

cho·line (ko′lēn) a quaternary amine, often classified as a member of the B vitamin complex; it occurs in phosphatidylcholine and acetylcholine, is an important methyl donor in intermediary metabolism, and prevents the deposition of fat in the liver 胆碱，

C

季胺，通常被归类为 B 族维生素复合物的一员；存在于磷脂酰胆碱和乙酰胆碱中，是中间代谢中的重要甲基供体，并防止脂肪在肝脏中沉积；**c. magnesium trisalicylate** 三水杨酸胆碱镁，见 *trisalicylate* 下词条。**c. salicylate** 水杨酸胆碱，见 *salicylate*

cho·line acet·y·lase (ko′lēn ə-set′ə-lās) choline acetyltransferase 胆碱乙酰转移酶

cho·line ac·e·tyl·trans·fer·ase (ko′lēn as″ĕtĕl-trans′fer-ās) an enzyme catalyzing the synthesis of acetylcholine; it is a marker for cholinergic neurons 胆碱乙酰化酶，催化乙酰胆碱合成的酶；是胆碱能神经元的标记物

cho·line ac·e·tyl·trans·fer·ase de·fi·cien·cy (ko′lēn as″ə-tēl-trans′fər-ās) a congenital autosomal recessive disorder characterized by generalized hypotonia, episodes of life-threatening apnea, feeding difficulty, ophthalmoparesis, and occasionally arthrogryposis; symptoms often improve with age 胆碱乙酰转移酶缺乏，先天性常染色体隐性遗传疾病，以全身性张力减退、危及生命的呼吸暂停、进食困难、眼肌瘫痪和偶尔关节挛缩为特征；症状常随年龄增长而改善

cho·lin·er·gic (ko″lin-ur′jik) 1. parasympathomimetic; stimulated, activated, or transmitted by choline (acetylcholine); said of the sympathetic and parasympathetic nerve fibers that liberate acetylcholine at a synapse when a nerve impulse passes 胆碱能，副交感神经的；由胆碱（乙酰胆碱）刺激、激活或传导的；交感神经和副交感神经纤维的一种，当神经冲动通过时在突触处释放乙酰胆碱；2. an agent that produces such an effect 产生上述效果的药物

cho·lin·es·ter·ase (ko″lin-es′tər-ās) serum cholinesterase, pseudocholinesterase; an enzyme that catalyzes the hydrolytic cleavage of the acyl group from various esters of choline and some related compounds; determination of activity is used to test liver function, succinylcholine sensitivity, and whether organophosphate insecticide poisoning has occurred 胆碱酯酶，血清胆碱酯酶，假性胆碱酯酶；催化不同的胆碱酯和相关化合物的酰基水解的酶；活性测定用于检测肝功能、琥珀酰胆碱敏感性以及是否发生有机磷杀虫剂中毒；**true c.,** acetylcholinesterase 真胆碱酯酶，乙酰胆碱酯酶

cho·li·no·cep·tive (ko″lin-o-sep′tiv) pertaining to the sites on effector organs that are acted upon by cholinergic transmitters 胆碱能受体的，胆碱能递质作用于效应器官上的部位

cho·li·no·cep·tor (ko″lin-o-sep′tər) cholinergic receptor 胆碱能受体

cho·li·no·lyt·ic (ko″lin-o-lit′ik) 1. blocking the action of acetylcholine, or of cholinergic agents. 胆碱酯化，阻断乙酰胆碱或胆碱能药物的作用；

2. an agent that blocks the action of acetylcholine in cholinergic areas, i.e., organs supplied by parasympathetic nerves, and voluntary muscles 阻止乙酰胆碱在胆碱能区（即副交感神经支配的器官和随意肌）作用的药剂

cho·li·no·mi·met·ic (ko″lin-o-mi-met′ik) having an action similar to acetylcholine; parasympathomimetic 拟胆碱的，具有类似乙酰胆碱的作用；副交感神经的

chol·uria (kol-u′re-ə) bile pigments or bile salts in the urine 胆汁尿，尿液中有胆色素或胆汁盐；**cholu′ric** adj.

cho·lyl·gly·cine (ko″ləl-gli′sēn) a bile salt, the glycine conjugate of cholic acid 甘氨胆酸，胆汁盐，胆酸的甘氨酸结合物

cho·lyl·tau·rine (ko″ləl-taw′rēn) a bile salt, the taurine conjugate of cholic acid 牛磺胆酸，胆汁盐，胆酸的牛磺酸共轭物

chon·dral (kon′drəl) pertaining to cartilage 软骨的

chon·dral·gia (kon-dral′jə) pain in a cartilage 软骨痛

chon·drec·to·my (kon-drek′tə-me) surgical removal of a cartilage 软骨切除术

chon·dri·fi·ca·tion (kon″drĭ-fĭ-ka′shən) the formation of cartilage; transformation into cartilage 软骨化，软骨的形成；转化为软骨

chon·dri·tis (kon-dri′tis) inflammation of a cartilage 软骨炎

chon·dro·an·gi·o·ma (kon″dro-an″je-o′mə) a benign mesenchymoma containing chondromatous and angiomatous elements 软骨血管瘤，含有软骨瘤和血管瘤成分的良性间质瘤

chon·dro·blast (kon′dro-blast) an immature cartilage-producing cell 成软骨细胞，又称 *chondroplast*

chon·dro·blas·to·ma (kon″dro-blas-to′mə) a usually benign tumor derived from immature cartilage cells, occurring primarily in the epiphyses of adolescents 软骨母细胞瘤，通常为良性肿瘤，来源于未成熟的软骨细胞，主要发生在青少年的骨骺

chon·dro·cal·cif·ic (kon″dro-kal-sif′ik) characterized by deposition of calcium salts in the cartilaginous structures of one or more joints 软骨钙化，以钙盐沉积在一个或多个关节的软骨结构中为特征

chon·dro·cal·ci·no·sis (kon″dro-kal″sī-no′sis) the presence of calcium salts, especially calcium pyrophosphate, in the cartilaginous structures of one or more joints 软骨钙质沉着症，钙盐存在于一个或多个关节的软骨结构中，特别是焦磷酸钙

chon·dro·cos·tal (kon″dro-kos′təl) pertaining to the ribs and costal cartilages 肋与肋软骨的

chon·dro·cra·ni·um (kon″dro-kra′ne-əm) that part of the neurocranium formed by endochondral ossification and comprising the bones of the base of the skull 软颅，脑颅的一部分包括颅底的骨骼由软骨内成骨形成

chon·dro·cyte (kon′dro-sīt) one of the cells embedded in the lacunae of the cartilage matrix 软骨细胞，软骨基质腔隙中的细胞；**chondrocyt′ic** adj.

chon·dro·dyn·ia (kon″dro-din′e-ə) pain in a cartilage 软骨痛

chon·dro·dys·pla·sia (kon″dro-dis-pla′zhə) dyschondroplasia 软骨发育不良，**c. puncta′ta,** a heterogeneous group of hereditary bone dysplasias, the common characteristic of which is stippling of the epiphyses in infancy 点状软骨发育不良，是遗传性骨发育不良的一个异质群体，其共同特点是婴儿期骨骺点彩

chon·dro·dys·tro·phia (kon″dro-dis-tro′fe-ə) chondrodystrophy 软骨发育不良

chon·dro·dys·tro·phy (kon″dro-dis′trə-fe) a disorder of cartilage formation 软骨发育异常

chon·dro·ec·to·der·mal (kon″dro-ek″todur′məl) of or pertaining to cartilaginous and ectodermal elements 软骨外胚层，属于或关于软骨和外胚层的

chon·dro·epi·phys·itis (kon″dro-ep″ĭ-fiz-i′tis) inflammation involving the epiphyseal cartilages 软骨骺炎，累及骨骺软骨的炎症

chon·dro·fi·bro·ma (kon″dro-fi-bro′mə) a fibroma with cartilaginous elements 软骨纤维瘤，含有软骨成分的纤维瘤

chon·dro·gen·e·sis (kon″dro-jen′ə-sis) formation of cartilage 软骨形成

chon·droid (kon′droid) 1. resembling cartilage 软骨样；2. hyaline cartilage 透明软骨

chon·dro·i·tin sul·fate (kon-dro′ ĭ-tin) 1. a glycosaminoglycan that predominates in connective tissue, particularly cartilage, bone, and blood vessels, and in the cornea 硫酸软骨素一种糖胺聚糖，主要存在于结缔组织，特别是软骨、骨和血管以及角膜中；2. a preparation of chondroitin sulfate from bovine tracheal cartilage, administered orally for the treatment of osteoarthritis and joint pain 从牛气管软骨中制备硫酸软骨素，口服用于治疗骨关节炎和关节痛

chon·dro·li·po·ma (kon″dro-lĭ-po′mə) a benign mesenchymoma with cartilaginous and lipomatous elements 软骨肉瘤，良性间质瘤，含有软骨和脂肪瘤成分

chon·dro·ma (kon-dro′mə) pl. *chondromas, chondro'mata.* A benign tumor or tumor-like growth of mature hyaline cartilage. It may remain centrally within the substance of a cartilage or bone (*enchondroma*) or may develop on the surface (*juxtacortical* or *periosteal c.*) 软骨瘤，成熟透明软骨的良性肿瘤或肿瘤样生长；可以在软骨或骨（内生软骨

瘤）的中心，也可以在表面（近皮质的或骨外膜表面的软骨瘤）形成；**joint c.,** a mass of cartilage in the synovial membrane of a joint 关节软骨瘤，关节滑膜中的软骨块；**synovial c.,** a cartilaginous body formed in a synovial membrane 滑膜软骨瘤，在滑膜中形成的软骨体

chon·dro·ma·la·cia (kon″dro-mə-la′shə) abnormal softening of cartilage 软骨软化症

chon·dro·ma·to·sis (kon″dro-mə-to′sis) formation of multiple chondromas 多发性软骨瘤形成；**synovial c.,** a rare condition in which cartilage is formed in the synovial membrane of joints, tendon sheaths, or bursae, sometimes being detached and producing a number of loose bodies 滑膜软骨瘤病，关节、肌腱鞘或囊的滑膜中形成软骨的一种罕见疾病，有时被分离并产生许多疏松的部分

chon·dro·mere (kon′dro-mēr) a cartilaginous vertebra of the fetal vertebral column 软骨节，胎儿脊柱的软骨性椎骨

chon·dro·meta·pla·sia (kon″dro-met″ə-pla′zhə) a condition characterized by metaplastic activity of the chondroblasts 软骨化生，软骨母细胞的化生

chon·dro·my·o·ma (kon″dro-mi-o′mə) a benign mesenchymoma of myomatous and cartilaginous elements 软骨肌瘤，良性的间质瘤，由肌瘤和软骨组成

chon·dro·myx·oid (kon″dro-mik′soid) of, pertaining to, or characterized by chondroid and myxoid elements 软骨黏液样的，以软骨样和黏液样成分为特征

chon·dro·myx·o·ma (kon″dro-mik-so′mə) chondromyxoid fibroma. 软骨黏液瘤，软骨黏液样纤维瘤

chon·dro·myxo·sar·co·ma (kon″dro-mik″sosahr-ko′mə) a malignant mesenchymoma containing cartilaginous and myxoid elements 软骨肉瘤，含有软骨和黏液成分的恶性间质瘤

chon·dro·os·se·ous (kon″dro-os′e-əs) composed of cartilage and bone 软骨与骨的

chon·drop·a·thy (kon-drop′ə-the) disease of cartilage 软骨病；又称 *chondrosis.*

chon·dro·phyte (kon′dro-fīt) a cartilaginous growth at the articular end of a bone 软骨疣，骨关节端的软骨生长

chon·dro·pla·sia (kon″dro-pla′zhə) the formation of cartilage by specialized cells (chondrocytes) 软骨生成

chon·dro·plas·ty (kon′dro-plas″te) plastic repair of cartilage 软骨成形术

chon·dro·po·ro·sis (kon″dro-po-ro′sis) the formation of sinuses or spaces in cartilage 软骨疏松

chon·dro·sar·co·ma (kon″dro-sahr-ko′mə) a malignant tumor derived from cartilage cells or their

C

precursors 软骨肉瘤，软骨细胞或其前体衍生的恶性肿瘤；**central c.**, one within a bone, usually not associated with a mass 内生软骨肉瘤

chon·dros·te·o·ma (kon-dros″te-o′mə) osteochondroma 骨软骨瘤

chon·dro·ster·nal (kon″dro-stur′nəl) pertaining to the costal cartilages and the sternum 肋软骨胸骨的

chon·dro·ster·no·plas·ty (kon″dro-stur′no-plas″te) surgical correction of funnel chest 漏斗胸矫正术

chon·drot·o·my (kon-drot′ə-me) the dissection or surgical division of cartilage 软骨切开术

chor·da (kor′də) pl. *chor′dae* [L.] a cord or sinew 腱索；**chor′dal** *adj.* **c. dorsa′lis**, notochord 脊索 c. **mag′na**, Achilles tendon 跟腱；**chor′dae tendi′neae cor′dis**, tendinous cords connecting the two atrioventricular valves to the appropriate papillary muscles in the heart ventricles 腱索，连接房室瓣膜和心室乳头肌的细索；**c. tym′pani**, a nerve originating from the intermediate nerve, distributed to the submandibular, sublingual, and lingual glands and anterior twothirds of the tongue; it is a parasympathetic and special sensory nerve 鼓索，起源于中间神经的神经，分布于下颌下、舌下、舌腺和舌前两翼；是副交感神经和特殊感觉神经

Chor·da·ta (kor-da′tə) a phylum of the animal kingdom comprising all animals having a notochord during some developmental stage 脊索动物类，动物的一个门，包括所有发育阶段的脊索动物

chor·date (kor′dāt) 1. an animal of the Chordata 脊索动物；2. having a notochord 有脊索的

chor·dee (kor′de) (kor′da) downward bowing of the penis, due to a congenital anomaly or to urethral infection 阴茎下弯畸形

chor·di·tis (kor-di′tis) inflammation of a vocal cord or spermatic cord 声带炎，精索炎

chor·do·ma (kor-do′mə) a malignant tumor arising from the embryonic remains of the notochord 脊索瘤，由脊索胚胎残体引起的恶性肿瘤

Chor·do·pox·vi·ri·nae (kor″do-poks″vir-i′ne) poxviruses of vertebrates: a subfamily of viruses of the family Poxviridae, containing the poxviruses that infect vertebrates. It includes the genus *Orthopoxvirus* 脊椎动物痘病毒亚科，痘病毒科的亚科，包含感染脊椎动物的痘病毒，包括正痘病毒属

chor·do·skel·e·ton (kor″do-skel′ə-ton) the part of the bony skeleton formed about the notochord 脊索骨骼，脊索四周的骨骼

chor·dot·o·my (kor-dot′ə-me) cordotomy 脊髓前侧柱切断术

cho·rea (kə-re′ə) [L.] the ceaseless occurrence of rapid, jerky, dyskinetic, involuntary movements 舞蹈症，快速、抽动性、运动障碍性的、非自主的运动持续发生；**chore′al, chore′ic** *adj.* **acute c.**, Sydenham c. 急性舞蹈病；**Huntington c.**, 亨廷顿舞蹈症，见 *disease* 下词条；**Sydenham c.**, a self-limited disorder, occurring between the ages of 5 and 15, or during pregnancy, linked with rheumatic fever, and marked by involuntary movements that gradually become severe, affecting all motor activities 小舞蹈症，自限性疾病，发生在 5—15 岁，或在怀孕期间，与风湿热有关，以逐渐加重的非自主性运动为特征，影响所有活动

cho·re·i·form (kə-re′ ĭ-form) resembling chorea 舞蹈症样的

cho·reo·acan·tho·cy·to·sis (kor″e-o-ə-kan″tho-si-to′sis) an autosomal recessive syndrome characterized by tics, chorea, and personality changes, with acanthocytes in the blood 神经棘红细胞增多症，常染色体隐性遗传综合征，以抽搐、舞蹈症和人格改变为特征，血液中有棘细胞

cho·reo·ath·e·to·sis (kor″e-o-ath″ə-to′sis) a condition characterized by choreic and athetoid movements 舞蹈徐动症，以舞蹈病样和手足徐动为特征；**choreoathetot′ic** *adj.*

cho·rio·ad·e·no·ma (kor″e-o-ad″ə-no′mə) adenoma of the chorion 绒毛膜腺瘤；**c. destru′ens**, a hydatidiform mole in which molar chorionic villi enter the myometrium or parametrium or, rarely, are transported to distant sites, most often the lungs 破坏性绒毛膜瘤，葡萄胎绒毛侵入子宫肌层或子宫旁组织，或有远处转移，通常是肺

cho·rio·al·lan·to·is (kor″e-o-ə-lan′to-is) an extraembryonic structure formed by union of the chorion and allantois, which by means of vessels in the associated mesoderm serves in gas exchange. In reptiles and birds, it is a membrane apposed to the shell; in many mammals, it forms the placenta 尿囊绒膜，绒毛膜与尿囊结合形成的胚胎外结构，通过中胚层中的血管进行气体交换；在爬行动物和鸟类中，它是一层紧贴外壳的膜，在多数哺乳动物中，其形成胎盘；**chorioallanto′ic** *adj.*

cho·rio·am·ni·o·ni·tis (kor″e-o-am″ne-o-ni′tis) inflammation of the chorion and amnion 绒毛膜羊膜炎

cho·rio·an·gi·o·ma (kor″e-o-an″je-o′mə) an angioma of the chorion 绒毛膜血管瘤

cho·rio·cap·il·la·ris (kor″e-o-kap″ĭ-lar′is) lamina choroidocapillaris 脉络膜毛细血管

cho·rio·car·ci·no·ma (kor″e-o-kahr″sĭ-no′mə) a malignant neoplasm of trophoblastic cells, formed by abnormal proliferation of the placental epithelium, without production of chorionic villi; most arise in the uterus 绒毛膜癌，滋养层细胞的恶性肿瘤，由胎盘上皮的异常增殖形成，不产生绒毛膜绒毛，大多数发生在子宫内

cho·rio·cele (kor′e-o-sēl″) protrusion of the chorion through an aperture 脉络膜膨出

cho·rio·epi·the·li·o·ma (kor″e-o-ep″ĭ-the″leo′mə) choriocarcinoma 绒毛膜上皮癌

cho·rio·gen·e·sis (kor″e-o-jen′ə-sis) the development of the chorion 绒毛膜形成

cho·rio·go·nad·o·tro·pin (kor″e-o-go″nə-do-tro″pin) chorionic gonadotropin 绒毛膜促性腺激素；**c. alfa,** human chorionic gonadotropin produced by recombinant technology, used to induce ovulation and pregnancy in certain infertile, anovulatory women, and to stimulate oocyte development and maturation in patients using assisted reproductive technologies 绒毛促性腺激素 α，采用重组技术生产的人绒毛膜促性腺激素，用于诱导不孕、无排卵妇女排卵和妊娠，并通过辅助生殖技术刺激患者卵母细胞发育和成熟

cho·ri·oid (kor′e-oid) choroid 脉络膜

cho·ri·o·ma (kor″e-o′mə) 1. any trophoblastic proliferation, benign or malignant 任何滋养层良性或恶性增生；2. choriocarcinoma 绒毛膜癌

cho·rio·men·in·gi·tis (kor″e-o-men″in-ji′tis) cerebral meningitis with lymphocytic infiltration of the choroid plexus 脉络丛脑膜炎，伴有脉络丛淋巴细胞浸润的脑膜炎；**lymphocytic c.,** viral meningitis, occurring in adults between the ages of 20 and 40, during the fall and winter 淋巴细胞（性）脉络丛脑膜炎，病毒性脑膜炎，发生于20—40岁的成人，秋季和冬季高发

cho·ri·on (kor′e-on) 1. in human embryology, the cellular, outermost extraembryonic membrane, composed of trophoblast lined with mesoderm; it develops villi, becomes vascularized by allantoic vessels, and forms the fetal part of the placenta 绒毛膜，人类胚胎学中，滋养细胞和中胚层组成的最外层的细胞外膜，它发育绒毛，通过尿囊血管化，形成胎盘的胎儿部分；2. in mammalian embryology, the cellular, outer extraembryonic membrane, not necessarily developing villi 哺乳动物胚胎学中，为细胞外胚膜，不一定发育成绒毛；3. in biology, the noncellular membrane covering eggs of various animals, e.g., fish and insects 卵壳，生物学中，覆盖各种动物（如鱼和昆虫）卵的非细胞膜；**chorial, chorion′ic** adj. **c. frondo′sum,** the part of chorion bearing villi 叶状绒毛膜，绒毛膜的绒毛部分；**c. lae′ve,** the nonvillous, membranous part of the chorion 平滑绒毛膜，绒毛膜无绒毛、膜性的部分；**shaggy c., villous c.,** c. frondosum 丛密绒毛膜，叶状绒毛膜

cho·rio·ret·i·nal (kor″e-o-ret′ ĭ-nəl) pertaining to the choroid and retina 脉络膜视网膜的

cho·rio·ret·i·ni·tis (kor″e-o-ret′ ĭ-ni′tis) inflammation of the choroid and retina 脉络膜视网膜炎

cho·rio·ret·i·nop·a·thy (kor″e-o-ret″ĭ-nop′ə-the) a noninflammatory process involving both the choroid and retina 脉络膜视网膜病变，涉及脉络膜和视网膜的非炎性病变

cho·ris·to·ma (kor″is-to′mə) a mass of histologically normal tissue in an abnormal location 迷芽瘤，迷离瘤，组织学上指器官或机体某部来源正常、只是不在其正常位置的组织块

cho·roid (kor′oid) 1. the middle, vascular coat of the eyeball, between the sclera and the retina 脉络膜，眼球的中层，血管膜，位于巩膜和视网膜之间；2. resembling the chorion 绒毛膜样的。Spelled also *chorioid.* **choroid′al** adj.

cho·roi·dea (kor-oid′e-ə) choroid 脉络膜

cho·roid·er·e·mia (kor″oid-ər-e′me-ə) an X-linked primary choroidal degeneration, which, in males, eventually leads to blindness as degeneration of the retinal pigment epithelium progresses to complete atrophy; in females, it is nonprogressive and vision is usually normal 无脉络膜，X-连锁原发性脉络膜退行性变；男性患者，随着视网膜色素上皮的退行性变逐渐完全萎缩，最终导致失明；女性患者，该病是无进展的，视力通常正常

cho·roid·itis (kor″oid-i′tis) inflammation of the choroid 脉络膜炎

cho·roi·do·cyc·li·tis (kor-oi″do-sik-li′tis) inflammation of the choroid and ciliary processes 脉络膜睫状体炎

chro·maf·fin (kro-maf′in) staining strongly with chromium salts, as the chromaffin cells 嗜铬的，铬盐染色深，如嗜铬细胞

chro·maf·fi·no·ma (kro-maf″ĭ-no′mə) any tumor containing chromaffin cells, such as pheochromocytoma 嗜铬瘤，任何含有嗜铬细胞的肿瘤，如嗜铬细胞瘤

chro·maf·fi·nop·a·thy (kro-maf″ĭ-nop′ə-the) disease of the chromaffin system 嗜铬系统疾病

chro·mate (kro′māt) any salt of chromic acid 铬酸盐

chro·mat·ic (kro-mat′ik) 1. pertaining to color; stainable with dyes 关于颜色的；可染色的；2. pertaining to chromatin 与染色质有关

chro·ma·tid (kro′mə-tid) one of the paired daughter strands, joined at the centromere, which make up a chromosome after it has replicated. After division of the centromere, each becomes a separate chromosome 染色单体，在着丝粒处连接的成对的子链中的一条，其在复制后形成一条染色体；在着丝粒分裂后，每一个都成为一个单独的染色体

chro·ma·tin (kro′mə-tin) the complex of nucleic acids and proteins (primarily histones) in the eukaryotic cell nucleus, that constitutes the chromosomes 染色质，真核细胞核内构成染色体的核酸和蛋

C

白质（主要是组蛋白）的复合体；**chromatin'ic** *adj.* sex c., Barr body 性染色质，巴氏小体

chro·ma·tin-neg·a·tive (kro″mə-tin-neg′ə-tiv) lacking sex chromatin (Barr body); characteristic of the somatic cell nuclei of normal human males or other individuals with only one X chromosome 性染色质阴性，缺乏性染色质（巴氏小体）；只有一条 X 染色体的正常男性或其他个体的体细胞核特征

chro·ma·tin-pos·i·tive (kro″mə-tin-poz′ ĭ-tiv) containing sex chromatin (Barr body); characteristic of the somatic cell nuclei of normal human females and other individuals with at least two X chromosomes 性染色质阳性，含有性染色质（巴氏小体）；至少含有两条 X 染色体的正常人类女性和其他个体的体细胞核特征

chro·ma·tism (kro′mə-tiz″əm) abnormal pigment deposits 色（像）差

chro·ma·tog·e·nous (kro″mə-toj′ə-nəs) producing color or coloring matter 产色的，产生颜色或染色物质

chro·mato·gram (kro-mat′o-gram) the record produced by chromatography 色谱图，层析谱

chro·mato·graph (kro-mat′o-graf) 1. the apparatus used in chromatography 色谱仪，用于色谱分析的仪器；2. to analyze by chromatography 用色谱法分析

chro·ma·tog·ra·phy (kro″mə-tog′rə-fe) a method of separating and identifying the components of a complex mixture by differential movement through a two-phase system, in which the movement is effected by a flow of a liquid or a gas (mobile phase), which percolates through an adsorbent (stationary phase) or a second liquid phase 色谱法，通过两相系统的微分运动和识别复杂混合物成分的一种方法，其中运动受液体或气体（流动相）的流动影响，该流动通过吸附剂（固定相）或第二液相渗透；**chromatograph'ic** *adj.* adsorption c., that in which the stationary phase is an adsorbent 吸附色谱法，吸附层析，其中固定相是一种吸附剂；affinity c., that based on a highly specific biologic interaction such as that between antigen and antibody or receptor and ligand, one such substance being immobilized and acting as the sorbent 亲和色谱法，亲和层析，基于抗原与抗体或受体与配体等高度特异性的生物体相互作用，其中一种物质被固定并作为吸附剂；column c., that in which the various solutes of a solution are allowed to travel down an absorptive column, the individual components being absorbed by the stationary phase 柱色谱法，柱层析，溶液中的各种溶质沿着吸收柱向下流动的色谱法，其中个别组分被固定相吸收；gas c. (GC), that in which an inert gas moves

the vapors of the materials to be separated through a column of inert material 气相色谱法（气相层析），惰性气体移动待分离物质的蒸汽通过惰性物质柱；gas-liquid c. (GLC), gas chromatography in which the sorbent is a nonvolatile liquid coated on a solid support 气 - 液色谱法，气液层析，一种气相色谱法，其中吸附剂是一种覆盖在固体载体上的不挥发液体；gas-solid c. (GSC), gas chromatography in which the sorbent is an inert porous solid 气 - 固色谱法，气固层析，吸附剂为惰性多孔固体的气相色谱法；gel filtration c., gel permeation c., that in which the stationary phase consists of gel-forming hydrophilic beads containing specifically sized pores that trap and delay molecules small enough to enter them. 凝胶过滤色谱法，凝胶渗透色谱法，其中固定相是由凝胶形成的亲水珠，其包含特定大小的孔，该法捕获并延迟小分子进入它们的分子；high-performance liquid c., high-pressure liquid c. (HPLC), a type of automated chromatography in which the mobile phase is a liquid that is forced under high pressure through a column packed with a sorbent 高效液相色谱法，高压液相色谱法，一种自动色谱法，其中流动相是一种液体，在高压下通过填充有吸附剂的柱强制流动；ion exchange c., that in which the stationary phase is an ion exchange resin 离子交换色谱法，其中固定相是离子交换树脂；molecular exclusion c., molecular sieve c., gel filtration c. 分子排阻色谱法、分子筛色谱法；paper c., that using a sheet of blotting paper, usually filter paper, for the adsorption column 纸色谱法，即用一张吸墨纸，通常是滤纸，作为吸附柱；partition c., a method using the partition of the solutes between two liquid phases (the original solvent and the film of solvent on the adsorption column) 分配色谱法，利用两个液相（吸附柱上的原始溶剂和溶剂膜）之间的溶质不同进行分离的方法；thin-layer c. (TLC), chromatography through a thin layer of inert material, such as cellulose 薄层色谱法，通过一薄层惰性物质，如纤维素进行色谱分析

chro·ma·toid (kro′mə-toid) dyeing or staining like, or otherwise resembling, chromatin 拟染色体；染色或染色样的，或其他类似染色质

chro·ma·tol·y·sis (kro″mə-tol′ə-sis) disintegration of Nissl bodies of a neuron as a result of injury, fatigue, or exhaustion 尼氏体溶解，神经元尼氏体由于损伤、疲劳、衰竭而崩解

chro·ma·to·phil (kro-mat′o-fil″) a cell or structure that stains easily 易染细胞，容易染色的细胞或结构；**chromatophil'ic** *adj.*

chro·mato·phore (kro-mat′o-for″) a pigment cell in animals or color-producing organelle in plant cells 色素细胞，动物中的色素细胞或植物细胞中

产生颜色的细胞器

chro·ma·top·sia (kro″mə-top′se-ə) a visual defect in which colorless objects appear to be tinged with color 色视症，视觉缺陷，无色物体似乎带有色彩

chro·ma·top·tom·e·try (kro″mə-top-tom′ə-tre) measurement of color perception 色觉检查

chro·ma·tu·ria (kro″mə-tu′re-ə) abnormal coloration of the urine 色素尿，尿液颜色异常

chro·mes·the·sia (kro″mes-the′zhə) association of imaginary color sensations with actual sensations of taste, hearing, or smell 假色觉，假想的颜色感觉与实际的味觉、听觉或嗅觉的联系

chrom·hi·dro·sis (kro″mī-dro′sis) secretion of colored sweat 色汗症，有色汗液分泌

chro·mic (kro′mik) of, pertaining to, or related to chromium 铬的；**c. phosphate P 32,** a radiolabeled phosphate salt of chromium used in the treatment of metastatic intrapleural or intraperitoneal effusions and of certain ovarian and prostate carcinomas 磷酸铬P32，一种放射性标记的含铬磷酸盐，用于治疗转移性胸膜内或腹膜内积液以及某些卵巢癌和前列腺癌

chro·mic ac·id (kro′mik) the common name for chromium trioxide (CrO₃), although the term strictly refers to the species H₂CrO₄, which exists only in aqueous solution. It is a highly toxic, corrosive, strong oxidizing agent 铬酸，三氧化铬（CrO₃）的通用名称，是一种剧毒、腐蚀性强的氧化剂

chro·mi·um (Cr) (kro′me-əm) a silver-white, lustrous, hard, metallic element; at. no. 24, at. wt. 51.996. In the trivalent state it is an essential dietary trace element, but hexavalent chromium is carcinogenic 铬（Cr），银白色，有光泽，坚硬，金属元素；原子序数24，原子质量51.996，三价态是必需的膳食微量元素，六价铬具有致癌作用；**c. 51,** a radioactive isotope of chromium having a half-life of 27.7 days and decaying by electron capture with emission of gamma rays (0.32 MeV); it is used to label red blood cells for measurement of mass or volume, survival time, and sequestration studies, for the diagnosis of gastrointestinal bleeding, and to label platelets to study their survival 铬51，铬的一种放射性同位素，半衰期为27.7天，通过释放伽马射线（0.32兆电子伏）捕获电子而衰变；用于标记红细胞，以测量其质量或体积、存活时间和整合作用，诊断胃肠道出血，并标记血小板以研究其存活率；**c. trioxide,** chromic acid 三氧化铬

Chro·mo·bac·te·ri·um (kro″mo-bak-tēr′e-əm) a genus of gram-negative, rod-shaped bacteria of the family Neisseriaceae, found in soil and water in tropical countries, and characteristically producing violet pigment. Members are usually nonpathogenic, but *C. viola'ceum* may cause abscesses, diarrhea, and urinary tract and systemic infections 色杆菌属，革兰阴性杆菌属，产于热带国家的土壤和水中，特征是被染成紫色；紫色杆菌成员通常是非致病性的，但可引起脓肿、腹泻、尿路和全身感染

chro·mo·blast (kro′mo-blast) an embryonic cell that develops into a pigment cell 成色素细胞，发育成色素细胞的胚胎细胞

chro·mo·blas·to·my·co·sis (kro″mo-blas″tomi-ko′sis) a chronic fungal infection of the skin, producing wartlike nodules or papillomas that may ulcerate 着色芽生菌病，皮肤的慢性真菌感染，产生疣状结节或乳头状瘤，可能溃烂

chro·mo·cys·tos·co·py (kro″mo-sis-tos′kə-pe) cystoscopy of the ureteral orifices after oral administration of a dye that is excreted in the urine 染色膀胱镜检查，膀胱镜检查口服染料后输尿管口的尿液排出情况

chro·mo·cyte (kro′mo-sīt) any colored cell or pigmented corpuscle 色素细胞，任何有色细胞或色素小体

chro·mo·dac·ry·or·rhea (kro″mo-dak″re-ore′ə) the shedding of bloody tears 血泪症

chro·mo·gen (kro′mo-jən) any substance giving origin to a coloring matter 色原，任何产生颜色的物质

chro·mo·gen·e·sis (kro″mo-jen′ə-sis) the formation of color or pigment 色素形成

chro·mo·gran·in (kro″mo-gran′in) any of a group of acidic polypeptides that are the major soluble protein constituents of the secretory granules of the chromaffin cells of the adrenal medulla; they are also widely distributed in endocrine tissues and tumor cells. Some are precursors of peptide hormones 嗜铬粒蛋白，一种酸性多肽，肾上腺髓质嗜铬细胞分泌颗粒中主要的可溶性蛋白成分，也广泛分布于内分泌组织和肿瘤细胞中，有些是肽类激素的前体

chro·mo·mere (kro′mo-mēr) one of the series of beadlike granules occurring along eukaryotic chromosomes, representing localized coiling and condensation of the chromatin 染色粒，真核细胞染色体上出现的一系列珠状颗粒，代表染色质的局部卷曲和凝集

chro·mo·my·co·sis (kro″mo-mi-ko′sis) chromoblastomycosis 着色芽生菌病

chro·mo·ne·ma (kro″mo-ne′mə) pl. *chromone'mata.* The central thread of a chromatid, along which lie the chromomeres 染色线，染色单体的中心线，染色单体沿其分布; **chromone'mal** adj.

chro·mo·phil (kro′mo-fil) any easily stainable cell or tissue 易染细胞; **chromophil'ic** adj.

chro·mo·phobe (kro′mo-fōb) any cell or tissue not readily stainable, such as the chromophobe cells in the anterior lobe of the pituitary 嫌色，不易染色的细胞或组织，如垂体前叶的嫌色细胞

chro·mo·pho·bia (kro″mo-fo′be-ə) the quality of staining poorly with dyes 嫌色性，难染色的；**chromopho′bic** adj.

chro·mo·phore (kro′mo-for) any chemical group whose presence gives a decided color to a compound and which unites with certain other groups (auxochromes) to form dyes 生色团，化学基团，其存在使化合物具有确定的颜色，并与某些其它基团（助色基团）结合形成染料

chro·mo·phor·ic (kro″mo-for′ik) 1. bearing color 承载颜色；2. pertaining to a chromophore 关于发色团的

chro·mo·phose (kro′mo-fōs) sensation of color 色幻视

chro·mos·co·py (kro-mos′kə-pe) diagnosis of renal function by color of the urine after administration of dyes 尿色检查法，观察给予染色剂后尿液颜色以对肾功能进行评断

chro·mo·some (kro′mə-sōm) 1. in eukaryotic cells, a structure in the nucleus consisting of chromatin (q.v.) and carrying the genetic information for the cell. Each organism of a species is normally characterized by the same number of chromosomes in its somatic cells; 46 is the number in humans, including the two (XX or XY) that determine the sex 染色体，真核细胞中，细胞核中的一种结构，由染色质组成，并携带细胞的遗传信息，种的每一个有机体在其细胞中的染色体数目通常相同；人类有 46 条染色体，包括决定性别的 XX 或 XY 染色体；2. the analogous structure carrying the genetic material in prokaryotes, mitochondria, and chloroplasts; a closed circle of double-stranded DNA 在原核生物、线粒体和叶绿体中携带遗传物质的类似结构；双链闭合环 DNA；**chromo′somal** adj. **homologous c′s**, a matching pair of chromosomes, one from each parent, with the same gene loci in the same order 同源染色体，一对配对的染色体，父母各提供一条，基因座序相同；**Ph¹ c.**, **Philadelphia c.**, an abnormality of chromosome 22 present in chronic myelogenous leukemia; generally a reciprocal translocation between chromosomes 9 and 22 that results in expression of an oncogenic fusion gene 费城染色体，存在于慢性粒细胞白血病中的 22 号染色体异常；通常是 9 号和 22 号染色体之间的相互易位，导致致癌融合基因的表达；**ring c. (r)**, a chromosome in which both ends have been lost (deletion) and the two broken ends have reunited to form a ring 环状染色体，染色体两端丢失（缺失），两个断端重新结合形成一个环；

sex c′s, those associated with sex determination, in mammals constituting an unequal pair, the X and Y chromosomes 性染色体，与性别决定有关的染色体，在哺乳动物中构成不相等的 X 和 Y 染色体；**somatic c.**, autosome 体细胞染色体，常染色体；**X c.**, the sex chromosome present in two copies in human female somatic cells; carried by half the male gametes and all female gametes X 染色体，存在于女性体细胞中的性染色体，一半雄性配子和所有雌性配子携带；**Y c.**, the sex chromosome present in human male somatic cells, but not female; carried by half the male gametes and none of the female gametes Y 染色体，存在于男性体细胞中的性染色体；由一半的雄性配子携带，雌性配子不携带

chro·naxy (kro′nak-se) the minimum time an electric current must flow at a voltage twice the rheobase to cause a muscle to contract. Spelled also *chronaxie* 时值，在阈值两倍的电压下，为引起肌肉收缩，流过电流必须的最短时间

chron·ic (kron′ik) persisting for a long time 慢性的

chron·o·bi·ol·o·gy (kron″o-bi-ol′ə-je) the scientific study of the effect of time on living systems and of biologic rhythms 时间生物学，研究时间对生物系统和生物节律影响的科学；**chronobiolog′ic, chronobiolog′ical** adj.

chron·og·no·sis (kron″og-no′sis) perception of the lapse of time 时觉，对时间流逝的感知

chron·o·graph (kron′o-graf) an instrument for recording small intervals of time 计时器，用于记录较短的时间

chron·o·phil·ia (kron′o-fil′e-ə) sexual attraction to those of a specific age range 年龄偏好症对特定年龄阶段的性偏好

chron·o·tar·ax·is (kron″o-tər-ak′sis) disorientation in relation to time 时间错觉

chron·not·ro·pism (kro-not′ro-piz-əm) interference with regularity of a periodical movement, such as the heart's action 变时现象，对周期性运动规律性（如心搏）的干扰；**chronotro′pic** adj.

chry·si·a·sis (krī-si′ə-sis) deposition of gold in living tissue 金沉着病

chryso·der·ma (kris″o-dur′mə) permanent pigmentation of the skin due to gold deposit 金沉着性皮变色，由于金沉积而造成的皮肤永久性色素沉着

Chryso·my·ia (kris″o-mi′yə) a genus of flies whose larvae may be secondary invaders of wounds or internal parasites of humans 金蝇，苍蝇属，其幼虫可能是人类伤口或内部寄生虫的第二入侵者

Chrys·ops (kris′ops) a genus of small bloodsucking horse flies, including *C. disca′lis*, a vector of tularemia in the western United States, and *C. sila′cea*, an intermediate host of *Loa loa* 斑虻，吸血小马蝇属，包括美国西部兔热病的媒介中室斑虻，及罗阿丝虫的中间宿主静斑虻

chryso·ther·a·py (kris″o-ther′ə-pe) treatment with gold salts 金疗法

chryso·tile (kris′o-tīl) the most widely used form of asbestos, a gray-green magnesium silicate in the serpentine class of asbestos; its dust may cause asbestosis or, rarely, mesotheliomas or other lung cancers 温石棉，石棉使用最广泛的一种形式，灰绿色硅酸镁蛇纹样石棉; 其粉尘可引起石棉病，或引起间皮瘤或其他肺癌

CHS cholinesterase 胆碱酯酶

chy·lan·gi·o·ma (ki-lan″je-o′mə) a tumor of intestinal lymph vessels filled with chyle 乳糜管瘤，充满乳糜的肠淋巴管肿瘤

chyle (kīl) the milky fluid taken up by the lacteals from food in the intestine, consisting of an emulsion of lymph and triglyceride fat (chylomicrons); it passes into the veins by the thoracic duct and mixes with blood 乳糜，食物被小肠乳糜管吸收形成的乳状液体，由淋巴乳剂和长链脂肪乳（乳糜微粒）组成；通过胸导管进入静脉与血液混合

chyl·ec·ta·sia (ki″lek-ta′zhah) dilatation of a lacteal 乳糜管扩张

chy·le·mia (ki-le′me-ə) chyle in the blood 乳糜血

chy·li·form (ki′lĭ-form) resembling chyle 乳糜样

chy·lo·me·di·as·ti·num (ki″lo-me″de-ə-sti′nəm) chyle in the mediastinum 纵隔乳糜

chy·lo·mi·cron (ki″lo-mi′kron) a class of lipoproteins that transport exogenous (dietary) cholesterol and triglycerides after meals from the small intestine to tissues for degradation to chylomicron remnants 乳糜微粒，脂蛋白的一种，在饭后将外源性（饮食性）胆固醇和甘油三酯从小肠输送到组织，以降解为乳糜微粒残余物

chy·lo·mi·cro·ne·mia (ki″lo-mi″kro-ne′me-ə) an excess of chylomicrons in the blood 乳糜微粒血症

chy·lo·peri·car·di·um (ki″lo-per″ĭ-kahr′de-əm) effused chyle in the pericardium 乳糜心包

chy·lo·peri·to·ne·um (ki″lo-per″ĭ-to-ne′əm) effused chyle in the peritoneal cavity 乳糜腹

chy·lo·pneu·mo·tho·rax (ki″lo-noo″ mothor′aks) chyle and air in the pleural cavity 乳糜气胸

chy·lo·tho·rax (ki″lo-thor′aks) pleural effusion of chyle or chylelike fluid 乳糜胸

chy·lous (ki′ləs) pertaining to or mixed with chyle 乳糜的

chy·lu·ria (kīl-u′re-ə) chyle in the urine, due to obstruction between the intestinal lymphatics and the thoracic duct and rupture of renal lymphatics into the renal tubules 乳糜尿，由于肠淋巴管和胸导管之间的阻塞以及肾淋巴管破裂进入肾小管，尿液中出现乳糜

chyme (kīm) the semifluid, creamy material produced by digestion of food 食糜，由食物消化产生的半流质、乳脂状物质

chy·mi·fi·ca·tion (ki″mĭ-fĭ-ka′shən) conversion of food into chyme 食糜生成，把食物变成食糜；gastric digestion 胃消化

chy·mo·pa·pain (ki″mo-pə-pān′) a cysteine endopeptidase from the tropical tree *Carica papaya*; it catalyzes the hydrolysis of proteins and polypeptides with a specificity similar to that of papain and is used in chemonucleolysis 凝乳蛋白酶，热带番木瓜树的半胱氨酸内肽酶，催化蛋白质和多肽的水解，具有与木瓜蛋白酶相似的特异性，用于化学溶解

chy·mo·sin (ki′mo-sin) rennin; an enzyme that catalyzes the cleavage of casein to form soluble paracasein, which then reacts with calcium to form a curd, insoluble paracasein. It is found in the fourth stomach of the calf and other ruminants. A commercial preparation, rennet, is used for making cheese and rennet custards 凝乳酶，催化酪蛋白分解形成可溶性副酪蛋白的酶，与钙反应形成凝乳，不溶性副酪蛋白；在小牛和其他反刍动物的第四个胃中发现；一种商业制剂，用于制作奶酪和蛋挞

chy·mo·tryp·sin (ki″mo-trip′sin) an endopeptidase with action similar to that of trypsin, produced in the intestine by activation of chymotrypsinogen by trypsin; a product crystallized from an extract of the pancreas of the ox is used clinically for enzymatic zonulolysis and debridement 糜蛋白酶，作用类似于胰蛋白酶的内肽酶，由胰蛋白酶在肠内激活糜蛋白酶原产生；临床上用从牛胰腺提取物中结晶的产品进行酶睫状小带松解和清创

chy·mo·tryp·sin·o·gen (ki″mo-trip-sin′o-jən) an inactive proenzyme secreted by the pancreas and cleaved by trypsin in the small intestine to yield chymotrypsin 胰凝乳蛋白酶原，由胰腺分泌并在小肠内被胰蛋白酶裂解生成胰凝乳蛋白酶的非活性酶原

CI cardiac index 心脏指数；Colour Index 颜色指数

Ci curie 居里，放射性强度单位

cib. [L.] ci′bus (food) 食品物

cic·a·trec·to·my (sik″ə-trek′tə-me) excision of a cicatrix 瘢痕切除术

cic·a·tri·cial (sik″ə-trish′əl) pertaining to or of the nature of a cicatrix 瘢痕性的

cic·a·trix (sĭ-ka′triks) (sik′ə-triks) pl. *cica′trices* [L.] scar 瘢痕；**vicious c.**, one causing deformity or impairing the function of a limb 恶性瘢痕，导致肢体畸形或损害肢体功能

cic·a·tri·za·tion (sik″ə-trĭ-za′shən) the formation

of a cicatrix or scar 瘢痕形成

cic·lo·pir·ox (si″klo-pēr′oks) (si″klo-pir′oks) a broad-spectrum antifungal with activity similar to that of the imidazoles; applied topically as the olamine salt 环吡酮, 广谱抗真菌药, 具有类似于咪唑类化合物的活性; 局部用药用其乙醇胺盐

ci·dof·o·vir (sī-dof′o-vir) an antiviral nucleoside analogue used in the treatment of cytomegalovirus retinitis in patients with acquired immunodeficiency syndrome 西多福韦, 用于治疗获得性免疫缺陷综合征患者巨细胞病毒视网膜炎的抗病核苷类似物

CIDP chronic inflammatory demyelinating polyneuropathy 慢性炎性脱髓鞘性多发性神经病

ci·gua·te·ra (se″gwǝ-ta′rǝ) a form of ichthyosarcotoxism, marked by gastrointestinal and neurologic symptoms due to ingestion of tropical or subtropical marine fish that have ciguatoxin in their tissues 鱼肉毒, 一种鱼肉中毒, 以消化道和神经系统症状为特征, 由于摄入了组织中含有雪卡毒素的热带或亚热带海鱼所致

ci·gua·tox·in (se′gwǝ-tok″sin) a heat-stable toxin originating in the dinoflagellate *Gambierdiscus toxicus* as a pretoxin and concentrated as the active form in the tissues of certain marine fish; it causes ciguatera 雪卡毒素, 热稳定毒素, 源于冈比亚鞭毛虫毒素, 作为前毒素, 在某些海洋鱼类的组织中以活性形式富集; 可引起雪卡食物中毒

ci·la·stat·in (si″lǝ-stat′in) a dipeptidase inhibitor used with imipenem to decrease the metabolism of imipenem in the kidneys and increase its concentration in the urine; administered as the sodium salt 西司他丁, 与亚胺培南一起使用的二肽酶抑制药, 用于降低亚胺培南在肾脏中的代谢并增加其在尿液中的浓度; 常用其钠盐

cil·ia (sil′e-ǝ) sing. *cil′ium*. [L.] 1. the eyelids or their outer edges 眼睑或其外缘; 2. the eyelashes 睫毛; 3. minute hairlike processes that extend from a cell surface, composed of nine pairs of microtubules around a core of two microtubules. They beat rhythmically to move the cell or to move fluid or mucus over the surface 纤毛, 从细胞表面延伸出来的微小的毛状突起, 由围绕两个微管核心的九对微管组成, 有节奏地跳动以移动其表面的细胞、液体或黏液

cil·i·ar·ot·o·my (sil″e-ǝ-rot′ǝ-me) surgical division of the ciliary zone 睫状体切开术

cil·i·ary (sil′e-ar″e) pertaining to or resembling cilia; used particularly in reference to certain eye structures, as the ciliary body or muscle 纤毛状的; 特别用于指某些眼睛结构, 如睫状体或睫状肌

cil·i·ate (sil′e-āt) 1. having cilia 有纤毛的; 2. any individual of the Ciliophora 纤毛虫

cil·i·ec·to·my (sil″e-ek′tǝ-me) 睫状体切除术 1. excision of a portion of the ciliary body 切除睫状体的一部分; 2. excision of the portion of the eyelid containing the roots of the lashes 切除包含睫毛根部的眼睑部分

cil·i·op·athy (sil-ee″op′athy) any of a group of human genetics disorders associated with mutations encoding defective proteins; the mutations result in abnormal formation or function of cilia; may manifest in various forms, including retinal degeneration, renal disease, cerebral anomalies, congenital fibrocystic diseases of the liver, diabetes, obesity, and skeletal dysplasias 纤毛病, 一组与编码缺陷蛋白的突变有关的人类遗传疾病; 突变导致纤毛的异常形成或功能异常; 可表现为多种形式, 包括视网膜变性、肾病、大脑异常、先天性肝纤维囊性疾病、糖尿病、肥胖和骨骼发育不良

Cil·i·oph·o·ra (sil″e-of′ǝ-rǝ) a phylum of protozoa whose members possess cilia during some developmental stage and usually have two kinds of nuclei (a micro- and a macronucleus); it includes the Kinetofragminophorea, Oligohymenophorea, and Polyhymenophorea 纤毛亚门, 原生动物中的一门, 在某些发育阶段具有纤毛, 通常有两种细胞核（微核和大核）; 包括动基裂纲、寡膜纲和多膜纲

cil·io·spi·nal (sil″e-o-spi′nǝl) pertaining to the ciliary body and the spinal cord 睫状体脊髓的

cil·i·um (sil′e-ǝm) [L.] *cilia.* 的单数形式, 纤毛

cil·o·sta·zol (sī-lo′stǝ-zol) a phosphodiesterase inhibitor that inhibits platelet aggregation and causes vasodilation; used in the treatment of intermittent claudication 西洛他唑, 抑制血小板聚集并引起血管扩张的磷酸二酯酶抑制药; 用于治疗间歇性跛行

cim·bia (sim′be-ǝ) a white band running across the ventral surface of the crus cerebri 大脑脚横束

ci·met·i·dine (si-met′ĭ-dēn) a histamine H₂ receptor antagonist, which inhibits gastric acid secretion; used as the base or the monohydrochloride salt in the treatment and prophylaxis of gastric or duodenal ulcers, gastroesophageal reflux disease, upper gastrointestinal bleeding, and conditions associated with gastric hypersecretion 西米替丁, 抑制胃酸分泌的组胺 H₂ 受体拮抗药, 其碱或单盐酸盐用于治疗和预防胃或十二指肠溃疡、胃食管反流病、上消化道出血以及与胃液分泌过多相关的疾病

Ci·mex (si′mǝks) [L.] a genus of blood-sucking insects (order Hemiptera), the bedbugs; it includes *C. boue′ti* of West Africa and South America, *C. lect·ula′rius*, the common bedbug of temperate regions and *C. rotunda′tus* of the tropics. 吸血昆虫的一个属（半翅目）, 臭虫; 包括西非和南美洲的卜氏臭虫、温带地区常见的温带臭虫（见 *bedbug* 图）和热带

的热带臭虫

CIN   cervical intraepithelial neoplasia 宫颈上皮内瘤变

cin·cho·na   (sin-ko′nə) the dried bark of the stem or root of various South American trees of the genus *Cinchona*; it is the source of quinine and other alkaloids and was used as an antimalarial 金鸡纳，南美金鸡纳树的茎或根的干树皮；其为奎宁和其他生物碱的来源，用作抗疟疾药

cin·cho·nism   (sin′ko-niz″əm) toxicity due to cinchona alkaloid overdosage; symptoms are tinnitus and slight deafness, photophobia and other visual disturbances, mental dullness, depression, confusion, headache, and nausea 金鸡钠中毒，因金鸡纳生物碱过量而产生的毒性反应；症状为耳鸣和轻微耳聋、畏光和其他视觉障碍、精神迟钝、抑郁、精神错乱、头痛和恶心

cine·an·gio·car·diog·ra·phy   (sin″ə-an″je-okahr″de-og′rə-fe) the photographic recording of fluoroscopic images of the heart and great vessels by motion picture techniques 心血管荧光电影照相术，用电影技术拍摄心脏和大血管的荧光图像

cine·an·gi·og·ra·phy   (sin″ə-an″je-og′rə-fe) the photographic recording of fluoroscopic images of the blood vessels by motion picture techniques 血管荧光电影照相术，用电影技术对血管的荧光图像进行摄影记录

cine·ra·di·og·ra·phy   (sin″ə-ra″de-og′rə-fe) the making of a motion picture record of successive images appearing on a fluoroscopic screen 射线电影照相术，对荧光屏上出现的连续影像进行动态记录

ci·ne′rea   (sĭ-nēr′e-ə) substantia grisea 灰质；**cine′real** *adj.*

cinesi-   见 kinesi-

cin·gu·late   (sing′gu-lāt) pertaining to a cingulum 扣带回

cin·gu·lec·to·my   (sing″gu-lek′tə-me) bilateral extirpation of the anterior half of the cingulate gyrus 扣带回切除术，摘除扣带回前半部的双侧

cin·gu·lot·o·my   (sing″gu-lot′ə-me) the creation of lesions in the cingulate gyrus for relief of intractable pain and in the treatment of certain psychiatric disorders 扣带回切开术，切开扣带回，以减轻顽固性疼痛和治疗某些精神疾病

cin·gu·lum   (sing′gu-ləm) pl. *cin′gula* [L.] 1. an encircling structure or part; a girdle 环绕的结构或部分；环绕物; 2. a bundle of association fibers deep to the cingulate gyrus and encircling the corpus callosum close to the median plane, interrelating the cingulate and hippocampal gyri 扣带，一束深至扣带回并环绕靠近正中面脑胼胝体的相关纤维，与扣带回和海马回相互连接; 3. the lingual lobe of an anterior tooth（牙）基嵴

cin·gu·lum·ot·o·my   (sing″gu-ləm-ot′ə-me) cingulotomy 扣带回切开术

C1   **INH** C1 inhibitor C1 抑制物

cip·ro·flox·a·cin   (sip″ro-flok′sə-sin) a synthetic antibacterial effective against many gram-positive and gram-negative bacteria; used as the hydrochloride salt 环丙沙星，对多种革兰阳性和革兰阴性细菌有效的合成抗生素；常用其盐酸盐

cir·ca·di·an   (sər-ka′de-ən) denoting a 24-hour period 昼夜节律；见 *rhythm* 下词条

cir·ci·nate   (sur′sĭ-nāt) 1. circular 圆形; 2. ring-shaped 环形

cir·cle   (sur′kəl) a round structure or part 圆形结构或部分；**Berry c′s,** charts with circles on them for testing stereoscopic vision 贝里环形立体视力表，上面有圈的图表，用于测试立体视觉; **cerebral arterial c.,** c. of Willis 大脑动脉环; **defensive c.,** the coexistence of two conditions that tend to have an antagonistic or inhibiting effect on each other 两种条件共存，往往对彼此有拮抗或抑制作用; **c. of Haller,** a circle of arteries in the sclera at the site of the entrance of the optic nerve 视神经血管环，视神经入口处巩膜内的一圈动脉环; **Minsky c′s,** a series of circles used for the graphic recording of eye lesions Minsky 环，记录眼损害的一种图表; **c. of Willis,** the anastomotic loop of vessels near the base of the brain Willis 环，靠近大脑底部的血管吻合环

cir·cuit   (sur′kət) [L.] the round or course traversed by an electric current 电流穿过的环或路线；**reentrant c.,** the circuit formed by the circulating impulse in reentry 折返环，循环脉冲反复折返形成的回路；**reverberating c.,** a neuronal pathway arranged in a circle so that impulses are recycled to cause positive feedback or reverberation 反响回路，排列成圆圈的神经通路，使脉冲被循环以产生正反馈或混响

cir·cu·la·tion   (sur″ku-la′shən) movement in a regular course, as the movement of blood through the heart and blood vessels 循环，有规律的运动，如血液通过心脏和血管的运动；**collateral c.,** that carried on through secondary channels after obstruction of the principal channel supplying the part 侧支循环，供血的主通道阻塞后，通过辅助血管进行供血；**enterohepatic c.,** the cycle in which bile salts and other substances excreted by the liver are absorbed by the intestinal mucosa and returned to the liver via the portal circulation 肠肝循环，肝脏排出的胆汁盐和其他物质被肠黏膜吸收并经过门静脉循环返回肝脏的循环；**extracorporeal c.,** circulation of blood outside the body, as through an artificial kidney or a heart-lung apparatus 体外循环，血液在体外的循环，

C

如通过人工肾或心肺装置；**fetal c.**, that propelled by the fetal heart through the fetus, umbilical cord, and placental villi 胎儿循环，胎儿心脏推动血液通过胎儿、脐带和胎盘绒毛；**first c., primordial c.; hypophysioportal c.**, that passing from the capillaries of the median eminence of the hypothalamus into the portal vessels to the sinusoids of the anterior lobe of the pituitary 垂体门脉循环，下丘脑正中隆起的毛细血管进入门静脉到垂体前叶的窦状体；**intervillous c.**, the flow of maternal blood through the intervillous space of the placenta 绒毛间循环，母体血液通过胎盘的绒毛间隙流动；肺循环，持续性胎儿循环；**lesser c., pulmonary c.; persistent fetal c.**, persistent pulmonary hypertension of the newborn 新 生 儿 持续性肺动脉高压；**placental c.**, 1. the circulation of blood through the placenta during prenatal life 胎 盘循环，产前通过胎盘的血液循环；绒毛间循环；2. intervillous c. **portal c.**, a general term denoting the circulation of blood through larger vessels from the capillaries of one organ to those of another; applied to the passage of blood from the gastrointestinal tract and spleen through the portal vein to the liver 门脉循环，指血液通过大血管从一个器官的毛细血管到另一个器官的毛细血管的循环；如血液从胃肠道和脾脏经门静脉进入肝脏；**primordial c.**, the earliest circulation by which nutrient material and oxygen are conveyed to the embryo 原始循环，营养物质和氧气被输送到胚胎的最早的循环；**pulmonary c.**, the flow of blood from the right ventricle through the pulmonary artery to the lungs, where carbon dioxide is exchanged for oxygen, and back through the pulmonary vein to the left atrium 肺循环，血流从右心室流经肺动脉到肺，二氧化碳被交换成氧气，然后通过肺静脉回到左心房；**systemic c.**, the general circulation, carrying oxygenated blood from the left ventricle to the body tissues, and returning venous blood to the right atrium 全身循环，左心室向身体组织输送含氧血，并将静脉血返回右心房的一般循环；**umbilical c.**, fetal circulation through the umbilical vessels 脐带循环，胎儿通过脐带血管的循环；**vitelline c.**, the circulation through the blood vessels of the yolk sac 卵黄囊循环，通过卵黄囊血管的循环

cir·cu·la·to·ry (sur′ ku-lə-tor″e) 1. pertaining to circulation, particularly that of the blood 血液循环，2. containing blood 含血的

cir·cu·lus (sur′ku-ləs) pl. *cir′culi* [L.] a circle 环

cir·cum·anal (sur″kəm-a′nəl) surrounding the anus 肛门周围的

cir·cum·cise (sur′kəm-sīz) to perform circumcision 环切

cir·cum·ci·sion (sur″kəm-sizh′ən) the removal of all or part of the prepuce of the penis in males 包 皮环切术，切除男性阴茎包皮的全部或部分；另见

female c. **female c.**, any of various procedures involving excision of some portion of the external female genitalia with or without infibulation 女子环切术，切除女性有无内翻的外生殖器某些部分的手术；**pharaonic c.**, a type of female circumcision comprising two procedures: a radical form comprising removal of the clitoris, labia minora, and labia majora followed by infibulation, and a modified form in which the prepuce and glans of the clitoris and adjacent labia minora are removed 法老割礼，一种阴蒂切开术，包括两种术式：一种根治性手术，包括切除阴蒂、小阴唇和大阴唇，然后进行阴部内翻；另一种为改良式手术，切除阴蒂的包皮和腺体以及相邻的小阴唇；**Sunna c.**, a form of female circumcision in which the prepuce of the clitoris is removed 伊斯兰教教规割礼，切除阴蒂包皮的女性包皮环切术

cir·cum·duc·tion (sur″kəm-duk′shən) circular movement of a limb or of the eye 肢体或眼睛的圆周运动

cir·cum·fer·en·tial (sur″kəm-fər-en′shəl) pertaining to a circumference 圆周的；encircling 环绕的；peripheral 外围的

cir·cum·flex (sur′kəm-fleks) curved like a bow 旋、弓样弯曲

cir·cum·in·su·lar (sur″kəm-in′su-lər) surrounding, situated, or occurring about the insula 脑岛周围的

cir·cum·len·tal (sur″kəm-len′təl) situated or occurring around the lens 晶状体周的

cir·cum·pul·pal (sur″kəm-pul′pəl) surrounding the pulp 牙髓周围

cir·cum·re·nal (sur″kəm-re′nəl) around the kidney 肾周

cir·cum·scribed (sur″kəm-skrībd″) bounded or limited; confined to a limited space 有限的；局限于有限的空间

cir·cum·stan·ti·al·i·ty (sur″kəm-stan″sheal′ĭ-te) a disturbed pattern of speech or writing characterized by delay in getting to the point because of the interpolation of unnecessary details and irrelevant parenthetical remarks 病理性赘述，由于插入不必要的细节和不相关的附加语而延迟达到目的的一种受干扰的语言或文字叙述

cir·cum·val·late (sur″kəm-val′āt) surrounded by a ridge or trench, as the vallate papillae 轮廓状的，如轮廓乳突

cir·rho·sis (sĭ-ro′sis) a group of liver diseases marked by interstitial inflammation of the liver, loss of normal hepatic architecture, fibrosis, and nodular regeneration 肝硬化，以肝间质炎症、肝脏正常结构丢失、纤维化和结节再生为特征的一组肝病；**cirrhot′ic** *adj.* **alcoholic c.**, a type in alcoholics, due to associated nutritional deficiency or chronic excessive exposure to alcohol as a hepatotoxin 酒精性肝硬化，酒精中毒的一种类型，由于相关的营养缺乏或长期过度饮酒所导致的肝细胞中毒；**biliary c.,** a type due to chronic bile retention after obstruction or infection of the major extra- or intrahepatic bile ducts (*secondary biliary c.*), or of unknown etiology (*primary biliary c.*), and sometimes occurring after administration of certain drugs 胆汁性肝硬化，梗阻或主要肝外或肝内胆管感染（继发性胆汁性肝硬化）或病因不明（原发性胆汁性肝硬化）的慢性胆汁淤积，有时在服用某些药物后发生；**cardiac c.,** fibrosis of the liver, probably following central hemorrhagic necrosis, in association with congestive heart disease 心源性肝硬化，中心出血性坏死之后的肝纤维化，与充血性心脏病有关；**fatty c.,** a form in which liver cells become infiltrated with fat 脂肪性肝硬化，肝细胞被脂肪浸润所致；**Laënnec c.,** a type associated with alcohol abuse Laënnec 肝硬化，与酗酒有关的肝硬化；**macronodular c.,** a type that follows subacute hepatic necrosis due to toxic or viral hepatitis 大结节性肝硬化，中毒性或病毒性肝炎引起的亚急性肝坏死；**metabolic c.,** a type associated with metabolic diseases, such as hemochromatosis, Wilson disease, glycogen storage disease, galactosemia, and disorders of amino acid metabolism 代谢性肝硬化，与代谢性疾病有关的类型，如血色素沉着病、Wilson 病、糖原贮积病、半乳糖血症和氨基酸代谢紊乱；**portal c.,** Laënnec c. 门脉性肝硬化，Laënnec 肝硬化；**posthepatitic c.,** a type (usually macronodular) that is a sequel to acute hepatitis 肝炎后肝硬化，急性肝炎的后遗症（通常为大结节性）；**postnecrotic c.,** macronodular c. 坏死后性肝硬化

cir·soid (sur'soid) resembling a varix 曲张的

cir·som·pha·los (sər-som'fə-los) caput medusae 脐周静脉曲张，海蛇头

cis (sis) [L.] 顺式 1. in organic chemistry, having certain atoms or radicals on the same side 有机化学中，某些原子或自由基在同一侧；2. in genetics, denoting two or more loci, especially pseudoalleles, occurring on the same chromosome of a homologous pair. Cf. *trans.* 遗传学中，指出现在同一对同源染色体上的两个或多个基因座，特别是假等位基因；另见 *test* 下的 *cis-trans* test

cis- a prefix denoting on this side, the same side, or the near side 表示这一侧、同一侧或近侧的前缀

cis·at·ra·cu·ri·um (sis″at-rə-kūr'e-əm) a nondepolarizing neuromuscular blocking agent administered intravenously as the besylate salt as an adjunct to general anesthesia or during mechanical ventilation 顺式阿曲库铵，非去极化神经肌肉阻滞药，其苯磺酸盐用于静脉注射，作为全麻或机械通气的辅助药物

cis·plat·in (sis'plat-in) DDP; a platinum coordination complex capable of producing inter- and intrastrand DNA crosslinks; used as an antineoplastic 顺铂，能够产生链间和链内 DNA 交联的铂配位化合物；用作抗肿瘤药

cis·tern (sis'tərn) a closed space serving as a reservoir for fluid, e.g., one of the enlarged spaces of the body containing lymph or other fluid 池，作为液体贮存器的封闭空间，例如，含有淋巴或其他液体的体内空间；**cister'nal** *adj.* **lumbar c.,** the enlargement of the subarachnoid space caudal to the conus medullaris, containing the cauda equina, filum terminale internum, and cerebrospinal fluid 腰大池，蛛网膜下腔尾至脊髓圆锥的扩大，包括马尾、终丝和脑脊液；**terminal c's,** pairs of transversely oriented channels that are confluent with the sarcotubules, which together with an intermediate T tubule constitute a triad of skeletal muscle 终末池，与肌小管汇合的一对横向通道，与中间 T 管一起构成骨骼肌三联体

cis·ter·na (sis-tur'nə) pl. *cister'nae* [L.] cistern 池；**c. cerebellomedulla'ris poste'rior,** posterior cerebellomedullary cistern; the enlarged subarachnoid space between the undersurface of the cerebellum and the posterior surface of the medulla oblongata 小脑延髓后池；小脑下表面和延髓后表面之间的蛛网膜下腔扩大；**c. chy'li,** the dilated part of the thoracic duct at its origin in the lumbar region 乳糜池，胸导管在腰部起始处的膨大部分

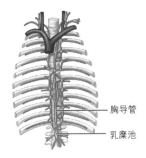

胸导管
乳糜池

cis·ter·nog·ra·phy (sis″tər-nog'rə-fe) radiography of the basal cistern of the brain after subarachnoid injection of a contrast medium 脑池显像术，蛛网膜下腔注射造影剂后，对大脑脚间池的放射照相术

ci·tal·o·pram (si-tal'o-pram) 西酞普兰 1. an antidepressant compound used in the treatment of major depressive disorder, administered orally as the hydrobromide 用于治疗严重抑郁症的抗抑郁化合物，其氢溴酸盐常用于口服；2. a selective serotonin reuptake inhibitor used as the hydrobromide salt as

224

an antidepressant 选择性血清素再摄取抑制药，其氢溴酸盐，作为抗抑郁药

cit·rate (sit′rāt) a salt of citric acid 柠檬酸盐，柯橡酸盐；**c. phosphate dextrose (CPD)**, anticoagulant citrate phosphate dextrose solution 柯橡酸盐磷酸盐右旋糖；**c. phosphate dextrose adenine (CPDA-1)**, anticoagulant citrate phosphate dextrose adenine solution 柠檬酸磷酸酸葡萄糖脉嘌呤

cit·ric ac·id (sit′rik) a tricarboxylic acid obtained from citrus fruits that is an intermediate in the tricarboxylic acid cycle; it chelates calcium ions and prevents blood clotting and functions as an anticoagulant for blood specimens and for stored whole blood and red cells. It is also used in the preparation of effervescent mixtures and as a synergist to enhance the action of antioxidants. 柠檬酸

Cit·ro·bac·ter (sit′ro-bak″tər) a genus of gramnegative, facultatively anaerobic, rod-shaped bacteria of the family Enterobacteriaceae. *C. amalona′ticus*, *C. freun′dii*, and *C. kos′eri* have been associated with nosocomial infection, particularly in debilitated patients, and in neonates have caused meningitis and brain abscess. 柠檬酸杆菌属

cit·ro·nel·la (sit′rə-nel′ə) a fragrant grass, the source of a volatile oil (citronella oil) used in perfumes and insect repellents 香茅

cit·rul·line (sit′rə-lēn) an alpha-amino acid involved in urea production; formed from ornithine and itself converted into arginine in the urea cycle 瓜氨酸

cit·rul·lin·emia (sit-rul″in-e′me-ə) 1. argininosuccinate synthase deficiency 瓜氨酸血症，精氨琥珀酸合成酶缺乏；2. a group of inherited disorders caused by deficient argininosuccinate synthase activity, characterized by elevated plasma levels of citrulline and ammonia and urinary excretion of citrulline and orotic acid, often with intellectual disability and neurologic abnormalities 瓜氨酸血症，精氨琥珀酸合成酶活性不足导致的一组遗传性疾病，造成瓜氨酸和乳清酸的血浆浓度过高，通常伴有智能障碍和神经系统畸形

cit·rul·lin·uria (sit-rul″in-u′re-ə) 瓜氨酸尿症；1. argininosuccinate synthase deficiency 精氨琥珀酸合成酶缺乏；2. excessive citrulline in the urine 尿中瓜氨酸过多

CK creatine kinase 肌酸激酶

Cl chlorine 氯

Clado·phi·a·loph·o·ra (klad″o-fi″ə-lof′ə-rə) a genus of chiefly saprobic, dematiaceous, anamorphic fungi, including species causing infections ranging from chromoblastomycosis and other skin infections to disseminated and cerebral infections 斑替枝孢属

Clado·spo·ri·um (klad″o-spor′e-əm) a genus of

ubiquitous, chiefly saprobic, dematiaceous, anamorphic fungi; they are common molds on dead organic matter and in air. Various species, notably *C. cladosporioi′des* and *C. herba′rum*, produce allergens and have been associated with asthma and other respiratory disorders 枝孢属

clad·ri·bine (kla′drī-bēn) a purine antimetabolite used as an antineoplastic in the treatment of hairy cell leukemia 克拉屈滨

clair·voy·ance (klār-voi′əns) [Fr.] extrasensory perception in which knowledge of objective events is acquired without the use of the senses 预见力，不依靠感觉就可感知客观事物

clamp (klamp) a surgical device for compressing a part or structure 夹钳，压迫机体结构的外科器械 **rubber dam c.**, a metallic device used to retain the dam on a tooth 橡皮障夹

clamp·ing (klamp′ing) in the measurement of insulin secretion and action, the infusion of a glucose solution at a rate adjusted periodically to maintain a predetermined blood glucose concentration 血糖固定，在胰岛素分泌和活性测定中，以定时调整的速率注射葡萄糖溶液，以维持预定的血浆葡萄糖浓度

cla·pote·ment (klah-pawt-maw′) [Fr.] a splashing sound, as in succussion 振水音

clar·if·i·cant (klar-if′ ĭ-kənt) a substance that clears a liquid of turbidity 净化剂，可使浑浊液体澄清

cla·rith·ro·my·cin (klə-rith″ro-mi′sin) a macrolide antibiotic effective against a wide spectrum of gram-positive and gram-negative bacteria; used in the treatment of respiratory tract, skin, and soft tissue infections and of *Helicobacter pylori*–associated duodenal ulcer 克拉霉素

class (klas) 1. a taxonomic category subordinate to a phylum and superior to an order 纲；2. a subgroup of a population for which certain variables fall between specific limits 一个群体的亚群，某些可变因素介于特定限度之间的个体的集合

clas·sic (klas′ik) standard, typical, or traditional 标准的，典型的，传统的

clas·si·cal (klas′ ĭ-kəl) classic 标准的，典型的，传统的

clas·si·fi·ca·tion (klas″ĭ-fĭ-ka′shən) the systematic arrangement of similar entities on the basis of certain differing characteristics 分类；**adansonian c.**, numerical taxonomy 数值分类学；**Angle c.**, a classification of dental malocclusion based on the mesiodistal position of the mandibular dental arch and teeth relative to the maxillary dental arch and teeth 安格尔分类法，一种错𬌗畸形的分类方法；**Bergey c.**, a system of classifying bacteria by

Gram reaction, metabolism, and morphology 一 种基于革兰染色、代谢、形态学的细菌分类系统；**Caldwell-Moloy c.**, classification of female pelves as gynecoid, android, anthropoid, and platypelloid Caldwell-Moloy 分类，将女性骨盆分为女性骨盆、男性骨盆、类人猿型骨盆和扁平骨盆；**FIGO c.**, any of the classification systems established by the International Federation of Gynecology and Obstetrics for the staging of gynecologic cancers 所有基于国际妇产科联盟妇科肿瘤分期的分类方法；**Gell and Coombs c.**, a classification of immune mechanisms of tissue injury, comprising four types: *type I*, immediate hypersensitivity reactions, mediated by interaction of IgE antibody and antigen and release of histamine and other mediators; *type II*, antibody-mediated hypersensitivity reactions, due to antibody-antigen interactions on cell surfaces; *type III*, immune complex–mediated hypersensitivity reactions, local or general inflammatory responses due to formation of circulating immune complexes and their deposition in tissues; and *type IV*, cell-mediated hypersensitivity reactions, initiated by sensitized T lymphocytes either by release of lymphokines or by T-cell–mediated cytotoxicity 一种组织损伤免疫机制的分类方法，包括4型：Ⅰ型、速发型超敏反应，Ⅱ型、细胞毒型超敏反应，Ⅲ型、免疫复合物型超敏反应，Ⅳ型、迟发型超敏反应；**Keith-Wagener-Barker c.**, a classification of hypertension and arteriolosclerosis based on retinal changes 一种基于视网膜改变的高血压和小动脉硬化分类方法；**Lancefield c.**, the classification of hemolytic streptococci into groups on the basis of serologic action 兰斯菲尔德分类法，一种基于血清学反应的溶血性链球菌分类方法；**New York Heart Association (NYHA) c.**, a functional and therapeutic classification for prescription of physical activity for cardiac patients 纽约心脏协会分类法，一种基于体力活动症状的心脏病分类方法；**Revised European American Lymphoma (REAL) c.**, a classification of lymphomas based on histologic criteria, dividing them into three main categories: B-cell neoplasms, T- or NK-cell neoplasms, and Hodgkin disease 修订后欧美淋巴瘤分类法，一种基于组织学标准的淋巴瘤分类方法，将其分为三大类：B 细胞淋巴瘤、T 细胞或 NK 细胞淋巴瘤和霍奇金病

clas·tic (klas′tik) 1. undergoing or causing division 分裂的；2. separable into parts 碎片化的

clas·to·gen·ic (klas″to-jen′ik) causing disruption or breakages, as of chromosomes 致染色体断裂的

clath·rate (klath′rāt) 1. having the shape of a lattice 网格状的；2. a clathrate compound, or pertaining or relating to a clathrate compound 包合物；见

compound 下词条

clau·di·ca·tion (klaw′dĭ-ka′shən) limping; lameness 跛行；**intermittent c.**, pain, tension, and weakness in the legs on walking, which intensifies to produce lameness and is relieved by rest; it is seen in occlusive arterial disease 间歇性跛行；**jaw c.**, a complex of symptoms like those of intermittent claudication but seen in the muscles of mastication in giant cell arteritis 颌跛行，巨细胞动脉炎引起咀嚼肌表现出类似于间歇性跛行的一组症状；**neurogenic c.**, that accompanied by pain and paresthesias in the back, buttocks, and legs that is relieved by stooping, caused by mechanical disturbances due to posture or by ischemia of the cauda equina 神经源性跛行，由姿势相关的机械压迫或马尾神经缺血导致，伴有背部、臀部和大腿的疼痛和感觉异常，弯腰可缓解；**venous c.**, intermittent claudication due to venous stasis 静脉性跛行，静脉血流停滞造成的间歇性跛行

claus·tro·pho·bia (klaws″tro-fo′be-ə) irrational fear of being shut in, of closed places 幽闭恐惧症

claus·trum (claws′trəm) pl. *claus′tra* [L.] the thin layer of gray matter lateral to the external capsule, separating it from the white matter of the insula 屏状核

cla·va (kla′və) gracile tubercle 薄束结节

Clav·i·ceps (klav′ĭ-seps) a genus of parasitic fungi that infest various plant seeds. *C. purpu′rea* is the source of ergot 麦角属

clav·i·cle (klav′ĭ-kəl) collar bone : a bone, curved like the letter f, that articulates with the sternum and scapula, forming the anterior portion of the pectoral girdle on either side 锁 骨；见 图 1；**clavic′ular** *adj.*

clav·i·cot·o·my (klav″ĭ-kot′ə-me) surgical division of the clavicle 锁骨切断术

cla·vic·u·la (klə-vik′u-lə) [L.] clavicle 锁骨

clav·u·la·nate (klav′u-lə-nāt) a β-lactamase inhibitor used as the potassium salt in combination with penicillins in treating infections caused by β-lactamase–producing organisms 克拉维酸

cla·vus (kla′vəs) pl. *cla′vi* [L.] corn 鸡眼

claw (klaw) a nail of an animal, particularly a carnivore, that is long and curved and has a sharp end 爪；**cat's c.**, a woody South American vine, *Uncaria tomentosa* or a preparation of its root bark, which has antiviral, immunostimulant, and antiinflammatory properties and is used in folk medicine 猫 爪 藤；**devil's c.**, a perennial herb, *Harpagophytum procumbens*, whose dried tubular secondary roots and lateral tubers are used for dyspepsia, loss of appetite, and rheumatism; also used in homeopathy for rheumatism and in folk medicine 南非钩麻

C

claw·foot (klaw'foot) a high-arched foot with the toes hyperextended at the metatarsophalangeal joint and flexed at the distal joints 爪形足

claw·hand (klaw'hand) flexion and atrophy of the hand and fingers 爪形手

clear (klēr) 1. to remove cloudiness from microscopic specimens by the use of a clearing agent 清洁，用清洁剂去除显微样本中的云状物；2. to remove a substance from the blood 清除，从血中清除某种物质；3. transparent; not cloudy, turbid, or opaque 透明的

clear·ance (C) (klēr'əns) 1. the act of clearing 清除；2. a quantitative measure of the rate at which a substance is removed from the blood, as by the kidneys, the liver, or hemodialysis; the volume of plasma cleared per unit time 清除率；3. the space between opposed structures 空　隙；**blood-urea c.,** urea c.; **creatinine c.,** the volume of plasma cleared of creatinine after parenteral administration of a specified amount of the substance 肌酐清除率；**inulin c.,** an expression of the renal efficiency in eliminating inulin from the blood 菊糖清除率；**mucociliary c.,** the clearance of mucus and other materials from the airways by the cilia of the epithelial cells 黏膜纤毛清除，通过上皮细胞纤毛将气道中的黏液和其他物质清除的过程；**urea c.,** the volume of the blood cleared of urea per minute by either renal clearance or hemodialysis. 尿素清除率

cleav·age (kle'vəj) 1. division into distinct parts 分　裂；2. the early successive splitting of a zygote into smaller cells (blastomeres) by mitosis 卵裂

cleaved (klēvd) split or separated, as by cutting 分开的

cleft (kleft) a fissure, especially one occurring during embryonic development 裂，特指胚胎发育过程中形成的；**anal c.,** gluteal c.; **branchial c's,** 1. the slitlike openings in the gills of fish, between the branchial arches 鳃　裂；2. pharyngeal grooves. 咽沟 **facial c.,** 1. any of the clefts between the embryonic prominences that normally unite to form the face 面裂；2. prosoposchisis: failure of union of a facial cleft, causing a developmental defect such as cleft cheek or lip 面裂联合不全造成发育缺陷，如颊裂、唇裂；**gluteal c.,** that which separates the buttocks 臀裂；**pudendal c.,** the space between the labia majora 女阴裂；**subneural c's,** evenly spaced lamella-like clefts within the primary synaptic cleft, formed by infoldings of the sarcolemma into the underlying muscle sarcolemma 神经下裂；**synaptic c.,** 1. a narrow extracellular cleft between the presynaptic and postsynaptic membranes 突触间隙；2. synaptic trough 突触窝；**visceral c.,** pharyngeal grooves 鳃裂，咽沟

clei·do·cra·ni·al (kli″do-kra′ne-əl) pertaining to the clavicle and the head 锁骨头颅的

clem·as·tine (klem′əs-tēn) an antihistamine with anticholinergic and sedative effects, used as the fumarate salt 氯马斯汀

click (klik) a brief, sharp sound, especially any of the short, dry, clicking heart sounds during systole, indicative of various heart conditions 喀喇音，一种短暂、尖锐、清脆的收缩期额外心音，见于多种情况

cli·din·i·um (kli-din′e-əm) an anticholinergic with pronounced antispasmodic and antisecretory effects in the gastrointestinal tract; used as the bromide salt 克利溴铵

cli·mac·ter·ic (kli-mak′tər-ik) 1. the syndrome of endocrine, somatic, and psychic changes occurring at menopause in women 更年期；2. similar changes occurring in men (andropause) 男性更年期

cli·max (kli′maks) the period of greatest intensity, as in the course of a disease (crisis), or in sexual excitement (orgasm) 高潮，如疾病极期、性高潮

clin·da·my·cin (klin″də-mi′sin) a semisynthetic derivative of lincomycin used systemically, topically, and vaginally as an antibacterial, primarily against gram-positive bacteria; used also as the hydrochloride and phosphate salts and as the hydrochloride salt of the ester of clindamycin and palmitic acid 克林霉素

clin·ic (klin′ik) 1. a clinical lecture; examination of patients before a class of students; instruction at the bedside 临　床；2. an establishment where patients are admitted for study and treatment by a group of physicians practicing medicine together 诊所；**ambulant c.,** one for patients not confined to the bed 门　诊；**dry c.,** a clinical lecture with case histories, but without patients present 仅提供病史，而无病人在场的临床课程

clin·i·cal (klin′ĭ-kəl) pertaining to a clinic or to the bedside; pertaining to or founded on actual observation and treatment of patients, as distinguished from theoretical or basic sciences 临床的

cli·ni·cian (klĭ-nish′ən) an expert clinical physician and teacher 临床医师

clin·i·co·patho·log·ic (klin″ĭ-ko-path″ə-loj′ik) pertaining to symptoms and pathology of disease 临床病理学的

Clin·i·stix (klin′ĭ-stiks) trademark for glucose oxidase reagent strips used to test for glucose in urine 尿糖试纸的一种品牌

Clin·i·test (klin′ĭ-test) trademark for alkaline copper sulfate reagent tablets used to test for reducing substances, e.g., sugars, in urine 碱性硫酸铜试剂片的一种品牌，用于检测尿糖等物质

cli·no·ceph·a·ly (kli″no-sef′ə-le) congenital flatness or concavity of the top of the head 鞍形头，头

颅顶部先天性扁平或凹陷

cli·no·dac·ty·ly (kli″no-dak′tə-le) permanent deviation or deflection of one or more fingers 手指弯曲变形

cli·noid (klī′noid) bed-shaped 床形的

clip (klip) a device for approximating the edges of a wound or for the prevention of bleeding from small individual blood vessels 钳，用于牵引创口边缘或阻止小血管出血的一类器材

clis·om·e·ter (klis″e-om′ə-tər) an instrument for measuring the angles between the axis of the body and that of the pelvis 骨盆斜度计

clit·i·on (klit′e-on) the midpoint of the anterior border of the clivus 斜坡前界的中点

Cli·to·cy·be (kli-tos′ĭ-be) a genus of mushrooms including many poisonous species, some containing the toxin muscarine 大杯蕈属

clit·o·ri·dec·to·my (klit″ə-rĭ-dek′tə-me) excision of the clitoris 阴蒂切除术

clit·o·ri·dot·o·my (klit″ə-rĭ-dot′ə-me) incision of the clitoris; female circumcision 阴蒂切开术

clit·o·ri·meg·a·ly (klit″ə-rĭ-meg′ə-le) enlargement of the clitoris 阴蒂肥大

clit·o·ris (klit′ə-ris) (kli′tə-ris) (klī-tor′is) the small, elongated, erectile body in the female, situated at the anterior angle of the rima pudendi and homologous with the penis in the male 阴蒂

clit·o·rism (klit′ə-riz″əm) (kli′tə-riz″əm) 1. hypertrophy of the clitoris 阴蒂肥大; 2. persistent erection of the clitoris 阴蒂异常勃起

clit·o·ri·tis (klit″ə-ri′tis) (kli′tə-ri′tis) inflammation of the clitoris 阴蒂炎

clit·o·ro·plas·ty (klit′ə-ro-plas″te) plastic surgery of the clitoris 阴蒂成形术

cli·vog·ra·phy (kli-vog′rə-fe) radiographic visualization of the clivus, or posterior cranial fossa 斜坡照相术，斜坡或颅前窝的放射性成像

cli·vus (kli′vəs) [L.] a bony surface in the posterior cranial fossa sloping upward from the foramen magnum to the dorsum sellae 斜坡，颅前窝的一处骨性表面，由枕骨大孔至鞍背

CLL chronic lymphocytic leukemia 慢性淋巴细胞白血病

clo·a·ca (klo-a′kə) pl. *cloa′cae* [L.] 1. a common passage for fecal, urinary, and reproductive discharge in most lower vertebrates 泄殖腔; 2. the terminal end of the hindgut before division into rectum, bladder, and genital primordia in mammalian embryos 哺乳动物胚胎中后肠的末端; 3. an opening in the involucrum of a necrosed bone 死骨包膜的开口; **cloa′cal** *adj.*

clo·a·co·gen·ic (klo″ə-ko-jen′ik) originating from the cloaca or from persisting cloacal remnants 泄殖

腔源性的

clo·be·ta·sol (klo-ba′tə-sol) a synthetic corticosteroid used topically as the propionate salt for the relief of inflammation and pruritus in corticosteroid-responsive dermatoses 氯倍他索

clock (klok) a device for measuring time 钟; **biologic c.**, the physiologic mechanism that governs the rhythmic occurrence of certain biochemical, physiologic, and behavioral phenomena in living organisms 生物钟

clo·cor·to·lone (klo-kor′to-lōn) a synthetic corticosteroid used topically as the pivalate ester for the relief of inflammation and pruritus in certain dermatoses 氯可托龙

clo·fi·brate (klo-fi′brāt) an antihyperlipidemic used to reduce serum lipids 安妥明，氯贝丁酯

clo·mi·phene (klo′mĭ-fēn) a nonsteroidal estrogen analogue, used as the citrate salt to stimulate ovulation 克罗米酚

clo·mip·ra·mine (klo-mip′rə-mēn) a tricyclic antidepressant with anxiolytic activity, also used in obsessive-compulsive disorder, panic disorder, bulimia nervosa, cataplexy associated with narcolepsy, and chronic, severe pain; used as the hydrochloride salt 氯丙咪嗪; 氯米帕明

clo·nal·i·ty (klo-nal′ĭ-te) the ability to be cloned 可克隆性

clo·naz·e·pam (klo-naz′ə-pam) a benzodiazepine used as an anticonvulsant and as an antipanic agent 氯硝西泮

clone (klōn) 1. one of a group of genetically identical (barring mutation) cells or organisms derived asexually from a single common ancestor 克隆，由同一祖先无性生殖产生的细胞或有机体的集合; 2. a DNA population derived from a single molecule by recombinant DNA technology DNA 克隆; 3. to establish such a progeny or population. 克隆，产生遗传信息完全相同的后代; **clo′nal** *adj.* 克隆的

clon·ic (klon′ik) pertaining to or of the nature of clonus 阵挛的

clo·ni·dine (klo′nĭ-dēn) a centrally acting antihypertensive agent, used as the hydrochloride salt; also used in the prophylaxis of migraine and the treatment of dysmenorrhea, anxiety, menopausal symptoms, opioid withdrawal, and cancer-related pain 可乐定

clon·ism (klon′iz-əm) a succession of clonic spasms 持续阵挛

clo·no·gen·ic (klo″no-jen′ik) giving rise to a clone of cells 克隆源性的

clo·nor·chi·a·sis (klo″nor-ki′ə-sis) infection of the biliary passages with the liver fluke *Clonorchis sinensis*, causing inflammation of the biliary tree, prolifer-

228

ation of the biliary epithelium, and progressive portal fibrosis; extension into the liver parenchyma causes fatty changes and cirrhosis 华支睾吸虫病

clono·spasm (klon′o-spaz″əm) clonic spasm 阵挛

clo·nus (klo′nəs) 1. alternate involuntary muscular contraction and relaxation in rapid succession 阵挛; 2. a continuous rhythmic reflex tremor initiated by the spinal cord below an area of spinal cord injury, set in motion by reflex testing 在神经反射检查中，由脊髓损伤节段下的脊髓始动的连续性、节奏性、反射性震颤; **clon′ic** *adj.* 阵挛的; **ankle c., foot c.,** a series of abnormal reflex movements of the foot, induced by sudden dorsiflexion, causing alternate contraction and relaxation of the triceps surae muscle 踝阵挛; **wrist c.,** spasmodic movement of the hand, induced by forcibly extending the hand at the wrist 腕阵挛

clo·pid·o·grel (klo-pid′o-grel) a platelet inhibitor used as an antithrombotic for the prevention of myocardial infarction, stroke, and vascular death in patients with atherosclerosis; used as the bisulfate salt 氯吡格雷

clor·az·e·pate (klor-az′ə-pāt) a benzodiazepine used as the dipotassium salt as an antianxiety agent, anticonvulsant, and aid in the treatment of acute alcohol withdrawal 氯氮䓬

Clos·tri·dia (klos-trid′e-ə) a class of bacteria of the phylum Firmicutes, consisting of grampositive or gram-negative, aerobic to anaerobic rods or cocci 梭菌纲

Clos·tri·di·a·ceae (klos-trid″e-a′se-e) a family of bacteria of the order Clostridiales, consisting of anaerobic organisms that vary widely in morphology, physiology, and metabolism 梭菌科

Clos·tri·di·a·les (klos-trid″e-a′lēz) a phenotypically diverse order of bacteria of the class Clostridia that includes many medically important bacteria 梭菌目

Clos·trid·i·um (klos-trid′e-əm) a large genus of anaerobic, spore-forming, rod-shaped bacteria of the family Clostridiaceae 梭菌属; *C. bifermen′tans,* a species common in feces, sewage, and soil and associated with gas gangrene 双酶梭菌; *C. botuli′num,* the species that causes botulism, divided into seven types (A through G) that elaborate immunologically distinct toxins 肉毒杆菌; *C. diffi′cile,* a species that is part of the normal colon flora in infants and some adults; it produces a toxin that can cause pseudomembranous enterocolitis in patients receiving antibiotic therapy 艰难梭菌; *C. histoly′ticum,* a species found in feces and soil and frequently associated with gas gangrene 溶组织梭菌; *C. kluy′veri,* a species used in the study of both microbial synthesis and microbial oxidation of fatty acids 克氏梭菌; *C. no′vyi,* a species, sep-

arable into three immunologic types (A to C), that is an important cause of gas gangrene 诺氏梭菌; *C. perfrin′gens,* the most common etiologic agent of gas gangrene, distinguishable as several different types; *type A* causes human gas gangrene, colitis, and food poisoning and *type C* causes enteritis 产气荚膜梭菌; *C. ramo′sum,* a species found in human and animal infections and feces and commonly isolated from clinical specimens 多枝梭菌; *C. sporo′genes,* a species widespread in nature, reportedly associated with pathogenic anaerobes in gangrenous infections 产芽孢梭菌; *C. ter′tium,* a species found in feces, sewage, and soil and associated with gas gangrene 第三芽孢梭菌; *C. te′tani,* a common inhabitant of soil and human and horse intestines, and the cause of tetanus in humans and domestic animals 破伤风梭菌

clos·trid·i·um (klos-trid′e-əm) pl. *clostri′dia* An individual of the genus *Clostridium* 梭菌; **clostrid′ial** *adj.* 梭菌的

clot (klot) 1. coagulum; a semisolid mass, as of blood or lymph 凝块; 2. coagulate 凝固; **agony c.,** a type of antemortem clot formed in the process of dying 濒死时产生的血块; **antemortem c.,** one formed in the heart or in a large vessel before death but found after death 死前血块, 死亡前心脏或大血管内形成的血块, 但在死亡后发现; **blood c.,** a coagulum in the bloodstream formed of an aggregation of blood factors, primarily platelets, and fibrin with entrapment of cellular elements 血块; **chicken fat c.,** a yellow-appearing blood clot, due to settling out of erythrocytes before clotting 鸡脂样血块, 因凝固前红细胞已沉降分离而产生的黄色血块; **currant jelly c.,** a reddish clot, due to the presence of erythrocytes enmeshed in it 果浆样血块, 因红细胞被网罗其中而产生的红色血块; **laminated c.,** a blood clot formed by successive deposits, giving it a layered appearance 层状血块; **passive c.,** one formed in the sac of an aneurysm through which the blood has stopped circulating 被动性血块, 在动脉瘤中因停止流动而产生的血块; **plastic c.,** one formed from the intima of an artery at the point of ligation, forming a permanent obstruction of the artery 成形性血块, 结扎时在动脉内膜处形成的血块, 永久成为动脉结构的一部分; **postmortem c.,** one formed in the heart or in a large blood vessel after death 死后血凝块, 死亡后在心脏或大动脉内形成的血块

clo·trim·a·zole (klo-trim′ə-zōl) an imidazole derivative used as a broad-spectrum antifungal agent 克霉唑

clot·ting (klot′ing) coagulation (1) 凝固

cloud·ing (kloud′ing) loss of clarity 模糊; **c. of consciousness,** a lowered level of consciousness

C

marked by loss of perception or comprehension of the environment, with loss of ability to respond properly to external stimuli 意识模糊，缺乏感知或对环境的理解力的低意识状态，对外来刺激缺乏反应能力

cloudy (clou′de) 1. murky; turbid; not transparent 浑浊的，不透明的；2. marked by indistinct streaks 有模糊条纹的

clove (klōv) the tropical tree *Syzygium aromaticum*, or its dried flower bud, which is used as a source of clove oil 丁香

clo·ver (klo′vər) a leguminous plant with trifoliate leaves, sometimes specifically a member of the genera *Trifolium* or *Melilotus* 三叶草；**red c.**, the leguminous plant *Trifolium pratense* or a preparation of its flower heads, which is used for coughs and respiratory symptoms and for chronic skin conditions; also used in traditional Chinese medicine 红三叶草

clox·a·cil·lin (klok″sə-sil′in) a semisynthetic penicillin; used as the sodium salt to treat staphylococcal infections due to penicillinase-positive organisms 氯唑西林

clo·za·pine (klo′zə-pēn) a sedative and antipsychotic agent; used in the treatment of schizophrenia 氯氮平

club·bing (klub′ing) proliferation of soft tissue around the ends of fingers or toes, without osseous change 杵状指

club·foot (klub′foot) a congenitally twisted foot 畸形足；见 *talipes*

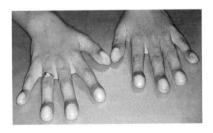

▲ 青少年法洛四联症患者的杵状指（**clubbing**）

club·hand (klub′hand) a deformity of the hand due to congenital absence of the radius (*radial c.*) or ulna (*ulnar c.*) in which the hand is twisted out of shape or position; talipomanus 因桡骨或尺骨先天性缺失导致的手畸形；畸形手

clump·ing (klump′ing) the aggregation of particles, such as bacteria, into irregular masses 凝集，颗粒样物质（如细菌）聚集成不规则团块

clu·nis (kloo′nis) pl. *clu′nes* [L.] buttock 臀；**clu′neal** *adj.*

cly·sis (kli′sis) 1. administration other than orally of a solution to replace lost body fluid, supply nutriment, or raise blood pressure 通过口服以外的方式进行补液，以补充体液、营养支持或升高血压，如灌肠、静脉滴注；2. the solution so administered 前述操作使用的溶液

CM [L.] Chiari malformation Chiari 畸形；Chirur′giae Magis′ter (Master of Surgery) 外科学硕士

Cm curium 锔，（放射性化学元素）

cm centimeter 厘米

cm³ cubic centimeter 立方厘米

CMA Canadian Medical Association 加拿大医学会；Certified Medical Assistant 执业助理医师

CMD cerebromacular degeneration 大脑黄斑变性症

CMHC community mental health center 社区精神健康中心

CMI cell-mediated immunity 细胞免疫

CML cell-mediated lympholysis 细胞免疫性淋巴细胞溶解；chronic myeloid leukemia 慢性髓细胞性白血病

CMT Certified Medical Transcriptionist 执业医疗录写员；Charcot-Marie-Tooth disease 夏科 - 马思 - 图思病；combined modality therapy 综合治疗

CMV cytomegalovirus 巨细胞病毒

CNA Canadian Nurses Association 加拿大护士协会

C3 NeF C3 nephritic factor C3 肾炎因子

Cni·da·ria (ni-dar′e-ə) a phylum of marine invertebrates including sea anemones, hydras, corals, jellyfish, and comb jellies, characterized by a radially symmetric body bearing tentacles around the mouth 刺胞动物门

cni·dar·i·an (ni-dar′e-ən) 1. pertaining or belonging to the phylum Cnidaria 刺胞动物的；2. an individual of the phylum Cnidaria 刺胞动物，又称 *coelenterate*

CNM Certified Nurse-Midwife 执业护理助产士；见 *nurse-midwife*

CNS central nervous system 中枢神经系统

CO cardiac output 心输出量；cervical orthosis. 颈椎矫正

Co cobalt 钴

COA Canadian Orthopaedic Association 加拿大整形外科协会

CoA 1. coenzyme A 辅酶 A；2. coarctation of the aorta 主动脉缩窄

co·ac·er·va·tion (ko-as″ər-va′shən) the separation of a mixture of two liquids, one or both of which are colloids, into two phases, one of which, the coacervate, contains the colloidal particles, the other being an aqueous solution, as when gum arabic is added to gelatin 凝聚，将两种液体的混合物（至少一种为胶体）分离成两个相，其中一个为含有胶体颗粒的凝聚层，另一个为水相溶液

co·ad·ap·ta·tion (ko-ad″ap-ta′shən) the correlated changes in two interdependent organs 共适应

co·ag·glu·ti·na·tion (ko″ə-gloo″tĭ-na′shən) the aggregation of particulate antigens combined with agglutinins of more than one specificity 协同凝集

co·ag·u·la·bil·i·ty (ko-ag″u-lə-bil′ĭ-te) the capability of forming or of being formed into clots 凝固性

co·ag·u·lant (ko-ag′u-lənt) promoting or accelerating coagulation of blood; an agent that so acts 促凝剂

co·ag·u·lase (ko-ag′u-lās) an antigenic substance of bacterial origin, produced by staphylococci, which may be causally related to thrombus formation 凝固酶

co·ag·u·late (ko-ag′u-lāt) to undergo coagulation 凝固

co·ag·u·la·tion (ko-ag″u-la′shən) 1. formation of a clot 凝固; 2. in surgery, the disruption of tissue by physical means to form an amorphous residuum, as in electrocoagulation and photocoagulation 在外科学中，指通过物理手段使阻止破坏而形成无定形残留物，如电凝固和光凝固; 3. in colloid chemistry, the solidification of a sol into a gelatinous mass 在胶体化学中，指溶胶固化为凝胶状物质; **blood c.**, the sequential process by which the multiple coagulation factors of blood interact in the coagulation cascade, resulting in formation of an insoluble fibrin clot 血液凝固; **disseminated intravascular c. (DIC)**, a bleeding disorder characterized by reduction in the elements involved in blood clotting due to their use in widespread clotting within the vessels. In the late stages, it is marked by profuse hemorrhaging 弥散性血管内凝血

co·ag·u·la·tive (ko-ag′u-lə-tiv) associated with, of the nature of, or promoting a process of coagulation 凝固性的

co·ag·u·la·tor (ko-ag′u-la″tər) a surgical device that utilizes electrical current or light to stop bleeding 促凝器，运用电流或光以阻止出血的一类外科器械; **argon beam c. (ABC)**, a device that uses a jet of argon gas carrying electrical energy from a needle electrode recessed inside a probe to effect hemostasis in bleeding tissue 氩气刀

co·ag·u·lop·a·thy (ko-ag″u-lop′ə-the) any disorder of blood coagulation; called also bleeding disorder 凝血病，又称出血性疾病; **consumption c.**, disseminated intravascular coagulation 消耗性凝血病

co·ag·u·lum (ko-ag′u-ləm) pl. *coa′gula* [L.] clot

(1) 凝块

co·a·les·cence (ko″ə-les′əns) the fusion or blending of parts 联合，各部分的融合或混合

co·a·li·tion (ko″ə-lish′ən) the fusion of parts that are normally separate 联合，正常情况下应是分离的部分的融合; **tarsal c.**, the fibrous, cartilaginous, or bony fusion of two or more of the tarsal bones, often resulting in talipes planovalgus 跗骨联合，两块或以上跗骨的纤维性、软骨性或骨性的融合，通常会造成外翻平跗足

co·apt (ko-apt′) to approximate, as the edges of a wound 使接合，如伤口的边缘

co·ap·ta·tion (ko-ap-ta′shən) the process of approximating, or joining together 接合

co·arc·tate (ko-ahrk′tāt) 1. to press close together; contract 使压紧; 2. pressed together; restrained 缩窄

co·arc·ta·tion (ko″ahrk-ta′shən) narrowing 缩窄; **c. of aorta**, a local malformation marked by deformed aortic media, causing narrowing of the lumen of the vessel 主动脉缩窄; **reversed c.**, Takayasu arteritis 反向缩窄，大动脉缩窄

coarse (kors) not fine; not microscopic 粗劣的; 非微观的

coat (kōt) 1. tunica; a membrane or other tissue covering or lining an organ or part 被膜; 2. the layer(s) of protein surrounding the nucleic acid in a virus 衣壳，病毒核酸外由蛋白质构成的保护层; **buffy c.**, the thin yellowish layer of leukocytes overlying the packed erythrocytes in centrifuged blood 血沉棕黄层，血液离心后红细胞层上方由白细胞形成的一淡黄色薄层

co·bal·a·min (ko-bal′ə-min) a compound comprising the substituted ring and nucleotide structure characteristic of vitamin B_{12}, either one lacking a ligand at the 6 position of cobalt or any substituted derivative, including cyanocobalamin, particularly one with vitamin B_{12} activity 钴胺素，维生素 B_{12}

co·balt (Co) (ko′bawlt) a hard, lustrous, silvergray metallic element; at. no. 27, at. wt. 58.933. It is an essential trace element, acting as the active center of cobalamin coenzymes, including the mammalian vitamin B_{12}. Inhalation of the dust can cause pneumoconiosis, and exposure to the powder can cause dermatitis 钴; **c. 60**, a radioisotope of cobalt used in radiation therapy 钴 60，用于放射治疗的一种放射性同位素

co·bra (ko′brə) any of several extremely poisonous elapid snakes commonly found in Africa, Asia, and India, which are capable of expanding the neck region to form a hood and have two comparatively short, erect, deeply grooved fangs. Most inject venom by biting, but some species, spitting c's, can eject a fine spray of venom several meters and cause severe eye irritation or blindness 眼镜蛇

co·caine (ko-kān′) an alkaloid obtained from leaves of various species of *Erythroxylon* (coca plants) or produced synthetically, used as a local anesthetic; also used as the hydrochloride salt. Abuse can lead to addiction 可卡因

co·car·cin·o·gen (ko-kahr-sin′ə-jən) 1. a type of epigenetic carcinogen that promotes neoplastic growth only after initiation by another substance 辅致癌原，在其他物质始动肿瘤生长后才能促进肿瘤生长的一类外源性致癌原；2. something that exacerbates the carcinogenic effects of another substance 辅致癌物质，能增强其他物质致癌性的一类物质

co·car·ci·no·gen·e·sis (ko-kahr″sī-no-jen′ə-sis) the development, according to one theory, of cancer only in preconditioned cells as a result of conditions favorable to its growth 辅致癌作用

coc·ci (kok′si) 球菌，*coccus* 的复数形式

Coc·cid·ia (kok-sid′e-ə) a subclass of parasitic protozoa comprising the orders Agamococcidiida, Protococcidiida, and Eucoccidiida 球虫亚纲

coc·cid·ia (kok-sid′e-ə) 球虫，coccidium 的复数形式

Coc·cid·i·oi·des (kok-sid″e-oi′dēz) a genus of pathogenic anamorphic fungi found in the soil, including *C. im′mitis* and *C. posada′sii*, which cause coccidioidomycosis 球孢子菌属；**coccidioi′dal** *adj.* 球孢子菌的

coc·cid·i·oi·din (kok-sid″e-oi′din) a sterile preparation containing byproducts of *Coccidioides immitis*, injected intracutaneously in a test for coccidioidomycosis 球孢子菌素

coc·cid·i·oi·do·my·co·sis (kok-sid″e-oi″domi-ko′sis) infection by inhaled spores of *Coccidioides* species, usually occurring as an acute, benign, often asymptomatic respiratory infection but potentially becoming a chronic, granulomatous pulmonary infection or disseminating to involve other organs, particularly the skin, bones and joints, or meninges 球孢子菌病

coc·cid·i·o·sis (kok″sid-e-o′sis) infection by coccidia. In humans, applied to the presence of *Isospora hominis* or *I. belli* in stools; it is often asymptomatic, rarely causing a severe watery mucous diarrhea 球虫病

coc·cid·i·um (kok-sid′e-əm) pl. *cocci′dia*. Any member of the subclass Coccidia 球虫

coc·ci·gen·ic (kok″sī-jen′ik) produced by cocci 球菌源性的

coc·co·ba·cil·lus (kok″o-bə-sil′əs) pl. *coccobacil′li*. An oval bacterial cell intermediate between the

coccus and bacillus forms 球杆菌；**coccobac′illary** *adj.* 球杆菌的

coc·co·bac·te·ria (kok″o-bak-tēr′e-ə) a common name for spheroid bacteria, or for bacterial cocci 球菌

coc·cus (kok′əs) pl. *coc′ci* [L.] a spherical bacterium, less than 1 μm in diameter 球菌；**coc′cal** *adj.* 球菌的

coc·cy·al·gia (kok″se-al′jə) coccygodynia 尾骨痛

coc·cyg·e·al (kok-sij′e-əl) pertaining to or located in the region of the coccyx 尾骨的

coc·cy·gec·to·my (kok″sī-jek′tə-me) excision of the coccyx 尾骨切除术

coc·cy·go·dyn·ia (kok″sī-go-din′e-ə) pain in the coccyx and neighboring region 尾骨痛

coc·cy·got·o·my (kok″sī-got′ə-me) incision of the coccyx 尾骨切开术

coc·cyx (kok′siks) tail bone; the small bone caudad to the sacrum, formed by union of four (sometimes five or three) rudimentary vertebrae, and forming the caudal extremity of the vertebral column 尾骨，见图 1

coch·i·neal (koch″ĭ-nēl′) dried female insects of *Coccus cacti*, enclosing young larvae; used as a coloring agent for pharmaceuticals and as a biologic stain 胭脂虫

coch·lea (kok′le-ə) 1. anything of a spiral form 任何螺旋形的事物；2. a spiral tube forming part of the inner ear, which is the essential organ of hearing 耳蜗，见图 29；**coch′lear** *adj.* 耳蜗的

coch·le·ar·i·form (kok″le-ar′ĭ-form) spoon-shaped 匙形的

coch·leo·sac·cu·lot·o·my (kok″le-o-sak″ulot′ə-me) creation of a fistula between the saccule and cochlear duct by means of a pick introduced through the cochlear window, in order to relieve endolymphatic hydrops 耳蜗球囊切开术

coch·leo·top·ic (kok″le-o-top′ik) relating to the organization of the auditory pathways and auditory area of the brain 与听觉通路和脑听觉区有关的

Coch·lio·my·ia (kok″le-o-mi′yə) a genus of flies, including *C. hominivo′rax*, the screw-worm fly, which deposits its eggs on animal wounds; after hatching, the larvae burrow into the wound and feed on living tissue 锥蝇属

coc·to·la·bile (kok″to-la′bəl) (-la′bīl) capable of being altered or destroyed by heating 不耐热的

coc·to·sta·bile (kok″to-sta′bəl) (-sta′bīl) not altered by heating to the boiling point of water 耐煮沸的

code (kōd) 1. a set of rules for regulating conduct 法则；2. a system by which information can be communicated 代码；**genetic c.,** the arrangement of consecutive nucleotide triplets (codons) in a nucleic acid that specifies the sequence of amino acids for synthesis of a protein 遗传密码；triplet c., the form taken by the genetic code, in which each amino acid or start or stop signal is encoded by a group of three nucleotides (codon) 三联体密码，密码子

co·deine (ko′dēn) a narcotic alkaloid obtained from opium or prepared from morphine by methylation and used as the base or as the phosphate or sulfate salt as an opioid analgesic, antitussive, and antidiarrheal 可待因

co·dom·i·nance (ko-dom′ĭ-nəns) the full phenotypic expression in a heterozygote of both alleles of a pair, with each contributing to the phenotype, as in a person with blood group AB 共显性；**codom′inant** adj. 共显性的

co·don (ko′don) a set of three adjacent bases on an mRNA that specifies an amino acid to be added to the growing polypeptide chain, or directs chain initiation or termination 密码子

co·ef·fi·cient (ko″ə-fish′ənt) 1. an expression of the change or effect produced by variation in certain factors, or of the ratio between two different quantities 系数；2. a number or figure put before a chemical formula to indicate how many times the formula is to be multiplied 化学方程式中的系数；**absorption c.**, 1. absorptivity 吸收系数；2. linear absorption c 线性吸收系数；3. mass absorption c 质量吸收系数；**biological c.**, the amount of potential energy consumed by the body at rest 生物系数；**correlation c.**, a measure of the relationship between two statistical variables, most commonly expressed as their covariance divided by the standard deviation of each 相关系数；**linear absorption c.**, in radiation physics, the fraction of a beam of radiation absorbed per unit thickness of the absorber 线性吸收系数；**mass absorption c.**, in radiation physics, the linear absorption coefficient divided by the density of the absorber 质量吸收系数；**phenol c.**, a measure of the bactericidal activity of a chemical compound in relation to phenol 石炭酸系数；**sedimentation c.**, the velocity at which a particle sediments in a centrifuge relative to the applied centrifugal field, usually expressed in Svedberg units (S), equal to 10^{-13} second, which are used to characterize the size of macromolecules 沉降系数；**c. of thermal conductivity**, a number indicating the quantity of heat passing in a unit of time through a unit thickness of a substance when the difference in temperature is 1℃热传导系数；**c. of thermal expansion**, the change in volume per unit volume of a substance produced by a 1℃ temperature increase 热膨胀系数

Coe·len·ter·a·ta (se-len″tər-a′tə) former name for a phylum of invertebrates that included the hydras, jellyfish, sea anemones, and corals, which are now assigned to the phylum Cnidaria 腔肠动物门

coe·len·ter·ate (se-len′tər-āt) cnidarian 腔肠动物

coe·lom (se′ləm) body cavity, especially the cavity in the mammalian embryo between the somatopleure and splanchnopleure, which is both intra- and extraembryonic; the principal cavities of the trunk arise from the intraembryonic portion 体腔；**coelom′ic** adj. 体腔的

coe·lo·mate (sēl′o-māt) 1. having a coelom 有体腔的；2. an individual of the Eucoelomata; eucoelomate 真体腔动物

coe·lo·zo·ic (se″lo-zo′ik) inhabiting the intestinal canal of the body; said of parasites 腔内寄生的

coe·nu·ro·sis (se″nu-ro′sis) infection by coenurus; a rare infection in humans is manifest as cysts in the central nervous system and increased intracranial pressure 多头蚴病

Coe·nu·rus (se-nu′rəs) a genus of tapeworm larvae, including *C. cerebra′lis*, the larva of *Taenia multiceps*, which causes coenurosis 多头蚴属

coe·nu·rus (se-nu′rəs) the larval stage of tapeworms of the genus *Taenia*, a semitransparent, fluid-filled, bladderlike organism that contains multiple scoleces attached to the inner surface of its wall and that does not form brood capsules. It develops in various parts of the host body, especially in the central nervous system 多头蚴

co·en·zyme (ko-en′zīm) an organic nonprotein molecule, frequently a phosphorylated derivative of a water-soluble vitamin, that binds with the protein molecule (apoenzyme) to form the active enzyme (holoenzyme) 辅酶；**c. A (CoA) (CoA-SH)**, a coenzyme containing among its constituents pantothenic acid and a terminal thiol group that forms high-energy thioester linkages with various acids, e.g., acetic acid (acetyl CoA) and fatty acids (acyl CoA); these thioesters play a central role in the tricarboxylic acid cycle, the transfer of acetyl groups, and the oxidation of fatty acids 辅酶 A；**c. Q, c. Q₁₀**, ubiquinone 辅酶 Q，泛醌

coeur (kur) [Fr.] heart 心脏，**c. en sabot**, (ah sä-bo′) a heart whose shape on a radiograph resembles that of a wooden shoe; seen in tetralogy of Fallot 靴形心，见于法洛四联症

co·fac·tor (ko′fak-tər) an element or principle, e.g., a coenzyme, with which another must unite in order to function 辅因子；**heparin c.** Ⅱ, a serine proteinase inhibitor of the serpin family that inhibits thrombin. 肝素辅因子Ⅱ，丝氨酸蛋白酶抑制药家族的一员，可抑制凝血酶

co·fi·lin (cō-fə′lin) a protein that acts as a mediator of actin dynamics, which promotes filament severing and depolymerization, facilitating the breakdown of existing filaments and the enhancement of filament growth from newly created barbed ends. Abnormalities in cofilin/actin-depolymerizing factor affect multiple pathologic conditions, such as neurologic and cardiovascular disorders or cancer metastasis 丝切蛋白

cog·ni·tion (kog-nish′ən) that operation of the mind process by which we become aware of objects of thought and perception, including all aspects of perceiving, thinking, and remembering 认知；**cog′nitive** adj. 认知的

co·he·sion (ko-he′zhən) the intermolecular attractive force causing various particles of a single material to unite 内聚力；**cohe′sive** adj. 内聚力的

co·hort (ko′hort) 1. in epidemiology, a group of individuals sharing a common characteristic and observed over time in the group（流行病学）队列；2. a taxonomic category approximately equivalent to a division, order, or suborder in various systems of classification 同生群

co·hosh (ko-hosh′) [Algonquian] any of various North American medicinal plants 升麻；**black c.,** the plant *Cimicifuga racemosa* or its fresh or dried root, which has estrogenic effects and is used in menopause and premenstrual syndrome; also used in folk medicine and traditional Chinese medicine 黑升麻；**blue c.,** the herb *Caulophyllum thalictroides* or its fresh roots or dried rhizome and roots, which have weak estrogenic effects; used for menstrual disorders and as an antispasmodic and uterine stimulant during labor; also used in homeopathy 蓝升麻

coil (koil) spiral (2) 螺旋形的

co·in·fec·tion (ko′in-fek″shən) simultaneous infection by separate pathogens, as by hepatitis B and hepatitis D viruses 混合感染

coi·no·site (koi′no-sīt) a free commensal organism 自由共生生物

co·i·to·pho·bia (ko″ī-to-fo′be-ə) irrational fear of coitus 性交恐怖症

co·i·tus (ko′ī-təs) sexual connection per vaginam between male and female. 性 交；**co′ital** adj. 性交的；**c. incomple′tus, c. interrup′tus,** coitus in which the penis is withdrawn from the vagina before ejaculation 体外射精，在射精前阴茎从阴道内抽出；**c. reserva′tus,** coitus in which ejaculation is intentionally suppressed 射精被有意抑制的性交

col (kol) a depression in the interdental tissues just below the interproximal contact area, connecting the buccal and lingual papillae 牙齿邻面下方牙间组织的一处凹陷，连接颊乳头与舌乳头

col·chi·cine (kol′chĭ-sēn) an alkaloid from the tree *Colchicum autumnale* (meadow saffron), used as a suppressant for gout 秋水仙碱

cold (kōld) 1. low in temperature, in physiologic activity, in radioactivity 冷 的，温度低的，生理活动低下的，放射活性低下的；2. common cold; a catarrhal disorder of the upper respiratory tract, which may be viral, a mixed infection, or an allergic reaction, and marked by acute rhinitis, slight temperature rise, and chilly sensations 普通感冒；**common c.,** cold (2)

co·lec·to·my (ko-lek′tə-me) excision of the colon or of a portion of it 结肠切除术

co·le·sev·e·lam (ko″lə-sev′ə-lam) a bile acid-binding polymer that decreases serum levels of total cholesterol, LDL cholesterol, and apolipoprotein B and increases levels of HDL cholesterol; used as the hydrochloride salt in the treatment of primary hypercholesterolemia 考来维仑

co·les·ti·pol (ko-les′tĭ-pol) an anion exchange resin that binds bile acids in the intestines to form a complex that is excreted in the feces; administered in the form of the hydrochloride salt as an antihyperlipoproteinemic 考来替泊，降胆宁

col·fos·e·ril (kol-fos′ə-ril) a synthetic pulmonary surfactant used as the palmitate ester, in combination with cetyl alcohol and tyloxapol, in the prophylaxis and treatment of neonatal respiratory distress syndrome 考福西利

co·li·bac·il·lo·sis (ko″lī-bas-ĭ-lo′sis) infection with *Escherichia coli* 大肠杆菌病

co·li·bac·il·lus (ko″lī-bə-sil′əs) *Escherichia coli.* 大肠杆菌

col·ic (kol′ik) 1. acute paroxysmal abdominal pain 腹绞痛；2. pertaining to the colon 结肠的；**appendicular c.,** pain in the vermiform appendix caused by inflammation 阑尾绞痛；**biliary c.,** colic due to passage of gallstones along the bile duct 胆绞痛；**gallstone c., hepatic c.,** biliary c.；**infantile c.,** a paroxysmal type seen during the first 3 months of life 婴儿腹绞痛；**lead c.,** colic due to lead poisoning 铅中毒性腹绞痛；**renal c.,** pain due to thrombosis of the renal vein or artery, dissection of the renal artery, renal infarction, intrarenal mass lesions, or passage of a stone within the collecting system 肾绞痛；**vermicular c.,** appendicular c.

col·i·cin (kol′ĭ-sin) a protein secreted by colicinogenic strains of *Escherichia coli* and other enteric bacteria; lethal to related, sensitive bacteria 大肠菌素

col·icky (kol′ik-e) pertaining to colic 腹绞痛的

col·i·form (ko′lĭ-form) pertaining to fermentative gram-negative enteric bacilli, sometimes restricted to those fermenting lactose, e.g., *Escherichia, Klebsiella,* or *Enterobacter* 大肠菌群

col·i·phage (kol'ĭ-fāj) any bacteriophage that infects *Escherichia coli* 大肠杆菌噬菌体，所有可感染大肠杆菌的噬菌体

col·is·ti·meth·ate (ko-lis″tĭ-meth′āt) a colistin derivative; the sodium salt is used as an antibacterial 多黏菌素

co·lis·tin (ko-lis'tin) an antibiotic produced by *Bacillus polymyxa* var. *colistinus,* related to polymyxin and effective against many gram-negative bacteria; used as the sulfate salt 黏菌素

co·li·tis (ko-li'tis) inflammation of the colon 结肠炎；见 *enterocolitis.* **amebic c.,** 阿米巴结肠炎见 *dysentery* 下词条。**antibiotic-associated c.,** 抗生素相关性结肠炎，见 *enterocolitis* 下词条；**collagenous c.,** a type of colitis of unknown etiology characterized by deposits of collagenous material beneath the epithelium of the colon, with crampy abdominal pain and watery diarrhea 胶原性结肠炎；**granulomatous c.,** transmural colitis with the formation of noncaseating granulomas 肉芽肿性结肠炎；**ischemic c.,** acute vascular insufficiency of the colon, affecting the portion supplied by the inferior mesenteric artery; symptoms include pain at the left iliac fossa, bloody diarrhea, low-grade fever, and abdominal distention and tenderness 缺血性结肠炎；**regional c., segmental c.,** transmural or granulomatous inflammatory disease of the colon; regional enteritis involving the colon. It may be associated with ulceration, strictures, or fistulas 节段性结肠炎；**transmural c.,** inflammation of the full thickness of the bowel, rather than just mucosa and submucosa, usually with formation of noncaseating granulomas. It may be confined to the colon (segmentally or diffusely) or be associated with regional enteritis in the small intestine. Clinically, it may resemble ulcerative colitis, but with deeper ulcerations, stricture formation, and fistulas, particularly in the perineum 透壁性结肠炎；**ulcerative c.,** chronic ulceration in the colon, chiefly of the mucosa and submucosa, manifested by cramping abdominal pain, rectal bleeding, and loose discharges of blood, pus, and mucus with scanty fecal particles 溃疡性结肠炎

co·li·tox·emia (ko″lĭ-tok-se'me-ə) toxemia due to infection with *Escherichia coli* 大肠杆菌毒血症

co·li·tox·in (ko'lĭ-tok″sin) a toxin from *Escherichia coli* 大肠杆菌毒素

col·la·gen (kol'ə-jən) any of a family of extracellular, closely related proteins occurring as a major component of connective tissue, giving it strength and flexibility; composed of molecules of tropocollagen 胶原，胶原蛋白；**collag'enous** *adj.* 胶原的

col·la·ge·nase (kə-laj'ə-nās) an enzyme that catalyzes the hydrolysis of peptide bonds in triple helical regions of collagen 胶原酶

col·lag·e·na·tion (kə-laj″ə-na'shən) the appearance of collagen in developing cartilage 胶原生成

col·lag·e·no·blast (kə-laj'ə-no-blast) a cell arising from a fibroblast and which, as it matures, is associated with collagen production; it may also form cartilage and bone by metaplasia 成胶原细胞

col·lag·e·no·cyte (kə-laj'ə-no-sīt″) a mature collagen-producing cell 胶原细胞，可产生胶原的成熟细胞

col·la·gen·o·gen·ic (kə-laj″ə-no-jen'ik) pertaining to or characterized by collagen production; forming collagen or collagen fibers 胶原源性的

col·la·gen·ol·y·sis (kol″ə-jən-ol'ə-sis) dissolution or digestion of collagen 胶原溶解；**collagenolyt'ic** *adj.* 胶原溶解的

col·lag·e·nous (kə-laj'ə-nəs) pertaining to, forming, or producing collagen 胶原的

col·lapse (kə-laps') 1. a state of extreme prostration and depression, with failure of circulation 极度虚脱、压抑的状态，伴有循环障碍；2. abnormal falling in of the walls of a part or organ 结构或器官的壁异常坍陷；**circulatory c.,** shock (2) 休克

col·lar (kol'ər) an encircling band, generally around the neck 领；**cervical c.,** 颈托，见 *orthosis* 下词条；**Philadelphia c.,** a type of cervical orthosis that restricts anterior-posterior cervical motion considerably but allows some normal rotation and lateral bending 一种颈部支具，限制颈部前后活动但允许一些正常的旋转和侧向活动

col·lar·ette (kol″ər-et') 1. a narrow rim of loosened keratin overhanging the periphery of a circumscribed skin lesion, attached to the normal surrounding skin 局限性皮肤病变外周松弛的角质贴附于正常皮肤上所形成的小环；2. an irregular jagged line dividing the anterior surface of the iris into two regions 将虹膜前表面分成两部分的异常齿状线

col·lat·er·al (ko-lat'ər-əl) 1. secondary or accessory; not direct or immediate 继发的，附属的；2. a small side branch, as of a blood vessel or nerve 侧支

col·lic·u·lec·to·my (kə-lik″u-lek'tə-me) excision of the seminal colliculus 精阜切除术

col·lic·u·lus (kə-lik'u-ləs) pl. *colli'culi* [L.] a small elevation 丘；**seminal c., c. semina'lis,** verumontanum; a portion of the male urethral crest on which are the openings of the prostatic utricle and the ejaculatory ducts 精阜

col·li·ma·tion (kol″ĭ-ma'shən) 1. in microscopy, the process of making light rays parallel; the adjustment or aligning of optical axes 准直，在显微镜技

术中，使光线平行的过程；光轴的调整或对准；2. in radiology, the elimination of the more divergent portion of an x-ray beam 在放射学中，指消除 X 线束发散的部分；3. in nuclear medicine, the use of a perforated absorber to restrict the field of view of a detector and reduce scatter 在核医学中，指使用穿孔吸收器以限制探测仪的视野，减少散射

col·liq·ua·tive (kə-lik′wə-tiv) characterized by excessive liquid discharge, or by liquefaction of tissue 液化的

col·lo·di·a·phys·e·al (kol″o-di″ə-fiz′e-əl) pertaining to the neck and shaft of a long bone, especially the femur 长骨颈和骨干的，特别指股骨

col·lo·di·on (kə-lo′de-ən) a syrupy liquid compounded of pyroxylin, ether, and alcohol, which dries to a transparent, tenacious film; used as a topical protectant, applied to the skin to close small wounds, abrasions, and cuts, to hold surgical dressings in place, and to keep medications in contact with the skin 火棉胶剂；**flexible c.**, a preparation of camphor, castor oil, and collodion, used as a topical protectant 弹性火棉胶剂；**salicylic acid c.**, flexible collodion containing salicylic acid; used topically as a keratolytic 水杨酸火棉胶剂

col·loid (kol′oid) 1. glutinous or resembling glue 胶状的；2. a chemical system composed of a continuous medium (continuous phase) throughout which are distributed small particles, 1 to 1000 nm in size (disperse phase), which do not settle out under the influence of gravity; the particles may be in emulsion or in suspension. The term may be used to denote either the particles or the entire system 胶体；**colloid′al** adj. 胶状的，胶体的；**dispersion c.**, colloid (2), sometimes specifically an unstable colloid system 分散胶体；**emulsion c.**, 1. lyophilic c. 2. rarely, emulsion 乳胶体；**lyophilic c.**, a colloid system in which the disperse phase is relatively liquid, usually comprising highly complex organic substances such as starch, which readily absorb solvent, swell, and distribute uniformly through the medium 亲液胶体；**lyophobic c.**, an unstable colloid system in which the disperse phase particles tend to repel liquids, are easily precipitated, and cannot be redispersed with additional solvent 疏液胶体；**stannous sulfur c.**, a sulfur colloid containing stannous ions; complexed with technetium 99m it is used in bone, liver, and spleen imaging 硫化亚锡胶体；**suspension c.**, lyophobic c. 悬浮胶体

col·lum (kol′əm) (kol′la [L.] the neck, or a necklike part 颈，颈部或颈样的部分

col·lu·to·ry (kol′u-tor″e) mouthwash or gargle 漱口液

col·lyr·i·um (kə-lir′e-əm) pl. colly′ria [L.] a lotion

for the eyes; an eye wash 洗眼剂

col·o·bo·ma (kol″o-bo′mə) pl. colobomas, colobo′mata [L.] 1. an absence or defect of tissue 组织缺损；2. a defect of ocular tissue, usually due to failure of part of the fetal fissure to close; it may affect the choroid, ciliary body, eyelid, iris, lens, optic nerve, or retina 眼组织缺损，通常是由于部分脉络裂未闭合；可累及脉络膜、睫状体、眼睑、虹膜、晶状体、视神经和视网膜；**bridge c.**, coloboma of the iris in which a strip of iris tissue bridges over the fissure 桥形缺损；**Fuchs c.**, a small, crescent-shaped defect of the choroid at the lower edge of the optic disk 在视盘下缘处脉络膜的新月形小型缺损；**c. lo′buli**, fissure of the ear lobe 耳垂裂

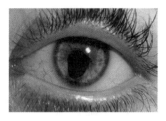

▲ 虹膜缺损（**coloboma of the iris**）

co·lo·cen·te·sis (ko″lo-sen-te′sis) surgical puncture of the colon 结肠穿刺术

co·lo·co·los·to·my (ko″lo-kə-los′tə-me) surgical anastomosis between two portions of the colon 结肠结肠吻合术

co·lo·cu·ta·ne·ous (ko″lo-ku-ta′ne-əs) pertaining to the colon and skin, or communicating with the colon and the cutaneous surface of the body 结肠皮肤的

co·lo·cys·to·plas·ty (ko″lo-sis′to-plas″te) augmentation cystoplasty using an isolated section of colon 结肠膀胱成形术

co·lo·fix·a·tion (ko″lo-fik-sa′shən) the fixation or suspension of the colon in cases of ptosis 结肠固定术

co·lon (ko′lən) [L.] the part of the large intestine extending from the cecum to the rectum 结肠，见插图及图 27；**ascending c.**, the portion of the colon passing cephalad from the cecum to the right colic flexure 升结肠；**congenital pouch c.**, a congenital malformation in which part or all of it is replaced by a dilated pouch and there is anorectal malformation with a fistula between the colon and the genitourinary tract 先天性袋状结肠；**descending c.**, the portion of the colon passing caudad from the left colic flexure to the sigmoid colon 降结肠；**iliac c.**, the part of the descending colon lying in the left iliac fossa and continuous with the sigmoid colon 结

肠髂部；**irritable c.,** irritable bowel syndrome 易激性结肠症；**left c.,** the distal portion of the large intestine, developed embryonically from the hindgut and functioning in the storage and elimination from the body of nonabsorbed residue of ingested material 左结肠，大肠的远端部分，由胚胎的后肠发育而来，具有储存、排出未消化的摄入物的功能；**pelvic c.,** sigmoid c.；**right c.,** the proximal portion of the large intestine, developed embryonically from the terminal portion of the midgut and functioning in absorption of ingested material 右结肠，大肠的近端部分，由胚胎的中肠发育而来，具有吸收的作用；**sigmoid c.,** that portion of the left colon situated in the pelvis and extending from the descending colon to the rectum 乙状结肠；**spastic c.,** irritable bowel syndrome 痉挛性结肠；**transverse c.,** the portion of the large intestine passing transversely across the upper part of the abdomen, between the right and left colic flexures 横结肠

co·lon·ic (ko-lon′ik) 1. pertaining to the colon 结肠的；2. colon hydrotherapy 结肠水疗

co·lon·og·ra·phy (ko″lən-og′rə-fe) imaging of the colon, as by computed tomography or magnetic resonance imaging 结肠造影

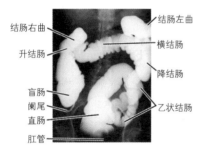

▲ 钡剂灌肠后的结肠（**colon**）X 线照片

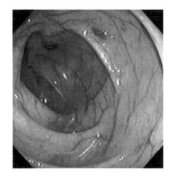

▲ 结肠镜（**colonoscopy**）示正常结肠

co·lon·op·a·thy (ko″lo-nop′ə-the) any disease or disorder of the colon 结肠病

co·lon·os·co·py (ko″lən-os′kə-pe) endoscopic examination of the colon. nnColonoscopy showing a normal colon 结肠镜

col·o·ny (kol′ə-ne) a discrete group of organisms, as a collection of bacteria in a culture 菌落，如培养的细菌集落

co·lo·pexy (ko′lo-pek″se) surgical fixation or suspension of the colon 结肠固定术

co·lo·pli·ca·tion (ko″lo-plĭ-ka′shən) the operation of infolding or taking tucks in the wall of the colon in cases of dilatation 结肠折叠术

co·lo·proc·tec·to·my (ko″lo-prok-tek′tə-me) surgical removal of the colon and rectum 结肠直肠吻合术

co·lo·proc·tos·to·my (ko″lo-prok-tos′tə-me) colorectostomy 结肠直肠吻合术

co·lo·punc·ture (ko′lo-pungk′chər) colocentesis. 结肠穿刺术

col·or (kul′ər) 1. a property of a surface or substance due to absorption of certain light rays and reflection of others within the range of wavelengths (roughly 370~760 nm) adequate to excite the retinal receptors 颜色；2. radiant energy within the range of adequate chromatic stimuli of the retina, i.e., between the infrared and ultraviolet 辐射能，视网膜所能感知的颜色光所含的辐射能；3. a sensory impression of one of the rainbow hues 对某种彩虹色的感觉印记；**complementary c's,** a pair of colors the sensory mechanisms for which are so linked that when they are mixed on the color wheel they cancel each other out, leaving neutral gray 互补色；**confusion c's,** different colors liable to be mistakenly matched by persons with defective color vision, and hence used for detecting different types of color vision defects 混淆色，可能被色觉障碍者混淆的不同颜色，因此被用于检查不同的色觉障碍；**primary c's,** a small number of fundamental colors; (*a*) in visual science, red, green, and blue, the colors specifically picked up by the retinal cones; (*b*) in painting and printing, blue, yellow, and red 原色；**pure c.,** one whose stimulus consists of homogeneous wavelengths, with little or no admixture of wavelengths of other hues 纯色

co·lo·rec·tos·to·my (ko″lo-rek-tos′tə-me) formation of an opening between the colon and rectum 结肠直肠吻合术

co·lo·rec·tum (ko″lo-rek′təm) the distal 10 inches (25 cm) of the bowel, including the distal portion of the colon and the rectum, regarded as a unit 结直肠，肠的末端25cm，包括结肠远端和直肠，通常被视为一个单位；**colorec′tal** *adj.* 结直肠的

col·or·im·e·ter (kul″ər-im′ə-tər) an instrument for measuring color or color intensity in a solution 色度计

co·lor·rha·phy (ko-lor′ə-fe) suture of the colon 结肠缝合术

co·lo·sig·moid·os·to·my (ko″lo-sig″moid-os″tə-me) surgical anastomosis of a formerly remote portion of the colon to the sigmoid 结肠乙状结肠吻合术

co·los·to·my (kə-los′tə-me) the surgical creation of an opening between the colon and the body surface; also, the opening (stoma) so created 结肠造口术；**dry c.,** colostomy performed in the left colon, the discharge from the stoma consisting of soft or formed fecal matter 左结肠的结肠造口术，造口的排泄物为软的或成形的粪便；**ileotransverse c.,** surgical anastomosis between the ileum and the transverse colon 回肠—横结肠吻合术；**wet c.,** colostomy in (*a*) the right colon, the drainage from which is liquid, or (*b*) the left colon following anastomosis of the ureters to the sigmoid or descending colon so that urine is also expelled through the same stoma (a) 右结肠的结肠造口术，造口的排泄物为液体；(b) 左结肠的结肠造口术，并有输尿管乙状结肠或降结肠吻合，尿液可从该造口排出

co·los·trum (kə-los′trəm) the thin, yellow, milky fluid secreted by the mammary gland a few days before or after parturition 初乳

co·lot·o·my (ko-lot′ə-me) incision of the colon 结肠切开术

co·lo·ves·i·cal (ko″lo-ves′ĭ-kəl) pertaining to or communicating with the colon and bladder 结肠膀胱的，结肠膀胱瘘的

col·pal·gia (kol-pal′jə) pain in the vagina 阴道痛

col·pec·ta·sia (kol″pek-ta′zhə) distention or dilatation of the vagina 阴道扩张

col·pec·to·my (kol-pek′tə-me) excision of the vagina 阴道切除术

col·peu·ry·sis (kol-pu′rĭ-sis) dilatation of the vagina 阴道扩张术

col·pi·tis (kol-pi′tis) vaginitis 阴道炎

col·po·clei·sis (kol″po-kli′sis) surgical closure of the vaginal canal 阴道闭合术

col·po·cy·to·gram (kol″po-si′to-gram) differential listing of cells observed in vaginal smears 阴道细胞涂片谱

col·po·cy·tol·o·gy (kol″po-si-tol′ə-je) the study of cells exfoliated from the epithelium of the vagina 阴道细胞学

col·po·hy·per·pla·sia (kol″po-hi″pər-pla′zhə) excessive growth of the mucous membrane and wall of the vagina 阴道黏膜增生

col·po·mi·cro·scope (kol″po-mi′kro-skōp) an instrument for microscopic examination of the tissues of the cervix in situ 阴道显微镜

col·po·per·i·neo·plas·ty (kol″po-per″ĭ-ne′o·plas″te) plastic repair of the vagina and perineum 阴道会阴成形术

col·po·per·i·ne·or·rha·phy (kol″po-per″ĭ-neor′ə-fe) suture of the ruptured vagina and perineum 阴道会阴缝合术

col·po·pexy (kol′po-pek″se) suture of a relaxed vagina to the abdominal wall 阴道固定术

col·pop·to·sis (kol″pop-to′sis) prolapse of the vagina 阴道下垂

col·por·rha·phy (kol-por′ə-fe) 1. suture of the vagina 阴道缝合术；2. the operation of denuding and suturing the vaginal wall to narrow the vagina 阴道缩窄术

col·por·rhex·is (kol″po-rek′sis) laceration of the vagina 阴道裂伤，阴道破裂

col·po·scope (kol′po-skōp) vaginoscope; a speculum for examining the vagina and cervix using a magnifying lens 阴道镜

col·po·spasm (kol′po-spaz″əm) vaginal spasm 阴道痉挛

col·po·ste·no·sis (kol″po-stə-no′sis) contraction or narrowing of the vagina 阴道狭窄

col·po·ste·not·o·my (kol″po-stə-not′ə-me) a cutting operation for stricture of the vagina 阴道狭窄切开术

col·po·sus·pen·sion (kol″po-səs-pen′shən) bladder neck suspension 膀胱颈悬吊术

col·pot·o·my (kol-pot′ə-me) incision of the vagina with entry into the cul-de-sac 阴道切开术

col·po·xe·ro·sis (kol″po-ze-ro′sis) abnormal dryness of the vulva and vagina 阴道干燥

Col·ti·vi·rus (kol′tī-vi″rəs) a genus of viruses of the family Reoviridae, containing the agent of Colorado tick fever 呼吸道肠道病毒属

col·u·mel·la (kol″u-mel′ə) pl. *columel′lae* [L.] 1. a little column 小柱；2. in certain fungi and protozoa, an invagination into the sporangium 在某些真菌和原虫中，指插入孢子囊繁殖区的孢子囊柄的非繁殖部分；**c. coch′leae,** modiolus 蜗轴，耳蜗轴；**c. na′si,** the fleshy external end of the nasal septum. 鼻小柱

col·umn (kol′əm) an anatomic part in the form of a pillar-like structure 柱；**anal c's,** vertical folds of mucous membrane at the upper half of the anal canal 肛柱；**anterior c. of spinal cord,** 1. the anterior portion of the gray substance of the spinal cord, in transverse section seen as a horn 前柱；2. palatoglossal arch 腭舌弓；**Bertin c's,** renal c's; **Burdach c.,** cuneate fasciculus of spinal cord 脊髓楔束；**enamel c's,** adamantine prisms 釉质柱；**Goll c.,** gracile fasciculus of spinal cord 脊髓薄束；

C

gray c's of spinal cord, the longitudinally oriented parts of the spinal cord in which the nerve cell bodies are found, comprising the gray substance of the spinal cord 脊髓灰柱; **lateral c. of spinal cord,** the lateral portion of the spinal cord, in transverse section seen as a horn; present only in the thoracic and upper lumbar regions 脊髓侧柱; **Morgagni c's, anal c's** 肛柱; **posterior c. of spinal cord,** 1. the posterior portion of gray substance of the spinal cord, in transverse section seen as a horn 脊髓后柱; 2. palatopharyngeal arch 腭咽弓; **rectal c's, anal c's.; renal c's,** inward extensions of the cortical substance of the kidney between contiguous renal pyramids 肾柱; **spinal c.,** vertebral c; **vertebral c.,** the rigid structure in the midline of the back, composed of the vertebrae 脊柱

co·lum·na (kə-lum′nə) pl. *colum′nae* [L.] column 柱

co·lum·nar (kə-lum′nər) having the shape of a column; arranged in or characterized by columns 柱状的

col·um·ni·za·tion (kol″əm-nī-za′shən) support of the prolapsed uterus by tampons 棉塞支托法

co·ma (ko′mə) [L.] a state of profound unconsciousness from which the patient cannot be aroused, even by powerful stimuli 昏迷; **co′matose adj. alcoholic c.,** stupor accompanying severe alcoholic intoxication 酒精中毒性昏迷; **diabetic c.,** the coma of severe diabetic acidosis 糖尿病昏迷; **hepatic c.,** coma accompanying hepatic encephalopathy 肝(性)昏迷; **irreversible c.,** brain death 脑死亡; **Kussmaul c.,** diabetic c; **metabolic c.,** the coma accompanying metabolic encephalopathy 代谢性昏迷; **uremic c.,** lethargic state due to uremia 尿毒症昏迷; **c. vigil,** locked-in syndrome 睁眼昏迷

com·bus·tion (kəm-bus′chən) rapid oxidation with emission of heat 燃烧

com·e·do (kom′ə-do) pl. *comedo′nes.* A plug of keratin and sebum within the dilated orifice of a hair follicle, frequently containing the bacteria *Propionibacterium acnes, Staphylococcus albus,* and *Pityrosporum ovale* 粉刺; **closed c.,** whitehead; a comedo whose opening is not widely dilated, appearing as a small, flesh-colored papule; it may rupture and cause an inflammatory lesion in the dermis 闭合性粉刺; **open c.,** blackhead; a comedo with a widely dilated orifice in which the pigmented impaction is visible at the skin surface 开放性粉刺

com·e·do·gen·ic (kom″ə-do-jen′ik) producing comedones 产生粉刺的，引起粉刺的

com·e·do·mas·ti·tis (kom″ə-do-mas-ti′tis) mammary duct ectasia 粉刺性乳痛，粉刺状乳腺炎

co·mes (ko′mēz) pl. *comi′tes* [L.] an artery or vein

accompanying another artery or vein or a nerve trunk 并行血管，伴行血管

com·frey (kom′fre) the perennial herb *Symphytum officinale,* or a preparation of its leaves and roots, which are demulcent and astringent and are used topically for bruises and sprains and to promote bone healing; also used in folk medicine 紫草科植物，聚合草

com·men·sal (ko-men′səl) 1. living on or within another organism, and deriving benefit without harming or benefiting the host 共生的，共栖的; 2. a parasite that causes no harm to the host 共栖寄生体

com·men·sal·ism (ko-men′səl-iz″əm) symbiosis in which one population (or individual) is benefited and the other is neither benefited nor harmed 共栖，共生生活

com·mi·nut·ed (kom′ī-noot′əd) broken or crushed into small pieces, as a comminuted fracture 捣碎的，粉碎的

com·mis·su·ra (kom″ī-su′rə) pl. *commissu′rae* [L.] commissure 连合

com·mis·sure (kom′ī-shər) a site of union of corresponding parts; specifically, the sites of junction between adjacent leaflets of the heart valves 连合; **commis′sural adj. anterior c.,** the band of fibers connecting the parts of the two cerebral hemispheres 前连合; **Gudden c.,** 见 *supraoptic c's*; **Meynert c.,** 见 *supraoptic c's*; **posterior c.,** a large fiber bundle crossing from one side of the cerebrum to the other, dorsal to where the aqueduct opens into the third ventricle 后连合; **supraoptic c's,** commissural fibers crossing the midline of the human brain dorsal to the caudal border of the optic chiasm, representing the combined commissures of Gudden and Meynert 视连合

com·mis·su·ror·rha·phy (kom″ī-shər-or′ə-fe) suture of the components of a commissure, to lessen the size of the orifice 连合部缝合术

com·mis·sur·ot·o·my (kom″ī-shər-ot′ə-me) surgical incision or digital disruption of the components of a commissure to increase the size of the orifice; commonly done to separate adherent, thickened leaflets of a stenotic left atrioventricular valve 连合部切开术

com·mon (kom′ən) 1. belonging to or shared by two or more entities 共同的，公共的; 2. usual; being frequent, prevalent, widespread, or habitual 通常的，普通的，普遍的，广泛的，习惯性的

com·mu·ni·ca·ble (kə-mu′nī-kə-bəl) contagious; capable of being transmitted from one individual to another 传染的，传播的

com·mu·ni·cans (kə-mu′nə-kanz) [L.] communicating 交通的

com·mu·ni·cat·ing (kə-mu′nə-ka″ting) 1. denoting spreading or transmission, as of a disease 传染，传播；2. being connected, one with another 相连的，相通的

com·mu·ni·ty (kə-mu′nĭ-te) a body of individuals living in a defined area or having a common interest or organization 团体，群落；**biotic c.**, an assemblage of populations living in a defined area 生物群落；**therapeutic c.**, a structured mental treatment center employing group and milieu therapy and encouraging the patient to function within social norms 治疗中心

co·mor·bid (ko-mor′bid) pertaining to a disease or other pathologic process that occurs simultaneously with another 共病

com·pact (kom′pakt) (kəm-pakt′) dense; having a dense structure 致密的，紧密的

com·pac·tion (kəm-pak′shən) 1. a complication of labor in twin births in which there is simultaneous full engagement of the leading fetal poles of both twins, so that the lesser pelvis is filled and further descent is prevented 双胎紧贴；2. in embryology, the process during which blastomeres change their shape and align themselves tightly against each other to form the compact morula 胚胎学中的一种过程，在此过程中，囊胚改变其形状并彼此紧密排列，形成紧密的桑椹胚

com·part·ment (kəm-pahrt′mənt) a small enclosure within a larger space 隔间，隔室，分隔空间 **endoplasmic reticulum–Golgi intermediate c. (ERGIC)**, a compartment of vesicles between the endoplasmic reticulum and the Golgi complex, formed by the fusion of transport vesicles from the endoplasmic reticulum 内质网 - 高尔基体中间室

com·pen·sat·ed (kom′pən-sa″təd) counterbalanced; offset 补偿的，代偿的

com·pen·sa·tion (kom″pən-sa′shən) 1. the counterbalancing of any defect 补偿，赔偿；2. the conscious or unconscious process by which a person attempts to make up for real or imagined physical or psychological deficiencies 代偿功能；3. in cardiology, the maintenance of an adequate blood flow without distressing symptoms, accomplished by cardiac and circulatory adjustments 征；(心) 代偿；**dosage c.**, the mechanism that regulates the expression of sex-linked genes in the sex carrying two or more copies of the same chromosome in those species in which the genes differ in dose between males and females 补偿量

com·pen·sa·to·ry (kəm-pen′sə-tor″e) making good a defect or loss; restoring a lost balance 代偿的

com·pe·ti·tion (kom″pə-tish′ən) the phenomenon in which two structurally similar molecules "compete" for a single binding site on a third molecule 竞争；**compet′itive** *adj.* **antigenic c.**, an altered response to an immunogen resulting from the simultaneous or close administration of two immunogens: the response to one is normal, while the response to the second is suppressed or diminished 抗原竞争

com·plaint (kəm-plānt′) a disease, symptom, or disorder 陈述，症状，疾病，不适；**chief c.**, the symptom or group of symptoms about which the patient first consults the doctor; the presenting symptom 主诉

com·ple·ment (kom′plə-mənt) a heat-labile cascade system of at least 20 serum glycoproteins that interact to provide many of the effector functions of humoral immunity and inflammation, including vasodilation and increase of vascular permeability, facilitation of phagocyte activity, and lysis of certain foreign cells. It can be activated via either the *classical* or *alternative complement pathways* (q.v.). 补体

com·ple·men·ta·ry (kom″plə-men′tə-re) 1. supplying a defect, or helping to do so; making complete; accessory 补偿的，补充的，附属的；2. in biochemistry, pertaining to the specific pairing between purine and pyrimidine bases in two nucleotide strands 互补的，配对的

com·ple·men·ta·tion (kom″plə-men-ta′shən) the interaction between two sets of genes within a cell such that the cell can function even though each set of genes carries a mutated, nonfunctional gene; indicates the defects are not identical 互补作用

com·plex (kom′pleks) 1. a combination of various things, e.g., a complex of symptoms; 见 *syndrome*. 复合体，络合物，复合症；2. sequence (2) 连续，序列；3. a group of interrelated ideas, mainly unconscious, that have a common emotional tone and strongly influence a person's attitudes and behavior 情结；4. that portion of an electrocardiogram representing the systole of an atrium or ventricle 复合波（心电图）；**AIDS dementia c.**, HIV encephalopathy 艾滋病相关痴呆综合征；**AIDS-related c. (ARC)**, former term for a complex of signs and symptoms representing a less severe stage of human immunodeficiency virus (HIV) infection 艾滋病相关综合征；**anomalous c.**, in electrocardiography, an abnormal atrial or ventricular complex resulting from aberrant conduction over accessory pathways 异常复合波；**antigen-antibody c.**, a complex formed by the binding of antigen to antibody 抗原抗体复合物；**anti-inhibitor coagulant c. (AICC)**, a concentrated fraction from pooled human plasma,

240

which includes various coagulation factors; used as an antihemorrhagic in hemophilic patients with factor VIII inhibitors 抗抑制剂凝血剂复合物；**atrial c.**, the P wave of the electrocardiogram, representing electrical activation of the atria 心 房 复 合 波；**atrial premature c. (APC),** a single ectopic atrial beat arising prematurely, which may be associated with structural heart disease 心房期前复合波；**atrioventricular (AV) junctional escape c.**, 房室交界性逸搏综合征，见 beat 下词条；**atrioventricular (AV) junctional premature c.**, an ectopic beat arising prematurely in the atrioventricular junction and traveling toward both the atria and ventricles if unimpeded, causing the P wave to be premature and abnormal or absent and the QRS complex to be premature 房室交界性期前复合波；**branched-chain α-keto acid dehydrogenase c.**, a multienzyme complex that catalyzes the oxidative decarboxylation of the keto acid analogues of the branched-chain amino acids; deficiency of any enzyme of the complex causes maple syrup urine disease 支链 α-酮酸脱氢酶复合物；**calcarine c.**, calcar avis 禽距；**castration c.**, in psychoanalytic theory, unconscious thoughts and motives stemming from fear of damage to or loss of sexual organs as punishment for forbidden sexual desires 阉割情节；**Eisenmenger c.**, a defect of the interventricular septum with severe pulmonary hypertension, hypertrophy of the right ventricle, and latent or overt cyanosis Eisenmenger 综合征；**Electra c.**, the counterpart in females of the Oedipus complex, involving the daughter's love for her father and jealousy or resentment toward her mother; now rarely used since *Oedipus complex* (q.v.) has come to be applied to both sexes 恋父情结；**extrophy-epispadias c.**, a spectrum of congenital defects of the anterior abdominal wall, ranging from epispadias to bladder exstrophy to cloacal exstrophy 膀胱外翻合并尿道上裂；**factor IX c.**, a partially purified factor IX fraction also including factor II, VII, and X fractions, from venous human plasma. It is used in the treatment of hemophilia B, replacement of factor VII, and treatment of anticoagulant-induced hemorrhage. IX因子复合物；**Ghon c.**, primary c. (1). **β-glycosidase c.**, the enzyme complex comprising lactase and phlorhizin hydrolase activities, occurring in the brush border membrane of the intestinal mucosa and hydrolyzing lactose as well as cellobiose and cellotriose β- 糖苷酶复合物；**Golgi c.**, Golgi apparatus; a complex cellular organelle consisting mainly of a number of flattened sacs (cisternae) and associated vesicles, involved in the synthesis of glycoproteins, lipoproteins, membrane-bound proteins, and lysosomal enzymes. The

sacs form primary lysosomes and secretory vacuoles 高尔基复合体；**immune c.**, antigen-antibody c. 免疫复合物；**inclusion c.**, one in which molecules of one type are enclosed within cavities in the crystalline lattice of another substance 包 合 物；**inferiority c.**, unconscious feelings of inadequacy, producing timidity or, as a compensation, exaggerated aggressiveness and expression of superiority 自卑情结；**junctional premature c.**, atrioventricular junctional premature c. LCMVLASV c., a group of antigenically related viruses comprising the Old World arenaviruses. Lassa virus (Lassa fever) and lymphocytic choriomeningitis virus are pathogenic for humans 淋巴细胞性脉络丛脑膜炎病毒和拉沙热病毒群；**Lutembacher c.**, 二尖瓣狭窄伴房间隔缺损；**major histocompatibility c. (MHC),** the chromosomal region containing genes that control the histocompatibility antigens. In humans, it controls the HLA antigens 主要组织相容性复合体；**membrane attack c. (MAC),** the pentamolecular complex of components C5b-6, -7, -8, and -9 formed in the final pathway of complement activation, inserting into the target cell membrane where it creates a pore and results in cytolysis 膜攻击复合物；*Mycobacterium avium-intracellulare* c., a complex of *M. avium* and *M. intracellulare* that is associated with pulmonary disease, lymphadenitis in children, and serious systemic disease in immunocompromised patients 鸟 - 胞内分枝杆菌复合菌组；**nuclear pore c.**, a nuclear pore (q.v.) and its associated glycoproteins, which regulates transport between the nucleus and the cytoplasm 核孔复合体；**Oedipus c.**, the feelings and conflicts occurring in a child that result from sexual attraction to the opposite-sex parent, including envious, aggressive feelings toward the same-sex parent 恋母情结；**primary c.**, 1. the combination of a Ghon focus and a corresponding lymph node focus in primary tuberculosis in children; similar lesions are seen with other mycobacterial and fungal infections 原发综合征；2. the primary cutaneous lesion at the site of skin infection, e.g., a chancre in syphilis or tuberculosis 皮肤感染部位的原发性皮肤病变；**primary inoculation c., primary tuberculous c.**, tuberculous chancre 原发性结核性复征；**pyruvate dehydrogenase c.**, a multienzyme complex that catalyzes the formation of acetyl coenzyme A from pyruvate and coenzyme A; deficiency of any component of the complex results in lactic acidemia, ataxia, and psychomotor retardation 丙酮酸脱氢酶复合物；**QRS c.**, the portion of the electrocardiogram comprising the Q, R, and S waves, together representing ventricular depolarization QRS 波群；

sucrase-isomaltase c., the enzyme complex comprising sucrase and isomaltase activities, occurring in the brush border of the intestinal mucosa and hydrolyzing maltose as well as maltotriose and some other glycosidic bonds 蔗糖酶 - 异麦芽糖酶复合体；**symptom c.**, syndrome 综合症状；**synaptonemal c.**, a ladderlike structure consisting of two lateral elements connected to a central element by transverse filaments that joins together homologous chromosomes in synapsis 联会复合体；**Tacaribe c.**, a group of antigenically related viruses comprising the New World arenaviruses, which cause hemorrhagic fever in South America 塔卡里布病毒组；**tuberous sclerosis c.**, an autosomal dominant disorder caused by mutation in either of two genes involved in tumor suppression; characterized by hamartomas of the brain, skin, and other vital organs 结节性硬化复合症；**VATER c.**, an association of congenital anomalies consisting of vertebral defects, imperforate anus, tracheoesophageal fistula, and radial and renal dysplasia 脊柱、肛门、肾脏、桡骨、气管畸形综合征；**ventricular c.**, the combined QRS complex and T wave, together representing ventricular electrical activity 心室复合波；**ventricular premature c. (VPC)**, an ectopic beat arising in the ventricles and stimulating the myocardium prematurely 心室期前复合波

com·plex·ion (kəm-plek′shən) the color and appearance of the skin of the face 面容，面色

com·pli·ance (kəm-pli′əns) the quality of yielding to pressure without disruption, or an expression of the ability to do so, as an expression of the distensibility of an air- or fluid-filled organ, e.g., lung or urinary bladder, in terms of unit of volume change per unit of pressure change. Symbol C. 依从，顺从，顺应性

com·pli·cat·ed (kom′plĭ-kāt′əd) involved; associated with other injuries, lesions, or diseases 复杂的

com·pli·ca·tion (kom″plĭ-ka′shən) 1. disease(s) concurrent with another disease 合并症；2. occurrence of several diseases in the same patient 并发症

com·po·nent (kom-po′nənt) 1. a constituent element or part 成分；2. in neurology, a series of neurons forming a functional system for conducting the afferent and efferent impulses in the somatic and splanchnic mechanisms of the body 组元；**M c.**, an abnormal monoclonal immunoglobulin occurring in the serum in plasma cell dyscrasias, formed by proliferating concentrations of immunoglobulin-producing cells 成分；**plasma thromboplastin c. (PTC)**, coagulation factor Ⅸ 血浆凝血激酶（凝血）因子Ⅸ

com·pos·ite (kəm-poz′it) 1. a solid containing two or more distinct constituent materials or phases 含有两种或两种以上不同组成物质或相的固体；2. made up of unlike parts 由不同的部分组成；**resin c.**, a reinforced polymer material comprising an organic polymer matrix, usually methacrylate-based, inorganic filler particles, and a coupling agent, chiefly used in dental restorations 复合树脂

com·pos men·tis (kom′pos men′tis) [L.] sound of mind; sane 精神健全

com·pound (kom′pound) 1. made up of two or more parts or ingredients 复合物；2. in chemistry, a substance consisting of two or more elements in union 杂合子；3. to combine to form a whole; unite 化合物；**clathrate c.**, a type of inclusion complex in which molecules of one type are trapped within cavities of another substance, as within a crystalline lattice structure or large molecule 笼形（化合）物；**inorganic c.**, a compound of chemical elements containing no carbon atoms 无机化合物；**organic c.**, a compound of chemical elements containing carbon atoms 有机化合物；**organometallic c.**, a compound in which carbon is linked to a metal 有机金属化合物；**quaternary ammonium c.**, an organic compound containing a quaternary ammonium group, a nitrogen atom carrying a single positive charge bonded to four carbon atoms, e.g., choline 季铵化合物

com·press (kom′pres) a pad or bolster of folded linen or other material, applied with pressure; sometimes medicated, it may be wet or dry, or hot or cold 敷布，压布

com·pres·sion (kəm-presh′ən) 1. the act of pressing upon or together; the state of being pressed together 压迫，压缩；2. in embryology, the shortening or omission of certain developmental stages 发育期缩短

com·pul·sion (kəm-pul′shən) 1. an overwhelming urge to perform an irrational act or ritual 强迫性冲动；2. the repetitive or stereotyped action that is the object of such an urge 强迫行为，强迫症；**compul′sive** adj. **repetition c.**, in psychoanalytic theory, the impulse to reenact earlier emotional experiences or traumatic behavior 强迫性重复行为

co·na·tion (ko-na′shən) in psychology, the power that impels effort of any kind; the conscious tendency to act 意志，意图，意欲；**con′ative** adj.

c-onc (se′onk″) [cellular oncogene] a protooncogene that has been activated within the host so that oncogenicity results 原癌基因

con·ca·nav·a·lin A (kon″kə-nav′ə-lin) a phytohemagglutinin isolated from the jack bean (*Canavalia ensiformis*); it is a hemagglutinin that agglutinates blood erythrocytes and a mitogen stimulating

C

predominantly T cells 伴刀豆球蛋白 A

con·cave (kon-kāv′) rounded and somewhat depressed or hollowed out 凹的，凹面的

con·ca·vo·con·cave (kən-ka″vo-kon′kāv) concave on each of two opposite surfaces 双凹的，对凹的

con·ca·vo·con·vex (kən-ka″vo-kon′veks) having one concave and one convex surface 凹凸的

con·ceive (kən-sēv′) 1. to become pregnant 受孕；2. take in, grasp, or form in the mind 接受，构思，拥有

con·cen·trate (kon′sən-trāt) 1. to bring to a common center; to gather at one point 集中，聚集；2. to increase the strength by diminishing the bulk of, as of a liquid; to condense 浓缩；3. a drug or other preparation that has been strengthened by evaporation of its nonactive parts 浓缩液；**activated prothrombin complex c. (APCC),** anti-inhibitor coagulant complex 活化凝血酶原复合物；**prothrombin complex c. (PCC),** factor IX complex 凝血因子IX制剂

con·cen·tra·tion (kon″sən-tra′shən) 1. increase in strength by evaporation 浓缩；2. the ratio of the mass or volume of a solute to the mass or volume of the solution or solvent 浓度；**hydrogen ion c.,** the degree of concentration of hydrogen ions in a solution; related inversely to the pH of the solution by the equation $[H^+] = 10^{-pH}$ 氢离子浓度；**mass c.,** the mass of a constituent substance divided by the volume of the mixture, as milligrams per liter (mg/L), etc 质量浓度；**mean corpuscular hemoglobin c. (MCHC),** the average hemoglobin concentration in erythrocytes, expressed in grams per deciliter of red cells 红细胞平均血红蛋白量；**molar c. (c),** the concentration of a substance expressed in terms of molarity 克分子浓度

con·cen·tric (kən-sen′trik) having a common center; extending out equally in all directions from a common center 同心的，同轴的

con·cept (kon′sept) the image of a thing held in the mind 概念，观念

con·cep·tion (kən-sep′shən) 1. an imprecise term denoting the formation of a viable zygote 妊娠，受孕，受精；2. concept 概念，观念，思想；**con·cep′tive** *adj.*

con·cep·tus (kən-sep′təs) the product of the union of oocyte and spermatozoon at any stage of development from fertilization until birth, including extraembryonic membranes as well as the embryo or fetus 孕体

con·cha (kong′kə) pl. *con′chae* [L.] a shellshaped structure 甲；**c. of auricle,** the hollow of the auricle of the external ear, bounded anteriorly by the tragus and posteriorly by the anthelix 耳甲；**c. bullo′sa, a**

cystic distention of the middle nasal concha 泡状鼻甲；**inferior nasal c.,** a thin, bony plate forming the lower part of the lateral wall of the nasal cavity, and the mucous membrane covering the plate 下鼻甲；**middle nasal c.,** the lower of two bony plates projecting from the inner wall of the ethmoid labyrinth and separating the superior from the middle meatus of the nose, and the mucous membrane covering the plate 中鼻甲；**sphenoidal c.,** a thin curved plate of bone at the anterior and lower part of the body of the sphenoid bone, on either side, forming part of the roof of the nasal cavity 蝶甲；**superior nasal c.,** the upper of two bony plates projecting from the inner wall of the ethmoid labyrinth and forming the upper boundary of the superior meatus of the nose, and the mucous membrane covering the plate 上鼻甲；**supreme nasal c.,** a thin bony plate occasionally found projecting from the inner wall of the ethmoid labyrinth, above the bony superior nasal concha, and the mucous membrane covering the plate 最上鼻甲

con·cli·na·tion (kon″klī-na′shən) inward rotation of the upper pole of the vertical meridian of each eye 两眼内旋

con·com·i·tant (kən-kom′ ī-tənt) accompanying; accessory; joined with another 伴行的，附带的，共同的

con·cor·dance (kən-kor′dəns) in genetics, the occurrence of a given trait in both members of a twin pair 和谐，一致性，协调；**concor′dant** *adj.*

con·cres·cence (kən-kres′əns) 1. a growing together of parts originally separate 愈合；2. in embryology, the flowing together and piling up of cells 结合，细胞合成

con·cre·tio (kən-kre′she-o) concretion 凝结物，结石，粘连，凝结；**c. cor′dis, c. pericar′dii,** adhesive pericarditis in which the pericardial cavity is obliterated 心包粘连

con·cre·tion (kən-kre′shən) 1. a calculus or inorganic mass in a natural cavity or in tissue 结石；2. abnormal union of adjacent parts 粘连；3. the process of becoming harder or more solid 结节

con·cus·sion (kən-kush′ən) a violent shock or jar, or the condition resulting from such an injury 震荡，震伤；**c. of the brain,** loss of consciousness, transient or prolonged, due to a blow to the head; there may be transient amnesia, vertigo, nausea, weak pulse, and slow respiration 脑震荡；**c. of the labyrinth,** deafness with tinnitus due to a blow on or explosion near the ear 迷路震荡；**pulmonary c.,** mechanical damage to the lungs caused by an explosion 肺震荡；**c. of the spinal cord,** transient spinal cord dysfunction caused by mechanical injury 脊髓震荡

con·den·sa·tion (kon″dən-sa′shən) 1. conversion from a gaseous to a liquid or solid phase 凝结；2. compression (1)；3. the packing of dental filling materials into a tooth cavity 将牙科填充材料填空到牙洞中；4. a mental process in which one symbol stands for a number of components all the emotions associated with them 精神分析中的凝缩是指以一个符号代表若干成分，并包含与此有关的全部情感

con·den·ser (kən-den′sər) 1. a vessel or apparatus for condensing gases or vapors 冷凝器，冷凝管；2. a device for illuminating microscopic objects 聚光器；3. an apparatus for concentrating energy or matter 电容器；4. a dental instrument used to pack plastic filling material into the prepared cavity of a tooth 充填器

con·di·tion (kən-dish′ən) to train; to subject to conditioning 训练，使成条件反射

con·di·tion·ing (kən-dish′ən-ing) 1. learning in which a stimulus initially incapable of evoking a certain response becomes able to do so by repeated pairing with another stimulus that does evoke the response 条件反射，条件形成；2. in physical medicine, improvement of the physical state with a program of exercise 健体；**aversive c.,** learning in which punishment or other unpleasant stimulation is used to reduce the frequency of an undesirable response 厌恶性条件反射；**instrumental c., operant c.,** learning in which the frequency of a particular voluntary response is altered by the application of positive or negative consequences 操作性条件反射；**pavlovian c.,** conditioning (1)

con·dom (kon′dəm) a sheath or cover worn over the penis during sexual activity to prevent impregnation or transmission of infection（男用）避孕套；**female c.,** a sheath worn inside the vagina, also extending outward to cover the vulva, to prevent pregnancy or transmission of infection 女用避孕套

con·duc·tance (kən-duk′təns) the capacity for conducting or ability to convey. Symbol G. 传导力，导电性电导符号"G"；**airway c.,** the reciprocal of airway resistance; the airflow divided by the mouth-to-alveoli pressure difference 气道交换阻力

con·duc·tion (kən-duk′shən) conveyance of energy, as of heat, sound, or electricity 传导；**conduc′tive adj. aberrant c.,** cardiac conduction through pathways not normally conducting cardiac impulses, particularly through ventricular tissue 差异性传导，异常传导；**aerotympanal c.,** conduction of sound waves to the ear through the air and the tympanum 气鼓传导；**air c.,** conduction of sound waves to the inner ear through the external auditory canal and middle ear 空气传导；**anterograde c.,** transmis-

sion of a cardiac impulse in the normal direction, from the sinus node to the ventricles, particularly forward conduction through the atrioventricular node 顺向传导；**bone c.,** conduction of sound waves to the inner ear through the bones of the skull 骨传导；**concealed c.,** incomplete penetration of a propagating impulse through the cardiac conducting system such that electrocardiograms reveal no evidence of transmission but the behavior of one or more subsequent impulses is somehow affected 隐匿性传导；**concealed retrograde c.,** retrograde conduction blocked in the atrioventricular node; it does not produce an extra P wave but leaves the node refractory to the next normal sinus beat 隐匿性逆向传导；**decremental c.,** delay or failure of propagation of an impulse in the atrioventricular node resulting from progressive decrease in the rate of the rise and amplitude of the action potential as it spreads through the node 递减传导；**retrograde c.,** transmission of a cardiac impulse backward in the ventricular to atrial direction, particularly conduction from the atrioventricular node into the atria 逆行性传导，逆向传导；**saltatory c.,** the passage of a potential from node to node of a nerve fiber, rather than along the membrane 跳跃式传导

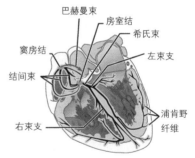

▲ 心脏冲动的顺向传导（anterograde conductioon）通路

con·duc·tiv·i·ty (kon″dək-tiv′ĭ-te) the capacity of a body to transmit a flow of electricity or heat; the conductance per unit area of the body 导电性，传导性

con·du·it (kon′doo-it) channel 管道；**ileal c.,** the surgical anastomosis of the ureters to one end of a detached segment of ileum, the other end being used to form a stoma on the abdominal wall 回肠膀胱术，回肠流出道术

con·dy·lar·thro·sis (kon″dəl-ahr-thro′sis) ellipsoid joint 髁状关节

con·dyle (kon′dīl) a rounded projection on a bone,

usually for articulation with another bone 髁, 髁突;
con′dylar, condylicus *adj.*

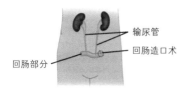

输尿管

回肠造口术

回肠部分

▲ 回肠膀胱术（**ileal conduit**）

con·dyl·i·on (kon-dil′e-ən) the most lateral point on the surface of the head of the mandible 髁状突外点

con·dy·loid (kon′də-loid) resembling a condyle or knuckle 髁状的

con·dy·lo·ma (kon″də-lo′mə) pl. *condylo′mata* [Gr.] an elevated lesion of the skin 湿疣; **condylo′matous** *adj.* **c. acumina′tum,** a papilloma with a central core of connective tissue covered with epithelium, caused by human papillomavirus, usually found on the mucous membrane or skin of the external genitals or in the perianal region 尖锐湿疣; **flat c.,** c. latum; **giant c.,** Buschke-Löwenstein tumor 巨尖锐湿疣扁平湿疣; **c. la′tum,** a broad, flat type seen on folds of moist skin, especially about the genitals and anus, in secondary syphilis 扁平

con·dy·lot·o·my (kon″də-lot′ə-me) transection of a condyle 髁切断术

con·dy·lus (kon′də-ləs) pl. *con′dyli* [L.] condyle 平髁突

cone (kōn) 1. a solid figure or body having a circular base and tapering to a point 锥, 圆锥, 锥体; 2. retinal c.; 3. in radiology, a conical or open-ended cylindrical structure used as an aid in centering the radiation beam and as a guide to source-tofilm distance 锥体术; 4. in root canal therapy, a solid substance with a tapered form, usually made of gutta-percha or silver, fashioned to conform to the shape of a root canal 电弧锥部; **c. of light,** the triangular reflection of light seen on the tympanic membrane 光锥; **retinal c.,** one of the specialized conical or flask-shaped outer segments of the visual cells, which, with the retinal rods, form the light-sensitive elements of the retina 视锥, 视锥细胞; **twin c's,** retinal cone cells in which two cells are blended 双锥（体）

con·fab·u·la·tion (kon″fab-u-la′shən) unconscious filling in of gaps in memory by telling imaginary experiences 虚构症

con·fi·den·ti·al·i·ty (kon″fi-den″she-al′ĭ-te) the principle in medical ethics that the information a patient reveals to a health care provider is private and has limits on how and when it can be disclosed to a third party 可信性

con·flict (kon′flikt) a mental struggle, often unconscious, arising from the clash of incompatible or opposing impulses, wishes, drives, or external demands 冲突, 矛盾, 心理冲突; **extrapsychic c.,** that between the self and the external environment 心理外冲突; **intrapsychic c.,** that between forces within the self 心理内冲突

con·flu·ence (kon′floo-əns) 1. a running together; a meeting of streams 汇合, 融合; 2. in embryology, the flowing of cells, a component process of gastrulation 胚胎学中原肠胚的形成过程; **con′fluent** *adj.* **c. of sinuses,** the dilated point of confluence of the superior sagittal, straight, occipital, and two transverse sinuses of the dura mater 窦汇

con·fron·ta·tion (kon″frən-ta′shən) a therapeutic technique constituting the act of facing or being made to face one's own attitudes and shortcomings, the way one is perceived, and the consequences of one's behavior, or of causing another to face these things 质对

con·fu·sion (kən-fu′zhən) disturbed orientation in regard to time, place, or person, sometimes accompanied by disordered consciousness 意识错乱

con·ge·ner (kon′jə-nər) something closely related to another thing, as a member of the same genus, a muscle having the same function as another, or a chemical compound closely related to another in composition and exerting similar or antagonistic effects, or something derived from the same source or stock 协同肌, 同源物; **congener′ic, congen′erous** *adj.*

con·gen·ic (kən-jen′ik) pertaining to two inbred strains of animals that are genetically identical except at a single locus or a small chromosomal segment 同基因系的, 异系同基因的

con·gen·i·tal (kən-jen′ĭ-təl) existing at, and usually before, birth; referring to conditions that are present at birth, regardless of their causation 先天的, 天生的, 生来俱有的

con·ges·tion (kən-jes′chən) abnormal accumulation of blood in a part 充血; **conges′tive** *adj.*; **hypostatic c.,** congestion of a dependent part of the body or an organ due to gravitational forces, as in venous insufficiency 沉积性充血; **passive c.,** that due to lack of vital power or to obstruction of escape of blood from the part 淤血, 被动充血; **pulmonary c.,** engorgement of pulmonary vessels with transudation of fluid into the alveolar and interstitial spaces, seen in cardiac disease, infections, and certain injuries 肺充血; **venous c.,** passive c. 静脉

淤血

con·glo·ba·tion (kon″glo-ba′shən) the act of forming, or the state of being formed, into a rounded mass 成团，团块；**conglo′bate** adj.

con·glu·ti·na·tion (kən-gloo″tĭ-na′shən) 1. adhesion 凝集；2. agglutination of erythrocytes that is dependent upon both complement and antibodies 胶固反应

con·i·cal (kon′ĭ-kəl) cone-shaped 圆锥形的

co·ni·dio·bo·lo·my·co·sis (kə-nid″e-o-bo″lomi-ko′sis) rhinoentomophthoromycosis; fungal infection caused by *Conidiobolus coronatus*, usually occurring in male adults in the tropics; it begins in the nasal submucosa and spreads slowly to involve subcutaneous tissues of the nose and perinasal regions 虫霉病，冠状分生孢子虫引起的真菌感染，通常发生于热带地区常见，成年男性；它开始于鼻黏膜下层，慢慢扩散到鼻和鼻周的皮下组织

Co·nid·io·bo·lus (ko-nid″e-ob′o-ləs) a genus of fungi of the family Entomophthoraceae, order Entomophthorales, having few septa in the mycelium and producing few zygospores but many chlamydospores and conidia. *C. corona'tus* causes conidiobolomycosis 耳霉属

co·nid·i·um (kə-nid′e-əm) pl. *conid'ia* [L.] an asexually produced fungal spore 分生孢子

co·nio·fi·bro·sis (ko″ne-o-fi-bro′sis) pneumoconiosis with overgrowth of lung connective tissue 肺尘性纤维变性，纤维性尘肺病

co·ni·o·sis (ko″ne-o′sis) a disease caused by inhalation of dust, such as byssinosis or pneumoconiosis 粉尘病，尘埃沉着病

co·nio·spo·ro·sis (ko″ne-o-spə-ro′sis) maple bark disease 梨孢霉菌

con·iza·tion (kon″ĭ-za′shən) the removal of a cone of tissue, as in biopsy of the cervix uteri 锥形切除术；**cold c.**, that done with a cold knife, as opposed to electrocautery, to better preserve the histologic elements 冷冻锥形切除术

con·joined (kən-joind′) joined together; united 联体的

con·ju·ga·ta (kon″jə-ga′tə) the conjugate diameter of the pelvis（骨盆）直径；**c. ve′ra pel′vis,** the true conjugate diameter of the pelvis 骨盆直径

con·ju·gate (kon′jə-gāt) 1. paired, or equally coupled; working in unison 共轭；2. a conjugate diameter of the pelvic inlet; used alone usually to denote the true conjugate diameter（骨盆）直径，见 *diameter* 下 *pelvic diameter*；3. the product of chemical conjugation 缀合物

con·ju·ga·tion (kon″jə-ga′shən) 1. the act of joining together 接合；2. in unicellular organisms, a form of sexual reproduction in which two cells join

in temporary union to transfer genetic material 接合（生殖）；3. in chemistry, the joining together of two compounds to produce another compound 接合作用

con·junc·ti·va (kən-junk′tĭ-və) pl. *conjunc'tivae* [L.] the delicate membrane lining the eyelids and covering the eyeball 结膜；**conjuncti′val** adj.

con·junc·ti·vi·tis (kən-junk″tĭ-vi′tis) inflammation of the conjunctiva 结膜炎；**acute contagious c., acute epidemic c.,** pinkeye; a highly contagious form of conjunctivitis caused by *Haemophilus aegyptius* 急性触染性结膜炎，急性流行性结膜炎；**acute hemorrhagic c.,** a contagious conjunctivitis due to infection with enteroviruses 急性出血性结膜炎；**allergic c.,** conjunctival inflammation, itching, tearing, and redness caused by allergens 过变应性结膜炎 **atopic c.,** allergic conjunctivitis of the immediate type, due to airborne allergens such as pollens, dusts, spores, and animal hair 特应性结膜炎；**giant papillary c.,** chronic inflammation of the conjunctiva lining the upper eyelid, with the formation of giant papillae on the tarsal conjunctiva, most often associated with contact lens wear 巨乳头结膜炎；**gonococcal c., gonorrheal c.,** a severe conjunctivitis due to infection with gonococci 淋球菌性结膜炎；**granular c.,** trachoma 颗粒性结膜炎；**inclusion c.,** a type of conjunctivitis seen primarily in newborn infants, caused by a strain of *Chlamydia trachomatis*, beginning as acute purulent conjunctivitis and leading to papillary hypertrophy of the palpebral conjunctiva 包涵体性结膜炎；**neonatal c.,** ophthalmia neonatorum 新生儿结膜炎；**phlyctenular c.,** conjunctivitis marked by small vesicles surrounded by a reddened zone 泡性结膜炎；**spring c., vernal c.,** a bilateral idiopathic conjunctivitis usually occurring in the spring in children 春季结膜炎

con·junc·ti·vo·ma (kən-junk″tĭ-vo′mə) a tumor of the eyelid composed of conjunctival tissue 结膜瘤

con·junc·ti·vo·plas·ty (kən-junk″tĭ-vo-plas″te) plastic repair of the conjunctiva 结膜成形术

con·nec·tion (kə-nek′shən) the act of connecting or the state of being connected 连接，接合，联系

con·nec·tive (kə-nek′tiv) serving as a link or binding 连接的

con·nec·tor (kə-nek′tər) anything serving as a link between two separate objects or units, as between the bilateral parts of a removable partial denture 连接体

con·nex·us (kə-nek′səs) pl. *connex'us* [L.] a connecting structure 结合质；Spelled also *conexus.*

Co·no·cy·be (ko″no-si′be) a genus of mushrooms 锥盖伞属，蘑菇的一种；*C. fila'ris,* a common lawn mushroom, contains amatoxins; several other species contain the hallucinogens psilocybin and psilocin 一种常见的草坪蘑菇，含有毒伞蕈毒素

co·noid (ko′noid) cone-shaped 锥形的，类锥形的

con·san·guin·i·ty (kon″sang-gwin′ ĭ-te) blood relationship; kinship 血亲，近亲；**consanguin′eous** adj.

con·science (kon′shəns) the nontechnical term for the moral faculty of the mind, corresponding roughly to the superego; differing in that the operations of the superego are often unconscious, unlike the ordinary conception of conscience 良心，道德心理

con·scious (kon′shəs) 1. having awareness of one's self, acts, and surroundings 意识；2. a state of alertness characterized by response to external stimuli 对外界刺激的警觉反应；3. in Freud's terminology, the part of the mind that is constantly within awareness（弗洛伊德术语）意识

con·scious·ness (kon′shəs-nəs) 1. the state of being conscious 清醒状态；2. subjective awareness of the aspects of cognitive processing and the content of the mind 认知的，主观意识；3. the current totality of experience of which an individual or group is aware at any time 知觉，感觉；4. the conscious 意识

con·ser·va·tive (kən-sur′və-tiv) designed to preserve health, restore function, and repair structures by nonradical methods 保存的，防腐的，保守的

con·sol·i·da·tion (kən-sol″ĭ-da′shən) solidification; the process of becoming or the condition of being solid; said especially of the lung as it fills with exudate in pneumonia 实变

con·stant (kon′stənt) 1. stable; not subject to change 固定的，不变的；2. a quantity that is not subject to change 常数；**association c.**, a measure of the extent of a reversible association between two molecular species 缔合常数；**Avogadro's c.**, 阿伏加德罗常数；**binding c.**, association c 结合常数；**Michaelis c.** (K_M) (K_m), a constant representing the substrate concentration at which the velocity of an enzyme-catalyzed reaction is half maximal 米氏常数；**sedimentation c.**, 沉降常数，见 *coefficient.* 下词条

con·sti·pa·tion (kon″stĭ-pa′shən) infrequent or difficult evacuation of feces 便秘；**constipa′ted** adj.

con·sti·tu·tion (kon″stĭ-too′shən) 1. the makeup or functional habit of the body 体质；2. the arrangement of atoms in a molecule 构造；**constitu′tional** adj.

con·sti·tu·tive (kon-stĭ-too′tiv) (kon-stich′utiv) produced constantly or in fixed amounts, regardless of environmental conditions or demand 组成的，基本的，要素的

con·stric·tion (kən-strik′shən) 1. a narrowing or compression of a part; a stricture 狭窄，缩窄；2. a diminution in range of thinking or feeling, associated with diminished spontaneity 压迫感；**constric′tive** adj.

con·sult[1] (kən-sult′) to confer with another physician about a case 会诊

con·sult[2] (kon′sult) consultation 会诊

con·sul·ta·tion (kon″səl-ta′shən) a deliberation by two or more physicians about diagnosis or treatment in a particular case 应诊，会商

con·sump·tion (kən-sump′shən) 1. the act of consuming, or the process of being consumed 消费的行为，或者被消耗的过程；2. a wasting away of the body 身体逐渐消瘦

con·tact (kon′takt) 1. a mutual touching of two bodies or persons 接触；2. an individual known to have been sufficiently near an infected person to have been exposed to the transfer of infectious material.（传染病）接触者 **balancing c.**, the contact between the upper and lower occlusal surfaces of the teeth on the side opposite the working contact 平衡接触；**complete c.**, contact of the entire adjoining surfaces of two teeth 全邻面接触；**direct c.**, the contact of a healthy person with a person having a communicable disease, the disease being transmitted as a result 直接接触；**indirect c.**, that achieved through some intervening medium, as prolongation of a communicable disease through the air or by means of fomites 间接接触；**occlusal c.**, contact between the upper and lower teeth when the jaws are closed 咬合接触；**proximal c.**, proximate c., touching of the proximal surfaces of two adjoining teeth 邻面接触；**working c.**, that between the upper and lower teeth on the side toward which the mandible has been moved in mastication 工作侧的咬触

con·tac·tant (kən-tak′tənt) an allergen capable of inducing delayed contact-type hypersensitivity of the epidermis after contact 接触物，接触性过敏原

con·ta·gion (kən-ta′jən) 1. the communication of disease from one individual to another（接触）传染；2. a contagious disease 传染病

con·ta·gious (kən-ta′jəs) communicable; capable of being transmitted from one individual to another 接触传染的

con·tam·i·nant (kən-tam′ ĭ-nənt) something that causes contamination 污染物

con·tam·i·na·tion (kən-tam″ĭ-na′shən) 1. the soiling or making inferior by contact or mixture 污染；2. the deposition of radioactive material in any place where it is not desired 沾污

con·tent (kon′tent) that which is contained within

a thing 内容物，内含物；**latent c.**, the hidden and unconscious true meaning of a symbolic representation such as a dream or fantasy 潜隐内容；**manifest c.**, the content of a dream or fantasy as it is experienced and remembered, and in which the latent content is disguised and distorted by various mechanisms 梦情显义

con·ti·gu·i·ty (kon″tĭ-gu′ ĭ-te) contact or close proximity 接触，接近

con·ti·nence (kon′tĭ-nəns) the ability to exercise voluntary control over natural impulses 节制，节欲；**con′tinent** adj.

con·ti·nu·i·ty (kon″tĭ-nu′ ĭ-te) the quality of being without interruption or separation 连续，持续

con·tin·u·ous (kən-tin′u-əs) not interrupted; having no interruption 连续的

con·tour (kon′toor) [Fr.] 1. the normal outline or configuration of the body or of a part 轮廓；2. to shape a solid along certain desired lines 成形

con·tra-an·gle (kon″trə-ang′gəl) an angulation by which the working point of a surgical instrument is brought close to the long axis of its shaft 反角

con·tra-ap·er·ture (kon″trə-ap′ər-chər) a second opening made in an abscess to facilitate the discharge of its contents 对口

con·tra·cep·tion (kon″trə-sep′shən) the prevention of conception or impregnation 避孕，节育

con·tra·cep·tive (kon″trə-sep′tiv) 1. diminishing the likelihood of or preventing conception 避孕；2. an agent that so acts 避孕药；**barrier c.**, a contraceptive device that physically prevents spermatozoa from entering the endometrial cavity and fallopian tubes 屏障，避孕器；**chemical c.**, a spermicidal agent inserted into the vagina before intercourse to prevent pregnancy 化学避孕剂；**emergency c.**, postcoital c. 紧急避孕药；**hormonal c.**, one that administers hormones to prevent pregnancy, usually by prevention of ovulation, e.g., oral contraceptives, transdermal patch, vaginal ring, implants, and injections 激素避孕药；**oral c.**, a hormonal compound taken orally to block ovulation and prevent the occurrence of pregnancy 口服避孕药；**postcoital c.**, one that blocks or terminates pregnancy after sexual intercourse 性交后避孕药

con·tract (kən-trakt′) 1. to reduce in size or shorten 缩短，缩小；2. in muscle physiology, to become activated and generate force; such a process does not necessarily result in the shortening of the muscle 在肌肉生理学中，被激活而产生力量，这样的过程并不一定导致肌肉缩短；3. to acquire or incur 获得

con·trac·tile (kən-trak′tīl) able to contract in response to a suitable stimulus 收缩的

con·trac·til·i·ty (kon″trak-til′ ĭ-te) capacity for contracting in response to a suitable stimulus 收缩性，收缩力

con·trac·tion (kən-trak′shən) a drawing together; a shortening or shrinkage 收缩；**Braxton Hicks c.'s**, light, usually painless, irregular uterine contractions during pregnancy, gradually increasing in intensity and frequency and becoming more rhythmic during the third trimester 妊娠期中的子宫无痛性收缩；**carpopedal c.**, the condition due to chronic shortening of the muscles of the fingers, toes, arms, and legs in tetany 手足挛缩；**cicatricial c.**, the shrinkage and spontaneous closing of open skin wounds 瘢痕收缩；**clonic c.**, clonus 阵挛性反缩；**hourglass c.**, contraction of an organ, such as the stomach or uterus, at or near the middle 葫芦状收缩；**isometric c.**, muscle contraction without appreciable shortening or change in distance between its origin and insertion 等长收缩；**isotonic c.**, muscle contraction without appreciable change in the force of contraction; the distance between the muscle's origin and insertion becomes lessened 等张收缩；**lengthening c.**, a muscle contraction in which the ends of the muscle move farther apart, as when the muscle is forcibly flexed 伸长收缩；**paradoxical c.**, contraction of a muscle caused by the passive approximation of its extremities 被动收缩；**postural c.**, the state of muscular tension and contraction that just suffices to maintain the posture of the body 体位性收缩；**shortening c.**, a muscle contraction in that the ends of the muscle move closer together, as when a flexed limb is extended 缩短性收缩；**tetanic c.**, sustained muscular contraction without intervals of relaxation 强直性收缩；**tonic c.**, tetanic c；**twitch c.**, twitch 单收缩；**uterine c.**, contraction of the uterus during labor. 子宫收缩，宫缩；**wound c.**, the shrinkage and spontaneous closure of open skin wounds 伤口收合，伤口缩合

con·trac·ture (kən-trak′chər) abnormal shortening of muscle tissue, rendering the muscle highly resistant to passive stretching 挛缩；**Dupuytren c.**, flexion deformity of the fingers or toes, due to shortening, thickening, and fibrosis of the palmar or plantar fascia 掌腱膜挛缩；**ischemic c.**, muscular contracture and degeneration due to interference with the circulation from pressure, or from injury or cold 缺血性肌挛缩；**organic c.**, permanent and continuous contracture 器质性挛缩；**Volkmann c.**, contraction of the fingers and sometimes of the wrist, or of analogous parts of the foot, with loss of power, after severe injury or improper use of a tourniquet 福尔克曼挛缩

con·tra·fis·sure (kon″trə-fish′ər) a fracture in a

part opposite the site of the blow 对裂

con·tra·in·ci·sion (kon″trə-in-sizh′ən) counterincision to promote drainage 对口切开

con·tra·in·di·ca·tion (kon″trə-in″dĭ-ka′shən) any condition that renders a particular line of treatment improper or undesirable 禁忌证

con·tra·lat·er·al (kon″trə-lat′ər-əl) pertaining to, situated on, or affecting the opposite side 对侧的

con·tra·sex·u·al (kon″trə-sek′shoo-əl) pertaining to or characteristic of the opposite sex 异性的，显示异性特征的

con·trast (kon′trast) 1. the degree to which light and dark areas of an image differ in brightness or in optical density 对比度；2. in radiology, the difference in optical density in a radiograph that results from a difference in radiolucency or penetrability of the subject 对比

con·tre·coup (kōn″trə-koo′) [Fr.] denoting an injury, as to the brain, occurring at a site opposite to the point of impact 对侧伤，对侧外伤

con·trol (kən-trōl′) 1. the governing or limitation of certain objects or events 控制；2. a standard against which experimental observations may be evaluated 对照；3. the conscious restraint, regulation, or suppression of impulses, instincts, and affects 对（照）组. **aversive c.**, in behavior therapy, the use of unpleasant stimuli to change undesirable behavior 厌恶控制；**birth c.**, deliberate limitation of childbearing by measures designed to control fertility and to prevent pregnancy 节育，生育控制；**motor c.**, the systematic transmission of impulses from the motor cortex to motor units, resulting in coordinated muscular contractions 运动控制；**stimulus c.**, any influence of the environment on behavior 刺激控制

Con·trolled Sub·stan·ces Act a federal law that regulates the prescribing and dispensing of psychoactive drugs, including narcotics, hallucinogens, depressants, and stimulants 药物控制条例

con·tuse (kən-tooz′) to bruise; to wound by beating 挫伤

con·tu·sion (kən-too′zhən) bruise; an injury of a part without a break in the skin 挫伤；**contrecoup c.**, one resulting from a blow on one side of the head with damage to the cerebral hemisphere on the opposite side by transmitted force 对侧挫伤

co·nus (ko′nəs) pl. *co′ni* [L.] 1. a cone or cone-shaped structure 锥，圆锥体；2. posterior staphyloma of the myopic eye 弧形斑；**c. arterio′sus**, infundibulum; the anterosuperior portion of the right ventricle of the heart, at the entrance to the pulmonary trunk 动脉圆锥；**c. medulla′ris**, the cone-shaped lower end of the spinal cord, at the level of

the upper lumbar vertebrae 脊髓圆锥；**c. termina′-lis**, conus medullaris；**co′ni vasculo′si**, lobules of epididymis 附睾小叶

con·va·les·cence (kon″və-les′əns) the stage of recovery from an illness, operation, or injury 恢复期

con·vec·tion (kən-vek′shən) the act of conveying or transmission, specifically transmission of heat in a liquid or gas by bulk movement of heated particles to a cooler area 对流；**convec′tive** *adj.*

con·ver·gence (kən-vur′jəns) 1. in evolution, the development of similar structures or organisms in unrelated taxa 趋同；2. in embryology, the movement of cells from the periphery to the midline in gastrulation 会聚，集合；3. coordinated inclination of the two lines of sight toward their common point of fixation, or that point itself 辐辏作用；4. the exciting of a single sensory neuron by incoming impulses from multiple other neurons 会聚；**conver′gent** *adj.* **negative c.**, outward deviation of the visual axes 负会聚，负集合；**positive c.**, inward deviation of the visual axes 正会聚，正集合

con·ver·sion (kən-vur′zhən) 1. a shift from one state to another 转化；2. an unconscious defense mechanism by which the anxiety that stems from intrapsychic conflict is converted and expressed in somatic symptoms 转换（一种无意识的防御机制）

con·ver·tase (kən-vur′tās) an enzyme of the complement system that activates specific components of the system 转换酶，转化酶

con·ver·tin (kən-vur′tin) the activated form of coagulation factor Ⅶ 转变素，转变加速因子

con·vex (kon-veks′) having a rounded, somewhat elevated surface 凸，凸起；**convex′ity** *adj.*

con·vexo·con·cave (kon-vek″so-kon′kāv) having one convex and one concave surface 凹凸的

con·vexo·con·vex (kon-vek″so-kon′veks) convex on two surfaces 双凸的，对凸的

con·vo·lut·ed (kon″vo-loot′əd) rolled together or coiled 卷曲的，回旋的

con·vo·lu·tion (kon″vo-loo′shən) a tortuous irregularity or elevation caused by the infolding of a structure upon itself 卷曲，回旋；回，脑回；**Broca c.**, the center of speech, occupying the inferior frontal gyrus, usually of the left hemisphere, of the cerebrum 左额下回

con·vul·sion (kən-vul′shən) 1. an involuntary contraction or series of contractions of the voluntary muscles 惊厥，抽搐；2. seizure (2) 癫痫发作；**convul′sive** *adj.*；**febrile c's**, those associated with high fever, usually in infants and children 热性惊厥，高热惊厥

co·op·er·a·tiv·i·ty (ko-op″ər-ə-tiv′ĭ-te) the phenomenon of alteration in binding of subsequent ligands upon binding of an initial ligand by an enzyme, receptor, or other molecule with multiple binding sites; the affinity for further binding may be enhanced (*positive c.*) or decreased (*negative c.*) 协同性，合作性

co·or·di·na·tion (ko-or″dǐ-na′shən) the harmonious functioning of interrelated organs and parts 协调，协同作用，协调功能，共济

COPD chronic obstructive pulmonary disease 慢性阻塞性肺疾病

cope (kōp) in dentistry, the upper or cavity side of a denture flask 根鞘根端盖（牙科用）

cop·ing (kōp′ing) a thin metal covering or cap, such as the plate of metal applied over the prepared crown or root of a tooth prior to attaching an artificial crown 盖，型合盖

co·poly·mer (ko-pol′ĭ-mər) a polymer containing monomers of more than one kind 共聚物

cop·per (Cu) (kop′ər) a reddish, malleable metallic element; at. no. 29, at. wt. 63.546. It is an essential dietary trace element, being a necessary component of several enzymes, but is toxic in excess 铜；**c. sulfate,** cupric sulfate 硫酸铜

cop·per·head (kop′ər-hed) 1. a venomous snake (a pit viper), *Agkistrodon contortrix,* of the United States, having a brown to copper-colored body with dark bands 铜头蛇；2. a very venomous elapid snake, *Denisonia superba,* of Australia, Tasmania, and the Solomon Islands 一种剧毒的眼镜蛇

cop·ro·an·ti·body (kop″ro-an′tǐ-bod″e) an antibody (chiefly IgA) present in the intestinal tract, associated with immunity to enteric infection 粪抗体

cop·ro·la·lia (kop″ro-la′le-ə) the compulsive utterance of obscene words, especially words relating to feces 秽语症；**coprolal′ic** *adj.*

cop·ro·lith (kop′ro-lith) fecalith 粪石

cop·ro·phil·ia (kop″ro-fil′e-ə) an absorbing interest in feces or filth, particularly a paraphilia in which sexual arousal or activity is linked to feces 嗜粪癖；**coprophil′iac, coprophil′ic** *adj.*

cop·ro·pho·bia (kop″ro-fo′be-ə) abnormal repugnance to defecation and to feces 粪便恐怖症，排便恐怖症

cop·ro·por·phy·ria (kop″ro-por-fir′e-ə) any of various types of porphyria characterized by elevated levels of coproporphyrin in the body 粪卟啉症；**hereditary c. (HCP),** a hepatic porphyria due to a defect in an enzyme involved in porphyrin synthesis, characterized by recurrent attacks of gastroenterologic and neurologic dysfunction, cutaneous photosensitivity, and excretion of coproporphyrin Ⅲ in the feces and urine and of δ -aminolevulinic acid and porphobilinogen in urine 遗传性粪卟啉症

cop·ro·por·phy·rin (kop″ro-por′fə-rin) a porphyrin occurring as several isomers; the Ⅲ isomer, an intermediate in heme biosynthesis, is excreted in the feces and urine in hereditary coproporphyria and variegate porphyria; the I isomer, a side product, is excreted in the feces and urine in congenital erythropoietic porphyria 粪卟啉

cop·ro·por·phy·rin·o·gen (kop″ro-por′fə-rin′o-jən) a porphyrinogen formed from uroporphyrinogen and existing naturally as two isomers, types I and Ⅲ 粪卟啉原

cop·ro·por·phy·rin·uria (kop″ro-por″fə-rinu′re-ə) coproporphyrin in the urine 粪卟啉尿

cop·ros·ta·sis (kop-ros′tə-sis) fecal impaction 便结，粪积

cop·ro·zoa (kop″ro-zo′ə) protozoa found in feces outside the body, but not in the intestines 粪内寄生动物

cop·u·la (kop′u-lə) 1. any connecting part or structure 介体，连接机构；2. a median ventral elevation on the embryonic tongue formed by union of the second pharyngeal arches and playing a role in tongue development 联合突

cop·u·la·tion (kop″u-la′shən) 1. sexual union; the transfer of the sperm from male to female; usually applied to the mating process in nonhuman animals 交配；2. joining together in coupling; sexual intercourse 性交

Co·quil·let·tid·ia (ko-kwil′ə-tid′e-ə) a genus of large, mostly yellow, viciously biting, freshwater mosquitoes; *C. pertur′bans* is a vector of eastern equine encephalitis in North America, and *C. venezuelen′sis* is a South American species that is the vector of several arboviruses, including Oropouche virus 轲蚊亚属

cor (kor) [L.] heart 心，心脏；**acute c. pulmonale,** acute overload of the right ventricle due to pulmonary hypertension, usually due to acute pulmonary embolism 急性肺源性心脏病；**c. adipo′sum,** fatty heart (2) 脂肪心；**c. bilocula′re,** a two-chambered heart with one atrium and one ventricle, and a common atrioventricular valve, due to failure of formation of the interatrial and interventricular septa 双腔心；**c. bovi′num,** a greatly enlarged heart resulting from a hypertrophied or dilated left ventricle 巨心，牛心症；**chronic c. pulmonale,** heart disease due to pulmonary hypertension secondary to disease of the lung or its blood vessels, with hypertrophy of the right ventricle 慢性肺源性心脏病；**c. triatria′tum,** a heart with three atrial chambers, the pulmonary veins emptying into an accessory chamber above the true left atrium and communicating with it by a small opening 三房心；

C

c. **trilocula′re**, three-chambered heart 三 腔 心；c. **trilocula′re biatria′tum**, a three-chambered heart with two atria communicating, by the tricuspid and left atrioventricular valve, with a single ventricle 三 腔 二 房 心；c. **trilocula′re biventricula′re**, a three-chambered heart with one atrium and two ventricles 三腔二室心

cor·a·cid·i·um (kor″ə-sid′e-əm) pl. *coraci'dia* [L.] the individual free-swimming or freecrawling, spherical, ciliated embryo of certain tapeworms, e.g., *Diphyllobothrium latum* 钩球蚴，纤毛蚴

cor·a·co·cla·vic·u·lar (kor″ə-ko-klə-vik′ulər) pertaining to the coracoid process and the clavicle 喙突锁骨的，喙锁的

cor·a·coid (kor′ə-koid) 1. like a crow's beak 喙状的；2. the coracoid process 喙突

cord (kord) any long, cylindrical, flexible structure 索，带。Spelled also *chord.*; **genital c.**, in the embryo, the midline fused caudal part of the two urogenital ridges, each containing a mesonephric and paramesonephric duct 生殖索；**gubernacular c.**, a portion of the gubernaculum testis or of the round ligament of the uterus that develops in the inguinal crest and adjoining body wall 睾丸引带；**sexual c's**, the seminiferous tubules of the early fetus 生殖索；**spermatic c.**, the structure extending from the abdominal inguinal ring to the testis, comprising the pampiniform plexus, nerves, ductus deferens, testicular artery, and other vessels 精索；**spinal c.**, that part of the central nervous system lodged in the vertebral canal, extending from the foramen magnum to the upper part of the lumbar region 脊髓 见 Plate & umbilical **c.**, the structure connecting the fetus and placenta, and containing the vessels through which fetal blood passes to and from the placenta 脐带；**vocal c's**, folds of mucous membrane in the larynx; the superior pair are called the *false vocal cords* and the inferior pair, the *true vocal cords* 声带；**Willis c's**, fibrous bands traversing the inferior angle of the superior sagittal sinus 上矢状窦横索

cor·dec·to·my (kor-dek′tə-me) excision of all or part of a cord, as of a vocal cord or the spinal cord 索带切除术

cor·di·tis (kor-di′tis) chorditis 精索炎

cor·do·cen·te·sis (kor″do-sen-te′sis) percutaneous puncture of the umbilical vein under ultrasonographic guidance to obtain a fetal blood sample 脐静脉穿刺术

cor·dot·o·my (kor-dot′ə-me) 1. section of a vocal cord 声带切开术；2. surgical division of the lateral spinothalamic tract of the spinal cord, usually in the anterolateral quadrant 脊髓束切断术。Spelled also *chordotomy*

cor·ec·ta·sis (kor-ek′tə-sis) dilation of the pupil 瞳孔扩大，瞳孔散大

cor·ec·tome (kor-ek′tōm) cutting instrument for iridectomy 虹膜刀

cor·ec·to·me·di·al·y·sis (ko-rek″to-me″deal′ə-sis) surgical creation of an artificial pupil by detaching the iris from the ciliary ligament 人造瞳孔术，假瞳孔术，造瞳术

cor·ec·to·pia (kor″ek-to′pe-ə) abnormal location of the pupil of the eye 瞳孔异位

core·di·al·y·sis (kor″ə-di-al′ə-sis) surgical separation of the external margin of the iris from the ciliary body 虹膜根部分离术

cor·el·y·sis (kə-rel′ə-sis) operative destruction of the pupil; especially detachment of adhesions of the pupillary margin of the iris from the lens 虹膜后粘连分离术

cor·e·mor·pho·sis (kor″ə-mor-fo′sis) surgical formation of an artificial pupil 瞳孔形成术

cor·eo·plas·ty (kor′e-o-plas″te) any plastic operation on the pupil 瞳孔成形术，造瞳术

co·re·pres·sor (ko″re-pres′ər) in genetic theory, a small molecule that combines with an aporepressor to form the complete repressor 辅助阻遏物

Co·rio·bac·te·ri·a·ceae (kor″e-o-bak-tēr″ea′se-e) a family of gram-positive, rod-shaped to coccoid bacteria of the order Coriobacteriales 红蜷杆菌科

Co·rio·bac·te·ri·a·les (kor″e-o-bak-tēr″e-a′lēz) an order of bacteria of the class Actinobacteria 红蜷杆菌目

co·ri·um (kor′e-əm) dermis 真皮

corn (korn) a horny induration and thickening of the stratum corneum of the epidermis, caused by friction and pressure and forming a conical mass pointing down into the dermis, producing pain and irritation 鸡眼；**hard c.**, one usually located on the outside of the little toe or the upper surfaces of the other toes 硬 鸡眼；**soft c.**, one between the toes, kept softened by moisture, often leading to painful inflammation under the corn 软鸡眼

cor·nea (kor′ne-ə) the transparent anterior part of the eye 角膜，见 图 30；**cor′neal** *adj.*；**conical c.**, keratoconus 圆锥形角膜

cor·neo·scle·ra (kor″ne-o-skler′ə) the cornea and sclera regarded as one organ 角巩膜

cor·ne·ous (kor′ne-əs) 1. horny 角样的；2. keratinous 角质的

cor·nic·u·late (kor-nik′u-lāt) shaped like a small horn 小角状的

cor·nic·u·lum (kor-nik′u-ləm) [L.] corniculate cartilage 小角软骨

cor·ni·fi·ca·tion (kor″nī-f ī-ka′shən) 1. keratinization 角质化；2. conversion of epithelium to the stratified squamous type 复层鳞状上皮

cor·nu (kor'noo) pl. *cor'nua* [L.] horn 角；c. **ammo'nis,** hippocampus proper 海 马；**sacral c., c. sacra'le,** either of two hook-shaped processes extending down from the arch of the last sacral vertebra 骶骨角

cor·nu·al (kor'noo-əl) pertaining to a horn, especially to the horns of the spinal cord 角的，角状突起的。又称 *cornuate.*

co·ro·na (kə-ro'nə) pl. *coro'nae, coronas* [L.] a crown; in anatomic nomenclature, a crownlike eminence or encircling structure 冠；c. **glan'dis pe'nis,** the rounded proximal border of the glans penis 阴茎头冠；c. **radia'ta,** 1. the radiating crown of projection fibers passing from the internal capsule to every part of the cerebral cortex 辐射冠；2. a superficial layer of radially elongated follicle cells surrounding the zona pellucida 放 射 冠；c. **ve'neris,** a ring of syphilitic sores around the forehead 额（发缘）梅毒疹，梅毒冠

co·ro·nad (kor'ō-nad) toward the crown of the head or any corona 向头冠，向冠

cor·o·nal (kor'ə-nəl) [L.] 1. pertaining to the crown of a structure 冠的，头冠的；2. of, relating to, or situated in the plane of the coronal suture or parallel to it 冠向的

co·ro·na·lis (kor"o-na'lis) [L.] coronal 冠的

cor·o·nary (kor'ə-nar"e) encircling like a crown; applied to vessels, ligaments, etc., especially to the arteries of the heart, and to pathologic involvement of them 冠状的

Co·ro·na·vi·ri·dae (kə-ro"nə-vir' ĭ-de) a family of RNA viruses; human disease is caused by the genus *Coronavirus* 冠状病毒科，日冕形病毒科

Co·ro·na·vi·rus (kə-ro'nə-vi"rus) the coronaviruses; a genus of RNA viruses of the family Coronaviridae that cause respiratory disease and sometimes gastroenteritis in humans and other animals 冠状病毒属，日冕形病毒属

co·ro·na·vi·rus (kə-ro'nə-vi"rəs) any virus belonging to the family Coronaviridae 冠状病毒，日冕形病毒

cor·o·ner (kor'ə-nər) a public official, elected or appointed, who holds inquests in regard to violent, sudden, or unexplained deaths within a given jurisdiction 验尸官

cor·o·noid (kor'ə-noid) 1. shaped like a crow's beak 喙状的；2. crown-shaped 冠状的

cor·o·noi·dec·to·my (kor"ə-noi-dek'tə-me) surgical removal of the coronoid process of the mandible（下颌）冠状突切除术

co·rot·o·my (kə-rot'ə-me) iridotomy 虹膜切开术

corpse (korps) a dead body; used to refer specifically to a human body in the early period after death 尸体。Cf. *cadaver.*

cor·pu·len·cy (kor'pu-len"se) obesity 肥胖

cor·pus (kor'pəs) pl. *cor'pora* [L.] body 体；c. **adipo'sum buc'cae,** sucking pad 颊脂体；c. **al'bicans,** white fibrous tissue that replaces the regressing corpus luteum in the human ovary in the latter half of pregnancy, or soon after ovulation when pregnancy does not supervene 白 体；c. **amygdaloi'deum,** a small mass of subcortical gray matter within the tip of the temporal lobe, anterior to the inferior horn of the lateral ventricle of the brain; it is part of the limbic system 杏仁核；**cor'pora amyla'cea,** small hyaline masses, of unknown pathologic significance and occurring more commonly with advancing age, derived from degenerate cells or thickened secretions and found in the prostate, neuroglia, and pulmonary alveoli 淀粉样体；**cor'pora arena'cea,** brain sand; gritty calcareous concretions deposited in the brain, particularly the extracellular matrix of the pineal body, and accumulating progressively with age 脑 干；**cor'pora bige'mina,** two bodies in the brain of the human fetus that later split to become the corpora quadrigemina 二叠体；c. **callo'sum,** an arched mass of white matter in the depths of the longitudinal fissure, composed of transverse fibers connecting the cerebral hemispheres 胼胝体；c. **caverno'sum,** either of the columns of erectile tissue forming the body of the clitoris (c. *caverno·sum clitoridis*) or penis (c. *cavernosum penis*) 海绵体；c. **hemorrha'gicum,** a blood clot formed in the cavity left by the mature ovarian follicle after its rupture during ovulation 黄体血块；c. **lu'teum,** a yellow glandular mass in the ovary, formed by an ovarian follicle that has matured and discharged its oocyte 黄 体；**cor'pora quadrige'mina,** four rounded eminences on the posterior surface of the midbrain 四叠体；c. **spongio'sum pe'nis,** a column of erectile tissue forming the urethral surface of the penis, in which the urethra is found 阴茎海绵体；c. **stria'tum,** a subcortical mass of gray and white substance in front of and lateral to the thalamus in each cerebral hemisphere 纹 状 体；c. **u'teri,** body of uterus: that part of the uterus above the isthmus and below the orifices of the uterine tubes 子宫体；c. **vi'treum,** vitreous body 玻璃体

cor·pus·cle (kor'pəs-əl) a small mass or body 小体，细胞；**corpus'cular** *adj.*; **blood c.,** 血细胞，见 *cell* 下词条；**corneal c's,** star-shaped connective tissue cells within the corneal stroma 角 膜 小体；**Hassall c's,** spherical or ovoid bodies found in the medulla of the thymus, composed of concentric arrays of epithelial cells that contain keratohyalin and bundles of cytoplasmic filaments 哈 索 耳 小 体；**malpighian c.**, 1. renal c.；2. aggregations of B lymphocytes that occur at intervals along the periarteriolar lymphoid sheaths in the white pulp of the spleen 马儿皮基体；**Meissner c.**, a rapidly adapting encapsulated nerve ending specialized for tactile discrimination and found in the dermal ridges of glabrous skin 触觉小体；**pacinian c.**, a large, ovoid, rapidly adapting, encapsulated nerve ending sensitive to pressure, touch, and vibration; found in the skin and deeper tissues. Its core contains the nonmyelinated nerve terminal and its Schwann cells, surrounded by concentric layers of modified fibroblasts, in cross-section resembling a sliced onion 帕奇尼小体，环层下体；**red c.**, erythrocyte. 红细胞；**renal c.**, a body that forms the beginning of a nephron, consisting of the glomerulus and glomerular capsule 肾小体；**white c.**, leukocyte 白细胞

cor·pus·cu·lum (kor-pus′ku-ləm) pl. *corpus′cula* [L.] corpuscle 小体，细胞

▲ 真 皮 中 的 帕 奇 尼 小 体（**pacinian corpuscle**）

cor·rec·tion (kə-rek′shən) a setting right, e.g., the provision of lenses for improvement of vision, or an arbitrary adjustment made in values or devices in performance of experiments 矫正，改正

cor·re·la·tion (kor″ə-la′shən) in statistics, the degree and direction of association of variable phenomena; how well one can be predicted from the other 相关

cor·re·spon·dence (kor″ə-spon′dəns) the condition of being in agreement or conformity 对 应，相 对；**anomalous retinal c.**, a condition in which disparate points on the retinas of the two eyes come to be associated sensorially 异常视网膜对应；**normal retinal c.**, the condition in which the corresponding points on the retinas of the two eyes are associated sensorially 正常视网膜对应；**retinal c.**, the state concerned with the impingement of image-producing stimuli on the retinas of the two eyes 视网膜对应

cor·rin (kor′in) a tetrapyrrole ring system resembling the porphyrin ring system. The cobalamins contain a corrin ring system 咕啉

cor·ro·sive (kə-ro′siv) 1. producing gradual destruction, as of a metal by electrochemical reaction or of tissues by the action of a strong acid or alkali 腐蚀的；2. an agent that so acts 腐蚀剂

cor·tex (kor′teks) pl. *cor′tices* [L.] the outer layer of an organ or other structure, as distinguished from its inner substance 皮质，皮层；**cor′tical** *adj.*；**adrenal c.**, the outer firm layer comprising the larger part of the suprarenal gland; it secretes many steroid hormones, including mineralocorticoids, glucocorticoids, androgens, 17-ketosteroids, and progestins 肾 上 腺 皮 质；**cerebellar c.**, **c. cerebella′ris**, the superficial gray matter of the cerebellum 小脑皮质；**cerebral c.**, **c. cerebra′lis**, the convoluted layer of gray substance covering each cerebral hemisphere; see *archicortex*, *paleocortex*, and *neocortex* 大 脑 皮质；**c. len′tis**, the softer, external part of the lens of the eye 晶状体皮质；**motor c.**, 运动皮质，见 *area* 下 词 条；**provisional c.**, the cortex of the fetal suprarenal gland that undergoes involution in early fetal life 临 时 皮 质；**renal c.**, **c. re′nis**, the outer part of the substance of the kidney, composed mainly of glomeruli and convoluted tubules 肾 皮质；**striate c.**, the part of the occipital lobe of the cerebral cortex that is the primary receptive area for vision 纹状皮质；**c. of thymus**, the outer part of each lobule of the thymus; it consists chiefly of closely packed lymphocytes (thymocytes) and surrounds the medulla 胸腺皮质；**visual c.**, the area of the occipital lobe of the cerebral cortex concerned with vision 视皮质

cor·ti·cate (kor′tĭ-kāt) having a cortex or bark 有皮质的，有树皮的

cor·ti·cec·to·my (kor″tĭ-sek′tə-me) topectomy 脑皮质切除术

cor·ti·cif·u·gal (kor″tĭ-sif′ə-gəl) efferent; proceeding or conducting away from the cerebral cortex 离皮质的，离皮层的

cor·ti·cip·e·tal (kor″tĭ-sip′ə-təl) proceeding or conducting toward the cerebral cortex 向皮质的，向皮层的。Cf. *afferent*

cor·ti·co·bul·bar (kor″tĭ-ko-bul′bər) pertaining to or connecting the cerebral cortex and the medulla oblongata or brainstem（脑）皮质延髓的

cor·ti·coid (kor′tĭ-koid) corticosteroid（肾上腺）类皮质激素

cor·ti·co·ster·oid (kor″tĭ-ko-ster′oid) any of the steroids elaborated by the adrenal cortex (excluding the sex hormones) or any synthetic equivalents; divided into two major groups, the *glucocorticoids* and *mineralocorticoids*; used clinically for hormonal replacement therapy, for suppression of ACTH secretion, as anti-inflammatory agents, and to suppress the immune response（肾上腺）皮质类固醇

cor·ti·cos·ter·one (kor″tĭ-kos′tər-ōn) a natural corticoid with moderate glucocorticoid activity, some mineralocorticoid activity, and actions similar to cortisol except that it is not antiinflammatory 皮质酮

cor·ti·co·ten·sin (kor″tĭ-ko-ten′sin) a polypeptide purified from kidney extract that exhibits a vasopressor effect when given intravenously 皮质加压素

cor·ti·co·troph (kor″tĭ-ko-trōf) an acidophil of the anterior lobe of the pituitary that secretes corticotropin 促（肾上腺）皮质激素细胞

cor·ti·co·tro·pin (kor″tĭ-ko-tro″pin) 1. a hormone secreted by the anterior lobe of the pituitary, having a stimulating effect on the adrenal cortex 促肾上腺皮质激素；2. a preparation of the hormone derived from animals, used for diagnostic testing of adrenocortical function and as an anticonvulsant in infantile spasms 促肾上腺皮质激素制剂。Spelled also *corticotrophin*

cor·ti·lymph (kor′tĭ-limf″) the fluid filling the intercellular spaces of the organ of Corti, similar in composition to perilymph. nnPacinian corpuscle in dermis 柯替淋巴

Cor·ti·na·ri·us (kor″tĭ-nar′e-əs) a large genus of mushrooms including *C. orella′nus* and other species containing the nephrotoxin orellanine 丝膜蕈属

cor·ti·sol (kor′tĭ-sol) the major natural glucocorticoid elaborated by the adrenal cortex; it affects the metabolism of glucose, protein, and fats and has mineralocorticoid activity. See *hydrocortisone* for therapeutic uses 皮质醇，氢化可的松

cor·ti·sone (kor′tĭ-sōn) a natural glucocorticoid that is metabolically convertible to cortisol; the acetate ester is used as an antiinflammatory and immunosuppressant and for replacement therapy in adrenocortical insufficiency 可的松

co·run·dum (ko-run′dəm) native aluminum oxide, Al_2O_3, used in dentistry as an abrasive and polishing agent 刚砂

cor·us·ca·tion (kor″əs-ka′shən) the sensation as of a flash of light before the eyes 闪光感

co·rym·bi·form (ko-rim′bĭ-form) clustered; said of lesions grouped around a single, usually larger, lesion 伞房花形的

Co·ry·ne·bac·te·ri·a·ceae (ko-ri″ne-bak-tēr″ea′se-e) a family of bacteria of the order Actinomycetales 棒状杆菌科

Co·ry·ne·bac·te·ri·um (ko-ri″ne-bak-tēr′e-əm) a genus of gram-positive, club-shaped bacteria of the family Corynebacteriaceae; it includes *C. diph-the′riae*, the etiologic agent of diphtheria, and *C. minutis′simum*, the etiologic agent of erythrasma 棒状杆菌属

co·ry·ne·form (ko-ri′nə-form) denoting or resembling organisms of the family Corynebacteriaceae 棒状的

Co·ry·nes·po·ra (kor″ĭ-nes′pə-rə) a widespread genus of imperfect fungi 棒孢属；*C. cassi′cola* is a cause of eumycotic mycetoma 丛梗孢菌属

co·ry·za (ko-ri′zə) [L.] acute rhinitis 卡他性鼻炎

COS Canadian Ophthalmological Society 加拿大眼科学会

cos·me·sis (koz-me′sis) 1. the preservation, restoration, or bestowing of bodily beauty 美容；2. the surgical correction of a disfiguring physical defect 整容

cos·met·ic (koz-met′ik) 1. pertaining to cosmesis 美容的，整容的；2. a beautifying substance or preparation 美容剂（品）

cos·ta (kos′tə) [L.] 1. a rib 肋（骨）；2. a thin, firm, rodlike structure running along the base of the undulating membrane of certain flagellates 肋（骨）的，缘，边的；**cos′tal** *adj.*

cos·tal·gia (kos-tal′jə) 1. pain in the ribs 肋痛；2. pain in the costal muscles 肋肌痛

cos·ta·lis (kos-ta′lis) [L.] costal 肋的

cos·to·chon·dral (kos″to-kon′drəl) pertaining to a rib and its cartilage 肋骨（肋）软骨

cos·to·cla·vic·u·lar (kos″to-klə-vik′u-lər) pertaining to the ribs and clavicle 肋锁的

cos·to·gen·ic (kos″to-jen′ik) arising from a rib, especially from a defect of the marrow of the ribs 肋骨性的

cos·to·scap·u·lar·is (kos″to-skap″u-lar′is) the serratus anterior muscle 前锯肌

cos·to·ster·no·plas·ty (kos″to-stur′no-plas″te) surgical repair of funnel chest, a segment of rib being used to support the sternum 肋骨胸骨成形术，漏斗胸成形术

cos·to·trans·ver·sec·to·my (kos″to-trans″ vərsek′tə-me) excision of a part of a rib along with the transverse process of a vertebra 肋骨横突切除术

cos·to·ver·te·bral (kos″to-vur′tə-brəl) pertaining to a rib and a vertebra 肋椎的

co·syn·tro·pin (ko″sin-tro′pin) a synthetic polypeptide identical with a portion of corticotropin, having its corticotropic activity but not its allergenicity; used in the screening of adrenal insufficiency on the basis of plasma cortisol response 促皮质素

co·trans·duc·tion (ko″trans-duk′shən) simultaneous transduction of two or more genes, indicating close linkage 共传导

co·trans·fec·tion (ko″trans-fek′shən) simultaneous transfection of two or more physically unlinked DNA fragments into eukaryotic target cells; generally one of the fragments contains a gene that is easily assayed and acts as a marker 共转染

co·trans·for·ma·tion (ko″trans-for-ma′shən) 1. simultaneous transformation of a single cell by two or more bacterial genes 共转化；2. cotransfection 同转染

co·trans·port (ko-trans′port) linking of the transport of one substance across a membrane with the simultaneous transport of a different substance in the same direction 协同转运

co·tri·mox·a·zole (ko″tri-moks′ə-zōl) a combination of trimethoprim and sulfamethoxazole, an antibacterial used primarily in the treatment of urinary tract infections and pneumocystis pneumonia 复方增效磺胺，增效磺胺甲基异噁唑

cot·ton (kot′ən) a plant of the genus *Gossypium*,or a textile material derived from its seeds 棉，棉花；**absorbable c.**, oxidized cellulose 氧化纤维素；**absorbent c., purified c.**, cotton freed from impurities, bleached, and sterilized; used as a surgical dressing 脱脂棉，吸水棉

cot·y·le·don (kot″ə-le′don) 1. the seed leaf of the embryo of a plant 子叶；2. any subdivision of the uterine surface of the placenta 胎盘小叶

cot·y·loid (kot′ə-loid) cup-shaped 杯状的；臼状的，髋臼的

cough (kawf) 1. sudden noisy expulsion of air from lungs 咳嗽；2. to produce such an expulsion 产生这样的驱逐；**dry c.**, cough without expectoration 干咳；**hacking c.**, a short, frequent, shallow and feeble cough 频咳；**productive c.**, cough with expectoration of material from the bronchi 排痰性咳；**reflex c.**, cough due to irritation of some remote organ 反射性咳；**wet c.**, productive c. 湿咳；**whooping c.**, pertussis 百日咳

cou·lomb (C) (koo′lom) the SI unit of electric charge, defined as the quantity of electric charge transferred across a surface by 1 ampere in 1 second 库（仑）

cou·ma·rin (koo′mə-rin) 1. a principle extracted from the tonka bean; it contains a factor, dicumarol, that inhibits hepatic synthesis of vitamin K–dependent coagulation factors, and a number of its derivatives are used as anticoagulants in treating disorders characterized by excessive clotting 香豆素；2. any of these derivatives or any synthetic compound with similar activity 类香豆素

count (kount) a numerical computation or indication 计数；**Addis c.**, determining the number of erythrocytes, leukocytes, epithelial cells, casts, and protein content in an aliquot of a 12-hour urine specimen 艾迪斯计数；**blood c., blood cell c.**, determining the number of formed elements in a cubic millimeter of blood; it may be a complete blood count or it may measure just one of the formed elements 血细胞计数；**complete blood c.**, a series of tests of the peripheral blood, including the hematocrit, the amount of hemoglobin, and counts of each type of formed element 全血细胞计数；**differential leukocyte c.**, a count on a stained blood smear of the proportion of different types of leukocytes, expressed in percentages 白细胞分类计数；**platelet c.**, determination of the total number of platelets per cubic millimeter of blood; the *direct platelet c.* simply counts the cells using a microscope, and the *indirect platelet c.* determines the ratio of platelets to erythrocytes on a peripheral blood smear and computes the number of platelets from the erythrocyte count 血小板计数

coun·ter (koun′tər) an instrument to compute numerical value; in radiology, a device for enumerating ionizing events 计数器；**Coulter c.**, an automatic instrument used in enumeration of formed elements in the peripheral blood 库尔特颗粒计数器；**Geiger c., Geiger-Müller c.**, an amplifying device that indicates the presence of ionizing particles, particularly β particles 盖格计数器；**scintillation c.**, a device for detecting ionization events, permitting determination of the concentration of radioisotopes in the body or other substance 闪烁计数器

coun·ter·cur·rent (koun′tər-kur′ənt) flowing in an opposite direction 逆流，反流

coun·ter·ex·ten·sion (koun″tər-eks-ten′shən) traction in a proximal direction coincident with traction in opposition to it 对抗牵伸术

coun·ter·im·mu·no·elec·tro·pho·re·sis (koun″tər-im″u-no-e-lek″tro-fə-re′sis) immunoelectrophoresis in which the antigen and antibody migrate in opposite directions 免疫双扩散法

coun·ter·in·ci·sion (koun″tər-in-sī′zhən) a second incision made to promote drainage or to relieve tension on the edges of a wound 对口切开

coun·ter·ir·ri·ta·tion (koun″tər-ir″ī-ta′shən) superficial irritation intended to relieve some other irritation 对抗刺激

coun·ter·open·ing (koun″tər-o′pən-ing) a second incision made across an earlier one to promote drainage 对口切开

coun·ter·pul·sa·tion (koun″tər-pəl-sa′shən) a technique for assisting the circulation and decreasing the work of the heart, by synchronizing the force of an external pumping device with cardiac systole and diastole 对抗搏动法，反搏法；**intra-aortic**

balloon (IAB) c., circulatory support provided by a balloon inserted into the descending thoracic aorta, inflated during diastole and deflated during systole 主动脉内球囊反搏

coun·ter·shock (koun′tər-shok″) a highintensity direct current shock delivered to the heart to interrupt ventricular fibrillation and restore synchronous electrical activity 对抗性电震法

coun·ter·stain (koun′tər-stān″) a stain applied to render the effects of another stain more discernible 复染色，对比染色

coun·ter·trac·tion (koun″tər-trak′shən) traction opposed to another traction; used in reduction of fractures 对抗牵引

coun·ter·trans·fer·ence (koun″tər-transfur′əns) a transference reaction of a psychoanalyst or other psychotherapist to a patient 反转移法，反移情作用

coun·ter·trans·port (koun″tər-trans′port) the simultaneous transport of two substances across a membrane in opposite directions, either by the same carrier or by two carriers that are biochemically linked to each other 反向运输

coup (koo) [Fr.] a blow or attack 反作，打击

c. de fouet, (də fwa′) rupture of the plantaris muscle accompanied by a sharp disabling pain 跖肌断裂；

c. de sabre, en c. de sabre, (də sahb′) a lesion of linear scleroderma on the forehead and scalp, sometimes associated with hemiatrophy of the face 军刀状头面伤

cou·ple (kup′əl) 1. to link together 联系在一起；join 加入；connect 连接；2. two equal forces operating on an object in parallel but opposite directions 力偶；3. an area of contact between two dissimilar metals, producing a difference in electrical potential 电偶

coup·let (kup′lət) pair (2) 偶联

coup·ling (kup′ling) 1. the joining together of two things 配对；2. in genetics, the occurrence on the same chromosome in a double heterozygote of the two mutant alleles of interest 联结；3. in cardiology, serial occurrence of a normal heartbeat followed closely by a premature beat 偶联

co·va·lence (ko-va′ləns) 共价 1. the number of electron pairs an atom can share with other atoms；2. one or more chemical bonds formed by sharing of electron pairs between atoms. **cova′lent** adj. 共价的

co·var·i·ance (ko-vār′e-əns) a measure of the tendency of two random variables to vary together 协方差

cov·er·glass (kuv′ər-glas″) a thin glass plate that covers a mounted microscopical object or a culture 盖玻片

cov·er·slip (kuv′ər-slip″) coverglass 盖玻片

cow·per·itis (kou″pər-i′tis) inflammation of the Cowper (bulbourethral) glands 尿道球腺炎

cow·pox (kou′poks) a mild eruptive disease of milk cows, confined to the udder and teats, due to cowpox virus, and transmissible to humans 牛痘

coxa (kok′sə) [L.] 1. hip 髋；2. hip joint 髋关节；**c. mag′na,** broadening of the head and neck of the femur 髋膨大；**c. pla′na,** osteochondrosis of the capitular epiphysis of the femur 扁平髋；**c. val′ga,** deformity of the hip with increase in the angle of inclination between the neck and shaft of the femur 髋外翻；**c. va′ra,** deformity of the hip with decrease in the angle of inclination between the neck and shaft of the femur 髋内翻

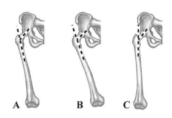

▲ **A. 正常髋关节（hip joint）。B. 髋内翻（coxa vara）。C. 髋外翻（coxa valga）**

cox·al·gia (kok-sal′jə) 1. hip-joint disease 髋关节（结核）病；2. pain in the hip 髋痛

cox·ar·throp·a·thy (kok″sahr-throp′ə-the) hip-joint disease 髋关节病

Cox·i·el·la (kok″se-el′ə) a genus of gramnegative, rod-shaped bacteria of the family Coxiellaceae, occurring only in the vacuoles of host cells. *C. burne′tii* is the etiologic agent of Q fever 柯克斯体

Cox·i·el·la·ceae (kok″se-el·a′se-e) a family of bacteria of the order Legionellales, consisting of intracellular parasites found only in cytoplasmic vacuoles of host cells 柯克斯体科

coxo·fem·o·ral (kok″so-fem′ə-rəl) pertaining to the hip and thigh 髋股的

cox·sack·ie·vi·rus (kok-sak′e-vi″rəs) any of a large group of viruses of the genus Enterovirus; some strains produce in humans a disease resembling poliomyelitis, but without paralysis 柯萨奇病毒

CPD citrate phosphate dextrose 枸橼酸盐磷酸盐右旋糖；见 *solution* 下 *anticoagulant citrate phosphate dextrose solution*

CPDA-1 citrate phosphate dextrose adenine 枸橼酸磷酸酸葡萄糖腺嘌呤；见 *solution* 下 *anticoagulant citrate phosphate dextrose adenine solution*

CPDD calcium pyrophosphate deposition disease

焦磷酸钙沉积症

C Ped Certified Pedorthist 注册足科矫形师

CPHA Canadian Public Health Association 加拿大公共卫生协会

CPK creatine kinase 肌酸激酶

cpm counts per minute, an expression of the rate of particle emission from a radioactive material 次/分

CPP cerebral perfusion pressure 脑灌注压；chronic pelvic pain 慢性骨盆疼痛

CPPS chronic pelvic pain syndrome 慢性盆腔疼痛综合征

CPR cardiopulmonary resuscitation 心肺复苏

cps cycles per second; see hertz 周/秒；见 hertz

CR conditioned reflex (response) 条件反射

Cr chromium 元素铬的符号

crack (krak) an incomplete split, break, or fissure 裂口，裂缝

crack·le (krak′əl) rale 湿啰音

cra·dle (kra′dəl) a frame placed over the body of a bed patient for application of heat or cold or for protecting injured parts from contact with bed covers 支架

cramp (kramp) a painful spasmodic muscular contraction 痛性痉挛；**heat c.**, spasm with pain, weak pulse, and dilated pupils; seen in workers in intense heat 热痉挛；**recumbency c′s**, cramping in legs and feet occurring while resting or during light sleep 躺卧性痉挛；**writers' c.**, a muscle cramp in the hand caused by excessive use in writing 书写痉挛

cra·ni·ad (kra′ne-ad) in a cranial direction; toward the anterior (in animals) or superior (in humans) end of the body 向颅，向颅的方向

cra·ni·al (kra′ne-əl) 1. pertaining to the cranium 颅骨的；2. toward the head end of the body; a synonym of *superior* in humans and other bipeds 颅侧的

cra·ni·a·lis (kra″ne-a′lis) [L.] cranial 颅侧的

cra·nio·cele (kra′ne-o-sēl″) encephalocele 脑膨出

cra·nio·fa·cial (kra″ne-o-fa′shəl) pertaining to the cranium and the face 颅面的

cra·nio·fe·nes·tria (kra″ne-o-fə-nes′tre-ə) defective development of the fetal cranium, with areas in which no bone is formed 颅顶骨多孔（畸形）

cra·nio·la·cu·nia (kra″ne-o-lə-koo′ne-ə) defective development of the fetal cranium, with depressed areas on the inner surface 颅顶骨内面凹陷

cra·nio·ma·la·cia (kra″ne-o-mə-la′shə) abnormal softness of the bones of the skull 颅骨软化

cra·ni·om·e·try (kra″ne-om′ə-tre) the scientific measurement of the dimensions of the bones of the skull and face 颅测量法；**craniomet′ric** *adj.*

cra·ni·op·a·thy (kra″ne-op′ə-the) any disease of the skull 颅病；**metabolic c.**, a condition characterized by lesions of the calvaria with multiple metabolic changes, and by headache, obesity, and visual disorders 代谢性颅病

cra·nio·pha·ryn·gi·o·ma (kra″ne-o-fə-rin″jeo′mə) a tumor arising from cell rests derived from the infundibulum of the hypophysis or Rathke pouch. 颅咽管瘤

cra·nio·plas·ty (kra′ne-o-plas″te) any plastic operation on the skull 颅成形术

cra·nio·ra·chis·chi·sis (kra″ne-o-rə-kis′kĭ-sis) congenital fissure of the cranium and vertebral column 颅脊柱裂（畸形）

cra·ni·os·chi·sis (kra″ne-os′kĭ-sis) cranium bifidum 颅裂（畸形）

cra·nio·scle·ro·sis (kra″ne-o-sklə-ro′sis) thickening of the bones of the skull 颅骨硬化

cra·nio·ste·no·sis (kra″ne-o-stə-no′sis) deformity of the skull caused by craniosynostosis, with consequent cessation of skull growth 颅狭（窄）症

cra·nio·os·to·sis (kra″ne-os-to′sis) craniosynostosis（先天性）颅缝骨化

cra·nio·syn·os·to·sis (kra″ne-o-sin″os-to′sis) premature closure of the sutures of the skull 颅缝骨接合，颅缝早闭

cra·nio·ta·bes (kra″ne-o-ta′bēz) reduction in mineralization of the skull, with abnormal softness of the bone, usually affecting the occipital and parietal bones along the lambdoidal sutures 颅骨软化

cra·ni·ot·o·my (kra″ne-ot′ə-me) any operation on the cranium 颅骨切开术

cra·ni·um (kra′ne-əm) pl. *cra′nia* [L.] the skeleton of the head, variously construed as including all of the bones of the head except the mandible, or as the eight bones forming the vault lodging the brain 颅；**cra′nial** *adj.*; **c. bi′fidum**, a congenitally incomplete skull, often with an incomplete brain 颅裂（畸形）

cra·ter (kra′tər) an excavated area surrounded by an elevated margin 火山口，喷火口

cra·vat (krə-vaht′) a triangular bandage 三角巾绷带

CRE carbapenem-resistant Enterobacteriaceae 碳青霉烯耐药肠杆菌科细菌

cream (krēm) 1. the fatty part of milk from which butter is prepared, or a fluid mixture of similar consistency 乳膏，霜；2. in pharmaceutical preparations, a semisolid dosage form being either an emulsion of oil and water or an aqueous microcrystalline dispersion of a long-chain fatty acid or alcohol 制药中指水包油或油包水的半固体乳剂，常作局部应用

crease (krēs) a line or slight linear depression 褶

痕，皱褶；**flexion c.,** any of the normal permanent skin furrows on flexor surfaces that accommodate flexion of a movable joint by separating folds of tissue 掌褶，屈褶；**simian c.,** a single transverse palmar flexion crease formed by fusion of the usual proximal and distal creases 猿线

cre·a·tine (kre′ə-tin) an amino acid occurring in vertebrate tissues, particularly in muscle; phosphorylated creatine is an important storage form of high-energy phosphate 肌酸；**c. phosphate,** phosphocreatine 磷酸肌酸

cre·a·tine ki·nase (kre′ə-tin ki′nās) an enzyme that catalyzes the phosphorylation of creatine by ATP to form phosphocreatine. It occurs as three isozymes (specific to brain, cardiac muscle, and skeletal muscle, respectively), each having two components composed of M (muscle) and/or B (brain) subunits. Differential determination of isozymes is used in clinical diagnosis 肌酸激酶

cre·at·i·nine (kre-at′ĭ-nin) an anhydride of creatine, the end product of phosphocreatine metabolism; measurements of its rate of urinary excretion are used as diagnostic indicators of kidney function and muscle mass 肌酸酐

crem·as·ter·ic (krem″as-ter′ik) pertaining to the cremaster muscle 提睾肌的

cre·na (kre′nə) pl. *cre′nae* [L.] a notch or cleft 裂，裂隙

cre·nat·ed (kre′nāt-id) scalloped or notched 扇形的，切迹的，钝锯齿的，有小裂口的（叶缘）

cre·na·tion (kre-na′shən) 1. the formation of abnormal notching around the edge of an erythrocyte 红细胞皱缩；2. the notched appearance of an erythrocyte due to its shrinkage after suspension in a hypertonic solution 红细胞在高渗溶液中皱缩

cre·no·cyte (kre′no-sīt) burr cell 皱缩红细胞

cre·o·sote (kre′o-sōt) an oily liquid obtained from distillation from coal tar, wood tar, or the resin from the creosote bush 木馏油；**coal tar c.,** that obtained by high-temperature carbonization of bituminous coal; a brown to black, oily liquid, a mixture of aromatic hydrocarbons, tar acids, and tar bases; mainly used as a wood preservative. It is toxic by contact, ingestion, or inhalation, and coal tar is a carcinogen 煤焦杂酚油

crep·i·ta·tion (krep″ĭ-ta′shən) a dry sound like that of grating the ends of a fractured bone 捻发音；**crep′itant** *adj.*

crep·i·tus (krep′ĭ-təs) 1. the discharge of flatus from the bowels 肠排气；2. crepitation 呷轧音；3. crepitant rale 捻发音

cres·cent (kres′ənt) 1. shaped like a new moon 新月形的；2. something with this shape 新月形结构；

crescen′tic *adj.*; **Giannuzzi c′s,** crescent-shaped patches of serous cells surrounding the mucous tubercles in seromucous glands 新月腺细胞；**myopic c.,** a crescentic staphyloma in the fundus of the eye in myopia 眼后葡萄肿，近视性圆锥；**sublingual c.,** the crescent-shaped area on the floor of the mouth, bounded by the lingual wall of the mandible and the base of the tongue 舌下新月体

cre·sol (kre′sol) a toxic, corrosive liquid with disinfectant and antiseptic actions, obtained from coal tar as a mixture of three isomeric forms and containing not more than 5 percent phenol; used for sterilizing items 甲酚，煤酚

crest (krest) a projection, or projecting structure or ridge, especially one surmounting a bone or its border 嵴，突出物或突出结构；**ampullar c.,** the most prominent part of a localized thickening of the membrane lining the ampullae of the semicircular ducts 壶腹嵴；**frontal c.,** a median ridge on the internal surface of the frontal bone 额嵴；**iliac c.,** the thickened, expanded upper border of the ilium 髂嵴；**intertrochanteric c.,** a ridge on the posterior femur connecting the greater and lesser trochanters 前转子间嵴；**lacrimal c., anterior,** the lateral margin of the groove on the posterior border of the frontal process of the maxilla 泪前嵴；**lacrimal c., posterior,** a vertical ridge dividing the lateral or orbital surface of the lacrimal bone into two parts 泪后嵴；**nasal c.,** 1. (of maxilla) a ridge, raised along the medial border of the palatine process of the maxilla, with which the vomer articulates 上颌骨鼻嵴；2. (of palatine) a thick ridge projecting superiorly from the horizontal plate of the palatine bone and articulating with the posterior part of the vomer （腭骨的）嵴顶；**neural c.,** a cellular band dorsolateral to the embryonic neural tube; it gives origin to the spinal ganglia and other structures 腭骨鼻嵴；**occipital c., external,** a ridge sometimes extending on the external surface of the occipital bone from the external protuberance toward the foramen magnum 枕外嵴；**occipital c., internal,** a median ridge on the internal surface of the occipital bone, extending from the midpoint of the cruciform eminence toward the foramen magnum 枕内嵴；**pubic c.,** the thick, rough anterior border of the body of the pubic bone 耻骨嵴；**sacral c.,** any of various ridges or tubercles on the dorsal surface of the sacrum, named for their location as *median* or as *lateral* or *medial* (relative to the dorsal sacral foramina); used alone it usually denotes the median sacral crest 骶嵴；**sphenoidal c.,** a median ridge on the anterior surface of the body of the sphenoid bone, articulating with the ethmoid bone 蝶骨嵴；**supramastoid c.,** the superior border of the posterior root of the zygomatic process of the temporal bone. 乳突上嵴; **supraventricular c.**, a ridge on the inner wall of the right ventricle, marking off the conus arteriosus 室上嵴; **temporal c. of frontal bone**, a ridge extending superiorly and posteriorly from the zygomatic process of the frontal bone 额骨颞嵴; **turbinal c.**, 1. (of maxilla) an oblique ridge on the maxilla, articulating with the nasal conchae 上颌骨鼻甲嵴; 2. (of palatine bone) a horizontal ridge on the internal surface of the palatine bone 上颌骨筛骨嵴; **urethral c.**, a prominent longitudinal mucosal fold along the posterior wall of the female urethra, or a median elevation along the posterior wall of the male urethra between the prostatic sinuses 女性尿道嵴; **vestibular c.**, a ridge between the spherical and elliptical recesses of the vestibule, dividing posteriorly to bound the cochlear recess 前庭嵴

cre·tin·ism (kre′tin-iz-əm) arrested physical and mental development with dystrophy of bones and soft tissues, due to congenital lack of thyroid secretion 克汀病，呆小病; **athyrotic c.**, cretinism due to thyroid aplasia or destruction of the thyroid of the fetus in utero 甲状腺功能缺失克汀病; **endemic c.**, a form occurring in regions of severe endemic goiter, marked by deaf-mutism, spasticity, and motor dysfunction in addition to, or instead of, the usual manifestations of cretinism 地方性克汀病; **sporadic goitrous c.**, a genetic disorder in which enlargement of the thyroid gland is associated with deficient circulating thyroid hormone 散发性甲状腺克汀病

cre·tin·oid (kre′tin-oid) resembling or suggestive of cretinism 克汀病样的

crev·ice (krev′is) fissure 缝，纵裂; **gingival c.**, the space between the cervical enamel of a tooth and the overlying unattached gingiva 龈缝，龈下隙

cre·vic·u·lar (krə-vik′u-lər) pertaining to a crevice, especially the gingival crevice 缝的

CRH corticotropin-releasing hormone 促肾上腺皮质释放激素

crib·ra·tion (krib-ra′shən) 1. the quality of being cribriform 多孔性; 2. the process or act of sifting or passing through a sieve 过筛

crib·ri·form (krib′rĭ-form) perforated like a sieve 筛状的，多孔的

cri·coid (kri′koid) 1. ring-shaped 环状的; 2. the cricoid cartilage 环状软骨

cri·co·thy·rot·o·my (kri″ko-thi-rot′ə-me) incision through the skin and cricothyroid membrane to secure a patent airway for emergency relief of upper airway obstruction 环甲软骨切开术

cri·co·tra·che·ot·o·my (kri″ko-tra″ke-ot′ə-me) incision of the trachea through the cricoid cartilage 环状软骨气管切开术

cri du chat (kre doo shah′) [Fr.] 猫叫声，见 *syndrome* 下词条

crin·oph·a·gy (krin-of′ə-je) the intracytoplasmic digestion of the contents (peptides, proteins) of secretory vacuoles, after the vacuoles fuse with lysosomes 分泌自噬

cri·sis (kri′sis) pl. *cri′ses* [L.] 1. the turning point of a disease for better or worse; especially a sudden change, usually for the better, in the course of an acute disease 疾病好转的转折点; 2. a sudden paroxysmal intensification of symptoms in the course of a disease 危象; **addisonian c., adrenal c.**, fatigue, nausea, vomiting, and weight loss accompanying an acute attack of Addison disease 艾迪生病危象; **aplastic c.**, a sickle cell crisis in which there is a temporary stop in the formation of bone marrow 再生障碍性危象; **blast c.**, a sudden, severe change in the course of chronic myelogenous leukemia with an increase in the proportion of myeloblasts 原始细胞危象; **genital c. of newborn**, estrinization of the vaginal mucosa and hyperplasia of the breast, influenced by transplacentally acquired estrogens 新生儿生殖器危象; **hemolytic c.**, acute red cell destruction leading to jaundice, occasionally seen with sickle cell disease 溶血危象; **identity c.**, a period in the psychosocial development of an individual, usually occurring during adolescence, manifested by confusion over one′s self, values, or perceived role expected by society 同一性危机，个性转变期; **sickle cell c.**, a broad term for several acute conditions occurring with sickle cell disease, including hemolytic crisis and vasoocclusive crisis 镰状细胞危象; **thyroid c., thyrotoxic c.**, thyroid storm; a sudden and dangerous increase of symptoms of thyrotoxicosis 甲状腺中毒危象; **vasoocclusive c.**, a type of sickle cell crisis in which there is severe pain due to infarctions, which may be in the bones, joints, lungs, liver, spleen, kidney, eye, or central nervous system 血管闭塞危象

CRISPR clustered regularly interspaced short palindromic repeats 短回文重复序列

cris·ta (kris′tə) pl. *cris′tae* [L.] crest 嵴; **cris′tae cu′tis**, dermal ridges; ridges of the skin produced by the projecting papillae of the dermis on the palm of the hand or sole of the foot, producing a fingerprint or footprint characteristic of the individual 皮嵴; **c. gal′li**, a thick, triangular process projecting superiorly from the cribriform plate of the ethmoid bone 鸡冠; **mitochondrial cristae**, numerous narrow transverse infoldings of the inner membrane of a mitochondrion 线粒体嵴

crit·i·cal (krit′ĭ-kəl) 1. pertaining to or of the nature of a crisis 危象的；2. pertaining to a disease or other morbid condition in which there is danger of death 极期的；3. in sufficient quantity as to constitute a turning point, as a critical mass 临界的

cri·zo·ti·nib (krī-zō′tĭ-nib) a tyrosine kinase inhibitor used to treat non–small-cell lung cancer, specifically ALK-positive and ROS1-positive tumors 克唑替尼

CRL crown-rump length 顶臀长度

CRNA Certified Registered Nurse Anesthetist 注册麻醉护士

cRNA complementary RNA 互补 RNA

cro·cid·o·lite (krə-sid′ə-līt) an amphibole type of asbestos that causes asbestosis as well as mesotheliomas and other cancers（矿）青石棉

cro·mo·lyn (kro′mə-lin) an inhibitor of the release of histamine and other mediators of immediate hypersensitivity from mast cells; used as the sodium salt for prophylaxis and treatment of allergic rhinitis, bronchial asthma associated with allergy, and allergen-induced inflammation of the conjunctiva or cornea, and for treatment of mastocytosis 色甘酸

cross (kros) 1. any figure or structure in the shape of a cross 十字；2. the production of progeny containing genetic information from two or more parents 杂交；3. the progeny so derived 如此衍生的后代；**back c.,** backcross 使回交，逆代杂交；**test c.,** mating of an individual with the dominant phenotype for a gene or genes, but unknown genotype, to a tester homozygous recessive for the genes in question, in order to reveal the unknown genotype 测交

cross·bite (kros′bīt″) malocclusion in which the mandibular teeth are in buccal version (or complete lingual version in posterior segments) to the maxillary teeth 反颌，反咬合

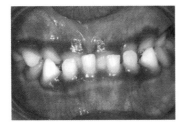

▲ 5 岁儿童的反咬合（**crossbite**）

cross·breed·ing (kros′brēd-ing) outbreeding 杂交育种

crossed (krost) shaped or arranged like a cross or the letter X 交叉的，十字的

cross·ing over (kros′ing o′vər) the reciprocal exchange of genetic material between homologous chromosomes, resulting in recombination; often specifically that between nonsister chromatids of paired homologous chromosomes during meiosis 交换

cross-link (kros′link″) a covalent bond formed between polymer chains, either within or across chains 交联，交叉结合

cross·match·ing (kros′mach″ing) determination of the compatibility of the blood of a donor and that of a recipient before transfusion by placing the donor's cells in the recipient's serum and the recipient's cells in the donor's serum; absence of agglutination, hemolysis, and cytotoxicity indicates compatibility 交叉配血

cross re·ac·tiv·i·ty (kros″re-ak-tiv′ĭ-te) the degree to which an antibody participates in cross reactions 交叉反应

cross-re·sis·tance (kros″re-zis′təns) multidrug resistance 交叉耐药性

cross-tol·er·ance (kros′tol″ər-əns) extension of the tolerance for a substance to others of the same class, even those to which the body has not been exposed previously 交叉耐受

cro·ta·lid (kro′tə-lid) 1. any snake of the family Crotalidae; a pit viper 响尾蛇；2. of or pertaining to the family Crotalidae 响尾蛇科的

Cro·tal·i·dae (kro-tal′ĭ-de) a family of venomous snakes, the pit vipers 响尾蛇科

cro·ta·line (kro′tə-lēn) crotalid 响尾蛇；响尾蛇科的

Cro·ta·lus (kro′tə-ləs) a genus of rattlesnakes 响尾蛇属

cro·ta·mi·ton (kro″tə-mi′ton) an acaricide used in the treatment of scabies and as an antipruritic 克罗米通，优乐散

cro·ton·ic ac·id (kro-ton′ik) an unsaturated fatty acid found in croton oil 巴豆酸

croup (kroop) acute partial obstruction of the upper airway, usually in young children and caused by a viral or bacterial infection, allergy, foreign body, or new growth; characteristics include barking cough, hoarseness, and stridor 哮吼；**croupous, croup′y** *adj.* **bacterial c.,** 细菌性哮吼；**membranous c.,** 膜性喉炎；**pseudomembranous c.,** bacterial tracheitis. 细菌性气管炎

crown (kroun) 1. the topmost part of an organ or structure, e.g., the top of the head 冠；2. artificial c.; **anatomic c.,** the upper, enamel-covered part of a tooth 解剖性冠；**artificial c.,** a reproduction of a crown affixed to the remaining natural structure of a tooth 人造冠；**clinical c.,** the portion of a tooth exposed beyond the gingiva 临床冠；**physiologic**

C

c., the portion of a tooth distal to the gingival crevice or to the gum margin 生理性冠

crown·ing (kroun′ing) the appearance of a large segment of the fetal scalp at the vaginal orifice in childbirth 儿头初露着冠

CRPS complex regional pain syndrome 复合性区域的疼痛综合征

cru·ci·ate (kroo′she-āt) cruciform 十字形

cru·ci·form (kroo′sĭ-form) cross-shaped 十字形的

cru·ra (kroo′rə) [L.] 小腿 *crus* 的复数形式

cru·ral (kroor′əl) pertaining to the lower limb or to a leglike structure (crus) 脚的，脚样结构的

cru·rot·o·my (kroo-rot′ə-me) the cutting of a crus of the stapes, usually the anterior one 镫脚切断术

crus (krus) pl. *cru′ra* [L.] 1. leg (1) 小腿; 2. a leglike part 脚; **c. ce′rebri,** a large bundle of nerve fiber tracts forming the part of the basis pedunculi anterior to the substantia nigra in the midbrain 大脑脚; **c. of clitoris,** the continuation of each corpus cavernosum of the clitoris, diverging posteriorly to be attached to the pubic arch 阴蒂脚; **crura of diaphragm,** two fibromuscular bands that arise from the lumbar vertebrae and insert into the central tendon of the respiratory diaphragm 膈肌脚; **c. of fornix,** either of two flattened bands of white substance that unite to form the body of the fornix 穹窿角; **c. of penis,** the continuation of each corpus cavernosum of the penis, diverging posteriorly to be attached to the pubic arch 阴蒂海绵体脚

crust (krust) a formed outer layer, especially of solid matter formed by drying of a bodily exudate or secretion 痂，壳; **milk c.,** crusta lactea 乳痂

crus·ta (krus′tah) pl. *crus′tae* [L.] a crust. 痂，壳; **c. lac′tea,** seborrhea of the scalp of nursing infants 乳痂

Crus·ta·cea (krəs-ta′she-ə) a class of arthropods including the lobsters, crabs, shrimps, wood lice, water fleas, and barnacles 甲壳纲

crutch (kruch) a staff, ordinarily extending from the armpit to the ground, with a support for the hand and usually also for the arm or axilla; used to support the body in walking 拐杖，腋杖

crux (kruks) pl. *cru′ces* [L.] cross 十字; **c. of heart,** the intersection of the walls separating the right and left sides and the atrial and ventricular heart chambers 心十字，房室交叉; **cru′ces pilo′rum,** crosslike patterns formed by hair growth, the hairs lying in opposite directions 毛十字

cry·al·ge·sia (kri′əl-je′ze-ə) pain on application of cold 冷痛觉

cry·an·es·the·sia (kri-an″es-the′zhə) loss of power of perceiving cold 冷觉缺失

cry·es·the·sia (kri″es-the′zhə) abnormal sensitiveness to cold 冷觉过敏

cryo·ab·la·tion (kri″o-ab-la′shən) the removal of tissue by destroying it with extreme cold 冷切除

cryo·an·al·ge·sia (kri″o-an″əl-je′ze-ə) the relief of pain by application of cold by cryoprobe to peripheral nerves 冷止痛

cryo·an·es·the·sia (kri″o-an″es-the′zhə) local anesthesia produced by chilling the part to near freezing temperature 冷冻麻醉

cryo·bank (kri′o-bank″) a facility for freezing and preserving semen at low temperatures (usually −196.5℃) for future use 精子冷藏室

cryo·bi·ol·o·gy (kri″o-bi-ol′ə-je) the science dealing with the effect of low temperatures on biologic systems 低温生物学

cryo·cau·tery (kri″o-kaw′tər-e) cauterization by freezing, using a substance such as carbon dioxide snow, or a very cold instrument 冻烙术，冷烙器

cryo·dam·age (cri″o-dam″əj) damage to tissues, cells, or other biologic substrates as a result of exposure to cold 冷冻损伤

cryo·ex·trac·tion (kri″o-ek-strak′shən) application of extremely low temperature for the removal of a cataractous lens 冷冻（内障）摘除术

cryo·ex·trac·tor (kri″o-ek-strak′tər) a cryoprobe used in cryoextraction 冷冻（内障）摘除器

cry·o·fi·brin·o·gen (kri″o-fi-brin′o-jən) an abnormal fibrinogen that precipitates at low temperatures and redissolves at 37℃ 冷沉（淀）纤维蛋白原

cryo·fi·brin·o·gen·emia (kri″o-fi-brin″o-jə-ne′me-ə) the presence of cryofibrinogen in the blood 冷沉淀纤维蛋白原

cry·o·gen·ic (kri″o-jen′ik) producing low temperatures 制冷的

cryo·glob·u·lin (kri″o-glob′u-lin) an abnormal globulin that precipitates at low temperatures and redissolves at 37℃ 冷球蛋白

cryo·glob·u·lin·emia (kri″o-glob″u-lĭ-ne′me-ə) the presence in the blood of cryoglobulin, which is precipitated in the microvasculature on exposure to cold 冷球蛋白血症

cryo·hy·po·phys·ec·to·my (kri″o-hi″po-fizek′tə-me) destruction of the pituitary gland by the application of cold 垂体冷凝破坏法

cry·op·a·thy (kri-op′ə-the) a morbid condition caused by cold 寒冷病

cryo·phil·ic (kri″o-fil′ik) psychrophilic 嗜冷的

cryo·pre·cip·i·tate (kri″o-pre-sip′ ĭ-tāt) any precipitate that results from cooling, sometimes specifically the one rich in coagulation factor Ⅷ obtained from cooling of blood plasma 冷沉淀物

cryo·pres·er·va·tion (kri″o-prez″ər-va′shən) maintenance of the viability of excised tissue or organs by storing at very low temperatures 低温储藏

cryo·probe (kri′o-prōb″) an instrument for applying extreme cold to tissue 冷冻探子

cryo·pro·tec·tion (kri″o-pro-tek′shən) protection, as of a tissue, cell, organism, or other substance, from cold-induced damage 冷冻防护，抗冻保护作用

cryo·pro·tec·tive (kri″o-pro-tek′tiv) capable of protecting against injury due to freezing, as glycerol protects frozen red blood cells 冷冻防护的

cryo·pro·tein (kri″o-pro′tēn) a blood protein that precipitates on cooling 冷沉蛋白

cry·os·co·py (kri-os′kə-pe) examination of fluids based on the principle that the freezing point of a solution varies according to the amount and nature of the solute 冰点下降法；**cryoscop′ic** *adj.*

cryo·stat (kri′o-stat″) 1. a device by which temperature can be maintained at a very low level 低温控制器；2. in pathology and histology, a chamber containing a microtome for sectioning frozen tissue 恒冷切片机

cryo·sur·gery (kri″o-sur′jər-e) the destruction of tissue by application of extreme cold 低温外科，冷冻破坏法

cryo·thal·a·mec·to·my (kri″o-thal′ə-mek′tə-me) destruction of a portion of the thalamus by application of extreme cold 丘脑冷冻切除术

cryo·ther·a·py (kri″o-ther′ə-pe) the therapeutic use of cold 冷冻疗法

crypt (kript) a blind pit or tube on a free surface 隐窝，小囊，**anal c's,** 肛门陷凹，肛窦，见 *sinus* 下词条；**bony c.,** the bony compartment surrounding a developing tooth 骨隐窝；**enamel c.,** a space bounded by dental ledges on either side and usually by the enamel organ, and filled with mesenchyma 釉囊；**c's of Fuchs, c's of iris,** pitlike depressions in the iris 肛膜隐窝；**c's of Lieberkühn,** intestinal glands 肠腺；**Luschka c's,** deep indentations of the gallbladder mucosa that penetrate into the muscular layer of the organ Luschka 隐窝；**c. of Morgagni, 1.** the lateral expansion of the urethra in the glans penis Morgagni 隐窝；**2.** 见 *anal sinuses*；**synovial c.,** a pouch in the synovial membrane of a joint 滑膜憩室；**c's of tongue,** deep, irregular invaginations from the surface of the lingual tonsil 舌滤泡隐凹；**tonsillar c's,** epithelium-lined clefts in the palatine, lingual, and pharyngeal tonsils 咽扁桃体隐窝

cryp·ta (krip′tə) pl. *cryp′tae* [L.] crypt 隐窝，小囊

cryp·tes·the·sia (krip″tes-the′zhə) subconscious perception of occurrences not ordinarily perceptible to the senses 潜在感觉

cryp·ti·tis (krip-ti′tis) inflammation of a crypt, especially the anal crypts 隐窝炎

crypt(o)- word element [Gr.], *concealed*; *crypt* 隐藏的，潜在的，隐窝

cryp·to·coc·co·sis (krip″to-kŏ-ko′sis) infection by *Cryptococcus,* usually *C. neoformans* or *C. gattii,* having a predilection for the brain and meninges but also invading the skin, lungs, and other organs 隐球菌病

Cryp·to·coc·cus (krip″to-kok′əs) a genus of yeast-like fungi, including *C. neofor′mans* and *C. gattii,* which cause cryptococcosis 隐球菌属；**cryptococ′cal** *adj.*

cryp·to·de·ter·min·ant (krip″to-de-tur′mĭnənt) hidden determinant 隐蔽决定簇，隐定子

cryp·to·gen·ic (krip″to-jen′ik) of obscure or doubtful origin 隐源性的，原因不明的

cryp·to·lith (krip′to-lith) a concretion in a crypt 隐窝结石

cryp·to·men·or·rhea (krip″to-men″o-re′ə) the occurrence of menstrual symptoms without external bleeding, as in imperforate hymen 隐经

cryp·toph·thal·mos (krip″tof-thal′mos) congenital absence of the palpebral fissure, the skin extending from the forehead to the cheek, with the eye malformed or rudimentary 隐眼（畸形）。又称 *cryptophthalmia, cryptophthalmus*

cryp·to·py·ic (krip″to-pi′ik) characterized by concealed suppuration 隐脓的

crypt·or·chid·ism (krip-tor′kĭ-diz″əm) failure of one or both testes to descend into the scrotum 隐睾病；**cryptor′chid** *adj.*

cryp·tor·chi·do·pexy (krip-tor″kĭ-do-pek′se) orchiopexy 隐睾固定术

cryp·to·spo·rid·i·o·sis (krip″to-spo-rid″eo′sis) infection with protozoa of the genus *Cryptosporidium*; in the immunocompetent it is a rare self-limited diarrhea syndrome, but in the immunocompromised it is a severe syndrome of prolonged diarrhea, weight loss, fever, and abdominal pain, sometimes spreading to the trachea and bronchial tree 隐孢子虫病

Cryp·to·spo·ri·di·um (krip″to-spo-rid′e-əm) a genus of parasitic protozoa found in the intestinal tracts of many different vertebrates and the etiologic agent of cryptosporidiosis in humans 隐孢子虫属

crys·tal (kris′təl) a homogeneous angular solid of definite form, with systematically arranged elemental units 晶体，结晶，**blood c's,** hematoidin crystals in the blood 血晶；**Charcot-Leyden c's,** elongated, diamond-shaped, birefringent crystals derived from disintegrating eosinophils, seen in the sputum in asthma, in the stool in some cases of intestinal parasitism, and in tissues infiltrated by eosinophils 夏科 - 莱登结晶

crys·tal·line (kris′tə-lēn) 1. pertaining to crystals 结晶的，晶状的，透明的；2. resembling a crystal in nature or clearness 结晶体的

crys·tal·lu·ria (kris″tal-u′re-ə) excretion of crystals in the urine, causing renal irritation 结晶尿症

CS cesarean section 剖宫产术；conditioned stimulus 条件刺激；coronary sinus 冠状窦

Cs cesium 元素铯的符号

CSAA Child Study Association of America 美国儿童研究协会

CSF cerebrospinal fluid 脑脊液

CSFP coronary slow flow phenomenon 冠状动脉慢血流现象

CSGBI Cardiac Society of Great Britain and Ireland 大不列颠及爱尔兰心脏学会

CSM cerebrospinal meningitis 脑脊膜炎

CSMLS Canadian Society of Medical Laboratory Science 加拿大医学实验科学学会

C-spine cervical spine 颈椎

CT computed tomography 计算机断层扫描

CTE chronic traumatic encephalopathy 慢性创伤性脑病

Cte·no·ce·phal·i·des (te″no-sə-fal′ĭ-dēz) a genus of fleas, including *C. ca′nis*, frequently found on dogs, which may transmit the dog tapeworm to humans, and *C. fe′lis*, commonly parasitic on cats 栉头蚤属

C-ter·mi·nal (tur′mĭ-nəl) the end of the peptide chain carrying the free alpha carboxyl group of the last amino acid, conventionally written to the rightC- 末端，羧基末端

CTHD conotruncal heart defect 圆锥动脉干发育畸形

CTIBL cancer treatment–induced bone loss 癌症治疗引起的骨质流失；castration treatment–induced bone loss 去势治疗引起的骨质流失

CTL cytotoxic T lymphocytes 细胞毒性 T 淋巴细胞

CTP cytidine triphosphate 胞苷三磷酸

Cu copper (L. *cu′prum*) 元素铜的符号

cu·bi·tus (ku′bĭ-təs) elbow 肘，肘关节；前臂；尺 骨；**cu′bital** *adj.*；c. val′gus, deformity of the elbow in which the forearm deviates away from the midline of the body when extended 肘外翻；c. va′rus, deformity of the elbow in which the forearm deviates toward the midline of the body when extended 肘内翻

cu·boid (ku′boid) 1. resembling a cube 骰状的；2. cuboid bone 骰骨

cu·boi·dal (ku-boi′dəl) resembling a cube 骰状的

cuff (kuf) a small, bandlike structure encircling a part or object 套；**musculotendinous c.**, one formed by intermingled muscle and tendon fibers

肌 腱 套；**rotator c.**, a musculotendinous structure encircling and giving strength to the glenohumeral joint 肩袖

cuff·ing (kuf′ing) formation of a cufflike surrounding border, as of leukocytes about a blood vessel, observed in some infections and in multiple sclerosis 成套

cul-de-sac (kul″də-sak′) [Fr.] a blind pouch 盲管，陷凹；**Douglas c.-de-s.**, rectouterine pouch 直肠子宫陷凹 **cul·do·cen·te·sis** (kul″do-sen-te′sis) transvaginal puncture of the Douglas cul-de-sac for aspiration of fluid 后穹隆穿刺术

cul·dos·co·py (kəl-dos′kə-pe) visual examination of the female viscera through an endoscope introduced into the pelvic cavity through the posterior vaginal fornix 后陷凹镜检查

Cu·lex (ku′ləks) a genus of mosquitoes found throughout the world, many species of which are vectors of disease-producing organisms 库蚊属

cu·li·cide (ku′lĭ-sīd) an agent that destroys mosquitoes 杀蚊剂

cu·lic·i·fuge (ku-lis′ ĭ-fūj) an agent that repels mosquitoes 驱蚊剂

cu·li·cine (ku′lĭ-sin) (ku′lĭ-sīn) 1. a member of the genus *Culex* or related genera 库蚊；2. pertaining to, involving, or affecting mosquitoes of the genus *Culex* or related species 库蚊属的

cul·men (kul′mən) pl. *cul′mina* [L.] the portion of the vermis of the anterior lobe of the cerebellum between the central lobule and the primary fissure 小脑山顶

cul·ti·va·tion (kul″tĭ-va′shən) the propagation of living organisms, especially the growing of cells in artificial media 培养

cul·ture (kul′chər) 1. the propagation of microorganisms or of living tissue cells in media conducive to their growth 培养 法；2. to induce such propagation 培养物；3. the product of such propagation 培 养；**cul′tural** *adj.*；**cell c.**, 1. the maintenance or growth of animal cells in vitro 动物细胞在体外的维持或生长；2. a culture of such cells 细胞培养；**continuous flow c.**, the cultivation of bacteria in a continuous flow of fresh medium to maintain bacterial growth in logarithmic phase 连续流动培养；**hanging-drop c.**, a culture in which the material to be cultivated is inoculated into a drop of fluid attached to a coverglass inverted over a hollow slide 悬滴培养；**plate c.**, a culture grown on a medium, usually agar or gelatin, on a Petri dish 平板培养；**primary c.**, a cell or tissue culture started from material taken directly from an organism, as opposed to that from an explant from an organism 初 代 培 养，原代培养；**pure c.**, a culture of a single cell species, without presence of any contaminants 纯培养（物）；**slant c.,** a culture made on the surface of solidified medium in a tube that has been tilted to provide a greater surface area for growth 斜面培养；**stab c.,** a culture in which the medium is inoculated by thrusting a needle deep into its substance 针刺培养；**streak c.,** a culture in which the medium is inoculated by drawing an infected wire across it 画线培养；**suspension c.,** a culture in which cells multiply while suspended in a suitable medium 悬浮培养；**tissue c.,** maintenance or growth of tissue, organ primordia, or the whole or part of an organ in vitro so as to preserve its architecture and function 组织培养；**type c.,** a culture of a species of microorganism usually maintained in a central collection of type or standard cultures 模式培养

cul·ture me·di·um (kul′chər me′de-əm) any substance used to cultivate living cells 培养基，培养液

cu·mu·la·tive (ku′mu-lə-tiv) increasing by successive additions, the total being greater than the expected sum of its parts 累积的，积蓄的

cu·mu·lus (ku′mu-ləs) pl. *cu′muli* [L.] a small elevation 丘；**c. oo′phorus,** a mass of follicular cells surrounding the oocyte in the vesicular ovarian follicle 卵丘

cu·ne·ate (ku′ne-āt) cuneiform 楔状的

cu·ne·i·form (ku-ne′ĭ-form) wedge-shaped 楔状的

cu·ne·us (ku′ne-əs) pl. *cu′nei* [L.] a wedgeshaped lobule on the medial aspect of the occipital lobe of the cerebrum 楔叶

cu·nic·u·lus (ku-nik′u-ləs) pl. *cuni′culi* [L.] 1. a tunnel 隧道；2. a burrow in the skin made by the itch mite 疥隧

cun·ni·lin·gus (kun′ĭ-ling′əs) oral stimulation of the female genitalia 舔阴

Cun·ning·ha·mel·la (kun″ing-ham-el′ə) a genus of fungi of the order Mucorales, characterized by a lack of a sporangium and by conidia that arise from a vesicle. *C. bertholle′tiae* causes opportunistic mucormycosis of the lung in immunocompromised or debilitated patients 毛霉菌

cup (kup) a depression or hollow 杯状部分，杯状结构；**glaucomatous c.,** a form of optic disk depression peculiar to glaucoma 青光眼杯；**optic c.,** 1. a depression in the center of the optic disk 视盘中央的凹陷；2. an indentation of the distal wall of the optic vesicle, brought about by rapid marginal growth and producing a double-layered cup 视杯，眼小泡的远端壁的凹陷，由边缘的快速生长和产生双层杯状物引起；**physiologic c.,** optic c. (1) 生理凹

cu·po·la (koo′pə-lə) cupula 顶

cup·ping (kup′ing) 1. the application of a small glass or bamboo cup to the skin, after exhausting the air from within it to create a vacuum, in order to draw blood and lymph to the surface of the body and increase local circulation 杯吸法，拔火罐，拔罐法；2. the formation of a cup-shaped depression 杯状陷凹形成

cu·pric (koo′prik) containing copper in its divalent form (=Cu), and yielding divalent ions (Cu^{2+}) in aqueous solution 二价铜的；**c. sulfate,** a crystalline salt of copper used as an emetic, astringent, and fungicide, as an oral antidote to phosphorus poisoning and a topical treatment of cutaneous phosphorus burns, and as a catalyst in iron deficiency anemia 硫酸铜

cu·pro·phane (koo′pro-fān) a membrane made of regenerated cellulose, commonly used in hemodialyzers 铜纺，再生纤维素制成的膜，是血透析中最常用的膜

cu·prous (koo′prəs) pertaining to or containing monovalent copper 亚铜的

cu·pru·re·sis (koo″proo-re′sis) hypercupriuria 尿铜排泄

cu·pu·la (koo″pu-lə) pl. *cu′pulae* [L.] a small, inverted cup or dome-shaped cap over a structure 壶腹帽；**cu′pular** *adj.*

cu·pu·li·form (koo′pu-lĭ-form″) shaped like a small cup 圆顶状的

cu·pu·lo·li·thi·a·sis (ku″pu-lo-lĭ-thi′ə-sis) the presence of calculi in the cupula of the posterior semicircular duct 嵴帽沉石病

cu·ran·de·ra (koo-rahn-da′rah) [Sp.] healer; a woman who practices curanderismo 治愈者

cu·ran·de·ris·mo (koo-ron″da-rēz′mo) a traditional Mexican-American healing system combining various theoretical elements into a holistic approach to illness and believing that disease may have not only natural but also spiritual causes 一种传统的墨西哥裔美国人的治疗系统，将各种理论因素结合成一个整体的方法来治疗疾病，并相信疾病可能不仅有自然的，而且有精神上的原因

cu·ran·de·ro (koo-rahn-da′ro) [Sp.] healer; a man who practices curanderismo 治愈者

cu·ra·re (koo-rah′re) any of a wide variety of highly toxic extracts from various botanical sources, used originally as arrow poisons in South America. An extract of the shrub *Chondodendron tomentosum* has been used as a skeletal muscle relaxant 箭毒

cu·ra·ri·mi·met·ic (koo-rah″re-mi-met′ik) producing effects similar to those of curare 箭毒样作用的

cu·rar·iza·tion (koo″rah-rī-za′shən) adminis-

C

tration of curare (usually tubocurarine) to induce muscle relaxation by its blocking activity at the myoneural junction 箭毒化

cur·a·tive (kūr′ə-tiv) tending to overcome disease and promote recovery 治疗的

cure (kūr) 1. the treatment of any disease, or of a special case 治愈；2. the successful treatment of a disease or wound 疾病和伤口的治愈；3. a system of treating diseases 疗法；4. a medicine effective in treating a disease（有治愈疗效的）药

cu·ret (ku-ret′) 1. a spoon-shaped instrument for cleansing a diseased surface 刮匙；2. to use a curet 刮除术

cu·ret·tage (ku″rə-tahzh′) [Fr.] the cleansing of a diseased surface, as with a curet 刮除术，**medical c.**, induction of bleeding from the endometrium by administration and withdrawal of a progestational agent 内科刮子宫法；**periapical c.**, removal with a curet of diseased periapical tissue without excision of the root tip 牙根周刮除法；**suction c., vacuum c.**, removal of tissue or the entire contents of the uterus by means of suction through a hollow curet; done for diagnosis or to induce abortion（子宫）吸刮术

cu·rette·ment (ku-ret′ment) curettage 刮除术；**physiologic c.**, enzymatic débridement 酶清创术

cu·rie (Ci) (ku′re) a unit of radioactivity, defined as the quantity of any radioactive nuclide in which the number of disintegrations per second is 3.7 × 10^{10} 居里（符号 Ci）

cu·rie-hour (kūr′e our′) a unit of dose equivalent to that obtained by exposure for 1 hour to radioactive material disintegrating at the rate of 3.7 × 10^{10} atoms per second 居里小时

cu·ri·um (Cm) (kūr′e-əm) a synthetic, hard, dense, silvery, heavy metal transuranium element; at. no. 96, at. wt. 247 锔（元素符号 Cm）

cur·rent (kur′ənt) 1. anything that flows 流；2. electric c 电流；**action c.**, the current generated in the cell membrane of a nerve or muscle by the action potential 动作电流；**alternating c.**, a current that periodically flows in opposite directions 交流电；**convection c.**, a current caused by movement by convection of warmer fluid into an area of cooler fluid 对流；**direct c.**, a current flowing in one direction only 直流电；**electric c.** (*I*), the stream of electricity that moves along a conductor 电流；**galvanic c.**, a steady direct current, especially one produced chemically 动电电流，化电流；**c. of injury**, a flow of current to (*systolic c. of injury*) or from (*diastolic c. of injury*) the injured region of an ischemic heart, due to regional alteration in transmembrane potential 损伤电流；**pacemaker c.**, the small net positive current flowing into certain cardiac cells, such as those of the sinoatrial node, causing them to depolarize 起搏器电流

cur·va·tu·ra (kur″və-tu′rə) pl. *curvatu′rae* [L.] curvature 弯，曲

cur·va·ture (kur′və-chər″) deviation from a rectilinear direction 弯，曲；**greater c. of stomach**, the left or lateral and inferior border of the stomach, marking the inferior junction of the anterior and posterior surfaces 胃大弯；**lesser c. of stomach**, the right or medial border of the stomach, marking the superior junction of the anterior and posterior surfaces 胃小弯；**Pott c.**, abnormal posterior curvature of the spine due to tuberculous caries 波特弯曲；**spinal c.**, 1. any of the normal curvatures that occur in the cervical, thoracic, pelvic, and lumbar regions of the vertebral column 脊柱的正常弯曲；2. abnormal deviation of the vertebral column 脊柱弯曲

curve (kurv) a line that is not straight, or that describes part of a circle, especially representing varying values in a graph 曲线，曲面；**Barnes c.**, the segment of a circle whose center is the sacral promontory, its concavity being directed posteriorly 巴恩斯曲线；**c. of Carus**, the normal axis of the pelvic outlet 卡鲁斯曲线；**dental c.**, c. of occlusion 牙列曲线；**dye dilution c.**, an indicator dilution curve in which the indicator is a dye, usually indocyanine green 燃料稀释曲线；**growth c.**, the curve obtained by plotting the increase in size or numbers against the elapsed time 生长曲线；**indicator dilution c.**, a graphic representation of the concentration of an indicator added in known quantity to the circulatory system and measured over time; used in studies of cardiovascular function 指示剂稀释曲线；**isodose c's**, lines delimiting body areas receiving the same quantity of radiation in radiotherapy 等量曲线；**c. of occlusion**, the curve of a dentition on which the occlusal surfaces lie 咬合曲线；**oxygen-hemoglobin dissociation c.**, a graphic curve representing the normal variation in the amount of oxygen that combines with hemoglobin as a function of the tension of oxygen and carbon dioxide 氧离曲线；**Price-Jones c.**, a graphic curve representing the variation in the size of the red blood corpuscles 普-琼二氏曲线；**Starling c.**, a graphic representation of cardiac output or other measure of ventricular performance as a function of ventricular filling for a given level of contractility 斯达林曲线；**strength-duration c.**, a graphic representation of the relationship between the intensity of an electric stimulus at the motor point of a muscle and the length of time it must flow to elicit a minimal contraction 力量-耐力曲线；**temperature**

C

c., a graphic tracing showing the variations in body temperature 温度曲线; **tension c's,** lines observed in cancellous tissue of bones, determined by the exertion of stress during development 张力曲线; **ventricular function c.,** Starling c. 心室功能曲线

Cur·vu·la·ria (kur″vu-lar′e-ə) a genus of imperfect fungi commonly found in soil and elsewhere; *C. luna'ta* is found in human mycetomas 曲腔菌

cush·ion (koosh′ən) a soft or padlike part 垫; **anal c's,** discrete masses of subepithelial tissue in the left lateral, right posterior, and right anterior quadrants of the anal canal, consisting of venous plexus, smooth muscle fibers, and elastic and connective tissue; they seal the anal canal and maintain continence 肛垫; **endocardial c's,** elevations on the atrioventricular canal of the embryonic heart that later help form the interatrial septum 心内膜垫; **intimal c's,** longitudinal thickenings of the intima of certain arteries, e.g., the penile arteries; they serve functionally as valves, controlling blood flow by occluding the lumen of the artery 内膜垫

cusp (kusp) a pointed or rounded projection, as on the crown of a tooth, or one of the triangular segments of a cardiac valve 尖; **semilunar c.,** any of the semilunar segments of the aortic valve (having posterior, right, and left leaflets) or the pulmonary valve (having anterior, right, and left leaflets) 半月性尖

cus·pid (kus′pid) 1. having one cusp or point 尖（端）的; 2. cuspid tooth 尖牙

cus·pis (kus′pis) pl. *cus′pides* [L.] a cusp 尖

cu·ta·ne·ous (ku-ta′ne-əs) pertaining to the skin 皮的，属于皮的

cut·down (kut′doun) creation of a small incised opening, especially over a vein (*venous c.*), to facilitate venipuncture and permit passage of a needle or cannula for withdrawal of blood or administration of fluids 静脉造口术

cu·ti·cle (ku′tĭ-kəl) 1. a layer of more or less solid substance covering the free surface of an epithelial cell 表皮，护膜; 2. eponychium (1) 甲上皮; 3. a horny secreted layer 角质层; **dental c.,** a film on the enamel and cement of some teeth, external to the primary cuticle, with which it combines, deposited by the epithelial attachment as it migrates along the tooth 牙小皮; **enamel c., primary c.,** a film on the enamel of unerupted teeth, consisting primarily of degenerating ameloblast remnants after completion of enamel formation 釉小皮，原发性护膜; **secondary c.,** dental c. 继发性釉护膜

cu·tic·u·la (ku-tik′u-lə) pl. *cuti′culae* [L.] cuticle 表皮，护膜

cu·ti·re·ac·tion (ku″tĭ-re-ak′shən) an inflamma-tory or irritative reaction on the skin, occurring in certain infectious diseases, or on application or injection of a preparation of the organism causing the disease 皮肤反应

cu·tis (ku′tis) skin 皮肤; **c. anseri′na,** transitory elevation of the hair follicles due to contraction of the arrectores pilorum muscles; a reflection of sympathetic nerve discharge 鸡皮; **c. hyperelas′tica,** Ehlers-Danlos syndrome 皮肤弹力过度症; **c. lax′a,** a group of disorders of the elastic fiber network, usually hereditary, in which the skin hangs in loose pendulous folds 皮肤松垂; **c. marmora′ta,** transient livedo reticularis occurring as a normal response to cold 大理石样皮; **c. rhomboida′lis nu′chae,** thickening of the skin of the neck with accentuation of its markings, giving an appearance of diamondshaped plaques 颈部菱形皮; **c. ver′ticis gyra′ta,** enlargement and thickening of the skin of the scalp, forming folds and furrows 头皮松垂，回状头皮

cu·vette (ku-vet′) [Fr.] a glass container generally having well-defined characteristics (dimensions, optical properties), to contain solutions or suspensions for study 小杯

CV cardiovascular 心血管的

CVID common variable immunodeficiency 常见变异型免疫缺陷病

CVP central venous pressure 中心静脉压

CVS cardiovascular system 心血管系统; chorionic villus sampling 绒毛活检术

cy·an·he·mo·glo·bin (si″an-he′mo-glo″bin) a compound formed by action of hydrocyanic acid on hemoglobin 氰血红蛋白

cy·a·nide (si′ə-nīd) 1. a compound containing the cyanide group (−CN) or ion (CN−) 氰化物; 2. hydrogen cyanide 氰化化合物

cy·an·met·he·mo·glo·bin (si″an-met-he′mo-glo″bin) a tightly bound complex of methemoglobin with the cyanide ion; the pigment most widely used in hemoglobinometry 氰化正铁血红蛋白

cy·an·met·myo·glo·bin (si″an-met-mi′oglo″bin) a compound formed from myoglobin by addition of the cyanide ion to yield reduction to the ferrous state 氰化正铁肌红蛋白

Cy·a·no·bac·te·ria (si″ə-no-bak-tēr′e-ə) a phylum of bacteria comprising the blue-green bacteria (formerly called blue-green algae), which are photosynthetic and also fix nitrogen 蓝细菌

cy·a·no·co·bal·a·min (si″ə-no″ko-bal′ə-min) a cobalamin in which the substituent is a cyanide ion; it is the form of vitamin B_{12} first isolated and, although an artifact, is used to denote the vitamin; preparations are used to treat vitaminassociated deficiencies, particularly pernicious anemia and other megaloblastic anemias 氰钴铵

cy·a·no·phil (si-an′o-fil) 1. stainable with blue dyes 嗜蓝的; 2. a cell or other histologic element readily stainable with blue dyes 嗜蓝细胞; **cyanoph′ilous** *adj.*

cy·a·nop·sia (si″ə-nop′se-ə) defect of vision in which objects appear tinged with blue 蓝视症

cy·a·no·sis (si″ə-no′sis) a bluish discoloration of skin and mucous membranes due to excessive concentration of reduced hemoglobin in the blood 发绀; **cyanosed, cyanot′ic** *adj.*; **central c.**, that due to arterial unsaturation, the aortic blood carrying reduced hemoglobin 中央性发绀; **enterogenous c.**, a syndrome due to absorption of nitrites and sulfides from the intestine, marked primarily by methemoglobinemia and/or sulfhemoglobinemia with cyanosis, as well as severe enteritis, constipation or diarrhea, headache, dyspnea, dizziness, syncope, and anemia 肠源性发绀; **peripheral c.**, that due to an excessive amount of reduced hemoglobin in the venous blood as a result of extensive oxygen extraction at the capillary level 外因性发绀; **pulmonary c.**, central cyanosis due to poor oxygenation of the blood in the lungs 肺性发绀; **c. re′tinae,** cyanosis of the retina, observable in certain congenital cardiac defects 视网膜发绀; **shunt c.,** central cyanosis due to the mixing of unoxygenated blood with arterial blood in the heart or great vessels 短路性发绀

cy·ber·net·ics (si″bər-net′iks) the science of the processes of communication and control in the animal and in the machine 控制论

cy·cla·mate (si′klə-māt) any salt of cyclamic acid; the sodium and calcium salts have been widely used as non-nutritive sugar substitutes 环己烷氨基磺酸盐

cyc·lar·thro·sis (sik″lahr-thro′sis) a pivot joint 车轴关节

cy·clase (si′klās) an enzyme that catalyzes the formation of a cyclic phosphodiester 环化酶

cy·cle (si′kəl) a succession or recurring series of events 周期, 循环; **carbon c.**, the steps by which carbon (in the form of carbon dioxide) is extracted from the atmosphere by living organisms and ultimately returned to the atmosphere. It comprises a series of interconversions of carbon compounds beginning with the production of carbohydrates by plants during photosynthesis, proceeding through animal consumption, and ending and beginning again in the decomposition of the animal or plant or in the exhalation of carbon dioxide by animals 碳循环; **cardiac c.**, a complete cardiac movement, or heart

beat, including systole, diastole, and intervening pause 心动周期; **cell c.**, the cycle of biochemical and morphologic events occurring in a reproducing cell population; it consists of the *S phase*, occurring toward the end of interphase, in which DNA is synthesized; the *G2 phase*, a relatively quiescent period; the M phase, consisting of the four phases of mitosis; and the *G1 phase* of interphase, which lasts until the *S phase* of the next cycle 细胞周期; **citric acid c.**, tricarboxylic acid c. 柠檬酸循环; **Cori c.**, the mechanism by which lactate produced by muscles is carried to the liver, converted back to glucose via gluconeogenesis, and returned to the muscles Cori 循环; **γ-glutamyl c.**, a metabolic cycle for transporting amino acids into cells γ谷氨酰胺循环; **hair c.**, the phases of the life of a hair, consisting of anagen, catagen, and telogen 头发生长的各个阶段, 包括生长期、生长期和休止期; **Krebs c.**, tricarboxylic acid c.; **Krebs-Henseleit c.**, urea c.; **menstrual c.**, the regular cycle of physiologic changes in the endometrium during the reproductive years; by convention, the menstrual cycle begins with the first day of menstruation. If pregnancy occurs, the menstrual cycles cease; otherwise, partial shedding of the endometrium with bleeding from the vagina (menstruation) occurs 月经周期; **mosquito c.**, that period in the life of a malarial parasite that is spent in the body of the mosquito host 蚊体内生环; **nitrogen c.**, the steps by which nitrogen is extracted from the nitrates of soil and water, incorporated as amino acids and proteins in living organisms, and ultimately reconverted to nitrates: (1) conversion of nitrogen to nitrates by bacteria; (2) the extraction of the nitrates by plants and the building of amino acids and proteins by adding an amino group to the carbon compounds produced in photosynthesis; (3) the ingestion of plants by animals; and (4) the return of nitrogen to the soil in animal excretions or on the death and decomposition of plants and animals 氮循环; **ornithine c.**, urea c. 鸟氨酸循环; **ovarian c.**, the sequence of physiologic changes in the ovary involved in ovulation 卵巢周期; **reproductive c.**, the cycle of physiologic changes in the female reproductive organs, from the time of fertilization of the oocyte through gestation and parturition. 生殖周期; **sex c., sexual c.**, 1. the physiologic changes recurring regularly in the genital organs of nonpregnant female mammals; in humans, the menstrual cycle 性周期; 2. the period of sexual reproduction in an organism that also reproduces asexually 生殖周期; **tricarboxylic acid c.**, the final common pathway for the oxidation to CO_2 of fuel molecules, most of which enter as acetyl coenzyme A; it also provides intermediates for biosynthetic reactions and generates ATP by providing electrons to the electron transport chain 三羧酸循环; **urea c.**, a series of metabolic reactions in the liver, by which ammonia is converted to urea using cyclically regenerated ornithine as a carrier 尿素循环; **uterine c.**, the phenomena occurring in the endometrium during the menstrual cycle, preparing it for implantation of the blastocyst 子宫周期; **visual c.**, the cyclic interconversion of 11-cis-retinal and all-*trans*-retinal and association with opsins, creating an electric potential and initiating the cascade generating a sensory nerve impulse in vision 视循环

cyc·lec·to·my (sik-lek′tə-me) 1. excision of a piece of the ciliary body 睫状体切除术; 2. excision of a portion of the ciliary border of the eyelid 睑缘切除术

cyc·lic (sik′lik) (si′klik) pertaining to or occurring in a cycle or cycles; applied to chemical compounds containing a ring of atoms in the nucleus 周期的，循环的，环的

cyc·li·tis (sik-li′tis) inflammation of the ciliary body 睫状体炎

cycl(o)- word element [Gr.], *round; recurring; ciliary body of the eye* 圆形；睫状体

cy·clo·ben·za·prine (si″klo-ben′zə-prēn) a skeletal muscle relaxant, used as the hydrochloride salt 胺苯环庚烯

cy·clo·cho·roid·itis (si″klo-kor″oid-i′tis) inflammation of ciliary body and choroid 睫状体脉络膜炎

cy·clo·cryo·ther·a·py (si″klo-kri″o-ther′ə-pe) freezing of the ciliary body; done in the treatment of glaucoma 睫状体冷冻疗法

cy·clo·di·al·y·sis (si″klo-di-al′ə-sis) surgical creation of a communication between the anterior chamber of the eye and the perichoroidal space, in glaucoma 睫状体分离术

cy·clo·di·a·ther·my (si″klo-di′ə-thur″me) destruction of a portion of the ciliary body by diathermy 睫状体透热凝固术

cy·cloid (si′kloid) characterized by alternating moods of elation and depression 循环性人格的，循环情感性的

cy·clo·ker·a·ti·tis (si″klo-ker″ə-ti′tis) inflammation of cornea and ciliary body 睫状体角膜炎

cy·clo·oxy·gen·ase (si″klo-ok′sə-jən-ās) a component of prostaglandin synthase (q.v.) 环氧合酶

cy·clo·pho·ria (si″klo-for′e-ə) heterophoria in which there is deviation of the eye from the anteroposterior axis in the absence of visual fusional stimuli 旋转隐斜; **minus c.**, incyclophoria 内旋转隐斜视; **plus c.**, excyclophoria 外旋转隐斜视

cy·clo·phos·pha·mide (si″klo-fos′fə-mīd) a cytotoxic alkylating agent of the nitrogen mustard group; used as an antineoplastic, as an immunosuppressant to prevent transplant rejection, and to treat some diseases characterized by abnormal immune function 环磷酰胺

cy·clo·pia (si-klo′pe-ə) a developmental anomaly marked by a single orbital fossa, with the globe absent, rudimentary, apparently normal, or duplicated, or the nose absent or present as a tubular appendix above the orbit 独眼

cy·clo·ple·gia (si″klo-ple′je-ə) paralysis of the ciliary muscles so as to prevent accommodation of the eye; called also *paralysis of accommodation* 睫状肌麻痹，又称调节麻痹

cy·clo·ple·gic (si″klo-ple′jik) pertaining to, characterized by, or causing cycloplegia; or an agent that so acts 睫状肌麻痹的，睫状肌麻痹剂

cy·clo·pro·pane (si″klo-pro′pān) a colorless, highly flammable and explosive gas, C_3H_6, used as an inhalation anesthetic 环丙烷

cy·clops (si′klops) a fetus exhibiting cyclopia 并眼症

cy·clo·ro·ta·tion (si″klo-ro-ta′shən) torsion (3) 扭转; **cycloro′tary** adj.

cy·clo·ser·ine (si″klo-ser′ēn) an antibiotic produced by *Streptomyces orchidaceus* or obtained synthetically; used as a tuberculostatic and in treatment of urinary tract infections 环丝氨酸

cy·clo·spo·ri·a·sis (si″klo-spə-ri′ə-sis) infection by protozoa of the genus *Cyclospora*, especially *C. cayetanen′sis*, seen especially in immunocompromised patients and occurring as recurrent gastrointestinal disease and watery diarrhea 圆孢球虫病

cy·clo·spor·in A (si″klo-spor′in) cyclosporine 环孢素 A

cy·clo·spor·ine (si″klo-spor′ēn) a cyclic peptide from an extract of soil fungi that selectively inhibits T-cell function; used as an immunosuppressant to prevent rejection in organ transplant recipients and to treat severe psoriasis and severe rheumatoid arthritis; also used topically to treat chronic dry eye 环孢霉素

cy·clo·thy·mia (si″klo-thi′me-ə) cyclothymic disorder 环性心境，（躁郁）环性气质

cy·clot·o·my (si-klot′ə-me) incision of the ciliary muscle 睫状肌切开术

cy·clo·tro·pia (si″klo-tro′pe-ə) permanent deviation of an eye around the anteroposterior axis in the presence of visional fusional stimuli, resulting in diplopia 旋转斜视

-cyesis word element [Gr.], *pregnancy* 妊娠

cyl·in·der (sil′in-dər) 1. a solid body shaped like a

C

column 圆柱管型；2. cylindrical lens 圆柱透镜；**cylin′drical, cylin′driform** *adj.*；axis c., axon (1) 轴突

cyl·in·droid (sil′in-droid) 1. shaped like a cylinder 圆柱状的；2. a urinary cast that tapers to a slender, sometimes curled or twisting, tail 圆柱状体

cyl·in·dro·ma (sil″in-dro′mə) 1. adenoid cystic carcinoma 圆柱瘤；2. a benign adnexal tumor on the face and scalp, consisting of cylindrical masses of epithelial cells surrounded by a thick band of hyaline material 腺样囊性癌；3. multiple trichoepithelioma 多发性毛发上皮瘤；**cylindrom′atous** *adj.*

cym·bo·ceph·a·ly (sim″bo-sef′ə-le) scaphocephaly 舟状头（畸形）的

cy·no·pho·bia (si′no-fo′be-ə) irrational fear of dogs 犬恐怖

cyp·i·o·nate (sip′e-o-nāt) USAN contraction for cyclopentanepropionate 环戊烷丙酸盐

cy·pro·hep·ta·dine (si″pro-hep′tə-dēn) an antihistamine with anticholinergic, sedative, and serotonin-blocking effects, used as the hydrochloride salt. It is also used in migraine prophylaxis 盐酸赛庚啶

cyr·to·sis (sir-to′sis) 1. kyphosis 驼背，脊柱后凸；2. distortion of the bones 骨弯曲

Cys cysteine 半胱氨酸

cyst (sist) 1. bladder 膀胱；2. an abnormal closed epithelium-lined cavity in the body, containing liquid or semisolid material 囊，孢囊；3. a stage in the life cycle of certain parasites, during which they are enveloped in a protective wall 胞囊；**adventitious c.**, one formed about a foreign body or exudate 异物周围囊肿；**alveolar c.**, dilatations of pulmonary alveoli, which may fuse by breakdown of their septa to form pneumatoceles 肺泡囊肿；**aneurysmal bone c.**, a benign, rapidly growing, osteolytic lesion, usually of childhood, characterized by blood-filled cystic spaces lined by bony or fibrous septa 动脉瘤样骨囊肿；**arachnoid c.**, a fluid-filled cyst between the layers of the leptomeninges, lined with arachnoid membrane, usually in the sylvian fissure 蛛网膜囊肿；**Baker c.**, a swelling behind the knee, caused by escape of synovial fluid that becomes enclosed in a membranous sac 腘窝囊肿；**Bartholin c.**, a mucus-filled cyst of a Bartholin gland, usually developing after obstruction of the duct by trauma, infection, epithelial hyperplasia, or congenital atresia or narrowing 前庭大腺囊肿；**Blessig c′s**, cystic spaces formed at the periphery of the retina 视网膜周囊样变性；**blue dome c.**, a benign, blue retention cyst of the breast 蓝顶囊肿；**Boyer c.**, an enlargement of the subhyoid bursa 舌骨下囊增生；

branchial c., one arising in the lateral aspect of the neck, from epithelial remnants of a branchial cleft (pharyngeal groove), usually between the second and third pharyngeal arches 鳃裂囊肿，颈囊肿；**bronchogenic c.**, a congenital cyst, usually in the mediastinum or lung, arising from anomalous budding during formation of the tracheobronchial tree, lined with bronchial epithelium that may contain secretory elements 支气管源性囊肿，支气管囊肿；**chocolate c.**, one having dark, syrupy contents, resulting from collection of hemosiderin following local hemorrhage 巧克力囊肿，卵巢子宫内膜异位症；**choledochal c.**, a congenital cystic dilatation of the common bile duct, which may cause pain in the right upper quadrant, jaundice, fever, or vomiting, or be asymptomatic 胆总管囊肿；**congenital preauricular c.**, one due to imperfect fusion of the first and second branchial arches in formation of the auricle, communicating with an ear pit on the surface 先天性耳前囊肿；**daughter c.**, a small parasitic cyst such as a hydatid cyst developed from the walls of a larger cyst 棘球子囊，子囊；**dentigerous c.**, a fluidcontaining odontogenic cyst surrounding the crown of an unerupted tooth 含牙囊肿；**dermoid c.**, a teratoma, usually benign, characterized by mature ectodermal elements, having a fibrous wall lined with stratified epithelium, and containing keratinous material, hair, and sometimes material such as bone, tooth, or nerve tissue; found most often in the ovary 皮样囊肿，颅壁表皮样囊肿；**duplication c.**, a congenital cystic malformation of the alimentary tract, consisting of a duplication of the segment to which it is adjacent, occurring anywhere from the mouth to the anus but most frequently affecting the ileum and esophagus 消化道的先天性囊性畸形，由消化道及其邻近组织的重复部分构成，可以见于全消化道的任意部位，但最常影响回肠和食管；**echinococcal c., echinococcus c.**, hydatid c.；**embryonic c.**, one developing from bits of embryonic tissue that have been overgrown by other tissues, or from developing organs that normally disappear before birth 胚胎囊肿；**enteric c., enterogenous c.**, a cyst of the intestine arising or developing from a fold or pouch along the intestinal tract 肠囊肿；**epidermal c.**, a benign cyst derived from the epidermis or the epithelium of a hair follicle; it is formed by cystic enclosures of epithelium within the dermis, filled with keratin and lipid-rich debris 表皮囊肿；**epidermal inclusion c.**, a type of epidermal cyst occurring on the head, neck, or trunk, formed by keratinizing squamous epithelium with a granular layer 表皮包涵性囊肿；**epidermoid c.**, 1. epidermal c.；2. a benign tumor formed by inclusion of epidermal elements, especially at the time of closure of the neural groove, and located in the skull, meninges, or brain 表皮肿瘤；**epithelial c.**, 1. any cyst lined by keratinizing stratified squamous epithelium, found most often in the skin 上皮囊肿；2. epidermal c.; **exudation c.**, one formed by an exudate in a closed cavity 渗出液囊肿；**follicular c.**, one due to occlusion of the duct of a follicle or small gland, especially one formed by enlargement of a graafian follicle as a result of accumulated transudate 毛囊囊肿，滤泡囊肿；**globulomaxillary c.**, one within the maxilla at the junction of the globular portion of the medial nasal process and the maxillary process 球颌突囊肿；**hydatid c.**, the larval cyst stage of the tapeworms *Echinococcus granulosus* and *E. multilocularis*, containing daughter cysts with many scoleces 棘球蚴囊；**keratinizing c.**, one arising in the pilosebaceous unit, lined by stratified squamous epithelium and containing largely macerated keratin and often sebum that renders the contents greasy or rancid 角质化囊肿；**lutein c.**, a cyst of the ovary developed from a corpus luteum. 黄体囊肿；**median anterior maxillary c.**, one in or near the incisive canal, arising from proliferation of epithelial remnants of the nasopalatine duct 上颌前正中囊肿；**median palatal c.**, one in the midline of the hard palate, between the lateral palatal processes 腭中囊肿；**meibomian c.**, a cyst of the meibomian gland, sometimes applied to a chalazion 睑板腺囊肿；**mucus retention c.**, a mucus-containing retention cyst caused by blockage of a salivary gland duct 黏液潴留囊肿；**multilocular c.**, 1. a cyst containing several loculi or spaces 多房性囊肿；2. a hydatid cyst with many small irregular cavities that may contain scoleces but generally little fluid 棘球囊；3. a thick-walled cyst in the kidney, found in clusters and usually unilaterally. In children it contains blastema and may develop into a Wilms tumor 肾内厚壁囊肿；**myxoid c.**, a nodular lesion usually overlying an interphalangeal finger joint, consisting of focal mucinous degeneration of collagen of the dermis; not a true cyst, it lacks an epithelial wall and does not communicate with the underlying synovial space 黏液囊肿；**nabothian c's**, 子宫颈腺囊肿，见 *follicle* 下词条；**nasoalveolar c., nasolabial c.**, a fissural cyst arising outside the bones at the junction of the globular portion of the medial nasal process, lateral nasal process, and maxillary process 鼻唇囊肿；**odontogenic c.**, a cyst in the jaw, derived from epithelium, usually containing fluid or semi-solid material, developing during any of various stages of odontogenesis; it is nearly always enclosed within bone 牙源性囊肿；**osseous hydatid c's**, hy-datid cysts formed by the larvae of *Echinococcus granulosus* in bone, which may become weakened and eroded by the exuberant growth 骨刺球囊；**parasitic c.**, a cyst formed by the larva of a parasite, such as a hydatid cyst 寄生虫包囊；**periapical c.**, a periodontal cyst involving the apex of an erupted tooth 根尖周囊肿；**periodontal c.**, one in the periodontal ligament and adjacent structures, usually at the apex of the tooth (*periapical c.*) 牙周囊肿；**pilar c.**, an epithelial cyst of the scalp, almost identical to an epidermal cyst, arising from the outer root sheath of the hair follicle 毛发囊肿；**pilonidal c.**, a haircontaining sacrococcygeal dermoid cyst or sinus, often opening at a postanal dimple 藏毛囊肿；**radicular c.**, an epithelium-lined sac at the apex of a tooth 根尖囊肿；**Rathke c's, Rathke cleft c's**, groups of epithelial cells forming small colloid-filled cysts in the pars intermedia of the pituitary gland; they are vestiges of the Rathke pouch and are closely related to craniopharyngiomas 颅颊裂囊肿；**retention c.**, one caused by blockage of the excretory duct of a gland, so that glandular secretions are retained 潴留囊肿；**sarcosporidian c.**, sarcocyst (2) 内孢子虫囊；**sebaceous c.**, a retention cyst of a sebaceous gland, containing cheesy yellow material, usually on the face, neck, scalp, or trunk 皮脂腺囊肿；**simple bone c.**, a pathologic bone space in the metaphyses of long bones of growing children; it may be either empty or filled with fluid and have a delicate connective tissue lining 单纯性骨囊肿；**subchondral c.**, a bone cyst within the fused epiphysis beneath the articular plate 软骨下囊肿；**tarry c.**, 1. one resulting from hemorrhage into a corpus luteum 柏油样囊肿；2. a bloody cyst resulting from endometriosis 子宫内膜异位囊肿；**tarsal c.**, chalazion 睑板腺囊肿；**thecalutein c.**, a cyst of the ovary in which the cystic cavity is lined with theca interna cells 膜胺黄素化红as；**traumatic bone c.**, a cystlike cavity formed in bone, particularly the mandible, in response to trauma. After a hematoma forms and then is resorbed, bone is not replaced and an empty space forms without epithelial lining 外伤性骨囊肿；**unicameral bone c.**, simple bone c.；**wolffian c.**, a cyst of the broad ligament developed from vestiges of the mesonephros 午非管囊肿

cys·tad·e·no·car·ci·no·ma (sis-tad″ə-nokahr″sĭ-no′mə) adenocarcinoma with tumorlined cystic cavities, usually in the ovaries but sometimes in the appendix, pancreas, thyroid, or elsewhere 囊腺癌；**mucinous c.**, 1. cystadenocarcinoma with cystic masses that produce a gelatinous, glycoprotein-rich fluid, usually in the ovary 黏液性囊腺癌；2. a malignant, usually bulky, exocrine pancreatic tumor,

containing cystic epithelium 胰腺黏液囊腺癌

cys·tad·e·no·ma (sis″tad-ə-no′mə) adenoma characterized by epithelium-lined cystic masses that contain secreted material, usually serous or mucinous, generally in the ovaries, salivary gland, or pancreas 囊 腺 瘤; **mucinous c.,** 1. a multilocular, usually benign, tumor produced by ovarian epithelial cells and having mucin-filled cavities 黏液性囊腺瘤; 2. a benign, usually bulky, exocrine pancreatic tumor, containing cystic epithelium 胰腺黏液囊腺瘤; **papillary c.,** 1. any tumor producing patterns that are both papillary and cystic 乳头状囊腺瘤; 2. a type of adenoma in which the acini are distended by fluids or outgrowths of tissue 乳腺腺瘤; **serous c.,** a cystic tumor of the ovary with thin, clear yellow serum and some solid tissue 浆液性囊腺瘤

cys·tal·gia (sis-tal′jə) pain in the bladder 膀胱痛

γ-cys·ta·thi·o·nase (sis″tə-thi′o-nās) a pyridoxal phosphate–containing enzyme that catalyzes the hydrolysis of cystathionine to cysteine, ammonia, and α-ketoglutarate; deficiency results in cystathioninuria 胱硫醚 γ- 裂解酶

cys·ta·thi·o·nine (sis″tə-thi′o-nēn) a thioester of homocysteine and serine; it serves as an intermediate in the transfer of a sulfur atom from methionine to cysteine 胱硫醚

cys·ta·thi·o·nine β-syn·thase (sis″tə-thi′onēn sin′thās) a pyridoxal phosphate–containing lyase that catalyzes a step in the catabolism of methionine; deficiency occurs in an aminoacidopathy characterized by homocystinuria, elevated blood methionine levels, and abnormalities in the eye and the skeletal, nervous, and vascular systems 胱硫醚 β- 合成酶

cys·ta·thi·o·nin·u·ria (sis″tə-thi″o-ne-nu′re-ə) 1. excess of cystathionine in the urine 胱硫醚尿; 2. a benign hereditary disorder of metabolism that causes an excess of cystathionine in urine and body tissues without other clinical manifestations 胱硫醚代谢紊乱

cys·tec·ta·sia (sis″tek-ta′zhah) slitting of the membranous portion of the urethra and dilation of the bladder neck for extraction of a calculus 膀胱扩张术

cys·tec·to·my (sis-tek′tə-me) 1. excision of a cyst 囊肿切除术; 2. excision or resection of the bladder 膀胱切除术

cys·te·ic ac·id (sis-te′ik) an intermediate product in the oxidation of cysteine to taurine 磺基丙氨酸

cys·te·ine (Cys, C) (sis′te-ēn) a sulfurcontaining, nonessential amino acid produced by enzymatic or acid hydrolysis of proteins, readily oxidized to cystine; sometimes found in urine 半胱氨酸

cys·tic (sis′tik) 1. pertaining to or containing cysts 囊的，囊肿的; 2. pertaining to the urinary bladder

or to the gallbladder 与膀胱或胆囊有关的

cys·ti·cer·co·sis (sis″tĭ-sər-ko′sis) infection with cysticerci. In humans, infection with the larval forms of *Taenia solium* 囊尾蚴病

cys·ti·cer·cus (sis″tĭ-sur′kəs) pl. *cysticer′ci* A larval form of tapeworm, consisting of a single scolex enclosed in a bladderlike cyst 囊尾蚴属; cf. *hydatid cyst*

cys·tig·er·ous (sis-tij′ər-əs) containing cysts 囊尾蚴

cys·tine (sis′tēn) (sis′tin) a sulfur-containing amino acid produced by digestion or acid hydrolysis of proteins, sometimes found in the urine and kidneys, and readily reduced to two molecules of cysteine 胱氨酸

cys·ti·no·sis (sis″tĭ-no′sis) a hereditary disorder of cystine metabolism; the most common and severe type appears in childhood with osteomalacia, aminoaciduria, phosphaturia, and deposition of cystine in tissues throughout the body, leading to renal failure 胱氨酸病

cys·tin·uria (sis″tĭ-nu′re-ə) a hereditary disorder of amino acid transport, characterized by excessive urinary excretion of cystine due to impaired renal tubular reabsorption, resulting in the formation of urinary cystine calculi 胱氨酸尿

cys·ti·tis (sis-ti′tis) inflammation of the urinary bladder 膀胱炎; **c. follicula′ris,** that in which the bladder mucosa is studded with nodules containing lymph follicles 滤泡性膀胱炎; **c. glandula′ris,** that in which the mucosa contains mucinsecreting glands 腺性膀胱炎; **hemorrhagic c.,** cystitis with severe hemorrhage, a dose-limiting toxic condition occurring with administration of cytotoxic alkylating agents or as a complication of stem cell transplantation 出血性膀胱炎; **interstitial c.,** a bladder condition with an inflammatory lesion, usually in the vertex, and involving the entire thickness of the wall 间质性膀胱炎; **radiation c.,** inflammatory changes in the bladder caused by ionizing radiation 放射性膀胱炎

cys·to·cele (sis′to-sēl) hernial protrusion of the urinary bladder, usually through the vaginal wall 膀胱膨出

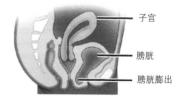

子宫

膀胱

膀胱膨出

cys·to·gas·tros·to·my (sis″to-gas-tros′tə-me) surgical anastomosis of a cyst to the stomach for drainage 囊肿胃吻合引流术

cys·to·gram (sis′to-gram) a radiograph of the bladder 膀胱平片

cys·tog·ra·phy (sis-tog′rə-fe) radiography of the urinary bladder 膀胱造影术; **voiding c.**, radiography of the bladder while the patient is urinating 排尿膀胱造影术

cys·toid (sis′toid) 1. resembling a cyst 囊肿样的; 2. a cystlike, circumscribed collection of softened material, having no enclosing capsule 类囊肿

Cys·to·i·sos·po·ra (sis″to-i-sos′pə-rə) a genus of coccidian protozoa that infects the intestines of mammals; formerly classified as part of *Isospora. C. bel′li* causes coccidiosis in humans 囊等孢球虫属

cys·to·je·ju·nos·to·my (sis″to-jə-joo-nos′tə-me) surgical anastomosis of a cyst to the jejunum 囊空肠造口吻合术

cys·to·li·thi·a·sis (sis″to-lĭ-thi′ə-sis) formation of vesical calculi 膀胱结石病

cys·to·li·thot·o·my (sis″to-lĭ-thot′ə-me) incision of the bladder for removal of a calculus 膀胱切开取石术

cys·tom·e·ter (sis-tom′ə-tər) an instrument for studying the neuromuscular mechanism of the bladder by means of measurements of pressure and capacity 膀胱内压测量器

cys·to·me·trog·ra·phy (sis″to-mə-trog′rə-fe) the graphic recording of intravesical volumes and pressures 膀胱内压描记法

cys·to·mor·phous (sis″to-mor′fəs) resembling a cyst or bladder 囊形的

cys·to·pa·re·sis (sis″to-pə-re′sis) paralysis of the urinary bladder 膀胱麻痹

cys·to·pexy (sis′to-pek″se) fixation of the bladder to the abdominal wall 膀胱固定术

cys·to·plas·ty (sis′to-plas″te) plastic repair of the bladder 膀胱成形; **augmentation c.**, enlargement of the bladder by grafting to it a detached segment of intestine (enterocystoplasty) or stomach (gastrocystoplasty) 膀胱扩大成形术; **sigmoid c.**, augmentation cystoplasty using an isolated segment of the sigmoid colon 使用乙状结肠的孤立段的膀胱扩大成形术

cys·to·ple·gia (sis″to-ple′jə) cystoparesis 膀胱麻痹

cys·to·pros·ta·tec·to·my (sis″to-pros-tə-tek′tə-me) surgical removal of the urinary bladder and prostate gland 膀胱前列腺切除术

cys·top·to·sis (sis″top-to′sis) prolapse of part of the inner bladder into the urethra 膀胱下垂

cys·to·py·eli·tis (sis″to-pi″ə-li′tis) pyelocystitis 肾盂膀胱炎

cys·tor·rha·phy (sis-tor′ə-fe) suture of the bladder 膀胱缝合

cys·to·sar·co·ma (sis″to-sahr-ko′mə) phyllodes tumor 囊性肉瘤

cys·tos·co·py (sis-tos′kə-pe) visual examination of the urinary tract with an endoscope 膀胱镜检查; **cystoscop′ic** *adj.*

cys·tos·to·my (sis-tos′tə-me) surgical formation of an opening into the bladder 膀胱造口术

cys·tot·o·my (sis-tot′ə-me) surgical incision of the urinary bladder 膀胱切开术

cys·to·ure·ter·itis (sis″to-u-re″tər-i′tis) inflammation of the urinary bladder and ureters 膀胱尿管炎

cys·to·ure·ter·og·ra·phy (sis″to-u-re″tər-og′rə-fe) radiography of the bladder and ureter 膀胱输尿管造影

cys·to·ure·throg·ra·phy (sis″to-u″rə-throg′rə-fe) radiography of the urinary bladder and urethra 尿道膀胱造影; **chain c.**, cystourethrography in which a sterile beaded metal chain is introduced via a modified catheter into the bladder and urethra; used in evaluating anatomic relationships of the bladder and urethra 链标膀胱尿道造影术

cys·to·ure·thro·scope (sis″to-u-re′thro-skōp″) an endoscope for examining the posterior urethra and bladder 膀胱尿道镜

cyt·a·phe·re·sis (sīt′ə-fə-re′sis) apheresis of blood cells 细胞单采法; 见 *erythrocytapheresis, leukapheresis,* and *thrombocytapheresis-*

cy·tar·a·bine (ara-C) (si-tar′ə-bēn) an antimetabolite that inhibits DNA synthesis and hence has antineoplastic properties; used in the treatment of acute myelogenous and other types of leukemia and of meningitis associated with leukemia or lymphoma 阿糖胞苷

cy·ti·dine (C) (si′tĭ-dēn) a purine nucleoside consisting of cytosine and ribose, a constituent of RNA and important in the synthesis of a variety of lipid derivatives 胞苷; **c. triphosphate (CTP),** an energy-rich nucleotide that acts as an activated precursor in the biosynthesis of RNA and other cellular constituents 胞苷三磷酸

cy·ti·dyl·ic ac·id (si″tĭ-dil′ik) phosphorylated cytidine, usually cytidine monophosphate 胞苷酸

cy·to·ar·chi·tec·ton·ic (si″to-ahr″kĭ-tekton′ik) pertaining to cellular structure or the arrangement of cells in tissue 关于细胞的结构或组织中细胞的排列

cy·to·chal·a·sin (si″to-kal′ə-sin) any of a group of fungal metabolites that interfere with the formation of microfilaments and thus disrupt cellular processes dependent on those filaments 细胞松弛素, 松胞菌素

cy·to·chem·is·try (si″to-kem′is-tre) the identification and localization of the different chemical compounds and their activities within the cell 细胞化学

cy·to·chrome (si'to-krōm) any of a class of hemoproteins, widely distributed in animal and plant tissues, whose main function is electron transport using the heme prosthetic group; distinguished according to their prosthetic groups, e.g., *a*, *b*, *c*, *d*, and P-450 细胞色素

cy·to·cide (si'to-sīd) an agent that destroys cells 杀细胞药；**cytoci'dal** *adj.*

cy·to·dif·fer·en·ti·a·tion (si″to-dif′ə-ren″shea'shən) the development of specialized structures and functions in embryonic cells 细胞分化

cy·to·dis·tal (si″to-dis'təl) denoting that part of an axon remote from the cell body 远离细胞的

cy·to·gen·e·sis (si″to-jen'ə-sis) the origin and development of cells 细胞发生

cy·to·ge·net·ic (si″to-jə-net'ik) 1. pertaining to chromosomes 关于染色体的；2. pertaining to cytogenetics 关于细胞遗传学

cy·to·ge·net·ics (si″to-jə-net'iks) the branch of genetics devoted to cellular constituents concerned in heredity, i.e., chromosomes 细胞遗传学；**clinical c.**, the branch of cytogenetics concerned with relations between chromosomal abnormalities and pathologic conditions 临床细胞遗传学

cy·to·gen·ic (si-to-jen'ik) 1. pertaining to cytogenesis 关于细胞发生的；2. forming or producing cells 形成或产生细胞

cy·tog·e·nous (si-toj'ə-nəs) producing cells 产生细胞的

cy·to·gly·co·pe·nia (si″to-gli″ko-pe'ne-ə) deficient glucose content of body or blood cells 体内或血细胞内葡萄糖含量不足

cy·to·his·to·gen·e·sis (si″to-his″to-jen'ə-sis) the development of the structure of cells 细胞发生

cy·to·his·tol·o·gy (si″to-his-tol'ə-je) the combination of cytologic and histologic methods 细胞组织学；**cytohistolog'ic** *adj.*

cy·toid (si'toid) resembling a cell 像细胞的，细胞状的

cy·to·kine (si'to-kīn) a generic term for nonantibody proteins released by one cell population on contact with a specific antigen; they act as intercellular mediators, as in the generation of an immune response 细胞因子

cy·to·ki·ne·sis (si″to-kī-ne'sis) the final stage of cell division, following telophase, during which the cell separates at the equator into two daughter cells and the nucleolus appears 胞质分裂

cy·tol·o·gy (si-tol'ə-je) cell biology 细胞学；**cytolog'ic** *adj.*；**aspiration biopsy c. (ABC),** the

microscopic study of cells obtained from superficial or internal lesions by suction through a fine needle 针吸活检细胞学；**exfoliative c.,** microscopic examination of cells desquamated from a body surface or lesion as a means of detecting malignancy and microbiologic changes, to measure hormonal levels, etc. Such cells are obtained by aspiration, washing, a smear, or scraping 脱落细胞学

cy·tol·y·sin (si-tol'ə-sin) a substance or antibody that produces cytolysis 溶细胞素

cy·tol·y·sis (si-tol'ə-sis) the dissolution of cells 细胞溶解；**cytolyt'ic** *adj.*；**immune c.,** cell lysis produced by antibody with the participation of complement 免疫细胞溶解

cy·to·ly·so·some (si″to-li'so-sōm) autophagosome 自噬体，细胞溶酶体

cy·to·me·gal·ic (si″to-mə-gal'ik) pertaining to the greatly enlarged cells with intranuclear inclusions seen in cytomegalovirus infections 巨细胞的

Cy·to·meg·a·lo·vi·rus (si″to-meg'ə-lo-vi″rəs) a genus of ubiquitous viruses of the family Herpesviridae that upon infection cause production of unique large cells with intranuclear inclusions; it includes the species human herpesvirus 5. See table at *herpesvirus*. 巨细胞病毒，参见疱疹病毒表

cy·to·meg·a·lo·vi·rus (CMV) (si″to-meg'ə-lovi″rəs) a virus of the genus *Cytomegalovirus* 巨细胞病毒

cy·tom·e·ter (si-tom'ə-tər) a device for counting cells, either visually or automatically 血细胞计数器

cy·tom·e·try (si-tom'ə-tre) the characterization and measurement of cells and cellular constituents 细胞计量术；**flow c.,** a technique for counting cells suspended in fluid as they flow one at a time past a focus of exciting light 流式细胞术

cy·to·mor·phol·o·gy (si″to-mor-fol'ə-je) the morphology of body cells 细胞形态学

cy·to·mor·pho·sis (si″to-mor-fo'sis) the changes through which cells pass in development 细胞变形

cy·to·patho·gen·e·sis (si″to-path″o-jen'ə-sis) production of pathologic changes in cells 细胞病理变化；**cytopathogenet'ic** *adj.*

cy·to·path·o·gen·ic (si″to-path″o-jen'ik) capable of producing pathologic changes in cells 致细胞病变的

cy·to·pa·thol·o·gist (si″to-pə-thol'ə-jist) an expert in cytopathology 细胞病理学家

cy·to·pa·thol·o·gy (si″to-pə-thol'ə-je) the study of cells in disease 细胞病理学

cy·top·a·thy (si-top'ə-the) a disorder of a cell or of its constituents 细胞病变；**cytopath'ic** *adj.*；**mitochondrial c's,** a diverse group of disorders characterized by decreased energy production by the mitochondria; they may be acquired, secondary to another disorder, or inherited. Symptoms develop gradually and manifestations are extremely variable and often resemble those of other diseases 线粒体细胞病

cy·to·pe·nia (si″to-pe′ne-ə) deficiency in the number of any of the cellular elements of the blood 血细胞减少症

cy·to·phago·cy·to·sis (si″to-fa″go-si-to′sis) cytophagy 细胞吞噬作用

cy·toph·a·gy (si-tof′ə-je) the ingestion of cells by phagocytes 细胞吞噬作用

cy·to·phil·ic (si-to-fil′ik) having an affinity for cells 亲细胞的

cy·to·phy·lax·is (si″to-fə-lak′sis) 1. the protection of cells against cytolysis 细胞防御；2. increase in cellular activity 细胞活性增强

cy·to·pi·pette (si″to-pi-pet′) a pipette for taking cytological smears 细胞吸管

cy·to·plasm (si′to-plaz″əm) the protoplasm of a cell exclusive of that of the nucleus (nucleoplasm) 细胞质；**cytoplas′mic** adj.

cy·to·pro·tec·tive (si″to-pro-tek′tiv) 1. protecting cells from noxious chemicals or other stimuli 保护细胞免受有毒化学品或其他刺激；2. an agent that so protects 细胞保护剂

cy·to·prox·i·mal (si″to-prok′sĭ-məl) denoting that part of an axon nearer to the cell body 近细胞的

cy·to·re·duc·tion (si″to-re-duk′shən) 1. decrease in number of cells, as in a tumor 细胞数量减少，如在肿瘤中；2. debulking 切除

cy·to·re·duc·tive (si″to-rə-duk′tiv) reducing the number of cells 减少细胞数量

cy·to·sine (C) (si′to-sēn) a pyrimidine base occurring in animal and plant cells, usually condensed with ribose or deoxyribose to form the nucleosides cytidine and deoxycytidine, major constituents of nucleic acids 胞嘧啶；**c. arabinoside,** cytarabine 阿糖胞苷

cy·to·skel·e·ton (si″to-skel′ə-tən) a conspicuous internal reinforcement in the cytoplasm of a cell, consisting of tonofibrils, filaments of the terminal web, and other microfilaments 细胞骨架；**cyto-skel′etal** adj.

cy·to·sol (si′to-sol) the liquid medium of the cytoplasm, i.e., cytoplasm minus organelles and nonmembranous insoluble components 胞质溶胶；**cytosol′ic** adj.

cy·to·some (si′to-sōm) the body of a cell apart from its nucleus 胞质体

cy·to·stat·ic (si″to-stat′ik) 1. suppressing the growth and multiplication of cells 抑制细胞生长和增殖；2. an agent that so acts 细胞生长抑制药

cy·to·stome (si′to-stōm) the cell mouth; the aperture through which food enters certain protozoa 胞口；食物进入某些原生动物的摄食孔

cy·to·tax·is (si-to-tak′sis) the movement and arrangement of cells with respect to a specific source of stimulation 细胞趋性；**cytotac′tic** adj.

cy·to·tox·ic·i·ty (si″to-tok-sis′ĭ-te) the degree to which an agent possesses a specific destructive action on certain cells or the possession of such action 细胞毒性；**cytotoxic** adj.; **antibody-dependent cell-mediated c. (ADCC),** lysis of antibodycoated target cells by effector cells with cytolytic activity and Fc receptors 依赖抗体的细胞毒性；**cell-mediated c.,** cytolysis of a target cell by effector lymphocytes, such as cytotoxic T lymphocytes or NK cells; it may be antibody-dependent or independent 细胞毒作用

cy·to·tox·in (si′to-tok″sin) a toxin or antibody having a specific toxic action upon cells of special organs 细胞毒素

cy·to·tropho·blast (si″to-trof′o-blast) the cellular (inner) layer of the trophoblast 细胞滋养层；**cytotrophoblas′tic** adj.

cy·to·tro·pism (si-tot′ro-piz-əm) 1. cell movement in response to external stimulation 细胞对外界刺激的反应；2. the tendency of viruses, bacteria, drugs, etc., to exert their effect upon certain cells of the body 病毒、细菌、药物等对人体某些细胞产生作用的趋势；**cytotro′pic** adj.

cy·to·zo·ic (si″to-zo′ik) living within or attached to cells; said of parasites 细胞内寄生的

cy·tu·ria (si-tu′re-ə) excessive or unusual cells in the urine 细胞尿症

D dalton 道尔顿；deciduous (tooth) 乳齿；density 密度；deuterium 氘；died 死亡；diopter 屈光度；distal 远端的；dorsal vertebrae (D1 to D12) 胸椎 (D1~12)；dose 剂量；duration 持续时间

D. [L.] da (give) 给予；de′tur (let it be given) 需给予；dex′ter (right) 右的；do′sis (dose) 剂量

2,4-D a toxic chlorphenoxy herbicide (2,4-dichlorophenoxyacetic acid), a component of Agent Orange 一种有毒的氯苯氧基除草剂（2,4- 二氯苯氧乙酸），一种试剂橙色成分

D- a chemical prefix specifying the relative configuration of an enantiomer, indicating a carbohydrate

D

with the same configuration at a specific carbon atom as d-glyceraldehyde or an amino acid having the same configuration as d-serine. Opposed to L-D（构）型的，对映体即镜像构型为 L- 的相对构型

d day 日，天；deci- 十分之一；deoxyribose (in nucleosides and nucleotides) 脱氧核酸

d. [L.] da (give) 给予；de′tur (let it be given) 需给予；dex′ter (right) 右的；do′sis (dose) 剂量

d density 密度；diameter 直径

d- dextro- (right or clockwise, dextrorotatory)Opposed to *l-* 右的，顺时针方向，右旋的；与 *l-* 相反

Δ- (capital delta, the fourth letter of the Greek alphabet) position of a double bond in a carbon chain (大写三角形, 希腊字母的第四个字母) 碳链中双键的位置

δ (delta, the fourth letter of the Greek alphabet) heavy chain of IgD; δ chain of hemoglobin (三角形, 希腊字母的第四个字母) IgD 的重链和血红蛋白的 δ 链的符号

δ- a prefix designating 一种前缀，表示 (1) the position of a substituting atom or group in a chemical compound 取代原子或基团在化学化合物中的位置；(2) fourth in a series of four or more related entities or chemical compounds 四种或四种以上相关连接或化合物中的第四种

Da dalton 道尔顿

da·big·a·tran (də-big′ə-tran) a thrombin inhibitor used as the etexilate ester to reduce the risk of stroke and systemic embolism in patients with atrial fibrillation 达比加群（凝血酶抑制药）

da·braf·e·nib (da-brəf′e-nib) an inhibitor of certain mutated forms of BRAF kinase, used alone or in combination to treat melanoma with *BRAF* V600E or V600K mutations; administered orally 达拉菲尼

DAC decitabine 地西他滨

da·car·ba·zine (də-kahr′bə-zēn) a cytotoxic alkylating agent used as an antineoplastic primarily for treatment of malignant melanoma and in combination chemotherapy for Hodgkin disease and sarcomas 达卡巴嗪；氮烯唑胺

dac·lat·as·vir (dək-lat′az-veer) an inhibitor of nonstructural protein 5A, a protein involved in the replication of hepatitis C virus 达卡他韦

da·cliz·u·mab (də-kliz′u-mab) an immunosuppressant used to prevent acute organ rejection in renal transplant patients 达利珠单抗

dac·ryo·ad·e·nal·gia (dak″re-o-ad″ə-nal′jə) pain in a lacrimal gland 泪腺痛

dac·ryo·ad·e·nec·to·my (dak″re-o-ad″ə-nek′tə-me) excision of a lacrimal gland 泪腺切除术

dac·ryo·blen·nor·rhea (dak″re-o-blen″ore′ə) mucous flow from the lacrimal apparatus 从泪道流出

的黏液

dac·ryo·cyst (dak′re-o-sist″) the lacrimal sac 泪囊

dac·ryo·cys·tec·to·my (dak″re-o-sis-tek′tə-me) excision of the wall of the lacrimal sac 泪囊壁切除术

dac·ryo·cys·to·blen·nor·rhea (dak″re-osis″toblen″o-re′ə) chronic catarrhal inflammation of the lacrimal sac, with constriction of the lacrimal gland 泪囊的慢性内障炎症，伴泪腺收缩

dac·ryo·cys·to·cele (dak″re-o-sis′to-sēl) hernial protrusion of the lacrimal sac 泪囊突出症

dac·ryo·cys·to·rhi·no·ste·no·sis (dak″re-osis″-to-ri″no-sis-no′sis) narrowing of the duct leading from the lacrimal sac to the nasal cavity 鼻泪管狭窄

dac·ryo·cys·to·rhi·nos·to·my (dak″re-osis″to-ri-nos′tə-me) surgical creation of an opening between the lacrimal sac and nasal cavity 泪囊鼻腔造口术

dac·ryo·cys·to·ste·no·sis (dak″re-o-sis″tostə-no′sis) narrowing of the lacrimal sac 泪囊狭窄

dac·ryo·cys·tos·to·my (dak″re-o-sis-tos′tə-me) creation of a new opening into the lacrimal sac 泪囊造口术

dac·ryo·hem·or·rhea (dak″re-o-hem″ore′ə) the discharge of tears mixed with blood 血泪症

dac·ryo·lith (dak′re-o-lith″) a lacrimal calculus 泪道结石

dac·ry·o·ma (dak″re-o′mə) a tumor-like swelling due to obstruction of the lacrimal duct 泪管肿大

dac·ry·ops (dak′re-ops) 1. a watery state of the eye 泪眼；2. distention of a lacrimal duct by contained fluid 泪管积液

dac·ryo·py·o·sis (dak″re-o-pi-o′sis) suppuration of the lacrimal apparatus 泪器化脓

dac·ryo·scin·tig·ra·phy (dak″re-o-sin-tig′rə-fe) scintigraphy of the lacrimal ducts 泪道闪烁显像术

dac·ryo·ste·no·sis (dak″re-o-stə-no′sis) stricture or narrowing of a lacrimal duct 泪管狭窄

dac·ti·no·my·cin (dak″tĭ-no-mi′sin) actinomycin D, an antibiotic derived from several species of *Streptomyces*; used as an antineoplastic 放线菌素 D

dac·tyl (dak′təl) a digit 指（趾）

dac·ty·log·ra·phy (dak″tə-log′rə-fe) the study of fingerprints 指纹学

dac·ty·lo·gry·po·sis (dak″tə-lo-grĭ-po′sis) permanent flexion of the fingers 弯指

dac·ty·lol·o·gy (dak″tə-lol′ə-je) signing 手语

dac·ty·lol·y·sis (dak″tə-lol′ĭ-sis) 1. surgical correction of syndactyly 合指外科矫治；2. loss or amputation of a digit 指缺失或截肢；d. sponta′nea, ainhum 自发性指（趾）脱落

dac·ty·los·co·py (dak″tə-los′kə-pe) examination of fingerprints for identification 指纹鉴定法

dac·ty·lus (dak′tə-ləs) [L.] a digit 指节

DAF decay accelerating factor 衰变加速因子

dal·fo·pris·tin (dal-fo′pris-tin) a semisynthetic antibacterial used in conjunction with quinupristin against various gram-positive organisms, including vancomycin-resistant *Enterococcus faecium* 达福普汀

dal·tep·a·rin (dal-tep′ə-rin) an antithrombotic used as the sodium salt in the prevention of pulmonary thromboembolism and deep venous thrombosis in at-risk abdominal surgery patients 达肝素钠，抗血栓形成药物

dal·ton (**D, Da**) (dawl′tən) an arbitrary unit of mass, being 1/12 the mass of the nuclide of carbon-12, equivalent to 1.657×10^{-24} g 道尔顿（原子和分子的质量单位）

dam (dam) 1. a barrier to obstruct the flow of fluid 阻碍流体流动的屏障；2. a thin sheet of latex used in surgical procedures to separate certain tissues or structures 一种薄薄的胶乳，用于外科手术以分离某些组织或结构；3. rubber d.；**rubber d.**, a thin sheet of latex rubber used to isolate teeth from mouth fluids during dental therapy 橡皮障

damp·ing (damp′ing) steady diminution of the amplitude of successive vibrations of a specific form of energy, as of electricity 衰减，阻尼，减幅

da·nap·a·roid (də-nap′ə-roid) an antithrombotic used as the sodium salt in the prophylaxis of pulmonary thromboembolism and deep vein thrombosis 低分子量肝素

dan·a·zol (dan′ə-zol) an anterior pituitary suppressant used in the treatment of endometriosis, fibrocystic breast disease, and gynecomastia and the prophylaxis of attacks of hereditary angioedema 达那唑

D and C dilatation and curettage 刮宫术，宫颈扩张及刮宫术

dan·de·li·on (dan′də-li″ən) a weedy herb, *Taraxacum officinale*, having deeply notched leaves and brilliant yellow flowers; used for dyspepsia, loss of appetite, urinary tract infections, and liver and gallbladder complaints 蒲公英

dan·der (dan′dər) small scales from the hair or feathers of animals, which may be a cause of allergy in sensitive persons 毛皮垢屑，羽毛垢屑

dan·druff (dan′drəf) 1. dry scaly material shed from the scalp; applied to that normally shed from the scalp epidermis as well as to the excessive scaly material associated with disease 头皮屑；2. seborrheic dermatitis of the scalp 头皮脂溢性皮炎

DANS 5-dimethylamino-1-naphthalenesulfonic acid; the acyl chloride is a fluorochrome employed in immunofluorescence studies of tissues and cells 5-二甲基氨基-1-萘磺酸

dan·tro·lene (dan′tro-lēn) a skeletal muscle relaxant, used as the sodium salt in the treatment of chronic spasticity and the treatment and prophylaxis of malignant hyperthermia 硝苯呋海音（骨骼肌松弛药）

da·pip·ra·zole (də-pip′rə-zōl) an alpha-adrenergic blocking agent used topically as the hydrochloride salt to reverse pharmacologically induced mydriasis 诺霉素

dap·sone (dap′sōn) an antibacterial bacteriostatic for a broad spectrum of gram-positive and gram-negative organisms; used as a leprostatic, as a dermatitis herpetiformis suppressant, and in the prophylaxis of falciparum malaria 氨苯砜

dar·tos (dahr′tos) either the dartos muscle or the tunica dartos 肉膜

dar·u·na·vir (dar-oo′nŭ-veer) an HIV protease inhibitor that blocks cleavage of polyproteins to prevent the formation of mature infectious viral particles; used in the treatment of human immunodeficiency virus infection 地瑞那韦，一种 HIV 蛋白酶抑制药

da·sat·i·nib (də-sat′ĭ-nib) a tyrosine kinase inhibitor used in the treatment of Philadelphia chromosome–positive chronic myelogenous leukemia and acute lymphoblastic leukemia 达沙替尼

dau·no·ru·bi·cin (daw″no-roo′bĭ-sin) an anthracycline (q.v.) antibiotic used as an antineoplastic; administered as the hydrochloride salt or as a liposome-encapsulated preparation of the citrate salt 道诺霉素，柔红霉素

DAy Doctor of Ayurvedic Medicine 阿育吠陀医学博士

dB, db decibel 分贝的符号

DBS deep brain stimulation 脑深部电刺激

DC direct current 直流电；Doctor of Chiropractic 按摩医师

D & C dilatation and curettage 刮宫术

DCIS ductal carcinoma in situ 乳腺导管原位癌

DDP, *cis*-DDP cisplatin 顺铂

DDS dapsone 二氨二苯砜；Denys-Drash syndrome Denys-Drash 综合征；Doctor of Dental Surgery 牙外科博士

DDT dichloro-diphenyl-trichloroethane, a powerful insect poison; used in dilution as a powder or in an oily solution as a spray 滴滴涕，二氯二苯三氯乙烷

de·acyl·ase (de-a′səl-ās) any hydrolase that catalyzes the cleavage of an acyl group in ester or amide linkage 脱酰酶

dead (ded) 1. destitute of life 贫苦的生活 2. anesthetic (1) 麻木的

deaf (def) lacking the sense of hearing or not having the full power of hearing 聋的

de·af·fer·en·ta·tion (de-af″ər-ən-ta′shən) the elimination or interruption of sensory nerve fibers 去传入

deaf·ness (def′nis) hearing loss 耳聋，耳闭；**word d.**, auditory aphasia 词聋

de·am·i·dase (de-am′ĭ-dās) an enzyme that splits amides to form a carboxylic acid and ammonia 脱酰胺酶

de·am·i·di·za·tion (de-am″ĭ-dī-za′shən) the removal of an amido group from a molecule 脱酰胺作用

de·am·i·nase (de-am′ĭ-nās) an enzyme causing deamination, or removal of the amino group from organic compounds, usually cyclic amidines 脱氨基酶

de·am·i·na·tion (de-am″ĭ-na′shən) removal of the amino group, —NH₂, from a compound 脱氨作用，脱氨基

death (deth) the cessation of life; permanent cessation of all vital bodily functions 生命的停止，死亡；**activation-induced cell d.** (AICD), recognition and deletion of T lymphocytes that have been induced to proliferate by receptor-mediated activation, preventing their overgrowth 激活诱导细胞死亡；**black d.**, bubonic plague 黑死病；**brain d.**, irreversible coma; irreversible brain damage as manifested by absolute unresponsiveness to all stimuli, absence of all spontaneous muscle activity, and an isoelectric electroencephalogram for 30 minutes, all in the absence of hypothermia or intoxication by central nervous system depressants 脑死亡；**cot d., crib d.**, sudden infant death syndrome 婴儿猝死；**programmed cell d.**, the theory that particular cells are programmed to die at specific sites and at specific stages of development 细胞程序性死亡；**somatic d.**, cessation of all vital cellular activity 整体死亡

de·bil·i·ty (də-bil′ĭ-te) asthenia 虚弱

de·branch·er en·zyme (de-branch′ər en′zīm) 脱支酶，见 *enzyme* 下词条

dé·bride·ment (da-brēd-maw′) [Fr.] the removal of foreign material or devitalized tissue from or adjacent to a traumatic or infected lesion until surrounding healthy tissue is exposed, either by cutting (*surgical d.*) or by application of an enzyme able to lyse devitalized tissue (*enzymatic d.*) 清创术

de·bris (də-bre′) fragments of devitalized tissue or foreign matter. In dentistry, soft foreign material loosely attached to a tooth surface 碎屑

debt (det) something owed 欠债；**oxygen d.**, the oxygen that must be used in the oxidative energy processes after strenuous exercise to reconvert lactic acid to glucose and decomposed ATP and creatine phosphate to their original states 氧债

de·bulk·ing (de-bulk′ing) cytoreduction; removal of the major portion of the material composing a lesion 缩小体积手术

de·cal·ci·fi·ca·tion (de-kal″sĭ-fĭ-ka′shən) 1. loss of calcium salts from a bone or tooth 脱钙作用；2. the process of removing calcareous matter 除石灰质

de·can·nu·la·tion (de-kan″u-la′shən) extubation of a cannula 拔管

de·can·ta·tion (de″kan-ta′shən) the pouring of a clear supernatant liquid from a sediment 倾泻

de·cap·i·ta·tion (de-kap″ĭ-ta′shən) the removal of the head, as of an animal, fetus, or bone 断头术

de·cap·su·la·tion (de-kap″su-la′shən) capsulectomy 被膜剥脱术；**renal d.**, removal of all or part of the renal capsule 肾被膜剥脱术

de·car·box·y·lase (de″kahr-bok′sə-lās) any enzyme of the lyase class that catalyzes the removal of a carbon dioxide molecule from carboxylic acids 脱羧酶

de·cay (de-ka′) 1. the decomposition of dead matter 腐烂，腐化；2. the process of decline, as in aging 衰变，蜕变；**beta d.**, disintegration of the nucleus of an unstable radionuclide in which the mass number is unchanged but the atomic number is changed by 1, as a result of emission of a negatively or positively charged (beta) particle（质点）衰变；**tooth d.**, dental caries 龋齿

de·ce·dent (də-se′dənt) a person who has recently died 死者

de·cel·er·a·tion (de-sel′ər-a″shən) decrease in rate or speed 减速；**early d.**, in fetal heart rate monitoring, a transient decrease in heart rate that coincides with the onset of a uterine contraction 早期减速；**late d.**, in fetal heart rate monitoring, a transient decrease in heart rate occurring at or after the peak of a uterine contraction, which may indicate fetal hypoxia 晚期减速；**variable d's**, in fetal heart rate monitoring, a transient series of decelerations that vary in intensity, duration, and relation to uterine contraction, resulting from vagus nerve firing in response to a stimulus such as umbilical cord compression in the first stage of labor 变异减速

de·cen·ter (de-sen′tər) in optics, to design or make a lens such that the visual axis does not pass through the optical center of the lens 偏心，在光学技术中，设计或制造一个透镜，使其视觉轴不穿过透镜的光学中心

de·cer·e·brate[1] (de-ser′ə-brāt) in experimental animals, to eliminate cerebral function, as by removal of the brain, transection of the brainstem, or ligation of the common carotid arteries and the basilar artery 在实验动物中，通过切除大脑、切断脑干或结扎颈总动脉和基底动脉来消除脑功能

de·cer·e·brate[2] (de-ser′ə-brət) 1. pertaining to an animal that has had cerebral function interrupted 脑功能受损的动物；2. resulting from decerebration or, in humans, exhibiting neurologic characteristics similar to those of a decerebrated animal 由去脑引起的，或在人类中表现出与去脑动物相似的神经学特征

deci- word element [L.], one-tenth; used in naming units of measurement to indicate onetenth of the unit designated by the root with which it is combined (10^{-1}); symbol d 十分之一，用来命名测量单位，表示它联用的词根单位的十分之一（10^{-1}）；符号为 d

dec·i·bel (des' ĭ-bəl) a unit used to express the ratio of two powers, usually electric or acoustic powers, equal to one-tenth of a bel; 1 decibel equals approximately the smallest difference in acoustic power the human ear can detect 分贝

de·cid·ua (də-sid′u-ə) the endometrium of the pregnant uterus, all of which, except the deepest layer, is shed at parturition 蜕膜；**decid′ual** *adj.*; **basal d., d. basa′lis,** that portion directly underlying the chorionic sac and attached to the myometrium 底蜕膜；**capsular d., d. capsula′ris,** that portion directly overlying the chorionic sac and facing the uterine cavity 包蜕膜；**parietal d., d. parieta′lis,** that portion lining the uterus elsewhere than at the site of attachment of the chorionic sac 壁蜕膜

de·cid·u·itis (də-sid″u-i′tis) a bacterial disease leading to changes in the decidua 蜕膜炎

de·cid·u·o·sis (də-sid″u-o′sis) the presence of decidual tissue or tissue resembling the endometrium of pregnancy in an ectopic site 蜕膜病

de·cid·u·ous (də-sid′u-əs) falling off or shed at maturity, as the teeth of the first dentition 脱落的，脱膜的

dec·i·li·ter (**dL**) (des′ĭ-le″tər) one-tenth (10^{-1}) of a liter; 100 milliliters 分升

de·ci·ta·bine (**DAC**) (de-si′tə-bēn″) a cytotoxic compound used as an antineoplastic in the treatment of acute leukemia 地西他滨

dec·li·na·tion (dek″lĭ-na′shən) cyclophoria 偏差，偏角，偏转

de·clive (de-kli′ve) the part of the vermis of the cerebellum just caudal to the primary fissure 山坡

de·cli·vis (de-kli′vis) [L.] declive 小脑山坡

de·col·or·a·tion (de-kul″ər-a′shən) 1. removal of color 脱色；bleaching 漂白；2. lack or loss of color 缺乏或失去颜色

de·com·pen·sa·tion (de-kom″pən-sa′shən) 1. inability of the heart to maintain adequate circulation, marked by dyspnea, venous engorgement, and edema 代偿失调；2. in psychiatry, failure of defense mechanisms resulting in progressive personality disintegration 防御功能失常

de·com·po·si·tion (de″kom-pə-zish′ən) the sep-

aration of compound bodies into their constituent principles 分解，腐解，腐败

de·com·pres·sion (de″kom-presh′ən) 1. removal of pressure, especially from deep-sea divers and caisson workers to prevent bends, and from persons ascending to great heights 减压；2. a surgical operation for the relief of pressure in a body compartment 体室减压手术；**cardiac d.,** decompression of heart 心减压术；**cerebral d.,** relief of intracranial pressure by removal of a skull flap and incision of the dura mater 脑减压术；**d. of heart,** pericardiotomy with evacuation of a hematoma 心减压术；**microvascular d.,** a microsurgical procedure for relief of trigeminal neuralgia 微血管减压术；**nerve d.,** relief of pressure on a nerve by surgical removal of the constricting fibrous or bony tissue 神经减压术；**d. of pericardium,** decompression of heart 心包减压术；**d. of spinal cord,** surgical relief of pressure on the spinal cord, which may be due to hematoma, bone fragments, etc 脊髓减压术

de·con·ges·tant (de″kən-jes′tənt) 1. tending to reduce congestion or swelling 减少充血或肿胀；2. an agent that so acts 减少充血或肿胀的介质

de·con·tam·i·na·tion (de″kən-tam″ĭ-na′shən) the freeing of a person or object of some contaminating substance, e.g., war gas, radioactive material 消毒，纯化，净化

de·cor·po·ra·tion (de-kor″pə-ra′shən) the removal of radionuclides internalized by the body to reduce contamination and the risk of acute or chronic damage by these agents 退去，排出，促排剂；**decorporation a.,** a drug product that increases the removal of radioactive contaminants from the body 去污剂

de·cor·ti·ca·tion (de-kor″tĭ-ka′shən) 1. removal of the outer covering from a plant, seed, or root 去皮；2. removal of portions of the cortical substance of a structure or organ 皮质剥除术，去皮质术

dec·re·ment (dek′rə-mənt) 1. subtraction, or decrease 减去或减少；the amount by which a quantity or value is decreased 减少数量或价值的数额；2. the stage of decline of a disease 疾病的衰退阶段；**decremen′tal** *adj.*

de·cru·des·cence (de″kroo-des′əns) diminution or abatement of the intensity of symptoms 减退

de·cu·bi·tus (de-ku′bĭ-təs) pl. *decu′bitus* [L.] 1. an act of lying down; the position assumed in lying down 卧位；2. decubitus ulcer 褥疮；**decu′bital** *adj.*; **dorsal d.,** lying on the back 仰卧位；**lateral d.,** lying on one side, designated *right lateral d.* when the subject lies on the right side and *left lateral d.* when lying on the left side 侧卧位；**ventral d.,** lying on the stomach 腹卧位，伏卧位

de·cus·sa·tio (de″kə-sa′she-o) pl. *decussatio′nes*

D

[L.] decussation 交叉

de·cus·sa·tion (de″kə-sa′shən) a crossing over; the intercrossing of fellow parts or structures in the form of an X 交叉；**Forel d.,** the ventral tegmental decussation of the rubrospinal and rubroreticular tracts in the midbrain 被盖前交叉；**fountain d. of Meynert,** the dorsal tegmental decussation of the tectospinal tract in the midbrain 被盖后交叉；**pyramidal d.,** the anterior part of the lower medulla oblongata in which most of the fibers of the pyramids intersect 锥体交叉

de·dif·fer·en·ti·a·tion (de-dif″ər-en″she-a′shən) anaplasia 脱分化

deep (dēp) situated far beneath the surface 表面之下的；not superficial 不肤浅的

de·epi·car·di·al·iza·tion (de-ep″ĭ-kahr″de-əl″ĭ-za′shən) a surgical procedure for the relief of intractable angina pectoris, in which epicardial tissue is destroyed by application of a caustic agent to promote development of collateral circulation 去心包作用

def·e·ca·tion (def″ə-ka′shən) the evacuation of fecal matter from the rectum 排泄物从直肠排出

def·e·cog·ra·phy (def″ə-kog′rə-fe) the recording, by videotape or high-speed radiographs, of defecation following barium instillation into the rectum; used in the evaluation of fecal incontinence 排粪摄影

de·fect (de′fekt) an imperfection, failure, or absence 缺损，缺陷；**defec′tive** *adj*；**acquired d.,** a nongenetic imperfection arising secondarily, after birth 后天缺损；**aortic septal d.,** a congenital anomaly in which there is abnormal communication between the ascending aorta and pulmonary artery just above the semilunar valves 主动脉隔缺损；**atrial septa·l d's, atrioseptal d's,** congenital anomalies in which there is persistent patency of the atrial septum due to failure of fusion between either the septum secundum or the septum primum and the endocardial cushions 房间隔缺损；**birth d.,** one present at birth, whether a morphologic defect (dysmorphism) or an inborn error of metabolism 先天缺损；**congenital d.,** birth d.；**cortical d.,** a benign, symptomless, circumscribed rarefaction of cortical bone, detected radiographically 皮质缺损；**endocardial cushion d's,** a spectrum of septal defects resulting from imperfect fusion of the endocardial cushions, and ranging from persistent ostium primum to persistent common atrioventricular canal 心内膜垫缺损；见 *atrial septal d.* 和 *atrioventricularis communis*；**fibrous cortical d.,** a small, asymptomatic, osteolytic, fibrous lesion occurring within the bone cortex, particularly in the metaphyseal region of long bones in childhood 纤维皮质缺损；**filling d.,** any localized defect in the contour of the stomach, duodenum, or intestine, as

seen in the radiograph after a barium enema 充盈缺损；**genetic d.,** 遗传缺陷，见 *disease* 下词条；**luteal phase d.,** inadequate secretory transformation of the endometrium during the luteal phase of the menstrual cycle; it can cause infertility and habitual abortion 黄体期缺损；**metaphyseal fibrous d.,** 1. fibrous cortical d.；2. nonossifying fibroma 非骨化性纤维瘤；**neural tube d.,** a developmental anomaly of failure of closure of the neural tube, resulting in conditions such as anencephaly or spina bifida 神经管缺陷；**retention d.,** a defect in the power of recalling or remembering names, numbers, or events 记忆缺损；**septal d.,** a defect in a cardiac septum resulting in an abnormal communication between the opposite chambers of the heart 中隔缺损；**ventricular septal d.,** a congenital cardiac anomaly in which there is persistent patency of the ventricular septum in either the muscular or fibrous portions, most often due to failure of the bulbar septum to completely close the interventricular foramen 室间隔缺损

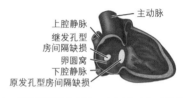

▲ 房间隔缺损（**atrial septal defects**），显示右心房内房间隔缺损和继发孔型缺损的可能位置

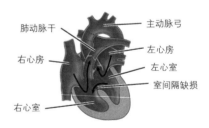

▲ 室间隔缺损（**ventricular septal defect**）心室间传导异常

de·fem·i·ni·za·tion (de-fem″ĭ-nĭ-za′shən) loss of female sexual characteristics 丧失女性特征

de·fense (de-fens′) behavior directed to protection of the individual from injury 防御；**character d.,** any character trait, e.g., a mannerism, attitude, or affectation, which serves as a defense mechanism 性格防御；**insanity d.,** a legal concept that a person cannot be convicted of a crime if the person lacked criminal responsibility by reason of insanity at the time of commission of the crime 精神病辨护

de·fen·sin (de-fen′sin) any of a group of small antimicrobial cationic peptides occurring in neutrophils and macrophages 防御素，防御肽

def·er·ens (def′ər-enz) [L.] deferent 输送的；见 ductus *deferens*

def·er·ent (def′ər-ənt) conveying anything away, as from a center 输运的，输出的

def·er·en·tial (def″ər-en′shəl) pertaining to the ductus deferens 输精管的

def·er·en·ti·tis (def″ər-ən-ti′tis) inflammation of the ductus deferens 输精管炎

de·fer·i·prone (də-fer′ ĭ-prōn) a synthetic iron chelator used in the treatment of transfusional iron overload in patients with thalassemia 去铁酮

de·fer·ox·amine (de″fər-oks′ə-mēn) an ironchelating agent isolated from *Streptomyces pilosus*; used as the mesylate salt as an antidote in iron poisoning 去铁胺

def·er·ves·cence (def″ər-ves′əns) 1. abatement of fever 退热；2. the period of abatement of fever 退热的过程

de·fib·ril·la·tion (de-fib″rĭ-la′shən) termination of atrial or ventricular fibrillation, usually by electroshock 心脏除颤，除颤

de·fib·ril·la·tor (de-fib″rĭ-la′tər) an electronic apparatus used to counteract atrial or ventricular fibrillation by application of a brief electric shock to the heart 除颤器；**automatic external d. (AED)**, a portable defibrillator designed to be automated such that it can be used by persons without substantial medical training who are responding to a cardiac emergency 自动体外除颤器；**automatic implantable cardioverter-d.**, 植入型心律转复除颤器，见 *cardioverter* 下词条

de·fi·bri·na·tion (de-fi″brĭ-na′shən) removal of fibrin from the blood 去纤维蛋白法

de·fi·brino·gen·a·tion (de″fi-brin′ə-jə-na′shən) induced defibrination, as in thrombolytic therapy 诱导降纤

de·fi·bro·tide (dee-fy′brō-tīd) as the sodium salt, a clotting inhibitor that protects endothelial cells from adhesion damage through unclear cellular mechanisms. Administered by intravenous injection in adults and children for the treatment of venoocclusive disease of the liver after hematopoietic stem-cell transplantation 去纤维蛋白多核苷酸

de·fi·cien·cy (de-fish′ən-se) a lack or shortage; a condition characterized by presence of less than normal or necessary supply or competence 缺乏或短缺；不足；**color vision d.**, color blindness; any deviation from normal perception of one or more colors 色盲；**disaccharidase d.**, less than normal

activity of the enzymes of the intestinal mucosa that cleave disaccharides, usually denoting a generalized deficiency of all such enzymes secondary to a disorder of the small intestine 二糖酶缺乏；**factor XⅠd.**, an autosomal disorder due to lack of coagulation factor XⅠ; seen predominantly in persons of Jewish ancestry and characterized by minor bleeding, mild bruising, severe prolonged postsurgical bleeding, and abnormal clotting test times 因子XⅠ缺乏；**familial apolipoprotein C-Ⅱ d.**, a form of familial hyperchylomicronemia due to lack of apo C-Ⅱ, a necessary cofactor for lipoprotein lipase 家族性载脂蛋白 c Ⅱ缺乏症；**familial high-density lipoprotein d.**, any of several inherited disorders of lipoprotein and lipid metabolism that result in decreased plasma levels of HDL, particularly Tangier disease 家族性高密度脂蛋白缺乏；**familial lipoprotein d.**, any inherited disorder of lipoprotein metabolism resulting in deficiency of one or more plasma lipoproteins 家族性脂蛋白缺乏；**molybdenum cofactor d.**, an inherited disorder in which deficiency of the molybdenum cofactor causes deficiency of a variety of enzymes, resulting in severe neurologic abnormalities, dislocated ocular lenses, intellectual disability, xanthinuria, and early death 钼辅因缺乏症；**plasma thromboplastin antecedent d., PTA d.**, factor Ⅸ deficiency 血浆凝血激酶前质；见 *factor Ⅸ*；**selective IgA d.**, the most common immunodeficiency disorder; deficiency of IgA but normal levels of other immunoglobulin classes and normal cellular immunity; it is marked by recurrent sinopulmonary infections, allergy, gastrointestinal disease, and autoimmune diseases 选择性 IgA 缺陷

def·i·cit (def′ĭ-sit) deficiency 缺乏；**oxygen d.**, 氧亏，见 *anoxia*, *hypoxemia* 和 *hypoxia*；**pulse d.**, the difference between the heart rate and the pulse rate in atrial fibrillation 脉搏短绌；**reversible ischemic neurologic d. (RIND)**, a type of cerebral infarction whose clinical course lasts between 24 and 72 hours 可逆性缺血性脑疾病

de·fin·i·tive (də-fin′ə-tiv) 1. established with certainty 有把握；2. in embryology, denoting acquisition of final differentiation or character 在胎儿学中，指最终分化或性状的获得；3. in parasitology, denoting the host in which a parasite reaches the sexual stage 在寄生虫学中，指寄生虫达到有性阶段的宿主

Def·i·tel·i·o (dĕf-ih-tel′ē-yo) trademark for a sodium salt preparation of defibrotide, an anticoagulant used to treat venoocclusive disease of the liver after hematopoietic stem-cell transplantation in adults and children 去纤维钠制剂的商标

de·flec·tion (de-flek′shən) deviation or movement

from a straight line or given course, such as from the baseline in electrocardiography 偏离，偏向

de·flu·vi·um (de-floo′ve-əm) [L.] 1. a flowing down 流下；2. a disappearance 失踪

de·flux·ion (de-fluk′shən) 1. a sudden disappearance 突然消失；2. a copious discharge, as of catarrh 大量排出；3. a falling out, as of hair 脱落

de·form·a·bil·i·ty (de-form″ə-bil′ĭ-te) ability of cells to change shape when passing through narrow spaces, such as erythrocytes might do when passing through the microvasculature 可变形性

de·for·ma·tion (de″for-ma′shən) 1. in dysmorphology, a type of structural defect characterized by the abnormal form or position of a body part, caused by a nondisruptive mechanical force 变形，畸形；2. the process of adapting in shape or form 变形性

de·form·i·ty (də-for′mĭ-te) distortion of any part or of the body in general 变形，畸形；**Åkerlund d.,** an indentation (in addition to the niche) in the duodenal bulb in a radiograph of a duodenal ulcer 阿克隆德变形；**Madelung d.,** radial deviation of the hand secondary to overgrowth of the distal ulna or shortening of the radius 马德隆畸形；**reduction d.,** congenital absence of a portion or all of a body part, especially of the limbs 短缺畸形；**silver fork d.,** the deformity seen in Colles fracture 银叉样畸形；**Sprengel d.,** congenital elevation of the scapula, due to failure of descent of the scapula to its normal thoracic position during fetal life 高位肩胛；**Volkmann d.,** 福尔克曼畸形，见 *disease* 下词条

Deg degeneration 退化，变性，（神经）溃变

de·gen·er·a·cy (de-jen′ər-ə-se) 1. the state of being degenerate 退化的状态；2. the process of degenerating 退化过程；3. d. of code；**d. of code,** the presence in the genetic code of more than one codon encoding a specific amino acid 密码简并

de·gen·er·ate[1] (de-jen′er-āt) to change from a higher to a lower form 退化

de·gen·er·ate[2] (de-jen′er-ət) characterized by degeneration 退化的

de·gen·er·a·tion (de-jen″er-a′shən) deterioration; change from a higher to a lower form, especially change of tissue to a lower or less functionally active form 变质，变性，退化；**degen′erative** *adj.*；**age-related macular d.,** that with onset between the ages of 50 and 60, the leading cause of blindness in the elderly. Most cases are *exudative* or *dry*, with gradual wearing out of retinal pigment cells and loss of central vision. A minority are *exudative* or *wet*, with formation of a neovascular membrane on or near the macula that interferes with vision 老年性黄斑变性；**ascending d.,** wallerian degeneration of centripetal nerve fibers that progresses toward the brain or spinal cord 上行性

变性；**calcareous d.,** degeneration of tissue with deposit of calcareous material 石灰变性；**caseous d.,** caseation (2) 干酪样变性；**cerebromacular d. (CMD), cerebroretinal d.,** 1. degeneration of brain cells and of the macula retinae 大脑黄斑变性；2. any lipidosis with cerebral lesions and degeneration of the macula retinae 大脑视网膜变性；3. any form of neuronal ceroid-lipofuscinosis 神经元蜡样脂褐质沉积症，沉积病；**Crooke hyaline d.,** Crooke hyalinization Crooke 透明变性；**descending d.,** wallerian degeneration that progresses peripherally along nerve fibers 下行性变性；**fatty d.,** deposit of fat globules in a tissue, a type of fatty change 脂肪变性；**fibrinous d.,** necrosis with deposit of fibrin within the cells of the tissue 纤维蛋白变性；**gray d.,** degeneration of the white substance of the spinal cord, in which it loses myelin and assumes a gray color 灰色变性；**hepatolenticular d.,** Wilson disease 肝豆状核变性；**hyaline d.,** a regressive change in cells in which the cytoplasm takes on a homogeneous, glassy appearance; also used loosely to describe the histologic appearance of tissues 玻璃样变性，透明变性；**lattice d. of retina,** an often bilateral, usually benign, asymptomatic condition, characterized by patches of fine gray or white intersecting lines in the peripheral retina, usually with numerous round punched-out areas of retinal thinning or retinal holes 视网膜格子样变性；**macular d.,** degenerative changes in the macula lutea, including *age-related macular d.* and several inherited forms (Best disease, Stargardt disease) 黄斑变性；**mucoid d.,** that with deposit of myelin and lecithin in the cells. 黏液样变；**myxomatous d.,** degeneration in which mucoid material accumulates in connective tissues. 黏液瘤样变性；**spongy d. of central nervous system, spongy d. of white matter,** a rare hereditary form of leukodystrophy of early onset in which widespread demyelination and vacuolation of cerebral white matter gives it a spongy appearance; there is intellectual disability, megalocephaly, atony of neck muscles, limb spasticity, and blindness, with death in infancy 中枢神经系统海绵状变性，白质海绵状变性；**striatonigral d.,** a form of multiple system atrophy with nerve cell degeneration mainly in the region of the substantia nigra and the neostriatum; symptoms are similar to those of parkinsonism 纹状体黑质变性；**subacute combined d. of spinal cord,** degeneration of posterior and lateral columns of the spinal cord, with various motor and sensory disturbances; it is due to vitamin B_{12} deficiency and usually associated with pernicious anemia 脊髓亚急性联合变性；**tapetoretinal d.,** degeneration of the pigmented layer of the retina 毯层视网膜变性；**transneuronal**

d., atrophy of certain neurons after interruption of afferent axons or death of other neurons to which they send their efferent output 跨神经元变性；**wallerian d.,** fatty degeneration of a nerve fiber that has been severed from its nutritive centers 沃勒变性；**Zenker d.,** hyaline degeneration and necrosis of striated muscle 蜡样坏死

de·glov·ing (de-gluv′ing) avulsion of skin from underlying structures 脱套

de·glu·ti·tion (deg″loo-tish′ən) swallowing 吞咽

deg·ra·da·tion (deg″rə-da′shən) conversion of a chemical compound to one less complex, as by splitting off one or more groups of atoms 降解

deg·ron (deg′rən) a sequence of amino acids that acts as a signal targeting unstable proteins for degradation. Those at the N-terminus of proteins, called N-degrons, are substrates of the N-end rule pathway (q.v.) 降解决定子

de·gus·ta·tion (de″gəs-ta′shən) tasting 尝味

de·his·cence (de-his′əns) a splitting open 裂开，劈开；**uterine d.,** rupture of the uterus following cesarean section, especially separation of the uterine scar prior to or during a subsequent labor 子宫破裂；**wound d.,** separation of the layers of a surgical wound 伤口裂开

de·hy·dra·tase (de-hi′drə-tās) a common name for a hydro-lyase 脱水酶

de·hy·drate (de-hi′drāt) to remove water from (a compound, the body, etc.) 脱水

de·hy·dra·tion (de″hi-dra′shən) 1. removal of water from a substance 脱水；2. the condition that results from excessive loss of body water 脱水作用；**hypernatremic d.,** a condition in which electrolyte losses are disproportionately smaller than water losses 高钠性失血

7-de·hy·dro·cho·les·ter·ol (de-hi″dro-kə-les′tər-ol) a sterol present in skin, which, on ultraviolet irradiation, produces vitamin D 7- 脱氢胆固醇；**activated 7-d.,** cholecalciferol 活化 7- 脱氢胆固醇

11-de·hy·dro·cor·ti·cos·ter·one (de-hi″dro-kor″tĭ-kos′tər-ōn) a steroid produced by the adrenal cortex 11- 脱氢皮质酮

de·hy·dro·epi·an·dros·ter·one **(DHEA)** (de-hi″dro-ep″e-an-dros′tər-ōn) a steroid secreted by the adrenal cortex, the major androgen precursor in females; often present in excessive amounts in patients with adrenal virilism 脱氢表雄酮

de·hy·dro·gen·ase (de-hi′dro-jən″ās) an enzyme that catalyzes the transfer of hydrogen or electrons from a donor, oxidizing it, to an acceptor, reducing it 脱氢酶

de·hy·dro·ret·i·nol (de-hi″dro-ret′ ĭ-nol) vitamin A₂, a form of vitamin A found with retinol (vitamin

A₁) in freshwater fish; it has one more conjugated double bond than retinol and approximately one-third its biologic activity 脱氢视黄醇

de·ion·iza·tion (de-i″on-ĭ-za′shən) the production of a mineral-free state by the removal of ions 去离子化，去离子（作用）

dé·jà vu (da′zhah voo′) [Fr.] an illusion that a new situation is a repetition of a previous experience 似曾相识

de·jec·tion (de-jek′shən) a mental state marked by sadness; the lowered mood characteristic of depression 沮丧，情绪低落

de·lam·i·na·tion (de-lam″ĭ-na′shən) separation into layers, as of the blastoderm 分层，如胚层

del·a·vir·dine (del″ə-vir′dēn) an antiretroviral, inhibiting reverse transcriptase; used as the mesylate salt in the treatment of HIV infection 地拉韦啶一种抗逆转录病毒，抑制逆转录酶；其甲磺酸盐用于治疗 HIV 感染

de·layed-re·lease (de-lād′ re-lēs′) releasing a drug at a time later than that immediately following its administration 缓控释

de-lead (de-led′) to induce the removal of lead from tissues and its excretion in the urine by the administration of chelating agents 除铅

del·e·te·ri·ous (del″ə-tēr′e-əs) injurious; harmful 有害的

de·le·tion (də-le′shən) in genetics, loss of genetic material from a chromosome 缺失

Delf·tia (delf′te-ə) a genus of aerobic, gramnegative, motile, rod-shaped bacteria; *D. acidovo′rans* (formerly classified in the genus *Pseudomonas*) is an opportunistic pathogen 代尔夫特菌属

de·lin·quent (də-ling′kwənt) 1. failing to do that which is required by law or obligation 失职的；2. a person who neglects a legal obligation 犯罪者

del·i·ques·cence (del″ĭ-kwes′əns) dampness or liquefaction from the absorption of water from air 潮解；**deliques′cent** *adj.*

de·lir·i·um (də-lēr′e-əm) pl. *deli′ria.* A mental disturbance of relatively short duration usually reflecting a toxic state, marked by illusions, hallucinations, delusions, excitement, restlessness, impaired memory, and incoherence 谵妄，发狂，妄想；**alcohol withdrawal d,** that caused by cessation or reduction in alcohol consumption, typically in alcoholics with many years of heavy drinking, characterized by autonomic hyperactivity, such as tachycardia, sweating, and hypertension; a coarse, irregular tremor; delusions, vivid hallucinations, wild, agitated behavior; and possible seizures 戒酒性谵妄；**d. tre′mens,** alcohol withdrawal d. 震颤性谵妄

de·liv·ery (de-liv′ər-e) expulsion or extraction of the child and fetal membranes at birth 分 娩; **abdominal d.**, delivery of an infant through an incision made into the intact uterus through the abdominal wall 剖宫产; **breech d.**, delivery in which the fetal buttocks present first 臀先露; **forceps d.**, extraction of the child from the maternal passages by application of forceps to the fetal head; designated *low* or *midforceps delivery* according to the degree of engagement of the fetal head and *high* when engagement has not occurred 产钳分娩; **postmortem d.**, delivery of a child after death of the mother 死后分娩; **spontaneous d.**, birth of an infant without any aid from an attendant 顺产，自然分娩

del·le (del′ə) the clear area in the center of a stained erythrocyte 小凹

del·ta (del′tə) 1. the fourth letter of the Greek alphabet 希腊字母的第四个字母；另见 δ-; 2. a triangular area 三角形区域

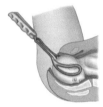

▲ 产钳分娩（**forceps delivery**）

Del·ta·ret·ro·vi·rus (del″tə-ret′ro-vi″rəs) a genus of the family Retroviridae; the species human T-lymphotropic viruses 1 and 2 can cause B- and T-cell leukemia and lymphoma and neurologic disease 丁型逆转录病毒属

del·toid (del′toid) 1. triangular 三角（形）的; 2. the deltoid muscle 三角肌

de·lu·sion (də-loo′zhən) an idiosyncratic false belief that is firmly maintained in spite of incontrovertible and obvious proof or evidence to the contrary 妄 想; **delu′sional** *adj.*; **bizarre d.**, one that is patently absurd, with no possible basis in fact 怪 异 妄 想; **d. of control,** the delusion that one's thoughts, feelings, and actions are not one's own but are being imposed by someone else or other external force 受控妄想; **depressive d.**, one that is congruent with a predominant depressed mood 抑郁性妄想; **erotomanic d.**, one associated with erotomania 爱恋妄想; **d. of grandeur, grandiose d.**, delusional conviction of one's own importance, power, or knowledge or that one is, or has a special relationship with, a deity or a famous person 夸大妄想; **d. of jealousy,** a delusional belief that one's spouse or lover is unfaithful, based on erroneous inferences drawn from innocent events imagined to be evidence 妒忌妄想; **mixed d.,** one in which no central theme predominates 混 合 妄 想; **d. of negation, nihilistic d.**, a depressive delusion that the self or part of the self, part of the body, other persons, or the whole world has ceased to exist 否认妄想; **d. of persecution,** a delusion that one is being attacked, harassed, persecuted, cheated, or conspired against 受迫害妄想; **d. of reference,** a delusional conviction that ordinary events, objects, or behaviors of others have particular and unusual meanings specifically for oneself 关系妄想，牵扯妄想; **systematized d's,** a group of delusions organized around a common theme 系统化妄想

De·man·sia (de-man′se-ə) a genus of venomous snakes of the family Elapidae, including the brown snake of Australia and New Guinea 褐眼镜蛇属

de·mat·i·a·ceous (de-mat″e-a′shəs) dark brown to black in color 暗色孢科真菌的

dem·e·ca·ri·um (dem″ə-kar′e-əm) an anticholinesterase agent used topically as the bromide salt in the treatment of glaucoma and accommodative esotropia 癸二胺苯酯（抗胆碱酯酶药）

dem·e·clo·cy·cline (dem″ə-klo-si′klēn) a broad-spectrum tetracycline antibiotic produced by a mutant strain of *Streptomyces aureofaciens* or semisynthetically; used as the hydrochloride salt 地美环素

de·men·tia (də-men′shə) a general loss of cognitive abilities, including impairment of memory as well as one or more of the following: aphasia, apraxia, agnosia, or disturbed planning, organizing, and abstract thinking abilities. It does not include decreased cognitive functioning due to clouding of consciousness, depression, or other functional mental disorder 痴 呆; **Alzheimer d.**, 阿尔茨海默病，见 *disease* 下词条; **d. of the Alzheimer type,** dementia of insidious onset and gradually progressive course, with histopathologic changes characteristic of Alzheimer disease, categorized as *early onset* or *late onset* depending on whether or not it begins by the age of 65 阿尔茨海默型痴呆; **arteriosclerotic d.**, multi-infarct dementia as a result of cerebral arteriosclerosis. 动脉硬化性痴呆; **Binswanger d.**, 宾斯万格氏痴呆，见 *disease* 下词条; **boxer's d.**, a syndrome due to cumulative cerebral injuries in football, boxing, and other sports, with forgetfulness, slowness in thinking, dysarthric speech, and slow uncertain movements, especially of the legs 拳击员痴呆; **multi-infarct d.**, vascular d. 多发梗死性痴呆; **paralytic d., d. paraly′tica,** general paresis 麻痹性痴呆; **presenile d.**, that occurring in younger persons, usually age 65 or younger; since most cases are due to Alzheimer disease, the term is sometimes used as a synonym of *d. of the Alzheimer type, early onset*, and has also been used to denote *Alzheimer disease* 早老性痴呆；**senile d.**, that occurring in older persons, usually over the age of 65; since most cases are due to Alzheimer disease, the term is sometimes used as a synonym of *d. of the Alzheimer type, late onset* 老年性痴呆；**subcortical d.**, any of a group of dementias thought to be caused by lesions particularly affecting subcortical brain structures, characterized by memory loss with slowness of information processing and of the formation of intellectual responses 皮质下痴呆；**substance-induced persisting d.**, that resulting from exposure to or use or abuse of a substance (e.g., alcohol, sedatives, anticonvulsants, or lead) but persisting long after exposure ends, usually with permanent and worsening deficits 物质诱导持久性痴呆；**vascular d.**, that with a stepwise deteriorating course and a patchy distribution of neurologic deficits caused by cerebrovascular disease 血管性痴呆

de·min·er·al·iza·tion (de-min″ər-əl-ī-za′shən) excessive elimination of mineral or organic salts from tissues of the body 去矿化

Dem·o·dex (dem′o-deks) a genus of mites parasitic within the hair follicles of the host, including the species *D. folliculo′rum* in humans 蠕螨属

de·mog·ra·phy (de-mog′rə-fe) the statistical science dealing with populations, including matters of health, disease, births, and mortality 人口学

de·mul·cent (de-mul′sənt) 1. soothing; bland 舒缓的，平淡，镇痛的；2. a soothing mucilaginous or oily medicine or application 镇痛药，润滑剂，缓和剂

de·my·elin·a·tion (de-mi″ə-lĭn-a′shən) destruction, removal, or loss of the myelin sheath of a nerve or nerves 脱髓鞘；**segmental d.**, degeneration of the myelin sheath in segments between successive nodes of Ranvier, with preservation of the axon 节段性脱髓鞘

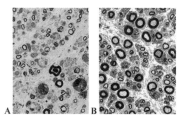

▲ 脱髓鞘多根神经根病变的腓肠神经横截面。**A.** 节段性脱髓鞘（**segmental demyelination**）。**B.** 相对不受影响的区域

de·na·sal·i·ty (de″na-zal′ĭ-te) hyponasality 鼻音过少

de·na·tur·a·tion (de-na″chər-a′shən) destruction of the usual nature of a substance, as by the addition of methanol or acetone to alcohol to render it unfit for drinking, or the change in the physical properties of a substance, as a protein or nucleic acid, caused by heat or certain chemicals that alter tertiary structure 变性

den·drite (den′drīt) one of the threadlike extensions of the cytoplasm of a neuron, which typically branch into treelike processes; they compose most of the receptive surface of a neuron 树突

den·drit·ic (den-drit′ik) 1. pertaining to or possessing dendrites 关于或拥有树突的；2. arborescent 具树状突的

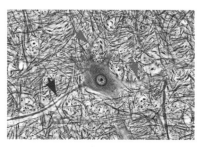

▲ 脊髓灰质染色制备过程中运动神经元的树突（**dendrite**）（浅箭）和轴突（深箭）

Den·dro·as·pis (den″dro-as′pis) a genus of extremely venomous African snakes of the family Elapidae, related to cobras but lacking a dilatable hood. *D. angus′ticeps* is the green mamba and *D. polyle′pis* is the black mamba 树眼镜蛇属

den·dro·den·drit·ic (den″dro-den-drit′ik) referring to a synapse between dendrites of two neurons 树突间的

den·dro·phago·cy·to·sis (den″dro-fa″gosi-to′sis) the absorption by microglial cells of broken portions of astrocytes 噬胞突作用

de·ner·va·tion (de″nər-va′shən) interruption of the nerve connection to an organ or part 失神经支配，去神经

den·gue (deng′ge) [Sp.] dān′ga an infectious, eruptive, febrile, viral disease of tropical areas, transmitted by *Aedes* mosquitoes, and marked by severe pains in the head, eyes, muscles, and joints, sore throat, catarrhal symptoms, and sometimes a skin eruption and painful swellings of parts 登革热；**hemorrhagic d.**, a severe form of dengue characterized by hemorrhagic manifestations such as thrombocytopenia and hemoconcentration 出血性登革热

de·ni·al (də-ni′əl) a type of defense mechanism in which the existence of unpleasant internal or external realities is kept out of conscious awareness 否认，否定

den·i·da·tion (den″ĭ-da′shən) degeneration and expulsion of the endometrium during the menstrual cycle 经期子宫内膜脱落

den·i·leu·kin dif·ti·tox (den″ĭ-loo′kin dif′tĭ-toks) a genetically engineered construct combining amino acid sequences for specific diphtheria toxin fragments linked to sequences for interleukin-2 (IL-2); used as an antineoplastic 一种将特定白喉毒素片段与白细胞介素 -2(IL-2) 连接的氨基酸序列组合的基因工程结构；用于抗肿瘤

dens (dens) pl. *den′tes* [L.] 1. tooth 牙齿；2. a toothlike structure 齿突；3. dens axis; the toothlike process that projects from the superior surface of the body of the axis, ascending to articulate with the atlas 牙轴；d. in den′te, a malformed tooth caused by invagination of the crown before it is calcified, giving the appearance of a "tooth within a tooth." 牙中牙

den·si·tom·e·try (den″sĭ-tom′ə-tre) determination of variations in density by comparison with that of another material or with a certain standard 密度测量法

den·si·ty (den′sĭ-te) 1. the quality of being compact or dense 密度；2. quantity per unit space, e.g., the mass of matter per unit volume. Symbol *d*. 物质密度；3. the degree of darkening of exposed and processed photographic or x-ray film 暗度

den·tal (den′təl) pertaining to a tooth or teeth 牙齿或与牙齿有关的

den·tal ce·ram·ics (den-tul suh-ram′icks) the use of porcelain and similar materials in restorative dentistry 牙科陶瓷

den·tal·gia (den-tal′jə) toothache 牙痛

den·tate (den′tāt) notched; tooth-shaped 有缺口的；齿状的

den·tes (den′tēz) [L.] plural of *dens* 牙，齿

den·tia (den′shə) a condition relating to development or eruption of the teeth 出牙；d. prae′cox, premature eruption of the teeth; presence of teeth in the mouth at birth 乳牙早出；d. tar′da, delayed eruption of the teeth, beyond the usual time for their appearance 迟出牙

den·ti·buc·cal (den″tĭ-buk′əl) pertaining to the cheek and teeth 牙颊的

den·ti·cle (den′tĭ-kəl) 1. a small toothlike process 小齿状突起；2. a distinct calcified mass within the pulp chamber of a tooth 牙髓石

den·ti·frice (den′tĭ-fris) a preparation for cleansing and polishing the teeth; it may contain a thera-

peutic agent, such as fluoride, to inhibit dental caries 洁牙剂

den·tig·er·ous (den-tij′ər-əs) bearing or having teeth 有牙齿的

den·ti·la·bi·al (den″tĭ-la′be-əl) pertaining to the teeth and lips 牙唇的

den·tin (den′tin) the chief substance of the teeth, surrounding the tooth pulp and covered by enamel on the crown and by cementum on the roots 牙本质。Spelled also *dentine*. **den′tinal** *adj*.; **adventitious d.**, secondary d.; **circumpulpal d.**, the inner portion of dentin, adjacent to the pulp, consisting of thinner fibrils 髓周牙质；**cover d.**, the peripheral portion of dentin, adjacent to the enamel or cementum, consisting of coarser fibers than the circumpulpal d. 罩牙本质；**irregular d.**, secondary d.; **mantle d.**, cover d.; **opalescent d.**, dentin giving an unusual translucent or opalescent appearance to the teeth, as occurs in dentinogenesis imperfecta 乳光牙本质；**primary d.**, dentin formed before the eruption of a tooth 原发性牙本质；**secondary d.**, new dentin formed in response to stimuli associated with the normal aging process or with pathologic conditions, such as caries or injury, or cavity preparation 继发性牙本质；**transparent d.**, dentin in which some dentinal tubules have become sclerotic or calcified, producing the appearance of translucency 透明牙本质

den·ti·no·ce·men·tal (den″tĭ-no-sə-men′təl) pertaining to the dentin and the cementum 齿骨质的

den·ti·no·enam·el (den″tĭ-no-ə-nam′əl) pertaining to the dentin and the enamel 齿本质和釉质的

den·ti·no·gen·e·sis (den″tĭ-no-jen′ə-sis) the formation of dentin 牙本质发生；d. imperfec′ta, a hereditary condition marked by imperfect formation and calcification of dentin, giving the teeth a brown or blue opalescent appearance 牙本质发生不全

den·ti·no·gen·ic (den″tĭ-no-jen′ik) forming or producing dentin 牙本质生成的

den·ti·no·ma (den″tĭ-no′mə) an odontogenic tumor consisting mainly of dysplastic dentin 牙本质瘤

den·tist (den′tist) a person with a degree in dentistry and authorized to practice dentistry 牙医

den·tis·try (den′tis-tre) 1. that branch of the healing arts concerned with the teeth, oral cavity, and associated structures, including prevention, diagnosis, and treatment of disease and restoration of defective or missing tissue 口腔医学；2. the work done by dentists, e.g., the creation of restorations, crowns, and bridges, and surgical procedures performed in and about the oral cavity 牙科技术；holistic d., dental practice that takes into account the effect of dental treatment and materials on the overall health of the individual 整体牙医学；**operative d.,** dentistry concerned with restoration of parts of the teeth that are defective as a result of disease, trauma, or abnormal development to a state of normal function, health, and esthetics 牙体修复学；**pediatric d.,** pedodontics 儿童牙科；**preventive d.,** dentistry concerned with maintenance of a normal masticating mechanism by fortifying the structures of the oral cavity against damage and disease 预防牙科学；**prosthetic d.,** prosthodontics 牙修复学；**restorative d.,** dentistry concerned with the restoration of existing teeth that are defective because of disease, trauma, or abnormal development to normal function, health, and appearance; it includes crowns and bridgework 牙修复学

den·ti·tion (den-tish′ən) the teeth in the dental arch; ordinarily used to designate the natural teeth in position in their alveoli 齿列，牙列；**deciduous d.,** 乳齿齿系，见 *tooth* 下词条；**mixed d.,** the complement of teeth in the jaws after eruption of some of the permanent teeth, but before all the deciduous teeth are shed 混合牙列；**permanent d.,** 恒牙列，见 *tooth* 下词条；**precocious d.,** abnormally accelerated appearance of the deciduous or permanent teeth 出牙过早；**primary d.,** deciduous teeth 乳牙列，见 *tooth* 下词条；**retarded d.,** abnormally delayed appearance of the deciduous or permanent teeth 出牙延迟

den·to·al·ve·o·lar (den″to-al-ve′ə-lər) pertaining to a tooth and its alveolus 牙槽的

den·to·fa·cial (den″to-fa′shəl) of or pertaining to the teeth and alveolar process and the face 牙面的

den·to·tro·pic (den″to-tro′pik) turning toward or having an affinity for tissues composing the teeth 亲牙的

den·tu·lous (den′tu-ləs) having natural teeth 有天然牙的

den·ture (den′chər) a complement of teeth, either natural or artificial; ordinarily used to designate an artificial replacement for the natural teeth and adjacent tissues 义齿，牙列；**complete d.,** an appliance replacing all the teeth of one jaw, as well as associated structures of the jaw 全口义齿；**implant d.,** one constructed with a metal substructure embedded within the underlying soft structures of the jaws 种植义齿；**interim d.,** a denture to be used for a short interval of time for reasons of esthetics, mastication, occlusal support, or convenience, or to condition the patient to the acceptance of an artificial substitute for missing natural teeth until more definitive prosthetic dental treatment can be provided 暂时义齿；**overlay d.,** a complete den-

ture supported both by soft tissue (mucosa) and by a few remaining natural teeth that have been altered, as by insertion of a long or short coping, to permit the denture to fit over them 覆盖义齿；**partial d.,** a dental appliance that is removable (*removable partial d.*) or permanently attached (*fixed partial d.* or *bridge*) and replaces one or more missing teeth, receiving support and retention from underlying tissues and some or all of the remaining teeth 部分义齿；**provisional d.,** an interim denture used for the purpose of conditioning the patient to the acceptance of an artificial substitute for missing natural teeth 临时托牙；**transitional d.,** a partial denture that is to serve as a temporary prosthesis; teeth will be added to it as more teeth are lost, and it will be replaced after postextraction tissue changes have occurred 过渡义齿

de·nu·da·tion (den″u-da′shən) the stripping or laying bare of any part 剥光或裸露任何部分

de·odor·ant (de-o′dər-ənt) 1. masking offensive odors 掩蔽进攻性气味；2. an agent that so acts 除臭剂

de·or·sum·duc·tion (de-or″səm-duk′shən) infraduction 下转（眼）

de·os·si·fi·ca·tion (de-os″ĭ-fĭ-ka′shən) loss or removal of the mineral elements of bone 除骨质，骨质缺损

deoxy- chemical prefix designating a compound containing one less oxygen atom than the reference substance 脱氧；另见 *desoxy-* 开头的词条

de·oxy·chol·ic ac·id (de-ok″se-ko′lik) a secondary bile acid formed from cholic acid in the intestine; it is a choleretic 脱氧胆酸

de·oxy·he·mo·glo·bin (de-ok″se-he′moglo″bin) hemoglobin not combined with oxygen, formed when oxyhemoglobin releases its oxygen to the tissues 去氧血红蛋白

de·oxy·ri·bo·nu·cle·ase (DNase) (de-ok″seri″bo-noo′kle-ās) any nuclease catalyzing the cleavage of phosphate ester linkages in deoxyribonucleic acids (DNA); separated by whether they cleave internal bonds or bonds at termini 脱氧核糖核酸酶，DNA 酶

de·oxy·ri·bo·nu·cle·ic ac·id (DNA) (de-ok″seri″bo-noo-kle′ik) the nucleic acid in which the sugar is deoxyribose; composed also of phosphoric acid and the bases adenine, guanine, cytosine, and thymine. It constitutes the primary genetic material of all cellular organisms and the DNA viruses and occurs predominantly in the nucleus, usually as a double helix (q.v.), where it serves as a template for synthesis of ribonucleic acid (transcription). It is duplicated by replication 脱氧核糖核酸

de·oxy·ri·bo·nu·cleo·pro·tein (de-ok″seri″bo-noo″kle-o-pro′tēn) a nucleoprotein in which the sugar is d-2-deoxyribose 脱氧糖核蛋白

de·oxy·ri·bo·nu·cleo·side (de-ok″se-ri″bonoo′kle-o-sīd) a nucleoside having a purine or pyrimidine base bonded to deoxyribose 脱氧核苷

de·oxy·ri·bo·nu·cleo·tide (de-ok″se-ri″-bonoo′kle-o-tīd) a nucleotide having a purine or pyrimidine base bonded to deoxyribose, which in turn is bonded to a phosphate group 脱氧核苷酸

de·oxy·ri·bose (de-ok″se-ri′bōs) a deoxypentose found in deoxyribonucleic acids (DNA), deoxyribonucleotides, and deoxyribonucleosides 脱氧核糖

de·oxy·ri·bo·vi·rus (de-ok″se-ri′bo-vi″rəs) DNA virus DNA 病毒

de·oxy·uri·dine (de-ok″se-ūr′ ī-dēn) a pyrimidine nucleoside, uracil linked to deoxyribose; its triphosphate derivative is an intermediate in the synthesis of deoxyribonucleotides 脱氧尿苷

de·pen·dence (de-pen′dəns) 1. a state of relying on or requiring the aid of something 依赖; 2. a state in which there is a compulsive or chronic need, as for a drug; 见 substance d.; **drug d.**, **psychoactive substance d.**, **substance d.**, 1. compulsive use of a substance despite significant problems resulting from such use. Although tolerance and withdrawal were previously defined as necessary and sufficient for dependence, they are currently only two of several possible criteria 作用于精神物质依赖; 2. substance abuse 药物依赖

de·pen·den·cy (de-pen′dən-se) reliance on others for love, affection, mothering, comfort, security, food, warmth, shelter, protection, and the like—the so-called dependency needs 依靠, 依赖, 附属

de·pen·dent (de-pen′dənt) 1. exhibiting dependence or dependency 依赖性或依赖性的; 2. hanging down 下垂的

De·pen·do·vi·rus (də-pen′do-vi″rəs) adenoassociated viruses; a genus of viruses of the family Parvoviridae that require coinfection with an adenovirus or herpesvirus to provide a helper function for replication; asymptomatic human infection is common 德佩多病毒, 依赖性病毒

de·per·son·al·iza·tion (de-pur″sən-əl-īza′shən) alteration in the perception of self so that the usual sense of one's own reality is temporarily lost or changed; it may be a manifestation of a neurosis or another mental disorder or can occur in mild form in normal persons 人格解体

dep·i·la·tion (dep″ī-la′shən) epilation; removal of hair by the roots 脱毛术

de·pil·a·to·ry (də-pil′ə-tor″e) 1. having the power to remove hair 有脱毛能力的; 2. an agent for removing

or destroying hair 脱毛药

de·ple·tion (də-ple′shən) the act or process of emptying or removing, as of fluid from a body compartment 排空或除去液体的行为或过程

de·po·lar·iza·tion (de-po″lər-ī-za′shən) 1. the process or act of neutralizing polarity 去极化; 2. in electrophysiology, reversal of the resting potential in excitable cell membranes when stimulated 退偏振; **atrial premature d. (APD)**, 房性早搏去极化; 见 complex 下词条; **ventricular premature d. (VPD)**, 室性期前收缩, 见 complex 下词条

de·po·lym·er·iza·tion (de″pə-lim″ər-ī-za′shən) the conversion of a polymer into its component monomers 解聚

de·pos·it (de-poz′it) 1. sediment or dregs 沉积物或渣; 2. extraneous inorganic matter collected in the tissues or in an organ of the body 沉淀

de·pot (de′po) (dep′o) a body area in which a substance, e.g., a drug, can be accumulated, deposited, or stored and from which it can be distributed 脂肪贮存

L-dep·re·nyl- (dep′rē-nil) selegiline 丙炔苯丙胺

de·pres·sant (de-pres′ənt) diminishing any functional activity; an agent that so acts 镇静作用的, 抑制药; **cardiac d.**, an agent that depresses the rate or force of contraction of the heart 心脏抑制药

de·pressed (de-prest′) 1. below the normal level 低于正常水平; 2. associated with psychological depression 与心理抑郁有关

de·pres·sion (de-presh′ən) 1. a hollow or depressed area; downward or inward displacement 凹陷; 2. a lowering or decrease of functional activity 压低, 阻抑; 3. a mental state of altered mood characterized by feelings of sadness, despair, and discouragement 抑郁症; **depres′sive adj.**; **agitated d.**, major depressive disorder accompanied by more or less constant activity 激越性抑郁; **anaclitic d.**, impairment of an infant's physical, social, and intellectual development resulting from absence of mothering 依赖性抑郁症; **congenital chondrosternal d.**, congenital deformity with a deep, funnel-shaped depression in the anterior chest wall 先天性肋软骨胸骨凹陷; **endogenous d.**, a type caused by an intrinsic biologic or somatic process rather than an environmental influence; in contrast to a reactive depression 内源性抑郁; **major d.**, major depressive disorder 重度抑郁症; **neurotic d.**, one that is not a psychotic depression (q.v.); used sometimes broadly to indicate any depression without psychotic features and sometimes more narrowly to denote only milder forms of depression 神经症性抑郁; **pacchionian d's**, small pits on the internal cranium on either side of the groove for the superior sagittal sinus, occupied by the arachnoid granulations 帕基奥尼凹陷；**psychotic d.**, major depressive disorder with psychotic features, such as hallucinations, delusions, mutism, or stupor 精神病性抑郁；**reactive d., situational d.**, a usually transient depression that is precipitated by a stressful life event or other environmental factor 反应性抑郁（症）；cf. *endogenous d.*；**unipolar d.**, depression that is not accompanied by episodes of mania or hypomania, as in major depressive disorder or dysthymic disorder; the term is sometimes used to denote the former specifically 单相抑郁（症）

de·pres·sor (de-pres′ər) 1. that which causes depression, as a muscle, agent, or instrument 抑制；2. depressor nerve 抑制药

dep·ri·va·tion (dep″rĭ-va′shən) loss or absence of parts, powers, or things that are needed 剥夺；**emotional d.**, deprivation of adequate and appropriate interpersonal or environmental experience in the early developmental years 情感剥夺；**sensory d.**, deprivation of usual external stimuli and the opportunity for perception 感觉剥夺

depth (depth) distance measured perpendicularly downward from a surface 深度；**focal d., d. of focus,** the measure of the power of a lens to yield clear images of objects at different distances 焦深

de·rail·ment (de-rāl′ment) disordered thought or speech characteristic of schizophrenia and marked by constant jumping from one topic to another before the first is fully realized 思维或语言紊乱

de·re·al·i·za·tion (de-re″əl-ĭ-za′shən) a loss of the sensation of the reality of one's surroundings 现实解体

de·re·ism (de′re-iz-əm) dereistic thinking 脱离现实

de·re·is·tic (de″re-is′tik) directed away from reality; not using normal logic 空想癖的；见 *thinking* 下词条

de·re·pres·sion (de″re-presh′ən) removal of repression of a gene or operon, leading to or enhancing gene expression 去阻遏作用

de·riv·a·tive (də-riv′ə-tiv) a chemical substance produced from another substance either directly or by modification or partial substitution 衍生物

Der·ma·bac·ter (dur″mə-bak″tər) a genus of gram-positive, facultatively anaerobic actinomycetes of the family Dermabacteraceae; *D. ho′minis* is a normal inhabitant of the human skin and an opportunistic pathogen 皮杆菌属

Der·ma·bac·te·ra·ceae (dur″mə-bak-tərə′se-e) a family of gram-positive, facultatively anaerobic, non–spore-forming bacteria of the suborder Micrococcineae 微球菌亚纲的革兰阳性、兼性厌氧菌，非孢子形成菌

derm·abra·sion (dur″mə-bra′zhən) planing of the skin by mechanical means, e.g., sandpaper, wire brushes 皮肤磨削术，见 *planing*

Der·ma·cen·tor (dur″mə-sen′tər) a genus of ticks that are important transmitters of disease. *D. ander-so′ni* is parasitic in various wild mammals and transmits Rocky Mountain spotted fever, Colorado tick fever, tularemia, and tick paralysis. *D. varia′bi-lis* is usually parasitic in dogs but also attacks cattle, horses, rabbits, and humans and is the chief vector of Rocky Mountain spotted fever in the central and eastern United States 革蜱

der·mal (dur′məl) pertaining to the dermis or to the skin 真皮的，皮肤的

Der·ma·nys·sus (dur″mə-nis′əs) a genus of mites. *D. galli′nae* is the bird or chicken mite, which sometimes infests humans 皮刺螨属

der·ma·ti·tis (dur″mə-ti′tis) pl. *dermati′tides.* Inflammation of the skin 皮炎；**actinic d.**, dermatitis due to exposure to actinic radiation, such as that from the sun, ultraviolet waves, or x- or gamma radiation 光化性皮炎；**allergic d.**, 1. atopic d.; 2. allergic contact d.；**allergic contact d.**, contact dermatitis due to allergic sensitization 变应性接触性皮炎；**atopic d.**, a chronic inflammatory, pruritic, eczematous skin disorder in individuals with a hereditary predisposition to cutaneous pruritus; often accompanied by allergic rhinitis, hay fever, and asthma 特应性皮炎；**berlock d.**, dermatitis of the neck, face, or chest, caused by exposure to a toilet article containing bergamot oil followed by exposure to sunlight 伯洛克皮炎；**cercarial d.**, an itching dermatitis due to penetration into the skin of larval forms (cercaria) of schistosomes, found in those who bathe in infested waters 尾蚴性皮炎；**chronic actinic d. (CAD)**, a long-term form of photosensitivity dermatitis with an eczematous reaction to sunlight; the etiology is unknown, but sometimes it may be a continuation of photoallergic contact dermatitis after the allergen has been removed 慢性光化性皮炎；**contact d.**, acute or chronic dermatitis caused by substances contacting the skin; it may involve allergic or nonallergic mechanisms 接触性皮炎；**diaper d.**, 尿布皮炎，见 *rash* 下词条；**d. exfoliati′va neonato′rum**, staphylococcal scalded skin syndrome 葡萄球菌烫伤样皮肤综合征；**exfoliative d.**, widespread erythema, desquamation, scaling, and itching of the skin, with loss of hair 剥脱性皮炎；**factitial d.**, any of various types of self-inflicted lesions, usually produced by mechanical means, burning, or application of chemical irritants or caustics 人工性皮

D

炎；**d. herpetifor′mis,** pruritic chronic dermatitis with successive groups of symmetrical, erythematous, papular, vesicular, eczematous, or bullous lesions, usually associated with asymptomatic gluten-sensitive enteropathy 疱疹样皮炎；**infectious eczematous d.,** a pustular eczematoid eruption arising from a primary lesion that is the source of an infectious exudate 传染性湿疹样皮炎；**insect d.,** a transient skin eruption caused by the toxin-containing irritant hairs of insects such as certain moths and their caterpillars昆虫皮炎；**irritant d.,** a nonallergic type of contact dermatitis due to exposure to a substance that damages the skin 刺激性皮炎；**livedoid d.,** local pain, swelling, livedoid changes, and increased temperature; due to temporary or prolonged local ischemia from vasculitis or from accidental arterial obliteration during intragluteal administration of medications 青斑状皮炎；**meadow d., meadow grass d.,** phytophotodermatitis with eruption of vesicles and bullae in streaks or other config-urations, caused by exposure to sunlight after contact with meadow grass 草地皮炎；**nickel d.,** a type of contact dermatitis from prolonged expo-sure to nickel, such as from jewelry 镍 皮 炎；**photoallergic contact d., photocontact d.,** allergic contact dermatitis caused by the action of sunlight on skin sensitized by contact with substances such as halogenated salicylanilides, sandalwood oil, or hexachlorophene 光变应性接触性皮炎，光接触性皮炎；**photosensitivity d.,** any dermatitis occurring as a manifestation of photosensitivity 光敏性皮炎；**phototoxic d.,** erythema followed by hyperpigmentation of sun-exposed areas of the skin due to exposure to agents containing photosensitizing substances, such as coal tar and psoralen-containing perfumes, drugs, or plants, and then to sunlight 光毒性皮炎；**poison ivy d.,** allergic contact dermatitis due to exposure to plants of the genus *Rhus*, which contain urushiol, a skin-sensitizing agent 野 葛 皮 炎；**radiation d.,** radiodermatitis 放射性皮炎；**rat mite d.,** that due to a bite of the rat-mite, *Ornithonyssus bacoti* 鼠螨性皮炎；**rhus d.,** poison ivy d. 漆树皮炎；**schistosome d.,** cercarial d. 血吸虫皮炎；**seborrheic d.,** chronic pruritic dermatitis with erythema, scal-ing, and yellow crust on areas such as the scalp, with exfoliation of excessive dandruff 脂 溢 性 皮 炎；**stasis d.,** chronic eczematous dermatitis due to venous insufficiency, initially on the inner as-pect of the lower leg above the internal malleolus, sometimes spreading over the lower leg, marked by edema, pigmentation, and often ulceratio 淤积性皮炎；**uncinarial d.,** ground itch 钩虫皮炎；**x-ray d.,** radiodermatitis X 射线皮炎

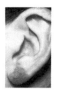

▲ 镍过敏引起的变应性接触性皮炎（**allergic contact dermatitis**）

der·ma·to·au·to·plas·ty (dur″mə-to-aw′toplas″te) autotransplantation of skin 自皮成形术

Der·ma·to·bia (dur″mə-to′be-ə) a genus of botflies. The larvae of *D. ho′minis* are parasitic in the skin of humans, mammals, and birds 皮蝇属

der·ma·to·fi·bro·ma (dur″mə-to-fi-bro′mə) a fibrous tumorlike nodule of the skin, usually on the leg. Its etiology is not known, but it is most likely a neoplastic disorder. Although it is benign, itching and pain can be a source of severe discomfort 皮肤纤维瘤

der·ma·to·fi·bro·sar·co·ma (dur″mə-to-fi″brosahr-ko′mə) a fibrosarcoma of the skin 皮肤纤维肉瘤；**d. protu′berans,** a locally aggressive, bulky, pro-tuberant, nodular, fibrotic neoplasm in the dermis, usually on the trunk, often extending into the subcu-taneous fat 隆突性皮肤纤维肉瘤

der·ma·to·glyph·ics (dur″mə-to-glif′iks) the study of fingerprints and similar skin patterns of hands and feet 皮纹学

der·ma·tog·ra·phism (dur″mə-tog′rə-fiz″əm) urticaria due to physical allergy, in which moder-ately firm stroking or scratching of the skin with a dull instrument produces a pale, raised welt or wheal, with a red flare on each side 皮肤划痕症；**dermograph′ic** *adj.*；**black d.,** black or greenish streaking of the skin caused by deposit of fine metallic particles abraded from jewelry by various dusting powders 黑色划皮现象；**white d.,** linear blanching of (usually erythematous) skin of persons with atopic dermatitis in response to firm stroking with a blunt instrument 白色划皮现象

der·ma·to·het·ero·plas·ty (dur″mə-to-het′ər-o-plas″te) the grafting of skin derived from an individ-ual of another species 异种皮肤移植

der·ma·tol·o·gy (dur″mə-tol′ə-je) the medical specialty concerned with the diagnosis and treatment of skin diseases 皮肤病学

der·ma·tol·y·sis (dur″mə-tol′ə-sis) cutis laxa 皮肤松弛症

der·ma·tome (dur′mə-tōm) 1. an instrument for cutting thin skin slices for grafting 取皮机；2. the area of skin supplied with afferent peripheral nerve fibers by a single posterior spinal root 皮区；3. the lateral part of an embryonic somite 生皮节

der·ma·to·mere (dur′mə-to-mēr″) any segment or metamere of the embryonic integument 皮节

der·ma·to·my·co·sis (dur″mə-to-mi-ko′sis) a superficial fungal infection of the skin or its appendages 皮肤真菌病

der·ma·to·my·o·ma (dur″mə-to-mi-o′mə) leiomyoma cutis 皮肤平滑肌瘤

der·ma·to·myo·si·tis (dur″mə-to-mi″ə-si′tis) polymyositis with skin changes such as discoloration and plaques on elbows, knees, and knuckles 皮肌炎

der·ma·to·path·ic (dur″mə-to-path′ik) pertaining or attributable to disease of the skin, as dermatopathic lymphadenopathy 皮肤病的

der·ma·to·pa·thol·o·gy (dur″mə-to-pə-thol′ə-je) the pathology of the skin, including both anatomic pathology and pathologic histology 皮肤病理学

Der·ma·toph·a·goi·des (dur″mə-tof″ə-goi′dēs) a genus of sarcoptiform mites, usually found on the skin of chickens. *D. pteronys′sinus* is the house dust mite, an antigenic species that produces allergic asthma in atopic persons 表皮螨属

der·ma·to·phar·ma·col·o·gy (dur″mə-tofahr″mə-kol′ə-je) pharmacology as applied to dermatologic disorders 皮肤药理学

Der·ma·to·phi·la·ceae (dur″mə-to-fi-la′se-e) a family of bacteria of the gram-positive, aerobic suborder Micrococcineae 嗜皮菌科

der·ma·to·phi·lo·sis (dur″mə-to-fī-lo′sis) an actinomycotic disease caused by *Dermatophilus congolensis*, affecting ruminants, horses, and sometimes humans. The human disease is marked by painless upper limb pustules that break down and form shallow red ulcers that later regress and leave scarring. 嗜皮菌病

Der·ma·toph·i·lus (dur″mə-tof′ ĭ-ləs) 1. *Tunga* 潜蚤属；2. a genus of pathogenic actinomycetes of the family Dermatophilaceae. *D. congolen′sis* is the etiologic agent of dermatophilosis 嗜皮菌属

der·ma·to·phyte (dur′mə-to-fīt″) any of the group of fungi of the genera *Microsporum*, *Epidermophyton*, and *Trichophyton* that colonize the stratum corneum of keratinized tissue and may cause infection, usually superficial 皮肤真菌，皮癣菌

der·ma·to·phy·tid (dur″mə-tof′ ī-tid) an id reaction expressing hypersensitivity to infection by a dermatophyte, especially *Epidermophyton*, occurring on an area remote from the site of infection 皮癣菌疹

der·ma·to·phy·to·sis (dur″mə-to-fi-to′sis) a superficial fungal infection caused by a dermatophyte

and involving the skin, hair, or nails; it broadly comprises onychomycosis and tinea 皮肤癣菌病

der·ma·to·plas·ty (dur″mə-to-plas″te) a plastic operation on the skin; operative replacement of destroyed or lost skin 皮肤成形术；**dermatoplas′tic** *adj.*

der·ma·to·sis (dur″mə-to′sis) pl. *dermato′ses*. Any skin disease, especially one not characterized by inflammation 皮肤病；**d. papulo′sa ni′gra**, a form of seborrheic keratosis seen chiefly in blacks, with multiple miliary pigmented papules usually on the cheek bones, but sometimes occurring more widely on the face and neck 黑色丘疹性皮肤病；**progressive pigmentary d.,** Schamberg disease 进行性色素性皮肤病；**subcorneal pustular d.,** a bullous dermatosis resembling dermatitis herpetiformis, with single and grouped vesicles and sterile pustular blebs beneath the stratum corneum of the skin 角层下脓疱性皮肤病

der·ma·to·spa·rax·is (dur″mə-to-spə-rak′sis) extreme fragility of the skin 皮肤脆裂症

der·ma·to·zo·on (dur″mə-to-zo′ən) any animal parasite on the skin; an ectoparasite 皮肤寄生虫

der·mis (dur′mis) corium; the layer of skin beneath the epidermis, consisting of a bed of vascular connective tissue, and containing sensory nerves and organs, hair roots, and sebaceous and sweat glands 真皮；**der′mal, der′mic** *adj.*

der·mo·blast (dur′mo-blast) the part of the mesoblast that develops into the dermis 成皮细胞

der′moid (dur′moid) 1. skinlike 皮肤样；2. dermoid cyst 皮样囊肿

der·moid·ec·to·my (dur″moid-ek′tə-me) excision of a dermoid cyst 皮样囊肿切除术

der·mo·myo·tome (dur″mo-mi′o-tōm) all but the sclerotome of a mesodermal somite; the primordium of skeletal muscle and, perhaps, of the dermis 皮肌节

der·mop·a·thy (dər-mop′ə-the) any skin disorder 皮肤病。又称 *dermatopathy*；**diabetic d.,** benign discolored lesions on the shins seen in diabetes mellitus 糖尿病皮肤病变

der·mo·vas·cu·lar (dur″mo-vas′ku-lər) pertaining to the blood vessels of the skin 皮肤血管的

DES diethylstilbestrol 己烯雌酚；drug-eluting stent 药物洗脱支架

de·sat·u·ra·tion (de-sach″ə-ra′shən) the process of converting a saturated compound to one that is unsaturated, such as the introduction of a double bond between carbon atoms of a fatty acid 去饱和作用

des·ce·me·to·cele (des″ə-met′o-sēl) hernia of the Descemet membrane 后弹力层膨出

des·cend·ing (de-send′ing) extending inferiorly 下行的

des·cen·sus (de-sen′səs) pl. *descen′sus* [L.] downward displacement or prolapse 下垂

de·sen·si·ti·za·tion (de-sen″sĭ-tĭ-za′shən) 1. the prevention or reduction of immediate hypersensitivity reactions by administration of graded doses of allergen 脱敏作用，脱敏；2. treatment of phobias and related disorders by intentionally exposing the patient, in imagination or in real life, to a hierarchy of emotionally distressing stimuli 脱敏治疗

de·ser·pi·dine (de-sur′pĭ-dēn) an alkaloid of *Rauwolfia canescens*, used as an antihypertensive 去甲氧利血平

des·fer·ri·ox·amine (des-fer″e-oks′ə-mēn) deferoxamine 去铁敏

des·flu·rane (des-floo′rān) an inhalational anesthetic used for induction and maintenance of general anesthesia 地氟醚

des·ic·cant (des′ĭ-kənt) 1. promoting dryness 促进干燥的；2. an agent that promotes dryness 干燥剂

de·sip·ra·mine (de-ip′rə-mēn) a tricyclic antidepressant of the dibenzazepine class; used as the hydrochloride salt 去甲丙咪嗪

des·lan·o·side (des-lan′o-sīd) a cardiotonic glycoside obtained from lanatoside C; used where digitalis is recommended 去乙酰毛花苷

des·min (dez′min) a protein that polymerizes to form the intermediate filaments of muscle cells; used as a marker of these cells 结蛋白

des·mi·tis (des-mi′tis) inflammation of a ligament 韧带炎

des·mo·cra·ni·um (des″mo-kra′ne-əm) the mass of mesoderm at the cranial end of the notochord in the early embryo, forming the earliest stage of the skull 膜颅

des·mog·e·nous (des-moj′ə-nəs) of ligamentous origin 韧带原的

des·mog·ra·phy (des-mog′rə-fe) a description of ligaments 韧带学

des·moid (dez′moid) 1. fibrous or fibroid 纤维性的；硬纤维瘤；2. 见 *tumor* 下词条；**periosteal d.**, a benign fibrous tumorlike proliferation of the periosteum, occurring particularly in the medial femoral condyle in adolescents 骨膜硬纤维瘤

des·mo·lase (dez′mo-lās) any enzyme that catalyzes the addition or removal of some chemical group to or from a substrate without hydrolysis 碳链裂解酶

des·mop·a·thy (des-mop′ə-the) any disease of the ligaments 韧带病

des·mo·pla·sia (des″mo-pla′zhə) the formation and development of fibrous tissue 结缔组织生成

desmoplas′tic *adj.*

des·mo·pres·sin (des″mo-pres′in) a synthetic analogue of vasopressin, used as the acetate salt as an antidiuretic in central diabetes insipidus and in primary nocturnal enuresis, and as an antihemorrhagic in hemophilia A and von Willebrand disease 去氧加压素

des·mo·some (dez′mo-sōm) a circular, dense body that forms the site of attachment between cells, especially those of stratified epithelium of the epidermis; it consists of local differentiations of the apposing cell membranes with a dense cytoplasmic plaque underlying each membrane, toward which numerous tonofilaments converge 桥粒

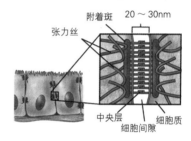

附着斑　20～30nm
张力丝
中央层　细胞质
细胞间隙

▲ 桥粒（**desmosome**）

des·mot·o·my (des-mot′o-me) incision or division of a ligament 韧带切开术

des·o·ges·trel (des″o-jes′trəl) a progestational agent with little androgenic activity; used in combination with an estrogen as an oral contraceptive 去氧孕烯

des·o·nide (des′ə-nīd) a synthetic corticosteroid used topically for the relief of inflammation and pruritus in corticosteroid-responsive dermatoses 丙缩羟强龙

de·sorb (de-sorb′) to remove a substance from the state of absorption or adsorption 解除吸附

des·ox·i·met·a·sone (des-ok″sĭ-met′ə-sōn) a synthetic corticosteroid used topically for the relief of inflammation and pruritus in corticosteroid-responsive dermatoses 去氧米松

de·spe·ci·ate (de-spe′she-āt) to undergo despeciation; to subject to (as by chemical treatment) or to undergo loss of species antigenic characteristics 种属特性丧失

des·qua·ma·tion (des″kwə-ma′shən) the shedding of epithelial elements, chiefly of the skin, in scales or sheets 脱屑；**desquam′ative, desquamatory** *adj.*

dest. [L.] destilla′ta (distilled) 蒸馏

de·sulf·hy·drase (de″səlf-hi′drās) an enzyme that removes a hydrogen sulfide molecule from a compound 脱巯基酶

DET diethyltryptamine 二乙色胺

de·tach·ment (de-tach′mənt) the condition of being separated or disconnected 脱落; **d. of retina, retinal d.,** separation of the inner layers of the retina from the pigment epithelium 视网膜脱落

de·tec·tor (de-tek′tər) an instrument or apparatus for revealing the presence of something 探测仪; **lie d.,** polygraph 测谎仪

de·ter·gent (de-tur′jənt) an agent that purifies or cleanses 清洁剂, 去污剂

de·ter·mi·nant (de-tur′mĭ-nənt) a factor that establishes the nature of an entity or event 决定子; **antigenic d.,** the structural component of an antigen molecule responsible for its specific interaction with antibody molecules elicited by the same or related antigen 抗原决定簇; **hidden d.,** an antigenic determinant in an unexposed region of a molecule so that it is prevented from interacting with receptors on lymphocytes, or with antibody molecules, and is unable to induce an immune response; it may appear following stereochemical alterations of molecular structure 隐蔽决定簇

de·ter·mi·na·tion (de-tur′mĭ-na′shən) the establishment of the exact nature of an entity or event 决定; **embryonic d.,** the loss of pluripotentiality in any embryonic part and its start on the way to an unalterable fate 胚胎决定; **sex d.,** the process by which the sex of an organism is fixed; associated, in humans, with the presence or absence of a particular gene (*SRY* gene) on the Y chromosome 性别决定

de·ter·min·ism (de-tur′mĭ-niz-əm) the theory that all phenomena are the result of antecedent conditions, nothing occurs by chance, and there is no free will 决定论

de·tox·i·fi·ca·tion (de-tok″sĭ-fĭ-ka′shən) 1. reduction of the toxic properties of poisons 解毒; 2. treatment designed to free an addict from a drug habit 戒毒; 3. in naturopathy, the elimination of toxic substances from the body, either by metabolic change or by excretion 解毒反应, 代谢解毒; **metabolic d.,** reduction of the toxicity of a substance by chemical changes induced in the body, producing a compound less poisonous or more readily eliminated 解毒代谢

de·tri·tion (de-trish′ən) the wearing away, as of teeth, by friction 磨损

de·tri·tus (de-tri′təs) particulate matter produced by or remaining after the wearing away or disintegration of a substance or tissue 腐质, 碎屑

de·tru·sor (de-troo′sər) [L.] 1. a body part that pushes down 逼尿肌; 2. detrusor muscle（膀胱）逼尿肌的

de·tu·mes·cence (de″too-mes′əns) the subsidence of congestion and swelling 消肿

deu·tan (doo′tən) a person exhibiting deuteranomalopia or deuteranopia 绿色觉异常者

deu·ter·anom·a·ly (doo″tər-ə-nom′ə-le) a type of anomalous trichromatic vision in which the second, green-sensitive cones have decreased sensitivity; the most common color vision deficiency 绿色弱视; **deuteranom′alous** *adj.*

deu·ter·an·o·pia (doo″tər-ə-no′pe-ə) a type of dichromatic vision with confusion of greens and reds, and retention of the sensory mechanism for two hues only—blue and yellow 绿色盲。又称 *deuteranopsia*; **deuteranop′ic** *adj.*

deu·te·ri·um (D) (doo-tēr′e-əm) 氘, 见 *hydrogen*

Deu·tero·my·co·ta (doo″tər-o-mi-ko′tə) 无性型真菌, 见 *fungus* 下 *anamorphic fungi*

deu·ter·op·a·thy (doo″tər-op′ə-the) a disease that is secondary to another disease 继发病

deu·tero·plasm (doo′tər-o-plaz″əm) the passive or inactive materials in protoplasm, especially reserve foodstuffs, such as yolk 滋养质

de·vas·cu·lar·iza·tion (de-vas″ku-lər-ĭ-za′shən) interruption of circulation of blood to a part due to obstruction of blood vessels supplying it 血行阻断

de·vel·op·ment (de-vel′əp-mənt) the process of growth and differentiation 发育; **developmen′tal** *adj.* **cognitive d.,** the development of intelligence, conscious thought, and problem-solving ability that begins in infancy 认知发展; **psychosexual d.,** 1. development of the individual's sexuality as affected by biologic, cultural, and emotional influences from prenatal life onward throughout life 性心理发育; 2. in psychoanalysis, libidinal maturation from infancy through adulthood (including the oral, anal, and genital stages) 性欲成熟; **psychosocial d.,** the development of the personality, and the acquisition of social attitudes and skills, from infancy through maturity 社会心理发育

de·vi·ant (de′ve-ənt) 1. varying from a determinable standard 偏离标准的; 2. a person with characteristics varying from what is considered standard or normal 不正常者

de·vi·a·tion (de″ve-a′shən) 1. variation from the regular standard or course 偏离常规标准或路线; 2. strabismus 斜视; 3. the difference between a sample value and the mean 离差, 偏差; **complement d.,** inhibition of complement fixation or complement-mediated immune hemolysis in the presence of excess antibody 补体偏离; **conjugate d.,** deflection of the eyes in the same direction at the same time 同向偏斜; **immune d.,** modification of the immune response to an antigen by previous inoculation of the same antigen 免疫偏离; **radial d.,** 1. a hand deformity sometimes seen in rheumatoid arthritis, in which the fingers are displaced to the radial side 桡侧偏斜；2. splinting of arthritic hands into this position to correct ulnar deviation 手关节夹板；**sexual d.**, sexual behavior or fantasy outside that which is morally, biologically, or legally sanctioned, often specifically one of the paraphilias 性偏离；**standard d. (SD)**, a measure of the amount by which each value deviates from the mean; equal to the square root of the variance 标准差；符号 σ；**ulnar d.**, a hand deformity of chronic rheumatoid arthritis and lupus erythematosus in which swelling of the metacarpophalangeal joints causes displacement of the fingers to the ulnar side 尺侧偏斜

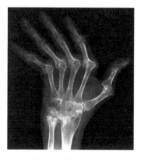

▲ 类风湿关节炎的尺侧偏斜（**ulnar deviation**）

de·vice (də-vīs′) something contrived for a specific purpose 仪器，设备；**biventricular assist d. (BVAD)**, a ventricular assist device with the combined functions of both left and right ventricular assist devices 双心室辅助装置；**contraceptive d.**, one used to prevent conception, such as a barrier contraceptive, an intrauterine device, or a means of preventing ovulation (e.g., birth control pill) 避孕用具，避孕品；**intrauterine d. (IUD)**, a plastic or metallic device inserted in the uterus to prevent pregnancy 宫内节育器；**ventricular assist d. (VAD)**, a circulatory support device that augments the function of the left ventricle, the right ventricle, or both, by providing mechanically assisted pulsatile blood flow 心室辅助装置

de·vi·om·e·ter (de″ve-om′ə-tər) an instrument for measuring the deviation in strabismus 斜视计

de·vi·tal·ize (de-vi′təl-īz) to deprive of life or vitality 失活

dex·a·meth·a·sone (deks″sə-meth′ə-sōn) a synthetic glucocorticoid used primarily as an antiinflammatory in various conditions, including collagen diseases and allergic states; it is the basis of a screening test in the diagnosis of Cushing syndrome; used also as the acetate or sodium phosphate salt 地塞米松

dex·brom·phen·ir·a·mine (deks″brom-fənir′ə-mēn) the dextrorotatory isomer of brompheniramine, used as the maleate salt as an antihistamine 右旋溴苯吡胺

dex·chlor·phen·ir·a·mine (deks″klor-fənir′ə-mēn) the dextrorotatory isomer of chlorpheniramine, used as the maleate salt as an antihistamine 右氯苯吡胺

dex·med·e·to·mi·dine (deks″med-ĕ-to′mĭdēn) a selective α₂-adrenergic receptor agonist, used as the hydrochloride salt as a sedative for patients in intensive care units 右美托咪啶

dex·meth·yl·phen·i·date (deks″meth-əlfen′ĭ-dāt) a central nervous system stimulant used as the hydrochloride salt in the treatment of attention-deficit/hyperactivity disorder 右哌醋甲酯（中枢神经系统兴奋药）

Dex·on (dek′son) trademark for a synthetic suture material, polyglycolic acid, a polymer that is completely absorbable and nonirritating 合成缝合材料聚乙醇酸的商标

dex·ra·zox·ane (deks″ra-zok′sān) a cardioprotectant used in chemotherapy to counteract doxorubicin-induced cardiomyopathy 右丙亚胺

dex·ter (dek′stər) [L.] right; on the right side 右；在右侧

dex·trad (dek′strad) to or toward the right side 向右，往右

dex·tral (dek′strəl) pertaining to the right side 与右侧有关的

dex·tral·i·ty (dek-stral′ ĭ-te) lateral dominance on the right side 右利

dex·tran (dek′strən) a high-molecular-weight polymer of d-glucose, produced by enzymes on the cell surface of certain lactic acid bacteria. Dextrans formed from sucrose by bacteria in the mouth adhere to the tooth surfaces and produce dental plaque. Commercially prepared, uniform-molecular-weight dextrans are used as plasma volume expanders, with specific preparations named for their average molecular weight 右旋糖苷

dex·trano·mer (dek-stran′o-mər) small beads of highly hydrophilic dextran polymers, used in débridement of secreting wounds, such as venous stasis ulcers; the sterilized beads are poured over secreting wounds to absorb wound exudates and prevent crust formation 聚糖苷

dex·trin (dek′strin) 1. any one, or the mixture, of the water-soluble, intermediate polysaccharides formed during the hydrolysis of starch to sugar 糊精；2. a preparation of such formed by boiling starch and used in pharmacy 糊剂，**limit d.**, any of the small polymers remaining after exhaustive digestion of glycogen or starch by enzymes that catalyze the removal of terminal sugar residues but that cannot cleave the linkages at branch points 极限糊精

α-dex·trin·ase (dek′strin-ās) isomaltase, limit dextrinase; an enzyme catalyzing the cleavage of linear and branched oligoglucosides and maltose and isomaltose, completing the digestion of starch or glycogen to glucose. It occurs in the brush border of the intestinal mucosa, as a complex with sucrase α - 糊精酶；另见 *sucrase-isomaltase deficiency*

dex·tri·no·sis (dek″strĭ-no′sis) accumulation in the tissues of an abnormal polysaccharide 糊精尿；limit d., glycogen storage disease, type Ⅲ 糖原贮积症Ⅲ型

dex·trin·uria (dek″strĭ-nu′re-ə) presence of dextrin in the urine 糊精尿

dex·tro·am·phet·amine (dek″stro-am-fet′ə-mēn) the dextrorotatory isomer of amphetamine; used as the sulfate salt in the treatment of narcolepsy and attention-deficit/hyperactivity disorder. Abuse of this drug may lead to dependence 右旋苯异丙胺

dex·tro·car·dia (dek″stro-kahr′de-ə) location of the heart in the right side of the thorax, the apex pointing to the right 右位心；isolated d., mirrorimage transposition of the heart without accompanying alteration of the abdominal viscera 孤立性右位心；mirror-image d., location of the heart in the right side of the chest, the atria being transposed and the right ventricle lying anteriorly and left of the left ventricle 镜影心

dex·tro·cli·na·tion (dek″stro-klĭ-na′shən) rotation of the upper poles of the vertical meridians of the eyes to the right 右旋眼

dex·tro·duc·tion (dek″stro-duk′shən) movement of an eye to the right 右转

dex·tro·gas·tria (dek″stro-gas′tre-ə) displacement of the stomach to the right 右位胃

dex·tro·gy·ra·tion (dek″stro-ji-ra′shən) rotation to the right 右转，右旋

dex·tro·man·u·al (dek″stro-man′u-əl) righthanded 右利手的

dex·tro·meth·or·phan (dek″stro-məthor′fan) a synthetic morphine derivative used as an antitussive; used in the form of the base or as the hydrobromide salt or sulfonated styrenedivinylbenzene (polistirex) copolymer 右甲吗喃

dex·tro·po·si·tion (dek″stro-pə-zish′ən) displacement to the right 右移位

dex·tro·ro·ta·to·ry (dek″stro-ro′tə-tor-e) turning the plane of polarization to the right 右旋性的

dex·trose (dek′strōs) a monosaccharide, d-glucose monohydrate; used chiefly as a fluid and nutrient replenisher, and also as a diuretic and for various other clinical purposes. Known as *D-glucose* in biochemistry and physiology 葡萄糖，右旋糖

dex·tro·sin·is·tral (dek″stro-sin′is-trəl) 1. extending from right to left 从右向左延伸；2. a left-handed person trained to use the right hand 训练用右手的左利手的人

dex·tro·ver·sion (dek″stro-vur′zhən) 1. version to the right, especially movement of the eyes to the right 右旋；2. location of the heart in the right chest, the left ventricle remaining in the normal position on the left, but lying anterior to the right ventricle 心脏右倾

dez·o·cine (dez′o-sēn) an opioid analgesic, having both agonist and antagonist activity, used for the short-term relief of pain 氨甲苯环癸醇

DGAC Dietary Guidelines Advisory Committee 膳食指引咨询委员会

DH delayed hypersensitivity 迟发型超敏反应

DHA docosahexaenoic acid 二十二碳六烯酸

dha·tu (thah′too) [Sanskrit] in ayurveda, the seven physical interconnected body tissues that are produced from metabolism and energy and anchor mind and spirit: plasma, blood, muscle, fat, bone, marrow, and reproductive tissue. Each tissue, though separate, is formed from another and depends upon its predecessor for its health 在阿育吠陀中，由新陈代谢、能量、锚定心灵和精神产生的七种相互联系的身体组织

DHEA dehydroepiandrosterone 脱氢表雄酮

DHF dihydrofolate or dihydrofolic acid 二氢叶酸

DHom Doctor of Homeopathic Medicine 顺势疗法医学博士

DHT dihydrotestosterone 双氢睾酮

di·a·be·tes (di″ə-be′tēz) any disorder characterized by excessive urine excretion. When used alone, the term refers to *diabetes mellitus.*多尿症，糖尿病；adult-onset d. mellitus, type 2 d. mellitus 成人型糖尿病；brittle d., type 1 d. mellitus characterized by wide, unpredictable fluctuations of blood glucose values and difficult to control 脆性糖尿病；bronze d., bronzed d., hemochromatosis 青铜色糖尿病；central d. insipidus, diabetes insipidus due to injury of the neurohypophyseal system, with a deficient quantity of antidiuretic hormone being released or produced, causing failure of renal tubular reabsorption of water 中枢性尿崩症；gestational d., gestational d. mellitus, that with onset or first recognition during pregnancy 妊娠糖尿病；growth-onset d. mellitus, type 1 d. mellitus 生长发育期糖尿病；d. insi′pidus, any of several types of polyuria in which the volume of urine exceeds 3 liters per day, causing dehydration and great thirst, as well as sometimes emaciation and great hunger 尿 崩 症；**insulin-dependent d. mellitus (IDD, IDDM),** type 1 d. mellitus 胰岛素依赖型糖尿病；**juvenile d. mellitus, juvenile-onset d. mellitus,** type 1 d. mellitus 幼年型糖尿病；**ketosis-prone d. mellitus,** type 1 d. mellitus 趋酮症性糖尿病；**maturity-onset d. mellitus,** type 2 d. mellitus 成熟期突发型糖尿病；**d. melli′tus (DM),** a chronic syndrome of impaired carbohydrate, protein, and fat metabolism due to insufficient secretion of insulin or to target tissue insulin resistance. It occurs in two major forms: *type 1 d. mellitus* and *type 2 d. mellitus*, which differ in etiology, pathology, genetics, age of onset, and treatment 糖尿病；**nephrogenic d. insipidus,** inherited or acquired diabetes insipidus caused by failure of the renal tubules to reabsorb water in response to antidiuretic hormone, without disturbance in the renal filtration and solute excretion rates 肾 性 尿 崩 症；**non–insulin-dependent d. mellitus (NIDD, NIDDM),** type 2 d. mellitus 非胰岛素依赖型糖尿病；**preclinical d.,** former name for *impaired glucose tolerance* 临床前期糖尿病；**renal d.,** 肾性糖尿病，见 *glycosuria* 下 词 条；**subclinical d.,** former name for *impaired glucose tolerance* 亚 临 床 型 糖 尿 病；**TypeⅠd. mellitus,** type 1 d. mellitus 1 型 糖 尿 病；**type 1 d. mellitus,** one of the two major types of diabetes mellitus, characterized by abrupt onset of symptoms (often in early adolescence), insulinopenia, and dependence on exogenous insulin; it is due to lack of insulin production by the pancreatic beta cells. With inadequate control, hyperglycemia, protein wasting, and ketone body production occur; the hyperglycemia leads to overflow glycosuria, osmotic diuresis, hyperosmolarity, dehydration, and diabetic ketoacidosis, which can progress to nausea and vomiting, stupor, and potentially fatal hyperosmolar coma. The associated angiopathy of blood vessels (particularly microangiopathy) affects the retinas, kidneys, and arteriolar basement membranes. Polyuria, polydipsia, polyphagia, weight loss, paresthesias, blurred vision, and irritability also occur 1 型糖尿病；**TypeⅡd. mellitus,** type 2 d. mellitus 2 型糖尿病；**type 2 d. mellitus,** one of the two major types of diabetes mellitus, peaking in onset between 50 and 60 years of age, characterized by gradual onset with few symptoms of metabolic disturbance (glycosuria and its consequences) and control by diet, with or without oral hypoglycemics but without exogenous insulin required. Basal insulin secretion is maintained at normal or reduced levels, but insulin release in response to a glucose load is delayed or reduced. Defective glucose recep-

tors on the pancreatic beta cells may be involved. It is often accompanied by disease of blood vessels, particularly the large ones, leading to premature atherosclerosis with myocardial infarction or stroke syndrome 2 型糖尿病

di·a·bet·ic (di″ə-bet′ik) 1. pertaining to or affected with diabetes 糖尿病的，受糖尿病影响的；2. a person with diabetes 糖尿病患者

di·a·be·to·gen·ic (di″ə-bet″o-jen′ik) producing diabetes 致糖尿病的

di·a·be·tog·e·nous (di″ə-be-toj′ə-nəs) caused by diabetes 糖尿病性的

di·a·brot·ic (di″ə-brot′ik) 1. ulcerative; caustic 腐蚀性的；苛性的；2. a corrosive or escharotic substance 腐蚀性物质

di·ac·e·tyl·mor·phine (di″ə-se″təl-mor′fēn) heroin 二乙酰吗啡

di·ac·la·sis (di-ak′lə-sis) osteoclasis 折骨术

di·ac·ri·sis (di-ak′rĭ-sis) 1. diagnosis 诊断；2. a disease marked by a morbid state of the secretions 分泌异常；3. a critical discharge or excretion；窘迫排泄

di·acyl·glyc·er·ol (di-a″səl-glis′ər-ol) any of various compounds of glycerol linked to two fatty acids; they are triglyceride and phospholipid degradation products and are second messengers in calcium-mediated responses to hormones 二酰甘油

di·ad·o·cho·ki·ne·sia (di-ad″ə-ko-kī-ne′zhə) the function of arresting one motor impulse and substituting one that is diametrically opposite, permitting sequential alternating movements 轮替运动

di·ag·nose (di′əg-nōs″) to identify or recognize a disease 诊断

di·ag·no·sis (di″əg-no′sis) the determination of the nature of a case of a disease or the distinguishing of one disease from another 诊断；**diagnos′tic** *adj.*；**clinical d.,** diagnosis based on signs, symptoms, and laboratory findings during life 临床诊断；**differential d.,** the determination of which one of several diseases may be producing the symptoms 鉴别判断；**physical d.,** diagnosis based on information obtained by inspection, palpation, percussion, and auscultation 物理诊断；**serum d.,** serodiagnosis 血清诊断

Di·ag·nos·tic and Sta·tis·ti·cal Man·u·al of Men·tal Dis·or·ders (DSM) a categorical system of classification of mental disorders, published by the American Psychiatric Association, that delineates objective criteria to be used in diagnosis 精神疾病诊断与统计手册

di·ag·nos·tics (di″əg-nos′tiks) the science and practice of diagnosis of disease 诊断学

di·a·gram (di′ə-gram) a graphic representation, in simplest form, of an object or concept, made up of lines and lacking pictorial elements 图表；**vector d.,**

in cardiology, a diagram representing the direction and magnitude of electromotive forces of the heart for one entire cycle, based on analysis of the scalar electrocardiogram 向量表，矢量表

di·a·ki·ne·sis (di'ə-kī-ne'sis) the fifth and final stage of prophase in meiosis I, during which the chromosomes condense and shorten, the nucleolus and nuclear envelope disappear, and the spindle fibers form 终变期

di·al·y·sance (di-al'ə-səns) the minute rate of net exchange of solute molecules passing through a membrane in dialysis 透析度

di·al·y·sate (di-al'ə-sāt) the fluid and solutes in a dialysis process that flow through the dialyzer, do not pass through the membrane, and are discarded along with removed toxic substances after leaving the dialyzer 透析液

di·al·y·sis (di-al'ə-sis) [Gr.] 1. the process of separating macromolecules from ions and lowmolecular-weight compounds in solution by the difference in their rates of diffusion through a semipermeable membrane, through which crystalloids pass readily but colloids pass slowly or not at all 溶液中大分子与离子和低分子化合物通过半透膜的扩散速度不同而分离的过程；2. hemodialysis 透析；**dialyt′ic** *adj.*；**equilibrium d.**, a technique of determination of the association constant of hapten-antibody reactions 平衡透析法；**peritoneal d.**, dialysis through the peritoneum, the dialyzing solution being introduced into and removed from the peritoneal cavity, as either a continuous or an intermittent procedure 腹膜透析

di·a·lyz·er (di'ə-līz″ər) hemodialyzer 透析器，渗析器

di·am·e·ter (d) (di-am′ə-tər) the length of a straight line passing through the center of a circle and connecting opposite points on its circumference 直径；**anteroposterior d.**, the distance between two points located on the anterior and posterior aspects, respectively, of the structure being measured, such as the true conjugate diameter of the pelvis or occipitofrontal of the skull 前后径；**Baudelocque d.**, externadiameterl conjugate d. 骨盆外直径；见 **pelvic d. conjugate d.**, 骨盆直径，见 *pelvic d.*；**cranial d., craniometric d.**, the distance between landmarks of the skull, such as the *biparietal* (between the two parietal eminences); *bitemporal* (between the two ends of the coronal suture); *cervicobregmatic* (between the center of the anterior fontanel and the junction of the neck with the floor of the mouth); *frontomental* (between the forehead and chin); *occipitofrontal* (between the external occipital protuberance and most prominent midpoint of the frontal bone); *occipitomental* (between the external occipital protuberance and the most prominent midpoint of the chin); and *suboccipitobregmatic* (between the lowest posterior point of the occiput and the center of the anterior fontanel) 头颅直径，测颅径；**pelvic d.**, any diameter of the pelvis, such as *diagonal conjugate*, joining the posterior surface of the pubis to the tip of the sacral promontory; *external conjugate*, joining the depression under the last lumbar spine to the upper margin of the pubis; *true (internal) conjugate*, the anteroposterior diameter of the pelvic inlet, measured from the upper margin of the pubic symphysis to the sacrovertebral angle; *oblique*, joining one sacroiliac articulation to the iliopubic eminence of the other side; *transverse* (of inlet), joining the two most widely separated points of the pelvic inlet; *transverse* (of outlet), joining the medial surfaces of the ischial tuberosities 骨盆径线

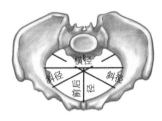

横径

斜径　斜径

前后径

▲　盆腔入口直径（**diameter**）

p-**di·ami·no·di·phen·yl** (di-ə-me″no-di-fen′əl) benzidine 对二氨基联苯

di·am·ni·ot·ic (di-am″ne-ot′ik) having or developing within separate amniotic cavities, as diamniotic twins 双羊膜腔的

di·a·pause (di'ə-pawz) a state of inactivity and arrested development accompanied by greatly decreased metabolism, as in many eggs, insect pupae, and plant seeds; it is a mechanism for surviving adverse winter conditions 滞育（指某些昆虫的发育停滞），间歇期

di·a·pe·de·sis (di″ə-pə-de′sis) the outward passage of cellular elements of the blood through intact vessel walls 血细胞渗出；**diapedet′ic** *adj.*

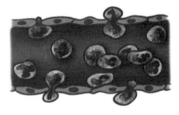

▲　白细胞渗出（**diapedesis of leukocytes**）

di·aph·e·met·ric (di-af'ə-met'rik) pertaining to measurement of the sense of touch 测量触觉的

di·a·pho·re·sis (di″ə-fə-re'sis) sweating, especially of a profuse type 出汗，尤指大量出汗

di·a·pho·ret·ic (di″ə-fo-ret'ik) 1. pertaining to, characterized by, or promoting sweating 促进发汗的；2. an agent that promotes sweating 发汗药

di·a·phragm (di'ə-fram) 1. the musculomembranous partition separating the abdominal and thoracic cavities and serving as a major muscle aiding inhalation 横膈；2. any separating membrane or structure 隔膜；3. a disk with one or more openings or with an adjustable opening, mounted in relation to a lens or source of radiation, by which part of the light or radiation may be excluded from the area 光阑；4. a shallow, dome-shaped latex or silicone disk fitted over the uterine cervix before intercourse to prevent entrance of spermatozoa 阴道隔膜；**diaphrag·mat'ic** adj.; **contraceptive d.,** diaphragm (4); **pelvic d.,** the portion of the floor of the pelvis formed by the coccygeal and levator ani muscles and their fasciae 盆膈；**polyarcuate d.,** one showing abnormal scalloping of the margins on radiographic visualization 多弓形光阑；**Potter-Bucky d.,** 波－布二氏 X 线滤器，见 *grid* 下词条；**respiratory d.,** diaphragm (1)；**urogenital d.,** traditional but no longer valid concept that fascial layers enclose the sphincter urethrae and deep transverse perineal muscles and together form a musculomembranous sheet that extends between the ischiopubic rami 泌尿生殖膈；**vaginal d.,** diaphragm (4)

di·a·phrag·ma (di″ə-frag'mə) pl. *diaphrag'mata* [Gr.] diaphragm (1) 横膈

di·a·phrag·mi·tis (de″ə-frag-mi'tis) phrenitis 膈炎

di·a·phy·se·al (di″ə-fiz'e-əl) pertaining to or affecting the shaft of a long bone (diaphysis) 骨干的

di·a·phys·ec·to·my (di″ə-fiz-ek'tə-me) excision of part of a diaphysis 部分骨干切除术

di·aph·y·sis (di-af'ə-sis) pl. *diaph'yses* [Gr.] 1. the shaft of a long bone, between the epiphyses 骨干；2. the portion of a long bone formed from a primary center of ossification 长骨

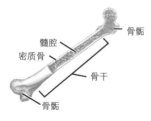

▲ 股骨的骨干（**diaphysis**）和骨骺

di·a·phys·itis (di″ə-fiz-i'tis) inflammation of a diaphysis 骨干炎

di·a·poph·y·sis (di″ə-pof'ə-sis) an upper transverse process of a vertebra 椎弓横突

di·ar·rhea (di″ə-re'ə) abnormally frequent evacuation of watery feces 腹泻，泄泻；**diarrhe'al, diarrhe'ic, diarrhet'ic** adj.; **familial chloride d.,** a type of severe watery diarrhea that begins in early infancy with feces containing excessive chloride because of impairment of chloride-bicarbonate exchange in the lower colon. Affected infants have a distended abdomen, lethargy, and retarded growth and mental development 家族性氯化物腹泻；**osmotic d.,** that due to the presence of osmotically active nonabsorbable solutes in the intestine, e.g., magnesium sulfate 渗透性腹泻；**parenteral d.,** diarrhea due to infections outside the gastrointestinal tract 肠外性腹泻；**secretory d.,** watery voluminous diarrhea resulting from increased stimulation of ion and water secretion, inhibi-tion of their absorption, or both; osmolality of the feces approximates that of plasma 分泌性腹泻；**toxigenic d.,** the watery voluminous diarrhea caused by enterotoxins from enterotoxigenic bacteria such as *Vibrio cholerae* and enterotoxigenic strains of *Escherichia coli* 产肠毒性腹泻；**traveler's d.,** diarrhea in travelers, especially those visiting tropical or subtropical areas where sanitation is poor; many different agents can cause it, the most common being enterotoxigenic *E. coli* 旅行者腹泻；**tropical d.,** 热带腹泻，见 *sprue* 下词条；**weanling d.,** diarrhea in an infant when put on food other than its mother's milk, usually due to inadequate sanitation and infection by enterotoxigenic *E. coli* or rotaviruses 断奶引起的婴儿腹泻

di·ar·rhe·o·gen·ic (di″ə-re″o-jen'ik) giving rise to diarrhea 致腹泻的

di·ar·thric (di-ahr'thrik) diarticular; pertaining to or affecting two different joints 两关节的

di·ar·thro·sis (di″ahr-thro'sis) pl. *diarthro'ses* [Gr.] a synovial joint 滑膜关节；**diarthro'dial** adj.

di·ar·tic·u·lar (di″ahr-tik'u-lər) diarthric 两关节的

di·as·chi·sis (di-as'kĭ-sis) loss of function and electrical activity due to cerebral lesions in areas remote from the lesion but neuronally connected to it 神经功能联系不能

di·a·scope (di'ə-skōp) a glass or clear plastic plate pressed against the skin for observing changes produced in the underlying skin after the blood vessels are emptied and the skin is blanched 透皮玻片

di·a·stase (di'ə-stās) a mixture of starch-hydrolyzing enzymes from malt; used to convert starch into simple sugars 淀粉酶

di·as·ta·sis (di-as'tə-sis) 1. dislocation or separation of two normally attached bones between which there is no true joint. Also, separation beyond the normal between associated bones, as between the ribs 脱离; 2. a relatively quiescent period of slow ventricular filling during the cardiac cycle, occurring just prior to atrial systole 舒张末期

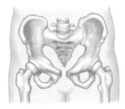

▲ 耻骨联合分离（**diastasis**）

di·a·ste·ma (di″ə-ste′mə) pl. *diaste′mata* [Gr.] 1. a space or cleft 空隙或裂缝; 2. a space between two adjacent teeth in the same dental arch 牙间隙，同一牙弓中两个相邻牙齿之间的空间; 3. a narrow zone in the equatorial plane through which the cytosome divides in mitosis 窄区

di·a·stem·a·to·cra·nia (di″ə-stem″ə-tokra′ne-ə) congenital longitudinal fissure of the cranium 先天性颅纵裂

di·a·stem·a·to·my·elia (di″ə-stem″ə-to-mie′le-ə) abnormal congenital division of the spinal cord by a bony spicule or fibrous band protruding from a vertebra or two, each half surrounded by a dural sac 脊髓纵裂

di·as·to·le (di-as′to-le) the dilatation, or the period of dilatation, of the heart, especially of the ventricles 心舒期; **diastol′ic** *adj.*

di·a·stroph·ic (di″ə-strof′ik) bent or curved; said of structures, such as bones, deformed in such manner 弯曲变形的

di·atax·ia (di″ə-tak′se-ə) ataxia affecting both sides of the body 两侧共济失调; **cerebral d.,** cerebral palsy with ataxia 大脑性双侧共济失调

di·a·ther·my (di′ə-thur″me) the heating of body tissues due to their resistance to the passage of high-frequency electromagnetic radiation, electric current, or ultrasonic waves 透热疗法; **short wave d.,** diathermy with high-frequency current, with frequency from 10 million to 100 million cycles per second and wavelength from 30 to 3 meters 短波疗法

di·ath·e·sis (di-ath′ə-sis) an unusual constitutional susceptibility or predisposition to a particular disease 素质，因素; **diathet′ic** *adj.*

di·a·tom (di′ə-tom) a unicellular microscopic form of alga having a cell wall of silica 硅藻属

di·a·to·ma·ceous (di″ə-to-ma′shəs) composed of diatoms; said of earth composed of the siliceous skeletons of diatoms 含硅藻的

dia·tri·zo·ate (di″ə-tri-zo′āt) the most commonly used water-soluble, iodinated, radiopaque medium; used in the form of its meglumine and sodium salts 泛影酸盐

di·az·e·pam (di-az′ə-pam) a benzodiazepine used as an antianxiety agent, sedative, antipanic agent, antitremor agent, skeletal muscle relaxant, or anticonvulsant, and in the management of alcohol withdrawal symptoms 安定，地西泮

di·a·zi·quone (AZQ) (di-a′zĭ-kwōn″) an alkylating agent that acts by cross-linking DNA; used as an antineoplastic in the treatment of primary brain malignancies 地吖醌

diaz(o)- the group —N ═ N—重氮基

di·az·o·tize (di-az′o-tīz) to introduce the diazo group into a compound 重氮化

di·az·ox·ide (di″ə-zok′sīd) an antihypertensive structurally related to chlorothiazide but having no diuretic properties; used for treatment of hypertensive emergencies. Because it inhibits release of insulin, it is also used in hypoglycemia due to hyperinsulinism 氯甲苯噻嗪，二氮嗪

di·ba·sic (di-ba′sik) containing two replaceable hydrogen atoms, or furnishing two hydrogen ions 二元的

di·ben·zaz·e·pine (di-ben-zaz′ə-pēn) any of a group of structurally related drugs including the tricyclic antidepressants clomipramine, desipramine, imipramine, and trimipramine 二苯卓嗪吡丁，一种结构相关药物，包括三环抗抑郁药氯丙胺、地普拉明、亚氨基丙胺和三吡嗪

di·ben·zo·cy·clo·hep·ta·di·ene (di-ben″zosi″klo-hep′tə-di′ēn) any of a group of structurally related drugs including the tricyclic antidepressants amitriptyline, nortriptyline, and protriptyline 三环抗抑郁药，阿米替林，去甲替林和普替林

di·ben·zo·di·az·e·pine (di-ben″zo-di-az′ə-pēn) any of a group of structurally related drugs including the antipsychotic agent clozapine 二苯二氮平

di·ben·zox·az·e·pine (di-ben″zok-az′ə-pēn) any of a class of structurally related heterocyclic drugs, including the antipsychotic loxapine and the antidepressant amoxapine 二苯氧氮平类

di·ben·zox·e·pine (di-ben-zok′sə-pēn) any of a group of structurally related drugs including the tricyclic antidepressant doxepin 一组与结构有关的药物，包括三环抗抑郁药多塞平

di·both·rio·ceph·a·li·a·sis (di-both″re-osef″ə-li′ə-sis) diphyllobothriasis 双槽头绦虫病

di·bro·mo·chlo·ro·pro·pane (di-bro″moklor″o-

D

pro′pān) a colorless, halogenated, carcinogenic hydrocarbon formerly used as a pesticide, fumigant, and nematocide but now restricted in usage 二溴氯丙烷

1,2-di·bro·mo·eth·ane (di-bro″mo-eth′ān) ethylene dibromide 1, 2- 二溴乙烷

di·bu·caine (di′bu-kān) a local anesthetic used topically on the skin and mucous membranes and rectally 辛可卡因

DIC disseminated intravascular coagulation 弥散性血管内凝血

di·cen·tric (di-sen′trik) 1. pertaining to, developing from, or having two centers 双着丝粒染色体；2. having two centromeres 具双着丝粒的

di·ceph·a·lus (di-sef′ə-ləs) a fetus with two heads 双头畸形

di·chlo·ral·phen·a·zone (di″klor-əl-fen′ə-zōn) a complex of chloral hydrate and antipyrine (phenazone); used in combination with isometheptene mucate and acetaminophen in the treatment of migraine and tension headache 二氯醛比林

o-di·chlo·ro·ben·zene (di-klor″o-ben′zēn) a solvent, fumigant, and insecticide toxic by ingestion or inhalation 邻二氯苯

di·chlor·phen·a·mide (di″klor-fen′ə-mīd) a carbonic anhydrase inhibitor; used as an adjunct to reduce intraocular pressure in the treatment of glaucoma 二氯苯二磺胺

di·cho·ri·al (di-kor′e-əl) dichorionic 双绒毛膜的

di·cho·ri·on·ic (di-kor″e-on′ik) having two distinct chorions; said of dizygotic twins 双绒毛膜的

di·chro·ism (di′kro-iz-əm) the quality or condition of showing one color in reflected light and another in transmitted light 二色性；**dichro′ic** *adj.*

di·chro·ma·cy (di-kro′mə-se) dichromatic vision 二色视觉

di·chro·mate (di-kro′māt) a salt containing the bivalent Cr_2O_7 radical 重铬酸盐

di·chro·mat·ic (di″kro-mat′ik) pertaining to or having dichromatic vision 具有二色视觉的

di·chro·ma·tism (di-kro′mə-tiz-əm) 1. the quality of existing in or exhibiting two different colors 二色性；2. dichromatic vision 二色视觉

di·clo·fen·ac (di-klo′fen-ak) a nonsteroidal anti-inflammatory drug used as the potassium or sodium salt in the treatment of rheumatic and nonrheumatic inflammatory conditions, and as the potassium salt to relieve pain and dysmenorrhea; also applied topically to the conjunctiva as the sodium salt to reduce ocular inflammation or photophobia after certain kinds of surgery and to the skin to treat actinic keratoses 双氯芬酸

di·clox·a·cil·lin (di-klok″sah-sil′in) a semisyn-thetic penicillinase-resistant penicillin; used as the sodium salt, primarily in the treatment of infections due to penicillinase-producing staphylococci 双氯青霉素，双氯西林，双氯苯甲异噁唑青霉素

di·coe·lous (di-se′ləs) 1. hollowed on each of two sides 双凹的；2. having two cavities 有两腔的

Dic·ro·coe·li·um (dik″ro-se′le-əm) a genus of flukes, including *D. dendri′ticum*, which has been found in human biliary passages 双腔属

di·cro·tism (di′krŏ-tiz-əm) the occurrence of two sphygmographic waves or elevations to one beat of the pulse 二波脉现象；**dicrot′ic** *adj.*

dic·tyo·tene (dik′te-o-tēn) the protracted stage resembling suspended prophase in which the primary oocyte persists from late fetal life until discharged from the ovary at or after puberty 核网期

di·cu·ma·rol (di-koo′mə-rol) a coumarin anticoagulant, which acts by inhibiting the hepatic synthesis of vitamin K–dependent coagulation factors 双香豆素

di·cy·clo·mine (di-si′klo-mēn) an anticholinergic, used as the hydrochloride salt as a gastrointestinal antispasmodic 双环胺

di·dan·o·sine (di-dan′o-sēn) an analogue of dideoxyadenosine; an antiretroviral agent used for the treatment of advanced HIV-1 infection and acquired immunodeficiency syndrome, administered orally 去羟肌苷

2′,3′-di·de·oxy·aden·o·sine (di″de-ok″se-ə-den′o-sēn) a dideoxynucleoside in which the base is adenine, used as an antiretroviral agent in the treatment of acquired immunodeficiency syndrome 2′, 3′- 二脱氧腺苷

di·de·oxy·nu·cleo·side (di″de-ok″se-noo′kleo-sīd″) any of a group of synthetic nucleoside analogues, several of which are used as antiretroviral agents 二脱氧腺苷

di·der·mo·ma (di″dər-mo′mə) a teratoma composed of cells and tissues derived from two cell layers 双胚叶畸胎瘤

did·y·mi·tis (did″ə-mi′tis) orchitis 睾丸炎

die (di) a form used in the construction of something, as a positive reproduction of the form of a prepared tooth in a suitable hard substance 模，模型

di·el·drin (di-el′drin) a chlorinated insecticide; inhalation, ingestion, or skin contact may cause poisoning 狄氏剂（杀虫药）

di·en·ceph·a·lon (di″ən-sef′ə-lon) 1. the posterior part of the forebrain, consisting of the hypothalamus, thalamus, metathalamus, and epithalamus; the subthalamus is often recognized as a distinct division 间脑，中脑；2. the posterior of the two brain vesicles formed by specialization in embryonic development 胚胎发育专门化形成的两个脑泡的后部，另见 *brainstem*；**diencephal'ic** *adj*.

di·en·es·trol (di″ən-es′trol) a synthetic estrogen administered intravaginally in the treatment of atrophic vaginitis and kraurosis vulvae 双烯雌酚

Di·ent·amoe·ba (di″ent-ə-me′bə) a genus of amebas commonly found in the human colon and appendix, including *D. fra'gilis*, a species that has been associated with diarrhea 双核阿米巴属

di·er·e·sis (di-er′ə-sis) 1. the division or separation of parts normally united 分开或分离；2. the surgical separation of parts 外科分离

di·et (di′ət) the customary amount and kind of food and drink taken by a person from day to day; more narrowly, a diet planned to meet specific requirements of the individual, including or excluding certain foods 饮食；**di'etary** *adj.* 饮食的；**acid-ash d.**, one of meat, fish, eggs, and cereals with few fruits or vegetables and no cheese or milk 酸化饮食；**alkaliash d.**, one of fruits, vegetables, and milk with as little as possible of meat, fish, eggs, and cereals 碱化饮食；**balanced d.**, one containing foods that furnish all the nutritive factors in proper proportion for adequate nutrition 均衡饮食；**bland d.**, one that is free of irritating or stimulating foods 清淡饮食；**diabetic d.**, one prescribed in diabetes mellitus, usually limited in the amount of sugar or readily available carbohydrate 糖尿病饮食；**elimination d.**, one for diagnosis of food allergy, based on sequential omission of foods that might cause the symptoms 排除饮食（不会致过敏性食物的饮食）；**Feingold d.**, a controversial diet for hyperactive children that excludes artificial colors, artificial flavors, preservatives, and salicylates 法因戈尔德饮食法；**gouty d.**, one for mitigation of gout, restricting nitrogenous, especially high-purine foods, and substituting dairy products, with prohibition of wines and liquors 痛风饮食；**high-calorie d.**, one furnishing more calories than needed to maintain weight, often more than 3500 to 4000 calories per day 高热量饮食；**high-fat d.**, ketogenic d. 高脂饮食；**high-fiber d.**, a diet relatively high in dietary fibers, which decreases transit time through the intestine and relieves constipation 高纤维饮食；**high-protein d.**, a diet containing large amounts of protein, such as from meat, fish, milk, legumes, and nuts 高蛋白饮食；**ketogenic d.**, one containing large amounts of fat, with minimal amounts of protein and carbohydrate 生酮饮食；**low-calorie d.**, one containing fewer calories than needed to maintain weight, e.g., less than 1200 calories per day for an adult 低热量饮食；**low-fat d.**, a diet that contains limited amounts of fat 低脂饮食；**low-purine d.**, one for mitigation of gout, omitting meat, fowl, and fish and substituting milk, eggs, cheese, and vegetable protein 低嘌呤饮食；**low-residue d.**, one giving the least possible fecal residue 少渣饮食，低渣饮食；**low-salt d.**, **low-sodium d.**, one containing very little sodium chloride; often prescribed for hypertension and edematous states 低盐饮食，低钠饮食；**protein-sparing d.**, one consisting only of liquid proteins or liquid mixtures of proteins, vitamins, and minerals, and containing no more than 600 calories; designed to maintain a favorable nitrogen balance 蛋白质节约饮食；**purine-free d.**, see *low-purine d.* 无嘌呤饮食；**salt-free d.**, low-salt d. 无盐饮食

di·e·tet·ic (di″ə-tet′ik) pertaining to diet or proper food 饮食的

di·e·tet·ics (di″ə-tet′iks) the science of diet and nutrition 饮食学；营养学

di·eth·yl·ene·tri·amine pen·ta·ace·tic ac·id (DTPA) (di-eth″əl-ēn-tri′ə-mēn pen″tə-ə-se′tik as′id) pentetic acid 二乙基三胺五乙酸

di·eth·yl·pro·pi·on (di-eth″əl-pro′pe-on) a sympathomimetic amine used as an anorectic in the form of the hydrochloride salt 二乙胺苯丙酮，安非拉酮

di·eth·yl·stil·bes·trol (DES) (di-eth″əl-stilbes′trol) a synthetic nonsteroidal estrogen, used as the base or the diphosphate salt for the palliative treatment of prostatic carcinoma and sometimes breast carcinoma; it is an epigenetic carcinogen and females exposed to it in utero are subject to increased risk of vaginal and cervical carcinomas 己烯雌酚

di·eth·yl·tryp·ta·mine (DET) (di-eth″əl-trip′tə-mēn) a synthetic hallucinogenic substance closely related to dimethyltryptamine 二乙基色胺

di·e·ti·tian (di″ə-tish′ən) one skilled in the use of diet in health and disease 营养学家

di·fe·nox·in (di″fə-nok′sin) an antiperistaltic used as the hydrochloride salt in the treatment of diarrhea 氰苯哌酸，地芬诺辛

dif·fer·ence (dif′ər-ens) the condition or magnitude of variation between two qualities or quantities 差异；**differen'tial** *adj.* 差别的；**arteriovenous oxygen d.**, the difference in the blood oxygen content between the arterial and venous systems 动静脉氧差

dif·fer·en·ti·ate (dif″ər-en′she-āt) 1. to distinguish, on the basis of differences 区分；2. to develop specialized form, character, or function differing from that surrounding it or from the original 分化

dif·fer·en·ti·a·tion (dif″ər-en″she-a′shən) 1. the distinguishing of one thing from another 区别；2. the act or process of acquiring completely individual characters, as occurs in progressive diversification

D

of embryonic cells and tissues 分化；3. increase in morphologic or chemical heterogeneity 异质化

dif·frac·tion (dĭ-frak′shən) the bending or breaking up of a ray of light into its component parts 衍射

dif·fu·sate (dĭ-fu′zāt) material that has diffused through a membrane, such as solutes that pass out of the blood into the dialysate fluid in a dialyzer 扩散

dif·fuse[1] (dĭ-fūs′) not definitely limited or localized; widely distributed 弥漫的

dif·fuse[2] (dĭ-fūz′) to pass through or to spread widely through a tissue or structure 扩散的

dif·fus·ible (dĭ-fūz′ĭ-bəl) susceptible of becoming widely spread 可扩散的

dif·fu·sion (dĭ-fu′zhən) 1. the process of becoming diffused, or widely spread 传播；2. the spontaneous movement of molecules or other particles in solution, owing to their random thermal motion, to reach a uniform concentration throughout the solvent, a process requiring no addition of energy to the system 分子扩散，弥散；3. in hemodialysis, the movement of solutes across semipermeable membranes down concentration gradients（血液）透析；4. immunodiffusion 免疫扩散；**double d.**, an immunodiffusion test in which both antigen and antibody diffuse into a common area so that, if the antigen and antibody are interacting, they combine to form bands of precipitate 双向扩散；**gel d.**, a test in which antigen and antibody diffuse toward one another through a gel medium to form a precipitate 凝胶扩散

Di·fi·cid (dih′-fih-sid) trademark for a preparation of fidaxomicin 非达霉素

di·flor·a·sone (di-flor′ə-sōn) a synthetic corticosteroid used topically as the diacetate salt in the treatment of inflammation and pruritus in certain dermatoses 二氟拉松

di·flu·cor·to·lone (di″floo-kor′tah-lōn″) a synthetic corticosteroid used topically as the valerate salt for the relief of inflammation and pruritus in corticosteroid-responsive dermatoses 二氟可龙

di·flu·ni·sal (di-floo′nĭ-səl) a nonsteroidal antiinflammatory drug that lacks antipyretic activity; used in the treatment of rheumatic and nonrheumatic inflammatory disorders, gout and calcium pyrophosphate deposition disease, dysmenorrhea, and vascular headaches 双氟尼酸

di·gas·tric (di-gas′trik) 1. having two bellies 二腹的；2. digastric muscle 二腹肌

di·ges·tion (di-jes′chən) 1. the act or process of converting food into chemical substances that can be absorbed and assimilated 消化；2. the subjection of a substance to prolonged heat and moisture, so as to

disintegrate and soften it 分解软化；**diges′tive** *adj.* 消化的；**artificial d.**, digestion outside the body. 人工消化；**gastric d.**, digestion by gastric juice 胃消化；**gastrointestinal d.**, the gastric and intestinal digestions together 胃肠消化；**intestinal d.**, digestion by intestinal juices 肠消化；**pancreatic d.**, digestion by pancreatic juice in the duodenum 胰消化；**salivary d.**, the change of starch into maltose by the saliva 唾液消化

dig·it (dij′it) a finger or toe 手指或足趾

dig·i·tal (dij′ĭ-təl) 1. of, pertaining to, or performed with, a finger 手指的；2. resembling the imprint of a finger 类似于手指印的；3. relating to data that are represented in the form of discrete numeric symbols 数据

Dig·i·tal·is (dij″ĭ-tal′is) a genus of herbs. *D. lana′ta* yields digoxin and lanatoside, and the leaves of *D. purpu′rea*, the purple foxglove, furnish digitalis 洋地黄属

dig·i·tal·is (dij″ĭ-tal′is) 1. the dried leaf of *Digitalis purpurea*; used as a cardiotonic agent 洋地黄的干叶；2. the digitalis glycosides or cardiac glycosides, collectively 洋地黄苷（一种强心药）

dig·i·tal·iza·tion (dij″ĭ-təl-ĭ-za′shən) the administration of digitalis or one of its glycosides in a dosage schedule designed to produce and then maintain optimal therapeutic concentrations of its cardiotonic glycosides 洋地黄化

dig·i·tate (dij′ĭ-tāt) having digit-like branches 指状的

dig·i·ta·tion (dij″ĭ-ta′shən) 1. a finger-like process 指状突起；2. surgical creation of a functioning digit by making a cleft between two adjacent metacarpal bones, after amputation of some or all of the fingers 手指再造术

dig·i·to·nin (dij″ĭ-to′nin) a saponin from *Digitalis purpurea* with no cardiotonic action; used as a reagent to precipitate cholesterol 洋地黄皂苷

di·gi·toxi·ge·nin (dij″ĭ-tok″sĭ-je′nin) the steroid nucleus that is the aglycone of digitoxin 洋地黄毒苷配基

dig·i·tox·in (dij″ĭ-tok′sin) a cardiotonic glycoside from *Digitalis purpurea* and other *Digitalis* species; used similarly to digitalis 洋地黄毒苷

dig·i·tus (dij″ĭ-təs) pl. *di′giti* [L.] a digit 趾

di·glyc·er·ide (di-glis′ər-īd) diacylglycerol 甘油二酯

di·goxi·ge·nin (dĭ-jok″sĭ-je′nin) the steroid nucleus that is the aglycone of digoxin 地高辛

di·gox·in (dĭ-jok′sin) a cardiotonic glycoside from the leaves of *Digitalis lanata*; used similarly to digitalis 地高辛；**d. immune Fab (ovine),** 地高辛免疫抗原结合片段，见 *Fab* 下词条

di·hy·dric (di-hi′drik) having two hydrogen atoms in each molecule 二羟基的

di·hy·dro·co·deine (di-hi″dro-ko′dēn) an opioid analgesic and antitussive; used as the acid tartrate for the relief of moderate to moderately severe pain; administered orally 双氢可待因

di·hy·dro·er·got·amine (di-hi″dro-ər-got′ə-mēn) an antiadrenergic derived from ergotamine; used as d. mesylate as a vasoconstrictor in the treatment of migraine 二氢麦角胺 (用于治疗偏头痛)

di·hy·dro·fo·late (DHF) (di-hi″dro-fo′lāt) an ester or dissociated form of dihydrofolic acid 二氢叶酸

di·hy·dro·fol·ic ac·id (di-hi″dro-fo′lik) any of the folic acids in which the bicyclic pteridine structure is in the dihydro, partially reduced form; they are intermediates in folate metabolism 二氢叶酸

di·hy·dro·py·rim·i·dine de·hy·dro·gen·ase (NADP⁺) (di-hi″dro-pə-rim′ĭ-dēn de-hi′drojən-ās) an enzyme catalyzing a step in the catabolism of pyrimidines; deficiency results in elevated plasma, urine, and cerebrospinal levels of pyrimidines, cerebral dysfunction in children, and hypersensitivity to 5-fluorouracil in adults 二氢嘧啶脱氢酶

di·hy·dro·tach·ys·te·rol (di-hi″dro-tak-is′tə-rol) an analogue of ergocalciferol that raises serum calcium levels, used in the treatment of hypocalcemia, hypophosphatemia, rickets, and osteodystrophy associated with a variety of disorders and the prophylaxis and treatment of postoperative or idiopathic tetany 二氢速甾醇

di·hy·dro·tes·tos·te·rone (DHT) (di-hi″drotes-tos′tə-rōn) an androgenic hormone formed in peripheral tissue by the action of 5α-reductase on testosterone; thought to be the androgen responsible for development of male primary sex characters during embryogenesis and of male secondary sex characters at puberty, and for adult male sexual function 双氢睾酮

di·hy·droxy (di″hi-drok′se) a molecule containing two molecules of the hydroxy (OH) radical; used also as a prefix (hydroxy-) to denote such a compound 二羟基

di·hy·droxy·ac·e·tone (di″hi-drok″se-as′ə-tōn) the simplest ketose, a triose; it is an isomer of glyceraldehyde. D. phosphate is an intermediate in glycolysis, the glycerol phosphate shuttle, and the biosynthesis of carbohydrates and lipids 二羟基丙酮

di·hy·droxy·alu·mi·num (di″hi-drok″se-ə-loo′mĭ-nəm) an aluminum compound having two hydroxyl groups in a molecule; available as d. aminoacetate and d. sodium carbonate, which are used as antacids 二羟化铝

di·hy·droxy·cho·le·cal·cif·er·ol (di″hidrok″se-ko″lə-kal-sif′ə-rol) a group of active metabolites of cholecalciferol (vitamin D₃). 1,25-Dihydroxycholecalciferol (1,25-dihydroxyvitamin D₃ or calcitriol) increases intestinal absorption of calcium and phosphate, enhances bone resorption, and prevents rickets, and, because of these activities at sites distant from the site of its synthesis, is considered to be a hormone 二羟胆钙化 (甾) 醇，二羟维生素 D₃，骨化三醇；另见 calcitriol 下词条

1,25-di·hy·droxy·vi·ta·min D (di″hi-drok″sevi′tə-min) 1,25-dihydroxycholecalciferol, the corresponding dihydroxy derivative of ergocalciferol, or both collectively 1,25- 二羟维生素 D

1,25-di·hy·droxy·vi·ta·min D₃ (di″hi-drok″sevi′tə-min) 1,25-dihydroxycholecalciferol 1,25- 二羟维生素 D₃，见 dihydroxycholecalciferol 下词条

di·io·do·ty·ro·sine (di″i-o″do-ti′ro-sēn) an organic iodine-containing precursor of thyroxine, liberated from thyroglobulin by hydrolysis 二碘酪氨酸

di·iso·cy·anate (di-i″so-si′ə-nāt) any of a group of compounds containing two isocyanate groups (—NCO), used in the manufacture of plastics and elastomers; they can cause sensitization and are eye and respiratory system irritants 二异氰酸酯

dik·ty·o·ma (dik″te-o′mə) a medulloepithelioma of the epithelium lining the basal lamina of the ciliary body 视网膜胚瘤

di·lac·er·a·tion (di-las″ər-a′shən) a tearing apart, as of a cataract. In dentistry, an abnormal angulation or curve in the root or crown of a formed tooth 弯曲牙

dil·a·ta·tion (dil″ə-ta′shən) 1. the condition, as of an orifice or tubular structure, of being dilated or stretched beyond normal dimensions 扩张过程，膨胀过程；2. the act of dilating or stretching 扩张，膨胀；d. and curettage (D & C), expanding of the ostium uteri to permit scraping of the walls of the uterus 刮宫术；d. of the heart, compensatory enlargement of the cavities of the heart, with thinning of its walls 心脏扩张；segmental d., dilatation of a portion of a tubular structure, such as the intestine, the segments on either side of the dilatation being of normal caliber 节段性扩张

di·late (di′lāt) to stretch an opening or hollow structure beyond its normal dimensions 膨胀，扩张

di·la·tion (di-la′shən) 1. the act of dilating or stretching 扩张过程；2. dilatation 扩张

di·la·tor (di-la′tər) (di′-la-tər) 1. a structure that dilates, or an instrument used to dilate 扩张器；2. dilator muscle 扩张肌

DILI drug-induced liver injury 药物性肝损伤

dil·ti·a·zem (dil-ti′ə-zəm) a calcium channel blocker

that acts as a vasodilator; used as the hydrochloride salt in the treatment of angina pectoris, hypertension, and supraventricular tachycardia 地尔硫草

dil·u·ent (dil'u-ənt) 1. causing dilution 稀释的；2. an agent that dilutes or renders less potent or irritant 稀释剂

di·lu·tion (di-loo'shən) 1. reduction of concentration of an active substance by admixture of a neutral agent 稀释；2. a substance that has undergone dilution 稀释液；3. in homeopathy, the diffusion of a given quantity of a medicinal agent in ten or one hundred times the same quantity of water 稀释度；**dilu′tional** *adj.*；**serial d.**, a set of dilutions in a mathematical sequence, as to obtain a culture plate with a countable number of separate colonies 连续稀释法

di·men·hy·dri·nate (di″mən-hi'drī-nāt) an antihistamine used as an antiemetic, particularly in the treatment of motion sickness 茶苯海明；晕海宁；乘晕宁

di·mer (di'mər) 1. a compound formed by combination of two identical molecules 二聚体；2. a capsomer having two structural subunits 2 个亚基组成的病毒衣壳

di·mer·cap·rol (di″mər-kap'rol) a metal complexing agent used as an antidote to poisoning by arsenic, gold, mercury, and lead 二巯基丙醇

di·meth·i·cone (di-meth' ī-kōn) a silicone oil used as a skin protective 二甲基硅油，另见 *simethicone*

di·meth·yl sulf·ox·ide (DMSO) (di-meth'əl sul-fok'sīd) a powerful solvent with the ability to penetrate plant and animal tissues and to preserve living cells during freezing; it is instilled into the bladder for relief of interstitial cystitis and has been proposed as a topical analgesic and antiinflammatory agent and for increasing penetrability of other substances 二甲基亚砜

di·meth·yl·tryp·ta·mine (DMT) (di-meth″əl-trip'tə-mēn) a hallucinogenic substance derived from the plant *Prestonia amazonica*, which is native to parts of South America and the West Indies 二甲基色胺

di·mor·phism (di-mor'fiz-əm) the quality of existing in two distinct forms 二态性；**dimor′phic, dimor′phous** *adj* 二态的；**sexual d.**, systematic physical or behavioral differences associated with gender within a species, e.g., color or size 两性异形，两性异型，性二态

dim·ple (dim'pəl) a slight depression, as in the flesh of the cheek, chin, or sacral region 笑靥，酒窝；**postanal d.**, a dermal pit near the tip of the coccyx, indicative of the site of attachment of the embryonic neural tube to the skin 尾小凹

di·ni·tro-o-cre·sol (DNOC) (di-ni″tro-kre'sol) a highly toxic pesticide that affects the central nervous system and energy-producing metabolic processes; metabolic rate is increased and fatal hyperpyrexia may occur 二硝基邻甲酚

di·ni·tro·tol·u·ene (di-ni″tro-tol'u-ēn) any of three highly toxic, possibly carcinogenic isomers used in organic synthesis and the manufacture of dyes and explosives 二硝基甲苯

di·no·flag·el·late (di″no-flaj'ə-lāt) 1. of or pertaining to the order Dinoflagellida 腰鞭毛虫的；2. any individual of the order Dinoflagellida 腰鞭毛目

Di·no·fla·gel·li·da (di″no-flə-jel' ī-də) an order of minute plantlike, chiefly marine protozoa, which are an important component of plankton. They may be present in sea water in such vast numbers that they cause a discoloration (red tide), which may result in the death of marine animals, including fish, by exhaustion of their oxygen supply. Some species secrete a powerful neurotoxin that can cause a severe toxic reaction in humans who ingest shellfish that feed on the toxin-producing organisms 双鞭毛虫目

di·no·prost (di'no-prost) name for prostaglandin $F_{2\alpha}$ when used as a pharmaceutical; used as the base or the tromethamine salt as an oxytocic for induction of abortion, for evacuation of the uterus in management of missed abortion, and in treatment of hydatidiform mole 地诺前列素，前列腺素 $F_{2\alpha}$

di·no·prost·one (di″no-pros'tōn) name given to prostaglandin E_2 when used pharmaceutically; used as an oxytocic for induction of abortion or labor, to aid ripening of the cervix, and in the treatment of missed abortion or hydatidiform mole 地诺前列酮，前列腺素 E_2

di·nu·cleo·tide (di-noo'kle-o-tīd) one of the cleavage products into which a polynucleotide may be split, itself composed of two mononucleotides 二核苷酸

Di·oc·to·phy·ma (di-ok″to-fi'mah) a genus of nematodes, including *D. rena'le*, the kidney worm, found in dogs, cattle, horses, and other animals, and rarely in humans; it is highly destructive to kidney tissue 膨结线虫属

di·op·ter (D) (di-op'tər) a unit for refractive power of lenses, being the reciprocal of the focal length expressed in meters 屈光度；**prism d. (Δ)**, a unit of prismatic deviation, being the deflection of 1 centimeter at a distance of 1 meter 棱镜屈光度

di·op·tom·e·try (di″op-tom'ə-tre) the measurement of ocular accommodation and refraction 屈光测量

di·op·tric (di-op'trik) pertaining to refraction or to transmitted and refracted light; refracting 屈光的

di·ov·u·la·to·ry (di-ov'u-lə-tor″e) discharging two

oocytes in one ovarian cycle 排双卵的

di·ox·ide (di-ok′sīd) an oxide with two oxygen atoms. 二氧化物

di·ox·in (di-ok′sin) any of the heterocyclic hydro-carbons present as trace contaminants in herbicides; many are oncogenic and teratogenic 二噁英

di·oxy·ben·zone (di-ok″se-ben′zōn) a topical sunscreening agent, absorbing UVB and some UVA light 二苯甲酮

di·pep·ti·dase (di-pep′tī-dās) any of a group of enzymes that catalyze the hydrolysis of the peptide linkage in a dipeptide 二肽酶

Di·pet·a·lo·ne·ma (di-pet″ə-lo-ne′mə) a genus of nematode parasites (superfamily Filarioidea), including *D. per′stans* and *D. streptocer′ca*, species primarily parasitic in humans, other primates serving as reservoir hosts 棘唇线虫属

di·pha·sic (di-fa′zik) having two phases 双相的

di·phen·hy·dra·mine (di″fen-hi′drə-mēn) a potent antihistamine, used as the hydrochloride salt in the treatment of allergic symptoms and for its anticholinergic, antitussive, antiemetic, antivertigo, and antidyskinetic effects, and as the hydrochloride or citrate salt as a sedative and hypnotic 苯海拉明

di·phen·ox·y·late (di″fə-nok′sə-lāt) an antiperi-staltic derived from meperidine; the hydrochloride salt is used as an antidiarrheal for 苯乙哌啶，地芬诺酯

di·phen·yl (di-fen′əl) a toxic compound compris-ing two linked benzene rings, used as a fungistat in containers for shipping citrus fruits 联苯

di·phen·yl·amine·chlor·ar·sine (DM) (difen′əl-ə-mēn″klor-ahr′sēn) phenarsazine chloride 二苯胺氯胂

di·phen·yl·bu·tyl·pi·per·i·dine (di-fen″əlbu″təl-pi-per′ī-dēn) any of a class of structurally related antipsychotic agents that includes pimozide 二苯丁哌啶

di·phos·pha·ti·dyl·glyc·er·ol (di″fos-fə-ti″dəlglis′ər-ol) glycerol linked to two molecules of phosphatid-ic acid; 1,3-diphosphatidylglycerol is cardiolipin 心磷脂

di·phos·pho·nate (di-fos′fə-nāt) 1. a salt, ester, or anion of a dimer of phosphonic acid, structurally similar to pyrophosphate but more stable 二磷酸盐; 2. any of a group of such compounds, having affin-ity for sites of osteoid mineralization and used as sodium salts to inhibit bone resorption as well as complexed with technetium Tc 99m for bone imag-ing 双膦酸酯

diph·the·ria (dif-thēr′e-ə) an acute infectious dis-ease caused by *Corynebacterium diphtheriae* and its toxin, affecting the membranes of the nose, throat, or larynx, and marked by formation of a gray-white

pseudomembrane, with fever, pain, and, in the la-ryngeal form, aphonia and respiratory obstruction. The toxin may also cause myocarditis and neuritis 白喉; **diphthe′rial, diphther′ic, diphtherit′ic** *adj.* 白喉的

diph·the·roid (dif′thə-roid) 1. resembling diphtheria 类白喉; 2. a bacterium resembling *Corynebacterium diphtheriae* but not causing diphtheria 类白喉棒状杆菌; 3. pseudodiphtheria 假白喉

di·phyl·lo·both·ri·a·sis (di-fil″o-both-ri′ə-sis) infection with *Diphyllobothrium* 裂头绦虫病

Di·phyl·lo·both·ri·um (di-fil″o-both′re-əm) a genus of large tapeworms, including *D.* la′tum (broad or fish tapeworm), found in the intestine of humans, cats, dogs, and other fish-eating mammals; its first intermediate host is a crustacean and the second a fish, the infection in humans being acquired by eat-ing inadequately cooked fish 裂头绦虫属

di·phy·odont (di-fi′o-dont″) having two denti-tions, a deciduous and a permanent 双套牙列的

di·piv·e·frin (di-piv′ə-frin) an ester converted in the eye to epinephrine, lowering intraocular pressure by decreasing the production and increasing the outflow of aqueous humor; the hydrochloride salt is applied topically in the treatment of open-angle or secondary glaucoma 地匹福林

dip·la·cu·sis (dip″lə-koo′sis) the perception of a single auditory stimulus as two separate sounds 复听; **binaural d.,** different perception by the two ears of a single auditory stimulus 双耳复听; **disharmonic d.,** binaural diplacusis in which a pure tone is heard differently in the two ears 不调和性复听; **echo d.,** binaural diplacusis in which a sound of brief dura-tion is heard at different times in the two ears 回声性复听; **monaural d.,** diplacusis in which a pure tone is heard in the same ear as a split tone of two frequencies 单耳复听

di·ple·gia (di-ple′je-ə) paralysis of like parts on either side of the body 双侧瘫痪; **diple′gic** *adj.* 双侧瘫痪的

dip·lo·ba·cil·lus (dip″lo-bə-sil′əs) pl. *diplobacil′li.* A short, rod-shaped organism occurring in pairs 双杆菌

dip·lo·coc·cus (dip″lo-kok′əs) pl. *diplococ′ci.* Any of the spherical, lanceolate, or coffee-bean–shaped bacteria occurring usually in pairs as a result of incomplete separation after cell division in a single plane 双球菌

dip·loid (dip′loid) having two sets of chromo-somes, as normally found in the somatic cells of eukaryotes ($2n$ or, in humans, 46) 二倍体

dip·lo·my·elia (dip″lo-mi-e′le-ə) complete or in-complete duplication of the spinal cord 脊髓纵裂

D

di·plo·pia (dǐ-plo′pe-ə) the perception of two images of a single object 复视；**binocular d.**, double vision in which the images of an object are formed on noncorresponding points of the retinas 双眼复视；**crossed d.**, diplopia in which the image belonging to the right eye is displaced to the left of the image belonging to the left eye 交叉复视；**direct d.**, that in which the image belonging to the right eye appears to the right of the image belonging to the left eye 同侧性复视；**heteronymous d.**, crossed d.; **homonymous d.**, direct d.；**horizontal d.**, that in which the images lie in the same horizontal plane, being either direct or crossed 水平复视；**monocular d.**, perception by one eye of two images of a single object 单眼复视；**paradoxical d.**, crossed d.; **torsional d.**, that in which the upper pole of the vertical axis of one image is inclined toward or away from that of the other 扭转复视；**vertical d.**, that in which one image appears above the other in the same vertical plane 垂直复视

dip·lo·some (dip′lo-sōm) the two centrioles of a mammalian cell 双中心体

dip·lo·tene (dip′lo-tēn) the fourth stage of prophase in meiosis I, during which the synaptonemal complex disintegrates and the homologous chromosomes separate, held together only by chiasmata （减数分裂）双线期

di·pole (di′pōl) 1. a molecule having separated charges of equal and opposite sign 偶极；2. a pair of electric charges or magnetic poles separated by a short distance 偶极子

dip·se·sis (dip-se′sis) thirst 病理性烦渴；**dipset′ic** adj. 烦渴的

dip·so·gen (dip′so-jən) an agent or measure that induces thirst and promotes ingestion of fluids 善渴原，致渴剂；**dipsogen′ic** adj. 致渴的

dip·so·sis (dip-so′sis) excessive thirst 烦渴

dip·stick (dip′stik) a strip of cellulose chemically impregnated to render it sensitive to protein, glucose, or other substances in the urine 纤维素试纸

Dip·tera (dip′tər-ə) an order of insects, including flies, gnats, and mosquitoes 双翅目

dip·ter·ous (dip′tər-əs) 1. having two wings 双翅；2. pertaining to insects of the order Diptera 双翅目的

Dip·y·lid·i·um (dip′ə-lid′e-əm) a genus of tapeworms. *D. cani′num*, the dog tapeworm, is parasitic in dogs and cats and is occasionally found in humans 复孔绦虫属

di·py·rid·a·mole (di″pī-rid′ə-mōl) a platelet inhibitor and coronary vasodilator used to prevent thromboembolism associated with mechanical heart valves, to treat transient ischemic attacks, and as an adjunct in preventing myocardial reinfarction and in myocardial perfusion imaging 双嘧达莫，商品名潘生丁

di·rect (dǐ-rekt′) 1. straight; in a straight line 笔直的；2. performed immediately and without the intervention of subsidiary means 直接地

di·rec·tor (dǐ-rek′tər) a grooved instrument for guiding a surgical instrument （手术）引导器

di·rith·ro·my·cin (di-rith″ro-mi′sin) a macrolide antibiotic used in the treatment of bacterial infections of the respiratory tract, streptococcal pharyngitis, and skin and soft tissue infections; administered orally 地红霉素

Di·ro·fi·la·ria (di″ro-fī-lar′e-ə) a genus of filarial nematodes (superfamily Filarioidea), including *D. immit′is*, the heartworm, found in the right heart and veins of the dog, wolf, and fox 恶丝虫属

di·ro·fil·a·ri·a·sis (di″ro-fil″ə-ri′ə-sis) infection with nematodes of genus *Dirofilaria*, common in dogs but rare in humans 恶丝虫病

dis·a·bil·i·ty (dis″ə-bil′ĭ-te) 1. an incapacity or inability to function normally, physically or mentally 残疾；2. anything that causes such an incapacity. 致残因素；3. as defined by the federal government: "inability to engage in any substantial gainful activity by reason of any medically determinable physical or mental impairment which can be expected to last or has lasted for a continuous period of not less than 12 months." 劳动能力丧失；**developmental d.**, any disorder in which developmental milestones are not reached on schedule, or may not be reached at all 发育障碍，发育性残疾

di·sac·cha·ri·dase (di-sak′ə-rĭ-dās″) an enzyme that catalyzes the hydrolysis of disaccharides 双糖酶

di·sac·cha·ride (di-sak′ə-rīd) any of a class of sugars yielding two monosaccharides on hydrolysis 二糖

di·sac·cha·rid·uria (di-sak″ə-rīd-u′re-ə) presence of excessive levels of a disaccharide in the urine, such as in a disaccharide intolerance 二糖尿

dis·ar·tic·u·la·tion (dis″ahr-tik″u-la′shən) exarticulation; amputation or separation at a joint 关节离断术

disc (disk) disk 圆盘；**bilaminar d., embryonic d., germinal d.**, a flat area in a blastocyst in which the first traces of the embryo are seen, visible early in the second week in human development 胚盘

dis·charge (dis′chahrj) 1. a setting free, or liberation 释放；2. matter or force set free 免责；3. an excretion or substance evacuated 排泄；4. release from a hospital or other course of care 出院；5. the passing of an action potential through a neuron, an axon, or muscle fibers 电位的传递，放电；**myokymic d.**, patterns of grouped or repetitive discharges of motor unit action potentials sometimes seen in myokymia 肌颤搐放电；**myotonic d.**, high-frequency repetitive discharges seen in myotonia and evoked by insertion of a needle electrode, percussion of a muscle, or stimulation of a muscle or its motor nerve 肌强直放电；**periodic lateralized epileptiform d.** (PLED), a pattern of repetitive paroxysmal slow or sharp waves seen on an electroencephalogram from just one side of the brain 周期性一侧癫痫样放电

dis·ci·form (dis′ĭ-form) in the form of a disk 盘状的

dis·cis·sion (dĭ-sizh′ən) incision, or cutting into, as of a soft cataract 挑开术

dis·cli·na·tion (dis″klī-na′shən) extorsion 外旋

dis·co·blas·tu·la (dis″ko-blas′tu-lə) the specialized blastula formed by cleavage of a fertilized telolecithal egg, consisting of a cellular cap (blastoderm) separated by the blastocoele from a floor of uncleaved yolk 盘状囊胚；**discoblas′tic** adj. 盘状囊胚的

dis·co·gen·ic (dis″ko-jen′ik) caused by derangement of an intervertebral disk 椎间盘性的

dis·coid (dis′koid) 1. disk-shaped 盘状的；2. a dental instrument with a disklike or circular blade 盘状牙科器械；3. a disk-shaped dental excavator designed to remove the carious dentin of a decayed tooth 盘型牙科电凿器

dis·con·tin·u·ous (dis″kən-tin′u-əs) 1. interrupted; intermittent; marked by breaks 中断，间歇；2. discrete; separate 分离的，离散的；3. lacking logical order or coherence 缺乏逻辑性

dis·cop·a·thy (dis-kop′ə-the) any disease of an intervertebral disk 椎间盘病

dis·co·pla·cen·ta (dis″ko-plə-sen′tə) a discoid placenta 盘状胎盘

dis·cor·dance (dis-kor′dəns) the occurrence of a given trait in only one member of a twin pair 不一致，双胞胎中仅有一人出现了某特征；**discor′dant** adj. 不一致的

dis·crete (dis-krēt′) made up of separated parts or characterized by lesions that do not become blended 离散的

dis·crim·i·na·tion (dis-krim″ĭ-na′shən) the making of a fine distinction 辨别

dis·cus (dis′kəs) pl. dis′ci [L.] disk 圆盘

dis·cu·ti·ent (dis-ku′shənt) scattering, or causing a disappearance; a remedy that so acts 消肿的

dis·ease (dĭ-zēz′) any deviation from or interruption of the normal structure or function of any body part, organ, or system that is manifested by a characteristic set of symptoms and signs and whose etiology, pathology, and prognosis may be known or un-known 疾病；另见 *syndrome* 下词条；**acquired cystic d. of kidney**, the development of cysts in the formerly noncystic failing kidney in end-stage renal disease 获得性肾囊肿；**Addison d.**, bronzelike pigmentation of the skin, severe prostration, progressive anemia, low blood pressure, diarrhea, and digestive disturbance, due to adrenal hypofunction 艾迪生病，肾上腺皮质功能不全 **Albers-Schönberg d.**, osteopetrosis 骨硬化病，一种罕见的遗传性骨骼疾病；**allogeneic d.**, graft-versus-host reaction occurring in immunosuppressed animals receiving injections of allogeneic lymphocytes 异源疾病；**alpha chain d.**, heavy chain disease characterized by plasma cell infiltration of the lamina propria of the small intestine, resulting in malabsorption with diarrhea, abdominal pain, and weight loss, possibly accompanied by pulmonary involvement α 链疾病；**Alzheimer d.**, progressive degenerative disease of the brain characterized by diffuse atrophy throughout the cerebral cortex with distinctive histopathological changes, including cortical atrophy and formation of plaques and neurofibrillary tangles; believed to be due to various inherited or sporadic defects in metabolism of a specific amyloid precursor protein 阿尔茨海默病；**Andersen d.**, glycogen storage d., type 糖原贮积症Ⅳ型；**apatite deposition d.**, a connective tissue disorder marked by deposition of hydroxyapatite crystals in one or more joints or bursae 磷灰石沉积病；**Aran-Duchenne d.**, spinal muscular atrophy 脊髓病性肌萎缩；**arteriosclerotic cardiovascular d. (ASCVD)**, atherosclerotic involvement of arteries to the heart and to other organs, resulting in debility or death; sometimes used specifically for ischemic heart disease 动脉硬化性心血管病；**arteriosclerotic heart d. (ASHD)**, ischemic heart d. 动脉硬化性心脏病；**autoimmune d.**, any of a group of disorders in which tissue injury is associated with humoral or cellmediated responses to the body's own constituents; they may be systemic or organ-specific 自身免

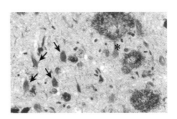

▲ 阿尔茨海默病（**Alzheimer disease**）（银染）神经元胞质中的神经原纤维缠结（箭）和神经炎斑块（NP）

疫 病；**Ayerza d.**, polycythemia vera with chronic cyanosis, dyspnea, bronchitis, bronchiectasis, hepatosplenomegaly, bone marrow hyperplasia, and pulmonary artery sclerosis Ayerza 病；**Banti d.**, congestive splenomegaly 充血性脾肿大；**Barlow d.**, scurvy in infants 巴洛病，婴儿坏血病；**Barraquer d.**, partial lipodystrophy 部分脂肪营养不良；**Basedow d.**, Graves d.; **Batten d.**, **Batten-Mayou d.**, 1. Vogt-Spielmeyer d.; 2. more generally, any or all of the group of disorders constituting neuronal ceroid lipofuscinosis 神经元蜡样质脂褐质沉积症；**Bayle d.**, general paresis 麻痹性痴呆；**Bazin d.**, erythema induratum 硬红斑；**Becker d.**, the autosomal recessive form of myotonia congenita. 贝 克症，常染色体隐性遗传的肌强直；**Benson d.**, asteroid hyalosis. 本逊病，星形玻璃体炎；**Berger d.**, IgA glomerulonephritis IgA 肾病；**Bernhardt d.**, **Bernhardt-Roth d.**, meralgia paresthetica 感觉异常性股痛；**Besnier-Boeck d.**, sarcoidosis 结节病；**Best d.**, an autosomal dominant form of macular degeneration, characterized by an orange cystlike lesion; it does not progress to blindness 卵 黄 状 黄 斑 变 性；**Bielschowsky-Janský d.**, Janský-Bielschowsky d.; **Binswanger d.**, a degenerative dementia of presenile onset caused by demyelination of the subcortical white matter of the brain 宾斯旺格病，皮下动脉硬化性脑病；**Blocq d.**, astasia-abasia 站立行走不能；**Blount d.**, tibia vara 胫骨内翻；**Boeck d.**, sarcoidosis 结节病；**Bornholm d.**, epidemic pleurodynia 博恩霍尔姆病；**Bowen d.**, a squamous cell carcinoma in situ, often due to prolonged exposure to arsenic; usually occurring on sun-exposed areas of skin. The corresponding lesion on the glans penis is termed erythroplasia of Queyrat 鲍 恩 病；**Brill d.**, Brill-Zinsser d.; **Brill-Symmers d.**, giant follicular lymphoma 巨滤泡性淋巴瘤；**Brill-Zinsser d.**, mild recrudescence of epidemic typhus years after the initial infection, because *Rickettsia prowazekii* has persisted in body tissue in an inactive state, with humans as the reservoir 复发性斑疹伤寒；**broad beta d.**, familial dysbetalipoproteinemia; named for the electrophoretic mobility of the abnormal chylomicron and very-low-density lipoprotein remnants produced 宽 β 脂蛋白病，Ⅲ型高脂蛋白血症；**Busse-Buschke d.**, cryptococcosis 隐球菌病；**Caffey d.**, infantile cortical hyperostosis 婴儿骨皮质增生症；**calcium hydroxyapatite deposition d.**, apatite deposition d.; **calcium pyrophosphate deposition d. (CPDD)**, an acute or chronic inflammatory arthropathy caused by deposition of calcium pyrophosphate dihydrate (CPPD) crystals in the joints, chondrocalcinosis, and crystals in the synovial fluid. Acute attacks are some-

times called *pseudogout* 焦磷酸钙沉积症；**Calvé-Perthes d.**, osteochondrosis of capitular epiphysis of femur 股骨头骨骺骨软骨病；**Camurati-Engelmann d.**, diaphyseal dysplasia 卡干骺端发育异常；**Canavan d.**, **Canavan-van Bogaert-Bertrand d.**, spongy degeneration of the central nervous system 海绵状白质脑病；**Carrión d.**, bartonellosis (2) 巴尔通体病；**Castleman d.**, a benign or premalignant condition resembling lymphoma but without recognizable malignant cells; there are isolated masses of lymphoid tissue and lymph node hyperplasia, usually in the abdominal or mediastinal area 卡 斯 尔 曼病；**catscratch d.**, a usually benign, self-limited disease of the regional lymph nodes, caused by *Bartonella henselae* and characterized by a papule or pustule at the site of a cat scratch, subacute painful regional lymphadenitis, and mild fever 猫抓病；**celiac d.**, an autoimmune malabsorption syndrome precipitated by ingestion of gluten-containing foods, with inflammation of the small bowel mucosa, atrophy of the intestinal villi, bulky, frothy diarrhea, abdominal distention, flatulence, weight loss, and vitamin and electrolyte depletion. Susceptibility is genetically determined 乳糜泻；**Chagas d.**, trypanosomiasis due to *Trypanosoma cruzi*; its course may be acute, subacute, or chronic 美洲锥虫病；**Charcot-Marie-Tooth d.**, progressive, symmetric muscular atrophy of variable inheritance, beginning in the muscles supplied by the fibular nerves and progressing to those of the hands and arms 进行性神经性腓骨肌萎缩症；**cholesteryl ester storage d. (CESD)**, a lysosomal storage disease due to deficiency of lysosomal cholesterol esterase, variably characterized by some combination of hepatomegaly, hyperbetalipoproteinemia, and premature atherosclerosis 胆固醇酯积累病；**Christmas d.**, hemophilia B 血友病 B；**chronic granulomatous d.**, frequent, severe infections of the skin, oral and intestinal mucosa, reticuloendothelial system, bones, lungs, and genitourinary tract associated with a genetically determined defect in the intracellular bactericidal function of leukocytes 慢性肉芽肿病；**chronic obstructive pulmonary d. (COPD)**, any disorder marked by persistent obstruction of bronchial air flow 慢性阻塞性肺疾病；**Coats d.**, a type of retinopathy marked by masses of white to yellow exudate and blood debris from hemorrhage in the posterior part of the fundus oculi, sometimes progressing to blindness 外层渗出性视网膜病变；**collagen d.**, any of a group of diseases characterized by widespread pathologic changes in connective tissue; they include lupus erythematosus, dermatomyositis, scleroderma, polyarteritis nodosa, thrombotic purpura, rheumatic fever, and rheumatoid arthritis 胶原性疾病。Cf. *collagen disorder.*; **communicable d.**, contagious disease; an infectious disease transmitted from one individual to another, either directly or indirectly 传染病; **Concato d.**, progressive malignant polyserositis with large effusions into the pericardium, pleura, and peritoneum 进行性多发性浆膜炎; **constitutional d.**, one involving a system of organs or one with widespread symptoms 体质性疾病; **contagious d.**, communicable d.; **Cori d.**, glycogen storage d., type Ⅲ糖原贮积症Ⅲ型; **coronary artery d. (CAD)**, atherosclerosis of the coronary arteries, which may cause angina pectoris, myocardial infarction, and sudden death; risk factors include hypercholesterolemia, hypertension, smoking, diabetes mellitus, and low levels of high-density lipoproteins 冠状动脉疾病; **coronary heart d. (CHD)**, ischemic heart d. 冠状动脉性心脏病; **Cowden d.**, a hereditary disease marked by multiple ectodermal, mesodermal, and endodermal nevoid and neoplastic anomalies 多发性错构瘤综合征; **Creutzfeldt-Jakob d.**, a rare prion disease existing in sporadic, familial, and infectious forms, with onset usually in middle life, and having a wide variety of clinical and pathological features. The most commonly seen are spongiform degeneration of neurons, neuronal loss, gliosis, and amyloid plaque formation, accompanied by rapidly progressive dementia, myoclonus, motor disturbances, and encephalographic changes, with death occurring usually within a year of onset 克罗伊茨费尔特-雅各布病; **Crohn d.**, regional enteritis; a chronic granulomatous inflammatory disease usually in the terminal ileum with scarring and thickening of the wall, often leading to intestinal obstruction and formation of fistulas and abscesses 克罗恩病; **Cruveilhier d.**, spinal muscular atrophy 脊髓性肌萎缩症; **Cushing d.**, Cushing syndrome in which the hyperadrenocorticism is secondary to excessive pituitary secretion of adrenocorticotropic hormone 库

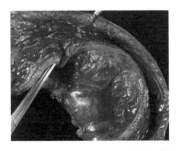

▲ 克罗恩病（Crohn disease）的小肠狭窄

欣病; **cystic d. of breast,** mammary dysplasia with formation of blue dome cysts 乳腺囊性增生病; **cytomegalic inclusion d., cytomegalovirus d.,** an infection due to cytomegalovirus and marked by nuclear inclusion bodies in enlarged infected cells. In the congenital form, there is hepatosplenomegaly with cirrhosis, and microcephaly with mental or motor retardation. Acquired disease may cause a clinical state similar to infectious mononucleosis. When acquired by blood transfusion, postperfusion syndrome results 巨细胞病毒感染; **deficiency d.,** a condition caused by dietary or metabolic deficiency, including all diseases due to an insufficient supply of essential nutrients 营养缺乏症; **degenerative joint d.,** osteoarthritis 骨关节炎，退行性关节病; **Dejerine-Sottas d.,** Dejerine-Sottas syndrome; a severe, progressive, degenerative peripheral neuropathy beginning in early life, marked by atrophy of distal parts of the lower limbs, and by diminution of tendon reflexes and of sensation; characterized by slowing of nerve conduction velocity, onion bulb formation, and segmental demyelination. It is associated with various mutations affecting proteins of the myelin sheath. Sometimes considered to be a subtype of Charcot-Marie-Tooth disease (type III) 德热里纳-索塔斯病; **demyelinating d.,** any condition characterized by destruction of the myelin sheaths of nerves 脱髓鞘性病变; **de Quervain d.,** overuse injury with painful tenosynovitis due to relative narrowness of the common tendon sheath of the abductor pollicis longus and extensor pollicis brevis 桡骨茎突狭窄性腱鞘炎症; **disappearing bone d.,** gradual resorption of a bone or group of bones, sometimes associated with multiple hemangiomas, usually in children or young adults and following trauma 消失性骨病; **diverticular d.,** a general term including the prediverticular state, diverticulosis, and diverticulitis 肠憩室; **Duchenne d.,** 1. spinal muscular atrophy 脊髓性肌萎缩; 2. progressive bulbar paralysis 进行性延髓性麻痹; 3. tabes dorsalis 运动性共济失调; 4. Duchenne muscular dystrophy 迪谢内肌营养不良; **Duchenne-Aran d.,** spinal muscular atrophy 脊髓性肌萎缩; **Duhring d.,** dermatitis herpetiformis 疱疹样皮炎; **Durand-Nicolas-Favre d.,** lymphogranuloma venereum性病淋巴肉芽肿; **Duroziez d.,** congenital mitral stenosis 先天性二尖瓣狭窄; **Ebola virus d.,** an acute, often fatal, type of hemorrhagic fever caused by Ebola virus, seen in Central Africa 埃博拉出血热; **Ebstein d.,** 埃布斯坦综合征，见 *anomaly* 下词条; **end-stage renal d.,** chronic irreversible renal failure 终末期肾病; **Erb d.,** Duchenne muscular dystrophy 进行性假肥大性

肌营养不良；**Erb-Goldflam d.**, myasthenia gravis 重症肌无力；**Eulenburg d.**, paramyotonia congenita 先天性肌强直；**Fabry d.**, an X-linked lysosomal storage disease of glycosphingolipid catabolism resulting from deficiency of α-galactosidase A and leading to accumulation of ceramide trihexoside in the cardiovascular and renal systems 法布里病，一种 X 连锁的溶酶体贮积症；**Farber d.**, a lysosomal storage disease due to defective acid ceramidase and characterized by granulomatous infiltration, painful swelling of joints, nodules over affected joints and pressure points, hoarseness, and feeding and respiratory problems 法伯病，一种溶酶体贮积症；**Fazio-Londe d.**, a rare type of progressive bulbar palsy occurring in childhood 进行性延髓麻痹；**Feer d.**, acrodynia 肢端痛；**fibrocystic d. of breast**, a form of mammary dysplasia with formation of cysts of various size containing a semitransparent, turbid fluid that imparts a brown to blue color to the unopened cysts; believed due to abnormal hyperplasia of the ductal epithelium and dilatation of the ducts of the mammary gland, resulting from exaggeration and distortion of normal menstrual cycle–related breast changes 维囊性乳腺纤病；**fifth d.**, erythema infectiosum 传染性红斑；**flint d.**, chalicosis 石末沉着病；**floating beta d.**, familial dysbetalipoproteinemia 家族性异常 β 脂蛋白血症；**focal d.**, a localized disease 局限性疾病；**foot-and-mouth d.**, an acute, contagious viral disease of wild and domestic cloven-footed animals and occasionally humans, marked by vesicular eruptions on the lips, buccal cavity, pharynx, legs, and feet 口蹄疫；**Forbes d.**, glycogen storage d., type III 糖原贮积症III型；**Fox-Fordyce d.**, a persistent and recalcitrant, itchy, papular eruption, chiefly of the axillae and pubes, due to inflammation of apocrine sweat glands 福克斯 - 福代斯病，汗腺毛囊角化病；**Freiberg d.**, osteochondrosis of the head of the second metatarsal bone 跖骨头骨软骨病；**Friedländer d.**, endarteritis obliterans 闭塞性动脉内膜炎；**Friedreich d.**, paramyoclonus multiplex 多发性肌阵挛；**functional d.**, functional disease, 见 *disorder* 下词条；**Garré d.**, sclerosing nonsuppurative osteomyelitis 硬化性非化脓性骨髓炎功能性疾病，**gastroesophageal reflux d. (GERD)**, any condition resulting from gastroesophageal reflux, characterized by heartburn and regurgitation 胃食管返流病；另见 *reflux esophagitis*；**Gaucher d.**, a hereditary lysosomal storage disease marked by glucocerebroside accumulation in cells of the reticuloendothelial system, with hepatosplenomegaly and skeletal involvement. There are three types, based on the presence and severity of central nervous system involvement. Type I is the mildest and most common, with onset at any age and no neurologic involvement; type II begins in infancy, with severe neurologic involvement and death by age 2; and type III is of later onset, with systemic and moderate neurologic involvement 戈谢病，一种溶酶体贮积症；**genetic d.**, a general term for any disorder caused by a genetic mechanism, comprising chromosome aberrations (or anomalies), mendelian (or monogenic or single-gene) disorders, and multifactorial disorders 遗传病；**gestational trophoblastic d.**, 滋养细胞疾病，见 *neoplasia* 下词条；**Glanzmann d.**, 血小板无力症，见 *thrombasthenia*；**glycogen storage d.**, a group of rare inborn errors of metabolism caused by defects in specific enzymes or transporters involved in the metabolism of glycogen 糖原贮积症；**type 0**, an autosomal recessive disorder caused by deficiency of glycogen synthase, most commonly of the liver isozyme and characterized by decreased hepatic glycogen stores; infants present with early morning drowsiness and fatigue with hypoglycemia and hyperketonemia 糖原贮积症 0 型，常染色体隐性疾病，糖原合成障碍；**type I**, a severe hepatorenal form due to deficiency of the catalytic subunit of glucose-6-phosphatase, resulting in liver, kidney, and intestinal mucosa involvement, with hepatomegaly, fasting hypoglycemia, hyperuricemia, hyperlacticacidemia, hyperlipidemia, xanthomas, bleeding, and adiposity 糖原贮积症 I 型，由于葡萄糖 -6- 磷酸酶催化亚单位缺乏而引起的严重肝肾型；**type IA**, glycogen storage d., type I 糖原贮积症 I a 型；**type IB**, a form resembling type I but additionally predisposing to infection due to neutropenia and to chronic inflammatory bowel disease; due to a defect in the transport system for glucose 6-phosphate 糖原贮积症 I b 型，葡萄糖 -6- 磷酸的运输系统缺陷引起；**type II**, a disorder due to deficiency of the lysosomal enzyme acid α-glucosidase (acid maltase), the severe infant form resulting in generalized glycogen accumulation, with cardiomegaly, cardiorespiratory failure, and death, a milder adult form being a gradual skeletal myopathy that sometimes causes respiratory problems, and a heterogeneous juvenile-onset form with lateonset myopathy and variable cardiac involvement 糖原贮积症 II 型，酸性 α - 葡萄糖苷酶缺乏引起；**type III**, an autosomal recessive disorder due to deficiency of debrancher enzyme (amylo-1,6-glucosidase), either of both liver and muscle isoforms, or of just one; defects in the liver isoform are characterized by hepatomegaly and hypoglycemia, whereas defects in the muscle isoform are characterized by progressive muscle wasting and weakness 糖原贮积症Ⅲ型，脱支酶缺陷引起；*type IV*, an autosomal recessive disorder due to deficiency of the glycogen brancher enzyme, characterized by cirrhosis of the liver, hepatosplenomegaly, progressive hepatic failure, and death in childhood 糖原贮积症Ⅳ型，糖原分支酶缺陷引起；*type V*, an autosomal recessive disorder due to deficiency of the skeletal muscle isozyme of glycogen phosphorylase (muscle phosphorylase), characterized by muscle cramps and fatigue during exercise 糖原贮积症Ⅴ型，糖原磷酸化酶的骨骼肌同工酶缺乏引起；*type VI*, an autosomal recessive disorder due to deficiency of the liver isozyme of glycogen phosphorylase (hepatic phosphorylase), characterized by hepatomegaly, mild to moderate hypoglycemia, and mild ketosis 糖原贮积症Ⅵ型，糖原磷酸化酶的肝同工酶缺乏引起；*type VII*, an autosomal recessive disorder due to deficiency of the muscle isozyme of 6-phosphofructokinase; characterized by muscle weakness and cramping after exercise. Erythrocyte isozyme activity is also decreased, causing increased hemolysis and a mild compensated hemolytic anemia 糖原贮积症Ⅶ型，6- 磷酸果糖激酶的肌同工酶缺乏引起；*type IX*, a disorder of glycogen storage due to deficiency of phosphorylase kinase. There are multiple subtypes depending on which enzyme subunit is affected; the most common affects the liver isoform, has X-linked inheritance, is characterized in affected males by hepatomegaly, occasional fasting hypoglycemia, and some growth retardation 糖原贮积症Ⅸ型，磷酸化酶激酶缺乏引起；**graft-versus-host (GVH) d.**, disease caused by the immune response of histoincompatible, immunocompetent donor cells against the tissue of immunocompromised host, as a complication of stem cell transplantation, or as a result of maternal-fetal blood transfusion, or therapeutic transfusion to an immunocompromised recipient 移植物抗宿主病；**Graves d.**, an association of hyperthyroidism, goiter, and exophthalmos, with accelerated pulse rate, profuse sweating, nervous symptoms, psychic disturbances, emaciation, and elevated basal metabolism 格雷夫斯病；**Greenfield d.**, former name for the late infantile form of metachromatic leukodystrophy 婴儿异染性脑白质营养不良；**Gull d.**, atrophy of the thyroid gland with myxedema 甲状腺萎缩伴黏液水肿；**Günther d.**, congenital erythropoietic porphyria 先天性红细胞生成性卟啉病；**H d.**, Hartnup disorder 哈氏遗传性疾病；**Hailey-Hailey d.**, benign familial pemphigus 家族性良性天疱疮；**Hallervorden-Spatz d.**, pantothenate kinase–associated neurodegeneration 哈勒沃登 - 施帕茨病，苍白球黑质红核色素变性；**Hal-**

tia-Santavuori d., a type of neuronal ceroid lipofuscinosis, with onset at about 1 year of age, characterized by intracellular accumulation of lipofuscin, failure to thrive, myoclonic seizures, hypotonia, psychomotor developmental delay and deterioration, and blindness; death occurs by the age of about 10 years 神经性神经鞘瘤性脂褐病；**hand-foot-and-mouth d.**, a mild, highly infectious viral disease of children, with vesicular lesions in the mouth and on the hands and feet 手足口病；**Hand-Schüller-Christian d.**, a chronic, progressive form of multifocal Langerhans cell histiocytosis, sometimes with accumulation of cholesterol, characterized by the triad of calvarial bone defects, exophthalmos, and diabetes insipidus 汉 - 许 - 克病；**Hansen d.**, leprosy 麻风；**Hashimoto d.**, a progressive disease of the thyroid gland with degeneration of its epithelial elements and replacement by lymphoid and fibrous tissue 桥本甲状腺炎；**heavy chain d's**, a group of malignant neoplasms of lymphoplasmacytic cells marked by the presence of immunoglobulin heavy chains or heavy chain fragments; they are classified according to heavy chain type, e.g., alpha chain disease 重链病；**Heine-Medin d.**, the major form of poliomyelitis 脊髓灰质炎；**hemolytic d. of newborn**, erythroblastosis fetalis 新生儿溶血病；**hemorrhagic d. of newborn**, a self-limited hemorrhagic disorder of the first few days of life, due to deficiency of vitamin K–dependent coagulation factors Ⅱ , Ⅶ , Ⅸ , and Ⅹ 新生儿出血病；**Hers d.**, glycogen storage d., type Ⅵ糖原贮积症Ⅵ型；**hip-joint d.**, tuberculosis of the hip joint 髋关节结核；**Hippel d.**, von Hippel d.; **Hirschsprung d.**, congenital megacolon 先天性巨结肠；**His d., His-Werner d.**, trench fever 战壕热；**Hodgkin d.**, a form of malignant lymphoma marked clinically by painless, progressive enlargement of lymph nodes, spleen, and general lymphoid tissue; other symptoms may include anorexia, lassitude, weight loss, fever, pruritus, night sweats, and anemia. Reed-Sternberg cells are characteristically present. Four types have been distinguished on the basis of histopathologic criteria 霍奇金病；**hoof-and-mouth d.**, foot-and-mouth d.; **hookworm d.**, infection with hookworms, usually *Ancylostoma duodenale* or *Necator americanus*. Larvae enter the body through the skin or in contaminated food or water and migrate to the small intestine, where they become adults, attach to the mucosa, and ingest blood; symptoms may include abdominal pain, diarrhea, colic or nausea, and anemia 钩虫病；**Huntington d. (HD)**, a triplet repeat disorder with autosomal dominant inheritance and characterized by variable age of onset, chronic progressive chorea, and mental deterioration terminating in dementia 亨廷顿病; **hyaline membrane d.**, a type of neonatal respiratory distress syndrome in which there is formation of a hyalinelike membrane lining the terminal respiratory passages; extensive atelectasis is attributed to lack of surfactant 透明膜病; **hydatid d.**, an infection, usually of the liver, due to larval forms of tapeworms of the genus *Echinococcus*, marked by development of expanding cysts 棘球蚴病，泌尿生殖系统包虫病; **immune complex d.**, local or systemic disease caused by the formation of circulating immune complexes and their deposition in tissue, due to activation of complement and to recruitment and activation of leukocytes in type III hypersensitivity reactions 免疫复合物病; **infantile Refsum d.**, an autosomal recessive disorder in which peroxisome biogenesis is defective and phytanic acid accumulates; characterized by early onset, moderate facial dysmorphism, severe intellectual disability, retinitis pigmentosa, sensorineural hearing deficit, hepatomegaly, and hypocholesterolemia 婴儿雷夫叙姆病; **infectious d.**, a disease caused by a pathogenic microorganism, including bacteria, viruses, fungi, protozoa, and multicellular parasites; it may be transmitted from another host or arise from the host's indigenous microflora 传染病，感染性疾病; **inflammatory bowel d.**, any idiopathic inflammatory disease of the bowel, such as Crohn disease and ulcerative colitis 炎（症）性肠病; **intercurrent d.**, one occurring during the course of another disease with which it has no connection 间发病，发生在另一疾病的过程中但与之无关; **iron storage d.**, hemochromatosis 铁贮积病; **ischemic bowel d.**, ischemic colitis 缺血性肠病; **ischemic heart d. (IHD)**, any of a group of acute or chronic cardiac disabilities resulting from insufficient supply of oxygenated blood to the heart 缺血性心脏病; **Janský-Bielschowsky d.**, a type of neuronal ceroid lipofuscinosis, with onset between 2 and 4 years of age, characterized by intracellular accumulation of lipofuscin, myoclonic seizures, and progressive neurologic and retinal deterioration; death occurs by age 10 to 15 比-杨病; **jumping d.**, any of several culture-specific disorders characterized by exaggerated responses to small stimuli, muscle tics including jumping, obedience even to dangerous suggestions, and sometimes coprolalia or echolalia 跳跃痉挛; **juvenile Paget d.**, hyperostosis corticalis deformans juvenilis 青少年佩吉特病; **Kashin-Bek (Kaschin-Beck) d.**, a disabling degenerative disease of the peripheral joints and spine, endemic in parts of northeastern Asia; believed to have a multifactorial cause,

with selenium deficiency predisposing chondrocytes to oxidative stress from free-radical carriers, such as mycotoxins in storage grain and organic matter in drinking water 大骨节病; **Katayama d.**, schistosomiasis japonica 日本血吸虫病; **Kawasaki d.**, a febrile illness usually affecting infants and young children, with conjunctival injection, changes to the oropharyngeal mucosa, changes to the peripheral extremities including edema, erythema, and desquamation, a primarily truncal polymorphous exanthem, and cervical lymphadenopathy. It is often associated with vasculitis of the large coronary vessels 川崎病; **Kennedy d.**, spinobulbar muscular atrophy 脊髓延髓性肌萎缩; **Kienböck d.**, slowly progressive osteochondrosis of the lunate bone; it may affect other wrist bones 月骨骨软化病; **Köhler bone d.**, 1. osteochondrosis of the tarsal navicular bone in children 跗骨舟骨骨软化病; 2. thickening of the shaft of the second metatarsal bone and changes about its articular head, with pain in the second metatarsophalangeal joint on walking or standing 第二跖骨病; **Krabbe d.**, an autosomal recessive lysosomal storage disease, usually beginning in infancy, due to deficiency of galactosylceramidase and characterized by seizures, convulsions, progressive mental deterioration, and early death. Pathologically, there is rapidly progressive cerebral demyelination and large globoid bodies in the white matter 克拉伯病，半乳糖神经酰胺脂质贮积症; **Kufs d.**, a type of neuronal ceroid lipofuscinosis, with onset prior to age 40, characterized by progressive neurologic deterioration but not blindness, intracellular accumulation of lipofuscin, and shortened life expectancy 库夫斯病，神经元蜡样脂褐质沉积症; **Kümmell d.**, compression fracture of vertebra, with symptoms a few weeks after injury, including spinal pain, intercostal neuralgia, lower limb motor disturbances, and kyphosis 陈旧性锥体骨折骨不连; **Kyrle d.**, a chronic disorder of keratinization marked by keratotic plugs that develop in hair follicles and eccrine ducts, penetrating the epidermis and extending down into the corium, causing foreign-body reaction and pain 基勒病，穿通性角化过度症; **Lafora d.**, an autosomal recessive progressive myoclonic epilepsy characterized by attacks of intermittent or continuous myoclonus resulting in difficulties in voluntary movement, by severe mental deterioration, and by intracellular inclusions (Lafora bodies) 拉福拉病; **legionnaires' d.**, an often fatal bacterial infection caused by *Legionella pneumophila*, not spread by person-toperson contact, characterized by high fever, gastrointestinal pain, headache, and pneumonia; there may also be involvement of the kidneys, liver, and nervous system 军团病；**Leiner d.**, a disorder of infancy characterized by generalized seborrhea-like dermatitis and erythroderma, severe intractable diarrhea, recurrent infections, and failure to thrive 脱屑性红皮病；**Leriche d.**, posttraumatic osteoporosis 创伤后骨萎缩；**Letterer-Siwe d.**, a Langerhans cell histiocytosis of early childhood, of autosomal recessive inheritance, characterized by cutaneous lesions resembling seborrheic dermatitis, hemorrhagic tendency, hepatosplenomegaly, lymphadenitis, and progressive anemia. If untreated it is rapidly fatal 莱特勒 - 西韦病，非类脂组织细胞增多症。又称 *acute disseminated Langerhans cell histiocytosis* 急性弥散性组织细胞增生症；**Libman-Sacks d.**, 疣状心内膜炎见 *endocarditis* 下词条；**Lindau d.**, **Lindau-von Hippel d.**, von Hippel-Lindau d.；**Little d.**, congenital spastic stiffness of the limbs, a form of cerebral palsy due to lack of development of the pyramidal tracts Little 病，脑性痉挛性双侧瘫痪；**Lou Gehrig d.**, amyotrophic lateral sclerosis 肌萎缩侧索硬化；**Lutz-Splendore-Almeida d.**, paracoccidioidomycosis 南美芽生菌病；**Lyme d.**, a recurrent multisystemic disorder caused by the spirochete *Borrelia burgdorferi*, the vectors being the ticks *Ixodes scapularis* and *I. pacificus*; usually beginning with erythema chronicum migrans, often accompanied by minor systemic symptoms, followed by variable manifestations including musculoskeletal pain, neurologic and cardiac abnormalities, and, in persistent infection, arthritis of the large joints 莱姆病；**lysosomal storage d.**, an inborn error of metabolism with (1) a defect in a specific lysosomal enzyme; (2) intracellular accumulation of an unmetabolized substrate; (3) clinical progression affecting multiple tissues or organs; (4) considerable phenotypic variation within a disease 溶酶体贮积症；**MAC d.**, *Mycobacterium avium* complex d. 鸟分枝杆菌复合菌组病；**McArdle d.**, glycogen storage d., type V 糖原贮积病 V 型；**mad cow d.**, bovine spongiform encephalopathy 疯牛病；**Madelung d.**, 1. 马德隆畸形，见 *deformity* 下词条；2. multiple symmetric lipomatosis 多发对称性脂肪瘤病；**maple bark d.**, hypersensitivity pneumonitis in logging and sawmill workers due to inhalation of spores of a mold, *Cryptostroma corticale*, growing under the maple bark 枫皮病；**maple syrup urine d. (MSUD)**, a hereditary enzyme defect in metabolism of branchedchain amino acids, marked clinically by mental and physical retardation, severe ketoacidosis, feeding difficulties, and a characteristic maple syrup odor in the urine and on the body 枫糖尿症，支链酮酸尿症；**Marburg d.**, **Marburg virus d.**, a rare, acute, often fatal type of hemorrhagic fever caused by the Marburg virus, occurring most often in central and southern Africa 马尔堡病；**Marchiafava-Micheli d.**, paroxysmal nocturnal hemoglobinuria 阵发性睡眠性血红蛋白尿症；**Marie-Bamberger d.**, hypertrophic pulmonary osteoarthropathy 肥大性肺性骨关节病；**Marie-Strümpell d.**, ankylosing spondylitis 强直性脊柱炎；**Marie-Tooth d.**, Charcot-Marie-Tooth d.；**Mediterranean d.**, thalassemia major 地中海病；**medullary cystic d.**, a progressive, autosomal dominant disorder of the kidneys characterized by adult onset, cyst formation, hypertension, hyperuricemia, anemia, gout, salt wasting, and impaired renal function progressing to end-stage renal disease 肾髓质囊性病；**Meige d.**, lymphedema praecox 早发性淋巴水肿；**Meniere d.**, deafness, tinnitus, and dizziness, in association with nonsuppurative disease of the labyrinth 梅尼埃病；**Menkes d.**, an X-linked recessive disorder of copper metabolism marked by sparse, brittle, twisted scalp hair; loose skin; hyperextensible joints; bladder diverticula; skeletal anomalies; and severe cerebral degeneration. Death occurs by 3 years of age in untreated patients 门克斯病；**mental d.**, 精神疾病 *disorder*. 下词条；**Merzbacher-Pelizaeus d.**, Pelizaeus-Merzbacher d.；**metabolic d.**, one caused by a disruption of a normal metabolic pathway because of a genetically determined enzyme defect 代谢病；**Meyer d.**, adenoid vegetations of the pharynx 腺样体肥大，扁桃体肥大；**Mikulicz d.**, benign, self-limited lymphocytic infiltration and enlargement of the lacrimal and salivary glands of uncertain etiology 米库利奇病；**Milroy d.**, familial primary lymphedema occurring at or soon after birth 遗传性淋巴水肿；**Minamata d.**, a severe neurologic disorder due to alkyl mercury poisoning, with permanent neurologic and mental disabilities or death; once prevalent among those eating contaminated seafood from Minamata Bay, Japan 水俣病；**minimal change d.**, subtle alterations in kidney function demonstrable by clinical albuminuria and the presence of lipid droplets in cells of the proximal tubules, seen primarily in young children 微小病变性肾小球病；**mixed connective tissue d.**, a combination of scleroderma, myositis, systemic lupus erythematosus, and rheumatoid arthritis, and marked serologically by the presence of antibody against extractable nuclear antigen 混合性结缔组织病；**Möbius d.**, ophthalmoplegic migraine 眼肌麻痹性偏头痛；**molecular d.**, any disease in which the pathogenesis can be traced to a single molecule, usually a protein, which is either abnormal in structure or present in reduced amounts 分子病；**Mondor d.**, phlebitis affecting the large subcutaneous veins normally crossing the lateral chest wall and breast from the epigastric or hypochondriac region to the axilla 蒙多病，胸壁浅表血栓性解脉炎；**Monge d.**, chronic mountain sickness 慢性高山病；**motor neuron d., motor system d.**, any disease of a motor neuron, including spinal muscular atrophy, progressive bulbar paralysis, amyotrophic lateral sclerosis, and lateral sclerosis 运动神经元病；*Mycobacterium avium* **complex d.**, MAC disease; systemic disease caused by infection with organisms of the *M. avium-intracellulare* complex in patients with human immunodeficiency virus infection 鸟分枝杆菌综合征；**Newcastle d.**, a viral disease of birds, including domestic fowl, transmissible to humans, characterized by respiratory, gastrointestinal or pulmonary, and encephalitic symptoms 鸡新城疫；**new variant Creutzfeldt-Jakob d. (nvCJD)**, a variant of Creutzfeldt-Jakob disease having a younger age of onset than is seen in Creutzfeldt-Jakob disease, and caused by the same agent that causes bovine spongiform encephalopathy 新变异型克罗伊茨费尔特 - 雅各布病；**Nicolas-Favre d.**, lymphogranuloma venereum 性病淋巴肉芽肿；**Niemann-Pick d.**, a clinically variable, autosomal recessive lysosomal storage disease characterized by accumulation of sphingomyelin in the reticuloendothelial system and the presence of characteristic Niemann-Pick cells. There are three types, designated *A*, *B*, and *C*, varying in age of onset, degree of CNS involvement, and genetic and biochemical defect 尼曼 - 皮克病；**nil d.**, minimal change d; **Norrie d.**, an X-linked disorder consisting of bilateral blindness from retinal malformation, intellectual disability, and deafness 早产儿视网膜病变综合征；**notifiable d.**, one required to be reported to federal, state, or local health officials when diagnosed, because of infectiousness, severity, or frequency of occurrence 应申报的传染病；**oasthouse urine d.**, methionine malabsorption syndrome 甲硫氨酸吸收不良综合征；**obstructive small airways d.**, chronic bronchitis with irreversible narrowing of the bronchioles and small bronchi with hypoxia and often hypercapnia 阻塞性支气管病；**occupational d.**, disease due to various factors involved in one's employment 职业病；**Oguchi d.**, a rare autosomal recessive form of congenital night blindness with slowed dark adaptation of rods and yellowishgold fundus discoloration that disappears in darkness; due to mutation involving either of two proteins of the visual cycle 静止型白点状眠底；**organic d.**, a disease associated with demonstrable change in a bodily organ or tissue 器质性疾病；**Osgood-Schlatter d.**, traction apoph-

ysitis of the tuber of the tibia with osteochondrosis 胫骨粗隆骨软骨病；**Osler d.**, 1. polycythemia vera 真性红细胞增多症；2. hereditary hemorrhagic telangiectasia 遗传性出血性毛细血管扩张；**Owren d.**, parahemophilia 类血友病；**Paget d.**, 1. (of bone) osteitis deformans 畸形性骨炎；2. (of breast) an intraductal inflammatory carcinoma of the breast, involving the areola and nipple 乳腺导管内炎性癌；3. an extramammary counterpart of Paget disease of the breast, usually involving the vulva, and sometimes other sites, as the perianal and axillary regions 乳头乳晕湿疹样癌；**Parkinson d.**, a slowly progressive disorder of the basal ganglia, usually occurring in late life, characterized by mask-like facies, resting tremor, slowing of voluntary movements, festinating gait, flexed posture, and muscle weakness, sometimes with excessive sweating and feelings of heat. There is degeneration of dopaminergic neurons of the pars compacta of the substantia nigra and dramatic decrease in the levels of dopamine in the substantia nigra and corpus striatum 帕金森病；**parrot d.**, psittacosis 鹦鹉热；**Parry d.**, Graves d.; **Pelizaeus-Merzbacher d.**, a progressive familial form of leukoencephalopathy, marked by nystagmus, ataxia, tremor, parkinsonian facies, dysarthria, and mental deterioration 佩利措伊斯 - 梅茨巴赫病；**Pellegrini d., Pellegrini-Stieda d.**, calcification of the medial collateral ligament of the knee due to trauma 内侧副韧带钙化；**pelvic inflammatory d. (PID)**, any pelvic infection involving the upper female genital tract beyond the cervix 盆腔炎；**periodontal d.**, any disease or disorder of the periodontium 牙周病；**Perthes d.**, osteochondrosis of capitular femoral epiphysis 儿童股骨头缺血性坏死；**Peyronie d.**, induration of the corpora cavernosa of the penis, producing a painful fibrous chordee and penile curvature 阴茎纤维性海绵体炎；**Pick d.**, 1. progressive atrophy of the cerebral convolutions in a limited area (lobe) of the brain, with clinical manifestations and course similar to Alzheimer disease 额颞（叶）痴呆；2. Niemann-Pick d. 尼曼 - 皮克病，鞘磷脂沉积病；**polycystic kidney d., polycystic renal d.**, either of two unrelated heritable disorders marked by cysts in both kidneys: the *autosomal dominant* or *adult* form is more common, appears in adult life, and is marked by loss of renal function that can be either rapid or slow; the *autosomal recessive* or *infantile* form is more rare, may be congenital or may appear later in childhood, and almost always progresses to renal failure 多囊肾病；**Pompe d.**, glycogen storage d., type Ⅱ 糖原贮积症Ⅱ型；**Pott d.**, spinal tuberculosis 波特病，脊柱结核；**primary electrical** d., serious ventricular tachycardia, and sometimes ventricular fibrillation, in the absence of recognizable structural heart disease 原发性心脏病；**prion d.**, any of a group of fatal, transmissible neurodegenerative diseases, which may be sporadic, familial, or acquired, caused by abnormalities of prion protein metabolism resulting from mutations in the prion protein gene or from infection with pathogenic forms of the protein 朊病毒病；**pulseless d.**, Takayasu arteritis 无脉病；**Raynaud d.**, a primary or idiopathic vascular disorder, most often affecting women, marked by bilateral attacks of Raynaud phenomenon 雷诺病，肢体动脉痉挛症；**Refsum d.**, an inherited disorder of lipid metabolism, characterized by accumulation of phytanic acid, chronic polyneuritis, retinitis pigmentosa, cerebellar ataxia, and persistent elevation of protein in cerebrospinal fluid 雷夫叙姆病，植烷酸贮积症；**remnant removal d.**, familial dysbetalipoproteinemia 家族性血β脂蛋白异常；**reversible obstructive airway d.**, a condition characterized by bronchospasm reversible by intervention, as in asthma 可逆阻塞性气道疾病；**rheumatic heart d.**, the most important manifestation and sequel to rheumatic fever, consisting chiefly of valvular deformities 风湿性心脏病；**rheumatoid d.**, a systemic condition best known by its articular involvement (rheumatoid arthritis) but emphasizing nonarticular changes, e.g., pulmonary interstitial fibrosis, pleural effusion, and lung nodules 风湿性疾病；**Ritter d.**, dermatitis exfoliativa neonatorum 新生儿剥脱性皮炎；**Roger d.**, a ventricular septal defect; the term is usually restricted to small, asymptomatic defects 室间隔缺损；**runt d.**, a graft-versus-host disease produced by immunologically competent cells in a foreign host that is unable to reject them, resulting in gross retardation of host development and in death 移植抗宿主疾病；**Salla d.**, an inherited disorder of sialic acid metabolism; characterized by accumulation of sialic acid in lysosomes and excretion in the urine, intellectual disability, delayed motor development, and ataxia 唾液酸贮积症；**Sandhoff d.**, a GM$_2$ gangliosidosis resembling Tay-Sachs d. but due to a defect in the β subunit of hexosaminidase, which is common to both A and B isozymes 桑德霍夫病；**Schamberg d.**, a slowly progressive purpuric and pigmentary disease of the skin affecting chiefly the shins, ankles, and dorsa of the feet 进行性色素性皮肤病；**Scheuermann d.**, osteochondrosis of vertebral epiphyses first manifesting in adolescence, with anterior wedging of vertebrae, resulting in a rigid thoracic or thoracolumbar kyphosis (Scheuermann kyphosis) 舒尔曼病；**Schilder d.**, subacute or chronic leukoencephalopathy in children and adolescents, similar to adrenoleukodystrophy; massive destruction of the white matter of the cerebral hemispheres leads to blindness, deafness, bilateral spasticity, and mental deterioration 希尔德病风温性紫癜；**Schönlein d.**, 见 *purpura*. 下词条；**secondary d.**, 继发病 1. one subsequent to or as a consequence of another disease. 2. one due to introduction of incompatible, immunologically competent cells into a host rendered incapable of rejecting them by heavy exposure to ionizing radiation; **self-limited d.**, one that runs a limited and definite course 自限性疾病；**serum d.**, 血清病，见 *sickness* 下词条；**Sever d.**, traction apophysitis of the calcaneus 跟骨骨骺炎；**severe combined immunodeficiency d. (SCID)**, 重度联合免疫缺陷病，见 *immunodeficiency* 下词条；**sexually transmitted d.**, venereal disease; any of a diverse group of infections transmitted by sexual contact; in some this is the only important mode of transmission, and in others transmission by nonsexual means is possible 性传播疾病；**sickle cell d.**, any disease associated with the presence of hemoglobin S 镰状细胞病；**Simmonds d.**, 全垂体功能减退症，见 *panhypopituitarism*；**sixth d.**, exanthema subitum 幼儿急疹；**small airways d.**, chronic obstructive bronchitis with irreversible narrowing of the bronchioles and small bronchi 小气道病变，另见 *obstructive small airways d.*；**Smith-Strang d.**, methionine malabsorption syndrome 甲硫胺酸吸收障碍综合征；**Spielmeyer-Vogt d.**, Vogt-Spielmeyer d.；**Stargardt d.**, an autosomal recessive form of macular degeneration that first appears between the ages of 6 and 20 and is marked by abnormal pigmentation and other changes in the macular area, with rapid loss of visual acuity 眼底黄色斑点症；**Steinert d.**, myotonic dystrophy 肌强直性营养不良；**Still d.**, systemic onset juvenile rheumatoid arthritis 斯蒂尔病；**storage d.**, a metabolic disorder in which a specific substance (a lipid, a protein, etc.) accumulates in certain cells in unusually large amounts 贮积症；**storage pool d.**, a blood coagulation disorder due to failure of the platelets to release adenosine diphosphate (ADP) in response to aggregating agents; characterized by mild bleeding episodes, prolonged bleeding time, and reduced aggregation response to collagen or thrombin 贮存池病；**Strümpell d.**, hereditary lateral sclerosis with the spasticity mainly limited to the legs 遗传性侧索硬化；**Strümpell-Leichtenstern d.**, hemorrhagic encephalitis 出血性脑炎；**Sutton d.**, 1. halo nevus 晕痣；2. periadenitis mucosa necrotica recurrens 复发坏死性黏膜腺周炎；3. granuloma fissuratum 裂隙肉芽肿；**Swift d.**, **Swift-Feer d.**, acrodynia 肢痛

314

症；**Takayasu d.**, 无脉病，见 *arteritis* 下词条；
Tangier d., a familial disorder characterized by a
deficiency of high-density lipoproteins in the blood
serum, with storage of cholesteryl esters in tissues
丹吉尔病；**Tarui d.**, glycogen storage d., type Ⅶ
糖原贮积症Ⅶ型；**Tay-Sachs d. (TSD)**, a GM₂
gangliosidosis caused by deficiency of activity of
hexosaminidase A, due to mutation affecting the α
subunit of the enzyme or an activator protein necessary for enzyme activity, and usually seen in Ashkenazi Jews. It occurs as a classic infantile-onset form,
characterized by doll-like facies, cherryred macular
spot, early blindness, hyperacusis, macrocephaly,
seizures, hypotonia, and death in early childhood,
and also as juvenile and adult forms, with greater
age at onset correlated with decreased severity 家族
性黑矇性痴呆；**Thomsen d.**, the autosomal dominant form of myotonia congenita 强直性白内障；
thyrotoxic heart d., heart disease associated with
hyperthyroidism, marked by atrial fibrillation, cardiac enlargement, and congestive heart failure 甲状腺
毒性心脏病；**transmissible neurodegenerative d.**,
prion d.; **trophoblastic d.**, gestational trophoblastic
neoplasia 滋养层疾病；**Unverricht d., Unverricht-Lundborg d.**, a slowly progressive autosomal
recessive form of myoclonic epilepsy with severe,
continuous, stimulus-triggered myoclonic seizures
and degenerative changes in the brain without presence of the Lafora bodies of Lafora disease 肌阵挛
性癫痫；**uremic bone d.**, renal osteodystrophy 尿
毒症骨病；**venereal d.**, sexually transmitted d; ve-
noocclusive d. of the liver, symptomatic occlusion
of the small hepatic venules caused by ingestion of
Senecio tea or related substances, by certain chemotherapy agents, or by radiation 肝小静脉闭塞病；
vinyl chloride d., acro-osteolysis resulting from exposure to vinyl chloride, characterized by Raynaud
phenomenon and skin and bony changes on the
limbs 氯乙烯病；**Vogt-Spielmeyer d.**, a type of
neuronal ceroid lipofuscinosis with onset between
ages 5 and 10 years, characterized by intracellular
accumulation of lipofuscin and rapid cerebroretinal
degeneration leading to blindness; death occurs between 20 and 40 years of age 家族黑矇性白痴；
Volkmann d., congenital deformity of the foot due
to tibiotarsal dislocation 胫骨脱位导致的先天性足
畸形；**von Hippel d.**, hemangiomatosis confined
principally to the retina; when associated with
hemangioblastoma of the cerebellum, it is known as
von Hippel-Lindau d. 视网膜血管瘤病；**von Hippel-Lindau d.**, a hereditary condition marked by
hemangiomas of the retina and hemangioblastomas
of the cerebellum, sometimes with similar lesions of

the spinal cord and cysts of the viscera; there may
be neurologic symptoms such as seizures and mental
retardation 希佩尔 - 林道病，脑视网膜血管瘤病；
von Recklinghausen d., 1. neurofibromatosis 神经
纤维瘤病；2. osteitis fibrosa cystica 纤维囊性骨
炎；**von Willebrand d.**, a mainly autosomal dominant bleeding disorder characterized by prolonged
bleeding time, deficiency of von Willebrand factor,
and often impairment of adhesion of platelets on
glass beads, associated with epistaxis and increased
bleeding after trauma or surgery, menorrhagia, and
postpartum bleeding 血管性血友病；**Walden-
ström d.**, osteochondrosis of the capitular femoral
epiphysis 股骨头骨骺骨软骨症；**Weber-Christian
d.**, nodular nonsuppurative panniculitis 复发性
结节性非化脓性脂膜炎；**Werlhof d.**, idiopathic
thrombocytopenic purpura 特发性血小板减少性紫
癜；**Wernicke d.**, 韦尼克病，见 *encephalopathy*
下词条；**Westphal-Strümpell d.**, hepatolenticular
degeneration 肝豆状核变性；**Whipple d.**, a malabsorption syndrome caused by infection with *Tro-
pheryma whiplei*, marked by diarrhea, steatorrhea,
skin pigmentation, arthralgia and arthritis, lymphadenopathy, central nervous system lesions, and infiltration of the intestinal mucosa with macrophages
containing PASpositive material 惠普尔病；**Wilson
d.**, a progressive autosomal recessive disorder of
copper transport, with accumulation of copper in
liver, brain, kidney, cornea, and other tissues; it is
characterized by cirrhosis, degenerative changes in
the brain, and a Kayser-Fleischer ring 肝豆状核变
性，威尔逊氏病；**Wolman d.**, a lysosomal storage
disease due to deficiency of the lysosomal sterol esterase, occurring in infants, and associated with hepatosplenomegaly, adrenal steatorrhea, calcification,
abdominal distention, anemia, and inanition 酸性脂
酶缺乏症；**woolsorter's d.**, inhalational anthrax 吸
入性炭疽

dis·en·gage·ment (dis″ən-gāj′mənt) emergence of
the fetus from the vaginal canal 分娩

dis·equi·lib·ri·um (dis-e″kwī-lib′re-əm) dysequilibrium 平衡失调；**linkage d.**, the occurrence
in a population of two linked alleles at a frequency
higher than expected by chance 连锁不平衡

dis·ger·mi·no·ma (dis-jur″mī-no′mə) dysgerminoma 无性细胞瘤

dish (dish) a shallow vessel of glass or other material for laboratory work 用于实验室工作的浅容器；
Petri d., a shallow glass dish for growing bacterial
cultures 细菌培养皿

dis·in·fec·tant (dis″in-fek′tənt) 1. an agent that
disinfects, particularly one used on inanimate objects 消毒剂；2. freeing from infection 消毒

dis·in·fes·ta·tion (dis″in-fəs-ta′shən) destruction of insects, rodents, or other animal forms present on the person or their clothes or in their surroundings, and which may transmit disease 杀虫

dis·in·te·grant (dis-in′tə-grənt) an agent used in pharmaceutical preparation of tablets that causes them to disintegrate and release their medicinal substances on contact with moisture 分解质，崩解剂

dis·in·te·gra·tion (dis-in″tə-gra′shən) 1. the process of breaking up or decomposing 分解，分解过程；2. disruption of integrative functions of personality in mental illness; disorganization of the psychic and behavioral processes 精神错乱

dis·in·te·gra·tive (dis-in′tə-gra″tiv) 1. being reduced to components, particles, or fragments; losing cohesion or unity 分解的；2. having disorganized psychic and behavioral processes 使崩溃的

dis·junc·tion (dis-junk′shən) 1. the act or state of being disjoined 分　离；2. in genetics, the moving apart of bivalent chromosomes during anaphase of meiosis or mitosis（染色体）分裂；**craniofacial d.,** Le Fort Ⅲ fracture 颅面关节分离

disk (disk) a circular or rounded flat plate 盘。Spelled also *disc*; **articular d.,** a pad of fibrocartilage or dense fibrous tissue present in some synovial joints 关节盘；**Bowman D's,** flat, disklike plates making up striated muscle fibers 鲍曼肌盘；**choked d.,** papilledema 视神经乳头水肿；**ciliary d.,** pars plana 睫状环；**contained d.,** protrusion of a nucleus pulposus in which the anulus fibrosus remains intact 髓核突出，纤维环完整；**cupped d.,** a pathologically depressed optic disk 病理性视盘凹陷；**epiphyseal d.,** the thin plate of cartilage between the epiphysis and the metaphysis of a growing long bone 骺盘；**extruded d.,** herniation of the nucleus pulposus through the anulus fibrosus, with the nuclear material remaining attached to the intervertebral disk 髓核通过纤维环突出；**gelatin d.,** a disk or lamella of gelatin variously medicated, used chiefly in eye diseases 明胶盘；**growth d.,** epiphyseal d.；**hair d.,** a vascularized and innervated area of skin in the connective tissue sheath of a hair follicle, acting as a mechanoreceptor 毛囊盘；**Hensen d.,** H band 横纹肌盘；**herniated d.,** herniation of intervertebral disk 椎间盘突出，见 *herniation* 下词条；**interarticular d.,** articular d.；**intervertebral d.,** the layer of fibrocartilage between the bodies of each pair of adjacent vertebrae 椎间板，椎间盘；**intraarticular d.,** articular d.；**Merkel d.,** 梅克尔触盘，见 *cell* 下词条；**noncontained d.,** herniation of the nucleus pulposus with rupture of the anulus fibrosus 髓核突出伴纤维环破裂；**optic d.,** the intraocular part of the optic nerve formed by fibers converging from the retina and appearing as a pink to white disk; because there are no sensory receptors in the region, it is not sensitive to stimuli 视盘；**Placido d.,** a disk marked with concentric circles, used in examining the cornea 角膜镜；**protruded d., ruptured d.,** herniation of intervertebral disk 椎间盘突出，见 *herniation* 下词条；**sequestered d.,** a free fragment of the nucleus pulposus that is in the spinal canal outside of the anulus fibrosus and no longer attached to the intervertebral disk 髓核的游离碎片；**slipped d.,** popular term for herniation of an intervertebral disk 椎间盘突出，见 *herniation* 下词条

dis·kec·to·my (dis-kek′tə-me) excision of an intervertebral disk 椎间盘切除术

dis·ki·tis (dis-ki′tis) inflammation of a disk, particularly of an articular disk 关节盘炎

dis·kog·ra·phy (dis-kog′rə-fe) radiography of the vertebral column after injection of radiopaque medium into an intervertebral disk 椎间盘造影术

dis·lo·ca·tion (dis″lo-ka′shən) displacement of a part 脱位，错位；**complete d.,** one completely separating the surfaces of a joint 全脱位；**compound d.,** one in which the joint communicates with the air through a wound 复合错位；**congenital d. of the hip,** developmental dysplasia of the hip 先天性髋关节脱位；**pathologic d.,** one due to paralysis, synovitis, infection, or other disease 病理性脱位；**simple d.,** one in which there is no communication with the air through a wound 单纯脱位；**subspinous d.,** dislocation of the head of the humerus into the space below the spine of the scapula 棘窝下脱位

dis·mem·ber·ment (dis-mem′bər-mənt) amputation of a limb or a portion of it 截肢

dis·oc·clude (dis″ō-klood′) to grind a tooth so that it does not touch its antagonist in the other jaw in any masticatory movements 使无咬合

di·so·my (di′so-me) the presence of two chromosomes of a homologous pair in a cell; in humans the normal state, with each pair usually comprising one chromosome from each parent 二倍体；**uniparental d.,** the abnormal state in which both chromosomes of the homologous pair are from the same parent 单亲二倍体

di·so·pyr·a·mide (di″so-pir′ə-mīd) a cardiac depressant with anticholinergic properties, used as the base or phosphate salt as an antiarrhythmic 丙吡胺

dis·or·der (dis-or′dər) a derangement or abnormality of function; a morbid physical or mental state 障碍；**46,XX d. of sex development, 46,XX DSD,** a condition in which a genetic female has female gonads but virilized external genitalia, due to excessive intrauterine exposure to endogenous or exoge-

316

nous androgens. Formerly called *female pseudohermaphroditism* 46,XX 性发育障碍；**46, XX testicular d.** of sex development, 46, XX testicular DSD, a condition in which a genetic female has male gonads, azoospermia, absence of müllerian structures, and normal to ambiguous male external genitalia; gender identity is male. It is usually due to translocation of the *SRY* (testis-determining) gene from the Y to the X chromosome 46, XX 睾丸性发育障碍；**46, XY d.** of sex development, 46, XY DSD, a heterogeneous condition in which a genetic male has slightly to significantly undervirilized external genitalia; if gonads are present, they vary from rudimentary to normal testes; causes include defects in androgen receptors and in testosterone production or metabolism. Formerly called *male pseudohermaphroditism* 46, XY 性发育障碍；**acute stress d.,** an anxiety disorder characterized by development of anxiety, dissociative, and other symptoms within 1 month following exposure to an extremely traumatic event. If persistent, it may become posttraumatic stress disorder 急性应激障碍；**adjustment d.,** maladaptive reaction to identifiable stress (e.g., divorce, illness), which is assumed to remit when the stress ceases or when the patient adapts 适应障碍；**affective d's,** mood d's.; **alcohol-related cognitive d.,** a condition associated with alcohol addiction, resulting in deficits in executive function processes, such as problem solving, planning, organizing, and working memory 酒精相关认知障碍；**amnestic d's,** mental disorders characterized by acquired impairment in the ability to learn and recall new information, sometimes accompanied by inability to recall previously learned information 遗忘症；**antisocial personality d.,** a personality disorder characterized by continuous and chronic antisocial behavior in which the rights of others or generally accepted social norms are violated 反社会人格障碍；**anxiety d's,** mental disorders in which anxiety and avoidance behavior predominate, i.e., panic disorder, agoraphobia, social phobia, specific phobia, obsessive-compulsive disorder, posttraumatic stress disorder, acute stress disorder, generalized anxiety disorder, and substance-induced anxiety disorder 焦虑症；**attention-deficit/hyperactivity d.,** a childhood neurodevelopmental disorder classification characterized by several inattentive (e.g., distractibility, forgetfulness, not appearing to listen) or hyperactive-impulsive (e.g., restlessness, excessive running or climbing, excessive talking, and other disruptive behavior) symptoms that were present before age 12. May be diagnosed along with autism spectrum disorder 多动症；**autism spectrum d.,** includes the conditions of autism, Asperger disorder, childhood disintegrative disorder, and pervasive developmental disorder not otherwise specified; these conditions are characterized by both deficits in social communication and social interaction and by restricted and repetitive behaviors, interests, and activities (RRBs) 孤独症谱系障碍；**autistic d.,** autism; a severe pervasive developmental disorder with onset usually before 3 years of age and a biologic basis; it is characterized by qualitative impairments in reciprocal social interactions, verbal and nonverbal communications, and the capacity for symbolic play; by a restricted and unusual repertoire of activities and interests; and often by cognitive impairment 孤独症；**avoidant personality d.,** a personality disorder characterized by social discomfort, hypersensitivity to criticism, low self-esteem, and an aversion to activities that involve significant interpersonal contact 回避型人格障碍；**behavior d.,** conduct d. 行为障碍；**binge-eating d.,** an eating disorder characterized by repeated episodes (on average, at least once per week for 3 months) of binge eating, as in bulimia nervosa, but not followed by inappropriate compensatory behavior such as purging, fasting, or excessive exercise; eating any amount of food that is larger than what most people would eat in a given period of time under similar circumstances; people who suffer from this condition feel they have no control while eating 暴食症；**bipolar d's,** mood disorders with a history of manic, mixed, or hypomanic episodes, usually with present or previous history of one or more major depressive episodes; included are *bipolar* I *d.,* characterized by one or more manic or mixed episodes, *bipolar* II *d.,* characterized by one or more hypomanic episodes but no manic episodes, and *cyclothymic disorder.* The term is sometimes used in the singular to denote either bipolar I or bipolar II disorder, or both 双相情感障碍；**body dysmorphic d.,** a somatoform disorder characterized by a normal-looking person's preoccupation with an imagined defect in appearance 躯体变形障碍；**borderline personality d.,** a personality disorder marked by a pervasive instability of mood, self-image, and interpersonal relationships, with fears of abandonment, chronic feelings of emptiness, threats, anger, and self-damaging behavior 边缘型人格障碍；**breathing-related sleep d.,** any of several disorders characterized by sleep disruption due to some sleep-related breathing problem, resulting in excessive sleepiness or insomnia 呼吸相关睡眠障碍；**brief psychotic d.,** an episode of psychotic symptoms with sudden onset, lasting less than 1 month 短暂精神性障碍；**cannabis

withdrawal d., a condition that occurs with the cessation of marijuana use that causes significant distress or impairment in social, occupational, or other important areas of functioning; characterized by the development of at least three signs or symptoms, which may include irritability, anger, or aggression; nervousness or anxiety; insomnia; decreased appetite or weight loss; or restlessness 大麻戒断障碍；**catatonic d.**, catatonia due to the physiologic effects of a general medical condition and neither better accounted for by another mental disorder nor occurring exclusively during delirium; formerly a classification of schizophrenia characterized by marked psychomotor disturbance, including some combination of motoric immobility (stupor, catalepsy), excessive motor activity, extreme negativism, mutism, echolalia, echopraxia, and peculiarities of voluntary movement, such as posturing, mannerisms, grimacing, or stereotyped behaviors 紧张性精神障碍；**character d's**, personality d's.；**childhood disintegrative d.**, pervasive developmental disorder characterized by marked regression in various developmental skills, including language, play, and social and motor skills, after 2 to 10 years of initial normal development 儿童瓦解性障碍；**childhood-onset fluency d.**, stuttering 儿童期发病的流畅性障碍；**circadian rhythm sleep d.**, a lack of synchrony between the schedule of sleeping and waking required by the external environment and that of a person's own circadian rhythm 昼夜节律性睡眠障碍；**collagen d.**, an inborn error of metabolism involving abnormal structure or metabolism of collagen, e.g., Marfan syndrome, cutis laxa 胶原代谢紊乱。Cf. *collagen disease*；**communication d's**, mental disorders characterized by difficulties with speech or language, severe enough to interfere academically, occupationally, or socially 沟通障碍；**conduct d.**, a type of disruptive behavior disorder of childhood and adolescence marked by persistent violation of the rights of others or of age-appropriate societal norms or rules 品行障碍；**conversion d.**, a somatoform disorder characterized by conversion symptoms (loss or alteration of voluntary motor or sensory functioning suggesting physical illness) with no physiological basis and not produced intentionally or feigned; a psychological basis is suggested by exacerbation of symptoms during psychological stress, relief from tension (primary gain), or gain of outside support or attention (secondary gains) 游离转换障碍；**cyclothymic d.**, a mood disorder characterized by alternating cycles of hypomanic and depressive periods with symptoms like those of manic and major depressive episodes but of lesser severity 循环性

心境障碍；**delusional d.**, a mental disorder marked by well-organized, logically consistent delusions of grandeur, persecution, or jealousy, with no other psychotic feature. There are seven types: persecutory, jealous, erotomanic, somatic, grandiose, mixed, and unspecified; for diagnosis, symptoms must not be better explained by other conditions, such as obsessive-compulsive disorder or body dysmorphic disorder 妄想性障碍；**dependent personality d.**, a personality disorder marked by an excessive need to be taken care of, with submissiveness and clinging, feelings of helplessness when alone, and preoccupation with fears of being abandoned 依赖型人格障碍；**depersonalization d.**, a dissociative disorder characterized by intense, prolonged, or otherwise troubling feelings of detachment from one's body or thoughts, not secondary to another mental disorder 人格解体障碍；**depressive d's**, mood disorders in which depression is unaccompanied by manic or hypomanic episodes 抑郁障碍；**depressive personality d.**, a persistent and pervasive pattern of depressive cognitions and behaviors, such as unhappiness, low self-esteem, pessimism, critical and derogatory attitudes, guilt or remorse, and an inability to relax or feel enjoyment 抑郁型人格障碍；**developmental coordination d.**, problematic or delayed development of gross and fine motor coordination skills, not due to a neurologic disorder or to general intellectual disability, resulting in the appearance of clumsiness 发展性协调障碍；**disruptive behavior d's**, a group of mental disorders of children and adolescents consisting of behavior that violates social norms and is disruptive 破坏性行为障碍；**disruptive mood dysregulation d.**, diagnosed in children ages 6 to 18 years; symptoms include abnormal irritability and explosive temper outbursts that are not in accord with the child's developmental level, that occur at least three times per week for more than 1 year, and that began to happen before the age of 10 破坏性情绪失调障碍；**dissociative d's**, mental disorders characterized by sudden, temporary alterations in identity, memory, or consciousness, segregating normally integrated parts of one's personality from one's dominant identity 分离性障碍；**dissociative identity d.**, a dissociative disorder characterized by the existence in an individual of two or more distinct personalities, with at least two of the personalities controlling the patient's behavior in turns. The host personality usually is totally unaware of the alternate personalities; alternate personalities may or may not have awareness of the others 分离性身份识别障碍；**dream anxiety d.**, nightmare d. 梦境焦虑障碍；**dysthymic d.**, a mood disorder characterized by depressed feeling, loss of interest or pleasure in one's usual activities, and other symptoms typical of depression but tending to be longer in duration and less severe than in major depressive disorder 情绪障碍；**eating d.**, abnormal feeding habits associated with psychological factors, including anorexia nervosa, bulimia nervosa, pica, and rumination disorder 进食障碍；**expressive language d.**, a communication disorder occurring in children and characterized by problems with the expression of language, either oral or signed 语言表达障碍；**factitious d.**, a mental disorder characterized by repeated, intentional simulation of physical or psychological signs and symptoms of illness for no apparent purpose other than obtaining treatment 做作性障碍；**factitious d. by proxy**, a form of factitious disorder in which one person (usually a mother) intentionally fabricates or induces physical (*Munchausen syndrome by proxy*) or psychological disorders in another person under their care (usually their child) and subjects that person to needless diagnostic procedures or treatment, without any external incentives for the behavior 代理人为疾患；**female orgasmic d.**, consistently delayed or absent orgasm in a female, even after a normal phase of sexual excitement and adequate stimulation 女性性高潮障碍；**female sexual arousal d.**, a sexual dysfunction involving inability of a female either to attain or maintain lubrication and swelling during sexual activity, after adequate stimulation 女性性唤起障碍；**functional d.**, a disorder of physiologic function having no known organic basis 功能障碍；**gender identity d.**, a disturbance of gender identification in which affected persons have an overwhelming desire to change their anatomic sex or insist that they are of the opposite sex, with persistent discomfort about their assigned sex or about filling its usual gender role 性别认同障碍；**generalized anxiety d. (GAD)**, an anxiety disorder characterized by excessive, uncontrollable worry about two or more life circumstances for 6 months or more 广泛性焦虑症；**Hartnup d.**, a usually asymptomatic, autosomal recessive defect of intestinal and renal transport of neutral amino acids; symptoms, when they occur, include a pellagra-like skin rash, intermittent cerebellar ataxia, and aminoaciduria restricted to neutral amino acids 哈氏遗传性疾病；**histrionic personality d.**, a personality disorder marked by excessive emotionality and attention-seeking behavior 表演型人格障碍；**hypersexual d.**, excessive, uncontrollable nonparaphilic sexual behavior that may cause significant personal distress; may stem from underlying or associated disorders

纵欲障碍；**hypoactive sexual desire d.**, a sexual dysfunction consisting of persistently or recurrently low level or absence of sexual fantasies and desire for sexual activity 性欲减退障碍；**impulse control d's**, a group of mental disorders characterized by repeated failure to resist an impulse to perform some act harmful to oneself or to others 冲动控制障碍；**induced psychotic d.**, shared psychotic d. 感应性精神障碍；**intermittent explosive d.**, an impulse control disorder characterized by multiple discrete episodes of loss of control of aggressive impulses resulting in serious assault or destruction of property that are out of proportion to any precipitating stressors 间歇性暴发性障碍；**language d.**, any disorder of normal languagebased communication, whether psychogenic or neurogenic; includes expressive and mixed receptive-expressive language disorders 语言障碍；**learning d's**, a group of disorders characterized by academic functioning that is substantially below the level expected on the basis of the patient's age, intelligence, and education 学习障碍；**lymphoproliferative d's**, a group of malignant neoplasms arising from cells related to the common multipotential lymphoreticular cell, including lymphocytic, histiocytic, and monocytic leukemias, multiple myeloma, plasmacytoma, and Hodgkin disease 淋巴增殖性疾病；**lymphoreticular d's**, a group of disorders of the lymphoreticular system, characterized by the proliferation of lymphocytes or lymphoid tissues 淋巴管疾病；**major depressive d.**, a mood disorder characterized by the occurrence of one or more major depressive episodes and the absence of any history of manic, mixed, or hypomanic episodes 重性抑郁障碍；**male erectile d.**, a sexual dysfunction involving inability of a male to attain or maintain an adequate erection until completion of sexual relations 男性勃起失能；**male orgasmic d.**, consistently delayed or absent orgasm in a male, even after a normal phase of sexual excitement and stimulation adequate for his age 男性性高潮障碍；**manic-depressive d.**, former name for a mood disorder now known as *bipolar I d.* or *bipolar II d.* and often called *bipolar d.* (q.v.) 躁狂抑郁症；**mendelian d.**, a genetic disease showing a mendelian pattern of inheritance, caused by a single mutation in the structure of DNA, which causes a single basic defect with pathologic consequences 孟德尔疾病；**mental d.**, any clinically significant behavioral or psychological syndrome characterized by the presence of distressing symptoms, impairment of functioning, or significantly increased risk of suffering death, pain, or other disability 精神障碍；**minor depressive d.**, a mood disorder closely resembling major depressive disorder and dysthymic disorder but intermediate in severity between the two 轻度抑郁症；**mixed receptive-expressive language d.**, a communication disorder involving both the expression and the comprehension of language, either spoken or signed 混合性感受 - 表达性语言障碍；**monogenic d.**, mendelian d. 单基因病；**mood d's**, mental disorders characterized by disturbances of mood manifested as one or more episodes of mania, hypomania, depression, or some combination, the two main subcategories being *bipolar disorders* and *depressive disorders* 情感障碍；**motor d.**, a classification that includes developmental coordination disorder, stereotypic movement disorder, Tourette syndrome, persistent (chronic) motor or vocal tic disorder, provisional tic disorder, other specified tic disorder, and unspecified tic disorder 运动障碍；**motor skills d.**, any disorder characterized by inadequate development of motor coordination severe enough to restrict locomotion or the ability to perform tasks, schoolwork, or other activities 运动技能障碍；**multifactorial d.**, one caused by the interaction of genetic, and sometimes also nongenetic, environmental factors, e.g., diabetes mellitus 多因病；**multiple personality d.**, dissociative identity d. 多人格症；**myeloproliferative d's**, a group of usually neoplastic diseases possibly related histogenetically, including granulocytic leukemias, myelomonocytic leukemias, polycythemia vera, and myelofibroerythroleukemia 骨髓增生性疾病；**narcissistic personality d.**, a personality disorder characterized by grandiosity (in fantasy or behavior), lack of social empathy combined with hypersensitivity to the judgments of others, interpersonal exploitativeness, a sense of entitlement, and a need for constant signs of admiration 自恋型人格障碍；**neuropsychologic d.**, any disorder in which brain dysfunction is manifested by disturbances in behavior or cognition 神经心理障碍；**neurotic d.**, neurosis 神经症性障碍；**nightmare d.**, repeated episodes of nightmares that awaken the sleeper, with full orientation and alertness and vivid recall of the dreams 梦魇症；**obsessive-compulsive and related d's**, a classification that includes obsessive-compulsive disorder, hoarding disorder, excoriation (skin-picking) disorder, body dysmorphic disorder, and trichotillomania (hair-pulling) 强迫症和相关疾病；**obsessive-compulsive d. (OCD)**, an anxiety disorder characterized by recurrent obsessions or compulsions, which are severe enough to interfere significantly with personal or social functioning 强迫症。Cf. *obsessive-compulsive personality d.*；**obsessive-compulsive personality d.**, a personality

disorder characterized by an emotionally constricted manner that is unduly rigid, stubborn, perfectionistic, and stingy, with preoccupation with trivial details, overconcern with having everything done one's own way, excessive devotion to work and productivity, and overconscientiousness 强迫型人格障碍。Cf. *obsessive-compulsive d.*；**oppositional defiant d.**, a type of disruptive behavior disorder characterized by a recurrent pattern of defiant, hostile, disobedient, and negativistic behavior directed toward those in authority 对立违抗性障碍；**organic mental d.**, a term formerly used to denote any mental disorder with a specifically known or presumed organic etiology. It was sometimes used synonymously with *organic mental syndrome* 器质性精神障碍；**orgasmic d's**, sexual dysfunctions characterized by inhibited or premature orgasm 性高潮障碍；见 *female orgasmic d., male orgasmic d.,* 和 *premature ejaculation*；**ovotesticular d. of sex development**, a genetically heterogeneous disorder in which ovarian and testicular tissue coexist, either separately or combined in an ovotestis. The karyotype is variable (46,XX, 46,XY, or 46,XX/46,XY) and the external genitalia are usually atypical with some virilization, but can appear male or female 卵睾性性发育异常，真两性畸形。Formerly called *true hermaphroditism*；**pain d.**, a somatoform disorder characterized by a chief complaint of severe chronic pain which is neither feigned nor intentionally produced, but in which psychological factors appear to play a major role in onset, severity, exacerbation, or maintenance 疼痛障碍；**panic d.**, an anxiety disorder characterized by attacks of panic (anxiety), fear, or terror, by feelings of unreality, or by fears of dying, or losing control, together with somatic signs such as dyspnea, choking, palpitations, dizziness, vertigo, flushing or pallor, and sweating. It may occur with or, rarely, without agoraphobia 惊恐障碍；**paranoid d.**, 1. delusional d.；2. a former classification of schizophrenia characterized by preoccupation with one or more systematized delusions or with frequent auditory hallucinations, but without disorganized speech, disorganized or catatonic behavior, or flat or inappropriate affect 偏执型精神分裂；**paranoid personality d.**, a personality disorder marked by a view of other people as hostile, devious, and untrustworthy and a combative response to disappointments or to events experienced as rebuffs or humiliations 偏执型人格障碍；**passive-aggressive personality d.**, a personality disorder characterized by indirect resistance to demands for adequate social or occupational performance and by negative, defeatist attitudes 被动 - 攻击型人格障碍；**per-**

oxisome biogenesis d's, a heterogeneous group of disorders caused by defects in the PEX genes, a large group of genes that encode proteins necessary for peroxisome biosynthesis, with consequent absence or reduction in the number of peroxisomes and deficient activity of multiple peroxisomal enzymes 过氧化物酶生物合成障碍；**persistent depressive d.**, dysthymic disorder 持续性抑郁障碍；**personality d's**, a category of mental disorders characterized by enduring, inflexible, and maladaptive personality traits that deviate markedly from cultural expectations and either generate subjective distress or significantly impair functioning 人格障碍；**pervasive developmental d's**, disorders in which there is impaired development in multiple areas, including reciprocal social interactions, verbal and nonverbal communications, and imaginative activity, as in autistic disorder 广泛性发育障碍；**phagocytic dysfunction d's**, a group of immunodeficiency conditions characterized by disordered phagocytic activity, occurring as both *extrinsic* and *intrinsic* types. Bacterial or fungal infections may range from mild skin infection to fatal systemic infection 吞噬功能紊乱；**phobic d's**, 恐惧症，见 *phobia.*；**phonological d.**, a communication disorder characterized by failure to use age- and dialect-appropriate sounds in speaking, with errors occurring in the selection, production, or articulation of sounds 语音障碍；**plasma cell d's**, 浆细胞功能紊乱，见 *dyscrasia* 下词条；**postconcussional d.**, 脑震荡后综合征，见 *syndrome* 下词条；**posttraumatic stress d. (PTSD)**, an anxiety disorder in adults and children caused by experiencing or witnessing an intensely traumatic event or suffering serious injuries or threats; characterized by mentally reexperiencing the trauma, avoidance of trauma-associated stimuli or situations, social withdrawal, numbing of emotional responsiveness, hyperalertness, and difficulty in sleeping, remembering, or concentrating 创伤后应激障碍；**premenstrual dysphoric d. (PMDD)**, a condition more serious than premenstrual syndrome; characterized by marked irritability, anger, anxiety, tension, or depressed mood and feelings of hopelessness 经前焦虑症；**psychoactive substance use d's**, substance use d's 精神活性物质使用障碍；**psychosomatic d.**, one in which the physical symptoms are caused or exacerbated by psychological factors, as in migraine headaches, lower back pain, or irritable bowel syndrome 心身障碍；**psychotic d.**, psychosis 精神病症；**reactive attachment d.**, a mental disorder of infancy or early childhood characterized by notably unusual and developmentally inappropriate social

relatedness, usually associated with grossly pathologic care 反应性依恋障碍；**rumination d.**, excessive rumination of food by infants, after a period of normal eating habits, potentially leading to death by malnutrition 反刍症；**sadistic personality d.**, a pervasive pattern of cruel, demeaning, and aggressive behavior; satisfaction is gained from intimidating, coercing, hurting, and humiliating others 施虐型人格障碍；**schizoaffective d.**, a mental disorder involving prominent psychotic symptoms characteristic of schizophrenia, which may be accompanied by symptoms of a mood disorder 分裂情感障碍；**schizoid personality d.**, a personality disorder marked by indifference to social relationships and a restricted range of emotional experience and expression 分裂样人格障碍；**schizophreniform d.**, a mental disorder with the signs and symptoms of schizophrenia but of less than 6 months' duration 类精神分裂症；**schizotypal personality d.**, a personality disorder characterized by marked deficits in interpersonal competence and eccentricities in ideation, appearance, or behavior 分裂型人格障碍；**seasonal affective d. (SAD)**, depression with fatigue, lethargy, oversleeping, overeating, and carbohydrate craving recurring cyclically during specific seasons, most commonly the winter months 季节性情感障碍；**self-defeating personality d.**, a persistent pattern of behavior detrimental to the self, including being drawn to problematic situations or relationships and failing to accomplish tasks crucial to life objectives 自我挫败型人格障碍；**separation anxiety d.**, prolonged, developmentally inappropriate, excessive anxiety and distress in a child concerning removal from parents, home, or familiar surroundings 分离性焦虑障碍；**d's of sex development (DSD)**, congenital conditions in which development of chromosomal, gonadal, or anatomic sex is atypical 性发育异常疾病；**sexual d's**, 1. any disorders involving sexual functioning, desire, or performance 性欲／功能障碍；2. specifically, any such disorder that is caused at least in part by psychological factors; divided into sexual dysfunctions and paraphilias 心理因素引起的性功能障碍；**sexual arousal d's**, sexual dysfunctions characterized by alterations in sexual arousal 性唤起障碍；见 *female sexual arousal d.* 和 *male erectile d.*；**sexual aversion d.**, feelings of repugnance for and active avoidance of genital sexual contact with a partner, causing substantial distress or interpersonal difficulty 性厌恶；**sexual desire d's**, sexual dysfunctions characterized by alteration in sexual desire 性欲障碍；见 *hypoactive sexual desire d.* 和 *sexual aversion d.*；**sexual pain d's**, sexual dysfunctions characterized by pain associated with intercourse; it includes dyspareunia and vaginismus not due to a general medical condition 性疼痛障碍; **shared psychotic d.**, a delusional system that develops in one or more persons as a result of a close relationship with someone who already has a psychotic disorder with prominent delusions 共有型精神障碍; **sleep d's**, chronic disorders involving sleep, either primary (dyssomnias, parasomnias) or secondary to factors including a general medical condition, mental disorder, or substance use 睡眠障碍; **sleep terror d.**, a sleep disorder of repeated episodes of pavor nocturnus 睡惊症; **sleepwalking d.**, a sleep disorder of the parasomnia group, consisting of repeated episodes of somnambulism 梦游症; **social anxiety d.**, social phobia 社交焦虑症; **social communication d.**, a condition marked by persistent difficulty in social uses of verbal and nonverbal communication 社交障碍; **somatization d.**, a somatoform disorder characterized by multiple somatic complaints, including a combination of pain, gastrointestinal, sexual, and neurologic symptoms, and not fully explainable by any known general medical condition or the direct effect of a substance, but not intentionally feigned or produced 躯体化障碍; **somatoform d's**, mental disorders characterized by symptoms suggesting physical disorders of psychogenic origin but not under voluntary control, e.g., body dysmorphic disorder, conversion disorder, hypochondriasis, pain disorder, somatization disorder, and undifferentiated somatoform disorder 躯体形式障碍; **somatoform pain d.**, pain d. 躯体形式疼痛障碍; **specific learning d.**, a disorder that comprises the conditions of reading disorder, mathematics disorder, disorder of written expression, and learning disorder not otherwise specified 学习障碍; **speech d.**, defective ability to speak; it may be either psychogenic (see *communication d.*) or neurogenic 语言障碍; 另见 *aphasia, aphonia, dysphasia* 和 *dysphonia.*; **speech sound d.**, phonologic disorder 语音障碍; **stereotypic movement d.**, a mental disorder characterized by repetitive nonfunctional motor behavior that often appears to be driven and can result in serious self-inflicted injuries 刻板运动障碍; **substance-induced d's**, a subgroup of the substance-related disorders comprising a variety of behavioral or psychological anomalies resulting from ingestion of or exposure to a drug of abuse, medication, or toxin 物质性障碍。Cf. *substance use d's*; **substance-related d's**, any of the mental disorders associated with excessive use of or exposure to psychoactive substances, including drugs of abuse, medications, and toxins. The group is divided

into *substance use d's* and *substance-induced d's* 物质相关障碍; **substance use d's**, a subgroup of the substance-related disorders, in which psychoactive substance use or abuse repeatedly results in significantly adverse consequences. The group comprises *substance abuse* and *substance dependence* 物质使用障碍; **temporomandibular d. (TMD), temporomandibular joint d. (TMJD)**, chronic facial pain associated with dysfunction of some combination of the temporomandibular joint, jaw muscles, and associated nerves. Symptoms include facial, neck, and shoulder pain, clicking or other sounds associated with jaw movement, limited jaw opening and locking of the jaw, headache, otalgia, neck and shoulder pain, and dizziness. There are *myogenous* and *arthrogenous* forms; the former is most often due to some combination of malocclusion, jaw clenching, bruxism, and physical and mental stress and anxiety; the latter is usually caused by disk displacement or by disease, dislocation, or congenital anomaly of the joint 颞下颌关节紊乱; **trauma and stressor-related d.**, a category of anxiety disorders that includes reactive attachment disorder, disinhibited social engagement disorder, posttraumatic stress disorder, acute stress disorder, and adjustment disorder 创伤和应激相关疾病; **triplet repeat d's**, disorders caused by unstable, dynamic mutations that result in expansion of triplet repeats within the affected gene, leading to abnormalities in gene expression and function 三联重复障碍; **undifferentiated somatoform d.**, one or more physical complaints, not intentionally produced or feigned and persisting for at least 6 months, that cannot be fully explained by a general medical condition or the direct effects of a substance 未分化躯体形式障碍; **unipolar d's**, depressive d's 单相抑郁障碍

dis·or·gan·iza·tion (dis-or″gən-ĭ-za′shən) 1. the process of destruction of any organic tissue 有机组织结构破坏; 2. any profound change in the tissues of an organ or structure that causes the loss of most or all of its proper characters 器官结构组织特征丧失

dis·or·i·en·ta·tion (dis-or″e-ən-ta′shən) the loss of proper bearings, or a state of mental confusion as to time, place, or identity 举止或精神混乱状态; **spatial d.**, the inability of a pilot or other air crew member to determine spatial attitude in relation to the surface of the earth; it occurs in conditions of restricted vision, and results from vestibular illusions 空间定向障碍

dis·pen·sa·ry (dis-pen′sə-re) 1. a place for dispensation of free or low-cost medical treatment（慈善机构的）医务室，诊所; 2. any place where drugs and medicines are actually dispensed（医院、商店等的）药房，配药处

dis·pen·sa·to·ry (dis-pen′sə-tor-e) a book that describes medicines and their preparation and uses 药典; **D. of the United States of America,** a collection of monographs on unofficial drugs and drugs recognized by the United States Pharmacopeia, the British Pharmacopoeia, and the National Formulary; also on general tests, processes, reagents, and solutions of the U.S.P. and N.F., as well as drugs used in veterinary medicine 美国药典

dis·pense (dis-pens′) to prepare medicines for and distribute them to their users 配药，发药

di·sper·my (di′spər-me) the penetration of two spermatozoa into one oocyte 双受精

dis·perse (dis-purs′) to scatter the component parts, as of a tumor or the fine particles in a colloid system; also, the particles so dispersed 分散

dis·per·sion (dis-pur′zhən) 1. the act of scattering or separating; the condition of being scattered 分散; 2. the incorporation of the particles of one substance into the body of another, comprising solutions, suspensions, and colloid systems; used particularly for an unstable colloid system 溶解; 见 *colloid* (2)

dis·per·sive (dis-pur′siv) 1. tending to become dispersed 趋向分散的; 2. promoting dispersion 促进分散

dis·place·ment (dis-plās′mənt) 1. removal from the normal position or place 移位; 2. percolation 渗滤; 3. a defense mechanism in which emotions, ideas, wishes, or impulses are unconsciously shifted from their original object to a more acceptable substitute 转移; 4. in a chemical reaction, the replacement of one atom or group in a molecule by another 取代

dis·pro·por·tion (dis″pro-por′shən) a lack of the proper relationship between two elements or factors 不相称; **cephalopelvic d.,** a condition in which the fetal head is too large for the mother's pelvis 头盆不称

dis·rup·tion (dis-rup′shən) a morphologic defect resulting from the extrinsic breakdown of, or interference with, a developmental process 发育过程受到干扰所致的形态缺陷

dis·rup·tive (dis-rup′tiv) 1. bursting apart; rending 破坏性的，扰乱性的; 2. causing confusion or disorder 引起混乱的

dis·sect (dĭ-sekt′) (di-sekt′) 1. to cut apart, or separate 把……分成小块; 2. to expose structures of a cadaver for anatomic study 解剖

dis·sec·tion (dĭ-sek′shən) 1. the act of dissecting 解剖，切开; 2. a part or whole of an organism prepared by dissecting 解剖下来的一部分; **aortic d.,** a dissecting aneurysm of the aorta, usually the de-

scending thoracic aorta 主动脉夹层; **axillary d., axillary lymph node d.; axillary lymph node d.,** surgical removal of axillary lymph nodes, done as part of radical mastectomy 腋窝淋巴结清扫术; **blunt d.,** dissection accomplished by separating tissues along natural cleavage lines, without cutting 钝性分离; **lymph node d.,** lymphadenectomy 淋巴结清扫术; **sharp d.,** dissection accomplished by incising tissues with a sharp edge 锐性分离

dis·sem·i·nat·ed (dĭ-sem′ ĭ-nāt″əd) scattered; distributed over a considerable area 扩散

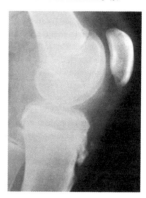

▲ 胫骨粗隆骨软骨病（**Osgood-Schlatter disease**）：图像显示胫骨结节不规则和碎裂

dis·so·ci·a·tion (dĭ-so″se-a′shən) 1. the act of separating or state of being separated 分离; 2. the separation of a molecule into two or more fragments produced by the absorption of light or thermal energy or by solvation 分解; 3. segregation of a group of mental processes from the rest of a person's usually integrated functions of consciousness, memory, perception, and sensory and motor behavior 解体; **atrial d.,** independent beating of the left and right atria, each with normal rhythm or with one or both having an abnormal rhythm 心房分离; **atrioventricular d.,** control of the atria by one pacemaker and of the ventricles by another, independent pacemaker 房室分离; **electromechanical d.,** continued electrical rhythmicity of the heart in the absence of effective mechanical function 电机械分离

dis·so·ci·a·tive (dĭ-so′se-ə-tiv) pertaining to or tending to produce dissociation 分离的

dis·so·lu·tion (dis″o-loo′shən) 1. the process in which one substance is passed in another 溶解; 2. separation of a compound into its components by chemical action 分解; 3. liquefaction 液化; 4. death 消亡，死亡

dis·solve (dĭ-zolv′) 1. to cause a substance to pass into solution 使（固体）溶解；2. to pass into solution 溶解

dis·tad (dis′tad) in a distal direction 在末梢，向远侧

dis·tal (dis′təl) remote; farther from any point of reference 远端的，末梢的

dis·ta·lis (dis-ta′lis) [L.] distal 远端，远侧

dis·tance (dis′təns) the measure of space intervening between two objects or two points of reference 距离，间距；**focal d.**, that from the focal point to the optical center of a lens or the surface of a concave mirror 焦距；**interarch d.**, the vertical distance between the maxillary and mandibular arches under certain specified conditions of vertical dimension 颌间距离；**interocclusal d.**, the distance between the occluding surfaces of the maxillary and mandibular teeth with the mandible in physiologic rest position 咬合间距；**interocular d.**, the distance between the eyes, usually used in reference to the interpupillary distance 瞳距；**working d.**, the distance between the front lens of a microscope and the object when the instrument is correctly focused 焦距，工作距离

dis·ti·chi·a·sis (dis″tĭ-ki′ə-sis) the presence of a double row of eyelashes, one or both of which are turned in against the eyeball 双行睫

dis·til·la·tion (dis″tĭ-la′shən) vaporization; the process of vaporizing and condensing a substance to purify it or to separate a volatile substance from less volatile substances 蒸馏；**destructive d.**, 分解蒸馏；**dry d.**, decomposition of a solid by heating in the absence of air, resulting in volatile liquid products 干馏；**fractional d.**, that attended by the successive separation of volatilizable substances in order of their respective volatility 分馏

dis·to·clu·sion (dis″to-kloo′zhən) malrelation of the dental arches with the lower jaw in a distal or posterior position in relation to the upper 远中错𬌗

dis·to·mo·lar (dis″to-mo′lər) a supernumerary molar; any tooth distal to a third molar 远中磨牙

dis·tor·tion (dis-tor′shən) 1. the state of being twisted out of normal shape or position 扭曲，变形；2. in psychiatry, the conversion of material offensive to the superego into acceptable form 转变，转化；3. deviation of an image from the true outline or shape of an object or structure 歪曲，失真

dis·trac·tion (dis-trak′shən) 1. diversion of attention 转移注意力；2. separation of joint surfaces without rupture of their binding ligaments and without displacement 关节表面分离；3. surgical separation of the two parts of a bone after the bone is transected 外科分离

dis·tri·bu·tion (dis″trĭ-bu′shən) 1. the specific location or arrangement of continuing or successive objects or events in space or time 分布，位置；2. the extent of a ramifying structure such as an artery or nerve and its branches（动脉或神经）分支的范围；3. the geographical range of an organism or disease 疾病的地理范围；**chi-square d.**, a distribution of sample differences using observations of a random sample drawn from a normal population 卡方分布；**normal d.**, a continuous probability density function roughly characterizing a random variable that is the sum of a large number of independent random events; usually represented by a smooth bell-shaped curve symmetric about the mean 正态分布

dis·tur·bance (dis-tur′bəns) a departure or divergence from that which is considered normal 偏离

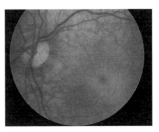

▲ 家族性黑矇性痴呆（Tay-Sachs disease），表现为特征性樱桃红黄斑

di·sul·fi·ram (di-sul′fi-ram) an antioxidant that inhibits the oxidation of the acetaldehyde metabolized from alcohol, resulting in high concentrations of acetaldehyde in the body. Used to produce aversion to alcohol in the treatment of alcoholism because extremely uncomfortable symptoms occur when its administration is followed by ingestion of alcohol 双硫仑

di·urese (di″u-rēs′) to bring about diuresis 利尿

di·ure·sis (di″u-re′sis) increased excretion of urine 利尿；**osmotic d.**, that resulting from the presence of nonabsorbable or poorly absorbable, osmotically active substances in the renal tubules 渗透性利尿；**pressure d.**, increased urinary excretion of water when arterial pressure increases, a compensatory mechanism to maintain blood pressure within the normal range 压力性利尿

di·uret·ic (di″u-ret′ik) 1. pertaining to or causing diuresis 利尿的；2. an agent that promotes diuresis 利尿药；**high-ceiling d's, loop d's**, those exerting their action on the sodium reabsorption mechanism of the thick ascending limb of the loop of Henle, resulting in excretion of urine isotonic with plasma 襻利尿药; **osmotic d's,** a group of low-molecular-weight substances that can remain in high concentrations in renal tubules, thus contributing to osmolality of glomerular filtrate 渗透性利尿药; **potassium-sparing d's,** those blocking exchange of sodium for potassium and hydrogen ions in the distal tubule, increasing sodium and chloride excretion without increasing potassium excretion 保钾利尿药; **thiazide d's,** a group of synthetic compounds that decrease reabsorption of sodium by the kidney and thereby increase loss of water and sodium; they enhance excretion of sodium and chloride equally 噻嗪类利尿药

di·ur·nal (di-ur′nəl) pertaining to or occurring during the daytime, or period of light 昼行性的

di·va·lent (di-va′lent) having a valence of two; bivalent 二价的

di·val·pro·ex (di-val′pro-eks) an anticonvulsant, used as **d. sodium,** a 1:1 compound of valproate sodium and valproic acid, in the treatment of migraine, manic episodes of bipolar disorder, and epileptic seizures, particularly absence seizures 双丙戊酸钠

di·ver·gence (di-vur′jəns) a moving apart from, or inclination away from, a common point 分歧, 差异; **diver′gent** *adj.* 分歧的

di·ver·sion (di-vur′zhən) a turning aside 转向, 转移; **urinary d.,** surgical creation of an alternate route for urine flow to replace an absent or diseased portion of the lower urinary tract in order to preserve renal function 尿路分流术

di·ver·tic·u·la (di″vər-tik′u-lə) [L.] 憩室, *diverticulum* 的复数形式

di·ver·tic·u·lar (di″vər-tik′u-lər) pertaining to or resembling a diverticulum 憩室的

di·ver·tic·u·lec·to·my (di″vər-tik″u-lek′tə-me) excision of a diverticulum 憩室切除术

di·ver·tic·u·li·tis (di″vər-tik″u-li′tis) inflammation of a diverticulum 憩室炎

di·ver·tic·u·lo·sis (di″vər-tik″u-lo′sis) the presence of diverticula in the absence of inflammation 憩室病

di·ver·tic·u·lum (di″vər-tik′u-ləm) pl. *diverti'cula* A circumscribed pouch or sac occurring normally or created by herniation of the lining mucous membrane through a defect in the muscular coat of a tubular organ 憩室; **allantoic d.,** the endodermal sacculation that becomes the allantois; in humans it is an outpouching of the caudal wall of the yolk sac that becomes the urachus 尿囊憩室; **ileal d.,** **Meckel d.,** an occasional sacculation or appendage of the ileum, derived from an unobliterated yolk

stalk 回肠憩室, 梅克尔憩室

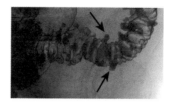

▲ 结肠憩室在双重对比灌肠中用箭表示（黑色部分为钡剂）

di·vi·sion (di-vizh′ən) 1. the act of separating into parts 分隔, 分配; 2. a section or part of a larger structure（分出来的）部分; 3. in the taxonomy of plants and fungi, a level of classification equivalent to the *phylum* of the animal kingdom 植物和真菌界相当于动物界中门这一级水平的分类类别; **cell d.,** fission of a cell 细胞分裂; 见 *meiosis* 和 *mitosis*; **direct cell d.,** 直接分裂, 见 *amitosis*; **indirect cell d.,** 间接分裂, 见 *meiosis* 和 *mitosis;* **maturation d.,** meiosis 减数分裂, 成熟分裂

di·vulse (dī-vuls′) to pull apart forcibly 撕开, 扯裂

di·vul·sion (dī-vul′shən) the act of separating or pulling apart 扯裂

di·zy·got·ic (di″zi-got′ik) pertaining to or derived from two separate zygotes 两受精卵的

diz·zi·ness (diz′e-nis) 1. a disturbed sense of relationship to space; a sensation of unsteadiness and a feeling of movement within the head; lightheadedness; dysequilibrium 头晕; 2. erroneous synonym for *vertigo* 眩晕

dL deciliter 分升

DL- chemical prefix (small capitals) used with d and l convention to indicate a racemic mixture of enantiomers 外消旋混合物的前缀

dl- chemical prefix used with the *d* and *l* convention to indicate a racemic mixture of enantiomers; the prefix (±)- is used with the same meaning 外消旋混合物的前缀

DLE discoid lupus erythematosus 盘状红斑狼疮

DLMO dim light melatonin onset 弱光褪黑素发作

DM diabetes mellitus; phenarsazine chloride (diphenylaminechlorarsine) 糖尿病

DMARD disease-modifying antirheumatic drug 改善疾病的抗风湿药物

DMD Doctor of Dental Medicine 牙科医生

DMDD disruptive mood dysregulation disorder 破坏性情绪失调

DMFO eflornithine 二氟甲基鸟氨酸

DMRD Diploma in Medical Radio-Diagnosis

(Brit.) 医学放射诊断文凭

DMRT Diploma in Medical Radio-Therapy (Brit.) 医学放射治疗文凭

DMSO dimethyl sulfoxide 二甲基亚砜

DNA deoxyribonucleic acid 脱氧核糖核酸 **complementary DNA, copy DNA (cDNA),** DNA transcribed from a specific RNA in vitro through the reaction of the enzyme reverse transcriptase 互补 DNA；**minisatellite DNA，小卫星 DNA。**见 *minisatellite*；**mitochondrial DNA (mtDNA),** the DNA of the mitochondrial genome (q.v.) 线粒体 DNA；**nuclear DNA (nDNA),** the DNA of the chromosomes found in the nucleus of a eukaryotic cell 核 DNA；**recombinant DNA,** a composite DNA molecule constructed in vitro by joining a fragment of foreign DNA with a vector DNA molecule capable of replicating in host cells 重组 DNA；**repetitive DNA,** eukaryotic DNA sequences occurring multiply (a few to a million copies) within a genome; it can be closely linked or dispersed, and most does not encode proteins 重复 DNA；**satellite DNA,** short, highly repeated eukaryotic DNA sequences, usually clustered in groups of many tandem repeats in heterochromatin and generally not transcribed 卫星 DNA；**single-copy DNA (scDNA),** nucleotide sequences present once in the haploid genome, as are most of those encoding polypeptides in the eukaryotic genome 单拷贝 DNA；**spacer DNA,** nontranscribed DNA sequences occurring between genes, usually containing highly repetitive DNA 间隔 DNA；**unique DNA,** single-copy DNA 单一（序列）DNA

DNA gy·rase (ji′rās) a type II DNA topoisomerase DNA 旋转酶

DNA li·gase (li′gās) a ligase that catalyzes the linkage between two free ends of doublestranded DNA chains by forming a phosphodiester bond between them, as in the repair of damaged DNA DNA 连接酶

DNA po·lym·er·ase (pə-lim′ər-ās) any of various enzymes catalyzing the templatedirected incorporation of deoxyribonucleotides into a DNA chain, particularly one using a DNA template DNA 聚合酶

DNA topo·isom·er·ase (to″po-i-som′ər-ās) either of two types of isomerase that catalyze the breakage, passage, and rejoining of one or both DNA strands. *Type* I *topoisomerases* are specific for single-strand passage, and *type* II *isomerases* are specific for double-strand passage, thus altering the topology of the molecule DNA 拓扑异构酶

DNase deoxyribonuclease 脱氧核糖核酸酶

DNOC dinitro-*o*-cresol 二硝基邻甲酚

DO Doctor of Osteopathy 骨病医生

DOA dead on admission (arrival) 入院时死亡

do·bu·ta·mine (do-bu′tə-mēn) a synthetic catecholamine having direct inotropic effects; used as the hydrochloride salt in the treatment of congestive heart failure and low cardiac output 多巴酚丁胺

do·ce·tax·el (do″sə-tak′səl) an antineoplastic agent used particularly in treating carcinoma of the breast and non–small cell lung carcinoma 多西他赛

do·co·sa·hexa·eno·ic ac·id (do-ko″sə-hek″sə-e-no′ik) an omega-3, polyunsaturated, 22-carbon fatty acid found almost exclusively in fish and marine animal oils 二十二碳六烯酸，DHA

do·co·sa·nol (do-ko′sə-nol) an antiviral effective against lipid-enveloped viruses, including herpes simplex virus; used in the treatment of recurrent herpes labialis 二十二烷醇

doc·tor (dok′tər) 1. a practitioner of the healing arts, as one graduated from a college of medicine, dentistry, chiropractic, optometry, podiatry, osteopathic medicine, or veterinary medicine, and licensed to practice 医生；2. a holder of a diploma of the highest degree from a university, qualified as a specialist in a particular field of learning 博士

doc·u·sate (dok′u-sāt) any of a group of anionic surfactants widely used as emulsifying, wetting, and dispersing agents; the calcium, potassium, and sodium salts are used as stool softeners 多库酯，通利妥

do·fet·i·lide (do-fet′ə-līd) an antiarrhythmic used in the treatment of atrial arrhythmias 多非利特

dol (dōl) a unit of pain intensity 疼痛强度的单位

do·las·e·tron (do-las′ē-tron) a selective serotonin receptor antagonist, used as the mesylate salt for the prevention of nausea and vomiting associated with chemotherapy or occurring after surgery; administered orally and intravenously 多拉司琼

dol·i·cho·ce·phal·ic (dol″ĭ-ko-sə-fal′ik) long headed; having a cephalic index of 75.9 or less 长头的

do·lor (do′lor) pl. *dolo′res* [L.] pain; one of the cardinal signs of inflammation 疼痛

dol·or·if·ic (do″lor-if′ik) producing pain 致痛的

dol·or·im·e·ter (do″lor-im′ə-tər) an instrument for measuring pain in dols 测痛计

dol·or·o·gen·ic (do-lor″o-jen′ik) dolorific 致痛的

do·lu·teg·ra·vir (dō-loo-tĕg′raw-vir) a secondgeneration integrase strand transfer inhibitor used as an antiretroviral agent in the treatment of human immunodeficiency virus infection; administered orally 度鲁特韦（抗艾滋病药）

do·main (do-mān′) 1. an area or region that is

defined or delimited in some way 域；2. one of the three broad divisions into which all living organisms may be classified: the Archaea, the Bacteria, and the Eukaryota; the first two consist of the prokaryotes, the last contains the eukaryotes 界；**interchromatin d., interchromosomal d.**, a compartment of the cell nucleus, consisting of a network of channels separating the chromosome territories; most events of RNA transcription, processing, and transport are believed to occur in this domain 染色质间区

dom·i·nance (dom′ĭ-nəns) 1. the state of being dominant 支配，控制，主导；2. in genetics, the phenotypic expression of a gene in both heterozygotes and homozygotes 显性（基因）；3. in coronary artery anatomy, the state of supplying the posterior diaphragmatic part of the interventricular septum and the diaphragmatic surface of the left ventricle 优势（冠状动脉）；**incomplete d.**, failure of one gene to be completely dominant, heterozygotes showing a phenotype intermediate between the two parents 不完全显性；**lateral d.**, the preferential use, in voluntary motor acts, of ipsilateral members of the major paired organs of the body 单侧性优势；**partial d.**, incomplete d.

dom·i·nant (dom′ĭ-nənt) 1. exerting a ruling or controlling influence 首要的；占支配地位的；2. in genetics, capable of expression when carried by only one of a pair of homologous chromosomes （基因）显性的

do·nep·e·zil (do-nep′ə-zil) an acetylcholinesterase inhibitor used as the hydrochloride salt for the treatment of mild to moderate symptoms of dementia of the Alzheimer type; administered orally 多奈哌齐

dong quai (doong kwa) (-kwi) *Angelica sinensis* (Chinese angelica), or its root, a preparation of which is used for gynecologic disorders 当归

do·nor (do′nər) 1. an organism that supplies living tissue to be used in another body, as a person who furnishes blood for transfusion, or an organ for transplantation 捐赠者，献血者，器官捐献者；2. a substance or compound that contributes part of itself to another substance (acceptor) 供体；**cadaveric d.**, an organ or tissue donor who has already died 遗体捐献者；**living nonrelated d.**, living unrelated d.；**living related d.**, a donor of a transplant who is a close biologic relative of the recipient 活体亲属供体；**living unrelated d.**, a donor of a transplant who is not a close biologic relative of the recipient 活体非亲属供者；**universal d.**, a person whose blood is type O in the ABO blood group system; such blood is sometimes used in emergency transfusion 万能献血者（O型血者）

do·pa (do′pə) 3,4-dihydroxyphenylalanine, produced by oxidation of tyrosine by monophenol monooxygenase; it is the precursor of dopamine and an intermediate product in the biosynthesis of norepinephrine, epinephrine, and melanin. l-dopa is the naturally occurring form 多巴；见 *levodopa*

do·pa·mine (do′pə-mēn) a catecholamine formed in the body by the decarboxylation of dopa; it is an intermediate product in the synthesis of norepinephrine, and acts as a neurotransmitter in the central nervous system. The hydrochloride salt is used to correct hemodynamic balance in the treatment of shock and is also used as a cardiac stimulant 多巴胺

do·pa·min·er·gic (do″pə-mēn-ur′jik) activated or transmitted by dopamine; pertaining to tissues or organs affected by dopamine 多巴胺能的

Dop·pler (dop′lər) 多普勒；见 *ultrasonography* 下词条；**color D.**, color flow Doppler imaging 彩色多普勒

dor·nase al·fa (dor′nāz al′fə) recombinant human deoxyribonuclease I (DNase I) used to reduce the viscosity of sputum in cystic fibrosis 重组人 DNA 酶 I

dor·sad (dor′sad) toward the back 背部地，朝向背面

dor·sal (dor′səl) 1. pertaining to the back or to any dorsum 背部的；2. denoting a position more toward the back surface than some other object of reference; opposite of ventral 背部

dor·sa·lis (dor-sa′lis) [L.] dorsal 背部的

dor·si·flex·ion (dor″sĭ-flek′shən) flexion or bending toward the extensor aspect of a limb, as of the hand or foot 背屈

dor·so·ceph·a·lad (dor″so-sef′ə-lad) toward the back of the head 向枕部

dor·so·lat·er·al (dor″so-lat′ər-əl) pertaining to the back and the side 背侧（面）的

dor·so·ven·tral (dor″so-ven′trəl) 1. pertaining to the back and belly surfaces of a body 背腹部的；2. passing from the back to the belly surface 由背向腹的

dor·sum (dor′səm) pl. *dor·sa* [L.] 1. the back 后面，2. the aspect of an anatomic structure or part corresponding in position to the back; posterior in the human 背侧

dor·zo·la·mide (dor-zo′lə-mīd) a carbonic acid anhydrase inhibitor, used as an antiglaucoma agent in the treatment of open-angle glaucoma and ocular hypertension; applied topically to the conjunctiva as the hydrochloride salt 多佐胺

dos·age (do′səj) the determination and regulation of the size, frequency, and number of doses 剂量

dose (dōs) the quantity to be administered at one time, as a specified amount of medication or a given quantity of radiation 剂量; **absorbed d.**, the amount of energy from ionizing radiation absorbed per unit mass of matter 吸收剂量; **air d.**, 辐射剂量; 见 *exposure* 下词条; **booster d.**, a dose of an active immunizing agent, usually smaller than the initial dose, given to maintain immunity 加强剂量; **divided d.**, fractional d.; **effective d. (ED)**, that quantity of a drug that will produce the effects for which it is given 有效剂量; **erythema d.**, the amount of radiation which, when applied to the skin, causes temporary reddening 红斑量; **fatal d.**, lethal d.; **fractional d.**, **fractionated d.**, a fraction of the total quantity of a prescribed drug or of radiation to be given at intervals 分次剂量; **infective d.**, that amount of pathogenic organisms that will cause infection in susceptible subjects 感染剂量; **infinitesimal d.**, 极小剂量, 见 *principle* 下词条; **lethal d.**, the amount of an agent that can cause death 致死剂量; **loading d.**, a dose of medication, often larger than subsequent doses, administered to establish a therapeutic level of the medication 负荷剂量; **maximal d.**, **maximum d.**, the largest dose consistent with safety 极量; **maximum permissible d. (MPD)**, the largest amount of ionizing radiation that can be safely received by a person in a given time period 最大容许剂量; **median curative d. (CD$_{50}$)**, a dose that abolishes symptoms in half the test subjects 半数治愈量; **median effective d. (ED$_{50}$)**, a dose that produces the desired effect in half of a population 半数有效量; **median immunizing d.**, the dose of vaccine or antigen sufficient to provide immunity in 50 percent of test subjects 半数免疫剂量; **median infective d. (ID$_{50}$)**, the amount of microorganisms that causes infection in half the test subjects 半数感染量; **median lethal d. (LD$_{50}$)**, the quantity of an agent or of radiation that will kill half the test subjects or half of any population 半数致死量; **median toxic d. (TD$_{50}$)**, the dose that produces a toxic effect in half the population 半数中毒量; **minimal d.**, the smallest dose that will produce an appreciable effect 最小剂量; **minimal erythema d. (MED)**, the smallest amount of ionizing radiation that causes erythema 最小红斑量; **minimum d.**, minimal d.; **minimum lethal d. (MLD)**, 最低（小）致死量 1. the smallest amount of toxin that will kill an experimental animal; 2. the smallest quantity of injected diphtheria toxin that will kill a guinea pig within a specified time; **reference d.**, an estimate of the daily exposure to a substance for humans that is assumed to be without appreciable risk, more conservative than the older margin of safety 参考剂量; **skin d. (SD)**, 1. the air exposure of ionizing radiation at the skin surface (radiation plus backscatter) 空气在皮肤表面的电离辐射暴露剂量; 2. the absorbed dose in the skin 皮肤吸收剂量; **threshold d.**, minimal d. 阈剂量; **threshold erythema d.**, a single skin dose that within 30 days produces a faint but definite erythema in 80 percent of those tested, and causes no detectable reaction in the other 20 percent 红斑阈量; **tolerance d.**, the largest amount of an agent that can be administered safely 容许剂量

dosha (dosh′ə) according to the principle of constitution of the physical body in ayurveda, one of the three vital bioenergies (vata, pitta, kapha) condensed from the five elements; the doshas are responsible for the physical and emotional tendencies in the mind and body, and, along with the seven dhatus (tissues) and three malas (waste products), they make up the human body. The attributes of the doshas and their specific combination within each individual help determine the individual's physical and mental characteristics, while imbalance among the doshas is the cause of disease 生命能量

do·sim·e·try (do-sim′ə-tre) scientific determination of amount, rate, and distribution of radiation emitted from a source of ionizing radiation, in *biological d.* measuring the radiation-induced changes in a body or organism, and in *physical d.* measuring the levels of radiation directly with instruments 剂量测定

dot (dot) a small spot 小点；小圆点; **Gunn d's**, white dots seen about the macula lutea of the normal eye on oblique illumination 遗传性视网膜小点, 斜照明时正常眼内可以看到的黄斑旁白色小点; **Maurer d's**, irregular dots, staining red with Leishman stain, seen in erythrocytes infected with *Plasmodium falciparum* 莫尔小点, 恶性疟红细胞内的红色不规则小点; **Mittendorf d.**, a congenital anomaly manifested as a small gray or white opacity just inferior and nasal to the posterior pole of the lens, representing the remains of the lenticular attachment of the hyaloid artery; it does not affect vision 晶状体后极下方和鼻侧的灰白色小浑浊; **Schüffner d's**, minute granules observed in erythrocytes infected with *Plasmodium vivax* when stained by certain methods 间日疟原虫染色时红细胞观察到的微小颗粒; **Trantas d's**, small, white calcareous-looking dots in the limbus of the conjunctiva in vernal conjunctivitis 春季结膜炎结膜缘有白色钙质小点

dou·ble blind (dub′əl blīnd) pertaining to an experiment in which neither the subject nor the person administering treatment knows which treatment any particular subject is receiving 双盲

douche (dōōsh) [Fr.] a stream of water directed against a part of the body or into a cavity (妇女阴道等) 冲洗；**air d.,** a current of air blown into a cavity, particularly into the tympanum to open the eustachian tube 空气灌入（鼓室等）

doug·la·si·tis (dug″lə-si′tis) inflammation of the rectouterine excavation (Douglas cul-de-sac) 直肠子宫陷凹炎

dow·el (dou′əl) a peg or pin for fastening an artificial crown or core to a natural tooth root, or affixing a die to a working model for construction of a crown, inlay, or partial denture 固定牙冠的钉子

down·reg·u·la·tion (doun″reg-u-la′shən) controlled decrease, particularly the attenuation of expression of a gene in response to cellular or environmental factors or the reduction in responsiveness of a cell to stimulatory factors after a first exposure 下调

down·stream (doun′strēm) a region of DNA or RNA that is located to the 3′ side of a gene or region of interest 下游

dox·a·cu·ri·um (dok″sə-ku′re-əm) a long-acting neuromuscular blocking agent used as the chloride salt as a skeletal muscle relaxant during surgery and endotracheal intubation 多库氯铵

dox·a·pram (dok′sə-pram) a respiratory stimulant, used after anesthesia or in chronic obstructive pulmonary disease; used as the hydrochloride salt 多沙普仑

dox·a·zo·sin (dok-sa′zo-sin) a compound that blocks α₁-adrenergic receptors; used as *d. mesylate* in the treatment of hypertension and of benign prostatic hyperplasia 多沙唑嗪

dox·e·pin (dok′sə-pin) a tricyclic antidepressant of the dibenzoxepine class; also used to treat chronic pain, peptic ulcer, pruritus, and idiopathic cold urticaria, administered as the hydrochloride salt 多塞平

dox·er·cal·cif·er·ol (dok″sər-kal-sif′ər-ol) a synthetic analogue of vitamin D2, used to reduce levels of circulating parathyroid hormone in the treatment of secondary hyperparathyroidism associated with chronic renal failure 度骨化醇

doxo·ru·bi·cin (dok″so-roo′bĭ-sin) an antineoplastic antibiotic, produced by *Streptomyces peucetius*, which binds to DNA and inhibits nucleic acid synthesis; used as the hydrochloride salt and as a liposome-encased preparation of the hydrochloride salt 阿霉素

doxy·cy·cline (dok″se-si′klēn) a semisynthetic broad-spectrum tetracycline antibiotic, active against a wide range of gram-positive and gramnegative organisms; used also as *d. calcium* and *d. hyclate* 多西环素

dox·yl·amine (dok-sil′ə-mēn) an antihistamine with anticholinergic and sedative effects, used as the succinate salt 多西拉敏

DP Doctor of Pharmacy 药学博士；Doctor of Podiatry 足病学博士

DPH Diploma in Public Health 公共卫生学文凭

DPM Diploma in Psychological Medicine 心理医学文凭；Doctor of Podiatric Medicine 足病医学博士

DR reaction of degeneration 变性反应

dra·cun·cu·li·a·sis (drə-kung″ku-li′ə-sis) infection by nematodes of the genus *Dracunculus* characterized by pruritic skin vesicles that may ulcerate 龙线虫病

dra·cun·cu·lo·sis (drə-kung″ku-lo′sis) dracunculiasis 龙线虫病

Dra·cun·cu·lus (drə-kung′ku-ləs) a genus of nematode parasites, including *D. medinen′sis* (guinea worm), a threadlike worm, 30 to 120 cm long, widely distributed in India, Africa, and Arabia, inhabiting subcutaneous and intermuscular tissues of humans and other animals 龙线虫属

drain (drān) any device by which a channel or open area may be established for exit of fluids or purulent material from a cavity, wound, or infected area 引流物；**controlled d.,** a square of gauze, filled with gauze strips, pressed into a wound, the corners of the square and ends of the strips left protruding 纱布引流；**Mikulicz d.,** a single layer of gauze, packed with several thick wicks of gauze, pushed into a wound cavity Mikulicz 引流；**Penrose d.,** a thin rubber tube, usually 0.5 to 1 inch in diameter 烟卷式引流；**stab wound d.,** one brought out through a small puncture wound at some distance from the operative incision, to prevent infection of the operation wound 侧创引流

drain·age (drān′əj) systematic withdrawal of fluids and discharges from a wound, sore, or cavity 引流；**capillary d.,** that effected by strands of hair, surgical gut, spun glass, or other material of small caliber which acts by capillary attraction 毛细管引流法；**closed d.,** drainage of an empyema cavity carried out with protection against the entrance of outside air into the pleural cavity 胸腔闭式引流；**manual lymph d.,** the application of light rhythmic strokes, similar to those of effleurage, in the direction of the heart to increase the drainage of lymph from the involved structures 手法淋巴引流；**open d.,** drainage of an empyema cavity through an opening in the chest wall into which one or more rubber drainage tubes are inserted, the opening not being sealed against the entrance of outside air 开放引流术；**postural d.,** therapeutic drainage in bronchiectasis and lung abscess by placing the patient head downward so that the trachea will be inclined below the affected area 体位引流；**through d.,** that achieved by passing a perforated tube through the cavity, so that irrigation may be effected by injecting fluid into one aperture and letting it escape out of another 贯穿引流法

dream (drēm) 1. a mental phenomenon occurring during REM sleep in which images, emotions, and thoughts are experienced with a sense of reality 梦，睡梦；2. to experience such a phenomenon 梦幻状态；**day d.,** wishful, purposeless reveries, without regard to reality 白日梦；**wet d.,** slang for *nocturnal emission* 梦遗

drep·a·no·cyt·ic (drep″ə-no-sit′ik) having or pertaining to sickle cells 镰状细胞的

dress·ing (dres′ing) any material used for covering and protecting a wound 敷料；**antiseptic d.,** gauze impregnated with antiseptic material 抗菌敷料；**occlusive d.,** one that seals a wound from contact with air or bacteria 密闭敷料；**pressure d.,** one by which pressure is exerted on the covered area to prevent collection of fluids in underlying tissues 加压敷料

drift (drift) 1. slow movement away from the normal or original position 缓缓移动；2. a chance variation, as in gene frequency between populations; the smaller the population, the greater the chance of random variations（基因）机会变异，随机变异；**radial d.,** 桡骨连续变异，见 *deviation* 下词条；**ulnar d.,** 尺骨连续变异，见 *deviation* 下词条

drip (drip) the slow, drop-by-drop infusion of a liquid（静脉）滴注；**postnasal d.,** drainage of excessive mucous or mucopurulent discharge from the postnasal region into the pharynx 鼻后滴涕

driv·en·ness (driv′ən-nis) hyperactivity (1) 活动亢进；**organic d.,** hyperactivity seen in brain-damaged individuals as a result of injury to and disorganization of cerebellar structures 小脑受损引起的多动

dromo·graph (drom′o-graf) a recording flowmeter for measuring blood flow 血流速度描记器

dro·mo·stan·o·lone (dro″mo-stan′o-lōn) an androgenic, anabolic steroid used as an antineoplastic agent in the palliative treatment of advanced metastatic, inoperable breast cancer in certain postmenopausal women; used as the propionate salt 屈他雄酮

drom·o·tro·pic (drom″o-tro′pik) affecting conductivity of a nerve fiber 影响（神经纤维）传导的

dro·nab·i·nol (dro-nab′in-ol) one of the major active substances in cannabis, used as an antiemetic for cancer chemotherapy and anorexia and weight loss in AIDS; it is subject to abuse because of its psychotomimetic activity 屈大麻酚

drop (drop) 1. a minute sphere of liquid as it hangs or falls 液珠；2. to descend or fall 使落下；3. a descent or falling below the usual position 下降，下跌

dro·per·i·dol (dro-per′ĭ-dol) a tranquilizer of the butyrophenone series, used as a preanesthetic and anesthesia adjunct, as postoperative antiemetic, and to produce conscious sedation. In combination with fentanyl citrate, it is used as a neuroleptanalgesic 氟哌利多

drop·sy (drop′se) edema 水肿

Dro·soph·i·la (dro-sof′ĭ-lə) a genus of fruit flies. *D. melanogas'ter* is a small species used extensively in experimental genetics 果蝇

dros·pi·re·none (dros-pi′rə-nōn) a spironolactone analogue that acts as a progestational agent; used in combination with an estrogen component as an oral contraceptive 屈螺酮

drown·ing (droun′ing) suffocation and death resulting from filling of the lungs with water or other substance 溺死

DrPH Doctor of Public Health 公共卫生医师；公共卫生学博士

drug (drug) 1. a chemical substance that affects the processes of the mind or body 药物；2. any chemical compound used in the diagnosis, treatment, or prevention of disease or other abnormal condition 用于诊断、治疗、疾病预防和其他非正常情况的任何化学物质；3. recreational d.；4. to administer such a substance to someone. 派发药物；**designer d.,** a new drug of abuse similar in action to an older abused drug and usually created by making a small chemical modification in the older one 特制药物（在已有滥用药物基出上进行小的修饰而产生的新型滥用药物）；**disease-modifying antirheumatic d. (DMARD),** a classification of antirheumatic agents referring to their ability to modify the course of disease, as opposed to simply treating symptoms 改变病情抗风湿药；**nonsteroidal antiinflammatory d. (NSAID),** any of a large, chemically heterogeneous group of drugs that inhibit the enzyme cyclooxygenase, resulting in decreased synthesis of prostaglandin and thromboxane precursors; they have analgesic, antipyretic, and antiinflammatory actions 非甾体抗炎药；**orphan d.,** one that has limited commercial appeal because of the rarity of the condition it is used to treat 罕用药；**psychoactive d., psychotropic**

D

d., 精神活性药物，见 *substance* 下词条；recre-ational d., a legal or illegal psychoactive substance that is used nonmedically for the satisfaction derived from it 消遣药，一种用于获得满足感而非医学用途的合法或不合法的精神活性物质

drug·gist (drug'ist) pharmacist 药剂师；药商

drum (drum) tympanic membrane 鼓膜

drum·stick (drum'stik) a nuclear lobule attached by a slender strand to the nucleus of some polymorphonuclear leukocytes of normal females but not of normal males 鼓槌体

drunk·en·ness (drung'kən-nis) inebriation 酩酊；醉态；醉；**sleep d.,** prolonged transition from sleep to waking, with partial alertness, disorientation, drowsiness, poor coordination, and sometimes excited or violent behavior 不完全睡眠状醉态

dru·sen (droo'zən) [Ger.] hyaline excrescences in the Bruch membrane of the eye, usually due to aging 玻璃疣

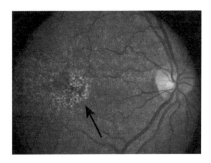

▲ 弥漫性点状的或表皮的玻璃疣（**drusen**），见于一名 56 岁男性

DS Duane syndrome 眼球后缩综合征

DSD disorders of sex development 性发育异常

DSM *Diagnostic and Statistical Manual of Mental Disorders* 精神障碍诊断与统计手册

DT diphtheria and tetanus toxoids 白喉和破伤风类毒素

DTaP diphtheria and tetanus toxoids and acellular pertussis vaccine 白喉和破伤风类毒素以及无细胞百日咳疫苗

DTP diphtheria and tetanus toxoids and pertussis vaccine 白喉和破伤风类毒素以及百日咳疫苗

DTPA diethylenetriamine pentaacetic acid 二乙基三胺五乙酸，见 *pentetic acid*

DUB dysfunctional uterine bleeding 功能失调性子宫出血

duct (dukt) a passage with well-defined walls, especially a tubular structure for the passage of excretions or secretions 导管；输送管；**duc'tal** *adj.*

导管的；aberrant d., any duct that is not usually present or that takes an unusual course or direction 迷管；**alveolar d's,** small passages connecting the respiratory bronchioles and alveolar sacs 肺泡管；**Bartholin d.,** the larger of the sublingual ducts, which opens into the submandibular duct 舌下腺大管；**Bellini d.,** papillary d.；**bile d.,** 1. any of the passages that convey bile in and from the liver 胆管；2. common bile d.；**biliary d.,** bile d.；**branchial d's,** the drawn-out branchial grooves that open into the temporary cervical sinus of the embryo 鳃管；**cochlear d.,** a spiral tube in the bony canal of the cochlea, divided into the scala tympani and scala vestibuli by the lamina spiralis 耳蜗管；**common bile d.,** the duct formed by the union of the cystic and hepatic ducts 胆总管；**d's of Cuvier,** common cardinal veins 居维叶管，总主静脉；**cystic d.,** the passage connecting the gallbladder neck and the common bile duct 胆囊管；**deferent d.,** ductus deferens 输精管；**efferent d.,** any duct that gives outlet to a glandular secretion 输出小管；**ejaculatory d.,** the duct formed by union of the ductus deferens and the duct of the seminal vesicle, opening into the prostatic urethra on the colliculus seminalis 射精管；**endolymphatic d.,** a canal connecting the membranous labyrinth of the ear with the endolymphatic sac 内淋巴管；**d. of epididymis,** the single tube into which the coiled ends of the efferent ductules of the testis open; its convolutions make up most of the epididymis 附睾管；**excretory d.,** a duct that is merely conductive and not secretory 排泄管；**genital d.,** 生殖管，见 *canal* 下词条；**hepatic d.,** the excretory duct of the liver (*common hepatic d.*), or one of its branches in the lobes of the liver (*left* and *right hepatic d's*). 肝管；**interlobular d's,** channels between different lobules of a gland 小叶间导管；**lacrimal d.,** 泪道，见 *canaliculus* 下词条；**lactiferous d's,** ducts conveying the milk secreted by the mammary lobes to and through the nipples 输乳管；**left lymphatic d.,** thoracic d. 左淋巴导管；**Luschka d's,** tubular structures in the wall of the gallbladder; some are connected with bile ducts, but none with the lumen of the gallbladder 胆囊壁管状结构；**lymphatic d's,** the main lymph channels, the right lymphatic duct, thoracic duct, and cisterna chyli (when present), into which the converging lymph vessels drain, which in turn empty into the bloodstream 淋巴导管；**mesonephric d.,** an embryonic duct of the mesonephros, which in the male develops into the epididymis, ductus deferens and its ampulla, seminal vesicles, and ejaculatory duct and in the female is largely obliterated 中肾管；**müllerian d.,** paramesonephric d；**nasolacrimal** d., the canal conveying the tears from the lacrimal sac to the inferior meatus of the nose 鼻泪管；**omphalomesenteric d.,** yolk stalk 脐肠系膜管；卵黄管；**pancreatic d.,** the main excretory duct of the pancreas, which usually unites with the common bile duct before entering the duodenum 胰管；**papillary d.,** a wide terminal tubule in the renal pyramid, formed by union of several straight collecting tubules and emptying into the renal pelvis 乳头管；**paramesonephric d.,** either of the paired embryonic ducts developing into the uterine tubes, uterus, and vagina in the female and becoming largely obliterated in the male 中肾旁管；**paraurethral d's of female urethra,** inconstantly present ducts in the female, which drain a group of the urethral glands, the paraurethral glands, into the vestibule 女性尿道旁腺管；**paraurethral d's of male urethra,** the ducts of the urethral glands situated in the spongy portion of the male urethra 男性尿道旁腺管；**parotid d.,** the duct by which the parotid gland empties into the mouth 腮腺管；**perilymphatic d.,** cochlear aqueduct 外淋巴管；蜗水管；**pronephric d.,** the duct of the pronephros, which later serves as the mesonephric duct 前肾管；**d's of prostate gland, prostatic d's,** 前列腺导管，见 *ductule* 下词条；**right lymphatic d.,** a vessel draining lymph from the upper right side of the body, receiving lymph from the right subclavian, jugular, and mediastinal trunks when those vessels do not open independently into the right brachiocephalic vein 右淋巴导管；**d. of Santorini,** a small inconstant duct draining a part of the head of the pancreas into the minor duodenal papilla 副胰管；**secretory d.,** a smaller duct that is tributary to an excretory duct of a gland and that also has a secretory function 分泌导管；**semicircular d's,** the long ducts of the membranous labyrinth of the ear 半规管；**seminal d's,** the passages for conveyance of spermatozoa and semen 输精管；Skene d's, paraurethral d's of female urethra；**spermatic d.,** ductus deferens 输精管；**Stensen d.,** parotid d.；**submandibular d.,** the duct that drains the submandibular gland and opens at the sublingual caruncle 下颌下腺管；**sudoriferous d., sweat d.,** the duct that leads from the body of a sweat gland to the surface of the skin 汗腺导管；**tear d.,** nasolacrimal d.；**thoracic d.,** the canal that ascends from the cisterna chyli to the junction of the left subclavian and left internal jugular veins 胸导管；**thyroglossal d., thyrolingual d.,** an embryonic duct extending between the thyroid primordium and the posterior tongue 甲状舌管；**Wharton d.,** submandibular d.；**d. of Wirsung,** pancreatic d.；**wolffian d.,** mesonephric d.

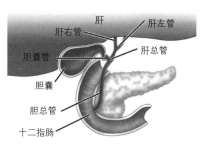

肝
肝左管
肝右管
肝总管
胆囊管
胆囊
胆总管
十二指肠

D

duc·tile (duk'til) susceptible of being drawn out without breaking 柔软的；有韧性的；易延展的

duc·tion (duk'shən) in ophthalmology, the rotation of an eye by the extraocular muscles around its horizontal, vertical, or anteroposterior axis（眼球）转动

duct·ule (duk'tūl) a minute duct 小管；**alveolar d's,** 肺泡小管，见 *duct* 下词条；**bile d's,** 1. the small channels that connect the interlobular ductules with the right and left hepatic ducts 胆小管；2. cholangioles 毛细胆管；**interlobular d's,** small channels between the hepatic lobules, draining into the bile ductules 小叶间胆管；**d's of prostate,** ducts from the prostate, opening into or near the prostatic sinuses on the posterior urethra 前列腺导管

duc·tu·lus (duk'tu-ləs) pl. *duc'tuli* [L.] ductule 小管

duc·tus (duk'təs) pl. *duc'tus* [L.] duct 导管；管道；**d. arterio'sus,** a fetal blood vessel that joins the descending aorta and left pulmonary artery 动脉导管；**d. chole'dochus,** common bile duct 胆总管；**d. de'ferens,** the excretory duct of the testis, which joins the excretory duct of the seminal vesicle to form the ejaculatory duct 输精管；**patent d. arteriosus (PDA),** abnormal persistence of an open lumen in the ductus arteriosus after birth, flow being from the aorta to the pulmonary artery and thus recirculating arterial blood through the lungs 动脉导管未闭；**d. veno'sus,** a major blood channel that develops through the embryonic liver from the left umbilical vein to the inferior vena cava 静脉导管

dull (dul) not resonant on percussion 钝的；沉闷的；呆滞的

dull·ness (dul'nis) diminished resonance on percussion; also a peculiar percussion sound that lacks the normal resonance 浊音

du·lox·e·tine (doo-lok'sə-tēn) a serotoninnorepinephrine reuptake inhibitor, used as the hydrochloride salt for the treatment of major depressive disorder and the relief of pain in diabetic neuropathy 度洛西汀

du·o·de·nal (doo″o-de'nəl) (doo-od'ə-nəl) of or pertaining to the duodenum 十二指肠的

du·o·de·nec·to·my (doo″o-də-nek′tə-me) excision of the duodenum, total or partial 十二指肠切除术

du·od·e·ni·tis (doo-od″ə-ni′tis) inflammation of the duodenal mucosa 十二指肠炎

du·o·de·no·cho·led·o·chot·o·my (doo″ode″no-ko-led″ə-kot′ə-me) incision of the duodenum and common bile duct 十二指肠胆总管切开术

du·o·de·no·en·ter·os·to·my (doo″o-de″noen″tər-os′tə-me) anastomosis of the duodenum to some other part of the small intestine 十二指肠小肠吻合术

du·o·de·no·gas·tric (doo″o-de′no-gas′trik) going from the duodenum to the stomach 从十二脂肠到胃

du·o·de·no·gram (doo″o-de′no-gram) a radiograph of the duodenum 十二指肠 X 线照片

du·o·de·nog·ra·phy (doo″o-də-nog′rə-fe) radiography of the duodenum using barium as a contrast medium 十二指肠造影

du·o·de·no·he·pat·ic (doo″o-de″no-hə-pat′ik) pertaining to the duodenum and liver 十二指肠肝相关的

du·o·de·no·je·ju·nal (doo″o-de″no-jə-joo′nəl) pertaining to the duodenum and the jejunum 十二指肠空肠相关的

du·o·de·no·je·ju·nos·to·my (doo″o-de″nojĕ″joo-nos′tə-me) anastomosis of the duodenum to the jejunum 十二指肠空肠吻合术

du·o·de·no·scope (doo″o-de′no-skōp) an enteroscope for examining the duodenum 十二指肠镜

du·o·de·nos·co·py (doo″o-də-nos′kə-pe) enteroscopy of the duodenum 十二指肠镜检查

du·o·de·nos·to·my (doo″o-də-nos′tə-me) surgical formation of a permanent opening into the duodenum 十二指肠造口术

du·o·de·num (doo″o-de′nəm) (doo-od″ə-nəm) the first or proximal portion of the small intestine, extending from the pylorus to the jejunum 十二指肠; **duode′nal** *adj.* 十二指肠的

du·pli·ca·tion (doo″plĭ-ka′shən) 1. the act or process of doubling, or the state of being doubled 复制、备份的过程或状态; 2. in genetics, the presence in the genome of additional genetic material (a chromosome or segment thereof, a gene or part thereof) 基因复制; 3. abnormal doubling of a part 某个部分异常的重复

dupp (dup) a syllable used to represent the second heart sound in auscultation 听诊中代表第二心音的音节

du·ral (doo′rəl) pertaining to the dura mater 硬脑膜的

du·rap·a·tite (door-ap′ə-tīt) a crystalline form of hydroxyapatite used as a prosthetic aid 用于假体、义肢的多晶型羟磷灰石

du·ro·ar·ach·ni·tis (doo″ro-ar″ak-ni′tis) inflammation of the dura mater and arachnoid 硬脑膜蛛网膜炎

DVM Doctor of Veterinary Medicine 兽医学博士

dwarf (dworf) an unusually short individual, particularly one of atypical proportions 侏儒，另见 *dwarfism*

dwarf·ism (dworf′iz-əm) unusually short stature, sometimes specifically that greater than three standard deviations below the mean; it may be subclassified as *short-limb d.* or *shorttrunk d.* and as *disproportionate d.* or *proportionate d.* 侏儒症，矮小; **acromelic d.,** that predominantly affecting the bones of the hands and feet 肢远端侏儒症; **hypophysial d.,** pituitary d; **Laron d.,** 拉伦侏儒症，见 *syndrome* 下词条; **mesomelic d.,** that predominantly affecting the bones of the leg and forearm 肢中间侏儒症; **pituitary d.,** a type with retention of infantile characteristics, due to undersecretion of growth hormone and gonadotropin deficiency 垂体性侏儒症; **primordial d.,** that characterized by a profound but proportionate decrease in size that is present at birth 原始侏儒症; **psychosocial d.,** severe growth retardation with functional hypopituitarism as a result of extreme emotional deprivation or stress; behavioral manifestations may include bizarre eating and drinking habits, social withdrawal, and primitive speech 社会心理性侏儒症; **rhizomelic d.,** that predominantly affecting the bones of the thigh and arm 肢近端侏儒症

DWI diffusion-weighted imaging 弥散加权成像

Dx diagnosis 诊断

Dy dysprosium 镝

dy·ad (di′ad) a double chromosome resulting from the halving of a tetrad 二分体

dy·clo·nine (di′klo-nēn) a bactericidal and fungicidal local anesthetic, used topically as the hydrochloride salt 达克罗宁，一种可以杀灭细菌和真菌的局部麻醉药

dye (di) any colored substance containing auxochromes and thus capable of coloring substances to which it is applied; used for staining and coloring, as a test reagent, and as a therapeutic agent 染料; 用于染色的诊断治疗试剂; **acid d., acidic d.,** one that is acidic in reaction and usually unites with positively charged ions of the material acted upon 酸性染料; **amphoteric d.,** a dye containing both reactive basic and reactive acidic groups, and staining both acidic and basic elements 两性染料; **anionic d.,** acid d.; **basic d.,** one that is basic in reaction and unites with negatively charged ions of the material acted upon 碱性染料; **cationic d.,** basic d.

dy·ing (di′ing) the final stage in life; the process

of approaching death 死亡状态，死亡过程

dy·nam·ic (di-nam′ik) 1. pertaining to or manifesting force 有活力的，强有力的；2. of or relating to energy or to objects in motion 动态的；3. characterized by or tending to produce change 不断变化的

dy·nam·ics (di-nam′iks) the scientific study of forces in action; a phase of mechanics 动力学；力学

dy·na·mom·e·ter (di″nə-mom′ə-tər) an instrument for measuring the force of muscular contraction 测力计

dyne (dīn) a unit of force; the amount that when acting continuously upon a mass of 1 g will impart to it an acceleration of 1 cm per second per second; equal to 10^{-5} newton 力的单位

dy·nein (di′nēn) 动力蛋白 1. an ATP-splitting enzyme essential to the motility of cilia and flagella because of its interactions with microtubules 一种与微管相互作用而为纤毛和鞭毛运动所必要的 ATP 裂解酶；2. any of a family of ATP-splitting enzymes that move along microtubules and act as motors to produce the beating of flagella and cilia and the movement of vesicles and chromosomes 沿微管运动并作为动力促进鞭毛和纤毛有节奏地摆动以及囊泡和染色体的运动的 ATP 裂解酶家族中的任何一种。Cf. *kinesin*

dy·nor·phin (di-nor′fin) any of a family of opioid peptides found throughout the central and peripheral nervous systems; most are agonists at opioid receptor sites. Some are probably involved in pain regulation and others in the hypothalamic regulation of eating and drinking 强啡肽

dy·phyl·line (di′fəl-in) a derivative of theophylline used as a bronchodilator in the treatment of asthma, chronic bronchitis, and emphysema 双羟丙茶碱

dys·acu·sis (dis″ə-koo′sis) 1. a hearing impairment in which the loss is not measurable in decibels, but in disturbances in discrimination of speech or tone quality, pitch, or loudness, etc 听觉损害；2. a condition in which sounds produce discomfort 因声音而产生不适的情况

dys·aphia (dis-a′fe-ə) paraphia 触觉障碍

dys·ar·te·ri·ot·o·ny (dis″ahr-tēr″e-ot′ə-ne) abnormality of blood pressure 血压异常

dys·ar·thria (dis-ahr′thre-ə) a speech disorder caused by disturbances of muscular control because of damage to the central or peripheral nervous system 由于中枢或外周神经系统病变引起肌肉控制紊乱而导致的构音障碍

dys·ar·thro·sis (dis″ahr-thro′sis) 1. deformity or malformation of a joint 关节变形；2. dysarthria 构音障碍

dys·au·to·no·mia (dis″aw-to-no′me-ə) malfunction of the autonomic nervous system 自主神经系统障碍；**familial d.**, an inherited disorder of childhood characterized by defective lacrimation, skin blotching, emotional instability, motor incoordination, absence of pain sensation, and hyporeflexia; it occurs almost exclusively in Ashkenazi Jews 家族性自主神经系统障碍

dys·bar·ism (dis′bər-iz-əm) any clinical syndrome due to difference between the surrounding atmospheric pressure and the total gas pressure in the tissues, fluids, and cavities of the body 气压病

dys·ba·sia (dis-ba′zhə) difficulty in walking, especially due to a nervous lesion 行走困难

dys·be·ta·lipo·pro·tein·emia (dis-ba″tə-lip″o-pro″te-ne′me-ə) 1. the accumulation of abnormal β-lipoproteins in the blood 异常 β 脂蛋白血症；2. familial d.；**familial d.**, an inherited disorder of lipoprotein metabolism caused by interaction of a defect in apolipoprotein E with genetic and environmental factors causing hypertriglyceridemia; its phenotype is that of a type Ⅲ hyperlipoproteinemia 家族性异常 β 脂蛋白血症

dys·ceph·a·ly (dis-sef′ə-le) malformation of the cranial and facial bones 颅面骨畸形

dys·che·zia (dis-ke′zhə) difficult or painful defecation 大便困难

dys·chi·ria (dis-ki′re-ə) loss of power to tell which side of the body has been touched 左右感觉障碍

dys·chon·dro·pla·sia (dis″kon-dro-pla′zhə) 1. enchondromatosis 软骨发育不良；2. formerly, a general term encompassing both enchondromatosis and exostosis, which has caused their synonyms to become tangled 过去为内生软骨瘤病和外生骨疣的通用术语

dys·chro·ma·top·sia (dis-kro″mə-top′se-ə) disorder of color vision 色觉障碍

dys·chro·mia (dis-kro′me-ə) any disorder of pigmentation of skin or hair 皮肤或头发着色异常

dys·con·trol (dis″kən-trōl′) inability to control one's behavior; 失控；另见 *syndrome* 下词条

dys·co·ria (dis-kor′e-ə) abnormality in the form or shape of the pupil or in the reaction of the two pupils 瞳孔变形；瞳孔反应异常

dys·cra·sia (dis-kra′zhə) [Gr.] a term formerly used to indicate an abnormal mixture of the four humors; in surviving usages it is now roughly synonymous with disease or pathologic condition 病态；失调；恶质；**plasma cell d's**, a diverse group of neoplastic diseases involving proliferation of a single clone of cells producing a serum M component (a monoclonal immunoglobulin or immunoglobulin

334

fragment) and usually having a plasma cell morphology; it includes multiple myeloma and heavy chain diseases 浆细胞病

dys·ejac·u·la·tion (dis″e-jak″u-la′shən) 1. any failure of normal ejaculation of semen 射精障碍; 2. a painful, burning sensation in the inguinal region during semen ejaculation 射精时腹股沟区域疼痛、烧灼感

dys·en·tery (dis′ən-ter″e) any of a number of disorders marked by inflammation of the intestine, especially of the colon, with abdominal pain, tenesmus, and frequent stools containing blood and mucus 痢疾; **dysenter′ic** adj. 痢疾的; **amebic d.,** dysentery due to ulceration of the bowel caused by severe amebiasis 阿米巴痢疾; **bacillary d.,** dysentery caused by *Shigella.* 细菌性痢疾; **viral d.,** dysentery caused by a virus, occurring in epidemics and marked by acute watery diarrhea 病毒性痢疾

dys·equi·lib·ri·um (dis″e-kwī-lib′re-əm) 1. any derangement of the state of equilibrium 感觉失衡、感觉混乱; 另见 *dizziness* 和 *vertigo* 下词条; 2. disturbance of a state of equilibrium 不平衡状态。Spelled also *disequilibrium*

dys·er·gia (dis-ur′jə) motor incoordination due to defect of efferent nerve impulse 传出性共济失调

dys·es·the·sia (dis″es-the′zhə) 1. distortion of any sense, especially of the sense of touch 感觉失真, 尤其是触觉; 2. an unpleasant abnormal sensation produced by normal stimuli 正常刺激引起的异常感觉; **dysesthet′ic** adj 感觉迟钝的, 感觉异常的; **auditory d.,** dysacusis (2) 听声不适

dys·fi·brin·o·ge·ne·mia (dis-fi-brin″o-jə-ne′me-ə) the presence in the blood of abnormal fibrinogen 异常纤维蛋白原血症

dys·func·tion (dis-funk′shən) disturbance, impairment, or abnormality of functioning of an organ 功能障碍; **dysfunc′tional** adj. 功能障碍的; **erectile d.,** impotence (2) 勃起功能障碍; **minimal brain d.,** former name for *attention-deficit/hyperactivity disorder* 注意缺陷障碍(伴多动), 注意力缺陷/多动症的曾用名; **sexual d.,** any of a group of sexual disorders characterized by disturbance either of sexual desire or of the psychophysiologic changes that usually characterize sexual response 性功能障碍

dys·gam·ma·glob·u·lin·emia (dis-gam″ə-glob″u-lin-e′me-ə) an immunologic deficiency state marked by selective deficiencies of one or more, but not all, classes of immunoglobulins 异常丙种球蛋白血症; **dysgammaglobuline′mic** adj. 异常丙种球蛋白血症的

dys·gen·e·sis (dis-jen′ə-sis) defective development; malformation 发育不良; **46,XY complete gonad-**

al d., a heterogeneous disorder in which a 46,XY karyotype is associated with normal female external genitalia and müllerian structures, streak gonads, absence of pubertal development of secondary sex characteristics, and primary amenorrhea 46,XY 单纯性腺发育不全; **gonadal d.,** defective development of the gonads; it comprises various disorders usually qualified at least on the basis of genotype (e.g., 46,XY) and sometimes on the basis of the state of underdevelopment of the gonads (e.g., complete) 性腺发育不全

dys·ger·mi·no·ma (dis″jər-mĭ-no′mə) a malignant ovarian neoplasm, thought to be derived from primordial germ cells of the sexually undifferentiated embryonic gonad; it is the counterpart of the classical testicular seminoma 无性细胞瘤

dys·geu·sia (dis-goo′zhə) parageusia 味觉障碍

dys·gna·thia (dis-na′the-ə) any oral abnormality extending beyond the teeth to involve the maxilla or mandible, or both 上下颌异常; **dysgnath′ic** adj. 上下颌异常的

Dys·go·no·mo·nas (dis-gon″o-mo′nəs) a genus of gram-negative, anaerobic, rod-shaped bacteria; *D. capnocytophagoi′des* is an opportunistic pathogen 微生长单胞菌属

dys·graph·ia (dis-graf′e-ə) difficulty in writing 书写困难, 书写障碍 cf. *agraphia*

dys·he·ma·to·poi·e·sis (dis-he″mə-to″poie′sis) defective blood formation 造血障碍; **dyshemato-poiet′ic** adj. 造血障碍的

dys·he·sion (dis-he′zhon) 1. disordered cell adherence 细胞黏附障碍; 2. loss of intercellular cohesion 细胞间连接丧失; a characteristic of malignancy 恶性的特征

dys·hi·dro·sis (dis″hĭ-dro′sis) 1. pompholyx 汗疱疹; 2. any disorder of eccrine sweat glands 出汗障碍

dys·kary·o·sis (dis-kar″e-o′sis) abnormality of form or staining characteristics of the cell nucleus 核异质; **dyskaryot′ic** adj. 核异质的

dys·ker·a·to·ma (dis-ker″ə-to′mə) a dyskeratotic tumor 角化不良瘤; **warty d.,** a solitary brownish red nodule with a soft, yellowish, central keratotic plug, occurring on the face, neck, scalp, or axilla, or in the mouth; histologically it resembles an individual lesion of keratosis follicularis 疣角化不良瘤

dys·ker·a·to·sis (dis-ker″ə-to′sis) abnormal, premature, or imperfect keratinization of the keratinocytes 角化不良; **dyskaryot′ic** adj. 角化不良的

dys·ki·ne·sia (dis″kĭ-ne′zhə) distortion or impairment of voluntary movement, as in tic or spasm 运动障碍; **dyskinet′ic** adj. 运动障碍的; **biliary d.,** derangement of the filling and emptying mechanism of the gallbladder 胆道运动障碍；d. intermit′tens, intermittent disability of the limbs due to impaired circulation 间歇性运动障碍；orofacial d., facial movements resembling those of tardive dyskinesia, seen in elderly, edentulous, demented patients 面部运动障碍；primary ciliary d., a genetically heterogeneous autosomal recessive disorder resulting from defects in the primary ciliary apparatus; characterized by impaired mucociliary clearance from the airways, with frequent respiratory, sinus, and ear infections 原发性纤毛运动不良症。Cf. *Kartagener syndrome*；**tardive d.**, an iatrogenic disorder of involuntary repetitive movements of facial, buccal, oral, and cervical muscles, induced by long-term use of antipsychotic agents, sometimes persisting after withdrawal of the agent 迟发性运动障碍

dys·la·lia (dĭs-la′le-ə) paralalia 言语困难

dys·lex·ia (dis-lek′se-ə) impairment of ability to read, spell, and write words, despite the ability to see and recognize letters 阅读障碍；**dyslex′ic** *adj.* 阅读障碍的

dys·lip·id·e·mia (dis-lip″id-e′me-ə) abnormality in, or abnormal amounts of, lipids and lipoproteins in the blood. 血脂异常

dys·lipo·pro·tein·emia (dis-lip″o-pro″tene′me-ə) the presence of abnormal concentrations of lipoproteins or abnormal lipoproteins in the blood 异常脂蛋白血症

dys·ma·tur·i·ty (dis-mə-choor′ĭ-te) 1. disordered development 发育障碍；2. postmaturity syndrome 过熟综合征；**dysmature′** *adj.* 成熟障碍的；**pulmonary d.**, Wilson-Mikity syndrome Wilson-Mikity 综合征

dys·me·lia (dis-me′le-ə) anomaly of a limb or limbs resulting from a disturbance in embryonic development 肢体发育不良，肢体畸形

dys·men·or·rhea (dis-men″ə-re′ə) painful menstruation 痛经；**dysmenorrhe′al, dysmenorrhe′ic** *adj.* 痛经的；**primary d.**, that not associated with pelvic pathology; usually beginning in adolescence with the onset of ovulatory cycles 原发性痛经；**secondary d.**, that associated with pelvic pathology; usually beginning after 20 years of age 继发性痛经

dys·me·tab·o·lism (dis″mə-tab′o-liz-əm) defective metabolism 代谢障碍

dys·me·tria (dis-me′tre-ə) disturbance of the power to control the range of movement in muscular action 动作幅度控制紊乱

dys·mor·phism (dis-mor′fiz-əm) 1. an abnormality in morphologic development 形态学发育异常；2. allomorphism 异形；畸形；3. the ability to appear in different morphologic forms 展现不同形态的能力；**dysmor′phic** *adj.* 异形的

dys·mor·phol·o·gy (dis″mor-fol′ə-je) the study of abnormal physical development 畸形学

dys·my·elin·a·tion (dis″mi-ə-lin-a′shən) breakdown or defective formation of a myelin sheath, usually involving biochemical abnormalities 髓鞘形成障碍

dys·odon·ti·a·sis (dis″o-don-ti′ə-sis) defective, delayed, or difficult eruption of the teeth 出牙不良

dys·on·to·gen·e·sis (dis″on-to-jen′ə-sis) defective embryonic development. 胚胎发育不良；**dysontogenet′ic** *adj.* 胚胎发育不良的

dys·orex·ia (dis″o-rek′se-ə) impaired or deranged appetite 食欲障碍

dys·os·teo·gen·e·sis (dis-os″te-o-jen′ə-sis) defective bone formation; dysostosis 成骨不良

dys·os·to·sis (dis″os-to′sis) defective ossification; defect in the normal ossification of fetal cartilages. 成骨不良；骨发育不全；**cleidocranial d.**, 颅骨锁骨发育不良，见 *dysplasia* 下词条；**craniofacial d.**, Crouzon syndrome. 颅面骨发育不全；**mandibulofacial d.**, a hereditary disorder occurring in a complete form (*Franceschetti syndrome*) and a less severe form (*Treacher Collins syndrome*), with antimongoloid slant of the palpebral fissures, coloboma of the lower lid, micrognathia and hypoplasia of the zygomatic arches, and microtia 下颌骨颜面发育不全，特雷彻·柯林斯综合征；**metaphyseal d.**, a skeletal abnormality in which the epiphyses are normal and the metaphyseal tissues are replaced by masses of cartilage, producing interference with enchondral bone formation 干骺端骨发育不良

dys·pa·reu·nia (dis″pə-roo′ne-ə) difficult or painful sexual intercourse 性交困难

dys·pep·sia (dis-pep′se-ə) impairment of the power or function of digestion; usually applied to epigastric discomfort after meals 消化不良；**dyspep′tic** *adj.* 消化不良的；**nonulcer d.**, dyspepsia with symptoms that resemble those of peptic ulcer, although no ulcer is detectable 非溃疡性消化不良

dys·pha·gia (dis-fa′je-ə) difficulty in swallowing 吞咽困难

dys·pha·sia (dis-fa′zhə) impairment of speech, consisting of lack of coordination and failure to arrange words in their proper order; due to a central lesion 言语障碍

dys·pho·nia (dis-fo′ne-ə) a voice impairment or speech disorder 发声困难；**dysphon′ic** *adj.* 发声困难的

dys·pho·ria (dis-for′e-ə) [Gr.] disquiet; restlessness; malaise 病理性心境恶劣，烦躁；**dysphoret′ic, dysphor′ic** *adj.* 烦躁不安的；**gender d.**, unhappiness with one's biologic sex or its usual gender role, with the desire for the body and role of the opposite sex 性别不安症，性别焦虑

dys·pig·men·ta·tion (dis-pig″mən-ta′shən) dyschromia 色素沉着异常

dys·pla·sia (dis-pla′zhə) 1. abnormality of development 发育异常; 2. in pathology, alteration in size, shape, and organization of adult cells 异型增生; **dysplas′tic** *adj.*; **anhidrotic ectodermal d.**, an inherited disorder characterized by ectodermal dysplasia associated with aplasia or hypoplasia of the sweat glands, hypothermia, alopecia, anodontia, conical teeth, and facial abnormalities 无汗性外胚层发育不良; **anteroposterior facial d.**, defective development resulting in abnormal anteroposterior relations of the maxilla and mandible to each other or to the cranial base 前后面部发育不良; **arrhythmogenic right ventricular d.**, a congenital cardiomyopathy in which transmural infiltration of adipose tissue results in weakness and bulging of regions of the right ventricle and leads to ventricular tachycardia arising in the right ventricle 致心律失常性右心室发育不良; **bronchopulmonary d.**, chronic lung disease of premature infants that results from disruption of immature lung structures and necessitates the use of supplemental oxygen for at least 28 days after birth; it is caused by injury during mechanical ventilation or antenatal exposure to factors that interfere with development of normal lung structure 支气管肺发育不良; **camptomelic d.**, an autosomal dominant disorder of severe skeletal dysplasia and dwarfism, with bowing of the tibia and fibula, spinal abnormalities, and often severe respiratory distress and tracheobronchial hypoplasia; (XY) males also often have ambiguous or female external genitalia 屈肢骨发育不良; **chondroectodermal d.**, achondroplasia with defective development of skin, hair, and teeth, polydactyly, and defect of cardiac septum 软骨外胚层发育不良; **cleidocranial d.**, a hereditary condition marked by defective ossification of the cranial bones, absence of the clavicles, and dental and vertebral anomalies 颅骨锁骨发育不良; **developmental d. of the hip (DDH)**, instability of the hip joint leading to dislocation in the neonatal period; it may be associated with various neuromuscular disorders or occur in utero but occurs most commonly in neurologically normal infants and is multifactorial in origin. Formerly called *congenital dislocation of the hip* 髋关节发育不良, 曾被称为先天性髋关节脱臼; **diaphyseal d.**, abnormal thickening of the cortex of the midshaft area of the long bones, progressing toward the epiphyses, and sometimes also in the flat bones 骨干发育不良; **ectodermal d.**, any of a group of hereditary disorders involving tissues and structures derived from embryonic ectoderm, including an-

hidrotic ectodermal dysplasia, hidrotic ectodermal dysplasia, and EEC syndrome 外胚层发育不良; **epiphyseal d.**, faulty growth and ossification of the epiphyses with radiographically apparent stippling and decreased stature, not associated with thyroid disease 骨骺发育不良; **fibromuscular d.**, dysplasia with fibrosis of the muscular layer of an artery wall, with collagen deposition and hyperplasia of smooth muscle, causing stenosis and hypertension; seen most often in renal arteries, it is a major cause of renovascular hypertension 纤维肌性发育不良; **fibrous d. of bone**, thinning of the cortex of bone and replacement of marrow by gritty fibrous tissue containing bony spicules, causing pain, disability, and gradually increasing deformity; only one bone may be involved (*monostotic fibrous d.*) or several to many (*polyostotic fibrous d.*) 骨纤维性结构不良, 可涉及单骨纤维性结构不良或多骨纤维性结构不良; **florid osseous d.**, an exuberant form of periapical cemental dysplasia resembling diffuse sclerosing osteomyelitis but not inflammatory 红骨性发育不良; **hidrotic ectodermal d.**, an inherited disorder characterized by hypotrichosis, cutaneous hyperpigmentation over joints, hyperkeratosis of the palms and soles, normal dentition, and normal sweat gland function 有汗性外胚层发育不良; **metaphyseal d.**, a disturbance in enchondral bone growth, failure of modeling causing the ends of the shafts to remain larger than normal in circumference 干骺端发育不良; **monostotic fibrous d.**, 见 *fibrous d. of bone*; **multiple epiphyseal d.**, an inherited developmental abnormality of various epiphyses, which appear late and are mottled, flattened, fragmented, and usually hypoplastic; digits are short, thick, and blunted, and stature may be diminished from flattening deformities at the hips, knees, and ankles. 多发性骨骺发育不良; **oculodentodigital d.**, a rare autosomal dominant condition, characterized by bilateral microphthalmos, abnormally small nose with anteverted nostrils, hypotrichosis, dental anomalies, camptodactyly, syndactyly, and missing phalanges of the toes 眼齿指发育不良; **periapical cemental d.**, a nonneoplastic condition characterized by formation of areas of fibrous connective tissue, bone, and cement around the apex of a tooth 根尖周牙骨质异常增生; **polyostotic fibrous d.**, 见 *fibrous d. of bone*; **septo-optic d.**, a syndrome of hypoplasia of the optic disk with other ocular abnormalities, absence of the septum pellucidum, and hypopituitarism leading to growth deficiency 视隔发育不良; **spondyloepiphyseal d.**, hereditary dysplasia of the vertebrae and extremities resulting in dwarfism of the short-trunk type, often with shortened limbs due

to epiphyseal abnormalities 脊椎骨骺发育不良；
thanatophoric d., a lethal skeletal dysplasia presenting as severe proximal shortening of the limbs, thoracic cage deformity, flattening of the vertebral bodies, and relative macrocephaly, sometimes with cloverleaf skull; due to de novo mutation of a fibroblast growth factor receptor 致死性骨发育不良
dysp·nea (disp-ne′ə) (disp′ne-ə) labored or difficult breathing 呼吸困难；**dyspne′ic** *adj.* 呼吸困难的；
paroxysmal nocturnal d., respiratory distress that awakens patients from sleep, related to posture (especially reclining at night), attributed to congestive heart failure with pulmonary edema or sometimes to chronic pulmonary disease 夜间阵发性呼吸困难
dys·prax·ia (dis-prak′se-ə) partial loss of ability to perform coordinated acts 运用障碍，应用障碍
dys·pro·si·um (Dy) (dis-pro′se-əm) a lustrous, silvery white, rare earth and heavy metal element; at. no. 66, at. wt. 162.50 镝；**d. 165,** a radioactive isotope of dysprosium, having an atomic mass of 165 and a half-life of 140 minutes, and emitting beta particles (1.287 MeV); used in radiation synovectomy 镝的放射性同位素
dys·pro·tein·emia (dis-pro″tēn-e′me-ə) 1. disorder of the protein content of the blood 异常蛋白血症；2. a plasma cell dyscrasia 一种浆细胞恶病质
dys·ra·phism (dis-rāf′iz-əm) incomplete closure of a raphe; defective fusion, particularly of the neural tube 脊管闭合不全；另见 *neural tube defect*
dys·rhyth·mia (dis-rith′me-ə) 1. disturbance of rhythm 节律障碍；2. an abnormal cardiac rhythm; the term *arrhythmia* is usually used, even for abnormal but regular rhythms 心脏节律；**dysrhyth′mic** *adj.*; **cerebral d., electroencephalographic d.,** a disturbance or irregularity in the rhythm of the brain waves as recorded by electroencephalography 脑电节律异常
dys·se·ba·cea (dis″se-ba′shə) disorder of sebaceous follicles; specifically, a condition seen (but not exclusively) in riboflavin deficiency, marked by greasy, branny seborrhea on the midface, with erythema in the nasal folds, canthi, or other skin folds 皮脂障碍症
dys·som·nia (dis-som′ne-ə) any of various disturbances in the quality, amount, or timing of sleep 睡眠障碍
dys·sper·mia (dis-spur′me-ə) impairment of the spermatozoa, or of the semen 精子异常；精液异常
dys·sta·sia (dis-sta′shə) difficulty in standing 站立困难；**dysstat′ic** *adj.* 站立困难的
dys·syn·er·gia (dis″sin-ur′je-ə) muscular incoordination 协同动作障碍；**d. cerebella′ris myoclo′nica,** dyssynergia cerebellaris progressiva associated with myoclonus epilepsy 肌痉挛性小脑协同障碍；**d. cerebella′ris**

progressi′va, a condition marked by generalized intention tremors associated with disturbance of muscle tone and of muscular coordination; due to disorder of cerebellar function 进行性小脑协同失调；
detrusor-sphincter d., contraction of the urethral sphincter muscle at the same time the detrusor muscle of the bladder is contracting, resulting in obstruction of normal urinary outflow; it may accompany detrusor hyperreflexia or instability 逼尿肌括约肌协同失调
dys·tax·ia (dis-tak′se-ə) difficulty in controlling voluntary movements 共济失调
dys·thy·mia (dis-thi′me-ə) dysthymic disorder 抑郁障碍
dys·thy·mic (dis-thi′mik) characterized by symptoms of mild depression 轻度抑郁
dys·thy·roid (dis-thi′roid) denoting defective functioning of the thyroid gland 甲状腺功能紊乱
dys·to·cia (dis-to′shə) abnormal labor or childbirth 难产
dys·to·nia (dis-to′ne-ə) dyskinetic movements due to disordered tonicity of muscle 肌张力失常，肌张力障碍；**dyston′ic** *adj.*; **action d.,** dystonia in which dyskinetic movements occur during voluntary action and are absent when the affected part is at rest 自主运动时肌张力异常而休息时缓解；**cervical d.,** spasmodic torticollis; a focal dystonia affecting the cervical muscles, causing abnormal movements or postures of the head, neck, and shoulders 颈部肌力障碍；**early-onset torsion d.,** a hereditary dystonia that appears in childhood or adolescence, beginning as an action dystonia in an arm or leg and spreading to affect the trunk and other limbs; when generalized, it results in severe disability 早发性扭转性肌张力障碍；**focal d.,** dystonia localized to a specific part of the body 局灶性肌张力障碍；
d. musculo′rum defor′mans, a hereditary disorder marked by involuntary, irregular, clonic contortions of the muscles of the trunk and limbs, which twist the body forward and sideways grotesquely 畸形性肌张力障碍；**d.-plus,** any of several syndromes consisting of a combination of dystonia with other neurologic signs, such as myoclonus or parkinsonism 肌张力障碍叠加综合征
dys·to·pia (dis-to′pe-ə) malposition; displacement 异位
dys·tro·phia (dis-tro′fe-ə) [Gr.] dystrophy 营养不良；**d. adiposogenita′lis,** adiposogenital dystrophy 肥胖性生殖无能性营养不良；**d. myoto′nica,** myotonic dystrophy 营养不良性肌强直；**d. un′guium,** nail dystrophy 甲营养不良
dys·tropho·neu·ro·sis (dis-trof″o-noo-ro′sis) 1. any nervous disorder due to poor nutrition 营养不

良性神经病；2. impairment of nutrition due to nervous disorder 神经紊乱性营养不良

dys·tro·phy (dis′trə-fe) any disorder due to defective or faulty nutrition 营养不良；**dystroph′ic** *adj.* 营养不良的；**adiposogenital d.**, a condition marked by adiposity of the feminine type, genital hypoplasia, changes in secondary sex characters, and metabolic disturbances; seen with lesions of the hypothalamus 肥胖性生殖无能性营养不良；**Becker muscular d.**, **Becker type muscular d.**, a form closely resembling *Duchenne muscular d.* but having a late onset and a slowly progressive course; it is transmitted as an X-linked trait and has been associated with mutations of the gene encoding the muscle protein dystrophin 贝克肌营养不良；**Duchenne muscular d.**, **Duchenne type muscular d.**, the most common and severe type of pseudohypertrophic muscular dystrophy; it begins in early childhood, is chronic and progressive, and is characterized by increasing weakness in the pelvic and pectoral girdles, pseudohypertrophy of muscles followed by atrophy, lordosis, and a peculiar swinging gait with the legs kept wide apart. It is transmitted as an X-linked trait and has been linked to mutations of the gene encoding the muscle protein dystrophin 迪谢内肌营养不良；**Emery-Dreifuss muscular d.**, a rare type of muscular dystrophy beginning early in life and involving slowly progressive weakness of the upper arm and pelvic girdle muscles, with cardiomyopathy and flexion contractures of the elbows; muscles are not hypertrophied. The two forms (X-linked and autosomal dominant) have been linked to mutations affecting proteins of the cytoskeleton, emerin and lamin A 埃默里-德赖赖弗斯肌营养不良；**facioscapulohumeral muscular d.**, a relatively benign form of muscular dystrophy, with marked atrophy of the muscles of the face, pectoral girdle, and arm 面肩胛肱肌营养不良；**Fukuyama type congenital muscular d.**, a form of muscular dystrophy with muscle abnormalities resembling those of *Duchenne muscular d.*; characterized also by intellectual disability with polymicrogyria and other cerebral abnormalities 福山型先天性肌营养不良；**Landouzy muscular d.**, **Landouzy-Dejerine d.**, **Landouzy-Dejerine muscular d.**, facioscapulohumeral muscular d. **Leyden-Möbius muscular d.**, **limb-girdle muscular d.**, slowly progressive muscular dystrophy, usually beginning in childhood, marked by weakness and wasting in the pelvic girdle (*pelvifemoral muscular dystrophy*) or pectoral girdle (*scapulohumeral muscular dystrophy*) 肢带型肌营养不良；**muscular d.**, a group of genetically determined, painless, degenerative myopathies marked by muscular weakness and atrophy without nervous system involvement. The three main types are *pseudohypertrophic muscular d.*, *facioscapulohumeral muscular d.*, and *limb-girdle muscular d.* 肌营养不良；**myotonic d.**, a rare, slowly progressive, hereditary disease, a triplet repeat disorder; marked by myotonia followed by muscular atrophy (especially of the face and neck), cataracts, hypogonadism, frontal balding, and cardiac disorders 强直性肌营养不良；**nail d.**, changes in the texture, structure, and/or color of the nails due to no demonstrable cause, but presumed to be attributable to some disturbance of nutrition 甲营养不良；**oculopharyngeal d.**, **oculopharyngeal muscular d.**, a form with onset in adulthood, characterized by weakness of the external ocular and pharyngeal muscles that causes ptosis, ophthalmoplegia, and dysphagia 眼咽型肌营养不良；**pseudohypertrophic muscular d.**, a group of muscular dystrophies characterized by enlargement (pseudohypertrophy) of muscles, most commonly *Duchenne muscular d.* or *Becker muscular d.* 假性肥大性肌营养不良；**reflex sympathetic d.**, complex regional pain syndrome type 1 反射性交感神经营养不良

dys·uria (dis-u′re-ə) painful or difficult urination 排尿困难，尿痛；**dysu′ric** *adj.* 排尿困难的

E enzyme 酶；**exa-** 表示 10^{18}

E elastance 弹回性；electromotive force 电动势；energy 能量；illumination 照度

e- word element [L.], *away from; without; outside* 离，外

ε (epsilon, the fifth letter of the Greek alphabet)（希腊字母表的第五个字母）；heavy chain of IgE IgE 的重链；the ε chain of hemoglobin 血红蛋白的 ε 链

ε- a prefix designating 前缀 (1) the position of a substituting atom or group in a chemical compound 取代原子或基团在化合物中的位置；(2) fifth in a series of five or more related entities or chemical compounds 表示五个或更多相关实体或化合物中的第五个

EAC an abbreviation used in studies of complement, in which E represents erythrocyte, A antibody, and C complement 红细胞、抗体和补体的符号

ear (ēr) the organ of hearing and of equilibrium, consisting of the external ear, the middle ear, and the internal ear 耳，听觉和平衡器官，包括外耳、中耳和内耳。见图 29；**Blainville e's,** asymmetry of the ears 双耳不对称；**cauliflower e.,** a partially deformed auricle due to injury and subsequent perichondritis 菜花状耳；**external e.,** the pinna and external meatus together 外耳；**glue e.,** a chronic condition marked by a collection of fluid of high viscosity in the middle ear, due to obstruction of the eustachian tube 胶耳；**inner e., internal e.,** the labyrinth; the vestibule, cochlea, and semicircular canals together 内耳；**middle e.,** the cavity in the temporal bone comprising the tympanic cavity, auditory ossicles, and auditory tube 中耳；**outer e.,** external e.；**swimmer's e., tank e.,** otitis externa 外耳道炎

ear·ache (ēr′āk) otalgia 耳痛

ear·drum (ēr′drəm) tympanic membrane 鼓膜

ear·lobe (ēr′lōb) the lower fleshy part of the external ear 耳屏

ear·wax (ēr′waks) cerumen 耵聍

eat·ing (ēt′ing) the act of ingestion 摄食；**binge e.,** uncontrolled ingestion of large quantities of food in a discrete interval, often with a sense of lack of control over the activity 暴食

ebur·na·tion (e″bər-na′shən) conversion of bone into a hard, ivory-like mass 骨质象牙化

EBV human herpesvirus 4 (Epstein-Barr virus)EB 病毒；人类疱疹病毒 4 型

ECAC expiratory central airway collapse 呼气中央气道塌陷

ecau·date (e-kaw′dāt) tail-less 无尾的

ec·bol·ic (ek-bol′ik) oxytocic 催产剂；催产的

ec·cen·tric (ek-sen′trik) situated or occurring or proceeding away from a center 古怪的；偏心的

ec·cen·tro·chon·dro·pla·sia (ek-sen″trokon″dro-pla′zhə) Morquio syndrome 离心性软骨发育不良

ec·chon·dro·ma (ek″on-dro′mə) pl. *ecchondromas, ecchondro'mata.* A hyperplastic growth of cartilaginous tissue on the surface of a cartilage or projecting under the periosteum of a bone 外生软骨瘤

ec·chy·mo·ma (ek-ĭ-mo′mə) swelling due to blood extravasation 瘀血；皮下血肿

ec·chy·mo·sis (ek″ĭ-mo′sis) pl. *ecchymo'ses* [Gr.] a small hemorrhagic spot in the skin or a mucous membrane, larger than a petechia, forming a nonelevated, rounded, or irregular blue or purplish patch 瘀斑；**ecchymot'ic** *adj.* 瘀斑的

ec·crine (ek′rin) exocrine, with special reference to ordinary sweat glands 外分泌的

ec·cy·e·sis (ek″si-e′sis) ectopic pregnancy 异位妊娠

ECF-A eosinophil chemotactic factor of anaphylaxis 过敏反应嗜酸性粒细胞趋化因子；a primary mediator of type Ⅰ hypersensitivity Ⅰ型超敏反应的主要介质

ECG electrocardiogram 心电图

ec·go·nine (ek′go-nin) the final basic product obtained by hydrolysis of cocaine and several related alkaloids; *e. methyl* ester is the major hydrolytic metabolite of cocaine detectable in blood by laboratory testing 芽子碱

Echi·na·cea (ek″ĭ-na′shə) a genus of North American flowering herbs. *E. purpu'rea* is used for colds and respiratory and urinary tract infections and for wounds and burns. *E. pal'lida* root is used for fevers and colds. *E. angustifo'lia* is used in folk medicine 紫锥花属

Echi·no·coc·cus (e-ki″no-kok′əs) a genus of small tapeworms, including *E. granulo'sus,* usually parasitic in dogs and wolves, whose larvae (hydatids) may develop in mammals, forming hydatid tumors or cysts chiefly in the liver, and *E. multilocula'ris,* whose larvae form alveolar or multilocular cysts and whose adult forms usually parasitize the fox and wild rodents, although humans are sporadically infected 棘球绦虫属

echi·no·coc·cus (e-ki″no-kok′əs) pl. *echinococ'ci.* An individual organism of the genus *Echinococcus* 棘球绦虫

echi·no·cyte (e-ki′no-sīt) burr cell 棘红细胞

echo (ek′o) a repeated sound, produced by reverberation of sound waves; also, the reflection of ultrasonic, radio, and radar waves 回声；**amphoric e.,** a resonant repetition heard on auscultation of the chest, at an interval after a vocal sound 空瓮音；**metallic e.,** a ringing repetition of heart sounds sometimes heard in patients with pneumopericardium or pneumothorax 金属音，部分气胸和心包积气的患者可及

echo·acou·sia (ek″o-ə-koo′zhə) the subjective experience of hearing echoes after normally heard sounds 正常心音后的回声感

echo·car·dio·gram (ek″o-kahr′de-o-gram″) the record—usually a video or photograph—produced by echocardiography 超声心动图

echo·car·di·og·ra·phy (ek″o-kahr″de-og′rə-fe) recording of the position and motion of the heart walls or internal structures of the heart by the echo obtained from beams of ultrasonic waves directed through the chest wall 超声心动图显像，超声心动图；**color Doppler e.,** color flow Doppler imaging 彩色多普勒超声检查；**contrast e.,** that in which the ultrasonic beam detects tiny bubbles produced by intravascular injection of a liquid or a small amount of carbon dioxide gas 心脏超声造影术；**Doppler**

e., a technique for recording the flow of red blood cells through the cardiovascular system by means of Doppler ultrasonography, either continuous wave or pulsed wave 多普勒超声心动图；**M-mode e.**, that recording the amplitude and rate of motion (M) in real time, yielding a monodimensional （"icepick"）view of the heart M 型超声心动描记术；**transesophageal e.** (TEE), the introduction of a transducer attached to a fiberoptic endoscope into the esophagus to provide two-dimensional cardiographic images or Doppler information 经食道超声心动图

echo·ge·nic·i·ty (ek″o-jen-is′ĭ-te) in ultrasonography, the extent to which a structure gives rise to reflections of ultrasonic waves 回声强度

echo·graph·ia (ek″o-graf′e-ə) agraphia in which the patient can copy writing but cannot write to express ideas 失写症

echog·ra·phy (ə-kog′rə-fe) ultrasonography 超声波检查法；超声波扫描术

echo·ki·ne·sis (ek″o-kĭ-ne′sis) echopraxia 模仿动作；模仿倾向

echo·la·lia (ek″o-la′le-ə) stereotyped repetition of another person's words and phrases 模仿言语

echo·lu·cent (ek″o-loo′sənt) permitting the passage of ultrasonic waves without echoes, the representative areas appearing black on the sonogram 无回声区

echop·a·thy (ĕ-kop′ə-the) automatic repetition by a patient of words or movements of others; echolalia or echopraxia 模仿病

echo·pho·no·car·di·og·ra·phy (ek″o-fo″nokahr″de-og′rə-fe) the combined use of echocardiography and phonocardiography 超声心音检查法

echo·prax·ia (ek″o-prak′se-ə) stereotyped imitation of the movements of others 模仿动作

echo-rang·ing (ek″o-rānj′ing) in ultrasonography, determination of the position or depth of a body structure on the basis of the time interval between the moment an ultrasonic pulse is transmitted and the moment its echo is received 回声定位

echo·thi·o·phate (ek″o-thi′o-fāt) an anticholinesterase agent used topically as the iodide salt in the treatment of glaucoma and accommodative esotropia 二乙氧膦酰硫胆碱

echo·vi·rus (ek′o-vi″rəs) any of numerous species and strains of the family Picornaviridae, some of which cause aseptic meningitis or a febrile rash; they have now been renamed and assigned to the genera *Enterovirus* and *Parechovirus* 埃柯病毒

eclamp·sia (ə-klamp′se-ə) convulsions and coma, rarely coma alone, occurring in a pregnant or puerperal woman, and associated with hypertension, edema, and/or proteinuria 子痫；**eclamp′tic** *adj.* 子痫的；**uremic e.**, that due to uremia 尿毒症性惊厥

eclamp·to·gen·ic (ə-klamp″to-jen′ik) causing convulsions 致惊厥的

ECLS extracorporeal life support 体外生命支持系统

ECMO extracorporeal membrane oxygenation 体外膜氧合；见 *support* 下 *extracorporeal life support*

econ·a·zole (ə-kon′ə-zōl) an imidazole derivative used as the nitrate salt as a broad-spectrum antifungal agent 益康唑

econ·o·my (e-kon′ə-me) the management of domestic affairs 经济；**token e.**, in behavior therapy, a program of treatment in which the patient earns tokens, exchangeable for rewards, for appropriate personal and social behavior and loses tokens for antisocial behavior（行为治疗中采用的）代币经济奖励制度

eco·tax·is (ek′o-tak″sis) the movement or "homing" of a circulating cell, e.g., a lymphocyte, to a specific anatomic compartment 生态趋向性

eco·tro·pic (e″ko-tro′pik) pertaining to a virus that infects and replicates in cells from only the original host species 单嗜性

ECT electroconvulsive therapy 电休克疗法

ec·tad (ek′təd) directed outward 向外

ec·ta·sia (ek-ta′zhə) dilatation, expansion, or distention 扩张，膨胀，延伸；**ectat′ic** *adj.*；**annuloaortic e.**, dilatation of the proximal aorta and the fibrous ring of the heart at the aortic orifice, marked by aortic regurgitation, and when severe by dissecting aneurysm; often associated with Marfan syndrome 主动脉环扩张；通常与马方综合征相关；**mammary duct e.**, benign dilatation of the collecting ducts of the mammary gland, with inspissation of gland secretion and inflammatory changes in the tissues, usually during or after menopause 乳管扩张症

ec·teth·moid (ek-teth′moid) ethmoidal labyrinth 筛骨外侧部

ec·thy·ma (ek-thi′mə) an ulcerative pyoderma caused by infection at the site of minor trauma, usually on the shins or feet 臁疮；**contagious e.**, orf; an endemic infectious vesiculopustular eruption of sheep and goats caused by a poxvirus, which can be transmitted to humans, usually as a few painless pustules on a finger, but potentially showing sytematic symptoms such as lymphadenitis and fever 传染性羊痘疮

ec·to·an·ti·gen (ek″to-an′tĭ-jən) 1. an antigen that seems to be loosely attached to the outside of bacteria 在细菌外附着松散的抗原；2. an antigen formed in the ectoplasm (cell membrane) of a bacterium 在细菌外质中形成的抗原

ec·to·blast (ek′to-blast) 1. ectoderm 外胚层；2. an external membrane 外膜；a cell wall 细胞壁

ec·to·car·dia (ek″to-kahr′de-ə) congenital displacement of the heart 异位心

ec·to·cer·vix (ek″to-sur′viks) portio vaginalis cervicis 子宫颈阴道部；**ectocer′vical** adj. 子宫颈阴道部的

ec·to·derm (ek′to-dərm) the outermost of the three primitive germ layers of the embryo; from it are derived the epidermis and epidermic tissues, such as the nails, hair, and glands of the skin, the nervous system, external sense organs, and mucous membrane of the mouth and anus 外胚层；**ectoder′mal, ectoder′mic** adj. 外胚层的

ec·to·der·mo·sis (ek″to-dər-mo′sis) a disorder based on congenital maldevelopment of organs derived from the ectoderm 外胚层形成异常

ec·to·en·zyme (ek″to-en′zīm) an extracellular enzyme（胞）外酶

ec·tog·e·nous (ek-toj′ə-nəs) exogenous 外源性的

ec·to·mere (ek′to-mēr) one of the blastomeres taking part in formation of the ectoderm 外胚层裂球

ec·to·mor·phy (ek′to-mor″fe) a type of body build in which tissues derived from the ectoderm predominate; relatively slight development of both visceral and body structures, the body being linear and delicate 外胚层体型；瘦型体质；**ectomor′phic** adj. 瘦型体质的

ec·to·my (ek′tə-me) [Gr.] resection 切除术

ec·to·par·a·site (ek″to-par′ə-sīt) a parasite that lives on the outside of the body of the host 体表寄生虫

ec·to·pia (ek-to′pe-ə) [Gr.] malposition, especially if congenital 异位，尤其是先天性的；**e. cor′dis,** congenital displacement of the heart outside the thoracic cavity 体外心；**e. len′tis,** abnormal position of the lens of the eye 晶状体异位；**e. pupil′lae conge′nita,** congenital displacement of the pupil 先天性瞳孔异位

ec·top·ic (ek-top′ik) 1. pertaining to ectopia 异位相关的；2. located away from normal position 远离正常位置；3. arising from an abnormal site or tissue 异常部位或组织引起的

ec·tos·te·al (ek-tos′te-əl) pertaining to or situated outside of a bone 骨骼以外的

ec·to·sto·sis (ek″to-sto′sis) ossification beneath the perichondrium of a cartilage or the periosteum of a bone 软骨膜下骨化

ec·to·thrix (ek′to-thriks) outside the hair; used to describe dermatophyte infections characterized by formation of a sheath of arthrospores on the outside of the hair 毛外癣菌。Cf. *endothrix*

ec·tro·dac·ty·ly (ek″tro-dak′tə-le) congenital absence of a digit or part of a digit 先天性缺指，先天性缺趾

ec·trog·e·ny (ek-troj′ə-ne) congenital absence or defect of a part 先天缺损；**ectrogen′ic** adj. 先天缺损的

ec·tro·me·lia (ek″tro-me′le-ə) gross hypoplasia or aplasia of one or more long bones of one or more limbs 缺肢畸形；**ectromel′ic** adj.

ec·tro·pi·on (ek-tro′pe-on) eversion or turning outward, as of the margin of an eyelid 外翻；睑外翻

ec·ze·ma (ek′zə-mə) a pruritic papulovesicular dermatitis characterized early by erythema, edema associated with a serous exudate in the epidermis and an inflammatory infiltrate in the dermis, oozing and vesiculation, and crusting and scaling; and later by lichenification, thickening, signs of excoriations, and altered pigmentation 湿疹；**eczem′atous** adj. 湿疹的；**asteatotic e.,** erythema, dry scaling, fine cracking, and pruritus of the skin, particularly of the limbs, in cold weather, as a result of excessive water loss from the stratum corneum 干性湿疹；**e. herpe′ticum,** Kaposi varicelliform eruption due to infection with herpes simplex virus superimposed on a pre-existing skin condition 疱疹样湿疹；**nummular e.,** that in which the patches are coin shaped; it may be a form of neurodermatitis 硬币样湿疹，**xerotic e.,** asteatotic e.

ec·zem·a·toid (ek-zem′ə-toid) resembling eczema 湿疹样

ED effective dose 有效剂量；emergency department 急诊室；erectile dysfunction 勃起功能障碍；erythema dose 红斑量

ED$_{50}$ median effective dose 半数有效量

EDAC excessive dynamic airway collapse 过度动态气道塌陷

ede·ma (ə-de′mə) an abnormal accumulation of fluid in intercellular spaces of the body 水肿；**edem′atous** adj. 水肿的；**angioneurotic e.,** angioedema 血管神经性水肿；**cardiac e.,** a manifestation of congestive heart failure, due to increased venous and capillary pressures and often associated with renal sodium retention 心源性水肿；**cytotoxic e.,** cerebral edema caused by hypoxic injury to brain tissue and decreased functioning of the cellular sodium pump so that the cellular elements accumulate fluid 细胞毒性水肿；**dependent e.,** edema in lower or dependent parts of the body 重力依赖性水肿；**e. neonato′rum,** a disease of premature and feeble infants resembling sclerema, marked by spreading edema with cold, livid skin（新生儿）硬肿症；**peripheral e.,** edema in a limb or limbs, most often the lower limbs 外周

性水肿；**pitting e.,** that in which pressure leaves a persistent depression in the tissues. 凹陷性水肿；**pulmonary e.,** diffuse edema in pulmonary tissues and air spaces due to changes in hydrostatic forces in capillaries or to increased capillary permeability, with intense dyspnea 肺水肿；**vasogenic e.,** cerebral edema in the area around tumors, often due to increased permeability of capillary endothelial cells 血管性水肿

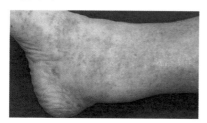

▲ 踝水肿 (edema of the ankle)

ede·ma·gen (ə-de′mə-jen) an irritant that elicits edema by causing capillary damage but not the cellular response of true inflammation 致水肿物

eden·tia (e-den′shə) absence of the teeth 缺齿

eden·tu·lous (e-den′tu-ləs) without teeth 无齿

ed·e·tate (ed′ə-tāt) USAN contraction for ethylenediaminetetraacetate, a salt of ethylenediaminetetraacetic acid (EDTA); the salts include *e. calcium disodium*, used in the diagnosis and treatment of lead poisoning, and *e. disodium*, used in the treatment of hypercalcemia because of its affinity for calcium 乙二胺四乙酸盐

edet·ic ac·id (ə-det′ik) ethylenediaminetetraacetic acid 乙二胺四乙酸

edis·y·late (ə-dis′ə-lāt) USAN contraction for 1,2-ethanedisulfonate 乙二磺酸盐

ed·ro·pho·ni·um (ed″ro-fo′ne-əm) a cholinergic used in the form of the chloride salt as a curare antagonist and as a diagnostic agent in myasthenia gravis 氯化腾喜龙

EDTA ethylenediaminetetraacetic acid 乙二胺四乙酸

EDV end-diastolic volume 舒张末期容积

Ed·ward·si·el·la (ed-wahrd″se-el′ə) a genus of gram-negative, facultatively anaerobic bacteria of the family Enterobacteriaceae; *E. tar'da* is an occasional opportunistic pathogen, causing diarrhea and sepsis 爱德华菌属

EEE eastern equine encephalomyelitis 东部马脑脊髓炎

EEG electroencephalogram 脑电图

EEJ electroejaculation 电刺激采精

EENT eye-ear-nose-throat 眼耳鼻喉

EFA essential fatty acid 必需脂肪酸

ef·a·vi·renz (ef′ah-vi″renz) an antiretroviral, inhibiting reverse transcriptase; used in the treatment of HIV infection 依法伟仑，用于 HIV 感染的治疗

ef·face·ment (ə-fās′mənt) the obliteration of features; said of the cervix during labor when it is so changed that only the external os remains 抹消；抹杀；宫颈管消失

ef·fect (ə-fekt′) the result produced by an action 效应；**Anrep e.,** abrupt elevation of aortic pressure results in a positive inotropic effect, augmented resistance to outflow in the heart 安莱普效应，主动脉压力突然升高引起正性肌力效应，增强了对心排增加的抵抗；**Bayliss e.,** increased perfusion pressure and subsequent stretch of vascular smooth muscle causes muscle contraction and increased resistance, which returns blood flow to normal in spite of the elevated perfusion pressure 贝利斯效应；**Bohr e.,** increase of carbon dioxide in blood causes decreased affinity of hemoglobin for oxygen 波尔效应；**Doppler e.,** the relationship of the apparent frequency of waves, as of sound, light, and radio waves, to the relative motion of the source of the waves and the observer, the frequency increasing as the two approach each other and decreasing as they move apart 多普勒效应；**experimenter e's,** demand characteristics 实验者效应；**founder e.,** an altered gene frequency in a particular derived population relative to the parental population, as a result of establishment of the derived population by a small number of founders carrying limited genetic diversity 奠基者效应，遗传漂变的一种形式；**Haldane e.,** increased oxygenation of hemoglobin promotes dissociation of carbon dioxide 霍尔丹效应，血红蛋白氧合作用的增加促进二氧化碳的解离；**placebo e.,** the total of all nonspecific effects, both good and adverse, of treatment; it refers primarily to psychological and psychophysiologic effects associated with the caregiver-patient relationship and the patient's expectations and apprehensions concerning the treatment 安慰剂效应；**position e.,** in genetics, the change in expression of a gene as a function of a change in its position relative to that of other genes. 位置效应；**pressure e.,** the sum of the changes that are due to obstruction of tissue drainage by pressure 压力效应；**side e.,** a consequence other than that for which an agent is used, especially an adverse effect on another organ system 副作用，不良反应；**Somogyi e.,** a rebound phenomenon occurring in diabetes: overtreatment with insulin induces hypoglycemia, which initiates the release of epinephrine, ACTH, glucagon, and growth hormone, which stimulate lipolysis, gluconeogenesis, and glycogenolysis, which, in turn, result in a rebound hyperglycemia and ketosis 索莫吉反应，低血糖后出现血糖反跳性增高的现象

ef·fec·tive·ness (ə-fek′tiv-nəs) 1. the ability to produce a specific result or to exert a specificmeasurable influence 作 用；效 应；2. the ability of an intervention to produce the desired beneficial effect in actual usage 效力；效能。Cf. *efficacy*; **effec′tive** *adj*. 有效的; **relative biological e. (RBE)**, an expression of the effectiveness of other types of radiation in comparison with that of gamma rays or x-rays 相对生物效应

ef·fec·tor (ə-fek′tər) 1. an agent that mediates a specific effect 效 应 物；2. an organ that produces an effect in response to nerve stimulation 效应器官; **allosteric e.**, an enzyme inhibitor or activator that has its effect at a site other than the catalytic site of the enzyme 变构效应体

ef·fem·i·na·tion (ə-fem″ĭ-na′shən) feminization (2) 女性化

ef·fer·ent (ef′ər-ənt) 1. conveying away from a center 输 出；2. something that so conducts, as an efferent nerve 输出管

ef·fi·ca·cy (ef′ĭ-kə-se) 1. the ability of an intervention to produce the desired beneficial effect in expert hands and under ideal circumstances 效力；效能；2. the ability of a drug to produce the desired therapeutic effect 药效

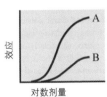

▲ 两种不同药效 **(efficacy)** 的药物的剂量效应曲线。药物 **A** 的药效强于药物 **B**

ef·fleu·rage (ef-loo-rahzh′) [Fr.] a stroking movement in massage 轻抚法

ef·flo·res·cent (ef″lo-res′ənt) 1. becoming powdery by losing the water of crystallization 风化; 2. developing into a rash 发展成皮疹

ef·flu·vi·um (ə-floo′ve-əm) pl. *efflu′via* [L.] 1. an outflowing or shedding, as of the hair 脱 发；2. an exhalation or emanation, especially one of noxious nature 呼出、散发出，尤其有害物质

ef·fu·sion (ə-fu′zhən) 1. escape of a fluid into a part; exudation or transudation 渗液；2. effused material; an exudate or transudate 渗 出 物; **pleural e.**, fluid in the pleural space 胸腔积液

ef·lor·ni·thine (DMFO) (ef-lor′nĭ-thēn″) an inhibitor of the enzyme catalyzing the decarboxylation of ornithine; used topically as the hydrochloride salt to inhibit growth of unwanted facial hair in females. It is also administered intravenously in the treatment of African trypanosomiasis 依氟乌氨酸

eges·tion (e-jes′chən) the casting out of undigestible material 排泄

egg (eg) ovum 卵

ego (e′go) that segment of the personality dominated by the reality principle, comprising integrative and executive aspects functioning to adapt the forces and pressures of the id and superego and the requirements of external reality by conscious perception, thought, and learning 自我

ego·ali·en (e″go-āl′e-ən) ego-dystonic 自我排斥的

ego·bron·choph·o·ny (e″go-brong-kof′ə-ne) egophony 羊鸣音，支气管咩音

ego·cen·tric (e″go-sen′trik) self-centered; preoccupied with one's own interests and needs; lacking concern for others 自我中心的

ego-dys·ton·ic (e″go-dis-ton′ik) denoting aspects of a person's thoughts, impulses, and behavior that are felt to be repugnant, distressing, unacceptable, or inconsistent with the self-conception 自我排斥的

ego·ism (e′go-iz-əm) 1. any of several ethical doctrines describing the relationship between morality, self-interest, and behavior 个人主义；2. excessive preoccupation with oneself, self-interest with disregard for the needs of others 利己的；3. egotism 自我中心

ego·ma·nia (e″go-ma′ne-ə) extreme self-centeredness; extreme egotism 自尊癖

egoph·o·ny (e-gof′ə-ne) increased resonance of voice sounds, with a high-pitched bleating quality, heard especially over lung tissue compressed by pleural effusion 羊鸣音，支气管咩音

ego-syn·ton·ic (e″go-sin-ton′ik) denoting aspects of a person's thoughts, impulses, attitudes, and behavior that are felt to be acceptable and consistent with the self-conception 自我协调的

ego·tism (e′go-tiz-əm) 1. conceit, selfishness, self-centeredness, with an inflated sense of one's importance 自私的，自我中心的；2. egoism (2) 利己的

EGTA egtazic acid; a chelator similar in structure and function to EDTA (ethylenediaminetetraacetic acid) but with a higher affinity for calcium than for magnesium 依他酸

Ehr·lich·ia (ār-lik′e-ə) a genus of gram-negative, nonmotile bacteria of the family Anaplasmataceae, transmitted by ticks and occurring in cytoplasmic vacuoles in mammalian host cells, often forming inclusion bodies. It includes the species *E. ca'nis*, *E. chaffeen'sis*, and *E. ewin'gii* 埃立克体属

ehr·lich·i·o·sis (ār-lik″e-o′sis) a febrile illness due to infection with bacteria of the genus *Ehrlichia* 埃立克体病；**human granulocytic e.**, a sometimes fatal human ehrlichiosis caused by an *Ehrlichia equi–* like species, characterized by flulike symptoms and involving predominantly neutrophils 人粒细胞埃立克体病；**human monocytic e.**, a sometimes fatal human ehrlichiosis caused by *Ehrlichia chaffeensis*, characterized by flulike symptoms and involving predominantly fixed tissue mononuclear phagocytes 人单核细胞埃立克体病

ei·co·nom·e·ter (i″kə-nom′ə-tər) eikonometer 影像计，眼光像测定计

ei·co·sa·pen·ta·eno·ic ac·id (EPA) (i-ko″sə-pen″tə-e-no′ik) an omega-3, polyunsaturated, 20-carbon fatty acid found almost exclusively in fish and marine animal oils 二十碳五烯酸，鱼油的主要成分

ei·det·ic (i-det′ik) denoting exact visualization of events or objects previously seen; a person having such an ability 遗觉的

ei·dop·tom·e·try (i″dop-tom′ə-tre) measurement of the acuteness of visual perception 视力测定法

ei·ko·nom·e·ter (i″kə-nom′ə-tər) an instrument for measuring the degree of aniseikonia 影像计

Ei·me·ria (i-mēr′e-ə) a genus of protozoa (order Eucoccidiida) found in the epithelial cells of humans and animals 艾美虫属

EIT erythrocyte iron turnover 红细胞铁周转率

ejac·u·late[1] (e-jak′u-lāt) to expel suddenly, especially semen 突然射精

ejac·u·late[2] (e-jak′u-lət) the semen discharged in a single ejaculation in the male, consisting of the secretions of the Cowper gland, epididymis, ductus deferens, seminal vesicles, and prostate, and containing the spermatozoa 精液

ejac·u·la·tio (e-jak″u-la′she-o) [L.] ejaculation 射精；**e. prae′cox**, premature ejaculation 早泄

ejac·u·la·tion (e-jak″u-la′shən) forcible, sudden expulsion; especially expulsion of semen from the male urethra 射精；**ejac′ulatory** *adj.* 射精的；**premature e.**, that consistently occurring either prior to, upon, or immediately after penetration and before it is desired 早泄；**retarded e.**, male orgasmic disorder 男性高潮障碍；**retrograde e.**, ejaculation in which semen travels up the urethra toward the bladder instead of to the outside of the body 逆行射精

ejec·tion (e-jek′shən) 1. the act of casting out or the state of being cast out, as of excretions, secretions, or other bodily fluids 射出，排出；2. something cast out 排出物；3. the discharge of blood from the heart 心脏射血；见 *period* 下词条

EKG electrocardiogram 心电图

EKY electrokymography 电记波照相术

elab·o·ra·tion (e-lab″ə-ra′shən) 1. the process of producing complex substances out of simpler materials 精心制作；2. in psychiatry, an unconscious mental process of expansion and embellishment of detail, especially of a symbol or representation in a dream. 意匠作用

el·a·pid (el′ə-pid) 1. any snake of the family Elapidae 眼镜蛇；2. of or pertaining to the family Elapidae 眼镜蛇科相关的

Elap·i·dae (e-lap′ĭ-de) a family of usually terrestrial, venomous snakes, which have cylindrical tails and front fangs that are short, stout, immovable, and grooved. It includes cobras, kraits, coral snakes, Australian copperheads, Australian blacksnakes, brown snakes, tiger snakes, death adders, and mambas 眼镜蛇科

elas·tance (*E*) (e-las′təns) the quality of recoiling without disruption on removal of pressure, or an expression of the measure of the ability to do so in terms of unit of volume change per unit of pressure change. It is the reciprocal of compliance 回弹性

elas·tase (e-las′tās) 弹性蛋白酶，见 *pancreatic elastase*

elas·tic (e-las′tik) able to resist and recover from stretching, compression, or distortion applied by a force 弹性的

elas·tin (e-las′tin) a scleroprotein that is the essential constituent of elastic connective tissue. It is arranged in fibers and discontinuous sheets in the extracellular matrix, particularly of the skin, lungs, and blood vessels 弹性蛋白。又称 *elasticin*

elas·to·fi·bro·ma (e-las″to-fi-bro′mə) a rare, benign, firm, unencapsulated tumor consisting of abundant sclerotic collagen and thick irregular elastic fibers 弹性纤维瘤

elas·tol·y·sis (e″las-tol′ə-sis) the digestion of elastic substance or tissue 弹性纤维松解

elas·to·ma (e″las-to′mə) a local tumorlike excess of elastic tissue fibers or abnormal collagen fibers of the skin 弹性组织瘤

elas·tom·e·try (e″las-tom′ə-tre) the measurement of elasticity 弹性测定法

elas·tor·rhex·is (e-las″to-rek′sis) rupture of fibers composing elastic tissue 弹性纤维断裂

elas·to·sis (e″las-to′sis) 1. degeneration of elastic tissue 弹性组织变性；2. degenerative changes in the dermal connective tissue with increased amounts of material having staining properties of elastin 伴随大量弹性蛋白增加的皮肤结缔组织变性；3. any disturbance of the dermal connective tissue 皮肤结

缔 组 织 病 变；**actinic e.,** photoaging of the skin with degeneration of the elastic tissue of the dermis 光化学弹性组织变性；**e. per′forans serpigino′sa, perforating e.,** an elastic tissue defect, occurring alone or in association with other disorders, including Down syndrome and Ehlers-Danlos syndrome, in which elastomas are extruded through small keratotic papules in the epidermis; the lesions are usually arranged in arcuate serpiginous clusters on the sides of the nape, face, or arms 穿孔性弹性组织病变

elas·tot·ic (e″las-tot′ik) 1. pertaining to or characterized by elastosis 弹性组织变性相关或以之为特征；2. resembling elastic tissue; having the staining properties of elastin 类弹性组织

ela·tion (e-la′shən) emotional excitement marked by acceleration of mental and bodily activity, with extreme joy and an overly optimistic attitude 情感高涨

el·bow (el′bo) 1. the bend in the upper limb between the arm and forearm 肘；2. any angular bend 弯角；**golfer′s e.,** medial epicondylitis 高 尔 夫 肘，肱骨内上髁炎；**Little Leaguer′s e.,** medial epicondylitis in a young baseball player 青少年棒球肘，肱骨内上髁炎；**miner′s e.,** enlargement of the bursa over the point of the elbow, due to resting the body weight on the elbow as in mining 矿工肘，尺骨鹰嘴滑囊炎；**pulled e.,** subluxation of the head of the radius distally under the round ligament 牵拉肘，桡骨头半脱位；**tennis e.,** lateral epicondylitis 网球肘，肱骨外上髁炎

elec·tro·acous·tic (e-lek″tro-ə-koos′tik) pertaining to the interaction or interconversion of electric and acoustic phenomena 电声的

elec·tro·acu·punc·ture (e-lek″tro-ak″upunk′chər) acupuncture in which the needles are stimulated electrically 电 针 疗 法；**e. after Voll (EAV),** a system of diagnosis and treatment based on the measurement of the electrical characteristics of acupoints, the results being used to determine a specific remedy 基于穴位电特性的治疗和诊断系统

elec·tro·an·al·ge·sia (e-lek″tro-an″əl-je′ze-ə) the reduction of pain by electrical stimulation of a peripheral nerve or the dorsal column of the spinal cord 电止痛法

elec·tro·bi·ol·o·gy (e-lek″tro-bi-ol′ə-je) the study of electric phenomena in living tissue 生物电学

elec·tro·car·dio·gram (ECG, EKG) (e-lek″tro-kahr′de-o-gram″) a graphic tracing of the variations in electrical potential caused by the excitation of the heart muscle and detected at the body surface. The normal electrocardiogram is a scalar representation that shows deflections resulting from cardiac activity

as changes in the magnitude of voltage and polarity over time and comprises the P wave, QRS complex, and T and U waves 心 电 图；另 见 *electrogram*；**scalar e.,** an electrocardiogram of one plane of the body 梯级心电图

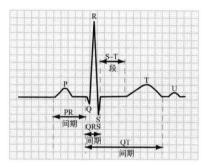

▲ 正常心电图（**electrocardiogram**）

elec·tro·car·di·og·ra·phy (e-lek″tro-kahr″deog′rə-fe) the making of graphic records of the variations in electrical potential caused by electrical activity of the heart muscle and detected at the body surface, as a method for studying the action of the heart muscle 心 电 描 记 术；另 见 *electrocardiogram* 和 *electrogram*；**electrocardiograph′ic** *adj.* 心电图的

elec·tro·cau·tery (e-lek″tro-kaw′tər-e) an apparatus for surgical dissection and hemostasis, using heat generated by a high-voltage, highfrequency alternating current passed through an electrode 电凝止血

elec·tro·chem·i·cal (e-lek″tro-kem′ĭ-kəl) pertaining to interaction or interconversion of chemical and electrical energies 电化学

elec·tro·co·ag·u·la·tion (e-lek″tro-ko-ag″ula′shən) coagulation of tissue by means of an electric current 电凝固

elec·tro·coch·le·og·ra·phy (e-lek″tro-kok″leog′rə-fe) measurement of electrical potentials of the eighth cranial nerve in response to acoustic stimuli applied by an electrode to the external acoustic canal, promontory, or tympanic membrane 耳蜗电 图 检查；**electrococh′leographic** *adj.* 耳蜗电图的

elec·tro·con·trac·til·i·ty (e-lek″tro-kon″traktil′ĭ-te) contractility in response to electrical stimulation 电刺激收缩

elec·tro·con·vul·sive (e-lek″tro-kən-vul′siv) inducing convulsions by means of electric shock 电休克痉挛

elec·tro·cor·ti·cog·ra·phy (e-lek″tro-kor″tĭkog′rə-fe) electroencephalography with the electrodes applied directly to the cerebral cortex 皮质脑电图描记法

elec·trode (e-lek′trōd) a conductor or medium by which an electric current is conducted to or from any medium, such as a cell, body, solution, or apparatus 电极; **active e.**, in electromyography, an exploring e. 活性电极; **calomel e.**, one capable of both collecting and giving up chloride ions in neutral or acidic aqueous media, consisting of mercury in contact with mercurous chloride; used as a reference electrode in pH measurements 甘汞电极; **esophageal e., esophageal pill e.**, a pill electrode that lodges in the esophagus at the level of the atrium to obtain electrograms and deliver pacing stimuli 食管电极; **exploring e.**, in electrodiagnosis, that placed nearest to the site of bioelectric activity being recorded, determining the potential in that localized area 探测电极; **ground e.**, an electrode that is connected to a ground 接地电极; **indifferent e.**, reference e.; **needle e.**, a thin, cylindrical electrode with an outer shaft beveled to a sharp point, enclosing a wire or series of wires 针状电极; **patch e.**, a tiny electrode with a blunt tip that is used in studies of membrane potentials 膜片电极; **pill e.**, an electrode usually encased in a gelatin capsule and attached to a flexible wire so that it can be swallowed 胶囊电极; **recording e.**, that used to measure electric potential change in body tissue; for recording, two electrodes must be used, the *exploring e.* and the *reference e.* 记录电极; **reference e.**, an electrode placed at a site remote from the source of recorded activity, so that its potential is assumed to be negligible or constant 参比电极; **stimulating e.**, an electrode used to apply electric current to tissue 刺激电极

elec·tro·der·mal (e-lek″tro-dur′məl) pertaining to the electrical properties of the skin, especially to changes in its resistance 皮肤电活动, 皮肤电反应

elec·tro·des·ic·ca·tion (e-lek″tro-des″ĭka′shən) destruction of tissue by dehydration, done by means of a high-frequency electric current 电干燥法

elec·tro·di·a·ly·zer (e-lek″tro-di′ə-li″zər) a blood dialyzer utilizing an applied electric field and semipermeable membranes for separating the colloids from the solution 电透析器

elec·tro·ejac·u·la·tion (EEJ) (e-lek″tro-ejak″u-la′shən) induction of ejaculation by application of a gradually increasing electrical current delivered through a probe inserted into the rectum 电刺激采精

elec·tro·en·ceph·a·lo·gram (EEG) (e-lek″troen-sef′ə-lo-gram″) a recording of the potentials on the skull generated by currents emanating spontaneously from nerve cells in the brain, with fluctuations in potential seen as waves 脑电图

elec·tro·en·ceph·a·log·ra·phy (e-lek″tro-ənsef′ə-log′rə-fe) the recording of changes in electric potential in various areas of the brain by means of electrodes placed on the scalp or on or in the brain itself 脑电图检查; **electroencephalograph′ic** *adj.* 脑电图的

elec·tro·ful·gu·ra·tion (e-lek″tro-ful″gə-ra′shən) a type of electrosurgery used to produce superficial desiccation of tissue 电灼

elec·tro·fo·cus·ing (e-lek″tro-fo′kəs-ing) isoelectric focusing 等电位聚焦

elec·tro·gas·trog·ra·phy (e-lek″tro-gastrog′rə-fe) the recording of the electrical activity of the stomach as measured between its lumen and the body surface 胃电图检查; **electrogastrograph′ic** *adj.* 胃电图的

elec·tro·gen·ic (e-lek″tro-jen′ik) pertaining to a process by which net charge is transferred to a different location so that hyperpolarization occurs 产电的, 生电的

elec·tro·gram (e-lek′tro-gram) any record produced by changes in electric potential 电描记图; **esophageal e.**, an electrogram recorded by an esophageal electrode, for enhanced detection of P waves and elucidation of complex arrhythmias 食管电描记图; **His bundle e. (HBE)**, an intracardiac electrogram of potentials in the lower right atrium, atrioventricular node, and His-Purkinje system, obtained by positioning intracardiac electrodes near the tricuspid valve 希氏束电图; **intracardiac e.**, a record of changes in the electric potentials of specific cardiac loci, as measured with electrodes placed within the heart via cardiac catheters; used for loci that cannot be assessed by body surface electrodes, such as the bundle of His or other regions within the cardiac conducting system. 心内电描记图

elec·tro·gus·tom·e·try (e-lek″tro-gəs-tom′ə-tre) the testing of the sense of taste by application of galvanic stimuli to the tongue 电味觉测定

elec·tro·he·mo·sta·sis (e-lek″tro-he-mos′tə-sis) arrest of hemorrhage by electrocautery 电止血

elec·tro·hys·ter·og·ra·phy (e-lek″tro-his″tərog′rə-fe) recording of changes in electric potential associated with uterine contractions 子宫电描记术

elec·tro·im·mu·no·dif·fu·sion (e-lek″troim″u-no-dī-fu′zhən) immunodiffusion accelerated by application of an electric current 电泳免疫扩散

elec·tro·ky·mog·ra·phy (e-lek″tro-ki-mog′rə-fe) the photography on x-ray film of the motion of the heart or of other moving structures that can be visualized radiographically 电子气流测量术

elec·trol·y·sis (e″lek-trol′ə-sis) destruction by

passage of a galvanic current, as in disintegration of a chemical compound in solution or removal of excessive hair from the body 电解；**electrolyt′ic** *adj.* 电解的
elec·tro·lyte (e-lek′tro-līt) a substance that dissociates into ions when fused or in solution, thus becoming capable of conducting electricity 电解质，电解液；**amphoteric e.**, ampholyte; a compound containing at least one group that can act as a base and at least one that can act as an acid 两性电解质
elec·tro·mag·net (e-lek″tro-mag′nət) a temporary magnet made by passing electric current through a coil of wire surrounding a core of soft iron 电磁
elec·tro·mag·net·ic (e-lek″tro-mag-net′ik) involving both electricity and magnetism 电磁的
elec·tro·me·chan·i·cal (e-lek″tro-mə-kan′ĭkəl) pertaining to interaction or interconversion of electrical and mechanical energies 电机械的
elec·tro·mo·tive (e-lek′tro-mo′tiv) causing electric activity to be propagated along a conductor 电动的
elec·tro·my·og·ra·phy (EMG) (e-lek″tro-miog′rə-fe) the recording and study of the electrical properties of skeletal muscle 肌电图检查；**electromyograph′ic** *adj.* 肌电图的
elec·tron (e-lek′tron) an elementary particle with the unit quantum of (negative) charge, constituting the negatively charged particles arranged in orbits around the nucleus of an atom and determining all of the atom's physical and chemical properties except mass and radioactivity 电子；**electron′ic** *adj.* 电子的
elec·tron-dense (e-lek′tron-dens″) in electron microscopy, having a density that prevents electrons from penetrating 电子致密的
elec·tro·neg·a·tive (e-lek″tro-neg′ə-tiv) bearing a negative electric charge 负电的
elec·tro·neg·a·tiv·i·ty (e-lek″tro-neg″ə-tiv′ ĭte) the relative power of an atom or molecule to attract electrons 负电性
elec·tro·neu·rog·ra·phy (e-lek″tro-noorog′rə-fe) the measurement of the conduction velocity and latency of peripheral nerves 神经电描记术
elec·tro·neu·ro·my·og·ra·phy (e-lek″tronoor″o-miog′rə-fe) electromyography in which the nerve of the muscle under study is stimulated by application of an electric current 神经肌电检查
elec·tro·nys·tag·mog·ra·phy (e-lek″tronis″tag-mog′rə-fe) electroencephalographic recordings of eye movements that provide objective documentation of induced and spontaneous nystagmus 眼震电图描记术
elec·tro·oc·u·lo·gram (EOG) (e-lek″tro-ok′ulogram″) the electroencephalographic tracings made while moving the eyes a constant distance between

two fixation points, inducing a deflection of fairly constant amplitude 眼电图
elec·tro·ol·fac·to·gram (EOG) (e-lek″tro-olfak′-to-gram) a recording of electrical potential changes detected by an electrode placed on the surface of the olfactory mucosa as the mucosa is subjected to an odorous stimulus 嗅电图
elec·tro·phile (e-lek′tro-fīl) an electron acceptor 亲电试剂；**electrophil′ic** *adj.* 亲电的
elec·tro·pho·re·sis (e-lek″tro-fə-re′sis) the separation of ionic solutes based on differences in their rates of migration in an applied electric field. Support media include paper, starch, agarose gel, cellulose acetate, and polyacrylamide gel, and techniques include zone, disc (discontinuous), two-dimensional, and pulsedfield 电泳；**electrophoret′ic** *adj* 电泳的；**counter e.**, counterimmunoelectrophoresis 对流电泳
elec·tro·pho·reto·gram (e-lek″tro-fə-ret′ogram) the record produced on or in a supporting medium by bands of material that have been separated by the process of electrophoresis 电泳图
elec·tro·phren·ic (e-lek″tro-fren′ik) pertaining to electrical stimulation of the phrenic nerve or respiratory diaphragm 电膈的
elec·tro·phys·i·ol·o·gy (e-lek″tro-fiz″e-ol′ə-je) 1. the study of the mechanisms of production of electrical phenomena, particularly in the nervous system, and their consequences in the living organism 电生理学；2. the study of the effects of electricity on physiologic phenomena 电生理学研究
elec·tro·pos·i·tive (e-lek″tro-poz′ĭ-tiv) bearing a positive electric charge 正电的
elec·tro·ret·in·o·graph (ERG) (e-lek″tro-ret′inograf) an instrument to measure the electrical response of the retina to light stimulation 视网膜电描记术
elec·tro·scis·sion (e-lek″tro-sizh′ən) cutting of tissue by means of electric cautery 电切术
elec·tro·scope (e-lek′tro-skōp) an instrument for measuring radiation intensity 验电器
elec·tro·shock (e-lek′tro-shok) shock produced by applying electric current to the brain 电休克
elec·tro·stat·ic (e-lek″tro-stat′ik) pertaining to static electricity 静电的
elec·tro·stri·a·to·gram (e-lek″tro-stri-āt′ogram) an electroencephalogram showing differences in electric potential recorded at various levels of the corpus striatum 纹状体电图
elec·tro·sur·gery (e-lek″tro-sur′jər-e) surgery performed by electrical methods; the active electrode may be a needle, bulb, or disk 电外科；**electrosur′gical** *adj.* 电外科的
elec·tro·tax·is (e-lek″tro-tak′sis) taxis in response

to electric stimuli 趋电性

elec·tro·ther·a·py (e-lek″tro-ther′ə-pe) treatment of disease by means of electricity 电治疗

elec·tro·ton·ic (e-lek″tro-ton′ik) 1. pertaining to electrotonus 电紧张的；2. denoting the direct spread of current in tissues by electrical conduction, without the generation of new current by action potentials 电传导的

elec·trot·o·nus (e-lek-trot′o-nəs) the altered electrical state of a nerve or muscle cell when a constant electric current is passed through it 电紧张

elec·tro·u·re·ter·og·ra·phy (e-lek″tro-u-re″tərog′rə-fe) electromyography in which the action potentials produced by peristalsis of the ureter are recorded 输尿管电描记术

elec·tro·va·lence (e-lek″tro-va′ləns) 1. the number of charges an atom acquires by the gain or loss of electrons in forming an ionic bond 形成离子键所需要获得或丢失的电子数；2. the ionic bonding resulting from such a transfer of electrons 电子转移所形成的离子键；**electrova′lent** adj. 电价的

el·e·doi·sin (el-ə-doi′sin) an endecapeptide from a species of octopus (*Eledone*), which is a precursor of a large group of biologically active peptides; it has vasodilator, hypotensive, and extravascular smooth muscle stimulant properties 章鱼唾腺精

el·e·i·din (el-e′ĭ-din) a protein related to keratin, found in the stratum lucidum of the skin 角母蛋白

El·e·ly·so (eh-leh-lī′sō) trademark for a preparation of taliglucerase alfa 药品商品名，活性成分 taliglucerase alfa

el·e·ment (el′ə-mənt) 1. any of the constituent parts of which a more complex entity is composed 组成部分；2. in chemistry, a simple substance that cannot be decomposed by chemical means and that is made up of atoms which are alike in their peripheral electronic configurations and so in their chemical properties and also in the number of protons in their nuclei, but which may differ in the number of neutrons in their nuclei and so in their mass number and in their radioactive properties. See *Chemical Elements* table 化学元素，见化学元素表；3. in the philosophies underlying some complementary medicine systems, a member of a group of basic substances that give rise to everything that exists 替代医学中的基本元素，**five e's**, 1. 五行，见 *phase* 下词条；2. in ayurvedic tradition, the basic entities (earth, air, fire, water, and space) whose interaction gives rise to material existence 阿育吠陀中的五大元素，**formed e's of the blood**, the blood cells 血细胞；**IS e.**, insertion sequence 插入序列；**trace e's**, chemical elements distributed throughout the tissues in very small amounts and that are either essential in nutrition, as cobalt, copper, etc., or harmful, as selenium 微量元素；**transposable e.**, a segment of DNA that can move from one genomic location to another, such as an insertion sequence, transposon, or certain bacteriophages. However, sometimes used interchangeably with *transposon* 转位子

el·e·men·ta·ry (el″ə-men′tə-re) not resolvable or divisible into simpler parts or components 基本的，初级的，元素的

el·e·phan·ti·a·sis (el″ə-fən-ti′ə-sis) 象皮肿。1. a chronic filarial disease, usually seen in the tropics, due to infection with *Brugia malayi* or *Wuchereria bancrofti*, marked by inflammation and obstruction of the lymphatics and hypertrophy of the skin and superficial fascia, chiefly affecting the legs and external genitals 慢性丝虫感染；2. hypertrophy and thickening of the tissues from any cause 任何原因引起的组织肥大和增生；**e. nos′tras**, swelling of a lower limb from chronic streptococcal erysipelas or chronic recurrent cellulitis 慢性链球菌性丹毒或慢性复发性蜂窝织炎引起的下肢肿胀；**e. scro′ti**, that affecting mainly the scrotum 阴囊象皮病

el·e·phan·toid (el″ə-fan′toid) relating to or resembling elephantiasis 类象皮肿或象皮肿相关的

el·e·trip·tan (el″ə-trip′tan) a selective serotonin receptor agonist, with actions similar to those of sumatriptan, used as the hydrobromide salt in the treatment of migraine; administered orally 依来曲普坦

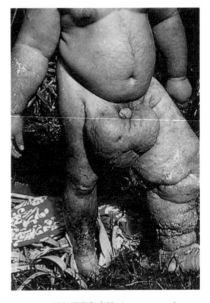

▲ 腿和阴囊象皮肿（**elephantiasis**）

化学元素 (Chemical Elements)

Name 元素名	Symbol 元素符号	At. No. 原子序数	At. Wt.* 原子量*	Name 元素名	Symbol 元素符号	At. No. 原子序数	At. Wt.* 原子量*
Actinium 锕	Ac	89	[227]	Mercury 汞	Hg	80	200.59
Aluminum 铝	Al	13	26.982	Molybdenum 钼	Mo	42	95.96
Americium 镅	Am	95	[243]	Moscovium‡ 镆‡	Mc	115	[288]
Antimony 锑	Sb	51	121.760	Neodymium 钕	Nd	60	144.242
Argon 氩	Ar	18	39.948	Neon 氖	Ne	10	20.180
Arsenic 砷	As	33	74.922	Neptunium 镎	Np	93	[237]
Astatine 砹	At	85	[210]	Nickel 镍	Ni	28	58.693
Barium 钡	Ba	56	137.327	Nihonium‡ 鿭‡	Nh	113	[286]
Berkelium 锫	Bk	97	[247]	Niobium 铌	Nb	41	92.906
Beryllium 铍	Be	4	9.012	Nitrogen 氮	N	7	14.007
Bismuth 铋	Bi	83	208.980	Nobelium 锘	No	102	[259]
Bohrium 𨨏	Bh	107	[270]	Oganesson‡ (鿫)‡	Og	118	[294]
Boron 硼	B	5	10.81	Osmium 锇	Os	76	190.23
Bromine 溴	Br	35	79.904	Oxygen 氧	O	8	15.999
Cadmium 镉	Cd	48	112.411	Palladium 钯	Pd	46	106.42
Calcium 钙	Ca	20	40.078	Phosphorus 磷	P	15	30.974

E

（续表）

Name 元素名	Symbol 元素符号	At. No. 原子序数	At. Wt.* 原子量*
Californium 锎	Cf	98	[251]
Carbon 碳	C	6	12.011
Cerium 铈	Ce	58	140.116
Cesium 铯	Cs	55	132.905
Chlorine 氯	Cl	17	35.45
Chromium 铬	Cr	24	51.996
Cobalt 钴	Co	27	58.933
Copernicium 鿔	Cn	112	[285]
Copper 铜	Cu	29	63.546
Curium 锔	Cm	96	[247]
Darmstadtium 鐽	Ds	110	[281]
Dubnium 𬭊	Db	105	[268]
Dysprosium 镝	Dy	66	162.50
Einsteinium 锿	Es	99	[252]
Erbium 铒	Er	68	167.259
Europium 铕	Eu	63	151.964
Fermium 镄	Fm	100	[257]

Name 元素名	Symbol 元素符号	At. No. 原子序数	At. Wt.* 原子量*
Platinum 铂	Pt	78	195.084
Plutonium 钚	Pu	94	[244]
Polonium 钋	Po	84	[209]
Potassium 钾	K	19	39.098
Praseodymium 镨	Pr	59	140.908
Promethium 钷	Pm	61	[145]
Protactinium 镤	Pa	91	231.036 †
Radium 镭	Ra	88	[226]
Radon 氡	Rn	86	[222]
Rhenium 铼	Re	75	186.207
Rhodium 铑	Rh	45	102.906
Roentgenium 錀	Rg	111	[280]
Rubidium 铷	Rb	37	85.468
Ruthenium 钌	Ru	44	101.07
Rutherfordium 𬬻	Rf	104	[265]
Samarium 钐	Sm	62	150.36
Scandium 钪	Sc	21	44.956

E

（续表）

E

Name 元素名	Symbol 元素符号	At. No. 原子序数	At. Wt.* 原子量*	Name 元素名	Symbol 元素符号	At. No. 原子序数	At. Wt.* 原子量*
Fluorine 氟	F	9	18.998	Seaborgium 𬭳	Sg	106	[271]
Francium 钫	Fr	87	[223]	Selenium 硒	Se	34	78.96
Gadolinium 钆	Gd	64	157.25	Silicon 硅	Si	14	28.085
Gallium 镓	Ga	31	69.723	Silver 银	Ag	47	107.868
Germanium 锗	Ge	32	72.63	Sodium 钠	Na	11	22.990
Gold 金	Au	79	196.967	Strontium 锶	Sr	38	87.62
Hafnium 铪	Hf	72	178.49	Sulfur 硫	S	16	32.06
Hassium 𬭶	Hs	108	[277]	Tantalum 钽	Ta	83	180.948
Helium 氦	He	2	4.003	Technetium 锝	Tc	43	[98]
Holmium 钬	Ho	67	164.930	Tellurium 碲	Te	52	127.60
Hydrogen 氢	H	1	1.008	Tennessine‡ 鿬‡	Ts	117	[294]
Indium 铟	In	49	114.818	Terbium 铽	Tb	65	158.925
Iodine 碘	I	53	126.904	Thallium 铊	Tl	81	204.38
Iridium 铱	Ir	77	192.217	Thorium 钍	Th	90	232.038 †
Iron 铁	Fe	26	55.845	Thulium 铥	Tm	69	168.934
Krypton 氪	Kr	36	83.798	Tin 锡	Sn	50	118.710

352

(续表)

Name 元素名	Symbol 元素符号	At. No. 原子序数	At. Wt.* 原子量*	Name 元素名	Symbol 元素符号	At. No. 原子序数	At. Wt.* 原子量*
Lanthanum 镧	La	57	138.905	Titanium 钛	Ti	22	47.867
Lawrencium 铹	Lw	103	[262]	Tungsten 钨	W	74	183.84
Lead 铅	Pb	82	207.2	Uranium 铀	U	92	238.029 †
Lithium 锂	Li	3	6.94	Vanadium 钒	V	23	50.942
Lutetium 镥	Lu	71	174.967	Xenon 氙	Xe	54	131.293
Magnesium 镁	Mg	12	24.305	Ytterbium 镱	Yb	70	173.054
Manganese 锰	Mn	25	54.938	Yttrium 钇	Y	39	88.906
Meitnerium 鿏	Mt	109	[276]	Zinc 锌	Zn	30	65.38
Mendelevium 钔	Md	101	[258]	Zirconium 锆	Zr	40	91.224

* Atomic weights are based on the 2009 values of the International Union of Pure and Applied Chemistry, rounded off to the nearest thousandth. For elements with no stable nuclides, the mass number of the longest-lived isotope of the element is shown in brackets 原子量数据来源于 2009 年国际理论与应用化学联合会。四舍五入到小数点后三位。对于没有稳定核素的元素，以寿命最长核素的同位素的原子量代替，并加方括号表示

† Although this element has no stable nuclides, it has a characteristic terrestrial composition upon which an atomic weight has been calculated. 虽然这些元素没有稳定核素，但其具有在地球上的代表性的成分，并且其原子量已经测定出来

‡ Names and symbols approved by International Union of Pure and Applied Chemistry, 28 November 2016 元素名称和符号已于 2016 年 11 月 28 日由国际理论与应用化学联合会通过

eleu·the·ro (ĕ-loo'thə-ro) Siberian ginseng 西伯利亚人参

el·e·va·tor (el'ə-va″tər) an instrument for lifting tissues or for removing bony fragments or roots of teeth 牙挺

elim·i·na·tion (e-lim″ĭ-na'shən) 1. the act of expulsion or extrusion, especially expulsion from the body 清除; 2. omission or exclusion 遗漏 或 排出

El·iq·uis (el'eh-kwis) trademark for a preparation of apixaban 艾乐妥，阿哌沙班

ELISA (e-li'sə) enzyme-linked immuno-sorbent assay; any enzyme immunoassay using an enzyme-labeled immunoreactant and an immunosorbent 酶联免疫吸附试验

elix·ir (e-lik'sər) a clear, sweetened, alcoholcontaining, usually hydroalcoholic liquid containing flavoring substances and sometimes active medicinal ingredients 酏剂

Eli·za·beth·king·ia (e-liz″ə-beth-king'e-ə) a genus of gram-negative, aerobic, non–spore-forming, nonmotile bacteria, including *E. meningosep'tica*, a major cause of nosocomial infections 一种革兰阴性菌属

el·lip·to·cyte (e-lip'to-sīt) an oval or elliptical erythrocyte 椭圆红细胞

el·lip·to·cy·to·sis (e-lip″to-si-to'sis) a hereditary disorder characterized by elliptocytes, with increased red cell destruction and anemia 椭圆红细胞增多症

elm (elm) any tree of the genus *Ulmus*; *Ulmus rubra* is the slippery elm, the source of slippery elm bark 榆木属

el·trom·bo·pag ol·amine (el-trom'bo-pag) a thrombopoietin receptor agonist that stimulates platelet production; used in the treatment of chronic idiopathic thrombocytopenic purpura insufficiently responsive to other treatments 艾曲波帕

el·u·ate (el'u-āt) the substance separated out by, or the product of, elution or elutriation 洗脱液

elu·tion (e-loo'shən) in chemistry, separation of material by washing; the process of pulverizing substances and mixing them with water in order to separate the heavier constituents, which settle out in solution, from the lighter 洗脱

elu·tri·a·tion (e-loo″tre-a'shən) purification of a substance by dissolving it in a solvent and pouring off the solution, thus separating it from the undissolved foreign material 淘析

el·ux·a·do·line (ə-lux-ə″doh'līn) a mu-opioid receptor agonist compound administered orally to treat patients with irritable bowel syndrome (IBS) and irritable bowel syndrome with diarrhea (IBS-D) 伊卢多啉

Em emmetropia 正视眼

ema·ci·a·tion (e-ma″she-a'shən) a wasted condition of the body 消瘦

emas·cu·la·tion (e-mas″ku-la'shən) bilateral orchiectomy 去雄，去势，阉割

em·balm·ing (em-bahm'ing) treatment of a dead body to retard decomposition 遗体保存技术

em·bar·rass (əm-bar'əs) to impede the function of; to obstruct 窘迫，扰乱，使受损

em·bed·ding (əm-bed'ing) fixation of tissue in a firm medium, in order to keep it intact during cutting of thin sections 埋入，植入

em·bo·lec·to·my (em″bə-lek'tə-me) surgical removal of an embolus 栓子切除术

em·bo·li (em'bə-li) *embolus* 的复数 栓子

em·bol·ic (em-bol'ik) pertaining to an embolus or to embolism 栓子的，栓塞的

em·bol·i·form (em-bol'ĭ-form) resembling an embolus 栓塞状

em·bo·lism (em'bə-liz-əm) the sudden blocking of an artery by a clot or foreign material which has been brought to its site of lodgment by the blood current 栓塞; **air e.,** that due to air bubbles entering the veins from trauma, surgical procedures, or severe decompression sickness 空气栓塞。Spelled also *aeroembolism*; **cerebral e.,** embolism of a cerebral artery 脑栓塞; **coronary e.,** embolism of a coronary artery 冠脉栓塞; **fat e.,** obstruction by a fat embolus, occurring especially after fractures of large bones 脂肪栓塞; **miliary e.,** embolism affecting many small blood vessels 粟粒状栓塞; **paradoxical e.,** blockage of a systemic artery by a thrombus originating in a systemic vein that has passed through a defect in the interatrial or interventricular septum 反常栓塞; **pulmonary e.,** obstruction of the pulmonary artery or one of its branches by an embolus 肺栓塞

em·bo·li·za·tion (em″bə-lĭ-za'shən) 1. the process or condition of becoming an embolus 栓塞形成; 2. therapeutic introduction of a substance into a vessel in order to occlude it 栓塞治疗

em·bo·lus (em'bo-ləs) pl. *em'boli* [L.] a mass of clotted blood or other material brought by the blood from one vessel and forced into a smaller one, obstructing the circulation 栓子，见 *embolism*; **fat e.,** an embolus composed of oil or fat 脂肪栓; **riding e., saddle e., straddling e.,** an embolus at the bifurcation of an artery, blocking both branches 血管分叉口栓子，鞍状栓子

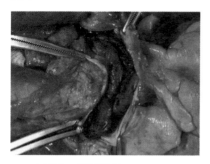

▲ 肺动脉分叉处的鞍状栓子(**saddle embolus**)

em·bo·ly (em′bə-le) invagination of the blastula to form the gastrula（胚胎）内陷

em·bra·sure (em-bra′zhər) the interproximal space occlusal to the area of contact of adjacent teeth in the same dental arch 楔状隙，外展隙

em·bry·ec·to·my (em″bre-ek′tə-me) excision of an extrauterine embryo or fetus 胚胎切除术

em·bryo (em′bre-o) 胚胎 1. in animals, those derivatives of the zygote that eventually become the offspring, during their period of most rapid growth, i.e., from the time the long axis appears until all major structures are represented 在动物中指受精卵发育至幼仔的阶段; 2. in humans, the developing organism from fertilization to the end of the eighth week 在人类中指从受精到第8周末。Cf. *fetus*; 3. in plants, the element of the seed that develops into a new individual. 在植物指从种子发育为新的个体的阶段; **em′bryonal, embryon′ic** *adj*. 胚胎的; **presomite e.,** the embryo at any stage before the appearance of the first somite 体节前期胚; **previllous e.,** the embryo before the placental chorionic villi develop 绒毛前期胚; **somite e.,** the embryo between the appearance of the first and the last somites 体节胚

em·bryo·blast (em′bre-o-blast″) inner cell mass; an aggregation of cells at the embryonic pole of the blastocyst, destined to form the embryo proper 成胚细胞

em·bryo·gen·e·sis (em″bre-o-jen′ə-sis) 1. the formation of an embryo 胚胎形成; 2. the development of a new individual by means of sexual reproduction, that is, from a zygote 从受精卵发育成新的个体; **embryoge′netic, embryogen′ic** *adj*. 胚胎形成的

em·bry·oid (em′bre-oid) resembling an embryo 胚胎状

em·bryo·le·thal·i·ty (em″bre-o-le-thal′ĭ-te) embryotoxicity that causes death of the embryo 致死胚胎毒性

em·bry·ol·o·gy (em″bre-ol′ə-je) the science of the origin and development of the individual from fertilization of an oocyte to the end of the embryonic and fetal periods 胚胎学

em·bry·o·ma (em″bre-o′mə) a neoplasm thought to be derived from embryonic cells or tissues, such as a dermoid cyst, teratoma, embryonal carcinoma or sarcoma, or a nephroblastoma 来源于胚胎组织的肿瘤

em·bry·op·a·thy (em″bre-op′ə-the) a morbid condition of the embryo or a disorder resulting from abnormal embryonic development 胚胎病; **rubella e.,** congenital rubella syndrome 先天性风疹综合征

em·bryo·plas·tic (em″bre-o-plas′tik) pertaining to or concerned in formation of an embryo 胚胎形成的

em·bry·ot·o·my (em″bre-ot′ə-me) 1. the dismemberment of a fetus in the uterus or vagina to facilitate delivery that is impossible by natural means 毁胎术; 2. the dissection of embryos and fetuses 解剖胚胎和胎儿

em·bryo·tox·ic·i·ty (em″bre-o-tok-sis′ĭ-te) developmental toxicity to an embryo 胚胎毒性

em·bryo·tox·on (em″bre-o-tok′son) a ringlike opacity at the margin of the cornea 角膜胚胎环; **anterior e.,** embryotoxon 角膜前胚胎环; **posterior e.,** Axenfeld anomaly 角膜后胚胎环

EMC emergency medical communication 紧急医疗通讯; encephalomyocarditis 脑心肌炎

eme·das·tine (em″ə-das′tēn) an antihistamine applied topically to the conjunctiva as *e. difumarate* in the treatment of allergic conjunctivitis 依美斯汀

emed·ul·late (e-med′u-lāt) to remove bone marrow 去除骨髓

emer·gen·cy (e-mur′jən-se) an unlooked for or sudden occurrence, often dangerous 突然发声

emer·gent (e-mur′jənt) 1. coming out from a cavity or other part 从腔内或其他部分出来; 2. pertaining to an emergency 紧急的

em·ery (em′ər-e) an abrasive substance consisting of corundum and various impurities, such as iron oxide 钢砂

em·e·sis (em′ə-sis) vomiting 呕吐

emet·ic (ə-met′ik) 1. causing vomiting 致呕吐的; 2. an agent that causes vomiting 致呕吐物

em·e·tine (em′ə-tēn) an alkaloid derived from ipecac or produced synthetically; its hydrochloride salt is used as an antiamebic 吐根碱，依米丁

em·e·to·ca·thar·tic (em″ə-to-kə-thahr′tik) both emetic and cathartic, or an agent that so acts 吐泻药

EMF electromotive force 电动势

em·i·gra·tion (em″ĭ-gra′shən) diapedesis 血细胞渗出; **leukocyte e.,** the escape (diapedesis) of leukocytes through the walls of small blood vessels 白细

胞渗出

em·i·nence (em′ĭ-nəns) a projection or boss 隆突，隆起；**caudal e.**, a taillike eminence in the early embryo, the remnant of the primitive node and the precursor of the hindgut, adjacent notochord and somites, and caudal part of the spinal cord 尾隆起

em·i·nen·tia (em″ĭ-nen′shə) pl. *eminen′tiae* [L.] eminence 隆突，隆起

em·is·sary (em′ĭ-sar″e) 1. affording an outlet, as an emissary vein 作为导静脉提供出口；2. emissary vein 导静脉

emis·sion (e-mish′ən) 1. discharge (1) 排放；2. an involuntary discharge of semen. 泄精；**nocturnal e.**, reflex emission of semen during sleep 梦遗；**positron e.**, a form of radioactive decay in which a positron (β⁺) and neutrino are ejected from the nucleus as a proton is transformed into a neutron. Collision of the positron with an electron causes annihilation of both particles and conversion of their masses into energy in the form of two 0.511-MeV gamma rays 正电子发射

em·men·a·gogue (ə-men′ə-gog) an agent or measure that induces menstruation 调经药；**emmenagog′ic** *adj.* 调经药的

em·me·nol·o·gy (em″ə-nol′ə-je) the sum of knowledge about menstruation and its disorders 月经学

em·me·tro·pia (E) (em″ə-tro′pe-ə) a state of proper correlation between the refractive system of the eye and the axial length of the eyeball, rays of light entering the eye parallel to the optic axis being brought to focus exactly on the retina 正视眼；**emmetrop′ic** *adj.* 正视眼的

Em·mon·sia (ĕ-mon′se-ə) a genus of Fungi Imperfecti, soil saprobes; two species, *E. cres′cens* and *E. par′va*, cause adiaspiromycosis in rodents and humans 金孢子菌属

emol·li·ent (e-mol′e-ənt) 1. softening or soothing 软化或舒缓；2. an agent that softens or soothes the skin, or soothes an irritated internal surface 软化剂；舒缓剂

emo·tion (e-mo′shən) a strong feeling state, arising subjectively and directed toward a specific object, with physiologic, somatic, and behavioral components 情绪；情感；**emo′tional** *adj.* 情感的

em·pa·thy (em′pə-the) intellectual and emotional awareness and understanding of another's thoughts, feelings, and behavior 移情，同理心，情感共鸣；**empath′ic** *adj.* 感同身受的

em·phy·se·ma (em″fə-se′mə) 1. a pathologic accumulation of air in tissues or organs 气肿；2. pulmonary e.；**emphysem′atous** *adj.* 气肿的；**atrophic e.**, senile e. 萎缩性肺气肿；**bullous e.**, single or mul-

tiple large cystic alveolar dilatations of lung tissue 大疱性肺气肿；**centriacinar e.**, **centrilobular e.**, focal dilatations of respiratory bronchioles rather than alveoli, throughout the lung among normal lung tissue 腺泡中央型肺气肿；**congenital lobar e.**, overinflation of a lung, usually in early life in one of the upper lobes, with respiratory distress 先天性肺叶性肺气肿；**hypoplastic e.**, pulmonary emphysema due to a developmental anomaly, with fewer and abnormally large alveoli 发育不全性肺气肿；**infantile lobar e.**, congenital lobar e. **interlobular e.**, air in the septa between lung lobules 叶间肺气肿；**interstitial e.**, air in the peribronchial and interstitial tissues of the lungs 间质性肺气肿；**intestinal e.**, pneumatosis cystoides intestinalis 肠道气肿；**lobar e.**, pulmonary emphysema involving less than all the lobes of the affected lung, such as unilateral emphysema 肺叶性气肿；**mediastinal e.**, pneumomediastinum 纵隔气肿；**obstructive e.**, that associated with partial bronchial obstruction that interferes with exhalation 阻塞性肺气肿；**panacinar e.**, **panlobular e.**, a type characterized by enlargement of air spaces throughout the acini 全腺泡型肺气肿；**pulmonary e.**, abnormal increase in size of lung air spaces distal to the terminal bronchioles 肺气肿；**pulmonary interstitial e. (PIE)**, a condition seen mostly in premature infants, in which air leaks from lung alveoli into interstitial spaces, often because of underlying lung disease or use of mechanical ventilation 间质性肺气肿；**senile e.**, overdistention and stretching of lung tissues due to atrophic changes 老年性肺气肿；**subcutaneous e.**, air or gas in subcutaneous tissues, usually caused by intrathoracic injury 皮下气肿；**surgical e.**, subcutaneous emphysema following surgery 外科后皮下气肿；**unilateral e.**, pulmonary emphysema affecting only one lung; it may be either congenital or acquired 单侧肺气肿；**vesicular e.**, panacinar e.

em·pir·i·cism (em-pir′ĭ-siz-əm) skill or knowledge based entirely on experience 经验主义；**empir′ic, empir′ical** *adj.* 经验主义的

em·pros·thot·o·nos (em″pros-thot′ə-nəs) tetanic forward flexure of the body 前弓反张

em·py·e·ma (em″pi-e′mə) 1. abscess 脓肿；2. a pleural effusion containing pus 脓胸；**empye′mic** *adj.* 脓胸的

EMS Emergency Medical Services 紧急医疗服务

EMT emergency medical technician 紧急医疗技师

em·tri·ci·ta·bine (em″tri-si′tə-bēn) a reverse transcriptase inhibitor used in the treatment of human immunodeficiency virus-1 infection 恩曲他滨

emul·gent (e-mul′jənt) causing a straining or purifying process 利泻药

emul·si·fi·er (e-mul′sĭ-fi″ər) an agent used to produce an emulsion 乳化剂

emul·sion (e-mul′shən) a mixture of two immiscible liquids, one being dispersed throughout the other in small droplets; a colloid system in which both the dispersed phase and the dispersion medium are liquids 乳剂

emul·soid (e-mul′soid) 1. lyophilic colloid 亲液胶体; 2. rarely, emulsion 乳液

ENA Emergency Nurses Association 急诊护士协会

enal·a·pril (ə-nal′ə-pril) an angiotensin-converting enzyme inhibitor used as the maleate salt in the treatment of hypertension, congestive heart failure, and asymptomatic left ventricular dysfunction 依那普利

enal·a·pril·at (ə-nal′ə-pril-at″) an angiotensinconverting enzyme inhibitor, the active metabolite of enalapril, used to treat hypertensive crisis and as an intravenous substitute for oral enalapril maleate 依那普利拉

enam·el (ə-nam′əl) 1. the glazed surface of baked porcelain, metal, or pottery 搪瓷, 金属或陶器的釉面; 2. any hard, smooth, glossy coating 釉质, 任何坚硬、光滑、有光泽的涂层; 3. dental enamel; the hard, thin, translucent substance covering and protecting the dentin of a tooth crown and composed almost entirely of calcium salts 牙釉质; **mottled e.**, dental fluorosis: hypoplasia of the dental enamel caused by drinking water with a high fluoride content during the time of tooth formation; characterized by defective calcification that gives a white chalky appearance to the enamel, gradually changing to a brown discoloration 氟斑牙

enam·el·o·ma (ə-nam″əl-o-mə) a small spherical nodule of enamel attached to a tooth at the cervical line or on the root 釉质瘤

enam·e·lum (ə-nam′əl-əm) [L.] enamel 釉质

en·an·thate (ə-nan′thāt) USAN contraction for *heptanoate*, the anionic form of the 7-carbon saturated fatty acid enanthic acid, which is producible by oxidation of fats 庚酸盐

en·an·the·ma (en″ən-the′mə) pl. *enanthe′mas, enanthe′mata*. An eruption on a mucous surface 黏膜疹

en·an·tio·bio·sis (en-an″te-o-bi-o′sis) commensalism in which the associated organisms are mutually antagonistic 对抗性共生

en·an·tio·mer (en-an′te-o″mər) one of a pair of compounds having a mirror image relationship 对映异构体

en·an·ti·om·er·ism (en-an″te-om′ər-iz-əm) the relationship between two stereoisomers having molecules that are mirror images of each other; they have identical chemical and physical properties in an achiral environment but form different products when reacted with other chiral molecules and exhibit optical activity. The enantiomer that rotates the plane of polarization of a beam of polarized light in the clockwise direction is indicated by the prefix (+)-, formerly *d*- or dextro-; that rotating the plane of polarization in the counterclockwise direction is indicated by the prefix (−)-, formerly *l*- or levo- 对映异构

en·an·tio·morph (en-an′te-o-morf″) 1. enantiomer 对映异构体; 2. either of two crystals exhibiting enantiomerism 对映异构体中的任何一个

en·ar·thro·sis (en″ahr-thro′sis) ball-andsocket joint. 球窝关节; **enarthro′dial** *adj.*

en·cai·nide (en-ka′nīd) a sodium channel blocker that acts on the Purkinje fibers and myocardium; used as the hydrochloride salt in treatment of life-threatening arrhythmias 恩卡胺

en·ceph·a·lat·ro·phy (en-sef″ə-lat′ro-fe) atrophy of the brain 脑萎缩

en·ce·phal·ic (en″sə-fal′ik) 1. pertaining to the encephalon 脑的; 2. within the skull 头颅内的

en·ceph·a·li·tis (en-sef″ə-li′tis) pl. *encephali′tides*. Inflammation of the brain 脑 炎; **acute disseminated e.,** 急性播散性脑炎, 见 *encephalomyelitis* 下词条; **California e.,** a usually mild form of mosquitoborne encephalitis, caused by a bunyavirus and primarily affecting children 加利福尼亚脑炎; **equine e.,** 马脑炎, 见 *encephalomyelitis* 下词条; **granulomatous amebic e.,** a rare, chronic, usually fatal opportunistic infection caused by species of *Acanthamoeba* or certain other amebae in debilitated, immunocompromised, diabetic, or alcoholic patients 肉芽肿性阿米巴脑炎; **hemorrhagic e.,** that in which there is inflammation of the brain with hemorrhagic foci and perivascular exudate 出血性脑炎; **herpes simplex e.,** that caused by herpesvirus, characterized by hemorrhagic necrosis of parts of the temporal and frontal lobes 单纯疱疹性脑炎; **HIV e.,** 人类免疫缺陷病毒性脑炎, 见 *encephalopathy* 下词条; **Japanese B e.,** a form of epidemic encephalitis of varying severity, caused by a flavivirus and transmitted by the bites of infected mosquitoes in eastern and southern Asia and nearby islands 日本乙型脑炎, 流行性乙型脑炎; **La Crosse e.,** that caused by the La Crosse virus, transmitted by *Aedes triseriatus* and occurring primarily in children 拉克罗斯病毒性脑炎; **lead e.,** 铅毒性脑炎, 见 *encephalopathy* 下词条; **postinfectious**

e., **postvaccinal e.**, acute disseminated encephalomyelitis 感染后脑炎，接种后脑炎；**St. Louis e.**, a viral disease resembling western equine encephalomyelitis, usually transmitted by mosquitoes 圣路易斯脑炎；**tick-borne e.**, any of several types of epidemic encephalitis usually spread by the bites of ticks infected with flaviviruses, sometimes accompanied by degenerative changes in other organs 蜱媒脑炎；**West Nile e.**, a usually mild, febrile form caused by the flavivirus West Nile virus, transmitted by *Culex* mosquitoes and first observed in Uganda; symptoms may include drowsiness, severe frontal headache, maculopapular rash, abdominal pain, loss of appetite, nausea, and generalized lymphadenopathy 西尼罗脑炎

en·ceph·a·lit·o·gen·ic (en-sef″ə-lit-o-jen′ik) causing encephalitis 致脑炎的

En·ce·phal·i·to·zo·on (en″sə-fal″ĭ-to-zo′on) a genus of parasitic protozoa, causing infection mainly in immunocompromised patients; *E. cuni'culi* affects predominantly the brain and kidney, *E. hel'lem* affects the eye, and *E. intestina'lis* affects the intestines 脑炎微孢子虫属

en·ceph·al·i·to·zoo·no·sis (en″sə-fal″ĭ-tozo″ono′sis) infection with protozoa of the genus *Encephalitozoon* 脑胞内原虫病

en·ceph·a·lo·cele (en-sef′ə-lo-sēl″) hernia of part of the brain and meninges through a congenital, traumatic, or postsurgical cranial defect 脑膨出，脑突出

en·ceph·a·lo·cys·to·cele (en-sef″ə-lo-sis′tosēl) hydroencephalocele 积水性脑膨出

en·ceph·a·log·ra·phy (en-sef″ə-log′rə-fe) radiography demonstrating the intracranial fluid-containing spaces after the withdrawal of cerebrospinal fluid and introduction of air or other gas; it includes pneumoencephalography and ventriculography 脑照相术

en·ceph·a·loid (en-sef′ə-loid) resembling the brain or brain substance 脑样的

en·ceph·a·lo·lith (en-sef′ə-lo-lith″) a brain calculus 脑石

en·ceph·a·lo·ma·la·cia (en-sef″ə-lo-mə-la′shə) softening of the brain 脑软化

en·ceph·a·lo·men·in·gi·tis (en-sef″ə-lomen″inji′tis) meningoencephalitis 脑膜脑膨出

en·ceph·a·lo·me·nin·go·cele (en-sef″ə-loməning′go-sēl) encephalocele 脑膨出

en·ceph·a·lo·mere (en-sef′ə-lo-mēr) one of the segments making up the embryonic brain 脑节

en·ceph·a·lom·e·ter (en-sef″ə-lom′ə-tər) an instrument used in locating certain of the brain regions 脑域测定器

en·ceph·a·lo·my·eli·tis (en-sef″ə-lo-mi″ə-li′tis)

inflammation of the brain and spinal cord 脑脊髓炎；**acute disseminated e.**, inflammation of the brain and spinal cord after infection (especially measles) or, formerly, rabies vaccination 急性播散性脑脊髓炎；**acute necrotizing hemorrhagic e.**, a rare, fatal postinfection or allergic demyelinating disease of the central nervous system, having a fulminating course; characterized by liquefactive destruction of the white matter and widespread necrosis of blood vessel walls 急性坏死出血性脑脊髓炎；**benign myalgic e.**, chronic fatigue syndrome 良性肌痛性脑脊髓炎；**eastern equine e. (EEE)**, a viral disease of horses and mules that can be spread to humans, seen in eastern North America and farther south; it usually affects children and the elderly and manifests as fever, headache, and nausea followed by drowsiness, convulsions, and coma 东方马脑炎；**equine e.**, 见 *eastern equine e.*, *western equine e.* 和 *Venezuelan equine e.*；**postinfectious e.**, postvaccinal e., acute disseminated e. **Venezuelan equine e. (VEE)**, a viral disease of horses and mules, communicable to humans, seen from Venezuela north to the southwestern United States; human infection resembles influenza, with little or no indication of nervous system involvement 委内瑞拉马脑炎；**western equine e. (WEE)**, a viral disease of horses and mules, communicable to humans, especially children, seen in western North America and farther south; symptoms include fever, drowsiness, and convulsions 西方马脑炎

en·ceph·a·lo·my·elo·neu·rop·a·thy (en-sef″ə-lo-mi″ə-lo-noo-rop′ə-the) a disease involving the brain, spinal cord, and peripheral nerves 脑脊髓神经病

en·ceph·a·lo·my·elo·ra·dic·u·li·tis (ensef″ə-lo-mi″ə-lo-rə-dik″u-li′tis) inflammation of the brain, spinal cord, and spinal nerve roots 脑脊髓脊神经根炎

en·ceph·a·lo·my·elo·ra·dic·u·lop·a·thy (en-sef″ə-lo-mi″ə-lo-rə-dik″u-lop′ə-the) a disease involving the brain, spinal cord, and spinal nerve roots 脑脊髓脊神经根病变

en·ceph·a·lo·myo·car·di·tis (en-sef″ə-lomi″o-kahr-di′tis) a viral disease marked by degenerative and inflammatory changes in skeletal and cardiac muscle and by central lesions resembling those of poliomyelitis 脑心肌炎

en·ceph·a·lon (en-sef′ə-lon) the brain 脑

en·ceph·a·lop·a·thy (en-sef′ə-lop′ə-the) any degenerative brain disease 脑病；**AIDS e.**, HIV e.；**anoxic e.**, hypoxic e.；**biliary e.**, bilirubin e., kernicterus 胆红素脑病；**bovine spongiform e.**, a transmissible spongiform encephalopathy of adult cattle, transmitted by feed containing protein in the form of meat and bone meal derived from infected animals. The etiologic agent is also the cause of new variant Creutzfeldt-Jakob disease 牛海绵状脑病; **boxer's e., boxer's traumatic e.,** slowing of mental function, confusion, and scattered memory loss due to continual head blows absorbed in the boxing ring 拳击手脑病综合征; **chronic traumatic e.,** a syndrome caused by repeated blows to the head; symptoms include a slowing of mental processes, confusion, and memory loss 慢性创伤性脑病。另见 *postconcussional syndrome*; **hepatic e.,** a condition, usually occurring secondarily to advanced liver disease, marked by disturbances of consciousness that may progress to deep coma (hepatic coma), psychiatric changes of varying degree, flapping tremor, and fetor hepaticus 肝性脑病; **HIV e., HIV-related e.,** AIDS encephalopathy; a progressive primary encephalopathy caused by human immunodeficiency virus type 1 infection, manifested by a variety of cognitive, motor, and behavioral abnormalities 人类免疫缺陷病毒性脑病; **hypoxic e.,** encephalopathy caused by hypoxia from decreased rate of blood flow or decreased oxygen in the blood; severe cases can cause permanent brain damage within 5 minutes 缺氧性脑病; **hypoxic-ischemic e.,** that resulting from fetal or perinatal asphyxia, characterized by feeding difficulties, lethargy, and convulsions 缺血缺氧性脑病; **lead e.,** edema and central demyelination caused by excessive ingestion of lead compounds, particularly in young children 铅中毒性脑病; **myoclonic e. of childhood,** a neurologic disorder of unknown etiology with onset between ages 1 and 3, characterized by myoclonus of trunk and limbs and by opsoclonus with ataxia of gait, and intention tremor; some cases have been associated with occult neuroblastoma 儿童肌阵挛脑病; **pancreatic e.,** metabolic encephalopathy occurring as a complication of pancreatitis 胰性脑病; **sepsis-associated e.,** altered brain function caused by infectious agents in the blood, along with effects of accompanying fever; mild to severe symptoms may include confusion, myopathy with rigidity, and possibly seizures and coma 脓毒症相关脑病; **subacute spongiform e., transmissible spongiform e.,** prion disease 传染性海绵状脑病; **Wernicke e.,** an inflammatory hemorrhagic form due to thiamine deficiency, usually associated with chronic alcoholism, with paralysis of the eye muscles, diplopia, nystagmus, ataxia, and usually accompanying or followed by Korsakoff syndrome 韦尼克脑病

en·ceph·a·lo·py·o·sis (en-sef″ə-lo-pi-o′sis) suppuration or abscess of the brain 脑脓肿

en·ceph·a·lor·rha·gia (en-sef″ə-lo-ra′jə) hemorrhage within or from the brain 脑出血

en·ceph·a·lo·sis (en-sef″ə-lo′sis) encephalopathy 器质性脑病

en·ceph·a·lot·o·my (en-sef″ə-lot′ə-me) incision of the brain 脑切开术

en·chon·dro·ma (en″kon-dro′mə) pl. *enchondromas, enchondro′mata.* A benign growth of cartilage arising in the metaphysis of a bone 内生软骨瘤; **enchondro′matous** *adj.*

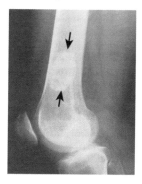

▲ 膝内生软骨瘤 (enchondroma)（侧面观）

en·chon·dro·ma·to·sis (en-kon″dro-mə-to′sis) hamartomatous proliferation of cartilage cells within the metaphysis of several bones, causing thinning of the overlying cortex and distortion of the growth in length; it may undergo malignant transformation 内生软骨瘤病

en·clave (en′klāv) (ahn-klahv′) tissue detached from its normal connection and enclosed within another organ 包体，与其正常连接脱离并被封闭在另一个器官中的组织

en·co·pre·sis (en-ko-pre′sis) fecal incontinence 大便失禁

en·cyo·py·eli·tis (en-si″o-pi″ə-li′tis) dilatation and edema of the ureters and renal pelvis during normal pregnancy, but seldom with all the classic signs of inflammation 妊娠肾盂炎

en·cyst·ed (en-sist′əd) enclosed in a sac, bladder, or cyst 被囊的

end·an·gi·itis (end-an″je-i′tis) intimitis; inflammation of the tunica intima of a vessel 血管内膜炎

end·aor·ti·tis (end″a-or-ti′tis) inflammation of the tunica intima of the aorta 主动脉内膜炎

end·ar·ter·ec·to·my (end-ahr″tər-ek′tə-me) excision of thickened atheromatous areas of the innermost coat of an artery 动脉内膜切除术

end·ar·ter·i·tis (end-ahr″tə-ri′tis) inflammation of the tunica intima of an artery 动脉内膜炎

end·au·ral (end-aw′rəl) within the ear 耳内的

end·brain (end′brān) cerebrum 端脑

en·dem·ic (en-dem′ik) present or usually prevalent in a population at all times 地区性

en·de·mo·ep·i·dem·ic (en″də-mo-ep″ĭ-dem′ik) endemic, but occasionally becoming epidemic 地方性流行的

end·er·gon·ic (end″ər-gon′ik) characterized or accompanied by the absorption of energy; requiring the input of free energy 吸能的

end-foot (end′foot) bouton terminal 终纽

en·do·an·eu·rys·mor·rha·phy (en″do-an″urizmor′ə-fe) opening of an aneurysmal sac and suture of the orifices 动脉瘤内缝术

en·do·ap·pen·di·ci·tis (en″do-ə-pen″dĭ-si′tis) inflammation of the mucous membrane of the vermiform appendix 阑尾黏膜炎

en·do·blast (en′do-blast) endoderm 内胚层

en·do·bron·chi·al (en″do-brong′ke-əl) within a bronchus or bronchi 支气管内的

en·do·bron·chi·tis (en″do-brong-ki′tis) inflammation of the epithelial lining of the bronchi 支气管黏膜炎

en·do·car·di·al (en″do-kahr′de-əl) 1. situated or occurring within the heart 心内的; 2. pertaining to the endocardium 心内膜的

en·do·car·di·tis (en″do-kahr-di′tis) exudative and proliferative inflammatory alterations of the endocardium, usually characterized by the presence of vegetations on the surface of the endocardium or in the endocardium itself, and most commonly involving a heart valve, but also affecting the inner lining of the cardiac chambers or the endocardium elsewhere 心内膜炎; **endocardit′ic** *adj.*; **atypical verrucous e.**, Libman-Sacks e. 非典型疣状心内膜炎; **bacterial e.**, infective endocarditis caused by bacteria, such as streptococci, staphylococci, enterococci, gonococci, or gram-negative bacilli 细菌性心内膜炎; **infectious e., infective e.**, that due to infection with microorganisms, especially bacteria and fungi; currently classified on the basis of etiology or underlying anatomy 感染性心内膜炎; **Libman-Sacks e.**, nonbacterial endocarditis found in association with systemic lupus erythematosus, usually occurring on the atrioventricular valves Libman-Sacks 心内膜炎; **Löffler e.**, Löffler fibroplastic parietal e., endocarditis associated with eosinophilia, marked by fibroplastic thickening of the endocardium, resulting in congestive heart failure, persistent tachycardia, hepatomegaly, splenomegaly, serous effusions into the pleural cavity, and edema of the limbs Löffler 嗜酸细胞增多性心内膜炎; **mycotic e.**, infective endocarditis, usually subacute, due to a fungal infection, most commonly by *Candida*, *Aspergillus*, or *Histoplasma* 霉菌性心内膜炎;

non-bacterial thrombotic e. (NBTE), that usually occurring in chronic debilitating disease, characterized by noninfected vegetations consisting of fibrin and other blood elements and susceptible to embolization 非细菌性血栓性心内膜炎; **prosthetic valve e.**, infective endocarditis as a complication of implantation of a prosthetic heart valve; the vegetations are usually along the line of suture 人工瓣膜心内膜炎; **rheumatic e.**, that associated with rheumatic fever; more accurately termed *rheumatic valvulitis* when an entire valve is involved 风湿性心内膜炎; **rickettsial e.**, endocarditis caused by invasion of the heart valves with *Coxiella burnetii*; is a sequela of Q fever, usually occurring in persons who have had rheumatic fever 立克次体心内膜炎; **vegetative e., verrucous e.**, endocarditis whose characteristic lesions are vegetations or verrucae on the endocardium; it may be either infective or some other type 疣状心内膜炎

en·do·car·di·um (en″do-kahr′de-əm) the endothelial lining membrane of the cavities of the heart and the connective tissue bed on which it lies 心内膜

en·do·cer·vi·ci·tis (en″do-sur″vĭ-si′tis) inflammation of the mucous membrane of the uterine cervix 宫颈内膜炎

en·do·cer·vix (en″do-sur′viks) 1. the mucous membrane lining the canal of the cervix uteri 宫颈内膜; 2. the region of the opening of the cervix into the uterine cavity 子宫颈; **endocer′vical** *adj.*

en·do·chon·dral (en″do-kon′drəl) situated, formed, or occurring within cartilage 软骨内的

en·do·co·li·tis (en″do-ko-li′tis) inflammation of the mucous membrane of the colon 结肠黏膜炎

en·do·cra·ni·um (en″do-kra′ne-əm) the endosteal layer of the dura mater of the brain 硬脑膜

en·do·crine (en′do-krin) (en′do-krīn) 1. secreting internally 内部分泌的; 2. pertaining to internal secretions; hormonal 内分泌. 另见 *system* 下词条

en·do·cri·nol·o·gist (en″do-krī-nol′ə-jist) a specialist in endocrinology 内分泌学家

en·do·cri·nol·o·gy (en″do-krī-nol′ə-je) 1. the study of hormones and the endocrine system 激素和内分泌系统; 2. a medical specialty concerned with the diagnosis and treatment of disorders of the endocrine system 内分泌学

en·do·cri·nop·a·thy (en″do-krī-nop′ə-the) any disease due to disorder of the endocrine system 内分泌病; **endocrinopath′ic** *adj.*

en·do·cy·to·sis (en″do-si-to′sis) the uptake by a cell of material from the environment by invagination of its plasma membrane; it includes both phagocytosis and pinocytosis 内吞

en·do·derm (en′do-dərm) the innermost of

the three primitive germ layers of the embryo; from it are derived the epithelium of the pharynx, respiratory tract (except the nose), digestive tract, bladder, and urethra 内胚层；**endoder′mal, endoder′mic** *adj.*

en·do·don·tics (en″do-don′tiks) the branch of dentistry concerned with the etiology, prevention, diagnosis, and treatment of conditions that affect the tooth pulp, root, and periapical tissues 牙髓病学

en·do·don·ti·um (en″do-don′she-əm) dental pulp 牙髓

en·do·don·tol·o·gy (en″do-don-tol′ə-je) endodontics 牙髓病学

en·do·en·ter·itis (en″do-en′tə-ri′tis) inflammation of the intestinal mucosa 肠黏膜炎

en·dog·a·my (en-dog′ə-me) fertilization by union of separate cells having the same genetic ancestry 近亲繁殖，同系交配；**endog′amous** *adj.*

en·dog·e·nous (en-doj′ə-nəs) produced within or caused by factors within the organism 内源，内生的

en·do·la·ryn·ge·al (en″do-lə-rin′je-əl) situated or occurring within the larynx 喉内的

en·do·lymph (en′do-limf) the fluid within the membranous labyrinth 内淋巴；**endolymphat′ic** *adj.*

en·dol·y·sin (en-dol′ĭ-sin) a bactericidal substance in cells, acting directly on bacteria 细胞内溶菌素

en·do·me·tri·al (en″do-me′tre-əl) pertaining to the endometrium 子宫内膜的

en·do·me·tri·oid (en″do-me′tre-oid) resembling endometrium 子宫内膜样的

en·do·me·tri·o·ma (en″do-me″tre-o′mə) a solitary non-neoplastic mass containing endometrial tissue 子宫内膜瘤

en·do·me·tri·o·sis (en″do-me″tre-o′sis) the aberrant occurrence of tissue containing typical endometrial granular and stromal elements, in various locations in the pelvic cavity or other areas of the body 子宫内膜异位症；**endometriot′ic** *adj.*；**e. exter′na**, endometriosis 子宫内膜异位症；**e. inter′na**, adenomyosis 子宫腺肌病；**ovarian e.**, that involving the ovary, in the form of either small superficial islands or epithelial ("chocolate") cysts of various sizes 卵巢子宫内膜异位症

en·do·me·tri·tis (en″do-me-tri′tis) inflammation of the endometrium 子宫内膜炎；**postpartum e., puerperal e.**, that following childbirth, often a precursor of puerperal fever 产后子宫内膜炎；**syncytial e.**, a benign tumor-like lesion with infiltration of the uterine wall by large syncytial trophoblastic cells 合体细胞性子宫内膜炎；**tuberculous e.**, inflammation of the endometrium, usually also involving the uterine tubes, due to infection by *Mycobacterium tuberculosis*, with the presence of tubercles 结核性

子宫内膜炎

en·do·me·tri·um (en″do-me′tre-əm) pl. *endome′tria*. The mucous membrane lining the uterus 子宫内膜

en·do·mi·to·sis (en″do-mi-to′sis) reproduction of nuclear elements within an intact nuclear envelope, not followed by chromosome movements and cytoplasmic division 核内有丝分裂，核内再复制；**endomitot′ic** *adj.*

en·do·morph (en′do-morf) an individual having the type of body build in which endodermal tissues predominate: soft roundness throughout, large digestive viscera, fat accumulations, large trunk and thighs, and tapering limbs 内胚层体型

en·do·myo·car·di·al (en″do-mi′o-kahr′de-əl) pertaining to the endocardium and the myocardium 心内膜心肌的

en·do·myo·car·di·tis (en″do-mi′o-kahr-di′tis) inflammation of the endocardium and myocardium 心肌心内膜炎

en·do·mys·i·um (en″do-mis′e-əm) the sheath of delicate reticular fibrils surrounding each muscle fiber 肌内膜

en·do·neu·ri·tis (en″do-noo-ri′tis) inflammation of the endoneurium 神经内膜炎

en·do·neu·ri·um (en″do-noor′e-um) the innermost layer of connective tissue in a peripheral nerve, forming an interstitial layer around each individual fiber outside the neurilemma 神经内膜；**endoneu′rial** *adj.*

en·do·nu·cle·ase (en″do-noo′kle-ās) any nuclease specifically catalyzing the hydrolysis of interior bonds of ribonucleotide or deoxyribonucleotide chains 内切核酸酶；**restriction e.**, an endonuclease that hydrolyzes DNA, cleaving it at an individual site of a specific base pattern 限制性内切核酸酶

en·do·pel·vic (en″do-pel′vik) intrapelvic 骨盆内的

en·do·pep·ti·dase (en″do-pep′tĭ-dās) protease; any peptidase that catalyzes the cleavage of internal bonds in a polypeptide or protein 内肽酶

en·do·peri·car·di·tis (en″do-per″ĭ-kahr-di′tis) inflammation of the endocardium and pericardium 心内膜心包炎

en·do·peri·to·ni·tis (en″do-per″ĭ-to-ni′tis) inflammation of the serous lining of the peritoneal cavity 腹膜内层炎

en·doph·thal·mi·tis (en″dof-thəl-mi′tis) inflammation of the ocular cavities and their adjacent structures 眼内炎

en·do·phyte (en′do-fīt) a parasitic plant organism living within its host's body 植物内生菌

en·do·phyt·ic (en″do-fit′ik) 1. pertaining to an endophyte 内生菌的；2. growing inward; proliferating on the interior of an organ or structure 内生的

en·do·plasm (en′do-plaz″əm) the central portion of the cytoplasm of a cell 内质; **endoplas′mic** *adj.*

en·do·poly·ploi·dy (en″do-pol″e-ploi′de) the occurrence in a diploid individual of cells containing 4, 8, 16, 32, etc., times the haploid number of chromosomes as the result of endomitosis 核内多倍性; **endopolyploid** *adj.*

en·do·pros·the·sis (en″do-pros-the′sis) 1. a prosthesis entirely inside the body 内假体; 2. a hollow stent, such as that placed in a bile duct for biliary drainage across an obstruction 内镜置管

en·do·py·elot·o·my (en″do-pi″ə-lot′ə-me) incision to correct a stenosed ureteropelvic junction, cutting from within using an instrument inserted through an endoscope 肾盂内切开术

en·do·re·du·pli·ca·tion (en″do-re-doo″plĭka′shən) replication of chromosomes without subsequent cell division 核内复制

end-or·gan (end-or′gən) one of the large encapsulated endings of sensory nerves 终末器

en·dor·phin (en-dor′fin) (en′dor-fin) any of three neuropeptides, α-, β-, and γ-*endorphins*; they are amino acid residues of β-lipotropin that bind to opiate receptors in various areas of the brain and have potent analgesic effect 内啡肽

en·do·sal·pin·gi·tis (en″do-sal″pin-ji′tis) inflammation of the endosalpinx 输卵管内膜炎

en·do·sal·pin·go·ma (en″do-sal″pin-go′mə) adenomyoma of the uterine tube 输卵管内膜瘤

en·do·sal·pinx (en″do-sal′pinks) the mucous membrane lining the uterine tube. 输卵管黏膜

en·do·scope (en′do-skōp) an instrument for examining the interior of a hollow viscus 内镜

en·dos·co·py (en-dos′kə-pe) visual examination by means of an endoscope 内镜检查术; **endoscop′ic** *adj.* peroral e., examination of organs accessible to observation through an endoscope passed through the mouth 经口内镜检查

en·do·skel·e·ton (en″do-skel′ə-ton) the cartilaginous and bony skeleton of the body, exclusive of that part of the skeleton of dermal origin 内骨骼

en·dos·mo·sis (en″dos-mo′sis) inward osmosis; inward passage of liquid through a membrane of a cell or cavity 内渗; **endosmot′ic** *adj.*

en·do·some (en′do-sōm) 1. in endocytosis, a vesicle that has lost its coat of clathrin 内（吞）体; 2. a nucleolus like, intranuclear, RNA-containing organelle of certain flagellate protozoa that persists during mitosis 核内体

en·dos·se·ous (en-dos′e-əs) endosteal (2) 骨内的

en·dos·te·al (en-dos′te-əl) 1. pertaining to the endosteum 骨内膜的; 2. occurring or located within a bone 骨内的

en·dos·te·o·ma (en-dos″te-o′mə) a tumor in the medullary cavity of a bone 骨髓腔肿瘤

en·dos·te·um (en-dos′te-əm) the tissue lining the medullary cavity of a bone 骨内膜

en·do·ten·din·e·um (en″do-tən-din′e-əm) the delicate connective tissue separating the secondary bundles (fascicles) of a tendon 腱内膜

en·do·the·lia (en″do-the′le-ə) [Gr.] 内皮 endothelium 的复数形式

en·do·the·li·al (en″do-the′le-əl) pertaining to or made up of endothelium 内皮的

en·do·the·lio·blas·to·ma (en″do-the″le-oblasto′mə) a tumor derived from primitive vasoformative tissue, it includes hemangioendothelioma, angiosarcoma, lymphangioendothelioma, and lymphangiosarcoma 成内皮细胞瘤

en·do·the·li·o·ma (en″do-the″le-o′mə) any tumor, particularly a benign one, arising from the endothelial lining of blood vessels 内皮瘤

en·do·the·li·o·ma·to·sis (en″do-the″le-o-mə-to′-sis) formation of multiple, diffuse endotheliomas 内皮瘤病

en·do·the·li·o·sis (en″do-the″le-o′sis) proliferation of endothelium 内皮增生; **glomerular capillary e.**, a renal lesion typical of eclampsia, characterized by deposition of fibrous material in and beneath the cells of the swollen glomerular capillary epithelium, occluding the capillaries 肾小球毛细血管内皮增生

en·do·ther·mic (en″do-thur′mik) characterized by or accompanied by the absorption of heat 吸热的。又称 *endothermal*

en·do·ther·my (en″do-thur′me) diathermy 透热法

en·do·tho·rac·ic (en″do-tho-ras′ik) within the thorax; situated internal to the ribs 胸内的

en·do·thrix (en′do-thriks) inside the hair; used to describe dermatophyte infections in which arthrospores are produced, and remain, within the hair shaft 毛内癣菌。Cf. *ectothrix*

en·do·tox·e·mia (en″do-tok-se′me-ə) the presence of endotoxins in the blood, which may result in shock 内毒素血症

en·do·tox·in (en′do-tok″sin) a heat-stable toxin present in the intact bacterial cell but not in cell-free filtrates of cultures of intact bacteria. Endotoxins are lipopolysaccharide complexes that occur in the cell wall; they are pyrogenic and increase capillary permeability 内毒素; **en′dotoxic** *adj.*

en·do·tra·che·al (en″do-tra′ke-əl) within or through the trachea 气管内的

en·do·urol·o·gy (en″do-u-rol′ə-je) the branch of urologic surgery concerned with closed procedures for visualizing or manipulating the urinary tract 腔

内泌尿外科学

en·do·vas·cu·li·tis (en″do-vas″ku-li′tis) endangiitis 血管内膜炎

end plate (end plāt) a flat termination 终板; **motor e. p.**, the discoid expansion of a terminal branch of the axon of a motor nerve fiber where it joins a skeletal muscle fiber, forming the neuromuscular junction 运动终板

en·drin (en′drin) a highly toxic insecticide of the chlorinated hydrocarbon group 彭德莱素

end-tidal (end-ti′dəl) pertaining to or occurring at the end of exhalation of a normal tidal volume 呼气末

en·e·ma (en′ə-mə) [Gr.] a solution introduced into the rectum to promote evacuation of feces or as a means of introducing nutrients, medicinal substances, or opaque material for radiologic examination of the lower intestinal tract 灌肠剂; **barium e.**, **contrast e.**, a suspension of barium injected into the intestine as a contrast medium 钡剂灌肠; 对比灌肠; **double-contrast e.**, injection and evacuation of a suspension of barium, followed by inflation of the intestines with air under light pressure 双重对比灌肠

en·er·gy (*E*) (en′ər-je) power that may be translated into motion, overcoming resistance, or effecting physical change; the ability to do work 能量; **free e.**, **Gibbs free e.** (*G*), that equal to the maximum amount of work that can be obtained from a process occurring under conditions of fixed temperature and pressure 自由能, 吉布斯自由能; **kinetic e.**, the energy of motion. 动能; **nuclear e.**, energy that can be liberated by changes in the nucleus of an atom (as by fission of a heavy nucleus or fusion of light nuclei into heavier ones with accompanying loss of mass) 核能; **potential e.**, energy at rest or not manifested in actual work 势能; **vital e.**, 生命力, 见 *force* 下词条

en·er·va·tion (en″ər-va′shən) 1. lack of nervous energy 神经无力; 2. neurectomy 神经切除

ENG electronystagmography. 眼震电流描记

en·gage·ment (en-gāj′mənt) the entrance of the fetal head or presenting part into the superior pelvic strait（胎头）衔接

en·gi·neer·ing (en″jĭ-nēr′ing) the application of physical, mathematical, and mechanical principles to practical purposes 工程学; **biomedical e.**, the use of engineering in biomedical technology, such as the analysis of movement of body parts or prosthetics 生物医学工程; **genetic e.**, the directed manipulation of the genome of a living organism for a variety of analytical, industrial, and medical applications; most methods involve use of recombinant DNA technology (q.v.) 基因工程; **tissue e.**, the application of methods and principles of engineering for understanding the relationship between structure and function of tissue and development of substitutes for pathologic, damaged, or missing tissue 组织工程

en·gorge·ment (en-gorj′mənt) 1. local congestion 局部充血; distention with fluids 液体膨胀; 2. hyperemia 充血

en·graft·ment (ən-graft′mənt) incorporation of grafted tissue into the body of the host 移植

en·hance·ment (en-hans′mənt) 1. the act of augmenting or the state of being augmented 增强; 2. immunologic enhancement; prolonged survival of tumor cells in animals immunized with antigens of the tumor because of "enhancing" or "facilitating" antibodies preventing an immune response against these antigens 免疫促进

en·keph·a·lin (en-kef′ə-lin) either of two pentapeptides (*leu-enkephalin* and *met-enkephalin*) occurring in the brain and spinal cord and also in the gastrointestinal tract; they have potent opiate-like effects and probably serve as neurotransmitters 脑啡肽

enol (e′nol) an organic compound in which one carbon of a double-bonded pair is also attached to a hydroxyl group, thus a tautomer of the ketone form; also used as a prefix or infix, often italicized 烯醇

eno·lase (e′no-lās) an enzyme that catalyzes the dehydration of 2-phosphoglycerate to form phospho*enol*pyruvate, a step in the pathway of glucose metabolism 烯醇化酶; **neuron-specific e.**, an isozyme of enolase found in normal neurons and all the cells of the neuroendocrine system; it is a marker for neuroendocrine differentiation in tumors 神经元特异性烯醇化酶

en·os·to·sis (en″os-to′sis) a morbid bony growth within a bone cavity or on the internal surface of the bone cortex 内生骨疣

enox·a·cin (ĕ-nok′sah-sin) a synthetic antibacterial effective against many gram-positive and gram-negative bacteria 依诺沙星

enox·a·par·in (e-nok″sə-par′in) a low-molecularweight heparin used as the sodium salt as an antithrombotic 依诺肝素

enox·i·mone (ə-nok′sī-mōn) a phosphodiesterase inhibitor similar to inamrinone; used as a cardiotonic in the short-term management of congestive heart failure, administered intravenously 依诺昔酮

en·si·form (en′sī-form) xiphoid (1) 剑形的

en·sul·i·zole (en-sul′ĭ-zōl) a water-soluble absorber of ultraviolet B radiation, used topically as a sunscreen 一种水溶性化学防晒剂

ENT ears, nose, and throat (otorhinolaryngology)

en·tac·a·pone (en-tak′ə-pōn) an antidyskinetic used in conjunction with levodopa and carbidopa in the treatment of idiopathic Parkinson disease 恩托卡朋

en·tad (en′tad) toward a center; inwardly 向内，向心

ent·ame·bi·a·sis (en″tə-me-bi′ə-sis) amebiasis caused by *Entamoeba* species 内阿米巴病

Ent·amoe·ba (en″tə-me′bə) a genus of amebas parasitic in the intestines of vertebrates, including three species commonly parasitic in humans: *E. co′li*, found in the intestinal tract; *E. gingiva′lis (E. bucca′lis)*, found in the mouth; and *E. histoly′tica*, the cause of amebic dysentery and tropical abscess of the liver 内阿米巴属

en·ter·al·gia (en″tər-al′jə) pain in the intestine 肠痛

en·ter·ic (en-ter′ik) within or pertaining to the small intestine 肠的，又称 enteral

en·ter·ic-coat·ed (en-ter′ik-kōt′əd) designating a special coating applied to tablets or capsules that prevents release and absorption of active ingredients until they reach the intestine 肠溶衣的

en·ter·i·tis (en″tər-i′tis) inflammation of the intestine, especially of the small intestine 肠炎; **regional e.**, Crohn disease 局限性肠炎

En·tero·bac·ter (en″tər-o-bak′tər) a genus of gram-negative, facultatively anaerobic, rodshaped bacteria of the family Enterobacteriaceae, widely distributed in nature and occurring in the intestinal tract of humans and animals; they frequently cause nosocomial infection, arising from contaminated medical devices and personnel. Species include *E. cloa′cae*, *E. gergo′viae*, and *E. sakaza′kii* 肠杆菌属

En·tero·bac·te·ri·a·ceae (en″tər-o-bakte″re-a′se-e) a large, widespread family of gram-negative, facultatively anaerobic, rodshaped bacteria of the order Enterobacteriales, consisting of saprophytes and plant and animal parasites; members frequently cause nosocomial infection and are opportunistic pathogens 肠杆菌科

En·tero·bac·te·ri·a·les (en″tər-o-bak-te″rea′lēz) an order of gram-negative, aerobic, rod-shaped bacteria of the class Gammaproteobacteria 肠杆菌目

en·tero·bi·a·sis (en″ter-o-bi′ə-sis) infection with nematodes of the genus *Enterobius*, especially *E. vermicularis* 蛲虫病

En·tero·bi·us (en″tər-o′be-əs) a genus of intestinal nematodes (superfamily Oxyuroidea), including *E. vermicula′ris*, the seatworm or pinworm, parasitic in the upper large intestine, and occasionally in the female genitals and bladder; infection is frequent in children, sometimes causing itching 蛲虫属

en·tero·cele (en′tər-o-sēl″) prolapse of the apex of the posterior vaginal wall, resulting in protrusion of the pouch of Douglas, with its intestinal contents, through the pelvic diaphragm 肠疝

en·tero·cen·te·sis (en″tər-o-sen-te′sis) surgical puncture of the intestine 肠穿刺术

en·ter·oc·ly·sis (en″tər-ok′lĭ-sis) 1. the injection of liquids into the intestine 灌肠; 2. introduction of barium into the small intestine through a nasogastric tube for radiographic examination 灌肠剂

En·tero·coc·ca·ceae (en″tər-o-kə-ka′se-e) a family of gram-positive, facultatively anaerobic to microaerophilic, nonmotile cocci of the order Lactobacillales 肠球菌科

En·tero·coc·cus (en″tər-o-kok′əs) a genus of gram-positive facultatively anaerobic cocci of the family Enterococcaceae; *E. faeca′lis* and *E. fae′cium* are normal inhabitants of the human intestinal tract that occasionally cause urinary tract infections, infective endocarditis, and bacteremia; *E. a′vium* is found primarily in the feces of chickens and may be associated with appendicitis, otitis, and brain abscesses in humans 肠球菌

en·tero·coc·cus (en″tər-o-kok′əs) pl. *enterococ′ci*. An organism belonging to the genus *Enterococcus* 肠球菌

en·tero·co·lec·to·my (en″tər-o-ko-lek′tə-me) resection of the intestine, including the ileum, cecum, and colon 肠切除术

en·tero·co·li·tis (en″tər-o-ko-li′tis) inflammation of the small intestine and colon. 小肠结肠炎; **antibiotic-associated e.**, that in which treatment with antibiotics alters the bowel flora and results in diarrhea or pseudomembranous enterocolitis 抗生素性小肠结肠炎; **hemorrhagic e.**, enterocolitis characterized by hemorrhagic breakdown of the intestinal mucosa, with inflammatory cell infiltration 出血性小肠结肠炎; **necrotizing e.**, acute inflammation of the bowel mucosa with formation of pseudomembranous plaques overlying an area of superficial ulceration, with passage of the pseudomembranous material in the feces 坏死性小肠结肠炎; **pseudomembranous e.**, an acute type with formation of pseudomembranous plaques that overlie superficial ulcerations and pass out in the feces; it may result from shock, ischemia, or aftereffects of antibiotic therapy (see *antibioticassociated e.*) 假膜性小肠结肠炎

en·tero·cu·ta·ne·ous (en″tər-o-ku-ta′ne-əs) pertaining to or communicating with the intestine and the skin, or surface of the body 肠皮肤的

en·tero·cyst (en′tər-o-sist″) enteric cyst 肠囊肿

en·tero·cys·to·ma (en″tər-o-sis-to′mə) enteric

cyst 肠囊瘤

en·tero·cys·to·plas·ty (en″tər-o-sis′to-plas″te) the most common type of augmentation cystoplasty, using a portion of intestine for the graft 肠膀胱成形术

en·tero·en·ter·os·to·my (en″tər-o-en″təros′tə-me) surgical anastomosis between two segments of the intestine 肠 - 肠吻合术

en·tero·gas·trone (en″tər-o-gas′trōn) anthelone E; a hormone of the duodenum that mediates the humoral inhibition of gastric secretion and motility produced by ingestion of fat 肠抑胃素

en·ter·og·e·nous (en″tər-oj′ə-nəs) 1. arising from the foregut 肠源性; 2. originating within the small intestine 小肠内发生的

en·tero·glu·ca·gon (en″tər-o-gloo′kə-gon) a glucagon-like hyperglycemic agent released by the mucosa of the upper intestine in response to the ingestion of glucose; immunologically distinct from pancreatic glucagon but with similar activities 肠高血糖素

en·tero·gram (en″tər-o-gram″) 1. a radiograph of the intestines 肠动图; 2. a tracing made by an instrument of the movements of the intestine 肠动描记图

en·ter·og·ra·phy (en″tər-og′rə-fe) radiographic examination of the intestines 肠动描记法

en·tero·he·pat·ic (en″tər-o-hə-pat′ik) pertaining to or connecting the liver and intestine 肠肝的

en·tero·hep·a·ti·tis (en″tər-o-hep″ə-ti′tis) inflammation of the intestine and liver 肠肝炎

en·tero·hep·a·to·cele (en″tər-o-hep′ə-to-sēl″) an umbilical hernia containing intestine and liver 肠肝脐疝

en·tero·lith (en′tər-o-lith″) a calculus in the intestine 肠石

en·ter·ol·o·gy (en″tər-ol′ə-je) scientific study of the intestine 肠病学

en·ter·ol·y·sis (en″tər-ol′ə-sis) surgical separation of intestinal adhesions 肠粘连松解术

en·tero·pa·re·sis (en″tər-o-pə-re′sis) relaxation of the intestine resulting in dilatation 肠麻痹

en·tero·patho·gen·e·sis (en″tər-o-path″ojen′ə-sis) the production of intestinal diseases or disorders 肠发病机制

en·ter·op·a·thy (en″tər-op′ə-the) any disease of the intestine 肠病; **enteropath′ic** adj.; gluten e., celiac disease 非热带口炎性腹泻

en·tero·pep·ti·dase (en″tər-o-pep′tĭ-dās) an endopeptidase, secreted by the small intestine, which catalyzes the cleavage of trypsinogen to the active form trypsin 肠肽酶

en·tero·pexy (en′tər-o-pek″se) surgical fixation of the intestine to the abdominal wall 肠固定术

en·tero·plas·ty (en′tər-o-plas″te) plastic repair of the intestine 肠成形术

en·ter·or·rha·gia (en″tər-o-ra′jə) intestinal hemorrhage 肠出血

en·ter·or·rhex·is (en″tər-o-rek′sis) rupture of the intestine 肠破裂

en·tero·scope (en′tər-o-skōp) an endoscope for inspecting the inside of the intestine 肠镜

en·ter·os·co·py (en″tər-os′kə-pe) examination of the intestine with an enteroscope 肠镜检查

en·tero·sep·sis (en″tər-o-sep′sis) sepsis developed from the intestinal contents 肠脓毒症

en·tero·ste·no·sis (en″tər-o-stə-no′sis) narrowing or stricture of the intestine 肠狭窄

en·ter·os·to·my (en″tər-os′tə-me) formation of a permanent opening into the intestine through the abdominal wall 肠造口术; **enterosto′mal** adj.

en·tero·tox·e·mia (en″tər-o-tok-se″me-ə) a condition characterized by the presence in the blood of toxins produced in the intestines 肠毒血症

en·tero·tox·in (en′tər-o-tok″sin) a toxin specific for the cells of the intestinal mucosa 肠毒素

en·tero·tro·pic (en″tər-o-tro′pik) affecting the intestine 向肠的

en·tero·vag·i·nal (en″tər-o-vaj′ĭ-nəl) pertaining to or communicating with the intestine and the vagina 肠阴道的

en·tero·ve·nous (en″tər-o-ve′nəs) communicating between the intestinal lumen and the lumen of a vein 肠静脉的

en·tero·ves·i·cal (en″tər-o-ves′ĭ-kəl) pertaining to or communicating with the urinary bladder and intestine 肠膀胱的

En·tero·vi·rus (en″tər-o-vi″rəs) the enteroviruses, a genus of the family Picornaviridae that preferentially inhabit the intestinal tract, with infection usually asymptomatic or mild. Human enteroviruses were originally classified as polioviruses, coxsackieviruses, or echoviruses 肠道病毒属

en·tero·vi·rus (en′tər-o-vi″rəs) any virus of the genus *Enterovirus* 肠道病毒; **enterovi′ral** adj.; human e., either of two species of the genus *Enterovirus* that infect humans; there are numerous different serogroups. Most strains cause only mild symptoms such as fever, but one causes acute hemorrhagic conjunctivitis and others cause aseptic meningitis, pericarditis, and pleurodynia 人类肠道病毒

en·thal·py (*H*) (en′thəl-pe) the heat content or chemical energy of a physical system; a thermodynamic function equal to the internal energy plus the product of the pressure and volume 焓, 热焓

en·the·sis (en-the′sis) the site of attachment of a muscle or ligament to bone 肌腱末端

en·the·sop·a·thy (en″thə-sop′ə-the) disorder of the muscular or tendinous attachment to bone 末端病

en·theto·bio·sis (en-thet″o-bi-o′sis) dependency on a mechanical implant, as on an artificial cardiac pacemaker 生命延续法

en·to·blast (en′to-blast) endoderm 内胚层

en·to·cor·nea (en″to-kor′ne-ə) Descemet membrane. 后弹性层（角膜）

en·to·derm (en′to-dərm) endoderm 内胚层; **entoder′mal, entoder′mic** adj.

en·to·mi·on (en-to′me-on) the tip of mastoid angle of parietal bone 乳突凸

en·to·mol·o·gy (en″tə-mol′ə-je) that branch of biology concerned with the study of insects 昆虫学

En·to·moph·tho·ra·les (en″to-mof″thə-ra′lēz) an order of fungi of the class Zygomycetes, typically parasites of insects but also causing human infections, often in apparently immunologically and physiologically normal people 虫霉目

en·to·moph·tho·ro·my·co·sis (en″tə-mof″thə-ro-mi-ko′sis) infection by *Basidiobolus* or *Conidiobolus* (fungi formerly grouped in Entomophthorales); usually occurring in the tropics as a chronic localized infection of the subcutaneous tissues in relatively immunocompetent individuals 虫霉病。Cf. *basidiobolomycosis* 和 *conidiobolomycosis*

en·top·ic (en-top′ik) occurring in the proper place 正常位置的

en·top·tic (en-top′tik) originating within the eye 眼内的，内视的

en·top·tos·co·py (en″tos-tos′ko-pe) inspection of the interior of the eye 眼内媒质检查

en·to·ret·i·na (en″to-ret′ĭ-nə) the nervous or inner layer of the retina 视网膜内层

en·to·zo·on (en″to-zo′on) pl. *entozo′a*. An internal animal parasite 内寄生动物; **entozo′ic** adj.

en·train (en-trān′) to modulate the cardiac rhythm by gaining control of the rate of the pacemaker with an external stimulus 起搏性心律调整

en·train·ment (en-trān′mənt) 1. a technique for identifying the slowest pacing necessary to terminate an arrhythmia, particularly atrial flutter 起搏性心律调整术; 2. the synchronization and control of cardiac rhythm by an external stimulus 以外源刺激同步控制心律

en·trap·ment (en-trap′mənt) compression of a nerve or vessel by adjacent tissue 神经或血管受周围组织压迫

en·tro·pi·on (en-tro′pe-on) inversion, or the turning inward, as of the margin of an eyelid 睑内翻

en·tro·py (en′tro-pe) 1. the measure of that part of the heat or energy of a system not available to perform work; it increases in all natural (spontaneous and irreversible) processes 熵，符号 S；2. the tendency of any system to move toward randomness or disorder 扩散；3. diminished capacity for spontaneous change 消失，衰退

en·ty·py (en′tə-pe) a method of gastrulation in which the endoderm lies external to the amniotic ectoderm 胚层反向

enu·cle·a·tion (e-noo″kle-a′shən) removal of an organ or other mass intact from its supporting tissues, as of the eyeball from the orbit 摘除

en·ure·sis (en″u-re′sis) urinary incontinence 遗尿

en·ve·lope (en′və-lōp) 1. an encompassing structure or membrane 包层，被膜; 2. in virology, the peplos, a coat surrounding the capsid and usually furnished at least partially by the host cell 包膜; 3. in bacteriology, the cell wall and the plasma membrane considered together 细菌学中指细胞壁和质膜; **nuclear e.,** the condensed double layer of lipids and proteins enclosing the cell nucleus and separating it from the cytoplasm; its two concentric membranes, inner and outer, are separated by a perinuclear space 核被膜

en·ven·om·a·tion (en-ven″o-ma′shən) poisoning by venom 螫刺毒作用

en·vi·ron·ment (en-vi′ron-mənt) the sum total of all the conditions and elements that make up the surroundings and influence the development of an individual 环境; **environmen′tal** adj.

en·vy (en′ve) a desire to have another's possessions or qualities for oneself 羡慕，妒忌; **penis e.,** the concept that the female envies the male his possession of a penis or, more generally, any of his characteristics 阴茎妒忌

en·za·cam·ene (en″zə-kam′ēn) an absorber of ultraviolet radiation, used topically as a sunscreen 一种防晒药

en·zy·got·ic (en″zi-got′ik) developed from the same zygote 同卵性的

en·zyme (E) (en′zīm) a protein that catalyzes chemical reactions of other substances without itself being destroyed or altered upon completion of the reactions. Enzymes are divided into six main groups: oxidoreductases, transferases, hydrolases, lyases, isomerases, and ligases 酶; **allosteric e.,** an enzyme whose catalytic activity is altered by binding of specific ligands at sites other than the substrate binding site 别构酶; **brancher e., branching e.,** 1,4-α-glucan branching enzyme; an enzyme that catalyzes the creation of branch points in glycogen (in plants, amylopectin); deficiency causes glycogen storage disease, type Ⅳ 分支酶; **constitutive e.,** an enzyme that is produced constantly, irrespective of environmental conditions or demand 组成酶;

debrancher e., debranching e., 1. amylo-1,6-glu-cosidase 淀粉 -1，6- 葡萄糖苷酶；2. any enzyme removing branches from macromolecules, usually polysaccharides, by cleaving at branch points 脱支酶；**induced e., inducible e.,** one whose production can be stimulated by another compound, often a substrate or a structurally related molecule 诱导酶；**proteolytic e.,** peptidase 蛋白水解酶；**repressible e.,** one whose rate of production is decreased as the concentration of certain metabolites is increased 抑制酶；**respiratory e.,** an enzyme that is part of an electron transport (respiratory) chain 呼吸酶；**stratum corneum tryptic e.,** an enzyme that is abundant in the stratum corneum and is important for the normal shedding of skin cells. An excess of this enzyme and of cathelicidin causes the formation of an abnormal peptide that is responsible for the lesions of rosacea 角质层胰蛋白酶

en·zy·mop·a·thy (en″zi-mop′ə-the) an inborn error of metabolism consisting of defective or absent enzymes, as in the glycogenoses or the mucopoly-saccharidoses 酶（不全）病

EOC epithelial ovarian cancer 上皮性卵巢癌

EOG electro-olfactogram 嗅电（流）图

eo·sin (e′o-sin) any of a class of rose-colored stains or dyes, all being bromine derivatives of flu-orescein; *eosin Y,* the sodium salt of tetrabromoflu-orescein, is much used in histologic and laboratory procedures 伊红

eo·sin·o·pe·nia (e″o-sin-o-pe′ne-ə) abnormal deficiency of eosinophils in the blood 嗜酸性粒细胞减少

eo·sin·o·phil (e″o-sin′o-fil) a granular leukocyte having a nucleus with two lobes connected by a thread of chromatin, and cytoplasm containing coarse, round granules of uniform size 嗜酸性粒细胞

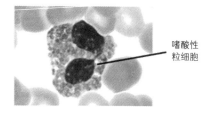

嗜酸性
粒细胞

eo·sin·o·phil·ia (e″o-sin″o-fil′e-ə) abnormally increased eosinophils in the blood 嗜酸性粒细胞增多症

eo·sin·o·phil·ic (e″o-sin″o-fil′ik) 1. readily stainable with eosin 嗜酸性的；2. pertaining to eosinophils 嗜酸性粒细胞的；3. pertaining to or characterized by eosinophilia 嗜酸性粒细胞增多的

EP evoked potential 诱发电位

EPA eicosapentaenoic acid 二十碳五烯酸

epac·tal (e-pak′təl) 1. supernumerary 多余的，额外的；2. sutural bone 缝间骨

ep·al·lo·bi·o·sis (əp-al″o-bi-o′sis) dependency on an external life-support system, as on a heartlung machine or hemodialyzer 体外生命支持法

ep·ax·i·al (əp-ak′se-əl) situated upon or above an axis 轴上的

epen·dy·ma (ə-pen′də-mə) the membrane lining the cerebral ventricles and the central canal of the spine 室管膜；**epen′dymal** *adj.*

epen·dy·mo·blast (ə-pen′də-mo-blast) an embryonic ependymal cell 成室管膜细胞

epen·dy·mo·cyte (ə-pen′də-mo-sīt″) an ependymal cell 室管膜细胞

epen·dy·mo·ma (ə-pen″də-mo′mə) a neoplasm, usually slow growing and benign, composed of differentiated ependymal cells 室管膜瘤

ephapse (e-faps′) electrical synapse 神经元间接触；**ephap′tic** *adj.*

ephe·bi·at·rics (ə-fe″be-at′riks) the branch of medicine that specializes in the diagnosis and treatment of diseases of youth 青春期医学

Ephed·ra (ə-fed′rə) a genus of low, branching shrubs indigenous to China and India. *E. equiseti′na* Bunge., *E. sini′ca* Stapf., *E. vulga′ris,* and other species (all called *ma huang* in China) are sources of ephedrine 麻黄属

ephed·rine (ə-fed′rin) (ef′ə-drin) an adrenergic extracted from several species of *Ephedra* or produced synthetically; used in the form of the hydrochloride, sulfate, or tannate salt as a bronchodilator, antiallergic, central nervous system stimulant, and antihypotensive. It has also been used in supplements, with benefits claimed to include weight loss, increased energy, and enhanced athletic performance 麻黄碱

ephe·lis (ə-fe′lis) pl. *ephe′lides* [Gr.] freckle 雀斑

epi·an·dros·ter·one (ep″e-an-dros′tər-ōn) an androgenic steroid less active than androsterone and excreted in small amounts in normal human urine 表雄（甾）酮

epi·blast (ep′ĭ-blast) 1. the upper layer of the bilaminar embryonic disc present during the second week; it gives rise to ectoderm 上胚层；2. ectoderm 外胚层；3. ectoderm, except for the neural plate 除神经板的外胚层；**epiblas′tic** *adj.*

epi·bleph·a·ron (ep″ĭ-blef′ə-ron) a developmental anomaly in which a horizontal fold of skin stretches across the border of the eyelid, pressing the eyelashes inward, against the eyelid 眼睑赘皮

epib·o·ly (e-pib′o-le) a process by which an outside cell layer spreads to envelope a yolk mass or deeper layer of cells 外包

epi·bul·bar (ep″ĭ-bul′bər) above the eyeball 眼球上的

epi·can·thus (ep″ĭ-kan′thəs) a vertical fold of skin on either side of the nose, sometimes covering the inner canthus; a normal characteristic in persons of certain races but anomalous in others 内眦赘皮；**epican′thal, epican′thic** adj.

epi·car·dia (ep″ĭ-kahr′de-ə) the portion of the esophagus below the respiratory diaphragm 横膈膜下食道部分

epi·car·di·um (ep″ĭ-kahr′de-əm) the visceral pericardium 心外膜

epi·cho·ri·on (ep″ĭ-kor′e-on) the portion of the uterine mucosa enclosing the implanted conceptus 包蜕膜

epi·con·dy·lal·gia (ep″ĭ-kon″də-lal′jə) pain in the muscles or tendons attached to the epicondyle of the humerus 上髁痛

epi·con·dyle (ep″ĭ-kon′dīl) an eminence upon a bone, above its condyle 上髁

epi·con·dy·li·tis (ep″ĭ-kon″də-li′tis) inflammation of an epicondyle of the humerus or of the tissues adjoining it, usually from an overuse injury 上髁炎；**lateral e.,** tennis elbow; an overuse injury of the lateral humeral epicondyle at the elbow, due to inflammation or irritation of the area where the extensor tendon attaches to it 肱骨外上髁炎；**medial e.,** golfer's elbow; an overuse injury with pain around the medial epicondyle of the humerus where the flexor muscles of the arm and hand attach 肱骨内上髁炎

epi·con·dy·lus (ep″ĭ-kon′də-ləs) pl. *epicon′dyli* [L.] epicondyle 上髁

epi·cra·ni·um (ep″ĭ-kra′ne-əm) the muscles, skin, and aponeurosis covering the skull 头盖，头皮

epi·cri·sis (ep″ĭ-kri″sis) a secondary crisis 第二次骤退

epi·crit·ic (ep″ĭ-krit′ik) determining accurately; said of cutaneous nerve fibers sensitive to fine variations of touch or temperature（皮肤神经纤维）精细觉的

epi·cys·tot·o·my (ep″ĭ-sis-tot′o-me) cystotomy by the suprapubic method 耻骨上膀胱切开术

epi·cyte (ep′ĭ-sīt) cell membrane 细胞膜

ep·i·dem·ic (ep″ĭ-dem′ik) occurring suddenly in numbers clearly in excess of normal expectancy 流行的

ep·i·de·mi·ol·o·gy (ep″ĭ-de″me-ol′ə-je) the science concerned with the study of the factors determining and influencing the frequency and distribution of disease, injury, and other healthrelated events and their causes in a defined human population.

Also, the sum of knowledge gained in such a study 流行病学

epi·der·mis (ep″ĭ-dur′mis) pl. *epider′mides.* The outermost and nonvascular layer of the skin, derived from the embryonic ectoderm, varying in thickness from 0.07 to 1.4 mm. On the palmar and plantar surfaces it comprises, from within outward, five layers: (1) *basal layer* (stratum basale), composed of columnar cells arranged perpendicularly; (2) *prickle cell* or *spinous layer* (stratum spinosum), composed of flattened polyhedral cells with short processes or spines; (3) *granular layer* (stratum granulosum), composed of flattened granular cells; (4) *clear layer* (stratum lucidum), composed of several layers of clear, transparent cells in which the nuclei are indistinct or absent; and (5) *horny layer* (stratum corneum), composed of flattened, cornified, non-nucleated cells. In the epidermis of the general body surface, the clear layer is usually absent 表皮, 真皮；**epider′mal, epider′mic** adj.

epi·der·mi·tis (ep″ĭ-dər-mi′tis) inflammation of the epidermis 表皮炎

epi·der·mo·dys·pla·sia (ep″ĭ-dur″mo-displa′zhə) faulty development of the epidermis 表皮发育异常；**e. verrucifor′mis,** a rare, autosomal recessive condition of widespread verruca plana, caused by infection with human papillomavirus, with a tendency to malignant degeneration 疣状表皮发育不良

epi·der·moid (ep″ĭ-dur′moid) 1. pertaining to or resembling the epidermis 表皮的，表皮状的；2. epidermoid cyst 表皮样囊肿

epi·der·moi·do·ma (ep″ĭ-dur″moi-do′mə) epidermoid cyst (2) 表皮样瘤

epi·der·mol·y·sis (ep″ĭ-dər-mol′ə-sis) a loosened state of the epidermis, with formation of blebs and bullae, either spontaneously or following trauma 表皮松解（症）；**epidermolyt′ic** adj.; **acquired e. bullosa,** an autoimmune condition with autoantibodies against collagen in fibrils at the dermal-epidermal junction; bullae and blisters are usually on pressure areas of the hands and feet 获得性大疱性表皮松解症；**e. bullo′sa,** a heterogeneous group of skin diseases in which bullae and vesicles develop at the site of trauma; there are hereditary and acquired forms. In the hereditary types there may be severe scarring after healing, or extensive denuded areas after rupture of the lesions 大疱性表皮松解；**e. bullo′sa dystro′phica,** hereditary epidermolysis bullosa with atrophy and scarring after blisters heal, and dystrophy or absence of the nails, due to defects in collagen. Autosomal dominant and recessive forms exist, with the recessive forms often being severely disabling or even fatal 营养不良性

大疱性表皮松解症；e. bullo′sa sim′plex, a group of hereditary nonscarring forms of epidermolysis bullosa mainly due to defects in basal layer keratins. The localized type may not be evident until adolescence or adulthood; generalized forms are seen in infants and vary widely from moderate to severe 单纯性大疱性表皮松解症；dystrophic e. bullosa, e. bullosa dystrophica.; junctional e. bullosa, a genetically heterogeneous, autosomal recessive type of epidermolysis bullosa, caused mainly by defects in laminin, with severe generalized blistering on the head, trunk, or lower limbs and often death from septicemia 交界型大疱性表皮松解症，致死性大疱性表皮松解症

Epi·der·moph·y·ton (ep″ĭ-dər-mof′ĭ-ton) a genus of fungi, including *E. flocco′sum*, which attacks skin and nails but not hair and is one of the causes of tinea cruris, tinea pedis (athlete's foot), and onychomycosis 表皮癣菌属

ep·i·did·y·mis (ep″ĭ-did′ə-mis) pl. *epididy′mides* [Gr.] an elongated cordlike structure along the posterior border of the testis; its coiled duct provides for storage, transit, and maturation of spermatozoa and is continuous with the ductus deferens 附睾；**epidid′ymal** *adj.*

epi·did·y·mi·tis (ep″ĭ-did′ə-mi′tis) inflammation of the epididymis 附睾炎

epi·did·y·mo-or·chi·tis (ep″ĭ-did″ə-mo-orki′tis) inflammation of the epididymis and testis 附睾睾丸炎

epi·did·y·mo·vas·os·to·my (ep″ĭ-did′ə-movə-sos′tə-me) vasoepididymostomy 输精管附睾吻合术

epi·du·ral (ep″ĭ-doo′rəl) situated upon or outside the dura mater 硬（脑）膜上的，硬膜外的

epi·du·rog·ra·phy (ep″ĭ-doo-rog′rə-fe) radiography of the spine after a radiopaque medium has been injected into the epidural space 硬膜外造影术

epi·es·tri·ol (ep″e-es′tre-ol) an estrogenic steroid found in pregnant women 表雌三醇

epi·gas·tri·um (ep″ĭ-gas′tre-əm) the upper and middle region of the abdomen, located within the sternal angle 上腹部；**epigas′tric** *adj.*

epi·gen·e·sis (ep″ĭ-jen′ə-sis) the development of an organism from an undifferentiated cell, consisting in the successive formation and development of organs and parts that do not preexist in the fertilized egg 后成说，渐成论

epi·ge·net·ic (ep″ĭ-jə-net′ik) 1. pertaining to epigenesis 渐成论的；2. altering the activity of genes without changing their DNA sequence 通过改变基因的 DNA 序列来改变基因的活性

epi·ge·net·ics (ep″ĭ-jə-net′iks) the study of heritable changes in gene function that occur without changes in the DNA sequence 表观遗传学

epi·ge·nome (ep″ĭ-je′nōm) the set of heritable modifications that interact with a genome to affect gene expression in a given differentiated cell without altering the nucleotide sequence 表观基因组

epi·ge·no·type (ep″ĭ-je′no-tīp) the pattern of gene expression in a differentiated cell, being a function of the combination of the genotype and epigenetic mechanisms such as DNA methylation 后生型，总发育体系

epi·glot·ti·dec·to·my (ep″ĭ-glot″ĭ-dek′tə-me) excision of the epiglottis 会厌切除术

epi·glot·tis (ep″ĭ-glot′is) the lidlike cartilaginous structure overhanging the entrance to the larynx, guarding it during swallowing 会厌；见图 31.；**epiglot′tic** *adj.*

epi·glot·ti·tis (ep″ĭ-glŏ-ti′tis) supraglottitis 会厌炎

ep·i·la·tion (ep″ĭ-la′shən) depilation 脱毛术

epil·a·to·ry (ə-pil′ə-tor″e) depilatory 脱毛药，脱毛的

ep·i·lem·ma (ep″ĭ-lem′ə) endoneurium 神经内膜

ep·i·lep·sia (ep″ĭ-lep′se-ə) [L.] epilepsy 癫痫；e. partia′lis conti′nua, a form of status epilepticus with focal motor seizures, marked by continuous clonic movements of a limited part of the body 部分性癫痫持续状态

ep·i·lep·sy (ep′ĭ-lep″se) any of a group of syndromes characterized by paroxysmal transient disturbances of brain function that may be manifested as episodic impairment or loss of consciousness, abnormal motor phenomena, psychic or sensory disturbances, or perturbation of the autonomic nervous system; symptoms are due to disturbance of the electrical activity of the brain 癫痫；absence e., that characterized by absence seizures, usually having its onset in childhood or adolescence 失神癫痫；Baltic myoclonic e., Unverricht-Lundborg disease Baltic 肌阵挛型癫痫；focal e., that consisting of focal seizures 局限型癫痫；generalized e., epilepsy in which the seizures are generalized; they may have a focal onset or be generalized from the beginning 全身型癫痫；grand mal e., a symptomatic form of epilepsy, often preceded by an aura, characterized by sudden loss of consciousness with tonic-clonic seizures 癫痫大发作；jacksonian e., epilepsy marked by focal motor seizures with unilateral clonic movements that start in one muscle group and spread systematically to adjacent groups, reflecting the march of epileptic activity through the motor cortex jacksonian 癫痫；juvenile myoclonic e., a syndrome of sudden myoclonic jerks, occurring particularly in the morning or under periods of stress or fatigue, primarily in children and adolescents 青少年肌阵挛性癫痫; **Lafora myoclonic e.**, Lafora disease Lafora 肌阵挛型癫; **myoclonic e., myoclonus e.**, any of a group of disorders, of varying etiologies, in which epilepsy is accompanied by muscle contractions (myoclonus); the group includes a benign idiopathic form, juvenile myoclonic e., and various other progressive inherited disorders 肌阵挛型癫; **petit mal e.**, absence e. 癫痫小发作; **photic e., photogenic e.**, reflex epilepsy in which seizures are induced by a flickering light 光敏性癫痫; **posttraumatic e.**, that occurring after head injury 创伤后癫痫; **psychomotor e.**, temporal lobe e. 精神运动型癫; **reflex e.**, epileptic seizures occurring in response to sensory stimuli 反射性癫痫; **rotatory e.**, temporal lobe epilepsy in which the automatisms consist of rotating body movements 旋转性癫痫; **sensory e.**, 1. seizures manifested by paresthesias or hallucinations of sight, smell, or taste 感觉性癫痫; 2. reflex e.; **somatosensory e.**, sensory epilepsy with paresthesias such as burning, tingling, or numbness 躯体感觉性癫痫; **temporal lobe e.**, a form characterized by complex partial seizures 颞叶癫痫; **visual e.**, sensory epilepsy in which there are visual hallucinations 视觉性癫痫

ep·i·lep·tic (ep″ĭ-lep′tik) 1. pertaining to or affected with epilepsy 癫痫样的; 2. a person affected with epilepsy 癫痫患者

ep·i·lep·ti·form (ep″ĭ-lep′tĭ-form) 1. resembling epilepsy or its manifestations 癫痫样; 2. occurring in severe or sudden paroxysms 严重或突然发作的

ep·i·lep·to·gen·ic (ep″ĭ-lep-to-jen′ik) causing an epileptic seizure 引起癫痫的, 致癫痫的

ep·i·lep·toid (ep″ĭ-lep′toid) epileptiform 癫痫样的

epi·man·dib·u·lar (ep″ĭ-man-dib′u-lər) situated on the lower jaw 下颌上的

epi·mas·ti·gote (ep″ĭ-mas′tĭ-gōt) a morphologic stage in the life cycle of certain trypanosomatid protozoa; the kinetoplast and basal body are located anterior to the central vesicular nucleus of the slender elongate cell, and the flagellum passes anteriorly attached to the body by an undulating membrane, becoming freeflowing at the anterior end 上鞭毛体

ep·i·mer (ep′ĭ-mər) either of two optical isomers that differ in the configuration around one asymmetric carbon atom in the configuration around one asymmetric carbon atom 差向异构体

epim·er·ase (ə-pim′ə-rās) an isomerase that catalyzes inversion of the configuration about an asymmetric carbon atom in a substrate having more than one center of asymmetry; thus epimers are interconverted 差向异构酶

ep·i·mere (ep′ĭ-mēr) the dorsal portion of a so-

mite, from which is formed muscles innervated by the dorsal ramus of a spinal nerve 轴上肌

epim·er·iza·tion (ə-pim″ər-ĭ-za′shən) the changing of one epimeric form of a compound into another, as by enzymatic action 差向异构化

epi·mor·pho·sis (ep″ĭ-mor-fo′sis) the regeneration of a part of an organism by proliferation at the cut surface 再生; **epimor′phic** adj.

epi·mys·i·ot·omy (ep″ĭ-mis″e-ot′ə-me) incision of the epimysium 肌外膜切开术

epi·mys·i·um (ep″ĭ-mis′e-əm) the fibrous sheath around an entire skeletal muscle 肌外膜, 见图 7

epi·neph·rine (ep″ĭ-nef′rin) a catecholamine hormone secreted by the adrenal medulla and a central nervous system neurotransmitter released by some neurons. It is stored in chromaffin granules and is released in response to hypoglycemia, stress, and other factors. It is a potent stimulator of the sympathetic nervous system (adrenergic receptors), and a powerful vasopressor, increasing blood pressure, stimulating the heart muscle, accelerating the heart rate, and increasing cardiac output. It is used as a topical vasoconstrictor, cardiac stimulant, systemic antiallergic, bronchodilator, and topical antiglaucoma agent; for the last two uses it is also administered as the bitartrate salt 肾上腺素。又称 adrenaline (Great Britain)

epi·neph·ryl bo·rate (ep″ĭ-nef′rəl) epinephrine complexed with borate; applied topically to the conjunctiva in the treatment of open-angle glaucoma 环硼肾上腺素

epi·neu·ri·um (ep″ĭ-noor′e-um) the outermost layer of connective tissue of a peripheral nerve 神经外膜; **epineu′rial** adj.

epi·ot·ic (ep″e-ot′ik) situated on or above the ear 耳上的

epi·phe·nom·e·non (ep″ĭ-fə-nom′ə-non) an accessory, exceptional, or accidental occurrence in the course of any disease 副现象, 偶发症状

epiph·o·ra (ə-pif′ə-rə) [Gr.] overflow of tears due to obstruction of a lacrimal duct 溢泪

epi·phys·e·al (ep″ĭ-fiz′e-əl) pertaining to or of the nature of an epiphysis 骺的

epi·phys·i·al (ep″ĭ-fiz′e-əl) epiphyseal 骺的

epiph·y·sis (ə-pif′ə-sis) pl. epi′physes [Gr.] the expanded articular end of a long bone, developed from a secondary ossification center, which during the period of growth is either entirely cartilaginous or is separated from the shaft by a cartilaginous disk 骺; **annular e.**, a raised ring of compact bone at the periphery of the superior and inferior surfaces of the vertebral body; generally considered to be a secondary ossification center 环状骺; **stippled e's**, chondrodysplasia punctata 斑点骺

epiph·y·si·tis (ə-pif″ə-si′tis) inflammation of an epiphysis or of the cartilage joining the epiphysis to a bone shaft 骺炎

ep·i·phyte (ep′ĭ-fīt) a plant ectoparasite 附生植物，附生菌；**epiphyt′ic** adj.

epi·pia (ep″ĭ-pi′ə) the part of the pia mater adjacent to the arachnoidea mater, as distinguished from the pia-glia 上软脑膜；**epipi′al** adj.

epip·lo·on (ə-pip′lo-on) [Gr.] omentum（大）网膜；**epiplo′ic** adj.

epi·ret·i·nal (ep″ĭ-ret′ĭ-nəl) overlying the retina 视网膜外层的

epi·ru·bi·cin (ep″ĭ-roo′bĭ-sin) an antineoplastic with action similar to doxorubicin; used in the treatment of various carcinomas, leukemia, lymphoma, and multiple myeloma 表阿霉素

epi·scle·ra (ep″ĭ-skler′ə) the loose connective tissue between the sclera and the conjunctiva 巩膜外层

epi·scle·ral (ep″ĭ-skler′əl) 1. overlying the sclera 巩膜上的；2. of or pertaining to the episclera 巩膜外层的

epi·scle·ri·tis (ep″ĭ-sklə-ri′tis) inflammation of the episclera and adjacent tissues 巩膜外层炎；**nodular e.**, that characterized by a mobile, tender, localized, injected nodule within the inflamed area 结节性巩膜外层炎

epis·io·per·i·neo·plas·ty (ə-piz″e-o-per″ĭne′o-plas″te) plastic repair of the vulva and perineum 外阴会阴修复成形术

epis·io·per·i·ne·or·rha·phy (ə-piz″e-o-per″ĭne-or′ə-fe) suture of the vulva and perineum 外阴会阴成形术

epis·i·or·rha·phy (ə-piz″e-or′ə-fe) 1. suture of the labia majora 大阴唇缝合术；2. suture of a lacerated perineum 撕裂会阴缝合术

epis·io·ste·no·sis (ə-piz″e-o-stə-no′sis) narrowing of the vulvar orifice 外阴狭窄

epis·i·ot·o·my (ə-piz″e-ot′o-me) surgical incision into the perineum and vagina to prevent traumatic tearing during delivery 外阴切开术

ep·i·sode (ep′ĭ-sōd) a noteworthy happening occurring in the course of a continuous series of events 发作；**hypomanic e.**, a period of elevated, expansive, or irritable mood resembling a manic episode but less severe 轻度躁狂发作；**major depressive e.**, a period of at least 2 weeks marked by depressed mood or loss of interest or pleasure in virtually all activities, associated with some combination of altered weight, appetite, or sleep patterns, psychomotor agitation or retardation, difficulty in thinking or concentration, fatigue, feelings of worthlessness and hopelessness, and thoughts of death

and suicide 严重抑郁发作；**manic e.**, a period of predominant mood elevation, expansiveness, or irritation together with some combination of inflated self-esteem or grandiosity, decreased need of sleep, talkativeness, flight of ideas, distractibility, hyperactivity, hypersexuality, and recklessness 躁狂发作；**mixed e.**, a period during which the symptoms of both a major depressive episode and of a manic episode occur nearly every day, with rapidly alternating moods 混合发作

ep·i·some (ep′ĭ-sōm) in bacterial genetics, any accessory extrachromosomal replicating genetic element that can exist either autonomously or integrated with the chromosome 附加体，游离体，游离基因

epi·spa·di·as (ep″ĭ-spa′de-əs) congenital absence of the upper wall of the urethra, occurring in both sexes, but more often in the male, with the urethral opening somewhere on the dorsum of the penis 尿道上裂；**epispa′diac, epispa′dial** adj.

epis·ta·sis (ə-pis′tə-sis) 1. suppression of a secretion or excretion 抑制分泌或排泄的；2. the interaction between genes at different loci that results in one gene masking the expresssion of the other 上位效应，基因在不同位点的相互作用，导致一个基因掩盖了另一个基因的表达

ep·i·stax·is (ep″ĭ-stak′sis) nosebleed; hemorrhage from the nose, usually due to rupture of small vessels overlying the anterior part of the cartilaginous nasal septum 鼻出血

epi·ster·num (ep″ĭ-stur′nəm) a bone present in reptiles and monotremes that may be represented as part of the manubrium, or first piece of the sternum 上胸骨

epi·thal·a·mus (ep″ĭ-thal′ə-məs) the part of the diencephalon just superior and posterior to the thalamus, comprising the pineal body and adjacent structures; considered by some to include the stria medullaris 丘脑上部，上丘脑

ep·i·the·li·al (ep″ĭ-the′le-əl) pertaining to or composed of epithelium 上皮的

ep·i·the·li·al·iza·tion (ep″ĭ-the″le-əl-ĭ-za′shən) healing by the growth of epithelium over a denuded surface 上皮形成

ep·i·the·li·a·lize (ep″ĭ-the′le-əl-īz″) to cover with epithelium 上皮覆盖

ep·i·the·li·itis (ep″ĭ-the″le-i′tis) inflammation of epithelium 上皮炎

ep·i·the·li·oid (ep″ĭ-the′le-oid) resembling epithelium 上皮样的

ep·i·the·li·ol·y·sin (ep″ĭ-the″le-ol′ə-sin) a cytolysin formed in the serum in response to injection of epithelial cells from a different species; it is capable of destroying epithelial cells of animals of the donor species 溶上皮素

ep·i·the·li·ol·y·sis (ep″ĭ-the″le-ol′ə-sis) destruction of epithelial tissue 上皮溶解；**epitheliolyt′ic** adj.

ep·i·the·li·o·ma (ep″ĭ-the″le-o′mə) 1. any tumor derived from epithelium 上皮瘤；2. loosely and incorrectly, carcinoma 癌；**epithelio′matous** adj.；**malignant e.**, carcinoma 恶性上皮瘤

ep·i·the·li·um (ep″ĭ-the″le-əm) pl. epithe′lia [Gr.] the cellular covering of internal and external body surfaces, including skin and the lining of vessels and small cavities. It consists of cells joined by small amounts of cementing substances and is classified according to the number of layers and the shape of the cells 上皮；**ciliated e.**, that bearing vibratile cilia on the free surface 纤毛上皮；**columnar e.**, that composed of columnar cells 柱状上皮；**cuboidal e.**, that composed of cuboidal cells 立方上皮；**glandular e.**, that composed of secreting cells 腺上皮；**olfactory e.**, pseudostratified epithelium lining the olfactory part of the nasal cavity and containing the receptors for the sense of smell 嗅上皮；**pseudostratified e.**, a type that looks stratified but is not, because its cells are arranged with their nuclei at different levels 假复层上皮；**sense e., sensory e.**, neuroepithelium (1) 感觉上皮；**simple e.**, that composed of a single layer of cells 单层上皮；**squamous e.**, that composed of squamous cells 扁平上皮；**stratified e.**, that composed of cells arranged in layers 复层上皮；**stratified squamous e.**, epithelium such as that of typical skin, having a basal layer of cuboidal cells and overlying layers of squamous cells 复层扁平上皮；**transitional e.**, a type often found lining hollow organs that are subject to great mechanical change due to contraction and distention; formerly thought to represent a transition between stratified squamous and columnar epithelium 变移上皮，移行上皮

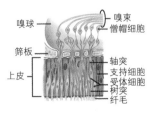

▲ 嗅上皮（**olfactory epithelium**）的受体

ep·i·tope (ep′ĭ-tōp) an antigenic determinant (see under determinant) of known structure 抗原表位，表位

ep·i·trich·i·um (ep″ĭ-trik′e-əm) periderm (1) 周皮

epi·troch·lea (ep″ĭ-trok′le-ə) the inner condyle of the humerus 肱骨内上髁

epi·tym·pan·ic (ep″ĭ-tim-pan′ik) 1. situated upon or over the tympanum 鼓室上的；2. pertaining to the epitympanum (epitympanic recess) 鼓室上隐窝的

epi·tym·pa·num (ep″ĭ-tim′pə-nəm) epitympanic recess 鼓室上隐窝

epler·e·none (ĕ-pler′ə-nōn) an aldosterone antagonist used for the treatment of hypertension 依普利酮

epo·e·tin (e-po′ə-tin) a recombinant form of human erythropoietin, used as an antianemic; in the United States the form used is e. alfa, but e. beta may be used elsewhere 红细胞生成素

ep·o·nych·i·um (ep″o-nik′e-əm) 1. cuticle; the narrow band of epidermis extending from the nail wall onto the nail surface 甲上皮；2. the horny fetal epidermis at the site of the future nail 胎儿角化皮层

ep·oöph·o·ron (ep″o-of′ə-rən) a vestigial structure associated with the ovary 卵巢冠

epo·pros·te·nol (e″po-pros′tə-nol) name for prostacyclin when used pharmaceutically; used in the form of the sodium salt as an inhibitor of platelet aggregation when blood contacts nonbiologic systems, a pulmonary antihypertensive, and a vasodilator 依前列醇

epox·ide (ə-pok′sīd) an organic compound containing a reactive group resulting from the union of an oxygen atom with two other atoms, usually carbon, that are themselves joined together 环氧化（合）物

epoxy (ə-pok′se) 1. epoxide 环氧化物；2. 环氧树脂，见 resin 下词条

EPP erythropoietic protoporphyria 红细胞生成性原卟啉病

ep·ro·sar·tan (ep″ro-sahr′tan) an angiotensin II antagonist used as the mesylate salt as an antihypertensive 依普沙坦

Ep·si·lon·pro·teo·bac·te·ria (ep″sĭ-lonpro″te-o-bak-tēr′e-ə) a class of bacteria of the Proteobacteria 变形菌纲

ep·ti·fib·a·tide (ep″tĭ-fib′ah-tīd) an inhibitor of platelet aggregation used for the prevention of thrombosis in patients with acute coronary syndrome or undergoing certain percutaneous coronary procedures 依替巴肽，血小板聚合抑制药

epu·lis (ə-pu′lis) pl. epu′lides [Gr.] 1. a nonspecific term used for tumors and tumorlike masses of the gingiva 龈瘤；2. peripheral ossifying fibroma 外周骨化纤维瘤；**giant cell e.**, a sessile or pedunculated lesion of the gingiva, representing an inflammatory reaction to injury or hemorrhage 巨细胞性牙龈瘤

equa·tion (e-kwa′zhən) an expression of equality

between two parts 方程；**Henderson-Hasselbalch e.**, a formula for calculating the pH of a buffer solution such as blood plasma Henderson-Hasselbalch 方程

equa·to·ri·al (e″kwə-tor′e-əl) 1. pertaining to an equator 赤道的；2. occurring at the same distance from each extremity of an axis 中纬线的

equi·ax·i·al (e″kwi-ak′se-əl) having axes of the same length 等轴的

equi·li·bra·tion (e-kwil″ĭ-bra′shən) the achievement of a balance between opposing elements or forces 平衡；**occlusal e.**, modification of the occlusal stress, to produce simultaneous occlusal contacts, or to achieve harmonious occlusion 殆平衡

equi·li·bri·um (e″kwĭ-lib′re-əm) 1. balance; harmonious adjustment of parts 平衡；2. sense of equilibrium 平衡感；**dynamic e.**, the condition of balance between varying, shifting, and opposing forces that is characteristic of living processes 动态平衡

equil·in (ek′wil-in) an estrogen in urine of pregnant mares 马烯雌酮

equine (e′kwīn) pertaining to, characteristic of, or derived from the horse 马的，似马的

equi·no·val·gus (e-kwi″no-val′gəs) talipes equinovalgus 马蹄外翻足

equi·no·va·rus (e-kwi″no-va′rəs) talipes equinovarus 马蹄内翻足

equi·po·ten·tial (e″kwĭ-po-ten′shəl) having similar and equal power or capability 等势的，等电位

equiv·a·lent (e-kwiv′ə-lent) 1. having the same value; neutralizing or counterbalancing each other 等量，2. 当量，见 *weight* 下词条；**migraine e.**, the presence of the aura associated with a migraine but in the absence of a headache 偏头痛等位发作

ER emergency room 急症室；endoplasmic reticulum 内质网；erythematotelangiectatic rosacea 红斑血管扩张玫瑰斑；estrogen receptor 雌激素受体

Er erbium 元素铒的符号

ERBF effective renal blood flow 有效肾血流量

er·bi·um (Er) (ur′be-əm) a silvery white, rare earth element; at. no. 68, at. wt. 167.259 铒（化学元素）

erec·tile (ə-rek′tīl) capable of erection 勃起

erec·tion (ə-rek′shən) the condition of being rigid and elevated, as erectile tissue when filled with blood 勃起

erec·tor (ə-rek′tər) [L.] a structure that erects, as a muscle that raises or holds up a part 勃起肌

erg (urg) a unit of work or energy, being the work performed when a force of 1 dyne moves its point of operation through a distance of 1 cm; equal to 10^{-7} joule 尔格，旧功或能量的单位，1 尔格等于 10^{-7} 焦耳

ERGIC endoplasmic reticulum–Golgi intermediate compartment 内质网 - 高尔基中间室

er·go·cal·cif·er·ol (ur″go-kal-sif′ər-ol) vitamin D_2; a sterol occurring in fungi and some fish oils or synthesized from ergosterol, with similar activity and metabolism to those of cholecalciferol; used as a dietary source of vitamin D and in the treatment of hypocalcemia, hypophosphatemia, rickets, and osteodystrophy associated with a variety of disorders 麦角钙化（固）醇，维生素 D_2

er·gom·e·ter (er-gom′ə-tər) a dynamometer 功率计；**bicycle e.**, an apparatus for measuring the muscular, metabolic, and respiratory effects of exercise 功率车

er·go·nom·ics (ur″go-nom′iks) the science relating to humans and their work, including the factors affecting the efficient use of human energy 工效学，人因学

er·go·no·vine (ur″go-no′vin) an alkaloid, from ergot or produced synthetically, used in the form of the maleate salt as an oxytocic and as a diagnostic aid in coronary vasospasm 麦角新碱

er·go·stat (ur′go-stat) a machine to be worked for muscular exercise 练肌器

er·gos·te·rol (ər-gos′tə-rol″) a sterol occurring mainly in yeast and forming ergocalciferol (vitamin D_2) on ultraviolet irradiation or electronic bombardment 麦角固醇

er·got (ur′got) a disease of cereals and other grasses caused by species of Claviceps, particularly that of rye caused by *C. purpurea*; also used to denote the causative fungus or its dried sclerotium. Ergot alkaloids have a variety of toxic and pharmaceutical effects 麦角

er·got·amine (ər-got′ə-min) an alkaloid of ergot; the tartrate salt is used for relief of migraine and cluster headaches 麦角胺

er·go·tism (ur′go-tiz-əm) poisoning from chronic excessive exposure to ergot alkaloids; occurring as a gangrenous form, affecting predominantly the lower limbs, and as a convulsive form, with spasms, cramps, and seizures; in both forms there initially may be gastrointestinal symptoms, paresthesias, and hallucinations 麦角中毒

eri·bu·lin (er″ĭ-bu′lin) a non taxane microtubule inhibitor used as the mesylate salt in the treatment of refractory, late-stage, metastatic carcinoma of the breast 一种非紫杉烷微管抑制药，其甲磺酸盐用于治疗难治性、晚期、转移性乳腺癌

er·lo·ti·nib (er-lo′tĭ-nib) a tyrosine kinase inhibitor used as the hydrochloride salt in the treatment of non–small-cell lung cancer and pancreatic cancer 埃罗替尼

erog·e·nous (ə-roj′ə-nəs) arousing erotic feelings 唤起情欲的

EROI epiphyseal region-of-interest 骨骺的
ero·sion (ə-ro′zhən) wearing away of a surface; a shallow or superficial ulceration; in dentistry, the wasting away or loss of tooth substance by a chemical process without known bacterial action 腐烂；腐蚀，侵蚀；**ero′sive** *adj.*
erot·ic (ə-rot′ik) 1. charged with sexual feeling 性爱的；2. pertaining to sexual desire 性欲的
er·o·tism (er′o-tiz″əm) a sexual instinct or desire; the expression of one's instinctual energy or drive, especially the sex drive 性兴奋，性爱倾向；**anal e.,** fixation of libido at (or regression to) the anal phase of infantile development; said to produce egotistic, dogmatic, stubborn, miserly character 肛欲；**genital e.,** achievement and maintenance of libido at the genital phase of psychosexual development, permitting acceptance of normal adult relationships and responsibilities 生殖器欲；**oral e.,** fixation of libido at the oral phase of infantile development; said to produce passive, insecure, sensitive character 口欲
ero·to·gen·ic (ə-rot″o-jen′ik) erogenous 动情的，引起性欲的
ero·to·ma·nia (ə-rot″o-ma′ne-ə) 1. a type of delusional disorder in which the subject harbors a delusion that a particular person is deeply in love with them; lack of response is rationalized, and pursuit and harassment may occur 钟情妄想；2. occasionally, hypersexuality 性欲过度；**erotoman′ic** *adj.*
ero·to·pho·bia (ə-rot″o-fo′be-ə) irrational fear of love, especially of sexual feelings and activities 爱情恐怖，性欲恐怖
ERP endocardial resection procedure 心内膜切除法
ERPF effective renal plasma flow 有效肾血浆流量
er·ror (er′ər) a defect in structure or function; a deviation 错误，结构功能紊乱，偏差；**inborn e. of metabolism,** a genetically determined biochemical disorder in which a specific enzyme defect causes a metabolic block that may have pathologic consequences at birth or in later life 先天性代谢缺陷；**refractive e.,** deviation from optimal focusing of light by the lens of the eye onto the retina 屈光不正
eru·cic ac·id (ə-roo′sik) a fatty acid occurring in rapeseed and mustard oils; because it has been linked to cardiac muscle damage, edible canola oil products are prepared from low erucic acid varieties of rapeseed plants（顺）芥子酸
eruc·ta·tion (ə-rək-ta′shən) belching; casting up wind from the stomach through the mouth 嗳气
erup·tion (ĕ-rup′shən) 1. the act of breaking out, appearing, or becoming visible, as eruption of the teeth 暴发；2. visible efflorescent lesions of the skin due to disease, with redness, prominence, or both; a

rash 发疹；**erup′tive** *adj.* **creeping e.,** cutaneous larva migrans 匐行疹；**drug e.,** an eruption or a solitary lesion caused by a drug taken internally 药疹；**fixed e.,** circumscribed inflammatory skin lesion(s) recurring at the same site(s) over a period of months or years; each attack lasts only a few days but leaves residual pigmentation, which is cumulative 固定疹
ERV expiratory reserve volume 补气量
er·y·sip·e·las (er″ə-sip′ə-ləs) an acute contagious type of cellulitis due to infection with *Streptococcus pyogenes*, with redness and swelling of affected areas, constitutional symptoms, and sometimes vesicular and bullous lesions 丹毒
er·y·sip·e·loid (er″ə-sip′ə-loid) a cellulitis of the hand seen in handlers of fish or meat products, caused by *Erysipelothrix insidiosa* 类丹毒
Ery·sip·e·lo·thrix (er″ə-sip′ə-lo-thriks″) a genus of gram-positive, non–spore-forming, rod-shaped bacteria of the family Erysipelotrichaceae, containing the single species *E. rhusiopath′iae*, which causes swine erysipelas and erysipeloid 丹毒丝菌属
Ery·si·pe·lo·tri·cha·ceae (er″ə-sip″ə-lo-trīka′se-e) a family of gram-positive, aerobic to anaerobic, rod-shaped bacteria of the class Mollicutes 丹毒丝菌科
er·y·the·ma (er″ə-the′mə) redness of the skin due to congestion of the capillaries 红斑；**erythem′a·tous, erythe′mic** *adj.* **e. annula′re,** a type of gyrate erythema with ring-shaped lesions 环形红斑；**e. annula′re centri′fugum,** a chronic variant of erythema multiforme usually affecting the thighs and lower legs, with single or multiple erythematousedematous papules that enlarge peripherally and clear in the center to produce annular lesions that may coalesce 离心性环状红斑；**e. chro′nicum mi′grans,** a deep form of gyrate erythema seen in Lyme disease. At the site of the tick bite a red papule develops and expands slowly, producing an annular lesion with central clearing 慢性游走性红斑；**cold e.,** a congenital hypersensitivity to cold seen in children, characterized by localized pain, widespread erythema, occasional muscle spasms, and vascular collapse on exposure to cold, and vomiting after drinking cold liquids 冷红斑；**gyrate e.,** erythema multiforme with lesions of different shapes that tend to spread peripherally with central clearing 回状红斑；**e. gyra′tum re′pens,** a superficial form of gyrate erythema, almost always associated with internal malignancy, characterized by migratory, elevated wavy bands over the entire body 匐行性回状红斑；**e. indura′tum,** a type of chronic necrotizing vasculitis, usually on the calves of young women and often associated with cutaneous tuberculosis 硬红斑；**e. infectio′sum,** a mildly contagious, sometimes

epidemic, disease of children between age 4 and 12, marked by a rose-colored, coarsely lacelike macular rash and caused by human parvovirus B19 传染性红斑; **e. margina′tum,** a superficial, often asymptomatic, form of gyrate erythema sometimes seen with rheumatic fever, characterized by a transient, slightly indurated eruption on the trunk and extensor surfaces of the limbs 边缘性红斑; **e. mi′grans,** 1. benign migratory glossitis 良性游走性舌炎; 2. e. chronicum migrans 慢性游走性环形红斑; **e. multifor′me,** a symptom complex with highly variable skin lesions, including macular papules, vesicles, and bullae; attacks are usually self-limited but recurrences are the rule 多形（性）红斑; **e. nodo′sum,** an acute inflammatory skin disease marked by tender red nodules, usually on the shins, due to exudation of blood and serum 结节性红斑; **e. nodo′sum lepro′sum,** a form of lepra reaction seen in lepromatous and sometimes borderline leprosy, marked by tender, inflamed subcutaneous nodules; the reactions resemble multifocal Arthus reactions 麻风结节性红斑; **e. tox′icum neonato′rum,** a self-limited urticarial condition affecting infants in the first few days of life 新生儿中毒性红斑

er·y·the·mo·gen·ic (er″ĭ-the″mo-jen′ik) producing erythema 引起红斑的

er·y·thras·ma (er″ə-thraz′mə) a chronic bacterial infection of the major skin folds due to *Corynebacterium minutissimum,* marked by red or brownish patches on the skin 红癣

er·y·thre·mia (er″ə-thre′me-ə) polycythemia vera 红细胞增多症

er·y·thre·mic (er″ə-thre′mik) pertaining to erythroid cells, particularly to those occurring in the blood in abnormal numbers or exhibiting abnormal development 红斑

eryth·ro·blast (ə-rith′ro-blast) originally, any nucleated erythrocyte, but now more generally used to designate a nucleated precursor cell in the erythrocytic series (q.v.). Four developmental stages in the series are recognized: the *proerythroblast* (q.v.), the *basophilic e.,* in which the cytoplasm is basophilic, the nucleus is large with clumped chromatin, and the nucleoli have disappeared; the *polychromatophilic e.,* in which the nuclear chromatin shows increased clumping and the cytoplasm begins to acquire hemoglobin and takes on an acidophilic tint; and the *orthochromatic e.,* the final stage before nuclear loss, in which the nucleus is small and ultimately becomes a blueblack, homogeneous, structureless mass 成红血细胞，成红细胞

eryth·ro·blas·to·ma (ə-rith″ro-blas-to′mə) a tumor-like mass composed of nucleated red blood cells 成红细胞瘤

eryth·ro·blas·to·pe·nia (ə-rith″ro-blas″tope′ne-ə) abnormal deficiency of erythroblasts 成红细胞减少症

eryth·ro·blas·to·sis (ə-rith″ro-blas-to′sis) the presence of erythroblasts in the circulating blood 成红细胞增多症; **erythroblastot′ic** *adj.*; **e. feta′lis,** 胎儿成红细胞增多症; **e. neonato′rum,** hemolytic anemia of the fetus or newborn due to transplacental transmission of maternally formed antibody against the fetus's erythrocytes, usually secondary to an incompatibility between the mother's Rh blood group and that of her offspring 新生儿成红细胞增多症

eryth·ro·chro·mia (ə-rith″ro-kro′me-ə) hemorrhagic, red pigmentation of the spinal fluid 脊（髓）液血色症

er·y·throc·la·sis (er″ə-throk′lə-sis) fragmentation of the red blood cells 红细胞破碎; **erythroclas′tic** *adj.*

eryth·ro·clast (ə-rith′ro-klast) ghost cell (2) 血影细胞

eryth·ro·cy·a·no·sis (ə-rith″ro-si″ə-no′sis) coarsely mottled bluish red discoloration on the legs and thighs, especially of girls; thought to be a circulatory reaction to exposure to cold 红绀病

eryth·ro·cy·ta·phe·re·sis (ə-rith″ro-si″tə-fə-re′sis) the withdrawal of blood, separation and retention of red blood cells, and retransfusion of the remainder into the donor 红细胞提取法

eryth·ro·cyte (ə-rith′ro-sīt) red blood cell; corpuscle; one of the formed elements in peripheral blood. Normally, in humans, the mature form is a non-nucleated, yellowish, biconcave disk, containing hemoglobin and transporting oxygen 红细胞; For immature forms, see *erythrocytic series,* under *series.* **basophilic e.,** an abnormal erythrocyte that takes basic stains, as seen in basophilia 嗜碱性红细胞; **hypochromic e.,** one that contains a less than normal concentration of hemoglobin and as a result appears paler than normal; it is usually also microcytic 低色素红细胞; **normochromic e.,** one of normal color with a normal concentration of hemoglobin 正常血色素红细胞; **polychromatic e.,** 多染性红细胞; **polychromatophilic e.,** one that, on staining, shows shades of blue combined with tinges of pink 嗜多染性红细胞; **target e.,** 靶红细胞，见 *cell* 下词条

eryth·ro·cy·the·mia (ə-rith″ro-si-the′me-ə) hypercythemia; an increase in the number of erythrocytes in the blood, as in erythrocytosis 红细胞增多症

eryth·ro·cyt·ic (ə-rith″ro-sit′ik) 1. pertaining to, characterized by, or of the nature of erythrocytes 红细胞的; 2. pertaining to the erythrocytic series 红

细胞系的

eryth·ro·cy·tol·y·sis (ə-rith″ro-si-tol′ə-sis) dissolution of erythrocytes and escape of the hemoglobin 红细胞溶解, 溶血

eryth·ro·cy·toph·a·gy (ə-rith″ro-si-tof′ə-je) erythrophagocytosis 噬红细胞现象

eryth·ro·cy·tor·rhex·is (ə-rith″ro-si″torek′sis) the escape from erythrocytes of round, shiny granules and the splitting off of particles 红细胞破碎

eryth·ro·cy·tos·chi·sis (ə-rith″ro-si-tos′kĭsis) degeneration of erythrocytes into plateletlike bodies 红细胞分裂

eryth·ro·cy·to·sis (ə-rith″ro-si-to′sis) increase in the total red cell mass secondary to any of a number of nonhematogenic systemic disorders in response to a known stimulus (*secondary polycythemia*), in contrast to primary polycythemia (*polycythemia vera*) 继发性红细胞增多症; **leukemic e.**, polycythemia vera 真性红细胞增多症; **stress e.**, 应激性红细胞增多, 见 *polycythemia* 下词条

eryth·ro·der·ma (ə-rith″ro-dur′mə) abnormal redness of the skin over widespread areas of the body 红皮病; **erythroder′mic** *adj.*; **congenital ichthyosiform e.**, a generalized hereditary dermatitis with scaling, which occurs in bullous (*epidermolytic hyperkeratosis*) and nonbullous (*lamellar ichthyosis*) forms 先天性鱼鳞状红皮病; **e. desquamati′vum**, Leiner disease 脱屑性红皮病; **psoriatic e.**, erythrodermic psoriasis 红皮病型银屑病

eryth·ro·don·tia (ə-rith″ro-don′shə) red to brown discoloration of the teeth 红牙

eryth·ro·gen·ic (ə-rith″ro-jen′ik) 1. producing erythrocytes 红细胞发生的; 2. producing a sensation of red 产生红色光觉的; 3. erythemogenic 引起红斑的

eryth·roid (ə-rith′roid) (er′ĭ-throid″) 1. of a red color; reddish 红色的; 2. pertaining to the cells of the erythrocytic series 红细胞系的

eryth·ro·ker·a·to·der·mia (ə-rith″ro-ker′ə-to-dur′me-ə) a reddening and hyperkeratosis of the skin 红角皮病; **e. varia′bilis**, a rare hereditary form of ichthyosis marked by transient, migratory areas of discrete, macular erythroderma as well as fixed hyperkeratotic plaques 可变性红角皮病

eryth·ro·ki·net·ics (ə-rith″ro-kĭ-net′iks) the quantitative, dynamic study of in vivo production and destruction of erythrocytes 红细胞动力学

eryth·ro·labe (ĕ-rith′ro-lāb) the pigment in retinal cones that is more sensitive to the red range of the spectrum than are the other pigments (chlorolabe and cyanolabe) 红敏素, 视红素

eryth·ro·leu·ke·mia (ə-rith″ro-loo-ke′me-ə) a malignant blood dyscrasia, one of the myeloproliferative disorders, with atypical erythroblasts and myeloblasts in the peripheral blood 红白血病

eryth·ro·mel·al·gia (ə-rith″ro-məl-al′jə) paroxysmal, bilateral vasodilation, particularly of the limbs, with burning pain and increased skin temperature and redness 红斑性肢痛病

eryth·ro·my·cin (ə-rith″ro-mi′sin) a broadspectrum antibiotic produced by *Streptomyces erythreus*; used against gram-positive bacteria and certain gram-negative bacteria, spirochetes, some rickettsiae, *Entamoeba*, and *Mycoplasma pneumoniae*; used in the form of the gluceptate, lactobionate, stearate, and other salts 红霉素

er·y·thron (er′ə-thron) the circulating erythrocytes in the blood, their precursors, and all the body elements concerned in their production 红细胞系

eryth·ro·neo·cy·to·sis (ə-rith″ro-ne″o-si-to′sis) presence of immature erythrocytes in the blood 幼稚红细胞（血）症

eryth·ro·pe·nia (ə-rith″ro-pe′ne-ə) deficiency in the number of erythrocytes 红细胞减少

eryth·ro·phage (ə-rith′ro-fāj) a phagocyte that ingests erythrocytes 噬红细胞

eryth·ro·phag·o·cy·to·sis (ə-rith″ro-fa″gosi-to′sis) the engulfment or consumption of erythrocytes 噬红细胞作用

eryth·ro·phil (ə-rith′ro-fil) 1. a cell or other element that stains easily with red 嗜红色的; 2. easily stained with red 红染细胞

eryth·ro·pho·bia (ə-rith″ro-fo′be-ə) 1. irrational fear of the color red, often accompanied by fear of blood (hematophobia) 害怕红色的; 2. fear of blushing; a distressing tendency to blush frequently 脸红恐怖症

eryth·ro·phose (ə-rith′ro-fōz) any red phose 红色幻视

eryth·ro·pla·kia (ə-rith″ro-pla′ke-ə) a slowgrowing, erythematous, velvety red lesion with well-defined margins, occurring on a mucous membrane, most often in the oral cavity 黏膜红斑病

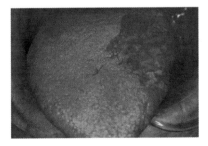

▲ 舌黏膜红斑（**erythroplakia**）

eryth·ro·pla·sia (ə-rith″ro-pla′zhə) a condition of the mucous membranes characterized by erythematous papular lesions 增殖性红斑；**e. of Queyrat**, penile intraepithelial neoplasia 凯拉增生性红斑

eryth·ro·poi·e·sis (ə-rith″ro-poi-e′sis) the formation of erythrocytes 红细胞发生；**erythropoiet′ic** adj.

eryth·ro·poi·e·tin (ə-rith″ro-poi′ə-tin) a glycoprotein hormone secreted by the kidney in the adult and by the liver in the fetus, which acts on stem cells of the bone marrow to stimulate red blood cell production (erythropoiesis) 红细胞生成素；**recombinant human e. (r-HuEPO)**, epoetin 重组人促红细胞生成素

eryth·ro·pros·o·pal·gia (ə-rith″ro-pros″opal′jə) a disorder similar to erythromelalgia, but with the redness and pain in the face 红斑性面痛

eryth·ror·rhex·is (ə-rith″ro-rek′sis) erythrocytorrhexis 红细胞（浆）进出

er·y·thro·sis (er″ə-thro′sis) 1. red to purple discoloration of the skin and mucous membranes, caused by capillary dilatation 皮肤红变；2. hyperplasia of the hematopoietic tissue 造红细胞组织增生

eryth·ro·sta·sis (ə-rith″ro-sta′sis) the stoppage of erythrocytes in the capillaries, as in sickle cell anemia 红细胞郁积

es·cape (əs-kāp′) the act of becoming free 脱逸；**atrioventricular junctional e.**, 房室交界区逸搏；**nodal e.**, one or more escape beats in which the atrioventricular node is the cardiac pacemaker 房室结性逸搏；**vagal e.**, the exhaustion of or adaptation to neural chemical mediators in the regulation of systemic arterial pressure 迷走神经脱逸；**ventricular e.**, the occurrence of one or more ectopic beats in which a ventricular pacemaker becomes effective before the pacemaker in the sinoatrial node 室性逸搏

es·char (es′kahr) 1. a slough produced by a thermal burn, by a corrosive application, or by gangrene 焦痂；2. tache noire 黑斑

es·cha·rot·ic (es″kə-rot′ik) an agent corrosive to tissue 腐蚀药

Esch·e·rich·ia (esh″ə-rik′e-ə) a widely distributed genus of gram-negative, facultatively anaerobic, rod-shaped bacteria of the family Enterobacteriaceae. Most species are nonpathogenic or opportunistic pathogens 埃希菌属；**E. co′li**, a species constituting the greater part of the normal intestinal flora of humans and other animals; most are nonpathogenic, but pathogenic strains causing pyogenic infections and diarrhea are common 大肠杆菌，大肠埃希菌

es·cutch·eon (es-kuch′ən) the pattern of distribution of the pubic hair 盾面

ESEM endoscopically suspected esophageal metaplasia 内镜检查怀疑食管化生

es·march (es′mahrk) Esmarch bandage 驱血绷带

es·mo·lol (es′mo-lol) a cardioselective β₁-blocker used as the hydrochloride salt as an antiarrhythmic in the short-term control of atrial fibrillation, atrial flutter, and noncompensatory sinus tachycardia 艾司洛尔

es·o·mep·ra·zole mag·ne·si·um (es″o-mep′rə-zōl) a proton pump inhibitor, administered orally as the magnesium salt in the treatment of gastroesophageal reflux disease and in the treatment of duodenal ulcer associated with *Helicobacter pylori* infection 埃索美拉唑镁

esoph·a·ge·al (ə-sof′ə-je′əl) of or pertaining to the esophagus 食管的

esoph·a·gism (ə-sof′ə-jiz-əm) spasm of the esophagus 食管痉挛

esoph·a·gi·tis (ə-sof′ə-ji′tis) inflammation of the esophagus 食管炎；**chronic peptic e.**, reflux e. 慢性消化性食管炎；**pill e.**, that resulting from irritation by a pill that passes too slowly through the esophagus 药物性食管炎；**reflux e.**, severe gastroesophageal reflux with damage to the esophageal mucosa, often with erosion and ulceration, and sometimes leading to stricture, scarring, and perforation 反流性食管炎

esoph·a·go·cele (ə-sof′ə-go-sēl″) abnormal distention of the esophagus; protrusion of the esophageal mucosa through a rupture in the muscular coat 食道疝

esoph·a·go·co·lo·plas·ty (ə-sof′ə-go-ko′loplas″te) excision of a portion of esophagus and its replacement by a segment of colon 食管结肠成形术

esoph·a·go·esoph·a·gos·to·my (ə-sof″ə-go-ə-sof″ə-gos′tə-me) anastomosis between two formerly remote parts of the esophagus 食管吻合术

esoph·a·go·gas·tric (ə-sof″ə-go-gas′trik) gastroesophageal (1) 食管和胃的

esoph·a·go·gas·tro·du·od·enos·co·py (EGD) (ə-sof″ə-go-gas″tro-doo″od-ə-nos′kə-pe) endoscopic examination of the esophagus, stomach, and duodenum 食道胃十二指肠镜检

esoph·a·go·gas·tro·plas·ty (ə-sof″ə-gogas′tro-plas″te) plastic repair of the esophagus and stomach 食管胃成形术

esoph·a·go·gas·tros·to·my (ə-sof″ə-go-gas-tros′tə-me) anastomosis of the esophagus to the stomach 食管胃吻合术

esoph·a·go·je·ju·nos·to·my (ə-sof-ə-goje′joo-nos′tə-me) anastomosis of the esophagus to the jejunum 食管空肠吻合术

esoph·a·go·my·ot·o·my (ə-sof″ə-go-miot′ə-me) incision through the muscular coat of the esophagus 食管肌层切开术

esoph·a·go·res·pi·ra·to·ry (ə-sof″ə-gores′pī-rə-tor″e) pertaining to or communicating with the esophagus and respiratory tract (trachea or a bronchus) 食管气道的

esoph·a·gos·co·py (ə-sof″ə-gos′ko-pe) endoscopic examination of the esophagus 食管镜检查（术）

esoph·a·go·ste·no·sis (ə-sof″ə-go-stə-no′sis) stricture of the esophagus 食管狭窄

esoph·a·got·o·my (ə-sof″ə-got′ə-me) incision of the esophagus 食管切开术

esoph·a·gus (ə-sof′ə-gəs) the musculomembranous passage extending from the pharynx to the stomach 食管

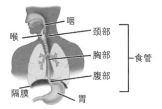

▲ 食管（esophagus），子宫颈，胸廓的和腹部

eso·pho·ria (es″o-fo′re-ə) deviation of the visual axis toward that of the other eye in the absence of visual fusional stimuli 内隐斜

eso·tro·pia (es″o-tro′pe-ə) cross-eye; deviation of the visual axis of one eye toward that of the other eye 内斜视；**esotrop′ic** *adj.*

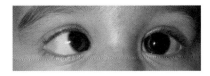

▲ 内斜视（esotropia）

ESR erythrocyte sedimentation rate 红细胞沉降率

ESRD end-stage renal disease 终末期肾病

es·sence (es′əns) 1. that which is or necessarily exists as the cause of the properties of a body 实质；2. in traditional Chinese medicine, jing (q.v.) 精气神（中医）；3. a solution of a volatile oil in alcohol 香精

es·sen·tial (ə-sen′shəl) 1. constituting the inherent part of a thing; giving a substance its peculiar and necessary qualities 本质；2. indispensable; required in the diet, as essential fatty acids 必需品；3. idiopathic; having no obvious external cause 特发性

EST electroshock therapy 电休克疗法

es·ter (es′tər) a compound formed from an alcohol and an acid by removal of water 酯

es·ter·ase (es′tər-ās) any enzyme that catalyzes the hydrolysis of an ester into its alcohol and acid 酯酶

es·ter·i·fy (es-ter′ĭ-fi) to combine with an alcohol with elimination of a molecule of water, forming an ester 酯化

es·ter·ol·y·sis (es″tər-ol′ə-sis) the hydrolysis of an ester into its alcohol and acid 灌肠；**esterolyt′ic** *adj.*

es·the·si·ol·o·gy (es-the″ze-ol′ə-je) the scientific study or description of the sense organs and sensations 感觉学

es·the·sod·ic (es″thə-zod′ik) conducting or pertaining to conduction of sensory impulses 感觉传导的

es·thet·ics (es-thet′iks) in dentistry, a philosophy concerned especially with the appearance of a dental restoration, as achieved through its color or form 牙科美学

es·ti·mate[1] (es′tĭ-mət) 1. a rough calculation or one based on incomplete data 估计；2. a statistic used to characterize the value of a population parameter 用来表示总体参数值的统计量

es·ti·mate[2] (es′tĭ-māt) 1. to produce or use a rough calculation 粗略计算产生或使用粗略的计算；2. to measure or calculate a statistic for characterization of a population parameter 测量或计算用于描述总体参数的统计量

es·ti·ma·tor (es′tĭ-ma″tər) estimate[1] (2)

es·tra·di·ol (es″trə-di′ol) (es-tra′de-ol) the most potent estrogen in humans; pharmacologically, it is often used in the form of its esters (e.g., e. cypionate, e. valerate) or as a semisynthetic derivative (ethinyl e.) 雌二醇，有关属性和用途见 *estrogen*

es·tra·mus·tine (es″trə-mus′tēn) an antineoplastic containing estradiol joined to mechlorethamine, used for palliative treatment of metastatic or progressive carcinoma of the prostate; used as *e. phosphate sodium* 雌二醇氮芥

es·trin (es′trin) estrogen 雌二醇

es·tri·ol (es′tre-ol) a relatively weak human estrogen (q.v.), being a metabolic product of estradiol and estrone found in high concentrations in urine, especially during pregnancy 雌三醇

es·tro·gen (es′trə-jen) a generic term for estrus-producing compounds; the female sex hormones, including estradiol, estriol, and estrone. In humans, the estrogens are formed in the ovary, adrenal cortex, testis, and fetoplacental unit; they are responsible for female secondary sex characteristic development and, during the menstrual cycle, act on the female genitalia to produce an environment suitable for fertilization, implantation, and nutrition of the early embryo. Uses for estrogens include oral contraceptives, hormone replacement therapy, advanced prostate or postmenopausal breast carcinoma treatment, and osteoporosis prophylaxis 雌激素；**conjugated e's,** a mixture of the sodium salts of the sulfate esters of estrone and equilin, having the actions and uses of estrogens 结合雌激素；**esterified e's,** a mixture of the sodium salts of esters of estrogenic substances, principally estrone; the uses are those of estrogens 酯化雌激素

es·tro·gen·ic (es-tro-jen′ik) 1. estrus-producing; having the properties of, or similar to, an estrogen 雌激素的；2. pertaining to, having the effects of, or similar to an estrogen 与雌激素有关的

es·trone (es′trōn) an estrogen isolated from pregnancy urine, human placenta, palm kernel oil, and other sources, also prepared synthetically 雌酮；有关属性和用途见 *estrogen*

es·tro·phil·in (es″tro-fil′in) a cell protein that acts as a receptor for estrogen, found in estrogenic target tissue and in estrogen-dependent tumors and metastases 亲雌激素蛋白

es·tro·pi·pate (es′tro-pī-pāt) a compound of estrone sulfate and piperazine; used as an estrogen 硫酸雌酮哌嗪

ESV end-systolic volume 收缩末期容积

eta·ner·cept (e-tan′ər-sept) a soluble tumor necrosis factor receptor that inactivates tumor necrosis factor, used in the treatment of rheumatoid arthritis etanercept，用于治疗类风湿关节炎

ETF electron-transferring flavoprotein 电子传送黄素蛋白

eth·a·cryn·ate (eth″ah-krin′āt) a salt, ester, or the conjugate base of ethacrynic acid; the sodium salt has the same actions as the acid 利尿酸盐

eth·a·cryn·ic ac·id (eth″ə-krin′ik) a loop diuretic used in the treatment of edema, including that associated with congestive heart failure or hepatic or renal disease, ascites, and hypertension 利尿酸

etham·bu·tol (ə-tham′bu-tol) an antibacterial, specifically effective against *Mycobacterium*; used with one or more other antituberculous drugs in the treatment of pulmonary tuberculosis, administered as the hydrochloride salt 乙胺丁醇片

eth·a·nol (eth′ə-nol) ethyl alcohol; a primary alcohol formed by microbial fermentation of carbohydrates or by synthesis from ethylene. Excessive ingestion results in acute intoxication, and ingestion during pregnancy can harm the fetus. The pharmaceutical preparation is called *alcohol* 乙醇

eth·a·nol·amine (eth″ə-nol′ə-mēn) monoethanolamine 乙醇胺；**e. oleate,** the oleate salt of monoethanolamine, used as a sclerosing agent in treatment of varicose veins and esophageal varices

乙醇胺油酸酯

ether (e′thər) 1. an organic compound having an oxygen atom bonded to two carbon atoms; R–O–R′ 醚，结构式为 R–O–R′ 的化合物；2. $C_2H_5OC_2H_5$ (*diethyl* or *ethyl e.*); the first inhalational anesthetic used for surgical anesthesia, now little used because of its flammability 乙醚

ethe·re·al (ə-the′re-əl) 1. pertaining to, prepared with, containing, or resembling ether 有关醚的，用醚制备的，含有醚的或类似醚的；2. evanescent; delicate 挥发性的

eth·i·nyl (eth′ī-nəl) the radical HC≡C–, derived from acetylene 乙炔基；**e. estradiol,** a semisynthetic derivative of estradiol; used in combination with a progestational agent as an oral contraceptive, in hormone replacement therapy, and as an antineoplastic in the treatment of advanced breast and prostate cancers 乙炔雌二醇

ethi·on·am·ide (ə-thi″ən-am′īd) an antibacterial, effective against *Mycobacterium tuberculosis*; used in the treatment of pulmonary tuberculosis 乙硫异烟胺

eth·mo·fron·tal (eth″mo-fron′təl) pertaining to the ethmoid and frontal bones 筛额的

eth·moid (eth′moid) 1. sievelike 筛骨；见 *bone* 下 *ethmoid bone*；2. ethmoidal 筛骨的

eth·moi·dal (eth-moi′dəl) of or pertaining to the ethmoid bone; *ethmoid* 筛骨的

eth·moid·ec·to·my (eth″moid-ek′tə-me) excision of ethmoidal cells or of a portion of the ethmoid bone 筛窦切除术

eth·moid·ot·o·my (eth″moi-dot′ə-me) incision into the ethmoid sinus 筛窦切开术

eth·mo·max·il·lary (eth″mo-mak′sī-lar-e) pertaining to the ethmoid and maxillary bones 筛颌的

eth·mo·tur·bi·nal (eth″mo-tur′bi-nəl) pertaining to the superior and middle nasal conchae 筛鼻甲的

eth·nic (eth′nik) pertaining to a group sharing cultural bonds or physical characteristics 种族的

eth·no·bi·ol·o·gy (eth″no-bi-ol′ə-je) the study of the interaction between cultural groups and the plant and animal life in their environment 人种生物学

eth·no·bot·a·ny (eth″no-bot′ə-ne) the systematic study of the interactions between a culture and the plants in its environment, particularly the knowledge about and use of such plants 民族植物学

eth·nol·o·gy (eth-nol′ə-je) the science dealing with the major cultural groups of humans, their descent, relationship, etc 人种学

eth·no·med·i·cine (eth″no-med′ī-sin) medical systems based on the cultural beliefs and practices of specific ethnic groups 民族药；**ethnomed′ical** *adj.*

eth·no·phar·ma·col·o·gy (eth″no-fahr″mə-kol′ə-je) the systematic study of the use of medicinal plants by specific cultural groups 传统药理学

ethol·o·gy (e-thol′ə-je) the scientific study of animal behavior, particularly in the natural state 习性学; **etholog′ical** *adj.*

etho·pro·pa·zine (eth″o-pro′pah-zēn) an antidyskinetic used as the hydrochloride salt in the treatment of parkinsonism and for the control of drug-induced extrapyramidal reactions 普罗吩胺

etho·sux·i·mide (eth″o-suk′sĭ-mīd) an anticonvulsant used in the treatment of seizures in absence epilepsy 乙琥胺

etho·to·in (eth′o-to″in) an anticonvulsant used in the treatment of grand mal epilepsy and temporal lobe epilepsy 乙基苯妥英

eth·yl (eth′əl) the monovalent radical, C_2H_5 乙烷基; **e. chloride,** a local anesthetic sprayed on intact skin to produce anesthesia by superficial freezing caused by its rapid evaporation 氯乙烷

eth·yl·cel·lu·lose (eth″əl-sel′u-lōs) an ethyl ether of cellulose; used as a pharmaceutical tablet binder 乙基纤维素

eth·y·lene (eth′ə-lēn) a colorless flammable gas, $CH_2=CH_2$, with a slightly sweet odor and taste; formerly used as an inhalation anesthetic 乙烯; **e. dibromide,** a fumigant and gasoline additive; it is a skin and mucous membrane irritant and is carcinogenic 二溴化乙烯; **e. dichloride,** a solvent, gasoline additive, and intermediate; it is irritating and toxic, and can be carcinogenic 二氯化乙烯; **e. glycol,** a solvent used as an antifreeze; ingestion can cause central nervous system depression, vomiting, hypotension, coma, convulsions, and death 乙二醇; **e. oxide,** a gas used in manufacturing organic compounds and as a fumigant, fungicide, and sterilizing agent; it is highly irritating to the eyes and mucous membranes and is carcinogenic 环氧乙烷

eth·y·lene·di·a·mine (eth″ə-lēn-di′ə-mēn) a clear liquid with an ammonialike odor and a strong alkaline reaction; complexed with theophylline it forms aminophylline 乙二胺

eth·y·lene·di·a·mine·tet·ra·a·ce·tic ac·id (EDTA) (eth″ə-lēn-di′ə-mēn-tet″rə-ə-se′tik) a chelating agent that binds calcium and other metals, used as an anticoagulant for preserving blood specimens; also used to treat lead poisoning and hypercalcemia (see *edetate*) 乙二胺四乙酸

eth·yl·i·dene (eth′əl-ĭ-dēn) the bivalent radical CH_3CH.; its chloride derivative is used as a solvent and fumigant and is toxic and irritant 亚乙基

eth·yl·nor·epi·neph·rine (eth″əl-nor-ep″ĭnef′rin) a synthetic adrenergic, used as the hydrochloride

salt in treatment of bronchial asthma 乙基去甲肾上腺素

ethy·no·di·ol (ə-thi″no-di′ol) a progestational agent used, as the diacetate salt, in combination with an estrogen component as an oral contraceptive 炔诺醇

eti·do·caine (ə-te′do-kān) a local anesthetic used as the hydrochloride salt for infiltration anesthesia, peripheral nerve block, retrobulbar block, and epidural block 依替卡因

eti·dro·nate (e-tĭ-dro′nāt) a diphosphonate compound used for treatment of osteitis deformans, heterotopic ossification, and neoplasmassociated hypercalcemia, usually as the disodium salt. Complexed with technetium 99m it is also used in bone scanning 羟乙二膦酸

eti·ol·o·gy (e″te-ol′ə-je) 1. the science dealing with causes of disease 病因学; 2. the cause of a disease 病原学; **etiolog′ic, etiolog′ical** *adj.*

ET-NANB enterically transmitted non-A, non-B 肠道传播性非甲非乙型肝炎; 见 *hepatitis* 下 *hepatitis* E

eto·do·lac (e-to-do′lak) a nonsteroidal antiinflammatory drug used as an analgesic and antiinflammatory, especially to treat arthritis 依托度酸

etom·i·date (ə-tom′ĭ-dāt) a sedative-hypnotic, administered intravenously for the induction and maintenance of anesthesia 依托咪酯

eto·po·side (e″to-po′sīd) a semisynthetic derivative of podophyllotoxin used as the base or the phosphate salt as an antineoplastic, particularly for treating testicular tumors and small cell lung carcinoma 依托泊苷

Eu europium 元素铕的符号

Eu″bac·te·ri·a·ceae (u″bak-tēr″e-a′se-e) a family of gram-positive, anaerobic, rod-shaped bacteria of the order Clostridiales 优杆菌科

Eu·bac·te·ri·um (u″bak-te′re-əm) a genus of gram-positive, anaerobic, rod-shaped bacteria of the family Eubacteriaceae, found as saprophytes in soil and water and as normal inhabitants of human skin and cavities, occasionally causing soft tissue infection 真细菌属

eu·ca·lyp·tol (u″kə-lip′tol) the chief constituent of eucalyptus oil, also obtained from other oils, and used as a flavoring agent, expectorant, and local anesthetic 桉树脑

eu·cap·nia (u-kap′ne-ə) normal carbon dioxide tension of the blood 血碳酸正常

eu·chlor·hy·dria (u″klor-hi′dre-ə) the presence of the normal amount of hydrochloric acid in the gastric juice 胃液盐酸正常

eu·cho·lia (u-ko′le-ə) normal condition of the bile

胆汁正常

eu·chro·ma·tin (u-kro′mə-tin) chromatin that is genetically active and constitutes the majority of the chromosomes; it is relatively uncoiled and stains lightly during interphase and condenses and stains more darkly during nuclear division 常染色质; **euchromat′ic** *adj.*

eu·cra·sia (u-kra′zhə) 1. a state of health; proper balance of different factors constituting a healthy state 健康状况; 2. a state in which the body reacts normally to ingested or injected drugs, proteins, etc 对摄入或注射的药物、蛋白质等作出正常反应的状态

eu·gen·ol (u′jən-ol) a dental analgesic and antiseptic obtained from clove oil or other natural sources; applied topically to dental cavities and also used as a component of dental protectives 丁香油酚

eu·glob·u·lin (u-glob′u-lin) one of a class of globulins characterized by being insoluble in water but soluble in saline solutions 优球蛋白

eu·gly·ce·mia (u″gli-se′me-ə) normal glucose content of the blood 血糖正常; **euglyce′mic** *adj.*

eu·gon·ic (u-gon′ik) growing luxuriantly; said of bacterial cultures 生长旺盛的

Eu·kar·ya (u-kar′e-ə) Eukaryota 真核生物

eu·kary·o·sis (u″kar-e-o′sis) the state of having a true nucleus 真核形成

Eu·kary·o·ta (u-kar″e-o′tə) the domain that includes all eukaryotic organisms: plants, animals, fungi, and protists; it excludes Archaea and Bacteria 真核生物

eu·kary·ote (u-kar′e-ōt) a member of the Eukaryota: plants, animals, fungi, and protists. Cells have a true nucleus bounded by a nuclear membrane, within which lie the chromosomes, and divide by mitosis; the cells contain membrane-bound organelles, in which cellular functions are performed, and are supported by a cytoskeleton 真核生物。Cf. *prokaryote*; **eukaryot′ic** *adj.*

eu·lam·i·nate (u-lam′ ĭ-nāt) having the normal number of laminae, as certain areas of the cerebral cortex 层数正常的

eu·men·or·rhea (u″mən-o-re′ə) normal menstruation 月经正常

eu·me·tria (u-me′tre-ə) [Gr.] a normal condition of nerve impulse, so that a voluntary movement just reaches the intended goal; the proper range of movement 神经冲动正常

Eu·my·co·ta (u″mi-ko′tə) in some systems of classification, a division of the Fungi, the true fungi; organisms whose trophic phase is not motile but whose reproductive cells may be motile 真菌门

eu·nuch (u′nək) a male deprived of the testes or external genitals, especially one castrated before puberty (so that male secondary sex characteristics fail to develop) 没有睾丸或外生殖器的男性，尤指青春期前被阉割的男性（因此男性的第二性征无法发育）

eu·nuch·oid·ism (u′nə-koi″diz-əm) hypogonadism in a male; deficiency of the testes or of their secretion, with deficient secondary sex characters 类无睾症; **female e.**, hypogonadism in which the ovaries fail to function at puberty, resulting in infertility, absence of development of secondary sex characteristics, infantile sexual organs, and excessive growth of the long bones 女性类无睾症; **hypergonadotropic e.**, 促性腺激素亢进性类无睾症; 见 *hypogonadism* 下词条; **hypogonadotropic e.**, 促性腺激素不足性类无睾症, 见 *hypogonadism* 下词条

eu·pep·sia (u-pep′se-ə) good digestion; the presence of a normal amount of pepsin in the gastric juice 消化正常; **eupep′tic** *adj.*

Eu·phor·bia (u-for′be-ə) a large genus of trees, shrubs, and herbs of the family Euphorbiaceae, whose sap is emetic and cathartic and in some species poisonous 大戟属

eu·pho·ria (u-for′e-ə) an exaggerated feeling of physical and mental well-being, especially when not justified by external reality 欣快; **euphor′ic** *adj.*

eu·plas·tic (u-plas′tik) readily becoming organized; adapted to the formation of tissue, as in embryonic development or wound healing 适于组织形成的

eu·ploid (u′ploid) having an exact multiple of the haploid number (*n*) of chromosomes 整倍体

eup·nea (ūp-ne′ə) normal respiration. **eupne′ic** *adj.* 平静呼吸

eu·rhyth·mia (u-rith′me-ə) harmonious relationships in body or organ development 发育均匀

eu·ro·pi·um (Eu) (u-ro′pe-əm) a bright, silvery, rare earth element; at. no. 63, at. wt. 151.964 铕

eu·ry·bleph·a·ron (u″re-blef′ə-ron) horizontally elongated palpebral aperture with decreased eyelid skin vertically, which may cause outward displacement of the eyelid and ectropion 睑赘皮

eu·ry·ce·phal·ic (u″re-sə-fal′ik) having a wide head 阔头的

eu·ry·on (u′re-on) a point on either parietal bone marking either end of the greatest transverse diameter of the skull 颅宽点, 颅侧点, 头侧点

eu·tha·na·sia (u″thə-na′zhə) 安乐死 1. an easy or painless death; 2. the deliberate ending of life of a person suffering from an incurable and painful disease

eu·thy·mia (u-thi′me-ə) [eu- + Gr. thymos mind] 1. a neutral mood, neither depressed nor manic, in

E

those with bipolar disorder 情感正常；2. a state of mental tranquility and well-being 一种精神上的安宁和幸福的状态

eu·to·cia (u-to′shə) normal labor, or childbirth 正常分娩

eu·top·ic (u-top′ik) situated normally; arising from the normal site or tissue 位置正常的，正位的

Eu·trom·bic·u·la (u″trom-bik′u-lə) a subgenus of *Trombicula; E. alfreddugèsi* is the most common chigger of the United States 真恙螨亚属

eu·tro·phia (u-tro′fe-ə) a state of normal (good) nutrition 富营养化；**eutroph′ic** *adj.*

eu·vo·le·mia (u-vo-le′me-ə) normovolemia 等容量；**euvolemic** *adj.*

eV electron volt 电子伏特

evac·u·ant (e-vak′u-ənt) 1. emptying 排空；2. cathartic (1, 2) 泻药；3. a remedy that empties any organ, such as a cathartic, emetic, or diuretic 排毒药，排空任何器官的药物，如泻药、止吐药或利尿药

evac·u·a·tion (e-vak″u-a′shən) 1. an emptying 排空；2. catharsis; emptying of the bowels 排泄

evag·i·na·tion (e-vaj″ĭ-na′shən) obtrusion of a layer or part to form a pouch 眼袋形成

even·tra·tion (e″ven-tra′shən) 1. protrusion of abdominal viscera 腹脏突出；2. removal of the abdominal viscera 腹脏除去法；**diaphragmatic e.**, a congenital anomaly characterized by failure of muscular development of part or all of one (or occasionally both) hemidiaphragms, resulting in superior displacement of abdominal viscera and altered lung development 膈膨升

ever·sion (e-vur′zhən) a turning inside out; a turning outward 外翻

evis·cer·a·tion (e-vis″ər-a′shən) 1. removal of viscera 除脏术；2. extrusion of viscera outside the body 将内脏挤出体外；3. removal of the contents of the eyeball while leaving the sclera 眼球内容物在离开巩膜时被摘除

evo·ca·tion (ev″o-ka′shən) the calling forth of morphogenetic potentialities through contact with organizer material 通过与组织材料的接触，激发形态发生潜能

evo·ca·tor (ev′o-ka″tər) a chemical substance emitted by an organizer that evokes a specific morphogenetic response from competent embryonic tissue in contact with it 诱发物

evo·lu·tion (ev″ə-loo′shən) a developmental process in which an organ or organism becomes more and more complex by differentiation of its parts; a continuous and progressive change according to certain laws and by means of resident forces 进化；**convergent e.**, the appearance of similar forms and/or functions in two or more lines not sufficiently related phylogenetically to account for the similarity 趋同进化；**organic e.**, the origin and development of species; the theory that existing organisms are the result of descent with modification from those of past times 生物进化

evul·sion (e-vul′shən) extraction by force 拔去

exa- a word element used in naming units of measurement to designate a quantity 10^{18} (a quintillion, or million million million) times the unit to which it is joined. Symbol E 一种单词元素，用于给度量单位命名，表示 10^{18}。符号 E

ex·am·i·na·tion (eg-zam″ĭ-na′shən) inspection or investigation, especially as a means of diagnosing disease 检查

ex·an·them (eg-zan′thəm) 皮疹 1. any eruptive disease or fever；2. an eruption characterizing an eruptive fever

ex·an·the·ma (eg″zan-the′mə) pl. *exanthemas, exanthem′ata* [Gr.] exanthem 疹；**e. su′bitum,** an acute but mild viral disease of children, with high fever for about 3 days, followed by a rash on the trunk; caused by human herpesvirus 6 幼儿急疹

ex·an·them·a·tous (eg″zan-them′ə-təs) characterized by or of the nature of an eruption or rash 发疹的

ex·ar·tic·u·la·tion (eks″ahr-tik″u-la′shən) disarticulation 脱臼

ex·ca·la·tion (eks″kə-la′shən) absence or exclusion of one member of a normal series, such as a vertebra 部分缺失

ex·ca·va·tio (eks″kə-va′she-o) pl. *excavatio′nes* [L.] excavation 陷凹

ex·ca·va·tion (eks″kə-va′shən) 1. the act of hollowing out 挖除；2. a hollowed-out space or pouchlike cavity 空腔；**dental e.**, removal of carious material from a tooth in preparation for filling 龋质挖除，去除牙齿上的龋病物质，以备充填

ex·cess (ek-ses′) (ek′ses) a surplus, an amount greater than that which is normal or that which is required 过量；**antigen e.**, the presence of more than enough antigen to saturate all available antibody binding sites 抗原过剩

ex·change (eks-chānj′) 1. the substitution of one thing for another 用一个东西替换另一个东西；2. to substitute one thing for another 用一种东西代替另一种东西；**plasma e.,** the removal of plasma from withdrawn blood, with retransfusion of the formed elements into the donor; done for removal of circulating antibodies or abnormal plasma constituents. The plasma removed is replaced by type-specific frozen plasma or by albumin 血浆置换

ex·chang·er (eks-chānj′ər) an apparatus by which something may be exchanged 交换器；**heat e.**, a device placed in the circuit of extracorporeal circulation to induce rapid cooling and rewarming of blood 热交换器

ex·cip·i·ent (ek-sip′e-ənt) any more or less inert substance added to a drug to give suitable consistency or form to the drug; a vehicle 赋形剂，辅料

ex·cise (ek-sīz′) to remove by cutting 切除

ex·ci·sion (ek-sizh′ən) resection; removal of a portion or all of an organ or other structure 切除；**excis′ional** *adj.*

ex·ci·ta·ble (ek-sīt′ə-bəl) irritable (1) 应激的

ex·ci·ta·tion (ek″si-ta′shən) 1. irritation or stimulation 刺激；2. the addition of energy, such as excitation of a molecule by absorption of photons 能量的增加，如通过吸收光子来激发分子；**direct e.**, electrostimulation of a muscle by placing the electrode on the muscle itself 直接激发；**indirect e.**, electrostimulation of a muscle by placing the electrode on its nerve 间接激发

ex·ci·tor (ek-si′tər) a nerve that stimulates a part to greater activity 刺激神经

ex·clave (eks′klāv) a detached part of an organ 器官游离部分

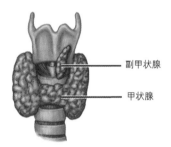

副甲状腺

甲状腺

▲ 副甲状腺是甲状腺的游离部分（**exclave**）

ex·clu·sion (eks-kloo′zhən) 1. a shutting out or elimination 排除或淘汰；2. surgical isolation of a part, as of a segment of intestine, without removal from the body 不从体内取出的外科分离部分，如肠的一部分

ex·coch·le·a·tion (eks-kok″le-a′shən) curettement of a cavity 刮除术

ex·co·ri·a·tion (eks-ko″re-a′shən) scratch (3) 抓痕

ex·cre·ment (eks′krə-mənt) 1. feces 粪便；2. excretion (2) 排泄物

ex·cres·cence (eks-kres′əns) an abnormal outgrowth; a projection of morbid origin 赘生物；**excres′cent** *adj.*

ex·cre·ta (eks-kre′tə) excretion (2) 排泄物

ex·crete (eks-krēt′) to throw off or eliminate by a normal discharge, such as waste matter 排泄；分泌

ex·cre·tion (eks-kre′shən) 1. the act, process, or function of excreting 排泄；2. material that is excreted 排泄物；**ex′cretory** *adj.*

ex·cur·sion (eks-kur′zhən) a range of movement regularly repeated in performance of a function, e.g., excursion of the jaws in mastication 移动，如咀嚼时下颌的偏移；**excur′sive** *adj.*

ex·cy·clo·pho·ria (ek-si″klo-for′e-ə) cyclophoria in which the upper pole of the visual axis deviates toward the temple 外旋转隐斜视

ex·cy·clo·tro·pia (ek-si″klo-tro′pe-ə) cyclotropia in which the upper pole of the visual axis deviates toward the temple 外旋转斜视

ex·cys·ta·tion (ek″sis-ta′shən) escape from a cyst or envelope, as in that stage in the life cycle of parasites occurring after the cystic form has been swallowed by the host 脱囊

exe·mes·tane (ek″sə-mes′tān) an aromatase inactivator related to androstenedione; used as an antineoplastic 依西美坦

ex·en·a·tide (ek-sen′ə-tīd) a glucagon-like peptide 1 receptor agonist that stimulates insulin secretion, used in the treatment of type 2 diabetes mellitus 艾塞那肽

ex·en·ter·a·tion (ek-sen″tər-a′shən) 1. extensive evisceration of organs and nearby structures 去脏术；2. in ophthalmology, removal of the entire contents of the orbit 在眼科学中，去除眼眶的全部内容物；**pelvic e.**, excision of the organs and adjacent structures of the pelvis 盆腔廓清术

ex·en·ter·a·tive (ek-sen′tər-ə-tiv) pertaining to or requiring exenteration, as exenterative surgery 去脏术的，挖出术的

ex·er·cise (ek′sər-sīz) performance of physical exertion for improvement of health or correction of physical deformity 运动；**active e.**, motion imparted to a part by voluntary contraction and relaxation of its controlling muscles 主动运动；**aerobic e.**, that designed to increase oxygen consumption and improve functioning of the cardiovascular and respiratory systems 有氧训练；**endurance e.**, one that involves the use of several large groups of muscles and is thus dependent on the delivery of oxygen to the muscles by the cardiovascular system 耐力运动；**isokinetic e.**, active exercise performed at a constant angular velocity; torque and tension remain constant while muscles shorten or lengthen 等速运动；**isometric e.**, active exercise performed against stable resistance, without change in the length of the muscle 等长运动；**isotonic e.**, active exercise without appreciable change in the force of muscular contraction, with shortening of the muscle 等 张 运 动；**Kegel e's,** exercises performed to strengthen the pubococcygeal muscle Kegel 运 动；**passive e.,** motion imparted to a part by another person or outside force, or produced by voluntary effort of another segment of the patient's own body 被动运动；**range-of-motion e.,** the putting of a joint through its full range of normal movements, either actively or passively 关节活动范围练习；**resistance e.,** 抗阻运动；**resistive e.,** that performed by the patient against resistance, as from a weight 阻力运动

ex·flag·el·la·tion (eks-flaj′ə-la′shən) the rapid formation in the gut of the insect vector of microgametes from the microgamont in *Plasmodium* and certain other sporozoan protozoa 出丝；小配子形成

ex·fo·li·a·tion (eks-fo″le-a′shən) 1. a falling off in scales or layers 表皮剥脱；2. the removal of scales or flakes from the surface of the skin 有质剥脱术；3. the normal loss of primary teeth after loss of their root structure 正常的乳牙脱落后，其根结构也随之脱落；**exfo′liative** *adj.*；**lamellar e. of newborn,** the condition in a minority of collodion babies when shedding of the membrane leaves relatively normal skin 新生儿表皮鳞样脱落

ex·ha·la·tion (eks″hə-la′shən) 1. the giving off of watery or other vapor 释放出水蒸气或其他蒸汽；2. a vapor or other substance exhaled or given off 呼出或释放出的蒸汽或其他物质；3. the act of breathing out 呼出的动作；又称 expiration

ex·hale (eks′hāl) to breathe out 呼出

ex·haus·tion (eg-zaws′chən) 1. a state of extreme mental or physical fatigue 极度的精神或身体疲劳的状态；2. the state of being drained, emptied, or consumed 被排干、排空或消耗的状态；**heat e.,** an effect of excessive exposure to heat, marked by subnormal body temperature with dizziness, headache, nausea, and sometimes delirium and/or collapse 热衰竭

ex·hi·bi·tion·ism (eg″zĭ-bish′ə-niz-əm) a paraphilia marked by recurrent sexual urges for and fantasies of exposing one's genitals to an unsuspecting stranger 露阴癖，露阴症

ex·hi·bi·tion·ist (eg″zĭ-bish′ə-nist) a person who indulges in exhibitionism 露阴癖患者

exo·crine (ek′so-krin) 外 分 泌 1. secreting externally via a duct 通过导管分泌的；2. denoting such a gland or its secretion 此类腺体或其分泌物

exo·cyc·lic (ek″so-sik′lik) (-si′klik) denoting one or more atoms attached to a ring but outside it 外环的

exo·cy·to·sis (ek″so-si-to′sis) 1. the discharge from a cell of particles that are too large to diffuse through the wall; the opposite of endocytosis 胞吐作用；2. the aggregation of migrating leukocytes in the epidermis as part of the inflammatory response 胞外分泌

exo·de·vi·a·tion (ek″so-de″ve-a′shən) a turning outward; in ophthalmology, exotropia 外斜视

ex·odon·tics (ek″so-don′tiks) that branch of dentistry dealing with extraction of teeth 拔牙学

exo·en·zyme (ek″so-en′zīm) an enzyme that acts outside the cell which secretes it 外酵素

exo·eryth·ro·cyt·ic (ek″so-ə-rith″ro-sit′ik) occurring outside the erythrocyte; applied to developmental stages of malarial parasites taking place in cells other than erythrocytes 红细胞外的

ex·og·a·my (ek-sog′ə-me) fertilization by union of cells not derived from the same parent cell 异系配合，异系配交；**exog′amous** *adj.*

ex·og·e·nous (ek-soj′ə-nəs) originating outside or caused by factors outside the organism 外生的，外成的

ex·om·pha·los (ek-som′fə-los) umbilical hernia 脐疝

ex·on (ek′son) a single uninterrupted coding sequence within a gene 外显子；cf. *intron*

exo·nu·cle·ase (ek″so-noo′kle-ās) any nuclease specifically catalyzing the hydrolysis of terminal bonds of deoxyribonucleotide or ribonucleotide chains, releasing mononucleotides 核酸外切酶，外切核酸酶

exo·pep·ti·dase (ek″so-pep′tĭ-dās) any peptidase that catalyzes the cleavage of the terminal or penultimate peptide bond, releasing a single amino acid or dipeptide from the peptide chain 外肽酶

Exo·phi·a·la (ek″so-fi′ə-lə) a widespread genus of saprobic, dematiaceous, anamorphic fungi. *E. dermati'tidis* (*Wangiella dermatitidis*) and other species are opportunistic pathogens, causing phaeohyphomycosis, eumycotic mycetoma, chromoblastomycosis, and other localized and systemic infections 分枝孢子菌属

exo·pho·ria (ek-so-for′e-ə) deviation of the visual axis of one eye away from that of the other eye in the absence of visual fusional stimuli 外隐斜；**exopho′ric** *adj.*

ex·oph·thal·mom·e·try (ek″sof-thəl-mom′ə-tre) measurement of the extent of protrusion of the eyeball in exophthalmos 眼球突出测量（法）；**exophthalmomet′ric** *adj.*

ex·oph·thal·mos (ek″sof-thal′mos) abnormal protrusion of the eye 突眼，眼球突出；**exophthal′mic** *adj.*

384

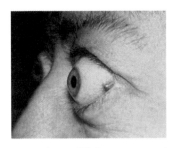

▲ Graves 病的眼球突出（exophthalmos）和眼睑回缩

exo·phyt·ic (ek″so-fit′ik) growing outward; in oncology, proliferating on the exterior or surface epithelium of an organ or other structure in which the growth originated 外部生长的，外寄生菌的

exo·skel·e·ton (ek″so-skel′ə-ton) a hard structure formed on the outside of the body, as a crustacean's shell; in vertebrates, applied to structures produced by the epidermis, such as the hair, nails, hoofs, and teeth 外骨骼

ex·os·mo·sis (ek″sos-mo′sis) osmosis or diffusion from within outward 外渗，渗入

ex·os·to·sis (ek″sos-to′sis) 1. a benign bony growth projecting outward from a bone surface 骨疣；2. osteochondroma 骨软骨瘤；**exostot′ic** adj.; **e. cartilagi′nea**, a variety of osteoma consisting of a layer of cartilage developing beneath the periosteum of a bone 软骨性外生骨疣；**ivory e.**, compact osteoma 象牙质样外生骨疣；**multiple e's, multiple cartilaginous e's**, an inherited condition in which multiple cartilaginous or osteocartilaginous excrescences grow out from the cortical surfaces of long bones 多发性外生骨疣；**subungual e.**, a cartilage-capped reactive bone spur occurring on the distal phalanx, usually of the great toe 甲下外生骨疣

exo·ther·mal (ek″so-thur′məl) exothermic 放热的，发热的

exo·ther·mic (ek″so-thur′mik) marked or accompanied by evolution of heat; liberating heat or energy 放热的

exo·tox·in (ek′so-tok″sin) a potent toxin formed and excreted by the bacterial cell, and free in the surrounding medium 外毒素；**ex′otoxic** adj.

exo·tro·pia (ek″so-tro′pe-ə) strabismus in which there is permanent deviation of the visual axis of one eye away from that of the other, resulting in diplopia 外斜视；**exotro′pic** adj.

ex·pan·der (ek-span′dər) [L.] extender 混合剂，添加物；**subperiosteal tissue e. (STE)**, a fillable tube inserted temporarily into the subperiosteal tissue and progressively inflated to expand the periosteal mucosa and create space for later reconstruction 骨膜下组织扩张器

ex·pan·sion (ek-span′shən) 扩张，膨胀，扩大 1. the process or state of being increased in extent, surface, or bulk；2. a region or area of increased bulk or surface；**clonal e.**, an immune response in which lymphocytes stimulated by antigen proliferate and amplify the population of relevant cells 克隆扩增；**dorsal digital e., extensor e.**, extensor aponeurosis, a triangular aponeurotic extension of the digital extensor tendon on the dorsum of the proximal phalanx of each digit, to which the tendons of the lumbrical and interosseous muscles are also attached, forming a movable hood around the metacarpophalangeal joint 伸指肌腱扩张部

ex·pec·to·rant (ek-spek′tə-rənt) 1. promoting expectoration 化痰的；2. an agent that promotes expectoration 除痰剂；**liquefying e.**, an expectorant that promotes the ejection of mucus from the respiratory tract by decreasing its viscosity 液化祛痰药

ex·pec·to·ra·tion (ek-spek″tə-ra′shən) 1. the coughing up and spitting out of material from the lungs, bronchi, and trachea 吐痰，咳痰；2. sputum 痰

ex·per·i·ment (ek-sper′ ī-mənt) a procedure done in order to discover or demonstrate some fact or general truth 实验，试验；**experimen′tal** adj.**control e.**, one made under standard conditions, to test the correctness of other observations 对照实验

ex·pi·rate (eks′pi-rāt) exhaled air or gas 呼气

ex·pi·ra·tion (ek″spī-ra′shən) 1. exhalation 呼气，2. termination or death 断气，死亡；**expi′ratory** adj.

ex·pi·ra·to·ry (ek-spi′rə-tor″e) pertaining to exhalation (expiration) 吐气的，呼气的

ex·pire (ek-spīr′) 1. to exhale 呼出; 2. to die 断气，死亡

ex·plant¹ (eks′plant) tissue taken from its original site and transferred to an artificial medium for growth 移植物

ex·plant² (eks-plant′) to remove something from the body, such as an implant, or tissue placed in an artificial medium for growth 移植，移出

ex·plo·ra·tion (ek″splə-ra′shən) investigation or examination for diagnostic purposes 探察，检查；**explo′ratory** adj.

ex·plo·sive (ek-splo′siv) 1. pertaining to or occurring in a sudden violent burst 爆炸的；2. tending to sudden violent outbursts 爆发的

ex·po·sure (ek-spo′zhər) 1. the act of laying open, as surgical exposure 暴露；2. the condition of being subjected to something that could have a harmful effect, such as an infectious agent or extremes of weather 暴 露；3. in radiology, a measure of the amount of ionizing radiation at the surface of the irradiated object, e.g., the body 照射；**air e.,** radiation exposure measured in a small mass of air, excluding backscatter from irradiated objects 空气照射

ex·pres·sion (ek-spresh′ən) 1. the aspect or appearance of the face as determined by the physical or emotional state 面容，（面部）表情；2. the act of squeezing out or evacuating by pressure 压出（法），压榨（法）；3. gene e. 基因表达；**gene e.,;** 1. the flow of genetic information from gene to protein. 2. the process, or the regulation thereof, by which the effects of a gene are manifested；3. the manifestation of a heritable trait

ex·pres·siv·i·ty (ek″sprĕ-siv′ĭ-te) in genetics, the level of phenotypic expression of an inherited trait in an individual 表现度，表达度

ex·san·gui·na·tion (ek-sang″wī-na′shən) extensive loss of blood due to internal or external hemorrhage 驱血法，放血

ex·sic·ca·tion (ek″sĭ-ka′shən) the act of drying out; in chemistry, the deprival of a crystalline substance of its water of crystallization 干燥法

ex·sorp·tion (ek-sorp′shən) the movement of substances out of the blood into the intestinal lumen 外吸渗

ex·stro·phy (ek′stro-fe) the turning inside out of an organ 外翻；**e. of bladder,** congenital absence of a portion of the lower anterior abdominal wall and the anterior bladder wall, with eversion of the posterior bladder wall through the defect, an open pubic arch, and widely separated ischia connected by a fibrous band 膀胱外翻；**e. of cloaca, cloacal e.,** a developmental anomaly in which two hemibladders are separated by an area of intestine with a mucosal surface, resembling a large red tumor in the midline of the lower abdomen 泄殖腔外翻

ext. extract 提取

ex·tend·ed-re·lease (ek-stend′əd-re-lēs′) allowing a twofold or greater reduction in frequency of administration of a drug in comparison with the frequency required by a conventional dosage form 缓释剂

ex·ten·der (ek-sten′dər) something that enlarges or prolongs 混合剂，添加物；**artificial plasma e.,** a substance that can be transfused to maintain fluid volume of the blood in event of great necessity, supplemental to the use of whole blood and plasma 人工血浆容量扩张剂

ex·ten·sion (ek-sten′shən) 1. the movement by which the two ends of any jointed part are drawn away from each other 牵伸术，使任何相连部分两端互相拉开的动作；2. the bringing of the members of a limb into or toward a straight condition. 伸

展，伸，使肢体某部分伸直的动作；**nail e.,** extension exerted on the distal fragment of a fractured bone by means of a nail or pin (Steinmann pin) driven into the fragment 导针牵伸术

ex·ten·sor (ek-sten′sor) [L.] 1. causing extension 引起兴奋；2. a muscle that extends a joint 伸肌

ex·te·ri·or·ize (ek-stēr′e-ə-rīz″) 1. to form a correct mental reference of the image of an object seen 赋予外形，具体化；2. in psychiatry, to turn one's interest outward（性格）外向化；3. to transpose an internal organ to the exterior of the body 外置术

ex·tern (ek′stərn) a medical student or graduate in medicine who assists in patient care in the hospital but does not reside there 实习医学生

ex·ter·nal (ek-stur′nəl) [externus L.] situated or occurring on the outside; farther from the center of a part or cavity 外的，外侧的

ex·tero·cep·tor (ek″stər-o-sep′tər) a sensory nerve ending stimulated by the immediate external environment, such as those in the skin and mucous membranes 外感受器；**exterocep′tive** *adj.* 外感受性的

ex·ti·ma (ek′stĭ-mə) [L.] outermost; the outermost coat of a blood vessel 外膜

ex·tinc·tion (ek-stink′shən) in psychology, the disappearance of a conditioned response as a result of nonreinforcement; also, the process by which the disappearance is accomplished 消退，在心理学中，指条件反应因未强化而消失

ex·tor·sion (ek-stor′shən) outward rotation of the upper pole of the vertical meridian of each eye 眼外转，眼外倾

ex·tor·tor (ek-stor′tər) 1. an outward rotator 外旋；2. an extraocular muscle that produces extorsion；外旋肌

ex·tra-ab·dom·i·nal (eks″trə-ab-dom′ĭ-nəl) outside the abdomen 腹外

ex·tra-an·a·tom·ic (eks″trə-an″ə-tom′ik) not following the normal anatomic path 解剖外

ex·tra·cap·su·lar (eks″trə-kap′su-lər) situated or occurring outside a capsule 囊外的

ex·tra·car·di·ac (eks″trə-kahr′de-ak) outside the heart 心外的

ex·tra·cel·lu·lar (eks″trə-sel′u-lər) outside a cell or cells（位于或发生于）细胞外的

ex·tra·chro·mo·so·mal (eks″trə-kro″moso′məl) outside or not involving the chromosome（位于或发生在）染色体外的

ex·tra·cor·po·re·al (eks″trə-kor-por′e-əl) situated or occurring outside the body 身体外的

ex·tract (ek′strakt) a concentrated preparation of a vegetable or animal drug 提取

ex·trac·tion (ek-strak′shən) 1. the process or act

E

of pulling or drawing out 取出，抽出；2. the preparation of an extract 提取（法），萃取（法）；**breech e.**, extraction of an infant from the uterus in breech presentation 胎臀牵引术；**flap e.**, extraction of a cataract by an incision that makes a flap of cornea 瓣状（白内障）摘出术；**serial e.**, the selective extraction of deciduous teeth during an extended period of time to allow autonomous adjustment 顺序拔牙；**testicular sperm e. (TESE)**, for men with obstructive azoospermia, extraction of spermatozoa directly from the testis through the skin 睾丸取精术

ex·trac·tive (ek-strak′tiv) any substance present in an organized tissue, or in a mixture in a small quantity, and requiring extraction by a special method 提取物，浸出物

ex·trac·tor (ek-strak′tər) an instrument for removing a calculus or foreign body 取出器，提取器；**basket e.**, a device for removal of calculi from the upper urinary tract 篮式提取器，篮式浸出器；**vacuum e.**, a device to assist delivery consisting of a metal traction cup that is attached to the fetus's head; negative pressure is applied and traction is made on a chain passed through the suction tube 真空提取（抽提）器

ex·tra·em·bry·on·ic (eks″trə-em″bre-on′ik) external to the embryo proper, as the extraembryonic coelom or extraembryonic membranes 胚外的

ex·tra·mal·le·o·lus (eks″trə-mə-le′o-ləs) the external malleolus 外踝

ex·tra·med·ul·lary (eks″trə-med′u-lar″e) situated or occurring outside a medulla, especially the medulla oblongata 髓外的，延髓外的

ex·tra·mu·ral (eks″trə-mu′rəl) situated or occurring outside the wall of an organ or structure 壁外的

ex·tra·nu·cle·ar (eks″trə-noo′kle-ər) situated or occurring outside a cell nucleus 细胞核外的

ex·tra·oc·u·lar (eks″trə-ok′u-lər) situated outside the eye 眼外的

ex·tra·pla·cen·tal (eks″trə-plə-sen′təl) outside of or independent of the placenta 胎盘外的

ex·trap·o·la·tion (ek-strap″o-la′shən) inference of a value on the basis of that which is known or has been observed 推断，推知

ex·tra·psy·chic (eks″trə-si′kik) occurring outside the mind; taking place between the mind and the external environment 心理外的，精神外的

ex·tra·pul·mo·nary (eks″trə-pool′mo-nar″e) not connected with the lungs 肺外的

ex·tra·py·ram·i·dal (eks″trə-pǐ-ram′ǐ-dəl) outside the pyramidal tracts 锥体束外的

ex·tra·re·nal (eks″trə-re′nəl) outside the kidney 肾外的

ex·tra·stim·u·lus (eks″strə-stim′u-ləs) a premature stimulus delivered, singly or in a group of several stimuli, at precise intervals during an extrasystole in order to terminate it 额外刺激

ex·tra·sys·to·le (eks″trə-sis′to-le) a premature cardiac contraction that is independent of the normal rhythm and arises in response to an impulse outside the sinoatrial node 期前收缩；**atrial e.**, atrial premature complex 房性期外收缩；**atrioventricular (AV) e.**, atrioventricular junctional premature complex（房室）结性期外收缩；**infranodal e.**, ventricular e. 结下性期外收缩；**interpolated e.**, 插入性期外收缩，见 *beat* 下词条；**junctional e.**, atrioventricular junctional premature complex 交界性早搏；**nodal e.**, atrioventricular e.; **retrograde e.**, a premature ventricular contraction, followed by a premature atrial contraction, due to transmission of the stimulus backward, usually over the bundle of His 逆行性期外收缩；**ventricular e.**, ventricular premature complex 室性期外收缩

ex·tra·thy·roi·dal (eks″trə-thi-roid′əl) outside or not involving the thyroid gland 甲状腺外的

ex·tra·uter·ine (eks″trə-u′tər-in) outside the uterus 子宫外的

ex·trav·a·sa·tion (ek-strav″ə-sa′shən) 1. a discharge or escape, as of blood, from a vessel into the tissues; blood or other substance so discharged 溢出，排出；2. the process of being extravasated 溢出作用

ex·tra·ver·sion (eks″trə-vur′zhən) extroversion 外向，外倾

ex·tra·vert (eks′trə-vərt) extrovert 外倾（性格）者

ex·trem·i·tas (ek-strem′ǐ-təs) pl. *extremita′tes* [L.] extremity 端

ex·trem·i·ty (ek-strem′ǐ-te) 1. the distal or terminal portion of an elongated or pointed structure 端；2. limb 四肢

ex·trin·sic (ek-strin′zik) of external origin 外部的，体外的，外源的

ex·tro·ver·sion (eks″tro-vur′zhən) 1. a turning inside out 外翻；2. direction of one's energies and attention outward from the self 外倾，外向

ex·tro·vert (eks′tro-vərt) 1. a person whose interest is turned outward 性格外向的人；2. to turn one's interest outward to the external world 使外向

ex·trude (ek-strood′) 1. to force out, or to occupy a position distal to that normally occupied 挤压出，挤压成，突出；2. in dentistry, to occupy a position occlusal to that normally occupied 挤占

ex·tu·ba·tion (eks″too-ba′shən) removal of a tube used in intubation 拔管

ex·u·ber·ant (eg-zoo′bər-ənt) copious or excessive in production; showing excessive proliferation 生长过多的，高度增生的

ex·u·date (eks′u-dāt) a fluid with a high content of protein and cellular debris that has escaped from blood vessels and has been deposited in tissues or on tissue surfaces, usually as a result of inflammation 渗出物，渗出液

ex·u·da·tion (eks″u-da′shən) 1. the escape of fluid, cells, and cellular debris from blood vessels and their deposition in or on the tissues, usually as the result of inflammation 渗出；2. an exudate 渗出的，渗出物，渗出液；**exu′dative** *adj.*

ex·um·bil·i·ca·tion (eks″əm-bil″ĭ-ka′shən) 1. marked protrusion of the navel 脐凸出；2. umbilical hernia 脐疝

ex·u·vi·a·tion (eks-u″ve-a′shən) shedding an epithelial structure, e.g., deciduous teeth 上皮脱落；乳牙脱落

ex vi·vo (eks ve′vo) outside the living body; denoting removal of an organ (e.g., the kidney) for reparative surgery, after which it is returned to the original site 在活体外

eye (i) the organ of vision 眼睛；见图30；**black e.**, a bruise of the tissue around the eye, marked by discoloration, swelling, and pain 眼圈青肿，眼眶淤青；**crossed e's**, esotropia 内斜视；**exciting e.**, the eye that is primarily injured and from which the influences start that involve the other eye in sympathetic ophthalmia 激发眼；**pink e.**, acute contagious conjunctivitis 传染性角膜炎；**shipyard e.**, epidemic keratoconjunctivitis 角膜结膜炎；**wall e.**, 1. leukoma of the cornea 角膜白斑；2. exophoria. 外斜视

eye·ball (i′bawl) the ball or globe of the eye 眼球

eye·brow (i′brou) 1. the transverse elevation at the junction of the forehead and the upper eyelid 眉，额和上睑连接处的横行隆凸；2. the hairs growing on this elevation 眉毛

eye·cup (i′kəp) 1. a small vessel for application of cleansing or medicated solution to the exposed area of the eyeball 洗眼杯，对眼球暴露部使用清洁液或治疗液的小器皿；2. optic cup (2) 视神经乳头凹陷

eye·glasses (i′glas-əz) glasses 眼镜

eye·ground (i′ground) the fundus of the eye as seen with the ophthalmoscope 眼底

eye·lash (i′lash) cilium; one of the hairs growing on the edge of an eyelid 睫毛

eye·lid (i′lid) either of two movable folds (upper and lower) protecting the anterior surface of the eyeball 眼睑

eye·piece (i′pēs) the lens or system of lenses of a microscope (or telescope) nearest the user's eye, serving to further magnify the image produced by the objective. 目镜

eye·strain (i′strān) fatigue of the eye from overuse or from an uncorrected defect in the focus of the eye 眼疲劳

Ey·lea (ī′lēə) trademark for a preparation of aflibercept Eylea 的商品名

e·zog·a·bine (e-zog′a-been) a potassium channel binder that opens and stabilizes channels to suppress neuronal excitability and that may augment GABA actions; used in combination to treat uncontrolled partial-onset seizures in adults 依佐加滨（抗癫痫药）

F

F Fahrenheit 华氏温标（见 *scale* 下词条）；farad 法拉（电容单位）；fertility 致育质粒（见 *plasmid* 下词条）；visual field 视野；fluorine 元素氟；formula 处方，药方；French 法兰西标度（见 *scale*）；phenylalanine 苯丙氨酸

F faraday 法拉第（电量单位）；force 力

F₁, F₂, F₃, etc. filial generation, with the generation specified by the subscript numeral 子代，用下标数字指定

f femto- 飞（母托）的符号

ƒ frequency (2) 频率的符号

Fab [*f*ragment, *a*ntigen-*b*inding] originally, either of two identical fragments, each containing an antigen-combining site, obtained by papain cleavage of the immunoglobulin G (IgG) molecule; now generally used as an adjective to refer to an "arm" of any immunoglobulin monomer Fab 片段，抗原结合片段（现在常用来指免疫球蛋白单体的"臂"）；**digoxin immune Fab (ovine)**, a preparation of antigen-binding fragments derived from specific antibodies produced against digoxin in sheep; used as an antidote to digoxin and digitoxin overdose 地高辛免疫抗原结合片段

fa·bel·la (fə-bel′ə) pl. *fabel′lae* [L.] a sesamoid fibrocartilage occasionally found on the gastrocnemius muscle, articulating with the femur 腓肠豆（腓肠肌内杆状纤维软骨）

FACD Fellow of the American College of Dentists 美国牙科医师学会会员

face (fās) 1. the anterior, or ventral, aspect of the head, usually from the forehead to the chin, inclusive, but sometimes excluding the forehead 脸；2. any presenting aspect or surface 方面；**moon f.**, 满月脸，见 *facies* 下词条

face-bow (fās′bo)面弓 1. a device used in dentistry to record the positional relations of the maxillary arch to the temporomandibular joints and to orient dental casts in this same relationship to the opening axis of the articulator; 2. an extraoral wire arch or bow used in orthodontics to connect an intraoral appliance to an extraoral anchorage

fac·et (fas′ət) (fə-set′) a small plane surface on a hard body, as on a bone 关节面

fac·e·tec·to·my (fas″ə-tek′tə-me) excision of the articular facet of a vertebra 椎骨关节面切除术

fa·cial (fa′shəl) pertaining to or directed toward the face 面部的

facies (fa′she-ēz) pl. *fa′cies* [L.] 1. the face (颜)面; 2. the surface or outer aspect of a body part or organ 身体、局部或器官的特定表面; 3. expression (1) 面容; **elfin f.**, facial features including wide-set eyes, low-set ears, and hirsutism; seen in children with congenital conditions such as Donohue syndrome and Williams syndrome 小精灵面容; **leonine f.**, a deeply furrowed, lionlike appearance of the face, seen in certain cases of advanced lepromatous leprosy and in other diseases associated with facial edema 狮面; **moon f.**, the rounded face, resulting from fat deposition in the cheeks and temporal regions, observed in Cushing syndrome 满月脸; **Parkinson f.**, a stolid masklike expression of the face, with infrequent blinking, pathognomonic of parkinsonism 帕金森相面容; **Potter f.**, the characteristic facial appearance seen with oligohydramnios sequence, including a flattened nose, receding chin, wide interpupillary space, and large, low-set ears 波特面容

fa·cil·i·ta·tion (fə-sil″ĭ-ta′shən) [L.] 1. hastening or assistance of a natural process 促进; 2. in neurophysiology, the effect of a nerve impulse acting across a synapse and resulting in increased postsynaptic potential of subsequent impulses in that nerve fiber or in other convergent nerve fibers 易化作用

fa·cil·i·ta·tive (fə-sil′ĭ-ta″tiv) in pharmacology, denoting a reaction arising as an indirect result of drug action, as development of an infection after the normal microflora has been altered by an antibiotic 促进的，助长的

fac·ing (fās′ing) a piece of porcelain cut to represent the outer surface of a tooth 牙面

fa·cio·bra·chi·al (fa″she-o-bra′ke-əl) pertaining to the face and the arm（神经痛等症状）面部与臂的

fa·cio·lin·gual (fa″she-o-ling′wəl) pertaining to the face and tongue（神经痛等症状）面部与舌的

fa·cio·plas·ty (fa′she-o-plas″te) restorative or plastic surgery of the face 面成形术

fa·cio·ple·gia (fa″she-o-ple′jə) facial paralysis 面神经麻痹，面瘫; **faciople′gic** *adj.*

FACOG Fellow of the American College of Obstetricians and Gynecologists 美国妇产科医师学会会员

FACP Fellow of the American College of Physicians 美国内科医师学会会员

FACS Fellow of the American College of Surgeons 美国外科医师学会会员

FACSM Fellow of the American College of Sports Medicine 美国运动医学学会会员

fac·ti·tious (fak-tish′əs) artificially induced; not natural 人工的，人造的。又称 *factitial*

fac·tor (fak′tər) an agent or element that contributes to the production of a result 因素，因子; **accelerator f.**, coagulation f. Ⅴ前加速因子; **angiogenesis f.**, a substance that causes the growth of new blood vessels, found in tissues with high metabolic requirements and also released by macrophages to initiate revascularization in wound healing 血管生长因子; **antihemophilic f. (AHF)**, 1. coagulation f. Ⅷ; 2. a preparation of f. Ⅷ used for the prevention or treatment of hemorrhage in patients with hemophilia A and the treatment of von Willebrand disease, hypofibrinogenemia, and f. ⅩⅢ deficiency, including preparations derived from human or porcine plasma or by recombinant technology 抗血友病因子; **antihemophilic f. A**, coagulation f. Ⅷ 抗血友病因子 A; **antihemophilic f. B**, coagulation f. Ⅸ 抗血友病因子 B; **antihemophilic f. C**, coagulation f. Ⅺ 抗血友病因子 C; **antinuclear f. (ANF)**, 抗核因子，见 *antibody* 下词条; **f. B**, a complement component that participates in the alternative complement pathway B 因子，补体旁路激活途径的固有成分之一; **B-cell differentiation f's (BCDF)**, factors derived from T cells that stimulate B cells to differentiate into antibody-secreting cells B 细胞分化因子; **B-lymphocyte stimulatory f's (BSF)**, a system of nomenclature for factors that stimulate B cells, replacing individual factor names with the designation BSF and an appended descriptive code B 淋巴细胞刺激因子; **Christmas f.** coagulation f. Ⅸ 凝血因子 Ⅸ; **clotting f's**, coagulation f's; **C3 nephritic f. (C3 NeF)** an autoantibody that stabilizes the alternative complement pathway C3 convertase, preventing its inactivation by factor H and resulting in complete consumption of plasma C3; it is found in the serum of many patients with type Ⅱ membranoproliferative glomerulonephritis C3 致肾炎因子; **coagulation f 's** substances in the blood that are essential to the clotting process and, hence, to the maintenance of normal hemostasis. They are designated by Roman numerals, to which the notation "a" is added to indicate the activated state 凝血因子, 另见 *platelet f's*; *f. I*, fibrinogen: a high-molecular-weight plasma protein converted to fibrin by the action of thrombin. Deficiency results in afibrinogenemia or hypofibrinogenemia. 凝血因子 I, 纤维蛋白原; *f. II*, prothrombin: a plasma protein converted to thrombin by activated f. X in the common pathway of coagulation. Deficiency leads to hypoprothrombinemia 凝血因子 II, 凝血酶原; *f. III*, tissue thromboplastin: a lipoprotein functioning in the extrinsic pathway of coagulation, activating f. X 凝血因子 III, 组织凝血激酶; *f. IV*, calcium 凝血因子 IV, 钙离子; *f. V*, proaccelerin: a factor functioning in both the intrinsic and extrinsic pathways of coagulation, catalyzing the cleavage of prothrombin to thrombin. Deficiency leads to parahemophilia 凝血因子 V, 前加速因子; *f. VII*, proconvertin: a factor functioning in the extrinsic pathway of blood coagulation, acting with f. III to activate factor X. Deficiency, either hereditary or associated with vitamin K deficiency, leads to hemorrhagic tendency 凝血因子 VII, 前转化因子; *f. VIII*, antihemophilic factor (AHF): a storage-labile factor participating in the intrinsic pathway of blood coagulation, acting as a cofactor in the activation of f. X. Deficiency, an X-linked recessive trait, causes hemophilia A 凝血因子 VIII, 抗血友病因子; *f. IX*, a relatively storage-stable substance involved in the intrinsic pathway of blood coagulation, activating f. X. Deficiency results in the hemorrhagic syndrome hemophilia B, resembling hemophilia A; it is treated with purified preparations of the factor, either from human plasma or recombinant, or with f. IX complex 凝血因子 IX, 血浆凝血活酶; *f. X*, Stuart factor: a storage-stable factor that participates in both the intrinsic and extrinsic pathways of blood coagulation, uniting them to begin the common pathway of coagulation; as part of the prothrombinase complex, activated f. X activates prothrombin. Deficiency may cause a systemic coagulation disorder. The activated form is called also thrombokinase 凝血因子 X, 斯图亚特因子; *f. XI*, plasma thromboplastin antecedent: a stable factor involved in the intrinsic pathway of blood coagulation, activating f. IX. Deficiency results in the blood-clotting defect hemophilia C 凝血因子 XI, 血浆凝血活酶前质; *f. XII*, Hageman factor: a stable factor activated by contact with glass or other foreign surfaces, which initiates the intrinsic process of blood coagulation by activating f. XI 凝血因子 XII, 哈格曼因子, 接触因子; *f. XIII*, fibrin-stabilizing factor: a factor that polymerizes fibrin monomers, enabling formation of a firm blood clot. Deficiency produces a clinical hemorrhagic diathesis 凝血因子 XIII, 纤维蛋白稳定因子; **colony-stimulating f's**, a group of glycoprotein lymphokines, produced by blood monocytes, tissue macrophages, and stimulated lymphocytes and required for the differentiation of stem cells into granulocyte and monocyte cell colonies; they stimulate the production of granulocytes and macrophages and have been used experimentally as cancer agents 集落刺激因子; **f. D**, a serine protease of the alternative complement pathway that cleaves f. B bound to C3b, releasing Ba while leaving Bb bound to C3b to form the C3 convertase C3bBb D 因子, 补体旁路中的一种蛋白质; **decay accelerating f. (DAF)**, a protein of most blood cells as well as endothelial and epithelial cells, CD55; it protects the cell membranes from attack by autologous complement 衰变加速因子; **endothelial- derived relaxing f., endothelium-derived relaxing f. (EDRF)**, nitric oxide 内皮细胞源性血管舒张因子; **epidermal growth f. (EGF)**, a mitogenic polypeptide produced by many cell types and made in large amounts by some tumors; it promotes growth and differentiation, is essential in embryogenesis, and is also important in wound healing 表皮生长因子; **extrinsic f.**, cyanocobalamin 外因子, 维生素 B$_{12}$ (氰钴胺); **F (fertility) f.**, F plasmid 致育因子, F 因子; **fibrin-stabilizing f. (FSF)**, coagulation f. XIII; **fibroblast growth f.**, a family of structurally related polypeptides that act as signaling molecules, regulating cellular proliferation, survival, migration, and differentiation 成纤维细胞生长因子; **Fitzgerald f.**, high-molecular-weight kininogen 高分子 (量) 激肽原; **Fletcher f.**, prekallikrein 前激肽释放酶, 激肽释放酶原; **glucose tolerance f.**, a biologically active complex of chromium and nicotinic acid that facilitates the reaction of insulin with receptor sites on tissues 葡萄糖耐量因子; **granulocyte colony-stimulating f. (G-CSF)**, a colony-stimulating factor that stimulates the production of neutrophils from precursor cells 粒细胞集落刺激因子; **granulocyte-macrophage colony- stimulating f. (GM-CSF)**, a colony-stimulating factor that binds to stem cells and most myelocytes and stimulates their differentiation into granulocytes and macrophages 粒细胞-巨噬细胞集落刺激因子; **growth f.**, any substance that promotes skeletal or somatic growth, usually a mineral, hormone, or vitamin 生长因子; **f. H**, a glycoprotein that acts as an inhibitor of the alternative pathway of complement activation H 因子, 一种补体活化替代途径的抑制药; **Hageman f. (HF)**, coagulation f. XII; **histamine-releasing f. (HRF)**, a lymphokine that induces the release of histamine by IgE-bound basophils in late-phase al-

F

lergic reaction 组胺释放因子; **homolo- gous restriction f. (HRF),** a regulatory protein that binds to the membrane attack complex in autologous cells, inhibiting the final stages of complement activation 同源限制因子; **f.** Ⅰ, a plasma enzyme that regulates both classical and alternative pathways of complement activation by inactivating their C3 convertases Ⅰ因子, 通过使补体 C3 转换酶失活来调节经典的和替代的补体激活途径的一种血浆酶; **inhibiting f's,** factors elaborated by one body structure that inhibit release of hormones by another structure; applied to substances of unknown chemical identity are called *inhibiting hormones* 抑制因子; **insulinlike growth f's (IGF),** insulin-like substances in serum that do not react with insulin antibodies; they are growth hormone–dependent and possess all the growthpromoting properties of the somatomedins 胰岛素样生长因子; **intrinsic f.,** a glycoprotein secreted by the parietal cells of the gastric glands, necessary for the absorption of vitamin B_{12}. Lack of intrinsic factor, with consequent deficiency of vitamin B_{12}, results in pernicious anemia 内（在）因子; **LE f.,** an antinuclear antibody having a sedimentation rate of 7S and reacting with leukocyte nuclei, found in the serum in systemic lupus erythematosus 红斑狼疮因子, LE 因子; **leukocyte inhibitory f. (LIF),** a lymphokine that prevents polymorphonuclear leukocytes from migrating 白细胞抑制因子; **lymph node permeability f. (LNPF),** a substance from normal lymph nodes that produces vascular permeability 淋巴结通透因子; **lymphocyte mitogenic f. (LMF),** a nondialyzable heat-stable macromolecule released by lymphocytes stimulated by a specific antigen; it causes blast transformation and cell division in normal lymphocytes 淋巴细胞有丝分裂因子; **lymphocyte- transforming f. (LTF),** a lymphokine causing transformation and clonal expansion of nonsensitized lymphocytes 淋巴细胞转化因子; **macrophage migration inhibitory f. (MIF),** a constitutively expressed lymphokine that inhibits macrophage migration in vitro; it regulates a variety of acute inflammatory and adaptive immune responses 巨噬细胞移动抑制因子; **myocardial depressant f. (MDF),** a peptide formed in response to a fall in systemic blood pressure; it has a negatively inotropic effect on myocardial muscle fibers 心肌抑制因子; **osteoclast-activating f. (OAF),** a lymphokine produced by lymphocytes that facilitates bone resorption 破骨细胞活化因子; **f. P,** properdin 备解素, P 因子; **platelet f's,** factors important in hemostasis that are contained in or attached to the platelets 血小板因子; *platelet f. 1,* adsorbed coagulation f. Ⅴ from the plasma. 血小板因子 1, 由血浆吸附的第五因子; *platelet f. 2,* an accelerator of the thrombin-fibrinogen reaction 血小板因子 2, 能加速凝血酶和纤维蛋白原反应; *platelet f. 3,* a lipoprotein with roles in the activation of both coagulation f. X and prothrombin 血小板因子 3, 能在血浆蛋白凝固时影响内源性凝血酶原的生成; *platelet f. 4,* an intracellular protein component of blood platelets capable of inhibiting the activity of heparin 血小板因子 4, 能抑制肝素的活性; **platelet- activating f. (PAF),** an immunologically produced substance that is a mediator of clumping and degranulation of blood platelets and of bronchoconstriction 血小板活化因子; **platelet-derived growth f.,** a substance contained in the alpha granules of blood platelets whose action contributes to the repair of damaged blood vessel walls 血小板生长因子; **R f.,** 抗性转移因子，见 *plasmid* 下词条; **releasing f's,** factors elaborated in one body structure that cause release of hormones from another structure; applied to substances of unknown chemical identity are called *releasing hormones* 释放因子; **resistance transfer f. (RTF),** the portion of an R plasmid containing the genes for conjugation and replication 抗药性转移因子; **Rh f., Rhesus f.,** genetically determined antigens present on the surface of erythrocytes; incompatibility for these antigens between mother and offspring is responsible for erythroblastosis fetalis Rh 因子; **rheumatoid f. (RF),** a protein (IgM) detectable by serologic tests, which is found in the serum of most patients with rheumatoid arthritis and in other related and unrelated diseases and sometimes in apparently normal persons 类风湿因子; **risk f.,** a clearly defined occurrence or characteristic that has been associated with the increased rate of a subsequently occurring disease 危险度, 危险因素; **Stuart f., Stuart-Prower f.,** coagulation f. X; **sun protection f.,** the ratio between the number of minimal erythema doses required to induce erythema through a film of sunscreen and that for unprotected skin 防晒系数; **tissue f.,** coagulation f. Ⅲ; **transforming growth f. (TGF),** any of several proteins secreted by transformed cells and causing growth of normal cells, although not causing transformation 转化生长因子; **tumor necrosis f. (TNF),** either of two lymphokines that cause hemorrhagic necrosis of certain tumor cells but do not affect normal cells; they have been used as experimental anticancer agents. *Tumor necrosis factor* α (formerly cachectin) is produced by macrophages, eosinophils, and NK cells. *Tumor necrosis factor* β is a lymphotoxin 肿瘤坏死因子;

F

vascular endothelial growth f. (VEGF), 血管内皮生长因子；**vascular permeability f. (VPF)**, a peptide factor that is a mitogen of vascular endothelial cells; it promotes tissue vascularization and is important in tumor angiogenesis 血管通透性因子；**von Willebrand f. (vWF)**, a glycoprotein that circulates complexed to coagulation f. Ⅷ, mediating adhesion of platelets to damaged epithelial surfaces. Deficiency results in von Willebrand disease 血管性假性血友病因子

fac·ul·ta·tive (fak′əl-ta″tiv) not obligatory; pertaining to the ability to adjust to particular circumstances or to assume a particular role 任意的，兼性的

fac·ul·ty (fak′əl-te) 1. a normal power or function, especially of the mind 能力，才能；2. the teaching staff of an institution of learning 全体教职员

FAD flavin adenine dinucleotide 黄素腺嘌呤二核苷酸

fae- for words beginning thus, see those beginning *fe-* 见 fe-

fail·ure (fāl′yər) inability to perform or to function properly 衰 竭；**acute congestive heart f.**, rapidly occurring cardiac output deficiency marked by venocapillary congestion, hypertension, and edema 急性充血性心力衰竭；**backward heart f.**, a concept of heart failure emphasizing the causative contribution of passive engorgement of the systemic venous system, as a result of dysfunction in a ventricle and subsequent pressure increase behind it 后向性心力衰竭；**bone marrow f.**, a failure of the hematopoietic function of the bone marrow 骨髓衰竭；**congestive heart f. (CHF)**, that characterized by breathlessness and abnormal sodium and water retention, resulting in edema, with congestion of the lungs or peripheral circulation, or both 充血性心力衰竭；**diastolic heart f.**, heart failure due to a defect in ventricular filling caused by an abnormality in diastolic function 舒张性心力衰竭；**forward heart f.**, a concept of heart failure that emphasizes the inadequacy of cardiac output relative to body needs and considers venous distention as secondary 前向性心力衰竭；**heart f.**, inability of the heart to pump blood at a rate adequate to fill tissue metabolic requirements or the ability to do so only at an elevated filling pressure; defined clinically as a syndrome of ventricular dysfunction with reduced exercise capacity and other characteristic hemodynamic, renal, neural, and hormonal responses 心力衰竭；**high-output heart f.**, that in which cardiac output remains high; associated with hyperthyroidism, anemia, arteriovenous fistulas, beriberi, osteitis deformans, or sepsis. 高输出性心力衰竭；

kidney f., renal f. 肾 衰；**left-sided heart f., left ventricular f.**, failure of adequate output by the left ventricle, marked by pulmonary congestion and edema 左侧心力衰竭；**low-output heart f.**, that in which cardiac output is decreased, as in most forms of heart disease, leading to manifestations of impaired peripheral circulation and vasoconstriction 低输出性心力衰竭；**premature ovarian f.**, primary ovarian insufficiency 卵巢功能早衰；**renal f.**, inability of the kidney to excrete metabolites at normal plasma levels under normal loading, or inability to retain electrolytes when intake is normal; in the acute form, it is marked by uremia and usually by oliguria, with hyperkalemia and pulmonary edema 肾 衰 竭；**right-sided heart f., right ventricular f.**, failure of adequate output by the right ventricle, marked by venous engorgement, hepatic enlargement, and pitting edema 右侧心力衰竭；**systolic heart f.**, heart failure due to a defect in the expulsion of blood that is caused by an abnormality in systolic function 收缩性心力衰竭；**f. to thrive**, physical and intellectual disability in infants and small children, sometimes from physical illness and sometimes from psychosocial effects such as maternal deprivation 成长受阻

faint (fānt) syncope 晕厥

fal·cate (fal′kāt) falciform 镰形的，镰状的

fal·cial (fal′shəl) pertaining to a falx 镰的

fal·ci·form (fal′sĭ-form) sickle-shaped 镰形的，镰状的

fal·lo·pos·co·py (fə-lo-pos′kə-pe) endoscopic visualization of the uterine tubes using a nonincisional transvaginal and transuterine approach 输卵管镜检查

false-neg·a·tive (fawls′ neg′ə-tiv) 1. denoting a test result that wrongly excludes an individual from a category 假阴性；2. an individual so excluded 被排除的个体；3. an instance of a false-negative result 一个假阴性结果的例子

false-pos·i·tive (fawls′ pos′ĭ-tiv) 1. denoting a test result that wrongly assigns an individual to a category 假阳性；2. an individual so categorized 按上述情况被归类的个体；3. an instance of a false-positive result 一个假阳性结果的例子

fal·si·fi·ca·tion (fawl″sĭ-fĭ-ka′shən) lying 错构；**retrospective f.**, unconscious distortion of past experiences to conform to present emotional needs 回溯性错构症

falx (falks) pl. *fal′ces* [L.] a sickle-shaped structure 镰；**f. cerebel′li**, a fold of dura mater separating the cerebellar hemispheres 小脑镰；**f. ce′rebri**, the fold of dura mater in the longitudinal fissure, separating the cerebral hemispheres 大脑镰；**inguinal f., f.**

inguina′lis, a lateral expansion of the lateral edge of the rectus abdominis that attaches to the pubic bone 腹股沟镰

fam·ci·clo·vir (fam-si′klo-vir) a prodrug of penciclovir used in the treatment of herpes zoster, of herpes genitalis, and of mucocutaneous herpes simplex in immunocompromised patients 泛昔洛韦（抗病毒药）

fa·mil·i·al (fə-mil′e-əl) occurring in or affecting more members of a family than would be expected by chance 家庭的，家族性。Cf. *genetic*

fam·i·ly (fam′ĭ-le) 1. a group descended from a common ancestor 家族，家属；2. a taxonomic subdivision subordinate to an order (or suborder) and superior to a tribe (or subfamily) 科（动植物分类学）

fam·o·ti·dine (fam-o′tĭ-dīn) a histamine H_2 receptor antagonist, which inhibits gastric acid secretion; used in the treatment and prophylaxis of gastric or duodenal ulcers, gastroesophageal reflux disease, upper gastrointestinal bleeding, and conditions associated with gastric hypersecretion 法莫替丁，组胺 H_2 受体拮抗药

F and R force and rhythm (of pulse) 力与节律（脉搏）

fang (fang) 1. a large canine tooth of a carnivore 尖牙；2. the envenomed tooth of a snake（蛇的）毒牙

Fan·nia (fan′e-ə) a genus of flies whose larvae cause intestinal and urinary myiasis in humans 厕蝇属

fan·ta·sy (fan′tə-se) an imagined sequence of events that can satisfy one′s unconscious wishes or express one's unconscious conflicts 幻想，臆想

FAPHA Fellow of the American Public Health Association 美国公共卫生（健康）协会会员

far·ad (F) (far′əd) the SI unit of electric capacitance; the capacitance of a condenser that charged with 1 coulomb gives a difference of potential of 1 volt 法拉（电容单位）

far·a·day (F) (far′ə-da) the electric charge carried by 1 mole of electrons or 1 equivalent weight of ions, equal to 9.649×10^4 coulombs 法拉第（电量单位）

far·cy (fahr′se) 鼻疽，见 *glanders*

far·sight·ed·ness (fahr′sīt-əd-nis) hyperopia 远视

fas·cia (fash′e-ə) pl. *fas′ciae* [L.] a sheet or band of fibrous tissue such as that which lies deep to the skin or invests muscles and various body organs 筋膜；**fas′cial** adj. **f. adhe′rens,** that portion of the junctional complex of the cells of an intercalated disk that is the counterpart of the zonula adherens of epithelial cells 筋膜附着的；**Camper f.,** the

fatty layer of the subcutaneous abdominal fascia, superficial to the membranous layer 坎珀尔筋膜（腹壁浅筋膜浅层）；**cribriform f.,** the superficial fascia of the thigh covering the saphenous opening 筛筋膜；**deep f.,** a dense, firm, fibrous membrane investing the trunk and limbs, and giving off sheaths to the various muscles; subdivided into fasciae of muscles and visceral fascia 深筋膜；**endothoracic f.,** that beneath the serous lining of the thoracic cavity 胸内筋膜；**extraperitoneal f.,** the thin layer of areolar connective tissue separating the parietal peritoneum from the transversalis fascia in the abdomen and pelvis 腹膜外筋膜；**extraserosal f.,** any fascial layer of the trunk lying inside the parietal fascia and outside the visceral fascia. 黏膜外筋膜；**investing f.,** a layer of fascia that extends internally from the deep fascia and invests structures such as muscles 封套筋膜，颈深部包围筋膜；**f. la′ta,** the investing fascia of the thigh 阔筋膜；**parietal f.,** any fascia that lies outside the parietal layer of a serosa and lines the wall of a body cavity 腔壁筋膜；**pharyngobasilar f.,** a strong fibrous membrane in the wall of the pharynx, blending with the periosteum at the base of the skull 咽颅底筋膜；**Scarpa f.,** the deep membranous layer of the subcutaneous tissue of the abdomen 斯卡帕筋膜（腹壁浅筋膜深层）；**superficial f.,** tela subcutanea 浅筋膜；**transversalis f.,** part of the inner superficial layer of the abdominal wall, continuous with the fascia of the other side behind the rectus abdominis muscle and its sheath 腹横筋膜；**visceral f.,** a general term including the fascia lying immediately outside the visceral layer of the serosae together with the fascia immediately surrounding the viscera 脏筋膜

fas·ci·cle (fas′ĭ-kəl) 1. a small bundle or cluster, especially of nerve, tendon, or muscle fibers 束，簇；2. a tract, bundle, or group of nerve fibers that are more or less associated functionally 神经纤维束

fas·cic·u·lar (fə-sik′u-lər) 1. pertaining to a fasciculus 束的；2. fasciculated 成束的

fas·cic·u·lat·ed (fə-sik′u-lāt-əd) clustered together or occurring in bundles, bundled, or fasciculi 成束的

fas·cic·u·la·tion (fə-sik″u-la′shən) 1. the formation of fascicles 成束；2. a small local involuntary muscular contraction visible under the skin, representing spontaneous discharge of fibers innervated by a single motor nerve filament 肌束震颤

fas·cic·u·lus (fə-sik′u-ləs) pl. *fasci′culi* [L.] fascicle 束；**cuneate f. of medulla oblongata,** the continuation into the medulla oblongata of the cuneate fasciculus of the spinal cord 延髓楔形束；**cuneate f. of spinal cord,** the lateral portion of the posterior funiculus of the spinal cord, composed of ascending fibers that end in the nucleus cuneatus 脊髓楔形束；**gracile f. of medulla oblongata,** the continuation into the medulla oblongata of the gracile fasciculus of the spinal cord 延髓纤细束；**gracile f. of spinal cord,** the median portion of the posterior funiculus of the spinal cord, composed of ascending fibers that end in the nucleus gracilis 脊髓薄束；**mammillothalamic f.,** a stout bundle of fibers from the mammillary body to the anterior nucleus of the thalamus 乳头丘脑束

fas·ci·itis (fas″e-i′tis) inflammation of a fascia 筋膜炎；**eosinophilic f.,** inflammation of fasciae of the limbs, with eosinophilia, edema, and swelling, often after strenuous exercise 嗜酸（细胞）性筋膜炎；**necrotizing f.,** a gas-forming, fulminating, necrotic infection of the superficial and deep fascia, resulting in thrombosis of subcutaneous vessels and rapidly spreading gangrene of underlying tissues; most closely associated with group A streptococci but often a polymicrobial (aerobic and anaerobic organisms) infection 坏死性筋膜炎；**nodular f.,** a benign, reactive proliferation of fibroblasts in the subcutaneous tissues, commonly affecting the deep fascia, usually in young adults 结节性筋膜炎；**proliferative f.,** a benign reactive proliferation of fibroblasts in superficial fascia, resembling nodular fasciitis but characterized also by basophilic giant cells and occurrence in the skeletal muscles in older adults 增生性筋膜炎；**pseudosarcomatous f.,** nodular f. 假肉瘤性筋膜炎

fas·ci·od·e·sis (fas″e-od′ə-sis) suture of a fascia to skeletal attachment 筋膜固定术

Fas·ci·o·la (fə-si′o-lə) a genus of flukes, including *F. hepa′tica,* the common liver fluke of herbivores, occasionally found in the human liver 片吸虫属

fas·ci·o·la (fə-si′o-lə) pl. *fasci′olae* [L.] 1. a small band or striplike structure 小片，小束；2. a small bandage 小绷带；**fasci′olar** *adj.*

fas·cio·li·a·sis (fas″e-o-li′ə-sis) infection with *Fasciola* 片形吸虫病

fas·ci·o·lop·si·a·sis (fas″e-o-lop-si′ə-sis) infection with *Fasciolopsis* 姜片虫病

Fas·ci·o·lop·sis (fas″e-o-lop′sis) a genus of trematodes, including *F. bus′ki,* the largest of the intestinal flukes, found in the small intestines of residents throughout Asia 姜片虫属

fas·ci·ot·o·my (fash″e-ot′ə-me) incision of a fascia 筋膜切开术

FASHP Federation of Associations of Schools of Health Professions 卫生专业学校协会联合会

fast (fast) 1. immovable, or unchangeable; resistant to the action of a specific agent, such as a stain or destaining agent 不动的，不变的；抵

抗某种特定物质的作用，如污渍或去污剂；2. abstention from food, or from food and liquid 绝食；3. to abstain from food, or from food and liquid 禁食

fas·tig·i·um (fas-tij′e-əm) [L.] 1. the highest point in the roof of the fourth ventricle of the brain 顶，尖顶（第四脑室顶的最高点）；2. the acme, or highest point 极度，顶点；**fastig′ial** *adj.*

fast·ing (fast′ing) abstinence from all food and drink except water for a prescribed period 禁食

fat(fat) 1. adipose tissue, forming soft pads between organs, smoothing and rounding out body contours, and furnishing a reserve supply of energy 脂肪（组织）；2. an ester of glycerol with fatty acids, usually oleic, palmitic, or stearic acid 酯；**polyunsaturated f.,** one containing polyunsaturated fatty acids 多不饱和脂肪；**saturated f.,** one containing saturated fatty acids 饱和脂肪；*trans* **f's,** 见 *fatty acid* 下词条；**unsaturated f.,** one containing unsaturated fatty acids 不饱和脂肪

fa·tal (fa′təl) mortal; lethal; causing death 致死的，致命的

fat·i·ga·bil·i·ty (fat″ĭ-gə-bil′ĭ-te) easy susceptibility to fatigue 易疲劳性

fa·tigue (fə-tēg′) a state of increased discomfort and decreased efficiency due to prolonged or excessive exertion; loss of power or capacity to respond to stimulation 疲劳，疲乏；**vocal f.,** phonasthenia 发声疲劳，嗓音疲劳

fat·ty (fat′e) pertaining to or characterized by fat 脂肪的

fat·ty **ac·id** (fat′e) any straight-chain monocarboxylic acid, especially those naturally occurring in fats 脂肪酸；**essential f. a. (EFA),** any fatty acid that cannot be synthesized by the body and must be obtained from dietary sources, e.g., linoleic acid and linolenic acid 必需脂肪酸；**free f. a's (FFA),** nonesterified f. a's 游离脂肪酸；**medium-chain f. a's (MCFA),** those having a chain length roughly 8 to 12 carbons long; absorbed directly into the portal blood, bypassing the lymphatic system 中链脂肪酸；**monounsaturated f. a's,** unsaturated fatty acids containing a single double bond, occurring predominantly as oleic acid, in peanut, olive, and canola oils 单不饱和脂肪酸；**nonesterifted f. a's (NEFA),** the fraction of plasma fatty acids not in the form of glycerol esters 非酯化脂肪酸；*ω*-3 **f. a's, omega-3 f. a's,** unsaturated fatty acids in which the double bond nearest the methyl terminus is at the third carbon from the end; present in marine animal fats and some vegetable oils and shown to affect leukotriene, prostaglandin, lipoprotein, and lipid levels and composition *ω*-3 脂肪酸；*ω*-6 **f. a's, omega-6 f. a's,** unsaturated fatty acids in which the double bond nearest the methyl terminus is at the sixth carbon from the end, present predominantly in vegetable oils ω-6 脂肪酸；**polyunsaturated f. a's (PUFA)**, unsaturated fatty acids containing two or more double bonds, occurring predominantly as linoleic, linolenic, and arachidonic acids, in vegetable and seed oils 多不饱和脂肪酸；**saturated f. a's**, those without double bonds, occurring predominantly in animal fats and tropical oils or produced by hydrogenation of unsaturated fatty acids 饱和脂肪酸；**short-chain f. a's (SCFA)**, those having a chain length up to roughly 6 carbon atoms long, produced by bacterial anaerobic fermentation, particularly of dietary carbohydrates, in the large intestine; readily absorbed and metabolized 短链脂肪酸；**trans–f. a's**, stereoisomers of the naturally occurring cis– fatty acids, produced by partial hydrogenation of unsaturated fatty acids in the manufacture of margarine and shortening 反式脂肪酸，又称 trans fats；**unsaturated f. a's**, those containing one or more double bonds, predominantly found in most plant-derived fats 不饱和脂肪酸

fau·ces (faw′sēz) the passage between the throat and pharynx 咽门；**fau′cial** *adj.*

fau·ci·tis (faw-si′tis) sore throat; inflammation of the fauces 咽喉炎

fau·na (faw′nə) the animal life present in or characteristic of a given location 动物区系

fa·ve·o·late (fa-ve′o-lāt) alveolate 蜂窝状的

fa·vism (fa′vis-əm) an acute hemolytic anemia precipitated by fava beans (ingestion, or inhalation of pollen), usually caused by deficiency of glucose-6-phosphate dehydrogenase in the erythrocytes 蚕豆病

fa·vus (fa′vəs) dermatophytosis, usually of the scalp but sometimes of glabrous skin, with formation of scutula, which may enlarge and coalesce to form prominent honeycomb-like masses, sometimes with hair loss, cutaneous atrophy, and scarring; due to infection by *Trichophyton*, usually *T. schoenleinii* 黄癣

Fc fragment, crystallizable; a fragment by papain digestion of immunoglobulin molecules. It contains most of the antigenic determinants 可结晶片段；作为免疫球蛋白分子的片段，能被木瓜蛋白酶消化，其含有大多数的抗原决定簇

Fc′ a fragment produced in minute quantities by papain digestion of immunoglobulin molecules. It contains the principal part of the C-terminal portion of two Fc fragments Fc′片段，通过木瓜蛋白酶消化免疫球蛋白分子产生的片段，其含有两个 Fc 片段的 C 末端部分的主要部分

Fd the heavy chain portion of a Fab fragment pro-duced by papain digestion of an IgG molecule Fd 片段通过木瓜蛋白酶消化 IgG 分子产生的 Fab 片段的重链部分

FDA Food and Drug Administration 食品及药物管理局

FDI Fédération Dentaire Internationale (International Dental Association) 国际牙科联合会

Fe iron (L. *fer′rum*) 元素铁的符号

fear (fēr) the unpleasant emotional state consisting of psychological and psychophysiologic responses to a real external threat or danger, including agitation, alertness, tension, and mobilization of the alarm reaction 恐惧

fe·cal (fe′kəl) pertaining to or of the nature of feces 排泄物的，与粪便相关的

fe·ca·lith (fe′kə-lith) coprolith; an intestinal concretion formed around a center of fecal matter 粪石

fe·cal·oid (fe′kəl-oid) resembling feces 粪便状的

fe·ces (fe′sēz) [L.] waste matter discharged from the intestine 粪便

fec·u·lent (fek′u-lənt) 1. having dregs or sediment 渣滓的、沉积物的；2. pertaining to or of the nature of feces 粪便的

fe·cun·da·bil·i·ty (fə-kun″də-bil′ĭ-te) the probability that conception will occur in a given population of couples during a specific time period 生育能力

fe·cun·da·tion (fe″kən-da′shən) fertilization 受精

fe·cun·di·ty (fə-kun′dĭ-te) 1. in demography, the physiologic ability to reproduce, as opposed to fertility 人口统计学中的再生育能力；2. ability to produce offspring rapidly and in large numbers 旺盛的生殖力

feed·back (fēd′bak) the return of some of the output of a system as input so as to exert some control in the process; feedback is *negative* when the return exerts an inhibitory control, *positive* when it exerts a stimulatory effect 反馈

feed·for·ward (fēd-for′wərd) the anticipatory effect that one intermediate in a metabolic or endocrine control system exerts on another intermediate further along in the pathway; such effect may be positive or negative 前馈

feed·ing (fēd′ing) the taking or giving of food 喂养；**artificial f.**, feeding of a baby with food other than mother's milk 人工喂养；**breast f.**, see under *B.* 母乳喂养；**forced f.**, administration of food by force to those who cannot or will not receive it 强迫喂食

FEF forced expiratory flow 用力呼气流量

fel·ba·mate (fel′bah-māt″) an anticonvulsant used in the treatment of epilepsy 非氨酯

fel·la·tio (fə-la′she-o) oral stimulation or manipulation of the penis 口交

fe·lo·di·pine (fə-lo′dĭ-pēn) a calcium channel blocker used as a vasodilator in the treatment of hypertension 非洛地平

fel·on (fel′ən) whitlow 瘭

felt·work (felt′wərk) a complex of closely interwoven fibers, as of nerve fibers 神经纤维网

fe·male (fe′māl) 1. an individual organism of the sex that bears young or produces ova or eggs 可以哺育幼代或产卵（蛋）的个体生物的性别；2. feminine 女性

fem·i·nine (fem′ĭ-nin) 1. pertaining to the female sex 女性的；2. having qualities normally associated with females 有女性气质的

fem·i·ni·za·tion (fem″ĭ-nī-za′shən) 女性化。1. the normal development of primary and secondary sex characters in females 女性第一或第二性征的正常发育；2. the induction or development of female secondary sex characters in the male 男性中的诱导或发育而出现女性第二性征；**testicular f.,** the complete form of androgen insensitivity syndrome 睾丸女性化

fem·o·ral (fem′ə-rəl) pertaining to the femur or to the thigh 股骨的，大腿的

fem·o·ro·cele (fem′ə-ro-sēl″) femoral hernia 股疝

femto- (fem′to) word element [Danish], *fifteen;* used in naming units of measurement to indicate one-quadrillionth (10-15) of the unit designated by the root with which it is combined; symbol f 飞（母托）（10⁻¹⁵）；符号 f

fe·mur (fe′mər) pl. *fem′ora, femurs* [L.] 1. thigh bone; the longest and largest bone in the body, extending from the pelvis to the knee; its head articulates with the coxal bone, and distally, along with the patella and tibia, it forms the knee joint 股骨，见图 1；2. thigh 大腿

fe·nes·tra (fə-nes′trə) pl. *fenes′trae* [L.] a windowlike opening 似窗的小开口；**f. coch′leae,** cochlear window 蜗窗，圆窗；**f. vesti′buli,** vestibular window 前庭窗，卵圆窗

fen·es·trat·ed (fen′əs-trāt″əd) pierced with one or more openings 有窗的，有孔的

fen·es·tra·tion (fen″əs-tra′shən) 1. the act of perforating or condition of being perforated 开窗法；2. the surgical creation of a new opening in the labyrinth of the ear for restoration of hearing in otosclerosis 外科开窗术；**aorticopulmonary f.,** aortic septal defect 主动脉开窗术

fen·flur·amine (fen-floor′ə-mēn) an amphetamine derivative, formerly used as an anorectic in the form of the hydrochloride salt 芬氟拉明，其盐酸盐曾用作食欲抑制药

fen·nel (fen′əl) the flowering herb F*oeniculum vulgare,* or its edible seeds, which are used as a source of fennel oil 茴香

fen·o·fi·brate (fen″o-fi′brāt) an antihyperlipidemic agent used to reduce elevated serum lipids 非诺贝特，降血脂药

fe·nol·do·pam (fe-nol′do-pam) a vasodilator used for short-term inpatient management of severe hypertension; used as the mesylate salt 非诺多泮，血管扩张药，用于严重高血压的短期住院治疗；用其甲磺酸盐

fen·o·pro·fen (fen″o-pro′fən) a nonsteroidal antiinflammatory drug used as the calcium salt in the treatment of rheumatic and nonrheumatic inflammatory disorders, pain, dysmenorrhea, and vascular headaches 非诺洛芬，非甾体抗炎药，其钙盐用于治疗风湿性和非风湿性炎症、疼痛、痛经和血管性头痛

fen·ta·nyl (fen′tə-nəl) an opioid analgesic; the citrate salt is used as an adjunct to anesthesia, in the induction and maintenance of anesthesia, in combination with droperidol (or similar agent) as a neuroleptanalgesic, and in the management of chronic severe pain 芬太尼阿片受体激动药

fen·u·greek (fen′u-grēk) the leguminous plant *Trigonella foenum-graecum,* or its seeds, which are used for loss of appetite and skin inflammations; also used in traditional Chinese medicine and in Indian medicine 胡芦巴

fer·ment (fər-ment′) to undergo fermentation; used for the decomposition of carbohydrates （使）发酵；用于分解碳水化合物

fer·men·ta·tion (fur″mən-ta′shən) the anaerobic enzymatic conversion of organic compounds, especially carbohydrates, to simpler compounds, especially to ethyl alcohol, producing energy in the form of ATP 发酵

fern·ing (furn′ing) the appearance of a fernlike pattern in a dried specimen of cervical mucus or vaginal fluid, an indication of the presence of estrogen 蕨样变

fer·re·dox·in (fer″ə-dok′sin) a nonheme ironcontaining protein having a very low redox potential; the ferredoxins participate in electron transport in photosynthesis, nitrogen fixation, and various other biologic processes 铁氧化还原蛋白

fer·ric (fer′ik) containing iron in its plus-three oxidation state, Fe(Ⅲ) (also written Fe³⁺) （化）（正）铁的，三价铁的，写作 Fe（Ⅲ）（或 Fe³⁺）；**f.chloride,** FeCl₃·6H₂O; used as a reagent and as a diagnostic aid in phenylketonuria 三氯化铁，在苯丙酮尿症中用作试剂和诊断辅助

fer·ri·tin (fer′ĭ-tin) the iron-apoferritin complex, one of the chief forms in which iron is stored in the body 铁蛋白

fer·ro·che·la·tase (fer″o-ke′lə-tās) a mitochondrial enzyme that catalyzes the insertion of ferrous iron into protoporphyrin IX to form the heme of hemoglobin. Inhibition of the enzyme in lead poisoning results in accumulation of protoporphyrin IX 铁螯合酶，亚铁螯合酶

fer·ro·ki·net·ics (fer″o-kĭ-net′iks) the turnover or rate of change of iron in the body; the rate at which it is cleared from the plasma and incorporated into red cells 铁循环

fer·ro·pro·tein (fer″o-pro′tēn) a protein combined with an iron-containing radical; ferroproteins are respiratory carriers 铁蛋白，一种含铁的蛋白质

fer·rous (fer′əs) containing iron in its plus-two oxidation state, Fe(Ⅱ) (sometimes designated Fe^{2+}). Various salts are used in iron deficiency, including *iron fumarate, iron gluconate*, and *iron sulfate* 亚铁的，写作 Fe（Ⅱ）（或 Fe^{2+}）

fer·ru·gi·nous (fə-roo′jĭ-nəs) 1. containing iron or iron rust 含铁的，铁锈的；2. of the color of iron rust 铁锈色的

fer·til·i·ty (fər-til′ĭ-te) 1. the capacity to conceive or induce conception 生育力；2. 生育率，见 *rate* 下词条；**fer′tile** *adj.*

fer·ti·li·za·tion (fur′tĭ-lĭ-za′shən) impregnation; union of male and female gametes to form the diploid zygote, leading to development of a new individual 受精；**external f.**, union of the gametes outside the bodies of the originating organisms, as in most fish 体外受精，如大部分鱼类是在自然条件下其配子在体外结合完成受精并发育成生物；**internal f.**, union of the gametes inside the body of the female, the sperm having been transferred into the body of the male by an accessory sex organ or other means 体内受精；**in vitro f.**, removal of a secondary oocyte, fertilization of it in a culture medium in the laboratory, and placement of the dividing zygote into the uterus 体外受精，从体内取出次级卵母细胞，在实验室的培养基中使其受精，再将分裂的受精卵置于子宫中

fer·ves·cence (fər-ves′əns) increase of fever or body temperature 发热或体温升高

FES functional electrical stimulation 功能性电刺激疗法

fes·ter (fes′tər) to suppurate superficially 化脓，溃烂

fes·ti·na·tion (fes″tĭ-na′shən) an involuntary tendency to take short accelerating steps in walking 慌张步态

fes·toon (fes-toon′) a carving in the base material of a denture that simulates the contours of the natural tissues being replaced 突彩，口腔医学中指假牙的基础材料上的雕刻，用于模拟被替换的天然

组织的轮廓

fe·tal (fe′təl) of or pertaining to a fetus or the period of its development 胎儿的

fe·tal·iza·tion (fe′təl-ĭ-za′shən) retention in the adult of characters that at an earlier stage of evolution were only infantile and were rapidly lost as the organism attained maturity 胎型（指出生后某些胎象的存留）

fe·ta·tion (fe-ta′shən) 1. development of the fetus 胎儿发育；2. pregnancy 妊娠

fe·ti·cide (fe′tĭ-sīd) the destruction of the fetus 堕胎

fet·id (fĕ′tid) (fe′tid) having a rank, disagreeable smell 恶臭的

fet·ish (fet′ish) (fe′tish) 1. a material object, such as an idol or charm, believed to have supernatural powers 迷信，偶像；2. an inanimate object used to obtain sexual gratification 恋物

fet·ish·ism (fet′ish-iz-əm) a paraphilia marked by recurrent sexual urges for and fantasies of using inanimate objects (fetishes) for sexual arousal or orgasm 恋物癖；**transvestic f.**, a paraphilia of heterosexual males, characterized by recurrent, intense sexual urges, arousal, or orgasm associated with fantasized or actual dressing in clothing of the opposite sex 异装癖

fe·tol·o·gy (fe-tol′ə-je) maternal-fetal medicine 胎儿学

fe·tom·e·try (fe-tom′ə-tre) measurement of the fetus, especially of its head 胎儿测量法

fe·top·a·thy (fe-top′ə-the) a disease or disorder seen in a fetus 胎儿病

α-fe·to·pro·tein (fe″to-pro′tēn) alpha fetoprotein 甲胎蛋白

fe·tor (fe′tor) stench, or offensive odor 恶臭；**f.hepa′ticus**, the peculiar odor of the breath characteristic of hepatic disease 肝病性口臭

fe·to·scope (fe′to-skōp) 1. a specially designed stethoscope for listening to the fetal heart beat 一种专门设计的听胎心心跳的听诊器；2. an endoscope for viewing the fetus in utero 胎儿镜，观察子宫内胎儿的内镜

fe·tus (fe′təs) [L.] the developing young in the uterus, specifically the unborn offspring in the postembryonic period, in humans from 9 weeks after fertilization until birth 胎儿，特指胚胎后期至出生前，在人类中指自受精后 9 周至出生之前；**harlequin f.**, an infant with a severe and usually lethal form of congenital ichthyosis, manifested by hyperkeratosis with rigid skin 花斑胎；**mummified f.**, a dried-up and shriveled fetus 木乃伊化胎儿；**f. papyra′ceus**, a dead fetus pressed flat by the growth of a living twin 纸样胎；**parasitic f.**, in asymmetric conjoined twins, an incomplete minor fetus attached to a larger, more completely developed twin 寄生胎 **Fet·zi·ma** (fĕt′zēmə) trademark for a preparation of levomilnacipran hydrochloride 盐酸左旋米那普仑的商品名

FEV forced expiratory volume 用力呼气量

fe·ver (fe′vər) 1. pyrexia; elevation of body temperature above the normal (37°C) 发热，体温超过正常值 37 ℃; 2. any disease characterized by elevation of body temperature 任何以体温升高为特征的疾病; **fe′brile, fe′verish** *adj.*; **African tick f.**, **African tick-bite f.**, 1. a type of spotted fever seen in southern Africa, caused by infection with *Rickettsia africae* and spread by the bites of ticks of the genus *Amblyomma* 非洲蜱传热; 2. a type of relapsing fever caused by *Borrelia duttonii* 非洲回归热; **aseptic f.**, fever associated with aseptic wounds, presumably due to the disintegration of leukocytes or to the absorption of avascular or traumatized tissue 无菌热; **blackwater f.**, a dangerous complication of falciparum malaria, with passage of dark red to black urine, severe toxicity, and high mortality 黑尿热; **boutonneuse f.**, a type of tick-bite fever endemic from the Mediterranean area across Central Asia to India, due to infection with *Rickettsia conorii*, with chills, fever, primary skin lesion (tache noire), and rash appearing on the second to fourth day 纽扣热; **cat-scratch f.**, 猫抓热，见 *disease* 下词条; **central f.**, sustained fever resulting from damage to the thermoregulatory centers of the hypothalamus 中枢性发热; **childbed f.**, puerperal f.; **Colorado tick f.**, a nonxanthematous tick-bite fever caused by an arenavirus and seen in the western United States and Canada 科罗拉多蜱传热; **continued f.**, one that varies only slightly in 24 hours 稽留热; **Crimean-Congo hemorrhagic f.**, a sometimes fatal hemorrhagic fever caused by a bunyavirus, transmitted by ticks and by contact with blood, secretions, or fluids from infected animals or humans; it occurs from southern Russia across Central Asia, as well as in sub-Saharan Africa 克里米亚 - 刚果出血热; **drug f.**, a febrile reaction to a therapeutic agent, such as a vaccine, antineoplastic, or antibiotic 药物热; **enteric f.**, any of a group of febrile illnesses with enteric symptoms caused by *Salmonella* species, especially typhoid fever and paratyphoid fever 肠热病，尤其是伤寒和副伤寒; **epidemic hemorrhagic f.**, an acute infectious disease characterized by fever, purpura, peripheral vascular collapse, and acute renal failure, caused by viruses of the genus *Hantavirus*, thought to be transmitted to humans by contact with saliva and excreta of infected rodents 流行性出血热; **famil-**

ial Mediterranean f., a hereditary disease usually seen in Armenians and Sephardic Jews, with short recurrent attacks of fever, pain in the abdomen, chest, or joints, and erythema like that of erysipelas; it may be complicated by amyloidosis 家族性地中海热; **Haverhill f.**, the bacillary form of ratbite fever contracted by ingestion of contaminated raw milk or its products 流行性关节红斑; **hay f.**, a seasonal form of allergic rhinitis, with acute conjunctivitis, lacrimation, itching, swelling of the nasal mucosa, nasal catarrh, and attacks of sneezing, an anaphylactic or allergic reaction excited by a specific allergen (such as pollen) 枯草热，花粉症，季节性变应性鼻炎; **hemorrhagic f′s**, viral hemorrhagic fevers; a group of diverse, severe viral infections seen around the world but mainly in the tropics, usually transmitted to humans by arthropod bites or contact with virus-infected rodents; common features include fever, hemorrhagic manifestations, thrombocytopenia, shock, and neurologic disturbances 出血热; **humidifier f.**, malaise, fever, cough, and myalgia caused by inhalation of air that has been passed through humidifiers, dehumidifiers, or air conditioners contaminated by fungi, amebas, or thermophilic actinomycetes 湿化器热; **intermittent f.**, an attack of malaria or other fever, with recurring fever episodes separated by times of normal temperature 间歇热; **Japanese spotted f.**, an acute infection occurring in Japan and caused by *Rickettsia japonica,* transmitted by ticks of the family Ixodidae;characterized by fever and headache and the appearance of an eschar and rash 日本斑点热; **Katayama f.**, fever associated with severe schistosomiasis, accompanied by hepatosplenomegaly and by eosinophilia 片山钉螺热; **Lassa f.**, an acute hemorrhagic fever caused by an arenavirus, endemic throughout West Africa but seen globally, transmitted via *Mastomys* rodents or occasionally between persons; most infections are mild or subclinical, but infection may progress to severe multisystem involvement, potentially fatal 拉沙热; **metal fume f.**, a disease of welders and others working with volatilized metals, marked by sudden thirst, metallic taste in the mouth, high fever with chills, sweating, and leukocytosis 金属烟雾热; **mud f.**, a type of leptospirosis seen in workers in flooded fields and swamps in Germany and Russia 泥热，泥疹; **nonseasonal hay f.**, nonseasonal allergic rhinitis 非季节性枯草热; **Oroya f.**, the first stage of bartonellosis, with frequently fatal hemolytic anemia 奥罗亚热，为巴尔通体病的第一阶段; **paratyphoid f.**, a febrile illness clinically indistinguishable from typhoid fever, but usually milder and caused by different species of *Salmonella* 副伤寒；**parrot f.,** psittacosis 鹦鹉热；**perennial hay f.,** nonseasonal allergic rhinitis 常年性枯草热；**pharyngoconjunctival f.,** an epidemic disease due to an adenovirus, seen mainly in schoolchildren, with fever, pharyngitis, conjunctivitis, rhinitis, and enlarged cervical lymph nodes 咽结膜热；**phlebotomus f.,** a febrile viral disease of short duration, transmitted by the bite of the sandfly *Phlebotomus papatasi,* with dengue-like symptoms, seen in Mediterranean and Middle Eastern countries 白蛉热；**polymer fume f.,** an occupational disorder due to exposure to the products of combustion of polymers such as Teflon; the manifestations are quite similar to those of metal fume fever 聚合物烟雾热；**Pontiac f.,** a self-limited disease marked by fever, cough, muscle aches, chills, headache, chest pain, confusion, and pleuritis, caused by a species of *Legionella* 庞蒂亚克热；**pretibial f.,** a type of leptospirosis marked by a rash on the pretibial region, with lumbar and postorbital pain, malaise, coryza, and fever 胫骨前皮疹热；**puerperal f.,** fever with septicemia after childbirth, with the focus of infection most often being in the uterus; it is usually due to a streptococcus 产褥热；**Q f.,** a febrile infection, usually respiratory, first described in Australia, caused by *Coxiella burnetii* Q 热；**rat-bite f.,** either of two clinically similar acute infectious diseases with high fever and a rash, usually transmitted through a rat bite. The *bacillary form* is caused by *Streptobacillus moniliformis* and the *spirillary form* is caused by *Spirillum minor* 鼠咬热；**recurrent f.,** 1. a paroxysmal fever that recurs, as in diseases such as malaria and tularemia 回归热，如疟疾和兔热病；2. relapsing f.; **relapsing f.,** either of two infectious diseases due to species of *Borrelia. Tick-borne relapsing f.* is endemic wherever certain ticks are found, and *louseborne relapsing f.* is spread by the human body louse when people live in crowded, unsanitary conditions. Both are marked by alternating periods of fever and apyrexia that last 5 to 7 days 蜱传或虱传的回归热（复发热）；**remittent f.,** one that shows significant variations in 24 hours but without return to normal temperature 弛张热；**rheumatic f.,** a febrile disease that is a sequela to Group A hemolytic streptococcal infections, with multiple focal inflammatory lesions of connective tissue structures, especially the heart, blood vessels, and joints; Sydenham chorea; and Aschoff bodies in the myocardium and skin 风湿热；**Rocky Mountain spotted f.,** infection with *Rickettsia rickettsii*, transmitted by ticks, marked by fever, muscle pain, and weakness followed by a macular petechial eruption that begins on the hands and feet and spreads to the trunk and face, with other symptoms in the central nervous system and elsewhere 落基山斑点热；**sandfly f.,** phlebotomus fever 白蛉热；**San Joaquin Valley f.,** coccidioidomycosis 圣华金谷热，球孢子菌病；**scarlet f.,** an acute disease caused by Group A β-hemolytic streptococci, marked by pharyngotonsillitis and a skin rash caused by an exotoxin produced by the streptococcus; the rash is diffuse and bright red and may be followed by desquamation 猩红热；**spotted f.,** any of various tick-bite fevers due to rickettsiae, characterized by skin eruptions, such as Rocky Mountain spotted fever or boutonneuse fever 斑点热；**tick f., tick-bite f.,** any febrile condition spread by a tick vector, such as relapsing fever 蜱热，蜱咬热，以蜱为媒介所致的发热；**trench f.,** a louse-borne rickettsial disease due to *Bartonella quintana,* transmitted by the body louse, *Pediculus humanus corporis,* and characterized by intermittent fever, generalized aches and pains, particularly severe in the shins, chills, sweating, vertigo, malaise, typhus-like rash, and multiple relapses 战壕热；**typhoid f.,** infection by *Salmonella typhi* chiefly involving the lymphoid follicles of the ileum, with chills, fever, headache, cough, prostration, abdominal distention, splenomegaly, and a maculopapular rash; perforation of the bowel may occur in untreated cases 伤寒；**f. of unknown origin (FUO),** a febrile illness of at least 3 weeks' duration (some authorities permit a shorter duration), with a temperature of at least 38.3℃ on at least three occasions and failure to establish a diagnosis in spite of intensive inpatient or outpatient evaluation (three outpatient visits or 3 days' hospitalization) 不明原因发热；**viral hemorrhagic f's,** hemorrhagic f's 病毒性出血性发热；**West Nile f.,** 西尼罗热，见 *encephalitis* 下词条；**yellow f.,** an acute, infectious, mosquito-borne viral disease, endemic in tropical Central and South America and Africa, marked by fever, jaundice due to necrosis of the liver, and albuminuria 黄热病

fe·ver·few (feʹvər-fu″) the dried leaves of the herb *Tanacetum parthenium,* used for migraine, arthritis, rheumatic diseases, and allergy, and for various uses in folk medicine 小白菊

fex·o·fen·a·dine (fek″so-fenʹə-dēn) an antihistamine (H1-receptor antagonist) used as the hydrochloride salt in the treatment of hay fever and chronic idiopathic urticaria 非索非那定

FFA free fatty acids 游离脂肪酸；fundus fluorescein angiography 荧光素眼底血管造影（术）

FIAC Fellow of the International Academy of Cytology 国际细胞学学会会员

fi·ber (fi'bər) 1. an elongated, threadlike structure 细长的线状结构；2. nerve f.；3. dietary f.；**A f's,** myelinated afferent or efferent fibers of the somatic nervous system having a diameter of 1 to 22 μm and a conduction velocity of 5 to 120 meters per second; they include the alpha, beta, delta, and gamma fibers A 类纤维 (神经)；**accelerating f's, accelerator f's,** adrenergic fibers that transmit the impulses that accelerate the heart beat 加速纤维，属肾上腺素能神经纤维，可传递冲动使心率增快；**adrenergic f's,** nerve fibers, usually sympathetic, that liberate epinephrine or related substances as neurotransmitters 肾上腺素能神经纤维；**afferent f's, afferent nerve f's,** 传入纤维，传入神经纤维 1. nerve fibers that convey sensory impulses from the periphery to the central nervous system 将感觉冲动从外周传递到中枢神经系统的神经纤维；2. fibers or axons that are projecting toward a nucleus, using that nucleus as a reference point 向细胞核投射的纤维或轴突，以细胞核为参照点；**alpha f's,** motor and proprioceptive fibers of the A type, having conduction velocities of 70 to 120 meters per second and ranging from 13 to 22 μm in diameter α 纤维；**alveolar f's,** fibers of the periodontal ligament extending from the cement of the tooth root to the walls of the alveolus 牙槽纤维；**arcuate f's,** the bow-shaped fibers in the brain, such as those connecting adjacent gyri in the cerebral cortex, or the external or internal arcuate fibers of the medulla oblongata 弓状纤维；**association f.,** one of the nerve fibers connecting different cortical areas within one hemisphere 联络纤维；**autonomic nerve f's,** nerve fibers that innervate smooth muscle, cardiac mucle, and glandular epithelium, either stimulating and activating the muscle or tissue *(autonomic efferent f's)* or receiving sensory impulses from them *(autonomic afferent f's)* 自主神经纤维；**B f's,** myelinated preganglionic autonomic axons having a fiber diameter of ≤ 3μm and a conduction velocity of 3 to 15 meters per second; these include only efferent fibers B 类 纤 维；**basilar f's,** those that form the middle layer of the zona arcuata and the zona pectinata of the organ of Corti (螺旋器) 基底纤维；**beta f's,** motor and proprioceptive fibers of the A type, having conduction velocities of 30 to 70 meters per second and ranging from 8 to 13 μm in diameter β 纤维；**C f's,** unmyelinated postganglionic fibers of the autonomic nervous system, also the unmyelinated fibers at the dorsal roots and at free nerve endings, having a conduction velocity of 0.6 to 2.3 meters per second and a diameter of 0.3 to 1.3 μm C 纤维；**collagen f's, collagenous f's,** the soft, flexible, white fibers that are the most characteristic constituent of all types of connective tissue, consisting of the protein collagen, and composed of bundles of fibrils that are in turn made up of smaller unit fibrils, which show a characteristic crossbanding 胶原纤维；**commissural f.,** one of the nerve fibers that pass between the cortex of opposite hemispheres of the brain, or between two sides of the brainstem or spinal cord 连合纤维；**dietary f.,** that part of whole grains, vegetables, fruits, and nuts that resists digestion in the gastrointestinal tract; it consists of carbohydrate (cellulose, etc.) and lignin 膳食纤维；**efferent f's, efferent nerve f's,** 传出纤维，传出神经纤维 1. nerve fibers that convey motor impulses away from the central nervous system toward the periphery 从中枢神经系统向周围传递运动冲动的神经纤维；2. fibers or axons that are projecting away from a nucleus, using that nucleus as a reference point 以细胞核为参照点，从细胞核向外投射的纤维或轴突；**elastic f's,** yellowish fibers of elastic quality traversing the intercellular substance of connectivetissue 弹性纤维；**fusimotor f's,** efferent A fibers that innervate the intrafusal fibers of the muscle spindle 肌梭运动纤维；**gamma f's,** any A fibers that conduct at velocities of 15 to 40 meters per second and range from 3 to 7μm in diameter, comprising the fusimotor fibers γ 纤 维；**gray f's,** unmyelinated nerve fibers found largely in the sympathetic nerves 灰纤维，多见于交感神经的无髓鞘纤维；**insoluble f.,** that not soluble in water, composed mainly of lignin, cellulose, and hemicelluloses and primarily found in the bran layers of cereal grains 不溶性纤维；**intrafusal f's,** modified muscle fibers that, surrounded by fluid and enclosed in a connective tissue envelope, compose the muscle spindle 梭 内 肌 纤 维；**Mahaim f's,** specialized tissue connecting components of the conduction system directly to the ventricular septum 马 海 姆 纤维；**motor f's,** efferent fibers 运动神经纤维，传出神经纤维；**Müller f's,** elongated neuroglial cells traversing all the layers of the retina, forming its principal supporting element 米勒纤维 (视网膜内神经胶质的支持纤维)；**muscle f.,** any of the cells of skeletal or cardiac muscle tissue. Skeletal muscle fibers are cylindrical multinucleate cells containing contracting myofibrils, across which run transverse striations. Cardiac muscle fibers have one or sometimes two nuclei, contain myofibrils, and are separated from one another by an intercalated disk; although striated, cardiac muscle fibers branch to form an interlacing network 肌纤维，见图 7；**myelinated f's,** grayish white nerve fibers whose axons are encased in a myelin sheath, which may in turn be enclosed by a neurilemma 有 髓 (神

F

经）纤维；**nerve f.**, a slender process of a neuron, especially the prolonged axon that conducts nerve impulses away from the cell; classified as either afferent or efferent according to the direction in which the impulses flow, and either myelinated or unmyelinated according to whether there is or is not a myelin sheath 神经纤维，见图 14；**osteogenetic f's, osteogenic f's**, precollagenous fibers formed by osteoclasts and becoming the fibrous component of bone matrix 成骨纤维；**preganglionic f's**, the axons of preganglionic neurons 节前纤维；**pressor f's**, nerve fibers that, when stimulated reflexly, cause or increase vasomotor tone 升压神经纤维；**projection f's, projection nerve f's**, one of the nerve fibers that connect the cerebral cortex with the subcortical centers, the brainstem, and the spinal cord 投射纤维；**Purkinje f's**, modified cardiac muscle fibers composed of Purkinje cells, occurring as an interlaced network in the subendothelial tissue and constituting the terminal ramifications of the cardiac conducting system 浦肯野纤维；**radicular f's**, fibers in the roots of the spinal nerves 根纤维；**reticular f's**, immature connective tissue fibers staining with silver, forming the reticular framework of lymphoid and myeloid tissue, and occurring in interstitial tissue of glandular organs, the papillary layer of the dermis, and elsewhere 网状纤维；**sensory f's**, afferent fibers 感觉神经纤维，传入神经纤维；**Sharpey f's**, 穿通纤维，沙比纤维；1. collagenous fibers that pass from the periosteum and are embedded in the outer circumferential and interstitial lamellae of bone 骨外膜中的胶原纤维穿入骨质形成的纤维；2. terminal portions of principal fibers that insert into the cement of a tooth 插入牙齿黏合剂的主要纤维的末端部分；**soluble f.**, that with an affinity for water, either dissolving or swelling to form a gel; it includes gums, pectins, mucilages, and some hemicelluloses and is primarily found in fruits, vegetables, oats, barley, legumes, and seaweed 可溶性纤维；**somatic nerve f's**, nerve fibers that stimulate and activate skeletal muscle and somatic tissues *(somatic efferent f's)* or receive impulses from them *(somatic afferent f's)* 躯体神经纤维；**spindle f's**, the microtubules radiating from the centrioles during mitosis and forming a spindle-shaped configuration 纺锤丝；**unmyelinated f's**, nerve fibers that lack the myelin sheath 无髓（神经）纤维；**vasomotor f's**, unmyelinated nerve fibers going chiefly to arteriolar muscles 血管舒缩纤维；**visceral nerve f's**, autonomic nerve f's 内脏神经纤维；**white f's**, collagenous f's 白纤维

fi·ber·il·lu·mi·nat·ed (fiʹbər-ĭ-looʹmĭ-nātʺəd) transmitting light by bundles of glass or plastic fi-bers, using a lens system to transmit the image; said of endoscopes of such design 纤维光束

fi·bra (fiʹbrə) pl. *fiʹbrae* [L.] fiber 纤维

fi·brates (fiʹbrāts) general term for fibric acid (q.v.) derivatives 苯氧酸类，贝特类，纤维酸衍生物的总称

fi·bric ac·id (fiʹbrik) any of a group of compounds structurally related to clofibrate that can reduce plasma levels of triglycerides and cholesterol; used to treat hypertriglyceridemia and hypercholesterolemia 神经纤维酸

fi·bril (fiʹbril) a minute fiber or filament 原纤维，原纤；**fiʹbrillar, fibʹrillary** *adj*；**collagen f's**, delicate fibrils of collagen in connective tissue, composed of molecules of tropocollagen aggregated in linear array. In some types of collagen, the fibrils are aggregated to form larger fibrils, which may themselves be aggregated to form collagen fibers 胶原原纤维；**dentinal f's**, component fibrils of the dentinal matrix 牙质原纤维；**muscle f.**, myofibril 肌原纤维

fi·bril·la (fi-brilʹə) pl. *fibrilʹlae* [L.] a fibril 原纤维，纤丝

fi·bril·la·tion (fibʺrĭ-laʹshən) 1. the quality of being made up of fibrils 纤维化，纤维形成；2. a small, local, involuntary muscular contraction, due to spontaneous activation of single muscle cells or muscle fibers whose nerve supply has been damaged or cut off 肌纤维震颤；3. the initial degenerative changes in osteoarthritis, marked by softening of the articular cartilage and development of vertical clefts between groups of cartilage cells 原纤维显现；**atrial f.**, atrial arrhythmia marked by rapid randomized contractions of small areas of the atrial myocardium, causing a totally irregular, and often rapid, ventricular rate 心房颤动；**ventricular f.**, cardiac arrhythmia marked by fibrillary contractions of the ventricular muscle due to rapid repetitive excitation of myocardial fibers without coordinated ventricular contraction and by absence of atrial activity 心室颤动，心室纤颤

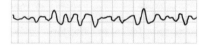

▲ 心室颤动（**ventricular fibrillation**）

fi·brin (fiʹbrin) an insoluble protein that is essential to clotting of blood, formed from fibrinogen by action of thrombin 纤维蛋白，血纤蛋白

fi·bri·no·cel·lu·lar (fiʺbrĭ-no-selʹu-lər) made up of fibrin and cells 纤维蛋白细胞的

fi·brin·o·gen (fi-brinʹo-jən) coagulation factor I

纤维蛋白原，血纤维蛋白原，即凝血因子 I

fi·bri·no·gen·ic (fi″brĭ-no-jen′ik) producing or causing the formation of fibrin 纤维蛋白原的

fi·bri·no·ge·nol·y·sis (fi″brĭ-no-jə-nol′ə-sis) the proteolytic destruction of fibrinogen in circulating blood 纤维蛋白原溶解；**fibrinogenolyt′ic** adj.

fi·brino·geno·pe·nia (fi-brin′o-jen″o-pe′ne-ə) hypofibrinogenemia 低纤维蛋白原血症

fi·brin·oid (fi′brin-oid) 1. resembling fibrin 纤维蛋白样的。2. a homogeneous, eosinophilic, relatively acellular refractile substance with some of the staining properties of fibrin 具有某些纤维蛋白染色特性的

fi·bri·nol·y·sin (fi″brĭ-nol′ĭ-sin) 1. plasmin 纤溶酶；2. a preparation of proteolytic enzyme formed from profibrinolysin (plasminogen); to promote dissolution of thrombi 纤维蛋白溶解酶

fi·bri·nol·y·sis (fi″brĭ-nol′ə-sis) dissolution of fibrin by enzymatic action 纤维蛋白溶解，血纤蛋白溶解；**fibrinolyt′ic** adj.

fi·bri·no·pep·tide (fi″brĭ-no-pep′tīd) either of two peptides (A and B) split off from fibrinogen during coagulation by the action of thrombin 血纤肽

fi·bri·no·pu·ru·lent (fi″brĭ-no-pu′roo-lənt) characterized by the presence of both fibrin and pus 脓性纤维蛋白的

fi·brin·ous (fi′brin-əs) pertaining to or of the nature of fibrin 纤维蛋白的

fi·brin·uria (fi″brĭ-nu′re-ə) the presence of fibrin in the urine 纤维蛋白尿

fi·bro·ad·e·no·ma (fi″bro-ad″ə-no′mə) adenofibroma 纤维腺瘤；**giant f. of breast,** phyllodes tumor 乳腺巨大纤维腺瘤

fi·bro·ad·i·pose (fi″bro-ad′ĭ-pōs) both fibrous and fatty 纤维脂肪性的

fi·bro·are·o·lar (fi″bro-ə-re′o-lər) both fibrous and areolar. 纤维蜂窝组织性的

fi·bro·blast (fi′bro-blast) 1. an immature fiber-producing cell of connective tissue capable of differentiating into chondroblast, collagenoblast, or osteoblast 成纤维细胞；2. collagenoblast; the collagenproducing cell. The cells also proliferate at the site of chronic inflammation 成胶原细胞；**fibroblas′tic** adj.

fi·bro·blas·to·ma (fi″bro-blas-to′mə) any tumor arising from fibroblasts, divided into fibromas and fibrosarcomas 成纤维细胞瘤

fi·bro·bron·chi·tis (fi″bro-brong-ki′tis) fi - brinous bronchitis 纤维蛋白性支气管炎

fi·bro·cal·cif·ic (fi″bro-kal-sif′ik) pertaining to or characterized by partially calcified fibrous tissue 纤维钙化性的

fi·bro·car·ci·no·ma (fi″bro-kahr″sĭ-no′mə) scirrhous carcinoma 纤维癌

fi·bro·car·ti·lage (fi″bro-kahr′tĭ-ləj) cartilage of parallel, thick, compact collagenous bundles, separated by narrow clefts containing the typical cartilage cells (chondrocytes) 纤维软骨；**fibrocartilag′inous** adj.；**elastic f.,** that containing elastic fibers 弹性纤维软骨；**interarticular f.,** articular disk 关节盘

fi·bro·car·ti·la·go (fi″bro-kahr″tĭ-lah′go) pl. fibrocartilag′ines [L.] fibrocartilage 纤维软骨

fi·bro·chon·dri·tis (fi″bro-kon-dri′tis) in - flammation of fibrocartilage 纤维软骨炎

fi·bro·col·lag·e·nous (fi″bro-ko-laj′ə-nəs) both fibrous and collagenous; pertaining to or composed of fibrous tissue mainly composed of collagen 纤维胶原性的

fi·bro·cys·tic (fi″bro-sis′tik) characterized by an overgrowth of fibrous tissue and development of cystic spaces, especially in a gland 纤维囊肿的

fi·bro·cyte (fi′bro-sīt) fibroblast 纤维原细胞；纤维组织细胞

fi·bro·dys·pla·sia (fi″bro-dis-pla′zhə) abnormality in development of fibrous connective tissue 纤维发育不良

fi·bro·elas·tic (fi″bro-e-las′tik) both fibrous and elastic 纤维（组织与）弹性组织的

fi·bro·elas·to·sis (fi″bro-e″las-to′sis) overgrowth of fibroelastic elements 纤维弹性组织增生；**endocardial f.,** diffuse patchy thickening of the mural endocardium, particularly in the left ventricle, due to proliferation of collagenous and elastic tissue; often associated with congenital cardiac malformations 心内膜弹力纤维增生症

fi·bro·ep·i·the·li·al (fi″bro-ep″ĭ-the′le-əl) having fibrous and epithelial elements 纤维上皮的

fi·bro·ep·i·the·li·o·ma (fi″bro-ep″ĭ-the″leo′mə) a tumor composed of both fibrous and epithelial elements 纤维上皮瘤

fi·bro·fol·lic·u·lo·ma (fi″bro-fə-lik″u-lo′mə) a benign adnexal tumor of perifollicular connective tissue, occurring as one or more yellow, dome-shaped papules, usually on the face 纤维毛囊瘤

fi·bro·his·tio·cyt·ic (fi″bro-his″te-o-sit′ik) having fibrous and histiocytic elements 纤维组织细胞的

fi·broid (fi′broid) 1. having a fibrous structure; resembling a fibroma 类纤维瘤的。2. fibroma 纤维瘤。3. leiomyoma 平滑肌瘤；4. (in the pl.) a colloquial term for leiomyoma of the uterus 子宫肌瘤（口语）

fi·broid·ec·to·my (fi″broid-ek′tə-me) uterine myomectomy 子宫肌瘤切除术

fi·bro·la·mel·lar (fi″bro-lə-mel′ər) characterized by the formation of fibers of collagen in layers 纤维板层

fi·bro·li·po·ma (fi″bro-lĭ-po′mə) a lipoma with

excessive fibrous tissue 纤维脂肪瘤; **fibrolipo′matous** *adj.*

fi·bro·ma (fi-bro′mə) pl. *fibromas, fibro′mata.* a tumor composed mainly of fibrous or fully developed connective tissue 纤维瘤; **ameloblastic f.,** an odontogenic tumor marked by simultaneous proliferation of both epithelial and mesenchymal tissue, without formation of enamel or dentin 成釉细胞纤维瘤; **cementifying f.,** a tumor of fibroblastic tissue containing masses of cement-like tissue, usually in the mandible of older persons 牙骨质化纤维瘤; **central odontogenic f.,** a rare, benign, unencapsulated odontogenic tumor of the jaw, usually the mandible, characterized by islands of odontogenic epithelium within fibrous connective tissue and sometimes by calcifications 中心性牙源性纤维瘤; **chondromyxoid f.,** a rare, benign, slowly growing tumor of bone of chondroblastic origin, usually affecting the large long bones of the lower limb 软骨黏液样纤维瘤; **cystic f.,** one that has undergone cystic degeneration 囊性纤维瘤; **f. mol′le, f. mollus′cum,** acrochordon 软性纤维瘤; **nonossifying f., nonosteogenic f.,** a degenerative, proliferative lesion of the medullary and cortical tissues of bone 非骨化性纤维瘤; **odontogenic f.,** 牙源性纤维瘤, 见 *central odontogenic f.* 和 *peripheral odontogenic f.*; **ossifying f., ossifying f. of bone,** a benign, slow-growing, central bone tumor, usually of the jaws, especially the mandible, composed of fibrous connective tissue within which bone is formed 骨化性纤维瘤; **perifollicular f.,** a type of benign, small, flesh-colored, papular, follicular adnexal tumor on the head or neck, sometimes found in groups 毛囊周围纤维瘤; **peripheral odontogenic f.,** an extraosseous counterpart to a central odontogenic fibroma; it is a gingival mass of vascularized fibrous connective tissue with strands of odontogenic epithelium 外周性牙源性纤维瘤; **peripheral ossifying f.,** epulis; a fibroma, usually of the gingiva, showing areas of calcification or ossification 外周性骨化性纤维瘤; **periungual f.,** one of multiple smooth, firm, protruding nodules occurring at the nail folds, pathognomonic of tuberous sclerosis 甲周纤维瘤; **soft f.,** acrochordon 软纤维瘤

fi·bro·ma·to·sis (fi-bro″mə-to′sis) 1. the presence of multiple fibromas 纤维瘤病; 2. the formation of a fibrous, tumor-like nodule arising from the deep fascia, with a tendency to local recurrence 纤维状肿瘤样结节; **aggressive f.,** desmoid tumor, particularly one that is extraabdominal 侵袭性纤维瘤病; **f. gingi′vae, gingival f.,** noninflammatory fibrous hyperplasia of the gingiva manifested as a dense, diffuse, smooth or nodular overgrowth of the gingi-

val tissues 牙龈纤维瘤病; **palmar f.,** fibromatosis of palmar fascia, resulting in Dupuytren contracture 掌部纤维瘤病; **plantar f.,** fibromatosis of plantar fascia, with single or multiple nodular swellings, sometimes with pain but usually without contractures 跖部纤维瘤病

fi·bro·mus·cu·lar (fi″bro-mus′ku-lər) composed of fibrous and muscular tissue 纤维肌性的

fi·bro·my·itis (fi″bro-mi-i′tis) inflammation of muscle with fibrous degeneration 纤维性肌炎

fi·bro·my·o·ma (fi″bro-mi-o′mə) a myoma containing fibrous elements 纤维肌瘤

fi·bro·myx·o·ma (fi″bro-mik-so′mə) myxofibroma 纤维黏液瘤

fi·bro·myx·o·sar·co·ma (fi″bro-mik″so-sahrko′mə) a sarcoma containing fibromatous and myxomatous elements 纤维黏液肉瘤

fi·bro·nec·tin (fi″bro-nek′tin) an adhesive glycoprotein: one form circulates in plasma and acts as an opsonin; another is a cell-surface protein that mediates cellular adhesive interactions 纤维粘连蛋白; 纤连蛋白

fi·bro·odon·to·ma (fi″bro-o″don-to′mə) a tumor containing both fibrous and odontogenic elements 纤维牙瘤

fi·bro·pap·il·lo·ma (fi″bro-pap″ĭ-lo′mə) fibroepithelial papilloma 纤维乳头状瘤

fi·bro·pla·sia (fi″bro-pla′zhə) the formation of fibrous tissue 纤维组织形成, 纤维组织增生; **fibroplas′tic** *adj;* **retrolental f. (RLF),** retinopathy of prematurity 晶体后纤维增生症, 早产儿视网膜病变综合征

fi·bro·sar·co·ma (fi″bro-sahr-ko′mə) a malignant, locally invasive, hematogenously spreading tumor derived from collagen-producing fibroblasts that are otherwise undifferentiated 纤维肉瘤; **ameloblastic f.,** an odontogenic tumor that is the malignant counterpart to an ameloblastic fibroma, within which it usually arises 成釉细胞纤维肉瘤; **odontogenic f.,** a malignant tumor of the jaws, originating from one of the mesenchymal components of the tooth or tooth germ 牙源性纤维肉瘤

fi·brose (fi′brōs) 1. to form fibrous tissue 纤维化; 2. fibrous 纤维的

fi·bro·sis (fi-bro′sis) formation of fibrous tissue 纤维化; **fibrot′ic** *adj.*; **congenital hepatic f.,** a developmental disorder of the liver marked by formation of irregular broad bands of fibrous tissue containing multiple cysts formed by disordered terminal bile ducts, resulting in vascular constriction and portal hypertension 先天性肝纤维化; **cystic f.,** a lethal autosomal recessive disorder in which there is widespread dysfunction of the exocrine glands, signs of chronic pulmonary disease, pancreatic deficiency, abnormally high levels of electrolytes in the sweat, and obstruction of pancreatic ducts by amorphous eosinophilic concretions with consequent deficiency of pancreatic enzymes. It is caused by mutations in the *CFTR* gene, which encodes the cystic fibrosis transmembrane regulator 囊性纤维化；**endomyocardial f.**, idiopathic myocardiopathy seen endemically in parts of Africa and less often in other areas, characterized by cardiomegaly, thickening of the endocardium with dense, white fibrous tissue that often extends to involve the inner third or half of the myocardium, and congestive heart failure. 心内膜心肌纤维化；**idiopathic pulmonary f.**, chronic inflammation and progessive fibrosis of the pulmonary alveolar walls, with progressive dyspnea and potentially fatal lack of oxygen or right heart failure. The acute form is called *Hamman-Rich syndrome.* 特发性肺纤维化；**mediastinal f.**, fibrous mediastinitis; development of white, hard fibrous tissue in the upper portion of the mediastinum, sometimes obstructing the air passages and large blood vessels 纵隔纤维变性；**nodular subepidermal f.**, 1. benign fibrous histiocytoma 良性纤维组织细胞瘤；2. a type of benign fibrous histiocytoma marked by subepidermal formation of fibrous nodules as a result of productive inflammation 结节性表皮下纤维化，为良性纤维组织细胞瘤的一种；**pleural f.**, fibrosis of the visceral pleura so that part or all of a lung becomes covered with a thick layer of nonexpansible fibrous tissue; fibrothorax is a more extensive form 胸膜纤维化；**proliferative f.**, that in which the fibrous elements continue to proliferate after the original causative factor has ceased to operate 增生性纤维化；**pulmonary f.**, idiopathic pulmonary fibrosis 肺纤维化；**retroperitoneal f.**, deposition of fibrous tissue in the retroperitoneal space, producing abdominal discomfort and often blockage of the ureters, with resultant hydronephrosis and impaired renal function, which may result in renal failure 腹膜后纤维化

fi·bro·si·tis (fi″bro-si′tis) inflammatory hyperplasia of the white fibrous tissue, especially of the muscle sheaths and fascial layers of the locomotor system 纤维组织炎

fi·bro·tho·rax (fi″bro-thor′aks) adhesion of the two layers of pleura, so that the lung is covered by a thick layer of nonexpansible fibrous tissue (see *fibrinous pleurisy*). It is often a consequence of traumatic hemothorax or of pleural effusion 纤维胸

fi·brous (fi′brəs) composed of or containing fibers 纤维的，纤维性的

fi·bro·xan·tho·ma (fi″bro-zan-tho′mə) a type of xanthoma containing fibromatous elements, sometimes described as synonymous with or a subtype of either benign or malignant fibrous histiocytoma 纤维黄（色）瘤；**atypical f. (AFX)**, a small cutaneous nodular neoplasm usually occurring on sun-exposed areas of the face and neck; sometimes described as related to or a subtype of either benign or malignant fibrous histiocytoma 非典型纤维黄（色）瘤

fi·bro·xan·tho·sar·co·ma (fi″bro-zan″thosahr-ko′mə) malignant fibrous histiocytoma 纤维黄（色）肉瘤

fib·u·la (fib′u-lə) [L.] the outer and smaller of the two bones of the leg, which articulates proximally with the tibia and distally is joined to the tibia in a syndesmosis 腓骨，见图1

fib·u·lar (fib′u-lər) pertaining to the fibula or to the lateral aspect of the leg 腓侧

fib·u·la·ris (fib′u-lar′is) [L.] fibular 腓骨

fib·u·lo·cal·ca·ne·al (fib″u-lo-kal-ka′ne-əl) pertaining to fibula and calcaneus 腓跟的

fi·cain (fi′kān) an enzyme derived from the sap of fig trees that catalyzes the cleavage of specific bonds in proteins; it enhances the agglutination of red blood cells with IgG antibodies and is therefore used in the determination of the Rh factor 无花果蛋白酶

FICD Fellow of the International College of Dentists 国际牙医师学会会员

fi·cin (fi′sin) ficain 无花果蛋白酶

FICS Fellow of the International College of Surgeons 国际外科医师学会会员

fi·dax·o·mi·cin (fi-dăx″o-mi′-sīn) a macrolide antibiotic that is used to treat diarrhea caused by *Clostridium difficile* 非达霉素

field (fēld) 1. an area or open space, as an operative field or visual field 视野，区域；2. a range of specialization in knowledge, study, or occupation（知识，学习或职业）的领域；3. in embryology, the developing region within a range of modifying factors（胚胎学的）发生场；**auditory f.**, the space or range within which stimuli may be perceived as sound 听阈，听觉范围；**individuation f.**, a region in which an organizer influences adjacent tissue to become a part of a total embryo（胚胎）个体形成区；**morphogenetic f.**, an embryonic region out of which definite structures normally develop 形态发生场；**visual f. (F) (vf)**, the area within which stimuli will produce the sensation of sight with the eye in a straightahead position 视野

FIGLU formiminoglutamic acid 甲氨基谷氨酸
fig·ure (fig′yər) 1. an object of particular form 特定形式的物体；2. a number, or numeral 数字；**mitotic f's**, stages of chromosome aggregation ex-

hibiting a pattern characteristic of mitosis 分裂象，核分裂象

fi·la (fi'lə) [L.] plural of *filum* 丝

fil·a·ment (fil'ə-mənt) a delicate fiber or thread 丝，组成原纤维的亚级线状结构; **actin f.,** one of the thin contractile myofilaments in a myofibril 肌动蛋白丝, **intermediate f's,** a class of cytoplasmic filaments that predominantly act as structural components of the cytoskeleton and also affect various movements in cellular processes 中间丝; **muscle f.,** myofilament 肌丝; **myosin f.,** one of the thick contractile myofilaments in a myofibril 肌球蛋白丝，粗肌丝; **thick f's,** bipolar myosin filaments occurring in striated muscle 粗肌丝; **thin f's,** actin filaments occurring, associated with troponin and tropomyosin, in striated muscle 细肌丝

fil·a·men·tous (fil"ə-men'təs) composed of long, threadlike structures 细丝状的，纤维所成的

fil·a·men·tum (fil"ə-men'təm) pl. *filamen'ta* [L.] filament 丝

fi·la·ria (fī-lar'e-ə) pl. *fila'riae* [L.] a nematode worm of the superfamily Filarioidea 丝虫; **fila'rial** *adj.*

fil·a·ri·a·sis (fil"ə-ri'ə-sis) infestation by filariae 丝虫病

fi·lar·i·cide (fī-lar'ĭ-sīd) an agent that destroys filariae 杀丝虫药

Fi·lar·i·oi·dea (fī-lar"e-oi'de-ə) a superfamily or order of parasitic nematodes, the adults being threadlike worms that invade the tissues and body cavities where the female deposits microfilariae (prelarvae) 丝虫目

fil·gras·tim (fil-gras'tim) a human granulocyte colony-stimulating factor produced by recombinant technology; used to enhance neutrophil function, stimulating hematopoiesis and decreasing neutropenia 非格司亭

fil·i·al (fil'e-al) 1. of or pertaining to a son or daughter 子女的; 2. in genetics, of or pertaining to those generations following the initial (parental) generation 子代的

fil·i·form (fil'ĭ-form) (fi'lĭ-form) 1. threadlike 细丝状的; 2. an extremely slender bougie 非常细长的探条

fil·let (fil'et) 1. a loop, as of cord or tape, for making traction on the fetus（胎儿）牵引环; 2. in the nervous system, a long band of nerve fibers 神经环路

fill·ing (fil'ing) 1. material inserted in a prepared tooth cavity（口腔）充填材料; 2. restoration of the crown with appropriate material after removal of carious tissue from a tooth 充填; **complex f.,** one for a complex cavity 复杂充填; **composite f.,** one

consisting of a resin composite 复合充填材料; **compound f.,** one for a cavity that involves two surfaces of a tooth 复合充填

film (film) 1. a thin layer or coating 薄膜，薄层，涂层; 2. a thin transparent sheet of cellulose acetate or similar material coated on one or both sides with an emulsion that is sensitive to light or radiation 醋酸纤维素系列膜，特指由醋酸纤维素及其衍生物为主体材料制成的膜; **absorbable gelatin f.,** a sterile, nonantigenic, absorbable, water-insoluble sheet of gelatin, used as an aid in surgical closure and repair of defects and as a local hemostatic 吸水明胶片; **bite-wing f.,** an x-ray film for radiography of oral structures, with a protruding tab to be held between the upper and lower teeth 咬合翼片; **plain f.,** a radiograph made without the use of a contrast medium 平片; **spot f.,** a radiograph of a small anatomic area obtained either by rapid exposure during fluoroscopy to provide a permanent record of a transiently observed abnormality or by limitation of radiation passing through the area to improve definition and detail of the image produced 点片; **x-ray f.,** film sensitized to x-rays, either before or after exposure X 线片

film badge (film baj) a pack of radiographic film or films, usually worn on the body during potential exposure to radiation in order to detect and quantitate the dosage of exposure 胶片剂量计

Fi·lo·vi·ri·dae (fi"lo-vir'ĭ-de) a family of RNA viruses that includes just one genus, *Filovirus* 纤丝病毒科

Fi·lo·vi·rus (fi'lo-vi"rəs) Marburg and Ebola viruses: a genus of viruses of the family Filoviridae that cause hemorrhagic fevers (Marburg disease, Ebola virus disease) 线状病毒（包括马尔堡病毒和埃博拉病毒）

fil·ter (fil'tər) 1. a device for eliminating or separating certain elements, as (1) particles of certain size from a solution, or (2) rays of certain wavelength from a stream of radiant energy 过滤器, 如滤液器，滤光器; 2. to cause such separation or elimination 过滤，滤除; **membrane f.,** a filter made up of a thin film of nylon, cellulose acetate, or other material, with a defined pore size 膜滤器

fil·ter·able (fil'tər-ə-bəl) capable of passing through the pores of a filter 可过滤的

fil·trate (fil'trāt) a liquid or gas that has passed through a filter 滤液

fil·tra·tion (fil-tra'shən) passage through a filter or other material that prevents passage of certain molecules, particles, or substances 过滤，滤过

fi·lum (fi'ləm) pl. *fi'la* [L.] a threadlike structure or part 丝状的结构或部分; **f. termina'le,** a slender threadlike filament of connective tissue that descends from the conus medullaris to attach to the inner aspect of the dural sac and from there to the base of the coccyx; divided into a filum terminale internum and a filum terminale externum, the dividing line being the lower border of the second sacral vertebra 终丝

fim·bria (fim′bre-ə) pl. *fim′briae* [L.] 1. a fringe, border, or edge; a fringelike structure 边缘，边界，边缘结构；2. pilus (2) 菌毛，伞毛；**f. hippocam′pi,** the band of white matter along the median edge of the ventricular surface of the hippocampus 海马伞；**ovarian f.,** the longest of the processes that make up the fimbriae of the uterine tube, extending along the free border of the mesosalpinx and fused to the ovary 卵巢伞；**fimbriae of uterine tube,** the numerous divergent fringelike processes on the distal part of the infundibulum of the uterine tube 输卵管伞

fim·bri·at·ed (fim′bre-āt″əd) fringed 伞状的

fim·bri·ec·to·my (fim″bre-ek′tə-me) surgical removal of the fimbriae of the uterine tube along with tubal ligation as a method of female sterilization 输卵管伞端切除术

fim·brio·cele (fim′bre-o-sēl″) hernia containing the fimbriae of the uterine tube 输卵管伞突出

fim·bri·o·plas·ty (fim′bre-o-plas″te) plastic surgery of the fimbriae of the uterine tube 输卵管伞端成形术

fi·nas·te·ride (fĭ-nas′tər-īd) an inhibitor of 5 α -reductase, used in the treatment of benign prostatic hyperplasia and as a hair growth stimulant in the treatment of androgenetic alopecia 非那雄胺

Fine·gol·dia (fĭn-gol′de-ə) a genus of grampositive, anaerobic, coccoid bacteria of the family Peptostreptococcaceae, occurring usually in masses and tetrads; *F. mag′na* is part of the normal flora of the gastrointestinal and female genitourinary tracts and causes septic arthritis and soft tissue infections 芬戈尔德菌属

fin·ger (fing′gər) one of the five digits of the hand 手指；**baseball f.,** mallet f. 垒球指；**clubbed f.,** a finger with clubbing 杵状指，槌状指；**index f.,** forefinger 示指，食指；**mallet f.,** partial permanent flexion of the terminal phalanx of a finger caused by an object striking the end or back of the finger, owing to rupture of the attachment of the extensor tendon 锤状指；**ring f.,** the fourth digit of the hand 环指；**webbed f's,** syndactyly of the fingers 蹼指

fin·ger·print (fing′gər-print) 1. an impression of the cutaneous ridges of the fleshy distal portion of a finger（手指的）指纹；2. the image obtained by fingerprinting (q.v.) of proteins or nucleic acids（蛋白质或核酸的）指纹图；3. the infrared absorption spectrum of a molecule（分子的）红外吸收光谱

fin·ger·print·ing (fing′gər-print″ing) a technique for determining the structure of or identifying a protein or nucleic acid (*DNA f.*) by cleavage of the molecule into defined fragments, chromatographic or electrophoretic separation of the fragments, and visualization of the resulting pattern（蛋白质或核酸的）指纹分析法

fin·gol·i·mod (fin-gol′ĭ-mod) a sphingosine 1-phosphate receptor antagonist that reduces the movement of T and B lymphocytes from lymphoid organs to peripheral inflammatory tissues; used as the hydrochloride salt for the treatment of relapsing forms of multiple sclerosis 芬戈莫德

Fir·a·zyr (feer′uh-zeer) trademark for a preparation of icatibant 艾替班特（icatibant）的商品名

Fir·mi·cu·tes (fər-mik′u-tēz) (fur″mĭ-ku′tēz) a phenotypically diverse phylum of mainly grampositive bacteria; with Bacteroidetes it is one of the two major constituents of the intestinal flora 厚壁菌门

first aid (furst ād) emergency care and treatment of an injured or ill person before complete medical and surgical treatment can be secured 急救

fis·sion (fish′ən) 1. the act of splitting 分裂；2. asexual reproduction in which the cell divides into two (*binary f.*) or more (*multiple f.*) daughter parts, each of which becomes an individual organism 无性生殖中的二分裂或复分裂；3. nuclear fission; the splitting of the atomic nucleus, with release of energy（原子的）核裂变

fis·sip·a·rous (fĭ-sip′ə-rəs) propagated by fission 有分裂能力的

fis·su·la (fis′u-lə) [L.] a small cleft 小裂缝

fis·su·ra (fis-u′rə) pl. *fissu′rae* [L.] fissure 裂隙；**f. in a′no,** anal fissure 肛裂

fis·sure (fish′ər) 1. any cleft or groove, normal or otherwise, especially a deep fold in the cerebral cortex involving its entire thickness 裂缝，凹槽，也指大脑褶皱之间的沟；2. a fault in the enamel surface of a tooth（牙体解剖学）裂隙，指牙釉质表面的缺陷；**abdominal f.,** a congenital cleft in the abdominal wall 腹裂；**anal f., f. in ano,** painful lineal ulcer at the margin of the anus 肛裂；**anterior median f.,** a longitudinal furrow along the midline of the anterior aspect of the spinal cord and medulla oblongata 前正中裂；**basisylvian f.,** the part of the sylvian fissure between the temporal lobe and the orbital surface of the frontal bone 大脑基底侧沟；**branchial f's,** 1. branchial clefts (1) 鳃裂；2. pharyngeal grooves 咽沟；**calcarine f.,** distal沟，见 *sulcus* 下词条；**central f.,** central cerebral sulcus 大脑中央沟；**collateral f.,** 侧副沟，

F

见 *sulcus* 下词条；**enamel f.,** fissure (2) 牙釉质裂隙；**hippocampal f.,** 海马裂，见 *sulcus* 下词条；**lateral cerebral f.,** sylvian f.; one extending laterally between the temporal and frontal lobes, and turning posteriorly between the temporal and parietal lobes 大脑外侧裂；**palpebral f.,** the longitudinal opening between the eyelids 睑裂；**portal f.,** porta hepatis 肝门；**posterior median f.,** 后正中沟，见 *sulcus* 下词条；**presylvian f.,** the anterior branch of the fissure of Sylvius 前水平支；**primary f. of cerebellum,** that separating the cranial and caudal lobes in the cerebellum 小脑原裂；**f. of Rolando,** central cerebral sulcus 罗朗多裂，大脑中央沟；**sphenooccipital f.,** the fissure between the basilar part of the occipital bone and the sphenoid bone 蝶枕裂；**sylvian f., Sylvius f.,** lateral cerebral f.；**transverse f.,** 1. porta hepatis 肝门；2. the transverse cerebral fissure between the diencephalon and the cerebral hemispheres 大脑横裂

fis·tu·la (fis'tu-lə) pl. *fistulas, fis'tulae* [L.] an abnormal passage between two internal organs or from an internal organ to the body surface 瘘；**anal f.,** one from the anus to the skin, sometimes communicating with the rectum 肛瘘；**arteriovenous f.,** 1. one between an artery and a vein 动静脉瘘；2. a surgically created arteriovenous connection that provides a site of access for hemodialysis tubing 动静脉瘘术；**blind f.,** one open at one end only, opening on the skin *(external blind f.)* or on an internal mucous surface *(internal blind f.).* 单口瘘，分单口外瘘和单口内瘘；**branchial f.,** a persistent pharyngeal groove (branchial cleft) 鳃瘘；**cerebrospinal fluid f.,** one between the subarachnoid space and a body cavity, with leakage of cerebrospinal fluid, usually as otorrhea or rhinorrhea 脑脊液漏，常为耳漏或鼻漏；**colonic f.,** one connecting the colon with the body surface or another organ 结肠瘘；**craniosinus f.,** one between the cerebral space and one of the sinuses, permitting escape of cerebrospinal fluid into the nose 鼻脑脊液漏；**enterovesical f.,** one connecting the urinary bladder with some part of the intestines 肠膀胱瘘；**fecal f.,** a colonic fistula that discharges feces on the body surface 粪瘘；**gastric f.,** one communicating with the stomach, either pathologically or surgically created through the abdominal wall 胃瘘；**genitourinary f.,** one between two organs of the urogenital system or between one of thosen organs and some other system 生殖尿道瘘；**incomplete f.,** blind f. 不完全瘘，即单口瘘；**intestinal f.,** one communicating with the intestine; sometimes surgically created through the abdominal wall 肠瘘；**perilymph f.,** rupture of the round window with

leakage of perilymph into the middle ear, causing sensorineural hearing loss 外淋巴瘘；**pulmonary arteriovenous f.,** a congenital fistula between the pulmonary arterial and venous systems, so that unoxygenated blood enters the systemic circulation 肺动静脉瘘；**salivary f.,** one communicating with a salivary duct 涎腺瘘；**tracheoesophageal f.,** one connecting the trachea and esophagus, either pathologically or created surgically to restore speech after laryngectomy 气管食管瘘；**umbilical f.,** one communicating with the colon or the urachus at the umbilicus 脐肠瘘

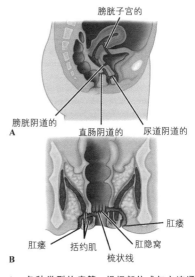

▲ 各种类型的瘘管，根据部位或与之连通的器官而命名。A. 生殖尿道瘘 (genitourinary fistulae)。B. 肛瘘 (analfistulae)

fis·tu·la·tome (fis'tu-lə-tōm) an instrument for cutting a fistula 瘘管刀

fis·tu·li·za·tion (fis″tu-lĭ-za'shən) 1. the process of becoming fistulous 瘘管形成；2. the surgical creation of a fistula 造瘘术

fis·tu·lot·o·my (fis″tu-lot'ə-me) incision of a fistula 瘘管切开术

fit (fit) 1. seizure (2) 癫痫单次发作；2. the adaptation of one structure into another 适合

fit·ness (fit'nis) 1. in genetics, the probability of transmitting one's genotype to the next generation relative to the average probability for the population （遗传学）适合度；2. physical f.；**aerobic f. cardiorespiratory f.,** the capacity of the cardiovascular and respiratory systems of an individual to supply oxygen and energy during sustained physical activity 有氧适能，心肺适能；**physical f.,** the capacity of an individual to perform physical activities requiring cardiorespiratory exertion, muscular endurance, strength, or flexibility. 体适能

five and five (fīv and fīv) an approach recommended by the Red Cross for delivering first aid to a choking person. First, five back blows are given between the person's shoulder blades with the heel of the hand, followed by five abdominal thrusts 五五交替法，指在对呼吸道异物窒息者采取急救时，用手掌击其背部（肩胛骨之间）5 次再对腹部挤压 5 次，如此循环直到异物去除

fix (fiks) to fasten or hold firm 固定，系牢；见 *fixation*

fix·a·tion (fik-sa′shən) 1. the act or operation of holding, suturing, or fastening in a fixed position （做出）固定（的操作或行为）；2. the condition of being held in a fixed position（位置上的）固定状态；3. in psychiatry, (a) arrest of development at a particular stage, or (b) a close suffocating attachment to another person, especially a childhood figure, such as a parent（精神病学）固着；4. the use of a fixative to preserve histologic or cytologic specimens（利用固定剂）固定（组织学或细胞学标本）；5. in chemistry, the process whereby a substance is removed from the gaseous or solution phase and localized 分离提纯；6. in ophthalmology, direction of the gaze so that the visual image of the object falls on the fovea centralis（眼科学）视觉成像；7. in film processing, removal of all undeveloped salts of the film emulsion, leaving only the developed silver to form a permanent image （胶片处理中的）定影；**complement f., f. of complement,** addition of another serum containing an antibody and the corresponding antigen to a hemolytic serum, making the complement incapable of producing hemolysis 补体结合

fix·a·tive (fik′sə-tiv) an agent used in preserving a histologic or pathologic specimen so as to maintain the normal structure of its constituent elements 固定剂

flac·cid (flak′sid) (flas′id) 1. weak, lax, and soft 虚弱的，松弛的，软弱的；2. atonic 失张力的

fla·gel·la (flə-jel′ə) [L.] 鞭毛，*flagellum* 的复数形式

fla·gel·lar (flə-jel′ər) pertaining to a flagellum 鞭毛的

flag·el·late (flaj′ə-lāt) 1. any microorganism having flagella 所有有鞭毛的微生物；2. mastigote 鞭毛虫；3. having flagella 有鞭毛的；4. to practice flagellation 鞭打

flag·el·la·tion (flaj″ə-la′shən) 1. whipping or being whipped to achieve erotic pleasure 鞭打或被鞭打（以获得性快感）；2. exflagellation 除毛；3. the formation or arrangement of flagella on an organism or surface 鞭毛形成或排列

fla·gel·lin (flə-jel′in) a protein of bacterial flagella; it is composed of subunits in severalstranded helical arrangement 鞭毛蛋白

fla·gel·lo·spore (flə-jel′o-spor) zoospore 鞭毛孢子

fla·gel·lum (flə-jel′əm) pl. *flagel′la* [L.] a long, mobile, whiplike appendage arising from a basal body at the surface of a cell, serving as a locomotor organelle; in eukaryotic cells, flagella contain nine pairs of microtubules arrayed around a central pair; in bacteria, they contain tightly wound strands of flagellin 鞭毛

flail (flāl) exhibiting abnormal or pathologic mobility, as flail chest or flail joint 连枷的

flame (flām) 1. the luminous, irregular appearance usually accompanying combustion, or an appearance resembling it 火焰；2. to render an object sterile by exposure to a flame 烧灼灭菌

flange (flanj) a projecting border or edge; in dentistry, the part of the denture base that extends from around the embedded teeth to the border of the denture 凸缘；（牙科学）义齿基托的一部分

flank (flank) the side of the body between ribs and ilium 胁腹

flap (flap) 1. a mass of tissue for grafting, usually including skin, only partially removed from one part of the body so that it retains its own blood supply during transfer to another site 皮瓣；2. an uncontrolled movement 不可控运动；**advancement f., sliding f.** 推进皮瓣；**axial pattern f.,** a myocutaneous flap containing an artery in its long axis 轴型皮瓣；**bipedicle f.,** a pedicle flap with two vascular attachments 双蒂皮瓣；**bone f.,** craniotomy involving elevation of a section of the skull 骨瓣；**free f.,** an island flap detached from the body and reattached at the distant recipient site by microvascular anastomosis 游离皮瓣；**island f.,** one consisting of skin and superficial fascia, with a pedicle made up of only the nutrient vessels 岛状皮瓣；**jump f.,** one cut from the abdomen and attached to a flap of the same size on the forearm; the forearm flap is transferred later to another part of the body to fill a defect 迁移皮瓣；**myocutaneous f.,** a compound flap of skin and muscle with adequate vascularity to permit sufficient tissue to be transferred to the recipient site 肌皮瓣；**pedicle f.,** a flap consisting of the full thickness of the skin and the superficial fascia, attached by tissue through which it receives its blood supply 带蒂皮瓣；**random pattern f.,** a myocutaneous flap with arandom pattern of arteries,

as opposed to an axial pattern flap 随意型皮瓣；
rope f., **tube f.**; **rotation f.**, a local pedicle flap whose width is increased by having the edge distal to the defect form a curved line; the flap is then rotated and a counterincision is made at the base of the curved line to increase mobility of the flap 旋转皮瓣；**skin f.**, a full-thickness mass or flap of tissue containing epidermis, dermis, and superficial fascia 皮瓣；**sliding f.**, a flap carried to its new position by a sliding technique 滑行皮瓣；**tube f.**, one made by elevating a long strip of tissue from its bed except at its two ends, the cut edges then being sutured together to form a tube 管状瓣

flare　(flār) a diffuse area of redness on the skin around the point of application of an irritant, due to a vasomotor reaction 红肿（区域）

flask　(flask) 1. a laboratory vessel, usually of glass and with a constricted neck 烧瓶，长颈瓶；2. a metal case in which materials used in making artificial dentures are placed for processing 用于制作假牙的金属盒；**Erlenmeyer f.**, a conical glass flask with a broad base and narrow neck 锥形烧瓶；**volumetric f.**, a narrow-necked vessel of glass calibrated to contain or deliver an exact volume at a given temperature 量瓶，容量瓶

flat　(flat) 1. lying in one plane; having an even surface 平坦的，光滑的；2. having little or no resonance（声音）单调的；3. slightly below the normal pitch of a musical tone 降音的

flat·foot　(flat'foot) a condition in which one or more arches of the foot have flattened out 扁平足

flat·ness　(flat'nis) a peculiar sound lacking resonance, heard on percussing an abnormally solid part 实音

flat·u·lence　(flat'u-ləns) excessive formation of gases in the stomach or intestine 气胀

fla·tus　(fla'təs) [L.] 1. gas or air in the gastrointestinal tract 胃肠道中的气体；2. gas or air expelled through the anus 屁

flat·worm　(flat'wərm) an individual organism of the phylum Platyhelminthes 扁形动物

fla·vin　(fla'vin) any of a group of water-soluble yellow pigments widely distributed in animals and plants, including riboflavin and yellow enzymes 黄素；**f. adenine dinucleotide (FAD)**, a coenzyme composed of riboflavin 5′-phosphate (FMN) and adenosine 5′-phosphate in pyrophosphate linkage; it forms the prosthetic group of certain enzymes, including d-amino acid oxidase and xanthine oxidase, serving as an electron carrier by being alternately oxidized (FAD) and reduced (FADH$_2$). It is important in electron transport in mitochondria 黄素腺嘌呤二核苷酸；**f. mononucleotide (FMN)**,

riboflavin 5′-phosphate; it acts as a coenzyme for a number of oxidative enzymes, including NADH dehydrogenase, serving as an electron carrier by being alternately oxidized (FMN) and reduced (FMNH$_2$) 黄素单核苷酸

Fla·vi·vi·ri·dae　(fla″vĭ-vir′ĭ-de) the flaviviruses: a family of RNA viruses that includes viruses that cause dengue, encephalitis, and hepatitis C. It includes the genera *Flavivirus* and *Hepacivirus* 黄病毒科

Fla·vi·vi·rus　(fla′vĭ-vi″rəs) a genus of viruses of the family Flaviviridae of worldwide distribution, including those that cause yellow fever, dengue, Japanese B encephalitis, St. Louis encephalitis, tick-borne encephalitis, and West Nile encephalitis. Mosquitoes are the most common vector, with some species being tick-borne and some having no known vector 黄病毒属

fla·vi·vi·rus　(fla′və-vi″rəs) any virus of the family Flaviviridae 黄病毒

Fla·vo·bac·te·ri·a·ceae　(fla″vo-bak-tēr″ea′se-e) a family of gram-negative, rod-shaped bacteria of the phylum Bacteroidetes; most are saprophytes, but some are pathogenic 黄杆菌科

Fla·vo·bac·te·ri·um　(fla″vo-bak-tēr′e-əm) a widespread genus of gram-negative, aerobic or facultatively anaerobic, rod-shaped soil and water bacteria of the family Flavobacteriaceae, characterized by production of a yellow pigment. Organisms are opportunistic pathogens in humans 黄杆菌属

fla·vo·en·zyme　(fla″vo-en′zīm) any enzyme containing a flavin nucleotide (FMN or FAD) as a prosthetic group 黄素酶

fla·vo·noid　(fla′və-noid) any of a group of compounds containing a characteristic aromatic nucleus and widely distributed in higher plants, often as a pigment; a subgroup with biologic activity in mammals is the bioflavonoids 黄酮类，类黄酮

fla·vox·ate　(fla-voks′āt) a smooth muscle relaxant; the hydrochloride salt is used in treatment of spasms of the urinary tract 黄酮哌酯，平滑肌松弛药，其盐酸盐用于治疗尿道痉挛

flax·seed　(flak′sēd) linseed 亚麻子

flea　(fle) a small, wingless, bloodsucking insect; many fleas are parasitic and may act as disease carriers 蚤

fle·cai·nide　(flə-ka′nīd) a sodium channel blocker that decreases the rate of cardiac conduction and increases the ventricular refractory period; used as the acetate salt in the treatment of life-threatening arrhythmias 氟卡尼

fleece　(flēs) a mass of interlacing fibrils 毛丛；**f. of Stilling**, the lacework of myelinated fibers surrounding the dentate nucleus 施提林毛丛，齿状核周围的白纤维网丛

flesh (flesh) 1. muscular tissue 肌组织；2. skin 皮肤；**goose f.**, cutis anserina 鹅皮；**proud f.**, exuberant amounts of soft, edematous granulation tissue developing during healing of large surface wounds 赘肉

fleshy (flesh′e) 1. pertaining to or resembling flesh(似) 肉的；2. characterized by abundant flesh 多肉的，肥胖的

fleur·ette (floor-et′) [Fr.] a type of cell found in clusters in retinoblastomas and retinocytomas, representing differentiation of tumor cells into photoreceptors 花状细胞，特指视网膜母细胞瘤和视网膜细胞瘤的一种组织学类型

flex·i·bil·i·tas (flek″sĭ-bil′ĭ-təs) [L.] flexibility 柔性；**ce′rea f.**, 蜡样屈曲，见 C 下词条

flex·i·bil·i·ty (flek″sĭ-bil′ĭ-te) the quality of being readily bent without tendency to break 柔性，灵活性；**waxy f.**, in certain mental disorders, mild resistance to movement of the limbs (as if they were made of soft wax), the patient tending to maintain whatever position the patient has been placed in 蜡样屈曲

flex·ion (flek′shən) the act of bending or the condition of being bent 屈；俯屈（妇产科学）

flex·or (flek′sor) 1. causing flexion 导致屈曲；2. a muscle that flexes a joint 屈肌；**f. retina′culum**, 屈肌支持带，见 retinaculum 下词条

flex·u·ra (flek-shoo′rə) pl. flexu′rae [L.] flexure. 曲

flex·ure (flek′shər) a bend or fold; a curvation 弯曲，折叠，折襞；**caudal f.**, the bend at the aboral end of the embryo（胚胎）骶曲；**cephalic f.**, the curve in the midbrain of the embryo（胚胎）头曲；**cervical f.**, a bend in the neural tube of the embryo at the junction of the brain and spinal cord（胚胎）颈曲；**cranial f.**, cephalic f. 头曲；**dorsal f.**, one of the flexures in the mid-dorsal region of the embryo（胚胎）背曲；**duodenojejunal f.**, the bend at the junction of duodenum and jejunum 十二指肠空肠曲；**lumbar f.**, the ventral curvature in the lumbar region of the back 腰曲；**mesencephalic f.**, cephalic f. 中脑曲；**nuchal f.**, nuchal f. 颈曲；**pontine f.**, a flexure of the hindbrain in the embryo（胚胎）脑桥曲；**sacral f.**, caudal f. 骶曲；**sigmoid f.**, 乙状结肠，见 colon 下词条

flight of ideas (flīt of i-de′əz) a nearly continuous flow of rapid speech that jumps from topic to topic, usually based on discernible associations, distractions, or plays on words, but sometimes disorganized and incoherent 意念飘忽

float·ers (flo′tərz) "spots before the eyes"; deposits in the vitreous of the eye, usually moving about and probably representing fine aggregates of vitreous protein occurring as a benign degenerative change 漂浮物，由于良性退行性变化所发生的玻璃体蛋白质的细微集合物

floc·cil·la·tion (flok″sĭ-la′shən) the aimless picking at bedclothes by a patient with delirium, dementia, fever, or exhaustion 摸空症

floc·cose (flok′ōs) woolly; said of bacterial growth of short, curved chains variously oriented 羊毛状的；絮状的

floc·cu·la·tion (flok″u-la′shən) 1. the formation of lumpy or fluffy masses 絮结产物；2. a colloid phenomenon in which the disperse phase separates in discrete, usually visible, particles rather than congealing into a continuous mass 絮凝

floc·cu·lus (flok′u-ləs) pl. floc′culi [L.] 1. a small tuft or mass, as of wool or other fibrous material 絮状物；2. a small lobule on the lower side of each cerebellar hemisphere, continuous by a small stalk of nerve fibers with the nodule of the vermis, part of the flocculonodular lobe（小脑）绒球；**floccular adj.**

flood·ing (flud′ing) a form of desensitization for treating phobias and anxieties by repeated exposure to highly distressing stimuli until the lack of reinforcement of the anxiety response causes its extinction. It is usually used for actual exposure to the stimuli, with implosion used for imagined exposure, but the two terms are sometimes used synonymously 冲击疗法

floor (flor) the inferior inner surface of a hollow organ or other space 内部底面；**pelvic f.**, the layer of tissue just below the outlet of the pelvis, formed by the coccygeus and levator ani muscles and the perineal fascia 骨盆底

flo·ra (flor′ə) [L.] 1. the plant life present in or characteristic of a given location 植物群；2. the bacteria and fungi, both normally occurring and pathologic, found in or on an organ 菌群；**enteric f., gut f., intestinal f.**, the bacteria normally residing within the lumen of the intestine 肠道菌群

flor·id (flor′id) 1. in full bloom; occurring in fully developed form 盛开的；2. having a bright red color 鲜红的

flow (flo) 1. the movement of a liquid or gas 流动；2. the rate at which a fluid passes through an organ or part, expressed as volume per unit of time 流量；**blood f.**, 1. circulation (of the blood) 血液循环；2. circulation rate 血流量；**effective renal blood f. (ERBF)**, that portion of the total blood flow through the kidneys that perfuses functional renal tissue 有效肾血流量；**effective renal plasma f. (ERPF)**, the amount of plasma that perfuses the renal tubules per unit time, generally measured by the clearance rate of *p*-aminohippurate 有效肾血浆流量；**forced expiratory f. (FEF),** the rate of airflow recorded in measurements of forced vital capacity 用力呼气流量；**maximum expiratory f.,** the rate of airflow during a forced vital capacity maneuver, often specified at a given volume 最大呼气流量；**maximum midexpiratory f.,** the average rate of airflow measured between exhaled volumes of 25 and 75 percent of the vital capacity during a forced exhalation 最大呼气中期流量；**peak expiratory f. (PEF),** the greatest rate of airflow that can be achieved during forced exhalation beginning with the lungs fully inflated 呼气流量峰值；**renal plasma f. (RPF),** the amount of plasma that perfuses the kidneys per unit time, approximately 10 percent greater than the effective renal plasma flow 肾血浆流量

flow·er (flou′ər) the blossom of a plant; preparations of the flowers of some plants are used medicinally 花；**passion f.,** 1. any plant of the genus *Passiflora* 西番莲；2. a preparation of the aerial parts of P. incarnata, having anxiolytic and sedative properties and used for anxiety and insomnia; also used in homeopathy 粉色西番莲提取物

flow·me·ter (flo′me-tər) an apparatus for measuring the rate of flow of liquids or gases, often named for the method employed, e.g., *ultrasound f.* 流量计

flox·uri·dine (floks-ūr′ĭ-dēn) a derivative of fluorouracil used as an antineoplastic 尿苷；氟尿核苷；氟尿嘧啶脱氧核苷

fl oz fluid ounce 液体盎司

flu (floo) colloquialism for *influenza* 流感（流行性感冒的俗称）

flu·con·a·zole (floo-kon′ə-zōl) a triazole antifungal used in the systemic treatment of candidiasis and cryptococcal meningitis 氟康唑

fluc·tu·a·tion (fluk″choo-a′shən) a variation, as about a fixed value or mass; a wavelike motion 波动

flu·cy·to·sine (floo-si′to-sēn″) an antifungal used in the treatment of severe candidal and cryptococcal infections 氟胞嘧啶

flu·dar·a·bine (floo-dar′ə-bēn) an adenine analogue and purine antimetabolite used as the phosphate salt as an antineoplastic in the treatment of chronic lymphocytic leukemia 氟达拉滨

flu·de·oxy·glu·cose F 18 (floo″de-ok″se-glo- o′kōs) radiolabeled 2-deoxy-d-glucose; used in positron emission tomography in the diagnosis of brain disorders, cardiac disease, and tumors of various organs 氟 [18F] 脱氧葡萄糖

flu·dro·cor·ti·sone (floo″dro-kor′tĭ-sōn) a synthetic adrenal corticoid with effects similar to those of hydrocortisone and desoxycorticosterone, admin-

istered as the acetate salt 氟氢可的松

flu·ent (floo′ənt) flowing effortlessly; said of speech 流利的，通畅的

flu·id (floo′id) 1. a liquid or gas; any liquid of the body（人体内的）液体、气体；体液；2. composed of molecules that freely change their relative positions without separation of the mass 流体；**amniotic f.,** the liquid within the amnion that bathes the developing fetus and protects it from mechanical injury 羊水；**cerebrospinal f. (CSF),** the fluid contained within the ventricles of the brain, the subarachnoid space, and the central canal of the spinal cord 脑脊液；**follicular f.,** the fluid in a developing ovarian follicle 卵泡液；**interstitial f.,** the extracellular fluid bathing most tissues, excluding the fluid within the lymph and blood vessels 组织间液；**intracellular f.,** the portion of the total body water with its dissolved solutes that is within the cell membranes 细胞内液；**prostatic f.,** the secretion of the prostate gland, which contributes to formation of the semen 前列腺液；**Scarpa f.,** Scarpa 液（内淋巴）；**seminal f.,** semen 精液；**synovial f.,** synovia; the transparent, viscid fluid secreted by the synovial membrane and found in joint cavities, bursae, and tendon sheaths 滑液

flu·id ex·tract (floo″id ek′strakt) a liquid preparation of a vegetable drug, containing alcohol as a solvent or preservative, of such strength that each milliliter contains the therapeutic constituents of 1 g of the standard drug it represents 流浸膏剂

fluke (flook) trematode 吸虫

flu·like (floo′līk) 1. resembling influenza 流感样的；2. having symptoms that resemble those of influenza 流感样症状的

flu·ma·ze·nil (floo′ma-zə-nil″) a benzodiazepine agonist used to reverse the effects of benzodiazepines after sedation, general anesthesia, or overdose 氟马西尼

flu·men (floo′mən) pl. *flu′mina* [L.] a stream 水流；**flu′mina pilo′rum,** the lines along which the hairs of the body are arranged as they grow 毛流

flu·nis·o·lide (floo-nis′o-līd″) a synthetic glucocorticoid used as the acetate salt in treatment of bronchial asthma and seasonal and nonseasonal allergic rhinitis 氟尼缩松

flu·ni·traz·e·pam (floo″nĭ-traz′ə-pam) a short-acting benzodiazepine similar to diazepam, used as a hypnotic and as an induction agent in anesthesia. It is not used legally in the United States 氟硝基安定

flu·o·cin·o·lone (floo″ə-sin′ə-lōn) a synthetic corticosteroid used topically as *f. acetonide* for the relief of inflammation and pruritus in certain dermatoses 二氟羟泼尼松龙

flu·o·cin·o·nide (floo″ə-sin′ə-nīd) a synthetic corticosteroid used topically for the relief of inflammation and pruritus in certain dermatoses 氟轻松醋酸酯

flu·o·res·ce·in (floo-res′ēn) a fluorescing dye; its sodium salt is used as a tracer in retinal angiography and as a diagnostic aid for revealing corneal trauma and fitting contact lenses 荧光素

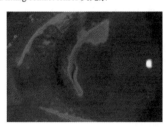

▲　角膜溃疡区域的荧光素（**fluorescein**）染色

flu·o·res·cence (floo-res′əns) the property of emitting light while exposed to light, the wavelength of the emitted light being longer than that of the absorbed light 荧光; **fluores′cent** *adj.*

flu·o·ri·da·tion (floor″ĭ-da′shən) treatment with fluorides; the addition of fluorides to a public water supply as a public health measure to reduce the incidence of dental caries 氟化

flu·o·rim·e·ter (floo-rim′ə-tər) fluorometer 荧光计

flu·o·rine (F) (floor′ēn) a yellow-green, nonmetallic, gaseous element of the halogen group; at. no. 9, at. wt. 18.998 氟

flu·o·ro·car·bon (floor′o-kahr″bən) any of the class of organic compounds consisting of carbon and fluorine only. Fluorocarbon emulsions dissolve oxygen and carbon dioxide and can be used in place of red blood cell preparations in the prevention and treatment of ischemia 碳氟化合物

flu·o·ro·chrome (floor′o-krōm) a fluorescent compound used as a dye to mark protein with a fluorescent label 荧光染料

flu·o·ro·do·pa F 18 (floor″o-do′pə) a radiolabeled compound of fluorine and levodopa, used for positron emission tomography of the cerebrum 氟和左旋多巴的放射性标记化合物

flu·o·rom·e·ter (floo-rom′ə-tər) the instrument used in fluorometry, consisting of an energy source (e.g., a mercury arc lamp or xenon lamp) to induce fluorescence, filters or monochromators for selection of the wavelength, and a detector 荧光计

flu·o·ro·meth·o·lone (floor″o-meth′ə-lōn) a syn-

thetic glucocorticoid used topically in the treatment of corticosteroid-responsive allergic and inflammatory conditions of the eye 氟米龙，氟甲松龙

flu·o·rom·e·try (floo-rom′ə-tre) an analytical technique for identifying and characterizing minute amounts of a substance by excitation of the substance with a beam of ultraviolet light and detection and measurement of the characteristic wavelength of fluorescent light emitted 荧光测定法

flu·o·ro·neph·e·lom·e·ter (floor″o-nef″ə- lom′ə-tər) an instrument for analysis of a solution by measuring the light scattered or emitted by it 荧光比浊计

flu·o·ro·pho·tom·e·try (floor″o-fo-tom′ə-tre) fluorometry 荧光光度法; **vitreous f.,** the measurement of light given off by intravenously injected fluorescein that has leaked through the retinal vessels into the vitreous; done to detect the breakdown of the blood-retinal barrier, an early ocular change in diabetes mellitus 玻璃体荧光光度测定（法）

flu·o·ro·quin·o·lone (floor″o-kwin′o-lōn) any of a subgroup of fluorine-substituted quinolones, having a broader spectrum of activity than nalidixic acid 氟喹诺酮类药物

flu·o·ro·scope (floor′o-skōp) an instrument for visual observation of the form and motion of the deep structures of the body by means of x-ray shadows projected on a fluorescent screen 荧光镜

flu·o·ros·co·py (floo-ros′kə-pe) examination by means of the fluoroscope 荧光透视法

flu·o·ro·sis (floo-ro′sis) a condition due to exposure to excessive amounts of fluorine or its compounds, resulting from accidental ingestion of certain insecticides and rodenticides, chronic inhalation of industrial dusts or gases, or prolonged ingestion of water containing large amounts of fluorides; characterized by skeletal changes such as osteofluorosis and by mottled enamel when exposure occurs during enamel formation 氟中毒; **chronic endemic f.,** fluorosis 慢性地方性氟中毒; **dental f.,** mottled enamel 氟斑牙，氟牙症

flu·o·ro·ura·cil (5-FU) (floor″o-ūr′ə-sil″) an antimetabolite activated like uracil, used as a systemic and topical antineoplastic 氟尿嘧啶

flu·ox·e·tine (floo-ok′sə-tēn) a selective serotonin reuptake inhibitor used as the hydrochloride salt in the treatment of depression, obsessivecompulsive disorder, bulimia nervosa, and premenstrual dysphoric disorder 氟西汀

flu·ox·y·mes·ter·one (floo-ok″se-mes′tər-ōn) an androgen used in the treatment of male hypogonadism and delayed male puberty and in palliation of metastatic breast carcinoma in postmenopausal

F

women 氟羟甲基睾丸素

flu·phen·a·zine (floo-fen′ə-zēn) a phenothiazine antipsychotic, used as *f. decanoate, f. enanthate,* and *f. hydrochloride* 羟哌氟丙嗪，吩噻嗪类抗精神病药

flur·an·dren·o·lide (floor″ən-dren′ə-līd) a synthetic corticosteroid used topically for relief of inflammation and pruritus in dermatoses 丙酮缩氟氢羟龙

flu·raz·e·pam (floo-raz′ĕ-pam) a benzodiazepine used as the hydrochloride salt as a sedative and hypnotic in the treatment of insomnia 氟胺安定

flur·bi·pro·fen (floor-bi′pro-fen) a nonsteroidal antiinflammatory drug administered orally in the treatment of arthritis and other inflammatory disorders and dysmenorrhea, and applied topically to the conjunctiva as the sodium salt to inhibit miosis during and treat inflammation following ophthalmic surgery 氟比洛芬

flush (flush) redness of the face and neck, seen with physical exertion, overheating, emotional stress, and certain disease and toxic conditions 潮红

flu·ta·mide (floo′tə-mīd) a nonsteroidal antiandrogen, used in the treatment of metastatic prostatic carcinoma 氟他胺

flu·tic·a·sone (floo-tik′ə-sōn″) a synthetic corticosteroid used as the propionate salt to treat inflammation in certain dermatoses, allergic rhinitis and other inflammatory nasal conditions, nasal polyps, and asthma 氟替卡松

flut·ter (flut′ər) a rapid vibration or pulsation 扑动，脉动；**atrial f.,** cardiac arrhythmia in which the atrial contractions are rapid (250 to 350 per minute) but regular 心房扑动；**diaphragmatic f.,** peculiar wavelike fibrillations of the respiratory diaphragm of unknown cause 膈扑动；**impure f.,** atrial flutter in which the electrocardiogram shows alternating periods of atrial flutter and fibrillation or periods not clearly one or the other 不纯（心房）扑动；**mediastinal f.,** abnormal motility of the mediastinum during respiration 纵隔扑动；**pure f.,** atrial f. 整齐扑动；**ventricular f. (VFl),** a possible transition stage between ventricular tachycardia and ventricular fibrillation, the electrocardiogram showing rapid, uniform, regular oscillations, 250 or more per minute 心室扑动

flut·ter-fi·bril·la·tion (flut′ər-fib″rĭ-la′shən) impure flutters constantly varying in their resemblance to flutter or fibrillation, respectively 扑动 - 纤颤

flu·va·stat·in (floo′və-stat″in) an inhibitor of cholesterol biosynthesis used as the sodium salt in the treatment of hyperlipidemia and to slow the progression of atherosclerosis associated with coronary heart disease 氟伐他汀

flu·vox·amine (floo-vok′sə-mēn) a selective serotonin reuptake inhibitor, used as the maleate salt to relieve the symptoms of obsessive-compulsive disorder 氟伏沙明

flux (fluks) 1. an excessive flow or discharge 流出；2. the rate of the flow of some quantity per unit area 通量；**magnetic f. (Φ),** a quantitative measure of a magnetic field 磁通量

flux·ion (fluk′shən) a flowing; especially an abnormal or excessive flow of fluid to a part 流动

fly (fli) a dipterous, or two-winged, insect that is often the vector of organisms causing disease 蝇；**tsetse f.,** any member of the genus *Glossina* 舌蝇属

FMN flavin mononucleotide 黄素单核苷酸

FMT fecal microbiota transplantation 粪便微生物群移植

fMTT first-moment mean transit time 第一时刻平均通过时间

FNH focal nodular hyperplasia 局灶性结节性增生

foam (fōm) 1. a dispersion of a gas in a liquid or solid 泡沫；2. frothy saliva 白沫（唾液）；3. to produce or cause production of such a substance 起泡沫，吐白沫；**foam′y** *adj.*

fo·cus (fo′kəs) pl. *fo′ci* [L.] 1. the point of convergence of light rays or sound waves 焦点；2. the chief center of a morbid process 病灶；**fo′cal** *adj.;* **epileptogenic f.,** the area of the cerebral cortex responsible for causing epileptic seizures 癫痫病灶；**Ghon f.,** the principal parenchymal lesion of primary pulmonary tuberculosis Ghon 病灶

fo·cus·ing (fo′kəs-ing) the act of converging at a point 集中，聚焦；**isoelectric f.,** electrophoresis in which the protein mixture is subjected to an electric field in a gel medium in which a pH gradient has been established; each protein then migrates until it reaches the site at which the pH is equal to its isoelectric point 等电聚焦

foe- for words beginning thus, see those beginning *fe-* 见以 fe- 开头的词

fog (fog) a colloid system in which the dispersion medium is a gas and the disperse particles are liquid 雾

fog·ging (fog′ing) in ophthalmology, a method of determining refractive error in astigmatism, the patient being first made artificially myopic in order to relax accommodation 雾视法

foil (foil) metal in the form of an extremely thin, pliable sheet 箔材

fo·late (fo′lāt) 1. the anionic form of folic acid 叶酸；2. more generally, any of a group of substances containing a form of pteroic acid conjugated with l-glutamic acid and having a variety of substitutions

蝶酰谷氨酸

fold (fōld) plica; a thin, recurved margin, or doubling over 褶 皱，皱 襞；**amniotic f.,** the folded edge of the amnion where it rises over and finally encloses the embryo 羊 膜 褶；**aryepiglottic f.,** a fold of mucous membrane extending on each side between the lateral border of the epiglottis and the summit of the arytenoid cartilage 杓 状 会 厌 襞；**Douglas f.,** a crescentic line marking the termination of the posterior layer of the sheath of the rectus abdominis muscle, just below the level of the iliac crest 道格拉斯襞；**gastric f's,** the series of folds in the mucous membrane of the stomach 胃襞；**gluteal f.,** the crease separating the buttocks from the thigh 臀沟；**head f.,** a crescentic, ventral fold of the embryonic disk at the cephalic end of the developing embryo(胚胎）头褶；**lacrimal f.,** a fold of mucous membrane in the nasal cavity next to the lower opening of the nasolacrimal duct 泪襞；**Marshall f.,** vestigial f. of Marshall；**medullary f.,** neural f. 髓 褶；**mesonephric f.,** 中肾褶，见 *ridge* 下词条；**nail f.,** 甲部，见 *wall* 下词条；**neural f.,** one of the paired folds lying on either side of the neural plate that form the neural tube 神经褶；**palmate f's,** a system of folds on the anterior and posterior walls of the cervical canal of the uterus 棕榈襞；**semilunar f. of conjunctiva,** a mucous fold at the medial angle of the eye 结膜半月襞；**skin f.,** 1. skinfold 皮褶厚度；2. a skin furrow deeper than a groove 皮肤皱襞；**synovial f.,** an extension of the synovial membrane from its free inner surface into the joint cavity 滑膜襞；**tail f.,** a crescentic, ventral fold of the embryonic disk at the future caudal end of the developing embryo 尾褶；**ventricular f., vestibular f.,** a false vocal cord 室襞；**vestigial f. of Marshall,** a pericardial fold enclosing the remnant of the embryonic left anterior cardinal vein 左 腔 静 脉 褶；**vocal f.,** the true vocal cord 声襞

fo·li·a·ceous (fo″le-a′shəs) foliate 多叶的，叶状的，薄层状的

fo·li·ate (fo′le-ət) 1. having, pertaining to, or resembling leaves 多叶的，叶状的；2. consisting of thin, leaflike layers 薄层状的

fo·lic   ac·id (fo′lik) a water-soluble vitamin of the B complex, pteroylglutamic acid or related derivatives, which is involved in hematopoiesis and the synthesis of amino acids and DNA; its deficiency causes megaloblastic anemia 叶酸，见 *tetrahydrofolic acid* 和 *folic acid antagonist*

fo·lie (fo-le′) [Fr.] psychosis; insanity 精 神 病，精 神 错 乱；**f. à deux,** (ah doo) mental disorder affecting two persons who share the same delusions; formally classified as *shared psychotic disorder* 二

联 性 精 神 病；**f. du pourquoi,** (doo poor-kwah′) psychopathologic constant questioning 问 难 癖；**f. gémellaire,** (zha″mĕ-lār′) psychosis occurring simultaneously in twins 孪生性精神病

fo·lin·ic   ac·id (fo-lin′ik) leucovorin; the 5-formyl derivative of tetrahydrofolic acid; it can act as a coenzyme carrier in certain folate-mediated reactions and is used, as the calcium salt leucovorin calcium, in the treatment of some disorders of folic acid deficiency 亚叶酸

fo·li·um (fo′le-əm) pl. *fo′lia* [L.] a leaflike structure, especially one of the leaflike subdivisions of the cerebellar cortex 小 叶，小 脑 小 叶；**f. ver″mis,** a lobule of the vermis of the cerebellum between the declive and the tuber vermis, continuous with the superior semilunar lobule on each side 蚓叶

fol·li·cle (fol′ĭ-kəl) a sac or pouchlike depression or cavity 滤泡，囊；**follic′ular** *adj.*；**atretic ovarian f.,** an involuted ovarian follicle 闭锁卵泡；**dominant ovarian f.,** the growing ovarian follicle in a given menstrual cycle that matures completely and forms the corpus luteum 卵 巢 优 势 卵 泡；**graafian f's,** vesicular ovarian f's; maturing ovarian follicles among whose cells fluid has begun to accumulate, leading to the formation of a single cavity and leaving the oocyte located in the cumulus oophorus 成熟卵泡；**hair f.,** one of the tubular invaginations of the epidermis enclosing the hairs, and from which the hairs grow 毛囊；**intestinal f's,** 肠 滤 泡，见 *gland* 下 词 条；nodular masses of lymphoid tissue at the root of the tongue, together constituting the lingual tonsil 舌 滤 泡；**lymphatic f., lymphoid f.,** lymphoid nodule 淋 巴 滤 泡；**nabothian f's,** cystlike formations due to occlusion of the lumina of glands in the mucosa of the uterine cervix, causing them to be distended with retained secretion 纳博特滤泡，子宫颈腺囊肿；**ovarian f.,** the oocyte and its encasing cells, at any stage in its development 卵巢 滤 泡；**primary ovarian f's,** immature ovarian follicles, each comprising an immature oocyte and the specialized epithelial cells (follicle cells) surrounding it 初级滤泡；**primordial ovarian f.,** an immature ovarian follicle that has not undergone recruitment and consists of an oocyte enclosed by a single layer of cells 原始卵巢滤泡；**solitary lymphoid f's,** 孤立淋巴滤泡，见 *nodule* 下词条；**thyroid f's,** discrete, cystlike units of the thyroid gland that are lined with cuboidal epithelium and are filled with a colloid substance, about 30 to each lobule 甲状腺滤泡；**vesicular ovarian f's,** graafian f's 囊状卵巢滤泡

fol·lic·u·li (fə-lik′u-li) [L.] plural of *folliculus* 卵泡的复数形式

fol·lic·u·li·tis (fə-lik″u-li′tis) inflammation of a follicle 滤泡炎；毛囊炎；**f. bar′bae**, sycosis barbae 须疮；**f. decal′vans**, suppurative folliculitis leading to scarring, with permanent hair loss on the involved area 毛囊炎性脱发；**gram-negative f.**, a superinfection complicating long-term treatment of acne vulgaris with tetracyclines or certain other antibiotics, usually caused by species of *Enterobacter, Klebsiella,* or *Proteus* 革兰阴性菌毛囊炎；**keloidal f., f. keloida′lis**, acne keloidalis 瘢瘤性毛囊炎

fol·lic·u·lus (fə-lik′u-ləs) pl. *folli′culi* [L.] follicle 滤泡

fol·li·tro·pin (fol′ĭ-tro″pin) follicle-stimulating hormone; *f. alfa* and *f. beta* are forms of follitropin produced by genetically modified hamster cells and used in the treatment of infertility 促卵泡（激）素

fo·men·ta·tion (fo″mən-ta′shən) treatment by warm moist applications; also, the substance thus applied 热敷；热湿敷（用）材料

fo·mite (fo′mīt) an inanimate object or material on which disease-producing agents may be conveyed 病媒，传染物

fo·mi·vir·sen (fo-miv′ər-sən) an antiviral agent used as the sodium salt in the treatment of cytomegalovirus retinitis associated with AIDS 福米韦生(抗病毒药)

Fon·se·caea (fon-se-se′ə) a genus of dematiaceous anamorphic fungi. *F. pedro′soi, F. compac′ta,* and *F. monoph′ora* cause chromoblastomycosis; the last also causes cerebral phaeohyphomycosis 着色真菌属

fon·ta·nelle (fon″tə-nel′) one of the membrane-covered spaces remaining at the junction of the sutures in the incompletely ossified skull of the fetus or infant 囟（门）。Spelled also *fontanel*

fon·tic·u·lus (fon-tik′u-ləs) pl. *fontic′uli* [L.] a fontanelle 囟（门）

foot (foot) 1. the distal portion of the leg, upon which an individual stands and walks; in humans, the tarsus, metatarsus, and phalanges, and the surrounding tissue 足，脚；2. something resembling this structure 类足结构；3. a unit of linear measure, 12 inches, equal to 0.3048 meter 英尺；**athlete's f.**, tinea pedis 足癣；**cleft f.**, a congenitally deformed foot in which the division between the third and fourth toes extends into the metatarsal region, often with ectrodactyly 裂足；**club f.**, 畸形足，见 *talipes*；**dangle f., drop f.**, footdrop 下垂足；**flat f.**, flatfoot 扁平足；**immersion f.**, damage to the skin of the feet of persons who have stood for long periods in warm or cold water 浸泡足；**Madura f.**, mycetoma of the foot 马杜拉足，足分枝菌病；**march f.**, painful swelling of the foot, usually with fracture of

a metatarsal bone, after excessive foot strain 行军足；**pericapillary end f., perivascular f., sucker f.**, a terminal expansion of the cytoplasmic process of an astrocyte against the wall of a capillary in the central nervous system 毛细血管周末足，血管周足，终足；**trench f.**, immersion foot from standing in cold water, resembling damage from frostbite 壕沟足

foot·drop (foot′drop) dropping of the foot from a fibular or tibial nerve lesion, a condition that causes paralysis of the anterior muscles of the leg 足下垂

foot·plate (foot′plāt) the flat portion of the stapes, which is set into the vestibular window on the labyrinthine wall of the middle ear 镫骨底

fo·ra·men (fo-ra′mən) pl. *fora′mina* [L.] a natural opening or passage, especially one into or through a bone 孔，骨孔；**aortic f.**, 主动脉裂孔，见 *hiatus* 下词条，**pical f. of tooth**, an opening at or near the apex of the root of a tooth, giving passage to the vascular, lymphatic, and neural structures supplying the pulp（牙）根尖孔；**f. of Bochdalek**, pleuroperitoneal hiatus 博赫达勒克孔，胸腹裂孔；**cecal f., f. ce′cum**, 1. a blind opening between the frontal crest and the crista galli（额骨）盲孔，位于额嵴和鸡冠之间；2. a small triangular expansion at the lower border of the pons, formed by the termination of the anterior median fissure of the medulla oblongata 延髓脑桥沟；3. a depression on the dorsum of the tongue at the median sulcus 舌盲孔；**conjugate f.**, a foramen formed by a notch in each of two opposed bones 接合孔；**costotransverse f.**, the narrow space between the posterior surface of the neck of a rib and the anterior surface of the transverse process of the corresponding vertebra 肋横突孔；**cribriform foramina**, the openings in the cribriform plate of the ethmoid bone for passage of the olfactory nerves 筛孔；**emissary f.**, any foramen in a cranial bone that gives passage to an emissary vein 蝶导静脉孔；**epiploic f.**, an opening connecting the two sacs of the peritoneum, below and behind the porta hepatis 网膜孔；**esophageal f.,**；食管裂孔，见 *hiatus* 下词条；**ethmoidal foramina**, small openings in the ethmoid bone at the junction of the labyrinthine wall with the roof of the orbit, the *anterior* transmitting the nasal branch of the ophthalmic nerve and the anterior ethmoid vessels, and the *posterior* transmitting the posterior ethmoid vessels 筛孔；**external auditory f.**, external acoustic meatus 外耳道；**frontal f.**, the frontal notch (q.v.) when it is bridged by osseous tissue 额孔；**greater palatine f.**, the lower opening of the greater palatine canal, found laterally on the horizontal plate of each palatine bone, transmitting a palatine nerve and artery 腭大孔；**incisive f.,** one of the openings of the incisive canals into the incisive fossa of the hard palate 切牙孔；**infraorbital f.,** a passage for the infraorbital nerve and artery 眶下孔；**internal auditory f.,** a passage for the auditory and facial nerves in the petrous bone 内耳门；**interventricular f.,** a communication between the lateral and third ventricles 室间孔；**intervertebral f.,** a passage for a spinal nerve and vessels that is formed by notches on pedicles of adjacent vertebrae 椎间孔；**jugular f.,** an opening formed by the jugular notches on the temporal and occipital bones 颈静脉孔；**f. of Key and Retzius,** an opening at the end of each lateral recess of the fourth ventricle that communicates with the subarachnoid space 基 - 雷二氏孔，第四脑室外侧孔；**lacerate f., anterior,** an elongated cleft between the wings of the sphenoid bone, transmitting nerves and vessels 眶上裂；**lacerate f., middle,** f. lacerum；**lacerate f., posterior,** jugular f.；**f. la′cerum,** a gap formed at the junction of the greater wing of the sphenoid bone, tip of the petrous part of the temporal bone, and basilar part of the occipital bone 破裂孔；**lesser palatine foramina,** the openings of the lesser palatine canals behind the palatine crest and the greater palatine foramina 腭小孔；**f. of Magendie,** an opening in the lower part of the roof of the fourth ventricle that communicates with the subarachnoid space Magendie 孔，第四脑室正中孔；**f. mag′num,** a large opening in the anterior part of the occipital bone, between the cranial cavity and vertebral canal 枕骨大孔；**mandibular f.,** the opening on the medial surface of the ramus of the mandible, leading into the mandibular canal 下颌孔；**mastoid f.,** an opening in the temporal bone behind the mastoid process 乳突孔；**medullary f.,** vertebral f.；**mental f.,** an opening on the lateral part of the body of the mandible, opposite the second bicuspid tooth, for passage of the mental nerve and vessels 颏孔；**Morgagni f.,** a small defect on either side of the inferior limit of the sternum, between the sternal and costal portions of the respiratory diaphragm, allowing passage of the superior epigastric blood vessels and a few lymphatic vessels Morgagni 孔，胸骨下界两侧的一个小缺口，位于呼吸隔膜的胸骨和肋部之间，允许上腹部血管和一些淋巴管通过；**nasal foramina,** openings on the outer surface of each nasal bone for the transmission of blood vessels 鼻骨孔；**nutrient f.,** any of the passages admitting nutrient vessels to the medullary cavity of bone 滋养孔；**obturator f.,** the large opening between the os pubis and ischium 闭孔；**olfactory foramina,** cribriform foramina 筛孔；**omental f.,** epiploic f.；**optic f.,** 视神经孔，见 *canal* 下词条；**f. ova′le,** 1. an opening between the atria in the fetal heart.（胎儿心房）卵圆孔；2. an aperture in the greater wing of the sphenoid bone for vessels and nerves（蝶骨大翼）卵圆孔；**patent f. ovale (PFO),** abnormal persistence after birth of the fetal foramen ovale, often resulting in a left-to-right or right-to-left shunt 卵圆孔未闭；**pterygopalatine f.** sphenopalatine f.；**f. rotun′dum** a round opening in the greater wing of the sphenoid bone for the maxillary branch of the trigeminal nerve 圆孔；**Scarpa f.,** an opening behind each upper medial incisor, for the nasopalatine nerve 斯卡尔帕孔，鼻腭神经孔；**sciatic f.,** either of two foramina, the greater and the lesser sciatic foramina, formed by the sacrotuberal and sacrospinal ligaments in the sciatic notch of the coxal bone 坐骨孔；**sphenoidal emissary f., f. of Vesalius** 蝶导静脉孔；**sphenopalatine f.,** a space between the orbital and sphenoidal processes of the palatine bone, opening into the nasal cavity, and transmitting the sphenopalatine artery and nasal nerves 蝶腭孔；**spinous f.,** an opening in the greater wing of the sphenoid bone for the middle meningeal artery 棘孔；**stylomastoid f.,** an opening between the styloid and mastoid processes for the facial nerve and the stylomastoid artery 茎乳孔；**supraorbital f.,** the supraorbital notch (q.v.) when it is bridged by osseous tissue 眶上孔；**thebesian foramina,** minute openings in the walls of the right atrium through which the smallest cardiac veins empty into the heart thebsian 孔，心最小静脉孔；**thyroid f.,** an inconstant opening in the thyroid cartilage, due to incomplete union of the fourth and fifth branchial cartilages 甲状软骨孔；**f. transversa′rium,** the passage in either process of a cervical vertebra that, in the upper six vertebrae, transmits the vertebral vessels; it is small or may be absent in the seventh（颈椎）横突孔；**f. ve′nae ca′vae,** an opening in the respiratory diaphragm for the inferior vena cava and some branches of the right vagus nerve 腔静脉孔；**venous f.,** 1. f. venae cavae 腔静脉孔；2. f. of Vesalius；**vertebral f.,** the large opening in a vertebra formed by its body and arch 椎孔；**f. of Vesalius,** an occasional opening medial to the foramen ovale of the sphenoid bone, for passage of a vein from the cavernous sinus Vesalius 孔（蝶骨卵圆孔内侧的小孔）；**Weitbrecht f.,** a foramen in the capsule of the glenohumeral joint. 魏特布雷希特孔，即肩关节囊孔 **f. of Winslow,** epiploic f. 温斯洛孔，网膜孔；**zygomaticofacial f.,** the opening on the anterior surface of the zygomatic bone for the zygomaticofacial nerves and vessels 颧面孔；**zygomatico-orbital f.,** either of the two openings on the orbital surface of each zygomatic bone, which transmit branches of the zygomatic branch of the trigeminal nerve and branches of the lacrimal artery 颧 眶 孔；**zygomaticotemporal f.**, an opening on the temporal surface of the zygomatic bone 颧颞孔

fo·ram·i·na (fo-ram'ĭ-nə) plural of *foramen* 孔，骨孔（复数）

force (*F*) (fors) energy or power; that which originates or arrests motion 力，势；**electromotive f. (E) (EMF)**, that which causes a flow of electricity from one place to another, giving rise to an electric current 电 动 势；**occlusal f.**, the force exerted on opposing teeth when the jaws are brought into approximation 𬌗力；**reserve f.**, energy above that required for normal functioning; in the heart, the power that will take care of the additional circulatory burden imposed by exertion 潜 力；心 力 储 备；**van der Waals f's**, the relatively weak, short-range forces of attraction existing between atoms and molecules and arising from brief shifts of orbital electrons; it results in the attraction of nonpolar organic compounds to each other 范德瓦耳斯力，范德华力；**vital f.**, the energy that characterizes a living organism; most systems of complementary medicine seek to affect or use it 生命力

for·ceps (for'seps) [L.] 1. a two-bladed instrument with a handle for compressing or grasping tissues in surgical operations and for handling sterile dressings, etc 镊子，钳子；2. any forcipate organ or part 钳状器官（或部分）；**alligator f.**, strong toothed forceps having a double clamp 鳄 牙 钳；**artery f.**, one for grasping and compressing an artery 动 脉 钳；**axis-traction f.**, specially jointed obstetrical forceps so made that traction can be applied in the line of the pelvic axis 轴牵引钳；**bayonet f.**, a forceps whose blades are offset from the axis of the handle 枪刺样牙钳，刺刀式钳；**Chamberlen f.**, the original form of obstetrical forceps Chamberlen 产钳；**clamp f.**, a forceps-like clamp with an automatic lock, for compressing arteries, etc 夹钳；**dental f.**, one for the extraction of teeth 拔牙钳；**dressing f.**, one with scissor like handles for grasping lint, drainage tubes, etc., used in dressing wounds 敷 料 钳；**fixation f.**, one for holding a part steady during operation 固 定 镊；**Kocher f.**, a strong forceps for holding tissues during operation or for compressing bleeding tissue 科赫尔钳；**Levret f.**, an obstetrical forceps curved to correspond with the curve of the parturient canal Levret 产钳；**Löwenberg f.**, one for removing adenoid growth Löwenberg 钳（增殖腺钳）；**f. ma′jor**, the terminal fibers of the corpus callosum that pass from the splenium into the occipital lobes 枕钳；

f. mi′nor, the terminal fibers of the corpus callosum that pass from the genu to the frontal lobes 额钳；**mouse-tooth f.**, one with one or more fine teeth at the tip of each blade 鼠牙钳；**obstetrical f.**, one for extracting the fetal head from the maternal passages 产 钳；**Péan f.**, a clamp for hemostasis Péan 钳；**rongeur f.**, one for use in cutting bone 骨钳，咬骨钳；**sequestrum f.**, one with small but strong serrated jaws for removing pieces of bone forming a sequestrum 腐骨钳，死骨钳；**speculum f.**, a long, slender forceps for use through a speculum 窥器钳；**tenaculum f.**, one having a sharp hook at the end of each jaw 持钩钳，单爪钳；**torsion f.**, one for making torsion on an artery to arrest hemorrhage 扭转钳；**volsella f.**, **vulsellum f.**, one with teeth for grasping and applying traction 双爪钳；**Willett f.**, a vulsellum for applying scalp traction to control hemorrhage in placenta previa 威勒特钳，头皮产引钳

for·ci·pate (for'sĭ-pāt) shaped like a forceps 镊状的

fore·arm (for'ahrm) antebrachium; the part of the arm between elbow and wrist 前臂

fore·brain (for'brān) prosencephalon 前脑

fore·con·scious (for'kon-shəs) preconscious 前意识的

fore·fin·ger (for'fing-gər) index finger; the second finger, counting the thumb as first 示指

fore·foot (for'foot) 1. one of the front feet of a quadruped(四足动物的)前脚；2. the fore part of the foot 足前段

fore·gut (for'gət) the endodermal canal of the embryo cephalic to the junction of the yolk stalk, giving rise to the pharynx, lung, esophagus, stomach, liver, and most of the small intestine 前肠

fore·head (for'hed) the anterior aspect of the head superior to the eyebrows and extending up to the hairline; usually considered to be part of the face but sometimes excluded 额

for·eign (for'ən) in immunology, pertaining to substances not recognized as "self" and capable of inducing an immune response 外源性的，异质的

fo·ren·sic (fə-ren'zik) pertaining to or applied in legal proceedings 法庭的，法医的

fore·play (for'pla) the sexually stimulating play preceding intercourse 性交前快感刺激，前期爱抚

fore·skin (for'skin) prepuce of the penis 包 皮；**hooded f.**, absence of the ventral prepuce, usually associated with hypospadias 头巾状包皮（腹侧包皮缺失）

fore·wa·ters (for'waw-tərz) the part of the amniotic sac that pouches into the uterine cervix in front of the presenting part of the fetus 前羊水

fork (fork) a pronged instrument, or something

resembling one 叉 或 叉 状 物 体 ； **replication f.**, a site on a DNA molecule at which unwinding of the helices and synthesis of daughter molecules are both occurring 复制叉 ； **tuning f.**, a device that produces harmonic vibration when its two prongs are struck; used to test hearing and bone conduction 音叉

for·mal·de·hyde (for-mal′də-hīd) a gas formerly used as a strong disinfectant; now used as an aqueous solution (见 solution 下 *formaldehyde solution*). The gas is toxic by inhalation or absorption and is carcinogenic 甲醛

for·ma·lin (for′mə-lin) formaldehyde solution 福尔马林（甲醛溶液）

for·mam·i·dase (for-mam′ĭ-dās) 1. an enzyme that catalyzes the hydrolytic deamination of formamide to produce formate; it also acts on similar amides 甲酰胺酶；2. arylformamidase 芳基甲酰胺酶

for·mate (for′māt) a salt of formic acid 甲酸盐

for·ma·tio (for-ma′she-o) pl. *formatio′nes* [L.] formation (2) 结构

for·ma·tion (for-ma′shən) 1. the process of giving shape or form; the creation of an entity or of a structure of definite shape 组成，形成（的过程）；2. a structure of definite shape 结构； **reaction f.**, a defense mechanism in which a person adopts conscious attitudes, interests, or feelings that are the opposites of their unconscious feelings, impulses, or wishes 反向形成； **reticular f.**, any of several diffuse networks of cells and fibers in the spinal cord and brainstem; generally subdivided into the reticular formations of the spinal cord, medulla oblongata, midbrain, and pons 网状结构

for·ma·tive (for′mə-tiv) concerned in the origination and development of an organism, part, or tissue 形成的，结构的

forme (form) pl. *formes* [Fr.] form 型； **f. fruste**, (froost) an atypical, especially a mild or incomplete, form, as of a disease 顿挫型； **f. tardive**, (tahrdēv′) a late-occurring form of a disease that usually appears at an earlier age 迟发型

for·mic ac·id (for′mik) an acid from the distillation of ants and derivable from oxalic acid and glycerin and from the oxidation of formaldehyde; its actions resemble those of acetic acid but it is much more irritating, pungent, and caustic to the skin. The acid and its sodium and calcium salts are used as food preservatives 甲酸

for·mi·ca·tion (for″mĭ-ka′shən) a sensation as if small insects were crawling on the skin 蚁走感

for·mim·i·no·glu·tam·ic ac·id (FIGLU) (formim″ĭ-no-gloo-tam′ik) an intermediate in the catabolic pathway from histidine to glutamate; it may be excreted in the urine in liver disease, vitamin B_{12} or folic acid deficiency, or glutamic formiminotransferase deficiency 亚胺甲基谷氨酸

for·mol (for′mol) formaldehyde solution 甲醛溶液

for·mu·la (for′mu-lə) pl. *formulas, for′mulae* [L.] an expression, using numbers or symbols, of the composition of, or of directions for preparing, a compound, such as a medicine, or of a procedure to follow to obtain a desired result, or of a single concept 分子式；方案，方法；公式； **chemical f.**, a combination of symbols used to express the chemical composition of a substance 化学式； **dental f.**, an expression in symbols of the number and arrangement of teeth in the jaws. Letters represent the various types of teeth: I, *incisor*; C, *canine*; P, *premolar*; M, *molar*. Each letter is followed by a horizontal line. Numbers above the line represent maxillary teeth; those below, mandibular teeth. The human dental formula is I22C11M22 = 10 (one side only) for deciduous teeth, and I22C11P22M33 = 16 (one side only) for permanent teeth 牙式（以符号表示上下颌牙齿的排列）； **empirical f.**, a chemical formula that expresses the proportions of the elements present in a substance 经验式； **molecular f.**, a chemical formula expressing the number of atoms of each element present in a molecule of a substance, without indicating how they are linked 分子式； **spatial f., stereochemical f.**, a chemical formula giving the number of atoms of each element present in a molecule of a substance, which atom is linked to which, the type of linkages involved, and the relative positions of the atoms in space 立体式，立体化学式； **structural f.**, a chemical formula showing the number of atoms of each element in a molecule, their spatial arrangement, and their linkage to each other 结构式； **vertebral f.**, an expression of the number of vertebrae in each region of the vertebral column; the human vertebral formula is C7 T12 L5 S5 Cd4 = 33 椎骨式（以数字表示各部椎骨）

for·mu·lary (for′mu-lar″e) a collection of recipes, formulas, and prescriptions 处方集； **National F.**, （美国）国家处方集，见 *N.*；

for·mu·late (for′mu-lāt) 1. to state in the form of a formula 列成公式，使公式化；2. to prepare in accordance with a prescribed or specified method 按处方或特定的方法制备

for·mu·la·tion (for″mu-la′shən) the act or product of formulating 配方；列成公式，公式化； **American Law Institute F.**, a section of the American Law Institute's Model Penal Code that states that "a person is not responsible for criminal conduct if at the time of such conduct as a result of mental disease or defect he lacks substantial capacity either to appreciate the criminality [wrongfulness] of his conduct or to conform his conduct to the requirements of the law." 美国法律学会案例集

for·myl (for′məl) the radical, HCO−, of formic acid 甲酰, 甲酸基

for·nix (for′niks) pl. *for′nices* [L.] 1. an archlike structure or the vaultlike space created by such a structure 穹; 2. fornix of brain; either of a pair of arched fiber tracts that unite under the corpus callosum, so that together they comprise two columns, a body, and two crura（端脑）穹窿, **f. vagi′nae,** vaginal fornix: the recess between the vaginal wall and the vaginal part of the cervix 阴道穹窿

fos·am·pren·a·vir (fos″am-pren′ə-vir) a prodrug of amprenavir (q.v.), used as the calcium salt in the treatment of human immunodeficiency virus infections 福沙那韦

fos·car·net (fos-kahr′net) a virostatic agent used as the sodium salt in the treatment of cytomegalovirus retinitis and herpes simplex in immunocompromised patients 膦甲酸

fos·fo·my·cin (fos-fo-mi′sin) an antibacterial agent active against a wide range of grampositive and gram-negative bacteria, used in the treatment of urinary tract infection; administered orally as the tromethamine salt 磷霉素

fo·sin·o·pril (fo-sin′o-pril) an angiotensin-converting enzyme inhibitor administered orally as the sodium salt to treat hypertension and congestive heart failure 福辛普利

fos·phen·y·to·in (fos′fen-ī-toin″) a prodrug of phenytoin used as the sodium salt in the treatment of epilepsy, excluding petit mal epilepsy 磷苯妥英

fos·sa (fos′ə) pl. *fos′sae* [L.] a trench or channel; in anatomy, a hollow or depressed area 沟, 凹陷, 窝; **acetabular f.,** a nonarticular area in the floor of the acetabulum 髋臼窝; **adipose fossae,** subcutaneous spaces in the female breast that contain fat 脂肪窝; **axillary f.,** the small hollow underneath the arm where it joins the body at the shoulder 腋窝; **canine f.,** a depression on the external surface of the maxilla superolateral to the canine tooth socket 尖牙窝; **condylar f.,** either of two pits on the lateral part of the occipital bone 髁窝; **coronoid f. of humerus,** a depression in the humerus for the coronoid process of the ulna 冠突窝; **cranial f.,** any one of three hollows (anterior, middle, and posterior) in the base of the cranium for the lobes of the brain 颅窝; **digastric f.,** 1. a depression on the inner surface of the mandible, giving attachment to the anterior belly of the digastric muscle 二腹肌窝; 2. mastoid

notch 乳突切迹; **digital f.,** 1. trochanteric f.; 2. femoral ring 股骨环; 3. the depression on the inside of the anterior abdominal wall lateral to the lateral umbilical fold 脐外侧襞; **duodenojejunal f.,** either of two peritoneal pockets, one behind the inferior and the other behind the superior duodenal fold 十二指肠空肠隐窝; **epigastric f.,** epigastrium 腹上窝; **ethmoid f.,** the groove in the cribriform plate of the ethmoid bones, for the olfactory bulb 筛沟; **hyaloid f.,** a depression in the front of the vitreous body, lodging the lens 玻璃体窝; **hypophysial f.,** a depression in the sphenoid bone that houses the pituitary gland 垂体窝; **iliac f.,** a concave area occupying much of the inner surface of the ala of the ilium, especially anteriorly; from it arises the iliac muscle 髂窝; **incisive f.,** 1. a depression in the midline of the bony palate, immediately posterior to the central incisors, into which the incisive canals open; 2. a shallow depression on the anterior surface of the maxilla above the incisor teeth, to which the depressor septi nasi muscle is attached; 3. a shallow depression on the body of the mandible, above the mental protuberance and below the alveolar border of the central and lateral incisors 切牙窝; **infraspinous f.,** the large, slightly concave area below the spinous process on the dorsal surface of the scapula 冈下窝; **infratemporal f.,** an irregularly shaped cavity medial or deep to the zygomatic arch 颞下窝; **ischioanal f., ischiorectal f.,** a potential space between the pelvic diaphragm and the skin below it; an anterior recess extends a variable distance between the pelvic and urogenital diaphragms 坐骨肛门窝; **Jobert f.,** a fossa in the popliteal region bounded by the adductor magnus and the gracilis and sartorius muscles Jobert 窝, 膝部内侧的窝, 其上至大收肌下至股薄肌与缝匠肌; **lacrimal f.,** a shallow depression in the roof of the orbit, lodging the lacrimal gland 泪腺窝; **lateral cerebral f.,** sylvian fossa; in the fetus, a depression on the lateral surface of each cerebral hemisphere; it becomes the sylvian fissure and its floor becomes the insula 大脑外侧窝; **mandibular f.,** a depression in the temporal bone in which the condyle of the mandible rests 下颌窝; **mastoid f.,** a small triangular area between the posterior wall of the external acoustic meatus and the posterior root of the zygomatic process of the temporal bone 乳突（三角）窝; **nasal f.,** the portion of the nasal cavity anterior to the middle meatus 鼻窝; **navicular f.,** 1. the vaginal vestibule between the vaginal orifice and the frenulum of the pudendal labia 阴道前庭窝; 2. the lateral expansion of the urethra of the glans penis 尿道舟状窝; 3. a depression on the internal pterygoid process of the sphenoid bone, giving attachment to the tensor veli palatini muscle 舟状窝（蝶骨内侧翼突上的凹陷）；**f. ova'lis,** a fossa in the right atrium of the heart; the remains of the fetal foramen ovale 卵圆窝；**ovarian f.,** a shallow pouch on the posterior surface of the broad ligament, in which the ovary is located 卵巢窝；**popliteal f.,** the depression in the posterior region of the knee 腘窝；**rhomboid f.,** the floor of the fourth ventricle, made up of the dorsal surfaces of the medulla oblongata and pons 菱 形 窝；**Rosenmüller f.,** pharyngeal recess 咽隐窝；**subarcuate f.,** a depression in the posterior inner surface of the petrous portion of the temporal bone 弓 状 下 窝；**subsigmoid f.,** a fossa between the mesentery of the sigmoid flexure and that of the descending colon 乙状结肠下窝；**supraspinous f.,** a depression above the spine of the scapula 冈上窝；**sylvian f.,** 1. lateral cerebral f.; 2. lateral cerebral fissure 大脑外侧裂；**tibiofemoral f.,** a space between the articular surfaces of the tibia and femur mesial or lateral to the inferior pole of the patella 胫股窝；**trochanteric f.,** a depression on the medial surface of the greater trochanter, receiving the tendon of the obturator externus muscle 转 子 窝；**Waldeyer f.,** the two duodenal fossae regarded as one Waldeyer 窝，十二指肠结肠系膜隐窝；**zygomatic f.,** infratemporal f. 颞下窝

fos·sette (fos-et′) [Fr.] 1. a small depression 窝，小凹陷；2. a small, deep, corneal ulcer 小而深的角膜溃疡

fos·su·la (fos′u-lə) pl. *fos′sulae* [L.] a small fossa 小窝

foun·da·tion (foun-da′shən) the structure or basis on which something is built 基础，地基；**denture f.,** the portion of the structures and tissues of the mouth available to support a denture 义齿承托区

four·chette (foor-shet′) [Fr.] frenulum of pudendal labia 阴唇系带

fo·vea (fo′ve-ə) pl. *fo′veae* [L.] a small pit or depression. Often used alone to indicate the central fovea of the retina 小凹，常特指视网膜中央凹；**f. centra′lis re′tinae, central f. of retina,** a small pit in the center of the macula lutea, the area of clearest vision, where the retinal layers are spread aside and light falls directly on the cones 视 网 膜 中 央凹；**submandibular f.,** a depression on the medial aspect of the mandible, lodging part of the submandibular gland 下颌下腺凹

fo·ve·a·tion (fo″ve-a′shən) formation of pits on a surface, as on the skin; a pitted condition 凹形，成凹

fo·ve·o·la (fo-ve′o-lə) pl. *fove′olae* [L.] a small pit or depression 小凹

Fr francium 元素钫的符号

frac·tion (frak′shən) 1. a portion of something larger 小部分，分数；2. in chemistry, one of the separable constituents of a substance 化学成分，组分；**frac′tional** *adj.*；**ejection f.,** the proportion of the volume of blood in the ventricles at the end of diastole that is ejected during systole; it is the stroke volume divided by the end-diastolic volume, often expressed as a percentage. It is normally 65 ± 8 percent; lower values indicate ventricular dysfunction 射血 分数；**plasma protein f.,** a preparation of serum albumin and globulin obtained by fractionating source blood, plasma, or serum from healthy human donors; used as a blood volume supporter 血浆蛋白组分

frac·tion·a·tion (frak″shən-a′shən) 1. in radiology, division of the total dose of radiation into small doses administered at intervals 辐射剂量分级；2. in chemistry, separation of a substance into components, as by distillation or crystallization 分馏；3. in histology, isolation of components of living cells by differential centrifugation 分级（分离）

frac·ture (frak′chər) 1. the breaking of a part, especially a bone 折断，使骨折；2. a break or rupture in a bone 骨折；**avulsion f.,** separation of a small fragment of bone cortex at the site of attachment of a ligament or tendon 撕脱性骨折；**axial compression f.,** fracture of a vertebra by excessive vertical force so that pieces of it move out in horizontal directions 轴向压缩性骨折；**Barton f.,** fracture of the distal end of the radius into the radiocarpal joint 巴顿骨折，即伸直型桡骨远端骨 折；**Bennett f.,** fracture of the base of the first metacarpal bone running into the carpometacarpal joint, complicated by subluxation 贝内特骨折，第1掌骨基底的斜形骨折；**blow-out f.,** fracture of the orbital floor caused by a sudden increase of intraorbital pressure due to traumatic force; the orbital contents herniate into the maxillary sinus so that the inferior rectus or inferior oblique muscle may become incarcerated in the fracture site, producing diplopia on looking up 爆裂性骨折；**burst f.,** axial compression f.；**capillary f.,** one that appears on a radiogram as a fine, hairlike line, the segments of bone not being separated; sometimes seen in fractures of the skull 线状骨折；**closed f.,** one that does not produce an open wound in the skin 闭 合性骨折；cf. *open f.*；**Colles f.,** fracture of the lower end of the radius, the lower fragment being displaced backward; if the lower fragment is displaced forward, it is *reverse Colles f.* 柯莱斯骨折，桡骨远端的背侧移位骨折；**comminuted f.,** one in which the bone is splintered or crushed 粉碎性骨折；

complete f., one involving the entire cross-section of the bone 完全骨折；compound f., open f.；depressed f., depressed skull f., fracture of the skull in which a fragment is depressed 凹陷性骨折，颅骨凹陷骨折；de Quervain f., fracture of the navicular bone together with a palmar luxation of the lunate bone 德凯尔万骨折，舟骨骨折伴月骨掌侧脱位；direct f., one at the site of injury 直接骨折；dislocation f., fracture of a bone near an articulation with concomitant dislocation of that joint 脱位骨折；Dupuytren f., Pott f. 迪皮特朗骨折，又称波特骨折，指内外踝骨折合并三角韧带断裂，踝关节完全失去稳定性并发生显著脱位；Duverney f., fracture of the ilium just below the anterior inferior spine Duverney 骨折，即髂前上棘骨折；fissure f., a crack extending from a surface into, but not through, a long bone 裂纹骨折；freeze f., 冷冻撕裂，见 *freeze-fracturing*；greenstick f., one in which one side of a bone is broken, the other being bent 青枝骨折；hangman's f., fracture through the pedicles of the axis (C2) with or without subluxation of the second cervical vertebra or the third 绞刑者骨折，又称创伤性枢椎滑脱，指第 2 颈椎（枢椎）椎弓根骨折；impacted f., one in which one fragment is firmly driven into the other 嵌插骨折；incomplete f., a fracture that does not entirely destroy the continuity of the bone 不完全骨折；insufficiency f., a stress fracture that occurs during normal stress on a bone of abnormally decreased density 不全骨折，骨密度异常降低的骨骼在正常应力期间发生的应力性骨折；intrauterine f., fracture of a fetal bone incurred in utero 子宫内骨折，胎儿在子宫内发生骨折；Jefferson f., fracture of the atlas (first cervical vertebra) 杰斐逊寰椎骨折；lead pipe f., one in which the bone cortex is slightly compressed and bulged on one side with a slight crack on the other side of the bone 铅管骨折；Le Fort f., bilateral horizontal fracture of the maxilla 上颌骨骨折，指上颌骨双侧水平骨折。Le Fort fractures are classified as follows: *Le Fort I f.*, a horizontal segmented fracture of the alveolar process of the maxilla, in which the teeth are usually contained in the detached portion of the bone 勒福 I 型骨折，上颌牙槽突的水平分段骨折，其中牙齿通常包含在骨的分离部分；*Le Fort II f.*, unilateral or bilateral fracture of the maxilla, in which the body of the maxilla is separated from the facial skeleton and the separated portion is pyramidal in shape; the fracture may extend through the body of the maxilla down the midline of the hard palate, through the floor of the orbit, and into the nasal cavity 勒福 II 型骨折，上颌单侧或双侧骨折，其中上颌体与面部骨骼分离，分离部分呈金字塔状；

骨折可通过上颌体向下延伸至硬腭中线，穿过眶底，进入鼻腔；*Le Fort III f.*, a fracture in which the entire maxilla and one or more facial bones are completely separated from the craniofacial skeleton; such fractures are almost always accompanied by multiple fractures of the facial bones 勒福 III 型骨折，整个上颌和一个或多个面部骨骼与颅面骨骼完全分离的骨折；常伴随面部骨骼的多处骨折；Monteggia f., one in the proximal half of the shaft of the ulna, with dislocation of the head of the radius 蒙泰齐骨折，蒙氏骨折，尺骨上 1/3 骨折合并桡骨小头脱位；open f., one in which a wound through the adjacent or overlying soft tissues communicates with the site of the break 开放性骨折；parry f., Monteggia f.；pathologic f., one due to weakening of the bone structure by pathologic processes, such as neoplasia, osteomalacia, or osteomyelitis 病理性骨折；pilon f., comminuted fracture of the inferior articular surface of the tibia and the malleoli, caused by axial compression of the ankle joint pilon 骨折，踝关节轴向压缩导致胫骨远端和踝关节下表面粉碎性骨折；ping-pong f., a type of depressed skull fracture usually seen in young children, resembling the indentation that can be produced with the finger in a ping-pong ball; when elevated, it resumes and retains its normal position 乒乓骨折，幼儿的凹陷性颅骨骨折，类似于用手指在乒乓球上产生的凹痕；Pott f., fracture of the lower part of the fibula, with serious injury of the lower tibial articulation, usually a chipping off of a portion of the medial malleolus, or rupture of the medial ligament Pott 骨折，内外踝骨折合并三角韧带断裂，踝关节完全失去稳定性并发生显著脱位；pyramidal f. (of maxilla), Le Fort II f. 上颌锥形骨折；sagittal slice f., fracture of a vertebra breaking it in an oblong direction; the vertebral column above is displaced horizontally, usually causing paraplegia（椎骨）矢状面骨折；silver fork f., Colles f. 银叉样骨折；simple f., closed f. 简单骨折；Smith f., reverse Colles f. 史密斯骨折，反柯莱斯骨折；spiral f., one in which the bone has been twisted apart 螺旋骨折；spontaneous f., pathologic f. 自发性骨折；sprain f., the separation of a tendon from its insertion, taking with it a piece of bone 扭伤骨折；Stieda f., fracture of the internal condyle of the femur Stieda 骨折，股骨内髁骨折；stress f., that caused by unusual or repeated stress on a bone 应力性骨折；transverse facial f., Le Fort III f. 上颌横型骨折；transverse maxillary f., a term sometimes used for horizontal maxillary fracture (Le Fort I f.) 上颌水平骨折；wedge-compression f., compression fracture of only the anterior part of a vertebra, leaving it wedge-shaped（椎骨）楔形压缩

性骨折

fra·gil·i·ty (frə-jil′ĭ-te) susceptibility, or lack of resistance, to influences capable of causing disruption of continuity or integrity 脆性，脆弱性，易碎性；**capillary f.**, abnormal susceptibility of capillary walls to rupture 毛细血管脆性；**erythrocyte f.**, susceptibility of erythrocytes to hemolysis 红细胞脆性；**osmotic f.**, susceptibility of erythrocytes to rupture when subjected to increasingly hypotonic saline solutions（红细胞）渗透脆性

fram·be·sia (fram-be′zhə) yaws 雅司病；**f. tro′pica**, yaws 雅司病

fram·be·si·o·ma (fram-be″ze-o′mə) mother yaw 雅司瘤

frame (frām) a rigid structure for giving support to or for immobilizing a part 框，支架；**Balkan f.**, an apparatus for continuous extension in treatment of fractures of the femur, consisting of an overhead bar, with pulleys attached, by which the leg is supported in a sling 巴尔干夹板，用于治疗股骨骨折；**Bradford f.**, a canvascovered, rectangular frame of pipe; used as a bed frame in disease of the spine or thigh Bradford 架，即大腿和脊柱疾病患者的床架；**quadriplegic standing f.**, a device for supporting in the upright position a patient whose four limbs are paralyzed 四肢麻痹站立支架；**Stryker f.**, one consisting of canvas stretched on anterior and posterior frames, on which the patient can be rotated around their longitudinal axis 翻身床；**trial f.**, an eyeglass frame designed to permit insertion of different lenses used in correcting refractive errors of vision 试镜架

Fran·ci·sel·la (fran-sĭ-sel′ə) a genus of gramnegative aerobic bacteria of the family Francisellaceae. *F. philomira′gia* is an opportunistic pathogen in humans, and *F. tularen′sis* causes tularemia 弗朗西斯菌属

Fran·ci·sel·la·ceae (fran″sis-el-a′-se-e) a family of gram-negative, aerobic, rod-shaped or coccoid bacteria of the order Thiotrichales 弗朗西斯菌科

fran·ci·um (Fr) (fran′se-əm) a rare, radioactive, alkali metal element; at. no. 87, at. wt. 223 钫

fra·ter·nal (frə-tur′nəl) 1. of or pertaining to brothers 兄弟的；2. derived from two zygotes; said of twins 双胞胎的

FRCP Fellow of the Royal College of Physicians 皇家内科医学院院士

FRCS Fellow of the Royal College of Surgeons 皇家外科医学院院士

freck·le (frek′əl) a pigmented spot on the skin due to accumulation of melanin resulting from exposure to sunlight 雀斑，小黑点；**Hutchinson f., melanotic f. of Hutchinson**, lentigo maligna 哈钦森雀斑，哈钦森黑素雀斑，即恶性雀斑样痣

freeze-dry·ing (frēz′dri′ing) a method of tissue preparation in which the tissue specimen is frozen and then dehydrated at low temperature in a high vacuum 冷冻干燥，冰冻干燥，冻干

freeze-etch·ing (frēz′ech″ing) a method used to study unfixed cells by electron microscopy, in which the object to be studied is placed in 20 percent glycerol, frozen at −100°C, and then mounted on a chilled holder 冷冻蚀刻，冰冻蚀刻

freeze-frac·tur·ing (frēz′frak″chər-ing) a method of preparing cells for electron microscopy: a tissue specimen is frozen at −150°C, inserted into a vacuum chamber, and fractured by a microtome; a platinum carbon replica of the exposed surfaces is made, freed of the underlying specimen, and then examined 冷冻撕裂

freeze-sub·sti·tu·tion (frēz′sub″stĭ-too′shən) a modification of freeze-drying in which the ice within the frozen tissue is replaced by alcohol or other solvents at a very low temperature 冰冻取代法，即冷冻干燥中的冰改用乙醇或其他试剂

frem·i·tus (frem′ĭ-təs) a vibration felt on palpation 震颤；**friction f.**, rub 肝区摩擦感；**rhonchal f.**, vibrations produced by passage of air through a large mucus-filled bronchus 鼾性震颤；**tactile f.**, vocal fremitus felt on the chest wall 触觉语颤；**tussive f.**, vibration felt on the chest when the patient coughs 咳嗽性震颤；**vocal f. (VF)**, one caused by speaking, perceived on auscultation 语音震颤

fre·no·plas·ty (fre′no-plas″te) the correction of an abnormally attached frenum by surgically repositioning it 系带成形术

fren·u·lum (fren′u-ləm) pl. *fren′ula* [L.] a small fold of integument or mucous membrane that limits the movements of an organ or part 系带；**f. of clitoris**, a fold formed by union of the labia minora with the clitoris 阴蒂系带；**labial f., f. of lip**; **lingual f.**, f. of tongue; **f. of lip, labial f.**; a median fold of mucous membrane connecting the inside of each lip to the corresponding gum 唇系带；**f. of prepuce of penis**, the fold under the penis connecting it with the prepuce 阴茎包皮系带；**f. of pudendal labia**, the posterior union of the labia minora, anterior to the posterior commissure 阴唇系带；**f. of superior medullary velum**, a band lying in the medullary velum at its attachment to the inferior colliculi 上髓帆系带；**f. of tongue**, lingual frenulum; the vertical fold of mucous membrane under the tongue, attaching it to the floor of the mouth 舌系带；**f. ve′li, f. of superior medullary velum**

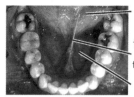

舌下表面

舌系带
（lingual
frenulum）

口腔底部

F

fre·num (fre′nəm) pl. *fre′na* [L.] a restraining structure or part 系带，见 *frenulum*；**fre′nal** *adj.*

fre·quen·cy (fre′kwən-se) 1. the number of occurrences of a periodic process in a unit of time 频率，符 号 ν ；2. in statistics, the number of occurrences of a determinable entity per unit of time or of population（统计学中的）频数，符号 *f*；**urinary f.**, urination at short intervals without increase in daily volume or urinary output, due to reduced bladder capacity 尿频

freud·i·an (froi′de-ən) 1. pertaining to Sigmund Freud, the founder of psychoanalysis, or his psychological theories and method of psychotherapy (psychoanalytic theory and technique) 弗洛伊德的，佛洛伊德学说的；2. an adherent or user of freudian theory or methods 佛洛伊德学说的拥护者或践行者

FRFSE fast recovery fast spin echo; fast relaxation fast spin echo 快速自旋回波脉冲序列

fri·a·ble (fri′ə-bəl) easily pulverized or crumbled 易碎的，脆弱的

fric·tion (frik′shən) 1. the act of rubbing 摩 擦；2. massage using a circular or back-and-forth rubbing movement, used especially for massage of deep tissues（医学上）按摩，尤其是深层组织的按摩

fri·gid·i·ty (fri-jid′ĭ-te) 1. coldness 寒冷；2. former name for *female sexual arousal disorder* 性冷淡，女性性唤起障碍的曾用名

frigo·la·bile (frig″o-la′bəl) (-la′bīl) easily affected or destroyed by cold 不耐寒的

frigo·sta·ble (frig″o-sta′bəl) resistant to cold or low temperatures 耐寒的

frit (frit) imperfectly fused material used as a basis for making glass and in the formation of porcelain teeth 熔块

frole·ment (frōl-maw′) [Fr.] a rustling sound often heard on auscultation in pericardial disease 轻擦音

frons (fronz) [L.] forehead 额

fron·tad (frun′tad) toward a front, or frontal aspect 向前，朝前

fron·tal (frun′təl) 1. pertaining to the forehead or frontal bone 额的，额骨的；2. denoting a longitudinal plane that divides the body into front and back parts 前面的，腹侧的

fron·ta·lis (frən-tal′is) [L.] 1. frontal 额的，额骨

的，前面的；2. the frontal belly of the occipitofrontalis muscle 枕额肌的前腹

fron·to·max·il·lary (frun″to-mak′sĭ-lar″e) pertaining to the frontal bone and maxilla 额上颌的

fron·to·tem·por·al (frun″to-tem′por-əl) pertaining to the frontal and temporal bones 额颞（骨）的

frost (frost) 1. frozen dew or vapor 霜；2. a deposit resembling this 类似霜的沉积物；**urea f.**, the appearance on the skin of salt crystals left by evaporation of the sweat in urhidrosis 尿素霜

frost·bite (frost′bīt) injury to tissues due to exposure to cold, ranging from superficial with full recovery to deep with gangrene 冻疮

frot·tage (fro-tahzh′) [Fr.] frotteurism 摩擦癖

frot·teur (fro-toor′) one who practices frotteurism 摩擦癖患者

frot·teur·ism (fro-toor′iz-əm) a paraphilia in which sexual arousal or orgasm is achieved by actual or fantasized rubbing up against another person, usually in a crowded place with an unsuspecting victim 摩擦癖，摩擦症

fro·zen (fro′zən) 1. turned into, covered by, or surrounded by ice 冷冻的，冷藏的，冰封的；2. very cold 严寒的；3. stiff or immobile, or rendered immobile 冻僵的

fruc·to·fu·ra·nose (frook″to-fu′rə-nōs) the combining and more reactive form of fructose 呋喃果糖

fruc·to·ki·nase (frook″to-ki′nās) an enzyme of the liver, intestine, and kidney cortex that catalyzes the transfer of a phosphate group from ATP to fructose as the initial step in its utilization. Deficiency causes essential fructosuria 果糖激酶

fruc·tose (frook′tōs) a sugar, $C_6H_{12}O_6$, found in honey and many sweet fruits; used as a fluid and nutrient replenisher 果糖

fruc·tose-1,6-bis·phos·pha·tase (frook″tōs bis-fos′fə-tās″) an enzyme catalyzing part of the route of gluconeogenesis in the liver and kidneys; deficiency causes apnea, hyperventilation, hypoglycemia, ketosis, and lactic acidosis and can be fatal in the neonatal period 果糖 -1,6- 二磷酸酶

fruc·to·se·mia (frook″to-se′me-ə) the presence of fructose in the blood, as in hereditary fructose intolerance and essential fructosuria 果糖血症

fruc·to·side (frook′to-sīd) a glycoside of fructose 果糖苷

fruc·to·su·ria (frook″to-su′re-ə) the presence of fructose in the urine 果糖尿症；**essential f.**, a benign hereditary disorder of carbohydrate metabolism due to a defect in fructokinase and manifested only by fructose in the blood and urine 实质性果糖尿

fruc·to·syl (frook′to-səl) a radical of fructose 果糖基

FSE febrile status epilepticus 发热性癫痫持续状态

FSF fibrin-stabilizing factor (coagulation factor XIII). 纤维蛋白稳定因子（凝血因子XIII）

FSH follicle-stimulating hormone 卵泡刺激素，促卵泡激素

FSH-RH follicle-stimulating hormone–releasing hormone 卵泡刺激素释放激素

FSMA Food Safety Modernization Act 食品安全现代化法案

5-FU 5-fluorouracil 氟尿嘧啶，见 *fluorouracil*

fuch·sin (fūk′sin) any of several red to purple dyes, sometimes specifically *basic f.* 品红；**acid f.**, a mixture of sulfonated fuchsins; used in various complex stains 酸性品红；**basic f.**, a histologic stain, containing predominantly pararosaniline and rosaniline 碱性品红

fuch·sin·o·phil·ia (fūk″sin-o-fil′e-ə) the property of staining readily with fuchsin dyes 嗜品红性；**fuchsinophil′ic, fuchsinophilous** *adj.*

fu·cose (fu′kōs) a monosaccharide occurring as l-fucose in a number of oligo- and polysaccharides and fucosides and in the carbohydrate portion of some mucopolysaccharides and glycoproteins, including the A, B, and O blood group antigens 岩藻糖

α-L-fu·co·si·dase (fu-ko′sĭ-dās) an enzyme that catalyzes the hydrolysis of fucose residues from fucosides; deficiency results in fucosidosis α-L- 岩藻糖苷酶

fu·co·si·do·sis (fu″ko-sĭ-do′sis) a lysosomal storage disease caused by deficient enzymatic activity of fucosidase and accumulation of fucosecontaining glycoconjugates in all tissues; it is marked by progressive psychomotor deterioration, growth retardation, hepatosplenomegaly, cardiomegaly, and seizures 岩藻糖苷贮积症

FUDR FUdR floxuridine 氟尿苷

fu·gac·i·ty (fu-gas′ĭ-te) a measure of the escaping tendency of a substance from one phase to another phase, or from one part of a phase to another part of the same phase 逸度

fugue (f ū g) a pathologic state of altered consciousness in which an individual may act and wander around as though conscious but their behavior is not directed by their complete normal personality and is not remembered after the fugue ends 神游，神游症；**dissociative f., psychogenic f.**, a dissociative disorder characterized by an episode of sudden, unexpected travel away from home or business, with amnesia for the past and partial to total confusion about identity or assumption of a new identity 解离性漫游症，分离性漫游症

ful·gu·rate (ful′gu-rāt) 1. to come and go like a flash of lightning 闪烁，闪光；2. to destroy by contact with electric sparks generated by a high-frequency current 电灼

ful·mi·nate (ful′mĭ-nāt) to occur suddenly with great intensity 暴发；**ful′minant** *adj.*

fu·ma·rase (fu′mə-rās) an enzyme that catalyzes the interconversion of fumarate and malate 延胡索酸酶

fu·ma·rate (fu′mə-rāt) a salt of fumaric acid 反丁烯二酸盐

fu·mar·ic ac·id (fu-mar′ik) an unsaturated dibasic acid, the *trans* isomer of maleic acid and an intermediate in the tricarboxylic acid cycle 富马酸，反丁烯二酸，延胡索酸

fu·mi·ga·tion (fu″mĭ-ga′shən) exposure to disinfecting fumes 熏蒸

fum·ing (fūm′ing) emitting a visible vapor 熏的，冒烟的

func·tio (funk′she-o) [L.] function 功能；**f. lae′sa**, loss of function; one of the cardinal signs of inflammation 功能丧失

func·tion (funk′shən) 1. the special, normal, or proper physiologic activity of an organ or part（器官的）功能；2. to perform such activity 起效，运转；3. in mathematics, a rule that assigns to each member of one set (the domain) a value in another set (the range) 函数

func·tion·al (funk′shən-əl) 1. pertaining to a function 功能的；2. affecting the function but not the structure 功能性的，非器质性的

fun·di·form (fun′dĭ-form) shaped like a loop or sling 吊带形的

fun·do·pli·ca·tion (fun″do-plĭ-ka′shən) mobilization of the lower end of the esophagus and plication of the fundus of the stomach up around it 胃底折叠术

fun·dus (fun′dəs) pl. *fun′di* [L.] the bottom or base of something, particularly an organ, or the part of a hollow organ farthest from its mouth 底，基底；**fun′dal, fun′dic** *adj.*; **f. of eye**, the back portion of the interior of the eyeball, visible through the pupil by use of the ophthalmoscope 眼底；**f. of gallbladder**, the inferior, dilated portion of the gallbladder 胆囊底；**f. of stomach**, the part of the stomach to the left and above the level of the opening of the esophagus 胃底；**f. tym′pani**, the floor of the tympanic cavity 鼓室底；**f. of urinary bladder**, the base or posterior surface of the urinary bladder 膀胱底；**f. of uterus**, the part of the uterus above the orifices of the uterine tubes 子宫底

fun·du·scope (fun′də-skōp) ophthalmoscope 检眼镜，眼底镜；**funduscop′ic** *adj.*

F

fun·gal (fung′gəl) pertaining to fungi 真菌的；
fun·gate (fung′gāt) 1. to produce fungus-like growths 真菌样生长；2. to grow rapidly, like a fungus 快速生长（速度似真菌）
Fun·gi (fun′ji) [L.] a kingdom of eukaryotic, heterotrophic organisms that live as saprobes or parasites, including mushrooms, yeasts, and molds; they have rigid cell walls but lack chlorophyll 真菌属；F.
Imperfec′ti, 见 *fungus* 下 *anamorphic fungi*
fun·gi (fun′ji) [L.] 真菌，*fungus* 的复数形式
fun·gi·cide (fun′jī-sīd) an agent that destroys fungi 杀真菌剂；**fungici′dal** *adj.*
fun·gi·form (fun′jī-form) shaped like a fungus 真菌状的
fun·gi·sta·sis (fun-jī-sta′sis) inhibition of the growth of fungi 抑真菌作用；**fungistat′ic** *adj.*
fun·gi·stat (fun′jī-stat) an agent that inhibits growth of fungi 抑真菌剂
fun·goid (fung′goid) resembling a fungus 真菌样的
fun·go·ma (fəng-go′mə) fungus ball 真菌球
fun·gu·ria (fung-gu′re-ə) the presence of fungi in the urine 真菌尿
fun·gus (fung′gəs) pl. *fun′gi* [L.] an organism belonging to the kingdom Fungi. Spelled also *fungous* 真菌；**anamorphic fungi,** the group of fungi with no known sexual (teleomorph) state; it is an artificial group, containing many fungi that do not share evolutionary relationships or morphologic or phylogenetic characteristics. Formerly considered an official taxon, variously *Fungi Imperfecti* and *Deuteromycota*; these terms are sometimes still used informally 无性型真菌；**dimorphic f.,** a fungus that can live as either a yeast or mold, depending on environmental conditions 双态真菌；**imperfect fungi, mitosporic fungi,** anamorphic fungi 半知菌，有丝分裂孢子真菌；**perfect fungi,** fungi for which both sexual (teleomorph) and asexual (anamorph) states are known 完全真菌
fu·nic (fu′nik) pertaining to a funis or to a funiculus 索的，脐带的
fu·ni·cle (fu′nī-kəl) funiculus 索
fu·nic·u·li·tis (fu-nik″u-li′tis) 1. inflammation of the spermatic cord 精索炎；2. inflammation of that portion of a spinal nerve root lying within the intervertebral canal 椎管内的脊髓神经根炎
fu·nic·u·lo·ep·i·did·y·mi·tis (fu-nik″u-lo-ep″ī-did″ī-mi′tis) inflammation of the spermatic cord and the epididymis 精索附睾炎
fu·nic·u·lus (fu-nik′u-ləs) pl. *funic′uli* [L.] a cord; a cordlike structure or part 索；**funic′ular** *adj.*；**anterior f. of spinal cord,** the white substance of the spinal cord lying on either side between the anterior median fissure and the ventral root 脊髓前索；**lateral**

f., 1. the white substance of the spinal cord lying on either side between the dorsal and ventral roots 外侧索；2. the continuation into the medulla oblongata of all the fiber tracts of the lateral funiculus of the spinal cord with exception of the lateral pyramidal tract 外侧索在延髓中的延伸；**posterior f. of spinal cord,** the white substance of the spinal cord lying on either side between the posterior median sulcus and the dorsal root 脊髓后索；**f. se′parans,** a narrow translucent ridge of thickened ependyma in the floor of the fourth ventricle that runs across the lower part of the trigone of the vagus nerve and separates it from the area postrema; the bloodbrain barrier may be modified in this area 分隔索
fu·ni·form (fu′nī-form) resembling a rope or cord 索状的
fu·nis (fu′nis) any cordlike structure, particularly the umbilical cord 绳索状结构，尤指脐带；**fu′nic** *adj.*
FUO fever of unknown origin 不明原因发热
fu·ra·nose (fu′rə-nōs) any sugar containing the four-carbon furan ring structure; it is a cyclic form that ketoses and aldoses may take in solution 呋喃糖
fu·ra·zol·i·done (fu″rə-zol′ī-dōn) an antibacterial and antiprotozoal effective against many gram-negative enteric organisms; used in the treatment of diarrhea and enteritis 呋喃唑酮
fur·cal (fur′kəl) shaped like a fork; forked 叉状的，分叉的
fur·ca·tion (fər-ka′shən) the anatomic area of a multirooted tooth where the roots divide 分叉，分支
fur·fu·ra·ceous (fur″fu-ra′shəs) fine and loose; said of scales resembling bran or dandruff 似麸的，糠状的，皮屑状的
fur·fu·ral (fur′fu-rəl) an aromatic compound from the distillation of bran, sawdust, etc., which irritates mucous membranes and causes photosensitivity and headaches 糠醛，呋喃甲醛
fu·ror (fu′ror) fury; rage 狂怒，躁狂；**f. epilep′ticus,** an attack of intense anger occurring in epilepsy 癫痫性狂怒
fu·ro·sem·ide (fu-ro′sə-mīd) a loop diuretic used in the treatment of edema and hypertension 呋塞米
fur·row (fur′o) sulcus 沟；**genital f.,** a groove that appears on the genital tubercle of the fetus at the end of the second month 生殖沟；**mentolabial f.,** the skin furrow between the lower lip and the chin 颏唇沟；**nympholabial f.,** a groove separating the labium majus and labium minus on each side 阴唇间沟；**skin f's,** sulci cutis 皮沟
fu·run·cle (fu′rung-kəl) a boil; a painful nodule formed in the skin by circumscribed inflammation of the dermis and superficial fascia after staphylococci

enter the skin through hair follicles 疖；**furun′cu-lar** *adj.*

fu·run·cu·lo·sis (fu-rung″ku-lo′sis) 1. the persistent sequential occurrence of furuncles over a period of weeks or months（长期、复发）疖病；2. the simultaneous occurrence of a number of furuncles 同时存在的多个疖

fu·run·cu·lus (fu-rung′ku-ləs) pl. *furun′culi* [L.] furuncle 疖

fu·sar·i·o·sis (fu-sar″e-o′sis) infection with fungi of the genus *Fusarium,* most often an opportunistic infection in an immunocompromised patient 镰刀菌病

Fu·sar·i·um (fu-sar′e-əm) a genus of anamorphic fungi originally recognized as plant pathogens; it is increasingly associated with invasive human disease, particularly the species *F. oxyspo′rum, F. so′lani,* and *F. verticillioi′des,* causing localized and systemic infections 镰刀菌属

fus·cin (fu′sin) a brown pigment of the retinal epithelium 暗褐菌素

fu·si·ble (fu′zĭ-bəl) capable of being melted 可熔的

fu·si·form (fu′zĭ-form) shaped like a spindle; tapered at each end 梭形的，纺锤状的

fu·si·mo·tor (fu″sĭ-mo′tər) innervating intrafusal fibers of the muscle spindle; said of motor nerve fibers of gamma motoneurons 肌梭运动神经的

fu·sion (fu′zhən) 1. the act or process of melting 熔融，熔化；2. the merging or coherence of adjacent parts or bodies 融合；3. the coordination of separate images of the same object in the two eyes into one 聚焦；4. the operative formation of an ankylosis or arthrosis 关节融合术；**anterior interbody f.,** spinal fusion in the lumbar region using a retroperitoneal approach, with immobilization by bone grafts on the anterior and lateral surfaces 前路椎体间融合术；**diaphysealepiphyseal f.,** operative estab lishment of bony union between the epiphysis and diaphysis of a bone 骨干骺融合术；**spinal f.,** operative immobilization or ankylosis of two or more vertebrae, often with diskectomy or laminectomy 脊椎融合术

Fu·so·bac·te·ria (fu″zo-bak-tēr′e-ə) 1. a phylum of gram-negative, anaerobic, non–sporeforming, rod-shaped bacteria 梭形杆菌门；2. the sole class of this phylum 梭形杆菌纲

Fu·so·bac·te·ri·a·ceae (fu″zo-bak-tēr″ea′se-e) a family of gram-negative, rod-shaped bacteria of the order Fusobacteriales 梭形杆菌科

Fu·so·bac·te·ri·a·les (fu″zo-bak-tēr″e-a′lēz) an order of bacteria of the class Fusobacteria 梭形杆菌目

Fu·so·bac·te·ri·um (fu″zo-bak-tēr′e-əm) a genus of gram-negative, anaerobic bacteria of the family Fusobacteriaceae, consisting of slender cells with tapered ends, that are normal inhabitants of the body cavities. Some species are pathogenic, causing purulent or gangrenous infections 梭形杆菌属

fu·so·bac·te·ri·um (fu″zo-bak-tēr′e-əm) pl. *fusobacte′ria* 1. A rod-shaped bacterium in which the cell is thicker in the center and tapers toward the ends 泛指形态为杆状的细菌；2. an organism of the genus *Fusobacterium* 梭形杆菌

fu·so·cel·lu·lar (fu″so-sel′u-lər) having spindle-shaped cells 梭形细胞的

fu·so·spi·ril·lo·sis (fu″so-spi″rĭ-lo′sis) necrotiz- ing ulcerative gingivitis 梭菌螺旋体病

fu·so·spi·ro·che·tal (fu″so-spi″ro-ke′təl) pertaining to or caused by fusobacteria and spirochetes 梭菌螺旋体性的

fu·so·spi·ro·che·to·sis (fu″so-spi″ro-ke-to′sis) infection with fusobacteria and spirochetes, as in acute necrotizing ulcerative gingivitis 梭菌螺旋体病

FVC forced vital capacity 用力肺活量

G

G gauss 高斯（磁通密度的单位）；giga- 吉（咖）；glycine 甘氨酸；gravida 孕妇；guanidine or guanosine 胍或鸟苷的符号

G conductance 电导；Gibbs free energy 吉布斯自由能

g gram 克的符号

g standard gravity 标准重力的符号

γ (gamma, the third letter of the Greek alphabet)（希腊字母表中的第 3 个字母）the heavy chain of IgG 免疫球蛋白 G 的重链；the γ chain of fetal hemoglobin 胎儿血红蛋白的 γ 链；formerly, mi- crogram 曾作为微克的符号

γ- [前缀]（1）the position of a substituting atom or group in a chemical compound 代表取代原子或基团在化合物中的位置；（2）a plasma protein migrating with the γ band in electrophoresis 蛋白电泳中与 γ 带移行的血浆蛋白质；（3）third in a series of three or more related entities or chemical compounds 3 个或以上的相关实体或化合物系列中的第 3 个

Ga gallium 镓

GABA γ-aminobutyric acid 氨基丁酸

GABA·er·gic (gab″ə-ur′jik) transmitting or secreting γ-aminobutyric acid γ-氨基丁酸能的
gab·a·pen·tin (gab″ə-pen′tin) an anticonvulsant related to γ-aminobutyric acid (GABA), used in the treatment of partial seizures and postherpetic neuralgia; as *g. enacarbil*, it is used in the treatment of restless legs syndrome 加巴喷丁
GAD generalized anxiety disorder 广泛性焦虑症
gad·o·lin·i·um (Gd) (gad″o-lin′e-əm) a silvery white, malleable, ductile, heavy metal, rare earth element; at. no. 64, at. wt. 157.25 钆; *g.* 153, an artificial isotope of gadolinium with a half-life of 241.6 days, used in dual-photon absorptiometry 钆-153(元素钆的人工同位素）
gad·o·pen·te·tate di·meg·lu·mine (gad″open′tə-tāt) a paramagnetic agent used as a contrast medium in magnetic resonance imaging of intracranial, spinal, and associated lesions 钆喷替酸二葡甲胺
gado·ver·set·a·mide (gad″o-vər-set′ə-mīd) a paramagnetic agent used as a contrast medium in magnetic resonance imaging of intracranial, liver, and spinal regions and associated lesions 钆弗塞胺
GAG glycosaminoglycan 糖胺聚糖
gag (gag) 1. a surgical device for holding the mouth open 张口器; 2. to retch, or to strive to vomit. 作呕
gain (gān) to acquire, obtain, or increase 获得，收获，增加; **antigen g.**, the acquisition by cells of new antigenic determinants not normally present or not normally accessible in the parent tissue 抗原获得; **primary g.**, the direct alleviation of anxiety by a defense mechanism; the relief from emotional conflict or tension provided by neurotic symptoms or illness 原发得益; **secondary g.**, external and incidental advantage derived from an illness, such as rest, gifts, personal attention, release from responsibility, and disability benefits 继发得益
gait (gāt) the manner or style of walking 步态; **antalgic g.**, a limp adopted so as to avoid pain on weight-bearing structures, characterized by a very short stance phase 减痛步态; **ataxic g.**, an unsteady, uncoordinated walk, employing a wide base and the feet thrown out 共济失调步态; **festinating g.**, a gait in which the patient involuntarily moves with short, accelerating steps, often on tiptoe, as in parkinsonism 慌张步态; **helicopod g.**, a gait in which the feet describe half circles, as in some conversion disorders 环形步态; **hip extensor g.**, a gait in which the heel strike is followed by throwing forward of the hip and throwing backward of the trunk and pelvis 髋伸肌步态; **myopathic g.**, exaggerated alternation of lateral trunk movements with an exaggerated elevation of the hip 肌病步态; **spastic g.**, spastic g. 截瘫痉挛步态; **quadriceps g.**, a gait in which at each step on the affected leg the knee hyperextends and the trunk lurches forward 股四头肌步态; **spastic g.**, a gait in which the legs are held together and move in a stiff manner, the toes seeming to drag and catch 痉挛步态; **steppage g.**, the gait in footdrop in which the advancing leg is lifted high so that the toes can clear the ground 跨阈步态; **stuttering g.**, one characterized by hesitancy that resembles stuttering 踌躇步态; **tabetic g.**, an ataxic gait that accompanies tabes dorsalis 脊髓痨步态; **waddling g.**, myopathic g 蹒跚步态
ga·lac·ta·cra·sia (gə-lak″tə-kra′zhə) abnormal condition of the breast milk 乳汁（组成）异常
ga·lac·ta·gogue (gə-lak′tə-gog) promoting milk flow; an agent that so acts 催乳药
ga·lac·tan (gə-lak′tən) any polymer composed of galactose residues and occurring in plants 半乳聚糖
ga·lac·to·cele (gə-lak′to-sēl) a milk-containing, cystic enlargement of the mammary gland 积乳囊肿
ga·lac·to·ce·re·bro·side (gə-lak″to-sə-re′bro-sīd″) any of the cerebrosides in which the head group is galactose; they are abundant in the cell membranes of nervous tissue 半乳糖脑苷脂
gal·ac·tog·ra·phy (gal″ak-tog′rə-fe) radiography of the mammary ducts after injection of a radio-opaque medium into the duct system 乳腺导管造影术
ga·lac·to·ki·nase (gə-lak″to-ki′nās) an enzyme that catalyzes the transfer of a high-energy phosphate group from a donor to d-galactose, the initial step of galactose utilization. Absence of enzyme activity results in galactokinase deficiency galactosemia 半乳糖激酶
ga·lac·to·phore (gə-lak′to-for) 1. galactophorous 乳腺; 2. a milk duct 乳腺管
gal·ac·toph·o·rous (gal″ak-tof′o-rəs) lactiferous 输乳的
ga·lac·to·poi·et·ic (gə-lak″to-poi-et′ik) 1. pertaining to, marked by, or promoting milk production 催乳的; 2. an agent that promotes milk flow 催乳药
ga·lac·tor·rhea (gə-lak″to-re′ə) excessive or spontaneous milk flow; persistent secretion of milk irrespective of nursing 乳溢
ga·lac·tose (gə-lak′tōs) a 6-carbon aldose epimeric with glucose but less sweet, occurring naturally in both d- and l- forms (the latter in plants). It is a component of lactose and other oligosaccharides, cerebrosides and gangliosides, and glycolipids and

glycoproteins 半乳糖

ga·lac·tos·e·mia (gə-lak″to-se′me-ə) any of three recessive disorders of galactose metabolism causing accumulation of galactose in the blood: the *classic* form, due to deficiency of the enzyme galactose 1-phosphate uridyltransferase, is marked by cirrhosis, hepatomegaly, cataracts, and intellectual disability in survivors. *Galactokinase deficiency* results in accumulation of galactitol in the lens, causing cataracts in infancy and childhood. *Galactose epimerase deficiency* results in benign accumulation of galactose 1-phosphate in the red blood cells 半乳糖血症

ga·lac·to·si·dase (gə-lak″to-si′dās) an enzyme that catalyzes the cleavage of terminal galactose residues from a variety of substrates; several such enzymes exist, each specific for α - or β -linked sugars and further specific for substrates, e.g., lactase 半乳糖苷酶

ga·lac·to·side (gə-lak′to-sīd) a glycoside containing galactose 半乳糖苷

gal·ac·to·sis (gal″ak-to′sis) the formation of milk by the lacteal glands 泌乳

gal·ac·tos·ta·sis (gal″ak-tos′tə-sis) 1. cessation of lactation 泌乳停止；2. abnormal collection of milk in the mammary glands 乳汁积滞

ga·lac·to·syl·ce·ram·i·dase (gə-lak″to-sələsə-ram′ĭ-dās) an enzyme that catalyzes the cleavage of galactose from galactocerebrosides to form ceramides, a reaction occurring in the lysosomal degradation of sphingolipids 半乳糖神经酰胺酶

ga·lac·to·syl·trans·fer·ase (gə-lak″to-səltrans′fər-ās) any of a group of enzymes that transfer a galactose radical from a donor to an acceptor molecule 半乳糖苷转移酶

ga·lan·ta·mine (gə-lan′tə-mēn) a reversible competitive inhibitor of acetylcholinesterase used as the hydrobromide salt in the treatment of Alzheimer disease 加兰他敏

ga·lea (ga′le-ə) [L.] a helmet-shaped structure 帽状（突起）物（体）；**g. aponeuro′tica,** the aponeurosis connecting the two bellies of the occipitofrontalis muscle 帽状腱膜

ga·len·i·cals (gə-len′ĭ-kəlz) medicines prepared according to Galen's formulas; now used to denote standard preparations containing one or several organic ingredients, as contrasted with pure chemical substances 盖伦制剂. 又称 *galenics*

ga·leo·pho·bia (ga″le-o-fo′be-ə) ailurophobia 惧猫症，恐猫症

Gal·er·i·na (gal-ə-ri′nə) a genus of mushrooms including *G. margina′ta* (also called *G. autumna′lis*), which contains amatoxins 盔孢伞属，蘑菇的一个属，含有毒伞毒素

gall (gawl) bile 胆汁

gal·la·mine tri·eth·io·dide (gal′ə-mēn tri″ə- thi′o-dīd) a quaternary ammonium compound used to induce skeletal muscle relaxation during surgery and other procedures, such as endoscopy or intubation. 三碘季铵酚，一种季铵盐化合物，用于手术和其他过程中诱导骨骼肌放松，如内镜检查或插管

gall·blad·der (gawl′blad′ər) the reservoir for bile on the posteroinferior surface of the liver 胆囊

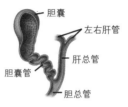

胆囊
左右肝管
肝总管
胆囊管
胆总管

gal·li·um (Ga) (gal′e-əm) a soft, silvery metal element, liquid at approximately room temperature; at. no. 31, at. wt. 69.723; some of its compounds are poisonous. The nitrate salt is an inhibitor of bone calcium resorption and is used to treat cancer-related hypercalcemia 镓；**g. citrate Ga 67,** a radiopharmaceutical imaging agent used to image neoplasms, particularly of soft tissues, and sites of inflammation and abscess 柠檬酸镓 Ga-67

gal·lon (gal′on) a measure of liquid volume, 4 quarts. A standard gallon (United States) is 3.785 liters; an imperial gallon (Great Britain) is 4.546 liters 加仑（容量单位）

gal·lop (gal′op) a disordered rhythm of the heart 奔马律；另见 *rhythm* 下词条；**atrial g.,** S_4 g. 房性奔马律；**diastolic g.,** S_3 g. 舒张期奔马律；**presystolic g.,** S_4 g. 收缩期前奔马律；**S3 g.,** an accentuated third heart sound in patients with cardiac disease characterized by pathologic alterations in ventricular filling in early diastole 第三心音奔马律；**S4 g.,** an accentuated, audible fourth heart sound usually associated with cardiac disease, often that with altered ventricular compliance 第四心音奔马律；**summation g.,** one in which the third and fourth sounds are superimposed, appearing as one loud sound; usually associated with cardiac disease 重叠型奔马律；**ventricular g.,** S_3 g. 室性奔马律

gall·stone (gawl′stōn) biliary calculus; a calculus formed in the gallbladder or bile duct 胆结石

GALT gut-associated lymphoid tissue 肠道相关淋巴组织

gal·va·nism (gal′və-niz-əm) 1. galvanic current

电流；2. the therapeutic use of this current, particularly for stimulation of nerves and muscle 直流电疗法；**galvan′ic** *adj.* **dental g.** production of galvanic current in the oral cavity due to the presence of two or more dissimilar metals in dental restorations that are bathed in saliva, or a single metal restoration and two electrolytes, saliva and pulp tissue fluid, thus producing an electrolytic cell and an electric current. When such restorations touch each other, the current may be high enough to irritate the dental pulp and cause sharp pain. The anodic restoration or areas of a restoration are subject to electrolytic corrosion 牙流电

gal·va·no·con·trac·til·i·ty (gal″va-no-kon″- traktil′ĭ-te) contractility in response to a galvanic stimulus 电流收缩性

gal·va·nom·e·ter (gal″va-nom′a-tar) an instrument for measuring current by electromagnetic action 检流计

gal·va·no·pal·pa·tion (gal″va-no-pal-pa′shan) testing of nerves of the skin by galvanic current 电触诊

gam·ete (gam′ēt) 1. one of two haploid reproductive cells, male *(spermatozoon)* and female *(oocyte)*, whose union is necessary in sexual reproduction to initiate the development of a new individual 配子；2. the malarial parasite in its sexual form in a mosquito's stomach, either male *(microgamete)* or female *(macrogamete);* the latter is fertilized by the former to develop into an ookinete 生殖型疟原虫；**gamet′ic** *adj.*

ga·me·to·cide (ga-me′to-sīd) an agent that destroys gametes or gametocytes 杀配子剂

ga·me·to·cyte (ga-me′to-sīt) 1. a cell capable of dividing to form gametes; an oocyte or spermatocyte 卵母细胞，精母细胞; 2. the sexual form, male or female, of certain sporozoa, such as malarial plasmodia, found in the erythrocytes, which may produce gametes when ingested by the secondary host 配子母细胞；另见 *macrogametocyte* 和 *microgametocyte*

gam·e·to·gen·e·sis (ga-me″to-jen′a-sis) the development of the male and female sex cells, or gametes 配子形成，配子发生；**gametogen′ic** *adj.*

gam·e·tog·o·ny (gam″a-tog′a-ne) 1. the development of merozoites of malarial plasmodia and other sporozoa into male and female gametes, which later fuse to form a zygote 疟原虫和其他孢子虫的裂殖子发育成雄性和雌性配子，以后融合形成合子；2. reproduction by means of gametes 配子生殖

gam·ma (gam′a) 1. third letter of the Greek alphabet 希腊字母表中的第 3 个字母（γ），另见 γ-; 2. obsolete equivalent for microgram 微克

gam·ma-ami·no·bu·tyr·ic ac·id (gam′a-a-me″no-

bu-tir′ik) γ -aminobutyric acid γ- 氨基丁酸

gam·ma ben·zene hex·a·chlo·ride (gam′aben′zēn hek″sa-klor′īd) lindane γ- 六氯化苯

gam·ma glob·u·lin (gam′a glob′u-lin) 丙种球蛋白，γ- 球蛋白，见 *globulin* 下词条；

gam·ma·glob·u·li·nop·a·thy (gam″a-glob″ulinop′a-the) gammopathy 丙种球蛋白病，γ- 球蛋白病

Gam·ma·pap·il·lo·ma·vi·rus (gam″a-pap″ĭ- lo′mavi″ras) a genus of viruses of the family Papillomaviridae that contains several of the human papillomaviruses 乳头瘤病毒科

Gam·ma·pro·teo·bac·te·ria (gam″a-pro″teobak-tēr′e-a) a class of bacteria of the Proteobacteria, including a large number of organisms of medical interest 丙型变形菌纲

gam·mop·a·thy (gam-op′a-the) abnormal proliferation of the lymphoid cells producing immunoglobulins; the gammopathies include multiple myeloma, macroglobulinemia, and Hodgkin disease 丙种球蛋白病，γ - 球蛋白病

gan·ci·clo·vir (gan-si′klo-vir) a derivative of acyclovir used in the form of the base or the sodium salt in the treatment of retinitis due to cytomegalovirus 更昔洛韦

gan·glia (gang′gle-a) plural of *ganglion* 神经节的复数形式

gan·gli·at·ed (gang′gle-āt″ad) ganglionated 有神经节的

gan·gli·form (gang′glĭ-form) having the form of a ganglion 神经节状的。Spelled also *ganglioform*

gan·gli·itis (gang″gle-i′tis) ganglionitis 神经节炎

gan·gli·o·blast (gang′gle-o-blast″) an embryonic cell of the cerebrospinal ganglia 成神经节细胞

gan·glio·cy·to·ma (gang″gle-o-si-to′ma) ganglioneuroma 神经节细胞瘤

gan·glio·gli·o·ma (gang″gle-o-gli-o′ma) a ganglioneuroma in the central nervous system 神经节细胞胶质瘤

gan·glio·glio·neu·ro·ma (gang″gle-o-gli″onooro′ma) ganglioneuroma 神经节胶质神经瘤

gan·gli·o·ma (gang″gle-o′ma) ganglioneuroma 神经节瘤

gan·gli·on (gang′gle-on) pl. *gan′glia, ganglions* [Gr.] 1. a knot, or knotlike mass; in anatomy, a group of nerve cell bodies, located outside the central nervous system; occasionally applied to certain nuclear groups within the brain 神经节；2. a form of benign cystic tumor on an aponeurosis or a tendon 腱鞘囊肿；**gan′glial, ganglion′ic** *adj.*

aberrant g., a small ganglion sometimes found on a dorsal cervical nerve root between the spinal ganglia and the spinal cord 迷走神经节；**Acrel g.,** a cystic tumor on an extensor tendon of the wrist Acrel 腱

鞘囊肿；**Andersch g.,** inferior g. (1)；**autonomic ganglia,** aggregations of cell bodies of neurons of the autonomic nervous system, divided into the *sympathetic* and *parasympathetic ganglia* 自主神经节；**basal ganglia,** 基底（神经）节，见 *nucleus* 下词条；**Bidder ganglia,** ganglia on the cardiac nerves, situated at the lower end of the atrial septum Bidder 神经节；**Bochdalek g.,** superior dental plexus 博赫达勒克神经节；**cardiac ganglia,** ganglia of the cardiac plexus near the arterial ligament 心 神 经节；**carotid g.,** an occasional small enlargement in the internal carotid plexus 颈动脉神经节；**celiac ganglia,** two irregularly shaped ganglia, one on each crus of the respiratory diaphragm within the celiac plexus 腹腔神经节；**cerebrospinal ganglia,** those associated with the cranial and spinal nerves 脑 脊神 经 节；**cervical,** 1. any of the three ganglia (inferior, middle, and superior) of the sympathetic trunk in the neck region 颈神经节；2. one near the cervix uteri 子宫颈神经节；**cervicothoracic g.,** one formed by fusion of the inferior cervical and the first thoracic ganglia 颈胸神经节，星状神经节；**cervicouterine g.,** cervical g. (2)；**ciliary g.,** a parasympathetic ganglion in the posterior part of the orbit 睫状神经节；**Cloquet g.,** a swelling of the nasopalatine nerve in the anterior palatine canal 克洛凯神经节，鼻腭神经节；**cochlear g.,** spiral g. 蜗神经节；**Corti g.,** spiral g. 科蒂神经节；**dorsal root g.,** spinal g. 背根神经节；**Ehrenritter g.,** superior g. (1) 舌咽神经上节；**false g.,** an enlargement on a nerve that does not have a true ganglionic structure 假神经节；**gasserian g.,** trigeminal g 半月神经节；**geniculate g.,** the sensory ganglion of the facial nerve, on the geniculum of the facial nerve 膝神经节；**g. im'par,** the ganglion commonly found in front of the coccyx, where the sympathetic trunks of the two sides unite 奇神经节；**inferior g.,** 1. the lower of two ganglia on the glossopharyngeal nerve as it passes through the jugular foramen（舌咽神经）下神经节；2. a ganglion of the vagus nerve, just below the jugular foramen（迷走神经）下神经节；**jugular g.,** superior g. 颈静脉神经节；**Lee g.,** cervical g. (2)；**Ludwig g.,** one near the right atrium of the heart, connected with the cardiac plexus Ludwig 神经节（心右房神经节）；**lumbar ganglia,** the ganglia on the lumbar part of the sympathetic trunk, usually four or five on either side 腰神经节；**Meckel g.,** pterygopalatine g. Meckel 神经节，蝶腭神经节；**Meissner g.,** one of the small groups of nerve cells in the Meissner plexus Meissner 神经节（肠黏膜下丛神经节）；**esenteric g., inferior,** a sympathetic ganglion near the origin of the inferior mesenteric artery 肠系膜下 神 经 节；**mesenteric g., superior,** one or more sympathetic ganglia at the sides of, or just below, the superior mesenteric artery 肠系膜上神经节；**otic g.,** a parasympathetic ganglion immediately below the foramen ovale; its postganglionic fibers supply the parotid gland 耳神经节；**parasympathetic g.,** one of the aggregations of cell bodies of cholinergic neurons of the parasympathetic nervous system; they are located near, on, or within the wall of the organs being innervated 副交感神经节；**phrenic g.,** a sympathetic ganglion often found within the phrenic plexus at its junction with the cardiac plexus 膈神经节；**posterior root g.,** spinal g 后根神经节；**pterygopalatine g.,** a parasympathetic ganglion in the pterygopalatine fossa; its preganglionic fibers are derived from the facial nerve via the greater petrosal nerve and the nerve of the pterygopalatine canal, and its postganglionic fibers supply the lacrimal, nasal, and palatine glands 蝶腭神经节；翼腭神经节；**Remak g.,** 1. a sympathetic ganglion on the heart wall near the superior vena cava 交感神经节位于上腔静脉附近的心壁上的交感神经节；2. one of the sympathetic ganglia in the diaphragmatic opening for the inferior vena cava 交感神经节下腔静脉膈肌开口中的交感神经节之一；3. one of the ganglia in the gastric plexus 胃神经丛中的神经节之一；**Ribes g.,** a small ganglion sometimes seen in the termination of the internal carotid plexus around the anterior communicating artery of the brain Ribes 神经节（大脑前交通动脉神经丛）；**sacral ganglia,** those of the sacral part of the sympathetic trunk, usually three or four on either side 骶神经节；**Scarpa g.,** vestibular g 斯卡尔帕神经节；**semilunar g.,** 1. trigeminal g.；2. (*in the pl.*) celiac ganglia 腹腔神经节；**sensory g.,** 1. spinal g.；2. (*in the pl.*) the ganglia on the roots of the cranial nerves, containing the cell bodies of sensory neurons 脑神经根上的神经节，包含感觉神经元的胞体；3. both of these considered together 感觉神经节；**simple g.,** a cystic tumor in a tendon sheath 单纯性腱鞘囊肿；**sphenomaxillary g.,** sphenopalatine g., pterygopalatine g 蝶腭神经节；**spinal g.,** one on the posterior root of each spinal nerve, composed of unipolar nerve cell bodies of the sensory neurons of the nerve 脊神经节；**spiral g.,** the ganglion on the cochlear nerve, located within the modiolus, sending fibers peripherally to the organ of Corti and centrally to the cochlear nuclei of the brainstem 螺旋神经节；**splanchnic g.,** one on the greater splanch nic nerve near the twelfth thoracic vertebra 胸内脏神经节；**submandibular g.,** a parasympathetic ganglion located superior to the deep part of the submandibular gland, on the lateral surface of

430

the hyoglossal muscle 下颌下神经节；**superior g.,** 1. the upper of two ganglia on the glossopharyngeal nerve as it passes through the jugular foramen（舌咽神经）上神经节；2. a small ganglion on the vagus nerve just as it passes through the jugular foramen（迷走神经）上神经节；**sympathetic g.,** any of the aggregations of cell bodies of adrenergic neurons of the sympathetic nervous system; they are arranged in chainlike fashion on either side of the spinal cord 交感神经节；**trigeminal g.,** one on the dorsal root of the fifth cranial nerve in a cleft in the dura mater on the anterior surface of the petrous part of the temporal bone, giving off the ophthalmic and maxillary nerves and part of the mandibular nerve 三叉神经节；**tympanic g.,** an enlargement on the tympanic branch of the glossopharyngeal nerve 鼓室神经节；**vagal g.,** 1. inferior g. (2); 2. superior g. (2)；**ventricular g.,** Bidder ganglia 心室神经节；**vestibular g.,** the sensory ganglion of the vestibular part of the eighth cranial nerve, located in the upper part of the lateral end of the internal acoustic meatus 前庭神经节；**Wrisberg ganglia,** cardiac ganglia 心神经节；**wrist g.,** cystic enlargement of a tendon sheath on the back of the wrist 腕部腱鞘囊肿

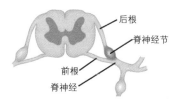

▲ 显示脊髓神经节的脊髓横截面

gan·gli·on·at·ed (gang′gle-ə-nāt″əd) provided with ganglia 有神经节的

gan·gli·on·ec·to·my (gang″gle-ə-nek′tə-me) excision of a ganglion 神经节切除术

gan·glio·neu·ro·ma (gang″gle-o-noo-ro′mə) a benign neoplasm composed of nerve fibers and mature ganglion cells 神经节瘤

gan·gli·on·ic (gang″gle-on′ik) pertaining to a ganglion 神经节的

gan·gli·on·itis (gang″gle-ə-ni′tis) inflammation of a ganglion 神经节炎

gan·gli·on·os·to·my (gang″gle-ə-nos′tə-me) surgical creation of an opening into a cystic tumor on a tendon sheath or aponeurosis 神经节切除术，腱鞘囊肿造口术

gan·glio·pleg·ic (gang″gle-o-ple′jik) 1. blocking transmission of impulses through the sympathetic and parasympathetic ganglia 神经节阻滞的；2. an agent that so acts 神经节阻滞药

gan·glio·side (gang′gle-o-sīd″) any of a group of glycosphingolipids found in the central nervous system tissues and having the basic composition ceramide-glucose-galactose-*N*-acetylneuraminic acid. The form GM$_1$ accumulates in tissues in GM$_1$ gangliosidoses and the form GM$_2$ in GM$_2$ gangliosidoses 神经节苷脂

gan·gli·o·si·do·sis (gang″gle-o-si-do′sis) pl. *gangliosido′ses.* Any of a group of lysosomal storage diseases marked by accumulation of gangliosides GM$_1$ or GM$_2$ and related glycoconjugates due to deficiency of specific lysosomal hydro lases, and by progressive psychomotor deterioration, usually beginning in infancy or childhood and usually fatal 神经节苷脂沉积病；**GM$_1$ g.,** that due to deficiency of lysosomal β -galactosidase activity, with accumulation of ganglioside GM$_1$, glycoproteins, and keratan sulfate GM$_1$ 神经节苷脂贮积症；**GM$_2$ g.,** that characterized by accumulation of ganglioside GM$_2$ and relatedglycoconjugates; due to deficiency of activity of specific hexosaminidase isozymes or of GM$_2$ activator protein necessary for activity. It occurs as three biochemically distinct variants, including Sandhoff disease and Tay-Sachs disease GM$_2$ 神经节苷脂沉积症

gan·grene (gang′grēn) death of tissue, usually in considerable mass, generally with loss of vascular (nutritive) supply and followed by bacterial invasion and putrefaction 坏疽；**gang′renous** *adj.*；**diabetic g.,** moist gangrene associated with diabetes 糖尿病坏疽；**dry g.,** that occurring without subsequent bacterial decomposition, the tissues becoming dry and shriveled 干性坏疽；**embolic g.,** a condition following cutting off of blood supply by embolism 栓塞性坏疽；**gas g.,** an acute, severe, painful condition in which the muscles and subcutaneous tissues become filled with gas and a serosanguineous exudate; due to infection of wounds by anaerobic bacteria, among which are various species of *Clostridium* 气性坏疽；**moist g.,** that associated with proteolytic decomposition resulting from bacterial action 湿性坏疽；**symmetric g.,** gangrene of corresponding digits on both sides, due to vasomotor disturbances 对称性坏疽

gan·gre·no·sis (gang″rə-no′sis) the development of gangrene 坏疽病

gan·i·re·lix (gan″ī-rel′iks) a synthetic decapeptide derived from, and an antagonist to, gonadotropinreleasing hormone; used as the acetate salt in the treatment of female infertility 药品名，促性腺激素释放激素拮抗药，其醋酸盐用于治疗女性不孕症

gan·o·blast (gan′o-blast) ameloblast 成釉细胞

gap (gap) an unoccupied interval in time; an opening or hiatus 隙 缝；**air-bone g.**, the lag between the audiographic curves for air- and bone-conducted stimuli, as an indication of loss of bone conduction of the ear 气骨导间距；**anion g.**, the concentration of plasma anions not routinely measured by laboratory screening, accounting for the difference between the measured anions and cations 阴离子隙；**auscultatory g.**, a period in which sound is not heard in the auscultatory method of sphygmomanometry 听诊无音间隙；**interocclusal g.**, 𬌗间距，见 *distance* 下词条

Gard·ner·el·la (gahrd″nər-el′ə) a genus of small, gram-negative, rod-shaped bacteria of the family Bifidobacteriaceae. It comprises a single species, *G. vagina'lis*, which is found in the normal female genital tract and is also a major cause of bacterial vaginitis 加德纳菌属

gar·gle (gahr′gəl) 1. a solution for rinsing mouth and throat 漱口剂；2. to rinse the mouth and throat by holding a solution in the open mouth and agitating it by expulsion of air from the lungs 漱口

gar·goyl·ism (gahr′goil-iz-əm) Hurler syndrome 脂肪软骨营养不良，软骨代谢障碍病

gar·lic (gahr′lik) the flowering plant *Allium sa'tivum*, or its bulbous stem base, which contains the antibacterial allicin; preparations of the bulbs are used for hyperlipidemia, hypertension, and arteriosclerosis; also used in folk medicine 大蒜

gas (gas) any elastic aeriform fluid in which the molecules are separated from one another and so have free paths 气体；**gas′eous** *adj.*；**alveolar g.**, the gas in the alveoli of the lungs, where gaseous exchange with the capillary blood takes place 肺泡气；**blood g's**, the partial pressures of oxygen and carbon dioxide in blood 血气的，血液中氧气和二氧化碳的分压；见 *analysis* 下词条；**laughing g.**, nitrous oxide 笑气，一氧化氮；**tear g.**, one that produces severe lacrimation by irritating the conjunctivae 催泪气

gas·o·met·ric (gas″o-met′rik) pertaining to the measurement of gases 气体定量的

gas·ter (gas′tər) [Gr.] stomach 胃

Gas·ter·oph·i·lus (gas″tər-of′ĭ-ləs) a genus of botflies the larvae of which develop in the gastrointestinal tract of horses and may sometimes infect humans, causing a creeping eruption 胃蝇属

gas·trad·e·ni·tis (gas″trad-ə-ni′tis) inflammation of the stomach glands 胃腺炎

gas·tral·gia (gas-tral′jə) pain in the stomach 胃痛

gas·trec·to·my (gas-trek′tə-me) excision of the stomach (*total g.*) or of a portion of it (*partial or subtotal g.*) 胃切除术

gas·tric (gas′trik) pertaining to, affecting, or originating in the stomach 胃的

gas·tric·sin (gas-trik′sin) a proteolytic enzyme isolated from gastric juice; its precursor is pepsinogen, but it differs from pepsin in molecular weight and in N-terminal amino acids 胃亚蛋白酶

gas·trin (gas′trin) a polypeptide hormone secreted by certain cells of the pyloric glands, which strongly stimulates secretion of gastric acid and pepsin and weakly stimulates secretion of pancreatic enzymes and gallbladder contraction 胃泌素

gas·tri·no·ma (gas″trī-no′mə) an islet cell tumor of non-beta cells that secretes gastrin; it is the usual cause of Zollinger-Ellison syndrome 胃泌素瘤

gas·tri·tis (gas-tri′tis) inflammation of the stomach 胃炎；**atrophic g.**, chronic gastritis with infiltration of the lamina propria, involving the entire mucosal thickness, by inflammatory cells 萎缩性胃炎；**eosinophilic g.**, that in which there is considerable edema and infiltration of all coats of the wall of the pyloric antrum by eosinophils 嗜酸（细胞）性胃炎；**erosive g.**, 糜烂性胃炎；**exfoliative g.**, that in which the gastric surface epithelium is eroded 剥脱性胃炎；**hypertrophic g.**, gastritis with infiltration and enlargement of the glands 肥厚性胃炎；**polypous g.**, hypertrophic gastritis with polypoid projections of the mucosa 息肉性胃炎；**pseudomembranous g.**, that in which a false membrane occurs in patches within the stomach 假膜性胃炎；**superficial g.**, chronic inflammation of the lamina propria, limited to the outer third of the mucosa in the foveolar area 浅表性胃炎；**toxic g.**, that due to action of a poison or corrosive agent 中毒性胃炎

gas·tro·anas·to·mo·sis (gas″tro-ə-nas″tomo′sis) gastrogastrostomy 胃吻合术

gas·tro·cele (gas′tro-sēl) hernial protrusion of the stomach or of a gastric pouch 胃膨出

gas·troc·ne·mi·us (gas″trok-) (gas″tro-ne′ me-əs) 腓肠肌，见 *muscle* 下词条

gas·tro·coele (gas′tro-sēl) archenteron 原肠，原肠腔

gas·tro·col·ic (gas″tro-kol′ik) pertaining to or communicating with the stomach and colon, as a fistula 胃结肠的

gas·tro·co·li·tis (gas″tro-ko-li′tis) inflammation of the stomach and colon 胃结肠炎

gas·tro·cu·ta·ne·ous (gas″tro-ku-ta′ne-əs) pertaining to the stomach and skin, or communicating with the stomach and the cutaneous surface of the body, as a gastrocutaneous fistula 胃皮肤的

gas·tro·cys·to·plas·ty (gas″tro-sis′to-plas″te) augmentation cystoplasty using a portion of the stomach 胃代膀胱术

Gas·tro·dis·coi·des (gas″tro-dis-koi′dēz) a genus of trematodes parasitic in the intestinal tract 似腹盘属

gas·tro·du·o·de·ni·tis (gas″tro-doo″o-də- ni′tis) inflammation of the stomach and duodenum 胃十二指肠炎

gas·tro·du·o·de·nos·to·my (gas″tro-doo″odə-nos′tə-me) gastroenterostomy between the stomach and duodenum 胃十二指肠吻合术

gas·tro·dyn·ia (gas″tro-din′e-ə) gastralgia 胃痛

gas·tro·en·ter·i·tis (gas″tro-en″tər-i′tis) inflammation of the stomach and intestine 胃肠炎; **bacterial g.,** any type caused by a bacterial toxin or bacterial infection, the most common agents being *Salmonella, Shigella,* and *Campylobacter* 细菌性肠胃炎; **eosinophilic g.,** a type usually associated with intolerance to specific foods, with infiltration of the mucosa of the small intestine (and often the stomach) by eosinophils; there is edema but no vasculitis; symptoms depend on the site and extent of the disorder 嗜酸细胞性胃肠炎; **Norwalk g., Norwalk virus g.,** a type caused by the Norwalk virus 诺沃克胃肠炎，诺沃克病毒性胃肠炎; **viral g.,** any type caused by a virus, the most common agents being rotaviruses and Norwalk virus 病毒性胃肠炎

gas·tro·en·tero·anas·to·mo·sis (gas″troen″tər-o-ə-nas′to-mo-sis) anastomosis between the stomach and small intestine 胃肠吻合术

gas·tro·en·ter·ol·o·gy (gas″tro-en″tərol′ə-je) the study of the stomach and intestine and their diseases 肠胃病学

gas·tro·en·ter·op·a·thy (gas″tro-en″tər-op′ ə-the) any disease of the stomach and intestines 胃肠病; **allergic g.,** eosinophilic gastritis of children with food allergies, particularly to cows' milk 变应性胃肠病

gas·tro·en·ter·os·to·my (gas″tro-en″təros′tə-me) surgical creation of an anastomosis between the stomach and the small intestine, or the opening so created 胃肠造口吻合术

gas·tro·en·ter·ot·o·my (gas″tro-en″tər-ot′ə-me) incision into the stomach and intestine 胃肠切开术

gas·tro·ep·i·plo·ic (gas″tro-ep″ĭ-plo′ik) pertaining to the stomach and epiploon (omentum) 胃网膜

gas·tro·esoph·a·ge·al (gas″tro-ə-sof″ə- je′əl) 1. pertaining to the stomach and esophagus 胃食道的; 2. proceeding from the stomach to the esophagus 胃到食管

gas·tro·esoph·a·gi·tis (gas″tro-ə-sof″ə- ji′tis) inflammation of the stomach and esophagus 胃食管炎

gas·tro·fi·ber·scope (gas″tro-fi′bər-skōp) fiberoptic gastroscope 胃纤维镜

gas·tro·gas·tros·to·my (gas″tro-gas-tros′ tə-me) surgical anastomosis of two previously remote portions of the stomach 胃胃吻合术

gas·tro·ga·vage (gas″tro-gə-vahzh′) artificial feeding through a tube passed into the stomach 胃管饲法

gas·tro·he·pat·ic (gas″tro-hə-pat′ik) pertaining to the stomach and liver 胃与肝脏的

gas·tro·hep·a·ti·tis (gas″tro-hep-ə-ti′tis) inflammation of the stomach and liver 胃肝炎

gas·tro·il·e·al (gas″tro-il′e-əl) pertaining to the stomach and ileum 胃回肠的

gas·tro·il·e·itis (gas″tro-il-e-i′tis) inflammation of the stomach and ileum 胃回肠炎

gas·tro·il·e·os·to·my (gas″tro-il″e-os′tə-me) gastroenterostomy between the stomach and ileum 胃回肠吻合术

gas·tro·in·tes·ti·nal (gas″tro-in-tes′tĭ-nəl) pertaining to or communicating with the stomach and intestine 胃肠的

gas·tro·je·ju·no·col·ic (gas″tro-jə-joo″no-kol′ik) pertaining to the stomach, jejunum, and colon 胃空肠结肠的

gas·tro·je·ju·nos·to·my (gas″tro-jə-joonos′tə-me) gastroenterostomy between the stomach and jejunum 胃空肠吻合术

gas·tro·li·e·nal (gas″tro-li′ən-əl) gastrosplenic 胃脾的

gas·tro·li·thi·a·sis (gas″tro-lĭ-thi′ə-sis) the presence or formation of calculi in the stomach 胃石症

gas·trol·y·sis (gas-trol′ə-sis) surgical division of perigastric adhesions to mobilize the stomach 胃松解术

gas·tro·ma·la·cia (gas″tro-mə-la′shə) softening of the wall of the stomach 胃软化

gas·tro·meg·a·ly (gas″tro-meg′ə-le) enlargement of the stomach 巨胃

gas·tro·pa·re·sis (gas″tro-pə-re′sis) paralysis of the stomach, which slows or stops its motility 胃轻瘫

gas·trop·a·thy (gas-trop′ə-the) any disease of the stomach 胃病

gas·tro·pexy (gas′tro-pek″se) surgical fixation of the stomach 胃固定术

Gas·troph·i·lus (gas-trof′ĭ-ləs) *Gasterophilus* 胃蝇属

gas·tro·phren·ic (gas″tro-fren′ik) pertaining to the stomach and respiratory diaphragm 胃膈的

gas·tro·pli·ca·tion (gas″tro-plĭ-ka′shən) treatment of gastric dilatation by stitching a fold in the stomach wall 胃折术

gas·trop·to·sis (gas″trop-to′sis) downward displacement of the stomach 胃下垂

gas·tror·rha·gia (gas″tro-ra′jə) hemorrhage from the stomach 胃出血

gas·tror·rhea (gas″tro-re′ə) excessive secretion by the glands of the stomach 胃溢液，胃液分泌过多

gas·tros·chi·sis (gas-tros′kĭ-sis) congenital fissure of the anterior abdominal wall 腹裂

gas·tro·scope (gas′tro-skōp) an endoscope for inspecting the interior of the stomach 胃镜；**gastroscop′ic** *adj.*; **fiberoptic g.**, one that uses fiberoptic technology 纤维胃镜

gas·tro·se·lec·tive (gas″tro-sə-lek′tiv) having an affinity for receptors involved in regulation of gastric activities 胃选择性的，嗜胃性的

gas·tro·spasm (gas′tro-spaz″əm) spasm of the stomach 胃痉挛

gas·tro·splen·ic (gas″tro-splen′ik) pertaining to the stomach and spleen 胃脾的

gas·tro·stax·is (gas″tro-stak′sis) the oozing of blood from the stomach mucosa 胃渗血，出血性胃炎

gas·tros·to·my (gas-tros′tə-me) surgical creation of an artificial opening into the stomach, or the opening so established 胃造口术

gas·trot·o·my (gas-trot′ə-me) incision into the stomach 胃切开术

gas·tro·tro·pic (gas″tro-tro′pik) having an affinity for or exerting a special effect on the stomach 亲胃的，对胃有亲和力或有特殊作用的

gas·tro·tym·pa·ni·tes (gas″tro-tim″pə- ni′tēz) tympanitic distention of the stomach 胃积气，胃鼓胀

gas·tru·la (gas′troo-lə) the embryo in the stage following the blastula or blastocyst; the simplest type consists of two layers of cells, the ectoderm and endoderm, which have invaginated to form the archenteron and an opening, the blastopore. In human embryos the gastrula stage occurs during the third week, as the embryonic disc becomes trilaminar, establishing the ectoderm, mesoderm, and endoderm 原肠胚，胚囊

gas·tru·la·tion (gas″troo-la′shən) the process by which a blastula becomes a gastrula or, in forms without a true blastula, the process by which three germ cell layers are acquired. In humans, the conversion of a bilaminar to a trilaminar embryonic disc (ectoderm, mesoderm, endoderm) 原肠胚形成

gat·i·flox·a·cin (gat″ĭ-flok′sə-sin) a fluoroquinolone antibacterial effective against many grampositive and gram-negative bacteria 加替沙星（氟喹诺酮类抗菌药）

gat·ing (gāt′ing) controlling access or passage through gates or channels 闸门开闭

ga·to·pho·bia (gat″o-fo′be-ə) ailurophobia 猫恐怖

gauss (gous) a unit of magnetic flux density, equal to 10^{-4} tesla 高斯，磁通密度的单位（$1G=10^{-4}T$）

gauze (gawz) a light, open-meshed fabric of muslin or similar material 纱布；**absorbable g.**, gauze made from oxidized cellulose 可吸收纱布；**absorbent g.**, white cotton cloth of various thread counts and weights, supplied in various lengths and widths and in different forms (rolls or folds) 脱脂纱布；**petrolatum g.**, a sterile material produced by saturation of sterile absorbent gauze with sterile white petrolatum 凡士林纱布；**zinc gelatin impregnated g.**, absorbent gauze impregnated with zinc gelatin 锌明胶浸渗纱布

ga·vage (gə-vahzh′) [Fr.] 1. forced feeding, especially through a tube passed into the stomach 管饲法；2. superalimentation 超量营养疗法

gaze (gāz) 凝视，注视；1. to look steadily in one direction. 2. the act of looking steadily at something；**conjugate g.**, the normal movement of the two eyes simultaneously in the same direction to bring something into view 共轭凝视

GBCA gadolinium-based contrast agent 钆对比剂

GC gas chromatography 气相色谱法

G-CSF granulocyte colony-stimulating factor 粒细胞集落刺激因子

Gd gadolinium 元素钆的符号

Ge germanium 元素锗的符号

ge·fit·i·nib (gə-fit′ĭ-nib) a tyrosine kinase inhibitor that acts on epidermal growth factor receptor; used in the treatment of non–small-cell lung cancer 吉非替尼

ge·gen·hal·ten (ga″gən-hahlt′ən) [Ger.] an involuntary resistance to passive movement, as may occur in cerebral cortical disorders 非自主抗拒

gel (jel) 1. a colloid in which the solid disperse phase forms a network in combination with the fluid continuous phase, resulting in a viscous semirigid sol 凝胶；2. to form such a compound or any similar semisolid material 胶滞体；**aluminum hydroxide g.**, a suspension of aluminum hydroxide and hydrated oxide used as a gastric antacid, especially in the treatment of peptic ulcer, and in the treatment of phosphate nephrolithiasis 氢氧化铝凝胶；**aluminium phosphate g.**, an aqueous suspension of aluminum phosphate, used as an antacid and to reduce excretion of phosphates in the feces 磷酸铝凝胶；**APF g.**, sodium fluoride and phosphoric acid g.；**basic aluminum carbonate g.**, an aluminum hydroxide–aluminum carbonate gel, used as an antacid, for treatment of hyperphosphatemia in renal insufficiency, and to prevent phosphate urinary calculi 碱性碳酸铝凝胶；**dried aluminum hydroxide g.**, an amorphous form of aluminum hydroxide prepared by drying aluminum hydroxide gel at a low temperature; used as an antacid 干燥氢氧化铝凝胶; **sodium fluoride and phosphoric acid g.,** a gel containing sodium fluoride, hydrofluoric acid, and phosphoric acid; applied topically to the teeth as a dental caries prophylactic 氟化钠和磷酸凝胶

gel·a·tin (jel′ə-tin) a substance obtained by partial hydrolysis of collagen derived from skin, white connective tissue, and bones of animals; used as a suspending agent, in manufacture of capsules and suppositories, and sometimes as an adjuvant protein food, and suggested for use as a plasma substitute 明胶; **zinc g.,** a preparation of zinc oxide, gelatin, glycerin, and purified water, used as a topical skin protectant 锌明胶

ge·lat·i·nous (jə-lat′ĭ-nəs) like jelly or softened gelatin 凝胶状的

ge·la·tion (jə-la′shən) conversion of a sol into a gel 胶凝（作用）

gem·cit·a·bine (jem-sit′ə-bēn) an antineoplastic agent used as the hydrochloride salt in the treatment of pancreatic adenocarcinoma and non–small-cell lung carcinoma 一种抗肿瘤药，其盐酸盐用于治疗胰腺癌和非小细胞肺癌

Ge·mel·la (jə-mel′ə) a genus of gram-positive, aerobic, or facultatively anaerobic cocci of the family Staphylococcaceae. Organisms, including *G. haemoly′sans* and *G. morbillo′rum,* are part of the normal oropharyngeal, gastrointestinal, and urogenital flora and are opportunistic pathogens, causing a variety of infectious illnesses, particularly in immunocompromised persons 兼性双球菌

gem·fib·ro·zil (jem-fib′ro-zil) a hypolipidemic agent used for treatment of patients with very high serum triglyceride levels (type IV hyperlipoproteinemia) who do not respond to dietary management 吉非贝齐，二甲苯氧庚酸（降血脂药）

gem·i·nate (jem′ĭ-nāt) paired; occurring in twos 成双的，成对发生的

gem·ma·tion (jə-ma′shən) budding; asexual reproduction in which a portion of the cell body is thrust out and then becomes separated, forming a new individual 芽生

gem·mule (jem′ūl) 1. a reproductive bud; the immediate product of gemmation 胚芽; 2. one of the many little spinelike processes on the dendrites of a neuron（神经细胞）芽突

gem·tu·zu·mab   ozo·ga·mi·cin (gem-too′zum-ab″ o″zo-gə-mi′sin) a recombinant DNA-derived monoclonal antibody conjugated with a cytotoxic antitumor antibiotic, used as an antineoplastic 一种抗肿瘤药，与细胞毒性抗肿瘤抗生素结合的重组DNA导向的单克隆抗体

gen·der (jen′dər) sex; the category to which an individual is assigned on the basis of sex 性别

gene (jēn) a segment of a DNA molecule (RNA in certain viruses) that contains all the information required for synthesis of a product (polypeptide chain or RNA molecule). It is the biologic unit of inheritance, self-reproducing, and transmitted from parent to progeny, and has a specific position (locus) in the genome 基因; **chimeric g.,** an artificial gene constructed by juxtaposition of fragments of unrelated genes or other DNA segments, which may themselves have been altered 嵌合基因; **complementary g's,** two or more nonallelic genes that act together to produce a phenotype that is produced by neither individually 互补基因; **H g.,** histocompatibility g., one that determines the specificity of tissue antigenicity (HLA antigens), and thus the compatibility of donor and recipient in tissue transplantation and blood transfusion 组织相容性基因; **holandric g.,** a gene that is located on the Y chromosome and thus appears only in males 限雄基因; **housekeeping g.,** one that encodes a protein needed for basic cell function and so is expressed in all cells 持家基因，管家基因; **immune response (Ir) g's,** genes of the major histocompatibility complex that govern the immune response to individual immunogens 免疫应答基因; **immune suppressor (Is) g's,** genes governing the ability of suppressor T cells to respond to certain antigens 免疫抑制基因; **lethal g.,** one whose expression brings about the death of the organism 致死基因; **regulator g., regulatory g.,** a gene whose product controls the activity of other, distant genes 调节基因; **split g.,** a gene containing multiple exons and at least one intron 割裂基因; **structural g.,** 结构基因 1. one that is transcribed into mRNA and thus encodes the amino acid sequence of a polypeptide chain; 2. one that encodes an mRNA, rRNA, or tRNA product; **X-linked g.,** one carried on the X chromosome 伴X染色体基因; **Y-linked g.,** one carried on the Y chromosome 伴Y染色体基因

gen·era (jen′ər-ə) plural of *genus* 属

gen·er·al (jen′ər-əl) affecting many parts or all parts of the organism; not local 全身的

gen·er·al·ize (jen′ər-əl-īz) 1. to spread throughout the body, as when local disease becomes systemic 泛化，扩散，全面化; 2. to form a general principle; to reason inductively 概括，综合，归纳

gen·er·a·tion (jen″ər-a′shən) 1. reproduction (1) 生殖; 2. a class composed of all individuals removed by the same number of successive ancestors from a common predecessor, or occupying positions on the same level in a pedigree chart 世代，一代;

alternate g., reproduction by alternate asexual and sexual means in an animal or plant species 世代交替；asexual g., 无性世代，见 *reproduction* 下词条；filial g., the offspring produced by the mating of the individuals of a given generation, with the offspring of the parental generation constituting the *first filial g.* (F₁), and their offspring the *second filial g.* (F₂), and so on 子代；parental g. (P₁), the generation with which a particular genetic study is begun 亲代；sexual g., 有性世代，见 *reproduction* 下词条

gen·er·a·tor (jen′ər-a″tər) 1. something that produces or causes to exist 生殖者，发生者；2. a machine that converts mechanical to electrical energy 发电机；pattern g., a network of neurons that produces a stereotyped form of complex movement, such as chewing or ambulation, that is almost invariable from one performance to the next 中枢模式发生器；pulse g., 1. an apparatus that delivers regular pulses of electricity for therapeutic purposes, such as the power source for a cardiac pacemaker system that supplies impulses to implanted electrodes either at a fixed rate or in some programmed pattern 脉冲发生器；2. a physiologic mechanism that yields regular pulses of a hormone or other substance within the body 脉冲式分泌

ge·ner·ic (jə-ner′ik) 1. pertaining to a genus 属的；2. nonproprietary; denoting a drug name not protected by a trademark, usually descriptive of the drug's chemical structure 非专利的

gen·e·sis (jən′ə-sis) [Gr.] creation; origination 起源，生殖

ge·net·ic (jə-net′ik) 1. pertaining to or determined by genes 遗传的；2. pertaining to reproduction or to birth or origin 起源的

ge·net·ics (jə-net′iks) the study of genes and their heredity 遗传学；biochemical g., the branch of genetics concerned with the chemical and physical nature of genes and the mechanisms by which they function at the molecular level, specifically the roles of genes in controlling steps in metabolic pathways 生物遗传学，clinical g., the application of genetics to diagnosis of genetic disorders and patient care 临床遗传学；developmental g., the branch of genetics concerned with how development is controlled by specific genes 发育遗传学；molecular g., that branch of genetics concerned with the molecular structure and functioning of genes, from DNA replication to protein product 分子遗传学；population g., the study of the distribution of genes in populations and of how genes and genotype frequencies are maintained or changed 群体遗传学；reproductive g., the use of a combination of clinical genetics, dysmorphology, maternal-fetal medicine, and assisted reproductive technologies for detection, understanding, and prevention of reproductive abnormalities 生殖遗传学

ge·ni·al (jə-ni′əl) mental (2) 颏的

gen·ic (jen′ik) pertaining to or caused by genes 基因的

ge·nic·u·lar (jə-nik′u-lər) pertaining to the knee 膝的

ge·nic·u·late (jə-nik′u-lāt) bent, like a knee 膝状的

ge·nic·u·lum (jə-nik′u-ləm) pl. *geni′cula* [L.] a little knee; used in anatomic nomenclature to designate a sharp kneelike bend in a small structure or organ 小膝，明显膝状弯曲的小结构或小器官的通称

gen·i·tal (jen′ĭ-təl) pertaining to reproduction or to the reproductive organs 生殖的；生殖器的

gen·i·ta·lia (jen″ĭ-ta′le-ə) [L.] the reproductive organs, particularly those that are external （外）生殖器；ambiguous g., atypical g., genital organs that are not congruent with chromosomal sex or that are not distinctly male or female, as in disorders of sex development 两性畸形，外生殖器畸形；external g., the reproductive organs external to the body, including pudendum, clitoris, and urethra in the female, and scrotum, penis, and urethra in the male 外生殖器；indifferent g., the reproductive organs of the embryo prior to the establishment of definitive sex 未分化生殖器；internal g., the reproductive organs within the body, including ovaries, uterine tubes, uterus, and vagina in the female, and testes, epididymides, ductus deferentes, seminal vesicles, ejaculatory ducts, prostate, and bulbourethral glands in the male 内生殖器

gen·i·tals (jen′ĭ-təlz) genitalia 生殖器

gen·i·tog·ra·phy (jen″ĭ-tog′rə-fe) radiography of the urogenital sinus and internal duct structures after injection of a contrast medium through the sinus opening 泌尿生殖窦 X 线造影术

gen·i·to·uri·nary (jen″ĭ-to-u′rĭ-nar-e) pertaining to the genital and urinary systems 泌尿生殖器的

ge·no·copy (je′no-kop″e) a phenotype that appears identical to another but that is caused by a different genetic mechanism 拟基因型

ge·no·der·ma·to·sis (je″no-dur″mə-to′sis) a genetic disorder of the skin, usually generalized 遗传性皮肤病

ge·nome (je′nōm) the entirety of the genetic information encoded by nucleotides of an organism, cell, organelle, or virus 基因组；**genom′ic** *adj.*；mitochondrial g., a circular double-stranded DNA molecule, 16.6 kb in size and containing 37 genes in humans, present in 5 to 10 copies within each mitochondrion, and thus in thousands of copies per cell, with a slightly different genetic code and a higher mutation rate than those of the nuclear genome. It is transmitted by maternal inheritance 线粒体基因组

ge·no·mics (je-no′miks) the study of the structure and function of the genome 基因组学

ge·no·tox·ic (je′no-tok″sik) damaging to DNA; said of agents such as radiation or chemical substances that do this and thereby cause mutations, sometimes resulting in cancer 遗传毒性的

ge·no·type (je′no-tīp) 1. the entire genetic constitution of an individual 基因型，遗传型；2. the alleles present at one or more specific loci 等位基因；**genotyp′ic** *adj.*

gen·ta·mi·cin (jen″tə-mi′sin) an aminoglycoside antibiotic complex isolated from bacteria of the genus *Micromonospora*, effective against many gram-negative bacteria as well as certain grampositive species; used as the sulfate salt 庆大霉素（氨基糖苷类抗生素）

gen·tian (jen′shən) the dried rhizome and roots of *Gentiana lutea;* used as a bitter tonic 龙胆；g. **violet**, an antibacterial, antifungal, and anthelmintic dye, applied topically in the treatment of infections of the skin and mucous membranes associated with gram-positive bacteria and molds; also used to treat blood collected in areas endemic for Chagas disease 龙胆紫（细胞染色剂）

gen·tian·o·phil·ic (jen′shən-o-fil′ik) staining readily with gentian violet 嗜龙胆紫的，易被龙胆紫染色的

gen·tian·o·pho·bic (jen″shən-o-fo′bik) not staining with gentian violet 拒龙胆紫的，不易用龙胆紫染色的

ge·nu (je′nu) pl. *ge′nua* [L.] 1. the knee 膝；2. any kneelike structure 膝状的；g. **extror′sum**, bowleg 膝内翻；g. **intror′sum**, knock-knee 膝外翻；g. **recurva′tum**, hyperextensibility of the knee joint 膝反屈；g. **val′gum**, knock-knee 膝外翻；g. **va′rum**, bowleg 膝内翻

ge·nus (je′nəs) pl. *gen′era* [L.] a taxonomic category subordinate to a tribe (or subtribe) and superior to a species (or subgenus) 属

Geo·ba·cil·lus (je″o-bə-sil′əs) a genus of thermophilic, gram-positive, rod-shaped bacteria of the family Bacillaceae. *G. stearothermo′philus,*which produces very resistant spores and is capable of growth at 65℃, is used to test for autoclave quality control 芽孢杆菌属

geo·graph·ic (je″o-graf′ik) in pathology, of or referring to a pattern that is well demarcated, resembling outlines on a map 界限的

geo·med·i·cine (je″o-med′ĭ-sin) the branch of medicine dealing with the influence of climatic and environmental conditions on health 地理医学

geo·pha·gia (je-o-fa′jə) the habitual eating of earth or clay, a form of pica 食土癖

geo·tri·cho·sis (je″o-trĭ-ko′sis) an opportunistic candidiasis-like infection due to *Geotrichum candidum*, which may cause mucocutaneous or disseminated disease 地丝菌病

Ge·ot·ri·chum (je-ot′rĭ-kəm) a genus of ascomycetous, yeastlike, anamorphic fungi, including the opportunistic pathogen *G. can′didum*, which causes geotrichosis. *G. capita′tum* is now *Saprochaete capitata* 地霉属

ge·ot·ro·pism (je-ot′ro-piz-əm) a tendency of growth or movement toward or away from the earth; the influence of gravity on growth 向地性

ge·phy·ro·pho·bia (jə-fi″rə-fō′bē-ə) fear of crossing bridges 过桥恐怖症

ge·rat·ic (jə-rat′ik) pertaining to old age 老年的

GERD gastroesophageal reflux disease 胃食管反流病

ger·i·at·ric (jer″e-at′riks) the department of medicine dealing especially with the problems of aging and diseases of the elderly 老年医学；dental g., gerodontics 老年牙科学

ger·i·at·rics (jer″e-at′rik) 1. pertaining to elderly persons or to the aging process 老年医学；2. pertaining to geriatrics 老年病学的

geri·odon·tics (jer″e-o-don′tiks) gerodontics 老年牙科学

germ (jurm) 1. a pathogenic microorganism 病菌，病原微生物；2. a living substance capable of developing into an organ, part, or organism as a whole; a primordium 胚，胚芽；dental g., collective tissues from which a tooth is formed 牙胚；enamel g., the epithelial rudiment of the enamel organ 釉胚；hair g., an ectodermal concentration in the basal layer of the embryonic epidermis, the precursor of a hair follicle and related structures 毛胚芽

ger·ma·ni·um (Ge) (jər-ma′ne-əm) a brittle gray metalloid element; at. no. 32, at. wt. 72.63 锗

ger·mi·cide (jur′mĭ-sīd) an agent that kills pathogenic microorganisms 杀菌剂；**germici′dal** *adj.*

ger·mi·nal (jur′mĭ-nəl) pertaining to or of the nature of a gamete (germ cell) or the primordial stage of development 胚的；发生的；原始的

ger·mi·na·tion (jur″mĭ-na′shən) the sprouting of a seed, spore, or plant embryo 萌发；发芽；**ger′minative** *adj.*

ger·mi·no·ma (jur″mĭ-no′mə) a type of germ cell tumor with large round cells with vascular nuclei, usually found in the ovary, undescended testis, anterior mediastinum, or pineal gland; in males called *seminoma* and in females called *dysgerminoma* 生殖细胞瘤

germ·line (jərm′līn) the sequence of cells in the line of direct descent from zygote to gamete, as opposed to somatic cells. Written also *germ line* 种系

gero·der·ma (jer″o-dur′mə) dystrophy of the skin and genitals, giving the appearance of old age 老年状皮肤

ger·odon·tics (jer″o-don′tiks) dentistry dealing with the dental problems of older people 老年牙医学; **gerodon′tic** *adj.*

gero·mor·phism (jer″o-mor′fiz-əm) premature aging of a body part 早衰状

geront (o)- word element [Gr.], *old age; the aged* [构词成分] 老人，老年

ger·on·tol·o·gy (jer″on-tol′ə-je) the scientific study of aging in all its aspects 老年学

ger·on·to·phil·ia (jer″on-toe-fil′e-ə) sexual attraction to old people 亲老人癖

gero·psy·chi·a·try (jer″o-si-ki′ə-tre) a subspecialty of psychiatry dealing with mental illness in the elderly 老年精神病学

ges·ta·gen (jes′tə-jen) progestational agent 孕激素

ge·stalt (gə-stawlt′)(gə-shtawlt′) [Ger.] form, shape; a whole perceptual configuration 完形的，格式塔的；见 *gestaltism*

ges·tal·tism (gə-stawl′tiz-əm) (gə-shtawl′tiz- əm) a theory in psychology that objects of the mind, as immediately presented to direct experience, come as complete unanalyzable wholes or forms (Gestalten) that cannot be split up into parts 完形心理学，格式塔主义

ges·ta·tion (jes-ta′shən) pregnancy 妊娠; **gesta′-tional** *adj.*

ges·to·sis (jes-to′sis) pl. *gesto′ses.* Any manifestation of preeclampsia in pregnancy 妊娠中毒

GeV gigaelectron volt; one billion (10^9) electron volts 吉（咖）电子伏，千兆电子伏（10^9 电子伏）

GFAP glial fibrillary acidic protein 胶质细胞原纤维酸性蛋白

GFR glomerular filtration rate 肾小球滤过率

GGF geniculate ganglion fossa 膝状神经节窝

GH growth hormone 生长激素

ghost (gōst) a faint or shadowy figure lacking the customary substance of reality 影; **red cell g.**, an erythrocyte membrane that remains intact after hemolysis 红细胞影

ghrel·in (grel′in) a peptide hormone related to motilin, expressed primarily by the stomach, that stimulates the secretion of growth hormone, stimulates the sensation of hunger, and has regulatory functions

in the gastrointestinal, cardiovascular, and immune systems and in weight maintenance 食欲刺激（激）素，胃生长激素释放素

GH-RH growth hormone–releasing hormone 生长素释放激素

GHT Glaucoma Hemifield Test 青光眼半视野分析

GI gastrointestinal 胃肠的

gi·ant·ism (ji′ənt-iz-əm) 1. gigantism 巨人症; 2. excessive size, as of cells or nuclei 细胞或核的体积过大

Gi·ar·dia (je-ahr′de-ə) a genus of flagellate protozoa parasitic in the intestinal tract of humans and other animals, which may cause giardiasis; *G. intestina′lis* (formerly *G. lam′blia*) is the species found in humans 贾第鞭毛虫属

gi·ar·di·a·sis (je″ahr-di′ə-sis) infection of the small intestine with the protozoan *Giardia lamblia,* spread via contaminated food or water or by direct person-to-person contact; symptoms are rare and range from nonspecific gastrointestinal discomfort to mild to profuse diarrhea, nausea, lassitude, anorexia, and weight loss 贾第鞭毛虫病

gib·bos·i·ty (gĭ-bos′ĭ-te) the condition of being humped; kyphosis 驼背，脊柱隆突的状态

gib·bus (gib′əs) hump 驼背

GIFT gamete intrafallopian transfer 配子输卵管内移植

giga- word element [Gr.], *huge;* used in naming units of measurement to designate an amount one billion (10^9) times the size of the unit to which it is joined; symbol G [构词成分] 巨大；吉（咖）(10^9)，符号为 G

gi·gan·ti·form (ji-gan′tĭ-form) very large 巨大

gi·gan·tism (ji-gan′tiz-əm) (ji′gan-tiz-əm) abnormal overgrowth; excessive size and stature 巨人症；巨大畸形; **cerebral g.**, gigantism in the absence of increased levels of growth hormone, attributed to a cerebral defect; infants are large, and accelerated growth continues for the first 4 or 5 years, the rate being normal thereafter. The hands and feet are large, the head is large and dolichocephalic, and the eyes have an antimongoloid slant, with hypertelorism. The child is clumsy, and mental retardation of varying degree is usually present 脑性巨大畸形; **pituitary g.**, that caused by oversecretion of growth hormone by the pituitary gland 垂体性巨人症

gi·gan·to·cel·lu·lar (ji-gan″to-sel′u-lər) pertaining to giant cells 巨细胞的

gi·gan·to·mas·tia (ji-gan″to-mas′te-ə) extreme macromastia 乳房过度肥大

gin·ger (jin′jər) the leafy herb *Zingiber officinale,* or the dried rhizome, which is used as a flavoring agent, in the treatment of digestive disorders, and to prevent motion sickness 姜

gin·gi·va (jin′jĭ-və) (jin-ji′və) pl. *gin′givae* [L.] the gum; the mucous membrane, with supporting fibrous tissue, covering the tooth-bearing border of the jaw 牙龈; **gin′gival** *adj.*; **alveolar g.**, the portion covering the alveolar process 牙槽龈; **areolar g.**, the portion attached to the alveolar process by loose areolar connective tissue, lying beyond the keratinized mucosa over the alveolar process 蜂窝状龈; **attached g.**, the portion of the gingiva that is firm, resilient, and bound to the underlying cementum and alveolar bone 附着龈; **free g.**, the unattached portion of the gingiva, forming the wall of the gingival crevice 游离龈; **marginal g.**, the crest of the free gingiva that surrounds the teeth in a collarlike fashion, often separated from the adjacent attached gingiva by the free gingival groove; it forms the wall of the gingival sulcus 龈缘

gin·gi·val·ly (jin′jī-vəl″e) toward the gingiva 向龈

gin·gi·vec·to·my (jin″jĭ-vek′tə-me) surgical excision of all loose infected and diseased gingival tissue 牙龈切除术

gin·gi·vi·tis (jin″jĭ-vi′tis) inflammation of the gingiva 龈炎; **acute necrotizing ulcerative g.(ANUG)**, **acute ulcerative g.**, **acute ulceromembranous g.**, **necrotizing ulcerative g.** 急性坏死性溃疡性龈炎; **atrophic senile g.**, inflammation, and sometimes atrophy, of the gingival and oral mucosa in menopausal and postmenopausal women, believed due to altered estrogen metabolism 老年性萎缩性龈炎; **fusospirochetal g.**, necrotizing ulcerative g. 梭菌螺旋体性龈炎; **herpetic g.**, infection of the gingivae by the herpes simplex virus 疱疹性龈炎; **necrotizing ulcerative g.**, trench mouth; a progressive painful infection,also seen in subacute and recurrent forms, marked by crateriform lesions of interdental papillae with pseudomembranous slough circumscribed by linear erythema; fetid breath; increased salivation; and spontaneous gingival hemorrhage 坏死性溃疡性龈炎; 见 *gingivostomatitis* 下词条; **pregnancy g.**, any of various gingival changes ranging from gingivitis to the so-called pregnancy tumor 妊娠期龈炎; **Vincent g.**, necrotizing ulcerative g 奋森龈炎

gin·gi·vo·sis (jin″jĭ-vo′sis) a chronic, diffuse inflammation of the gingivae, with desquamation of the papillary epithelium and mucous membrane 龈变性

gin·gi·vo·sto·ma·ti·tis (jin″jĭ-vo-sto″mə-ti′tis) inflammation of the gingivae and oral mucosa 龈口炎; **herpetic g.**, that due to infection with herpes simplex virus, with redness of the oral tissues, for-

mation of multiple vesicles and painful ulcers, and fever 疱疹性龈口炎; **necrotizing ulcerative g.**, pseudomembranous angina; a type due to extension of necrotizing ulcerative gingivitis to other areas of the oral mucosa 坏死性溃疡性龈口炎

gin·gly·moid (jin′glə-moid) resembling a hinge; pertaining to a ginglymus 屈戌样的

gin·gly·mus (jin′glĭ-məs) a joint that allows movement in only one plane, forward and backward, as does a door hinge 屈戌关节

gink·go (ging′ko) the dried leaves of the deciduous tree *Ginkgo biloba*, used for symptomatic relief of brain dysfunction, for intermittent claudication, and for tinnitus and vertigo of vascular origin; also used in traditional Chinese medicine and in homeopathy 银杏

gin·seng (jin′seng) 1. any herb of the genus *Panax,* especially *P. ginseng* (Chinese g.) and *P. quinquefolius* (American g.) 人参; 2. the root of Chinese or American g., used as a tonic and stimulant 人参根或西洋参根用作滋补药和兴奋药; 3. Siberian g.; **eleuthero g.**, **Siberian g.**, the shrub *Eleutherococcus senticosus,* or a preparation of its root, which is used to improve general well-being and for various indications in traditional Chinese medicine 西伯利亚人参

gir·dle (gur′dəl) cingulum; an encircling structure or part; anything encircling a body 环带; **pectoral g.**, **shoulder g.**; **pelvic g.**, the encircling bony structure supporting the lower limbs 下肢带骨, 髋带骨; **shoulder g.**, **thoracic g.**, the encircling bony structure supporting the upper limbs 上肢带骨

gla·bel·la (glə-bel′ə) 1. the most prominent point in the median plane between the superciliary arches; also used for the smooth area encompassing this point 眉间点; 2. more broadly, the smooth area on the frontal bone between the superciliary arches 眉间

gla·brous (gla′brəs) smooth and bare 光滑的, 光秃的

GLAD glenolabral articular disruption 关节盂孟唇囊内撕裂

gla·di·o·lus (glə-di′o-ləs) body of sternum 胸骨体

glairy (glār′e) resembling egg white 卵白状的; 蛋白状的

gland (gland) an aggregation of cells specialized to secrete or excrete materials not related to their ordinary metabolic needs 腺（体）; **accessory g.**, a minor mass of glandular tissue near or at some distance from a gland of similar structure 副腺; **accessory adrenal g's**, adrenal glandular tissue, usually either cortical or medullary, found in the abdomen or pelvis 副肾上腺; **adrenal g.**, suprarenal gland; a flattened body above either kidney, consisting of a cortex and a medulla, the former elaborating steroid hormones and the latter epinephrine and norepinephrine 肾 上 腺；**apocrine g.,** one whose discharged secretion contains part of the secreting cells; particularly used to denote an apocrine sweat gland 顶质分泌腺；**apocrine sweat g.,** a type of large, branched, specialized sweat gland, after puberty producing a viscous secretion that is acted on by bacteria to produce a characteristic acrid odor 顶泌汗腺；**axillary g's,** lymph nodes situated in the axilla 腋 腺；**Bartholin g.,** greater vestibular g.,；**biliary g's, g's of biliary mucosa,** tubuloalveolar glands in the mucosa of the bile ducts and the neck of the gallbladder 胆黏膜腺；**Blandin g's,** anterior lingual g's. 舌 前 腺；**bronchial g's,** seromucous glands in the mucosa and submucosa of bronchial walls 支气管腺；**Bruch g's,** lymph follicles in the conjunctiva of the lower lid 布鲁赫腺；**Brunner g's,** duodenal g's 布伦纳腺；**bulbocavernous g., bulbourethral g.,** one of two glands embedded in the substance of the sphincter of the urethra, posterior to the membranous part of the urethra 尿道球腺；**cardiac g's,** mucin-secreting glands of the cardiac part (cardia) of the stomach 贲 门 腺 的；**celiac g's,** lymph nodes anterior to the abdominal aorta 腹腔淋巴 结；**ceruminous g's,** cerumen-secreting glands in the skin of the external auditory canal 耵聍腺；**cervical g's of uterus,** compound clefts in the wall of the uterine cervix 子宫颈腺；**ciliary g's,** sweat glands that have become arrested in their development, located at the edges of the eyelids 睫状腺；**circumanal g's,** specialized sweat and sebaceous glands around the anus 肛周腺；**closed g's,** endocrine g's；**coccygeal g.,** glomus coccygeum 尾骨腺；**compound g.,** a gland made up of a number of smaller units whose excretory ducts combine to form ducts of progressively higher order 复 腺；**Cowper g.,** bulbourethral g.；**ductless g.,** one without a duct, of internal secretion 无管腺；见 *endocrine g's.***duodenal g's,** glands in the submucosa of the duodenum, opening into the glands of the small intestine 十二指肠腺；**Ebner g's,** serous glands at the back of the tongue near the taste buds 味腺；**eccrine g., eccrine sweat g.,** one of the ordinary, or simple, sweat glands, which is of the merocrine type 外分泌腺；**endocrine g's,** organs whose secretions (hormones) are released directly into the circulatory system; they include the pituitary, thyroid, parathyroid, and suprarenal glands, the pineal body, and the gonads 内 分 泌 腺；**exocrine g.,** one whose secretion is discharged through a duct opening on an internal or external surface of the body 外分泌腺；**fundic g's, fundus g's,** tubular glands in the mucosa of the fundus and body of the stomach, containing acid- and pepsin-secreting cells 胃底腺；**Galeati g's,**

duodenal g's.；**gastric g's,** the secreting glands of the stomach, including the fundic, cardiac, and pyloric glands 胃腺；**Gay g's,** circumanal g's.；**glossopalatine g's,** mucous glands at the posterior end of the smaller sublingual glands 舌腭腺；**greater vestibular g.,** Bartholin gland: either of two small reddish yellow bodies in the vestibular bulbs, one on each side of the vaginal orifice 前庭大腺；**haversian g's,** synovial villi 哈弗斯腺，滑液腺；**holocrine g.,** one whose discharged secretion contains complete secreting cells 全质分泌腺；**intestinal g's,** straight tubular glands in the mucous membrane of the intestine, opening, in the small intestine, between the bases of the villi, and containing argentaffin cells 肠 腺；**jugular g.,** accessory lacrimal glands deep in the conjunctival connective tissue, mainly near the upper fornix 颈静脉淋巴结；**lacrimal g.,** either of a pair of glands that secrete tears 泪 腺；**lesser vestibular g's,** small mucous glands opening upon the vestibular mucous membrane between the urethral orifice and the vaginal orifice 前庭小腺；**g's of Lieberkühn,** intestinal g's；**lingual g's,** the seromucous glands on the surface of the tongue 舌 腺；**lingual g's, anterior,** the deeply placed seromucous glands near the apex of the tongue 浆液腺的；**Littre g's,** 1. preputial g's；2. urethral g's (male)；**lymph g.,** 淋巴腺，见 *node* 下 词 条；**mammary g.,** the specialized gland of the skin of female mammals, which secretes milk for nourishment of the young 乳 腺；**meibomian g's,** sebaceous follicles between the cartilage and conjunctiva of eyelids 迈 博 姆 腺；**merocrine g.,** a gland in which the secretory cells maintain their integrity throughout the secretory cycle 局浆分泌腺；**mixed g's,** 1. seromucous g's 混 合 腺；2. glands that have both exocrine and endocrine portions 同时具有外分泌和内分泌功能的腺体；**monoptychial g.,** one in which the tubules or alveoli are lined with a single layer of secreting cells 扁桃体腺；**Morgagni g's,** urethral g's (male)；**mucous g.,** a gland that secretes mucus 黏 液 腺；**Nuhn g's,** anterior lingual g's；**olfactory g's,** small mucous glands in the olfactory mucosa 嗅腺；**parathyroid g's,** small bodies in the region of the thyroid gland, developed from the endoderm of the branchial clefts, occurring in a variable number of pairs, commonly two; they secrete parathyroid hormone and are concerned chiefly with the metabolism of calcium and phosphorus 甲状旁腺；**paraurethral g's,** a group of urethral glands of the female urethra that are drained by the paraurethral ducts 尿道旁腺；**parotid g.,** the largest of the three paired salivary glands, located in front of the ear 腮 腺；**pharyngeal g's,** mucous glands beneath the tunica mucosa of the pharynx 咽腺；**pineal g.**, pineal body; a small conical structure attached by a stalk to the mastoid wall of the third ventricle; it secretes melatonin 松果体，松果腺；**pituitary g.**, hypophysis; the epithelial body of dual origin at the base of the brain in the sella turcica, attached by a stalk to the hypothalamus. It consists of two main lobes, the *anterior lobe*, secreting most of the hormones, and the *posterior lobe*, which stores and releases neurohormones received from the hypothalamus 垂体；**preputial g's**, small sebaceous glands of the corona of the penis and the inner surface of the prepuce, which secrete smegma 包皮腺；**proper gastric g's**, fundic g's; **prostate g.**, prostate 前列腺；**pyloric g's**, the mucin-secreting glands of the pyloric part of the stomach 幽门腺；**racemose g's**, glands composed of acini arranged like grapes on a stem 葡萄状腺；**saccular g.**, one consisting of one or more sacs lined with glandular epithelium 囊状腺；**salivary g's**, glands of the oral cavity whose combined secretion constitutes the saliva, including the parotid, sublingual, and submandibular glands and numerous small glands in the tongue, lips, cheeks, and palate 唾液腺；**sebaceous g.**, one of the holocrine glands in the dermis that secrete sebum 皮脂腺；**seromucous g.**, one containing both serous and mucous secreting cells 浆液黏液腺；**serous g.**, a gland that secretes a watery albuminous material, commonly but not always containing enzymes 浆液腺；**sex g.**, gonad 性腺；**simple g.**, a gland with a nonbranching duct 单腺；**Skene g's**, paraurethral g's; **submandibular g.**, submaxillary g., a salivary gland on the inner side of each ramus of the lower jaw 颌下腺；**suprarenal g.**, adrenal g.; **Suzanne g.**, a mucous gland of the mouth, beneath the alveolingual groove Suzanne 腺，口腔黏膜腺；**sweat g.**, a gland that secretes sweat, found in the dermis or superficial fascia, opening by a duct on the body surface. The ordinary or *eccrine* sweat glands are distributed over most of the body surface and promote cooling by evaporation of the secretion; the *apocrine* sweat glands empty into the upper portion of a hair follicle instead of directly onto the skin and are found only in certain body areas, as around the anus and in the axilla 汗腺；**target g.**, one specifically affected by a pituitary hormone 靶腺；**tarsal g's**, tarsoconjunctival g's, meibomian g's. 睑板腺；**thymus g.**, 胸腺，见 *thymus*；**thyroid g.**, an endocrine gland consisting of two lobes, one on each side of the trachea, joined by a narrow isthmus, producing hormones (thyroxine and triiodothyronine), which require iodine for their elaboration and which are concerned in regulating the metabolic rate; it also secretes calcitonin 甲状腺；**Tyson g's**, preputial g's; **unicellular g.**, a single cell that functions as a gland, e.g., a goblet cell 单细胞腺；**urethral g's**, mucous glands in the wall of the urethra 尿道腺；**uterine g's**, simple tubular glands found throughout the endometrium 子宫腺；**vesical g's**, mucous glands sometimes found in the wall of the urinary bladder, especially in the area of the trigone 膀胱腺；**Virchow g.**, sentinel node 前哨淋巴结；**vulvovaginal g.**, Bartholin g. 外阴阴道腺；**Waldeyer g's**, glands in the attached edge of the eyelid Waldeyer 腺；**Weber g's**, the tubular mucous glands of the tongue Weber 腺；**g's of Zeis**, modified rudimentary sebaceous glands attached directly to the eyelash follicles 睑缘腺

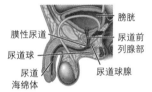

▲ 尿道球腺

glan·ders (glan′dərz) a contagious disease of horses, communicable to humans, due to *Pseudomonas mallei*, and marked by purulent inflammation of the mucous membranes and cutaneous eruption of nodules that coalesce and break down, forming deep ulcers, which may end in necrosis of cartilage and bone; the more chronic and constitutional form is known as *farcy* 鼻疽

glan·di·lem·ma (glan″dĭ-lem′ə) the capsule or outer envelope of a gland 腺被囊

glan·du·la (glan′du-lə) pl. *glan′dulae* [L.] a gland 腺

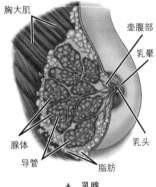

▲ 乳腺

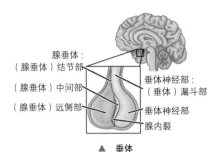

▲ 垂体

腺垂体：
（腺垂体）结节部
（腺垂体）中间部
（腺垂体）远侧部

垂体神经部：
（垂体）漏斗部
垂体神经部
腺内裂

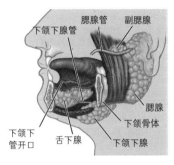

▲ 唾液腺

腮腺管　副腮腺
下颌下腺管
腮腺
下颌骨体
下颌下
管开口　舌下腺　下颌下腺

glan·du·lar (glan′du-lər) 1. pertaining to or of the nature of a gland 腺的，腺性的；2. glanular 阴茎头的，阴蒂头的

glans (glanz) pl. *glan′des* [L.] a small, rounded mass or glandlike body 小圆体或腺状体；**g. clito′ridis, g. of clitoris,** erectile tissue on the free end of the clitoris 阴蒂头；**g. pe′nis,** the cap-shaped expansion of the corpus spongiosum at the end of the penis 阴茎头

glan·u·lar (glan′u-lər) pertaining to the glans penis or glans clitoridis 阴茎头的，阴蒂头的

glan·u·lo·plas·ty (glan′u-lo-plas″te) plastic surgery on a glans 阴茎头成形术

glare (glār) discomfort in the eye and depression of central vision produced when a bright light enters the field of vision, particularly when the eye is adapted to dark. It is *direct g.* when the image of the light falls on the fovea and *indirect g.* when it falls outside the fovea 眩光

glass (glas) 1. a hard, brittle, often transparent material, usually consisting of the fused amorphous silicates of potassium or sodium, and of calcium, with silica in excess 玻璃；2. a container, usually cylindrical, made from glass 玻璃杯；**cupping g.,** a small vessel from which the air has been or can be exhausted; used in cupping 拔罐

glass·es (glas′əz) spectacles; lenses arranged in a frame holding them in the proper position before the eyes, as an aid to vision 眼镜；**bifocal g.,** those with bifocal lenses 双焦眼镜；**trifocal g.,** those with trifocal lenses 三焦点眼镜

gla·tir·a·mer (glə-tir′ə-mər) an immunomodulator used as the acetate ester to reduce relapses in multiple sclerosis 一种免疫调节药，其醋酸酯用于减少多发性硬化症的病发

glau·co·ma (glaw-) (glou-ko′mə) a group of eye diseases characterized by an increase in intraocular pressure, causing pathologic changes in the optic disk and typical visual field defects 青光眼；**glauco′matous** *adj*；**angle-closure g.,** glaucoma in which obstruction to outflow of aqueous humor is caused by closure of the anterior angle due to contact between the iris and the inner surface of the trabecular meshwork 闭角型青光眼；**congenital g.,** that due to defective development of the structures in and around the anterior chamber of the eye and resulting in impairment of aqueous humor; seen first at birth or up to age 3 years 先天性青光眼；**infantile g.,** congenital g. 婴幼儿型青光眼；**narrow-angle g.,** angle-closure g. 狭角性青光眼；**open-angle g.,** glaucoma in which the angle of the anterior chamber remains open but filtration is gradually diminished because of the tissues of the angle 开角型青光眼；**primary g.,** increased intraocular pressure occurring in an eye without previous disease 原发性青光眼；**pseudoexfoliation g.,** characterized by flakes of granular material at the pupillary margin of the iris and throughout the inner surface of the anterior chamber 假性剥脱性青光眼

glaze (glāz) in dentistry, a ceramic veneer added to a porcelain restoration, to simulate enamel 釉料

GLC gas-liquid chromatography 气液层析，气液色谱法

gle·no·hu·mer·al (gle″no-hu′mər-əl) pertaining to the glenoid fossa and the humerus 盂肱的

gle·noid (gle′noid) (glen′oid) resembling a pit or socket 关节盂的

glia (gli′ə) neuroglia 神经胶质

glia·cyte (gli′ə-sīt) a cell of the neuroglia 神经胶质细胞

gli·a·din (gli′ə-din) a protein present in wheat; it contains the toxic factor associated with celiac disease 麦溶蛋白

gli·al (gli′əl) of or pertaining to the neuroglia 神经胶质的

gli·mep·i·ride (gli-mep′ĭ-rīd) a sulfonylurea compound used as a hypoglycemic in the treatment of type 2 diabetes mellitus 一种磺脲类降血糖药，用于治疗2型糖尿病

glio·blas·to·ma (gli″o-blas-to′mə) the most malignant type of astrocytoma, composed of spongioblasts, astroblasts, and astrocytes; it usually occurs in the brain but may occur in the brainstem or spinal cord 胶质母细胞瘤。又称 glioblastoma multiforme

gli·o·ma (gli-o′mə) a tumor composed of neuroglia in any of its states of development; sometimes extended to include all intrinsic neoplasms of the brain and spinal cord, such as astrocytomas, ependymomas, etc.（神经）胶质瘤; **glio′matous** *adj.*; **g. re′tinae,** retinoblastoma 视网膜母细胞瘤

gli·o·ma·to·sis (gli″o-mə-to′sis) diffuse formation of gliomas 神经胶质瘤病

gli·o·sis (gli-o′sis) an excess of astroglia in damaged areas of the central nervous system 神经胶质增生

glip·i·zide (glip′ĭ-zīd) a sulfonylurea used as a hypoglycemic in the treatment of type 2 diabetes mellitus 一种用于治疗 2 型糖尿病的降血糖药

glis·sade (glĭ-sād′) [Fr.] a gliding involuntary movement of the eye in changing the point of fixation; it is a slower, smoother movement than is a saccade（眼）滑动; **glissad′ic** *adj.*

glis·so·ni·tis (glis″o-ni′tis) inflammation of the Glisson capsule 肝纤维囊炎

glo·bi (glo′bi) plural of *globus* 麻风球

glo·bin (glo′bin) 1. the protein constituent of hemoglobin 珠蛋白; 2. any of a group of proteins similar to the typical globin 任何一种类似典型珠蛋白的蛋白

glo·boid (glo′boid) spheroid 球状的

glo·o·side (glob′o-sīd) a glycosphingolipid containing acetylated amino sugars and simple hexoses that accumulates in tissues in Sandhoff disease but not in Tay-Sachs disease 红细胞糖苷脂

glob·ule (glob′ūl) 1. a small spherical mass or body 小球; 2. a small spherical drop of fluid or semifluid substance 小体; 3. a little globe or pellet, as of medicine 球剂; **glob′ular** *adj.*

glob·u·lin (glob′u-lin) any of a class of proteins, most of which are insoluble in water but soluble in saline solutions (euglobulins), but some of which are water-soluble (pseudoglobulins) with their other physical properties resembling those of the euglobulins 球蛋白; **α-g′s,** serum globulins with the most rapid electrophoretic mobility, further subdivided into faster α1- and slower α2-globulins 甲种球蛋白; **AC g., accelerator g.,** coagulation factor Ⅴ 促凝血球蛋白, 凝血因子Ⅴ; **alpha g′s, α-g′s; antihemophilic g. (AHG),** coagulation factor Ⅷ 抗血友病球蛋白, 凝血因子Ⅷ; **antilymphocyte g. (ALG),** the γ-globulin fraction of antilymphocyte serum (q.v.), used as an immunosuppressant

in organ transplantation 抗淋巴细胞球蛋白; **antithymocyte g. (ATG),** the γ-globulin fraction of antiserum derived from animals (e.g., rabbits) that have been immunized against human thymocytes; it causes specific destruction of T lymphocytes, used in treatment of allograft rejection 抗胸腺细胞球蛋白; **β-g′s,** globulins in plasma that, in neutral or alkaline solutions, have an electrophoretic mobility between those of the α- and γ-globulins β- 球蛋白; **bacterial polysaccharide immune g. (BPIG),** a human immune globulin derived from the blood plasma of adult human donors immunized with *Haemophilus influenzae* type b, pneumococcal, and meningococcal polysaccharide vaccines; used for the passive immunization of infants under 18 months of age 细菌多糖免疫球蛋白; **beta g′s, β-g′s; cytomegalovirus immune g.,** a purified immunoglobulin derived from pooled adult human plasma selected for high titers of antibody against cytomegalovirus; used for the treatment and prophylaxis of cytomegalovirus disease in transplant recipients 巨细胞病毒免疫球蛋白; **γ-g′s, gamma g′s,** γ -serum globulins having the least rapid electrophoretic mobility; the fraction is composed almost entirely of immunoglobulins 丙种球蛋白; **hepatitis B immune g.,** a specific immune globulin derived from blood plasma of human donors with high titers of antibodies against hepatitis B surface antigen; used as a passive immunizing agent 乙型肝炎免疫球蛋白; **hyperimmune g.,** any of various immunoglobulin preparations especially high in antibodies against certain specific diseases 超免疫球蛋白; **immune g.,** 1. immunoglobulin 免疫球蛋白; 2. a concentrated preparation of γ -globulins, predominantly IgG, from a large pool of human donors; used for passive immunization against measles, hepatitis A, and varicella and for replacement therapy in patients with immunoglobulin deficiencies 人免疫血清球蛋白; **immune human serum g.,** immune g. (2); **immune g. intravenous (human),** a preparation of immune globulin suitable for intravenous administration; used in the treatment of primary and secondary immunodeficiency states, idiopathic thrombocytopenic purpura, and Kawasaki disease 免疫球蛋白静脉注射; **immune serum g.,** immune g. (2); **pertussis immune g.,** a specific immune globulin derived from the blood plasma of human donors immunized with pertussis vaccine; used for the prophylaxis and treatment of pertussis 百日咳免疫球蛋白; **rabies immune g.,** a specific immune globulin derived from blood plasma or serum of human donors who have been immunized with rabies vaccine and have high titers of rabies antibody;

used as a passive immunizing agent 狂犬病免疫球蛋白；**respiratory syncytial virus immune g.**

intravenous, a preparation of IgG from pooled adult human plasma selected for high titers of antibodies against respiratory syncytial virus; used for passive immunization of infants and young children 呼吸道合胞病毒免疫球蛋白静脉注射；**Rh₀(D) immune g.,** a specific immune globulin derived from human blood plasma containing antibody to the erythrocyte factor Rh₀(D); used to prevent Rh-sensitization of Rh-negative females and thus prevent erythroblastosis fetalis in subsequent pregnancies; administered within 72 hours after exposure to Rh-positive blood resulting from delivery of an Rh-positive child, abortion or miscarriage of an Rh-positive fetus, or transfusion of Rh-positive blood; also used to stimulate the platelet count in idiopathic thrombocytopenic purpura Rh₀ (D) 免疫球蛋白；**serum g's,** all plasma proteins except albumin, which is not a globulin, and fibrinogen, which is not in the serum; they are subdivided into α-, β-, and γ-globulins 血清球蛋白；**sex hormone–binding g. (SHBG),** a β-globulin in plasma that binds to and transports testosterone and, to a lesser degree, estrogens 性激素结合球蛋白；**specific immune g.,** a preparation of immune globulin derived from a donor pool preselected for a high antibody titer against a specific antigen 特异性免疫球蛋白；**tetanus immune g.,** a specific immune globulin derived from the blood plasma of human donors who have been immunized with tetanus toxoid; used in the prophylaxis and treatment of tetanus 破伤风免疫球蛋白；**varicella-zoster immune g. (VZIG),** a specific immune globulin derived from plasma of human donors with high titers of varicellazoster antibodies; used as a passive immunizing agent 水痘-带状疱疹免疫球蛋白

glo·bus (glo′bəs) pl. *glo′bi* [L.] 1. a sphere or spherical structure 球；2. eyeball 球状感；3. one of the encapsulated globular masses containing bacilli, seen in smears of lepromatous leprosy lesions 麻风球，**g. hyste′ricus,** globus pharyngeus resulting from a conversion disorder 癔球症；**g. pal′lidus,** the smaller and more medial part of the lentiform nucleus 苍白球；**g. pharyn′geus,** sensation of a lump in the throat when none is there; it may be psychogenic *(g. hystericus)* or due to some disorder of the esophagus or nearby cervical structures 咽部异感症

glo·man·gi·o·ma (glo-man″je-o′mə) glomus tumor (1) 血管球瘤

glom·era (glom′ər-ə) plural of *glomus* 球

glo·mer·u·lar (glo-mer′u-lər) pertaining to or of the nature of a glomerulus, especially a renal

glomerulus 肾小球的

glo·mer·u·lo·ne·phri·tis (glo-mer″u-lo-nə-fri′tis) nephritis with inflammation of the capillary loops in the renal glomeruli 肾小球肾炎；**acute g.,** an acute form characterized by proteinuria, edema, hematuria, renal failure, and hypertension, sometimes preceded by tonsillitis or febrile pharyngitis 急性肾小球肾炎；**chronic g.,** a slowly progressive glomerulonephritis generally leading to irreversible renal failure 慢性肾小球肾炎；**diffuse g.,** a severe form with proliferative changes in more than half the glomeruli, often with epithelial crescent formation and necrosis; often seen in advanced systemic lupus erythematosus 弥漫性肾小球肾炎；**IgA g.,** IgA nephropathy; a chronic form marked by hematuria and proteinuria and by deposits of IgA in the mesangial areas of the renal glomeruli, with subsequent reactive hyperplasia of mesangial cells IgA 肾小球肾炎；**lobular g., membranoproliferative g.,** a chronic, slowly progressive glomerulonephritis in which the glomeruli are enlarged as a result of proliferation of mesangial cells and irregular thickening of the capillary walls, which narrows the capillary lumina 小叶性肾小球肾炎，膜增殖性肾小球肾炎；**membranous g.,** a form characterized histologically by proteinaceous deposits on the glomerular capillary basement membrane or by thickening of the membrane; clinically resembling chronic glomerulonephritis, occasionally with transient nephrotic syndrome 膜性肾小球肾炎；**mesangiocapillary g.,** membranoproliferative g. 系膜毛细血管性肾小球肾炎

glo·mer·u·lop·a·thy (glo-mer″u-lop′ə-the) any disease of the renal glomeruli 肾小球病；**diabetic g.,** intercapillary glomerulosclerosis 糖尿病性肾小球病

glo·mer·u·lo·scle·ro·sis (glo-mer″u-losklə-ro′sis) fibrosis and scarring resulting in senescence of the renal glomeruli 肾小球硬化症；**diabetic g.,** intercapillary g. 糖尿病肾小球硬化症；**focal segmental g.,** a syndrome of focal sclerosing lesions of the renal glomeruli with proteinuria, hematuria, hypertension, and nephrosis, with variable progression to end-stage renal disease 局灶性节段性肾小球硬化症；**intercapillary g.,** a degenerative complication of diabetes, manifested as albuminuria, nephrotic edema, hypertension, renal insufficiency, and retinopathy 毛细血管间肾小球硬化症

glo·mer·u·lus (glo-mer′u-ləs) pl. *glomer′uli* [L.] a small tuft or cluster, as of blood vessels or nerve fibers; often used alone to designate one of the renal glomeruli 神经纤维球，血管小球，肾小球；**olfactory g.,** one of the small globular masses of dense neuropil in the olfactory bulb, containing the first synapse in the olfactory pathway 嗅小球; **renal g.**, globular tufts of capillaries, one projecting into the expanded end or capsule of each of the uriniferous tubules, which together with the glomerular capsule constitute the renal corpuscle 肾小球

glo·mus (glo′məs) pl. **glom′era** [L.] 血管球 1. a small histologically recognizable body composed of fine arterioles connecting directly with veins and having a rich nerve supply; 2. glomus body; **glo′mera aor′tica**, aortic bodies 主动脉小球; **g. caro′ticum**, carotid bodies 颈动脉小球; **choroid g.**, **g. choroi′deum**, an enlargement of the choroid plexus of the lateral ventricle 脉络球; **coccygeal g.**, **g. coccy′geum**, a collection of arteriovenous anastomoses near the tip of the coccyx, formed by the middle sacral artery 尾骨球; **jugular g.**, **g. jugula′re**, jugular (tympanic) body 颈静脉球

glos·sal (glos′əl) lingual 舌的

glos·sec·to·my (glos-ek′tə-me) excision of all or a portion of the tongue 舌截除术

Glos·si·na (glŏ-si′nə) the tsetse flies, a genus of African biting flies that are vectors of trypanosomiasis in humans and other animals 舌蝇

glos·si·tis (glos-i′tis) inflammation of the tongue 舌炎; **g. area′ta exfoliati′va, benign migratory g.**, an inflammatory disease of the tongue characterized by multiple annular areas of desquamation of the filiform papillae, presenting as reddish lesions outlined in yellow that shift from area to area every few days 地图样舌; **median rhomboid g.**, a congenital anomaly of the tongue, with a reddish patch or plaque on the midline of the dorsal surface 正中菱形舌炎

glos·so·cele (glos′o-sēl) swelling and protrusion of the tongue 巨舌

glos·so·graph (glos′o-graf) an apparatus for registering tongue movements in speech 舌动描记器

glos·so·la·lia (glos′′o-la′le-ə) gibberish that simulates coherent speech 荒诞言语

glos·sol·o·gy (glos-ol′ə-je) the sum of knowledge regarding the tongue 舌学

glos·so·pal·a·tine (glos′′o-pal′ə-tīn) palatoglossal 舌腭的

glos·so·pha·ryn·ge·al (glos′′o-fə-rin′je-əl) pertaining to the tongue and pharynx 舌咽的

glos·so·plas·ty (glos′o-plas′′te) plastic surgery of the tongue 舌成形术

glos·sor·rha·phy (glos-or′ə-fe) suture of the tongue 舌缝合术

glos·so·trich·ia (glos′′o-trik′e-ə) hairy tongue 毛舌术

glot·tis (glot′is) pl. **glot′tides** [Gr.] the vocal appa-ratus of the larynx, consisting of the true vocal cords and the opening between them 声门; **glot′tal, glot′tic** adj.

glot·tog·ra·phy (glŏ-tog′rə-fe) the recording of the movements of the vocal cords during respiration and phonation 声门描记（法）

GLP glucagon-like peptide 胰高血糖素样肽

Glu glutamic acid 谷氨酸

glu·ca·gon (gloo′kə-gon) a polypeptide hormone secreted by the alpha cells of the islets of Langerhans in response to hypoglycemia or to stimulation by growth hormone, which stimulates glycogenolysis in the liver; used as the hydrochloride salt as an antihypoglycemic and as an adjunct in gastrointestinal radiography 胰高血糖素

glu·ca·gon·o·ma (gloo′′kə-gon-o′mə) an islet cell tumor of the alpha cells that secretes glucagon 胰高血糖素瘤

glu·can (gloo′kan) any polysaccharide composed only of recurring units of glucose; a homopolymer of glucose 葡聚糖

glu·car·pi·dase (gloo-kahr′pĭ-dās) a carboxypeptidase that hydrolyzes folic acid and methotrexate and other folic acid antagonists; used for elimination of methotrexate in patients with delayed clearance due to renal dysfunction 羧肽酶

glu·cep·tate (gloo-sep′tāt) USAN contraction for glucoheptonate, a 7-carbon carbohydrate derivative 葡庚糖酸盐

glu·ci·tol (gloo′sĭ-tol) sorbitol 葡糖醇，山梨醇

glu·co·cer·e·bro·si·dase (gloo′′ko-sə-re′′brosi′dās) glucosylceramidase 葡糖脑苷脂酶

glu·co·cer·e·bro·side (gloo′′ko-sə-re′brosīd′′) a cerebroside with a glucose sugar 葡糖脑苷脂

glu·co·cor·ti·coid (gloo′′ko-kor′tĭ-koid) 1. any of the group of corticosteroids predominantly involved in carbohydrate metabolism and also in fat and protein metabolism and many other activities (e.g., alteration of connective tissue response to injury and inhibition of inflammatory and allergic reactions); some also exhibit varying degrees of mineralocorticoid activity. In humans, the most important glucocorticoids are cortisol (hydrocortisone) and cortisone 肾上腺皮质激素; 2. of, pertaining to, or resembling a glucocorticoid 糖皮质激素的

glu·co·fu·ra·nose (gloo′′ko-fu′rə-nōs) glucose in the cyclic furanose configuration, a minor constituent of glucose solutions 呋喃葡萄糖

glu·co·ki·nase (gloo′′ko-ki′nās) 1. an enzyme of invertebrates and microorganisms that catalyzes the phosphorylation of glucose to glucose 6-phosphate 葡萄糖激酶; 2. the liver isozyme of hexokinase 肝己糖激酶同工酶

glu·co·ki·net·ic (gloo″ko-kǐ-net′ik) activating sugar so as to maintain the sugar level of the body 激动糖质的

glu·co·nate (gloo′ko-nāt) a salt, ester, or anionic form of gluconic acid 葡糖酸盐

glu·co·neo·gen·e·sis (gloo″ko-ne″o-jen′ə-sis) the synthesis of glucose from molecules that are not carbohydrates, such as amino and fatty acids 糖异生

glu·con·ic ac·id (gloo-kon′ik) the hexonic acid derived from glucose by oxidation of the C-1 aldehyde to a carboxyl group 葡糖酸

glu·co·phore (gloo′ko-for) the group of atoms in a molecule that gives the compound a sweet taste 生甜味基

glu·co·py·ra·nose (gloo″ko-pir′ə-nōs) glucose in the cyclic pyranose configuration, the predominant form 吡喃葡萄糖

glu·co·reg·u·la·tion (gloo″ko-reg′u-la′shən) regulation of glucose metabolism 糖代谢调节

glu·co·sa·mine (gloo-kōs′ə-mēn) an amino derivative of glucose, occurring in glycosaminoglycans and a variety of complex polysaccharides such as blood group substances. The sulfate salt is used as a nutritional supplement and as a popular remedy for osteoarthritis 氨基葡糖，葡糖胺

glu·co·san (gloo′ko-san) glucan 葡聚糖

glu·cose (gloo′kōs) 1. a 6-carbon aldose occurring as the d- form and found as a free monosaccharide in fruits and other plants or combined in glucosides and di-, oligo-, and polysaccharides. It is the end product of carbohydrate metabolism and is the chief source of energy for living organisms, its utilization being controlled by insulin. Excess glucose is converted to glycogen and stored in the liver and muscles for use as needed and, beyond that, is converted to fat and stored as adipose tissue. Glucose appears in the urine in diabetes mellitus. In pharmaceuticals, called *dextrose* 葡萄糖; 2. liquid g. liquid g., a thick, sweet, syrupy liquid obtained by incomplete hydrolysis of starch and consisting chiefly of dextrose, with dextrins, maltose, and water; used as a pharmaceutical aid 液状葡萄糖; g. 1-phosphate, an intermediate in carbohydrate metabolism 葡糖1-磷酸; g. 6-phosphate, an intermediate in carbohydrate metabolism 葡糖 6-磷酸

glu·cose me·ter (gloo′kōs me-tur) a device used to measure and display the amount of glucose in the blood 血糖仪

glu·cose-6-phos·pha·tase (gloo″kōs fos′fə- tās″) an enzyme that catalyzes the hydrolytic dephosphorylation of glucose 6-phosphate, the principal route for hepatic gluconeogenesis; deficiency causes glycogen storage disease, type Ⅰ 葡糖 6-磷酸酶

glu·cose-6-phos·phate de·hy·dro·gen·ase (G6PD) (gloo″kōs fos′fāt de-hi′dro-jən-ās) an enzyme of the pentose phosphate pathway that, with NADP+ as coenzyme, catalyzes the oxidation of glucose 6-phosphate to a lactone. Deficiency of the enzyme causes severe hemolytic anemia 葡糖 -6- 磷酸脱氢酶

glu·co·si·dase (gloo-ko′sǐ-dās) any of a group of enzymes of the hydrolase class that hydrolyze glucose residues from glucosides; they are specific for α - or β - configurations as well as for particular substrate configurations, e.g., maltase 葡 (萄) 糖苷酶

glu·co·side (gloo′ko-sīd) a glycoside in which the sugar constituent is glucose 葡 (萄) 糖苷

glu·co·syl·cer·am·i·dase (gloo″ko-səl-sə- ram′ǐ-dās) an enzyme that catalyzes the hydrolytic cleavage of glucose from glucocerebrosides to form ceramides in the lysosomal degradation of sphingolipids. Deficiency of enzyme activity, an autosomal recessive trait, results in Gaucher disease 葡糖脑苷脂酶

glu·cu·ron·ic ac·id (gloo″ku-ron′ik) the uronic acid derived from glucose; it is a constituent of several glycosaminoglycans and also forms conjugates (glucuronides) with drugs and toxins in their biotransformation 葡糖醛酸

β-glu·cu·ron·i·dase (gloo″ku-ron′ǐ-dās) an enzyme that attacks terminal glycosidic linkages in natural and synthetic glucuronides and that has been implicated in estrogen metabolism and cell division; it occurs in the spleen, liver, and endocrine glands; deficiency results in Sly syndrome β 葡糖醛酸糖苷酶

glu·cu·ron·ide (gloo″ku-ron′ǐd) any glycosidic compound of glucuronic acid; they are common soluble conjugates formed as a step in the metabolism and excretion of many toxins and drugs, such as phenols and alcohols 葡 (萄) 糖苷酸

glu·cu·ron·o·syl·trans·fer·ase (gloo″kuron′o-səl-trans′fər-ās) an enzyme that catalyzes a step in the conversion of bilirubin to its more soluble glucuronide conjugates, which are then secreted into the bile 葡糖醛酸基转移酶

glu·ta·mate (gloo′tə-māt) a salt of glutamic acid; in biochemistry, the term is often used interchangeably with glutamic acid 谷氨酸盐

glu·ta·mate for·mim·i·no·trans·fer·ase (gloo′tə-māt for-mim″ǐ-no-trans′fər-ās) a transferase catalyzing a step in the degradation of histidine; decreased enzyme activity has been associated with urinary excretion of formiminoglutamate and intellectual disability 谷氨酸亚胺甲基转移酶

glu·tam·ic ac·id (Glu, E) (gloo-tam′ik) a dibasic, nonessential amino acid widely distributed in proteins, a neurotransmitter that inhibits neural excitation in the central nervous system; its hydrochloride salt is used as a gastric acidifier 谷氨基酸, 氨基戊二酸

glu·tam·i·nase (gloo-tam′ĭ-nās) an enzyme that catalyzes the deamination of glutamine to form glutamate and an ammonium ion; most of the latter are converted to urea via the urea cycle 谷氨酰胺酶

glu·ta·mine (Gln, Q) (gloo′tə-mēn) the monoamide of glutamic acid, a nonessential amino acid occurring in proteins; it is an important carrier of urinary ammonia and is broken down in the kidney by the enzyme glutaminase 谷氨酰胺

glu·ta·ral (gloo′tə-rəl) glutaraldehyde 戊二醛

glu·ta·ral·de·hyde (gloo″tə-ral′də-hīd) a disinfectant used in aqueous solution for sterilization of non–heat-resistant equipment; also used as a tissue fixative for light and electron microscopy 戊二醛

glu·tar·ic ac·id (gloo-tar′ik) a dicarboxylic acid intermediate in the metabolism of tryptophan and lysine 戊二酸

glu·tar·ic·ac·i·de·mia (gloo-tar″ik-as″ĭ-de′me-ə) 1. glutaricaciduria (1) 戊二酸尿症; 2. an excess of glutaric acid in the blood 戊二酸血症

glu·tar·ic·ac·id·uria (gloo-tar″ik-as″ĭ-du′re-ə) 1. an aminoacidopathy characterized by accumulation and excretion of glutaric acid; there are three types (Ⅰ, Ⅱ, and Ⅲ) due to different enzyme deficiencies, with spectra of manifestations 戊二酸尿症; 2. excretion of glutaric acid in the urine 尿中戊二酸排泄

glu·ta·thi·one (gloo″tə-thi′ōn) a tripeptide of glutamic acid, cysteine, and glycine, existing in reduced (GSH) and oxidized (GSSG) forms and functioning in various redox reactions: in the destruction of peroxides and free radicals, as a cofactor for enzymes, and in the detoxification of harmful compounds. It is also involved in the formation and maintenance of disulfide bonds in proteins and in transport of amino acids across cell membranes 谷胱甘肽

glu·ta·thi·one syn·the·tase (gloo″tə-thi′ōn sin′thə-tās) a ligase catalyzing the formation of glutathione; autosomal recessive defects in activity cause decreased levels of glutathione and increased levels of 5-oxoproline and cysteine. If confined to erythrocytes, deficiency results in well-compensated hemolytic anemia; if generalized, metabolic acidosis and neurologic dysfunction may also occur 谷胱甘肽合成酶

glu·te·al (gloo′te-əl) pertaining to the buttocks 臀的

gluten (gloo′tən) the protein of wheat and other grains that gives to the dough its tough, elastic character 谷蛋白

glu·ti·nous (gloo′tĭ-nəs) adhesive; sticky 黏性的

Gly glycine 甘氨酸

gly·bur·ide (gli′būr-īd) a sulfonylurea used as a hypoglycemic in the treatment of type 2 diabetes mellitus 格列本脲

gly·can (gli′kan) polysaccharide 聚糖

gly·ce·mia (gli-se′me-ə) the presence of glucose in the blood 血糖

glyc·er·al·de·hyde (glis″ər-al′də-hīd) an aldose, the aldehyde form of the 3-carbon sugar derived from the oxidation of glycerol; isomeric with dihydroxyacetone. The 3-phosphate derivative is an intermediate in the metabolism of glucose, in both the Embden-Meyerhof and pentose phosphate pathways 甘油醛

gly·cer·ic ac·id (gli-sēr′ik) $CH_2OHCHOH-COOH$, an intermediate product in the transformation in the body of carbohydrate to lactic acid, formed by oxidation of glycerol 甘油酸

glyc·er·ide (glis′ər-īd) acylglycerol; an organic acid ester of glycerol, designated, according to the number of ester linkages, as mono-, di-, or triglyceride 甘油酯

glyc·er·in (glis′ər-in) a clear, colorless, syrupy liquid used as a laxative, an osmotic diuretic to reduce intraocular pressure, a demulcent in cough preparations, and a humectant and solvent for drugs 甘油。 Cf. *glycerol*.

glyc·er·ol (glis′ər-ol) a trihydroxy sugar alcohol that is the backbone of many lipids and an important intermediate in carbohydrate and lipid metabolism. Pharmaceutical preparations are called *glycerin* 甘油

glyc·er·ol·ize (glis′ər-ol-īz″) to treat with or preserve in glycerol, as in the exposure of red blood cells to glycerol solution so that glycerol diffuses into the cells before they are frozen for preservation 甘油化

glyc·er·yl (glis′ər-əl) the mono-, di-, or trivalent radical formed by the removal of hydrogen from one, two, or three of the hydroxy groups of glycerol 甘油基; **g. monostearate,** an emulsifying agent 单硬脂酸甘油酯; **g. trinitrate,** nitroglycerin 三硝酸甘油酯

gly·cine (Gly, G) (gli′sēn) a nonessential amino acid occurring as a constituent of proteins and functioning as an inhibitory neurotransmitter in the central nervous system; used as a gastric antacid and dietary supplement and as a bladder irrigation in transurethral prostatectomy 甘氨酸

gly·co·cal·yx (gli″ko-kal′iks) the glycoprotein-polysaccharide covering that surrounds many cells 糖被

gly·co·cho·late (gli″ko-ko′lāt) a salt of glycocholic acid 甘氨胆酸盐

gly·co·cho·lic ac·id (gli″ko-ko′lik) cholylglycine 甘氨胆酸

gly·co·con·ju·gate (gli″ko-kon′jə-gət) any of the complex molecules containing glycosidic linkages, such as glycolipids, glycopeptides, oligosaccharides, or glycosaminoglycans 糖结合物

gly·co·gen (gli′ko-jən) a highly branched polysaccharide of glucose chains, the chief carbohydrate storage material in animals, stored primarily in liver and muscle; it is synthesized and degraded for energy as demanded 糖原；**glycogen′ic** adj.

gly·co·gen·e·sis (gli″ko-jen′ə-sis) the conversion of glucose to glycogen for storage in the liver 糖生成的；**glycogenet′ic** adj.

gly·co·ge·nol·y·sis (gli″ko-jə-nol′ə-sis) the splitting up of glycogen in the liver, yielding glucose 糖原分解；**glycogenolyt′ic** adj.

gly·co·ge·no·sis (gli″ko-jə-no′sis) glycogen storage disease 糖原病，糖原贮积病

gly·co·gen phos·phor·y·lase (gli′ko-jən fosfor′ə-lās) 糖原磷酸化酶，见 phosphorylase

gly·co·gen syn·thase (gli′ko-jən sin′thās) an enzyme that catalyzes the synthesis of glycogen; the reaction is highly regulated by allosteric effectors, by kinases and phosphatases, and by insulin. Deficiency of the enzyme causes glycogen storage disease, type 0 (q.v.) 糖原合成酶

gly·co·geu·sia (gli″ko-goo′zhə) a sweet taste in the mouth 甘味症，甘幻味

gly·col (gli′kol) any of a group of aliphatic dihydric alcohols, with marked hygroscopic properties and useful as solvents and plasticizers 乙 二 醇；polyethylene g., 聚乙二醇，见 polyethylene 下词条

gly·col·ic ac·id (gli-kol′ik) an intermediate in the conversion of serine to glycine; it is accumulated and excreted in primary hyperoxaluria (type Ⅰ) 乙醇酸，羟基乙酸

gly·co·lip·id (gli″ko-lip′id) a lipid containing carbohydrate groups, usually galactose but also glucose, inositol, or others; although it can describe those lipids derived from either glycerol or sphingosine, with or without phosphates, the term is usually used to denote the sphingosine derivatives lacking phosphate groups (glycosphingolipids) 糖脂

gly·col·y·sis (gli-kol′ə-sis) the anaerobic enzymatic conversion of glucose to the simpler compounds lactate or pyruvate, resulting in energy stored in the form of ATP, as occurs in muscle 糖酵解；**glycolyt′ic** adj.

gly·co·neo·gen·e·sis (gli″ko-ne″o-jen′ə-sis) gluconeogenesis 糖异生

gly·co·pe·nia (gli″ko-pe′ne-ə) a deficiency of sugar in the tissues 低血糖

gly·co·pep·tide (gli″ko-pep′tīd) any of a class of peptides that contain carbohydrates, including those that contain amino sugars 糖肽

gly·co·phil·ia (gli″ko-fil′e-ə) a condition in which a small amount of glucose produces hyperglycemia 血糖敏感症

gly·co·phor·in (gli″ko-for′in) 血型糖蛋白 1. any of several related proteins that can project through the thickness of the cell membrane of erythrocytes; they attach to oligosaccharides at the outer cell membrane surface and to contractile proteins (spectrin and actin) at the cytoplasmic surface; 2. any of a group of transmembrane glycoproteins of erythrocytes that help anchor the network of spectrin and actin to the plasma membrane; some carry blood group antigens

gly·co·pro·tein (gli″ko-pro′tēn) a conjugated protein covalently linked to one or more carbohydrate groups; technically those with less than 4 percent carbohydrate but often expanded to include the mucoproteins and proteoglycans 糖蛋白

gly·co·pyr·ro·late (gli″ko-pir′o-lāt) a synthetic anticholinergic used as a gastrointestinal antispasmodic, an antisialagogue, and an antiarrhythmic for anesthesia- or surgery-associated arrhythmias 一种合成的抗胆碱能药物

gly·cor·rhea (gli″ko-re′ə) any sugary discharge from the body 糖溢

gly·cos·ami·no·gly·can (GAG) (gli″kōs-ə-me″-no-gli′kan) any of several high-molecular-weight linear polysaccharides having various disaccharide repeating units and generally occurring in proteoglycans, including the chondroitin sulfates, dermatan sulfates, heparan sulfate and heparin, keratan sulfates, and hyaluronan 糖胺聚糖

gly·co·se·cre·to·ry (gli″ko-se-kre′to-re) concerned in secretion of glycogen 糖原分泌的

gly·co·se·mia (gli″ko-se′me-ə) glycemia 糖血症

gly·co·si·a·lia (gli″ko-si-a′le-ə) sugar in the saliva 糖涎症

gly·co·si·a·lor·rhea (gli″ko-si″ə-lo-re′ə) excessive flow of saliva containing glucose 糖涎溢

gly·co·si·dase (gli-ko′sī-dās) any of a group of hydrolytic enzymes that catalyze the cleavage of hemiacetal bonds of glycosides 糖苷酶；β-g., 1. a glycosidase specifically cleaving β-linked sugar residues from glycosides; 2. 见 complex 糖苷酶

G

gly·co·side (gli′ko-sīd) any compound containing a carbohydrate molecule (sugar), particularly any such natural product in plants, convertible, by hydrolytic cleavage, into a sugar and a nonsugar component (aglycone), and named specifically for the sugar contained, as glucoside (glucose), pentoside (pentose), fructoside (fructose), etc. 糖苷；**cardiac g.**, any of a group of glycosides occurring in certain plants (e.g., *Digitalis, Strophanthus, Urginea*), acting on the contractile force of cardiac muscle; some are used as cardiotonics and antiarrhythmics 强心苷；**digitalis g.**, any of a number of cardiotonic and antiarrhythmic glycosides derived from *Digitalis purpurea* and *D. lanata,* or any drug chemically and pharmacologically related to these glycosides 洋地黄苷

gly·co·sphingo·lip·id (gli″ko-sfing″o-lip′id) any sphingolipid in which the head group is a mono- or oligosaccharide; included are the cerebrosides, sulfatides, and gangliosides 鞘糖脂

gly·co·stat·ic (gli″ko-stat′ik) tending to maintain a constant sugar level 维持糖量恒定的

gly·cos·uria (gli″ko-su′re-ə) the presence of glucose in the urine 糖尿；**renal g.**, that due to the inherited inability of the renal tubules to reabsorb glucose completely 肾性糖尿

gly·co·syl (gli′ko-sil″) a radical derived from a carbohydrate by removal of the anomeric hydroxyl group 糖基

gly·co·syl·a·tion (gli-ko″sə-la′shən) the formation of linkages with glycosyl groups 糖基化

gly·co·syl·cer·am·i·dase (gli″ko-sil″sə-ram′ĭ-dās) an enzyme that catalyzes the hydrolytic cleavage of β-linked sugar residues from β-glycosides with large hydrophobic aglycons; such activity occurs as part of the β-glycosidase complex, along with lactase, in the intestinal brush border membrane 糖基酰基鞘氨醇酶

gly·co·tro·pic (gli″ko-tro′pik) having an affinity for sugar; antagonizing the effects of insulin; causing hyperglycemia 亲糖的

glyc·yr·rhi·za (glis″ə-ri′zə) licorice 甘草

gly·ox·y·late (gli-ok′sə-lāt) a salt, anion, or ester of glyoxylic acid 乙醛酸盐

gly·ox·yl·ic ac·id (gli″ok-sil′ik) a keto acid formed in the conversion of glycolic acid to glycine; it is the primary precursor of oxalic acid 乙醛酸

gm gram 克

GM-CSF granulocyte-macrophage colony-stimulating factor 粒细胞 - 巨噬细胞集落刺激因子

GMP guanosine monophosphate 鸟苷 - 磷酸；**3′,5′-GMP, cyclic GMP,** cyclic guanosine monophosphate 环磷酸鸟苷

gnat (nat) a small dipterous insect. In Great Britain, the term is applied to mosquitoes; in America, to insects smaller than mosquitoes 蚊，蚋

gnath·i·on (nath′e-on) the lowest median point on the inferior border of the mandible 颏下点

gnath·itis (nath-i′tis) inflammation of the jaw 颌炎

gnatho·dy·na·mom·e·ter (nath″o-di″nə- mom′ə-tər) an instrument for measuring the force exerted in closing the jaws 颌力计

gnath·ol·o·gy (nath-ol′ə-je) a science dealing with the masticatory apparatus as a whole, including morphology, anatomy, histology, physiology, pathology, and therapeutics 颌学；**gnatholog′ic** *adj.*

gnath·os·chi·sis (nath-os′kĭ-sis) cleft jaw 颌裂

Gnath·os·to·ma (nath-os′to-mə) a genus of nematodes parasitic in cats, swine, cattle, and sometimes humans 颚口虫属

gnatho·sto·mi·a·sis (nath″o-sto-mi′ə-sis) infection with the nematode *Gnathostoma spinigerum*, acquired from eating undercooked fish infected with the larvae 颚口线虫病

gno·sia (no′se-ə) the faculty of perceiving and recognizing 认识，感知；**gnos′tic** *adj.*

gno·to·bi·ol·o·gy (no″to-bi-ol′ə-je) gnotobiotics 悉生生物学

gno·to·bio·ta (no″to-bi-o′tə) the specifically and entirely known microfauna and microflora of a specially reared laboratory animal 限菌区系

gno·to·bi·ote (no″to-bi′ōt) a specially reared laboratory animal whose microflora and microfauna are specifically known in their entirety 悉生生物；**gnotobiot′ic** *adj*

Gn-RH gonadotropin-releasing hormone 促性腺激素释放激素

goi·ter (goi′tər) enlargement of the thyroid gland, causing a swelling in the front part of the neck 甲状腺肿；**goi′trous** *adj.*；**aberrant g.**, goiter of a supernumerary thyroid gland 异常的甲状腺肿；**adenomatous g.**, that caused by adenoma or multiple colloid nodules of the thyroid gland 腺瘤性甲状腺肿；**Basedow g.**, a colloid goiter that has become hyperfunctioning after administration of iodine 基多甲状腺肿；**colloid g.**, a large, soft goiter with distended spaces filled with colloid 胶样甲状腺肿；**diffuse toxic g.**, Graves disease 毒性弥漫性甲状腺肿；**diving g.**, a goiter that is movable, sometimes above and sometimes below the sternal notch 游动性甲状腺肿；**exophthalmic g.**, one accompanied by exophthalmos 突眼性甲状腺肿；**fibrous g.**, one in which the thyroid capsule and stroma are hyperplastic 纤维性甲状腺肿；**follicular g.**, parenchymatous g.；**intrathoracic g.**, one in which a portion is in the thoracic cavity 胸内甲状腺肿; **iodide g.,** that occurring in reaction to iodides at high concentrations, due to inhibition of iodide organification 高碘性甲状腺肿; **lingual g.,** enlargement of the upper end of the thyroglossal duct, forming a tumor at the posterior part of the dorsum of the tongue 甲状腺舌管囊肿; **lymphadenoid g.,** Hashimoto disease 淋巴瘤性甲状腺肿; **multinodular g.,** goiter with circumscribed nodules within the gland 多结节性甲状腺肿; **nontoxic g.,** that occurring sporadically and not associated with hyperthyroidism or hypothyroidism 非毒性甲状腺肿; **parenchymatous g.,** one marked by an increase in follicles and a proliferation of epithelium 实质性甲状腺肿; **simple g.,** simple hyperplasia of the thyroid gland 单纯性甲状腺肿; **suffocative g.,** one that causes dyspnea by pressure 窒息性甲状腺肿; **wandering g.,** diving g.

goi·trin (goi′trin) a goitrogenic substance isolated from rutabagas and turnips 甲状腺肿因子

gold (Au) (gōld) a yellow, very malleable and ductile, metallic element; at. no. 79, at. wt. 196.967. Gold compounds (all of which are poisonous) are used in medicine, chiefly in treating arthritis 金; **g. 198,** a radioisotope of gold with a half-life of 2.69 days; it has been used as an intracavitary and interstitial antineoplastic and as a scintiscanning agent. 金 -198, 元素金的一种放射性同位素; **cohesive g.,** chemically pure gold that forms a solid mass when properly condensed into a tooth cavity 黏性金; **g. sodium thiomalate,** a monovalent gold salt used in treatment of rheumatoid arthritis 硫代苹果酸金钠

gol·den·seal (gōl′dən-sēl″) the North American herb *Hydrastis canadensis*, or its dried rhizome, a preparation of which is used in folk medicine and in homeopathy 白毛茛

go·mit·o·li (go-mit′o-li) a network of capillaries in the upper infundibular stem (of the hypothalamus) that surround terminal arterioles of the superior hypophyseal arteries and that lead into portal veins to the anterior lobe 下丘脑漏斗部毛细血管网

gom·pho·sis (gom-fo′sis) 嵌合 1. a type of fibrous joint in which a conical process is inserted into a socketlike portion; 2. specifically, one of the fibrous joints by which a tooth is held in its socket

go·nad (go′nad) a gamete-producing gland; an ovary or testis 性腺; **gonad′al** adj.; **indifferent g.,** the sexually undifferentiated gonad of the early embryo 未分化性腺; **streak g's,** undeveloped gonadal structures in the broad ligament below the fallopian tube, composed of whorled connective-tissue stroma without germinal or secretory cells; seen most often in Turner syndrome 条纹性腺

go·nad·ar·che (go″nə-dahr′ke) the onset of gonadal functioning 性腺功能初现

go·nad·ec·to·my (go″nə-dek′tə-me) surgical removal of an ovary or testis 性腺切除术

go·na·do·rel·in (gə-nad′o-rel′in) synthetic luteinizing hormone–releasing hormone; used as the acetate or hydrochloride salt in the evaluation of hypogonadism and as the acetate salt in the treatment of delayed puberty, infertility, and amenorrhea 戈那瑞林

go·na·do·tox·ic (gə-nad′o-tok″sik) having a deleterious effect on the gonads 性腺毒性

go·nado·trope (go-nad′o-trōp) 同 gonadotroph

go·nado·troph (go-nad′o-trōf) 1. a basophilic cell of the anterior pituitary specialized to secrete follicle-stimulating hormone and luteinizing hormone 促性腺激素细胞; 2. a substance that stimulates the gonads 促性腺物质

go·na·do·tro·phic (go″nə-do-tro′fik) gonadotropic 促性腺的

go·nado·tro·pic (go″nə-do-tro′pik) stimulating the gonads; applied to hormones of the anterior pituitary 促性腺的

go·nado·tro·pin (go″nə-do-tro′pin) any hormone that stimulates the gonads, especially follicle-stimulating hormone and luteinizing hormone 促性腺激素; **chorionic g., human chorionic g. (HCG, hCG),** a glycopeptide hormone produced by the fetal placenta syncytiotrophoblasts that maintains the function of the corpus luteum during the first few weeks of pregnancy; the basis for most commonly used pregnancy tests. It is used pharmaceutically to treat certain cases of cryptorchidism and male infertility, to induce ovulation and pregnancy in certain infertile, anovulatory women, and to stimulate oocyte development and maturation in patients using assisted reproductive technologies 人绒毛膜促性腺激素; 另见 *choriogonadotropin alfa*; **human menopausal g. (hMG),** menotropins 绝经促性腺素

go·nal·gia (go-nal′jə) pain in the knee 膝痛

gon·ar·thri·tis (gon″ahr-thri′tis) inflammation of the knee joint 膝关节炎

go·ni·om·e·ter (go″ne-om′ə-tər) 1. an instrument for measuring angles 角度计, 测角计; 2. a plank that can be tilted at one end to any height, used in testing for labyrinthine disease 测向器（检迷路病）; **finger g.,** one for measuring the limits of flexion and extension of the interphalangeal joints of the fingers 指角度计

go·ni·om·e·try (go″ne-om′ə-tre) the measurement of angles, particularly those of range of motion of a joint 测角术

go·ni·on (go′ne-on) pl. *go′nia* [Gr.] the most inferior, posterior, and lateral point on the external angle of the mandible 下颌角点；**go′nial** *adj.*

go·nio·punc·ture (go″ne-o-punk′chər) insertion of a knife blade through the clear cornea, just within the limbus, across the anterior chamber of the eye and through the opposite corneoscleral wall, in treatment of glaucoma 前房角穿刺

go·nio·scope (go′ne-o-skōp″) an optical instrument for examining the anterior chamber of the eye and for demonstrating ocular motility and rotation 前房角镜

go·ni·ot·o·my (go″ne-ot′ə-me) an operation for glaucoma; it consists of opening the venous sinus of the sclera under direct vision 前房角切开术

gono·coc·ce·mia (gon″o-kok-se′me-ə) the presence of gonococci in the blood 淋球菌（菌）血症

gono·coc·cus (gon″o-kok′əs) pl. *gonococ′ci.* An individual of the species *Neisseria gonorrhoeae,* the etiologic agent of gonorrhea 淋球菌；**gonococ′cal, gonococ′cic** *adj.*

gono·cyte (gon′o-sīt) primordial germ cell 生殖母细胞

gon·or·rhea (gon″o-re′ə) infection with *Neisseria gonorrhoeae,* most often transmitted venereally, marked in males by urethritis with pain and purulent discharge; commonly asymptomatic in females, but may extend to produce salpingitis, oophoritis, tubo-ovarian abscess, and peritonitis. Bacteremia may occur in both sexes, causing skin lesions, arthritis, and rarely meningitis or endocarditis 淋病；**gonorrhe′al** *adj.*

Gony·au·lax (gon″e-aw′laks) a genus of dinoflagellates found in fresh, salt, or brackish waters, having yellow to brown chromatophores; it includes *G. catenel′la,* a poisonous species, which helps to form the destructive red tide in the ocean 膝沟藻属，另见 *poison* 下词条

Gor·do·nia (gor-do′ne-ə) a genus of actinomycetes of the family Nocardiaceae, occurring widely in soil and water; some species, chiefly *G. bronchia′lis,* have been associated with human infections in immunocompromised patients 戈登菌属

go·se·rel·in (go′sə-rel″in) a synthetic gonadotropin-releasing hormone; on prolonged administration it suppresses release of gonadotropins and is used as the acetate salt to treat breast and prostate carcinomas and endometriosis and to thin the endometrium prior to endometrial ablation 戈舍瑞林

gos·sy·pol (gos′ə-pol) a toxin found in cottonseed and detoxified by heating; it has male antifertility properties, apparently having its effects in the seminiferous tubules 棉酚

GOT aspartate transaminase (glutamic-oxaloacetic transaminase) 天冬氨酸转氨酶（谷草转氨酶）

go·tu ko·la (go′too ko′lə) the creeping, umbelliferous plant *Centella asiatica* or preparations of its leaves and stems, which are used to promote wound healing and to treat the lesions of leprosy; also widely used in ayurveda, traditional Chinese medicine, and Asian folk medicine 雷公根

gouge (gouj) a hollow chisel for cutting and removing bone 圆凿

goun·dou (gōōn-doo′) a sequel of yaws and endemic syphilis, marked by headache, purulent nasal discharge, and formation of bony exostoses at the side of the nose 鼻骨增殖性骨膜炎，雅司病和地方性梅毒的晚期后遗症

gout (gout) a group of disorders of purine metabolism, manifested by various combinations of (1) hyperuricemia and uric acid calculi; (2) recurrent acute inflammatory arthritis induced by crystals of sodium urate; and (3) tophaceous deposits of these crystals in and around the joints of the extremities, sometimes causing joint destruction 痛风；**gout′y** *adj.*

GP general paresis 全身麻痹症，麻痹性痴呆；general practitioner 普通开业医师

G6PD glucose-6-phosphate dehydrogenase 葡萄糖-6-磷酸脱氢酶

GPT glutamic-pyruvic transaminase 谷（氨酸）-丙（酮酸）转氨酶；见 *alanine transaminase*

grac·ile (gras′il) slender or delicate 薄的，细的

gra·di·ent (gra′de-ənt) rate of increase or decrease of a variable value, or its graphic representation 阶度，梯度；**electrochemical g.,** a difference in ion concentration between two points so that ions tend to move passively along it 电化学梯度

grad·u·at·ed (graj′oo-āt″əd) marked by a succession of lines, steps, or degrees 有刻度的

graft (graft) 1. any tissue or organ for implantation or transplantation 移植物，移植片；2. to implant or transplant such tissues 移植；另见 *implant*；**accordion g.,** a full-thickness graft in which slits have been made so that it may be stretched to cover a larger area 手风琴样移植物，成折移植片；**arteriovenous g.,** an arteriovenous fistula consisting of a venous autograft or xenograft or a synthetic tube grafted onto the artery and vein 动静脉移植物；**avascular g.,** a graft of tissue in which not even transient vascularization is achieved 无血管移植片；**Blair-Brown g.,** a split-skin graft of intermediate thickness 布-布二氏移植片；**bone g.,** a piece of bone used to take the place of a removed bone or bony defect 骨移植物；**cable g.,** a nerve graft made up of several sections of nerve in the manner of a cable 电缆式神经移植物；**coronary artery bypass g. (CABG),** 冠状动脉旁路搭桥术，见 *bypass* 下词条；**delayed g.,** a skin graft sutured back into its bed and subsequently shifted to a new recipient site 延迟移植片；**dermal g.**, skin from which epidermis and subcutaneous fat have been removed; used instead of fascia in various plastic procedures 真皮移植片；**fascia g.**, one taken from the fascia lata or the lumbar fascia 筋膜移植片；**fascicular g.**, a nerve graft in which bundles of nerve fibers are approximated and sutured separately 神经束移植物；**free g.**, a graft of tissue completely freed from its bed, in contrast to a flap 游离移植物；**full-thickness g.**, a skin graft consisting of the full thickness of the skin, with little or none of the superficial fascia 全层皮移植片；**heterodermic g.**, a skin graft taken from a donor of another species 异体皮移植片；**heterologous g.**, **heteroplastic g.**, xenograft 异种移植物，异种移植；**homologous g.**, **homoplastic g.**, allograft （同种）异基因移植物，同种（异体）移植；**isogeneic g.**, **isologous g.**, **isoplastic g.**, syngraft 同基因移植物；**Krause-Wolfe g.** full-thickness g. Krause-Wolfe 移植片；**lamellar g.**, replacement of the superficial layers of an opaque cornea by a thin layer of clear cornea from a donor eye 角膜板层移植片；**nerve g.**, replacement of an area of defective nerve with a segment from a sound one 神经移植物；**omental g's**, free or attached segments of omentum used to cover suture lines following gastrointestinal or colonic surgery 网膜移植；**pedicle g.**, 蒂状移植片，见 *flap* 下词条；**periosteal g.**, a piece of periosteum to cover a denuded bone 骨膜移植物；**pinch g.**, a free skin graft 2 to 4 mm in diameter, obtained by elevating the skin with a needle and slicing it off with a knife 颗粒状移植皮片；**sieve g.**, a skin graft from which tiny circular islands of skin are removed so that a larger denuded area can be covered, the sievelike portion being placed over one area, and the individual islands over surrounding or other denuded areas 筛状移植片；**split-skin g.**, a skin graft consisting of only a portion of the skin thickness 分层皮移植片；**thick-split g.**, a skin graft cut in pieces, often including about two-thirds of the full thickness of the skin 厚分层皮移植片；**white g.**, avascular g. 无血管移植物

gram (g) (gram) a unit of mass in the SI system; one-thousandth of a kilogram 克

gram·i·ci·din (gram″i-si′din) an antibacterial polypeptide produced by *Bacillus brevis*; it is applied topically in infections due to susceptible gram-positive organisms 短杆菌肽

gram-neg·a·tive (gram-neg′ə-tiv) losing the stain or decolorized by alcohol in the Gram method of staining, characteristic of bacteria having a cell wall surface more complex in chemical composition than the gram-positive bacteria 革兰阴性的

gram-pos·i·tive (gram-poz′ĭ-tiv) retaining the stain or resisting decolorization by alcohol in the Gram method of staining, a primary characteristic of bacteria whose cell wall is composed of peptidoglycan and teichoic acid 革兰阳性的

gram-var·i·a·ble (gram-var′e-ə-bəl) appearing to be a mixture of gram-positive and gramnegative organisms, said of gram-positive bacteria that lose the stain easily, so that some bacteria in a sample are decolorized and others retain the stain 革兰染色不定

gra·na (gra′nə) dense green, chlorophyll-containing bodies in chloroplasts of plant cells （叶绿体）基粒

gran·di·ose (gran′de-ōs″) in psychiatry, pertaining to exaggerated beliefs or claims of one's importance or identity, often manifested by delusions of great wealth, power, or fame 夸大的（精神医学）

grand mal (grahn mahl) [Fr.] see under *epilepsy*. 癫痫大发作，强直阵挛（性癫痫）发作

gran·is·e·tron (grā-nis′ə-tron) an antiemetic used in conjunction with cancer chemotherapy or radiotherapy, administered as the hydrochloride salt （格拉司琼）

gran·u·lar (gran′u-lər) made up of or marked by the presence of granules or grains 颗粒的

gran·u·la·tio (gran″u-la′she-o) pl. *granulatio'nes* [L.] a granule or granular mass 颗粒

gran·u·la·tion (gran″u-la′shən) 1. the division of a hard substance into small particles 颗粒化；2. the formation in wounds of small, rounded masses of tissue during healing; also the mass so formed 肉芽形成；**arachnoidal g's**, **cerebral g's**, enlarged arachnoid villi projecting into the venous sinuses and creating slight depressions on the surface of the cranium 蛛网膜颗粒；**exuberant g's**, excessive proliferation of granulation tissue in healing wounds 过度生长的肉芽组织

gran·ule (gran′ūl) 1. a small particle or grain 颗粒；2. a small pill made from sucrose 颗粒剂；**acidophil g's**, granules staining with acid dyes 嗜酸颗粒；**acrosomal g.**, a large globule contained within a membranebounded acrosomal vesicle, which enlarges further to become the core of the acrosome of a spermatozoon 顶体颗粒；**alpha g's**, 1. oval granules found in blood platelets; they are lysosomes containing acid phosphatase 血小板卵形颗粒；2. large granules in the alpha cells of the islets of Langerhans; they secrete glucagon 胰岛α细胞大颗粒；3. granules found in the acidophils of the anterior lobe of the pituitary 腺垂体α细胞嗜酸性颗粒；**azurophil g.**, one staining easily with azure dyes; they are coarse reddish granules seen in many lymphocytes 嗜苯胺蓝颗粒；**basal g.,** 基体，见 *body* 下词条；**basophil g.,** 嗜碱粒。 1. any granule staining with basic dyes; 2. one of the coarse bluish-black granules found in basophils (2); 3. *(in the pl.)* 同 beta g's (2)；**beta g's,** β 颗粒 1. granules in the beta cells of the islets of Langerhans, which contain insulin; 2. granules found in the basophils of the anterior lobe of the pituitary；**Birbeck g's,** membrane-bound rod- or tennis racquet–shaped structures with a central linear density, found in the cytoplasm of Langerhans cells 伯贝克颗粒；**chromaffin g's,** organelles in the chromaffin cells of the adrenal medulla, where epinephrine and norepinephrine are synthesized, stored, and released 嗜铬颗粒；**elementary g's,** hemoconia 基本粒；**eosinophil g.,** one of the coarse round granules that stain with eosin and are found in eosinophils 嗜曙红粒；**iodophil g's,** granules staining brown with iodine, seen in polymorphonuclear leukocytes in various acute infectious diseases 嗜碘颗粒；**keratohyalin g's,** irregularly shaped granules, representing deposits of keratohyalin on tonofibrils in the stratum granulosum of the epidermis 透明角质颗粒；**lamellar g.,** 板状颗粒，见 *body* 下词条；**Langerhans g's,** Birbeck g's 郎格罕斯颗粒；**metachromatic g.,** a granular cell inclusion present in many bacterial cells, having an avidity for basic dyes and causing irregular staining of the cell 异染（颗）粒；**Nissl g's** 尼斯尔小体，见 *body* 下词条；**oxyphil g's,** 同 acidophil g's；**pigment g's,** small masses of coloring matter in pigment cells 色素颗粒；**proacrosomal g.,** one of the small, dense bodies found inside one of the vacuoles of the Golgi body, which fuse to form an acrosomal granule 前顶体粒；**seminal g's,** the small granular bodies in the spermatic fluid 精液粒；**specific atrial g's,** membrane-bound spherical granules with a dense homogeneous interior that are concentrated in the core of sarcoplasm of the atrial cardiac muscle, extending in either direction from the poles of the nucleus, usually near the Golgi complex; they are the storage site of atrial natriuretic peptide 心房特殊颗粒

gran·u·lo·ad·i·pose (gran″u-lo-ad′ĭ-pōs) showing fatty degeneration containing granules of fat 颗粒状脂变的

gran·u·lo·cyte (gran′u-lo-sīt″) granular leukocyte 颗粒细胞；**granulocyt′ic** *adj.*；**band-form g.,** band cell 带状粒细胞

gran·u·lo·cy·to·pe·nia (gran″u-lo-si″to-pe′ne-ə) reduction in the number of granular leukocytes in the blood 粒细胞减少症

gran·u·lo·cy·to·poi·e·sis (gran″u-lo-si″to-poie′sis)

granulopoiesis 粒细胞发生；**granulocytopoiet′ic** *adj.*

gran·u·lo·cy·to·sis (gran″u-lo-si-to′sis) an excess of granulocytes in the blood 粒细胞增多症

gran·u·lo·ma (gran″u-lo′mə) pl. *granulomas, granulo′mata.* An imprecise term for (1) any small nodular delimited aggregation of mononuclear inflammatory cells or (2) such a collection of modified macrophages resembling epithelial cells, usually surrounded by a rim of lymphocytes 肉芽肿；**actinic g.,** a round lesion with a raised border seen on skin chronically exposed to sunlight 光线性肉芽肿；**g. annula′re,** a benign, self-limited disease consisting of round granulomas of the dermis in groups, with papules or nodules, mainly seen in young girls 环状肉芽肿；**apical g.,** periapical g. 齿根尖肉芽肿；**eosinophilic g.,** 1. the mildest form of Langerhans cell histiocytosis, affecting primarily children, adolescents, and young adults. There may be a single cranial lesion or a few foci, most often in the skull, spine, pelvis, ribs, or mandible and less commonly in the long bones 嗜酸细胞肉芽肿；2. a disorder similar to eosinophilic gastroenteritis, with nodular or pedunculated lesions of the submucosa and muscle walls, especially in the pyloric region, caused by infiltration of eosinophils, but without peripheral eosinophilia or allergic symptoms 嗜酸细胞肉芽肿性息肉；3. anisakiasis 异尖线虫病；**g. fissure′tum,** a firm, red, fissured, fibrotic granuloma of the gum and buccal mucosa of an edentulous alveolar ridge between the ridge and cheek; caused by an illfitting denture 裂隙性肉芽肿；**infectious g.,** one due to a specific microorganism, such as tubercle bacilli 感染性肉芽肿；**g. inguina′le,** a granulomatous disease seen in the tropics and subtropics, spread by uncleanliness and sometimes sexually transmitted, marked by ulceration of the external genitals, caused by *Klebsiella granulomatis* 腹股沟肉芽肿；**lethal midline g.,** a rare lethal necrotizing granuloma that destroys the midface; it is nearly always preceded by longstanding nonspecific inflammation of the nose or nasal sinuses, with purulent, often bloody discharge 致命性中线性肉芽肿；**lipoid g.,** xanthoma 类脂性肉芽肿；**lipophagic g.,** granuloma with loss of subcutaneous fat 耗脂肉芽肿；**midline g.,** lethal midline g. 中线性肉芽肿；**periapical g.,** modified granulation tissue adjacent to the root apex of a tooth, containing elements of chronic inflammation with infected, necrotic pulp 根尖周肉芽肿；**peripheral giant cell reparative g.,** giant cell epulis 巨细胞性牙龈瘤；**pyogenic g.,** a solitary polypoid type of capillary hemangioma, usually found on the skin or oral mucous membranes; it often represents a vasoprolif-erative inflammatory response to trauma or irritation 化脓性肉芽肿；**reticulohistiocytic g.,** a solitary reticulohistiocytoma that is not associated with sys-temic involvement 网状组织细胞肉芽肿；**sarcoid g.,** the granuloma seen with sarcoidosis 肉样瘤性肉芽肿；**swimming pool g.,** one that complicates injuries sustained in swimming pools, attributed to *Mycobacterium* marinum, often healing sponta-neously over time 游泳池肉芽肿

gran·u·lo·ma·to·sis (gran″u-lo″mə-to′sis) any condition with formation of granulomas 肉芽肿病；**eosinophilic g.,** see eosinophilic granuloma 嗜酸性肉芽肿；**Langerhans cell g.,** 朗格汉斯细胞肉芽肿病，见 *histiocytosis* 下词条；**lymphomatoid g.,** a multisystem disease involving predominant-ly the lungs, skin, central nervous system, and kidneys, caused by invasion and destruction of vessels by atypical lymphoreticular cells; many patients develop frank lymphoma 淋巴瘤样肉芽肿病；**g. sidero′tica,** a condition in which brownish nodules are seen in the enlarged spleen 铁质沉着性肉芽肿病；**Wegener g.,** a progressive disease, with necrotizing granulomatous vasculitis involving the upper and lower respiratory tracts, glomerulone-phritis, and variable degrees of systemic, small-ves-sel vasculitis 韦氏肉芽肿病

gran·u·lom·a·tous (gran″u-lom′ə-təs) containing granulomas 肉芽肿的

gran·u·lo·mere (gran′u-lo-mēr″) the center portion of a platelet in a dry, stained blood smear, apparently filled with fine, red granules 颗粒区

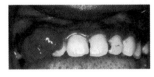

▲ 化脓性肉芽肿

gran·u·lo·pe·nia (gran″u-lo-pe′ne-ə) granulocyto-penia 粒细胞减少

gran·u·lo·plas·tic (gran″u-lo-plas′tik) forming granules 颗粒形成的

gran·u·lo·poi·e·sis (gran″u-lo-poi-e′sis) the formation of granulocytes 粒细胞生成；**granulopoiet′ic** *adj.*

gran·u·lo·sa (gran″u-lo′sə) pertaining to cells of the cumulus oophorus 粒层，粒膜

grape·seed (grāp′sēd) 葡萄籽，见 *seed* 下词条

graph (graf) a diagram or curve representing varying relationships between sets of data（曲线图，图解，图表）

grat·tage (grah-tahzh′) [Fr.] removal of granulations

by scraping 刷除术

grav·el (grav′əl) calculi occurring in small parti-cles 沙砾，尿砂

grav·id (grav′id) pregnant 妊娠的，怀孕的

grav·i·da (G) (grav′ĭ-də) a pregnant woman; called *g. I (primigravida)* during the first pregnancy, *g. II (secundigravida)* during the second, and so on 孕妇。Cf. *para*

grav·i·do·car·di·ac (grav″ĭ-do-kahr′de-ak) per-taining to heart disease in pregnancy 妊娠心脏病的

grav·i·met·ric (grav″ĭ-met′rik) pertaining to measurement by weight; performed by weight, as a gravimetric method of drug assay 比重测定的，重量分析的

grav·i·ty (grav′ĭ-te) 1. the phenomenon by which two bodies having mass are attracted to each other 重力；2. the gravitational attraction near a large body having mass, particularly near or on the sur-face of a planet or star 引力；**specific g.,** the ratio of the density of a substance to that of a reference sub-stance at a specified temperature 比重；**standard g.** *(g),* the acceleration due to gravity at mean sea level on earth, 9.80616 meters per second squared 标准重力

gray (gra) 1. of a hue between white and black 灰色；2. a unit of absorbed radiation dose equal to 100 rads. Abbreviated Gy 戈瑞，符号为 Gy

green (grēn) 1. a color between yellow and blue, produced by energy with wavelengths between 490 and 570 nm 绿色；2. a dye or stain with this color 绿色染料；**indocyanine g.,** a dye used intrave-nously in determination of blood volume and flow, cardiac output, and hepatic function 吲哚花青绿，靛氰绿

GRH growth hormone–releasing hormone 生长素释放激素

grid (grid) 1. a grating; in radiology, a device consisting of a series of narrow lead strips closely spaced on their edges and separated by spacers of low-density material; used to reduce the amount of scattered radiation reaching the x-ray film 滤线栅；2. a chart with horizontal and perpendicular lines for plotting curves 图表纸；**baby g.,** a direct-reading chart on infant growth 婴儿发育表；**Potter-Bucky g.,** a grid used in radiography; it prevents scattered radiation from reaching the film, thereby securing better contrast and definition, and moves during exposure so that no lines appear in the radiograph. 波 - 布二氏活动（X 线）滤线栅；**Wetzel g.,** a di-rect-reading chart for evaluating physical fitness in terms of body build, developmental level, and basal metabolism 韦策尔网格

grief (grēf) the normal emotional response to an

454

external and consciously recognized loss 悲伤
grip (grip) 1. grippe 流行性感冒；2. a grasping
or seizing 抓住
grippe (grip) [Fr.] influenza 流行性感冒
gris·eo·ful·vin (gris″e-o-ful′vin) an antibiotic
produced by *Penicillium griseofulvum;* used as an
antifungal in dermatophytoses 灰黄霉素
groin (groin) inguinal region 腹股沟
groove (groov) a narrow, linear hollow or depression 沟 **atrioventricular g.,** coronary sulcus 房 室
沟；**branchial g's,** pharyngeal g's 鳃沟；**Harrison
g.,** a horizontal groove along the lower border of the
thorax corresponding to the costal insertion of the
respiratory diaphragm; seen in advanced rickets in
children 哈里森沟；**medullary g., neural g.,** that
formed by beginning invagination of the neural plate
of the embryo to form the neural tube 髓沟，神经沟；
pharyngeal g's, the embryonic ectodermal clefts
between successive pharyngeal arches 咽沟；**primitive g.,** a lengthwise median furrow in the primitive
streak of the embryo 原 沟；**venous g's,** grooves
on the internal surfaces of the cranial bones for the
meningeal veins 静脉沟
gross (grōs) 1. coarse or large 粗的，大的；2. visible
to the naked eye without the use of magnification 肉
眼的
group (groop) 1. an assemblage of objects having
certain things in common 类，属，组，型，族，
群，团，具有若干共同性的物体的集合；2. a
number of atoms forming a recognizable and usually transferable portion of a molecule 化学簇，基，
分子中可辨认又常可转移的一群原子；**azo g.,** a
bivalent chemical group composed of two nitrogen
atoms, −N:N− 偶氮基；**blood g.,** 血型，见 *blood*
下词条；**Diagnosis-Related G's,** groupings of diagnostic categories used as a basis for hospital payment schedules by Medicare and other third-party
payment plans 诊断相关分组；**dorsal respiratory
g.,** a part of the medullary respiratory center that
controls the basic rhythm of respiration 背侧呼吸
组；**encounter g.,** a sensitivity group in which the
members strive to gain emotional rather than intellectual insight, with emphasis on the expression of
interpersonal feelings in the group situation 会心团
队；**prosthetic g.,** a low-molecular-weight, nonprotein compound that binds with a protein component
(apoprotein, specifically apoenzyme) to form a protein (e.g., holoenzyme) with biologic activity 辅基；
sensitivity training g., T-g., training g., a nonclini-
cal group, not intended for persons with severe emotional problems, which focuses on self-awareness
and understanding and on interpersonal interactions
in an effort to develop the assets of leadership, man-

agement, counseling, or other roles 敏感性训练小
组；**ventral respiratory g.,** a part of the medullary
respiratory center whose neurons function during
strong respiration, moving voluntary muscles to
control inhalation and exhalation or modify behavior of other respiratory motoneurons 腹侧呼吸组
growth (grōth) 1. a normal process of increase in
size of an organism as a result of accretion of tissue
similar to that originally present 生 长，生 物 体
和其各种组织结构体积的增大；2. an abnormal
formation, such as a tumor 一种异常的形成，如
肿瘤；3. the proliferation of cells, as in a bacterial
culture 生长，细胞的增殖，如在细菌培养中；
appositional g., growth by addition at the periphery
of a particular part 附加生长；**interstitial g.,** that
occurring in the interior of structures already formed
间质生长
gru·mous (groo′məs) lumpy or clotted 凝块的
gry·po·sis (grī-po′sis) [Gr.] abnormal curvature,
as of the nails 异常弯曲
GSC gas-solid chromatography 气固色谱法，气
固层析
GSH reduced glutathione 还原型谷胱甘肽
GSSG oxidized glutathione 氧化型谷胱甘肽
gt. [L.] gutta (drop) 滴（下降）
GTN gestational trophoblastic neoplasia 妊 娠 滋
养细胞肿瘤
GTP guanosine triphosphate 鸟苷三磷酸
gtt. [L.] guttae (drops) 滴
GU genitourinary 泌尿生殖系（的）
guai·ac (gwi′ək) a resin from the wood of trees of
the genus *Guajacum,* used as a reagent and formerly
in treatment of rheumatism 愈创木脂
guai·fen·e·sin (gwi-fen′ə-sin) an expectorant believed to act by reducing sputum viscosity 愈 创 木
酚甘油醚（祛痰药）
gua·na·benz (gwah′nə-benz) an α₂-adrenergic agonist used in the form of the base or the acetate ester
as an antihypertensive 氯压胍，胍那苄（抗高血
压药）
gua·na·drel (gwah′nə-drel) an adrenergic neuron–
blocking agent, used in the treatment of hypertension;
used as the sulfate salt 胍那决尔，胍环定，胍脱，
胍缩酮（抗高血压药）
guan·eth·i·dine (gwahn-eth′ĭ-dēn) an adrener-
gic-blocking agent, used as the monosulfate salt as
an antihypertensive 胍乙啶（肾上腺素阻滞药）
guan·fa·cine (gwahn′fə-sēn) an α 2-adrenergic
agonist used in the form of the hydrochloride salt as
an antihypertensive 胍法辛（抗高血压药）
gua·ni·dine (gwah′nĭ-dēn) the compound
NH=C(NH₂)₂, a strong base found in the urine as a
result of protein metabolism and used in the labora-

tory as a protein denaturant. The hydrochloride salt is used in the treatment of myasthenia gravis 胍

gua·ni·di·no·a·ce·tic ac·id (gwah″ni-de″no- ə-se′tik) an intermediate product formed enzymatically in the liver, pancreas, and kidney in the synthesis of creatine 胍乙酸

gua·nine (G) (gwah′nēn) a purine base, in animal and plant cells usually occurring condensed with ribose or deoxyribose to form guanosine and deoxyguanosine, constituents of nucleic acids 鸟嘌呤

gua·no·sine (G) (gwah′no-sēn) a purine nucleoside, guanine linked to ribose; it is a component of RNA and its nucleotides are important in metabolism 鸟苷，鸟嘌呤核苷；**cyclic g. monophosphate,** 3′,5′- GMP, cGMP, cyclic GMP; a cyclic nucleotide that acts as a second messenger similar in action to cyclic adenosine monophosphate but generally producing opposite effects on cell function 环磷酸鸟苷；**g. monophosphate (GMP),** a nucleotide important in metabolism and RNA synthesis 鸟苷一磷酸；**g. triphosphate (GTP),** an energy-rich compound involved in several metabolic reactions and an activated precursor in the synthesis of RNA 鸟苷三磷酸

gua·ra·na (gwə-rah′nə) [Tupi-Guarani] the Brazilian woody vine *Paullinia cupana*, or a dried paste prepared from its seeds that is used as a stimulant and tonic in folk medicine and for the treatment of headache in homeopathy 瓜拉那，巴西可可

gu·ber·nac·u·lum (goo″bər-nak′u-ləm) pl. *guberna'cula* [L.] a guiding structure 引带；**gubernac′ular** *adj.*；**g. tes′tis,** the fetal ligament attached at one end to the lower end of the epididymis and testis and at its other end to the bottom of the scrotum; it is present during the descent of the testis into the scrotum and then atrophies 睾丸引带

guide (gīd) a device by which another object is led in its proper course 导（子），标

guide·wire (gīd′wīr″) a thin, usually flexible wire that can be inserted into a confined or tortuous space to act as a guide for subsequent insertion of a stiffer or bulkier instrument 导丝

guil·lo·tine (ge′o-tēn) [Fr.] an instrument with a sliding blade for excising a tonsil or the uvula 环状刀

gul·let (gul′ət) the esophagus 食管

gum (gum) 1. a mucilaginous excretion from various plants 树胶; 2. gingiva 牙龈; **gum′my** *adj.*；**guar g.,** a gum obtained from the ground endosperms of the leguminous tree *Cyamopsis tetragonolobus;* used in pharmaceutical preparations and as a source of soluble dietary fiber 瓜尔胶，古尔胶；**karaya g.,** sterculia g., the dried gummy exudation from Sterculia

species, which becomes gelatinous when moisture is added; used as a bulk laxative. It is also adhesive and is used in dental adhesives and skin adhesives and protective barriers around stomas 刺梧桐胶

gum·boil (gum′boil) parulis 龈脓肿

gum·ma (gum′ə) pl. *gummas, gum′mata.* A chronic focal area of inflammatory destruction in tertiary syphilis from localization of *Treponema pallidum* in tissue 树胶样肿，梅毒瘤；**gummatous** *adj.*

gu·na (goo′nah) [Sanskrit] according to ayurveda, any of the three attributes of the universe and self that compose mind and body: sattva (equilibrium), rajas (activity), and tamas (inertia) 古纳（阿育吠陀中的三种生理特性）

gur·ney (gur′ne) a wheeled cot used in hospitals 医院里使用的轮床

gus·ta·tion (gəs-ta′shən) taste 味觉；**gus′tatory** *adj.*

gut (gut) 1. intestine 肠; 2. the primordial digestive tube, consisting of the fore-, mid-, and hindgut 原肠; 3. 同 surgical g.; **blind g.,** cecum 盲肠; **chromic g., chromicized g.,** surgical gut treated with a chromic salt to increase its resistance to absorption in tissues 铬肠线; **postanal g.,** a temporary extension of the embryonic gut caudal to the cloaca 肛后肠; **preoral g.,** Seessel pouch 口前肠; **primordial g.,** archenteron 原肠; **surgical g.,** catgut; an absorbable sterile strand made from collagen of a mammal; used in absorbable sutures 羊肠线; **tail g.,** 同 postanal g.

gut·ta (gut′ə) pl. *gut′tae* [L.] drop 滴，滴剂

gut·ta-per·cha (gut″ə-pur′chə) the coagulated latex of a number of trees of the family Sapotaceae; used as a dental cement and in splints 古塔胶；牙胶

Guttat. [L.] 同 guttatim (drop by drop)

gut·ta·tim (gə-ta′tim) [L.] drop by drop 逐滴地

gut·tur·al (gut′ər-əl) faucial; pertaining to the throat 咽喉的

Gy 同 gray (2)

Gym·no·din·i·um (jim″no-din′e-əm) a genus of dinoflagellates, most species of which have many colored chromatophores, found in water; when present in great numbers, they help to form the destructive red tide in the ocean 裸甲藻属

Gym·no·pi·lus (jim″no-pi′ləs) a genus of mushrooms; several species contain the hallucinogens psilocybin and psilocin 裸伞属

gy·nan·dro·blas·to·ma (gi-) (jə-nan″dro-blas-to′mə) an ovarian tumor containing elements of both arrhenoblastoma and granulosa cell tumor 腺性母细胞瘤

gy·ne·co·gen·ic (gi″nə-) (jin″ə-ko-jen′ik) producing female characteristics 女性化的

gy·ne·coid (gi′nə) (jin′ə-koid) womanlike 女性外

观特征的

gy·ne·co·log·ic (gi″nə-) (jin″ə-kə-loj′ik) pertaining to the female reproductive tract or to gynecology 妇科学的

gy·ne·co·log·i·cal (gi″nə-) (jin″ə-kə-loj′ĭ-kəl) 同 gynecologic

gy·ne·col·o·gist (gi″nə-) (jin″ə-kol′ə-jist) a person skilled in gynecology 妇科学家，妇科医生

gy·ne·col·o·gy (gi″nə-) (jin″ə-kol′ə-je) the branch of medicine dealing with diseases of the genital tract in women 妇科学

gy·ne·co·mas·tia (gi″nə-) (jin″ə-ko-mas′te-ə) excessive development of the male mammary glands, even to the functional state 男性乳房发育症

gy·ne·phil·ia (gī′-nə-fil″e-ə) (jĭn′fil″e-ə) sexual attraction to adult females or femininity 爱女人癖

gy·ne·pho·bia (gi″nə-) (jin″ə-fo′be-ə) irrational fear of or aversion to women 恐女症

gy·noid (gi′-) (jī′noid) 同 gynecoid

gyno·plas·ty (gi′no-) (jin′o-plas″te) plastic or reconstructive surgery of the female reproductive organs 女生生殖器成形术

gyp·sum gans. gyp·sum (jip′səm) native calcium sulfate dihydrate; when calcined, it becomes *plaster of Paris* 硫酸钙

gy·ra·tion (ji-ra′shən) revolution about a fixed center 回旋，螺层

gy·rec·to·my (ji-rek′tə-me) excision or resection of a cerebral gyrus, or a portion of the cerebral cortex 脑回切除术

Gy·ren·ceph·a·la (ji″rən-sef′ə-lə) a group of higher mammals, including humans, having cerebral hemispheres marked by convolutions 多脑回动物类

gy·ri (ji′ri) *gyrus* 的复数

Gy·ro·mi·tra (ji′ro-mi′trə) a genus of mushrooms including several toxic species, notably *G. esculen'-ta* (the false morel), which causes gastrointestinal and neurologic symptoms and hepatic failure 鹿花菌属

gy·rose (ji′rōs) marked by curved lines or circles 回状的，环形的

gy·rous (ji′rəs) gyrose 回状的，环形的

gy·rus (ji′rəs) pl. *gy′ri* [L.] cerebral g. 脑 回；**angular g.**, one arching over the superior temporal sulcus, continuous with the middle temporal gyrus 角回；**anterior paracentral g.**, the anterior portion of the paracentral lobule, medial to and continuous with the precentral gyrus; the primary somatomotor cortex for the lower extremities and genitalia 前中央旁回；**gy′ri bre′ves in′sulae**, the short, rostrally placed gyri on the surface of the insula 岛短回；**Broca g.**, 布罗卡回，见 *convolution* 下词条；**central g., anterior,** 同 precentral g.；**central g.,**

posterior, 同 postcentral g.；**cerebral g.**, any of the tortuous convolutions on the surface of the cerebral hemispheres, caused by infolding of the cortex and separated by fissures or sulci 大脑回；**cingulate g.**, an arch-shaped convolution just above the corpus callosum 扣 带 回；**dentate g.**, a serrated strip of gray matter under the medial border of the hippocampus proper and in its depths; a subregion of the hippocampus 齿状回；**frontal g.**, any of four gyri (inferior, medial, middle, and superior) of the frontal lobe 额回；**fusiform g.**, one on the inferior surface of the hemisphere between the inferior temporal and parahippocampal gyri, consisting of a lateral *(lateral occipitotemporal g.)* and a medial *(medial occipitotemporal g.)* part 梭 状 回；**g. geni'culi,** a vestigial gyrus at the anterior end of the corpus callosum 膝回；**hippocampal g.**, parahippocampal g. 海 马 回；**infracalcarine g.**, 同 lingual g.；**interlocking gyri**, small gyri in the opposing walls of the central sulcus that interlock with each other like gears 连接回；**lingual g.**, one on the occipital lobe, forming the inferior lip of the calcarine sulcus and, with the cuneus, the visual cortex 舌回；**g. lon'gus in'sulae**, the long, occipitally directed gyrus on the surface of the insula 岛长回；**occipital g.**, either of the two (superior and inferior) gyri of the occipital lobe 枕回；**occipitotemporal g., lateral,** the lateral portion of the fusiform gyrus 枕颞回外侧；**occipitotemporal g., medial,** the medial portion of the fusiform gyrus 枕颞回内侧；**orbital gyri,** irregular gyri on the orbital surface of the frontal lobe 眶回；**parahippocampal g.**, a convolution on the inferior surface of each cerebral hemisphere, lying between the hippocampal and collateral sulci 海 马 旁 回；**paraterminal g.**, a thin sheet of gray substance in front of and ventral to the genu of the corpus callosum 终板旁回；**postcentral g.**, the convolution of the frontal lobe between the postcentral and central sulci; the primary sensory area of the cerebral cortex for the face, upper extremity, trunk, and hip 中央后回；**posterior paracentral g.**, the posterior portion of the paracentral lobule, medial to and continuous with the postcentral gyrus; the primary somatosensory cortex for the lower extremities and genitalia 后中央旁回；**precentral g.**, the convolution of the frontal lobe between the precentral and central sulci; the primary motor area of the cerebral cortex for the face, upper extremity, trunk, and hip 中央前回；**g. rec'tus,** one on the orbital surface of the frontal lobe 直 回；**supramarginal g.**, that part of the inferior parietal convolution that curves around the upper end of the sylvian fissure 缘 上 回；**temporal g.**, any of the gyri of the temporal lobe, including the inferior, middle, superior, and transverse temporal gyri; the more prominent of the latter *(anterior transverse temporal g.)*, when two exist, represents the cortical center for hearing 颞回; **gy′ri transiti′vi ce′rebri,** various small folds on the cerebral surface that are too inconstant to bear individual names 过渡回

H

H[符号] henry 亨（利）; histidine 组氨酸; hydrogen 元素氢; hyperopia 远视

H[符号] enthalpy. 焓, 热焓

h[符号] hecto- 百; hour 小时

HAART highly active antiretroviral therapy 高效抗反转录病毒治疗

ha·be·na (hə-be′nə) pl. *habe′nae* [L.] any straplike anatomic structure 系带; 丘脑背侧表面的一个小隆起; **habe′nal, habe′nar** *adj.*

ha·ben·u·la (hə-ben′u-lə) pl. *haben′ulae* [L.] 1. a frenulum, or reinlike structure, such as one of a set of structures in the cochlea 系带; 2. a small eminence on the dorsomedial surface of the thalamus, just in front of the posterior commissure 缰核 **haben′ular** *adj.*

hab·it (hab′it) 1. an action that has become automatic or characteristic by repetition 瘾, 癖; 2. predisposition or bodily temperament 体型, 型

ha·bit·u·al (hə-bich′u-əl) 习惯性的; 1. according to or of the nature of a habit; 2. established through long use or frequent repetition

ha·bit·u·a·tion (hə-bich″u-a′shən) 1. the gradual adaptation to a stimulus or to the environment, with a decreasing response 习惯化; 2. an older term denoting sometimes tolerance and sometimes a psychological dependence due to repeated consumption of a drug, with a desire to continue its use, but with little or no tendency to increase the dose 习惯性

hab·i·tus (hab′ĭ-təs) [L.] 1. 同 attitude (2); 2. physique 体型

HABP hospital-acquired bacterial pneumonia 医院获得性细菌性肺炎

Hae·ma·dip·sa (he′mə-dip′sə) a genus of leeches 山蛭属

Hae·ma·phys·a·lis (he″mə-fis′ə-lis) a genus of hard-bodied ticks, species of which are important vectors of diseases such as Q fever and tularemia 血蜱属

Hae·moph·i·lus (he-mof′ĭ-ləs) a genus of hemophilic gram-negative, aerobic or facultatively anaerobic bacteria of the family Pasteurellaceae 嗜血杆菌属; *H. ducre′yi,* a species that causes chancroid 杜克雷嗜血杆菌; *H. influen′zae,* a species existing as several biovars and once thought to be the cause of epidemic influenza. Some are normal inhabitants of the human nasopharynx, while others cause conjunctivitis, bacterial meningitis, and acute epiglottitis, as well as pneumonia in children and immunocompromised patients 流感嗜血杆菌

Haf·nia (haf′ne-ə) a genus of gram-negative facultatively anaerobic, rod-shaped bacteria of the family Enterobacteriaceae 哈夫尼菌属; *H. al′vei,* a species that is part of the normal fecal flora, causes infection in patients with severe underlying illness and is associated with diarrhea 蜂房哈夫尼菌

haf·ni·um (Hf) (haf′ne-əm) a silvery gray, heavy metal element; at. no. 72, at. wt. 178.49 铪

hair (hār) pilus 菌毛, 纤毛; a threadlike structure, especially the specialized epidermal structure composed of keratin and developing from a papilla sunk in the dermis, produced only by mammals and characteristic of that group of animals. Also, the aggregate of such hairs 毛, 毛发; **hair′y** *adj.*; **beaded h.,** hair marked with alternate swellings and constrictions, as in monilethrix 念珠状发; **club h.,** one whose root is surrounded by a bulbous enlargement composed of keratinized cells, prior to normal loss of the hair from the follicle 杵状毛; **ingrown h.,** one that emerges from the skin but curves and reenters it 向内生毛; **lanugo h.,** lanugo 胎毛; **pubic h.,** pubes (1) 阴毛 **resting h.,** 静息毛, 见 *telogen;* **sensory h's,** hairlike projections on the cells of sensory epithelium 感觉毛; **taste h's,** clumps of microvilli that form short hairlike processes projecting into the lumen of a taste pore from the peripheral ends of the taste cells 味觉毛; **terminal h.,** the coarse hair on various areas of the body during adult years 终毛; **twisted h.,** one that at spaced intervals is twisted through an axis of 180 degrees and abnormally flattened 扭发, 弯曲发; **vellus h.,** vellus (1) 毫毛

hal·a·tion (hal-a′shən) indistinctness of the image caused by illumination coming from the same direction as the object being viewed 晕影

hal·cin·o·nide (hal-sin′ə-nīd) a synthetic corticosteroid used topically as an antiinflammatory and antipruritic 哈西奈德, 氯氟松

half-life ($T_{1/2}$) ($t_{1/2}$) (haf′līf″) the time required for the decay of half of a sample of particles of

a radionuclide or elementary particles 半 衰 期；
antibody h.-l., a measure of the mean survival time of antibody molecules following their formation, usually expressed as the time required to eliminate 50 percent of a known quantity of immunoglobulin from the animal body. Half-life varies from one immunoglobulin class to another 抗体半存留期；
biologic h.-l., the time required for a living tissue, organ, or organism to eliminate one-half of a radioactive substance that has been introduced into it 生物学半衰期（一个活组织器官或机体将已引入的放射性物质排出一半所需的时间）

half·way house (haf'wa hous') a residence for patients (e.g., mental patients, drug addicts, alcoholics) who do not require hospitalization but who need an intermediate degree of care until they can return to the community 中间站

hal·i·to·sis (hal″ĭ-to′sis) offensive odor of the breath 口臭

hal·lu·ci·na·tion (hə-loo″sĭ-na′shən) a sense perception (sight, touch, sound, smell, or taste) that has no basis in external stimulation 幻觉；**hallu′cinative, hallu′cinatory** *adj.*；**haptic h.**, 同 tactile h.；**hypnagogic h.**, one occurring just at the onset of sleep 入睡前幻觉；**hypnopompic h.**, one occurring during awakening 醒后幻觉；**kinesthetic h.**, a hallucination involving the sense of bodily movement 运动性幻觉；**somatic h.**, a hallucination involving the perception of a physical experience with the body 躯体幻觉；**tactile h.**, one involving the sense of touch 触幻，触幻觉

hal·lu·ci·no·gen (hə-loo′sĭ-no-jen″) an agent that is capable of producing hallucinations 致幻剂；**hallucinogen′ic** *adj.*

hal·lu·ci·no·sis (hə-loo″sĭ-no′sis) a state characterized by the presence of hallucinations without other impairment of consciousness 幻觉症；**hallucinot′ic** *adj.*；**organic h.**, a term used in a former classification system, denoting an organic mental syndrome characterized by hallucinations caused by a specific organic factor and not associated with delirium 器质性幻觉症

hal·lux (hal'əks) pl. *hal'luces* [L.] the great toe 踇趾；**h. doloro′sus**, a painful condition of the great toe, usually associated with flatfoot 踇趾疼痛，通常与扁平足有关；**h. flex′us**, 同 h. rigidus；**h. mal′leus**, hammer toe affecting the great toe 杵状趾；**h. ri′gidus**, painful flexion deformity of the great toe with limitation of motion at the metatarsophalangeal joint 踇僵症，趾疼痛性弯曲畸形，足跖关节活动受限；**h. val′gus**, angulation of the great toe toward the other toes 踇外翻，踇趾外翻；**h. va′rus**, angulation of the great toe away from the other toes 踇内翻，踇趾内翻

ha·lo (ha′lo) 1. a luminous or colored circle, as the colored circle seen around a light in glaucoma 晕轮；2. a ring seen around the macula lutea in ophthalmoscopic examinations 在检眼镜检查中看到黄斑周围的圆环；3. the imprint of the ciliary processes on the vitreous body 睫状体在玻璃体上的印痕；4. a metal or plastic band that encircles the head or neck, providing support and stability to an orthosis 环绕头部或颈部的金属或塑料带，为矫形器提供支撑和稳定性；**Fick h.**, a colored circle appearing around a light due to the wearing of contact lenses 由于戴隐形眼镜而出现在灯光周围的彩色圆圈；**h. glaucoma′sus, glaucomatous h.**, peripapillary atrophy seen in severe or chronic glaucoma 青光眼晕轮，在严重或慢性青光眼中观察到的毛细血管周围萎缩；**senile h.**, a zone of variable width around the optic papilla, due to exposure of various elements of the choroid as a result of senile atrophy of the pigmented epithelium 衰老性晕斑

hal·o·be·ta·sol (hal″o-ba′tə-sol) a very high potency synthetic corticosteroid used topically in the form of the propionate salt as an antiinflammatory and antipruritic agent 丙酸卤素倍他素，一种高效的合成皮质类固醇，其丙酸盐作为抗炎和止痒药局部使用

hal·o·fan·trine (hal″o-fan′trēn) an antimalarial used as the hydrochloride salt in the treatment of acute malaria due to *Plasmodium falciparum* and *P. vivax* 氯氟菲醇，其盐酸盐常作为抗疟药

hal·o·gen (hal'ə-jən) (ha′lə-jən) any of the nonmetallic elements of the seventh group of the periodic system: chlorine, iodine, bromine, fluorine, and astatine 卤素

ha·lom·e·ter (hə-lom′ə-tər) 1. an instrument for measuring ocular halos 眼晕测定器；2. an instrument for estimating the size of erythrocytes by measuring the halos formed around them when a beam of light shines on them and is diffracted 红细胞衍射晕测量器

hal·o·peri·dol (hal″o-per′ ĭ-dol) an antipsychotic agent of the butyrophenone group with antiemetic, hypotensive, and hypothermic actions; used especially in the management of psychoses and to control vocal utterances and tics of Gilles de la Tourette syndrome; used also as the decanoate ester in maintenance therapy for psychotic disorders 氟哌啶醇

hal·o·thane (hal′o-thān) an inhalational anesthetic used for induction and maintenance of general anesthesia 氟烷（吸入麻醉药）

HALP hand-assisted laparoscopic proctocolectomy 手辅助腹腔镜直肠结肠切除术

ham·ar·tia (ham-ahr′shə) defect in tissue combination during development 组织构成缺陷; **hamar′tial** *adj.*

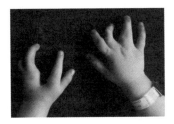

▲ 分裂手

ham·ar·to·ma (ham″ahr-to′mə) a benign tumorlike nodule composed of an overgrowth of mature cells and tissues normally present in the affected part, but with disorganization and often with one element predominating 错构瘤

ham·ate (ham′āt) shaped like a hook 钩状的

ham·mer (ham′ər) 1. an instrument with a head designed for striking blows 锤子; 2. malleus 锤骨; **percussion h.**, a small hammer, usually with a rubber head, for performing percussion 叩诊锤

ham·string (ham′string) one of the tendons bounding the popliteal space laterally and medially 腘绳肌腱; **inner h′s**, the tendons of the gracilis, sartorius, and two other muscles of the leg 内侧腘绳肌腱; **outer h.**, tendon of the biceps flexor femoris 外侧腘绳肌腱

ham·u·lus (ham′u-ləs) pl. *ham′uli* [L.] hook 钩 **ham′ular** *adj.*

hand (hand) the distal part of the upper limb, consisting of the carpus, metacarpus, and fingers 手; **ape h.**, one with the thumb permanently extended 猿手畸形; **claw h.**, 爪形手, 见 *clawhand*; **cleft h.**, a malformation in which the division between the fingers extends into the metacarpus; often with just two large digits, one on either side of the cleft 分裂手; **club h.**, 杵状手, 见 *clubhand*; **drop h.**, wristdrop 垂腕; **lobster-claw h.**, 同 cleft h.; **mitten h.**, the appearance the hand can assume in pseudosyndactyly or syndactyly when the epidermis encases it so that it resembles a mitten 并指畸形; **writing h.**, a hand in Parkinson disease, with the position by which a pen is commonly held 握笔状手, 帕金森病患者的手, 通常呈持笔姿势

H and E hematoxylin-eosin (stain) 苏木精 - 伊红 (染色)

hand·ed·ness (hand′əd-nis) the preferential use of the hand of one side in voluntary motor acts 用手习惯, 在随意运动行为优先使用的一侧手

hand·i·cap (han′dĭ-kap) any physical or mental defect, congenital or acquired, preventing or restricting a person from participating in normal life or limiting the capacity to work 障碍, 残障

hand·piece (hand′pēs″) that part of a dental engine held in the operator's hand and engaging the bur or working point while it is being revolved 手机, 牙科引擎的一部分, 握在操作员的手中, 并在旋转时接合钻头或工作点

hang·nail (hang′nāl) a shred of eponychium on a proximal or lateral nail fold 手足逆胪, 倒刺

Han·ta·vi·rus (han′tə-vi″rəs) a genus of viruses of the family Bunyaviridae that cause epidemic hemorrhagic fever or pneumonia; members include Hantaan, Puumala, and Seoul viruses 汉坦病毒属

hap·loid (hap′loid) having a single set of chromosomes, representing the normal complement of the species, as found in prokaryotes and in eukaryotic gametes (*n* or, in humans, 23) 单倍体

hap·lo·iden·ti·cal (hap″lo-i-den′tĭ-kəl) sharing a haplotype; having the same alleles at a set of closely linked genes on one chromosome 单倍同一性的(具有一个单倍型的; 具有相同等位基因的)

hap·lo·iden·ti·ty (hap″lo-i-den′tĭ-te) the condition of being haploidentical 单倍同一性

hap·lo·scope (hap′lo-skōp) a stereoscope for testing the visual axis 视轴计, 视轴测定器

hap·lo·type (hap′lo-tīp) 1. a set of alleles of a group of closely linked genes, such as the HLA complex, on one chromosome; usually inherited as a unit 单体型; 2. the genetic constitution of an individual at such a set of closely linked genes 个体在一组密切联系的基因上的遗传构成

hap·ten (hap′tən) partial antigen; a specific nonprotein substance that does not itself elicit antibody formation but does elicit the immune response when coupled with a carrier protein 半抗原, 不完全抗原; **hapten′ic** *adj.*

hap·tic (hap′tik) tactile 触觉的

hap·tics (hap′tiks) the study of the sense of touch 触觉学

hap·to·glo·bin (hap″to-glo′bin) a plasma glycoprotein with alpha electrophoretic mobility that irreversibly binds free hemoglobin, resulting in removal of the complex by the liver and preventing free hemoglobin from being lost in the urine; it has two major genetic variants, Hp 1 and Hp 2 触珠蛋白

hare·lip (hār′lip) former name for *cleft lip* 唇裂

har·le·quin (hahr′lə-kwin) 1. having a pattern of diamond shapes, particularly in bright colors (常为菱形图案组成的) 斑色的; 2. coral snake. 花斑眼镜蛇

har·ness (hahr′nis) the combination of straps,

bands, and other pieces that forms the working gear of a draft animal, or a device resembling such gear 马具；挽具；**Pavlik h.,** a device used to correct hip dislocations in infants with developmental dysplasia of the hip, consisting of a set of straps that hold the hips in flexion and abduction Pavlik 吊带，一种用于矫正髋关节发育不良的婴儿髋关节脱位的装置

har·vest (hahr′vəst) to remove tissues or cells from a donor and preserve them for transplantation 收获，采集，从供者取下组织或细胞，保存供移植用

Har·vo·ni (har″voh′nee) trademark for a preparation of ledipasvir and sofosbuvir ledipasvir 和 sofosbuvir 的商标

hash·ish (hă-shēsh′) [Arabic] a preparation of the unadulterated resin scraped from the flowering tops of female hemp plants *(Cannabis sativa),* smoked or chewed for its intoxicating effects. It is far more potent than marijuana 印度大麻（麻醉品）

hash·i·tox·i·co·sis (hash″ĭ-tok″sĭ-ko′sis) hyperthyroidism in patients with Hashimoto disease 桥本甲亢；桥本甲状腺毒症

haus·tel·lum (haw-stel′əm) pl. *haustel′la* [L.] a hollow tube with an eversible set of five stylets, by which certain ectoparasites, e.g., bedbugs and lice, attach themselves to the host and through which blood is drawn up 中喙

haus·tra·tion (haws-tra′shən) 1. the formation of a haustrum 袋形成；2. a haustrum 袋

haus·trum (haws′trəm) pl. *haus′tra* [L.] a recess or sacculation 袋；凹陷或囊状；**haus′tral** *adj.* **haus′tra co′li,** sacculations in the wall of the colon produced by adaptation of its length to the taeniae coli, or by the arrangement of the circular muscle fibers 结肠袋

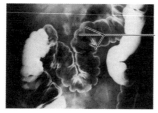

▲ 钡灌肠后的双重造影中的结肠袋（前后视图）

HAV hepatitis A virus 甲型肝炎病毒

haw·kin·sin·u·ria (haw″kin-sin-u′re-ə) a rare autosomal dominant inherited disorder of tyrosine catabolism, with urinary excretion of hawkinsin, a cyclic amino acid metabolite of tyrosine, metabolic acidosis, and failure to thrive 乙酸尿。Cf. *tyrosinemia*

haw·thorn (haw′thorn″) a shrub or tree of the genus *Crataegus,* or a preparation of the flowers, fruit, and leaves of certain of its species, having a mechanism of action similar to that of digitalis; used to decrease output in congestive heart failure; also used in traditional Chinese medicine, homeopathy, and folk medicine 山楂

HB hepatitis B 乙型肝炎

Hb hemoglobin 血红蛋白

HBcAg hepatitis B core antigen 乙型肝炎核心抗原

HbCV *Haemophilus* b conjugate vaccine 嗜血杆菌 b 结合疫苗

HBeAg hepatitis B e antigen 乙型肝炎 e 抗原

HBsAg hepatitis B surface antigen 乙型肝炎表面抗原

HBV hepatitis B virus 乙型肝炎病毒

HC Hospital Corps 医务队

HCG hCG human chorionic gonadotropin 人绒毛膜促性腺激素

HCM hypertrophic cardiomyopathy 肥厚型心肌病

HD hemodialysis 血液透析；Huntington disease 亨廷顿病

HDCV human diploid cell (rabies) vaccine 人二倍体细胞（狂犬病）疫苗，见 *vaccine* 下 *vaccine rabies*

HDL high-density lipoprotein 高密度脂蛋白

HDL-C high-density-lipoprotein cholesterol 高密度脂蛋白胆固醇

He helium 氦气

head (hed) caput; the upper, anterior, or proximal extremity of a structure, especially the part of an organism containing the brain and organs of special sense 头

head·ache (hed′āk″) pain in the head 头痛；**cluster h.,** a migraine-like disorder marked by attacks of unilateral intense pain over the eye and forehead, with flushing and watering of the eyes and nose; attacks last about an hour and occur in clusters 丛集性头痛；**cough h.,** severe, stabbing, bilateral head pain brought on by coughing or some other Valsalva maneuver 咳嗽性头痛；**exertional h.,** one occurring after exercise 劳累性头痛；**histamine h.,** cluster h. 组胺性头痛；**lumbar puncture h.,** the headache occurring after lumbar puncture as part of the post–lumbar puncture syndrome 腰椎穿刺后头痛；**migraine h.,** migraine 偏头痛；**organic h.,** a headache due to intracranial disease or other organic disease 器质性头痛；**postcoital h.,** one occurring during or after sexual activity, usually in males 性交后头痛；**primary h.,** one of the two broad categories of headache, comprising headaches that occur without a discernible underlying cause;

it includes cluster headache, tension headache, and migraine 原发性头痛，包括丛集性头痛、紧张性头痛和偏头痛。Cf. *secondary h.*; **secondary h.**, one of the two broad categories of headache, comprising headaches caused by an underlying pathologic condition 继发性头痛。Cf *primary h.* **sick h.**, migraine 呕吐性头痛；**tension h.**, a type due to prolonged overwork, emotional strain, or both, affecting especially the occipital region 紧张性头痛；**toxic h.**, headache caused by systemic poisoning or certain illnesses 中毒性头痛；**vascular h.**, a classification for certain types of headaches, based on a proposed etiology involving abnormal functioning of the blood vessels or vascular system of the brain; included are migraine, cluster headache, toxic headache, and headache caused by elevated blood pressure 血管性头痛

heal (hēl) 1. to restore wounded parts or to make healthy 治愈，愈合，痊愈；2. to become well or healthy 恢复健康的状态；使（某人）恢复健康

heal·ing (hēl′ing) a process of cure; the restoration of integrity to injured tissue 愈合，痊愈；**h. by first intention**, that in which union or restoration of continuity occurs directly without intervention of granulations 一期愈合；**h. by second intention**, union by closure of a wound with granulations 二期愈合；**spiritual h.**, the use of spiritual practices, such as prayer, for the purpose of effecting a cure of or an improvement in an illness 精神治疗；**h. by third intention**, treatment of a grossly contaminated wound by delaying closure until after contamination has been markedly reduced and inflammation has subsided 三期愈合

health (helth) a state of physical, mental, and social well-being 健康；**public h.**, the field of medicine concerned with safeguarding and improving the health of the community as a whole 公共卫生

hear·ing (hēr′ing) 1. the sense by which sounds are perceived 听，听觉；2. audition; the capacity to perceive sound 听力；**color h.**, a form of chromesthesia in which sounds cause sensations of color 色听，听觉性色感

hear·ing loss (hēr′ing los′) deafness; partial or complete loss of the sense of hearing 耳聋，听力损失，听力减退；**acoustic trauma h. l.**, noise-induced hearing loss caused by a single loud noise such as a blast 损伤性听力损失；**conductive h. l.**, that due to a defect of the soundconducting apparatus, i.e., of the external auditory canal or middle ear 传导性听力损失，传音性听力障碍；**functional h. l.**, hearing loss that lacks any organic lesion 功能性听力损失；功能性耳聋；**high- frequency h. l.**, sensorineural hearing loss of tones at high frequen-

cies, most commonly seen with noise-induced h. l.高频听力损失；**low-frequency h. l.**, sensorineural hearing loss of tones at low frequencies 低频听力损失；**mixed h. l.**, hearing loss that is both conductive and sensorineural 混合性听力损失，混合听觉丧失；**noise-induced h. l.**, sensorineural hearing loss caused by either a single loud noise or prolonged exposure to high levels of noise 噪声性听力减退；**ototoxic h. l.**, that caused by ingestion of toxic substances 耳毒性耳聋；**paradoxic h. l.**, that in which the hearing is better during loud noise 听觉倒错性聋；**postlingual h. l.**, hearing loss that occurs after the person has learned to speak 语言发展后听力损伤；**prelingual l.**, hearing loss that occurs before the person has learned to speak 语言发展前听力损伤；**sensorineural h. l.**, that due to a defect in the inner ear or the acoustic nerve 感觉神经性耳聋

heart (hahrt) cor; the viscus of cardiac muscle that maintains the circulation of the blood 心，心脏；见图24；**artiftcial h.**, a pumping mechanism that duplicates the rate, output, and blood pressure of the natural heart; it may replace the function of a part or all of the heart 人工心脏；**athletic h.**, hypertrophy of the heart without valvular disease, sometimes seen in athletes 运动员心（脏），无瓣膜疾病的心脏肥大；**extracorporeal h.**, an artificial heart located outside the body and usually performing pumping and oxygenating functions 体外人工心；**fatty h.**, 1. one that has undergone fatty degeneration; 2. a condition in which fat has accumulated around and in the heart muscle 脂肪心；**ftbroid h.**, one in which fibrous tissue replaces portions of the myocardium, as may occur in chronic myocarditis 心肌纤维变性；**horizontal h.**, a counterclockwise rotation of the electrical axis (deviation to the left) of the heart 横位心；**left h.**, the left atrium and ventricle, which propel the blood through the systemic circulation 左心，左心房和左心室；**right h.**, the right atrium and ventricle, which propel the venous blood into the pulmonary circulation 右心，右心房和右心室；**stone h.**, massive contraction band necrosis in an irreversibly noncompliant hypertrophied heart, occurring as a complication of cardiac surgery; believed to be due to low levels of ATP and to calcium overload 石头心，心脏手术的并发症，由于低水平的 ATP 和钙超载引起；**three-chambered h.**, a developmental anomaly in which the heart is missing the interventricular or interatrial septum and so has only three compartments 三腔心，心脏缺少室间隔或房间隔，只有三个隔室的发育异常；**water-bottle h.**, a radiographic sign of pericardial effusion, in which the cardiopericardial silhouette is enlarged and assumes the shape of a flask or water bottle 烧瓶状心

heart·beat (hahrt′bēt) a complete cardiac cycle, during which the electrical impulse is conducted and mechanical contraction occurs 心跳，心搏

heart block (hahrt blok) impairment of conduction of an impulse in heart excitation; often applied specifically to atrioventricular block. For specific types, see under *block* 心脏传导阻滞

heart·burn (hahrt′bərn) pyrosis; a retrosternal sensation of burning occurring in waves and rising toward the neck; it may be accompanied by a reflux of fluid into the mouth and is often associated with gastroesophageal reflux 胃灼热，胸骨后的灼烧感

heart fail·ure (hahrt fāl′yer) 心功能不全，心力衰竭，见 *failure* 下词条

heart rhy·thm the rhythm of the heartbeat 心律。又称 *cardiac rhythm*

heart valve (hahrt valv) a valve that controls the flow of blood through or from the heart, including the aortic, mitral, pulmonary, and tricuspid valves 心瓣膜，心脏瓣膜。又称 *cardiac valve*

heart·worm (hahrt′wərm) an individual of the species *Dirofilaria immitis* 犬恶丝虫

heat (hēt) 1. the sensation of an increase in temperature 热；高温；2. the energy producing such a sensation; it exists in the form of molecular or atomic vibration and may be transferred, as a result of a gradient in temperature 热度，符号 Q 或 q；3. to become, or to cause to become, warmer or hotter 加热；变热；（使）变暖；conductive h., heat transmitted by direct contact, as with a hot water bottle 传导热；convective h., heat transmitted by direct contact, as with a hot water bottle 对流热；conversive h., heat conveyed by currents of a warm medium, such as air or water 转换热；prickly h., miliaria rubra 汗疹；痱子

heat·stroke (hēt′strōk) 中暑，见 *stroke* 下词条

he·bet·ic (hə-bet′ik) pubertal 青春期的

heb·e·tude (heb′ə-tood) dullness; apathy 迟钝；精神迟钝；感觉迟钝

hect(o)- word element [Fr.], *hundred*; used in naming units of measurements to designate an amount 100 times (10^2) the size of the unit to which it is joined; symbol h.[构词成分] 百（10^2，符号为 h）

hedge·hog (hej′hog) any of a family of proteins homologous to that encoded by the *hedgehog* gene of *Drosophila* and part of a highly conserved developmental signaling pathway; the three in mammals are *desert H.*, *Indian H.*, and *Sonic H* 一种分节极性基因，因突变致胚胎呈多毛团状，酷似受到惊刺猬；刺猬

heel (hēl) calx; the hindmost part of the foot 脚跟

height (hīt) the vertical measurement of an object or body 高，高度；顶点；高地；海拔；**h. of contour,** 1. a line encircling a tooth representing its greatest circumference; 2. the line encircling a tooth in a more or less horizontal plane and passing through the surface point of greatest radius; 3. the line encircling a tooth at its greatest bulge or diameter with respect to a selected path of insertion 外形高点；外廓高隆线；外形高点线

hel·coid (hel′koid) like an ulcer 溃疡状的

hel·i·cal (hel′ĭ-kəl) spiral (1) 螺旋的，螺旋形的

he·li·cal branch de·vice (hē′lĭ-cul brănch dē-vīs) a flexible implantable device used to perform minimally invasive surgery to treat multiple aneurysms 螺旋分支装置

hel·i·cine (hel′ĭ-sēn) 同 spiral (1) 螺旋状的

He·li·co·bac·ter (hel″ĭ-ko-bak′tər) a genus of gram-negative, microaerophilic bacteria of the family Helicobacteraceae; *H. cinae'di* and *H. fennel'liae* have been associated with lower gastrointestinal disease, particularly in immunocompromised individuals; *H. pylo'ri* has been associated with gastritis, peptic ulcers, and gastric cancer 螺杆菌

He·li·co·bac·ter·a·ceae (hel″ĭ-ko-bak″təra′se-e) a morphologically, metabolically, and ecologically diverse family of bacteria of the order Campylobacterales 螺杆菌科

hel·i·co·pod (hel′ĭ-ko-pod″) denoting a peculiar dragging gait 螺旋形步态的，环形步态的，见 *gait* 下词条

hel·i·co·tre·ma (hel″ĭ-ko-tre′mə) a foramen between the scala tympani and scala vestibuli 蜗孔

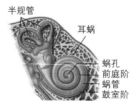

半规管
耳蜗
蜗孔
前庭阶
蜗管
鼓室阶

▲ 蜗孔，见于右侧骨迷路

he·li·um (He) (he′le-əm) a colorless, odorless, tasteless, inert gaseous element, which is not combustible and does not support combustion; at. no. 2; at. wt. 4.003. Used as a diluent for other gases, particularly with oxygen in the treatment of certain cases of respiratory obstruction, and as a vehicle for general anesthetics 氦气

he·lix (he′liks) pl. *he'lices*, helixes [Gr.] 1. 同 spiral (2)；2. the superior and posterior free margin of the pinna of the ear 耳轮；**α-h., alpha h.,** the structural arrangement of parts of protein molecules in which a single polypeptide chain forms a right-handed helix stabilized by intrachain hydrogen bonds α 螺旋；**double h.**, **Watson-Crick h.**, the usual configuration of double-stranded DNA in vivo, being two complementary antiparallel polynucleotide chains coiled into a helix, the sugar-phosphate backbone on the outside and the chains held together by hydrogen bonds between pairs of bases 双螺旋

hel·minth (hel′minth) a parasitic worm 蠕虫

hel·min·tha·gogue (hel-min′thə-gog) 同 anthelmintic (2)

hel·min·thol·o·gy (hel″min-thol′ə-je) the scientific study of parasitic worms 蠕虫学

he·lo·ma (he-lo′mə) corn 鸡眼，钉胼，脚或手上的角质硬粒或硬皮；**h. du′rum**, hard corn 硬鸡眼；**h. mol′le**, soft corn 软鸡眼

hema·cy·tom·e·ter (he″mə-si-tom′ə-tər) an apparatus used for making manual blood counts with a counting chamber 血细胞计数器，血球计数器

he·mad·sorp·tion (he″mad-zorp′shən) the adherence of red cells to other cells, particles, or surfaces 血细胞吸附；**hemadsor′bent** adj.

he·mag·glu·ti·na·tion (he″mə-gloo″tĭ-na′shən) agglutination of erythrocytes 血凝反应，血细胞凝集

he·mag·glu·ti·nin (he″mə-gloo′tĭ-nin) an antibody that causes agglutination of erythrocytes 血凝素，血细胞凝聚素；**cold h.**, one that acts only at temperatures near 4℃冷血凝素；**warm h.**, one that acts only at temperatures near 37℃温血凝素

he·mal (he′məl) 1. ventral to the spinal axis, where the heart and great vessels are located, as, e.g., the hemal arches 脊柱腹侧的；2. hemic 血液的；3. pertaining to blood vessels 血管的；见 *vascular* 下词条

hem·al·um (he′mə-ləm) a mixture of hematoxylin and alum used as a nuclear stain 苏木精明矾，矾紫

hem·a·nal·y·sis (he″mə-nal′ə-sis) analysis of the blood 血液分析

he·man·gio·amelo·blas·to·ma (he-man″jeo-ə-mel″o-blas-to′mə) a highly vascular ameloblastoma 血管性成釉细胞瘤

he·man·gio·blast (he-man′je-o-blast) a mesodermal cell that gives rise to both vascular endothelium and hemocytoblasts 成血管细胞

he·man·gio·blas·to·ma (he-man″je-o-blasto′mə) a benign blood vessel tumor of the cerebellum, spinal cord, or retina, consisting of proliferated blood vessel cells and angioblasts 血管母细胞瘤，血管网状细胞瘤

he·man·gio·en·do·the·li·al (he-man″je-oen″do-the′le-əl) pertaining to the vascular endothelium 血管内皮细胞

he·man·gio·en·do·the·lio·blas·to·ma (heman″je-o-en″do-the′le-o-blas-to′mə) a hemangioendothelioma with embryonic elements of mesenchymal origin 成血管内皮细胞瘤

he·man·gio·en·do·the·lio·ma (he-man″je-oen″do-the′le-o′mə) 1. a true neoplasm of vascular origin, with proliferation of endothelial cells around the vascular lumen 血管内皮细胞瘤；2. hemangiosarcoma 血管肉瘤

he·man·gi·o·ma a (he-man″je-o′mə) 1. a benign vascular malformation, usually in infants or children, made up of newly formed blood vessels and resulting from malformation of angioblastic tissue of fetal life 血管瘤，一种良性血管畸形；2. a benign or malignant vascular malformation resembling the classic type but occurring at any age 恶性血管瘤；**ameloblastic h.**, hemangioameloblastoma 成釉细胞血管瘤；**capillary h.**, 1. the most common type, having closely packed aggregations of capillaries, usually of normal caliber, separated by scant connective stroma 毛细血管瘤；2. 同 strawberry h.；**cavernous h.**, a red-blue spongy tumor with a connective tissue framework enclosing large, cavernous vascular spaces containing blood 海绵状血管瘤；**sclerosing h.**, a form of benign fibrous histiocytoma having numerous blood vessels and hemosiderin deposits 硬化性血管瘤；**strawberry h.**, 1. a red, firm, dome-shaped hemangioma seen at birth or soon after, usually on the head or neck, that grows rapidly and usually regresses and involutes without scarring 草莓状血管瘤；2. vascular nevus 血管痣；**venous h.**, a cavernous hemangioma in which the dilated vessels have thick, fibrous walls 静脉性血管瘤，静脉瘤

he·man·gio·peri·cy·to·ma (he-man″je-oper″ĭ-si-to′mə) a tumor composed of spindle cells with a rich vascular network, which apparently arises from pericytes 血管外皮细胞瘤

he·man·gio·sar·co·ma (he-man″je-o-sahrko′mə) a malignant tumor of vascular origin, formed by proliferation of endothelial tissue lining irregular vascular channels 血管肉瘤

he·ma·phe·re·sis (he″mə-fə-re′sis) apheresis 血成分提出

he·mar·thro·sis (he″mahr-thro′sis) extravasation of blood into a joint or its synovial cavity 关节积血，关节血肿

he·ma·tem·e·sis (he″mə-tem′ə-sis) the vomiting of blood 呕血，吐血

he·mat·ic (he-mat′ik) 1. 同 hemic；2. 同 hematinic

he·ma·ti·dro·sis (he″mə-) (hem″ə-tĭ-dro′sis) excretion of bloody sweat 血汗症。又称 *hematohidrosis*

he·ma·tin (he′mə-tin) 1. the hydroxide of heme; it stimulates the synthesis of globin, inhibits the synthesis of porphyrin, and is a component of cytochromes and peroxidases; it is also used as a reagent 高铁血红素；2. 同 hemin (1)

he·ma·tin·ic (he″mə-tin′ik) 1. pertaining to hematin 正铁血红素的；2. an agent that increases the hemoglobin level and the number of erythrocytes in the blood 补血药的

he·ma·tin·uria (he″mə-tĭ-nu′re-ə) the presence of hematin in the urine 正铁血红素尿，血红素尿

he·ma·to·cele (he′mə-to-) (hem′ə-to-sēl″) an effusion of blood into a cavity, especially into the tunica vaginalis testis 积血，鞘膜积血；**parametric h., pelvic h., retrouterine h.,** a swelling formed by effusion of blood into the pouch of Douglas 盆腔积血

he·ma·to·che·zia (he″mə-to-) (hem″ə-to-ke′-zhə) defecation in which feces are bloody 便血

he·ma·to·chy·lu·ria (he″mə-to-) (hem″ə-toki-lu′re-ə) the discharge of blood and chyle with the urine, as seen in filaria infections 乳糜性血尿，血性乳糜尿

he·ma·to·col·po·me·tra (he″mə-to-) (hem″ə- tokol″po-me′trə) accumulation of menstrual blood in the vagina and uterus 阴道子宫积血

he·ma·to·col·pos (he″mə-to-) (hem″ə-tokol′pəs) blood in the vagina 阴道积血

he·mat·o·crit (he-mat′ə-krit) the volume percentage of erythrocytes in whole blood; also, the apparatus or procedure used in its determination 红细胞比容，血细胞比容；血细胞比容管，血流比容计

he·ma·to·gen·ic (he″mə-to-) (he-mat″o-jen′ik) 1. hematopoietic 生血的；2. hematogenous 血源性的

he·ma·tog·e·nous (he″mə-toj′ə-nəs) 1. produced by or derived from the blood 血源性的；2. disseminated through the bloodstream 通过血液传播的

he·ma·toid·in (he-mə-toid′in) a hematogenous pigment apparently chemically identical with bilirubin but formed in the tissues from hemoglobin, particularly under conditions of reduced oxygen tension 橙色血质

he·ma·tol·o·gy (he″mə-tol′ə-je) the branch of medical science dealing with the blood and blood-forming tissues, including morphology, physiology, and pathology 血液学

he·ma·to·lymph·an·gi·o·ma (he″mə-to-) (hem″ə-to-lim″fan-je-o′mə) a benign tumor composed of blood and lymph vessels 血管淋巴管瘤

he·ma·tol·y·sis (he″mə-tol′ə-sis) hemolysis 溶血，血细胞溶解；**hematolyt′ic** *adj.*

he·ma·to·ma (he″mə-to′mə) a localized collection of extravasated blood, usually clotted, in an organ, space, or tissue 血肿；**subdural h.,** a massive blood clot beneath the dura mater that causes neurologic symptoms by pressure on the brain 硬脑膜下血肿

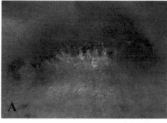

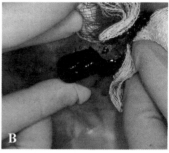

▲ 血肿。A. 术后形成。B. 排出

he·ma·to·me·di·as·ti·num (he″mə-to-) (hem″ə-to-me″de-ə-sti′nəm) hemomediastinum 纵隔积血

he·ma·to·me·tra (he″mə-to-) (hem″ə-tome′trə) blood in the uterus 子宫积血

he·ma·tom·e·try (he″mə-tom′ə-tre) measurement of various parameters of the blood, such as the complete blood count 血成分测定法

he·ma·to·my·e·lia (he″mə-to-) (hem″ə-tomie′le-ə) hemorrhage into the spinal cord 脊髓出血

he·ma·to·my·eli·tis (he″mə-to-) (hem″ə-tomi″ə-li′tis) acute myelitis with bloody effusion into the spinal cord 出血性脊髓炎

he·ma·to·my·elo·pore (he″mə-to-) (hem″ə- tomi″əl-o-por″) formation of canals in the spinal cord due to hemorrhage 出血性脊髓空洞

he·ma·to·pa·thol·o·gy (he″mə-to-) (hem″ə- topə-thol′ə-je) hemopathology 血液病理学

he·ma·to·pha·gia (he″mə-to-) (hem″ə-to-fa′jə) 1. blood drinking 吸血；2. subsisting on blood 血液寄生；**hematoph′agous** *adj.*

he·ma·to·poi·e·sis (he″mə-to-) (hem″ə-to-poie′sis)

the formation and development of blood cells 造血；血细胞生成；造血作用；**extramedullary h.**, that occurring outside the bone marrow, as seen normally in the fetus 骨髓外造血

he·ma·to·poi·et·ic　(he″mə-to-) (hem″ə-topoi-et′ik) 1. pertaining to hematopoiesis 造血的；2. an agent that promotes hematopoiesis 补血药

he·ma·to·por·phy·rin　(he″mə-to-) (hem″ə- to-por′fə-rin) an iron-free derivative of heme, a product of the decomposition of hemoglobin 血卟啉

he·ma·to·sal·pinx　(he″mə-to-) (hem″ə-tosal′pinks) blood in the uterine tube 输卵管积血

he·ma·to·sper·mato·cele　(he″mə-to-) (hem″ə-to-spər-mat′o-sēl) a spermatocele containing blood 阴囊积血

he·ma·to·sper·mia　(he″mə-to-) (hem″ə-tospur′me-ə) the presence of blood in the semen 血精

he·ma·tos·te·on　(he″mə-) (hem″ə-tos′te-on) hemorrhage into the medullary cavity of a bone 骨髓腔积血

he·ma·to·tox·ic　(he″mə-to-) (hem′ə-to-tok″sik) 1. pertaining to blood poisoning 血中毒的；2. poisonous to the blood and hematopoietic system 毒害血液及造血系统的

he·ma·to·tro·pic　(he″mə-to-) (hem″ə-to-tro′ pik) having a specific affinity for or exerting a specific effect on the blood or blood cells 亲血细胞的，亲血的

he·ma·tox·y·lin　(he″mə-tok′sĭ-lin) an acid coloring matter from the heartwood of the tree *Haematoxylon campechianum*; used as a histologic stain and also as an indicator 苏木素，苏木精

he·ma·tu·ria　(he″mə-) (he″mə-tu′re-ə) blood (erythrocytes) in the urine 血尿；**endemic h.**, urinary schistosomiasis 地方性血尿；**essential h.**, that for which no cause has been determined 特发性血尿病；**false h.**, pseudohematuria 假性血尿；**renal h.**, that in which the blood comes from the kidney 肾性血尿；**urethral h.**, that in which the blood comes from the urethra 尿道性血尿；**vesical h.**, that in which the blood comes from the bladder 膀胱性血尿

heme　(hēm) an iron compound of protoporphyrin that constitutes the pigment portion or protein-free part of the hemoglobin molecule and is responsible for its oxygen-carrying properties 血红素，亚铁血红素

hem·er·a·lo·pia　(hem″ər-ə-lo′pe-ə) day blindness; defective vision in bright light 昼盲症

hemi·achro·ma·top·sia　(hem″e-ə-kro″mə- op′se-ə) color vision deficiency in half, or in corresponding halves, of the visual field（偏）侧色盲

hemi·ageu·sia　(hem″e-ə-goo′zhə) ageusia on one side of the tongue 偏侧味觉缺失，半侧味觉丧乏

hemi·amy·os·the·nia　(hem″e-ə-mi″os-the′ne-ə) lack of muscular power on one side of the body 偏身肌无力

hemi·an·al·ge·sia　(hem″e-an″əl-je′ze-ə) analgesia on one side of the body 偏身痛觉缺失

hemi·an·es·the·sia　(hem″e-an″es-the′zhə) anesthesia of one side of the body 偏身麻木，偏侧感觉缺失；**crossed h.**, 交叉性偏身麻木；**h. crucia′ta**, loss of sensation on one side of the face and loss of pain and temperature sense on the opposite side of the body 交叉性偏身麻木

hemi·an·o·pia　(hem″e-ə-no′pe-ə) defective vision or blindness in half of the visual field of one or both eyes; loosely, scotoma in less than half of the visual field of one or both eyes 偏盲；**hemianop′ic** *adj*；**absolute h.**, blindness to light, color, and form in half of the visual field 完全偏盲；**bilateral h.**, hemianopia affecting both eyes 双侧偏盲；**binasal h.**, that in which the defect is in the nasal half of the visual field in each eye 两鼻侧偏盲，内侧偏盲；**binocular h.**, 同 bilateral h.；**bitemporal h.**, that in which the defect is in the temporal half of the visual field in each eye 颞侧偏盲，两外侧偏盲；**complete h.**, that affecting an entire half of the visual field in each eye 完全偏盲；**congruous h.**, that in which the defect is approximately the same in each eye 对称性偏盲，同侧偏盲；**crossed h.**, heteronymous h. 交叉偏盲；**heteronymous h.**, that affecting both nasal or both temporal halves of the field of vision 异侧偏盲；**homonymous h.**, that affecting the nasal half of the field of vision of one eye and the temporal half of the other 同侧偏盲；**nasal h.**, that affecting the medial half of the visual field, i.e., the half nearer the nose 鼻侧偏盲，内侧偏盲；**quadrant h.**, **quadrantic h.**, quadrantanopia 象限偏盲；**temporal h.**, that affecting the lateral vertical half of the visual field, i.e., the half nearest the temple 颞侧偏盲

hemi·aprax·ia　(hem″e-ə-prak′se-ə) apraxia on one side of the body only 偏侧失用症，单侧运用不能

hemi·atax·ia　(hem″e-ə-tak′se-ə) ataxia on one side of the body 偏身共济失调，偏身运动失调

hemi·ath·e·to·sis　(hem″e-ath″ə-to′sis) athetosis of one side of the body 偏身性手足徐动症

hemi·at·ro·phy　(hem″e-at′ro-fe) atrophy of one side of the body or one-half of an organ or part 偏侧萎缩，单侧萎缩

hemi·ax·i·al　(hem″e-ak′se-əl) at any oblique angle to the long axis of the body or a part 半轴的，与身体或某部的长轴呈斜角的

hemi·bal·lis·mus　(hem″e-bə-liz′məs) a violent form of dyskinesia involving one side of the body, most marked in the upper limb 偏身颤搐，偏身投掷（症），偏身挥舞（症）

hemi·blad·der (hem′e-blad′ər) a half bladder, as in exstrophy of the cloaca; the urinary bladder is formed as two physically separated parts, each with its own ureter 半膀胱（畸形），膀胱发育成两个分开的部分，各自接受一条输尿管

hemi·block (hem′e-blok) failure in conduction of the cardiac impulse in either of the two main divisions of the left branch of the bundle of His; the interruption may occur in either the anterior (superior) or posterior division 半支传导阻滞

he·mic (he′mik) (hem′ik) pertaining to blood 血的

hemi·car·dia (hem″e-kahr′de-ə) 1. a congenital anomaly characterized by the presence of only one side of a four-chambered heart 半心畸形；2. either lateral half of a normal heart 正常心脏的半侧部分

hemi·cen·trum (hem″e-sen′trəm) either lateral half of a vertebral centrum 半侧椎（骨）体

hemi·cho·rea (hem″e-kə-re′ə) chorea affecting only one side of the body 偏侧舞蹈症

hemi·cra·nia (hem″e-kra′ne-ə) 1. unilateral headache 偏头痛；2. incomplete anencephaly 半无脑畸形；**chronic paroxysmal h.**, a type of one-sided headache resembling a cluster headache but occurring in paroxysms of half an hour or less, several times a day, sometimes for years 慢性发作性半边头痛，慢性发作性偏头痛

hemi·cra·ni·o·sis (hem″e-kra″ne-o′sis) hyperostosis of one side of the cranium and face 偏侧颅骨肥大，单侧颅骨肥厚

hemi·des·mo·some (hem″e-des′mo-sōm) a structure representing half of a desmosome, found on the basal surface of some epithelial cells, forming the site of attachment between the basal surface of the cell and the basement membrane 半桥粒

hemi·dia·phragm (hem″e-di′ə-fram) one half of the respiratory diaphragm 偏侧膈

hemi·dys·es·the·sia (hem″e-dis″es-the′zhə) dysesthesia on one side of the body 偏身感觉障碍，偏身感觉迟钝

hemi·epi·lep·sy (hem″e-ep′ĭ-lep-se) epilepsy affecting one side of the body 偏身癫痫

hemi·fa·cial (hem″e-fa′shəl) pertaining to or affecting half of the face 偏侧（颜）面的，半面的

hemi·gas·trec·to·my (hem″e-gas-trek′tə-me) excision of half of the stomach 半胃切除术

hemi·geu·sia (hem″e-goo′zhə) hemiageusia 半侧味觉缺失

hemi·glos·sec·to·my (hem″e-glos-ek′tə-me) excision of one side of the tongue 半侧舌切除术

hemi·glos·si·tis (hem″e-glos-i′tis) inflammation of one-half of the tongue 半侧舌炎

hemi·hi·dro·sis (hem″e-hĭ-dro′sis) sweating on one side of the body only 半身出汗，偏身出汗

hemi·hy·pal·ge·sia (hem″e-hi″pəl-je′ze-ə) diminished sensitivity to pain on one side of the body 偏身痛觉减退

hemi·hy·per·es·the·sia (hem″e-hi″pər-esthe′zhə) increased sensitiveness of one side of the body 偏身感觉过敏

hemi·hy·per·hi·dro·sis (hem″e-hi″pər-hĭ- dro′sis) excessive perspiration on one side of the body 偏身多汗

hemi·hy·per·tro·phy (hem″e-hi-pur′trə-fe) overgrowth of one side of the body or of a part 偏身肥大

hemi·hy·pes·the·sia (hem″e-hi″pes-the′zhə) diminished sensitivity on one side of the body 偏身感觉迟钝

hemi·hy·po·to·nia (hem″e-hi″po-to′ne-ə) diminished muscle tone of one side of the body 偏身张力减退

hemi·in·at·ten·tion (hem″e-in-ə-ten′shən) unilateral neglect 偏侧不注意

hemi·lam·i·nec·to·my (hem″e-lam″ĭ-nek′tə- me) removal of a vertebral lamina on one side only 偏侧椎板切除术

hemi·lar·yn·gec·to·my (hem″e-lar″in-jek′tə- me) excision of one lateral half of the larynx 偏侧喉切除术，半喉切除术

hemi·lat·er·al (hem″e-lat′ər-əl) affecting one lateral half of the body only 偏侧的

hemi·me·lia (hem″e-me′le-ə) a developmental anomaly characterized by absence of all or part of a forearm 半肢畸形

he·min (he′min) 1. a porphyrin chelate of iron, derived from red blood cells; the chloride of heme. It is used to treat the symptoms of various porphyrias 氯高铁血红素；2. 同 hematin (1)

hemi·ne·phrec·to·my (hem″e-nə-frek′tə-me) excision of part (half) of a kidney 肾部分切除术

hemi·opia (hem″e-o′pe-ə) hemianopia 偏盲；一侧视野缺失；**hemiop′ic** adj.

hemi·par·a·ple·gia (hem″e-par″ə-ple′jə) paralysis of the lower half of one side 偏侧下身麻痹

hemi·pa·re·sis (hem″e-pə-re′sis) paresis affecting one side of the body. 轻偏瘫

hemi·pa·ret·ic (hem″e-pə-ret′ik) 1. pertaining to hemiparesis 轻偏瘫的；2. one affected with hemiparesis 轻偏瘫者

hemi·ple·gia (hem″e-ple′jə) paralysis of one side of the body 偏瘫，半身不遂；**hemiple′gic** adj.; **alternate h.**, paralysis of one side of the face and the opposite side of the body 交替性瘫痪；**cerebral h.**, that due to a brain lesion 脑性偏瘫；

crossed h., 同 alternate h.; **facial h.**, paralysis of one side of the face 面偏瘫, 偏侧面瘫; **spastic h.**, hemiplegia with spasticity of the affected muscles and increased tendon reflexes 痉挛性偏瘫; **spinal h.**, that due to a lesion of the spinal cord 脊髓性偏瘫

He·mip·tera (he-mip′tər-ə) an order of insects, winged or wingless, including ordinary bugs and lice, having mouth parts adapted for piercing and sucking 半翅目

hemi·ra·chis·chi·sis (hem″e-rə-kis′kǐ-sis) rachischisis without prolapse of the spinal cord 隐性脊柱裂

hemi·sec·tion (hem″e-sek′shən) 1. division into two equal parts 一半切除; 对切; 2. surgical division of a multiple rooted tooth from the crown to the furcation with removal of a root and part of the crown 半切牙术

hemi·spasm (hem′e-spaz″əm) spasm affecting one side only 偏侧痉挛, 半侧痉挛

hemi·sphere (hem′ĭ-sfēr) half of a spherical or roughly spherical structure or organ 半球; **cerebellar h.**, either of two lobes of the cerebellum lateral to the vermis 小脑半球; **cerebral h.**, one of the paired structures forming the bulk of the human brain, which together comprise the cerebral cortex, centrum semiovale, basal ganglia, and rhinencephalon and contain the lateral ventricles 大脑半球; **dominant h.**, the cerebral hemisphere that is more concerned than the other in the integration of sensations and the control of voluntary functions 优势（大脑）半球

hemi·sphe·ri·um (hem″ĭ-sfēr′e-əm) pl. *hemi-sphe′ria* [L.] either cerebral hemisphere 半球

hemi·ver·te·bra (hem″e-vur′tə-brə) 1. a developmental anomaly in which one side of a vertebra is incompletely developed 半脊椎畸形; 2. a vertebra that is incompletely developed on one side 半脊椎体

hemi·zy·gos·i·ty (hem″e-zi-gos′ĭ-te) the state of having only one of a pair of alleles transmitting a specific character, particularly the state of the male for X-linked genes 半合子状态; **hemizy′gous** adj.

he·mo·blast (he′mo-blast) blast cell 血原细胞, 成血细胞

He·moc·cult (he′mo-kəlt) trademark for a guaiac reagent strip test for occult blood 潜血检测试纸

he·mo·cho·ri·al (he″mo-kor′e-əl) denoting a type of placenta in which maternal blood comes in direct contact with the chorion, as in humans 血性绒毛膜的, 绒毛膜受血的

he·mo·chro·ma·to·sis (he″mo-kro″mə-to′sis) abnormal deposition of hemosiderin in the hepatic cells, causing tissue damage; dysfunction of the liver, pancreas, heart, and pituitary; and bronze skin.

It is usually an autosomal recessive condition but is occasionally acquired 血色素沉着病, 血色素沉积症; **hemochromatot′ic** adj.

he·mo·con·cen·tra·tion (he″mo-kon″sən′tra′shən) decrease of the fluid content of the blood, with increased concentration of formed elements 血浓缩

he·mo·co·nia (he″mo-ko′ne-ə) pl. *hemoco′niae* [L.] small bodies exhibiting brownian movement, observed in blood platelets in darkfield microscopy of a wet film of blood 血尘

he·mo·cy·a·nin (he″mo-si′ə-nin) a blue copper-containing respiratory pigment occurring in the blood of mollusks and arthropods 血蓝蛋白, 血青素

he·mo·cyte (he′mo-sīt) blood cell 血细胞

he·mo·cy·to·blast (he″mo-si′to-blast) blast cell 成血细胞

he·mo·cy·tom·e·ter (he″mo-si-tom′ə-tər) hemacytometer 血细胞计数器

he·mo·cy·to·trip·sis (he″mo-si″to-trip′sis) disintegration of blood cells by pressure 血细胞压碎, 通过压力解体血细胞

he·mo·di·a·fil·tra·tion (he″mo-di″ə-filtra′shən) hemofiltration with a dialytic component, so that blood flow is accelerated 血液透析滤过

he·mo·di·ag·no·sis (he″mo-di″əg-no′sis) diagnosis by examination of the blood 验血诊断法

he·mo·di·al·y·sis (he″mo-di-al′ə-sis) removal of certain elements from the blood by virtue of the difference in rates of their diffusion through a semipermeable membrane while being circulated outside the body; the process involves both diffusion and ultrafiltration 血液透析

he·mo·di·a·lyz·er (he″mo-di″ə-līz″ər) an apparatus for performing hemodialysis 血液透析器

he·mo·di·lu·tion (he″mo-di-loo′shən) increase in fluid content of blood, resulting in lowered concentration of formed elements 血液稀释

he·mo·dy·nam·ics (he″mo-di-nam′iks) the study of the movements of blood and of the forces concerned 血流动力学, 血液动力学; **hemodynam′ic** adj.

he·mo·fil·tra·tion (he″mo-fil-tra′shən) removal of waste products from blood by passing it through extracorporeal filters 血液滤过

he·mo·flag·el·late (he″mo-flaj′ə-lāt) any flagellate protozoan parasite of the blood; the term includes the genera *Trypanosoma* and *Leishmania* 血鞭毛虫

he·mo·fus·cin (he″mo-fūs′in) a brownishyellow hematogenous pigment resulting from hemoglobin decomposition, sometimes seen in the urine 血褐素, 血棕色素

he·mo·glo·bin (Hb) (he′mo-glo″bin) the oxygencarrying pigment of erythrocytes, formed by developing erythrocytes in the bone marrow; a hemoprotein made up of four different polypeptide globin chains that contain between 141 and 146 amino acids. Hemoglobin A is normal adult hemoglobin and hemoglobin F is fetal hemoglobin. Many abnormal hemoglobins have been reported; the first were given capital letters such as hemoglobin E, H, M, and S, and later ones have been named for the place of discovery. Homozygosity for hemoglobin S results in sickle cell anemia, and heterozygosity results in sickle cell trait 血红蛋白；**fetal h.**, that forming more than half of the hemoglobin of the fetus, present in minimal amounts in adults and abnormally elevated in certain blood disorders 胎儿血红素，胎血红蛋白；**mean corpuscular h. (MCH)**, the average hemoglobin content of an erythrocyte 红细胞平均血红蛋白；**muscle h.**, myoglobin 肌红蛋白；**reduced h.**, that not combined with oxygen 还原血红蛋白；**h. S**, the most common abnormal hemoglobin, with valine substituted for glutamic acid at position six of the beta chain, resulting in the abnormal erythrocytes called sickle cells, and causing sickle cell anemia 血红蛋白 S

he·mo·glo·bin·emia (he″mo-glo′bin-e′me-ə) excessive hemoglobin in blood plasma 血红蛋白血症

he·mo·glo·bin·ol·y·sis (he″mo-glo″bin-ol′ə- sis) the splitting up of hemoglobin 血红蛋白分解

he·mo·glo·bin·om·e·ter (he″mo-glo″binom′ə-tər) an instrument for colorimetric determination of hemoglobin content of blood 血红蛋白计数

he·mo·glo·bin·op·a·thy (he″mo-glo″bin-op′-ə-the) 1. a hematologic disorder due to alteration in the genetically determined molecular structure of hemoglobin, such as sickle cell anemia, hemolytic anemia, or thalassemia 遗传性分子结构变异性血红蛋白病；2. sometimes more specifically, a hemoglobin disorder due to alterations in a globin chain, as opposed to the reduced or absent synthesis of normal chains in thalassemia 氨基酸序列改变性血红蛋白病

he·mo·glo·bin·uria (he″mo-glo″bĭ-nu′re-ə) free hemoglobin in the urine 血红蛋白尿；**hemoglobinu′ric adj.**；**march h.**, that seen after prolonged exercise 行军性血红蛋白尿症；**paroxysmal cold h.**, an autoimmune or postviral disease marked by episodes of hemoglobinemia and hemoglobinuria after exposure to cold, caused by complement-dependent hemolysis due to Donath-Landsteiner antibody 阵发性冷性血红蛋白尿症；**paroxysmal nocturnal h. (PNH)**, a chronic acquired blood cell abnormality with episodes of intravascular hemolysis and venous thrombosis 阵发性睡眠性血红蛋白尿症；**toxic h.**, that caused by ingestion of a poison 中毒性血红蛋白尿

he·mo·ki·ne·sis (he″mo-kī-ne′sis) circulation 血液流动；**hemokinet′ic adj.**

he·mo·lymph (he′mo-limf″) 1. blood and lymph 血淋巴；2. the bloodlike fluid of those invertebrates having open blood-vascular systems 血液（无脊椎动物）

he·mol·y·sin (he-mol′ə-sin) a substance that liberates hemoglobin from erythrocytes by interrupting their structural integrity 溶血素

he·mol·y·sis (he-mol′ə-sis) the liberation of hemoglobin, consisting of separation of the hemoglobin from the red cells and its appearance in the plasma 溶血（作用），溶血现象；**hemolyt′ic adj.**；**immune h.**, lysis by complement of erythrocytes sensitized as a consequence of interaction with specific antibody to the erythrocytes 免疫溶血

he·mo·lyze (he′mo-līz) 1. to subject to hemolysis 使溶血；2. to undergo hemolysis 发生溶血

he·mo·me·di·as·ti·num (he″mo-me″di-ə-sti′nəm) an effusion of blood into the mediastinum 纵隔血肿，纵隔积血

he·mo·me·tra (he″mo-me′trə) hematometra 子宫积血

he·mo·pa·thol·o·gy (he″mo-pə-thol′ə-je) the study of diseases of the blood 血液病理学

he·mop·a·thy (he-mop′ə-the) any disease of the blood 血液病；**hemopath′ic adj.**

he·mo·per·fu·sion (he″mo-pər-fu′zhən) the passing of large volumes of blood over an extracorporeal adsorbent substance in order to remove toxic substances 血液灌流

he·mo·peri·car·di·um (he″mo-per″ĭ-kahr′de- əm) an effusion of blood within the pericardium 心包积血

he·mo·pex·in (he″mo-pek′sin) a heme-binding serum glycoprotein 血色素结合蛋白

he·mo·phago·cyte (he″mo-fa′go-sīt) a phagocyte that destroys blood cells 噬红细胞

he·mo·phil (he′mo-fil) 1. an organism thriving on blood 嗜血的；2. a microorganism that grows best in media containing hemoglobin 嗜血菌

he·mo·phil·ia (he″mo-fil′e-ə) a hereditary hemorrhagic diathesis due to deficiency of a blood coagulation factor 血友病；**h. A**, classical h.; an X-linked recessive form due to deficiency of coagulation factor Ⅷ血友病 A；**h. B**, Christmas disease; an X-linked recessive form due to deficiency of coagulation factor Ⅸ血友病 B；**h. C**, factor Ⅺ deficiency 血友病 C；**classical h.**, h. 典型性血友病；**vascular h.**, von Willebrand disease. 血管性

血友病

he·mo·phil·ic (he-mo-fil′ik) 1. having an affinity for blood; in bacteriology, growing well in culture media containing blood or having a nutritional affinity for constituents of fresh blood 嗜血的；2. pertaining to or characterized by hemophilia 血友病的

he·mo·pho·bia (he″mo-fo′be-ə) irrational fear of blood 恐血症，血恐怖

he·mo·plas·tic (he″mo-plas′tik) hematopoietic 成血的

he·mo·pneu·mo·peri·car·di·um (he″monoo″mo-per″ī-kahr′de-əm) pneumohemopericardium 血气心包

he·mo·pneu·mo·tho·rax (he″mo-noo″mothor′aks) pneumothorax with hemorrhagic effusion 血气胸

he·mo·pre·cip·i·tin (he″mo-pre-sip′ī-tin) a blood precipitin 血沉淀素

he·mo·pro·tein (he′mo-pro″tēn) a conjugated protein containing heme as the prosthetic group, such as catalase, cytochrome, hemoglobin, or myoglobin 血红素蛋白

he·mop·so·nin (he″mop-so′nin) an opsonin making erythrocytes more liable to phagocytosis 血调理素，红细胞调理素（使血细胞易被吞噬的调理素）

he·mop·ty·sis (he-mop′tĭ-sis) the spitting of blood or of blood-stained sputum 咯血；**parasitic h.,** lung infection with flukes of genus *Paragonimus,* with cough, spitting of blood, and slow deterioration 寄生虫性咯血

he·mo·rhe·ol·o·gy (he″mo-re-ol′ə-je) the study of the deformation and flow properties of cellular and plasmatic components of blood and the rheologic properties of vessel structures it comes in contact with 血液流变学

hem·or·rhage (hem′ə-rəj) the escape of blood from the vessels; bleeding 出血；**hemorrhag′ic** adj.; **capillary h.,** the oozing of blood from the minute vessels 毛细血管出血；**cerebral h.,** hemorrhage into the cerebrum 脑出血；见 *stroke syndrome*；**concealed h.,** internal h. 隐匿性出血；**Duret h's,** small, linear hemorrhages in the midline of the brainstem and upper pons caused by traumatic downward displacement of the brainstem 脑干出血，桥脑出血；**fibrinolytic h.,** that due to abnormalities of fibrinolysis 纤溶出血；**internal h.,** that in which the extravasated blood remains within the body 内出血；**intracranial h.,** bleeding within the cranium, which may be extradural, subdural, subarachnoid, or cerebral (parenchymatous); all types can cause brain damage because of increased intracranial pressure 颅内出血；**petechial h.,** the tiny capillary hemorrhage that causes a petechia 点状出血；**splinter h.,** a linear hemorrhage beneath the nail 裂片形出血

hem·or·rha·gin (hem″ə-ra′jin) a cytolysin in certain venoms and poisons that is destructive to endothelial cells and blood vessels 出血蛇毒素，出血素

hem·or·rhoid (hem′ə-roid) prolapse of an anal cushion, resulting in bleeding and painful swelling in the anal canal 痔；**hemorrhoi′dal** adj.; **external h.,** a hemorrhoid distal to the pectinate line, covered with modified anal skin 外痔；**internal h.,** a hemorrhoid originating above the pectinate line, covered by mucous membrane 内痔；**mixed h.,** prolapse of an anal cushion on both sides of the pectinate line, forming an external and an internal hemorrhoid in continuity 混合痔；**prolapsed h.,** an internal hemorrhoid that has descended below the pectinate line and protruded outside the anal sphincter 脱痔，翻花痔；**strangulated h.,** a prolapsed hemorrhoid whose blood supply has become occluded by constriction of the anal sphincter 绞窄性痔；**thrombosed h.,** a hemorrhoid containing clotted blood 血栓性痔

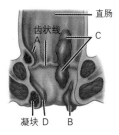

▲ 痔 **A.** 内痔。**B.** 外痔。**C.** 混合痔。**D.** 血栓性痔

hem·or·rhoid·ec·to·my (hem″ə-roid-ek′tə- me) excision of hemorrhoids 痔切除术

he·mo·sid·er·in (he″mo-sid′ər-in) an insoluble form of tissue storage iron, visible microscopically both with and without the use of special stains 含铁血黄素，血铁黄素蛋白

he·mo·sid·er·in·uria (he″mo-sid″ər-ĭ-nu′- re-ə) hemosiderin in the urine, as in hemochromatosis 含铁血黄素尿

he·mo·sid·er·o·sis (he″mo-sid″ər-o′sis) a focal or general increase in tissue iron stores without associated tissue damage 含铁血黄素沉着症；**pulmonary h.,** the deposition of abnormal amounts of hemosiderin in the lungs, due to bleeding into the lung interstitium 肺含铁血黄素沉着症

he·mo·sta·sis (he″mo-sta′sis) (he-mos′tə-sis) 1. the arrest of bleeding by the physiologic properties of vasoconstriction and coagulation or by surgical means 止血；2. interruption of blood flow through any vessel or to any anatomic area 中断止血

he·mo·stat (he′mo-stat) 1. a small surgical clamp for constricting blood vessels 止血钳；2. an antihemorrhagic agent 止血药

he·mo·stat·ic (he″mo-stat′ik) 1. causing hemostasis, or an agent that so acts 止血药；2. due to or characterized by stasis of the blood 止血性

he·mo·tho·rax (he″mo-thor′aks) a pleural effusion containing blood 血胸

he·mo·tox·ic (he′mo-tok″sik) hematotoxic 血中毒的

he·mo·tox·in (he′mo-tok″sin) an exotoxin characterized by hemolytic activity 血毒素

Hen·i·pa·vi·rus (hen′ĭ-pə-vi″rəs) a genus of viruses of the family Paramyxoviridae, subfamily Paramyxovirinae; it includes Hendra virus 尼帕病毒属

hen·ry (H) (hen′re) the SI unit of electric inductance, equivalent to 1 weber per ampere 亨（利）（电感单位）

HEP hepatoerythropoietic porphyria 肝性红细胞生成性卟啉症

Hep·a·ci·vi·rus (hep-as′ĭ-vi″rəs) the hepatitis C viruses, a genus of the family Flaviviridae that causes hepatitis C 丙型肝炎病毒属

Hep·ad·na·vi·ri·dae (hep-ad″nə-vir′ĭ-de) the hepatitis B–like viruses, a family of DNA viruses that cause infections, including hepatitis B, in humans and other animals. The human pathogens are in the genus *Orthohepadnavirus* 嗜肝病毒科

he·par (he′pahr) [Gr.] liver 肝

hep·a·ran sul·fate (hep′ə-ran) a glycosaminoglycan occurring in the cell membrane of most cells, consisting of a repeating disaccharide unit of glucosamine and uronic acid residues, which may be acetylated and sulfated; it accumulates in several mucopolysaccharidoses 硫酸乙酰肝素

hep·a·rin (hep′ə-rin) a sulfated glycosaminoglycan of mixed composition, released by mast cells and by blood basophils in many tissues, especially the liver and lungs, and having potent anticoagulant properties. It also has lipotrophic properties, promoting transfer of fat from blood to the fat depots by activation of lipoprotein lipase. It is used as the calcium or sodium salt in the prophylaxis and treatment of disorders in which there is excessive or undesirable clotting and to prevent clotting during extracorporeal circulation, blood transfusion, and blood sampling 肝素

hep·a·ri·nize (hep′ə-rĭ-nīz″) to render blood incoagulable with heparin 肝素化

hep·a·ta·tro·phia (hep″ə-tə-tro′fe-ə) atrophy of the liver 肝萎缩

he·pat·ic (hə-pat′ik) pertaining to the liver 肝的

he·pat·i·co·du·o·de·nos·to·my (hə-pat″ĭ-kodoo″o-də-nos′tə-me) anastomosis of the hepatic duct to the duodenum 肝管十二指肠吻合术

he·pat·i·co·gas·tros·to·my (hə-pat″ĭ-ko-gastros′tə-me) anastomosis of the hepatic duct to the stomach 肝管胃吻合术

he·pat·i·co·li·thot·o·my (hə-pat″ĭ-ko-lĭ- thot′ə-me) incision of the hepatic duct, with removal of calculi 肝管（切开）取石术

he·pat·i·cos·to·my (hə-pat″ĭ-kos′tə-me) fistulization of the hepatic duct 肝管造口术

he·pat·ic phos·phor·y·lase (hə-pat′ik fosfor′ə-lās) the liver isozyme of glycogen phosphorylase; deficiency causes glycogen storage disease, type VI 肝磷酸化酶（糖原磷酸化酶的肝同工酶）

hep·a·ti·tis (hep″ə-ti′tis) pl. *hepati′tides*. Inflammation of the liver 肝炎；**h. A,** a self-limited viral disease of worldwide distribution, usually transmitted by oral ingestion of infected material but sometimes transmitted parenterally; most cases are clinically inapparent or have mild flulike symptoms; any jaundice is mild 甲型肝炎；**anicteric h.,** viral hepatitis without jaundice 无黄疸型肝炎；**h. B,** an acute viral disease transmitted mainly parenterally (sometimes orally) by intimate personal contact, or from mother to neonate. Prodromal symptoms of fever, malaise, anorexia, nausea, and vomiting decline with onset of clinical jaundice, angioedema, urticarial skin lesions, and arthritis. After 3 to 4 months most patients recover completely, but some may become carriers or remain ill chronically 乙型肝炎；**h. C,** a viral disease caused by the hepatitis C virus, commonly occurring after transfusion or parenteral drug abuse; it frequently progresses to a chronic form that is usually asymptomatic but that may involve cirrhosis 丙型肝炎；**cholangiolitic h.,** cholestatic h. (1) 毛细胆管性肝炎；**cholestatic h.,** 1. inflammation of the bile ducts of the liver associated with obstructive jaundice 淤胆型肝炎；2. hepatic inflammation and cholestasis resulting from a reaction to drugs such as estrogens or chlorpromazines 药物性肝炎及胆汁淤积；**h. D, delta h.,** infection with hepatitis D virus, occurring either simultaneously with or as a superinfection in hepatitis B, whose severity it may increase 丁型肝炎；**h. E,** a type transmitted by the oral-fecal route, usually via contaminated water; chronic infection does not occur, but acute infection may be fatal in pregnant women 戊型肝炎；**enterically transmitted non-A, non-B h. (ET-NANB),** 同 h. E.；**h. G,** a post-transfusion disease caused by hepatitis G virus, ranging from asymptomatic infection to fulminant hepatitis 庚

型肝炎；**infectious h.**, **h. A** 传染性肝炎；**lupoid h.**, chronic active hepatitis with autoimmune manifestations 狼疮样肝炎；**neonatal h.**, a type with an uncertain etiology, occurring soon after birth, marked by prolonged persistent jaundice that may progress to cirrhosis 新生儿肝炎；**non-A, non-B h.**, acute viral hepatitis without the serologic markers of hepatitis A or B; usually hepatitis C or hepatitis E 通常是丙型肝炎或戊型肝炎；**posttransfusion h.**, viral hepatitis, now usually hepatitis C, transmitted via transfusion of blood or blood products, especially multiple pooled donor products such as clotting factor concentrates 输血后肝炎；**serum h.**, **h. B** 血清肝炎；**transfusion h.**, posttransfusion h. 输血性肝炎；**viral h.**, h. A, h. B, h. C, h. D, and h. E 病毒性肝炎

hep·a·ti·za·tion (hep″ə-tĭ-za′shən) consolidation of tissue into a liverlike mass, as in the lung in lobar pneumonia. The early stage, in which pulmonary exudate is blood stained, is called *red h*. The later stage, in which *red* cells disintegrate and a fibrinosuppurative exudate persists, is called *gray h*. 肝样变

hep·a·to·blas·to·ma (hep″ə-to-blas-to′mə) a malignant intrahepatic tumor consisting chiefly of embryonic tissue, occurring in infants and young children 肝母细胞瘤

hep·a·to·car·ci·no·ma (hep″ə-to-kahr″sĭ- no′mə) hepatocellular carcinoma 肝癌

hep·a·to·cele (hə-pat′o-sēl) hernia of the liver 肝膨出，肝突出

hep·a·to·cel·lu·lar (hep″ə-to-sel′u-lər) pertaining to or affecting liver cells 肝细胞的

hep·a·to·cho·lan·gio·car·ci·no·ma (hep″ə- to-ko-lan″je-o-kahr″sĭ-no′mə) cholangiohepatoma 胆管肝细胞癌

hep·a·to·cyte (hep′ə-to-sīt) a hepatic cell 肝（实质）细胞

hep·a·to·gas·tric (hep″ə-to-gas′trik) pertaining to the liver and stomach 肝胃的

hep·a·to·gen·ic (hep″ə-to-jen′ik) 1. giving rise to or forming liver tissue 生肝的；2. originating in the liver 肝源性的

hep·a·tog·e·nous (hep″ə-toj′ə-nəs) 同 hepatogenic

hep·a·to·gram (hep′ə-to-gram) a radiograph of the liver 肝 X 线（照）片

hep·a·toid (hep′ə-toid) resembling the liver 肝样的

hep·a·to·jug·u·lar (hep″ə-to-jug′u-lər) pertaining to the liver and jugular vein 肝颈静脉的；见 *reflux* 下词条

hep·a·to·lith (hep′ə-to-lith″) a calculus in the liver 肝石

hep·a·to·li·thi·a·sis (hep″ə-to-lĭ-thi′ə-sis) formation

or presence of calculi in the liver 肝石病

hep·a·tol·o·gy (hep″ə-tol′ə-je) the scientific study of the liver and its diseases 肝脏病学，肝脏学

hep·a·tol·y·sin (hep″ə-tol′ĭ-sin) a cytolysin destructive to liver cells 溶肝素

hep·a·tol·y·sis (hep″ə-tol′ ĭ-sis) destruction of the liver cells 肝细胞溶解；**hepatolyt′ic** *adj.*

hep·a·to·ma (hep″ə-to′mə) 1. a tumor of the liver 肝癌；2. hepatocellular carcinoma (malignant h.) 肝细胞癌

hep·a·to·meg·a·ly (hep″ə-to-meg′ə-le) enlargement of the liver 肝（肿）大

hep·a·to·mel·a·no·sis (hep″ə-to-mel″ə-no′- sis) melanosis of the liver 肝黑变病

hep·a·tom·pha·lo·cele (hep″ə-tom′fə-lo-sēl) umbilical hernia with liver involvement in the hernial sac 脐部肝突出

hep·a·to·pexy (hep″ə-to-pek′se) surgical fixation of a displaced liver 肝固定术

hep·a·to·pneu·mon·ic (hep″ə-to-noo-mon′ik) pertaining to, affecting, or communicating with the liver and lungs 肝肺的

hep·a·to·por·tal (hep″ə-to-por′təl) pertaining to the portal system of the liver 肝门静脉的

hep·a·to·re·nal (hep″ə-to-re′nəl) pertaining to the liver and kidneys 肝肾的

hep·a·tor·rhex·is (hep″ə-to-rek′sis) rupture of the liver 肝破裂

hep·a·to·sis (hep″ə-to′sis) any functional disorder of the liver 肝病，肝功能障碍；**serous h.**, veno-occlusive disease of the liver 浆液性肝功能障碍

hep·a·to·sple·ni·tis (hep″ə-to-splə-ni′tis) inflammation of the liver and spleen 肝脾炎

hep·a·to·sple·no·meg·a·ly (hep″ə-to-sple″nomeg′ə-le) enlargement of the liver and spleen 肝脾（肿）大

hep·a·to·tox·in (hep″ə-to-tok″sin) a toxin that destroys liver cells 肝毒素；**hep′atotoxic** *adj.*

Hep·a·to·vi·rus (hep′ə-to-vi″rəs) a genus of viruses of the family Picornaviridae that contains just one species, hepatitis A virus 肝炎病毒属；**hepatoviral** *adj.*

Hep·e·vi·rus (hep-e′vi-rəs) a genus of viruses that includes hepatitis E virus; it has not yet been assigned to a family 肝炎病毒属；戊型肝炎病毒属

hep·ta·chro·mic (hep″tə-kro′mik) 1. pertaining to or exhibiting seven colors 七色的；2. able to distinguish all seven colors of the spectrum 能辨七色光谱的

-hep·ta·ene a suffix denoting a chemical compound in which there are seven conjugated double bonds [后缀] 七烯化合物

hep·ta·no·ate (hep″tə-no′āt) enanthate 庚酸盐

hep·tose (hep′tōs) a sugar whose molecule contains seven carbon atoms 庚糖

herb (urb) (hurb) any leafy plant without a woody

stem, especially one used medicinally or as a flavoring 草药；草本；**her′bal** *adj.*

her·bal·ism (ur′-) (hur′bəl-iz-əm) the medical use of preparations containing only plant material 草药疗法，草药学

her·biv·o·rous (ər-) (hər-biv′ə-rəs) subsisting upon plants 草食性

he·red·i·tary (hə-red′ĭ-tar-e) genetically transmitted from parent to offspring 遗传的

he·red·i·ty (hə-red′ĭ-te) the genetic transmission of a particular quality or trait from parent to offspring 遗传

her·i·ta·bil·i·ty (her″ĭ-tə-bil′ĭ-te) 1. the capacity to be inherited 遗传力；2. a measure of the extent to which a phenotype is influenced by the genotype 遗传力；**her′itable** *adj.*

her·maph·ro·dite (hər-maf′ro-dīt) an individual with hermaphroditism 雌雄同体

her·maph·ro·di·tism (hər-maf′rə-dī-tiz″əm) co-existence of both ovarian and testicular tissue in an individual 雌雄同体，两性畸形；另见 *true h.*；**hermaphrodit′ic** *adj.*；**true h.**, former name for *ovo-testicular disorder of sex development* 真两性畸形

her·met·ic (hər-met′ik) impervious to air 密封的，不透气的

her·nia (hur′ne-ə) [L.] protrusion of a portion of an organ or tissue through an abnormal opening 疝，疝气；**her′nial** *adj.*；**Amyand h.**, an inguinal hernia containing the vermiform appendix 包含阑尾的腹股沟疝；**Bochdalek h.**, congenital diaphragmatic hernia through the pleuroperitoneal hiatus 胸腹膜裂孔疝；**cerebral h.**, protrusion of brain substance through the cranium 脑疝；**complete h.**, one in which the sac and its contents have passed through the defect 全疝；**congenital diaphragmatic h.**, congenital protrusion of abdominal viscera into the thorax through an opening in the respiratory diaphragm resulting from defective development of the pleuroperitoneal membrane 先天性膈疝；**diaphragmatic h.**, one through the respiratory diaphragm into the thorax 膈疝；**epigastric h.**, one above the umbilicus in the midline 上腹疝；**external h.**, one that protrudes through an opening or defect in the muscle wall 外疝；**fat h.**, hernial protrusion of preperitoneal fat through the abdominal wall 脂肪疝；**femoral h.**, one protruding through the femoral ring into the femoral canal 股疝；**hiatal h.**, one protruding through the esophageal hiatus into the respiratory diaphragm 裂孔疝；**incarcerated h.**, one that cannot be returned or reduced by manipulation 嵌顿性疝；**incomplete h.**, one that has not passed entirely through the defect 不全疝；**inguinal h.**, one into the inguinal canal; classified as *indirect* if it passes through the deep inguinal ring and into the inguinal canal and is thus lateral to the inferior epigastric vessels and *direct* if it passes directly through the muscular and fascial wall of the abdomen and is thus medial to the inferior epigastric vessels 腹股沟疝；**internal h.**, one that protrudes through an opening or defect within the abdominal cavity into another abdominal compartment 内疝；**interparietal h.**, one lying between layers of the abdominal wall 腹壁间层疝；**irreducible h.**, incarcerated h. 难复性疝；**Littre h.**, one containing Meckel diverticulum 憩室疝；**lumbar h.**, one through defects in the lumbar muscles or the posterior fascia, below the twelfth rib and above the iliac crest 腰疝；**mesocolic h.**, paraduodenal h. 结肠系膜疝；**Morgagni h.**, congenital diaphragmatic hernia with extrusion of tissue into the thorax through the foramen of Morgagni 先天性胸骨后膈疝；**obturator h.**, one protruding through the obturator foramen 闭孔疝；**pantaloon h.**, inguinal hernia in which there are both direct and indirect hernial sacs 腹股沟疝；**paraduodenal h.**, internal hernia in which abnormal rotation of the midgut during development results in herniation of the small intestine behind the mesocolon 十二指肠旁疝；**paraesophageal h.**, hiatal hernia in which part of the stomach protrudes into the thorax but the esophagogastric junction remains in place 食管旁疝；**perineal h.**, one into the perineum through a defect in the pelvic diaphragm musculature and fascia 会阴疝；**preperitoneal h.**, one lying between the parietal peritoneum and the transversalis fascia 腹膜前间隙疝；**reducible h.**, one that can be returned by manipulation 可复性疝；**Richter h.**, a hernia in which only the antimesenteric side of the bowel is involved, rather than the entire lumen 肠壁疝；**rolling h.**, 同 paraesophageal h.；**sciatic h.**, one through the sciatic foramen 坐骨疝；**sliding h.**, one in which the serosa of an intra-abdominal organ, usually the colon or urinary bladder, forms part of the hernia sac 滑疝；**sliding hiatal h.**, hiatal hernia with the upper stomach and the esophagogastric junction protruding into the posterior mediastinum; the protrusion may be fixed or intermittent and is partially covered by a peritoneal sac 滑动性食管裂孔疝；**spigelian h.**, one through a defect at the lateral border of the rectus abdominis muscle at the level of the semilunar line 半月线疝；**strangulated h.**, incarcerated hernia so tightly constricted as to compromise the blood supply of the hernial sac, leading to gangrene of the sac and its contents 绞窄性疝；**synovial h.**, protrusion of the inner lining membrane through the fibrous membrane of a joint capsule 滑膜疝；**umbilical h.**, protrusion of part of the intestine at the umbilicus, the abdominal wall defect and protruding intestine covered by skin and superficial fascia 脐疝；**h. u′teri inguina′lis,** 见 *syndrome* 下 *persistent müllerian duct syndrome*；**ventral h.**, one in the anterior or lateral abdominal wall 腹壁疝

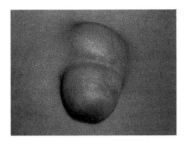

▲ 脐疝

her·ni·at·ed (hur′ne-āt″əd) protruding like a hernia; enclosed in a hernia 突出的，成疝的

her·ni·a·tion (hur″ne-a′shən) abnormal protrusion of an organ or other body structure through a defect or natural opening in a covering, membrane, muscle, or bone 疝出；**h. of intervertebral disk,** herniated disk; protrusion of the nucleus pulposus or anulus fibrosus of the disk, which may impinge on nerve roots 椎间盘突出；**h. of nucleus pulposus,** 髓核突出，见 *h. of intervertebral disk*；**tentorial h., transtentorial h.,** protrusion of brain structures through the tentorial notch; downward displacement *(descending transtentorial h.)* from a supratentorial mass is more common. *Ascending transtentorial h.* is when the cerebellum or nearby structures protrude upward 天幕裂孔疝，小脑幕裂孔疝

her·nio·plas·ty (hur′ne-o-plas″te) surgical repair of a hernia; sometimes specifically that using a mesh patch or plug for reinforcement 疝根治术。Cf. *herniorrhaphy*

her·ni·or·rha·phy (hur″ne-or′ə-fe) surgical repair of a hernia, sometimes specifically by apposition and suturing of the edges of the defect 疝修补术。Cf. *hernioplasty*

her·ni·ot·o·my (hə-r″ne-ot′ə-me) incision of a hernia for repair 疝切开术

her·o·in (her′o-in) diacetylmorphine; a highly addictive morphine derivative; the importation of heroin and its salts into the United States, as well as its use in medicine, is illegal 二乙酰吗啡，海洛因

herp·an·gi·na (hur″pən-ji′nə) herpes angina; an infectious febrile disease due to a coxsackievirus, marked by vesicular or ulcerated lesions on the fau-ces or soft palate 疱疹性咽峡炎

her·pes (hur′pēz) any inflammatory skin disease marked by the formation of small vesicles in clusters; the term is usually restricted to such diseases caused by herpesviruses and is used alone to refer to *h. simplex* or to *h. zoster.* 疱疹；由疱疹病毒引起的疾病；**h. febri′lis,** herpes simplex caused mainly by human herpesvirus 1, and primarily spread by oral secretions; it usually occurs as a concomitant of fever, and commonly involves the facial region, especially the vermilion border of the lips *(h. labialis)* and the nares; the vesicular lesions are self-limited 发热性疱疹；又称 *cold sore* 和 *fever blister*；**genital h., h. genita′lis,** herpes simplex in the genital region; it is mainly due to human herpesvirus 2 and is transmitted primarily sexually via genital secretions, and contact with viroids. Although symptoms in the female are more severe than in the male, the vesicular lesions are self-limited. Genital herpes at term in the pregnant female can lead to potentially fatal infection of the neonate 生殖器疱疹；**h. gestatio′nis,** a rare, self-limited, intensely pruritic, blistering skin disorder seen in pregnant women during the second and third trimesters and often recurring in subsequent pregnancies, resembling cutaneous herpes but not due to a herpesvirus; it may be an autoimmune disease 妊娠疱疹；**h. labia′lis,** herpes simplex on the vermilion border of the lips 唇疱疹；**h. sim′plex,** a group of acute infections caused by human herpesviruses 1 and 2, characterized by small fluidfilled vesicles on the skin or a mucous membrane with a raised erythematous base; it may be a primary infection or recurrent because of reactivation of a latent infection. Type 1 herpesvirus infections usually involve nongenital regions of the body, whereas type 2 infections are primarily on or around the genitals, although there is overlap between the two types. Precipitating factors include fever, exposure to cold temperature or ultraviolet rays, sunburn, cutaneous or mucosal abrasions, emotional stress, and nerve injury 单纯疱疹；**h. zos′ter,** shingles; an acute, unilateral, self-limited inflammatory disease of cerebral ganglia and the ganglia of posterior nerve roots and peripheral nerves in a segmented distribution, believed to represent activation of latent human herpesvirus 3 in those who have been rendered partially immune after a previous attack of chickenpox, and characterized by groups of small vesicles in the cutaneous areas along the course of affected nerves, and associated with neuralgic pain 带状疱疹；**h. zos′ter ophthal′micus,** herpes zoster involving the ophthalmic nerve, with a vesicular erythematous rash along the nerve path (forehead, eyelid, and cornea) preceded by lancinating pain; there is iridocyclitis, and corneal involvement may lead to keratitis and corneal anesthesia 眼带状疱疹；

h. zos′ter o′ticus, Ramsay Hunt syndrome (1) 耳带状疱疹

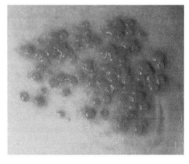

▲ 单纯疱疹，以簇集性的表皮小泡和真皮红斑为特征

Her·pes·vi·ri·dae (hur″pēz-vi′rī-de) the herpesviruses, a large family of DNA viruses that includes the genera *Cytomegalovirus, Lymphocryptovirus, Rhadinovirus, Roseolovirus, Simplexvirus,* and *Varicellovirus* 疱疹病毒科

her·pes·vi·rus (hur′pēz-vi″rəs) any virus of the family Herpesviridae 疱疹病毒属，见下表；**herpesvi′ral** *adj.*

her·pet·ic (hər-pet′ik) 1. pertaining to or of the nature of herpes 疱疹性的；2. pertaining to or caused by herpesviruses 疱疹病毒的

her·pet·i·form (hər-pet′ ĭ-form) resembling herpes; having grouped vesicles 疱疹样的

her·sage (ār-sahzh′) [Fr.] surgical separation of the fibers in a scarred area of a peripheral nerve 神经松解术

hertz (Hz) (hurts) the SI unit of frequency, equal to 1 cycle per second 赫，赫兹（频率单位）

hes·per·i·din (hes-per′ĭ-din) a bioflavonoid predominant in lemons and oranges 橙皮苷，橘皮苷

het·a·starch (het′ə-stahrch) an esterified amylopectin-containing starch, used as a plasma volume expander; administered by infusion 羟乙基淀粉

het·er·e·cious (het″ər-e′shəs) parasitic on different hosts in various stages of its existence 异栖的，异种寄生性的

het·er·er·gic (het″ər-ur′jik) having different effects; said of two drugs one of which produces a particular effect and the other does not 异效的，不同影响的

Human Herpesviruses 人类疱疹病毒科

Genus 属	Species 分类	Associated Disease 相关疾病
Simplexvirus 单纯疱疹病毒属	Human herpesvirus 1 人类疱疹病毒 1 型	Herpes simplex 单纯疱疹
Simplexvirus 单纯疱疹病毒属	Human herpesvirus 2 人类疱疹病毒 2 型	Herpes simplex 单纯疱疹
Varicellovirus 水痘病毒属	Human herpesvirus 3 人类疱疹病毒 3 型	Chickenpox, herpes zoster 水痘，带状疱疹
Lymphocryptovirus 淋巴隐病毒属	Human herpesvirus 4 (Epstein-Barr virus) 人类疱疹病毒 4 型 (E-B 病毒)	Infectious mononucleosis 传染性单核细胞增多症
Cytomegalovirus 巨细胞病毒属	Human herpesvirus 5 人类疱疹病毒 5 型	Cytomegalic inclusion disease 巨细胞包涵体病
Roseolovirus 玫瑰疹病毒属	Human herpesvirus 6 人类疱疹病毒 6 型	Exanthema subitum 幼儿急疹
Roseolovirus 玫瑰疹病毒属	Human herpesvirus 7 人类疱疹病毒 7 型	None known 未知
Rhadinovirus 猴病毒属	Human herpesvirus 8 人类疱疹病毒 8 型	Kaposi sarcoma, primary effusion lymphoma, multicentric plasma cell-type Castleman disease 卡波西肉瘤，原发性渗出性淋巴瘤，多中心卡斯尔曼病的大 B 细胞淋巴瘤

het·er·es·the·sia (het″ər-es-the′zhə) variation of cutaneous sensibility on adjoining areas 差异感觉

het·ero·ag·glu·ti·na·tion (het″ər-o-ə-gloo″tĭ-na′shən) agglutination of particulate antigens of one species by agglutinins derived from another species 异种凝集，异种凝集反应

het·ero·an·ti·body (het″ər-o-an″tĭ-bod′e) an antibody combining with antigens originating from a species foreign to the antibody producer 异种抗体

het·ero·an·ti·gen (het″ər-o-an″tĭ-jən) an antigen originating from a species foreign to the antibody producer 异种抗原

het·ero·blas·tic (het″ər-o-blas′tik) originating in a different kind of tissue 异形胚芽的，异生的

het·ero·cel·lu·lar (het″ər-o-sel′u-lər) composed of cells of different kinds 异型细胞的，异种细胞的

het·ero·chro·ma·tin (het″ər-o-kro′mə-tin) the form of chromatin that is dark-staining, genetically inactive, and tightly coiled; it can be constitutive or facultative 异染色质

het·ero·chro·mia (het″ər-o-kro′me-ə) diversity of color in a part normally of one color 异色性；**heterochro′mic** adj.; **iris h.**, difference of color in the two irides (h. iridum), or in different areas in the same iris (h. iridis) 虹膜异色，虹膜异色症

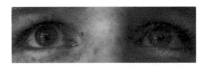

▲ 虹膜异色

het·ero·clad·ic (het″ər-o-klad′ik) pertaining to or characterized by an anastomosis between terminal branches from different arteries 动脉分支吻合的

het·ero·clit·ic (het″ər-o-klit′ik) irregular; said of a kind of antibody (see under *antibody*) 异偏态的

het·ero·crine (het′ər-o-krin) secreting more than one kind of matter 多种分泌的

het·ero·cyc·lic (het″ər-o-sik′lik) (-si′klik) having a closed chain or ring formation including atoms of different elements 杂环化合物

het·ero·cy·to·tro·pic (het″ər-o-si″to-tro′pik) having an affinity for cells from different species 亲异种细胞的

het·ero·der·mic (het″ər-o-dur′mik) denoting a skin graft from an individual of another species 异体皮肤移植的

het·ero·dont (het′ər-o-dont) having teeth of different shapes, such as molars, incisors, etc 异型齿，异齿型

het·er·od·ro·mous (het″ər-od′ro-məs) moving,

acting, or arranged in the opposite direction 异向旋转的，反向运动的

het·ero·erot·i·cism (het″ər-o-ə-rot′ ĭ-siz-əm) 1. sexual feeling directed toward someone of the opposite sex 性冲动；2. 同 alloeroticism (1) 异体性欲；3. a stage in which the erotic energy is directed toward objects other than oneself, specifically to those of the opposite sex 异体恋；**heteroerot′ic** adj.

het·ero·gam·e·ty (het″ər-o-gam′ə-te) the production of unlike gametes by an individual of one sex, as the production of X- and Y-bearing gametes by the human male 异型配子；**heterogamet′ic** adj.

het·er·og·a·my (het″ər-og′ə-me) 异配生殖 1. reproduction resulting from the union of two dissimilar gametes, particularly in higher organisms; 2. alternation of generations in which the two types of sexual reproduction alternate, as bisexual and parthenogenetic; **heterog′amous** adj.

het·ero·ge·ne·i·ty (het″ər-o-jə-ne′ ĭ-te) the state or quality of being heterogeneous 异质（原）性；**genetic h.**, the production of identical or similar phenotypes by more than one mutation, either by different mutant alleles at the same locus (allelic h.) or by mutations at two or more loci (locus h.) 遗传异质性

het·ero·ge·ne·ous (het″ər-o-je′ne-əs) 1. not of uniform composition, quality, or structure 不均匀的；2. in genetics, pertaining to a phenotype that can be produced by different mutations 异种的

het·er·og·e·nous (het″ər-oj′ə-nəs) 1. xenogeneic 异种；2. 同 heterogeneous

het·ero·geu·sia (het″ər-o-goo′zhə) any parageusia in which all gustatory stimuli are distorted in a similar way 异型味觉

het·ero·graft (het′ər-o-graft″) xenograft 异种移植物

het·ero·he·mag·glu·ti·na·tion (het″ər-ohe″mə-gloo″tĭ-na′shən) agglutination of erythrocytes of one species by a hemagglutinin derived from an individual of a different species 异种血凝反应，异种红细胞凝集

het·ero·he·mol·y·sin (het″ər-o-he-mol′ə-sin) a hemolysin that destroys red blood cells of animals of species other than that of the animal in which it is formed; it may occur naturally or be induced by immunization 异种溶血素

het·ero·im·mu·ni·ty (het″ə-ro-ĭ-mu′nĭ-te) 1. an immune state induced in an individual by immunization with cells of an animal of another species 异种免疫；2. a state in which an immune response to exogenous antigen (e.g., drugs or pathogens) results in immunopathologic changes 外源性抗原免疫；**heteroimmune′** adj.

het·ero·ker·a·to·plas·ty (het″ər-o-ker′ə-toplas″te) grafting of corneal tissue taken from an individual of another species 异种角膜形成术，异种角膜移植术

het·er·ol·o·gous (het″ər-ol′ə-gəs) 1. made up of tissue not normal to the part 异源的；2. xenogeneic 异种

het·er·ol·y·sis (het″ər-ol′ĭ-sis) lysis of the cells of one species by lysin from a different species 异种(细胞)溶解；**heterolyt′ic** adj.

het·ero·mer·ic (het″ər-o-mer′ik) sending processes through one of the commissures to the white matter of the opposite side of the spinal cord; said of neurons 异侧的（神经细胞突），神经细胞异侧的

het·ero·meta·pla·sia (het″ər-o-met″o-pla′zhə) formation of tissue foreign to the part where it is formed 异型发育

het·ero·met·ric (het″ər-o-met′rik) involving or dependent on a change in size 异原体；cf. *homeometric*

het·ero·me·tro·pia (het″ər-o-mə-tro′pe-ə) the state in which the refraction in the two eyes differs 屈光不等，双眼屈光差异

het·ero·mor·phic (het″ər-o-mor′fik) 1. of abnormal shape or structure 异形的；2. morphologically dissimilar 异态的

het·ero·mor·pho·sis (het″ər-o-mor-fo′sis) the development, particularly through regeneration, of an organ or structure inappropriate to the location 异形再生

het·er·on·o·mous (het″ər-on′ə-məs) 1. in biology, subject to different laws of growth; specialized along different lines 受不同生长规律支配的；2. in psychology, subject to another's will 异律的

het·er·on·y·mous (het″ər-on′ ī-məs) standing in opposite relations 异侧的

het·ero-os·teo·plas·ty (het″ər-o-os′te-o-plas″te) osteoplasty with bone taken from an individual of another species 异种骨成形术

het·er·oph·a·gy (het″ər-of′ə-je) the taking into a cell of exogenous material by phagocytosis or pinocytosis and the digestion of the ingested material after fusion of the newly formed vacuole with a lysosome 异体吞噬

het·ero·phil (het′ər-o-fil″) 1. a granular leukocyte represented by neutrophils in humans, but characterized in other mammals by granules that have variable sizes and staining characteristics 异嗜白细胞；2. 同 heterophilic

het·ero·phil·ic (het″ər-o-fil′ik) 1. having affinity for antigens or antibodies other than the one for which it is specific 异嗜性的（指对抗原或抗体）；2. staining with a type of stain other than the usual one 异染性的

het·ero·pho·ria (het″ər-o-for′e-ə) failure of the visual axes to remain parallel after elimination of visual fusional stimuli 隐斜视；**heterophor′ic** adj.

het·er·oph·thal·mia (het″ər-of-thal′me-ə) difference in the direction of the visual axes, or in the color, of the two eyes 两眼异色；两眼轴向不等

Het·er·oph·y·es (het″ər-of′e-ēz) a genus of minute trematode worms parasitic in the intestine of fish-eating mammals 异形吸虫属

het·ero·pla·sia (het″ər-o-pla′zhə) replacement of normal by abnormal tissue; malposition of normal cells 发育异常，再生异常；**heteroplas′tic** adj.; **progressive osseous h.**, progressive dermal ossification during childhood, inherited as an autosomal dominant loss of function mutation on the paternal allele, with development of islands of heterotopic bone within the dermis or subcutis, coalescence of the lesions into plaques, and invasion of deep connective tissues 进行性骨发育异常

het·ero·ploi·dy (het′ər-o-ploi″de) the state of having an abnormal number of chromosomes 异倍性

het·er·op·sia (het″ər-op′se-ə) unequal vision in the two eyes 双眼不等视

het·ero·sex·u·al (het″ər-o-sek′shoo-əl) 1. pertaining to, characteristic of, or directed toward the opposite sex 异性的，向异性的；2. one who is sexually attracted to or sexually active with the opposite sex 异性恋者

het·er·o·sis (het″ər-o′sis) the existence, in a first-generation hybrid, of greater vigor than is shown by either parent strain 杂种优势

het·er·os·po·rous (het″ər-os′pə-rəs) having two kinds of spores, which reproduce asexually 具异形孢子的

het·ero·sug·ges·tion (het″ər-o-səg-jes′chən) suggestion received from another person, as opposed to autosuggestion 他人暗示

het·ero·to·nia (het″ər-o-to′ne-ə) a state characterized by variations in tension or tone 异张性，张力不等；**heteroton′ic** adj.

het·ero·to·pia (het″ər-o-to′pe-ə) displacement or misplacement of parts; the presence of a tissue in an abnormal location 异位；**heterotop′ic** adj.

het·ero·trans·plan·ta·tion (het″ər-otrans-″plan-ta′shən) xenogeneic transplantation 异种移植术，异种移植

het·ero·tro·phic (het″ər-o-tro′fik) not selfsustaining; said of microorganisms requiring a reduced form of carbon for energy and synthesis 异养的

het·ero·tro·pia (het″ər-o-tro′pe-ə) strabismus 斜视，斜眼

het·ero·typ·ic (het″ə-ro-tip′ik) pertaining to, characteristic of, or belonging to a different type 异型的
het·ero·typ·i·cal (het″ər-o-tip′ĭ-kəl) heterotypic 异型的

het·er·ox·e·nous (het″ər-ok′sə-nəs) requiring more than one host to complete the life cycle 异种（宿主）寄生的，异栖

het·ero·zy·gos·i·ty (het″ər-o-zi-gos′ĭ-te) the state of possessing pairs of different alleles at one or more loci 杂合性，异型结合性（在某一位点上具有不同的等位基因）; **heterozy′gous** *adj.*

het·ero·zy·gote (het″ər-o-zi′gōt) an individual exhibiting heterozygosity 杂合子，异核合子; **manifesting h.**, a female heterozygous for an X-linked disorder in whom, because of unfavorable X inactivation, the trait is expressed clinically with the same severity as in hemizygous affected males 显示杂合子（一种女性杂合子的 X 连锁遗传病）

heu·ris·tic (hu-ris′tik) encouraging or promoting investigation; conducive to discovery 启发式的；鼓励或促使研究的，诱导发明的

hexa·chlo·ro·phene (hek″sə-klor′o-fēn) an antibacterial effective against gram-positive organisms; used as a local antiseptic and detergent for application to the skin 六氯酚

hex·ad (hek′sad) 1. a group or combination of six similar or related entities 六个一组; 2. an element with a valence of six 六价元素，六价基

hexa·dac·ty·ly (hek″sə-dak′tə-le) the occurrence of six digits on one hand or foot 六指（趾）畸形

hex·ane (hek′sān) a saturated hydrogen obtained by distillation from petroleum 己烷

hexo·ki·nase (hek″so-ki′nās) an enzyme that catalyzes the transfer of a high-energy phosphate group to a hexose, the initial step in the cellular utilization of free hexoses. The enzyme occurs in all tissues as various isozymes with varying specificities; the liver isozyme (type Ⅳ) is specific for glucose and is often called *glucokinase* 己糖激酶

hex·os·amine (hek-sōs′ə-mēn) any of a class of hexoses in which the hydroxyl group is replaced by an amino group 己糖胺

hex·os·amin·i·dase (hek″sōs-ə-min′ ĭ-dās) 1. any of the enzymes that cleave hexosamines or acetylated hexosamines from gangliosides or other glycosides 氨基己糖苷酶; 2. a specific hexosaminidase acting on keratan sulfate and ganglioside GM₂ and related compounds; occurring in several isoforms 一种特定己糖胺酶，特定氨基己糖酶

hex·ose (hek′sōs) a monosaccharide containing six carbon atoms in a molecule 己醣

hex·uron·ic ac·id (hek″su-ron′ik) any uronic acid formed by oxidation of a hexose 己糖醛酸

hex·yl·re·sor·ci·nol (hek″səl-rə-sor′sĭ-nol) a substituted phenol with bactericidal properties used as an antiseptic in mouthwashes and skin wound cleansers 己雷琐辛，己基间苯二酚

HF Hageman factor (coagulation factor Ⅻ) 哈格曼因子（凝血因子Ⅻ）

Hf hafnium 元素铪的符号

HFPEF heart failure with preserved ejection fraction 射血分数保留的心力衰竭

HFREF heart failure with reduced ejection fraction 射血分数降低的心力衰竭

Hg mercury (L. *hydrargy′rum*) 元素汞的符号

Hgb hemoglobin 血红蛋白

HGH hGH human growth hormone 人生长激素

HHPA hexahydrophthalic anhydride 六氢邻二甲酸酐

HHS Department of Health and Human Services （美国）卫生与人类服务部

hi·a·tus (hi-a′təs) [L.] an opening, gap, or cleft 裂孔，孔; **hia′tal** *adj.*; **aortic h.**, the opening in the respiratory diaphragm through which the aorta and thoracic duct pass 主动脉裂孔; **esophageal h.**, the opening in the respiratory diaphragm for the passage of the esophagus and the vagus nerves 食管裂孔; **pleuroperitoneal h.**, foramen of Bochdalek; a posterolateral opening in the fetal respiratory diaphragm; its failure to close leaves a congenital posterolateral defect that may become a site for congenital diaphragmatic hernia 胸膜裂孔; **sacral h.**, the opening at the inferior end of the sacral canal formed by failure of the laminae of the fifth and sometimes the fourth sacral vertebrae to meet in the midline 骶管裂孔; **saphenous h.**, the depression in the fascia lata bridged by the cribriform fascia and perforated by the great saphenous vein 隐静脉裂孔; **semilunar h., h. semiluna′ris**, the groove in the ethmoid bone through which the anterior ethmoidal air cells, the maxillary sinus, and sometimes the frontonasal duct drain via the ethmoid infundibulum 半月裂孔; **urogenital h.**, an opening in the pelvic diaphragm between the medial borders of the levator ani muscles of each side, which gives passage to the urethra and, in females, the vagina 泌尿生殖裂孔; **vena caval h.**, foramen venae cavae 腔静脉孔

hi·ber·na·tion (hi″bər-na′shən) 1. the dormant state in which certain animals pass the winter, marked by narcosis and by sharp reductions in body temperature and metabolism 动物冬眠; 2. an analogous temporary reduction in function, such as that of an organ（器官）冬眠; **artificial h.**, a state of reduced metabolism, muscle relaxation, and a twilight sleep resembling narcosis, produced by controlled inhibition of the sympathetic nervous system and causing attenuation of the homeostatic reactions of the organism 人工冬眠; **myocardial h.,** chronic but potentially reversible cardiac dysfunction caused by chronic myocardial ischemia, persisting at least until blood flow is restored 心肌冬眠

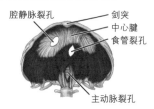

▲ 横膈膜的下视图，显示主动脉、食道和腔静脉通过的开口

hi·ber·no·ma (hi″bər-no′mə) a rare benign lipoma of soft tissue arising from vestiges of brown fat resembling that in hibernating animals; it is a small, lobulated, nontender lesion usually on the mediastinum or intrascapular region 蛰伏脂肪瘤，冬眠瘤，一种罕见的软组织良性脂肪瘤

hic·cup (hik′up) sharp sound of inhalation with spasm of the glottis and the respiratory diaphragm 呃逆，打嗝

hi·drad·e·ni·tis (hi″drad-ə-ni′tis) inflammation of the sweat glands 汗腺炎; **h. suppurati′va,** a severe, chronic, recurrent suppurative infection of the apocrine sweat glands 化脓性汗腺炎

hi·drad·e·no·car·ci·no·ma (hi-drad″ə-nokahr″sĭ-no′mə) a type of adnexal carcinoma arising in a sweat gland 汗腺癌

hi·drad·e·noid (hi-drad′ə-noid) resembling a sweat gland; having components resembling elements of a sweat gland 汗腺样的，类汗腺的

hi·drad·e·no·ma (hi-drad″ə-no′mə) a benign adnexal tumor originating in sweat gland epithelium; subtypes are named according to histologic pattern 汗腺腺瘤，汗腺瘤

hi·dro·ac·an·tho·ma (hi″dro-ak″an-tho′mə) a type of adenoma of an eccrine gland 汗腺棘皮瘤

hi·dro·cys·to·ma (hi″dro-sis-to′mə) a retention cyst of a sweat gland 汗腺囊瘤

hi·drot·ic (hi-drot′ik) 1. sudoriparous 出汗的，发汗的; 2. diaphoretic 发汗药

high-grade (hi′grād′) occurring near the high end of a range, as of a malignancy 优质的

hill·ock (hil′ək) a small prominence or elevation 丘，阜

hi·lum (hi′ləm) pl. *hi′la* [L.] a depression or pit on an organ, giving entrance and exit to vessels and nerves 门，脐。又称 *hilus*; **hi′lar** *adj.*

HIMSS Healthcare Information and Management Systems Society 医疗卫生信息与管理系统协会

hind·brain (hīnd′brān″) rhombencephalon 菱脑

hind·foot (hīnd′foot″) the back of the foot, comprising the region of the talus and calcaneus 足后段，包括距骨和跟骨

hind·gut (hīnd′gut″) the embryonic structure from which the caudal intestine, chiefly the colon, is formed 后肠

hip (hip) coxa; the region of the body around the joint between the femur and pelvis 髋关节; 髋(部)，臀部; **snapping h.,** a condition characterized by an audible or palpable snapping sensation that occurs during hip movement associated with exercise or normal daily activities, often accompanied by pain 髋关节弹响，弹响髋

hip·po·cam·pus (hip″o-kam′pəs) [L.] a convoluted elevation of gray matter in the floor of the temporal horn of the lateral ventricle; it is part of the limbic system and plays major roles in short-term memory and spatial navigation. The term often denotes the entire structure, including the hippocampus proper, dentate gyrus, and subiculum, but it can also be used more restrictively, most often denoting the hippocampus proper 海马; **hippocam′pal** *adj.*; **h. proper,** cornu ammonis; the tightly curved region of the hippocampus between the dentate gyrus and the subiculum; often used more broadly to denote the entire hippocampus (q.v.) 海马体

Hip·poc·ra·tes (hĭ-pok′rə-tēz) the Greek physician (5th century b.c.) regarded as the "Father of Medicine." Many of his writings and those of his school have survived, among which appears the Hippocratic Oath, the ethical guide of the medical profession 希波克拉底，希腊名医（公元前5世纪），被尊为"医学之父"; **hippocrat′ic** *adj.*

hip·pu·ric ac·id (hĭ-pūr′ik) $C_6H_5 \cdot CO \cdot NH \cdot C H_2COOH$, formed by conjugation of benzoic acid and glycine 马尿酸，N-苯甲酰甘氨酸

hip·pus (hip′əs) abnormal exaggeration of the rhythmic contraction and dilation of the pupil, independent of changes in illumination or in fixation of the eyes 虹膜震颤

hir·ci (hur′si) sing. *hir′cus.* [L.] the hairs growing in the axilla 腋毛

hir·sut·ism (hur′soot-iz-əm) abnormal hairiness, especially in women 多毛症，尤指妇女多毛

hi·ru·di·cide (hĭ-roo′dī-sīd) an agent that is destructive to leeches 杀水蛭药; **hirudici′dal** *adj.*

hi·ru·din (hĭ-roo′din) the active principle of the buccal secretion of leeches; it prevents coagulation by acting as an antithrombin 水蛭素

Hir·u·din·ea (hir″oo-din′e-ə) a class of annelids,

the leeches 蛭纲

Hi·ru·do (hĭ-roo′do) [L.] a genus of leeches, including *H. medicina′lis,* which have been used extensively for drawing blood 水蛭属

his·ta·mine (his′tə-mēn) an amine, $C_5H_9N_3$, produced by decarboxylation of histidine, found in all body tissues. It induces capillary dilation, which increases capillary permeability and lowers blood pressure; contraction of most smooth muscle tissue; increased gastric acid secretion; and acceleration of the heart rate. It is also a mediator of immediate hypersensitivity. There are three types of cellular receptors of histamine. H_1 receptors mediate the contraction of smooth muscle and capillary dilation, and H_2 receptors mediate acceleration of heart rate and promotion of gastric acid secretion. Both H_1 and H_2 receptors mediate the contraction of vascular smooth muscle. H3 receptors are believed to play a role in regulation of the release of histamine and other neurotransmitters from neurons. Histamine is used as an aid in the diagnosis of asthma and a positive control in skin testing 组胺；**histamin′ic** *adj.*

his·ta·min·er·gic (his″tə-min-ur′jik) pertaining to the effects of histamine at histamine receptors of target tissues 组织能的，被组胺激活的

his·ti·dase (his′tĭ-dās) an enzyme of the liver that converts histidine to urocanic acid 组氨酸酶

his·ti·dine (His, H) (his′tĭ-dēn) an essential amino acid obtainable from many proteins by the action of sulfuric acid and water; it is necessary for optimal growth in infants. Its decarboxylation results in formation of histamine 组氨酸

his·ti·din·emia (his″tĭ-dĭ-ne′me-ə) a hereditary aminoacidopathy marked by excessive histidine in the blood and urine due to deficient histidase activity; it is usually benign but may cause mild central nervous system dysfunction 组氨酸血症

his·ti·din·uria (his″tĭ-dĭ-nu′re-ə) an excess of histidine in the urine, usually associated with histidinemia or pregnancy 组氨酸尿

his·tio·cyte (his′te-o-sīt″) macrophage 组织细胞；**histiocyt′ic** *adj.*

his·tio·cy·to·ma (his″te-o-si-to′mə) a tumor containing histiocytes (macrophages) 皮肤纤维瘤；**benign fibrous h.,** any of a group of benign neoplasms in the dermis containing histiocytes and fibroblasts; the term sometimes encompasses types such as dermatofibroma, nodular subepidermal fibrosis, and sclerosing hemangioma, or may be used as a synonym for one of these 良性纤维组织细胞瘤；**malignant fibrous h.,** any of a group of malignant neoplasms containing cells resembling histiocytes and fibroblasts 恶性纤维组织细胞瘤

his·tio·cy·to·sis (his″te-o-si-to′sis) a condition marked by an abnormal appearance of histiocytes in the blood 组织细胞增生症，组织细胞增多病；**acute disseminated Langerhans cell h.,** Letterer-Siwe disease 急性播散性朗格汉斯细胞组织细胞增生症；莱特勒 - 西韦病；**Langerhans cell h.,** a generic term for a group of disorders characterized by proliferation of Langerhans cells (q.v.), believed to arise from disturbances in regulation of the immune system. Lesions may be unifocal or multifocal and may involve the bone marrow, endocrine system, or lungs 朗格汉斯细胞组织细胞增生症；**sinus h.,** a disorder of the lymph nodes in which the distended sinuses are filled by histiocytes, as a result of active multiplication of the littoral cells 窦组织细胞增多病；**h. X,** former name for *Langerhans cell h.* 组织细胞增多症 X

his·ti·o·gen·ic (his″te-o-jen′ik) histogenous 组织源的

his·to·blast (his′to-blast) a tissue-forming cell 成组织细胞

his·to·chem·is·try (his″to-kem′is-tre) that branch of histology dealing with the identification of chemical components in cells and tissues 组织化学；**histochem′ical** *adj.*

his·to·clin·i·cal (his″to-klin′ĭ-kəl) combining histologic and clinical evaluation 组织临床的

his·to·com·pat·i·bil·i·ty (his″to-kəm-pat″ĭ-bil′ĭ-te) that quality of being accepted and remaining functional; said of that relationship between the genotypes of donor and host in which a graft generally will not be rejected, a relationship determined by the presence of compatible HLA antigens 组织相容性；**histocompat′ible** *adj.*

his·to·dif·fer·en·ti·a·tion (his″to-dif″ər-en″shea′shən) the acquisition of tissue characteristics by cell groups 组织分化

his·to·gen·e·sis (his″to-jen′ə-sis) the formation or development of tissues from the undifferentiated cells of the germ layers of the embryo 组织发生；**histogenet′ic** *adj.*

his·tog·e·nous (his-toj′ə-nəs) formed by the tissues 组织原的

his·to·gram (his′to-gram) a graph in which values found in a statistical study are represented by vertical bars or rectangles 直方图，柱形图，矩形图

his·toid (his′toid) 1. developed from but one kind of tissue 单一组织的；2. like one of the tissues of the body 组织样的

his·to·in·com·pat·i·bil·i·ty (his″to-in″kəm-pat″ĭ-bil′ĭ-te) the quality of not being accepted or not remaining functional; said of that relationship between the genotypes of donor and host in which a graft generally will be rejected 组织不相容性；**histoincompat′ible** adj.

his·to·ki·ne·sis (his″to-kĭ-ne′sis) movement in the tissues of the body 组织运动

his·tol·o·gy (his-tol′ə-je) that department of anatomy dealing with the minute structure, composition, and function of tissues 组织学；**histolog′ic, histolog′ical** adj.；**pathologic h.**, the science of diseased tissues 病理组织学

his·tol·y·sis (his-tol′ə-sis) dissolution or breaking down of tissues 组织分解；**histolyt′ic** adj.

his·tone (his′tōn) a simple protein, soluble in water and insoluble in dilute ammonia, found combined as salts with acidic substances, e.g., the protein combined with nucleic acid or the globin of hemoglobin 组蛋白

his·to·phys·i·ol·o·gy (his″to-fiz″e-ol′ə-je) the correlation of function with the microscopic structure of cells and tissues 组织生理学

His·to·plas·ma (his″to-plaz′mə) a genus of anamorphic fungi containing the single species *H. capsula′tum*, which causes histoplasmosis. It occurs in soil, especially that contaminated with bird or bat excrement; it is found globally and in the United States is endemic in the Ohio and Mississippi River valleys 组织胞浆菌属

his·to·plas·min (his″to-plaz′min) a skin test antigen prepared from mycelial phase *Histoplasma capsulatum*, used primarily in epidemiologic surveys and in testing for cutaneous anergy in diagnosis of immunodeficiency 组织胞浆菌素

his·to·plas·mo·ma (his″to-plaz-mo′mə) a rounded granuloma of the lung due to infection with *Histoplasma capsulatum* 组织胞浆菌瘤

his·to·plas·mo·sis (his″to-plaz-mo′sis) infection with *Histoplasma capsulatum*, usually asymptomatic but in the immunocompromised sometimes causing more serious symptoms such as acute pneumonia, an influenzalike illness, disseminated reticuloendothelial hyperplasia with hepatosplenomegaly and anemia, or other organ damage 组织胞浆菌病，组织胞质菌病；**ocular h.**, disseminated choroiditis with scars in the periphery of the fundus near the optic nerve, and disciform macular lesions, probably due to *Histoplasma capsulatum* infection 眼组织胞浆菌病

his·to·throm·bin (his″to-throm′bin) thrombin derived from connective tissue 组织凝血酶

his·tot·o·my (his-tot′ə-me) dissection of tissues; microtomy 组织切开术

his·to·tox·ic (his′to-tok″sik) poisonous to tissue 毒害组织的，组织毒的

his·to·tro·pic (his″to-tro′pik) having affinity for tissue cells 向组织的

his·trel·in (his-trel′in) a synthetic preparation of gonadotropin-releasing hormone, used as the acetate ester in the treatment of precocious puberty 组胺瑞林，一种垂体激素释放兴奋药

his·tri·on·ic (his″tre-on′ik) excessively dramatic or emotional, as in histrionic personality disorder 表演样的；见 *personality* 下词条

HIV human immunodeficiency virus 人类免疫缺陷病毒

hives (hīvz) urticaria 荨麻疹

H⁺,K⁺-ATP·ase (a-te-pe′ās) a membrane-bound enzyme occurring on the surface of the parietal cells; it uses the energy derived from ATP hydrolysis to drive the exchange of ions (protons, chloride ions, and potassium ions) across the cell membrane, secreting acid into the gastric lumen H⁺,K⁺-腺苷三磷酸酶

Hl latent hyperopia 隐性远视

HLA human leukocyte antigens 人类白细胞抗原

Hm manifest hyperopia 显性远视

hMG menotropins (human menopausal gonadotropin) 人类绝经期促性腺激素

HMO health maintenance organization 健康维护组织

HMPV human metapneumovirus 人偏肺病毒

HMSN hereditary motor and sensory neuropathy 遗传性运动感觉神经病

HNPCC hereditary nonpolyposis colorectal cancer 遗传性非息肉病性结直肠癌

hnRNA heterogeneous nuclear RNA 核不均一RNA，核内异质 RNA，不均一核 RNA

Ho holmium 元素钬的符号

HOCM hypertrophic obstructive cardiomyopathy 肥厚型梗阻性心肌病

ho·do·neu·ro·mere (ho″do-noor′o-mēr) a segment of the embryonic trunk with its pair of nerves and their branches 神经分支节（胚胎）

hol·an·dric (hol-an′drik) inherited exclusively through the male descent; transmitted through genes located on the Y chromosome 限雄性的

ho·lis·tic (ho-lis′tik) considering the person as a functioning whole, or relating to the conception of a human being as a functioning whole 机体整体性的

hol·mi·um (Ho) (hōl′me-əm) a silvery white, ductile, rare earth element; at. no. 67, at. wt. 164.930（化学元素）钬

holo·blas·tic (hōl″o-blas′tik) undergoing cleavage in which the entire zygote participates; dividing completely 卵全裂的

holo·crine (ho′lo-krin) exhibiting glandular secretion in which the entire secretory cell laden with its secretory products is cast off 全浆分泌，全质分泌

holo·di·a·stol·ic (hōl″o-di″ə-stol′ik) pertaining to the entire diastole 全舒张（期）的

holo·en·dem·ic (hōl″o-en-dem′ik) endemic at a high level in a population, affecting most of the children and so affecting the adults in the same population less often 全地方病的

holo·en·zyme (hōl″o-en′zīm) the active compound formed by a combination of a coenzyme and an apoenzyme 全酶

hol·og·ra·phy (hōl-og′rə-fe) the lensless recording of three-dimensional images on film by means of laser beams 全息摄影术，全息术，全息摄影

holo·phyt·ic (hōl″o-fit′ik) obtaining food like a plant; said of certain protozoa 植物式营养的，自养植物的（指某些原虫）

holo·pros·en·ceph·a·ly (hōl″o-pros″ən-sef′ə-le) developmental failure of cleavage of the forebrain with a deficit in midline facial development, with cyclopia and other facial dysmorphisms in severe cases; due to a variety of chromosomal abnormalities, single-gene disorders, and environmental factors 前脑无裂畸形

holo·ra·chis·chi·sis (hōl″o-rə-kis′kĭ-sis) fissure of the entire spinal cord 脊柱全裂

holo·sys·tol·ic (hōl″o-sis-tol′ik) pertaining to the entire systole 全收缩（期）的

holo·zo·ic (hōl″o-zo′ik) having the nutritional characters of an animal, i.e., digesting protein 动物式营养性的

ho·mat·ro·pine (ho-mat′ro-pēn) an anticholinergic similar to atropine; *h. hydrobromide* is used as an ophthalmic mydriatic and cycloplegic, and *h. methylbromide* is used as an inhibitor of gastric spasm and secretion 后马托品

ho·max·i·al (ho-mak′se-əl) having axes of the same length 等轴的

ho·meo·met·ric (ho″me-o-met′rik) independent of a change in size; cf. *heterometric* 等距

ho·me·op·a·thy (ho″me-op′ə-the) a system of therapeutics based on the administration of minute doses of drugs that are capable of producing in healthy persons symptoms like those of the disease treated 顺势疗法；**homeopath′ic** *adj.*

ho·meo·pla·sia (ho″me-o-pla′zhə) formation of new tissue like that normal to the part 同质新生，同质形成；**homeoplas′tic** *adj.*

ho·meo·sta·sis (ho″me-o-sta′sis) a tendency to equilibrium or stability in the normal physiologic states of the organism 体内稳态，内环境稳定；**homeostat′ic** *adj.*

ho·meo·ther·a·py (ho″me-o-ther′ə-pe) treatment or prevention of disease with a substance similar to the causative agent of the disease 顺势疗法

ho·meo·ther·my (ho′me-o-thur″me) the maintenance of a constant body temperature despite changes in the environmental temperature 恒温性；**homeother′mal, homeother′mic** *adj.*

hom·er·gic (hōm-ur′jik) having the same effect; said of two drugs each of which produces the same overt effect 同效的

Ho·mo (ho′mo) [L.] the genus of primates containing the single species *H. sapiens* (humans) 人属

ho·mo·bio·tin (ho″mo-bi′o-tin) a homologue of biotin having an additional CH_2 group in the side chain and acting as a biotin antagonist 高生物素

ho·mo·car·no·sine (ho″mo-kahr′no-sēn) a dipeptide consisting of γ-aminobutyric acid and histidine, found in brain tissue 高肌肽

ho·mo·cit·rul·line (ho″mo-sit′roo-lēn) an unusual amino acid not normally present in urine but excreted in hyperornithinemia-hyperammonemiahomocitrullinuria syndrome 高瓜氨酸

ho·mo·cit·rul·lin·uria (ho″mo-sit″roo-lĭ-nu′re-ə) excess of homocitrulline in urine, seen in hyperornithinemia-hyperammonemia-homocitrullinuria syndrome 同型瓜氨酸尿

ho·mo·clad·ic (ho″mo-klad′ik) formed between small branches of the same artery; said of such an anastomosis 同脉吻合的，同支吻合的

ho·mo·cys·te·ine (ho″mo-sis′te-ēn) a sulfurcontaining amino acid homologous with cysteine and produced by demethylation of methionine; it can form cystine or methionine 高半胱氨酸，同型半胱氨酸

ho·mo·cys·tine (ho″mo-sis′tēn) a homologue of cystine formed from two molecules of homocysteine; it is a source of sulfur in the body 高胱氨酸

ho·mo·cys·tin·uria (ho″mo-sis″tin-u′re-ə) excessive homocystine in the urine, having various causes, some genetic; symptoms include developmental delay, failure to thrive, neurologic abnormalities, and others, depending on the cause. Sometimes the term refers specifically to the disorder due to lack of the enzyme cystathionine β-synthase 高胱氨酸尿，同型胱氨酸尿症

ho·mo·cy·to·tro·pic (ho″mo-si″to-tro′pik) having an affinity for cells of the same species 亲同种细胞的

ho·mod·ro·mous (ho-mod′ro-məs) moving or acting in the same or in the usual direction 同向的，同向运动的

ho·mo·erot·i·cism (ho″mo-ə-rot′ĭ-siz-əm) sexual feeling directed toward a member of the same sex 同性恋；**homoerot′ic** *adj.*

ho·mo·gam·ete (ho″mo-gam′ēt) one of two gametes

of the same size and structure, such as the X chromosome in the human female 同型配子

ho·mo·ga·met·ic (ho″mo-gə-met′ik) pertaining to production of gametes containing only one kind of sex chromosome, as in the human female 同型配子的

ho·mog·e·nate (ho-moj′ə-nāt) material obtained by homogenization 匀浆

ho·mo·ge·ne·ous (ho″mo-je′ne-əs) of uniform quality, composition, or structure throughout 同 种的，纯一的；同质的，均一的

ho·mo·gen·e·sis (ho″mo-jen′ə-sis) reproduction by the same process in each generation 同型生殖，纯一生殖；**homogenet′ic** adj.

ho·mog·e·nize (ho-moj′ə-nīz) to render homogeneous 使均匀，使均质

ho·mo·gen·tis·ic ac·id (ho″mo-jen-tis′ik) an aromatic hydrocarbon formed as an intermediate in the metabolism of tyrosine and phenylalanine and accumulated and excreted in the urine in alkaptonuria 尿黑酸，2，5-二羟苯乙酸

ho·mo·graft (ho′mo-graft) allograft 同种（异体）移植

ho·mo·log·ic (ho″mə-loj′ik) 同 homologous

ho·mol·o·gous (ho-mol′ə-gəs) 1. corresponding in structure, position, origin, etc.（结构，位置，起源）相应的；2. allogeneic 同种异体的

ho·mo·logue (ho′mo-log) 1. any homologous organ or part(细胞) 同源染色体；同系器官；相应物；2. in chemistry, one of a series of compounds distinguished by addition of a CH_2 group in successive members 同系（化合）物

ho·mol·y·sin (ho-mol′ə-sin) a lysin produced by injection into the body of an antigen derived from an individual of the same species 同种溶素，同族溶素

ho·mon·o·mous (ho-mon′ə-məs) designating homologous serial parts, such as somites 同律的，同列的，同系的（部分）

ho·mon·y·mous (ho-mon′ī-məs) 1. having the same or corresponding sound or name 同名的，同声的；2. pertaining to the corresponding vertical halves of the visual fields of both eyes 双眼视野各自垂直部分的

ho·mo·phil·ic (ho″mo-fil′ik) reacting only with a specific antigen 嗜同种的（与某一特异性抗原有亲合力或起反应的）

ho·mo·plas·tic (ho″mo-plas′tik) 1. allogeneic 同种异体的；2. denoting organs or parts, such as the wings of birds and insects, that resemble one another in structure and function but not in origin or development 非同源相似的

ho·mo·poly·sac·cha·ride (ho″mo-pol″esak′ə-rīd) a polysaccharide consisting of a single recurring monosaccharide unit 同多糖

hom·or·gan·ic (hom″or-gan′ik) produced by the same organ or by homologous organs 同种器官的

ho·mo·sal·ate (ho″mo-sal′āt) a sunscreen effective against ultraviolet B; applied topically to the skin 水杨酸三甲环己酯

ho·mo·sex·u·al (ho″mo-sek′shoo-əl) 1. pertaining to, characteristic of, or directed toward the same sex 同性的，同性恋的，同性性欲的；2. one who is sexually attracted to the same sex 同性恋者

ho·mo·top·ic (ho″mo-top′ik) occurring at the same place upon the body 等位（的）

ho·mo·type (ho′mo-tīp) a part having reversed symmetry with its mate, as the hand 同型，身体左右对称的部分，如手；**homotyp′ic** adj.

ho·mo·va·nil·lic ac·id (ho″mo-və-nil′ik) a major terminal urinary metabolite, converted from dopa, dopamine, and norepinephrine 高香草酸

ho·mo·zy·gos·i·ty (ho″mo-zi-gos′ī-te) the state of possessing a pair of identical alleles at a given locus 纯合性，在一定位点上具有一对相同等位基因的情况；**homozy′gous** adj.

ho·mo·zy·gote (ho″mo-zi′gōt) an individual exhibiting homozygosity 纯合子

hook (hook) 1. a long, thin, curved instrument for traction or holding 钩；针 钩；2. something with that shape 钩 状 物；**palate h.**, one for raising the palate in posterior rhinoscopy 提腭钩；**Tyrrell h.**, a slender hook used in eye surgery 提勒耳钩

hook·worm (hook′wurm″) a nematode parasitic in the intestines of humans and other vertebrates; two species that commonly cause human infection (*hookworm disease*) are *Necator americanus* (American, or New World, h.) and *Ancylostoma duodenale* (Old World h.) 钩虫

hops (hops) the dried flowers and cones of *Humulus lupulus*, the hop plant, used for nervousness and insomnia 啤酒花，用于神经紧张和失眠

hor·de·o·lum (hor-de′o-ləm) stye; a localized, purulent, inflammatory infection of a sebaceous gland (meibomian or zeisian) of the eyelid; *external h.* occurs on the skin surface at the edge of the lid, *internal h.* on the conjunctival surface 睑腺炎

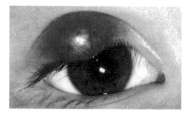

▲ 睑腺炎

hor·i·zon·tal (hor″ĭ-zon′təl) 1. parallel to the plane of the horizon 水平的，平行的；2. occupying or confined to a single level in a hierarchy 同一层次的

hor·i·zon·ta·lis (hor″ĭ-zon-ta′lis) 同 horizontal (1)

hor·mi·on (hor′me-on) point of union of the sphenoid bone with the posterior border of the vomer 蝶枕点，犁蝶点，顶冠穴

hor·mone (hor′mōn) a chemical substance produced in the body that has a specific regulatory effect on the activity of certain cells or a certain organ or organs 激素，荷尔蒙；**hormo′nal, hormon′ic** adj.；**adrenocortical h.**, 1. any of the corticosteroids elaborated by the adrenal cortex, the major ones being the glucocorticoids and mineralocorticoids, and including some androgens, progesterone, and perhaps estrogens 肾上腺皮质激素；2. corticosteroid 皮质类固醇；**adrenocorticotropic h. (ACTH)**, corticotropin 促肾上腺皮质激素；**adrenomedullary h's**, substances secreted by the adrenal medulla, including epinephrine and norepinephrine 肾上腺髓质激素；**androgenic h.**, androgen 雄激素；**anterior pituitary h's**, those produced in the adenohypophysis (anterior pituitary), including corticotropin, follicle-stimulating hormone, growth hormone, luteinizing hormone, prolactin, and thyrotropin 垂体前叶激素；**antidiuretic h.**, vasopressin 抗利尿激素，血管升压素；**cortical h.**, 同 adrenocortical h.；**corticotropin releasing h. (CRH)**, a neuropeptide elaborated mainly by the median eminence of the hypothalamus, but also by the pancreas and brain, that stimulates the secretion of corticotropin 促肾上腺皮质素释放激素；**ectopic h.**, one released from a neoplasm or cells outside the usual source of the hormone 异位激素；**eutopic h.**, one released from its usual site or from a neoplasm of that tissue 同位激素；**folliclestimulating h. (FSH)**, one of the gonadotropic hormones of the anterior lobe of the pituitary; it stimulates ovarian follicle growth and maturation, estrogen secretion, and endometrial changes characteristic of the first portion of the menstrual cycle in females, and stimulates spermatogenesis in males 促卵泡(激)素；**follicle-stimulating h.–releasing h. (FSH-RH)**, luteinizing hormone–releasing h. 促卵泡激素释放激素；**gonadotropic h.**, gonadotropin 促性腺激素；**gonadotropin-releasing h. (Gn-RH)**, 1. luteinizing hormone–releasing h. 促性腺激素释放激素；2. any hypothalamic factor that stimulates release of both follicle-stimulating hormone and luteinizing hormone 刺激卵泡刺激激素和黄体生成素释放的任何下丘脑因子；**growth h. (GH)**, any of several related hormones secreted by the anterior lobe of the pituitary that directly influence protein, carbohydrate, and lipid metabolism and control the rate of skeletal and visceral growth; used pharmaceutically as *somatrem* and *somatropin* 促生长素，生长激素；**growth h.–releasing h. (GH-RH)**, one elaborated by the hypothalamus, stimulating release of growth hormone from the anterior lobe of the pituitary 生长激素释放激素；**inhibiting h's**, hormones elaborated by one body structure that inhibit release of hormones from another structure; applied to substances of established clinical identity, while those whose chemical structure is still unknown are called *inhibiting factors* 抑制激素；**interstitial cell–stimulating h.**, luteinizing h. 间质细胞刺激素；**lactation h.**, lactogenic h., prolactin 催乳素；**local h.**, a substance with hormonelike properties that acts at an anatomically restricted site 局部激素；**luteinizing h. (LH)**, a gonadotropin of the anterior lobe of the pituitary, acting with follicle-stimulating hormone in females to promote ovulation as well as secretion of androgens and progesterone. It instigates and maintains the secretory portion of the menstrual cycle and is concerned with the corpus luteum formation. In males, it stimulates the development and functional activity of testicular Leydig cells 黄体生成素；**luteinizing h.–releasing h. (LH-RH)**, a glycoprotein gonadotropic hormone of the adenohypophysis that acts with follicle-stimulating hormone to promote ovulation and promotes secretion of androgen and progesterone. A preparation of the salts is used in the differential diagnosis of hypothalamic, pituitary, and gonadal dysfunction and in the treatment of some forms of infertility and hypogonadism 促黄体素释放激素；**melanocyte-stimulating h.**, melanophore-stimulating h. **(MSH)**, one of several peptides secreted by the anterior pituitary in humans and in the rhomboid fossa in lower vertebrates, influencing melanin formation and its deposition in the body 促黑(细胞激)素；**neurohypophysial h's**, 同 posterior pituitary h's；**ovarian h's**, those secreted by the ovary, such as estrogens and progestational agents 卵巢激素；**parathyroid h.**, a polypeptide hormone secreted by the parathyroid glands, which influences calcium and phosphorus metabolism and bone formation 甲状旁腺激素；**placental h's**, those produced by the placenta during pregnancy, including chorionic gonadotropin and other substances having estrogenic, progestational, or adrenocorticoid activity 胎盘激素；**posterior pituitary h's**, those released from the posterior lobe of the pituitary, including oxytocin and vasopressin 垂体后叶激素，神经垂体激素；**progestational h.**, 1. progesterone 孕激

素；2. 见 *agent* 下词条；**releasing h's,** hormones elaborated in one structure that cause the release of hormones from another structure; applied to substances of established chemical identity, while those whose chemical structure is unknown are called *releasing factors* 释放激素，释放因子；**sex h's,** the estrogens and androgens considered together 性激素；**somatotrophic h., somatotropic h.,** 同 growth h.；**somatotropinreleasing h. (SRH),** 同 growth hormone–releasing h.；**steroid h's,** those that are biologically active steroids; they are secreted by the adrenal cortex, testis, ovary, and placenta and include the progestogens, glucocorticoids, mineralocorticoids, androgens, and estrogens 类固醇激素；**thyroid h's,** thyroxine, calcitonin, and triiodothyronine; in the singular, thyroxine and/or triiodothyronine 甲状腺激素；**thyroid-stimulating h. (TSH), thyrotropic h.,** thyrotropin 促甲状腺激素；**thyrotropin-releasing h. (TRH),** a tripeptide hormone of the hypothalamus, which stimulates release of thyrotropin from the anterior lobe of the pituitary and also acts as a prolactin-releasing factor. It is used in the diagnosis of mild hyperthyroidism and Graves disease, and in differentiating among primary, secondary, and tertiary hypothyroidism. A synthetic preparation is called *protirelin* 促甲状腺激素释放激素

horn (horn) 1. cornu; a pointed projection such as the paired processes on the head of certain animals 角；2. something shaped like the horn of an animal 角状物；**horn'y** *adj.*；**cicatricial h.,** a hard, dry outgrowth from a scar 瘢痕角；**cutaneous h.,** a horny excrescence on the skin, commonly on the face or scalp; it often overlies premalignant or malignant lesions 皮角；**h. of pulp,** an extension of the pulp into an accentuation of the roof of the pulp chamber directly under a cusp or lobe of the tooth 牙髓角；**h. of spinal cord,** the horn-shaped structure, anterior or posterior, seen in transverse section of the spinal cord; the anterior horn is formed by the anterior column of the cord and the posterior by the posterior column 脊髓角

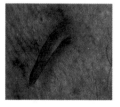

▲　光化性角化病引起的皮角（**Cutaneous horn arising from an actinic keratosis**）

ho·rop·ter (ho-rop′tər) the sum of all points seen in binocular vision with the eyes fixed 双眼单视界
hor·rip·i·la·tion (hor″ĭ-pĭ-la′shən) piloerection; erection of fine hairs of the skin 立毛状态；鸡皮疙瘩
Hor·taea (hor-te′ə) a genus of dematiaceous fungi containing the species *H. wernec′kii,* a halophilic yeast that causes tinea nigra 暗色真菌属，包括 *H. wernec′kii* 种，一种引起黑癣病的真菌
hos·pice (hos′pis) a facility that provides palliative and supportive care for terminally ill patients and their families, in the facility or at home, either directly or on a consulting basis 临终关怀
hos·pi·tal (hos′pĭ-təl) an institute for the treatment of the sick 医院；**lying-in h., maternity h.,** one for the care of obstetric patients 产院；**teaching h.,** one that conducts formal educational programs or courses of instruction that lead to granting of recognized certificates, diplomas, or degrees, or that are required for professional certification or licensure 教学医院；**voluntary h.,** a private, not-for-profit hospital that provides uncompensated care to the poor 慈善医院
hos·pi·tal·iza·tion (hos″pĭ-təl-ĭ-za′shən) 1. the placing of a patient in a hospital for treatment 入院，住院；2. the term of confinement in a hospital 住院期；**partial h.,** a psychiatric treatment program for patients who do not need full-time hospitalization, involving a special facility or an arrangement within a hospital setting to which the patient may come for treatment during the days, the nights, or the weekends only 部分住院
host (hōst) 寄主，宿主 1. an organism that harbors or nourishes another organism (the parasite) 寄生另一机体的动物或植物；2. the recipient of an organ or other tissue derived from another organism (the donor) 接受其他机体器官或组织移植的接受者；**accidental h.,** one that accidentally harbors an organism that is not ordinarily parasitic in the particular species 偶然宿主；**definitive h., final h.,** a host in which a parasite either attains sexual maturity (helminths) or undergoes sexual stages of development (protozoa) 终宿主；**intermediate h.,** a host in which a parasite passes through one or more of its asexual stages (protozoa) or larval stages (helminths); if there is more than one, the stages may be designated first, second, and so on 中间宿主；**paratenic h.,** an animal acting as a substitute intermediate host of a parasite, usually having acquired the parasite by ingestion of the original host 转续宿主；**primary h.,** definitive h. 主要宿主，原始寄主；**reservoir h.,** reservoir (2) 储存宿主
hot (hot) 1. characterized by high temperature 热的；2. radioactive; particularly used for the pres-

ence of significantly or dangerously high levels of radioactivity 放射性的

hot line (hot līn) telephone assistance for those in need of crisis intervention, generally roundthe-clock and staffed by nonprofessionals, with mental health professionals serving as advisors or in a back-up capacity 热线

HPL **hPL** human placental lactogen 人胎盘催乳素

HPLC high-performance liquid chromatography 高效液相色谱法

HPV human papillomavirus 人乳头瘤病毒

HRCT high-resolution computed tomography 高分辨力计算体层摄影（术）

HRF histamine-releasing factor 组胺释放因子；homologous restriction factor 同源限制因子

HRS Heart Rhythm Society（美国）心律协会

HRSA Health Resources and Services Administration, an agency of the United States Department of Health and Human Services 卫生资源与卫生事业管理局

HSAN hereditary sensory and autonomic neuropathy 遗传性感觉和自主神经病变

HSCT hematopoietic stem-cell transplantation 造血干细胞移植

HSR homogeneously staining regions 均匀染色区

HSV herpes simplex virus 单纯疱疹病毒

5-HT 5-hydroxytryptamine 5- 羟色胺；见 *serotonin*

HTLV-1 human T-lymphotropic virus 人类嗜 T（淋巴）细胞病毒 -1

HTLV-2 human T-lymphotropic virus 2 人类嗜 T（淋巴）细胞病毒 -2

hum (hum) a low, steady, prolonged sound 哼鸣，嗡嗡声；**venous h.**, a continuous blowing, singing, or humming murmur heard on auscultation over the right jugular vein in the sitting or erect position; it is an innocent sign that is obliterated on assumption of the recumbent position or on exerting pressure over the vein 静脉哼鸣

hu·mec·tant (hu-mek′tənt) 1. moistening 润湿；2. a moistening or diluent medicine 保湿剂，润湿剂

hu·mer·us (hu′mər-əs) pl. *hu′meri* [L.] the bone that extends from the shoulder to the elbow, articulating proximally with the scapula and distally with the radius and ulna 肱骨，见图 1；**hu′meral** *adj.*

hu·mor (hu′mər) pl. humors, humo′res [L.] any fluid or semifluid of the body 体液；**hu′moral** *adj.*；**aqueous h.**, the fluid produced in the eye, filling the spaces (anterior and posterior) in front of the lens and its attachments; it provides nutrients to the avascular cornea and lens and maintains intraocular pressure 房水；**ocular h.**, either of the humors (aqueous and vitreous) of the eye 眼液（眼房水或玻璃体液）；**vitreous h.**, the watery substance within the

interstices of the stroma in the vitreous body; the two are sometimes erroneously equated 玻璃体液

hump (hump) a rounded eminence 圆形隆起，驼背；**dowager's h.**, popular name for dorsal kyphosis caused by multiple wedge fractures of the thoracic vertebrae seen in osteoporosis.dowager 驼背，骨质疏松时多发胸椎楔形骨折所致

hump·back (hump′bak) kyphosis 驼背，脊柱后凸

hunch·back (hunch′bak) kyphosis 驼背，脊柱后凸

hun·ger (hung′gər) a craving, as for food 饥饿；**air h.**, Kussmaul respiration 空气饥

husk (husk) an outer covering or shell, as of some fruits and seeds 外皮；**psyllium h.**, the cleaned,dried seed coat from the seeds of *Plantago* species; used as a bulk-forming laxative; also used for various purposes in ayurveda and folk medicine 车前子壳

HVAD HeartWare ventricular assist device 心室辅助装置

hy·a·lin (hi′ə-lin) a translucent albuminoid product of amyloid degeneration 透明蛋白

hy·a·line (hi′ə-lēn) glassy and transparent or translucent 透明的，玻璃样的

hy·a·lin·i·za·tion (hi″ə-lin″ĭ-za′shən) conversion to hyalin 玻璃样变，透明化；**Crooke h.**, degeneration of corticotrophs of the pituitary gland, in which they lose their specific granulations and the cytoplasm becomes hyalinized; seen in Cushing syndrome and Addison disease Crooke 玻璃样变，垂体产生皮质激素的腺体细胞变性，失去特定的颗粒，胞质变得透明，常见于库欣综合征和艾迪生病

hy·a·li·no·sis (hi″ə-lin-o′sis) hyaline degeneration 透明变性

hy·a·li·tis (hi″ə-li′tis) inflammation of the vitreous body or the vitreous (hyaloid) membrane 玻璃体炎；**asteroid h.**, 星形玻璃体炎，见 *hyalosis* 下词条；**suppurative h.**, purulent inflammation of the vitreous body 化脓性玻璃体炎

hy·al·o·gen (hi-al′o-jən) an albuminous substance occurring in the cartilage, vitreous body, etc., and convertible into hyalin 透明蛋白原

hy·a·lo·hy·pho·my·co·sis (hi″ə-lo-hi″fo-miko′-sis) any of a group of infections caused by mycelial fungi with colorless walls; most are opportunistic 透明丝孢霉病

hy·a·loid (hi′ə-loid) hyaline 透明的

hy·a·lo·mere (hi′ə-lo-mēr″) the pale, homogeneous portion of a blood platelet in a dry, stained blood smear（血涂片中血小板的）透明区

Hy·a·lom·ma (hi″ə-lom′ə) a genus of ticks found on humans and other animals, primarily in hot and dry regions of Southern Europe, Africa, and Asia, serving as vectors for numerous diseases 璃眼蜱，

一种在南欧及亚非地区传播多种疾病的虫媒

hy·a·lo·mu·coid (hi″ə-lo-mu′koid) the mucoid of the vitreous body 玻璃体黏液质

hy·a·lo·nyx·is (hi″ə-lo-nik′sis) puncturing of the vitreous body 玻璃体穿刺术

hy·a·lo·plasm (hi′ə-lo-plaz″əm) the more fluid, finely granular substance of the cytoplasm of a cell 透明质

hy·a·lo·se·ro·si·tis (hi″ə-lo-se″ro-si′tis) inflammation of serous membranes, with hyalinization of the serous exudate into a pearly investment of the affected organ 透明性浆膜炎; **progressive multiple h.,** Concato disease 进行性多发性透明性浆膜炎

hy·a·lo·sis (hi″ə-lo′sis) degenerative changes in the vitreous humor 玻璃体变性; **asteroid h.,** the presence of spherical or star-shaped opacities in the vitreous humor 星形玻璃体退变，玻璃体液中存在球形或星形混浊

hy·a·lu·ron·an (hi″ə-loo-ron′an) a glycosaminoglycan found in lubricating proteoglycans of synovial fluid, vitreous humor, cartilage, blood vessels, skin, and the umbilical cord. A preparation from chicken combs is used for the treatment of pain in osteoarthritis. It is also used as an adjunct during surgical procedures on the eye to maintain the shape of the eye, to manipulate and separate tissues by hydraulic pressure, and to protect intraocular structures from trauma 透明质酸。又称 *hyaluronate* and *hyaluronic acid*

hy·a·lu·ro·nate (hi″ə-loo′rə-nāt) hyaluronan 透明质酸盐

hy·a·lu·ron·ic ac·id (hi″ə-loo-ron′ik) hyaluronan 透明质酸

hy·a·lu·ron·i·dase (hi″ə-loo-ron′ ĭ-dās) any of three enzymes that catalyze the hydrolysis of hyaluronan and similar glycosaminoglycans. They are found in snake and spider venom and in mammalian testicular and spleen tissue, and are produced by various pathogenic bacteria, enabling them to spread through tissues. A preparation from mammalian testes is used to aid absorption and dispersion of other injected drugs and fluids, for hypodermoclysis, and for improving resorption of radiopaque media 透明质酸酶

hy·brid (hi′brid) 1. an offspring of genetically different parents 杂种; 2. something of mixed origin or composition 复合

hy·brid·iza·tion (hi″brid-ī-za′shən) 1. the act or process of producing hybrids（生物）杂交; 2. 同 nucleic acid h.; 3. in chemistry, a procedure whereby orbitals of intermediate energy and desired directional character are constructed 杂化; **in situ h.,** nucleic acid hybridization in which a labeled (e.g., fluorescence, radioactivity), single-stranded

nucleic acid probe is applied to prepared cells or histologic sections and annealing occurs in situ 原位杂交; **molecular h., nucleic acid h.,** formation of a partially or wholly complementary DNA-RNA, DNA-DNA, or RNA-RNA duplex by association of single-stranded nucleic acids, sometimes specifically from different sources; used as the basis of a wide variety of analytical techniques 分子杂交，核酸分子杂交

hy·brid·o·ma (hi″brid-o′mə) a somatic cell hybrid formed by fusion of normal lymphocytes and tumor cells 杂交瘤

hy·dan·to·in (hi-dan′to-in) 1. a five-membered heterocyclic organic compound containing two nitrogens in the ring (C1 and C3) and two carbonyl groups (C2 and C4) 乙内酰脲; 2. any of a group of anticonvulsants containing such a ring structure, including phenytoin and ethotoin 海因类，包括含有该环的苯妥英和乙妥英

hy·da·tid (hi′də-tid) 1. hydatid cyst 棘球蚴囊; 2. any cystlike structure 囊; **h. of Morgagni,** 1. a cystlike remnant of the müllerian duct on the upper end of the testis 睾丸附件; 2. one of the small pedunculated structures attached to the uterine tubes near their fimbriated end; remnants of the mesonephric ducts（卵巢冠）囊状附件; **sessile h.,** 同 h. of Morgagni (1)

hy·da·tid·i·form (hi″də-tid′ ĭ-form) resembling a hydatid cyst 包虫囊状的，见 *mole* 下词条

hy·da·tid·o·sis (hi″də-tĭ-do′sis) hydatid disease 包虫病，棘球蚴病

hy·da·tid·os·to·my (hi″də-tĭ-dos′tə-me) incision and drainage of a hydatid cyst 棘球囊切开引流术

hy·dra·gogue (hi′drə-gog) 1. producing watery discharge, especially from the bowels 致水泻的; 2. a cathartic that causes watery purgation 水泻剂

hy·dral·a·zine (hy-dral′ə-zēn) a peripheral vasodilator used in the form of the hydrochloride salt as an antihypertensive 肼苯哒嗪

hy·dram·ni·os (hi-dram′ne-os) polyhydramnios 羊水过多

hy·dran·en·ceph·a·ly (hi″dran-ən-sef′ə-le) complete or almost complete absence of the cerebral hemispheres, their normal site being occupied by cerebrospinal fluid 积水性无脑畸形; **hydranencephal′ic** *adj.*

hy·drar·thro·sis (hi″drahr-thro′sis) an accumulation of effused watery fluid in a joint cavity 关节积水; **hydrarthro′dial** *adj.*

hy·dra·tase (hi′drə-tās) a hydro-lyase that catalyzes a reaction in which the equilibrium lies toward hydration 水化酶

hy·drate (hi′drāt) 1. any compound of a radical

with water 水化物；2. any salt or other compound containing water of crystallization 水合物

hy·dra·tion (hi-dra′shən) the absorption of or combination with water 水合（作用），水化（作用）

hy·drau·lics (hi-draw′liks) the science dealing with the mechanics of liquids 水力学

hy·dra·zine (hi′drə-zēn) a toxic, irritant, carcinogenic, gaseous diamine, $H_2N·NH_2$, or any of its substitution derivatives 肼，联胺

hy·dri·od·ic ac·id (hi″dri-o′dik) a gaseous haloid acid, HI; its aqueous solution and syrup have been used as alteratives 氢碘酸

hy·droa (hi-dro′ə) a vesicular eruption with intense itching and burning on skin exposed to sunlight 水疱病

hy·dro·al·co·hol·ic (hi″dro-al″kə-hol′ik) pertaining to or containing both water and alcohol 含水酒精的，水醇的

hy·dro·bro·mic ac·id (hi-dro-bro′mik) a gaseous haloid acid, HBr 氢溴酸

hy·dro·bro·mide (hi″dro-bro′mīd) an addition salt of hydrobromic acid 氢溴酸盐

hy·dro·ca·ly·co·sis (hi″dro-ka″lĭ-ko′sis) a usually asymptomatic cystic dilatation of a major renal calyx, lined by transitional epithelium and due to obstruction of the infundibulum 肾盏积水

hy·dro·car·bon (hi′dro-kahr″bən) an organic compound that contains carbon and hydrogen only 碳氢化合物；alicyclic h., one that has a cyclic structure and aliphatic properties 脂肪族环烃；aliphatic h., one in which no carbon atoms are joined to form a ring 脂肪族烃；aromatic h., one that has a cyclic structure and a closed conjugated system of double bonds 芳香烃；chlorinated h., any of a group of toxic compounds used mainly as refrigerants, industrial solvents, and dry cleaning fluids, and formerly as anesthetics 氯代烃

hy·dro·cele (hi′dro-sēl) a circumscribed collection of fluid, especially in the tunica vaginalis of the testis or along the spermatic cord 鞘膜积液，阴囊积液

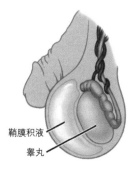

鞘膜积液
睾丸

hy·dro·ceph·a·lo·cele (hi″dro-sef′ə-lo-sēl″) hydroencephalocele 积水性脑突出

hy·dro·ceph·a·lus (hi″dro-sef′ə-ləs) a congenital or acquired condition marked by dilatation of the cerebral ventricles, usually occurring secondary to obstruction of the cerebrospinal fluid pathways, and accompanied by an accumulation of cerebrospinal fluid within the skull; typically, there is enlargement of the head, prominence of the forehead, brain atrophy, mental deterioration, and convulsions 脑积水；hydrocephal′ic adj. 脑积水的；communicating h., that in which there is free access of fluid between the ventricles of the brain and the spinal canal 交通性脑积水；h. ex va′cuo, compensatory replacement by cerebrospinal fluid of the volume of tissue lost in atrophy of the brain 脑外积水；noncommunicating h., obstructive h. 非交通性脑积水；normal-pressure h., normal-pressure occult h., dementia, ataxia, and urinary incontinence with enlarged ventricles associated with inadequacy of the subarachnoid spaces, but with normal cerebrospinal fluid pressure 正常压力脑积水；obstructive h., that due to obstruction of the flow of cerebrospinal fluid within the brain ventricles or through their exit foramina 梗阻性脑积水；otitic h., that caused by spread of inflammation of otitis media to the cranial cavity 耳源性脑积水；posthemorrhagic h., hydrocephalus in an infant following intracranial hemorrhage that has distended the ventricles and obstructed normal pathways for cerebrospinal fluid 出血后脑积水

hy·dro·chlo·ric ac·id (hi″dro-klor′ik) hydrogen chloride in aqueous solution, HCl, a highly corrosive mineral acid; it is used as a laboratory reagent and is a constituent of gastric juice, secreted by the gastric parietal cells 盐酸，氢氯酸

hy·dro·chlo·ride (hi″dro-klor′īd) a salt of hydrochloric acid 氢氯化物，盐酸化物，盐酸盐

hy·dro·chlo·ro·thi·a·zide (hi″dro-klor″othi′ə-zīd) a thiazide diuretic, used for treatment of hypertension and edema 氢氯噻嗪，双氢克尿塞，双氢氯噻嗪

hy·dro·cho·le·cys·tis (hi″dro-ko″lə-sis′tis) distention of the gallbladder with watery fluid 胆囊积水

hy·dro·cho·le·re·sis (hi″dro-ko″lə-re′sis) choleresis with excretion of watery bile (low in specific gravity, viscosity, and total solid content) 稀胆液排出增多

hy·dro·co·done (hi″dro-ko′dōn) a semisynthetic opioid analgesic similar to but more active than codeine; used as the bitartrate salt or polistirex complex as an analgesic and antitussive 氢可酮，二氢可待因酮

hy·dro·col·loid (hi″dro-kol′oid) a colloid system

in which water is the dispersion medium 水胶体

hy·dro·cor·ti·sone (hi″dro-kor′tĭ-sōn) the name given to natural or synthetic cortisol when it is used as a pharmaceutical. The base and its salts, including *h. acetate, h. butyrate, h. cypionate, h. probutate, h. sodium phosphate, h. sodium succinate,* and *h. valerate,* are used as replacement therapy in adrenocortical insufficiency and as antiinflammatory and immunosuppressant agents in the treatment of a wide variety of disorders 氢化可的松皮质醇

hy·dro·cy·an·ic ac·id (hi″dro-si-an′ik) hydrogen cyanide 氢氰酸，氰化氢；见 *hydrogen* 下词条

hy·dro·de·lin·e·a·tion (hi″dro-de-lin″e-a′shən) injection of fluid between the layers of the nucleus of the lens using a blunt needle; done to delineate the nuclear zones during cataract surgery 注液划区（白内障手术时，用钝针在晶状体核层之间注射液体，以便划出核区）

hy·dro·dis·sec·tion (hi″dro-dĭ-sek′shən) injection of a small amount of fluid into the capsule of the lens for dissection and maneuverability during extracapsular or phacoemulsification surgery 水分离术（眼科手术一）

hy·dro·en·ceph·a·lo·cele (hi″dro-en-sef′ə-lo-sēl) encephalocele into a distended sac containing cerebrospinal fluid 积水性脑突出

hy·dro·flu·me·thi·a·zide (hi″dro-floo″mə-thi′ə-zīd) a thiazide diuretic used for treatment of hypertension and edema 氢氟噻嗪

hy·dro·flu·o·ric ac·id (hi″dro-floor′ik) a gaseous haloid acid, HF, extremely poisonous and corrosive 氢氟酸

hy·dro·gen (H) (hi′dro-jən) the lightest element, an odorless, tasteless, colorless gas, inflammable and explosive when mixed with air; at. no. 1, at. wt. 1.008. It is found in water and in almost all organic compounds, and its ion is the active constituent of all acids in the water system. It exists as the mass 1 isotope *(protium, light* or *ordinary h.),* mass 2 isotope *(deuterium, heavy h.),* and mass 3 isotope *(tritium)* 氢；**h. cyanide,** an extremely poisonous liquid or gas, HCN, used as a rodenticide and insecticide 氰化氢；**h. peroxide,** a strongly disinfectant cleansing and bleaching liquid, H_2O_2, used in dilute solution in water 过氧化氢；**h. sulfide,** an ill-smelling, colorless, poisonous gas, H_2S 硫化氢

hy·dro·ki·net·ic (hi″dro-kĭ-net′ik) relating to movement of water or other fluid, as in a whirlpool bath 流体动力的

hy·dro·ki·net·ics (hi″dro-kĭ-net′iks) the science treating of fluids in motion 液体动力学

hy·dro·lase (hi′dro-lās) one of the six main classes of enzymes, comprising those that catalyze the hydrolytic cleavage of a compound 水解酶

hy·dro·ly·ase (hi″dro-li′ās) a lyase that catalyzes the removal of water from a substrate by breakage of a carbon-oxygen bond, leading to formation of a double bond 水裂解酶

hy·drol·y·sate (hi-drol′ə-zāt) any compound produced by hydrolysis 水解产物；**protein h.,** a mixture of amino acids prepared by splitting a protein with an acid, alkali, or enzyme; used as a fluid and nutrient replenisher 蛋白水解物，水解蛋白

hy·drol·y·sis (hi-drol′ə-sis) pl. *hydrol′yses.* The cleavage of a compound by the addition of water, the hydroxyl group being incorporated in one fragment and the hydrogen atom in the other 水解（作用）；**hydrolyt′ic** *adj.*

hy·dro·ma (hi-dro′mə) hygroma 水囊瘤

hy·dro·me·nin·go·cele (hi″dro-mə-ning′gosēl) a meningocele forming a sac containing cerebrospinal fluid but no brain or spinal cord substance 积水性脑膜突出

hy·drom·e·ter (hi-drom′ə-tər) an instrument for determining the specific gravity of a fluid 液体比重计

hy·dro·me·tro·col·pos (hi″dro-me″tro-kol′pos) a collection of watery fluid in the uterus and vagina 子宫阴道积水

hy·drom·e·try (hi-drom′ə-tre) measurement of specific gravity with a hydrometer 液体比重测定法；**hydromet′ric** *adj.*

hy·dro·mi·cro·ceph·a·ly (hi″dro-mi″kro-sef′ə-le) smallness of the head with an abnormal amount of cerebrospinal fluid 积水性小头

hy·dro·mor·phone (hi″dro-mor′fōn) a morphine alkaloid having opioid analgesic effects similar to but greater and of shorter duration than those of morphine; used as the hydrochloride salt as an analgesic, antitussive, and anesthesia adjunct 氢化吗啡酮，二氢吗啡酮

hy·dro·my·elia (hi″dro-mi-e′le-ə) dilatation of the central canal of the spinal cord with an abnormal accumulation of fluid 脊髓积水

hy·dro·my·elo·me·nin·go·cele (hi″dro-mi″ə-lo-mə-ning′go-sēl) myelomeningocele containing both cerebrospinal fluid and spinal cord tissue 积水性脑脊膜膨出

hy·dro·my·o·ma (hi″dro-mi-o′mə) uterine leiomyoma with cystic degeneration 水囊性肌瘤

hy·dro·ne·phro·sis (hi″dro-nə-fro′sis) distention of the renal pelvis and calices with urine, due to obstruction of the ureter, with atrophy of the kidney parenchyma 肾（盂）积水；**hydronephrot′ic** *adj.*

hy·dro·ni·um (hi-dro′ne-əm) the hydrated proton H_3O^+; it is the form in which the proton (hydrogen ion, H$^+$) exists in aqueous solution, a combination of H$^+$ and H$_2$O 水合氢离子

hy·dro·peri·car·di·tis (hi″dro-per″ĭ-kahr-di′tis) pericarditis with watery effusion 积水性心包炎

hy·dro·peri·to·ne·um (hi″dro-per″ĭ-to-ne′əm) ascites 腹水

Hy·dro·phi·idae (hi″dro-fi′ĭ-de) the sea snakes, a family of venomous snakes adapted for living in the ocean, found in the Indian and Pacific Oceans and characterized by an oarlike tail and immovable hollow fangs 海蛇科

hy·dro·phil·ic (hi″dro-fil′ik) readily absorbing moisture; hygroscopic; having strongly polar groups that readily interact with water 亲水（的）

hy·dro·pho·bia (hi″dro-fo′be-ə) 1. irrational fear of water 恐水; 2. choking, gagging, and fear on attempts to drink in the paralytic phase of rabies 恐水症; 3. former term for *rabies* 狂犬病

hy·dro·pho·bic (hi″dro-fo′bik) 1. pertaining to hydrophobia (rabies) 狂犬病的; 2. not readily absorbing water, or being adversely affected by water 疏水的; 3. lacking polar groups and therefore insoluble in water 斥水性的

hy·droph·thal·mos (hi″drof-thal′mos) distention of the eyeball in infantile glaucoma 水眼

hy·drop·ic (hi-drop′ik) edematous 水肿的

hy·dro·pneu·ma·to·sis (hi″dro-noo″mə-to′sis) a collection of fluid and gas in the tissues 水气肿症

hy·dro·pneu·mo·tho·rax (hi″dro-noo″mothor′aks) fluid and gas within the pleural cavity 液气胸

hy·drops (hi′drops) [L.] edema 积液; **fetal h., h. fetalis**, gross edema of the entire body, with severe anemia, occurring in hemolytic disease of the newborn 胎儿水肿

hy·dro·quin·one (hi″dro-kwĭ-nōn′) the reduced form of quinone, used topically as a skin depigmenting agent 对苯二酸

hy·dror·rhea (hi″dro-re′ə) a copious watery discharge 液溢; **h. gravidarum**, watery discharge from the vagina during pregnancy 妊娠溢液

hy·dro·sal·pinx (hi″dro-sal′pinks) a collection of watery fluid in a uterine tube, occurring as the end stage of pyosalpinx 输卵管积水

hy·dro·sol (hi′dro-sol) a sol in which the dispersion medium is water 水溶胶

hy·dro·stat·ics (hi″dro-stat′iks) science of equilibrium of fluids and the pressures they exert 流体静力学; **hydrostat'ic** *adj.*

hy·dro·tax·is (hi″dro-tak′sis) taxis in response to the influence of water or moisture 趋水性

hy·dro·ther·a·py (hi″dro-ther′ə-pe) the application of water, usually externally, in the treatment of disease 水治疗法; **colon h.**, an extension of the ene-

ma, used for cleansing and detoxification; the entire colon is irrigated with water, which may contain enzymes or herbs, introduced through the rectum 结肠水疗

hy·dro·thio·ne·mia (hi″dro-thi″o-ne′me-ə) hydrogen sulfide in the blood 硫化氢血症

hy·dro·tho·rax (hi″dro-thor′aks) a pleural effusion containing serous fluid 胸腔积液

hy·drot·ro·pism (hi-drot′ro-piz-əm) a growth response of a nonmotile organism to the presence of water or moisture 向水性

hy·dro·tu·ba·tion (hi″dro-too-ba′shən) introduction into the uterine tube of hydrocortisone in saline solution followed by chymotrypsin in saline solution to maintain its patency 输卵管通液术

hy·dro·ure·ter (hi″dro-u-re′tər) distention of the ureter with urine or watery fluid, due to obstruction 输尿管积水

hy·drox·ide (hi-drok′sīd) any compound containing a hydroxyl group 氢氧化物

hy·droxo·co·bal·a·min (hi-drok″so-ko-bal′ə-min) a hydroxyl-substituted cobalamin derivative, the naturally occurring form of vitamin B$_{12}$ and sometimes used as a source of that vitamin 羟钴胺

hydroxy- chemical prefix indicating the presence of the univalent radical OH [前缀] 羟（基），表示含一价根 OH

hy·droxy·am·phet·amine (hi-drok″se-amfet′ə-mēn) a sympathomimetic amine; its hydrobromide salt is used as a nasal decongestant, pressor, and mydriatic 羟苯丙胺，拟交感神经药，其氢溴酸盐用作鼻内减轻充血药、加压素和散瞳药

hy·droxy·ap·a·tite (hi-drok″se-ap′ə-tīt) an inorganic calcium-containing constituent of bone matrix and teeth, imparting rigidity to these structures. Synthetic compounds with similar structure are used as calcium supplements and prosthetic aids (see *durapatite*) 羟基磷灰石

hy·droxy·bu·ty·rate (hi-drok″se-bu′tī-rāt) a salt or anionic form of hydroxybutyric acid 羟基丁酸盐

hy·droxy·bu·tyr·ic ac·id (hi-drok″se-bu′tə-rik) any of several hydroxy derivatives of butyric acid; β *-h.a. (3-h.a.)* is a ketone body and is elevated in the blood and urine in ketosis, and γ *-h.a. (4-h.a.)* is elevated in some body fluids in semialdehyde dehydrogenase deficiency 羟（盐）丁酸

4-hy·droxy·bu·tyr·ic·ac·id·uria γ-hy·droxy·bu·tyr·ic·ac·id·uria (hi-drok″se-bu-tir″ikas″ĭ-du′re-ə) succinic semialdehyde dehydrogenase deficiency 4-羟丁酸尿（症），γ-羟丁酸尿（症），琥珀酸半醛脱氢酶缺乏症; 见 *succinate-semialdehyde dehydrogenase*

hy·droxy·chlo·ro·quine (hi-drok″se-klor′okwin)

an antiinflammatory and antiprotozoal used as the sulfate salt in the treatment of malaria, lupus erythematosus, and rheumatoid arthritis 羟化氯喹

25-hy·droxy·cho·le·cal·cif·e·rol (hi-drok″seko″lə-kal-sif′ə-rol) an intermediate in the hepatic activation of cholecalciferol; as the pharmaceutical preparation *calcifediol*, it is used in the treatment of hypocalcemia, hypophosphatemia, rickets, and osteodystrophy associated with various medical conditions 25- 羟胆钙化醇，25- 羟维生素 D_3

hy·droxy·cor·ti·co·ste·roid (hi-drok″sekor″tī-koster′oid) a corticosteroid bearing a hydroxyl substitution; *17-h's* are intermediates in the biosynthesis of steroid hormones and are accumulated and excreted abnormally in various disorders of steroidogenesis 羟皮质类固醇

hy·droxy·glu·tar·ic ac·id (hi-drok″se-glootar′ik) any of several hydroxylated derivatives of glutaric acid, some of which are accumulated and excreted in specific forms of glutaricaciduria 羟戊二酸

5-hy·droxy·in·dole·ace·tic ac·id (hi-drok″sein″dōl-ə-se′tik) a product of serotonin metabolism present in increased amounts in the urine of patients with carcinoid tumors 5- 羟基吲哚乙酸

3-hy·droxy·iso·va·ler·ic ac·id (hi-drok″sei″-so-və-ler′ik) a methylated form of isovaleric acid accumulated and excreted in the urine in some disorders of leucine catabolism 3- 羟基异戊酸

hy·drox·yl (hi-drok′səl) the univalent radical OH 羟（基），氢氧基

hy·drox·yl·ap·a·tite (hi-drok″səl-ap′ə-tīt) hydroxyapatite 羟基磷灰石

hy·drox·y·lase (hi-drok″sə-lās) any of a group of enzymes that catalyze the formation of a hydroxyl group on a substrate by incorporation of one atom (monooxygenases) or two atoms (dioxygenases) of oxygen from O_2 羟化酶；**11β-h.,** an enzyme that catalyzes the hydroxylation of steroids at the 11 position, a step in the synthesis of steroid hormones; deficiency causes a form of congenital adrenal hyperplasia 11β - 羟化酶，一种催化类固醇在 11 位羟基化的酶，缺乏会导致先天性肾上腺增生；**17α-h.,** an enzyme that catalyzes the oxidation of steroids at the 17 position, a step in the synthesis of steroid hormones; deficiency causes a form of congenital adrenal hyperplasia, and if it occurs during gestation can cause congenital undervirilization of external genitalia in males, with postnatal impairment of sexual development in both sexes 17α - 羟化酶，一种催化 17 位类固醇氧化的酶，缺乏会导致一种先天性肾上腺增生，如果在妊娠期间，可能会导致男性外生殖器先天性不足，产后两性性发育受损；**18-h.,** an enzyme that catalyzes

several steps in the biosynthesis of aldosterone from corticosteroids; deficiency causes salt wasting 18- 羟化酶，一种催化皮质类固醇生物合成醛固酮过程中几个步骤的酶，缺乏将导致体内盐丢失；**21-h.,** an enzyme that catalyzes the hydroxylation of steroids at the 21 position, a step in the synthesis of steroid hormones; deficiency impairs the ability to produce all glucocorticoids and causes a form of congenital adrenal hyperplasia 21- 羟化酶，一种催化 21 位类固醇羟基化的酶，缺乏会影响所有糖皮质激素的产生，并导致先天性肾上腺增生

hy·droxy·preg·nen·o·lone (hi-drok″se-pregnēn′ə-lōn) an intermediate in the biosynthesis of steroid hormones, accumulated and excreted abnormally in some disorders of steroidogenesis 羟孕烯醇酮

hy·droxy·pro·ges·ter·one (hi-drok″sepro-jes′tər-ōn) 1. 17α -hydroxyprogesterone; an intermediate formed in the conversion of cholesterol to cortisol, androgens, and estrogens 17α - 羟孕酮; 2. a synthetic preparation of the caproate ester, used in treatment of dysfunctional uterine bleeding and menstrual cycle abnormalities, and in the diagnosis of endogenous estrogen production 己酸酯的合成制剂

hy·droxy·pro·line (hi-drok″se-pro′lēn) a hydroxylated form of proline, occurring in collagen and other connective tissue proteins 羟脯氨酸

hy·droxy·pro·li·ne·mia (hi-drok″se-pro″līne′me-ə) 1. excess of hydroxyproline in the blood 羟脯氨酸过多; 2. a disorder of amino acid metabolism characterized by an excess of free hydroxyproline in the plasma and urine, due to a defect in the enzyme hydroxyproline oxidase; it may be associated with intellectual disability 羟脯氨酸血症，与羟脯氨酸氧化酶的缺陷相关

hy·droxy·pro·pyl cel·lu·lose (hi-drok″sepro′pəl sel′u-lōs) a partially substituted, watersoluble cellulose ether, used as a pharmaceutical aid and as a topical ophthalmic protectant and lubricant 羟丙基纤维素

hy·droxy·pro·pyl meth·yl·cel·lu·lose (hi-drok″se-pro′pəl meth″əl-sel′u-lōs) hypromellose 羟丙甲纤维素

8-hy·droxy·quin·o·line (hi-drok″se-kwin′olēn) oxyquinoline 8- 羟基喹啉，羟喹啉

hy·droxy·ste·roid (hi-drok″se-ster′oid) a steroid carrying a hydroxyl group 羟类固醇

17β-hy·droxy·ste·roid de·hy·dro·gen·ase de·fi·cien·cy (hi-drok″se-ster′oid de-hi′drojən-ās) any of several hereditary syndromes caused by a deficiency of enzymes of the 17β -hydroxysteroid dehydrogenase family. One is characterized in males by congenital undervirilization of external genitalia with variable gynecomastia, another resembles Zellweger syndrome, and a third is characterized by intellectual disability, choreoathetosis, and other neurologic abnormalities 17β- 羟基类固醇脱氢酶缺陷症；17- 酮类固醇还原酶缺陷

5-hy·droxy·tryp·ta·mine (5-HT) (hi-drok″setrip′tə-mēn) serotonin 5- 羟色胺

hy·droxy·urea (hi-drok″se-u-re′ə) an antineoplastic that inhibits a step in DNA synthesis, used in treatment of chronic myelogenous leukemia, some carcinomas, malignant melanoma, and polycythemia vera. It is also used to reduce the frequency of painful sickle cell crisis 羟基脲

25-hy·droxy·vi·ta·min D (hi-drok″se-vi′tə-min) either 25-hydroxycholecalciferol or the corresponding hydroxy- derivative of ergocalciferol, or both together 25- 羟基维生素 D

hy·droxy·zine (hi-drok′sə-zēn) a central nervous system depressant having antispasmodic, antihistaminic, and antifibrillatory actions; used as *h. hydrochloride* or *h. pamoate* as an antianxiety agent, antihistamine, antiemetic, and sedative 羟嗪

hy·dru·ria (hi-droo′re-ə) excretion of urine of low osmolality or low specific gravity 稀尿症；**hydrur′ic** *adj.*

hy·giene (hi′jēn) science of health and its preservation 卫生学；**hygien′ic** *adj.*；*oral h.*, proper care of the mouth and teeth 口腔卫生

hy·gien·ist (hi-jen′ist) (hi-je′nist) a specialist in hygiene 卫生学家；*dental h.*, an auxiliary member of the dental profession, trained in the art of removing calcareous deposits and stains from surfaces of teeth and in providing additional services and information on prevention of oral disease 牙科保健员

hy·gro·ma (hi-gro′mə) pl. *hygromas, hygro′- mata.* An accumulation of fluid in a sac, cyst, or bursa 水囊瘤；**hygrom′atous** *adj.*；*h. col′li,* a watery tumor of the neck 颈部水囊瘤；*cystic h., h. cys′ticum,* a lymphangioma usually occurring in the neck and composed of large, multilocular, thin-walled cysts 水囊状淋巴管瘤

hy·grom·e·try (hi-grom′ə-tre) measurement of moisture in the atmosphere 湿度测定法

hy·gro·scop·ic (hi″gro-skop′ik) readily absorbing moisture 吸湿的，收湿的；湿度计的

hy·men (hi′mən) the membranous fold partially or wholly occluding the external vaginal orifice 处女膜；**hy′menal** *adj.*

hy·me·no·lep·i·a·sis (hi″mə-no-lep-i′ə-sis) infection with *Hymenolepis* 膜壳绦虫病

Hy·me·nol·e·pis (hi″mə-nol′ə-pis) a genus of tapeworms, including *H. na′na,* found in rodents, rats, and humans, especially children 膜壳绦虫属

hy·men·ol·o·gy (hi″mən-ol′ə-je) the science dealing with the membranes of the body 膜学

Hy·men·op·tera (hi″mən-op′tər-ə) an order of insects with two pairs of well-developed membranous wings, like bees and wasps 膜翅目（昆虫）

hyo·epi·glot·tic (hi″o-ep″ĭ-glot′ik) pertaining to the hyoid bone and the epiglottis 舌骨会厌的

hyo·epi·glot·tid·e·an (hi″o-ep″ĭ-glŏ-tid′e-ən) hyoepiglottic 舌骨会厌的

hyo·glos·sal (hi″o-glos′əl) pertaining to the hyoid bone and tongue or to the hyoglossus muscle 舌骨舌的

hy·oid (hi′oid) shaped like the Greek letter upsilon (υ); pertaining to the hyoid bone 舌骨形的，（希腊字母）υ 形的；舌骨的

hyo·scine (hi′o-sēn) scopolamine 东莨菪碱

hyo·scy·amine (hi″o-si′ə-mēn) an anticholinergic alkaloid that is the levorotatory component of racemic atropine and has similar actions but twice the potency; used as an antispasmodic in gastrointestinal and urinary tract disorders, as the base or hydrobromide or sulfate salt 莨菪碱

hyp·al·ge·sia (hi″pal-je′ze-ə) decreased pain sense 痛觉减退；**hypalge′sic** *adj.*

hyp·ana·ki·ne·sis (hi-pan″ə-kī-ne′sis) 同 hypokinesia

hyp·ar·te·ri·al (hi″pahr-tēr′e-əl) beneath an artery 动脉下的

hyp·ax·i·al (hi-pak′se-əl) ventral to the long axis of the body 体轴下的

hy·per·ac·id (hi″pər-as′id) excessively acid 酸过多的

hy·per·ac·tiv·i·ty (hi″pər-ak-tiv′ ĭ-te) 1. excessive or abnormally increased muscular function or activity 活动亢进；2. former name for *attentiondeficit/hyperactivity disorder;* **hyperac′tive** *adj.*

hy·per·acu·sis (hi″pər-ə-koo′sis) an exceptionally acute sense of hearing, the threshold being very low 听觉过敏

hy·per·ad·e·no·sis (hi″pər-ad″ə-no′sis) enlargement of glands 腺增大

hy·per·ad·i·po·sis (hi″pər-ad″ĭ-po′sis) extreme fatness 肥胖过度

hy·per·ad·re·nal·ism (hi″pər-ə-dre′nəl-iz-əm) overactivity of the suprarenal glands 肾上腺功能亢进

hy·per·adre·no·cor·ti·cism (hi″pər-ə-dre″-nokor′tĭ-siz-əm) hypersecretion by the adrenal cortex 肾上腺皮质功能亢进

hy·per·al·dos·ter·on·ism (hi″pər-al-dos′tə- roniz″əm) aldosteronism 醛固酮过多症

hy·per·al·ge·sia (hi″pər-al-je′ze-ə) abnormally increased pain sense 痛觉过敏；**hyperalge′sic,**

hyperalget′ic *adj.*

hy·per·al·i·men·ta·tion (hi″pər-al″ĭ-menta′shən) the ingestion or administration of a greater than optimal amount of nutrients 饮食过度; **parenteral h.**, total parenteral nutrition 胃肠外高营养, 静脉高营养

hy·per·al·pha·lipo·pro·tein·emia (hi″pəral″fə-lip″o-pro″te-ne′me-ə) the presence of abnormally high levels of high-density lipoproteins in the serum 血 α- 脂蛋白过多, 高 α- 脂蛋白血 (症)

hy·per·am·mo·ne·mia (hi″pər-am″o-ne′me-ə) a metabolic disturbance marked by elevated levels of ammonia in the blood 高血氨 (症), 血氨过多

hy·per·am·mo·nu·ria (hi″pər-am″o-nu′re-ə) excessive ammonia in the urine 尿氨过多, 高氨尿

hy·per·an·dro·gen·ism (hi″pər-an′dro-jən-iz- əm) the state of having excessive secretion of androgens, as in congenital adrenal hyperplasia 雄激素过多症

hy·per·aphia (hi″pər-a′fe-ə) tactile hyperesthesia 触觉过敏; **hyperaph′ic** *adj.*

hy·per·arou·sal (hi″pər-ə-rou′səl) a state of increased psychological and physiologic tension marked by such effects as reduced pain tolerance, anxiety, exaggeration of startle responses, insomnia, fatigue, and accentuation of personality traits 觉 醒过度

hy·per·azo·te·mia (hi″pər-az″o-te′me-ə) an excess of nitrogenous matter in the blood 血氮过多, 高氮血 (症)

hy·per·bar·ic (hi″pər-bar′ik) having greater than normal pressure or weight; said of gases under greater than atmospheric pressure, or of a solution of greater specific gravity than another used as a reference standard 高压的; 高比重的

hy·per·bar·ism (hi″pər-bar′iz-əm) a condition due to exposure to ambient gas pressure or atmospheric pressures exceeding the pressure within the body 高气压病

hy·per·be·ta·lipo·pro·tein·emia (hi″pərba″tə-lip″o-pro″te-ne′me-ə) increased accumulation of low-density lipoproteins in the blood 高 β- 脂蛋白血症

hy·per·bil·i·ru·bin·emia (hi″pər-bil″ĭ-roo″bĭ-ne′me-ə) excess of bilirubin in the blood; classified as conjugated or unconjugated, according to the predominant form of bilirubin present 高胆红素血 (症)

hy·per·brady·ki·nin·ism (hi″pər-brad″e-ki′nĭ-niz-əm) a syndrome of high plasma bradykinin associated with a fall in systolic blood pressure on standing, increased diastolic pressure and heart rate, and ecchymoses of lower limbs 缓激肽过多症

hy·per·cal·ce·mia (hi″pər-kal-se′me-ə) an excess of calcium in the blood 高钙血症, 高血钙; **id-**

iopathic h., a condition of infants, associated with vitamin D intoxication, characterized by elevated serum calcium levels, increased density of the skeleton, mental deterioration, and nephrocalcinosis 特发性血钙过多; **h. of malignancy,** abnormal elevation of serum calcium associated with malignant tumors, resulting from osteolysis caused by bone metastases or by the action of circulating cytokines released from tumor cells 恶性高钙血症

hy·per·cal·ci·uria (hi″pər-kal″se-u′re-ə) excess of calcium in the urine 高钙尿症

hy·per·cap·nia (hi″pər-kap′ne-ə) excessive carbon dioxide in the blood 高碳酸血 (症); **hypercap′nic** *adj.*

hy·per·car·bia (hi″pər-kahr′be-ə) hypercapnia 高碳酸血

hy·per·car·o·ten·emia (hi″pər-kar″ə-tə-ne′me-ə) excessive carotene in the blood, often with yellowing of the skin (carotenosis) 高胡萝卜素血症

hy·per·ca·thar·sis s (hi″pər-kə-thahr′sis) excessive catharsis 腹泻过度; **hypercathar′tic** *adj.*

hy·per·cel·lu·lar·i·ty (hi″pər-sel″u-lar′ ĭ-te) abnormal increase in the number of cells present, as in bone marrow 细胞过多; **hypercell′ular** *adj.*

hy·per·chlor·emia (hi″pər-klor-e′me-ə) an excess of chlorides in the blood 高氯血症; **hyperchlore′mic** *adj.*

hy·per·chlor·hy·dria (hi″pər-klor-hi′dre-ə) excessive hydrochloric acid in gastric juice 胃酸过多 (症)

hy·per·cho·les·ter·ol·emia (hi″pər-kə-les″tərol-e′me-ə) an excess of cholesterol in the blood 高胆固醇血症; **hypercholesterole′mic** *adj.*; **familial h.**, an inherited disorder of lipoprotein metabolism due to defects in the receptor for lowdensity lipoprotein (LDL), with xanthomas, corneal arcus, premature corneal atherosclerosis, and a type II-a hyperlipoproteinemia biochemical phenotype with elevated plasma LDL and cholesterol 家族性高胆固醇血症

hy·per·chro·ma·sia (hi″pər-kro-ma′zhə) hyperchromatism 染色过深

hy·per·chro·ma·tism (hi″pər-kro′mə-tiz-əm) unusually intense or excessive coloration or staining 着色过度, 色素过多; **hyperchromat′ic** *adj.*

hy·per·chro·mia (hi″pər-kro′me-ə) 同 hyperchromatism; **hyperchromic** *adj.*

hy·per·chy·lo·mi·cro·ne·mia (hi″pər-ki″lomi″kro-ne′me-ə) presence in the blood of an excessive number of chylomicrons 高乳糜微粒血症; **familial h.**, an inherited disorder of lipoprotein metabolism characterized by elevated plasma chylomicrons and triglycerides, pancreatitis, cutaneous xanthomas, and hepatosplenomegaly; it is usually due to deficiency of lipoprotein lipase or its cofactor apolipoprotein

C-Ⅱ家族性高乳糜微粒血症

hy·per·cry·al·ge·sia (hi″pər-kri′al-je′ze-ə) 同 hypercryesthesia

hy·per·cry·es·the·sia (hi″pər-kri′es-the′zhə) excessive sensitivity to cold 冷觉过敏

hy·per·cu·pre·mia (hi″pər-ku-pre′me-ə) an excess of copper in the blood 高铜血症

hy·per·cu·pri·uria (hi″pər-ku-pre-u′re-ə) excessive copper in the urine 高铜尿

hy·per·cy·a·not·ic (hi″pər-si″ə-not′ik) extremely cyanotic 高度发绀的

hy·per·cy·the·mia (hi″pər-si-the′me-ə) erythrocythemia 血红细胞增多症

hy·per·di·crot·ic (hi″pər-di-krot′ik) markedly dicrotic 强二波脉的

hy·per·dis·ten·tion (hi″pər-dis-ten′shən) excessive distention 膨胀过度

hy·per·dy·na·mia (hi″pər-di-na′me-ə) hyperactivity (1) 肌力过度，肌活动过度；**hyperdynam′ic** adj.

hy·per·em·e·sis (hi″pər-em′ə-sis) excessive vomiting 剧吐；**hyperemet′ic** adj; **h. gravida′rum,** the pernicious vomiting of pregnancy 妊娠剧吐；**h. lacten′tium,** excessive vomiting in nursing babies 乳儿剧吐

hy·per·emia (hi″pər-e′me-ə) engorgement; an excess of blood in a part 充血；**hypere′mic** adj.; **active h., arterial h.,** that due to local or general relaxation of arterioles 主动性充血，动脉性充血；**exercise h.,** vasodilation of the capillaries in muscles in response to the onset of exercise, proportionate to the force of the muscular contractions 运动性充血；**passive h.,** that due to obstruction to flow of blood from the area 被动性充血；**reactive h.,** that due to an increase in blood flow after its temporary interruption 反应性充血；**venous h.,** passive h. 静脉性充血

hy·per·eo·sin·o·phil·ia (hi″pər-e″o-sin″ofil′e-ə) extreme eosinophilia 嗜曙红细胞增多症；**hypereosinophil′ic** adj.

hy·per·equi·lib·ri·um (hi″pər-e′kwī-lib′re- əm) excessive tendency to vertigo 平衡觉过敏，易晕性

hy·per·eso·pho·ria (hi″pər-es″o-for′e-ə) deviation of the visual axes upward and inward 上内（向）隐斜视

hy·per·es·the·sia (hi″pər-es-the′zhə) increased sensitivity to stimulation, particularly to touch 感觉过敏；**hyperesthet′ic** adj.; **acoustic h.,**; **auditory h.,** hyperacusis 听觉过敏；**cerebral h.,** hyperesthesia due to a cerebral lesion 大脑性感觉过敏；**gustatory h.,** hypergeusia 味觉过敏；**muscular h.,** muscular oversensitivity to pain or fatigue 肌觉过敏；**olfactory h.,** hyperosmia 嗅觉过敏；**oneiric h.,** increased sensitivity or pain during sleep and dreams 睡梦性感觉过敏；**optic h.,** abnormal sensitivity of the eye to light 光感过敏，对光感过敏，视觉过敏；**tactile h.,** excessive sensitivity of the sense of touch 触觉过敏

hy·per·es·tro·gen·ism (hi″pər-es′tro-jən-iz- əm) excessive amounts of estrogens in the body 雌激素过多（症）

hy·per·ex·ci·ta·tion (hi″pər-ex-cī-tā′shun) heightened states of electrical activity, such as depolarization block and depolarized lowamplitude membrane oscillation, observed in neurons of the suprachiasmatic nuclei 兴奋过度

hy·per·exo·pho·ria (hi″pər-ek″so-for′e-ə) deviation of the visual axes upward and outward 上外（向）隐斜视

hy·per·fer·re·mia (hi″pər-fer-e′me-ə) an excess of iron in the blood 高铁血症；**hyperferre′mic** adj.

hy·per·fi·bri·no·ge·ne·mia (hi″pər-fi-brin″ojə-ne′me-ə) excessive fibrinogen in the blood 高纤维蛋白原血症

hy·per·fil·tra·tion (hi″pər-fil-tra′shən) an increase in the glomerular filtration rate, often a sign of early type 1 diabetes mellitus 超滤

hy·per·frac·tion·a·tion (hi″pər-frak″shənə′shən) a subdivision of a radiation treatment schedule with some reduction of dose per exposure so as to decrease side effects while still delivering an equal or greater total dose of radiation over the course 高剂量分次疗法

hy·per·func·tion (hi″pər-funk′shən) excessive functioning of a part or organ 功能亢进

hy·per·ga·lac·tia (hi″pər-gə-lak′she-ə) excessive secretion of milk 乳汁过多

hy·per·gal·ac·to·sis (hi″pər-gal″ak-to′sis) 同 hypergalactia

hy·per·gam·ma·glob·u·lin·emia (hi″pərgam″ə-glob″u-lī-ne′me-ə) increased gamma globulins in the blood 高丙种球蛋白血症；**hypergammaglobuline′mic** adj.; **monoclonal h's,** plasma cell dyscrasias 单克隆高丙种球蛋白血症，浆细胞病

hy·per·gen·e·sis (hi″pər-jen′ə-sis) excessive development 发育过度；**hypergenet′ic** adj.

hy·per·geus·es·the·sia (hi″pər-goos″esthe′zhə) 同 hypergeusia

hy·per·geu·sia (hi″pər-goo′zhə) abnormal acuteness of the sense of taste 味觉过敏

hy·per·glu·ca·gon·emia (hi″pər-gloo″kə- gone′me-ə) abnormally high levels of glucagon in the blood 高血糖素症

hy·per·gly·ce·mia (hi″pər-gli-se′me-ə) abnormally increased content of glucose in the blood 高血糖症

hy·per·gly·ce·mic (hi″pər-gli-se′mik) 1. pertaining to, characterized by, or causing hyperglycemia 高血

糖的；2. an agent that increases the glucose level of the blood

hy·per·glyc·er·i·de·mia (hi″pər-glis″ər-ide′me-ə) excess of glycerides in the blood 高甘油酯血症

hy·per·glyc·er·ol·emia (hi″pər-glis″ər-ole′me-ə) 1. accumulation and excretion of glycerol due to deficiency of an enzyme catalyzing its phosphorylation; the infantile form is due to a chromosomal deletion that may also involve the loci causing Duchenne muscular dystrophy or congenital adrenal hyperplasia, or both 高甘油血症，由于缺乏催化磷酸化的酶而导致甘油的积累和排泄障碍，由于染色体缺失，也可能涉及引起 Duchenne 肌营养不良症或先天性肾上腺增生的基因座；2. excess of glycerol in the blood 血（内）甘油过多

hy·per·gly·cin·e·mia (hi″pər-gli″sī-ne′me-ə) excess of glycine in the blood or other body fluids; *ketotic h.* includes ketotic disorders secondary to a variety of organic acidemias; *nonketotic h.* is a hereditary disorder of neonatal onset, due to a defect in the glycine cleavage system, with lethargy, absence of cerebral development, seizures, myoclonic jerks, and frequently coma and respiratory failure 高甘氨酸血症，分为酮症高甘氨酸血症和非酮症高甘氨酸血症，前者包括继发于各种有机酸血症的酮症，后者由于甘氨酸裂解系统缺陷，出现嗜睡、脑发育不良、癫痫发作、肌阵挛性抽搐、经常昏迷和呼吸衰竭，是新生儿遗传性疾病

hy·per·gly·cin·uria (hi″pər-gli″sī-nu′re-ə) an excess of glycine in the urine 高甘氨酸尿，尿内甘氨酸过多；见 *hyperglycinemia*

hy·per·gly·co·gen·ol·y·sis (hi″pər-gli″kojən-ol′ə-sis) excessive glycogenolysis, resulting in excessive glucose in the body 糖原分解过度

hy·per·gly·cor·rha·chia (hi″pər-gli″ko-ra′ke- ə) excessive sugar in the cerebrospinal fluid 脑脊液糖分过多

hy·per·go·nad·ism (hi″pər-go′nad-iz-əm) abnormally increased functional activity of the gonads, with accelerated growth and precocious sexual development 性腺功能亢进

hy·per·go·nado·tro·pic (hi″pər-gon″ə-dotro′pik) relating to or caused by excessive amounts of gonadotropins 促性腺激素分泌过多的

hy·per·hi·dro·sis (hi″pər-hī-dro′sis) excessive perspiration 多汗，多汗症；**hyperhidrot′ic** *adj.* **compensatory h.**, excessive sweating on one part of the body to compensate for damage and inactivity of nearby sweat glands 代偿性多汗症；**emotional h.**, 1. hyperhidrosis due to emotional stimuli 精神性多汗症；2. an inherited disorder of the eccrine sweat glands in which emotional stimuli cause axillary or palmar sweating 情绪多汗症，情绪刺激引起腋窝

或手掌出汗

hy·per·hy·dra·tion (hi″pər-hi-dra′shən) overhydration; excessive fluids in the body 水分过多

Hy·per·i·cum (hi-per′ĭ-kum) a genus of herbs, including several types of St. John's wort 金丝桃属；*H. perfora′tum,* the species of St. John's wort whose above-ground parts are used medicinally 贯叶连翘

hy·per·im·mune (hi″pər-ĭ-mūn′) possessing very large quantities of specific antibodies in the serum 超免疫的

hy·per·im·mu·no·glob·u·lin·emia (hi″pərim″u-no-glob″u-lĭ-ne′me-ə) abnormally high levels of immunoglobulins in the serum 高免疫球蛋白血症

hy·per·su·lin·ism (hi″pər-in′sə-lin-iz″əm) 1. excessive secretion of insulin 高胰岛素血症；2. insulin shock 胰岛素休克

hy·per·ir·ri·ta·bil·i·ty (hi″pər-ir″ĭ-tə-bil′ ĭ-te) pathologic responsiveness to slight stimuli 应激性过高

hy·per·iso·ton·ic (hi″pər-i″so-ton′ik) denoting a solution containing more than 0.45% salt, in which erythrocytes become crenated as a result of exosmosis 高渗的

hy·per·ka·le·mia (hi″pər-kə-le′me-ə) an excess of potassium in the blood; hyperpotassemia 高钾血症；**hyperkale′mic** *adj.*

hy·per·ker·a·tin·iza·tion (hi″pər-ker″ə-tin″ī-za′shən) excessive development or retention of keratin in the epidermis 角化过度

hy·per·ker·a·to·sis (hi″pər-ker″ə-to′sis) hypertrophy of the stratum corneum of the skin, or any disease so characterized 角化过度，过度角化；**epidermolytic h.**, an autosomal dominant skin disease, with hyperkeratosis, blisters, and erythema; at birth the skin is entirely covered with thick, horny, armorlike plates that are soon shed, leaving a raw surface on which scales then reform 表皮松解性角化过度；**h. follicula′ris in cu′tem pe′netrans**, Kyrle disease 皮肤穿通性毛囊角化过度症；**palmoplantar h.**, 掌距角化病，见 *keratoderma* 下词条

hy·per·ke·ton·emia (hi″pər-ke″to-ne′me-ə) ketonemia 高酮血症

hy·per·ki·ne·mia (hi″pər-kī-ne′me-ə) abnormally high cardiac output; increased rate of blood flow through the circulatory system 心输出量过多

hy·per·ki·ne·mic (hi″pər-kī-ne′mik) increasing blood flow through a tissue, or an agent that causes such an increased blood flow 组织血流增多的；促组织血流增多药

hy·per·ki·ne·sia (hi″pər-kī-ne′zhə) hyperactivity 运动过度（症）

hy·per·ki·ne·sis (hi″pər-kī-ne′sis) hyperactivity

运动过度；**hyperkinet′ic** *adj*.

hy·per·lac·ta·tion (hi″pər-lak-ta′shən) lactation in greater than normal amount or for a longer than normal period 泌乳期过久，乳汁过多

hy·per·leu·ko·cy·to·sis (hi″pər-loo″ko-sito′sis) abnormally excessive numbers of leukocytes in the blood 白细胞过多症

hy·per·li·pe·mia (hi″pər-lĭ-pe′me-ə) hyperlipidemia 高脂血症；**carbohydrate-induced h.**, elevated blood lipids, particularly triglycerides, after carbohydrate ingestion; sometimes used synonymously with hyperlipoproteinemia type Ⅳ or Ⅴ phenotypes, or the genetic disorders causing them 糖诱导的血脂过多症；**combined fat- and carbohydrate induced h.**, persistently elevated blood levels of very-low-density lipoproteins and chylomicrons after ingestion of fat or carbohydrates; sometimes used synonymously with a type Ⅴ hyperlipoproteinemia or the genetic disorders causing it 联合脂肪和碳水化合物引起的高脂血症；**endogenous h.**, elevated plasma lipids derived from body stores (i.e., very-lowdensity lipoproteins) rather than from dietary sources; used as a generic descriptor of the type Ⅳ hyperlipoproteinemia phenotype 内源性高脂血症；**essential familial h.**, an inherited disorder causing a type Ⅰ hyperlipoproteinemia phenotype, or the phenotype itself 原发性家族性高脂血症；**exogenous h.**, elevated plasma levels of lipoproteins derived from dietary sources (i.e., chylomicrons); used as a generic descriptor of the type Ⅰ hyperlipoproteinemia phenotype 外源性高脂血症；**familial fat-induced h.**, persistently elevated blood chylomicrons after fat ingestion; sometimes used synonymously with hyperlipoproteinemia type Ⅰ phenotype or the genetic disorders causing it 家族性脂肪引起的高脂血症；**mixed h.**, generic designation for a hyperlipoproteinemia in which several classes of lipoproteins are elevated; usually used to denote a type Ⅴ phenotype, but sometimes used for a type Ⅱ -b phenotype 混合型高脂血症

hy·per·lip·id·emia (hi″pər-lip″ĭ-de′me-ə) elevated concentrations of any or all of the lipids in the plasma, including hypertriglyceridemia, hypercholesterolemia, etc. 高脂血症 **hyperlipide′mic** *adj*.；**combined h.**, a generic designation for a hyperlipidemia in which several classes of lipids are elevated; usually used to denote the phenotype of a type Ⅱ -b hyperlipoproteinemia 复合性高脂血症；**familial combined h.**, an inherited disorder of lipoprotein metabolism manifested in adulthood as hypercholesterolemia or hypertriglyceridemia, or a combination, with elevated plasma apolipoprotein B and premature coronary atherosclerosis 家族性复

合性高脂血症；**mixed h.**, 混合性高脂血症，见 *hyperlipemia* 下词条；**remnant h.**, a form in which the accumulated lipoproteins are normally transient intermediates, chylomicron remnants, and intermediate-density lipoproteins; a generic descriptor for the type Ⅲ hyperlipoproteinemia phenotype 残余性高脂血症

hy·per·lipo·pro·tein·emia (hi″pər-lip″o-pro″tene′me-ə) an excess of lipoproteins in the blood, due to a disorder of lipoprotein metabolism; it may be acquired or familial. It has been subdivided on the basis of biochemical phenotype, each type having a generic description and a variety of causes: *type Ⅰ*, exogenous hyperlipemia; *type Ⅱ -a*, hypercholesterolemia; *type Ⅱ -b*, combined hyperlipidemia; *type Ⅲ*, remnant hyperlipidemia; *type Ⅳ*, endogenous hyperlipemia; *type Ⅴ*, mixed hyperlipemia 高脂蛋白血症，Ⅰ型，外源性高脂血症；Ⅱ -a 型，高胆固醇血症；Ⅱ -b 型，联合性高脂血症；Ⅲ型，残余性高脂血症；Ⅳ型，内源性高脂血症；Ⅴ型，混合性高脂血症

hy·per·lu·cen·cy (hi″pər-loo′sən-se) excessive radiolucency 超射线透射性

hy·per·ly·sin·emia (hi″pər-li″se-ne′me-ə) 1. excess of lysine in the blood 血中赖氨酸过多；2. an aminoacidopathy characterized by an excess of lysine, and sometimes of saccharopine, in the blood and urine, possibly associated with intellectual disability 高赖氨酸血症，其特征是血液和尿液中有过量的赖氨酸或酵母氨酸，可能与智力障碍有关

hy·per·mag·ne·se·mia (hi″pər-mag″nə-se′me- ə) an abnormally large magnesium content of the blood plasma 高镁血症

hy·per·mas·tia (hi″pər-mas′te-ə) 1. presence of supernumerary mammary glands 多乳腺；2. macromastia 乳房肥大

hy·per·ma·ture (hi″pər-mə-choor′) past the stage of maturity 成熟过度的

hy·per·men·or·rhea (hi″pər-men″o-re′ə)menstruation with an excessive flow but at regular intervals and of usual duration 月经过多

hy·per·me·tab·o·lism (hi″pər-mə-tab′o-liz- əm) increased metabolism 高代谢；**extrathyroidal h.**, abnormally elevated basal metabolism unassociated with thyroid disease 非甲状腺性代谢亢进

hy·per·me·tria (hi″pər-me′tre-ə) ataxia in which movements overreach the intended goal 伸展过度

hy·per·me·tro·pia (hi″pər-me-tro′pe-ə) hyperopia 远视（眼）

hy·per·mo·bil·i·ty (hi″pər-mo-bil′ĭ-te) greater than normal range of motion in a joint 关节过度活动综合征；**hypermo′bile** *adj*.

hy·per·morph (hi′pər-morf) a mutant gene that

shows an increase in the activity it influences 超效等位基因；**hypermor′phic** *adj.*

hy·per·mo·til·i·ty (hi″pər-mo-til′ĭ-te) abnormally increased motility, as of the gastrointestinal tract（胃肠道）运动过强

hy·per·my·ot·ro·phy (hi″pər-mi-ot′rə-fe) excessive development of muscular tissue 肌肥大

hy·per·na·sal·i·ty (hi″pər-na-zal′ĭ-te) a quality of voice in which the emission of air through the nose is excessive due to velopharyngeal insufficiency; it causes deterioration of intelligibility of speech 鼻音过强

hy·per·na·tre·mia (hi″pər-nə-tre′me-ə) an excess of sodium in the blood 高钠血症；**hypernatre′mic** *adj.*

hy·per·neo·cy·to·sis (hi″pər-ne″o-si-to′sis) hyperleukocytosis with an excessive number of immature forms 幼稚白细胞过多性白细胞增多症

hy·per·ne·phro·ma (hi″pər-nə-fro′mə) renal cell carcinoma 肾上腺样瘤

hy·per·nu·tri·tion (hi″pər-noo-trish′ən) hyperalimentation 营养过度

hy·per·ope (hi′pər-ōp) an individual exhibiting hyperopia 远视者

hy·per·opia (H) (hi″pər-o′pe-ə) farsightedness; an error of refraction in which rays of light entering the eye parallel to the optic axis are brought to a focus behind the retina, as a result of the eyeball being too short from front to back 远视（眼）；**hypero′pic** *adj.*; **absolute h.**, that which cannot be corrected by accommodation 绝对远视；**axial h.**, that due to shortness of the anteroposterior diameter of the eye 轴性远视；**facultative h.**, that which can be entirely corrected by accommodation 兼性远视，条件性远视；**latent h.**, that degree of the total hyperopia corrected by the physiologic tone of the ciliary muscle, revealed by cycloplegic examination 隐性远视；**manifest h.**, that degree of the total hyperopia not corrected by the physiologic tone of the ciliary muscle, revealed by cycloplegic examination 显性远视；**relative h.**, facultative h. 相对远视；**total h.**, manifest and latent hyperopia combined 总远视，隐性远视和显性远视同时发生

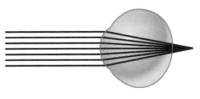

▲ 远视

hy·per·orex·ia (hi″pər-o-rek′se-ə) excessive appe-

tite 食欲过旺，善饥

hy·per·or·ni·thin·emia (hi″pər-or″nĭ-thĭ-ne′me-ə) excess of ornithine in the plasma 高鸟氨酸血，血中鸟氨酸过多

hy·per·or·tho·cy·to·sis (hi″pər-or″tho-sito′sis) hyperleukocytosis with a normal proportion of the various forms of leukocytes 正比例性白细胞增多症

hy·per·os·mia (hi″pər-oz′me-ə) increased sensitivity of smell 嗅觉过敏

hy·per·os·mo·lal·i·ty (hi″pər-oz″mo-lal′ ĭ-te) an increase in the osmolality of the body fluids（体液）重量渗克分子浓度过高

hy·per·os·mo·lar·i·ty (hi″pər-oz″mo-lar′ ĭ-te) abnormally increased osmolar concentration 容积渗克分子浓度过高

hy·per·os·to·sis (hi″pər-os-to′sis) hypertrophy of bone 骨质厚，骨质增生症；**hyperostot′ic** *adj.*; **h. cortica′lis defor′mans juveni′lis**, an inherited disorder of limb fractures and bowing, thickening of skull bones, osteoporosis, and elevated levels of serum alkaline phosphatase and urinary hydroxyproline 幼年畸形骨皮质肥厚症；**h. cortica′lis generalisa′ta**, a hereditary disorder manifesting during puberty, marked chiefly by osteosclerosis of the skull, mandible, clavicles, ribs, and diaphyses of long bones, associated with elevated blood alkaline phosphatase 弥漫性骨皮质增多症；**h. cra′nii**, hyperostosis involving the cranial bones 颅骨增生；**h. fronta′lis inter′na**, thickening of the inner table of the frontal bone, which may be associated with hypertrichosis and obesity, most commonly affecting women near menopause 额骨内板增生症；**infantile cortical h.**, an autosomal dominant, self-limited disorder of young infants, with soft tissue swelling over affected bones, fever, irritability, and periods of remission and exacerbation 婴儿骨皮质增生症

hy·per·ox·al·uria (hi″pər-ok″sə-lu′re-ə) an excess of oxalates in the urine 高草酸尿（症）；**enteric h.**, formation of calcium oxalate calculi in the urinary tract after resection or disease of the ileum, due to excessive absorption of oxalate from the colon 肠源性高草酸尿症；**primary h.**, an inborn error of metabolism with defective glyoxylate metabolism, excessive urinary excretion of oxalate, nephrolithiasis, nephrocalcinosis, early onset of renal failure, and often a generalized deposit of calcium oxalate 原发性高草酸尿症

hy·per·ox·ia (hi″pər-ok′se-ə) an excess of oxygen in the system 高氧；**hyperox′ic** *adj.*

hy·per·par·a·site (hi″pər-par′ə-sīt) a parasite that preys on a parasite 超寄生物，重寄生物；**hyper-**

parasit′ic *adj.*

hy·per·para·thy·roid·ism (hi″pər-par″ə- thi′roid-iz-əm) excessive activity of the parathyroid glands. *Primary h.* is associated with neoplasia or hyperplasia; the excess of parathyroid hormone leads to alteration in function of bone cells, renal tubules, and gastrointestinal mucosa. *Secondary h.* occurs when the serum calcium tends to fall below normal, as in chronic renal disease, etc. *Tertiary h.* refers to that due to a parathyroid adenoma arising from secondary hyperplasia caused by chronic renal failure 甲状旁腺功能亢进症，分为原发性、继发性和三级性 甲状旁腺功能亢进

hy·per·peri·stal·sis (hi″pər-per″ĭ-stawl′sis) excessively active peristalsis 蠕动过强

hy·per·pha·gia (hi″pər-fa′jə) polyphagia 饮食过多；**hyperpha′gic** *adj.*

hy·per·phen·yl·al·a·nin·emia (hi″pər-fen″əlal″ə-nī-ne′me-ə) 1. any of several inherited defects in the hydroxylation of phenylalanine, causing it to be accumulated and excreted; some are relatively benign whereas others cause phenylketonuria 高苯丙氨酸血症，苯丙氨酸羟基化过程中几种遗传缺陷，造成其累积和排泄，部分导致苯丙酮尿症；2. excess of phenylalanine in the blood 血苯丙氨酸过多

hy·per·pho·ne·sis (hi″pər-fo-ne′sis) intensification of the sound in auscultation or percussion（听诊或叩诊）声响过强

hy·per·pho·ria (hi′pər-for′e-ə) upward deviation of the visual axis of one eye in the absence of visual fusional stimuli 上隐斜

hy·per·phos·pha·ta·se·mia (hi″pər-fos″fə- tase′me-ə) high levels of alkaline phosphatase in the blood 高磷酸酯酶血，血内磷酸酯酶过多

hy·per·phos·pha·ta·sia (hi″pər-fos″fə-ta′zhə) hyperphosphatasemia 血内磷酸酯酶过多

hy·per·phos·pha·te·mia (hi″pər-fos″fə- te′me-ə) an excessive amount of phosphates in the blood 高磷（酸盐）血症

hy·per·phos·pha·tu·ria (hi″pər-fos″fə-tu′re- ə) an excess of phosphates in the urine 高磷酸盐尿，尿内磷酸盐过多

hy·per·pig·men·ta·tion (hi″pər-pig″mənta′shən) abnormally increased pigmentation 色素沉着

hy·per·pi·tu·i·ta·rism (hi″pər-pĭ-too″ĭ-tə- riz″əm) a condition due to pathologically increased activity of the pituitary gland, either of the basophilic cells, resulting in basophil adenoma causing compression of the pituitary gland, or of the eosinophilic cells, producing overgrowth, acromegaly, and gigantism *(true h.)* 垂体功能亢进

hy·per·pla·sia (hi″pər-pla′zhə) abnormal increase in the number of normal cells in normal arrangement in an organ or tissue, which increases its volume 增生，超常增生；**hyperplas′tic** *adj.*；**adrenal cortical h., adrenocortical h.,** 肾上腺皮质增生（症）；hyperplasia of adrenal cortical cells, as in adrenogenital syndrome and Cushing syndrome.**benign prostatic h. (BPH),** age-associated enlargement of the prostate resulting from proliferation of both stromal and glandular elements; it may cause urethral obstruction and compression 良性前列腺增生；**C-cell h.,** a premalignant stage in the development of the familial forms of medullary thyroid carcinoma, characterized by multicentric patches of parafollicular cells (C cells) 滤泡旁细胞增生（C细胞增生），甲状腺髓样癌的癌前病变；**congenital adrenal h. (CAH),** a group of inherited disorders of cortisol biosynthesis that result in compensatory hypersecretion of corticotropin and subsequent adrenal hyperplasia, excessive androgen production, and a spectrum of phenotypes 先天性肾上腺皮质增生症；**cutaneous lymphoid h.,** a group of benign cutaneous disorders with lesions clinically and histologically resembling those of malignant lymphoma 皮肤淋巴样组织增生；**focal nodular h. (FNH),** a benign, firm, nodular, highly vascular tumor of the liver, resembling cirrhosis 局灶性结节增生；**intravascular papillary endothelial h.,** a benign vascular tumor usually occurring as a solitary nodule of the head, neck, or finger and resembling angiosarcoma 血管内乳头状内皮增生；**nodular h. of the prostate,** benign prostatic h. 前列腺结节性增生；**sebaceous h.,** a type of pale, round lesion consisting of malformed sebaceous glands, usually on the face of an older adult 皮脂腺增生；**verrucous h.,** a superficial, typically white, hyperplastic lesion of the oral mucosa, usually occurring in older men and believed to be a precursor to verrucous carcinoma 疣状增生

hy·per·ploi·dy (hi″pər-ploi′de) the state of having more than the typical number of chromosomes in unbalanced sets, as in Down syndrome 超倍性

hy·per·pnea (hi″pərp-ne′ə) abnormal increase in depth and rate of respiration 呼吸过度，呼吸增强；**hyperpne′ic** *adj.*

hy·per·po·lar·iza·tion (hi″pər-po″lər-ĭ-za′shən) any increase in the amount of electrical charge separated by the cell membrane and, hence, in the strength of the transmembrane potential 超极化

hy·per·po·ne·sis (hi″pər-po-ne′sis) excessive action-potential output from the motor and premotor areas of the cortex 皮质运动区活动过度；**hyperponet′ic** *adj.*

hy·per·po·sia (hi″pər-po′zhə) abnormally in-

H

creased ingestion of fluids for relatively brief periods 饮水过多，进液过多

hy·per·po·tas·se·mia (hi″pər-po″tə-se′me-ə) hyperkalemia 高钾血症

hy·per·prax·ia (hi″pər-prak′se-ə) abnormal activity; restlessness 精神活动异常，精神兴奋过度

hy·per·pre·be·ta·lipo·pro·tein·emia (hi″pərpre-ba″tə-lip″o-pro″te-ne′me-ə) an excess of prebeta lipoproteins (very-low-density lipoproteins) in the blood 高前 β - 脂蛋白血症

hy·per·pro·in·su·lin·emia (hi″pər-pro-in″sə- lĭ-ne′me-ə) elevated levels of proinsulin or proinsulin-like material in the blood 高胰岛素原血，血胰岛素原过多

hy·per·pro·lac·tin·emia (hi″pər-pro-lak″tĭ-ne′me-ə) an elevated level of circulating prolactin, often associated with prolactinoma 高催乳素血症; **hyperprolactine′mic** adj.

hy·per·pro·lin·emia (hi″pər-pro″lĭ-ne′me-ə) 1. any of several benign aminoacidopathies marked by an excess of proline in the body fluids 高脯氨酸血（症）; 2. excess of proline in the blood 血脯氨酸过多

hy·per·pro·sex·ia (hi″pər-pro-sek′se-ə) preoccupation with one idea to the exclusion of all others 注意增强

hy·per·pro·te·o·sis (hi″pər-pro″te-o′sis) a condition due to an excess of protein in the diet 蛋白摄食过多

hy·per·py·rex·ia (hi″pər-pi-rek′se-ə) hyperthermia 高热; **hyperpyrex′ial, hyperpyret′ic** adj.; **malignant h.,** 恶性高热，见 hyperthermia 下词条

hy·per·re·ac·tio lu·te·in·a·lis (hi″pər-reak′she-o loo″te-ĭ-na′lis) benign, bilateral ovarian enlargement during pregnancy, which regresses after delivery, due to the presence of numerous theca-lutein cysts, caused by increased production of human chorionic gonadotropin 卵巢高反应性黄素化

hy·per·re·ac·tive (hi″pər-re-ak′tiv) showing a greater than normal response to stimuli 反应过度的

hy·per·re·flex·ia (hi″pər-re-flek′se-ə) disordered response to stimuli characterized by exaggeration of reflexes 反射亢进; **autonomic h.,** paroxysmal hypertension, bradycardia, forehead sweating, headache, and gooseflesh due to distention of the bladder and rectum, associated with lesions above the outflow of the splanchnic nerves 自主反射亢进; **detrusor h.,** increased contractile activity of the detrusor muscle of the bladder, resulting in urinary incontinence 逼尿肌反射亢进

hy·per·re·nin·emia (hi″pər-re″nĭ-ne′me-ə) elevated levels of renin in the blood, which may lead to

aldosteronism and hypertension 血（内）紧张肽原酶过多，高血管紧张肽原酶血症，高肾素血症

hy·per·res·o·nance (hi″pər-rez′o-nəns) exaggerated resonance on percussion 过清音

hy·per·re·spon·sive (hi″pər-rə-spon′siv) hyperreactive 高反应性

hy·per·sal·i·va·tion (hi″pər-sal″ĭ-va′shən) ptyalism 多涎

hy·per·sar·co·sin·e·mia (hi″pər-sahr″ko-sĭ-ne′me-ə) elevated plasma concentration of sarcosine 血肌氨酸过多，高肌氨酸血症，见 sarcosinemia

hy·per·se·cre·tion (hi″pər-se-kre′shən) excessive secretion 分泌过度

hy·per·sen·si·tiv·i·ty (hi″pər-sen″sĭ-tiv′ĭ-te) a state of altered reactivity in which the body reacts with an exaggerated immune response to what is perceived as a foreign substance. The hypersensitivity states and resulting reactions are usually subclassified by the Gell and Coombs classification (q.v.) 超敏反应，超敏性; **hypersen′sitive** adj.; **antibody mediated h.,** 1. 同 type Ⅱ h.; 2. occasionally, any form of hypersensitivity in which antibodies, rather than T lymphocytes, are the primary mediators, i.e., types Ⅰ to Ⅲ 抗体介导的超敏反应; **cell-mediated h.,** 同 type Ⅳ h. 细胞介导的超敏反应; **contact h.,** a type Ⅳ hypersensitivity produced by contact of the skin with a chemical substance having the properties of an antigen or hapten 接触性超敏反应; **cytotoxic h.,** 同 type Ⅱ h. 细胞毒性过敏反应; **delayed h. (DH), delayed-type h. (DTH),** that which takes 24 to 72 hours to develop and is mediated by T lymphocytes rather than by antibodies; usually used to denote the subset of type Ⅳ hypersensitivity involving cytokine release and macrophage activation, as opposed to direct cytolysis, but sometimes used more broadly, even as a synonym for *type Ⅳ h.* 迟发型超敏反应; **immediate h.,** 1. 同 type Ⅰ h.; 2. occasionally, any form of hypersensitivity mediated by antibodies and developing rapidly, generally in minutes to hours (i.e., *types Ⅰ to Ⅲ*), as distinguished from that mediated by T lymphocytes and macrophages and requiring days to develop (*type Ⅳ,* or *delayed h.*) 速发型超敏反应; **immune complex-mediated h.,** 同 type Ⅲ h. 免疫复合物介导的超敏反应; **T cell-mediated h.,** T 细胞介导的超敏反应; **type Ⅰ h., type Ⅱ h., type Ⅲ h., type Ⅳ h.,** Ⅰ 至Ⅳ型超敏反应见 *classification* 下 *Gell and Coombs classification*

hy·per·sex·u·al·i·ty (hi″pər-sek″shoo-al′ĭ-te) abnormally increased sexual desire or activity; involves recurrent and intense sexual fantasies, sexual urges 性欲亢进; 见 *nymphomania* 和 *satyriasis*

hy·per·som·nia (hi″pər-som′ne-ə) excessive

sleeping or sleepiness 睡眠过度，嗜睡

hy·per·som·no·lence (hi″pər-som′no-lens) 同 hypersomnia

hy·per·splen·ism (hi″pər-splen′iz-əm) exaggeration of the hemolytic function of the spleen, resulting in deficiency of peripheral blood elements, hypercellularity of bone marrow, and splenomegaly 脾功能亢进

hy·per·sthe·nia (hi″pər-sthe′ne-ə) great strength or tonicity 体力过盛；**hypersthen′ic** *adj.*

hy·per·stim·u·la·tion (hi″pər-stim″u-la′shən) excessive stimulation of an organ or part 刺激过度；**controlled ovarian h.,** monitored administration of agents designed to induce ovulation by a greater number of ovarian follicles and thus increase the probability of fertilization 控制性超促排卵

hy·per·telo·rism (hi″pər-te′lor-iz-əm) abnormally increased distance between two organs or parts （两器官间）距离过远；**ocular h., orbital h.,** increase in the interorbital distance, often associated with cleidocranial or craniofacial dysostosis and sometimes with mental deficiency 眼距过宽，眶距过宽

hy·per·ten·sion (hi″pər-ten′shən) persistently high arterial blood pressure; it may have no known cause *(essential, idiopathic,* or *primary h.)* or may be associated with other diseases *(secondary h.)* 高血压；**accelerated h.,** progressive hypertension with the funduscopic vascular changes of malignant hypertension but without papilledema 急进性高血压；**adrenal h.,** hypertension associated with an adrenal tumor that secretes mineralocorticoids 肾上腺（缺血）性高血压；**borderline h.,** a condition in which the arterial blood pressure is sometimes within the normotensive range and sometimes within the hypertensive range 临界性高血压；**Goldblatt h.,** that caused experimentally by a Goldblatt kidney Goldblatt 高血压；**labile h.,** 同 borderline h.；**malignant h.,** a severe hypertensive state with papilledema of the ocular fundus and vascular hemorrhagic lesions, thickening of the small arteries and arterioles, left ventricular hypertrophy, and a poor prognosis 恶性高血压；**ocular h.,** persistently elevated intraocular pressure in the absence of any other signs of glaucoma; it may or may not progress to open-angle glaucoma 高眼压症；**persistent pulmonary h. of the newborn,** a condition in newborns in which blood continues to flow through the foramen ovale and a patent ductus arteriosus, bypassing the lungs and resulting in hypoxemia 新生儿持续性肺动脉高压；**portal h.,** abnormally increased pressure in the portal circulation 门静脉高压（症）；**pulmonary h.,** abnormally increased

pressure in the pulmonary circulation 肺动脉高压；**renal h.,** that associated with or due to renal disease with a factor of parenchymatous ischemia 肾性高血压；**renovascular h.,** that due to occlusive disease of the renal arteries 肾血管性高血压；**systemic venous h.,** elevation of systemic venous pressure, usually detected by inspection of the jugular veins 系统性静脉高压

hy·per·ten·sive (hi″pər-ten′siv) 1. characterized by increased tension or pressure 高血压的；2. an agent that causes hypertension 血压升高药；3. a person with hypertension 高血压患者

hy·per·the·co·sis (hi″pər-the-ko′sis) hyperplasia and excessive luteinization of the cells of the inner stromal layer of the ovary 卵泡膜细胞增殖症

hy·per·ther·mal·ge·sia (hi″pər-thur″məlje′ze-ə) abnormal sensitivity to heat 热觉过敏

hy·per·ther·mia (hi″pər-thur′me-ə) hyperpyrexia; greatly increased body temperature 体温过高；**hyperther′mal, hyperther′mic** *adj.*; **malignant h.,** an autosomal dominant condition affecting patients undergoing general anesthesia, marked by a sudden, rapid rise in body temperature, associated with signs of increased muscle metabolism and, usually, muscle rigidity 恶性高热

hy·per·thy·mia (hi″pər-thi′me-ə) 1. excessive emotionalism 情感增盛；2. excessive activity, verging on hypomania 情感高涨；**hyperthy′mic** *adj.*

hy·per·thy·mism (hi″pər-thi′miz-əm) excessive activity of the thymus gland 胸腺功能亢进

hy·per·thy·roid·ism (hi″pər-thi′roid-iz-əm) excessive thyroid gland activity, marked by an increased metabolic rate, goiter, and disturbances in the autonomic nervous system and in creatine metabolism 甲状腺功能亢进（症）；**hyperthy′roid** *adj.*

hy·per·to·nia (hi″pər-to′ne-ə) a condition of excessive tone of the skeletal muscles; increased resistance of muscle to passive stretching 肌张力过高

hy·per·ton·ic (hi″pər-ton′ik) 1. denoting increased tone or tension 紧张过度的；2. denoting a solution having greater osmotic pressure than the solution with which it is compared 高渗的，高张的

hy·per·to·nic·i·ty (hi″pər-to-nis′ĭ-te) the state or quality of being hypertonic 高渗性，高张性

hy·per·tri·cho·sis (hi″pər-trĭ-ko′sis) excessive growth of hair 多毛（症）。Cf. *hirsutism*

hy·per·tri·glyc·er·i·de·mia (hi″pər-tri-glis′ə-ride′me-ə) an excess of triglycerides in the blood 高甘油三脂血脂，高三酰甘油血症

hy·per·tro·phy (hi-pur′trə-fe) enlargement or overgrowth of an organ or part due to an increase in size of its constituent cells 肥大；**hypertro′phic**

adj.; **asymmetric septal h. (ASH)**, hypertrophic cardiomyopathy, sometimes specifically that in which the hypertrophy is localized to the interventricular septum 非对称性心室间隔肥厚; **benign prostatic h.**, 良性前列腺肥大, 见 *hyperplasia* 下词条; **ventricular h.**, hypertrophy of the myocardium of a ventricle due to chronic pressure overload 心室肥大

hy·per·tro·pia (hi″pər-tro′pe-ə) strabismus in which there is permanent upward deviation of the visual axis of an eye 上斜视

hy·per·ty·ro·sin·emia (hi″pər-ti″ro-sĭ-ne′me-ə) 1. an elevated concentration of tyrosine in the blood 血内酪氨酸过多; 2. tyrosinemia 高酪氨酸血症

hy·per·uri·ce·mia (hi″pər-u″rĭ-se′me-ə) uricemia; an excess of uric acid in the blood 高尿酸血症, 血尿酸过多; **hyperurice′mic** *adj.*

hy·per·u·ri·co·su·ria (hi″pər-u″rĭ-ko-su′re-ə) an excess of urates or uric acid in the urine 高尿酸尿症

hy·per·u·ric·uria (hi″pər-u″rĭ-ku′re-ə) 同 hyperuricosuria

hy·per·ven·ti·la·tion (hi″pər-ven″tĭ-la′shən) 1. abnormally increased pulmonary ventilation, resulting in reduction of carbon dioxide tension, which, if prolonged, may lead to alkalosis 通气过度; 2. 见 *syndrome* 下词条

hy·per·vig·i·lance (hi″pər-vij′ĭ-ləns) abnormally increased arousal, responsiveness to stimuli, and scanning of the environment for threats 过度警觉

hy·per·vis·cos·i·ty (hi″pər-vis-kos′ĭ-te) excessive viscosity, as of the blood 黏滞性过高

hy·per·vi·ta·min·o·sis (hi″pər-vi″tə-mĭ-no′sis) a condition due to ingestion of an excess of one or more vitamins; symptom complexes are associated with excessive intake of vitamins A and D 维生素过多症; **hypervitaminot′ic** *adj.*

hy·per·vo·le·mia (hi″pər-vo-le′me-ə) abnormal increase in the plasma volume in the body 血容量过多

hyp·es·the·sia (hīp″es-the′zhə) hypoesthesia 感觉减退

hy·pha (hi′fə) pl. *hy′phae* [L.] 1. one of the filaments composing the mycelium of a fungus. 菌丝 2. branching filamentous outgrowths produced by some bacteria, sometimes forming a mycelium 菌丝体 **hy′phal** *adj.*

hyp·he·do·nia (hīp″hə-do′ne-ə) diminution of power of enjoyment 快感减少

hy·phe·ma (hi-fe′mə) hemorrhage within the anterior chamber of the eye 前房积血

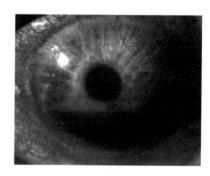

▲ **30%的前房积血**

hy·phe·mia (hi-fe′me-ə) 同 hyphema

hyp·hi·dro·sis (hīp″hĭ-dro′sis) 同 hypohidrosis

Hy·pho·my·ce·tes (hi″fo-mi-se′tēz) formerly, a class of anamorphic fungi comprising the molds producing conidia and hyphae; still used informally 丝孢菌

hyp·na·gog·ic (hip″nə-goj′ik) 1. 同 hypnotic (1, 2); 2. occurring just before sleep; applied to hallucinations occurring at sleep onset 入睡前的

hyp·nal·gia (hip-nal′jə) pain during sleep 睡发性疼痛

hyp·no·anal·y·sis (hip″no-ə-nal′ə-sis) a method of psychotherapy combining psychoanalysis with hypnosis 催眠分析

hyp·no·don·tics (hip″no-don′tiks) the application of hypnosis and controlled suggestion in the practice of dentistry 牙科催眠术

hyp·noid (hip′noid) resembling hypnosis or sleep 似睡的, 催眠状态样的

hyp·nol·o·gy (hip-nol′ə-je) scientific study of sleep or of hypnotism 催眠学

hyp·no·pom·pic (hip″no-pom′pik) persisting after sleep; applied to hallucinations occurring on awakening 半睡前的; 睡意朦胧（状态）的

hyp·no·sis (hip-no′sis) an altered state of consciousness characterized by focusing of attention, suspension of disbelief, increased amenability and responsiveness to suggestions and commands, and the subjective experience of responding involuntarily 催眠; 催眠状态

hyp·no·ther·a·py (hip″no-ther′ə-pe) the use of hypnosis in the treatment of disease 催眠疗法

hyp·not·ic (hip-not′ik) 1. inducing sleep 催眠的; 2. an agent that induces sleep 催眠药, 安眠药; 3. pertaining to or of the nature of hypnosis or hypnotism 催眠术的

hyp·no·tism (hip′no-tiz-əm) the study of or the method or practice of inducing hypnosis 催眠性的

hyp·no·tize (hip′no-tīz) to induce a state of hypnosis 催眠

hy·po (hi′po) 1. colloquialism for a hypodermic inoculation or syringe 皮下注射；皮下注射器（俗语）；2. sodium thiosulfate 海波，硫代硫酸钠

hy·po·ac·tiv·i·ty (hi″po-ak-tiv′ĭ-te) 1. abnormally diminished activity, as of peristalsis 活动减退；2. abnormally decreased motor and cognitive activity, with slowing of thought, speech, and movement 活动减少；**hypoac′tive** *adj.*

hy·po·acu·sis (hi″po-ə-ku′sis) slightly diminished auditory sensitivity 听觉减退

hy·po·adre·nal·ism (hi″po-ə-dre′nəl-iz-əm) adrenal insufficiency (1) 肾上腺素功能减退

hy·po·adre·no·cor·ti·cism (hi″po-ə-dre″nokor′tĭ-siz-əm) adrenocortical insufficiency 肾上腺皮质功能减退

hy·po·al·bu·min·o·sis (hi″po-al-bu″mĭ-no′sis) abnormally low level of albumin 白蛋白过少（症）

hy·po·al·i·men·ta·tion (hi″po-al″ĭ-mən-ta′shən) insufficient nourishment 营养不足

hy·po·al·pha·lipo·pro·tein·emia (hi″poal′fə-lip″o-pro″te-ne′me-ə) 1. deficiency of highdensity (alpha) lipoproteins in the blood 低 α - 脂蛋白血症；2. Tangier disease 丹吉尔病

hy·po·azo·tu·ria (hi″po-az″o-tu′re-ə) diminished nitrogenous material in the urine 尿氮过少，低氮尿

hy·po·bar·ic (hi″po-bar′ik) having less than normal pressure or weight; said of gases under less than atmospheric pressure or of a solution of a lower specific gravity than another taken as a standard of reference 低压的，低比重的

hy·po·bar·ism (hi″po-bar′iz-əm) the condition resulting when ambient gas or atmospheric pressure is below that within the body tissues 低气压病

hy·po·bar·op·a·thy (hi″po-bar-op′ə-the) 1. the disturbances experienced in high altitudes due to reduced air pressure, as in high-altitude sickness and mountain sickness 高空病；2. 同 hypobarism

hy·po·blast (hi′po-blast) the embryonic precursor to the endoderm 内胚层；**hypoblas′tic** *adj.* 内胚层的

hy·po·cal·ce·mia (hi″po-kal-se′me-ə) reduction of the blood calcium below normal 低钙血症；**hypocalce′mic** *adj.*

hy·po·cap·nia (hi″po-kap′ne-ə) deficiency of carbon dioxide in the blood 低碳酸血症；**hypocap′nic** *adj.*

hy·po·car·bia (hi″po-kahr′be-ə) hypocapnia 低碳酸血

hy·po·chlor·emia (hi″po-klor-e′me-ə) diminished chloride in the blood 低氯血症；**hypochlore′mic** *adj.*

hy·po·chlor·hy·dria (hi″po-klor-hi′dre-ə) lack of hydrochloric acid in the gastric juice 胃酸过少

hy·po·chlo·rite (hi″po-klor′īt) any salt of hypochlorous acid; used as a medicinal agent with disinfectant action, particularly as a diluted solution of sodium hypochlorite 次氯酸盐

hy·po·chlo·rous ac·id (hi″po-klor′əs) an unstable compound with disinfectant and bleaching action 次氯酸

hy·po·cho·les·te·re·mia (hi″po-kə-les″tə-re′me-ə) 同 hypocholesterolemia

hy·po·cho·les·ter·ol·emia (hi″po-kə-les″tərole′me-ə) diminished cholesterol in the blood 低胆固醇血症；**hypocholesterole′mic** *adj.*

hy·po·chon·dria (hi″po-kon′dre-ə) 1. plural of *hypochondrium;* the upper lateral abdominal region 季肋部, hypochondrium 的复数形式；2. 同 hypochondriasis

hy·po·chon·dri·ac (hi″po-kon′dre-ak) 1. pertaining to the hypochondrium 季肋部的；2. pertaining to hypochondriasis 疑病（症）的；3. a person with hypochondriasis 疑病症患者

hy·po·chon·dri·a·sis (hi″po-kon-dri′ə-sis) a somatoform disorder characterized by a preoccupation with bodily functions and the interpretation of normal sensations or minor abnormalities as indications of serious problems needing medical attention 疑病症；**hypochon′driac, hypochondri′acal** *adj.*

hy·po·chon·dri·um (hi″po-kon′dre-əm) pl. *hypochon′dria.* The upper lateral abdominal region, overlying the costal cartilages, on either side of the epigastrium 季肋部；**hypochon′drial** *adj.*

hy·po·chro·ma·sia (hi″po-kro-ma′zhə) 1. the condition of staining less intensely than normal 染色过浅；2. 同 hypochromia (1)

hy·po·chro·ma·tism (hi″po-kro′mə-tiz-əm) 1. abnormally deficient pigmentation, especially a deficiency of chromatin in a cell nucleus 着色不足；2. 同 hypochromia (1)

hy·po·chro·mia (hi″po-kro′me-ə) 1. abnormal decrease in the hemoglobin content of the erythrocytes 血红蛋白过少（尤指细胞核内染色质过少）；2. 同 hypochromatism (1)；**hypochro′mic** *adj.*

hy·po·cit·ra·tu·ria (hi″po-sĭ-tra-tu′re-ə) diminished citrates in the urine 低枸橼酸尿

hy·po·com·ple·men·te·mia (hi″po-kom″plə-men-te′me-ə) diminution of complement levels in the blood 低补体血症

Hypo·crea (hi″po-kre′ə) a genus of fungi of the family Hypocreaceae, found in soil, wood, and decaying vegetation; its anamorphs belong to *Trichoderma* 肉座菌属

H

hy·po·cy·clo·sis (hi″po-si-klo′sis) insufficient accommodation in the eye 调视功能减退

hy·po·cy·the·mia (hi″po-si-the′me-ə) deficiency in the number of erythrocytes in the blood 红细胞减少症

Hy·po·der·ma (hi″po-dur′mə) a genus of ox warble or heel flies whose larvae cause disease in cattle and a creeping eruption in humans 皮蝇属，皮下蝇属

hy·po·der·mi·a·sis (hi″po-dər-mi′ə-sis) a creeping eruption of the skin caused by larvae of *Hypoderma* 皮下蝇蛆病

hy·po·der·mic (hi″po-dur′mik) subcutaneous; beneath the skin 皮下的

hy·po·der·mis (hi″po-dur′mis) superficial fascia 皮下组织

hy·po·der·mo·cly·sis (hi″po-dər-mok′lĭ-sis) subcutaneous infusion of fluids, e.g., saline solution 皮下输液

hy·po·dip·sia (hi″po-dip′se-ə) abnormally diminished thirst 渴感减退

hy·po·don·tia (hi″po-don′shə) partial anodontia 牙发育不全，部分无齿畸形

hy·po·dy·na·mia (hi″po-di-na′me-ə) abnormally diminished power 力不足，乏力; **hypodynam′ic** *adj.*

hy·po·echo·ic (hi″po-ə-ko′ik) in ultrasonography, giving off few echoes; said of tissues or structures that reflect relatively few of the ultrasound waves directed at them 低回声的，弱回声的

hy·po·eso·pho·ria (hi″po-es″o-for′e-ə) deviation of the visual axes downward and inward 下内（向）隐斜视

hy·po·es·the·sia (hi″po-es-the′zhə) abnormally decreased sensitivity, particularly to touch 感觉迟钝; **hypoesthet′ic** *adj.*

hy·po·exo·pho·ria (hi″po-ek″so-for′e-ə) deviation of the visual axes downward and laterally 下外（向）隐斜视

hy·po·fer·re·mia (hi″po-fer-e′me-ə) deficiency of iron in the blood 血（内）铁过少

hy·po·fer·til·i·ty (hi″po-fər-til′ĭ-te) subfertility 生殖力减低; **hypofer′tile** *adj.*

hy·po·fi·brin·o·gen·emia (hi″po-fi-brin″o-jə-ne′me-ə) deficiency of fibrinogen in the blood 低纤维蛋白原血症

hy·po·ga·lac·tia (hi″po-gə-lak′she-ə) deficiency of milk secretion 乳汁减少; **hypogalac′tous** *adj.*

hy·po·gam·ma·glob·u·lin·emia (hi″po-gam″ə-glob″u-lĭ-ne′me-ə) deficiency of all classes of immunoglobulins, as in agammaglobulinemia, dysglobulinemia, and immunodeficiency. This is normal for a short period in infants but should not be prolonged 低丙（种）球蛋白血症; **hypogammaglobuline′mic** *adj.*; **common variable h.,** 普通

可变性低丙种球蛋白血症，见 *immunodeficiency* 下词条

hy·po·gan·gli·o·no·sis (hi″po-gang″gle-ə- no′sis) lessened number of myenteric ganglion cells in the distal large bowel, with constipation; a congenital type of megacolon 神经节细胞减少症

hy·po·gas·tric (hi″po-gas′trik) 1. inferior to the stomach 下腹的; 2. pertaining to the hypogastrium. 下腹部的; 3. pertaining to the internal iliac artery 髂内动脉的

hy·po·gas·tri·um (hi″po-gas′tre-əm) the pubic region, the lowest middle abdominal region 下腹部

hy·po·gas·tros·chi·sis (hi″po-gas-tros′kĭ-sis) congenital fissure of the hypogastrium 下腹裂（畸形）

hy·po·gen·e·sis (hi″po-jen′ə-sis) defective embryonic development 胚胎生长不良; **hypogenet′ic** *adj.*

hy·po·gen·i·tal·ism (hi″po-jen′ĭ-təl-iz″əm) hypogonadism 性腺功能减退（症）

hy·po·geus·es·the·sia (hi″po-goos″es-the′zhə) 同 hypogeusia

hy·po·geu·sia (hi″po-goo′zhə) abnormally diminished sense of taste 味觉减退

hy·po·glos·sal (hi″po-glos′əl) sublingual 舌下的

hy·po·glu·ca·gon·emia (hi″po-gloo″kə-gone′me-ə) abnormally reduced levels of glucagon in the blood 血内高血糖素过少，低高血糖素血

hy·po·gly·ce·mia (hi″po-gli-se′me-ə) deficiency of glucose concentration in the blood, which may lead to hypothermia, headache, and more serious neurologic symptoms 低血糖（症）

hy·po·gly·ce·mic (hi″po-gli-se′mik) 1. pertaining to, characterized by, or causing hypoglycemia 血糖过低的; 2. an agent that lowers blood glucose levels 降血糖药

hy·po·gly·cor·rha·chia (hi″po-gli″ko-ra′ke-ə) abnormally low sugar content in the cerebrospinal fluid 脑脊液糖分过少

hy·po·go·nad·ism (hi″po-go′nad-iz-əm) decreased functional activity of the gonads, with retardation of growth, sexual development, and secondary sex characters 性腺功能减退症; **hypergonadotropic h.,** that associated with high levels of gonadotropins, as in Klinefelter syndrome 高促性腺素性功能减退症; **hypogonadotropic h.,** that due to lack of gonadotropin secretion 低促性腺素性功能减退症

hy·po·go·na·do·tro·pic (hi″po-go″nə-do-tro′pik) relating to or caused by deficiency of gonadotropin 促性腺激素分泌不足的

hy·po·hi·dro·sis (hi″po-hĭ-dro′sis) abnormally diminished perspiration 少汗; **hypohidrot′ic** *adj.*

hy·po·ka·le·mia (hi″po-kə-le′me-ə) abnormally low potassium levels in the blood, which may lead to neuromuscular and renal disorders 低钾血症

hy·po·ka·le·mic (hi″po-kə-le′mik) 1. pertaining to or characterized by hypokalemia 低钾血的; 2. an agent that lowers blood potassium levels 降血钾药

hy·po·ki·ne·sia (hi″po-kĭ-ne′zhə) abnormally diminished motor function or activity 运动功能减退; 运动减少（症）; **hypokinet′ic** adj.

hy·po·lac·ta·sia (hi″po-lak-ta′zhə) deficiency of lactase activity in the intestines 肠乳糖酶缺乏症; 见 lactase deficiency

hy·po·ley·dig·ism (hi″po-li′dig-iz-əm) abnormally diminished secretion of androgens by Leydig cells 睾丸 Leydig 间质细胞功能减退, 雄激素分泌过少

hy·po·lip·i·de·mia (hi″po-lip″ĭ-de′me-ə) an abnormally decreased amount of fat in the blood 低脂血症; **hypolipide′mic** adj.

hy·po·mag·ne·se·mia (hi″po-mag″nə-se′me-ə) abnormally low magnesium content of the blood 血镁过少, 低镁血（症）

hy·po·ma·nia (hi″po-ma′ne-ə) an abnormality of mood resembling mania but of lesser intensity 轻躁狂; **hypoman′ic** adj.

hy·po·mel·a·no·sis (hi″po-mel″ə-no′sis) a deficiency of melanin in the tissues, especially in the skin 黑色素过少症

hy·po·men·or·rhea (hi″po-men″o-re′ə) diminution of menstrual flow or duration 月经过少

hy·po·mere (hi′po-mēr) 1. the ventrolateral portion of a myotome, innervated by an anterior ramus of a spinal nerve 肌节腹侧段, 为脊神经前支所支配; 2. the lateral plate of mesoderm that develops into the walls of the body cavities 轴外中胚层

hy·po·meth·yl·a·tion (hi″po-meth″əl-a′shən) presence of fewer methylated nucleotides in DNA than is usual for that DNA; localized or global, and related to DNA expression 低甲基化作用

hy·po·me·tria (hi″po-me′tre-ə) ataxia in which movements fall short of the intended goal 伸展不足, 运动范围不足

hy·po·morph (hi′po-morf″) hypomorphic allele 亚效等位基因

hy·po·myx·ia (hi″po-mik′se-ə) decreased secretion of mucus 黏液（分泌）减少

hy·po·na·sal·i·ty (hi″po-na-zal′ĭ-te) a quality of voice in which there is a complete lack of nasal emission of air and nasal resonance, so that speakers sound as if they have a cold 鼻音过少, 低鼻音

hy·po·na·tre·mia (hi″po-nə-tre′me-ə) deficiency of sodium in the blood 低钠血症; **depletional h.,** hyponatremia in which a low concentration of sodium in plasma is associated with a low concentration of total body sodium 失水失钠性低钠血（症）; **dilutional h.,** hyponatremia in which a

low concentration of sodium in plasma results from a loss of sodium from the body, with nonosmotic retention of water 稀释性低钠血症

hy·po·neo·cy·to·sis (hi″po-ne″o-si-to′sis) leukopenia with immature leukocytes in the blood 幼稚（白）细胞性白细胞过少（症）

hy·po·noia (hi″po-noi′ə) slow mental activity 精神迟钝, 精神活动不足

hy·po·nych·i·um (hi″po-nik′e-əm) the thickened epidermis beneath the free distal end of the nail 甲下皮; **hyponych′ial** adj.

hy·po·or·tho·cy·to·sis (hi″po-or″tho-si-to′sis) leukopenia with a normal proportion of the various forms of leukocytes 正比例性血细胞减少（症）

hy·po·os·mot·ic (hi″po-oz-mot′ik) containing a lower concentration of osmotically active components than a standard solution 低渗透性

hy·po·para·thy·roid (hi″po-par″ə-thi′roid) pertaining to or characterized by reduced function of the parathyroid glands 甲状旁腺功能减退

hy·po·para·thy·roid·ism (hi″po-par″ə-thi′roidiz-əm) greatly reduced function of the parathyroid glands, with hypocalcemia that may lead to tetany, hyperphosphatemia with decreased bone resorption, and other symptoms 甲状旁腺功能减退症

hy·po·per·fu·sion (hi″po-pər-fu′zhən) decreased blood flow through an organ, as in hypovolemic shock; if prolonged, it may result in permanent cellular dysfunction and death 低灌注, 灌注不足

hy·po·peri·stal·sis (hi″po-per″ĭ-stawl′sis) abnormally sluggish peristalsis 蠕动迟缓

hy·po·phar·ynx (hi″po-far′inks) laryngopharynx 下咽

hy·po·pho·ne·sis (hi″po-fo-ne′sis) diminution of the sound in auscultation or percussion 音响过弱

hy·po·pho·nia (hi″po-fo′ne-ə) a weak voice due to incoordination of the vocal muscles 发音过弱

hy·po·pho·ria (hi″po-for′e-ə) downward deviation of the visual axis of one eye in the absence of visual fusional stimuli 下隐斜

hy·po·phos·pha·ta·sia (hi″po-fos″fə-ta′zhə) an inborn error of metabolism with abnormally low serum alkaline phosphatase activity and phosphoethanolamine in the urine, most severe in babies before age 6 months. Affected infants and children have rickets and adults have osteomalacia 低磷酸酯酶症, 磷酸酶过少症

hy·po·phos·pha·te·mia (hi″po-fos″fə-te′me-ə) abnormally decreased level of phosphates in the blood 低磷（酸盐）血症; 另见 hypophosphatasia; **hypophosphate′mic** adj.; **familial h.,** familial hypophosphatemic rickets 家族性低磷（酸盐）血症; **X-linked h.,** a form of familial hypophosphatemic rickets X 连锁低磷酸血症，家族性低磷酸血症佝偻病

hy·po·phos·pha·tu·ria (hi″po-fos″fə-tu′re-ə) deficiency of phosphates in the urine 尿内磷酸盐过少，低磷酸盐尿

hy·po·phos·phor·ous ac·id (hi″po-fos-for′əs) a toxic, monobasic acid with strong reducing properties, H_3PO_2, which forms hypophosphites 次磷酸

hy·po·phren·ic (hi″po-fren′ik) subphrenic 低能的

hy·po·phys·e·al (hi″po-fiz′e-əl) 同 hypophysial

hy·po·phys·ec·to·my (hi-pof″ə-sek′tə-me) excision of the pituitary gland (hypophysis) 垂体切除术

hy·po·phys·i·al (hi″po-fiz′e-əl) pertaining to the hypophysis 垂体的

hy·po·phys·io·por·tal (hi″po-fiz″e-o-por′təl) denoting the portal system of the pituitary gland, in which hypothalamic venules connect with capillaries of the anterior pituitary 垂体门脉

hy·po·phys·io·priv·ic (hi″po-fiz″e-o-priv′ik) pertaining to deficiency of hormonal secretion of the pituitary gland (hypophysis) 垂体分泌缺乏的

hy·po·phys·io·tro·pic (hi″po-fiz″e-o-tro′pik) acting on the pituitary gland (hypophysis), as certain hormones 促垂体的

hy·poph·y·sis (hi-pof′ə-sis) [Gr.] pituitary gland 垂体；**h. ce′rebri**, pituitary gland 脑垂体; **pharyngeal h.**, a mass in the pharyngeal wall with a structure similar to that of the pituitary gland 咽垂体

hy·po·pig·men·ta·tion (hi″po-pig″mən-ta′shən) diminished pigmentation, such as of melanin in the skin 色素减退

hy·po·pi·tu·i·ta·rism (hi″po-pī-too′ĭ-tə-riz″əm) diminished hormonal secretion by the pituitary gland, especially the anterior pituitary 垂体功能减退（症）

hy·po·pla·sia (hi″po-pla′zhə) incomplete development or underdevelopment of an organ or tissue 发育不全，低常增生; **hypoplas′tic** *adj.*; **enamel h.**, incomplete or defective development of the enamel of the teeth; it may be hereditary or acquired 釉质发育不全（症）; **oligomeganephronic renal h.**, oligomeganephronia 肾单位稀少巨大症性肾发育不全，肾单位稀少巨大症

hy·pop·nea (hi-pop′ne-ə) diminished depth and rate of respiration 呼吸不足，呼吸减弱; **hypopne′ic** *adj.*

hy·po·po·ro·sis (hi″po-po-ro′sis) deficient callus formation after bone fracture 骨痂形成不全

hy·po·po·tas·se·mia (hi″po-pot″tə-se′me-ə) hypokalemia 低钾血症，血钾过少

hy·po·pros·o·dy (hi″po-pros′o-de) diminution of the normal variation of stress, pitch, and rhythm of speech 言语韵调减少

hy·po·pty·al·ism (hi″po-ti′əl-iz″əm) abnormally decreased secretion of saliva 涎液过少

hy·po·py·on (hi-po′pe-on) pus in the anterior chamber of the eye 眼前房积脓

hy·po·sal·i·va·tion (hi″po-sal″ĭ-va′shən) hypoptyalism 唾液（分泌）过少

hy·po·se·cre·tion (hi″po-se-kre′shən) diminished secretion, as by a gland 分泌过少

hy·po·sen·si·tive (hi″po-sen′sĭ-tiv) 1. exhibiting abnormally decreased sensitivity 低敏感的; 2. less sensitive to a specific allergen after repeated and gradually increasing doses of the offending substance 敏感减轻的

hy·pos·mia (hi-poz′me-ə) diminished sense of smell 嗅觉减退

hy·po·so·ma·to·tro·pism (hi″po-so-mat″otro′piz″əm) growth hormone deficiency; in children this causes pituitary dwarfism 生长激素过少症

hy·po·som·nia (hi″po-som′ne-ə) reduced time of sleep 失眠症

hy·po·spa·di·as (hi″po-spa′de-əs) a developmental anomaly in which the urethra opens inferior to its normal location; usually seen in males, with the opening on the underside of the penis or on the perineum 尿道下裂; **hypospadi′ac** *adj.*; **female h.**, a developmental anomaly in the female in which the urethra opens into the vagina 女性尿道下裂

hy·po·sper·ma·to·gen·e·sis (hi″po-spur″mə-to-jen′ə-sis) abnormally decreased production of spermatozoa 精子生成不足

hy·po·splen·ism (hi″po-splen′iz-əm) diminished functioning of the spleen, resulting in an increase in peripheral blood elements 脾功能减退症

hy·pos·ta·sis (hi-pos′tə-sis) poor or stagnant circulation in a dependent part of the body or an organ （血液）坠积

hy·po·stat·ic (hi″po-stat′ik) 1. pertaining to, due to, or associated with hypostasis 本质的; 2. pertaining to certain inherited traits that are particularly liable to be suppressed by other traits 下位的

hy·pos·the·nia (hi″pos-the′ne-ə) weakness 衰弱; **hyposthen′ic** *adj.*

hy·po·syn·er·gia (hi″po-sī-nur′jə) dyssynergia 协同（动作）不足

hy·po·te·lo·rism (hi″po-tel′ə-riz-əm) abnormally decreased distance between two organs or parts 两器官间距离过近; **ocular h., orbital h.**, abnormal decrease in the interorbital distance 两眼距离过近，两眶距离过近

hy·po·ten·sion (hi″po-ten′shən) abnormally low blood pressure 低血压; **orthostatic h.**, a fall in blood pressure associated with dizziness, blurred vision, and sometimes syncope, occurring upon standing or when standing motionless in a fixed position 体位性低血压

hy·po·ten·sive (hi″po-ten′siv) marked by low blood pressure or serving to reduce blood pressure 低血压的

hy·po·thal·a·mus (hi″po-thal′ə-məs) the part of the diencephalon forming the floor and part of the lateral wall of the third ventricle, including the optic chiasm, mammillary bodies, tuber cinereum, and infundibulum; the pituitary gland is also in this region but is physiologically distinct. Hypothalamic nuclei help activate, control, and integrate peripheral autonomic mechanisms, endocrine activities, and many somatic functions 下丘脑，丘脑下部；**hypothalam′ic** adj.

hy·poth·e·nar (hi-poth′ə-nər) (hi″po-the′nahr) 1. the fleshy eminence along the ulnar side of the palm 小鱼际；2. relating to this eminence 小鱼际的

hy·po·ther·mia (hi″po-thur′me-ə) 1. low body temperature, caused by cold weather or artificially induced to decrease the metabolism and need for oxygen during surgical procedures 低温；2. a reduction of core body temperature to 32℃ (95 ℉) or lower; may be caused by exposure to cold weather or induced as a means of decreasing metabolism of tissues, and thereby the need for oxygen, e.g., in various surgical procedures 低体温，降温；**hypother′mal, hypother′mic** adj.；**accidental h.**, unintentional reduction of the core body temperature, as in a cold environment 偶然性低温，意外体温过低

hy·poth·e·sis (hi-poth′ə-sis) a supposition that appears to explain a group of phenomena and is advanced as a basis for further investigation 假设，假说；**alternative h.**, one that is compared with the null hypothesis in a statistical test 备择假设；**biogenic amine h.**, the hypothesis that depression is associated with a deficiency of biogenic amines, especially norepinephrine, at functionally important receptor sites in the brain and that elation is associated with an excess of such amines 生物胺假说；**jelly roll h.**, a theory explaining the formation of nerve myelin, which states that it consists of several layers of the plasma membrane of a Schwann cell wrapped spirally around the axon in a jelly roll fashion 胶质卷假说；**lattice h.**, a theory of the nature of the antigen-antibody reaction that postulates it is the reaction between a multivalent antigen and a divalent antibody that gives an antigen-antibody complex its latticelike structure 晶格假说；**Lyon h.**, in mammalian somatic cells, all X chromosomes in excess of one are inactivated (in the form of sex chromatin) on a random basis at an early stage of

embryogenesis, leading to mosaicism of paternal and maternal X chromosomes in the female 莱昂假说，哺乳动物体细胞中，只有一个X染色体激活，其他X染色体被灭活；**null h.**, the particular one under investigation, which frequently asserts a lack of effect or of difference 无效假设；**one gene–one polypeptide chain h.**, a gene contains the DNA sequence that codes for the production of one polypeptide chain. Antibodies are an exception; separate genes for variable and constant regions are rearranged to code for a single polypeptide 一基因一多肽假说；**response–to–injury h.**, one explaining the development of atherogenesis as beginning with an injury to the endothelial cells lining an artery wall, which causes endothelial dysfunction and abnormal cellular interactions; atherogenesis then progresses 伤害反应假说（动脉粥样硬化发生机制的假说）；**sliding filament h.**, the stretching of individual muscle fibers raises the number of tension-developing bridges between the sliding contractile protein elements (actin and myosin) and thus augments the force of the next muscle contraction 肌丝滑动学说；**Starling h.**, the direction and rate of fluid transfer between blood plasma in a capillary and fluid in the tissue spaces depend on the hydrostatic pressure on each side of the capillary wall, on the osmotic pressure of protein in plasma and in tissue fluid, and on the properties of the capillary walls as a filtering membrane 斯塔灵假说；**wobble h.**, the third base of a tRNA anticodon does not have to pair with a complementary codon (as do the first two) but can form base pairs with any of several mRNA codons; explains how a specific transfer RNA (tRNA) molecule can translate different codons in a messenger RNA (mRNA) template 摆动假说

hy·po·thy·mia (hi″po-thi′me-ə) abnormally diminished emotional tone, as in depression 情感减退，情调低落；**hypothy′mic** adj.

hy·po·thy·mism (hi″po-thi′miz-əm) diminished thymus activity 胸腺功能减退

hy·po·thy·roid·ism (hi″po-thi′roid-iz-əm) deficiency of thyroid activity, a cause of cretinism in children and myxedema in adults, with a decreased metabolic rate, tiredness, and lethargy 甲状腺功能减退（症）；**hypothy′roid** adj.

hy·po·to·nia (hi″po-to′ne-ə) diminished tone of the skeletal muscles 肌张力低下，张力过低

hy·po·ton·ic (hi-po-ton′ik) 1. denoting decreased tone or tension 张力减退的；2. denoting a solution having less osmotic pressure than one with which it is compared 低渗的

hy·po·tri·cho·sis (hi″po-trī-ko′sis) presence of less than the normal amount of hair 稀毛症

hy·pot·ro·phy (hi-pot′rə-fe) 同 abiotrophy

hy·po·tro·pia (hi″po-tro′pe-ə) strabismus with permanent downward deviation of the visual axis of one eye 下斜视

hy·po·tym·pa·not·o·my (hi″po-tim″pə-not′ə- me) surgical opening of the hypotympanum 鼓室下部切开术，下鼓室开口术

hy·po·tym·pa·num (hi″po-tim′pə-nəm) the lower part of the cavity of the middle ear, in the temporal bone 下鼓室

hy·po·uri·ce·mia (hi″po-u″rī-se′me-ə) diminished uric acid in the blood, along with xanthinuria, due to deficiency of xanthine oxidase, the enzyme required for conversion of hypoxanthine to xanthine and of xanthine to uric acid 血内尿酸不足

hy·po·ven·ti·la·tion (hi″po-ven″tĭ-la′shən) reduction in the amount of air entering the pulmonary alveoli 通气不足；**primary alveolar h.**, 原发性肺泡通气不足

hy·po·vo·le·mia (hi″po-vo-le′me-ə) diminished volume of circulating blood in the body 血容量不足，血容量减少；**hypovole′mic** *adj.*

hy·po·vo·lia (hi″po-vo′le-ə) diminished water content or volume, as of extracellular fluid 液量过少，水含量过少

hy·po·xan·thine (hi″po-zan′thēn) a purine base formed as an intermediate in the degradation of purines and purine nucleosides to uric acid and in the salvage of free purines. Complexed with ribose, it is inosine 次黄嘌呤

hy·pox·emia (hi″pok-se′me-ə) deficient oxygenation of the blood 低氧血（症）

hy·pox·ia a tissue below physiologic levels despite adequate perfusion of the tissue by blood 缺氧，低氧；**hypox′ic** *adj.*；**anemic h.**, that due to reduction of the oxygen-carrying capacity of the blood owing to decreased total hemoglobin or altered hemoglobin constituents 贫血性缺氧；**fetal h.**, hypoxia in utero, caused by conditions such as inadequate placental function (often abruptio placentae), preeclamptic toxicity, prolapse of the umbilical cord, or complications from anesthetic administration 胎儿缺氧；**histotoxic h.**, that due to impaired use of oxygen by tissues 组织中毒性缺氧；**hypoxic h.**, that due to insufficient oxygen reaching the blood 氧分压过低性缺氧；**stagnant h.**, that due to failure to transport sufficient oxygen because of inadequate blood flow 淤血性缺氧

hy·pro·mel·lose (hi-pro′mə-lōs) a propylene glycol ether of methylcellulose, supplied in differing degrees of viscosity; used as a suspending and viscosity-increasing agent and tablet binder, coating, and excipient in pharmaceutical preparations and applied topically to the conjunctiva to protect and lubricate the cornea 羟丙基甲基纤维素，又称 *hydroxypropyl methylcellulose*；**h. phthalate**, a phthalic acid ester of hydroxypropyl methylcellulose, used as a coating agent for tablets and granules 邻苯二甲酸羟丙甲基纤维素酯

hyp·sar·rhyth·mia (hip″sə-rith′me-ə) an electroencephalographic abnormality commonly associated with jackknife seizures, with random, high-voltage slow waves and spikes spreading to all cortical areas 高度节律失调

hyp·so·ki·ne·sis (hip″so-kī-ne′sis) a backward swaying or falling when in erect posture; seen in paralysis agitans, Wilson disease, and similar conditions 后仰

hys·ter·al·gia (his″tər-al′jə) pain in the uterus 子宫痛

hys·ter·ec·to·my (his″tər-ek′tə-me) excision of the uterus 子宫切除术；**abdominal h.**, that performed through the abdominal wall 腹式子宫切除术；**cesarean h.**, cesarean section followed by removal of the uterus 剖宫产子宫切除术；**complete h.**, 同 total h.；**partial h.**, 同 subtotal h.；**radical h.**, excision of the uterus, upper vagina, and parametrium 根治性子宫切除术；**subtotal h.**, that in which the cervix is left in place 次全子宫切除术；**total h.**, that in which the uterus and cervix are completely excised 全子宫切除术；**vaginal h.**, that performed through the vagina 阴道子宫切除术

hys·te·re·sis (his″tə-re′sis) [Gr.] 1. a time lag in the occurrence of two associated phenomena, as between cause and effect 滞后；2. in cardiac pacemaker terminology, the number of pulses per minute below the programmed pacing rate that the heart must drop in order to cause initiation of pacing 磁滞

hys·ter·ia (his-ter′e-ə) a term formerly used widely in psychiatry. Its meanings have included (1) classical hysteria (now *somatization disorder*); (2) hysterical neurosis (now divided into *conversion disorder* and *dissociative disorders*); (3) anxiety hysteria; and (4) hysterical personality (now *histrionic personality*) 癔症，包括躯体化障碍、转换障碍和解离性障碍、焦虑型、戏剧性人格；**hyster′ic, hyster′ical** *adj.*；**fixation h.**, conversion disorder with symptoms based on an existing or previous organic disease or injury 固定性癔病

hys·ter·ics (his-ter′iks) popular term for an uncontrollable emotional outburst 癔症发作，歇斯底里的

hys·ter·og·ra·phy (his″tər-og′rə-fe) 1. the graphic recording of the strength of uterine contractions in labor 子宫收缩描记术；2. radiography of the uterus after instillation of a contrast medium 子宫造

影术

hys·ter·oid (his′tər-oid) resembling hysteria 癔病样的，类歇斯底里的

hys·ter·ol·y·sis (his″tər-ol′ə-sis) freeing of the uterus from adhesions 子宫松解术

hys·tero·myo·ma (his″tər-o-mi-o′mə) leiomyoma of the uterus 子宫肌瘤

hys·tero·myo·mec·to·my (his″tər-o-mi″omek′tə-me) uterine myomectomy 子宫肌瘤切除术

hys·tero·my·ot·o·my (his″tər-o-mi-ot′ə-me) incision of the uterus for removal of a solid tumor 子宫肌切开术

hys·ter·op·a·thy (his″tə-rop′ə-the) any disease of the uterus 子宫病

hys·tero·pexy (his′tər-o-pek″se) surgical fixation of a displaced uterus 子宫固定术

hys·ter·op·to·sis (his″tər-op-to′sis) uterine prolapse 子宫脱垂

hys·ter·or·rha·phy (his″tər-or′ə-fe) 1. suture of the uterus 子宫缝合术；2. 同 hysteropexy

hys·ter·or·rhex·is (his″tər-o-rek′sis) metrorrhexis 子宫破裂

hys·tero·sal·pin·gec·to·my (his″tər-o-sal″pinjek′tə-me) excision of the uterus and uterine tubes 子宫输卵管切除术

hys·tero·sal·pin·gog·ra·phy (his″tər-osal″pinggog′rə-fe) radiography of the uterus and uterine tubes 子宫输卵管造影（术）

hys·tero·sal·pin·go-ooph·o·rec·to·my (his″tər-o-sal-ping″go-o-of″ə-rek′tə-me) excision of the uterus, uterine tubes, and ovaries 子宫输卵管卵巢切除术

hys·tero·sal·pin·gos·to·my (his″tər-o-sal″pinggos′tə-me) anastomosis of a uterine tube to the uterus 子宫输卵管造口术

hys·tero·scope (his′tər-o-skōp″) an endoscope for direct visual examination of the cervical canal and uterine cavity 宫腔镜

hys·tero·spasm (his′tər-o-spaz″əm) spasm of the uterus 子宫痉挛

hys·ter·ot·o·my (his″tər-ot′ə-me) incision of the uterus, performed either transabdominally *(abdominal h.)* or vaginally *(vaginal h.)* 子宫切开术

Hz hertz 赫（兹）

I

I[符号] incisor 切牙；inosine (in nucleotides) 肌苷（核苷酸）；iodine 碘；isoleucine 异亮氨酸
I[符号] electric current 电流
IABP intra-aortic balloon pump 主动脉内球囊反搏
IAEA International Atomic Energy Agency 国际原子能机构
iat·ric (i-at′rik) pertaining to medicine or to a physician 医学的，医师的
iat·ro·gen·ic (i-at″ro-jen′ik) resulting from the activity of physicians; said of any adverse condition in a patient resulting from treatment by a physician or surgeon 由医生活动引起的，医源性的
ib·an·dro·nate (i-ban′drə-nāt) a bisphosphonate calcium-regulating agent used as the sodium salt to inhibit the resorption of bone in the prevention and treatment of osteoporosis 伊班膦酸盐
i·bru·ti·nib (eye-broo′tih-nib) an antineoplastic targeted therapy inhibitor of Bruton's tyrosine kinase 依鲁替尼
ibu·pro·fen (i″bu-pro′fən) a nonsteroidal antiinflammatory drug used in the treatment of pain, fever, dysmenorrhea, osteoarthritis, rheumatoid arthritis, other rheumatic and nonrheumatic inflammatory disorders, and vascular headaches 布洛芬
ibu·ti·lide (i-bu′tĭ-līd) a cardiac depressant used as an antiarrhythmic agent in the treatment of atrial

arrhythmias; administered by intravenous infusion as the fumarate salt 依布利特
IBX abbreviation for Independence Blue Cross health insurance company 美国独立蓝十字保险公司
IC inspiratory capacity 吸气容量；irritable colon 激惹性结肠，结肠过敏
i·cat·i·bant (eye-kat′i-bănt) a bradykinin β₂ receptor antagonist used to treat acute hereditary angioedema attacks in adults 艾替班特
ICD International Classification of Diseases (of the World Health Organization) 国际疾病分类法（世界卫生组织）；intrauterine contraceptive device 宫内节育器
ice (īs) the solid state of water occurring at or below 0℃ and 1 atmosphere 冰；dry i., carbon dioxide snow 干冰
ich·thy·oid (ik′the-oid) fishlike 鱼状的
ich·thyo·sar·co·tox·in (ik″the-o-sahr′kotok″sin) a toxin found in the flesh of poisonous fish 鱼肉毒素
ich·thyo·sar·co·tox·ism (ik″the-o-sahr″kotok″siz-əm) poisoning from eating of poisonous fish, marked by gastrointestinal and neurologic disturbances 鱼肉毒素中毒
ich·thyo·si·form (ik″the-o′sĭ-form) resembling ichthyosis 鱼鳞癣样的

ich·thy·o·sis (ik″the-o′sis) any in a group of cutaneous disorders characterized by increased or aberrant keratinization, resulting in noninflammatory scaling of the skin; most are genetically determined; often used to denote *i. vulgaris* 鱼鳞病，鱼鳞癣；**ichthyot′ic** *adj*.; *i.* **hys′trix**, a rare form of epidermolytic hyperkeratosis, marked by generalized, dark brown, linear verrucoid ridges somewhat like porcupine skin 豪猪样鱼鳞病；**lamellar i.**, a congenital autosomal recessive form; the affected infant is born encased in a collodionlike membrane *(collodion baby).* The membrane is soon shed, and the skin becomes covered with large, coarse scales, including on the flexures, palms, and soles 层板状鱼鳞病；**i.** **sim′plex**, **i. vulgaris** 单纯鱼鳞病；**i. vulga′ris**, hereditary ichthyosis present at or shortly after birth, with large, thick, dry scales on the neck, ears, scalp, face, and flexural surfaces 寻常性鱼鳞病

I·clu·sig (eye-clu′sig) trademark for a preparation of ponatinib 普纳替尼

ICN International Council of Nurses 国际护士会

ICP intracranial pressure 颅内压

ICS International College of Surgeons 国际外科医师协会

ICSH interstitial cell–stimulating hormone 促间质细胞激素，促黄体生成激素（黄体化激素）

ICSI intracytoplasmic sperm injection 卵质内单精子注射

ic·tal (ik′təl) pertaining to, marked by, or due to a stroke or an acute epileptic seizure 发作的，猝发性的

ic·tero·gen·ic (ik″tər-o-jen′ik) causing jaundice 致黄疸的

ic·tero·hep·a·ti·tis (ik″tər-o-hep″ə-ti′tis) inflammation of the liver with marked jaundice 黄疸性肝炎

ic·ter·us (ik′tər-əs) [L.] jaundice 黄疸；**icter′ic** *adj*.; *i.* **neonato′rum**, jaundice in newborn children 新生儿黄疸

ic·tus (ik′təs) pl. *ic′tus* [L.] a seizure, stroke, blow, or sudden attack 暴发，发作，猝发；搏动，冲击；**ic′tal** *adj*.

ICU intensive care unit（重症）监护室

ID₅₀ median infective dose 半数感染量，平均感染量

id (id) in psychoanalytic theory, the innate, unconscious, primitive aspect of the personality dominated by the pleasure principle and seeking immediate gratification 本我，伊底（精神分析法的术语）

-id word element [Gr.][构词成分]1. having the shape of, resembling 形式，样子，类似；2. an id reaction associated with the disorder specified by the root word 疹

ida·ru·bi·cin (i″dah-roo′bĭ-sin) an anthracycline antineoplastic used as the hydrochloride salt in the treatment of acute myelogenous leukemia 伊达比星

IDD IDDM 1. insulin-dependent diabetes (mellitus) 胰岛素依赖型糖尿病；见 *diabetes* 下 *type 1 diabetes mellitus*, 2. intellectual and developmental disabilities 精神发育迟缓

-ide a suffix indicating a binary chemical compound [后缀] 二元化合物

idea (i-de′ə) a mental impression or conception 想法 **autochthonous i.**, a persistent idea originating within the mind but seeming to have come from an outside source and often therefore felt to be of malevolent origin 自发观念；**dominant i.**, one that controls or colors every action and thought 优势观念；**fixed i.**, a persistent morbid impression or belief that cannot be changed by reason 固定观念；**overvalued i.**, a false or exaggerated belief sustained beyond reason or logic but with less rigidity than a delusion, also often being less patently unbelievable 超价观念；**i. of reference**, the incorrect idea that words and actions of others refer to oneself or the projection of the causes of one's own imaginary difficulties upon someone else 牵连观念

ide·al (i-de′əl) a pattern or concept of perfection 理想的；**ego i.**, the component of the superego comprising the standard of perfection unconsciously created by people for themselves 自我理想

ide·al·iza·tion (i-de″əl-ĭ-za′shən) a conscious or unconscious mental mechanism in which the individual overestimates an admired aspect or attribute of another person 理想化

ide·a·tion (i″de-a′shən) the formation of ideas or images 思想作用，观念作用；**idea′tional** *adj*.

idée fixe (e-da′ fĕks) [Fr.] fixed idea 固定观念

iden·ti·fi·ca·tion (i-den″tĭ-fi-ka′shən) a largely unconscious process, sometimes a defense mechanism, by which one person patterns himself after another 认同，自居

iden·ti·ty (i-den′tĭ-te) the aggregate of characteristics by which individuals are recognized by themselves and others 认同；**gender i.**, a person's self-conception as male and masculine or female and feminine, or ambivalent 性别认同

ideo·ge·net·ic (i″de-o-jə-net′ik) related to mental processes in which images of sense impressions are used, rather than ideas ready for verbal expression 观念性的

ide·ol·o·gy (i″de-ol′ə-je) (id″e-ol′ə-je) 1. the science of the development of ideas 思想（体系）；2. the body of ideas characteristic of an individual or of a social unit 意识形态

ideo·mo·tion (i″de-o-mo′shən) motion or muscular action induced by a dominant idea rather than by reflex or volition 意想性动作，观念性动作

ideo·mo·tor (i″de-o-mo′tər) aroused by an idea or thought; said of involuntary motion so aroused 意想性动作的，观念运动的

id·io·glos·sia (id″e-o-glos′e-ə) extremely defective articulation, with the utterance of virtually unintelligible vocal sounds 自解（言）语症；**idioglot′tic** *adj.*

id·io·gram (id′e-o-gram″) a diagrammatic representation of a karyotype (q.v.) 核型模式图，染色体组型图

id·io·path·ic (id″e-o-path′ik) self-originated; occurring without known cause 自发的；特发的

id·io·ret·i·nal (id″e-o-ret′ĭ-nəl) pertaining to the retina alone; applied to a visual sensation occurring without a visual stimulus 视网膜自感性的

id·io·syn·cra·sy (id″e-o-sin′krə-se) 1. a habit peculiar to an individual 特质；2. an abnormal susceptibility to an agent (e.g., a drug) peculiar to an individual 特异体质；**idiosyncrat′ic** *adj.*

id·io·tro·phic (id″e-o-tro′fik) capable of selecting its own nourishment 自选食物的

id·i·ot sa·vant (id′e-ət sə-vahnt′) (e-dyo′ sahvahn′) [Fr.] a person who is severely mentally limited in some respects, yet has a particular mental faculty that is developed to an unusually high degree 低能特才

id·io·ven·tric·u·lar (id″e-o-vən-trik′u-lər) pertaining to the cardiac ventricles alone 心室自身的，只影响心室的

IDL intermediate-density lipoprotein 中密度脂蛋白

idox·ur·i·dine (i-doks-ūr′ĭ-dēn) an analogue of pyrimidine that inhibits viral DNA synthesis; used as an antiviral agent in the treatment of herpes simplex keratitis 碘苷，碘脱氧尿苷

IDU 同 idoxuridine

idu·ron·ic ac·id (i″du-ron′ik) a uronic acid that is a constituent of dermatan sulfate, heparan sulfate, and heparin 艾杜糖醛酸

L-id·uron·i·dase (i″du-ron′ĭ-dās) a hydrolase that catalyzes a step in the degradation of the glycosaminoglycans dermatan sulfate and heparan sulfate; deficiency leads to mucopolysaccharidosis I 左旋艾杜糖苷酶

IED immune-enhancing diet 免疫增强饮食；inflammatory eye disease 炎症性眼病；intermittent explosive disorder 间歇性暴发性疾病

IF interstitial fibrosis 间质纤维化；intrinsic factor 内（在）因子

ifos·fa·mide (i-fos′fə-mīd) a cytotoxic alkylating agent of the nitrogen mustard group, in structure and actions similar to cyclophosphamide; used in the treatment of solid tumors of the testis, ovary, and lung, as well as sarcomas 异环磷酰胺

Ig immunoglobulin of any of the five classes: IgA, IgD, IgE, IgG, and IgM 免疫球蛋白

IGF insulin-like growth factor 胰岛素样生长因子

IGRA interferon-gamma release assay 干扰素释放实验

IGT impaired glucose tolerance 糖耐量减低

IHD ischemic heart disease 缺血性心脏病

IHPC intraperitoneal hyperthermic chemotherapy 腹腔热灌注化疗

IHSS idiopathic hypertrophic subaortic stenosis 特发性肥厚性主动脉下狭窄

IL interleukin 白（细胞）介素

Ile isoleucine 异亮氨酸

il·e·ac (il′e-ak) 1. of the nature of ileus 肠梗阻的；2. ileal 回肠的

il·e·al (il′e-əl) pertaining to the ileum 回肠的

il·e·itis (il″e-i′tis) inflammation of the ileum 回肠炎；**distal i., regional i.,** Crohn disease affecting the ileum 回肠末端炎，节段性回肠炎

il·eo·a·nal (il″e-o-a′nəl) pertaining to or connecting the ileum and the anus 回肠肛管的

il·eo·ce·cal (il″e-o-se′kəl) pertaining to the ileum and cecum 回盲肠的

il·eo·ce·cos·to·my (il″e-o-se-kos′tə-me) 1. surgical creation of a new opening between the ileum and the cecum 回肠直肠吻合术；2. the opening so created 回肠盲肠吻合口

il·eo·col·ic (il″e-o-kol′ik) pertaining to the ileum and colon 回结肠的

il·eo·co·li·tis (il″e-o-ko-li′tis) inflammation of the ileum and colon 回肠结肠炎

il·eo·co·los·to·my (il″e-o-kə-los′tə-me) surgical anastomosis of the ileum to the colon 回肠结肠吻合术

il·eo·cys·to·plas·ty (il″e-o-sis′to-plas″te) augmentation cystoplasty using an isolated segment of the ileum. 回肠膀胱成形术

il·eo·cys·tos·to·my (il″e-o-sis-tos′tə-me) ileovesicostomy 回肠膀胱吻合术

il·eo·ile·os·to·my (il″e-o-il″e-os′tə-me) 1. surgical creation of an opening between two different parts of the ileum 回肠回肠吻合术；2. the opening so created 回肠回肠吻合口

il·e·or·rha·phy (il″e-or′ə-fe) suture of the ileum 回肠缝合术

il·eo·sig·moi·dos·to·my (il″e-o-sig″moidos′tə-me) 1. surgical creation of an opening between the ileum and the sigmoid colon 回肠乙状结肠吻合术；2. the opening so created 回肠乙状结肠吻合口

il·e·os·to·my　(il″e-os′tə-me) surgical creation of an opening into the ileum, with a stoma on the abdominal wall 回肠造口术

il·e·ot·o·my　(il″e-ot′ə-me) incision of the ileum 回肠切开术

il·eo·trans·verse　(il″e-o-trans-vərs′) pertaining to or connecting the ileum and the transverse colon 回肠横结肠的

il·eo·ves·i·cos·to·my　(il″e-o-ves″ĭ-kos′tə-me) use of a section of ileum to create a channel leading from the urinary bladder upward to the abdominal surface 回肠膀胱造瘘术

il·e·um　(il′e-m) the distal portion of the small intestine, extending from the jejunum to the cecum 回肠；**duplex i.**, congenital duplication of the ileum 双回肠

il·e·us　(il′e-əs) intestinal obstruction due to a nonmechanical cause such as paralysis 肠梗阻；**adynamic i.**, that due to inhibition of bowel motility 麻痹性肠梗阻；**dynamic i.**；**hyperdynamic i.**, 同 spastic i.；**meconium i.**, ileus in the newborn due to blocking of the bowel with thick meconium, as in cystic fibrosis 胎粪性肠梗阻；**paralytic i.**, 同 adynamic i.；**spastic i.**, a type due to persistent contracture of a bowel segment 痉挛性肠梗阻

il·i·ac　(il′e-ak) pertaining to the ilium 髂的

il·io·cos·tal　(il″e-o-kos′təl) connecting or pertaining to the ilium and ribs 髂肋的

il·io·fem·or·al　(il″e-o-fem′ə-rəl) pertaining to the ilium and femur 髂股的

il·io·lum·bar　(il″e-o-lum′bər) pertaining to the iliac and lumbar regions 髂腰的

il·io·pec·tin·e·al　(il″e-o-pek-tin′e-al) pertaining to the ilium and pubes 髂耻的

il·io·tib·i·al　(il″e-o-tib′e-əl) pertaining to or extending between the ilium and tibia 髂胫的

il·io·tro·chan·ter·ic　(il″e-o-tro-kan-ter′ik) pertaining to the ilium and a trochanter 髂转子的

il·i·um　(il′e-əm) pl. *i'lia* [L.] the expansive superior portion of the coxal bone 髂骨，见图 1

ill·ness　(il′nis) disease 病；**mental i.**, 心理疾病，见 *disorder* 下词条

il·lu·mi·na·tion　(*E*) (ĭ-loo″mĭ-na′shən) 1. the lighting up of a part, organ, or object for inspection. 照明；2. the luminous flux per unit area of a given surface; SI unit, lux 照度；**darkfield i., dark-ground i.**, the casting of peripheral light rays upon a microscopic object from the side, the center rays being blocked out; the object appears bright on a dark background 暗（视）野照明

il·lu·sion　(ĭ-loo′zhən) a mental impression derived from misinterpretation of an actual experience 错觉；**illu′sional** *adj.*

ilo·prost　(i′lo-prost) a synthetic analogue of prostacyclin that is a systemic and pulmonary arterial dilator, used in the treatment of primary pulmonary hypertension 伊洛前列素

IM　intramuscular 肌内的

im-　a prefix, replacing *in-* before words beginning with *b, m,* and *p*[前辍] 不，非，无（表示否定）放置在以 b，m，p 开始的词之前代替 in-

im·age　(im′əj) a picture or concept with likeness to an objective reality（映）像，影像，图像；**body i.**, the threedimensional concept of one's self, recorded in the cortex by perception of ever-changing body postures, and constantly changing with them 体像；**false i.**, that formed by the deviating eye in strabismus 虚像；**mirror i.**, one with right and left relations reversed, as in the reflection of an object in a mirror 镜像；**motor i.**, the organized cerebral model of the possible movements of the body 动态意象；**Purkinje-Sanson mirror i's**, three reflected images of an object seen in observing the pupil of the eye: two on the posterior and anterior surfaces of the lens and one on the anterior surface of the cornea 浦肯野 - 桑松像；**real i.**, an image formed where the emanating rays are collected, in which the object is pictured as being inverted 实像；**virtual i.**, a picture from projected light rays that are intercepted before focusing 虚像

im·age·ry　(im′əj-re) 1. the formation of a mental representation of something perceived by the senses 意象；2. any of a number of therapeutic techniques that use the formation of such representations to elicit changes in attitudes, behaviors, or physiologic reactions 表象；**guided i.**, a therapeutic technique in which the patient enters a relaxed state and focuses on an image related to the issue being confronted, which the therapist uses as the basis of an interactive dialogue to help resolve the issue 意象导引

imag·ing　(im′ə-jing) the production of diagnostic images, e.g., radiography, ultrasonography, or scintillation photography 成像；**color flow Doppler i.**, a method for visualizing direction and velocity of movement using Doppler ultrasonography and coding them as colors and shades, respectively 彩色多普勒血流成像；**echo planar i.**, a technique for obtaining a magnetic resonance image in less than 50 msec 平面回波成像；**electrostatic i.**, a method of visualizing deep structures of the body, in

I

which an electron beam is passed through the patient and the emerging beam strikes an electrostatically charged plate, dissipating the charge according to the strength of the beam. A film is then made from the plate 静电成像; **gated cardiac blood pool i.,** equilibrium radionuclide angiocardiography 门控心血池显像; **gated magnetic resonance i.,** a method for magnetic resonance imaging in which signal acquisition is gated to minimize motion or other artifacts 门控磁共振成像; **hot spot i., infarct avid i.,** 热区显像, 亲心肌梗死显像, 见 *scintigraphy* 下词条; **magnetic resonance i. (MRI),** a method of visualizing soft tissues of the body by applying an external magnetic field that makes it possible to distinguish between hydrogen atoms in different environments 磁共振成像; **myocardial perfusion i.,** 心肌灌注显像, 见 *scintigraphy* 下词条; **pyrophosphate i.,** infarct avid scintigraphy 闪烁扫描成像; **technetium Tc 99m pyrophosphate i.,** 1. infarct avid scintigraphy 梗死闪烁扫描法; 2. any type of imaging using Tc 99m pyrophosphate as an imaging agent 锝 Tc 99m 焦磷酸盐成像

ima·go (ĭ-ma'go) pl. *ima'goes, ima'gines* [L.] 1. the adult or definitive form of an insect 成虫（昆虫）; 2. a usually idealized, unconscious mental image of a key person in one's early life 意象（心理）

im·at·i·nib (ĭ-mat'ĭ-nib) a tyrosine kinase inhibitor acting on several abnormal protein-tyrosine kinases, inhibiting cell proliferation and inducing apoptosis. It is used as the mesylate salt in the treatment of Philadelphia chromosome–positive chronic myelogenous leukemia and gastrointestinal stromal tumors 伊马替尼

im·bal·ance (im-bal'əns) 1. lack of balance, such as that between two opposing muscles or between electrolytes in the body 不平衡; 2. dysequilibrium (2); **autonomic i.,** defective coordination between the sympathetic and parasympathetic nervous systems, especially with respect to vasomotor activities 自主神经共济失调; **vasomotor i.,** autonomic i. 血管运动功能失调

im·bi·bi·tion (im″bĭ-bish'ən) absorption of a liquid 浸润, 吸涨作用, 吸液

im·bri·cat·ed (im'brĭ-kāt″əd) overlapping like shingles 叠瓦状的

ImD₅₀ median immunizing dose 半数免疫剂量

im·id·az·ole (im″id-az'ōl) 1. a heterocyclic organic compound in which two of five ring atoms are nitrogen; used as an insecticide 咪唑; 2. any of a class of antifungal compounds containing this structure 咪唑类抗真菌药物

im·ide (im'īd) any compound containing the bi-

valent group, =NH, to which are attached only acid radicals 酰亚胺, 二酰亚胺

imido- a prefix denoting the presence of the bivalent group =NH attached to two acid radicals [前缀] 亚氨基

imi·do·di·pep·tide (im″ĭ-do-di-pep'tīd) a dipeptide in which the C-terminal amino acid is an imino acid 亚氨二肽, C 末端氨基酸是亚氨基酸的二肽

im·i·glu·cer·ase (im″ĭ-gloo'sər-ās) an analogue of glucosylceramidase, for which it is used as an enzyme replenisher in type 1 Gaucher disease 伊米苷酶

imine (ĭ-mēn') an organic compound containing an imino group; in a *substituted imine,* a nonacyl group replaces the imino hydrogen 亚胺

imino- a prefix denoting the presence of the bivalent group =NH attached to nonacid radicals [前缀] 亚氨基酸

im·i·no ac·id (im'ĭ-no) an organic acid containing the bivalent group =NH; e.g., proline 亚氨基酸

im·i·no·di·pep·tide (im″ĭ-no-di-pep'tīd) a dipeptide in which the N-terminal amino acid is an imino acid 亚氨基二肽, N 末端氨基酸为亚氨基酸的二肽

im·i·no·gly·cin·uria (im″ĭ-no-gli″sin-u're-ə) a benign hereditary disorder of renal tubular reabsorption of glycine and the imino acids proline and hydroxyproline, with an excess of all three in urine 亚氨基甘氨酸尿

im·i·no·stil·bene (im″ĭ-no-stil'bēn) a class of anticonvulsants used in the treatment of epilepsy 亚氨基芪

im·i·pen·em (im″ĭ-pen'əm) a β-lactam antibiotic with a broad spectrum of activity against both gram-positive and gram-negative organisms 亚胺培南

imip·ra·mine (ĭ-mip'rə-mēn) a tricyclic antidepressant of the dibenzazepine class, used as *i. hydrochloride* or *i. pamoate* 丙咪嗪

im·i·quim·od (im″ĭ-kwim'od) a biologic response modifier used topically in the treatment of condyloma acuminatum 咪喹莫特

im·ma·ture (im″ə-choor') unripe or not fully developed 不成熟的

im·mer·sion (ĭ-mur'zhən) 1. the plunging of a body into a liquid 浸; 2. the use of the microscope with the object and object glass both covered with a liquid 浸泡

im·mis·ci·ble (ĭ-mis'ĭ-bəl) not susceptible to being mixed 不可混合的

im·mo·bil·iza·tion (ĭ-mo″bĭ-lĭ-za'shən) the act of rendering immovable, as by a cast or splint 固定术,

制动术

im·mor·tal·i·za·tion (ĭ-mor″təl-ĭ-za′shən) the gaining of immunity to normal limitations on growth or life span, sometimes achieved by animal cells in vitro or by tumor cells 无限增殖化，永生化

im·mune (ĭ-mūn′) 1. resistant to a disease because of the formation of humoral antibodies or the development of cellular immunity, or both, or from some other mechanism, such as interferon activity in viral infections 免疫；2. characterized by the development of humoral antibodies or cellular immunity, or both, following antigenic challenge 有免疫应答的；3. produced in response to antigenic challenge, as is immune serum globulin 免疫系统的

im·mu·ni·ty (ĭ-mu′nĭ-te) the condition of being immune; the protection against infectious disease conferred either by the immune response generated by immunization or previous infection or by other nonimmunologic factors 免疫（力），免疫性；**acquired i.,** that occurring as a result of prior exposure to an infectious agent or its antigens *(active i.),* or of passive transfer of antibody or immune lymphoid cells *(passive i.)* 获得免疫；**active i.,** 主动免疫，见 *acquired i.;* **artificial i.,** acquired (active or passive) immunity produced by deliberate exposure to an antigen, as in vaccination 人工免疫；**cell-mediated i. (CMI), cellular i.,** acquired immunity in which the role of T lymphocytes is predominant 细胞免疫；**genetic i., innate i.** 遗传免疫；**herd i.,** the resistance of a group to attack by a disease to which a large proportion of the members are immune 群体免疫；**humoral i.,** acquired immunity in which the role of circulating antibodies is predominant 体液免疫；**inherent i., innate i.,** immunity determined by the genetic constitution of the individual 固有免疫，先天免疫；**maternal i.,** humoral immunity passively transferred across the placenta from mother to fetus 母源性免疫；**natural i.,** the resistance of the normal animal to infection 天然免疫，固有免疫；**nonspecific i.,** that which does not involve humoral or cell-mediated immunity, but includes lysozyme and interferon activity, etc. 非特异性免疫；**passive i.,** 被动免疫，见 *acquired i.;* **specific i.;** immunity against a particular disease or antigen 特异性免疫，适应性免疫

im·mu·ni·za·tion (im″u-nĭ-za′shən) the process of rendering a subject immune, or of becoming immune 免疫接种；**active i.,** stimulation with a specific antigen to induce an immune response 主动免疫接种；**passive i.,** the conferral of specific immune reactivity on previously nonimmune individuals by administration of sensitized lymphoid cells or serum from immune individuals 被动免疫接种

im·mu·no·ad·ju·vant (im″u-no-aj′ə-vənt) a nonspecific stimulator of the immune response, e.g., BCG vaccine or Freund's complete and incomplete adjuvants 免疫佐剂

im·mu·no·ad·sor·bent (im″u-no-ad-sor′bənt) a preparation of antigen attached to a solid support or antigen in an insoluble form, which adsorbs homologous antibodies from a mixture of immunoglobulins 免疫吸附剂

im·mu·no·as·say (im″u-no-as′a) quantitative determination of antigenic substances (e.g., hormones, drugs, vitamins) by serologic means, as by immunofluorescent techniques, radioimmunoassay, etc. 免疫测定法，免疫分析

im·mu·no·bead (im′u-no-bēd″) a minute plastic bead coated with antigen or antibody so that it aggregates or agglutinates in the presence of the corresponding antibody or antigen 免疫微珠

im·mu·no·bio·log·i·cal (im″u-no-bi″o-loj′ ĭ- kəl) an antigenic or antibody-containing preparation derived from a pool of human donors and used for immunization and immune therapy 免疫生物制品

im·mu·no·bi·ol·o·gy (im″u-no-bi-ol′ə-je) that branch of biology dealing with immunologic effects on such phenomena as infectious disease, growth and development, recognition phenomena, hypersensitivity, heredity, aging, cancer, and transplantation 免疫生物学

im·mu·no·blas·tic (im″u-no-blas′tik) pertaining to or involving the stem cells (immunoblasts) of lymphoid tissue 免疫母细胞的，成免疫细胞的，淋巴母细胞的

im·mu·no·blot (im′u-no-blot″) to transfer proteins onto an immobilizing matrix, analyzing or identifying them via antigen-antibody specific reactions, or the resulting blot, as in a Western blot; sometimes used synonymously with that term 免疫印迹

im·mu·no·chem·is·try (im″u-no-kem′is-tre) the study of the physical chemical basis of immune phenomena and their interactions 免疫化学

im·mu·no·che·mo·ther·a·py (im″u-no-ke″mother′ə-pe) a combination of immunotherapy and chemotherapy 免疫化学疗法

im·mu·no·com·pe·tence (im″u-no-kom′pə- təns) immunoresponsiveness; the capacity to develop an immune response after exposure to an antigen 免疫活性，**immunocom′petent** *adj.***im·mu·no·com·plex** (im″u-no-kom′pləks) antigen-antibody complex 免疫复合物

im·mu·no·com·pro·mised (im″u-no-kom′- prə-mīzd) having the immune response attenuated by administration of immunosuppressive drugs,

513

by irradiation, by malnutrition, or by certain disease processes (e.g., cancer) 免疫减弱的, 免疫缓和的

im·mu·no·con·glu·ti·nin (im″u-no-kən-gloo′- tĭ-nin) antibody formed against complement components that are part of an antigen-antibody complex, especially C3 免疫胶固素

im·mu·no·cyte (im′u-no-sīt″) any cell of the lymphoid series that can react with an antigen to produce antibody or to participate in cellmediated reactions 免疫细胞

im·mu·no·cy·to·ad·her·ence (im″u-no-si″toad-hēr′əns) the aggregation of red cells to form rosettes around lymphocytes with surface immunoglobulins 免疫细胞粘连

im·mu·no·de·fi·cien·cy (im″u-no-də-fish′ən-se) a deficiency of immune response or a disorder characterized by a deficient immune response; classified as *antibody* (B cell), *cellular* (T cell), or *combined immunodeficiency*, or *phagocytic dysfunction disorders* 免疫缺陷; **immunodefi′cient** *adj.*; **common variable i. (CVID)**, a heterogeneous group of disorders characterized by hypogammaglobulinemia, decreased antibody production, and recurrent pyogenic infections, and often associated with hematologic and autoimmune disorders. Most patients appear to have an intrinsic defect of B cell differentiation 常见变异型免疫缺陷病; **severe combined i. (SCID)**, a group of rare congenital disorders, occurring in both autosomal recessive and X-linked forms; characterized by gross impairment of both humoral and cell-mediated immunity, absence of T lymphocytes, and, in some forms, lack of B lymphocytes. Immunoglobulins are usually absent and there is marked lymphocytopenia. Unless treated with bone marrow or fetal tissue transplant, infants manifest persistent diarrhea, chronic mucocutaneous candidiasis, and failure to thrive, and die from opportunistic infection 重症联合免疫缺陷

im·mu·no·der·ma·tol·o·gy (im″u-no-dur″mə-tol′ə-je) the study of immunologic phenomena as they affect skin disorders and their treatment or prophylaxis 免疫皮肤学

im·mu·no·dif·fu·sion (im″u-no-dĭ-fu′zhən) any technique involving diffusion of antigen or antibody through a semisolid medium, usually agar or agarose gel, resulting in a precipitin reaction 免疫扩散, 免疫扩散试验

im·mu·no·dom·i·nance (im″u-no-dom′ĭ- nəns) the degree to which a subunit of an antigenic determinant is involved in binding or reacting with antibody 免疫优势

im·mu·no·elec·tro·pho·re·sis (im″u-no-elek″trofə-re′sis) a method of distinguishing proteins and other materials on the basis of their electrophoretic mobility and antigenic specificities 免疫电泳（法）; **rocket i.**, electrophoresis in which antigen migrates from a well through agar gel containing antiserum, forming cone-shaped (rocket) precipitin bands 火箭电泳（法）

im·mu·no·flu·o·res·cence (im″u-no-floores′əns) any immunohistochemical method using antibody labeled with a fluorescent dye; called *direct* if a specific antibody or antiserum is conjugated with a fluorochrome and used as a specific fluorescent stain, and called *indirect* if the fluorochrome is attached to an antiglobulin and a tissue constituent is stained using an unlabeled specific antibody and the labeled antiglobulin, which binds the unlabeled antibody 免疫荧光（法）

I

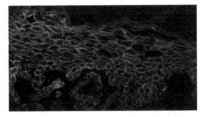

▲ 免疫荧光（绿色）用于检测寻常型天疱疮

im·mu·no·gen (im′u-no-jən) any substance capable of eliciting an immune response 免疫原, 抗原

im·mu·no·ge·net·ic (im″u-no-jə-net′ik) pertaining to immunology and genetics 免疫遗传的

im·mu·no·ge·net·ics (im″u-no-jə-net′iks) the study of the genetics of the immune response 免疫遗传学

im·mu·no·ge·nic·i·ty (im″u-no-jə-nis′ĭ-te) the property enabling a substance to provoke an immune response, or the degree to which a substance possesses this property 免疫原性; **immunogen′ic** *adj.*

im·mu·no·glob·u·lin (Ig) (im″u-no-glob′u-lin) any of the structurally related glycoproteins that function as antibodies, synthesized by lymphocytes and plasma cells and found in serum and in other body fluids and tissues. There are five distinct classes based on structural and antigenic properties: IgA, IgD, IgE, IgG, and IgM 免疫球蛋白, 见下表; See accompanying; **secretory i. A**, immunoglobulin in which two IgA molecules are linked by a polypeptide (secretory piece) and by a J chain; it is the predominant immunoglobulin 分泌型免疫球蛋白 A

Human Immunoglobulins 人类免疫球蛋白

	Mol Wt (kD) 分子量 (kD)	Number of Subclasses 亚类数目	Function 功能
IgM	900	2	Activation of classic complement pathway; opsonization 经典补体途径激活；调理作用
IgG	150	4	Activation of classic and alternative complement pathways; opsonization (IgG1 and IgG3 only); only class transferred across placenta, thus providing fetus and neonate with protection against infection 经典和替代补体途径激活；调理作用（仅限 IgG1 和 IgG3）；只有一类可转运至胎盘，保护胎儿和新生儿免受感染
IgA	155 (serum IgA) 155(血浆型 IgA) 400 (secretory IgA) 400(分泌型 IgA)	2	Activation of alternative complement pathway; secretory IgA is the predominant immunoglobulin in secretions 替代补体途径激活；分泌型 IgA 是分泌物中的主要免疫球蛋白
IgD	180	—	Along with IgM, appears to signal B cell activation in immune defense; may also help activate basophils and mast cells to produce antimicrobial factors that aid in human respiratory immune defense 与 IgM 一起，在免疫防御中标志 B 细胞活化；可能有助于激活嗜碱性粒细胞和肥大细胞，产生有助于人体呼吸道免疫防御的抗菌因子
IgE	190	—	Mediation of immediate hypersensitivity reactions 速发型超敏反应的介导

I

im·mu·no·glob·u·lin·op·a·thy (im″u-noglob″u-lin-op′ə-the) gammopathy 免疫球蛋白病

im·mu·no·hem·a·tol·o·gy (im″u-no-hēm″ə- tol′ə-je) the study of antigen-antibody reactions as they relate to blood disorders 免疫血液学

im·mu·no·his·to·chem·i·cal (im″u-no-his″tokem′ĭ-kəl) denoting the application of antigenantibody interactions to histochemical techniques, as in the use of immunofluorescence 免疫组织化学的

im·mu·no·in·com·pe·tent (im″u-in-kom′- pə-tent) lacking the ability or capacity to develop an immune response to an antigenic challenge 无免疫活性的，免疫功能不全的

im·mu·nol·o·gy (im″u-nol′ə-je) the branch of biomedical science concerned with the response of the organism to antigenic challenge, the recognition of self and not self, and all the biologic, serologic, and physical chemical effects of immune phenomena 免疫学；**immunolog′ic** adj.

im·mu·no·lym·pho·scin·tig·ra·phy (im″uno-lim″fos-in-tig′rə-fe) immunoscintigraphy used to detect metastatic tumor in lymph nodes 免疫淋巴闪烁扫描术

im·mu·no·mod·u·la·tion (im″u-no-mod″ula′shən) adjustment of the immune response to a desired level, as in immunopotentiation, immunosuppression, or induction of immunologic tolerance 免疫调节

im·mu·no·mod·u·lat·or (im″u-no-mod′ula″tər) an agent that augments or diminishes immune responses 免疫调节药

im·mu·no·patho·gen·e·sis (im″u-no-path″ojen′ə-sis) the process of development of a disease in which an immune response or the products of an immune reaction are involved 免疫发病机制

im·mu·no·pa·thol·o·gy (im″u-no-pə-thol′ə-je) 1. the branch of biomedical science concerned with immune reactions associated with disease, whether the reactions be beneficial, without effect, or harmful 免疫病理学；2. the structural and functional manifestations associated with immune responses to disease 免疫病理；**immunopatholog′ic** adj

im·mu·no·phe·no·type (im″u-no-fe′no-tīp) a phenotype of cells of hematopoietic neoplasms defined according to their resemblance to normal T cells and B cells 免疫表型，免疫显型

im·mu·no·po·ten·cy (im″u-no-po′tən-se) the immunogenic capacity of an individual antigenic determinant on an antigen molecule to initiate antibody synthesis（致）免疫力免疫放价，免疫效能

im·mu·no·po·ten·ti·a·tion (im″u-no-poten″shea′shən) accentuation of the response to an immunogen by administration of another substance 免疫强化

im·mu·no·pre·cip·i·ta·tion (im″u-no-presip″ĭta′shən) precipitation resulting from the interaction of a specific antibody and antigen 免疫沉淀反应

im·mu·no·pro·lif·er·a·tive (im″u-no-prolif″ərə-tiv) characterized by the proliferation of the lymphoid cells producing immunoglobulins, as in the gammopathies 免疫增生的

im·mu·no·ra·di·om·e·try (im″u-no-ra″deom′ə-tre) the use of radiolabeled antibody (in the place of radiolabeled antigen) in radioimmunoassay techniques 免疫放射测定；**immunoradiomet′ric** *adj.*

im·mu·no·reg·u·la·tion (im″u-no-reg″ula′shən) the control of specific immune responses and interactions between B and T lymphocytes and macrophages 免疫调节

im·mu·no·re·spon·sive·ness (im″u-no-respon′-siv-nis) immunocompetence 免疫应答

im·mu·no·scin·tig·ra·phy (im″u-no-sintig′rə-fe) scintigraphic imaging of a lesion using radiolabeled monoclonal antibodies or antibody fragments specific for antigen associated with the lesion 免疫闪烁法

im·mu·no·se·nes·cence (im″u-no-sə-nes′əns) decline of immune system function with advancing age 免疫衰老；**immunosenes′cent** *adj.*

im·mu·no·sor·bent (im″u-no-sor′bənt) an insoluble support for antigen or antibody used to absorb homologous antibodies or antigens, respectively, from a mixture; the antibodies or antigens so removed may then be eluted in pure form. 免疫吸附剂

im·mu·no·stim·u·la·tion (im″u-no-stim″ula′shən) stimulation of an immune response, e.g., by use of BCG vaccine 免疫刺激

im·mu·no·sup·pres·sant (im″u-no-sə-pres′- ənt) an agent capable of suppressing immune responses 免疫抑制药

im·mu·no·sup·pres·sion (im″u-no-sə- presh′ən) prevention or diminution of the immune response, such as by radiation, antimetabolites, or specific antibody 免疫抑制；**immunosuppres′sive** *adj.*

im·mu·no·ther·a·py (im″u-no-ther′ə-pe) passive immunization of an individual by administration of preformed antibodies (serum or gamma globulin)

actively produced in another individual; by extension, the term has come to include the use of immunopotentiators, replacement of immunocompetent lymphoid tissue (e.g., bone marrow or thymus), etc. 免疫疗法

im·mu·no·tox·in (im′u-no-tok″sin) any antitoxin 免疫毒素

im·mu·no·trans·fu·sion (im″u-no-transfu′zhən) transfusion of blood from a donor previously rendered immune to a disease to a patient with that disease 免疫输血法

im·pact·ed (im-pak′təd) being wedged in firmly or closely, as an impacted tooth or impacted twins 嵌入的

im·pac·tion (im-pak′shən) 1. the condition of being impacted 嵌入；2. in obstetrics, the indentation of any fetal parts of one twin onto the surface of its co-twin, so that the simultaneous partial engagement of both twins is permitted 阻生；**bony i.,** a dental impaction with blockage consisting of both bone and soft tissue 骨性嵌塞；**dental i.,** prevention of eruption, normal occlusion, or routine removal of a tooth because of its being locked in position by bone, dental restoration, or surfaces of adjacent teeth 牙阻生；**fecal i.,** a collection of hardened feces in the rectum or sigmoid 粪便嵌塞；**soft tissue i.,** a dental impaction with blockage consisting of soft tissue only 软组织嵌塞

im·pair·ment (im-pār′mənt) any abnormality of, partial or complete loss of, or loss of the function of, a body part, organ, or system, hearing loss 缺陷，损伤；**hearing i.,** hearing loss 听力损失

im·pal·pa·ble (im-pal′pə-bəl) not detectable by touch 感触不到的

im·ped·ance (Z) (im-pēd′əns) obstruction or opposition to passage or flow, as of an electric current or other form of energy 阻抗；**acoustic i.,** an expression of the opposition to passage of sound waves, being the product of the density of a substance and the velocity of sound in it 声阻抗；**aortic i.,** the sum of the external factors that resist ventricular ejection 主动脉阻抗

im·per·fect (im-pur′fəkt) of a fungus, capable of reproducing only by means of conidia (asexual spores) 无性孢子繁殖的真菌

im·per·fo·rate (im-pur′fə-rāt) not open; abnormally closed 闭锁的（通常指不正常的情况）

im·per·me·a·ble (im-pur′me-ə-bəl) not permitting passage, as of fluid 不透水的

im·pe·ti·go (im″pə-ti′go) [L.] a usually staphylococcal skin infection marked by vesicles that become pustular, rupture, and form crusts 脓疱病；**impetig′inous** *adj.*; **i. bullo′sa, bullous i.,**

a type usually seen in neonates; small vesicles progress to form large bullae that collapse and are covered with light crusts 大疱性脓疱病; **i. conta·gio′sa,** impetigo 传染性脓疱病; **i. herpetifor′mis,** a rare, acute dermatitis with symmetrically ringed, pustular lesions, seen chiefly in pregnant women with severe constitutional symptoms 疱疹样脓疱病; **i. neonato′rum, i. bullosa** 新生儿脓疱病; **nonbullous i.,** the most common type, caused by infection at sites of minor trauma; discrete fragile vesicles with erythematous borders become pustular, rupture, and discharge a thin yellow seropurulent fluid that dries and forms a thick crust 大疱性鱼鳞癣

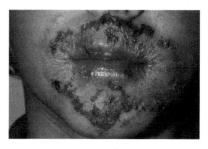

▲ 大疱性鱼鳞癣

im·plant¹ (im-plant′) to insert or to graft (tissue, or inert or radioactive material) into intact tissues or a body cavity 植入

im·plant² (im′plant) an object or material inserted or grafted into the body for prosthetic, therapeutic, diagnostic, or experimental purposes 植入体; **cochlear i.,** a mechanical alternative to hearing for deaf persons, consisting of a microphone, signal processor, external transmitter, and implanted receiver 人工耳蜗; **endosseous i., endosteal i.,** a dental implant consisting of a blade, screw, pin, or vent, inserted into the jaw bone through the alveolar or basal bone, with a post protruding through the mucoperiosteum into the oral cavity to serve as an abutment for dentures or orthodontic appliances, or to serve in fracture fixation 骨内植入物; **penile i.,** 阴茎植入物，见 *prosthesis* 下词条; **subperiosteal i.,** a metal frame implanted under the periosteum and resting on the bone, with a post protruding into the oral cavity 骨膜下种植体; **transmandibular i.,** a dental implant for patients with severe mandibular alveolar atrophy; it is fixed to the symphyseal border and traverses the mandible to attach directly to a denture 下颌外植体

im·plan·ta·tion (im″plan-ta′shən) 1. attachment of the blastocyst to the epithelial lining of the uterus, its penetration through the epithelium, and, in humans, its embedding in the endometrium, occurring 6 or 7 days after fertilization of the oocyte 植入物; 2. the insertion of an organ or tissue in a new site in the body 将有机体或组织植入人体某一部位; 3. the insertion or grafting into the body of biologic, living, inert, or radioactive material 将生物学的、活的、惰性的或放射性的物质植入

im·plo·sion (im-plo′zhən) 内爆疗法，见 *flooding*

im·po·tence (im′pə-təns) 1. lack of power 无力; 2. specifically, lack of copulative power in the male due to inability to initiate or to maintain an erection until ejaculation; usually considered to be due to a physical disorder (*organic i.*) or an underlying psychological condition (*psychogenic i.*, usually called *male erectile disorder*) 阳痿

im·preg·na·tion (im″prəg-na′shən) 1. fertilization 受精; 2. saturation (1) 饱和

im·pres·sio (im-pres′e-o) pl. *impressio′nes* [L.] 同 impression (1)

im·pres·sion (im-presh′ən) 1. a slight indentation, as one produced in the surface of one organ by pressure exerted by another 压痕; 2. a negative imprint of an object made in some plastic material that later solidifies 塑料材质的模具; 3. an effect produced upon the mind, body, or senses by some external stimulus or agent 印象; **basilar i.,** 1. platybasia 扁平颅底; 2. basilar invagination 基底印迹; **cardiac i.,** an impression made by the heart on another organ 心脏压痕; **dental i.,** one made of the jaw and/or teeth in some plastic material, which is later filled in with plaster of Paris to produce a facsimile of the oral structures present 牙齿印痕

im·print·ing (im-print′ing) rapid learning of species-specific behavior patterns that occurs with exposure to the proper stimulus at a sensitive period of early life 印记，印痕; **genomic i.,** differential expression of a gene or genes as a function of inheritance from the male versus the female parent 基因组印迹

im·pulse (im′pəls) 1. a sudden pushing force 推动，冲力; 2. a sudden uncontrollable determination to act 冲动; 3. 同 nerve i.; **cardiac i.,** movement of the chest wall caused by the heartbeat 心脏冲动; **ectopic i.,** 1. the impulse that causes an ectopic beat 异位搏动; 2. a pathologic nerve impulse that begins in the middle of an axon and proceeds simultaneously toward the cell body and the periphery 病理性神经冲动; **nerve i.,** the electrochemical process propagated along nerve fibers 神经冲动

im·pul·sion (im-pul′shən) blind obedience to internal drives, without regard for acceptance by others or pressure from the superego; seen in children and in adults with weak defensive organization 冲动；癖

In indium 元素铟的符号

INA International Neurological Association 国际神经病学协会

in·ac·ti·va·tion (in-ak″tĭ-va′shən) the destruction of biologic activity, as of a virus, by the action of heat or other agent 失活，灭活；**X-chromosome i.,** lyonization. X 染色体失活

in·am·ri·none (in-am′rĭ-nōn) a vasodilator and positive inotropic agent used as the lactate for the short-term management of congestive heart failure 氨力农

in·an·i·mate (in-an′ĭ-mət) 1. without life 无生命的；2. lacking in animation 无生机的

in·a·ni·tion (in″ə-nish′ən) the exhausted state due to prolonged undernutrition; starvation 营养不足，食物不足

in·ap·pe·tence (in-ap′ə-təns) lack of appetite or desire 食欲不振

in·ar·tic·u·late (in″ahr-tik′u-lət) 1. not having joints; disjointed 无关节的；脱臼的；2. uttered so as to be unintelligible; incapable of articulate speech （言语）无音节的，口齿不清的

in ar·tic·u·lo mor·tis (in ahr-tik′u-lo mor′tis) [L.] at the moment of death 濒于死亡

in·born (in′born) 1. genetically determined and present at birth 生来的；2. congenital 先天的

in·breed·ing (in′brēd-ing) the mating of closely related individuals or of individuals having closely similar genetic constitutions 近交

in·car·cer·at·ed (in-kahr′sər-āt″əd) imprisoned; constricted; subjected to incarceration 禁闭的；狭窄的；箝紧的

in·car·cer·a·tion (in-kahr″sər-a′shən) unnatural retention or confinement of a part 幽闭

in·cest (in′sest) sexual activity between persons so closely related that marriage between them is legally or culturally prohibited 近亲通婚，（性）乱伦

in·ci·dence (in′sĭ-dəns) the rate at which a certain event occurs, e.g., the number of new cases of a specific disease occurring during a certain period in a population at risk 发病率

in·ci·dent (in′sĭ-dənt) impinging upon, as incident radiation 入射的

in·ci·sal (in-si′zəl) 1. cutting 切（开）的；2. pertaining to the cutting edge of an anterior tooth 切缘

in·cised (in-sīzd′) cut; made by cutting 切开的

in·ci·sion (in-sizh′ən) 1. a cut or a wound made by cutting with a sharp instrument 切口；2. the act of cutting 切开；**incis′ional** adj.

▲ 各种腹部切口

肋缘下切口
上腹（正中）切口
麦氏克伯尼切口
旁正中切口
腹直肌旁切口
正中切口
腹部低横位切口
普芬南施蒂尔切口

in·ci·sive (in-si′siv) 1. having the power or quality of cutting 锐利的；2. pertaining to the incisor teeth 切牙的

in·ci·sor (**I**) (in-si′zər) 1. adapted for cutting 适宜切割的；2. incisor tooth 切牙

in·ci·su·ra (in-si-su′rə) pl. *incisu′rae* [L.] notch 切迹

in·ci·sure (in-si′zhər) notch 切迹；**Schmidt-Lanterman i′s,** channels of cytoplasm appearing as oblique lines or slashes in the myelin sheath of neurons and leading back to the body of the Schwann cell 施-兰切迹，髓鞘切迹

in·cli·na·tio (in″klĭ-na′she-o) pl. *inclinatio′nes* [L.] inclination 倾斜

in·cli·na·tion (in″klĭ-na′shən) a sloping or leaning; the angle of deviation from a particular line or plane of reference; in dentistry, the deviation of a tooth from the vertical 倾斜；**pelvic i.,** the angle between the plane of the pelvic inlet and the horizontal plane 骨盆斜度

in·clu·sion (in-kloo′zhən) 1. the act of enclosing or the condition of being enclosed 包括，包含；2. anything that is enclosed; a cell inclusion 内含物，**cell i.,** a usually lifeless, often temporary, constituent in the cytoplasm of a cell 细胞内含物；**dental i.,** 牙包埋 1. a tooth so surrounded with bony tissue that it is unable to erupt 被骨质包裹不会被腐蚀的牙；2. a cyst of oral soft tissue or bone 口腔软组织或骨头的囊肿

in·co·bot·u·li·num tox·in A (in″ko-boch″uli′nəm-tok″sin) a preparation of botulinum toxin type A, used to treat spasticity, cervical dystonia, blepharospasm, and glabellar lines A 型肉毒毒素

in·com·pat·i·ble (in″kəm-pat′ĭ-bəl) not suitable for combination, simultaneous administration, or transplantation; mutually repellent 不相容的；配伍禁忌的；相互排斥的

in·com·pe·tence (in-kom′pə-təns) 1. insufficiency 不充分；2. mental inadequacy 心理上没准备好；3. the legal status of a person determined by the court to be unable to manage his own affairs 无行为能力，（法律上）无资格；**atrial chronotropic i.,** inability to increase the heart rate to levels capable ot satisfying the needs of the body 心房变时性功能不全；**valvular i.**, 瓣膜关闭不全，见 *insufficiency* 下词条

in·com·pe·tent (in-kom′pə-tənt) 1. unable to function properly 无能力的；2. a person who is unable to perform the required functions of daily living 无能力者；3. a person determined by the courts to be unable to manage his or her own affairs（法律上）无行为能力者

in·con·ti·nence (in-kon′tĭ-nəns) 1. inability to control excretory functions 失禁；2. immoderation or excess 过度；**incon′tinent** *adj.*; **fecal i.**, involuntary passage of feces and flatus 大便失禁；**overflow i.**, urinary incontinence due to pressure of retained urine in the bladder after the bladder has contracted to its limits, with dribbling of urine 溢出性尿失禁；**passive i.**, urinary or fecal incontinence in which the bladder or colon is full and cannot be emptied in the usual way but can be induced by pressure 被动性失禁；**stress i.**, involuntary escape of urine due to strain on the orifice of the bladder, as in coughing or sneezing 压力性尿失禁；**urge i., urgency i.**, urinary or fecal incontinence preceded by a sudden, uncontrollable impulse to evacuate 急迫性尿失禁；**urinary i.**, inability to control the voiding of urine 尿失禁

in·con·ti·nen·tia (in-kon″tĭ-nen′shə) [L.] incontinence 失禁；**i. pigmen′ti**, a hereditary disorder in which early vesicular and later verrucous and bizarrely pigmented skin lesions are associated with eye, bone, and central nervous system defects 色素失调症

in·cor·di·na·tion (in″ko-or″dĭ-na′shən) ataxia 动作失调，协调运动障碍

in·cor·po·ra·tion (in-kor″por-a′shən) 1. the union of a substance with another, or with others, in a composite mass 掺合，混合；2. a primitive, unconscious defense mechanism in which aspects of another person are assimilated into the self 合一（一种原始的同化防御机制）

in·cre·ment (in′krə-mənt) increase or addition; the amount by which a value or quantity is increased 增加，增大；增值，增量；**incremen′tal** *adj.*

in·cre·tin (in-kre′tin) any of various gastrointestinal hormones and factors that act as potent stimulators of insulin secretion 肠促胰岛素，肠降血糖素

in·crus·ta·tion (in″krəs-ta′shən) 1. the formation of a crust 结痂；2. a crust, scab, or scale 痂

in·cu·bate (in′ku-bāt) 1. to subject to or to undergo incubation 孵育，孵化；2. material that has undergone incubation 经历过孵化的材料

in·cu·ba·tion (in″ku-ba′shən) 1. the provision of proper conditions for growth and development, as for bacterial or tissue cultures 提供适合的发育

条件；2. the development of an infectious disease from entrance of the pathogen to the appearance of clinical symptoms 潜伏期；3. the development of the embryo in the eggs of oviparous animals 孵化；4. the maintenance of an artificial environment for an infant, especially a premature infant 为婴儿（特别是早产儿）提供的人造环境

in·cu·ba·tor (in′ku-ba″tər) an apparatus for maintaining optimal conditions (temperature, humidity, etc.) for growth and development, as one used in the early care of premature infants or one used for cultures 孵化器

in·cu·dal (ing′ku-dəl) pertaining to the incus 砧骨的

in·cu·do·mal·le·al (ing″ku-do-mal′e-əl) pertaining to the incus and malleus 砧锤（骨）的

in·cur·a·ble (in-kūr′ə-bəl) not susceptible of being cured 不可治愈的

in·cus (ing′kəs) [L.] anvil; the middle of the three ossicles of the ear, which, with the stapes and malleus, serves to conduct vibrations from the tympanic membrane to the inner ear 砧骨，见图 29

in·cy·clo·pho·ria (in-si″klo-for′e-ə) cyclophoria in which the upper pole of the visual axis deviates toward the nose 内旋转隐斜

in·cy·clo·tro·pia (in-si″klo-tro′pe-ə) cyclotropia in which the upper pole of the vertical axis deviates toward the nose 内旋转斜视

in·dane·di·one (in″dān-di′ōn) any of a group of related synthetic anticoagulants, e.g., anisindione, which impairs the hepatic synthesis of the vitamin K–dependent coagulation factors (prothrombin, factors Ⅶ, Ⅸ, and Ⅹ) 茚满二酮

in·dap·a·mide (in-dap′ə-mīd) an antihypertensive and diuretic with actions and uses similar to those of chlorothiazide 吲达帕胺，茚磺苯酰胺(抗高血压药，利尿药)

in·dex (in′deks) pl. *indexes*, *in′dices* [L.] 1. forefinger 示指；2. a unitless quantity, usually a ratio of two measurable quantities having the same dimensions, or such a ratio multiplied by 100 指数；**body mass i. (BMI)**, the weight in kilograms divided by the square of the height in meters, used in the assessment of underweight and obesity 体重指数，体重 (kg) 除以身高 (m) 的平方，用于评估体重不足和肥胖；**cardiac i. (CI)**, cardiac output per unit time divided by body surface area 心脏指数，单位时间血液输出量除以体表面积；**Colour I.**, a publication of the Society of Dyers and Colourists and the American Association of Textile Chemists and Colorists containing an extensive list of dyes and dye intermediates. Each chemically distinct compound is identified by a specific number, the C.I.

number, avoiding the confusion of trivial names used for dyes in the dye industry 血色指数；**I. Medicus,** a monthly publication of the National Library of Medicine in which the world's leading biomedical literature is indexed by author and subject 医学文献索引；**mitotic i.,** an expression of the number of cells in a population undergoing mitosis 有丝分裂指数，在进行有丝分裂的群体中细胞数量的一种表述形式；**opsonic i.,** a measure of opsonic activity determined by the ratio of the number of microorganisms phagocytized by normal leukocytes in the presence of serum from an individual infected by the microorganism, to the number phagocytized in serum from a normal individual 调理指数，一种光活动的量度，由正常白细胞在感染该微生物的血清存在时被正常白细胞吞噬的微生物数量与正常个体血清中吞噬的微生物数量之比确定；**phagocytic i.,** the average number of bacteria ingested per leukocyte of the patient's blood 吞噬指数，患者血液中每个白细胞平均摄取的细菌数量；**Quetelet i.,** body mass i. 凯特勒指数；**refractive i. (n) (n),** the refractive power of a medium compared with that of air (assumed to be 1) 折射率；**short increment sensitivity i. (SISI),** a hearing test in which randomly spaced, 0.5-second tone bursts are superimposed at 1- to 5-decibel increments in intensity on a carrier tone having the same frequency and an intensity of 20 decibels above the speech recognition threshold 短增量敏感指数；**therapeutic i.,** originally, the ratio of the maximum tolerated dose to the minimum curative dose; now defined as the ratio of the median lethal dose (LD_{50}) to the median effective dose (ED_{50}). It is used in assessing the safety of a drug 治疗指数，曾指最大耐受剂量与最小治疗剂量之比；现在定义为中位致死剂量 (LD_{50}) 与中位有效剂量 (ED_{50}) 之比，用于评估药物的安全性；**vital i.,** the ratio of births to deaths within a given time in a population 出生死亡比率

in·di·can (in′dĭ-kən) potassium indoxyl sulfate, formed by decomposition of tryptophan in the intestines and excreted in the urine 尿蓝母

in·di·ca·tor (in′dĭ-ka″tər) 1. the index finger, or the extensor muscle of the index finger 示指伸肌；2. any substance that indicates the appearance or disappearance of a chemical by a color change or attainment of a certain pH 指示剂

in·dif·fer·ent (in-dif′ər-ənt) not tending one way or another; neutral; having no preponderating affinity 不关心的，淡漠的；中性的；无亲和力的

in·di·ges·tion (in″dĭ-jes′chən) lack or failure of digestion; commonly used to denote vague abdominal discomfort after meals 消化不良；**acid i.,** hyperchlorhydria 胃酸过多性消化不良；**fat i.,** steatorrhea 脂

肪消化不良；**gastric i.,** that taking place in, or due to a disorder of, the stomach 胃消化不良；**intestinal i.,** disorder of the digestive function of the intestine 肠消化不良；**sugar i.,** defective ability to digest sugar, resulting in fermental diarrhea 糖消化不良

in·dig·i·ta·tion (in-dij″ĭ-ta′shən) 同 intussusception (1)

in·di·go (in′dĭ-go) 1. a blue dyeing material from various leguminous and other plants, being the aglycone of indican and also made synthetically; sometimes found in the sweat and urine 靛蓝染料；2. a color between blue and violet, produced by energy of wavelengths between 420 and 450 nm 靛蓝色，波长在 420～450nm 之间

in·dig·o·tin (in″dĭ-go′tin) a neutral, tasteless, insoluble, dark blue powder, the principal ingredient of commercial indigo 靛蓝

in·di·go·tin·di·sul·fon·ate so·di·um (in″dĭ-go″tin-di-sul′fo-nāt) a dye, occurring as a dusky, purplish blue powder or blue granules, used as a diagnostic aid in cystoscopy 靛蓝二磺酸钠

in·din·a·vir (in-din′nə-vir) an HIV protease inhibitor that causes formation of immature, noninfectious viral particles; used as the sulfate salt in the treatment of HIV infection and AIDS 茚地那韦

in·di·rect (in″di-rekt′) 1. not immediate or straight 不直接的；2. acting through an intermediary agent 通过中介的

in·di·um (**In**) (in′de-əm) a rare, very soft, silvery, malleable metallic element; at. no. 49, at. wt. 114.818 铟；**i. 111,** an artificial isotope having a half-life of 2.81 days and emitting gamma rays; it is used to label a variety of compounds for nuclear medicine 一种人造同位素

in·di·vid·u·a·tion (in″dĭ-vid″u-a′shən) 1. the process of developing individual characteristics 个性发生；2. differential regional activity in the embryo occurring in response to organizer influence 个体化

in·dole (in′dōl) a compound obtained from coal tar and indigo and produced by decomposition of tryptophan in the intestine, where it contributes to the peculiar odor of feces. It is excreted in the urine in the form of indican 吲哚

in·do·lent (in′do-lənt) 1. causing little pain 无痛的；2. slow growing 缓慢增长的

in·do·meth·a·cin (in″do-meth′ə-sin) a nonsteroidal antiinflammatory drug; used in the treatment of various rheumatic and nonrheumatic inflammatory conditions, dysmenorrhea, and vascular headache. The trihydrated sodium salt is used to induce closure in certain cases of patent ductus arteriosus 吲哚美辛

in·dox·yl (in-dok′səl) an oxidation product of

indole, formed in tryptophan decomposition and excreted in the urine as indican 吲哚酚

in·duced (in-doost′) 1. produced artificially 人工制造的; 2. produced by induction 诱导产生的

in·duc·er (in-doos′ər) a molecule that causes a cell or organism to accelerate synthesis of an enzyme or sequence of enzymes in response to a developmental signal 诱导剂

in·du·ci·ble (in-doo′sī-bəl) produced because of stimulation by an inducer 可诱导的

in·duc·tance (in-duk′təns) that property of a circuit whereby changing current generates an electromotive force (EMF) in the same or a neighboring circuit; the EMF is proportional to the rate of change of the current, and inductance is quantitated as the ratio of these two 电感

in·duc·tion (in-duk′shən) 1. the act or process of inducing or causing to occur 诱导的过程; 2. the production of a specific morphogenetic effect in the embryo through evocators or organizers 大脑感应; 3. the production of anesthesia or unconsciousness by use of appropriate agents 使麻醉或昏迷的过程; 4. the generation of an electric current or magnetic properties in a body because of its proximity to another electric current or magnetic field 电磁感应

in·duc·tor (in-duk′tər) a tissue elaborating a chemical substance that acts to determine growth and differentiation of embryonic parts 诱导者

in·du·ra·tion (in″du-ra′shən) 1. sclerosis or hardening 变硬; 2. hardness 硬度; 3. an abnormally hard spot or place 不寻常的硬块; **indur′ative** adj.; **black i.**, hardening and pigmentation of lung tissue in coal workers' pneumoconiosis 黑色硬结, 煤工尘肺病肺组织硬化和色素沉着; **brown i.**, 1. a deposit of altered blood pigment in the lung 肺褐色硬结, 含铁血黄素沉积于肺部; 2. an increase of pulmonary connective tissue, dark colored due to anthracosis or chronic congestion from valvular heart disease 肺褐色硬化, 由于煤肺或瓣膜性心脏病慢性充血引起; **cyanotic i.**, hardening of the kidney from chronic venous congestion 紫绀硬结, 肾脏因慢性静脉淤血而硬化; **gray i.**, induration of lung tissue in or after pneumonia, without the pigmentation of brown induration 灰色硬结, 肺炎或肺炎后肺组织硬化, 无棕色硬结色素沉着; **penile i.**, Peyronie disease 阴茎硬结; **red i.**, red, congested lung tissue seen in idiopathic pulmonary fibrosis 红色硬结, 特发性肺纤维化中见红色充血的肺组织

in·du·si·um gris·e·um (in-doo′ze-əm gris′e-əm) [L.] a thin layer of gray matter on the dorsal surface of the corpus callosum 灰被（胼胝体上回）

in·dwell·ing (in′dwel-ing) pertaining to a catheter or other tube left within an organ or body passage for drainage, to maintain patency, or for the administration of drugs or nutrients 留置, 在器官或身体通道内用于引流、维持通畅或用于给药或营养等物质的导管或其他管

in·e·bri·a·tion (in-e″bre-a′shən) drunkenness; intoxication with, or as if with, alcohol 醉状, 酩酊状态

in·ert (in-urt′) inactive 无活力的; 惰性的, 不活泼的; 无作用的, 无效的

in·er·tia (in-ur′shə) [L.] inactivity; inability to move spontaneously 不活动, 无力; **colonic i.**, weak muscular activity of the colon, leading to distention of the organ and constipation 结肠无力, 结肠肌肉活动减弱, 导致器官膨胀和便秘; **uterine i.**, sluggishness of uterine contractions in labor 子宫收缩乏力, 分娩时子宫收缩迟缓

in ex·tre·mis (in ek-stre′mis) [L.] at the point of death 临终时

in·fan·cy (in′fən-se) the early period of life 婴儿期, 见 *infant*

in·fant (in′fənt) the human young from the time of birth to 1 year of age 婴儿（从出生到1岁）; **dysmature i.**, 同 postmature i.; **extremely low birth weight (ELBW) i.**, an infant weighing less than 1000 g at birth 超低出生体重儿, 通常指出生体重低于1000g的婴儿; 另见 *low-birth-weight i.*; **floppy i.**, 松软婴儿, 见 *syndrome* 下词条; **immature i.**, one usually weighing less than 2500 g at birth and not physiologically well developed 不成熟儿, 通常指出生体重不于2500g的婴儿; **low-birth-weight (LBW) i.**, one weighing less than 2500 g at birth 低出生体重儿, 通常指出生体重低于2500g的婴儿; **mature i.**, one weighing 2500g or more at birth, usually born at or near full term, is physiologically fully developed, and has an optimal chance of survival 成熟儿, 通常指出生体重高于2500g, 足月或近足月, 生理发育完全的婴儿; **oderately low birth weight (MLBW) i.**, one weighing at least 1500 g but less than 2500 g at birth 中度低出生体重儿, 通常指出生体重在1500～2500g的婴儿; **newborn i.**, the human young during the first 4 weeks after birth 新生儿; **postmature i.**, 1. one with postmaturity syndrome 过度成熟婴儿; 2. 同 postterm i.; **postterm i.**, one born at or after the fortysecond completed week (294 days) of gestation 过熟儿; **premature i.**, 1. one usually born after the twentieth completed week and before full term, defined as weighing 500 to 2499 g at birth; the chance of survival depends on the weight. In countries where adults are smaller than in the United States, the upper limit may be lower 未成熟儿; 2. 同 preterm i.; **preterm i.**, one born before the thirty-seventh completed week (259 days) of gestation 早产儿；**term i.,** one born in the interval from the thirty-seventh completed week to the forty-second completed week of gestation (259 to 293 days), inclusive 预产期；**very low birth weight (VLBW) i.,** one weighing less than 1500 g at birth 极低出生体重儿，通常指出生体重低于1500g

in·fan·tile (in′fən-tīl) pertaining to an infant or to infancy 婴儿（期）的

in·fan·ti·lism (in′fən-tī-liz″əm) (in-fan′tī- liz″əm) persistence of childhood characteristics into adult life, marked by intellectual disability, underdevelopment of sex organs, and often dwarfism 幼稚型，婴儿型；**sexual i.,** continuance of prepubertal sex characters and behavior after the usual age of puberty 性幼稚症；**universal i.,** short stature with absence of secondary sex characteristics 全身性幼稚症

in·farct (in′fahrkt) a localized area of ischemic necrosis produced by occlusion of the arterial supply or the venous drainage of the part 梗死；**anemic i.,** one due to the sudden arrest of circulation in a vessel, or to decoloration of hemorrhagic blood 贫血性梗死；**hemorrhagic i.,** one that is red owing to oozing of erythrocytes into the injured area 出血性梗死

in·farc·tion (in-fahrk′shən) 1. the formation of an infarct 梗死形成；2. 同 infarct；**acute myocardial i. (AMI),** that occurring during the period when circulation to a region of the heart is obstructed and necrosis is occurring 急性心肌梗死；**cardiac i.,** 同 myocardial i.；**cerebral i.,** an ischemic condition of the brain, causing a persistent focal neurologic deficit in the area affected 脑梗死；**mesenteric i.,** coagulation necrosis of the intestines due to a decrease in blood flow in the mesenteric vasculature 肠系膜梗死；**migrainous i.,** a focal neurologic defect that constituted part of a migrainous aura but that has persisted for a long period and may be permanent 偏头痛性脑梗死；**myocardial i. (MI),** gross necrosis of the myocardium, due to interruption of the blood supply to the area 心肌梗死；**non–Q wave i.,** myocardial infarction not characterized by abnormal Q waves 无Q波心肌梗死；**pulmonary i.,** localized necrosis of lung tissue, due to obstruction of the arterial blood supply 肺梗死；**Q wave i.,** myocardial infarction characterized by Q waves that are abnormal in character or number, or both Q波心肌梗死；**silent myocardial i.,** myocardial infarction occurring without pain or other symptoms; often detected only by electrographic or postmortem examination 无症状心肌梗死；**watershed i.,** cerebral infarction in a watershed area during a time of prolonged systemic hypotension 脑分水岭梗死

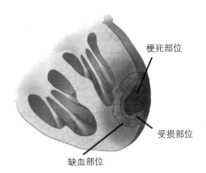

▲ 心肌梗死时的心室横截面

in·fect (in-fekt′) 1. to invade and produce infection in 感染；2. to transmit a pathogen or disease to 传染

in·fec·tion (in-fek′shən) 1. invasion and multiplication of microorganisms in body tissues, especially that causing local cellular injury due to competitive metabolism, toxins, intracellular replication, or antigen-antibody response 感染；2. infectious disease 传染性疾病；**airborne i.,** one that is contracted by inhalation of microorganisms or spores suspended in air on water droplets or dust particles 空气传播传染；**cross i.,** infection transmitted from one individual to another 交叉感染；**droplet i.,** airborne infection from inhalation of respiratory pathogens suspended on droplet nuclei 飞沫传染；**dustborne i.,** airborne infection by inhalation of pathogens attached to particles of dust 尘埃传播感染；**endogenous i.,** that due to reactivation of organisms present in a dormant focus, as occurs in tuberculosis, etc 内源性感染；**exogenous i.,** that caused by organisms not normally present in the body that have gained entrance from the environment 外源性感染；**HIV i., human immunodeficiency virus i.,** an epidemic, transmissible retroviral disease due to infection with human immunodeficiency virus (HIV), which attacks CD4 cells. The primary method of transmission is transfer from one person to another of bodily fluids that contain the virus. In its most severe manifestation, it is classified as acquired immunodeficiency syndrome (AIDS) 人类免疫缺陷病毒感染；**opportunistic i.,** infection by an organism that does not ordinarily cause disease but under certain circumstances (e.g., immunodeficiency disorders) becomes pathogenic 机会性感染；**pyogenic i.,** infection by pus-producing organisms, such as species of *Staphylococcus* or *Streptococcus* 化脓性感染；**secondary i.,** infection by a second pathogen after infection by one of another kind 继发感染；**terminal i.,** an acute infection near the end of a disease, sometimes ending in death 临终感染；**tunnel i.**, subcutaneous infection of an artificial passage into the body that has been kept patent 管道感染；**vector-borne i.**, one caused by microorganisms transmitted from one host to another by a carrier such as a biting insect 虫传感染；**water-borne i.**, one caused by microorganisms transmitted in water 水源性传染

in·fec·tious (in-fek′shəs) 1. caused by or capable of being communicated by infection, as an infectious disease 可被传染的；2. 同 infective (1)

in·fec·tive (in-fek′tiv) 1. capable of producing infection 有传染性的；2. 同 infectious (1)

in·fe·ri·or (in-fēr′e-ər) situated below, or directed downward; in anatomy, used in reference to the lower surface of a structure, or to the lower of similar structures 下

in·fer·til·i·ty (in″fər-til′ĭ-te) diminution or absence of ability to produce offspring 不孕（症），不 育 **infer′tile** *adj.*；**immunologic i.**, any of several types believed to be caused by presence in the female of antibodies that interfere with functioning of the sperm 免疫性不孕

in·fes·ta·tion (in-fes-ta′shən) parasitic attack or subsistence on the skin and/or its appendages, as by insects, mites, or ticks; sometimes used to denote parasitic invasion of the organs and tissues, as by helminths 叮咬，螨虫或蜱虫等对皮肤和其附属物的寄生性攻击，有时用于表示寄生虫对器官和组织的侵袭

in·fib·u·la·tion (in-fib″u-la′shən) the act of buckling or fastening as if with buckles, particularly the practice of fastening the prepuce or labia minora together to prevent coitus 锁阴术，阴部扣锁法

in·fil·trate (in-fil′trāt) 1. to penetrate the interstices of a tissue or substance 渗入，透过；2. the material or solution so deposited 沉积的材料或溶液

in·fil·tra·tion (in″fil-tra′shən) 1. the pathologic diffusion or accumulation in a tissue or cells of substances not normal to it or in amounts in excess of the normal 组织或细胞中不正常的物质病理积聚；2. 同 infiltrate (2)；3. the deposition of a solution directly into tissue 浸润，见 *anesthesia* 下词条；**adipose i.**, 同 fatty i.；**calcareous i.**, deposit of lime and magnesium salts in the tissues 石灰质浸润；**cellular i.**, the migration and accumulation of cells within the tissues 细胞浸润；**fatty i.**, 脂肪浸润 1. a deposit of fat in tissues, especially between cells; the term describes an older concept now included in *fatty change* 组织中，特别是细胞之间的脂肪沉积；2. the presence of fat vacuoles in the cell cytoplasm 细胞质中存在脂肪空泡

in·fil·tra·tive (in′fil-tra″tiv) pertaining to or characterized by infiltration 浸润性的

in·firm (in-firm′) weak; feeble, as from disease or old age 虚弱的

in·fir·ma·ry (in-fur′mə-re) a hospital or place where the sick or infirm are maintained or treated 医务室

in·flam·ma·gen (in-flam′ə-jən) an irritant that elicits both edema and the cellular response of inflammation 炎症刺激剂

in·flam·ma·tion (in″flə-ma′shən) a protective tissue response to injury or destruction of tissues, which serves to destroy, dilute, or wall off the injurious agent and the injured tissues. The classical signs of acute inflammation are pain (dolor), heat (calor), redness (rubor), swelling (tumor), and loss of function (functio laesa) 炎症；**inflam′matory** *adj.*；**acute i.**, inflammation, usually of sudden onset, marked by the classical signs (see *inflammation*), in which vascular and exudative processes predominate 急性炎症；**catarrhal i.**, a form affecting mainly a mucous surface, marked by a copious discharge of mucus and epithelial debris 卡他性炎；**chronic i.**, prolonged and persistent inflammation marked chiefly by new connective tissue formation; it may be a continuation of an acute form or a prolonged low-grade form 慢性炎；**exudative i.**, inflammation in which the prominent feature is an exudate 渗出性炎；**fibrinous i.**, one marked by an exudate of coagulated fibrin 纤维蛋白性炎；**granulomatous i.**, a form, usually chronic, marked by granuloma formation 肉芽肿性炎（症）；**hyperplastic i.**, one leading to the formation of new connective tissue fibers 增生性炎；**interstitial i.**, one affecting chiefly the stroma of an organ 间质性炎；**parenchymatous i.**, one affecting chiefly the essential tissue elements of an organ 实质炎；**productive i., proliferative i.**, 同 hyperplastic i.；**pseudomembranous i.**, an acute inflammatory response to a powerful necrotizing toxin, e.g., diphtheria toxin, with formation, on a mucosal surface, of a false membrane composed of precipitated fibrin, necrotic epithelium, and inflammatory white cells 假膜性炎；**purulent i.**, 同 suppurative i.；**serous i.**, one producing a serous exudate 浆液性炎；**subacute i.**, a condition intermediate between chronic and acute inflammation, exhibiting some of the characteristics of each 亚急性炎症；**suppurative i.**, one marked by pus formation 化脓性炎（症）；**ulcerative i.**, that in which necrosis on or near the surface leads to loss of tissue and creation of a local defect (ulcer) 溃疡性炎

in·fla·tion (in-fla′shən) distention, or the act of distending, with air, gas, or fluid 充气；膨胀；吹张，

吹张法

in·flec·tion (in-flek′shən) the act of bending inward, or the state of being bent inward 内曲，屈曲

in·flix·i·mab (in-flik′sĭ-mab) an anti–tumor necrosis factor antibody used in treatment of Crohn disease and rheumatoid arthritis 英夫利昔单抗

in·flu·en·za (in″floo-en′zə) [Ital.] an acute viral infection of the respiratory tract, occurring in isolated cases, epidemics, and pandemics, caused by *Influenzavirus A, B*, or *C*, usually with inflammation of the nasal mucosa, pharynx, and conjunctiva, headache, myalgia, fever, chills, and prostration 流行性感冒，流感; **influen′zal** *adj.*; **avian i.**, a highly contagious disease of birds caused by an influenza A virus, ranging in severity from mild to fulminating and highly fatal. It may be transmitted to humans through contact with bird droppings or contaminated surfaces or through intermediate hosts such as pigs, with person-toperson transmission occurring rarely. Symptoms in humans range from influenza-like symptoms to eye infections, pneumonia, acute respiratory distress, and other severe and life-threatening complications 禽流感

In·flu·en·za·vi·rus *A* (in″floo-en′zə-vi″rəs) a genus of viruses of the family Orthomyxoviridae, containing the agent of influenza A 甲型流感病毒属，见 *virus* 下 *influenza virus*

In·flu·en·za·vi·rus *B* (in″floo-en′zə-vi″rəs) a genus of viruses of the family Orthomyxoviridae containing the agent of influenza B 乙型流感病毒属，见 *virus* 下 *influenza virus*

In·flu·en·za·vi·rus *C* (in″floo-en′zə-vi″rəs) a genus of viruses of the family Orthomyxoviridae containing the agent of influenza C 丙型流感病毒属，见 *virus* 下 *influenza virus*

in·fold·ing (in-fōld′ing) 1. the folding inward of a layer of tissue, as in the formation of the neural tube in the embryo 内折; 2. the enclosing of redundant tissue by suturing together the walls of the organ on either side of it 折叠缝合术

in·fra·bulge (in′frə-bəlj) the surfaces of a tooth gingival to the height of contour, or sloping cervically 倒凹区

in·fra·cal·ca·rine (in″frə-kal′kə-rīn) inferior to the calcarine sulcus 舌回

in·fra·cla·vic·u·lar (in″frə-klə-vik′u-lər) subclavian 锁骨下的

in·fra·clu·sion (in″frə-kloo′zhən) a condition in which the occluding surface of a tooth does not reach the normal occlusal plane and is out of contact with the opposing tooth 低咬合，低𬌗

in·frac·tion (in-frak′shən) incomplete bone fracture without displacement 不全骨折

in·fra·den·ta·le (in″frə-dən-ta′le) a cephalometric landmark, being the highest anterior point on the gingiva between the mandibular medial (central) incisors 牙下点，龈下点，为下颌骨中切牙之间齿龈前面的最高点

in·fra·di·an (in″frə-de′ən) pertaining to a period longer than 24 hours; applied to the cyclic behavior of certain phenomena in living organisms (infradian rhythm) 超昼夜的

in·fra·duc·tion (in″frə-duk′shən) downward rotation of an eye around its horizontal axis 眼下转

in·fra·no·dal (in″frə-no′dəl) below a node 节下的

in·fra·or·bi·tal (in″frə-or′bĭ-təl) suborbital; under, or on the inferior surface of, the orbit 眶下的

in·fra·pa·tel·lar (in″frə-pə-tel′ər) subpatellar; below or beneath the patella 髌下的

in·fra·red (in-frə-red′) denoting electromagnetic radiation of wavelength greater than that of the red end of the spectrum, having wavelengths of 0.75 to 1000 μm; sometimes subdivided into *long-wave* or *far i.* (about 3.0–1000 μm) and *short-wave* or *near i.* (about 0.75–3.0 μm) 红外线

in·fra·son·ic (in″frə-son′ik) below the frequency range of sound waves 听域下的，次声的，亚声频的，亚声速的

in·fra·spi·nous (in″frə-spi′nəs) beneath the spine of the scapula 冈下的

in·fra·tem·po·ral (in″frə-tem′pə-rəl) inferior to the temple 颞下的

in·fra·ver·gence (in″frə-vur′jəns) rotation of one eye downward while the other one remains still 下转（眼）

in·fra·ver·sion (in″frə-vur′zhən) 1. 同 infraclusion; 2. the downward deviation of one eye 眼下斜; 3. conjugate downward rotation of both eyes 下转（两眼共轭性下转）

in·fun·dib·u·lar (in″fən-dib′u-lər) 1. pertaining to an infundibulum 漏斗的; 2. funnel-shaped 漏斗状的

in·fun·dib·u·lec·to·my (in″fən-dib″u-lek′tə-me) excision of the infundibulum of the heart 漏斗切除术

in·fun·dib·u·li·form (in″fən-dib′u-lĭ-form) 同 infundibular (2)

in·fun·dib·u·lo·ma (in″fən-dib″u-lo′mə) a tumor of the stalk (infundibulum) of the hypophysis（下丘脑）漏斗瘤

in·fun·dib·u·lum (in″fən-dib′u-ləm) pl. *infundib′ula* [L.] 1. a funnel-shaped structure 漏斗状; 2. conus arteriosus 动脉圆锥; 3. i. of posterior lobe of pituitary 垂体后叶; **infundib′ular** *adj.*; **ethmoidal i.**, 筛漏斗 1. a passage connecting the nasal cavity with anterior ethmoidal cells and frontal sinus 连接鼻腔与前筛窦细胞和额窦的通道；2. a sinuous passage connecting the middle nasal meatus with the anterior ethmoidal cells and often with the frontal sinus 连接中鼻道与前筛窦细胞并通常与额窦相连的蜿蜒通道；i. of hypothalamus, i. of neurohypophysis, a hollow, funnel-shaped mass in front of the tuber cinereum, extending to the posterior lobe of the pituitary 下丘脑漏斗；i. of uterine tube, the distal, funnel-shaped portion of the uterine tube 输卵管漏斗

in·fu·sion (in-fu′zhən) 1. the steeping of a substance in water to obtain its soluble principles 浸，浸出，将物质浸泡在水中以获得其可溶性成分；2. the product obtained by this process 浸液；3. the therapeutic introduction of fluid other than blood into a vein 输液

in·ges·tant (in-jes′tənt) a substance that is or may be taken into the body by mouth or through the digestive system 食入物，摄食物

in·ges·tion (in-jes′chən) the taking of food, drugs, etc., into the body by mouth 口服

in·gra·ves·cent (in″grə-ves′ənt) gradually becoming more severe 渐重的

in·grown (in′grōn) having grown inward, into the flesh 向内长的，长入肌肉内的

in·growth (in′grōth) an inward growth; something that grows inward or into 向内生长；向内生长物

in·guen (ing′gwən) pl. in′guina [L.] groin: the junctional region between the abdomen and thigh 腹股沟；**in′guinal** adj.

in·gui·nal (ing′gwĭ-nəl) pertaining to the groin 腹股沟的

in·hal·ant (in-ha′lənt) 1. something meant to be inhaled 吸入的；见 inhalation (3)；2. a class of psychoactive substances whose volatile vapors are subject to abuse 吸入剂，**antifoaming i.,** an agent that is inhaled as a vapor to prevent the formation of foam in the respiratory passages of a patient with pulmonary edema 止泡吸入剂

in·ha·la·tion (in″hə-la′shən) 1. the drawing of air or other substances into the lungs 吸入；2. the drawing of an aerosolized drug into the lungs with the breath 吸入法；3. any drug or solution of drugs administered (as by means of nebulizers or aerosols) by the nasal or oral respiratory route 吸入剂；**inhala′tional** adj.

in·hal·er (in-hāl′er) 1. an apparatus for administering vapor or volatilized medications by inhalation 吸入器；2. ventilator (2) 呼吸器

in·her·ent (in-her′ənt) implanted by nature; intrinsic; innate 内在的，固有的，生来的

in·her·i·tance (in-her′ĭ-təns) 1. the acquisition of characters or qualities by transmission from parent to offspring 遗传；2. that which is transmitted from

parent to offspring 遗传特征；**cytoplasmic i.,** inheritance of traits carried by genes not located on chromosomes of the nucleus, e.g., those of mitochondria 细胞质遗传；**dominant i.,** the inheritance of a trait that is expressed in both heterozygotes and homozygotes 显性遗传；**extrachromosomal i.,** 同 cytoplasmic i.；**maternal i.,** transmission of characters only from the maternal parent, as is characteristic of genes carried on the mitochondrial genome or other cytoplasmic organelle 母体（影响）遗传；**mendelian i.,** that which follows Mendel's laws (q.v.) 孟德尔遗传；**mitochondrial i.,** the inheritance of traits controlled by genes on the DNA of mitochondria in the ooplasm; thus the genes are inherited entirely from the maternal side, segregate randomly at meiosis or mitosis, and are variably expressed 线粒体遗传；**recessive i.,** the inheritance of a trait that is only expressed in homozygotes, not in a heterozygote also possessing a dominant allele for that locus 隐性遗传；**sex-linked i.** the pattern of inheritance shown by genes carried on a sex (X or Y) chromosome, which is different for males and females 伴性遗传，性连锁遗传；**X-linked i.,** the pattern of inheritance shown by X-linked genes; affected males always express the phenotype and transmit the gene to all their daughters but none of their sons X 连锁遗传；**Y-linked i.,** the pattern of inheritance shown by Y-linked genes; only males are affected, and they always express the phenotype and transmit the gene to all of their sons Y 连锁遗传

in·hib·it (in-hib′it) to retard, arrest, or restrain 抑制

in·hi·bi·tion (in″hĭ-bish′ən) 1. restraint or termination of a process 抑制；2. in psychoanalytic theory, the conscious or unconscious restraining of an impulse or desire 在精神分析理论中，对冲动或欲望有意识或无意识的抑制；**competitive i.,** inhibition of enzyme activity in which the inhibitor (a substrate analogue) competes with the substrate for binding sites on the enzymes 竞争性抑制；**contact i.,** the inhibition of cell division and motility in normal cells when in close contact with each other; loss of inhibition of cell division is a step in carcinogenesis 接触抑制；**end product i., feedback i.,** inhibition of the initial steps of a process by an end product of the reaction 反馈抑制；**noncompetitive i.,** inhibition of enzyme activity by substances that combine with the enzyme at a site other than that utilized by the substrate 非竞争性抑制

in·hib·i·tor (in-hib′ĭ-tər) 1. any substance that interferes with a chemical reaction, growth, or other biologic activity 抑制药；2. a chemical substance that inhibits or checks the action of a tissue organizer or the growth of microorganisms 抑制微生物生长的化学物质；3. an effector that reduces the catalytic activity of an enzyme 抑制基因；**ACE i's,** 同 angiotensin-converting enzyme i's；**alpha₁-proteinase i.,** alpha1-antitrypsin α1蛋白酶抑制药；**angiogenesis i.,** any of a group of drugs that prevent neovascularization of solid tumors 血管生成抑制药；**angiotensin-converting enzyme i's,** competitive inhibitors of angiotensin-converting enzyme; used as antihypertensives, usually in conjunction with a diuretic, and also as vasodilators in the treatment of congestive heart failure 血管紧张素转换酶抑制药；**aromatase i's,** a class of drugs that inhibit aromatase activity and thus block production of estrogens; used to treat breast cancer and endometriosis 芳香化酶抑制药；**C1 i. (C1 INH),** an inhibitor of activated C1, the initial component of the classic complement pathway. Deficiency of or defect in the protein causes hereditary angioedema C1 抑制物；**carbonic anhydrase i.,** any of a class of agents that inhibit carbonic anhydrase activity; used chiefly for the treatment of glaucoma, and for epilepsy, familial periodic paralysis, mountain sickness, and uric acid renal calculi 碳酸酐酶抑制药；**cholinesterase i.,** a compound that prevents the hydrolysis of acetylcholine by acetylcholinesterase, so that high levels of acetylcholine accumulate at reactive sites 胆碱酯酶抑制药；**COX-2 i., cyclooxygenase-2 i.,** any of a group of nonsteroidal antiinflammatory drugs (NSAIDs) that act by inhibiting cyclooxygenase-2 (COX-2) activity; they have fewer gastrointestinal side effects than other NSAIDs 环氧合酶-2 抑制药；**gastric acid pump i.,** 同 proton pump i.；**HIV protease i.,** any of a group of antiretroviral drugs active against the human immunodeficiency virus, preventing protease-mediated cleavage of viral polyproteins and so causing production of immature noninfectious viral particles HIV 蛋白酶抑制药；**MAO i.,** monoamine oxidase inhibitor 单胺氧化酶抑制药；**membrane i. of reactive lysis (MIRL),** protectin 膜反应性溶解抑制物；**monoamine oxidase i. (MAOI),** any of a group of antidepressant drugs that act by blocking the action of the enzyme monoamine oxidase; believed to act by thus increasing the level of catecholamines in the central nervous system 单胺氧化酶抑制药；**α₂-plasmin i.,** α₂-antiplasmin α₂-纤溶酶抑制药；**plasminogen activator i. (PAI),** any of several regulators of fibrinolysis that act by binding to and inhibiting free plasminogen activator; the most important are *PAI-1* and *PAI-2* 纤溶酶原激活物抑制物；**platelet i.,** any of a group of agents that inhibit the clotting activity of platelets 血小板抑制药；

protease i., 1. a substance that blocks the activity of an endopeptidase (protease) 蛋白酶抑制药；2. 同 HIV protease i.；**protein C i.,** the primary inhibitor of activated anticoagulant protein C; it is a type of protease inhibitor that also inhibits other proteins involved in coagulation 蛋白C抑制药；**proton pump i.,** an agent that inhibits the proton pump by blocking the action of H⁺, K⁺-ATPase at the secretory surface of gastric parietal cells, thus limiting hydrochloric acid secretion 质子泵抑制药；**reverse transcriptase i.,** a substance that blocks activity of the retroviral enzyme reverse transcriptase; used as an antiretroviral agent 反转录酶抑制药；**selective norepinephrine reuptake i. (NRI),** any of a group of drugs that inhibit the inactivation of norepinephrine by blocking its absorption in the central nervous system; used to treat attention-deficit/hyperactivity disorder and depression. Note: sometimes abbreviated SNRI, which, however, also denotes *serotonin-norepinephrine reuptake i.* 选择性去甲肾上腺素重摄取抑制药；**selective serotonin reuptake i. (SSRI),** any of a group of drugs that inhibit the inactivation of serotonin by blocking its absorption in the central nervoussystem; used to treat depressive, obsessive-compulsive, and panic disorders 5-羟色胺选择性重摄取抑制药；**serotonin-norepinephrine reuptake i. (SNRI),** any of a group of drugs that inhibit the inactivation of serotonin and norepinephrine by blocking their absorption in the central nervous system; used in the treatment of depression, anxiety disorders, obsessive-compulsive disorder, attention-deficit/hyperactivity disorder, and chronic neuropathic pain 去甲肾上腺素重摄取抑制药；**topoisomerase i.,** any of a group of antineoplastic drugs that interfere with the arrangement of DNA in cells 拓扑异构酶抑制药；**tyrosine kinase i.,** any of a class of compounds that inhibit one or more receptor protein-tyrosine kinases; because they interfere with cellular proliferation and differentiation, specific compounds have been used to inhibit the activity of tyrosine kinases associated with neoplasia 酪氨酸激酶抑制药

in·hib·i·to·ry (in-hib′ĭ-tor″e) restraining or arresting any process; causing a stay or arrest, partial or complete 抑制的

in·i·on (in′e-on) the external occipital protuberance 枕外隆凸尖；**in′iac, in′ial** *adj.*

ini·ti·a·tion (ĭ-nĭ″she-a′shən) the creation of a small alteration in the genetic coding of a cell by a low level of exposure to a carcinogen, priming the cell for neoplastic transformation upon later exposure to a carcinogen or a promoter 引发，通过将低水平的致癌物暴露在细胞遗传编码中产生微小的

改变，引发细胞的肿瘤转化

in·i·tis (in-i′tis) myositis 肌炎

in·jec·tion(in-jek′shən) 1. the forcing of a liquid into a part, as into the subcutaneous tissues, the vascular tree, or an organ 注射；2. a substance so forced or administered; in pharmacy, a solution of a medicament suitable for injection 注射液；**hypodermic i.,** 同 subcutaneous i.；**intracutaneous i.,** 同 intradermal i.；**intracytoplasmic sperm i.** (ICSI), a micromanipulation technique used in male factor infertility, with insertion of a spermatocyte directly into an oocyte 卵质内单精子注射，单精子卵细胞质内注射；**intradermal i.,** one made into the dermis or substance of the skin 皮内注射；**intramuscular i.,** one made into the substance of a muscle 肌内注射；**intrathecal i.,** injection of a substance through the theca of the spinal cord into the subarachnoid space 鞘内注射；**intravenous i.,** one made into a vein 静脉注射；**jet i.,** one made through the intact skin by an extremely fine jet of the solution under high pressure 喷射注射；**lactated Ringer i.,** a sterile solution of calcium chloride, potassium chloride, sodium chloride, and sodium lactate in water for injection, given as a fluid and electrolyte replenisher 乳酸盐林格注射液；**Ringer i.,** a sterile solution of sodium chloride, potassium chloride, and calcium chloride in water for injection, used as a fluid and electrolyte replenisher 林格注射液；**subcutaneous i.,** one made into the superficial fascia 皮下注射

in·ju·ry (in′jə-re) wound or trauma; harm or hurt; usually applied to damage inflicted on the body by an external force 损伤；**birth i.,** impairment of body function or structure due to adverse influences to which the infant has been subjected at birth 产伤；**Goyrand i.,** pulled elbow 牵引肘；**overuse i.** injury, such as to a muscle, nerve, or bone, caused by repetitive motion in certain occupations or sports 过度劳损；**straddle i.,** injury to the distal urethra from falling astride a blunt object 骑跨伤；**whiplash i.,** a popular nonspecific term applied to injury to the spine and spinal cord due to sudden extension of the neck 挥鞭伤

in·lay (in′la) material laid into a defect in tissue; in dentistry, a filling made outside the tooth to correspond with the cavity form and then cemented into the tooth 嵌体

in·let (in′lət) a means or route of entrance 入口；**laryngeal i.,** the aperture by which the pharynx communicates with the larynx 喉口；**pelvic i.,** the upper limit of the pelvic cavity 盆上口；**thoracic i.,** the elliptical opening at the summit of the thorax 胸腔入口。Cf. inferior thoracic aperture

INN International Nonproprietary Name 国际非专有药名

in·nate (ĭ-nāt′) inborn 天生的

in·ner·va·tion (in″ər-va′shən) 1. the distribution or supply of nerves to a part 神经支配；2. the supply of nervous energy or of nerve stimulation sent to a part 供给神经能量到一部位

in·nid·i·a·tion (ĭ-nid″e-a′shən) development of cells in a part to which they have been carried by metastasis 移生，移地发育

in·no·cent (in′o-sənt) not malignant; benign; not tending of its own nature to a fatal issue 良性的

in·nom·i·nate (ĭ-nom′ĭ-nāt) nameless 无名的；匿名的

ino·chon·dri·tis (in″o-kon-dri′tis) inflammation of a fibrocartilage 纤维软骨炎

in·oc·u·la·ble (ĭ-nok′u-lə-bəl) 1. susceptible to being inoculated 可接种的；2. transmissible by inoculation 可接种的

in·oc·u·late (ĭ-nok′u-lāt) 1. to implant infective materials into culture media 接种；2. to introduce immune serum, vaccines, or other antigenic material into a healthy individual to produce mild disease followed by immunity 预防注射；3. to spread a disease by inserting its etiologic agent 通过插入其病原体来传播疾病

in·oc·u·la·tion (ĭ-nok″u-la′shən) 1. introduction of microorganisms, infective material, serum, or other substances into tissues of living organisms, or culture media; introduction of a disease agent into a healthy individual to produce a mild form of the disease followed by immunity 接种；2. the process of inoculating something 接种的过程

in·oc·u·lum (ĭ-nok′u-ləm) pl. *inoc′ula.* Material that is inoculated 接种物

Ino·cy·be (i-nos′ĭ-be) a genus of mushrooms common in North America; many species contain the toxin muscarine and some contain the hallucinogen psilocybin 丝盖伞属

ino·di·la·tor (in″o-di′la-tər) (-di-la′tər) an agent with both positive inotropic and vasodilator effects 血管扩张药，具有加强肌力作用和血管扩张作用的药剂

in·op·er·a·ble (in-op′ər-ə-bəl) not susceptible to treatment by surgery 不能手术的，不宜手术的

in·or·gan·ic (in″or-gan′ik) 1. having no organs. 无器官的；2. not of organic origin 无机的

in·os·co·py (in-os′ko-pe) the diagnosis of disease by artificial digestion and examination of the fibers or fibrinous matter of sputum, blood, effusions, etc. 纤维质消化检查

in·o·se·mia (in″o-se′me-ə) 1. the presence of inositol in the blood 肌醇血；2. an excess of fibrin in the blood 纤维蛋白血

in·o·sine (I) (in′o-sēn) a purine nucleoside containing the base hypoxanthine and the sugar ribose, which occurs in transfer RNAs and as an intermediate in the degradation of purines and purine nucleosides to uric acid and in pathways of purine salvage 肌苷；**i. monophosphate (IMP),** a nucleotide produced by the deamination of adenosine monophosphate (AMP); it is the precursor of AMP and GMP in purine biosynthesis and an intermediate in purine salvage and in purine degradation 肌苷一磷酸

ino·si·tol (ī-no′sī-tol) a cyclic sugar alcohol, the fully hydroxylated derivative of cyclohexane; usually referring to the most abundant isomer, *myo*-inositol, which occurs in many plant and animal tissues and microorganisms and is often classified as a member of the vitamin B complex 肌醇，环己六醇；**i. 1,4,5-triphosphate (InsP₃, IP₃),** a second messenger that causes the release of calcium from certain intracellular organelles 肌醇三磷酸

in·o·tro·pic (in″o-tro′pik) affecting the force of muscular contractions 影响（肌）收缩力的

in·pa·tient (in′pa-shənt) a patient who comes to a hospital or other health care facility for diagnosis or treatment that requires an overnight stay 住院病人

in·quest (in′kwest) a legal inquiry before a coroner or medical examiner, and usually a jury, into the manner of death 死因审理

INRT involved node radiation therapy 累及淋巴结放射治疗

in·sa·lu·bri·ous (in″sə-loo′bre-əs) injurious to health 有碍健康的，有碍卫生的

in·san·i·ty (in-san′ĭ-te) a legal term for mental illness of such degree that the individual is not responsible for his or her acts 精神错乱；**insane′** *adj.*

in·scrip·tio (in-skrip′she-o) pl. *inscriptio′nes* [L.] 同 inscription；**i. tendi′nea,** 见 *intersectio* 下词条

in·scrip·tion (in-skrip′shən) 1. a mark, or line 划；2. that part of a prescription containing the names and amounts of the ingredients 药量记载

In·sec·ta (in-sek′tə) a class of arthropods whose members are characterized by division into three parts: head, thorax, and abdomen 昆虫纲

in·sem·i·na·tion (in-sem″ĭ-na′shən) the deposit of seminal fluid within the vagina or cervix 授精；**artificial i. (AI),** that done by artificial means 人工授精；**artificial i. by donor (AID),** 同 donor i.；**artificial i. by husband (AIH),** artificial insemination in which the semen used is from the woman's partner 夫精人工授精；**donor i.,** artificial insemination in which the semen used is not from the woman's partner 供精人工授精

in·sen·si·ble (in-sen′sĭ-bəl) 1. devoid of sensibility or consciousness 昏迷，不省人事的；2. not perceptible to the senses 无感觉的

in·ser·tion (in-sur′shən) 1. the act of implanting, or the condition of being implanted 插入；2. the site of attachment, as of a muscle to the bone that it moves 附着的部位；3. in genetics, a rare nonreciprocal type of translocation in which a segment is removed from one chromosome and then inserted into a broken region of a nonhomologous chromosome 一种罕见的非互易型易位；**velamentous i.,** attachment of the umbilical cord to the membranes rather than to the placenta 脐带帆状附着

in·sid·i·ous (in-sid′e-əs) coming on stealthily; of gradual and subtle development 隐袭的，隐伏的

in·sight (in′sīt) 1. in psychiatry, the patient's awareness and understanding of their attitudes, feelings, behavior, and disturbing symptoms; self-understanding 自知力；2. in problem solving, the sudden perception of the appropriate relationships of things that results in a solution 顿悟，领悟

in si·tu (in si′tu) [L.] in its normal place; confined to the site of origin 原位

in·sol·u·ble (in-sol′u-bəl) not susceptible of being dissolved 不能解释的

in·som·nia (in-som′ne-ə) inability to sleep; abnormal wakefulness 失眠，**insom″niac, insom′nic** *adj.*；**fatal familial i.,** an inherited prion disease affecting primarily the thalamus and characterized by progressive insomnia, hallucinations, stupor, and coma ending in death; autonomic and motor disturbances are also present 致死性家族型失眠；**primary i.,** a dyssomnia characterized by persistent difficulty initiating or maintaining sleep or by persistently nonrestorative sleep; not due to any other condition 原发性失眠

in·so·nate (in-so′nāt) to expose to ultrasound waves （使）接受超声波

in·sorp·tion (in-sorp′shən) movement of a substance into the blood, especially from the gastrointestinal tract into the circulating blood 内吸渗（指胃肠道的内含物进入循环血液内）

in·sper·sion (in-spur′zhən) the act of sprinkling, as with a powder 撒粉法，扑粉法

in·spi·ra·tion (in″spī-ra′shən) inhalation 吸气；**inspi′ratory** *adj.*

in·spis·sat·ed (in-spis′āt-əd) being thickened, dried, or made less fluid by evaporation 浓缩的，蒸浓的

in·sta·bil·i·ty (in-stə-bil′ĭ-te) lack of steadiness or stability 不稳定性；**detrusor i.,** involuntary contraction of the detrusor muscle of the bladder caused by nonneurologic problems 逼肌不稳定。Cf. *detrusor* *hyperreflexia*

in·star (in'stahr) any stage of an arthropod between molts 龄期，节肢动物两次蜕皮之间的时期

in·step (in'step) the dorsal part of the arch of the foot 足弓，足背

in·stil·la·tion (in″stĭ-la'shən) administration of a liquid drop by drop 滴注法

in·stinct (in'stinkt) a complex of unlearned responses characteristic of a species 本能; **instinc′-tive** *adj.*; **death i.**, in psychoanalysis, the latent instinctive impulse toward dissolution and death 死亡本能; **herd i.**, the instinct or urge to be one of a group and to conform to its standards of conduct and opinion 群集（居）本能; **life i.**, in psychoanalysis, all of the constructive tendencies of the organism aimed at maintenance and perpetuation of the individual and species 生的本能

in·sti·tu·tion·al·iza·tion (in-stĭ-too″shən-əl-ī-za'shən) 1. commitment of a patient to a health care facility for treatment, often psychiatric 收容入院(常为精神病治疗); 2. in patients hospitalized for a long period, the development of excessive dependency on the institution and its routines 长期住院患者过度依赖医疗机构及其常规

in·stru·ment (in'strə-mənt) any tool, appliance, or apparatus 器具

in·stru·men·tal (in″strə-men'təl) 1. pertaining to or performed by instruments 器械的; 2. serving as a means to a particular result 作为手段的

in·stru·men·ta·tion (in″strə-mən-ta'shən) 1. the use of instruments; work performed with instruments 器械用法，器械操作法; 2. a group of instruments used for a specific purpose 测试设备

in·su·date (in-soo'dāt) the substance accumulated in insudation 蓄积物

in·su·da·tion (in″soo-da'shən) the accumulation, as in the kidney, of substances derived from the blood 蓄积（ 如血液来的某些物质蓄积的肾脏）

in·suf·fi·cien·cy (in″sə-fish'ən-se) inability to perform properly an allotted function 不充分，不足; 功能不全; 闭锁不全，关闭不全; **adrenal i.**, 1. hypoadrenalism; abnormally diminished activity of the adrenal gland 肾上腺功能减退，肾上腺功能不全; 2. 同 adrenocortical i.; **adrenocortical i.**, abnormally diminished secretion of corticosteroids by the adrenal cortex, as in Addison disease 肾上腺皮质功能减退症; **aortic i., aortic valve i.**, defective functioning of the aortic valve, with incomplete closure resulting in aortic regurgitation 主动脉瓣关闭不全; **cardiac i.**, heart failure 心功能不全; **coronary i.**, decrease in flow of blood through the coronary blood vessels 冠状动脉供血不足; **i. of the externi**, deficient power in the externi muscles of the eye, resulting

in esophoria 眼外直肌功能不全; **i. of the interni**, deficient power in the interni muscles of the eye, resulting in exophoria. 眼内直肌功能不全; **mitral i., left atrioventricular valve i.**, defective functioning of the left atrioventricular valve, with incomplete closure causing mitral regurgitation 二尖瓣关闭不全，左房室瓣闭锁不全; **primary ovarian i.**, absence or irregularity of menses lasting at least 4 months, with menopausal levels of serum gonadotropins, in an adolescent girl or woman under 40 years of age 原发性卵巢功能不全; **pulmonary i.**, 1. 同 respiratory i.; 2. pulmonary valve i. 肺动脉瓣关闭不全; **pulmonary valve i.**, defective functioning of the pulmonary valve, with incomplete closure causing pulmonic regurgitation 肺动脉瓣关闭不全; **respiratory i.**, inability of the lungs to provide adequate oxygen intake or carbon dioxide expulsion as needed by the body and its cells 呼吸功能不全; **thyroid i.**, hypothyroidism 甲状腺功能减退; **tricuspid i., right atrioventricular valve i.**, defective functioning of the right atrioventricular valve, with incomplete closure causing tricuspid regurgitation; it is usually secondary to systolic overload 三尖瓣关闭不全，右房室瓣膜闭锁不全; **valvular i.**, dysfunction of a valve, with incomplete closure resulting in backward flow of blood across the valve 瓣膜关闭不全; **velopharyngeal i.**, failure of velopharyngeal closure due to cleft palate, muscular dysfunction, etc., resulting in defective speech 腭咽关闭不全，腭咽闭合不良; **venous i.**, impairment of venous drainage, resulting in edema, erythema, and stasis ulcers; caused by inadequacy of the venous valves or obstruction, or both 静脉功能不全; **vertebrobasilar i.**, transient ischemia of the brainstem and cerebellum due to stenosis of the vertebral or basilar artery 椎 - 基底动脉供血不足

in·suf·fla·tion (in″sə-fla'shən) 1. the act of blowing a powder, vapor, or gas into a body cavity 吹入法，注气法; 2. finely powdered or liquid drugs carried into the respiratory passages by such devices as aerosols 吹入剂，通过雾化器材进入呼吸道的细小药末或药液; **perirenal i.**, injection of air around the kidney for radiographic examination of the suprarenal glands 肾周注气法; **tubal i.**, Rubin test (1) 输卵管通气术

in·su·la (in'sə-lə) pl. *in'sulae* [L.] 1. an islandlike structure 岛状结构; 2. a triangular area of the cerebral cortex forming the floor of the lateral cerebral fossa 脑岛

in·su·lar (in'sə-lər) pertaining to the insula or to an island, as the islands (islets) of Langerhans 岛的，脑岛的，胰岛的

in·su·la·tion (in″sə-la'shən) 1. the surrounding of a space or body with material designed to prevent the entrance or escape of radiant or electrical energy 绝缘；2. the material so used 绝缘体，绝缘材料

in·su·lin (in′sə-lin) 1. a protein hormone formed from proinsulin in the beta cells of the pancreatic islets of Langerhans. The major fuel-regulating hormone, it is secreted into the blood in response to a rise in concentration of blood glucose or amino acids. Insulin promotes the storage of glucose and the uptake of amino acids, increases protein and lipid synthesis, and inhibits lipolysis and gluconeogenesis 胰岛素；2. a preparation of insulin, either of porcine or bovine origin or a recombinant form with a sequence the same as or similar to that in humans, used in the treatment of diabetes mellitus; classified as *rapid-acting*, *intermediate-acting*, or *long-acting* on the basis of speed of onset and duration of activity 胰岛素制剂；3. regular insulin; a rapid-acting, unmodified form of insulin prepared from crystalline bovine or porcine insulin 普通短效胰岛素；**i. aspart,** a rapid-acting analogue of human insulin created by recombinant DNA technology 门冬胰岛素；**buffered i. human,** insulin human buffered with phosphate; used particularly in continuousinfusion pumps 人胰岛素磷酸盐缓冲液，特别用于连续泵注；**extended i. zinc suspension,** a long-acting insulin consisting of porcine or human insulin in the form of large zinc-insulin crystals 长效胰岛素锌混悬液；**i. glargine,** an analogue of human insulin produced by recombinant DNA technology, having a slow, steady release over 24 hours 甘精胰岛素；**i. human,** a protein corresponding to insulin elaborated in the human pancreas, derived from pork insulin by enzymatic action or produced synthetically by recombinant DNA techniques; sometimes used specifically to denote a rapidacting regular insulin preparation of this protein 人胰岛素；**isophane i. suspension,** an intermediate-acting insulin consisting of porcine or human insulin reacted with zinc chloride and protamine sulfate 低精蛋白锌胰岛素；**Lente i.,** insulin zinc suspension 胰岛素锌混悬液；**i. lispro,** a rapid-acting analogue of human insulin synthesized by means of recombinant DNA technology 赖脯胰岛素；**NPH i.,** 同 isophane i. suspension；**prompt i. zinc suspension,** a rapid-acting insulin consisting of porcine insulin with zinc chloride added to produce a suspension of amorphous insulin 速效胰岛素锌混悬液；**regular i.,** 同 insulin (3)；**Semilente i.,** prompt insulin zinc suspension 速效胰岛素锌混悬液；**Ultralente i.,** extended insulin zinc suspension 特慢胰岛素；**i. zinc suspension,** an intermediate-acting insulin consisting of porcine or human insulin with a zinc salt added such that the solid phase of the suspension contains a 7∶3 ratio

of crystalline to amorphous insulin 中效胰岛素锌混悬液

in·su·lin·o·gen·e·sis (in″sə-lin-o-jen′ə-sis) the formation and release of insulin by the islets of Langerhans 胰岛素生成

in·su·li·no·ma (in″sə-lin-o′mə) an islet cell tumor of the beta cells, usually benign, that secretes insulin and is one of the chief causes of hypoglycemia 胰岛瘤

in·su·lin·o·pen·ic (in″sə-lin-o-pe′nik) diminishing, or pertaining to a decrease in, the level of circulating insulin 胰岛素分泌减少的

in·su·li·tis (in″sə-li′tis) lymphocytic infiltration of the islets of Langerhans, suggesting an inflammatory or immunologic reaction 胰岛炎

in·sus·cep·ti·bil·i·ty (in″sə-sep″tĭ-bil′ĭ-te) the state of being unaffected; immunity 不易感受性，无感受性；免疫性

in·take (in′tāk) the substances, or the quantities thereof, taken in and utilized by the body 吸入，纳入；摄取（量）

in·te·gra·tion (in″tə-gra′shən) 1. anabolism 合成代谢；2. coordination 协调，协同作用；3. assimilation 同化（作用）；4. the covalent insertion of one segment of DNA into another, such as the incorporation of viral or prophage DNA or a transposable element into genomic DNA 整合

in·te·grin (in-teg′rin) any of a family of transmembrane glycoproteins, consisting of two noncovalently linked polypeptide chains, designated α and β, that mediate cell-to-cell and cell-to- extracellular matrix interactions 整合素，整联蛋白

in·teg·u·ment (in-teg′u-mənt) 1. a covering or investment 覆盖物；2. the covering of the body; the skin with its various layers and accessory structures 体被，皮

in·teg·u·men·ta·ry (in-teg-u-men′tə-re) 1. pertaining to or composed of skin 外皮的，皮肤的，由皮肤构成的；2. serving as a covering 用作覆盖物的

in·teg·u·men·tum (in-teg″u-men′təm) [L.] integument 体被，皮；珠被，包膜

in·tel·lect (in′tə-lekt) the mind, thinking faculty, or understanding 智力，才智，理解力

in·tel·lec·tu·al·iza·tion (in″tə-lek″choo-əl-ĭ-za′shən) an unconscious defense mechanism in which reasoning is used to avoid confronting an objectionable impulse, emotional conflict, or other stressor and thus to defend against anxiety 理智化

in·ten·tion (in-ten′shən) 1. a manner of healing 愈合，见 *healing* 下词条；2. a goal or desired end 意图，目的

in·ter·ac·tion (in″tər-ak′shən) the quality, state, or process of (two or more things) acting on each other

相互作用，交互作用；**drug i.**, alteration of the effects of a drug by reaction with another drug or drugs, with foods or beverages, or with a preexisting medical condition 药物相互作用

in·ter·al·ve·o·lar (in″tər-al-ve′ə-lər) between alveoli 小泡间的

in·ter·ar·tic·u·lar (in″tər-ahr-tik′u-lər) situated between articular surfaces 关节间的

in·ter·atri·al (in″tər-a′tre-əl) situated between the atria of the heart 心房间的

in·ter·brain (in′tər-brān″) diencephalon 间脑

in·ter·ca·lat·ed (in-tur′kə-lāt″əd) inserted between; interposed 插入的，间介的；又称 *intercalary*

in·ter·cap·il·lary (in″tər-kap′ĭ-lar-e) among or between capillaries 毛细（血）管间的

in·ter·car·pal (in″tər-kahr′pəl) between the carpal bones 腕骨间的

in·ter·car·ti·lag·i·nous (in″tər-kahr″tĭ-laj′ĭ- nəs) between, or connecting, cartilages 软骨间的

in·ter·cav·er·nous (in″tər-kav′ər-nəs) between two cavities 腔间的

in·ter·cel·lu·lar (in″tər-sel′u-lər) between or among cells 细胞间的

in·ter·cos·tal (in″tər-kos′təl) between two ribs 肋间的

in·ter·course (in′tər-kors) 1. mutual exchange 交际，往来；2. 同 sexual i.; **sexual i.**, 1. coitus 性交；2. any physical contact between two individuals involving stimulation of the genital organs of at least one 两个人之间对至少一个人生殖器刺激的任何身体接触

in·ter·cri·co·thy·rot·o·my (in″tər-kri″ko-thirot′o-me) cricothyrotomy 环甲膜切开术

in·ter·crit·i·cal (in″tər-krit′ĭ-kəl) denoting the period between attacks, as of gout 发作间期的

in·ter·cur·rent (in″tər-kur′ənt) occurring during and modifying the course of another disease 并发的，间发的

in·ter·cusp·ing (in″tər-kusp′ing) the occlusion of the cusps of the teeth of one jaw with the depressions in the teeth of the other jaw 牙尖吻合的

in·ter·den·tal (in″tər-den′təl) between the proximal surfaces of adjacent teeth in the same arch 牙间的

in·ter·den·ti·um (in″tər-den′she-əm) interproximal space 牙间隙

in·ter·dig·i·ta·tion (in″tər-dij″ĭ-ta′shən) 1. an interlocking of parts by finger-like processes 交错结合，指状突起把各部分相连；2. one of a set of finger-like processes 指状突起

in·ter·face (in′tər-fās″) the boundary between two systems or phases 界面，接触面；**interfa′cial** *adj.*

in·ter·fas·cic·u·lar (in″tər-fə-sik′u-lər) between adjacent fascicles 束间的

in·ter·fem·o·ral (in″tər-fem′ə-rəl) between the thighs 股间的

in·ter·fer·on (IFN) (in″tər-fēr′on) any of a family of glycoproteins, production of which can be stimulated by viral infection, by intracellular parasites, by protozoa, and by bacteria and bacterial endotoxins, that exert antiviral activity and have immunoregulatory functions; they also inhibit the growth of nonviral intracellular parasites. Interferons are designated α, β, γ, and ω on the basis of association with certain producer cells and functions; all animal cells, however, can produce interferons and some cells can produce more than one type. Pharmaceutical preparations of natural or synthetic interferons (e.g., *i. alfa-2a, i. alfa-2b, i. alfa-n1, i. alfa-n3, i. alfacon-1, i. beta-1a, i. beta-1b, i. gamma-1b*) are used as antineoplastics and biologic response modifiers 干扰素

in·ter·glob·u·lar (in″tər-glob′u-lər) between or among globules, as of the dentin 球间的，如小球间牙本质

in·ter·glu·te·al (in″tər-gloo′te-əl) internatal; between the buttocks 臀间的

in·ter·ic·tal (in″tər-ik′təl) occurring between attacks or paroxysms 发作间期的

in·ter·ki·ne·sis (in″tər-kī-ne′sis) the period between the first and second divisions in meiosis, similar to mitotic interphase but without DNA replication 减数分裂间期（减数分裂中第一和第二次分裂之间的时期）

in·ter·leu·kin (in″tər-loo″kin) a generic term for a group of multifunctional cytokines that are produced by a variety of lymphoid and nonlymphoid cells and whose effects occur at least partly within the lymphopoietic system 白（细胞）介素；**i.-1 (IL-1)**, a predominantly macrophage-produced interleukin that mediates the host inflammatory response in innate immunity; two principal forms exist, designated α and β, with apparently identical biologic activity. At low concentrations, IL-1 principally acts to mediate local inflammation; at high concentrations, IL-1 enters the bloodstream and acts as an endocrine hormone, in some actions resembling tumor necrosis factor 白细胞介素 1；**i.-2 (IL-2)**, one produced by T cells in response to antigenic or mitogenic stimulation, acting to regulate the immune response. It stimulates the proliferation of T cells and the synthesis of other T cell–derived cytokines, stimulates the growth and cytolytic function of NK cells to produce lymphokine-activated killer cells, is a growth factor for and stimulates antibody synthesis in B cells, and may promote apoptosis in antigenactivated T cells; it is used pharmaceutically as an antineoplastic 白细胞介素 2

in·ter·lo·bar (in″tər-lo′bər) situated or occurring between lobes 叶间的

in·ter·lo·bi·tis (in″tər-lo-bi′tis) interlobular pleurisy 叶间胸膜炎

in·ter·lob·u·lar (in″tər-lob′u-lər) situated or occurring between lobules 小叶间的

in·ter·lock·ing (in″tər-lok′ing) closely joined, as by hooks or dovetails; locking into one another 交锁，紧密连接

in·ter·me·di·ate (in″tər-me′de-ət) 1. between; intervening; resembling, in part, each of two extremes 中间的，居间的；2. a substance formed in a chemical process that is essential to formation of the end product of the process 中间体，媒介物

in·ter·me·di·us (in″tər-me′de-əs) [L.] intermediate; in anatomy, denoting the middle structure of three in terms of their positions relative to the midline of the body or part 中间的；中间部

in·ter·men·stru·al (in″tər-men′stroo-əl) occurring between the menstrual periods 月经间期的

in·ter·mit·tent (in″tər-mit′ənt) marked by alternating periods of activity and inactivity 间歇的，周期性的

in·ter·mu·ral (in-tər-mu′rəl) between the walls of organs 壁间的

in·ter·mus·cu·lar (in″tər-mus′ku-lər) situated between muscles 肌间的

in·tern (in′tərn) a medical graduate serving in a hospital preparatory to being licensed to practice medicine 实习医师

in·ter·nal (in-tur′nəl) situated or occurring on the inside; nearer the center of a part or cavity 内部的，在内部的

in·ter·nal·iza·tion (in-tur″nəl-ī-za′shən) a mental mechanism whereby certain external attributes, attitudes, or standards of others are unconsciously taken as one's own 内在化

in·ter·na·tal (in″tər-na′təl) intergluteal 臀间的

in·ter·neu·ron (in″tər-noor′on) 中间神经元 1. a neuron between the primary sensory neuron and the final motoneuron 处于感觉神经元和运动神经元之间的神经元；2. any neuron whose processes are entirely confined within a specific area, as within the olfactory lobe, and which synapse with neurons extending into that area 突起完全限于特定区域（如嗅叶）并与进入该区的神经元建立突触联系的神经元

in·tern·ist (in-tur′nist) a specialist in internal medicine 内科医师

in·tern·ship (in′tərn-ship) the position or term of service of an intern in a hospital 实习医师职位；实习医师期

in·ter·nu·cle·ar (in″tər-noo′kle-ər) situated between nuclei or between nuclear layers of the retina 核间的，视网膜核层间的

in·ter·nun·ci·al (in″tər-nun′she-əl) transmitting impulses between two different parts 联络的（中枢间或神经元间）

in·ter·nus (in-tur′nəs) [L.] 同 internal

in·ter·oc·clu·sal (in″tər-o-kloo′zəl) situated between the occlusal surfaces of opposing teeth in the two dental arches（上下齿）咬合面间的

in·tero·cep·tor (in″tər-o-sep′tər) a sensory nerve ending that is located in and transmits impulses from the viscera 内部感受器；**interocep′tive** *adj.*

in·ter·oc·u·lar (in″tər-ok′u-lər) between the eyes 眼间的

in·ter·os·se·ous (in″tər-os′e-əs) between bones 骨间的

in·ter·pa·ri·e·tal (in″tər-pə-ri′ə-təl) 1. 同 intermural；2. between the parietal bones 顶骨间的

in·ter·pe·dun·cu·lar (in″tər-pə-dunk′u-lər) situated between two peduncles, as between two cerebellar peduncles（脑）脚间的

in·ter·phase (in′tər-fāz) the portion of the cell cycle between two successive cell divisions, during which normal cellular metabolism occurs and DNA is synthesized; chromosomes are not individually distinguishable but occupy chromosomal territories（细胞）分裂间期

in·ter·pleu·ral (in″tər-ploor′əl) between two layers of the pleura 胸膜间的

in·ter·po·lat·ed (in-tur′po-la″təd) inserted between other elements or parts 插入的

in·ter·po·la·tion (in-tur″po-la′shən) the determination of intermediate values in a series on the basis of observed values 内插法（根据观察到的数据决定数列的中间值）

in·ter·pre·ta·tion (in-tur″prə-ta′shən) in psychotherapy, the therapist's explanation to the patient of the latent or hidden meanings of what the patient says, does, or experiences 解释（在精神疗法上，医生用根据病人的行为等解释其潜在含义）

in·ter·prox·i·mal (in″tər-prok′sĭ-məl) between two adjoining surfaces 邻间的，邻接近端间的

in·ter·ra·dic·u·lar (in″tər-rə-dik′u-lər) between or among roots or radicles 根间的

in·ter·sec·tio (in″tər-sek′she-o) pl. *intersectio′nes* [L.] 同 intersection；**i. tendi′nea,** a fibrous band traversing the belly of a muscle, dividing it into two parts 腱划

in·ter·sec·tion (in″tər-sek′shən) a site at which one structure crosses another 交集，交叉点

in·ter·sex (in′tər-seks) former name for *disorders of sex development* 雌雄间体，间性体（性发育障

碍的曾用名）**intersex′ual** *adj.*

in·ter·space (in′tər-spās) a space between similar structures 间隙，中间，空间

in·ter·stice (in-tur′stis) a small interval, space, or gap in a tissue or structure 小间隙，裂缝

in·ter·sti·tial (in″tər-stish′əl) pertaining to parts or interspaces of a tissue 空隙的，裂缝的

in·ter·sti·ti·um (in″tər-stish′e-əm) 1. 同 interstice; 2. stroma 间质组织

in·ter·tha·lam·ic (in″tər-thə-lam′ik) between thalami, particularly the optic thalami 丘脑间的

in·ter·trans·verse (in″tər-trans-vərs′) between transverse processes of the vertebrae 椎骨横突间的

in·ter·tri·go (in″tər-tri′go) an erythematous skin eruption occurring on apposed skin surfaces 擦烂

in·ter·tro·chan·ter·ic (in″tər-tro″kan-ter′ik) situated in or pertaining to the space between the greater and lesser trochanters 转子间的，粗隆间的

in·ter·ure·ter·al (in″tər-u-re′tər-əl) 同 interureteric

in·ter·ure·ter·ic (in″tər-u″rə-ter′ik) between ureters 输尿管间的

in·ter·vag·i·nal (in″tər-vaj′ĭ-nəl) between sheaths 鞘间的

in·ter·val (in′tər-vəl) the space between two objects or parts; the lapse of time between two events 间隔，间距；间期；**atrioventricular i., AV i.,** the time between the start of atrial systole and the start of ventricular systole, equivalent to the P–R interval of electrocardiography 房室收缩间期；**cardioarterial i.,** the time between the apex beat and arterial pulsation 心搏动脉间期；**confidence i.,** an estimated statistical interval for a parameter, giving a range of values that may contain the parameter and the degree of confidence that it is in fact there 置信区间；**coupling i.,** the length of time between an ectopic beat and the sinus beat preceding it; in an arrhythmia characterized by such beats, the intervals may be constant *(fixed coupling i's)* or inconstant *(variable coupling i's)* 偶联间期，配对间期；**escape i.,** the interval between an escape beat and the normal beat preceding it 脱逸间期；**interdischarge i.,** the time between two discharges of the action potential of a single muscle fiber 释放间期，单一肌纤维两次动作电位放电的间期；**interpotential i.,** the time between discharges of action potentials of two different fibers from the same motor unit 波间期；**lucid i.,** 中间清醒期；1. a brief period of remission of symptoms in a psychosis 精神病症状的短暂缓解期；2. a brief return to consciousness after loss of consciousness in head injury 颅脑损伤昏迷后的短暂神志清醒期；**pacemaker escape i.,** the period between the last sensed spontaneous cardiac activity and the first beat stimulated by the artificial pacemaker 起搏点脱逸间期；**P–P i.,** the time from the beginning of one P wave to that of the next P wave, representing the length of the cardiac cycle P-P 间期（两次 P 波开始之间的间期）；**P–R i.,** the portion of the electrocardiogram between the onset of the P wave (atrial depolarization) and the QRS complex (ventricular depolarization) P-R 间期；**QRS i.,** the interval from the beginning of the Q wave to the termination of the S wave, representing the time for ventricular depolarization QRS 间期（Q 波开始到 S 波结束的间期）；**QRST i., Q–T i.,** the time from the beginning of the Q wave to the end of the T wave, representing the duration of ventricular electrical activity QRST 间期（Q 波开始到 T 波结束的间期）；**systolic time i's (STI),** any of several intervals measured for assessing left ventricular performance, particularly left ventricular ejection time, electromechanical systole, and preejection period 收缩时间间期；**V–A i.,** the time between a ventricular stimulus and the atrial stimulus following its V-A 间期

in·ter·ve·nous (in″tər-ve′nəs) between veins 静脉间的

in·ter·ven·tion (in″tər-ven′shən) 1. the act or fact of interfering so as to modify 干涉，干预；2. any measure whose purpose is to improve health or alter the course of disease 任何旨在改善健康或疾病进程的措施；**crisis i.,** 1. an immediate, short-term, psychotherapeutic approach, the goal of which is to help resolve a personal crisis within the individual's immediate environment 危机干预（心理疗法）；2. the procedures involved in responding to an emergency 应急性措施；**percutaneous coronary i. (PCI),** the management of coronary artery occlusion by any of various catheter-based techniques, such as percutaneous transluminal coronary angioplasty, atherectomy, excimer laser angioplasty, and implantation of coronary stents and related devices 经皮冠状动脉介入治疗

in·ter·ven·tric·u·lar (in″tər-vən-trik′u-lər) situated between ventricles（心）室间的

in·ter·ver·te·bral (in″tər-vur′tə-brəl) situated between two contiguous vertebrae 椎（骨）间的；见 *disk* 下词条

in·ter·vil·lous (in″tər-vil′əs) between or among villi 绒毛间的

in·tes·tine (in-tes′tin) the part of the alimentary canal extending from the pyloric opening of the stomach to the anus 肠，见图 27；**intes′tinal** *adj.*；**large i.,** the distal portion of the intestine, about 5 feet long, extending from its junction with the small intestine to the anus and comprising the cecum, colon, rectum, and anal canal 大肠；**small**

i., the proximal portion of the intestine, about 20 feet long, smaller in caliber than the large intestine, extending from the pylorus to the cecum and comprising the duodenum, jejunum, and ileum 小肠

in·tes·ti·num (in″tes-ti′nəm) pl. *intesti′na* [L.] 同 intestine

in·ti·ma (in′tĭ-mə) 1. innermost 内膜；2. tunica intima vasorum 膜；**n′timal** *adj.*

in·ti·mi·tis (in″tĭ-mi′tis) endangiitis 内膜炎

in·tol·er·ance (in-tol′ər-əns) inability to withstand or consume; inability to absorb or metabolize nutrients 不耐受，不耐性；**congenital sucrose i.**, a disaccharide intolerance specific for sucrase, usually due to a congenital defect in the sucrase-isomaltase enzyme complex 先天性蔗糖不耐受；见 *sucrase-isomaltase deficiency*；**disaccharide i.**, a complex of abdominal symptoms after ingestion of normal quantities of dietary carbohydrates, including diarrhea, flatulence, distention, and pain; it is usually due to deficiency of one or more disaccharidases but may be due to impaired absorption or other causes 双糖不耐受；**drug i.**, 药物耐受不良 1. inability to continue taking, or difficulty in continuing to take, a medication because of an adverse side effect that is not immune mediated 因非免疫介导的不良反应而不能或难以继续服用药物；2. the state of reacting to the normal pharmacologic doses of a drug with the symptoms of overdosage 对药物的正常药理学剂量有过量症状的反应状态；**hereditary fructose i.**, an autosomal recessive disorder of fructose metabolism due to an enzymatic deficiency, with onset in infancy, characterized by hypoglycemia with variable manifestations of fructosuria, fructosemia, anorexia, vomiting, failure to thrive, jaundice, splenomegaly, and an aversion to fructose-containing foods 遗传性果糖不耐受症；**lactose i.**, a disaccharide intolerance specific for lactose, usually due to an inherited deficiency of lactase activity in the intestinal mucosa, which may not be manifest until adulthood. *Congenital lactose i.* may be due to an inherited immediate deficiency of lactase activity or may be a more severe disorder with vomiting, dehydration, failure to thrive, disacchariduria, and cataracts, probably due to abnormal permeability of the gastric mucosa 乳糖耐受不良

in·tor·sion (in-tor′shən) inward rotation of the upper pole of the vertical meridian of each eye toward the midline of the face 内旋，内扭转

in·tox·i·ca·tion (in-tok″sĭ-ka′shən) 1. stimulation, excitement, or stupefaction caused by a chemical substance, or as if by one（疑似）化学物质造成的刺激、兴奋或昏迷；2. substance i., especially that due to ingestion of alcohol 精神活性物质（特别是酒精）中毒；3. poisoning; the state of being poisoned 中毒，中毒状态；**substance i.**, reversible, substance-specific, maladaptive behavioral or psychological changes directly resulting from the physiologic effects on the central nervous system of recent ingestion of or exposure to a psychoactive substance, particularly alcohol 精神活性物质（特别是酒精）中毒

in·tra·aor·tic (in″trə-a-or′tik) within the aorta 主动脉内的

in·tra·ar·te·ri·al (in″trə-ahr-tēr′e-əl) within an artery or arteries 动脉内的

in·tra·ar·tic·u·lar (in″trə-ahr-tik′u-lər) within a joint 关节内的

in·tra·can·a·lic·u·lar (in″trə-kan″ə-lik′u-lər) within canaliculi 小管内的

in·tra·cap·su·lar (in″trə-kap′su-lər) within a capsule 囊内的，被膜内的

in·tra·car·di·ac (in″trə-kahr′de-ak) within the heart 心脏内的

in·tra·cav·er·no·sal (in″trə-kav″ər-no′səl) within the corpus cavernosum 海绵体内的

in·tra·cel·lu·lar (in″trə-sel′u-lər) within a cell or cells 细胞内的

in·tra·cer·vi·cal (in″trə-sur′vĭ-kəl) within the canal of the cervix uteri 子宫颈内的

in·tra·cor·po·re·al (in″trə-kor-por′e-əl) situated or occurring within the body 体内的

in·tra·cra·ni·al (in″trə-kra′ne-əl) within the cranium 颅内的

in·tra·crine (in′trə-krin) denoting a type of hormone function in which a regulatory factor acts within the cell that synthesizes it by binding to intracellular receptors（细）胞内分泌

in·trac·ta·ble (in-trak′tə-bəl) resistant to cure, relief, or control 难治疗的，难控制的

in·tra·cu·ta·ne·ous (in″trə-ku-ta′ne-əs) within the skin 皮内的

in·tra·cys·tic (in″trə-sis′tik) within the bladder or a cyst 囊内的

in·tra·cy·to·plas·mic (in″trə-si″to-plaz′mik) within the cytoplasm of a cell 胞质内的

in·tra·der·mal (in″trə-dur′məl) 1. within the dermis 真皮内的；2. intracutaneous 皮内的

in·tra·duc·tal (in″trə-duk′təl) situated or occurring within the duct of a gland 管内的（位于或发生于腺管内的）

in·tra·du·ral (in″trə-doo′rəl) within or beneath the dura mater 硬膜内的

in·tra·ep·i·the·li·al (in″trə-ep″ĭ-the′le-əl) situated among the cells of the epithelium 上皮内的

in·tra·fal·lo·pi·an (in″trə-fə-lo′pe-ən) within the uterine (fallopian) tube 输卵管内的

in·tra·fat (in″trə-fat′) situated in or introduced into fatty tissue, as the superficial fascia 脂肪内的

in·tra·fu·sal (in″trə-fu′zəl) pertaining to the striated fibers within a muscle spindle 肌梭内的

in·tra·lig·a·men·ta·ry (in″trə-lig″ə-men′tə-re) 同 intraligamentous

in·tra·lig·a·men·tous (in″trə-lig″ə-men′təs) within a ligament 韧带内的

in·tra·lob·u·lar (in″trə-lob′u-lər) within a lobule 小叶内的

in·tra·med·ul·lary (in″trə-med′u-lar″e) within (1) the spinal cord, (2) the medulla oblongata, or (3) the medullary cavity of a bone 髓内的（指脊髓内的，延髓内的，骨髓腔内的）

in·tra·mem·bra·nous (in″trə-mem′brə-nəs) within a membrane 膜内的

in·tra·mu·ral (in″trə-mu′rəl) within the wall of an organ 壁内的

in·tra·mus·cu·lar (in″trə-mus′ku-lər) within the muscular substance 肌内的

in·tra·oc·u·lar (in″trə-ok′u-lər) within the eye 眼内的

in·tra·op·er·a·tive (in″trə-op′ər-ə-tiv) occurring during a surgical operation 手术期（中）的

in·tra·oral (in″trə-or′əl) within the mouth 口内的

in·tra·pa·ri·e·tal (in″trə-pə-ri′ə-təl) 1. 同 intramural；2. within the parietal region of the brain 脑顶区内的

in·tra·par·tal (in″trə-pahr′təl) 同 intrapartum

in·tra·par·tum (in″trə-pahr′təm) occurring during childbirth or during delivery 分娩期（内）的，产时的

in·tra·pel·vic (in″trə-pel′vik) within the pelvis 骨盆内的

in·tra·peri·to·ne·al (in″trə-per″ĭ-to-ne′əl) within the peritoneal cavity 腹膜腔内的

in·tra·psy·chic (in″trə-si′kik) arising, occurring, or situated within the mind 内心的

in·tra·re·nal (in″trə-re′nəl) within the kidney 肾内的

in·tra·spi·nal (in″trə-spi′nəl) within the vertebral column 脊柱内的

in·tra·the·cal (in″trə-the′kəl) within a sheath; through the theca of the spinal cord into the subarachnoid space 鞘内的

in·tra·tho·rac·ic (in″trə-thə-ras′ik) endothoracic 胸内的，胸廓内的

in·tra·tra·che·al (in″trə-tra′ke-əl) endotracheal 气管内的

in·tra·tym·pan·ic (in″trə-tim-pan′ik) within the tympanic cavity 鼓室内的

in·tra·uter·ine (in″trə-u′tər-in) within the uterus 子宫内的

in·trav·a·sa·tion (in-trav″ə-sa′shən) the entrance of foreign material into vessels 进入血管（异物），内渗

in·tra·vas·cu·lar (in″trə-vas′ku-lər) within a vessel 血管内的

in·tra·ve·nous (in″trə-ve′nəs) within a vein or veins 静脉内的；**intrave′nously** adj.

in·tra·ven·tric·u·lar (in″trə-ven-trik′u-lər) within a ventricle 心室内的

in·tra·ves·i·cal (in″trə-ves′ĭ-kəl) within the urinary bladder 膀胱内的

in·tra·vi·tal (in″trə-vi′təl) occurring during life 活体（内）的，生活期内的

in·tra vi·tam (in′trə vi′təm) [L.] during life 生存期间，生活期间

in·trin·sic (in-trin′sik) situated entirely within or pertaining exclusively to a part 固有的，内部的，内在的

in·troi·tus (in-tro′ĭ-təs) pl. *intro′itus* [L.] an entrance or opening 入口，口

in·tro·jec·tion (in″trə-jek′shən) a mental mechanism in which the standards and values of other persons or groups are unconsciously and symbolically taken within oneself 内向投射

in·tro·mis·sion (in″tro-mish′ən) the entrance of one part into another 插入

in·tron (in′tron) a noncoding sequence between two coding sequences within a gene, spliced out in the formation of mature mRNA 内含子

in·tro·spec·tion (in″tro-spek′shən) contemplation or observation of one's own thoughts and feelings; self-analysis 内省，自省；**introspec′tive** adj.

in·tro·sus·cep·tion (in″tro-sə-sep′shən) 同 intussusception 肠套叠

in·tro·ver·sion (in″tro-vur′zhən) 1. the turning outside in, more or less completely, of an organ, or the resulting condition 内翻，内倾；2. preoccupation with oneself, with reduction of interest in the outside world 内向

in·tro·vert (in′tro-vərt) 1. a person whose interest is turned inward to the self 内向的人；2. to turn one's interest inward to the self 内省；3. a structure that can be turned or drawn inward 可内翻（或内弯）的结构；4. to turn a part or organ inward upon itself. 使内翻，使内倾

in·tu·ba·tion (in″too-ba′shən) the insertion of a tube into a body canal or hollow organ, as into the trachea 插管法；**endotracheal i.**, insertion of a tube into the trachea for purposes of anesthesia, airway maintenance, aspiration of secretions, lung ventilation, or prevention of entrance of foreign material into the airway; the tube goes through the nose (*nasotracheal i.*) or mouth (*orotracheal i.*) 气

管内插管法；**nasal i.**, insertion of a tube into the respiratory or gastrointestinal tract through the nose 鼻插管法；**oral i.**, insertion of a tube into the respiratory or gastrointestinal tract through the mouth 口插管法

in·tu·mes·cence (in-too-mes′əns) 1. a swelling, normal or abnormal 肿大，隆起；2. the process of swelling 膨胀，肿胀的过程；**intumes′cent** *adj.*

in·tu·mes·cen·tia (in-too-mə-sen′she-ə) pl. *intumescen′tiae* [L.] 同 intumescence

in·tus·sus·cep·tion (in″tə-sə-sep′shən) prolapse of one part of the intestine into the lumen of an immediately adjacent part 肠套叠

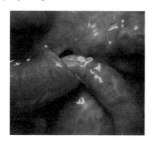

▲ 小肠套叠

in·tus·sus·cep·tum (in″tə-sə-sep′təm) the portion of intestine that has prolapsed in intussusception 肠套叠套入部

in·tus·sus·cip·i·ens (in″tə-sə-sip′e- əns) the portion of intestine containing the intussusceptum 肠套叠鞘部

in·u·lin (in′u-lin) a starch occurring in the rhizome of certain plants, yielding fructose on hydrolysis, and used in tests of renal function 菊粉，菊糖

in·unc·tion (in-ungk′shən) the act of anointing or applying an ointment by rubbing 涂擦，涂油

in utero (in u′tər-o) [L.] within the uterus 在子宫内

in vac·uo (in vak′u-o) [L.] in a vacuum 在真空中

in·vag·i·na·tion (in-vaj″ĭ-na′shən) 1. the infolding of one part within another part of a structure, as of the blastula during gastrulation 内陷，内折；2. intussusception；**basilar i.**, a developmental deformity of the occipital bone and upper end of the cervical spine in which the latter appears to have pushed the floor of the occipital bone upward 扁后脑，颅底凹陷症

in·va·sion (in-va′zhən) 1. the attack or onset of a disease 发病，发作；2. the simple, harmless entrance of bacteria into the body or their deposition in tissue, as opposed to infection 侵入；3. the infiltration and destruction of surrounding tissue, characteristic of malignant tumors 侵袭，侵害邻近组织

in·va·sive (in-va′siv) 1. pertaining to or characterized by invasion 入侵的，侵袭的；2. involving puncture of the skin or insertion of an instrument or foreign material into the body; said of diagnostic techniques 侵入性诊断技术

in·ven·to·ry (in′vən-tor″e) a comprehensive list of personality traits, aptitudes, and interests; some of the most popular include the *California Personality I. (CPI), Millon Clinical Multiaxial I. (MCMI)*, and *Minnesota Multiphasic Personality I. (MMPI)* 清单，调查表（有关个性特征、才能和兴趣等方面的综合调查表）

in·verse (in′vərs) 1. reversed in order, effect, or nature 倒转的，相反的；2. the reciprocal of a particular quantity 倒数

in·ver·sion (in-vur′zhən) 1. a turning inward, inside out, or other reversal of the normal relation of a part 内翻；反向，倒向；2. a chromosomal aberration due to the inverted reunion of an internal segment after breakage of a chromosome at two points, resulting in a change in sequence of genes or nucleotides 倒位（染色体畸变）；**i. of uterus**, a turning of the uterus whereby the fundus is forced through the cervix, protruding into or completely outside of the vagina 子宫内翻；**visceral i.**, the more or less complete right and left transposition of the viscera 内脏（左右）易位，内脏反向

in·ver·te·brate (in-vur′tə-brāt) 1. any animal that has no vertebral column 无脊椎动物；2. having no vertebral column 无脊椎的

in·vest·ment (in-vest′mənt) material in which a denture, tooth, crown, or model for a dental restoration is enclosed for curing, soldering, or casting, or the process of such enclosure（牙）包埋料，包埋法

in·vet·er·ate (in-vet′ər-ət) confirmed and chronic; long-established and difficult to cure 慢性顽固的，痼疾的，绵延难治的

in vi·tro (in ve′tro) [L.] within a glass; observable in a test tube; in an artificial environment 体外，离体

in vi·vo (in ve′vo) [L.] within the living body 体内

In·vo·ka·na (in″vō-kaw′naw) trademark for a preparation of canagliflozin 卡格列净（canagliflozin）的商品名

in·vo·lu·crum (in″vo-loo′krəm) pl. *involu′cra* [L.] a covering or sheath, as of a sequestrum 总苞，包壳

in·vol·un·tary (in-vol′ən-tar″e) 1. independent of the will 无意识的，不自觉的；2. contrary to the will 非自愿的，非本意的

in·vo·lu·tion (in″vo-loo′shən) 1. a rolling or turning inward 内转，内卷；2. a retrograde change of the body or of an organ, as the retrograde changes in size of the female genital organs after delivery 复旧，复原；3. the progressive degeneration occurring naturally with age, resulting in shriveling of organs or tissues 衰退，退化；**involu′tional** *adj.*

io·ben·guane (i″o-ben′gwān) a norepinephrine analogue that is taken up by the neuroendocrine cells and concentrated in the hormone storage vesicles; labeled with radioactive iodine, it is used for diagnostic imaging of neuroendocrine tumors and disorders of the adrenal medulla 碘苄胍

iod·ic ac·id (i-o′dik) a monobasic acid, HIO3, formed by oxidation of iodine with nitric acid or chlorates, which has strong acid and reducing properties 碘酸

io·dide (i′o-dīd) a binary compound of iodine 碘化物

io·din·a·tion (i″o-din-a′shən) the incorporation or addition of iodine in a compound 碘化作用

io·dine (I) (i′o-dīn) a halogen element of peculiar odor and acrid taste; a bluish black solid somewhat volatile at room temperature, forming a violet vapor; at. no. 53, at. wt. 126.904. It is essential in nutrition, being necessary for synthesis of thyroid hormones (thyroxine and triiodothyronine). Iodine solution is used as a topical antiinfective 碘；另见 *radioiodine*；**protein-bound i.,** iodine firmly bound to protein in the serum, determination of which constitutes one test of thyroid function 蛋白结合碘；**radioactive i.,** radioiodine 放射性碘

io·din·oph·i·lous (i″o-din-of′ī-ləs) easily stainable with iodine 嗜碘的

io·dism (i′o-diz-əm) chronic poisoning by iodine or iodides, with coryza, ptyalism, frontal headache, emaciation, weakness, and skin eruptions 碘中毒

io·do·der·ma (i-o″do-dur′mə) any skin lesion resulting from iodism 碘疹

io·do·hip·pu·rate so·di·um (i-o″do-hip′u-rāt) an iodine-containing compound that has been used as a radiopaque medium in pyelography. When labeled with radioactive iodine, it may be used as a diagnostic aid in determination of renal function and in renal imaging 碘马尿酸钠

io·do·phil (i-o′do-fil) 1. any cell or other element readily stainable with iodine 嗜碘体；2. iodinophilous 嗜碘的

io·do·phil·ia (i-o″do-fil′e-ə) a reaction shown by leukocytes in certain pathologic conditions, as in toxemia and severe anemia, in which the polymorphonuclears show diffuse brownish coloration when treated with iodine or iodides 嗜碘性

io·dop·sin (i″o-dop′sin) a photosensitive violet pigment found in the retinal cones of some animals

and important for color vision 视紫蓝质，视青质

io·do·quin·ol (i-o″do-kwin′ol) an amebicide used in the treatment of amebic dysentery; also used topically as an antibacterial and antifungal 双碘喹啉

io·hex·ol (i″o-hek′sol) a nonionic, water-soluble, low-osmolality radiopaque medium 碘海醇，碘酰六醇

ion (i′on) an atom or molecule that has gained or lost one or more electrons and acquired a positive charge (a cation) or negative charge (an anion) 离子；**ion′ic** *adj.*；**dipolar i.,** zwitterion 偶极离子，两性离子

ion·iza·tion (i″on-ī-za′shən) 1. any process by which a neutral atom or molecule gains or loses electrons, acquiring a net charge 电离，离子化；2. 同 iontophoresis

ion·o·phore (i-on′ə-for″) any molecule, as of a drug, that increases the permeability of cell membranes to a specific ion 离子载体

ion·to·pho·re·sis (i-on″to-fə-re′sis) the introduction of ions of soluble salts into the body by means of electric current 电离子透入疗法；**iontophoret′ic** *adj.*

IOP intensive outpatient 重症门诊；intraocular pressure 眼内压

io·pa·no·ic ac·id (i″o-pə-no′ik) a radiopaque medium used in cholecystography 碘番酸（胆囊造影剂）

io·phen·dy·late (i″o-fen′də-lāt) a radiopaque medium used in myelography 碘苯酯（脊髓造影剂）

io·pro·mide (i″o-pro′mīd) a nonionic, low-osmolality radiopaque medium used for cardiovascular imaging, excretory urology, and contrast enhancement in computed tomography 碘普罗胺（优维显溶液）

io·thal·a·mate (i″o-thal′ə-māt) a radiopaque medium for a variety of radiographic procedures, including angiography, arthrography, urography, cholangiography, and computed tomographic imaging; used as the meglumine or sodium salt, or a combination 碘酞酸盐

io·ver·sol (i″o-vur′sol) a nonionic contrast medium used in angiography and urography and for contrast enhancement in computed tomography 碘佛醇

iox·ag·late (i″ok-sag′lāt) a low-osmolality radiopaque medium, used as the meglumine or sodium salt 碘格仑酸盐

iox·i·lan (i-ok′sī-lan) a low-viscosity, lowosmolality, nonionic contrast medium used in arteriography, excretory urography, and computed tomography 碘昔兰（低渗造影剂）

IP intraperitoneal 腹腔内；isoelectric point 等电点

IPAA International Psychoanalytical Association 国际精神分析协会

IPD intermittent peritoneal dialysis 间歇性腹膜透析

ip·e·cac (ip′ə-kak) the dried rhizome and roots of *Cephaelis ipecacuanha* or *C. acuminata;* used as an emetic or expectorant 吐根

IPOIC immediate postoperative instillation of intravesical chemotherapy 术后即时膀胱灌注化疗

IPPB intermittent positive pressure breathing 间歇性正压通气

ipra·tro·pi·um (ip″rə-tro′pe-əm) a synthetic congener of atropine that acts as an anticholinergic agent; used as the bromide salt by inhalation as a bronchodilator and intranasally to relieve rhinorrhea 异丙托溴铵

ip·si·lat·er·al (ip″sĭ-lat′ər-əl) situated on or affecting the same side 同侧的

IPV poliovirus vaccine inactivated 灭活脊髓灰质炎病毒疫苗

IQ intelligence quotient 智商，智力商数

Ir iridium 元素铱的符号

ir·be·sar·tan (ir″bə-sahr′tan) an angiotensin Ⅱ receptor antagonist used as an antihypertensive 厄贝沙坦

ir·id·aux·e·sis (ir″id-awk-se′sis) thickening of the iris 虹膜肥厚

iri·dec·to·me·so·di·al·y·sis (ir″ĭ-dek″to-me″sodi-al′ə-sis) excision and separation of adhesions around the inner edge of the iris 虹膜分离切除术

iri·dec·to·my (ir″ĭ-dek′tə-me) excision of part of the iris 虹膜切除术

iri·dec·tro·pi·um (ir″ĭ-dek-tro′pe-əm) eversion of the iris 虹膜外翻

iri·de·mia (ir″ĭ-de′me-ə) hemorrhage from the iris 虹膜出血

iri·den·clei·sis (ir″ĭ-dən-kli′sis) surgical incarceration of a slip of the iris within a corneal or limbal incision to act as a wick for aqueous drainage in glaucoma 虹膜箝顿术

iri·den·tro·pi·um (ir″ĭ-dən-tro′pe-əm) inversion of the iris 虹膜内翻

iri·des (i′rĭ-dēz) (ir′ĭ-dēz) [Gr.] *iris* 的复数

iri·des·cence (ir″ĭ-des′əns) the condition of gleaming with bright and changing colors 彩虹色，晕色；**irides′cent** *adj.*

irid·e·sis (i-rid′ə-sis) repositioning of the pupil by fixation of a sector of iris in a corneal or limbal incision 虹膜固定术

irid·i·al (i-rid′e-əl) 同 iridic

irid·ic (i-rid′ik) pertaining to the iris 虹膜的

irid·i·um (**Ir**) (ĭ-rid′e-əm) a very hard, brittle, silvery white metallic element; at. no. 77, at. wt. 192.217 铱；**i. 192,** an artificial radioactive isotope with a half-life of 75 days, used in radiotherapy 铱

192

iri·do·avul·sion (ir″ĭ-ə-vul′shən) complete tearing away of the iris from its periphery 虹膜撕脱

iri·do·cele (i-rid′o-sēl) hernial protrusion of part of the iris through the cornea 虹膜突出

iri·do·con·stric·tor (ir″ĭ-do-kən-strik′tər) a muscle element or an agent that acts to constrict the pupil of the eye 虹膜收缩肌；缩瞳剂

iri·do·cor·ne·al (ir″ĭ-do-kor′ne-əl) pertaining to the iris and cornea 虹膜角膜的

iri·do·cy·cli·tis (ir″ĭ-do-si-kli′tis) inflammation of the iris and ciliary body 虹膜睫状体炎；**heterochromic i.,** a unilateral low-grade form leading to depigmentation of the iris of the affected eye 异色性虹膜睫状体炎

iri·do·cys·tec·to·my (ir″ĭ-do-sis-tek′tə-me) excision of part of the iris to form an artificial pupil. 虹膜囊切除术

irid·od·e·sis (ir″ĭ-dod′ə-sis) 同 iridesis

iri·do·di·al·y·sis (ir″ĭ-do-di-al′ə-sis) the separation or loosening of the iris from its attachments 虹膜根部断离

iri·do·di·la·tor (ir″ĭ-do-di′la-tər) (-di-la′tər) 1. a muscle element or an agent that acts to dilate the pupil of the eye 虹膜扩大肌；2. mydriatic 虹膜扩大剂

iri·do·do·ne·sis (ir″ĭ-do-do-ne′sis) tremulousness of the iris on movement of the eye, occurring in subluxation or loss of the lens 虹膜震颤

iri·do·ker·a·ti·tis (ir″ĭ-do-ker″ə-ti′tis) inflammation of the iris and cornea 虹膜角膜炎

iri·do·ki·ne·sis (ir″ĭ-do-kĭ-ne′sis) contraction and expansion of the iris 虹膜伸缩，又称 *iridokinesia;* **iridokinet′ic** *adj.*

iri·do·lep·tyn·sis (ir″ĭ-do-ləp-tin′sis) thinning or atrophy of the iris 虹膜萎缩，虹膜薄缩

iri·do·ma·la·cia (ir″ĭ-do-mə-la′shə) softening of the iris 虹膜软化

iri·do·me·so·di·al·y·sis (ir″ĭ-do-me″so-dial′ə-sis) surgical loosening of adhesions around the inner edge of the iris 虹膜内缘粘部分离

iri·do·mo·tor (ir″ĭ-do-me″so-dial′ə-sis) surgical loosening of adhesions around the inner edge of the iris 虹膜伸缩的，虹膜运动的

iri·don·cus (ir″ĭ-dong′kəs) tumor or swelling of the eye 虹膜肿，虹膜瘤

iri·do·ple·gia (ir″ĭ-do-ple′jə) paralysis of the sphincter of the iris 虹膜麻痹

iri·dop·to·sis (ir″ĭ-dop-to′sis) prolapse of the iris 虹膜脱垂

iri·do·rhex·is (ir″ĭ-do-rek′sis) 1. rupture of the iris 虹膜破裂；2. the tearing away of the iris 虹膜撕裂法

iri·dos·chi·sis (ir″ĭ-dos′kĭ-sis) splitting of the mesodermal stroma of the iris into two layers,with fibrils of the anterior layer floating in the aqueous 虹膜劈裂症

iri·do·ste·re·sis (ir″ĭ-do-stə-re′sis) removal of all or part of the iris 虹膜（部分或全部）切除术

iri·dot·o·my (ir″ĭ-dot′ə-me) incision of the iris 虹膜切开术

iri·no·te·can (i″rĭ-no-te′kan) a DNA topoisomerase inhibitor used as the hydrochloride salt as an antineoplastic in the treatment of colorectal carcinoma 伊立替康（抗肿瘤药）

iris (i′ris) pl. i′rides [Gr.] the circular pigmented membrane behind the cornea, perforated by the pupil 虹膜，见图 30

iri·tis (i-ri′tis) inflammation of the iris 虹膜炎；**irit′ic** adj.；**serous i.,** iritis with a serous exudate 浆液性虹膜炎

iri·to·ec·to·my (ir″ĭ-to-ek′tə-me) surgical excision of deposits of after-cataract on the iris, together with iridectomy, to form an artificial pupil 虹膜部分切除术

irit·o·my (i-rit′ə-me) 同 iridotomy

iron (Fe) (i′ərn) an abundant, hard, lustrous, grayish metallic element; at. no. 26; at. wt. 55.845. It is an essential constituent of hemoglobin, cytochromes, and other components of respiratory enzyme systems. Depletion of iron stores may result in iron-deficiency anemia, and various salts or complexes of iron are used as hematinics, including i. dextran, i. polysaccharide, i. sorbitex, and i. sucrose 铁

irot·o·my (i-rot′o-me) 同 iridotomy

ir·ra·di·ate (ĭ-ra′de-āt) to treat with radiant energy 放射治疗

ir·ra·di·a·tion (ĭ-ra′de-a′shən) 1. radiotherapy 放射治疗法；2. the dispersion of nervous impulse beyond the normal path of conduction 扩散；3. the application of rays, such as ultraviolet rays, to a substance to increase its vitamin efficiency 照射，辐射

ir·re·duc·i·ble (ir″e-doos′ĭ-bəl) not susceptible to reduction, as a fracture, hernia, or chemical substance 不能复位的

ir·ri·ga·tion (ir″ĭ-ga′shən) 1. washing by a stream of water or other fluid 冲洗，灌洗；2. a liquid used for such washing 冲洗剂，灌洗剂；**Ringer i.,** Ringer injection packaged for irrigation and used as a topical physiologic salt solution 林格液

ir·ri·ta·bil·i·ty (ir″ĭ-tə-bil′ĭ-te) the quality of being irritable 易激惹；**myotatic i.,** the ability of a muscle to contract in response to stretching 肌牵张应激性

ir·ri·ta·ble (ir′ĭ-tə-bəl) 1. capable of reacting to a stimulus 应激性的；2. abnormally sensitive to stimuli 过敏的；3. prone to excessive anger, annoyance, or

impatience 激怒的

ir·ri·ta·tion (ir″ĭ-ta′shən) 1. the act of stimulating 刺激；2. a state of overexcitation and undue sensitivity 兴奋；**ir′ritative** adj.

IRV inspiratory reserve volume 补吸气容积，补吸气量

IS insertion sequence 插入序列

is·che·mia (is-ke′me-ə) deficiency of blood in a part, usually due to functional constriction or actual obstruction of a blood vessel 局部缺血；**ische′mic** adj.；**silent i.,** cardiac ischemia without pain or other symptoms 无症状性心肌缺血

is·chi·al (is′ke-əl) ischiatic; pertaining to the ischium 坐骨的

is·chi·at·ic (is″ke-at′ik) 同 ischial

is·chio·anal (is″ke-o-a′nəl) pertaining to the ischium and anus 坐骨肛门的

is·chio·cap·su·lar (is″ke-o-kap′su-lər) pertaining to the ischium and the capsular ligament of the hip joint 坐骨囊韧带的

is·chio·coc·cyg·e·al (is″ke-o-kok-sij′e-əl) pertaining to the ischium and coccyx 坐骨尾骨的

is·chio·dyn·ia (is″ke-o-din′e-ə) pain in the ischium 坐骨神经痛

is·chio·glu·te·al (is″ke-o-gloo′te-əl) pertaining to the ischium and the buttocks 坐骨臀部的

is·chio·pu·bic (is″ke-o-pu′bik) pertaining to the ischium and pubes 坐骨耻骨的

is·chio·rec·tal (is″ke-o-rek′təl) pertaining to the ischium and rectum 坐骨直肠的

is·chi·um (is′ke-əm) pl. is′chia [L.] the inferior dorsal portion of the coxal bone. 坐骨，见图 1

isch·uria (is-ku′re-ə) retention of the urine 尿闭；**ischuret′ic** adj.

ISDP International Society of Dermatopathology 国际皮肤病理学会

is·ei·ko·nia (i″si-ko′ne-ə) the normal condition in which an image is the same in both eyes. 双眼等像 **iseikon′ic** adj.

is·eth·i·o·nate (i″sə-thi′ə-nāt) USAN contraction for 2-hydroxyethanesulfonate 羟乙基磺酸盐

is·land (i′lənd) a cluster of cells or isolated piece of tissue 岛；**blood i's,** aggregations of mesenchymal cells in the angioblast of the early embryo, developing into vascular endothelium and blood cells 血岛；**bone i.,** a benign focus of mature cortical bone within trabecular bone on a radiograph 骨岛；**i's of Langerhans,** 见 islet 下词条；**i's of pancreas,** 同 islets of Langerhans；**i. of Reil,** 同 insula (2)

is·let (i′let) an island 岛，小岛；**i's of Langerhans,** irregular microscopic structures scattered throughout the pancreas and comprising its endocrine portion. They contain the alpha cells, which secrete the hyperglycemic factor glucagon; the *beta cells,* which secrete insulin; the *delta cells,* which secrete somatostatin; and the *PP* (or *F*) *cells,* which secrete pancreatic polypeptide. Degeneration of the beta cells is one of the causes of diabetes mellitus 朗格汉斯岛，胰岛

iso·ag·glu·ti·nin (i″so-ə-gloo′tĭ-nin) an isoantigen that acts as an agglutinin 同种凝集素

iso·al·lele (i″so-ə-lēl′) an allele that appears phenotypically identical to another, but that can be distinguished at the protein or DNA level 同等位基因

iso·an·ti·body (i-so-an′tĭ-bod″e) an antibody produced by one individual that reacts with isoantigens of another individual of the same species 同种抗体，同系抗体

iso·an·ti·gen (i″so-an′tĭ-jən) an antigen existing in alternative (allelic) forms, thus inducing an immune response when one form is transferred to members who lack it; typical isoantigens are the blood group antigens 同种抗原

iso·bar (i′so-bahr) one of two or more chemical species with the same atomic weight but different atomic numbers 同量异位素

iso·bar·ic (i″so-bar′ik) having equal or constant pressure or weight across space or time 等比重的

iso·car·box·a·zid (i″so-kahr-bok′sə-zid) a monoamine oxidase inhibitor used as an antidepressant and in the prophylaxis of migraine 异唑肼，异噁唑酰肼

iso·cel·lu·lar (i″so-sel′u-lər) made up of identical cells 等细胞的，相同细胞（构成）的

iso·chro·mat·ic (i″so-kro-mat′ik) of the same colour throughout 等色的

iso·chro·mo·some (i″so-kro′mə-sōm) an abnormal chromosome having a median centromere and two identical arms, formed by transverse, rather than normal longitudinal, splitting of a replicating chromosome 等臂染色体

iso·chron·ic (i″so-kron′ik) 同 isochronous

isoch·ro·nous (i-sok′rə-nəs) performed in equal times; said of motions and vibrations occurring at the same time and being equal in duration 等时的

iso·ci·trate (i″so-sī′trāt) a salt of isocitric acid 异柠檬酸盐

iso·cit·ric ac·id (i″so-sit′rik) an intermediate in the tricarboxylic acid cycle, formed from oxaloacetic acid and converted to ketoglutaric acid 异柠檬酸

iso·co·ria (i″so-kor′e-ə) equality of size of the pupils of the two eyes 两瞳孔等大

iso·cor·tex (i″so-kor′teks) the neocortex as opposed to the allocortex 同形皮质，新（脑）皮质

iso·cy·tol·y·sin (i″so-si-tol′ə-sin) an isoantigen that acts as a cytolysin 同种细胞溶素

iso·cy·to·sis (i″so-si-to′sis) equality of size of cells, especially of erythrocytes 细胞等大，尤指红细胞等大

iso·dac·tyl·ism (i-so-dak′təl-iz-əm) relatively even length of the fingers 指等长

iso·dose (i′so-dōs″) a radiation dose of equal intensity to more than one body area 同等（辐射）量

iso·elec·tric (i″so-e-lek′trik) showing no variation in electric potential 等电的，等电势的

iso·en·er·get·ic (i″so-en′ər-jet′ik) exhibiting equal energy 等能的

iso·en·zyme (i″so-en′zīm) 同 isozyme

iso·eth·a·rine (i″so-eth′ə-rēn) a β 2-adrenergic receptor agonist, administered by inhalation in the form of the hydrochloride or mesylate salt as a bronchodilator 乙基异丙肾上腺素

isog·a·my (i-sog′ə-me) reproduction resulting from union of two gametes identical in size and structure, as in protozoa 同配生殖; **isog′amous** *adj.*

iso·ge·ne·ic (i″so-jə-ne′ik) syngeneic 同基因的，同系的，同源的

iso·gen·e·sis (i″so-jen′ə-sis) similarity in the processes of development 同源，同式发育

iso·gen·ic (i″so-jen′ik) syngeneic 同基因的，同系的，同源的

isog·e·nous (i-soj′ə-nəs) developed from the same cell 同源的

iso·graft (i′so-graft″) syngraft 同基因移植物，同系移植物；同系移植，同型移植

iso·he·mag·glu·ti·nin (i″so-he″mə-gloo′tĭ-nin) an isoantigen that agglutinates erythrocytes 同种血细胞凝集素，同族血凝素

iso·he·mol·y·sin (i″so-he-mol′ə-sin) an isoantigen that causes hemolysis 同种溶血素，同族溶血素

iso·ico·nia (i″so-i-ko′ne-ə) 同 iseikonia; **isoicon′ic** *adj.*

iso·im·mu·ni·za·tion (i″so-im″u-nĭ-za′shən) development of antibodies in response to isoantigens 同种免疫，同族免疫

iso·ki·net·ic (i″so-kĭ-net′ik) maintaining constant torque or tension as muscles shorten or lengthen 等动力的；见 exercise 下 isokinetic exercise

iso·late (i′so-lāt) 1. to separate from others 分离；2. a group of individuals prevented by geographic, genetic, ecologic, social, or artificial barriers from interbreeding with others of their kind 隔离群

iso·la·tion (i″so-la′shən) 1. the process of isolating, or the state of being isolated 孤立；2. physical separation of a part, as by tissue culture or by interposition of inert material 隔绝，绝缘；3. the extraction and purification of a chemical substance of unknown structure from a natural source 化学物质提取纯化；4. the separation of infected individuals from those uninfected for the communicable period 隔离；5. the successive propagation of a growth of microorganisms until a pure culture is obtained（微生物）分离；6. a defense mechanism in which emotions are detached from the ideas, impulses, or memories to which they usually connect 隔离，一种心理防御性机制

iso·lec·i·thal (i″so-les′ĭ-thəl) having small amounts of yolk evenly distributed throughout the cytoplasm, as in the eggs of mammals 等（卵）黄的，均（卵）黄的

iso·leu·cine (Ile, I) (i″so-loo′sēn) an essential amino acid produced by hydrolysis of fibrin and other proteins; necessary for optimal infant growth and for nitrogen equilibrium in adults 异亮氨酸

isol·o·gous (i-sol′o-gəs) characterized by an identical genotype 同基因的，同系的

isol·y·sin (i-sol′ə-sin) a lysin acting on cells of animals of the same species as that from which it is derived 同种溶素，同族溶素

iso·mal·tase (i″so-mawl′tās) α-dextrinase 异麦芽糖酶

iso·mer (i′so-mər) any compound exhibiting, or capable of exhibiting, isomerism（同分）异构体；**isomer′ic** *adj.*

isom·er·ase (i-som′ər-ās) a major class of enzymes comprising those that catalyze the process of isomerization（同分）异构酶

isom·e·rism (i-som′ə-riz-əm) the possession by two or more distinct compounds of the same molecular formula, each molecule having the same number of atoms of each element but in a different arrangement（同分）异构（现象）；**constitutional i.**, structural i.; that in which the compounds have the same molecular but different structural formulas, the linkages of the atoms being different 结构异构；**geometric i.**, stereoisomerism in which isomers differ in the arrangement of substituents of a rigid structure, such as double-bonded carbon atoms or a ring 立体异构；**optical i.**, stereoisomerism in which isomers differ in the arrangement of substituents at one or more asymmetric carbon atoms; thus some, but not necessarily all, are optically active 旋光异构；**structural i.**, 同 constitutional i.

isom·er·iza·tion (i-som″ər-ĭ-za′shən) the process whereby any isomer is converted into another isomer, usually requiring special conditions of temperature, pressure, or catalysts（同分）异构化（作用）

iso·meth·ep·tene mu·cate (i″so-mə-thep′tēn mu′kāt) an indirect-acting sympathomimetic amine that constricts dilated carotid and cerebral vessels, used in combination with dichloralphena zone and acetaminophen in the treatment of migraine and ten-

sion headache 半乳糖二酸甲异辛烯胺

iso·met·ric (i″so-met′rik) maintaining, or pertaining to, the same measure of length; of equal dimensions 等长的；等尺寸的

iso·me·tro·pia (i″so-mə-tro′pe-ə) equality in refraction of the two eyes 两眼屈光相等

iso·ni·a·zid (i″so-ni′ə-zid) an antibacterial used as a tuberculostatic 异烟肼

iso·pho·ria (i″so-for′e-ə) equality in the tension of the vertical muscles of each eye 两眼视线等平

iso·plas·tic (i″so-plas′tik) syngeneic 同基因的，同系的

iso·pre·cip·i·tin (i″so-pre-sip′ĭ-tin) an isoantigen that acts as a precipitin 同种沉淀素

iso·prene (i′so-prēn) an unsaturated, branchedchain, 5-carbon hydrocarbon that is the molecular unit of the isoprenoid compounds 异戊二烯

iso·pre·noid (i″so-pre′noid) any compound biosynthesized from or containing isoprene units, including terpenes, carotenoids, fat-soluble vitamins, ubiquinone, rubber, and some steroids 类异戊烯

iso·pro·pa·nol (i″so-pro′pə-nol) isopropyl alcohol 异丙醇

iso·pro·te·re·nol (i″so-pro-ter′ə-nol) a sympathomimetic used in the form of the hydrochloride and sulfate salts as a bronchodilator, and in the form of the hydrochloride salt as a cardiac stimulant 异丙肾上腺素

isop·ter (i-sop′tər) a curve representing areas of equal visual acuity in the field of vision 等视力线

iso·sen·si·ti·za·tion (i″so-sen″sĭ-tĭ-za′shən) allosensitization 同族致敏作用

iso·sex·u·al (i″so-sek′shoo-əl) pertaining to or characteristic of the same sex 同性的

isos·mot·ic (i″soz-mot′ik) having the same osmotic pressure 等渗的

iso·sor·bide (i″so-sor′bīd) an osmotic diuretic used to reduce intraocular pressure; its dinitrate and mononitrate esters are used as coronary vasodilators to treat coronary insufficiency and angina pectoris 异山梨醇

Isos·po·ra (i-sos′pə-rə) a genus of sporozoan parasites. Species that infect mammals, formerly classified here, are now classified in *Cystoisospora* 等孢子球虫属

iso·spore (i′so-spor) 1. an isogamete of organisms that reproduce by spores 同形孢子；2. an asexual spore produced by a homosporous organism 同形孢子产生的无性孢子

isos·then·uria (i″sos-thə-nu′re-ə) excretion of urine that has not been concentrated by the kidneys and has the same osmolality as that of plasma 等渗尿，等张尿

iso·tone (i′so-tōn″) one of several nuclides having the same number of neutrons, but differing in number of protons in their nuclei 同中子（异位）素

iso·to·nia protons in their nuclei. iso·to·nia (i″-so-to′ne-ə) 1. a condition of equal tone, tension, or activity 等张性; 2. equality of osmotic pressure between two elements of a solution or between two different solutions 等渗性

iso·ton·ic (i″so-ton′ik) 1. denoting a solution in which body cells can be bathed without net flow of water across the semipermeable cell membrane 等压的; 2. denoting a solution having the same tonicity as another solution with which it is compared 等渗的; 3. maintaining uniform tonus 等张的

iso·tope (i′so-tōp″) a chemical element having the same atomic number as another (i.e., the same number of nuclear protons) but having a different atomic mass (i.e., a different number of nuclear neutrons) 同位素

iso·trans·plan·ta·tion (i″so-trans″plan-ta′-shən) syngeneic transplantation 同系移植，同基因移植术

iso·tret·i·noin (i″so-tret′ĭ-no-in) (-noin) a synthetic form of retinoic acid, used orally to clear cystic and conglobate acne 异维甲酸

iso·tro·pic (i″so-tro′pik) 1. having the same value of a property, e.g., refractive index, in all directions 各向同性的; 2. being singly refractive 单折射的，单折光的

iso·va·ler·ic ac·id (i″so-və-ler′ik) a carboxylic acid occurring in excess in the plasma and urine in isovalericacidemia 异戊酸

iso·va·ler·ic ac·i·de·mia (i″so-və-ler″ik-as″ĭ-de′me-ə) an aminoacidopathy due to a defect in the pathway of leucine catabolism, characterized by elevated levels of isovaleric acid in the plasma and urine, causing a characteristic odor of sweaty feet, severe acidosis and ketosis, lethargy, convulsions, pernicious vomiting, and psychomotor retardation; in severe cases, coma and death may occur 异戊酸血（症）

iso·vo·lu·mic (i″so-və-loo′mik) maintaining the same volume 等容的

isox·su·prine (i-sok′su-prēn) an adrenergic used as a vasodilator in the form of the hydrochloride salt 异克舒令，苯氧丙酚胺

iso·zyme (i′so-zīm) one of the multiple forms in which an enzyme may exist in an organism or in different species, the various forms differing chemically, physically, or immunologically, but catalyzing the same reaction 同工酶

is·rad·i·pine (is-rad′ĭ-pēn) a calcium channel blocking agent used alone or with a thiazide diuretic for the treatment of hypertension 依拉地平

ISRT involved site radiation therapy 受累部位放疗

is·sue (ish′oo) a discharge of pus, blood, or other matter; a suppurating lesion emitting such a discharge 流出，流出物; 脓疮口

isth·mec·to·my (is-mek′tə-me) excision of an isthmus, especially the isthmus of the thyroid 峡部切除术，尤指甲状腺峡部切除术

isth·mo·pa·ral·y·sis (is″mo-pə-ral′ə-sis) 同 isthmoplegia

isth·mo·ple·gia (is″mo-ple′jə) paralysis of the isthmus of the fauces 咽峡麻痹，咽峡瘫痪

isth·mus (is′məs) pl. isth′mi. a narrow connection between two larger bodies or parts 峡; **isth′mian, isth′mic** adj.; **i. of auditory tube, i. of eustachian tube,** the narrowest part of the auditory tube at the junction of its bony and cartilaginous parts 咽鼓管峡; **i. of fauces, oropharyngeal i.,** the constricted aperture between the cavity of the mouth and the pharynx 咽峡; **i. of hindbrain,** the narrow segment of the fetal brain, forming the plane of separation between the hindbrain and cerebrum 后脑峡部; **i. of thyroid gland,** the band of tissue joining the lobes of the thyroid gland 甲状腺峡; **i. of uterine tube,** the narrower, thicker-walled portion of the uterine tube closest to the uterus 输卵管峡; **i. of uterus,** the constricted part of the uterus between the cervix and the body of the uterus 子宫峡

itch (ich) a skin disorder marked by itching 痒; **barber's i.,** 1. tinea barbae 触染性须疮; 2. sycosis barbae 寻常须疮; **grain i.,** itching dermatitis due to a mite, *Pyemotes ventricosus,* that preys on insect larvae living on straw, grain, and other plants 谷痒症; **ground i.,** the itching eruption caused by the entrance into the skin of the larvae of *Ancylostoma duodenale* or *Necator americanus* in hookworm disease 钩虫痒病; **jock i.,** tinea cruris 股癣; **seven-year i.,** popular name for *scabies* 疥疮, 疥螨病; **swimmer's i.,** cercarial dermatitis 游泳者痒诊，尾蚴性皮炎; **winter i.,** asteatotic eczema 冬令瘙痒

itch·ing (ich′ing) pruritus; an unpleasant cutaneous sensation, provoking the desire to scratch or rub the skin 痒，瘙痒

iter (i′tər) a tubular passage 导管，通路; **i′teral** adj.

it·ra·co·na·zole (it″rə-kon′ə-zōl) a triazole antifungal used in a variety of infections 依曲康唑

IU international unit (on The Joint Commission "Do Not Use" List) 国际单位

IUD intrauterine device 宫内节育器

IUGR intrauterine growth retardation (or restriction) 宫内发育迟缓

IV   intravenous 静脉内（静脉注射）

iva·caf·tor (i″və-kaf′tor) a potentiator of the cystic fibrosis transmembrane regulator (CFTR), used in the treatment of cystic fibrosis associated with impaired ability to transport chloride through the CFTR ion channel 依伐卡托

IVECSS   International Veterinary Emergency and Critical Care Society 国际兽医急救与重症监护学会

IVF   in vitro fertilization 体外受精

Ix·o·des (ik-so′dēz) a common genus of parasitic ticks (family Ixodidae); some species are vectors for diseases such as Lyme disease and tick-borne encephalitis 硬蜱属

ix·o·di·a·sis (ik″so-di′ə-sis) infestation with ixodid ticks, or a disease or lesion caused by their bites 蜱病

ix·o·did (ik′so-did) a tick, or pertaining to a tick, of the genus *Ixodes* 硬蜱（的）

Ix·od·i·dae (ik-sod′ĭ-de) a family of ticks (superfamily Ixodoidea), comprising the hard-bodied ticks 硬蜱科

Ix·od·i·des (ik-sod′ĭ-dēz) the ticks, a suborder of Acarina, including the superfamily Ixodoidea 蜱亚目

Ix·o·doi·dea (ik″so-doi′de-ə) a superfamily of arthropods (suborder Ixodides), comprising both the hard- and soft-bodied ticks 蜱总科

J

J   joule 焦耳的符号

jack·et (jak′ət) an enveloping structure or garment for the trunk or upper part of the body 背心，背夹；**plaster-of-Paris j.**, a casing of plaster of Paris enveloping the body, to support or correct deformities 石膏背心；**strait j.**, straitjacket 约束衣

jack·screw (jak′skroo″) a screw-turned device to expand the dental arch and move individual teeth 螺旋正牙器

jac·ti·ta·tion (jak″tĭ-ta′shən) restless tossing to and fro in acute illness（急性病期间）辗转不安

Ja·ka·fi (juh-kah′fi) trademark for a preparation of ruxolitinib 鲁索替尼（ruxolitinib）的商标名

jaun·dice (jawn′dis) icterus; yellowness of the skin, scleras, mucous membranes, and excretions due to hyperbilirubinemia and deposition of bile pigments 黄疸；**acholuric j.**, jaundice without bilirubinemia, associated with elevated unconjugated bilirubin that is not excreted by the kidney 无胆色素尿性黄疸；**breastfeeding j.**, jaundice occurring in breastfed infants within the first week of life, most commonly caused by inadequate intake 母乳喂养性黄疸；**breast milk j.**, jaundice occurring in breastfed infants after the first 3 to 5 days of life, with serum bilirubin generally peaking at approximately 2 weeks and falling gradually over the next several months 母乳性黄疸；**cholestatic j.**, that resulting from abnormal bile flow in the liver 胆汁淤积性黄疸；**hemolytic j.**, that due to increased production of bilirubin from hemoglobin under conditions causing accelerated degradation of erythrocytes 溶血性黄疸；**hepatocellular j.**, that due to injury to or disease of liver cells 肝细胞性黄疸；**hepa-**

togenic j., **hepatogenous j.**, that due to disease or disorder of the liver 肝源性黄疸；**leptospiral j.**, Weil syndrome 钩端螺旋体性黄疸；**mechanical j.**, 同 obstructive j.；**neonatal j.**, **j. of the newborn**, icterus neonatorum 新生儿黄疸；**nuclear j.**, kernicterus 核黄疸；**obstructive j.**, that due to blocking of bile flow 阻塞性黄疸，梗阻性黄疸；**physiologic j.**, mild icterus neonatorum lasting the first few days of life 生理性黄疸；**retention j.**, that due to inability of the liver to dispose of the bilirubin provided by the circulating blood 潴留性黄疸

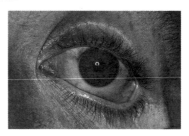

▲ 黄疸

jaw (jaw) either of the two bony tooth-bearing structures of the head, the mandible or the maxilla 颌，颌骨；**cleft j.**, a cleft between the median nasal and maxillary prominences through the alveolus 颌裂；**Hapsburg j.**, a mandibular prognathous jaw, often accompanied by Hapsburg lip 哈普斯堡型突颌；**phossy j.**, phosphorus necrosis 磷毒性颌骨坏死

JCAHO (ja′ko) Joint Commission on Accreditation of Healthcare Organizations. Now known as the Joint Commission 医疗机构评审联合委员会

je·ju·nal (jə-joo′nəl) pertaining to the jejunum 空肠的

je·ju·nec·to·my (jĕ″joo-nek′tə-me) excision of the jejunum 空肠切除术

je·ju·no·ce·cos·to·my (jə-joo″no-se-kos′tə-me) anastomosis of the jejunum to the cecum 空肠盲肠吻合术

je·ju·no·il·e·itis (jə-joo″no-il″e-i′tis) inflammation of the jejunum and ileum 空肠回肠炎

je·ju·no·je·ju·nos·to·my (jə-joo″no-jĕ″joo-nos′tə-me) anastomosis between two portions of the jejunum 空肠间吻合术

je·ju·nos·to·my (jĕ″joo-nos′tə-me) the creation of a permanent opening between the jejunum and the surface of the abdominal wall 空肠造口术

je·ju·not·o·my (jĕ″joo-not′ə-me) incision of the jejunum 空肠切开术

je·ju·num (jə-joo′nəm) that part of the small intestine extending from the duodenum to the ileum 空肠

jel·ly (jel′e) a soft substance that is coherent, tremulous, and more or less translucent; generally, a colloidal semisolid mass 凝胶，胶冻；胶状物。**cardiac j.**, a gelatinous substance present between the endothelium and myocardium of the embryonic heart, which transforms into the connective tissue of the endocardium 心胶质（胚胎）；**contraceptive j.**, a nongreasy jelly used in the vagina for prevention of conception 避孕胶冻；**petroleum j.**, petrolatum 石油凝胶，凡士林；**Wharton j.**, the intracellular mucoid connective tissue of the umbilical cord 脐带胶质

jerk (jurk) a sudden reflex or involuntary movement 急拉，急推；急跳；反射；**jer′ky** *adj.*；**Achilles j.**, **ankle j.**, triceps surae reflex 跟腱反射；**biceps j.**, 二头肌反射，见 *reflex* 下词条；**elbow j.**, triceps reflex 肘反射，肱三头肌反射；**jaw j.**, 下颌反射，见 *reflex* 下词条；**knee j.**, quadriceps j., patellar reflex 膝反射；**tendon j.**, 腱反射，见 *reflex* 下词条；**triceps surae j.**, 小腿三头肌反射，见 *reflex* 下词条

Jet·rea (jĕt′ree) trademark for a preparation of ocriplasmin 奥克纤溶酶（ocriplasmin）的商品名

JIA juvenile idiopathic arthritis 幼年特发性关节炎

JIF·SAN Joint Institute for Food Safety and Applied Nutrition 食品安全和应用营养联合研究所

jim·son weed (jim′sən wēd) stramonium 曼陀罗

jing (jing) [Chinese] one of the basic substances that according to traditional Chinese medicine pervade the body, usually translated as "essence"; the body reserves or constitutional makeup, replenished by food and rest, that supports life and is associated with developmental changes in the organism （中医）精，精华（人体生命的本原，构成人体和维持人体生命活动和生长发育的最基本物质）

joint (joynt) the place of junction or union between bones, especially one that allows motion of one or more of the bones 接合，接缝；关节。**amphidiarthrodial j.**, amphidiarthrosis 屈戌动关节；**ankle j.**, the joint formed between the tibia, fibula, and talus 踝关节；**arthrodial j.**, plane j 摩动关节；**ball-and-socket j.**, spheroidal j.; a synovial joint in which a round surface on one bone ("ball") moves within a concavity ("socket") on the other bone 球窝关节，杵臼关节；**biaxial j.**, one with two chief axes of movement, at right angles to each other 双轴关节；**bicondylar j.**, an ellipsoid joint with a meniscus between the articular surfaces 双髁状关节；**bilocular j.**, one with two synovial compartments separated by an interarticular cartilage 双腔关节；**bony j's**, the places of junction between two or more bones of the skeleton, which may be fibrous, cartilaginous, or synovial 骨关节；**carpal j's**, intercarpal j's; the joints between the carpal bones 腕关节；**cartilaginous j.**, a joint in which the bones are united by cartilage, subdivided into synchondroses and symphyses 软骨性关节；**Charcot j.**, neuropathic arthropathy 神经源性关节病；**cochlear j.**, a hinge joint that permits some lateral motion 蜗状关节；**complex j.**, **composite j.**, **compound j.**, one in which more than two bones articulate 复合关节；**condylar j.**, **condyloid j.**, ellipsoid j.; one in which an ovoid head of one bone moves in an elliptical cavity of another, permitting movements except axial rotation 髁状关节；**diarthrodial j.**, 同synovial j.；**elbow j.**, the joint between the humerus, ulna, and radius 肘关节；**ellipsoid j.**, condylar j. 椭圆关节，髁状关节；**facet j's**, the joints between the articular processes of the vertebrae 脊柱关节；**false j.**, pseudarthrosis 假关节；**fibrocartilaginous j.**, symphysis 纤维软骨联合；**fibrous j.**, a type of joint in which the bones are united by continuous intervening fibrous tissue; the group includes sutures, gomphoses, and syndesmoses 纤维连接；**flail j.**, an unusually mobile joint 连枷状关节；**ginglymoid j.**, ginglymus 屈戌关节；**glenohumeral j.**, shoulder j.; the joint formed by the head of the humerus and the glenoid fossa of the scapula 肩关节；**gliding j.**, plane j. 摩动关节；**hinge j.**, ginglymus 屈戌关节；**hip j.**, the ball and socket joint between the head of the femur and the acetabulum of the coxal bone 髋

关节；**immovable j.**, synarthrosis 不动关节；**intercarpal j's**, 同 carpal j's；**intertarsal j's**, tarsal j's 跗骨间关节；**knee j.**, the compound joint between the femur, patella, and tibia 膝关节；**Lisfranc j's**, the joints between the tarsal and metatarsal bones 跗跖关节；**multiaxial j.**, ball-and-socket j. 多轴关节；**neurocentral j.**, a synchondrosis between the body of a vertebra and either half of the vertebral arch 椎体弓连接；**peg-and-socket j.**, gomphosis 钉状关节，嵌合；**pivot j.**, a uniaxial joint in which one bone pivots within a bony or an osseoligamentous ring 车轴关节；**plane j.**, a synovial joint in which the opposed surfaces are flat or only slightly curved 平面关节；**polyaxial j.**, ball-and-socket j. 多轴关节，杵臼关节；**rotary j.**, pivot j. 车轴关节，旋转关节；**saddle j., sellar j.**, one having two saddle-shaped surfaces at right angles to each other 鞍状关节；**shoulder j.**, 同 glenohumeral j.；**simple j.**, one in which only two bones articulate 单关节；**spheroidal j.**, 同 ball-andsocket j.；**spiral j.**, 同 cochlear j.；**synarthrodial j.**, synarthrosis 不动关节；**synovial j.**, diarthrosis; a joint that permits more or less free motion, the union of the bony elements being surrounded by an articular capsule enclosing a cavity lined by synovial membrane 滑膜关节，动关节；**talocrural j.**, ankle j 踝关节，距小腿关节；**tarsal j's**, intertarsal j's; the joints between the various tarsal bones 跗关节；**temporomandibular j.**, a bicondylar joint formed by the head of the mandible and the mandibular fossa and the articular tubercle of the temporal bone 颞下颌关节；**transverse tarsal j.**, a compound joint running across the middle of the foot, comprising a joint connecting the calcaneus and the cuboid bone and one connecting the talus, calcaneus, and navicular bone 跗横关节；**uniaxial j.**, one that permits movement in one axis only 单轴关节；**unilocular j.**, a synovial joint having only one cavity 单腔关节；**zygapophyseal j's**, facet j's 关节突关节，髁状关节（腕部）

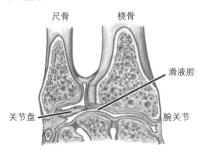

尺骨　　桡骨

滑液腔

关节盘　　腕关节

▲　髁状关节（腕部）

Joint Com·mis·sion　(joynt com′ishən) an independent, not-for-profit organization that accredits and certifies health care organizations; formerly known as Joint Commission on Accreditation of Healthcare Organizations (JCAHO) 联合委员会，曾称为国际医疗卫生机构认证联合委员会

joule　(**J**) (jōol) the SI unit of energy, being the work done by a force of 1 newton acting over a distance of 1 meter 焦耳

ju·gal　(joo′gəl) pertaining to the cheek 轭的，颧骨的

ju·ga·le　(joo-ga′le) jugal point 颧点

jug·u·lar　(jug′u-lər) 1. cervical 颈的；2. pertaining to a jugular vein 颈静脉的；3. a jugular vein 颈静脉

ju·gum　(joo′gəm) pl. *ju′ga* [L.] yoke; a depression or ridge connecting two structures 轭，隆凸

juice　(jōos) any fluid from animal or plant tissue 汁液；**gastric j.**, the secretion of the gastric glands 胃液；**intestinal j.**, the secretion of the intestinal glands 肠液；**pancreatic j.**, the enzyme-containing secretion of the pancreas, conducted through its ducts to the duodenum 胰液

jump·ing　(jump′ing) 1. the skipping of several steps in a series 跳跃的；2. 跳跃病，见 *disease* 下词条

junc·tio　(junk′she-o) pl. *junctio′nes* [L.] 同 junction

junc·tion　(junk′shən) the place of meeting or coming together 接点；接（合）处；**junc′tional** *adj.*；**adherens j.**, a type of adhesive junction that links cell membranes and cytoskeletal elements within and between cells by homophilic interactions between cadherins 黏着连接；**adhesive j.**, a type of intercellular junction that links cell membranes and cytoskeletal elements within and between cells, connecting adjacent cells mechanically 黏附连接；**amelodentinal j.**, 同 dentinoenamel j.；**atrioventricu lar j., AV j.**, part or all of the region comprising the atrioventricular node and the bundle of His, with the bundle branches sometimes specifically excluded 房室交界；**cementoenamel j.**, the line at which the cement covering the root of a tooth and the enamel covering its crown meet, designated anatomically as the cervical line 牙骨质釉质界；**dentinocemental j.**, the line of meeting of the dentin and cement on the root of a tooth（牙根）牙（本）质牙骨质界；**dentinoenamel j.**, the plane of meeting between dentin and enamel on the crown of a tooth（牙冠）牙本质釉质界；**dermal-epidermal j., dermoepidermal j.**, the plane of meeting between the dermis and epidermis 真皮表皮交界部；**esophagogastric j.**, the site of transition from the stratified squamous epithelium of the esophagus to the simple

columnar epithelium of the cardia of the stomach
食管胃交界处；**gap j.**, a narrowed portion of the
intercellular space containing channels linking adjacent cells and through which pass ions, most sugars,
amino acids, nucleotides, vitamins, hormones, and
cyclic AMP. In electrically excitable tissues, these
gap junctions transmit electrical impulses via ionic
currents and are known as *electrotonic synapses*
缝 隙 连 接；**gastroesophageal j.**, esophagogastric
j. 胃食管连接部；**ileocecal j.**, the junction of the
ileum and cecum, located at the lower right side of
the abdomen and fixed to the posterior abdominal
wall 回盲肠连接；**intercellular j's**, specialized
regions on the borders of cells that provide connections between adjacent cells 胞间连接；**mucocutaneous j.**, the site of transition between skin and
mucous membrane 黏膜皮肤连接；**mucogingival
j.**, the histologically distinct line marking the separation of the gingival tissue from the oral mucosa 黏
膜龈界；**myoneural j., neuromuscular j.**, the site
of apposition between a nerve fiber and the motor
end plate of the skeletal muscle that it innervates 肌
神经接点；**occluding j.**, 同 tight j.；**sclerocorneal
j.**, corneal limbus 角膜巩膜缘；**tight j.**, an intercellular junction at which adjacent plasma membranes
are joined tightly together by interlinked rows of
integral membrane proteins, limiting or eliminating
the intercellular passage of molecules 紧密连接；
ureteropelvic j., the junction between the ureter and
the renal pelvis 输尿管肾盂连接

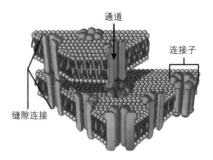

▲　相邻细胞内部之间提供通道的缝隙连接

junc·tu·ra　(junk-too′rə) pl. *junctu′rae* [L.] 同 joint

jur·is·pru·dence　(joor″is-proo′dəns) the science
of the law 法理学；**medical j.**, the science of the
law as applied to the practice of medicine 法医学

ju·ve·nile　(joo′və-nīl) 1. pertaining to youth or childhood 青年的；2. a youth or child; a young animal
青少年；3. a cell or organism intermediate between
immature and mature forms 介于发育未全和成熟
之间的细胞或有机体

jux·ta·ar·tic·u·lar　(juks″tə-ahr-tik′u-lər) situated
near or in the region of a joint 关节旁的，近关节的

jux·ta·glo·mer·u·lar　(juks″tə-glo-mer′u-lər) near
or next to a renal glomerulus 近肾小球的

Jux·ta·pid　(jux-tə′pid) trademark for a preparation
of lomitapide mesylate 甲磺酸洛美他派的商品名

jux·ta·po·si·tion　(juks″tə-pə-zish′ən) apposition
并置，并列，对合

K

K　[L. *ka′lium*] [符号] kelvin 开（开尔文温度标
的计量单位）；kerf 切口；lysine 赖氨酸；potas-
sium 钾

K_m　K_m Michaelis constant 米氏常数的符号

k kilo- 千的符号

κ　(kappa, the tenth letter of the Greek alphabet)
one of the two types of immunoglobulin light chains
（kappa, 希腊字母表的第 10 个字母）两种免疫
球蛋白轻链中的一个符号

ka·la·azar　(kah′lah-ah-zahr′) [Hindi] visceral
leishmaniasis 黑热病，内脏利什曼病

ka·li·ure·sis　(ka″le-u-re′sis) the excretion of potassium
in the urine 尿钾（排出）增多；**kaliuret′ic** *adj.*

kal·li·din　(kal′ĭ-din) lysyl-bradykinin, a decapeptide kinin produced by the action of tissue and
glandular kallikreins on LMW kininogen and having
physiologic effects similar to those of bradykinin 赖
氨酰缓激肽

kal·li·kre·in　(kal″ĭ-kre′in) any of several serine
proteinases that cleave kininogens to form kinins
血管舒缓素，激肽释放酶；**plasma k.**, a plasma
hydrolase that cleaves HMW kininogen to produce
bradykinin and also activates blood coagulation
factors Ⅻ and Ⅶ and plasminogen 血浆激肽释放
酶；**tissue k.**, a hydrolase of tissues and various
glandular secretions that cleaves LMW kininogen to
form kallidin 组织激肽释放酶

kal·li·kre·in·o·gen　(kal″ĭ-kre-in′ə-jən) prekallikrein 激肽释放酶原，血管舒缓素原

kam·po　(kahm′po) [Japanese] herbal medicine as
practiced in Japan, having its origin in traditional
Chinese medicine 汉方草药；Spelled also *kanpo*

kan·a·my·cin　(kan″ə-mi′sin) an aminoglycoside
antibiotic derived from *Streptomyces kanamyceticus,*
effective against aerobic gram-negative bacilli and
some gram-positive bacteria, including mycobacteria; used as the sulfate salt 卡那霉素

ka·o·lin　(ka′o-lin) native hydrated aluminum silicate, powdered and freed from gritty particles by elutriation; used as an adsorbent and, often with pectin, as an antidiarrheal 白陶土，高岭土

ka·o·lin·o·sis (ka″o-lin-o′sis) pneumoconiosis from inhaling particles of kaolin 肺白陶土沉着病

ka·pha (kah′fah) [Sanskrit] in ayurveda, one of the three doshas, condensed from the elements water and earth. It is the principle of stabilizing energy, governs growth in the body and mind, is concerned with structure, stability, lubrication, and fluid balance, and is eliminated from the body through the urine（梵语）kapha（在阿育吠陀中，由水和土两种元素浓缩而成，稳定能量，控制身体和精神的生长）

kar·ma (kahr′mə) [Sanskrit] in Indian philosophy, the total effect of a person's actions, both mental and physical, on his or her existence; a person's present state, including health, is determined by actions from a previous existence, and present actions determine their destiny for future existence（梵语）因果报应，因缘

kary·og·a·my (kar″e-og′ə-me) cell conjugation with union of nuclei 核配合，核融合

karyo·gram (kar′e-o-gram″) an image of a systematized array of a chromosome complement, with the expanded implication that the chromosomes of a single cell can typify an individual or even a species 核型（模式）图，染色体组型图；另见 *karyotype*

karyo·ki·ne·sis (kar″e-o-kī′ne′sis) division of the cell nucleus 核分裂；**karyokinet′ic** *adj.*

kary·ol·y·sis (kar″e-ol′ə-sis) 核溶解 1. the swelling of the nucleus of a necrotic cell and fading of the chromatin as it becomes less basophilic; 2. dissolution of the cell nucleus 细胞核溶解；cf. *karyorrhexis*；**karyolyt′ic** *adj.*

karyo·mor·phism (kar″e-o-mor′fiz-əm) the shape of a cell nucleus 核形

karyo·phage (kar′e-o-fāj″) a protozoan that phagocytizes the nucleus of the cell it infects 噬核细胞；噬核体

karyo·pyk·no·sis (kar″e-o-pik-no′sis) shrinkage of a cell nucleus, with condensation of the chromatin 核固缩；**karyopyknot′ic** *adj.*

kary·or·rhex·is (kar″e-o-rek′sis) fragmentation of a cell nucleus into formless granules; it is followed by dissolution *(karyolysis)* 核碎裂；**karyorrhec′tic** *adj.*

karyo·type (kar′e-o-tīp) formally, the symbolic (e.g., numbers, letters) representation of the chromosome set of an individual, tissue, or cell line. In practice, it is often used interchangeably with idiogram and karyogram 染色体组型，核型；**karyotyp′ic** *adj.*

kat katal 开特的符号

kat·al (kat) (kat′əl) a unit of measurement proposed to express activities of all catalysts, being that amount of a catalyst that catalyzes a reaction rate of 1 mole of substrate per second 开 特（表示酶活力的单位，指在特定条件下，每秒转化 1 mol 底物所需要的酶量）

ka·va **ka·va** (kah′və kah′və) a preparation of the rhizome of *Piper methysticum* (kava plant), having muscle-relaxing, anticonvulsive, anxiolytic, and sedative effects; used for the relief of stress and restlessness, and for sleep induction; also used in homeopathy and folk medicine 卡法根

kcal kilocalorie 千卡，大卡

kD, kDa kilodalton; 1000 daltons 千道尔顿

ke·loid (ke′loid) a sharply elevated, irregularly shaped, progressively enlarging scar due to excessive collagen formation in the dermis during connective tissue repair 瘢痕疙瘩；**keloid′al** *adj.*

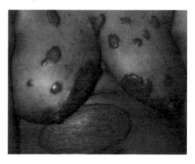

▲ 瘢痕疙瘩

kel·vin **(K)** (kel′vin) the base SI unit of temperature, equal to 1/273.16 of the absolute temperature of the triple point of water 开（开尔文温标的计量单位）

ker·a·tan **sul·fate** (ker′ə-tan) either of two glycosaminoglycans（Ⅰ and Ⅱ）, consisting of repeating disaccharide units of N-acetylglucosamine and galactose, but differing slightly in carbohydrate content and localization. It occurs in cartilage, the cornea, and the nucleus pulposus and is also an accumulation product in Morquio syndrome 硫酸角质素

ker·a·tec·ta·sia (ker″ə-tek-ta′zhə) protrusion of a thinned, scarred cornea 角膜扩张，角膜突出

ker·a·tec·to·my (ker″ə-tek′tə-me) excision of a portion of the cornea; kerectomy 角膜切除术；**photorefractive k.**, the correction of ametropia by using an excimer laser to remove a portion of the anterior corneal stroma in order to create a new radius of curvature 屈光性角膜切除术

ke·rat·ic (kə-rat′ik) 1. keratinous 角蛋白的；2. corneal 角膜的

ker·a·tin (ker′ə-tin) any of a family of scleroproteins that are the main constituents of epidermis, hair, nails, and horny tissues. The high-sulfur keratin polypeptides of ectodermally derived structures, e.g., hair and nails, are also called *hard k's* 角蛋白

ker·a·tin·ase (ker′ə-tĭ-nās) any of a group of proteolytic enzymes that catalyze the cleavage of keratin 角蛋白酶

ker·a·tin·i·za·tion (ker″ə-tin″ĭ-za′shən) conversion into keratin 角蛋白化

ke·rat·i·no·cyte (kə-rat′ĭ-no-sīt) the epidermal cell that synthesizes keratin, known in its successive stages in the layers of the skin as basal cell, prickle cell, and granular cell 角质化细胞

ke·rat·i·no·some (kə-rat′ĭ-no-sōm″) lamellar body 角质白小体

ke·rat·in·ous (kə-rat′ĭ-nəs) pertaining to or containing keratin 角质的；角蛋白的

ker·a·ti·tis (ker″ə-ti′tis) inflammation of the cornea 角膜炎；k. bullo′sa, presence of blebs upon the cornea 大疱性角膜炎；dendriform k., dendritic k., herpetic keratitis that results in a branching ulceration of the cornea 树枝状角膜炎；herpetic k., 1. that, commonly with dendritic ulceration *(dendriform* or *dendritic k.),* due to infection with herpes simplex virus（单纯疱疹病毒）疱疹性角膜炎；2. that occurring in herpes zoster ophthalmicus（带状疱疹病毒）疱疹性角膜炎；interstitial k., chronic keratitis with deep deposits in the cornea, which becomes hazy 间质性角膜炎，深层角膜炎；lattice k., bilateral hereditary corneal dystrophy with formation of interwoven filamentous lesions 格状角膜炎；microbial k., that resulting from bacterial or fungal infection of the cornea, usually associated with soft contact lens wear 细菌性角膜炎；neuroparalytic k., keratitis due to injury to the trifacial nerve that prevents closing of the eyelids, marked by dryness and fissuring of the corneal epithelium 神经麻痹性角膜炎；phlyctenular k., 泡性角膜炎，见 *keratoconjunctivitis* 下词条；sclerosing k., keratitis with scleritis 硬化性角膜炎；trachomatous k., pannus trachomatosus 沙眼性角膜炎；ulcerative k., keratitis with ulceration of the corneal epithelium, frequently a result of bacterial invasion of the cornea 溃疡性角膜炎

ker·a·to·ac·an·tho·ma (ker″ə-to-ak″an-tho′mə) a benign, locally destructive, epithelial tumor closely resembling squamous cell carcinoma but usually resolving spontaneously; lesions have craters, each filled with a keratin plug 角膜棘皮瘤

ker·a·to·cele (ker′ə-to-sēl″) hernial protrusion of the Descemet membrane 角膜后层膨出

ker·a·to·cen·te·sis (ker″ə-to-sen-te′sis) puncture of the cornea 角膜穿刺术

ker·a·to·con·junc·ti·vi·tis (ker″ə-to-kənjunk″tĭ-vi′tis) inflammation of the cornea and conjunctiva 角膜结膜炎；epidemic k., a highly infectious form, commonly with regional lymph node involvement, occurring in epidemics; an adenovirus has been repeatedly isolated from affected patients 流行性角膜结膜炎；phlyctenular k., a form marked by formation of a small, gray, circumscribed lesion at the corneal limbus 小泡性角膜结膜炎；k. sic′ca, a condition marked by hyperemia of the conjunctiva, thickening and drying of the corneal epithelium, itching and burning of the eye and, often, reduced visual acuity 角结膜干燥症，干眼症；viral k., epidemic k. 病毒性角膜结膜炎

ker·a·to·co·nus (ker″ə-to-ko′nəs) conical protrusion of the central part of the cornea 圆锥形角膜

ker·a·to·cyst (ker′ə-to-sist) an odontogenic cyst lined with a layer of keratinized squamous epithelium and commonly associated with a primordial cyst 角膜囊肿

ker·a·to·der·ma (ker″ə-to-dur′mə) 1. hypertrophy of the stratum corneum of the skin 皮肤角化病；2. a horny skin or covering 皮肤角质层；k. climacte′ricum, an acquired form of palmoplantar keratoderma seen in perimenopausal women 经绝期角化症；diffuse palmoplantar k., any of several hereditary types of palmoplantar keratoderma having well-demarcated, usually symmetric areas of scaling on the palms and soles; most types also have epidermolysis 弥漫性掌跖角化病；k. palma′re et planta′re, palmoplantar k., thickening of the skin of the palms and soles, sometimes with painful fissuring, often associated with other anomalies; most types are hereditary, but there are also acquired forms, e.g., with drug reactions, malignant conditions 掌跖角化病；punctate k., k. puncta′tum, an autosomal dominant form of palmoplantar keratoderma in which lesions are in multiple points on the palms and soles 点状皮肤角化病

ker·a·tog·e·nous (ker″ə-toj′ə-nəs) giving rise to a growth of horny material 角质增生的

ker·a·to·glo·bus (ker″ə-to-glo′bəs) a bilateral anomaly in which the cornea is enlarged and globular in shape 球形角膜

ker·a·to·hy·a·lin (ker″ə-to-hi′ə-lin) a substance in the granules in the stratum granulosum of the epidermis, possibly involved in keratinization, and also in Hassall corpuscles in the thymus 角质透明蛋白

ker·a·to·hy·a·line (ker″ə-to-hi′ə-līn) 1. both horny and hyaline 角质透明的；2. pertaining to keratohyalin or to the keratohyalin granules or the stratum granulosum of the epidermis 角质透明蛋白的；3. 同 keratohyalin

K

ker·a·to·i·ri·tis (ker″ə-to-i-ri′tis) inflammation of the cornea and iris 角膜虹膜炎

ker·a·to·lep·tyn·sis (ker″ə-to-lep-tin′sis) removal of the anterior portion of the cornea and replacement with bulbar conjunctiva 结膜遮盖角膜术

ker·a·to·leu·ko·ma (ker″ə-to-loo-ko′mə) a white opacity of the cornea 角膜白斑

ker·a·tol·y·sis (ker″ə-tol′ə-sis) softening and separation of the stratum corneum of the epidermis 角质层分离; **pitted k., k. planta′re sulca′tum,** a tropical disease marked by thickening and deep fissuring of the skin of the soles, occurring during the rainy season 跖沟状角化病

ker·a·to·lyt·ic (ker″ə-to-lit′ik) pertaining to, characterized by, or producing keratolysis, or an agent that so acts 角质层分离的

ker·a·to·ma (ker″ə-to′mə) pl. *keratomas, kerato·mata.* A callus or callosity 角化瘤

ker·a·to·ma·la·cia (ker″ə-to-mə-la′shə) softening and necrosis of the cornea associated with vitamin A deficiency 角膜软化

ker·a·tome (ker′ə-tōm) a knife for incising the cornea 角膜刀

ker·a·tom·e·try (ker″ə-tom′ə-tre) measurement of corneal curves 角膜曲率测量（法）; **keratomet′ric** *adj.*

ker·a·to·mi·leu·sis (ker″ə-to-mī-loo′sis) keratoplasty in which a slice of the patient's cornea is removed, shaped to the desired curvature, and then sutured back on the remaining cornea to correct optical error 角膜磨削术; **laser-assisted in-situ k. (LASIK),** keratoplasty in which the excimer laser and microkeratome are combined for vision correction; the microkeratome is used to shave a thin slice and create a hinged flap in the cornea, the exposed cornea is reshaped by the laser, and the flap is replaced, without sutures, to heal back into position 准分子激光原位角膜磨镶术

ker·a·to·my·co·sis (ker″ə-to-mi-ko′sis) fungal infection of the cornea 角膜真菌病

ker·a·top·a·thy (ker″ə-top′ə-the) noninflammatory disease of the cornea 非炎性角膜病; **band k.,** a condition characterized by an abnormal gray circumcorneal band 带状角膜病

ker·a·to·pha·kia (ker″ə-to-fa′ke-ə) keratoplasty in which a slice of the donor's cornea is shaped to a desired curvature and inserted between layers of the recipient's cornea to change its curvature 角膜移植成形术

ker·a·to·plas·ty (ker″ə-to-plas′te) plastic surgery of the cornea; corneal transplantation 角膜成形术，角膜移植术; **optic k.,** keratoplasty with removal and replacement of scar tissue that interferes with vision 复明角膜成形术; **refractive k.,** procedure in which a section of cornea from a patient or donor is removed, shaped to the desired curvature, and inserted either between (keratophakia) layers of the patient's cornea or on (keratomileusis) the patient's cornea to change its curvature and correct optical errors 屈光性角膜成形术; **tectonic k.,** transplantation of corneal material to replace tissue that has been lost 整复性角膜成形术

ker·a·to·rhex·is (ker″ə-to-rek′sis) rupture of the cornea 角膜破裂

ker·a·tor·rhex·is (ker″ə-to-rek′sis) 同 keratorhexis

ker·a·tos·co·py (ker″ə-tos′kə-pe) inspection of the cornea 角膜镜检查

ker·a·to·sis (ker″ə-to′sis) pl. *kerato′ses.* Anyhorny growth, such as a wart or callosity 角化病; **kera-tot′ic** *adj.*; **actinic k.** a sharply outlined verrucous or keratotic growth that may develop into a cutaneous horn or become malignant; it usually occurs in the middle-aged or elderly and is due to excessive exposure to the sun 光线性角化病; **k. follicula′ris,** a hereditary form marked by areas of crusting, itching, or warty or papular growths that may fuse to form plaques 毛囊角化病; **inverted follicular k.,** a benign, usually solitary, epithelial tumor originating in a hair follicle and occurring as a flesh-colored nodule or papule 倒置性毛囊角化症; **palmoplantar k.,** 见 *keratoderma* 下词条; **k. pharyn′gea,** that characterized by horny projections from the tonsils and the orifices of the lymph follicles in the pharyngeal walls 咽部角化病; **k. pila′ris,** hyperkeratosis limited to the hair follicles 毛发角化病; **k. puncta′ta, punctate k.,** 见 *keratoderma* 下词条; **seborrheic k.,** a benign tumor of epidermal origin, marked by soft friable plaques with slight to intense pigmentation, most often on the face, trunk, or limbs 脂溢性角化病; **solar k.,** actinic k. 日光角化病，光线性角化病

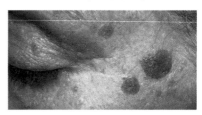

▲ 脂溢性角化病

ker·a·to·sul·fate (ker″ə-to-sul′fāt) 同 keratan sulfate

ker·a·tot·o·my (ker″ə-tot′ə-me) incision of the cornea 角膜切开术; **radial k.,** a series of incisions made in the cornea from its outer edge toward its center in spokelike fashion; done to flatten the cornea and thus to correct myopia 放射性角膜切开术

ker·a·to·to·rus (ker″ə-to-to′rəs) a vaultlike protrusion of the cornea 角膜隆凸

kerf (kirf) 1. a slit made by cutting 劈痕，切缝，锯口；2. the width of a cut made by a saw 锯缝宽度

ke·ri·on (kēr′e-on) a boggy, exudative tumefaction covered with pustules; associated with tinea infections 脓癣

ker·nic·ter·us (kər-nik′tər-əs) [Ger.] a condition with severe neural symptoms, associated with high levels of bilirubin in the blood 核黄疸

keta·mine (ke′tə-mēn) a rapid-acting general anesthetic, used as the hydrochloride salt 氯胺酮

ke·ta·zo·lam (kē-ta′zo-lam) a benzodiazepine used to treat anxiety disorders and to provide short-term relief of anxiety symptoms 凯他唑仑

ke·to ac·id (ke′to) a carboxylic acid containing a carbonyl group 酮酸

ke·to·ac·i·do·sis (ke″to-as″ĭ-do′sis) acidosis accompanied by the accumulation of ketone bodies in the body tissues and fluids 酮症酸中毒；**diabetic k.**, metabolic acidosis produced by accumulation of ketones in uncontrolled diabetes mellitus 糖尿病酮症酸中毒

ke·to·ac·id·uria (ke″to-as″ĭ-du′re-ə) the presence of keto acids in the urine 酮酸尿症；**branched-chain k.**, maple syrup urine disease 支链酮酸尿症

ke·to·a·mi·no·ac·i·de·mia (ke″to-ə-me″no-as″ĭ-de′me-ə) maple syrup urine disease 酮氨基酸血症，槭糖浆尿病

β-ke·to·bu·tyr·ic ac·id (ke″to-bu-tēr′ik) acetoacetic acid β- 酮丁酸，乙酰乙酸

ke·to·co·na·zole (ke″to-kon′ə-zōl) a derivative of imidazole used as an antifungal agent 酮康唑

ke·to·gen·e·sis (ke″to-jen′ə-sis) the production of ketone bodies 生酮作用；**ketogenet′ic** *adj.*

α-ke·to·glu·ta·rate (ke″to-gloo′tə-rāt) a salt or anion of α -ketoglutaric acid α - 酮戊二酸的阴离子形式

α-ke·to·glu·tar·ic ac·id (ke″to-gloo-tar′ik) a metabolic intermediate involved in the tricarboxylic acid cycle, in amino acid metabolism, and in transamination reactions as an amino group acceptor α - 酮戊二酸

ke·tol·y·sis (ke-tol′ə-sis) the splitting up of ketone bodies 解酮（作用）；**ketolyt′ic** *adj.*

ke·tone (ke′tōn) any of a class of organic compounds containing the carbonyl group, C=O, whose carbon atom is joined to two other carbon atoms, i.e., with the carbonyl group occurring within the carbon chain 酮；甲酮

ke·to·ne·mia (ke″to-ne′me-ə) excessive ketone

bodies in the blood 酮血（症）

ke·ton·uria (ke″to-nu′re-ə) an excess of ketone bodies in the urine 酮尿（症）

ke·to·pro·fen (ke″to-pro′fən) a nonsteroidal anti-inflammatory drug used in the treatment of various rheumatic and nonrheumatic inflammatory disorders, pain, dysmenorrhea, and vascular headaches 酮基布洛芬，苯酮苯丙酸

ke·to·ro·lac (ke″to-ro′lak) a nonsteroidal anti-inflammatory drug available as the tromethamine salt; used systemically for short-term management of pain; also applied topically to the conjunctiva in the treatment of allergic conjunctivitis and of ocular inflammation following cataract surgery 酮咯酸（氨丁三醇）

ke·tose (ke′tōs) a subgroup of the monosaccharides, being those having a nonterminal carbonyl (keto) group 酮糖

ke·to·sis (ke-to′sis) accumulation of excessive amounts of ketone bodies in body tissues and fluids, occurring when fatty acids are incompletely metabolized 酮症；**ketot′ic** *adj.*

ke·to·ster·oid (ke″to-ster′oid) a steroid having ketone groups on functional carbon atoms. The *17-ketosteroids*, found in normal urine and in excess in certain tumors and in congenital adrenal hyperplasia, have a ketone group on the 17th carbon atom and include certain androgenic and adrenocortical hormones 甾酮类，酮甾类，酮类固醇

ke·to·ti·fen (ke″to-ti′fen) a noncompetitive H1-receptor antagonist and mast cell stabilizer; used topically as the fumarate salt as an antipruritic in the treatment of allergic conjunctivitis 酮替芬，甲哌噻庚酮

keV kiloelectron volt; 1000 electron volts 千电子伏特

key·note (ke′nōt) in homeopathy, the characteristic property of a drug that indicates its use in treating a similar symptom of disease 同治药性

Key·tru·da (kee′troo-duh) trademark for a preparation of pembrolizumab pembrolizumab 的商品名

kg kilogram 千克，公斤

kHz kilohertz; 1000 hertz 千赫兹

ki (ke) [Japanese] qi [日语] 気

kid·ney (kid′ne) either of the two organs in the lumbar region that filter the blood, excreting the end products of body metabolism in the `form of urine and regulating the concentrations of hydrogen, sodium, potassium, phosphate, and other ions in the extracellular fluid 肾；**abdominal k.,** an ectopic kidney just above the iliac crest 腹肾；**amyloid k.,** a kidney with renal amyloidosis 淀粉样肾；**cake k.,** a solid, irregularly lobed organ of bizarre shape,

550

formed by fusion of the two renal anlagen 块状肾，饼状肾；**cicatricial k.**, a shriveled, irregular, and scarred kidney due to suppurative pyelonephritis 疤痕肾；**fatty k.**, one with fatty degeneration 脂肪肾；**flea-bitten k.**, one with scattered petechiae on its surface 蚤咬状肾；**floating k.**, nephroptosis 游动肾，浮游肾；**fused k.**, a single anomalous organ developed as a result of fusion of the renal anlagen 融合肾；**head k.**, pronephros 前肾；**horseshoe k.**, an anomaly in which the right and left kidneys are linked at one end by tissue 马蹄肾，蹄铁形肾；**hypermobile k.**, nephroptosis 游动肾，浮游肾；**lumbar k.**, an ectopic kidney found opposite the sacral promontory in the iliac fossa, anterior to the iliac vessels 腰肾；**lump k.**, 见 cake k.; **medullary sponge k.**, a usually asymptomatic, congenital condition in which small cystic dilatations of the collecting tubules of the renal medulla give the kidney a spongy feeling and appearance 髓质海绵肾，髓状海绵样肾；**middle k.**, mesonephros 中肾；**pelvic k.**, an ectopic kidney found opposite the sacrum and below the aortic bifurcation 骨盆肾；**polycystic k's,** 多囊肾，见 *disease* 下 *polycystic kidney disease*；**primordial k.**, pronephros 前肾；**sigmoid k.**, an anomaly in which the two kidneys are fused in the form of a capital Greek letter sigma 乙状肾；**sponge k.**, medullary sponge k. 海绵肾；**thoracic k.**, an ectopic kidney that protrudes above the respiratory diaphragm into the posterior mediastinum 胸肾；**waxy k.**, 同 amyloid k.

kilo·cal·o·rie (kcal) (kil′o-kal″ə-re) a unit of heat equal to 1000 calories 千卡，大卡

kilo·gram (kil′o-gram) the basic SI unit of mass, being 1000 g, or 1 cubic decimeter of water; equivalent to 2.205 pounds avoirdupois 千克，公斤

ki·nase (ki′nās) 1. a subclass of the transferases, comprising the enzymes that catalyze the transfer of a high-energy group from a donor (usually ATP) to an acceptor 激酶；2. a suffix used in the names of some enzymes that convert an inactive or precursor form 用于构成激酶的后缀

kin·e·plas·ty (kin′ə-plas″te) use of the stump of an amputated limb to produce motion of the prosthesis 运动成形切断术

kine·scope (kin′ə-skōp) an instrument for ascertaining ocular refraction 眼折射计，（电子）显像管

ki·ne·sia (kǐ-ne′zhə) motion sickness 晕动病

ki·ne·si·at·rics (kǐ-ne″se-at′riks) 同 kinesitherapy

ki·ne·sics (kǐ-ne′siks) the study of body movement as a part of the process of communication 运动学

ki·ne·si·gen·ic (kǐ-ne″sǐ-jen′ik) caused by movement 运动诱发的

kine·sim·e·ter (kin″ə-sim′ə-tər) an instrument for quantitative measurement of movements 运动测量器

ki·ne·sin (ki-ne′sin) any of a family of ATP-splitting cytoplasmic proteins that bind vesicles and particles and transport them along microtubules; they are also important in spindle formation in mitosis 驱动蛋白

ki·ne·si·ol·o·gy (kǐ-ne″se-ol′ə-je) 1. the sum of what is known regarding human motion; the study of motion of the human body 运动学；2. a system of diagnosis based on the theory that muscle dysfunction is secondary to subclinical structural, chemical, or mental dysfunction in other parts of the body; using manual muscle testing to help identify the primary dysfunction and treating by attempting to correct the underlying state 运动疗法

ki·ne·si·ol·o·gy tape (kǐ-ne″se-ol′ə-je tāp) elastic tape used to alleviate discomfort and decrease inflammation from physical injury 肌内效贴布，弹性治疗胶带；又称 *elastic therapeutic tape*

ki·ne·sio·neu·ro·sis (kǐ-ne″se-o-noo-ro′sis) a functional nervous disorder marked by motor disturbances 运动性神经功能病

Kin·es·io Tape (kǐ-nēz′ēo tāp) trademark for a brand of elastic therapy tape 一种弹性治疗胶带的商标名

ki·ne·sis (kǐ-ne″sis) (ki-ne′sis) [Gr.] 1. movement 运动，动作；2. stimulus-induced motion responsive only to the intensity of the stimulus, not the direction 对刺激反应的活动，反应方向不受刺激方向的控制；cf. *taxis*

ki·ne·si·ther·a·py (kǐ-ne″sǐ-ther′ə-pe) the treatment of disease by movements or exercise 运动疗法

kin·es·the·sia (kin″es-the′zhə) 1. the awareness of position, weight, tension, and movement 运动感；2. movement sense 动觉；**kinesthet′ic** *adj.*

kin·es·the·sis (kin″əs-the′sis) 同 kinesthesia

ki·net·ic (kǐ-net′ik) pertaining to or producing motion 动力的，运动的

ki·net·ics (kǐ-net′iks) the scientific study of the turnover, or rate of change, of a specific factor in the body, commonly expressed as units of amount per unit time 动力学；**chemical k.**, the study of the rates and mechanisms of chemical reactions 化学动力学

ki·ne·to·car·dio·gram (kǐ-ne″to-kahr′de-o-gram) the graphic record obtained by kinetocardiography 心动图

ki·ne·to·car·di·og·ra·phy (kǐ-ne″to-kahr″deog′rə-fe) the graphic recording of slow vibrations of the anterior chest wall in the region of the heart, the vibrations representing the absolute motion at a given point on the chest 心振动描记术，运动心动描记法

ki·ne·to·chore (kǐ-ne′to-kor) a structure embedded

in the surface of the centromere to which the spindle fibers are attached 动粒

ki·ne·to·gen·ic (kī-ne″to-jen′ik) causing or producing movement 促动的，引起运动的

ki·ne·to·plast (kī-ne′to-plast) a structure associated with the basal body in many protozoa, primarily the Mastigophora; it is rich in DNA and, like the basal body, it replicates independently 动基体

ki·net·o·sis (kin″ə-to′sis) pl. *kineto'ses.* Any disorder due to unaccustomed motions 晕动病；见 *motion sickness*

king·dom (king′dəm) in the traditional classification of living organisms, the highest of the categories; there are usually considered to be these six: Archaea, Bacteria, Protista, Fungi, Plantae (plants), and Animalia (animals); some systems now add a higher level (e.g., domain) 界；领域

ki·nin (ki′nin) any of a group of vasoactive straight-chain polypeptides formed by kallikrein-catalyzed cleavage of kininogens; causing vasodilation and also altering vascular permeability 肌肽

ki·nin·ase II (ki′nin-ās) 激肽酶Ⅱ，见 *peptidyl-dipeptidase A*

ki·nin·o·gen (ki-nin′o-jen″) either of two plasma α₂-globulins that are kinin precursors, *HMW (high-molecular-weight) k.,* precursor to bradykinin, and *LMW (low-molecular-weight) k.,* precursor to kallidin 激肽原

ki·no·cil·i·um (ki″no-sil′e-əm) pl. *kinocil'ia.* A motile, protoplasmic filament on the free surface of a cell 动纤毛

kin·ship (kin′ship) the state or fact of descent from a common ancestor 血缘关系

Kleb·si·el·la (kleb″se-el′ə) a widespread genus of gram-negative anaerobic bacteria of the family Enterobacteriaceae, frequently causing nosocomial urinary and pulmonary infections and wound infections 克雷伯菌属；*K. granulo'matis,* a species that causes granuloma inguinale 肉芽肿杆菌，又称 *Donovan body; K. mo'bilis,* a species that causes nosocomial pneumonia in debilitated patients 产气肠杆菌；*K. oxyto'ca,* a species that is similar to *K. pneumoniae* and causes nosocomial infections 催产克雷伯菌；*K. pneumo'niae,* an encapsulated species that includes several subspecies and causes infections of the urinary and respiratory tracts 肺炎克雷伯菌，见 *pneumonia* 下 *Klebsiella pneumonia*

klee·blatt·schä·del (kla″blaht-sha′dəl) [Ger.] cloverleaf skull; a congenital anomaly in which there is intrauterine synostosis of all cranial sutures except the metopic and squamosal, giving the head a trilobed appearance [德] 苜蓿状颅，三叶草叶形头颅

klep·to·ma·nia (klep″to-ma′ne-ə) compulsive stealing of objects unnecessary for personal use or monetary value 偷窃狂

Kluy·vera (kli′vər-ə) a genus of gram-negative, facultatively anaerobic, rod-shaped bacteria of the family Enterobacteriaceae; it is an occasional opportunistic pathogen, causing respiratory and urinary infections 克罗非菌属

knee (nee) 1. genu; the area around the articulation of the femur and tibia 膝；2. any structure resembling this part of the leg 膝状物；*housemaid's k.,* inflammation of the bursa of the patella, with fluid accumulating within it 髌前囊炎，膝盖黏液囊肿炎；*knock k.,* 同 knock-knee；*trick k.,* a popular term for a knee joint susceptible to locking in position, most often due to longitudinal splitting of the medial meniscus 膝关节交锁

knock-knee (nok′ne″) genu valgum; a deformity of the thigh or leg, or both, in which the knees are abnormally close together and the space between the ankles is increased 膝外翻

knot (not) 1. an intertwining of the ends or parts of one or more threads, sutures, or strips of cloth 结；2. in anatomy, a knoblike swelling or protuberance 解剖学中指结样肿胀或隆凸；*primitive k.,* 原结，见 *node* 下词条；*surgeon's k., surgical k.,* a knot in which the thread is passed twice through the first loop 外科结

knuck·le (nuk′əl) the dorsal aspect of any phalangeal joint, or any similarly bent structure 膨出部；指节

koi·lo·cyte (koi′lo-sīt″) a concave or hollow cell 中空细胞

koi·lo·cy·to·sis (koi″lo-si-to′sis) the presence of abnormal koilocytes that are vacuolated with clear cytoplasm or perinuclear halos and nuclear pyknosis 挖空细胞病；**koilocytot'ic** *adj.*

koil·onych·ia (koi″lo-nik′e-ə) dystrophy of the fingernails in which they are thinned and concave, with raised edges 反甲，匙状甲

koi·lor·rhach·ic (koi″lo-rak′ik) having a vertebral column in which the lumbar curvature is anteriorly concave 腰椎后凸的

koi·lo·ster·nia (koi″lo-stur′ne-ə) pectus excavatum 漏斗胸

Kr krypton 化学元素氪的符号

Krait (krāt) any member of the genus *Bungarus,* extremely venomous crotalid snakes found from India across Southeast and East Asia 金环蛇

krau·ro·sis (kraw-ro′sis) a dried, shriveled condition 干皱；*k. vul'vae,* lichen sclerosus of the female external genitalia, characterized by atrophy, leukoplakic patches on the mucosa, and intense itching 外阴干皱

kryp·ton (Kr) (krip′ton) a colorless, odorless, tasteless, nontoxic element of the noble gas group; at. no. 36, at. wt. 83.798 氪（化学元素）；**k. 81m,** an unstable radioactive isotope of krypton having a half-life of 13 seconds and emitting gamma rays (0.19 MeV); used in pulmonary ventilation studies 氪 81 m

kun·da·li·ni (koon″də-le′ne) 1. in Hindu tradition, psychospiritual energy that lies dormant in the lowest chakra 印度传统中休眠在最低脉轮中的精神能量；2. 见 *yoga* 下词条

ku·ru (koo′roo) an infectious form of prion disease with a long incubation period found only in New Guinea and thought to be associated with ritual cannibalism 库鲁病

kV kilovolt; 1000 volts 千伏（特）

kVp kilovolts peak 千伏峰位

kwash·i·or·kor (kwahsh″e-or′kor) a form of protein-energy malnutrition produced by severe protein deficiency; caloric intake is usually also deficient. Symptoms include retarded growth, changes in skin and hair pigment, edema, immune deficiency, and pathologic changes in the liver 水肿型营养不良，**marasmic k.,** a condition in which there is a deficiency of both calories and protein, with severe tissue wasting, loss of subcutaneous fat, and usually dehydration 消瘦型夸希奥科症

Ky·lee·na (kī′lee-nə) trademark for a levonorgestrel-releasing intrauterine system used for contraception 一种左炔诺孕酮宫内释放系统的商品名

kyn·uren·ic ac·id (kin″u-ren′ik) a bicyclic aromatic compound formed from kynurenine in a pathway of tryptophan catabolism and excreted in the urine in several disorders of tryptophan catabolism 犬尿烯酸

kyn·ure·nine (kin-u′rə-nēn″) an aromatic amino acid, first isolated from dog urine; it is an intermediate in the catabolism of tryptophan 犬尿素，犬尿氨酸

ky·phos (ki′fos) the hump in the spine in kyphosis 驼背，脊柱后凸

ky·pho·sco·li·o·sis (ki″fo-sko″le-o′sis) backward and lateral curvature of the vertebral column 脊柱后侧凸

ky·pho·sis (ki-fo′sis) abnormally increased convexity in the curvature of the thoracic spine as viewed from the side 驼背，脊柱后凸；**kyphot′ic adj.; juvenile k., Scheuermann k.,** the rigid thoracic or thoracolumbar kyphosis occurring in Scheuermann disease; sometimes used loosely to refer to the disease itself 幼年期脊柱后凸

Ky·pro·lis (kī′prō′lis) trademark for a preparation of carfilzomib carfilzomib 的商品名

kyr·tor·rhach·ic (kir″to-rak′ik) having a vertebral column in which the lumbar curvature is convex anteriorly 腰椎前凸的

Ky·to·coc·cus (ki″to-kok′əs) a genus of grampositive coccoid bacteria, including *K. sedenta′rius,* a species that produces keratin-degrading enzymes and is a cause of pitted keratolysis 包括不动盖球菌的革兰阳性球菌的一个属，可产生角蛋白降解酶

L

L left 左；leucine 亮氨酸；liter 升；lumbar vertebrae (L1 to L5) 肺，腰椎（L₁~L₅）；lung 肺

L- chemical prefix specifying the relative configuration of an enantiomer, indicating a carbohydrate with the same configuration around a specific carbon atom as L-glyceraldehyde or an amino acid having the same configuration as L-serine 左旋。Opposed to D-

l former symbol for *liter,* now replaced by L 升

l. [L.] ligamen′tum (ligament) 韧带的符号

l length 长度的符号

l- levo- (left, counterclockwise, levorotatory)，左旋。Opposed to *d-*

λ (lambda, the eleventh letter of the Greek alphabet) （希语的第 11 个字母）[符号]。wavelength 波长；one of the two types of immunoglobulin light chains 两种免疫球蛋白轻链之一

La lanthanum 镧（化学元素）

la·bel (la′bəl) 1. a mark, tag, or other characteristic that identifies something 标签；2. to provide something with such a characteristic 标记；**radioactive l.,** a radioisotope that is incorporated into a compound to mark it 放射性标记

la·bet·a·lol (lə-bet′ə-lol) a beta-adrenergic blocking agent with some alpha-adrenergic blocking activity; used in the form of the hydrochloride salt as an antihypertensive 拉贝洛尔，柳氨苄心定

la·bia (la′be-ə) plural of *labium* 唇（复数）

la·bi·al (la′be-əl) 1. pertaining to a lip or labium 唇的，阴唇的；2. in dental anatomy, pertaining to the tooth surface that faces the lip 在牙齿解剖学中，指面向嘴唇的牙齿表面

la·bi·al·ly (la′be-əl-e) toward the lips 向唇

la·bile (la′bəl) (la′bīl) 1. gliding; moving from mpoint to point over the surface; unstable; fluctuating 不稳定的，易变的，波动的；2. chemically unstable 化学上不稳定的

la·bil·i·ty (lə-bil′ə-te) 1. the quality of being labile

易变性，不稳定性；2. in psychiatry, emotional instability 情绪不稳定

la·bio·al·ve·o·lar (la″be-o-al-ve′o-lər) 1. pertaining to the lip and dental alveoli 唇牙槽的；2. pertaining to the labial side of a dental alveolus 牙槽唇侧的

la·bio·cho·rea (la″be-o-kə-re′ə) a choreic stiffening of the lips in speech, with stammering 唇肌痉挛性口吃

la·bio·cli·na·tion (la″be-o-klī-na′shən) deviation of an anterior tooth from the vertical, in the direction of the lips 唇侧倾斜

la·bio·graph (la′be-o-graf″) an instrument for recording lip motions in speaking 唇动描记器

la·bio·men·tal (la″be-o-men′təl) pertaining to the lip and chin 唇颏的

la·bio·place·ment (la″be-o-plās′mənt) displacement of a tooth toward the lip（牙）唇向移位

la·bio·ver·sion (la″be-o-vur′zhən) labial displacement of a tooth from the line of occlusion 唇侧移位

la·bi·um (la′be-əm) pl. *la′bia* [L.] 1. lip 唇；2. a fleshy border or edge; a liplike structure 唇状结构；3. in the plural, often used to denote the *labia majora* and *minora pudendi* 阴唇；**la′bial** *adj.*

la′bia majo′ra puden′di, elongated folds running downward and backward from the mons pubis in the female, one on either side of the rima pudendi 大阴唇；**la′bia mino′ra puden′di,** small skin folds, one on each side, running backward from the clitoris between the labia majora and the vaginal opening 小阴唇；**la′bia o′ris,** the lips of the mouth 口唇

la·bor (la′bər) [L.] the function of the female by which the infant is expelled through the vagina to the outside world: the *first stage* begins with onset of regular uterine contractions and ends when the os is completely dilated and flush with the vagina; the *second* extends from the end of the first stage until the expulsion of the infant is completed; the *third* extends from expulsion of the infant until the placenta and membranes are expelled; the *fourth* denotes the hour or two after delivery, when uterine tone is established 分娩，生产；**artificial l.,** 同 induced l.；**dry l.,** that in which the amniotic fluid escapes before the onset of uterine contractions 干产；**false l.,** 假临产，见 *pain* 下词条；**induced l.,** that brought on by mechanical or other extraneous means, usually by the intravenous infusion of oxytocin 引产；**missed l.,** that in which contractions begin and then cease, the fetus being retained for weeks or months 死胎不下，滞留死胎；**postmature l., postponed l.,** that occurring 2 weeks or more after the expected date of confinement 逾期分娩，过期分娩；**precipitate l.,** that occurring with undue rapidity 急产；**pre-**

mature l., preterm l., labor before the normal end of gestation; usually meaning between the twentieth and thirty-seventh weeks 早产

lab·o·ra·to·ry (lab′rə-tor″e) a place equipped for making tests or doing experimental work 实验室，化验室；**clinical l.,** one for examination of materials derived from the human body for the purpose of providing information on diagnosis, prognosis, prevention, or treatment of disease 临床实验室

la·brum (la′brəm) pl. *la′bra* [L.] an edge, rim, or lip 唇，上唇，缘

lab·y·rinth (lab′ə-rinth) 1. a system of interconnecting channels 迷路，互相联系的管道系统；2. inner ear 内耳迷路；**labyrin′thine** *adj.*；**bony l.,** the bony part of the inner ear 骨迷路；**cochlear l.,** the part of the membranous labyrinth that includes the perilymphatic space and the cochlear duct 耳蜗迷路，**endolymphatic l.,** membranous l. 膜迷路，内淋巴迷路；**ethmoidal l.,** either of the paired lateral masses of the ethmoid bone, which contain many thin-walled cellular cavities 筛骨迷路；**membranous l.,** a system of communicating epithelial sacs and ducts within the bony labyrinth, containing the endolymph 膜迷路；**osseous l.,** 同 bony l.；**perilymphatic l.,** perilymphatic space 外淋巴迷路；**vestibular l.,** the part of the membranous labyrinth that includes the utricle, saccule, and semicircular ducts 前庭迷路

lab·y·rin·thi·tis (lab″ə-rin-thi′tis) otitis interna; inflammation of the inner ear 迷路炎；**acute serous l.,** a type caused by chemical or toxic irritants that invade the labyrinth, usually from the middle ear 急性浆液性迷路炎；**acute suppurative l.,** a type in which pus enters the labyrinth, usually either through a fistula after infection of the middle ear or through temporal bone erosion from meningitis 急性化脓性迷路炎；**circumscribed l.,** perilabyrinthitis; acute serous labyrinthitis in a discrete area, due to erosion of the bony wall of a semicircular canal with exposure of the membranous labyrinth 局限性迷路炎

lab·y·rin·thus (lab″ə-rin′thəs) pl. *labyrin′thi* [L.] 同 labyrinth

lac (lak) [L.] 1. milk 乳；2. any milklike medicinal preparation 乳剂

La·ca·zia (lə-ka′ze-ə) a genus of anamorphic fungi comprising the single species *L. lo′boi,* which causes lacaziosis 洛博拉卡斯菌

la·ca·zi·o·sis (lə-ka′ze-o-sis) lobomycosis; a tropical fungal infection of humans and dolphins, mainly in South America; it is caused by *Lacazia loboi* and is characterized by red, smooth, hard cutaneous nodules resembling keloids 瘢痕疙瘩性芽生菌病

lac·er·at·ed (las′ər-āt″əd) torn; mangled; wounded

by a jagged instrument 撕裂的，裾状的，弄伤的

lac·er·a·tion (las″ər-a′shən) 1. the act of tearing 撕裂；2. a torn, ragged, mangled wound 裂伤

la·cer·tus (lə-sur′təs) [L.] a name given certain fibrous attachments of muscles（肌）纤维束

lac·ri·mal (lak′rĭ-məl) pertaining to the tears 泪的

lac·ri·ma·tion (lak″rĭ-ma′shən) secretion and discharge of tears 流泪

lac·ri·ma·tor (lak′rĭ-ma″tər) an agent, such as a gas, that induces the flow of tears 催泪剂

lac·ri·mot·o·my (lak″rĭ-mot′ə-me) incision of the lacrimal gland, duct, or sac 泪器切开术，泪囊切开术

lact·ac·id·e·mia (lak-tas″ĭ-de′me-ə) excess of lactic acid in the blood 乳酸血

lac·ta·gogue (lak′tə-gog) galactagogue 催乳药

lac·tam (lak′təm) a cyclic amide formed from aminocarboxylic acids by elimination of water；lactams are isomeric with lactims, which are enol forms of lactams 内酰胺，见 *antibiotic* 下词条

β-lac·ta·mase (lak′tə-mās) any of a group of enzymes, produced by almost all gram-negative bacteria, that hydrolyze the β-lactam ring of penicillins and cephalosporins, destroying their antibiotic activity. Individual enzymes may be called *penicillinases* or *cephalosporinases* based on their specificities β-内酰胺酶

lac·tase (lak′tās) a β-galactosidase occurring in the brush border membrane of the intestinal mucosa that catalyzes the cleavage of lactose to galactose and glucose；it is part of the β-glycosidase enzyme complex 乳糖酶

lac·tase de·fi·cien·cy (lak′tās) reduced or absent lactase activity in the intestinal mucosa；the hereditary adult form is the normal state in most populations other than white Northern Europeans and may be characterized by abdominal pain, flatulence, and diarrhea after milk ingestion (lactose intolerance)；the rare congenital form (congenital lactose intolerance) is characterized by diarrhea, vomiting, and failure to thrive 乳糖酶缺乏症

lac·tate (lak′tāt) 1. any salt or ester of lactic acid 乳酸（阴离子形成）；2. to secrete milk 分泌乳汁

l-lac·tate de·hy·dro·gen·ase (LDH) (lak′tāt de-hi′dro-jən-ās) an enzyme that catalyzes the interconversion of lactate and pyruvate. It is widespread in tissues and is abundant in the kidney, skeletal muscle；liver, and myocardium, appearing in elevated concentrations in the blood when these tissues are injured L-乳酸脱氢酶

lac·ta·tion (lak-ta′shən) 1. the secretion of milk 授乳，哺乳；2. the period of milk secretion 哺乳期

lac·te·al (lak′te-əl) any of the intestinal lymphatic vessels that transport chyle 乳糜管

lac·tes·cence (lak-tes′əns) resemblance to milk 乳状

lac·tic (lak′tik) pertaining to milk 乳的

lac·tica c·id (lak′tik) CH₃CHOHCOOH, a compound formed in the body in anaerobic metabolism of carbohydrate and also produced by bacterial action in milk. The sodium salt of racemic or inactive lactic acid *(sodium lactate)* is used as an electrolyte and fluid replenisher 乳酸

lac·tic·ac·i·de·mia (lak″tik-as″ĭ-de′me-ə) 同 lactacidemia

lac·ti·ce·mia (lak″tĭ-se′me-ə) 同 lacticacidemia

lac·tif·er·ous (lak-tif′ər-əs) conveying milk 输乳的，生乳的，又称 *lactigerous*

lac·ti·fuge (lak′tĭ-fūj) 同 antigalactic

lac·tim (lak′tim) 内酰亚胺，见 *lactam*

lac·ti·tol (lak′tĭ-tol) a disaccharide analogue of lactulose used as a bulk sweetener；it is also laxative and is used to treat constipation 乳糖醇

lac·tiv·o·rous (lak-tiv′ə-rəs) feeding or subsisting upon milk 哺乳的，乳食的

Lac·to·bac·il·la·ceae (lak″to-bas″ĭ-la′se-e) a family of gram-positive, non–spore-forming, rod-shaped bacteria of the order Lactobacillales 乳杆菌科

Lac·to·ba·cil·la·les (lak″to-ba-sĭ-la′lēz) an order of lactic acid–producing bacteria of the class Bacilli that ferment sugars to produce energy 乳杆菌目

Lac·to·bac·il·lus (lak″to-ba-sil′əs) a genus of the family Lactobacillaceae. They are anaerobic or microaerophilic and occur widely in nature and in the human mouth, vagina, and intestinal tract. In the oral cavity, they are found associated with dental caries but have no known etiologic ole. Some produce only lactic acid and others produce other end products of fermentation 乳杆菌属；*L. acido philus,* a lactobacillus producing the fermented product, acidophilus milk；preparations are used as digestive aids, for the production of B-complex vitamins, and to help prevent infections after antibiotic treatment 嗜酸乳杆菌

lac·to·bac·il·lus (lak″to-bə-sil′əs) pl. *lactobacil′li.* An organism of the genus *Lactobacillus* 乳杆菌

lac·to·cele (lak′to-sēl) galactocele 积乳囊肿

Lac·to·coc·cus (lak″to-kok′əs) a genus of bacteria of the family Streptococcaceae, found in dairy products and sometimes in opportunistic infections 乳球菌属

lac·to·gen (lak′to-jən) any substance that enhances lactation 催乳素；**human placental l.,** a hormone secreted by the placenta；it has lactogenic, luteotropic, and growth-promoting activity, and inhibits maternal insulin activity 人胎盘催乳素

lac·to·gen·ic (lak″to-jen′ik) galactopoietic 催乳的，催乳药

lac·to·glob·u·lin (lak″to-glob′u-lin) a globulin occurring in milk 乳球蛋白

lac·tone (lak′tōn) a cyclic organic compound in which the chain is closed by ester formation between a carboxyl and a hydroxyl group in the same molecule 内酯

lac·to·ovo·ve·ge·ta·ri·an (lak″to-o″vo-vej′ə-tar′e-ən) ovolactovegetarian 乳蛋素食者

lac·tor·rhea (lak″to-re′ə) galactorrhea 溢乳，乳溢

lac·tose (lak′tōs) a disaccharide occurring in mammalian milk, which on hydrolysis yields glucose and galactose; used as a tablet and capsule diluent, a powder bulking agent, and a component of infant feeding formulas 乳糖

lac·to·side (lak′to-sīd) glycoside in which the sugar constituent is lactose 乳苷，乳糖苷

lac·tos·uria (lak″to-su′re-ə) excessive lactose in the urine 乳糖尿

lac·to·trope (lak′to-trōp) 同 lactotroph

lac·to·troph (lak′to-trōf) an acidophil of the anterior lobe of the pituitary that secretes prolactin（垂体）催乳素细胞，泌乳细胞

lac·to·veg·e·tar·i·an (lak″to-vej″ə-tar′e-ən) 1. one who practices lactovegetarianism 乳品素食者；2. pertaining to lactovegetarianism 乳与蔬菜的

lac·to·veg·e·tar·i·an·ism (lak″to-vej″ə-tar′e- ən-iz″əm) restriction of the diet to vegetables and dairy products, eschewing other foods of animal origin 乳品素食主义

lac·tu·lose (lak′tu-lōs) a synthetic disaccharide used as a laxative and to enhance excretion or formation of ammonia in the treatment of hepatic encephalopathy 乳果糖

la·cu·na (lə-ku′nə) pl. lacu′nae [L.] 1. a small pit or hollow cavity 腔隙，陷窝；2. a defect or gap, as in the field of vision (scotoma) 缺损，裂隙（如视野中的暗点）；lacu′nar adj.; absorption l., 同 resorption l.; bone l., a small cavity within the bone matrix, containing an osteocyte; from it slender canaliculi radiate and penetrate the adjacent lamellae to anastomose with the canaliculi of neighboring lacunae, thus forming a system of cavities interconnected by minute canals 骨陷窝；cartilage l., any of the small cavities within the cartilage matrix, containing a chondrocyte 软骨陷窝；Howship l., resorption l. 豪希普陷窝，吸收陷窝；intervillous l., one of the blood spaces of the placenta in which the fetal villi are found 绒毛间腔隙，滋养层腔隙；lateral lacunae, venous meshworks within the dura mater on either side of, and continuous with, the superior sagittal sinus 窦外侧陷窝；osseous l., 同 bone l.;

l. pharyn′gis, a depression at the pharyngeal end of the eustachian tube 咽鼓窝；resorption l., a pit or groove in developing bone that is undergoing resorption; frequently found to contain osteoclasts 吸收陷窝；trophoblastic l., 同 intervillous l.

la·cu·nule (lə-ku′nūl) a minute lacuna 小陷窝，小腔隙

la·cus (la′kəs) pl. la′cus [L.] lake 湖

La·e·trile (la′ə-tril) trademark for l-mandelonitrile-β -glucuronic acid, a semisynthetic derivative of amygdalin; it is alleged to have antineoplastic properties L- 扁桃腈 -β - 葡萄糖醛酸的商品名；Cf. laetrile

la·e·trile (la′ə-tril) amygdalin (l-mandelonitrile-β -gentiobioside) derived from crushed pits of certain fruits, usually apricots, and alleged to have antineoplastic properties. Cf. Laetrile. 苦杏仁苷，L-扁桃腈 - β - 葡糖醛酸

lae·ve (le′və) [L.] nonvillous 无绒毛的

lag (lag) 1. the time between application of a stimulus and the reaction 迟滞期；2. the period after inoculation of bacteria into a culture medium, in which growth or cell division is slow 迟滞期；anaphase l., delayed movement during anaphase of one homologous chromosome in mitosis or of one chromatid in meiosis, so that the chromosome is not incorporated into the nucleus of one of the daughter cells; the result is one normal cell and one cell with monosomy 后期迟滞

la·ge·na (lə-je′nə) 1. a part of the upper end of the cochlear duct（蜗管）顶盲端；2. the organ of hearing in nonmammalian vertebrates 听壶（低等动物的听器）

la·gen·i·form (lə-jen′ĭ-form) flask-shaped 瓶形的，烧瓶形的

lag·oph·thal·mos (lag″of-thal′məs) inability to shut the eyes completely 兔眼

LAIV live, attenuated influenza vaccine 流感减毒活疫苗

lake (lāk) 1. to undergo separation of hemoglobin from erythrocytes 血细胞溶解；2. a circumscribed collection of fluid in a hollow or depressed cavity 湖；lacrimal l., the triangular space at the medial angle of the eye, where the tears collect 泪湖；marginal l's, discontinuous venous lacunae, relatively free of villi, near the edge of the placenta, formed by merging of the marginal portions of the intervillous space with the subchorial lake 缘湖，缘窦

lal·la·tion (lə-la′shən) a babbling, infantile form of speech 婴儿样语，言语不清

lal·or·rhea (lal″ə-re′ə) 同 logorrhea

lamb·da (lam′də) point of union of the lambdoid and sagittal sutures 人字缝尖

lamb·doid (lam′doid) shaped like the Greek letter lambda, Λ or λ 人字形的

Lam·blia (lam′ble-ə) *Giardia* 蓝氏鞭毛虫属，贾第虫属

lame (lām) incapable of normal locomotion; deviating from normal gait 跛的，跛行的

la·mel·la (lə-mel′ə) pl. *lamel′lae* [L.] 1. a thin leaf or plate, as of bone 薄片，薄板；2. a medicated disk or wafer to be inserted under the eyelid 眼片；**circumferential l.,** one of the layers of bone that underlie the periosteum and endosteum 环骨板；**concentric l.,** 同 haversian l.；**endosteal l.,** one of the bony plates lying beneath the endosteum 骨内板，内环骨板；**ground l.,** 同 interstitial l.；**haversian l.,** one of the concentric bony plates surrounding a haversian canal 哈弗斯骨板，同心性骨板；**intermediate l., interstitial l.,** one of the bony plates that fill in between the haversian systems 间骨板

la·mel·lar (lə-mel′ər) 1. pertaining to or resembling lamellae 板的，层状的，片状的；2. 同 lamellated (1)

lam·el·lat·ed (lam′ə-lāt″əd) 1. having, composed of, or arranged in lamellae 片层状的；2. 同 lamelliform

la·mel·li·form (lə-mel′ĭ-form) resembling lamellae 薄片形的，片层状的

la·mel·li·po·dia (lə-mel″ĭ-po′de-ə) sing. *lamellipo′dium.* Delicate sheetlike extensions of cytoplasm that form transient adhesions with the cell substrate and wave gently, enabling the cell to move along the substrate 薄片状伪足

lam·i·na (lam′ĭ-nə) pl. *la′minae* [L.] 1. layer; a thin, flat plate of a larger composite structure 层，板；2. 同 l. of vertebra；**basal l.,** 1. the layer of the basement membrane lying next to the basal surface of the adjoining cell layer, comprising two layers, the electron-lucent lamina lucida and the electron-dense lamina densa 基板，致密板；2. sometimes, the entire basement membrane 基底膜；3. 同 l. basalis (1)；**l. basa′lis,** 1. either of the pair of longitudinal zones of the embryonic neural tube, from which develop the ventral gray columns of the spinal cord and the motor centers of the brain(胚胎神经管)基底层；2. 同 basal l. (1)；**l. basila′ris,** the mastoid wall of the cochlear duct, separating it from the scala tympani 蜗管基底层；**bony spiral l.,** spiral l. 骨螺旋板；**Bowman l.,** 鲍曼层，角膜前界层，见 *membrane* 下 词 条；**l. choroidocapilla′ris,** the inner layer of the choroid, composed of a single-layered network of small capillaries 脉络膜毛细管层；**l. cribro′sa,** 1. *(of ethmoid bone)* the horizontal plate of ethmoid bone forming the roof of the nasal cavity, and perforated by many foramina for passage of olfactory nerves. 2. *(of sclera)* the perforated part of the sclera through which pass the axons of the retinal ganglion cells 筛 板；**l. den′sa,** see *basal l.* (1). 致 密 板；**episcleral l.,** loose connective and elastic tissue covering the sclera and anteriorly connecting it with the conjunctiva 巩 膜 上 层；**epithelial l.,** the layer of ependymal cells covering the choroid plexus 上皮层；**l. lu′cida,** 透明板，见 *basal l.* (1)；**nuclear l.,** a tightly woven meshwork that lines the nuclear side of the inner nuclear membrane; it is believed to control the shape of the nucleus and mediates interaction between the inner nuclear membrane and chromatin 核纤层；**l. pro′pria,** the connective tissue coat of a mucous membrane just deep to the epithelium and basement membrane(黏膜)固有层；**l. ra′ra,** lamina lucida; see *basal l.* (1). In the lung alveoli and renal glomeruli, one may occur on each side of the lamina densa 透明板，基底层；**reticular l.,** 1. a layer of the basement membrane, adjacent to the connective tissue, seen in some epithelia 网状板；2. the perforated hyaline membrane covering the organ of Corti 透明膜；**Rexed laminae, spinal laminae,** an architectural scheme used to classify the structure of the spinal cord, based on the cytologic features of the neurons in different regions of the gray substance; it consists of nine laminae (Ⅰ to Ⅸ) that extend throughout the cord and a tenth region (area Ⅹ) that surrounds the central canal 脊板；**spiral l.,** a double plate of bone winding spirally around the modiolus, dividing the spiral canal of the cochlea into the scala tympani and scala vestibuli 螺旋板；**l. termina′lis,** the thin plate derived from the cerebrum, forming the anterior wall of the third ventricle 终板；**l. of vertebra, l. of vertebral arch,** either of the pair of broad plates of bone flaring out from the pedicles of the vertebral arches and fusing together at the midline to complete the posterior part of the arch and provide a base for the spinous process 椎骨板，椎弓板

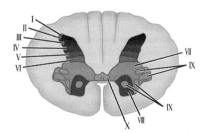

▲ 在脊髓横截面上，脊板大约与第 7 颈椎（C_7）水平

lam·i·nag·ra·phy (lam″ĭ-nag′rə-fe) tomography 体层照相术，断层照相术

lam·i·na·plas·ty (lam′ĭ-nə-plas″te) relief of compression of the spinal cord or nerve roots by incision completely through one lamina of a vertebral arch, creation of a trough in the contralateral lamina, and opening of the arch like a door 椎板成形术

lam·i·nar (lam′ĭ-nər) 1. pertaining to a lamina or laminae 板状的，层状的；2. 同 laminated；3. of, pertaining to, or being a streamlined, smooth fluid flow 层流

lam·i·nat·ed (lam′ĭ-nāt″ed) having, composed of, or arranged in layers or laminae 层状的，分层的，叠层的，层压的

lam·i·nec·to·my (lam″ĭ-nek′tə-me) excision of the posterior arch of a vertebra 椎板切除术

lam·i·not·o·my (lam″ĭ-not′ə-me) transection of a lamina of a vertebra 椎板切开术

la·miv·u·dine (lə-miv′u-dēn) a nucleoside analogue that inhibits reverse transcriptase, used as an antiviral agent in the treatment of chronic hepatitis B and, in combination with zidovudine, the treatment of HIV infection and AIDS 拉米夫定

la·mo·tri·gine (lə-mo′trī-jēn) an anticonvulsant used in the treatment of certain forms of epilepsy; also used to stabilize mood in bipolar I disorder 拉莫三嗪

lamp (lamp) an apparatus for furnishing heat or light 灯；**mercury arc l., mercury vapor l., quartz l.,** one in which the arc is in mercury vapor, enclosed in a quartz burner; used in photodynamic therapy; it may be air- or watercooled 水银弧光灯；**slit l.,** one having a diaphragm with a slitlike opening through which a narrow flat beam of intense light may be projected into the eye for microscopic study of the conjunctivae, cornea, iris, lens, and vitreous 裂隙灯；**sun l.,** a lamp that gives off radiation, especially ultraviolet, in ranges similar to those of the sun's rays 太阳灯；**Wood l.,** a medium-pressure mercury arc lamp that transmits Wood light for diagnosis of skin conditions such as erythrasma and fungus infections, as well as porphyrins or fluorescent minerals in the skin, scalp, and hair 伍德灯；**xenon arc l.,** one producing light of high intensity in a wide continuum of wavelengths; used with optical filters to simulate solar radiation 氙弧灯

lance (lans) 1. 同 lancet 柳叶刀；2. to cut or incise with a lancet 用柳叶刀切

lan·cet (lan′sət) a small, pointed, two-edged surgical knife 柳叶刀

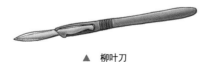

▲ 柳叶刀

lan·ci·nat·ing (lan′sĭ-nāt″ing) tearing, darting, or sharply cutting; said of pain 撕裂的

lan·o·lin (lan′o-lin) a purified, waxlike substance from the wool of sheep, *Ovis aries*, occurring in an anhydrous form and also a form containing 25 to 30 percent water; used as a water-in-oil ointment or cream base. *Modified l.* has been additionally processed to reduce the amount of free lanolin alcohols and detergent and pesticide residues 羊毛脂

lan·so·pra·zole (lan-so′prə-zōl) a proton pump inhibitor used to inhibit gastric acid secretion for the treatment of duodenal or gastric ulcer, gastroesophageal reflux disease, and hyperchlorhydria 兰索拉唑

lan·tha·num (La) (lan′thə-nəm) a silvery white, ductile, heavy metal, rare earth element; at. no. 57, at. wt. 138.905 镧（化学元素）；**l. carbonate,** the carbonate salt of lanthanum, used as a phosphate binder in the treatment of chronic kidney disease 碳酸镧

la·nu·go (lə-noo′go) the fine hair on the body of the fetus 胎毛，胎毳毛

lap·a·ro·hys·ter·ec·to·my (lap″ə-ro-his″tə- rek′tə-me) abdominal hysterectomy 剖腹子宫切除术

lap·a·ro·hys·ter·ot·o·my (lap″ə-ro-his″tərot′ə-me) abdominal hysterotomy 剖腹子宫切开术

lap·a·ro·scope (lap′ə-ro-skōp″) an endoscope for examining the peritoneal cavity 腹腔镜

lap·a·ro·scop·ic (lap″ə-ro-skop′ik) 1. pertaining to a laparoscope 腹腔镜；2. performed using a laparoscope 腹腔镜检查的

lap·a·ros·co·py (lap″ə-ros′kə-pe) examination or treatment of the interior of the abdomen by means of a laparoscope 腹腔镜检查

lap·a·rot·o·my (lap″ə-rot′ə-me) incision through the abdominal wall 剖腹术

lap·in·iza·tion (lap″in-ĭ-za′shən) serial passage of a virus or vaccine through rabbits to modify its characteristics 兔化法

LAR long-acting release 长效释放

LARC long-acting reversible contraceptive 长效可逆避孕药

lard (lahrd) purified internal fat of the abdomen of the hog 豚脂，猪脂

lar·va (lahr′və) pl. *lar′vae* [L.] an independent, motile, nonfeeding, developmental stage in the life history of an animal 幼虫，蚴；**l. cur′rens,** an extremely rapidly progressive, urticarial, creeping eruption of the anal region or trunk caused by migration of *Strongyloides stercoralis* larvae 肛周匍行疹；**cutaneous l. migrans,** creeping eruption caused by subcutaneous migration of larval nematodes, particularly *Ancylostoma braziliense*; also used for similar disease caused by other larval nematode parasites, e.g., gnathostomiasis. Occasionally it is used

L

broadly to denote any creeping eruption 皮肤幼虫移行症；**l. mi′grans** 1. a life stage of certain parasitic larvae in which they wander through the body of their host 幼虫体内移行期；2. infestation of a human or other animal by such a wandering parasitic larva 幼虫移行症；**ocular l. migrans,** infection of the eye with nematode larvae, usually *Toxocara canis* or *T. cati*, which may lodge in the choroid or retina or migrate to the vitreous; larvae death leads to a granulomatous inflammation, the lesion varying from a translucent elevation of the retina to massive retinal detachment and pseudoglioma 眼幼虫移行症；**visceral l. migrans,** a condition due to prolonged migration of nematode larvae in human tissue other than skin; commonly caused by the larvae of *T. canis* or *T. cati*, which do not complete their life cycle in humans 内脏幼虫移行症

lar·vate (lahr′vāt) masked; concealed; said of a disease or symptom of disease 隐蔽的，潜在的

lar·yn·ge·al (lə-rin′je-əl) pertaining to the larynx 喉的

lar·yn·gec·to·my (lar″in-jek′tə-me) surgical removal of the larynx 喉切除术

lar·yn·gis·mus (lar″in-jiz′məs) 同 laryngo-spasm；**laryngis′mal** *adj.*；**l. stri′dulus,** pseudocroup; sudden laryngeal spasm with crowing inhalation and cyanosis, usually seen in children at night 喘鸣性喉痉挛

lar·yn·gi·tis (lar″in-ji′tis) inflammation of the larynx 喉炎；**laryngit′ic** *adj.*；**subglottic l.,** inflammation of the undersurface of the vocal cords 声门下喉炎

la·ryn·go·cele (lə-ring′go-sēl) a congenital anomalous air sac communicating with the cavity of the larynx, which may bulge outward on the neck 喉囊肿

la·ryn·go·fis·sure (lə-ring″go-fish′ər) median laryngotomy 喉正切开术

lar·yn·gog·ra·phy (lar″ing-gog′rə-fe) radiography of the larynx 喉造影术

lar·yn·gol·o·gy (lar″ing-gol′ə-je) the branch of medicine dealing with the throat, pharynx, larynx, nasopharynx, and tracheobronchial tree 喉科学

lar·yn·gop·a·thy (lar-ing-gop′ə-the) any disorder of the larynx 喉病

la·ryn·go·pha·ryn·ge·al (lə-ring″go-fə-rin′je-əl) pertaining to the larynx and pharynx or to the laryngopharynx 咽喉的

la·ryn·go·phar·yn·gec·to·my (lə-ring″gofar″ən-jek′tə-me) excision of the larynx and pharynx 喉咽切除术

la·ryn·go·phar·ynx (lə-ring″go-far′inks) the portion of the pharynx below the upper edge of the epiglottis, opening into the larynx and esophagus 咽喉部；**laryngopharyn′geal** *adj.*

lar·yn·goph·o·ny (lar″ing-gof′ə-ne) a voice sound heard over the larynx 喉听诊音

la·ryn·go·plas·ty (lə-ring′go-plas″te) plastic repair of the larynx 喉成形术

la·ryn·go·ple·gia (lə-ring″go-ple′jə) paralysis of the larynx 喉麻痹

la·ryn·go·pto·sis (lə-ring″gop-to′sis) lowering and mobilization of the larynx, as is sometimes seen in the aged 喉下垂

la·ryn·gos·co·py (lar″ing-gos′kə-pe) visual examination of the interior larynx 喉镜检查；**laryngoscop′ic** *adj.*

la·ryn·go·spasm (lə-ring′go-spaz″əm) spasmodic closure of the larynx 喉痉挛

la·ryn·go·ste·no·sis (lə-ring″go-stə-no′sis) narrowing or stricture of the larynx 喉狭窄

lar·yn·gos·to·my (lar″ing-gos′tə-me) surgical fistulization of the larynx 喉造口术

la·ryn·got·o·my (lar″ing-got′ə-me) incision of the larynx 喉切开术；**inferior l.,** laryngotomy through the cricothyroid membrane 喉下部切开术；**median l.,** laryngotomy through the thyroid cartilage 喉正中切开术；**subhyoid l., superior l.,** laryngotomy through the thyrohyoid membrane 喉上部切开术

la·ryn·go·tra·che·itis (lə-ring″go-tra″ke-i′tis) inflammation of the larynx and trachea 喉气管炎

la·ryn·go·tra·che·ot·o·my (lə-ring″go-tra″keot′o-me) incision of the larynx and trachea 喉气管切开术

lar·ynx (lar′inks) pl. *laryn′ges* [L.] the organ of voice; the air passage between the lower pharynx and the trachea, containing the vocal cords and formed by nine cartilages: the thyroid, cricoid, and epiglottis and the paired arytenoid, corniculate, and cuneiform cartilages 喉，见图 25

LASEK (lay′sĕk) laser-assisted subepithelial keratomileusis 准分子激光上皮下角膜磨镶术

la·ser (la′zər) a device that transfers light of various frequencies into an extremely intense, small, and nearly nondivergent beam of monochromatic radiation in the visible region, with all the waves in phase; capable of mobilizing immense heat and power when focused at close range, it is used as a tool in surgery, in diagnosis, and in physiologic studies 激光；激光器；**argon l.,** a laser with ionized argon as the active medium, whose beam is in the blue and green visible light spectrum; used for photocoagulation 氩激光器；**carbondioxide l.,** a laser with carbon dioxide gas as the active medium, which produces infrared radiation at 10 600 nm; used to excise and incise tissue and to vaporize 二氧化碳激光器；**dye l.,** a laser with organic dye as the

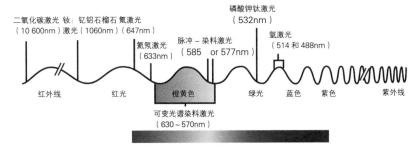

二氧化碳激光　钕：钇铝石榴石　氪激光
（10 600nm）激光（1060nm）（647nm）

磷酸钾钛激光
（532nm）

氦氖激光
（633nm）

脉冲 – 染料激光
（585 or 577nm）

氩激光
（514 和 488nm）

红外线　　　　红光　　　　橙黄色　　　　绿光　蓝色　紫色　　　　紫外线

可变光谱染料激光
（630～570nm）

▲　不同类型激光在电磁波谱上的相对位置

active medium, whose beam is in the visible light spectrum 染料激光；**excimer l.**, a laser with rare gas halides as the active medium, whose beam is in the ultraviolet spectrum and penetrates tissues only a short distance; used in ophthalmologic procedures and laser angioplasty 准分子激光器；**helium-neon l.**, a laser with a mixture of ionized helium and neon gases as the active medium, whose beam is in the red visible light spectrum; used as a guiding beam for lasers operating at nonvisible wavelengths 氦氖激光器；**krypton l.**, a laser with krypton ionized by electric current as the active medium, whose beam is in the yellow-red visible light spectrum; used for photocoagulation 氪激光器；**KTP l.**, one in which a beam generated by a neodymium:YAG laser is directed through a potassium titanyl phosphate crystal to produce a beam in the green visible spectrum; used for photoablation and photocoagulation 磷酸钾钛激光器；**neodymium: yttrium- aluminum-garnet (Nd:YAG) l.**, a laser whose active medium is a crystal of yttrium, aluminum, and garnet doped with neodymium ions, and whose beam is in the near infrared spectrum at 1060 nm; used for photocoagulation and photoablation. 钕：钇铝石榴石激光器；**potassium titanyl phosphate l.**, 同 KTP l.；**pulsed dye l.**, a dye laser in which excitation of the dye by pulses of intense light from a flashlamp produces a beam in the yellow visible light spectrum, with alternating on and off phases of a few microseconds each; used to decolorize pigmented lesions 脉冲 - 染料激光器；**tunable dye l.**, a dye laser whose active medium can be altered so that the beam has any of several wavelengths 可变光谱染料激光器
LASIK　laser-assisted in-situ keratomileusis 准分子激光原位角膜磨镶术
las·si·tude　(las′ĭ-tood) weakness; exhaustion 乏力，衰竭
la·tan·o·prost　(lə-tan′o-prost″) an antiglaucoma agent applied topically to the conjunctiva in the treatment of open-angle glaucoma and ocular hypertension 拉坦前列素（前列腺素类药，治疗青光眼的药物）
la·ten·cy　(la′tən-se) 1. a state of seeming inactivity 潜伏状态；2. the time between the instant of stimulation and the beginning of a response 潜伏期；3. 阶段，时期，见 *stage*
la·tent　(la′tənt) concealed; not manifest; potential; dormant; quiescent 潜伏的，隐蔽的
la·ten·ti·a·tion　(la-ten″she-a′shən) the process of making latent; in pharmacology, chemical modification of a biologically active compound to affect its absorption, distribution, etc., the modified compound being transformed after administration to the active compound by biologic processes 伏化（作用）
lat·er·ad　(lat′ər-ad) toward the lateral aspect 侧向
lat·er·al　(lat′ər-əl) 1. denoting a position farther from the median plane or midline of the body or a structure 侧的，外侧的；2. pertaining to a side 旁边的
lat·er·a·lis　(lat″ər-a′lis) [L.] 同 lateral
lat·er·al·i·ty　(lat″ər-al′ĭ-te) a tendency to use preferentially the organs (hand, foot, ear, eye) of the same side in voluntary motor acts 偏利，偏侧化；**crossed l.**, the preferential use of contralateral members of the different pairs of organs in voluntary motor acts, e.g., right eye and left hand 交叉偏利；**dominant l.**, lateral dominance 同侧偏利
lat·ero·col·lis　(lat″ər-o-kol′is) lateral hyperextension of the neck associated with increased tonicity of the ipsilateral cervical muscles in cervical dystonia 侧颈（颈肌张力障碍中一种与侧颈肌张力增加相关的颈外侧过伸）
lat·ero·dor·sal　(lat″ər-o-dor′səl) denoting a position farther from the median plane or midline and more toward the back surface 侧背面的，侧背的
lat·ero·duc·tion　(lat″ər-o-duk′shən) movement of an eye to either side 侧转，侧展
lat·ero·flex·ion　(lat″ər-o-flek′shən) flexion to one

side 侧屈，旁屈

lat·ero·tor·sion (lat″ər-o-tor′shən) twisting of the vertical meridian of the eye to either side 侧旋，外旋

lat·ero·ver·sion (lat″ər-o-vur′zhən) abnormal turning to one side 侧倾

la·tex (la′teks) a viscid, milky juice secreted by some seed plants（植物）乳汁、胶乳

lath·y·rism (lath′ə-riz-əm) spastic paraplegia, pain, hyperesthesia, and paresthesia due to excessive ingestion of the seeds of leguminous plants of the genus *Lathyrus,* which includes many kinds of peas. 山黧豆中毒；**lathyrit′ic** *adj.*

la·tis·si·mus (lə-tis′ĭ-məs) [L.] widest; in anatomy, denoting a broad structure 最阔的，最广泛的

lat·ro·dec·tism (lat″ro-dek′tiz-əm) intoxication due to venom of spiders of the genus *Latrodectus* 毒蛛中毒

Lat·ro·dec·tus (lat″ro-dek′təs) a genus of poisonous spiders, including *L. mac′tans,* the black widow spider, whose bite may cause severe symptoms or even death 毒蛛属

LATS long-acting thyroid stimulator 长效甲状腺刺激因子

La·tu·da (lə-too′də) trademark for a preparation of lurasidone hydrochloride 盐酸鲁拉西酮的商品名

la·tus[1] (la′təs) [L.] broad, wide 宽的，阔的

la·tus[2] (la′təs) pl. *la′tera* [L.] the side or lateral region 侧；胁腹

lau·rate (law′rāt) a salt, ester, or anionic form of lauric acid 月桂酸盐（酯或阴离子型）

lau·ric ac·id (law′rik) a 12-carbon saturated fatty acid found in many vegetable fats, particularly coconut oil and palm kernel oil 月桂酸

la·vage (lah-vahzh′) 1. the irrigation or washing out of an organ, as of the stomach or bowel 冲洗或灌洗；2. to wash out, or irrigate 洗出，冲洗

lav·en·der (lav′ən-dər) 1. any plant of the genus *Lavandula* 薰衣草；2. a preparation of the flowers of *L. angustifolia* or of the lavender oil extracted from them; used for loss of appetite, dyspepsia, nervousness, and insomnia; also widely used in folk medicine 干薰衣草花，薰衣草油

law (law) a uniform or constant fact or principle 法规，法律，定律；**Allen's l.,** the more sugar a normal person is given the more is utilized; the reverse is true in diabetics 艾伦反常定律；**all-or-none l.,** 全或无定律，见 *all or none;* **Beer's l., Beer-Lambert l.,** in spectrophotometry, the absorbance of a solution is proportional to the concentration of the absorbing solute and to the path length of the light beam through the solution 比 尔定律，比尔－朗伯特定律；**Boyle's l.,** at a constant temperature the volume of a perfect gas varies inversely as the pressure, and the pressure varies inversely as the volume 玻意耳定律；**Charles' l.,** at a constant pressure the volume of a given mass of a perfect gas varies directly with the absolute temperature 查理定律；**l. of conservation of energy,** in any given system the amount of energy is constant; energy is neither created nor destroyed, but only transformed from one form to another 能量守能定律；**l. of conservation of mass, l. of conservation of matter,** mass (or matter) can be neither created nor destroyed; this law can be violated on the microscopic level 质量守恒定律；**Dalton's l.,** the pressure exerted by a mixture of nonreacting gases is equal to the sum of the partial pressures of the separate components; it holds true only at very low pressures 道尔顿定律；**Hellin's l., Hellin-Zeleny l.,** one in about 89 pregnancies ends in the birth of twins; one in 89 × 89 (7921), of triplets; one in 89 × 89 × 89 (704,969), of quadruplets 海林定律；**Henry's l.,** the solubility of a gas in a liquid solution at a constant temperature is proportional to the partial pressure of the gas above the solution 亨利定律；**l. of independent assortment,** genes that are not alleles are distributed to the gametes independently of one another; one of Mendel's laws 自 由 组 合 定 律；**Mendel's l's, mendelian l's,** two laws of inheritance of single-gene traits that form the basis of genetics; the *law of segregation* and the *law of independent assortment* 孟德尔定律；**Nysten's l.,** rigor mortis affects first the muscles of mastication, next those of the face and neck, then those of the trunk and arms, and last those of the legs and feet Nysten 定律；**Ohm's l.,** the strength of an electric current varies directly as the electromotive force and inversely as the resistance 欧姆定律；**Raoult's l.,** the vapor pressure of a volatile component of an ideal solution is equal to the mole fraction of that substance in solution times its vapor pressure in the pure state at the temperature of the solution; it is true only for ideal solutions and ideal gases 拉乌耳定律；**l. of segregation,** the members of a pair of allelic genes segregate from one another and pass to different gametes; one of Mendel's laws 分离定律；孟德尔第一定律；**l. of similars,** in homeopathy, the principle that a substance that in large doses will produce symptoms of a specific disease will, in extremely small doses, cure it 类似定律；**l's of thermodynamics,** *Zeroth law:* two systems in thermal equilibrium with a third are in thermal equilibrium with each other. *First law:* energy is conserved in any process. *Second law:* there is always an increase in entropy in any naturally occurring (spontaneous) process.*Third law:*absolute zero is unattainable 热力学定律

lax·a·tive (lak′sə-tiv) 1. mildly cathartic 缓泻药; 2. a cathartic or purgative 泻药; **bulk l.**, **bulk-forming l.**, one promoting bowel evacuation by increasing fecal volume 容积性泻药; **contact l.**, one that increases the motor activity of the intestinal tract 接触性泻药; **lubricant l.**, one that promotes softening of the stool and facilitates passage of the feces through the intestines by its lubricant effect 润滑性泻药; **saline l.**, a salt administered in hypertonic solution to draw water into the intestinal lumen by osmosis, distending it and promoting peristalsis and evacuation 盐类泻药; **stimulant l.**, contact l. 刺激性泻药

lax·i·ty (lak′sĭ-te) 1. slackness or looseness; a lack of tautness, firmness, or rigidity 松弛，松懈; 2. slackness or displacement in the motion of a joint 关节运动中的松弛或移位; **lax** *adj.*

lay·er (la′ər) 1. a sheetlike mass of substance of nearly uniform thickness, several of which may be superimposed, one above another 层; 2. a female bird of the age when it is laying eggs 产蛋禽; **ameloblastic l.**, the inner layer of cells of the enamel organ, which forms the enamel prisms of the teeth 成釉细胞层; **bacillary l.**, 同 l. of rods and cones; **basal l.**, stratum basale 基底层; **basal cell l.**, the stratum basale of the epidermis 基底细胞层，表皮生发层; **blastodermic l.**, 同 germ l.; **l's of cerebral cortex**, six anatomic divisions (I to Ⅵ) of the cerebral cortex (specifically the neocortex), distinguished according to the types of cells and fibers they contain 大脑皮质; **clear l.**, stratum lucidum 透明层; **columnar l.**, mantle l. 柱状层; **enamel l.**, either of two walls, the inner concave wall or the outer convex wall, of the enamel organ 釉质层; **functional l. of endometrium**, stratum functionale 子宫内膜功能层; **ganglionic l. of cerebellum,** 同 Purkinje l.; **germ l.**, any of the three primary layers of cells of the embryo (ectoderm, endoderm, and mesoderm), from which the tissues and organs develop 胚层; **germinative l.**, stratum germinativum（组织）生发层; **granular l.**, 1. stratum granulosum 颗粒层; 2. the deep layer of the cortex of the cerebellum 小脑皮质深层; **half-value l.**, the thickness of a given substance that, when introduced in the path of a given beam of rays, will reduce its intensity by one-half 半价层; **Henle l.**, the outermost layer of the inner root sheath of the hair follicle 亨勒层（内根鞘的最外层）; **horny l.**, stratum corneum 角质层; **malpighian l.**, stratum germinativum 生发层; **mantle l.**, the mid-

dle layer of the wall of the primordial neural tube, containing primordial nerve cells and later forming the gray matter of the central nervous system 套层; **marginal l.**, the outermost layer of the wall of the primordial neural tube, a fibrous mesh into which the nerve fibers later grow, forming the white matter of the central nervous system 边缘层; **odontoblastic l.**, the epithelioid layer of odontoblasts in contact with the dentin of teeth 成牙质细胞层; **prickle cell l.**, stratum spinosum 棘（细胞）层; **Purkinje l.**, the layer of Purkinje neurons situated internal to the molecular layer and external to the granular layer of the cerebellar cortex 浦肯野细胞层; **l. of rods and cones,** a layer of the retina, located between the pigmented part and the external limiting membrane, containing the sensory elements, the rods and cones 视杆视锥层; **spinous l.**, stratum spinosum 棘层; **subendocardial l.**, the layer of loose fibrous tissue uniting the endocardium and myocardium and containing the vessels and nerves of the conducting system of the heart 心内膜下层; **subepicardial l.,** the layer of loose connective tissue uniting the epicardium and myocardium 心外膜下层

lb [L.] pound (L. *libra*) 磅

LBBB left bundle branch block 左束支传导阻滞; *block* 下 *bundle branch block*

LCAT lecithin-cholesterol acyltransferase 卵磷脂 - 胆固醇酰基转移酶

LCIS lobular carcinoma in situ 原位小叶癌

LD$_{50}$ median lethal dose 半数致死量

LDH l-lactate dehydrogenase 乳酸脱氢酶

LDL low-density lipoprotein 低密度脂蛋白

LDL-C low-density-lipoprotein cholesterol 低密度脂蛋白胆固醇

L-dopa (el″do′pə) 同 levodopa

LE left eye 左眼; lupus erythematosus 红斑狼疮

lead^1 (Pb) (led) a soft, grayish blue, heavy metal element with poisonous salts; at. no. 82, at. wt. 207.2. Absorption or ingestion causes poisoning, which affects the brain, nervous and digestive systems, and blood 铅

lead^2 (l ē d) any of the conductors connected to the electrocardiograph, each comprising two or more electrodes that are attached at specific body sites and used to examine electrical activity by monitoring changes in the electrical potential between them 导联，导程; **l. I**, the standard bipolar limb lead attached to the right and left arms 心电图 I 导联，即左右臂; **l. II**, the standard bipolar limb lead attached to the right arm and left leg 心电图 II 导联，即右臂左腿; **l. III**, the standard bipolar limb lead attached to the left arm and left leg 心电图Ⅲ导联，即左臂左腿; **augmented unipolar limb l.**, a mod-

L

ified unipolar limb lead; the three standard leads are aVF (left leg), aVL (left arm), and aVR (right arm) 加压单极肢体导联；aV_F l., an augmented unipolar limb lead in which the positive electrode is on the left leg aV_F 导联；aV_L l., an augmented unipolar limb lead in which the positive electrode is on the left arm aV_L 导联；aV_R l., an augmented unipolar limb lead in which the positive electrode is on the right arm aV_R 导联；**bipolar l.,** an array involving two electrodes placed at different body sites 双极导联；**limb l.,** an array in which any registering electrodes are attached to limbs 肢体导联；**pacemaker l., pacing l.,** the connection between the heart and the power source of an artificial cardiac pacemaker 起搏器导联；**precordial l's,** leads in which the exploring electrode is placed on the chest and the other is connected to one or more limbs; usually used to denote one of the V leads 心前导联；**standard l's,** the 12 leads used in a standard electrocardiogram, comprising the standard bipolar limb leads Ⅰ to Ⅲ, the augmented unipolar limb leads, and the standard precordial leads 标准导联；**unipolar l.,** an array of two electrodes, only one of which transmits potential variation 单极导联；**V l's,** the series of six standard unipolar leads in which the exploring electrode is attached to the chest, designated V_1 to V_6 胸导联，包括 V_1 到 V_6 导联；**XYZ l's,** leads used in one system of spatial vectorcardiography XYZ 导联

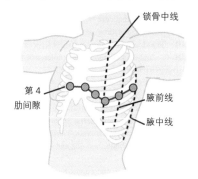

锁骨中线

第 4
肋间隙

腋前线

腋中线

▲ 胸导联 (V_1~V_6) 的位置

learn·ing (lur′ning) a long-lasting adaptive behavioral change due to experience 学 习；学 问，知识；**latent l.,** that which occurs without reinforcement, becoming apparent only when a reinforcement or reward is introduced 潜伏学习

lec·i·thal (les′ĭ-thəl) having a yolk; used especially as a word termination (*isolecithal,* etc.) 卵黄的

lec·i·thin (les′ĭ-thin) phosphatidylcholine 卵磷脂，磷脂酰胆碱

lec·i·thin–cho·les·ter·ol ac·yl·trans·fer·ase (LCAT) (les′ĭ-thin kə-les′tər-ol ə″səl-trans′fər- ās) an enzyme that catalyzes the formation of cholesteryl esters in high-density lipoproteins; deficiency of enzyme activity, an inherited disorder, results in accumulation of cholesterol and phosphatidylcholine in plasma and tissues, which causes corneal opacities, anemia, and often proteinuria 卵磷脂－胆固醇酰基转移酶

lec·tin (lek′tin) any of a group of hemagglutinating proteins found primarily in plant seeds, which bind specifically to the branching sugar molecules of glycoproteins and glycolipids on the surface of cells（植物）凝集素

le·dip·as·vir (lĕ-dip′as-veer) an antiviral inhibitor of the nonstructural protein 5A replication complex; it is used in combination therapy to treat hepatitis C virus 一种抗丙型肝炎病毒药

leech (lēch) any of the annelids of the class Hirudinea, especially *Hirudo medicinalis;* some species are bloodsuckers. Leeches have been used for drawing blood 水蛭，蚂蟥

le·flu·no·mide (lə-floo′no-mīd) an immunomodulator used in treatment of rheumatoid arthritis 来氟米特（一种抗类风湿关节炎的免疫调节剂）

leg (leg) 1. the part of the lower limb between the knee and ankle 小腿；2. in common usage, the entire lower limb, with the part below the knee being called the *lower leg* 下肢，包括小腿；3. any of the four limbs of a quadruped 四足动物的四肢；**bandy l.,** 同 bowleg；**bayonet l.,** ankylosis of the knee after backward displacement of the tibia and fibula 枪刺形腿；**bow l.,** 膝内翻，弓形腿，见 *bowleg*；**restless l's,** a disagreeable, creeping, irritating sensation in the legs, usually the lower legs, relieved only by walking or keeping the legs moving 多动腿；**scissor l.,** deformity with crossing of the legs in walking 剪形腿

Le·gio·nel·la (le″jə-nel′ə) a genus of gramnegative, aerobic, rod-shaped bacteria of the family Legionellaceae, normal inhabitants of lakes, streams, and moist soil; they have often been isolated from cooling-tower water, evaporative condensers, tap water, shower heads, and treated sewage. *L. micda'dei* causes Pittsburgh pneumonia. *L. pneumo'phila* causes legionnaires' disease 军团菌属

Le·gio·nel·la·ceae (le″jə-nel-a′se-e) a family of gram-negative, aerobic, non–spore-forming, rod-shaped bacteria of the order Legionellales 军团菌科

Le·gio·nel·la·les (le″jə-nel-a′-lēz) an order of bacteria of the class Gammaproteobacteria, whose members are intracellular parasites 军团菌目

le·gion·el·lo·sis (le″jə-nel-o′sis) disease caused by infection with *Legionella pneumophila;* see *legion-*

naires' disease and *Pontiac fever* 军团菌病

le·gume (leg'ūm) (lə-gūm') 1. any plant of the large family Leguminosae 豆科植物; 2. the pod or fruit of one of these plants, such as a pea or bean 豆荚, 豆

leio·myo·fi·bro·ma (li″o-mi″o-fi-bro′mə) leiomyoma 平滑肌纤维瘤

leio·myo·ma (li″o-mi-o′mə) a benign tumor derived from smooth muscle 平滑肌瘤; l. cu'tis, one or more smooth, firm, painful, often waxy nodules arising from cutaneous or subcutaneous smooth muscle fibers 皮肤平滑肌瘤; epithelioid l., leiomyoma, usually of the stomach, in which the cells are polygonal rather than spindle shaped 上皮样平滑肌瘤; l. u'teri, uterine l., leiomyoma of the uterus, the most common of all tumors found in women; it is usually in the body of the organ but may be elsewhere 子宫平滑肌瘤

leio·my·o·ma·to·sis (li″o-mi″o-mə-to′sis) the occurrence of multiple leiomyomas throughout the body 平滑肌瘤病

leio·myo·sar·co·ma (li″o-mi″o-sahr-ko′mə) a sarcoma containing spindle cells of smooth muscle 平滑肌肉瘤

Leish·ma·nia (lēsh-ma′ne-ə) a genus of parasitic protozoa, including several species pathogenic for humans; divided into two subgenera, *Leishmania* and *Viannia,* based on development in the sandfly vector; with species in the latter restricted to the New World. Species and complexes have been distinguished on the basis of geographic origin, clinical syndrome produced, and ecologic characteristics, or on the basis of association with specific leishmaniases, but increasingly are separated by phylogenetic relationships. Important pathogenic species include *L. donova'ni, L. infantum, L. ma'jor, L. tro'pica, L. mexica'na,* and *L. brazilien'sis* 利什曼原虫属; **leishma'nial** *adj.*

leish·ma·ni·a·sis (lēsh″mə-ni′ə-sis) infection with *Leishmania* 利什曼病; cutaneous l., any of the types that have cutaneous symptoms, often disfiguring; distinguished as either the *Old World* form caused mainly by *Leishmania major, L. tropica,* or *L. aethiopica* and the *New World* form caused mainly by *L. mexicana, L. amazonensis,* or *L. braziliensis* 皮肤利什曼病; **diffuse cutaneous l.,** a variant of cutaneous leishmaniasis in which a localized, nonulcerative lesion disseminates to form multiple cutaneous nodules or plaques resistant to treatment; usually occurring in immunocompromised patients and associated with *Leishmania amazonensis, L. mexicana,* or *L. aethiopica* 弥漫性皮肤利什曼病; **mucocutaneous l.,** a form in which a primary cuta-neous lesion is followed by secondary mucosal involvement, causing widespread destruction of tissue with marked deformity; occurring in the New World and usually caused by *Leishmania braziliensis* 黏膜皮肤利什曼病; **post-kala-azar dermal l.,** a condition associated with visceral leishmaniasis, characterized by hypopigmented or erythematous macules on the face and sometimes also the trunk and limbs, the facial lesions progressing to papules and nodules resembling those of lepromatous leprosy; usually caused by *Leishmania donovani* 黑热病后皮肤利什曼病; **l. reci'divans,** a prolonged, relapsing form of cutaneous leishmaniasis resembling lupus vulgaris; usually caused by *Leishmania tropica* in the Old World and occasionally by *L. braziliensis* in the New World 复发性利什曼病; **visceral l.,** a chronic infectious disease, highly fatal if untreated, caused by *Leishmania donovani,* characterized by hepatosplenomegaly, fever, chills, vomiting, anemia, leukopenia, hypergammaglobulinemia, and a gray color to the skin 黑热病, 内脏利什曼病

lem·mo·blas·tic (lem″o-blas′tik) forming or developing into neurilemma tissue 成神经膜的

lem·nis·cus (lem-nis′kəs) pl. *lemnis'ci* [L.] 1. a ribbon or band 带, 系带; 2. a band or bundle of fibers in the central nervous system 丘系, 蹄系

length (l) (length) the longest dimension of an object, or of the measurement between the two ends 长, 长度; **crown-heel l. (CHL),** the distance from the crown of the head to the heel in embryos, fetuses, and infants; the equivalent of standing height in older persons 冠－踵长; **crown-rump l. (CRL),** the distance from the crown of the head to the breech in embryos, fetuses, and infants; the equivalent of sitting height in older persons 冠－臀长; **focal l.,** the distance between a lens and an object from which all rays of light are brought to a focus 焦距

lens (lenz) 1. a piece of glass or other transparent material so shaped as to converge or scatter light rays 透镜, 镜片, 另见 *glasses*; 2. crystalline l.; the transparent, biconvex body separating the posterior chamber and vitreous body, and constituting part of the refracting mechanism of the eye 晶状体, 见图30; **achromatic l.,** a lens corrected for chromatic aberration 消色差透镜; **aplanatic l.,** one for correcting spherical aberrations 消球(面)差透镜; **bandage l.,** a soft contact lens worn on a diseased or injured cornea to protect or treat it 绷带透镜; **biconcave l.,** one concave on both faces 双凹透镜; **biconvex l.,** one convex on both faces 双凸透镜; **bifocal l.,** one with two parts of different refracting powers, the upper for distant and the lower for near vision 双焦点透镜; **concavoconvex l,** one with one concave and one convex face 凹凸透镜；**contact l.**, a curved shell of glass or plastic applied directly over the globe or cornea to correct refractive errors. It may be a *soft (hydrophilic) contact l.*, flexible and water absorbent, or a *hard (hydrophobic) contact l.*, rigid and not water absorbent; the latter type is subdivided into gas permeable and non–gas permeable, usually polymethylmethacrylate (PMMA), lenses 接触镜；**convexoconcave l.**, one with one convex and one concave face 凸凹透镜；**crystalline l.**, 同 lens (2)；**cylindrical l. (C)**, one for correcting astigmatism, with one plane surface and one cylindrical, or one spherical surface and one toroidal 柱面透镜；**decentered l.**, one whose optical axis does not pass through the center 轴偏透镜；**honeybee l.**, a magnifying lens resembling the multifaceted eye of the honeybee, consisting of three or six small telescopes mounted in the upper part of the lens and directed toward the center and right and left visual fields. Prisms are included to provide a continuous, unbroken magnified field of view 蜜蜂透镜；**omnifocal l.**, one whose power increases continuously and regularly in a downward direction, avoiding the discontinuity of bifocal and trifocal lenses 全焦距透镜；**planoconvex l.**, a lens with one plane and one convex side 平凸透镜；**spherical l. (S) (sph)**, one that is a segment of a sphere 球面透镜；**trial l.**, one used to test vision 试镜片；**trifocal l.**, one with three parts of different refracting powers, the upper for distant, the middle for intermediate, and the lower for near vision 三焦点镜片

len·ti·co·nus (len″ti-ko′nəs) a congenital conical bulging, anteriorly or posteriorly, of the lens of the eye 圆锥形晶状体

len·tic·u·lar (len-tik′u-lər) 1. pertaining to or shaped like a lens 透镜的；2. pertaining to the lens of the eye 晶状体的；3. pertaining to the lenticular nucleus 豆状核的

len·ti·form (len″tī-form) lens-shaped 透镜状的

len·tig·i·nes (len-tij′ĭ-nēz) *lentigo* 的复数

len·tig·i·no·sis (len-tij″ĭ-no′sis) a condition marked by multiple lentigines 雀斑样痣病，着色斑病；**progressive cardiomyopathic l.**, multiple symmetric lentigines, hypertrophic obstructive cardiomyopathy, and retarded growth, sometimes with intellectual disability 进行性心肌病变性着色斑病

len·ti·glo·bus (len″tī-glo′bəs) exaggerated curvature of the lens of the eye, producing an anterior spherical bulging 球形晶状体

len·ti·go (len-ti′go) pl. *lentig′ines* [L.] a flat brownish pigmented spot on the skin, due to increased deposition of melanin and an increased number of melanocytes 雀斑痣；**l. malig′na**, a circumscribed macular patch of hyperpigmentation, with shades of brown or black, that enlarges slowly and may be a precursor to malignant melanoma 恶性雀斑样痣；**senile l.**, **l. seni′lis**, solar l. 老年性雀斑样痣；**l. sim′plex**, the most common type, found on mucous membranes and skin, usually associated with a congenital syndrome 单纯性雀斑痣；**solar l.**, a benign, discrete type found on chronically sun-exposed skin in lightskinned adults, such as the forehead or back of the hand 日光性黑子

Len·ti·vi·rus (len′tĭ-vi″rəs) a genus of viruses of the family Retroviridae that cause persistent infection that typically results in chronic, progressive, sometimes fatal disease; it includes the human immunodeficiency viruses 慢病毒属，属于逆转录病毒科

len·ti·vi·rus (len′tĭ-vi″rəs) any virus of the subfamily Lentivirinae 慢病毒

le·on·ti·a·sis (le″on-ti′ə-sis) leonine facies 狮面；**l. os′sea, l. os′sium**, leonine facies due to hypertrophy of the bones of the cranium and face 骨性狮面

lep·er (lep′ər) a person with leprosy; a term now in disfavor 麻风患者；别人避之唯恐不及的人

Lep·i·o·ta (lep″e-o′tə) a genus of mushrooms with many toxic species; some cause only mild gastrointestinal symptoms, while others contain potentially lethal hepatotoxic amatoxins 环柄菇属

lep·i·ru·din (lep″ĭ-roo′din) a recombinant form of hirudin used as an anticoagulant in patients with heparin-induced thrombocytopenia 重组水蛭素，来匹芦定（抗血栓药）

lep·ra (lep′rə) 同 leprosy

lep·re·chaun·ism (lep′rə-kon″iz-əm) Donohue syndrome 矮妖精貌综合征

lep·ro·ma (ləp-ro′mə) a superficial granulomatous nodule rich in *Mycobacterium leprae, the* characteristic lesion of lepromatous leprosy 麻风结节

lep·ro·ma·tous (ləp-ro′mə-təs) pertaining to or containing lepromas 麻风结节的；见 *leprosy* 下的 *lepromatous leprosy*

lep·ro·min (lep′ro-min) a repeatedly boiled, autoclaved, gauze-filtered suspension of finely triturated lepromatous tissue and leprosy bacilli, used in the skin test for tissue resistance to leprosy 麻风菌素

lep·ro·stat·ic (lep″ro-stat′ik) inhibiting the growth of *Mycobacterium leprae,* or an agent that so acts 抑制麻风菌的，抗麻风药

lep·ro·sy (lep′rə-se) a chronic communicable disease caused by *Mycobacterium leprae* and characterized by the production of granulomatous lesions of the skin, mucous membranes, and peripheral nervous system. Two principal, or polar, types are recognized: lepromatous and tuberculoid 麻风；**leprot′ic, lep′rous** *adj.*；**lepromatous l.**, that form marked by the development of lepromas and by an abundance of leprosy bacilli from the onset; nerve damage occurs only slowly, and the skin reaction to lepromin is negative. It is the only form that regularly serves as a source of infection 瘤型麻风; **tuberculoid l.,** the form in which leprosy bacilli are few or lacking and nerve damage occurs early, so that all skin lesions are denervated from the onset, often with dissociation of sensation; the skin reaction to lepromin is positive, and the patient is rarely a source of infection to others 结核样麻风

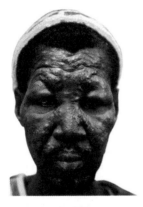

▲ 麻风

lep·to·ceph·a·lus (lep″to-sef′ə-ləs) a person with an abnormally tall, narrow skull 狭长头者

lep·to·cyte (lep′to-sīt) target cell (1) 薄红细胞

lep·to·me·nin·ges (lep″to-mə-nin′jēz) sing. *leptome′ninx.* The pia mater and arachnoid mater taken together; the pia-arachnoid 软脑（脊）膜，软脑膜; **leptomenin′geal** *adj.*

lep·to·me·nin·gi·tis (lep″to-men″in-ji′tis) inflammation of the leptomeninges 软脑膜炎

lep·to·men·in·gop·a·thy (lep″to-men″ingop′ə-the) any disease of the leptomeninges 软脑（脊）膜病

lep·to·mo·nad (lep″to-mo′nad) of or pertaining to *Leptomonas* 细滴虫，细滴虫属的

Lep·to·mo·nas (lep″to-mo′nəs) a genus of protozoa of the family Trypanosomatidae, parasitic in the digestive tract of insects 细滴虫属

lep·to·mo·nas (lep″to-mo′nəs) any protozoan of the genus *Leptomonas* 细滴虫

lep·to·pel·lic (lep″to-pel′ik) having a narrow pelvis 狭骨盆的

Lep·to·spi·ra (lep″to-spi′rə) a genus of aerobic spirochete bacteria of the family Leptospiraceae; all pathogenic strains (i.e., those that cause leptospi-

rosis) are contained in the species *L. inter′rogans,* which is divided into several serogroups, which are in turn divided into serovars 钩端螺旋体属

lep·to·spi·ra (lep″to-spi′rə) an individual organism belonging to the genus *Leptospira* 钩端螺旋体; **leptospi′ral** *adj.*

Lep·to·spi·ra·ceae (lep″to-spi-ra′se-e) a family of aerobic bacteria of the order Spirochaetales, consisting of flexible helical cells 钩端螺旋体科

lep·to·spi·ro·sis (lep″to-spi-ro′sis) any infectious disease due to a serovar of *Leptospira interrogans,* manifested by lymphocytic meningitis, hepatitis, and nephritis, separately or in combination; types vary in severity from a mild carrier state to fatal disease 钩端螺旋体病

lep·to·tene (lep′to-tēn) the first stage of prophase in meiosis I, in which the chromosomes are threadlike 细线期

les·bi·an (lez′be-ən) 1. pertaining to homosexuality between women 女性同性恋的; 2. a female homosexual 女同性恋者

les·bi·an·ism (lez′be-ən-iz″əm) homosexuality between women. 女性同性恋

le·sion (le′zhən) any pathologic or traumatic discontinuity of tissue or loss of function of a part 病变，损伤; **angiocentric immunoproliferative l.,** a multisystem disease consisting of invasion and destruction of body tissues and structures by atypical lymphocytoid and plasmacytoid cells resembling a lymphoma, often progresssing to lymphoma 血管中心性免疫增生性病损; **Armanni-Ebstein l.,** vacuolization of the renal tubular epithelium in diabetes 阿-埃二氏病变（糖尿病患者肾小管上皮的空泡化）; **benign lymphoepithelial l.,** enlargement of salivary glands with infiltration of parenchyma by polyclonal B and T cells, atrophy of acini, and formation of lymphoepithelial islands 良性淋巴上皮病变; **Blumenthal l.,** a proliferative vascular lesion in the smaller arteries in diabetes Blumenthal 病变（糖尿病患者小动脉增生性血管损害）; **bull's-eye l.,** 1. a shadow seen on a radiogram, usually of the duodenal wall, with a dark circle surrounding a central light circle; it represents tumor metastasis in which a mass has central ulceration 牛眼征; 2. 同 target l. (3); **central l.,** any lesion of the central nervous system 中枢性损害; **Ghon primary l.,** Ghon focus 高恩原发病损（肺原发结核病灶）; **Janeway l.,** a small erythematous or hemorrhagic lesion, usually on the palms or soles, in bacterial endocarditis Janeway 病变（细菌性心内膜炎患者出现的小红斑或出血性病变，通常在手掌或脚掌）; **Kimmelstiel-Wilson l.,** a microscopic, spherical, hyaline mass surrounded by capillaries, found in the

L

kidney glomerulus in the nodular form of intercapillary glomerulosclerosis Kimmelstiel-Wilson 病变（肾小球硬化症患者肾小球毛细血管间出现硬化的球状玻璃样物质）; **primary l.**, the original lesion manifesting a disease, as a chancre 原发病灶，原发性损害; **skip l.**, a lesion that is discontinuous; the most common occurrence is in two different segments of intestine affected by inflammatory bowel disease 跳跃性病变; **target l.**, 1. 同 bull's-eye lesion; 2. a small, circumscribed focus of necrosis with a gray center surrounded by erythema, seen in the lungs in invasive aspergillosis 侵袭性曲霉菌病时肺部出现的局限性坏死性小病灶; 3. a skin lesion characteristic of erythema multiforme, having a central bulla or crust surrounded by concentric zones of changed colors 靶形红斑

le·thal (le'thəl) fatal 致死的

leth·ar·gy (leth'ər-je) 1. a lowered level of consciousness, with drowsiness, listlessness, and apathy 嗜睡，昏睡; 2. a condition of indifference 呆滞

let·ro·zole (let'rah-zōl) an antineoplastic used in the treatment of advanced breast cancer in postmenopausal women 来曲唑（抗肿瘤药）

Leu 同 leucine

leu·cine (Leu, L) (loo'sēn) an essential amino acid necessary for optimal growth in infants and for nitrogen equilibrium in adults 亮氨酸

leu·co·vo·rin (loo″ko-vo'rin) folinic acid; the calcium salt is used as an antidote for folic acid antagonists, e.g., methotrexate, and in the treatment of megaloblastic anemias due to folic acid deficiency and colorectal carcinoma 甲酰四氢叶酸

leu·ka·phe·re·sis (loo″kə-fə-re'sis) the selective separation and removal of leukocytes from withdrawn blood, the remainder of the blood then being retransfused into the donor 白细胞清除术，白细胞去除术

leu·ke·mia (loo-ke'me-ə) a progressive, malignant disease of the blood-forming organs, marked by distorted proliferation and development of leukocytes and their precursors in the blood and bone marrow 白血病; **leuke'mic** *adj.*; **acute l.**, leukemia in which the involved cell line shows little or no differentiation, usually consisting of blast cells; it comprises two types, acute lymphocytic leukemia and acute myelogenous leukemia 急性白血病; **acute granulocytic l.**, acute myelogenous l. 急性粒细胞白血病; **acute lymphoblastic l. (ALL), acute lymphocytic l.**, one of the two major categories of acute leukemia, characterized by anemia, fatigue, weight loss; easy bruising, thrombocytopenia, granulocytopenia with bacterial infections, bone pain, lymphadenopathy, hepatosplenomegaly, and

sometimes spread to the central nervous system. It is subclassified on the basis of the surface antigens expressed, e.g., *B-cell type, T-cell type* 急性淋巴细胞白血病; **acute megakaryoblastic l., acute megakaryocytic l.**, a form of acute myelogenous leukemia in which megakaryocytes are predominant and platelets are increased in the blood 急性巨核细胞白血病; **acute monocytic l.**, an uncommon form of acute myelogenous leukemia in which the predominating cells are monocytes 急性单核细胞白血病; **acute myeloblastic l.**, 1. a common type of acute myelogenous leukemia in which myeloblasts predominate; it is divided into two types on the basis of degree of cell differentiation 急性髓母细胞白血病; 2. acute myelogenous l.; **acute myelocytic l.**, 同 acute myelogenous l.; **acute myelogenous l. (AML)**, one of the two major categories of acute leukemia, with symptoms including anemia, fatigue, weight loss, easy bruising, thrombocytopenia, and granulocytopenia 急性髓细胞性白血病; **acute myelomonocytic l.**, a common type of acute myelogenous leukemia, with both malignant monocytes and monoblasts 急性髓单核细胞白血病; **acute promyelocytic l.**, acute myelogenous leukemia in which more than half the cells are malignant promyelocytes 急性早幼粒细胞白血病; **acute undifferentiated l. (AUL)**, acute myelogenous leukemia in which the predominating cell is so immature it cannot be classified 急性未分化细胞白血病; **adult T-cell l./lymphoma (ATL)**, an adult onset, subacute or chronic malignancy of mature T lymphocytes, believed to be caused by human lymphotropic virus type I 成人 T 细胞性白血病; **aleukemic l.**, a form in which the total white blood cell count in the peripheral blood is not elevated; it may be lymphocytic, monocytic, or myelogenous 非白血性白血病，白细胞不增多性白血病; **basophilic l.**, leukemia in which the basophilic leukocytes predominate 嗜碱性粒细胞性白血病; **chronic l.**, leukemia in which the involved cell line is well differentiated, usually made up of B lymphocytes, but immunologically incompetent 慢性白血病; **chronic granulocytic l.**, 同 chronic myelogenous l. 慢性粒细胞白血病; **chronic lymphocytic l. (CLL)**, chronic leukemia of the lymphoblastic type, characterized by lymphadenopathy, fatigue, renal involvement, and pulmonary leukemic infiltrates 慢性淋巴细胞白血病; **chronic myelocytic l., chronic myelogenous l., chronic myeloid l.**, chronic leukemia of the myeloid type, usually associated with the Philadelphia chromosome abnormality and occurring in adulthood 慢性粒细胞白血病，慢性髓细胞性白血病; **chronic myelomonocytic l.**, a chronic, slowly progressing form characterized by malignant monocytes and myeloblasts, splenomegaly, and thrombocytopenia 慢性粒 - 单核细胞白血病；**l. cu′tis**, a cutaneous manifestation of leukemia resulting from infiltration of the skin by malignant leukocytes 皮肤白血病；**eosinophilic l.**, a form in which eosinophils are the predominating cells 嗜酸粒细胞白血病；**granulocytic l.**, myelogenous l. 粒细胞性白血病；**hairy cell l.**, chronic leukemia marked by splenomegaly and an abundance of large, mononuclear abnormal cells with numerous irregular cytoplasmic projections that give them a flagellated or hairy appearance in the bone marrow, spleen, liver, and peripheral blood 毛细胞白血病；**lymphatic l., lymphoblastic l., lymphocytic l.**, a form associated with hyperplasia and overactivity of the lymphoid tissue, with increased levels of circulating malignant lymphocytes or lymphoblasts 淋巴细胞白血病；**lymphogenous l., lymphoid l.**, 同 lymphatic l.；**lymphosarcoma cell l.**, (B-cell type) acute lymphoblastic l. 急性 B 淋巴（母）细胞白血病；**mast cell l.**, a rare form marked by overwhelming numbers of tissue mast cells in the peripheral blood 肥大细胞白血病；**megakaryoblastic l.**, 同 acute megakaryocytic l.；**megakaryocytic l.**, 1. 同 acute megakaryocytic l.；2. hemorrhagic thrombocythemia 出血性血小板增多症；**micromyeloblastic l.**, a form of myelogenous leukemia in which the immature nucleoli-containing cells are small and similar to lymphocytes 小原粒细胞性白血病；**monocytic l.**, acute monocytic l. 单核细胞性白血病；**myeloblastic l.**, 1. myelogenous l. 髓母细胞性白血病；2. 同 acute myeloblastic l.；**myelocytic l., myelogenous l., myeloid granulocytic l.**, a form arising from myeloid tissue in which the granular polymorphonuclear leukocytes and their precursors predominate 髓性白血病；另见 *acute myelogenous l.* 和 *chronic myelogenous l.* myelomonocytic l., acute myelomonocytic l. 慢性骨髓单核细胞性白血病；**plasma cell l.**, a form in which the predominating cell in the peripheral blood is the plasma cell 浆细胞白血病；**promyelocytic l.**, acute promyelocytic l. 早幼粒细胞白血病；**stem cell l.**, acute undifferentiated l. 干细胞白血病

leu·ke·mid (loo-ke′mid) any of the polymorphic skin eruptions associated with leukemia; clinically, they may be nonspecific (i.e., papular, macular, purpuric), but histopathologically they may represent true leukemic infiltrations 白血病疹

leu·ke·mo·gen (loo-ke′mo-jən) any substance that produces leukemia 致白血病物质；**leukemogen′ic** *adj.*

leu·ke·moid (loo-ke′moid) exhibiting blood and

sometimes clinical findings resembling those of leukemia, but due to some other cause 白血病样的

leu·kin (loo′kin) a bactericidal substance from leukocyte extract 白细胞素，白细胞溶菌素

leu·ko·ag·glu·ti·nin (loo″ko-ə-gloo′tĭ-nin) an agglutinin that acts upon leukocytes 白细胞凝集素

leu·ko·blas·to·sis (loo″ko-blas-to′sis) abnormal proliferation of leukocytes, as seen in leukemia 白细胞组织增生

leu·ko·ci·din (loo″ko-si′din) a substance produced by some pathogenic bacteria that is toxic to polymorphonuclear leukocytes (neutrophils) 杀白细胞素

leu·ko·cyte (loo′ko-sīt) white cell, white blood cell; a colorless blood corpuscle capable of ameboid movement the chief function of which is to protect the body against microorganisms causing disease and which may be classified in two main groups: *granular* and *nongranular* 白细胞，白血球；**leukocy′tal, leukocyt′ic** *adj.*；**agranular l.**, 同 nongranular l.；**basophilic l.**, basophil 嗜碱性粒细胞；**eosinophilic l.**, eosinophil 嗜酸性粒细胞；**granular l.**, granulocyte; a leukocyte containing abundant granules in the cytoplasm, such as a neutrophil, eosinophil, or basophil 粒细胞；**neutrophilic l.**, neutrophil (1) 嗜中性粒细胞；**nongranular l.**, a leukocyte without specific granules in the cytoplasm, such as a lymphocyte or monocyte 无粒白细胞

leu·ko·cy·to·gen·e·sis (loo″ko-si″to-jen′ə-sis) 同 leukopoiesis

leu·ko·cy·tol·y·sis (loo″ko-si-tol′ə-sis) 同 leukolysis；**leukocytolyt′ic** *adj.*

leu·ko·cy·to·ma (loo″ko-si-to′mə) a tumorlike mass of leukocytes 白细胞瘤

leu·ko·cy·to·pe·nia (loo″ko-si″to-pe′ne-ə) 同 leukopenia

leu·ko·cy·to·pla·nia (loo″ko-si″to-pla′ne-ə) wandering of leukocytes; passage of leukocytes through a membrane 白细胞游出

leu·ko·cy·to·poi·e·sis (loo″ko-si″to-poi-e′sis) 同 leukopoiesis

leu·ko·cy·to·sis (loo″ko-si-to′sis) a transient increase in the number of leukocytes in the blood, due to various causes 白细胞增多；**basophilic l.**, basophilia (1) 嗜碱性白细胞增多；**eosinophilic l.**, eosinophilia 嗜酸性粒细胞增多；**mononuclear l.**, mononucleosis 单核细胞增多；**neutrophilic l.**, neutrophilia 中性粒细胞增多；**pathologic l.**, that due to some morbid condition, such as infection or trauma 病理性白细胞增多；**physiologic l.**, that due to a nonpathologic condition such as strenuous exercise 生理性白细胞增多

leu·ko·cy·to·sper·mia (loo″ko-si″to-spur′me-ə)

L

excessive leukocytes in the seminal fluid 白细胞精液症

leu·ko·cy·to·tax·is (loo″ko-si″to-tak′sis) 同 leukotaxis

leu·ko·cy·to·tox·ic·i·ty (loo″ko-si″to-tok-sis′ĭ- te) lymphocytotoxicity 白细胞毒性

leu·ko·der·ma (loo″ko-dur′mə) an acquired condition with localized loss of pigmentation of the skin 白斑病；**syphilitic l.**, indistinct coarsely mottled hypopigmentation, usually on the sides of the neck, in late secondary syphilis 梅毒性白斑病

leu·ko·dys·tro·phy (loo″ko-dis′trə-fe) disturbance of the white substance of the brain 脑白质营养不良；另见 *leukoencephalopathy*；**adult-onset demyelinating l.**, an inherited leukoencephalopathy characterized by progressive degeneration of the white matter, with motor disturbances, bowel and bladder incontinence, and orthostatic hypotension 成人脱髓鞘性白质营养不良；**globoid cell l.**, Krabbe disease 球形细胞脑白质营养不良；**metachromatic l.**, an inherited disorder due to accumulation of sulfatide in tissues with a diffuse loss of myelin in the central nervous system; it occurs in several forms, with increasing age of onset correlated with decreasing severity, all initially presenting as mental regression and motor disturbances 异染性脑白质营养不良

leu·ko·ede·ma (loo″ko-ə-de′mə) a variant condition of the buccal mucosa, consisting of an increase in thickness of the epithelium and intracellular edema of the stratum spinosum or stratum germinativum 白色水肿

leu·ko·en·ceph·a·li·tis (loo″ko-ən-sef″ə-li′- tis) inflammation of the white substance of the brain 白质脑炎

leu·ko·en·ceph·a·lop·a·thy (loo″ko-ən-sef″ə- lop′ə-the) any of a group of diseases affecting the white substance of the brain. The term *leukodystrophy* is used to denote such disorders due to defective formation and maintenance of myelin in infants and children 白质脑病；**progressive multifocal l.**, opportunistic infection of the central nervous system by the JC virus, with demyelination occurring usually in the cerebral hemispheres and rarely in the brainstem and cerebellum 进行性多灶性白质脑病

leu·ko·eryth·ro·blas·to·sis (loo″ko-ə-rith″ ro-blas-to′sis) anemia associated with spaceoccupying lesions of the bone marrow that cause bone marrow suppression with a variable number of immature cells of the erythrocytic and granulocytic series in the circulation 幼白成红细胞增多病

leu·ko·ker·a·to·sis (loo″ko-ker″ə-to′sis)leukoplakia 白斑角化症

leu·ko·ko·ria (loo″ko-kor′e-ə) any condition marked by the appearance of a whitish reflex or mass in the pupillary area behind the lens 白瞳症

leu·ko·krau·ro·sis (loo″ko-kraw-ro′sis) kraurosis vulvae 外阴干皱

leu·kol·y·sis (loo-kol′ə-sis) destruction or disintegration of leukocytes 白细胞溶解；**leukolyt′ic** *adj.*

leu·ko·ma (loo-ko′mə) pl. *leuko′mata* [Gr.] 1. a dense, white corneal opacity 角膜白斑；2. leukoplakia of the buccal mucosa 颊白斑；**leuko′matous** *adj.*；**adherent l.**, a white tumor of the cornea enclosing a prolapsed adherent iris 粘连性角膜白斑

leu·ko·my·eli·tis (loo″ko-mi″ə-li′tis) inflammation of the white matter of the spinal cord 脊髓白质炎

leu·ko·nych·ia (loo″ko-nik′e-ə) abnormal whiteness of the nails, either total or in spots or streaks 白甲

leu·ko·path·ia (loo″ko-path′e-ə) 1. 同 leukoderma；2. disease of the leukocytes 白细胞疾病；**l. un′guium**, 同 leukonychia

leu·ko·pe·de·sis (loo″ko-pə-de′sis) leukocyte emigration 白细胞渗出

leu·ko·pe·nia (loo″ko-pe′ne-ə) reduction of the number of leukocytes in the blood below about 5000 per cubic millimeter 白细胞减少；**leukope′nic** *adj.*；**basophilic l.**, basophilopenia 嗜碱性白细胞减少；**malignant l., pernicious l.**, agranulocytosis 恶性白细胞减少

leu·ko·pla·kia (loo″ko-pla′ke-ə) 1. a white patch on a mucous membrane that will not rub off 黏膜白斑病；2. 同 oral l.；**hairy l.**, a white, filiform to flat patch on the tongue or the buccal mucosa, caused by infection with human herpesvirus 4 and associated with human immunodeficiency virus (HIV) infection 毛状白斑；**oral l.**, white, thick patches on the oral mucosa due to hyperkeratosis of the epithelium, producing favorable conditions for development of epidermoid carcinoma; often occurring on the cheeks (*l. bucca′lis*), gums, or tongue (*l. lingua′lis*) 口白斑病；**oral hairy l.**, hairy l. 口腔毛状白斑

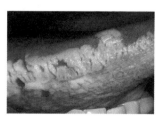

▲ 毛状白斑

leu·ko·poi·e·sis (loo″ko-poi-e′sis) production of

leukocytes 白细胞生成

leu·kor·rhea (loo″ko-re′ə) a whitish, viscid discharge from the vagina and uterine cavity 白带

leu·ko·sis (loo-ko′sis) pl. *leuko′ses.* Proliferation of leukocyte-forming tissue 造白细胞组织增生

leu·ko·tax·is (loo″ko-tak′sis) cytotaxis of leukocytes; the tendency of leukocytes to collect in regions of injury and inflammation 白细胞趋向性；**leukotac′tic** *adj.*

leu·ko·tome (loo′ko-tōm) a neurosurgical tool in which a wire loop on one end of a rigid shaft is used to cut tissue 脑白质切断器

leu·kot·o·my (loo-kot′ə-me) prefrontal lobotomy 脑白质切断术

leu·ko·tox·in (loo″ko-tok′sin) a cytotoxin destructive to leukocytes 白细胞毒素

leu·ko·trich·ia (loo″ko-trik′e-ə) whiteness of the hair in a circumscribed area 白发

leu·ko·tri·ene (loo″ko-tri′ēn) any of a group of biologically active compounds derived from arachidonic acid that function as regulators of allergic and inflammatory reactions. They are identified by the letters A, B, C, D, and E, with subscript numerals indicating the number of double bonds in each molecule 白细胞三烯，白三烯

leu·pro·lide (loo-pro′līd) a synthetic analogue of gonadotropin-releasing hormone, used in the form of the acetate ester as an antiendometriotic agent, antineoplastic, and gonadotropin inhibitor 亮丙瑞林（促性腺激素释放激素类似物）

lev·al·bu·ter·ol (lev″al-bu′tər-ol) R-albuterol; a β-adrenergic agent used as the hydrochloride salt as a bronchodilator for the treatment and prophylaxis of reversible bronchospasm 左旋沙丁胺醇

le·vam·i·sole (le-vam′ĭ-sōl) an immunomodulator used with fluorouracil in the treatment of colon cancer, administered as the hydrochloride salt 左旋咪唑

lev·ar·te·re·nol (lev″ahr-tēr′ə-nol) the levorotatory isomer of norepinephrine, a much more potent pressor agent than the natural dextrorotatory isomer 左旋去甲肾上腺素

le·va·tor (lə-va′tor) pl. *levato′res.* 1. a muscle that elevates an organ or structure 提肌；2. an instrument for raising depressed osseous fragments in fractures 骨片提位器

lev·el (lev′əl) relative position, rank, or concentration 水平、等级，浓度；**confidence l.,** the probability that a confidence interval does not contain the population parameter 置信水平，置信度；**l. of significance,** the probability of incorrectly rejecting the null hypothesis 显著性水平

le·ve·ti·rac·e·tam (le″və-ti-ras′ə-tam) an anticonvulsant used in the treatment of some forms of epilepsy 抗惊厥药，用于治某种类型的癫痫

lev·i·ga·tion (lev″ĭ-ga′shən) the grinding to a powder of a moist or hard substance 研磨，研碎

le·vo·be·tax·o·lol (le″vo-ba-tak′sə-lol) a cardioselective β-adrenergic blocking agent, used topically in the form of the hydrochloride salt in the treatment of glaucoma and ocular hypertension 左倍他洛尔（β受体阻滞药）

le·vo·bu·no·lol (le″vo-bu′no-lol) a nonspecific beta-adrenergic blocking agent used as the hydrochloride salt in the treatment of glaucoma and ocular hypertension 左布诺洛尔（β受体阻滞药）

le·vo·bu·piv·a·caine (le″vo-bu-piv′ə-kān) the S enantiomer of bupivacaine; a local anesthetic used as the hydrochloride salt for local infiltration anesthesia, peripheral nerve block, and epidural anesthesia 左布比卡因

le·vo·cab·as·tine (le″vo-kab′ə-stēn) an antihistamine applied topically to the conjunctiva as the hydrochloride salt to treat seasonal allergic conjunctivitis 左卡巴斯汀

le·vo·car·dia (le″vo-kahr′de-ə) a term denoting the normal position of the heart associated with transposition of other viscera (situs inversus) 左位心

le·vo·car·ni·tine (le″vo-kahr′nĭ-tēn) a preparation of the biologically active l-isomer of carnitine used in the treatment of carnitine deficiency 左旋肉毒碱

le·vo·cli·na·tion (le″vo-klĭ-na′shən) rotation of the upper poles of the vertical meridians of the two eyes to the left 左旋眼

le·vo·do·pa (le″vo-do′pə) l-dopa; the levorotatory isomer of dopa, used as an antiparkinsonian agent 左旋多巴

le·vo·flox·a·cin (le″vo-flok′sə-sin) a broadspectrum antibacterial agent for systemic and ophthalmic use 左氧氟沙星

le·vo·me·fo·late (le″vo-mə-fo′lāt) l-5- methyltetrahydrofolate; used as *l. calcium* as a source of folic acid L-5- 甲基四氢叶酸

le·vo·mil·na·ci·pran (lee″vō-mil-na′si-pran) a selective serotonin-norepinephrine reuptake inhibitor approved to treat major depressive disorder; administered orally as the hydrochloride salt 左旋米那普伦

le·vo·nor·ges·trel (le′vo-nor-jes′trel) the levorotatory form of norgestrel; used as an oral or subdermal contraceptive 左炔诺孕酮

le·vo·ro·ta·to·ry (le″vo-ro′tə-tor″e) turning the plane of polarization of polarized light to the left (counterclockwise) 左旋的

le·vor·pha·nol (le-vor′fə-nol) an opioid analgesic with properties and actions similar to those of morphine; used as the bitartrate salt as an analgesic and an anesthesia adjunct 左啡诺，左吗喃

le·vo·thy·rox·ine (le″vo-thi-rok′sēn) l-thyroxine, obtained from the thyroid gland of domesticated food animals or prepared synthetically; used as the sodium salt in the treatment of hypothyroidism and the treatment and prophylaxis of goiter and thyroid carcinoma 左甲状腺素

le·vo·tor·sion (le″vo-tor′shən) 同 levoclination

le·vo·ver·sion (le″vo-vur′zhən) a turning toward the left 左转，左倒转

LFA left frontoanterior (position of the fetus) 左额前位（胎位）

LFP left frontoposterior (position of the fetus) 左额后位（胎位）

LFT left frontotransverse (position of the fetus) 左额横位（胎位）

LH luteinizing hormone 促黄体（生成）激素

LH-RH luteinizing hormone–releasing hormone 促黄体激素释放激素

Li lithium 锂

li·bi·do (lĭ-be′do) (lĭ-bi′do) pl. *libid′ines* [L.] 1. sexual desire 性欲；2. the psychic energy derived from instinctive biologic drives; in early freudian theory it was restricted to the sexual drive, then expanded to all expressions of love and pleasure, but has evolved to include also the death instinct 力比多. **libid′inal** *adj.*

lice (līs) *louse* 的复数

li·cen·ti·ate (li-sen′she-āt) one holding a license from an authorized agency giving the right to practice a particular profession 执照持有人

li·chen (li′kən) 1. any of certain plants formed by the mutualistic combination of an alga and a fungus 地衣；2. any of various popular skin diseases in which the lesions are typically small, firm papules set close together 苔藓. **l. amyloido′sus,** 淀粉样变性苔藓，见 *amyloidosis* 下词条；**l. myxedemato′sus,** a condition resembling myxedema but unassociated with hypothyroidism, marked by a fibrocystic proliferation, increased deposition of acid mucopolysaccharides in the skin, and the presence of a circulating paraprotein; it may present as lichenoid papules or urticaria-like plaques and nodules 黏液水肿性苔藓；**l. ni′tidus,** a chronic inflammatory eruption consisting of many pinheadsized, pale, flat, sharply marginated, glistening, discrete papules, scarcely raised above the skin level 光泽苔藓；**l. planopila′ris,** a variant of lichen planus characterized by pointed, horny papules around hair follicles, as well as typical lesions of lichen planus 毛发扁平苔藓；**l. pla′nus, l. ru′ber pla′nus,** an inflammatory skin disease with wide, flat, viola-

ceous, shiny papules in circumscribed patches; it may also involve hair follicles, nails, or buccal mucosa 扁平苔藓；**l. sclero′sus,** a chronic atrophic skin disease marked by white papules with erythematous halos and keratotic plugging, usually around the external genitalia or in the perianal region 硬化性苔藓；**l. scrofuloso′rum, l. scrofulo′sus,** an eruption of minute reddish lichenoid follicular papules seen in children and young adults with tuberculosis 瘰疬性苔藓；**l. sim′plex chro′nicus,** a dermatosis caused by excessive scratching or rubbing of itches, marked by discrete or confluent papular eruptions, usually in a localized area 单纯慢性苔藓；**l. spinulo′sus,** a condition in which there is a horn or spine in the center of each hair follicle 小棘苔藓；**l. stria′tus,** a self-limited condition characterized by a linear lichenoid eruption, usually in children 条纹状苔藓

li·chen·i·fi·ca·tion (li-ken″ĭ-fĭ-ka′shən) thickening and hardening of the skin, with exaggeration of its normal markings 苔藓样变

lic·o·rice (lik′ə-ris) glycyrrhiza; the dried rhizome, roots, and stolons of various species of the perennial herb *Glycyrrhiza,* used as an expectorant and for the treatment of gastritis; also used in traditional Chinese medicine, ayurveda, and folk medicine 甘草

li·do·caine (li′do-kān) an anesthetic with sedative, analgesic, and cardiac depressant properties, applied topically in the form of the base or hydrochloride salt as a local anesthetic; also used in the latter form as a cardiac antiarrhythmic and to produce infiltration anesthesia and various nerve blocks 利多卡因

lie (li) the relation of the long axis of the fetus with respect to that of the mother 产式；cf. *presentation* and *position*；**oblique l.,** the situation during labor when the long axis of the fetal body crosses the long axis of the maternal body at an angle close to 45 degrees 斜产式；**transverse l.,** the situation during labor when the long axis of the fetus crosses the long axis of the mother 横产式；见 *position*

li·en (li′ən) [L.] spleen 脾；**lien′al** *adj.*；**l. accesso′rius,** accessory spleen 副脾

li·en·tery (li′ən-ter″e) diarrhea with passage of undigested food 消化不良性腹泻；**lienter′ic** *adj.*

LIF left iliac fossa 左髂窝；leukocyte inhibitory factor 白细胞抑制因子

life (līf) the aggregate of vital phenomena; the quality or principle by which living things are distinguished from inorganic matter, as manifested by such phenomena as metabolism, growth, reproduction, adaptation, etc. 生命；生物；生活

lig·a·ment (lig′ə-mənt) 1. a band of fibrous tissue connecting bones or cartilages, serving to support and strengthen joints 韧 带; 2. a double layer of peritoneum extending from one visceral organ to another 双层腹膜; 3. cordlike remnants of fetal tubular structures that are nonfunctional after birth 出生后无功能的胎儿管状结构的束状残余物; **liga-men'tous** *adj.*; **accessory l.,** one that strengthens or supports another 副韧带; **alar l's,** 1. two bands passing from the apex of the dens to the medial side of each occipital condyle 翼 状 韧 带; 2. a pair of folds of the synovial membrane of the knee joint 膝关节滑膜的一对皱褶; **annular l. of stapes,** a ring of fibrous tissue that attaches the base of the stapes to the vestibular window of the middle ear 镫骨环状 韧 带; **anococcygeal l.,** a fibrous band connecting the posterior fibers of the sphincter of the anus to the coccyx 肛尾韧带; **arcuate l's,** 1. the arched ligaments connecting the respiratory diaphragm with the lowest ribs and the first lumbar vertebra 弓状韧带; 2. ligamenta flava 黄韧带; **Bérard l.,** the suspensory ligament of the pericardium 心包悬韧带; **Bertin l., Bigelow l.,** iliofemoral l.; **l. of Botallo,** a strong thick fibromuscular cord extending from the pulmonary artery to the aortic arch; it is the remains of the ductus arteriosus 博塔洛韧带, 动脉韧带; **Bourgery l.,** oblique popliteal ligament; a broad band of fibers extending from the medial condyle of the tibia across the back of the knee joint to the lateral epicondyle of the femur 腘斜韧带; **broad l.,** 1. a broad fold of peritoneum supporting the uterus, extending from the uterus to the wall of the pelvis on either side 阔 韧 带; 2. a sickle-shaped sagittal fold of perineum helping attach the liver to the respiratory diaphragm and separating the left and right hepatic lobes 肝镰状韧带; **Brodie l.,** 同 transverse humeral l.; **Burns l.,** falciform process (1)Burns 韧带; **Campbell l.,** suspensory l. (2)Campbell 韧 带; **cardinal l.,** part of a thickening of the visceral pelvic fascia beside the cervix and vagina, passing laterally to merge with the upper fascia of the pelvic diaphragm 主韧带; **Colles l.,** a triangular band of fibers arising from the lacunar ligament and pubic bone and passing to the linea alba Colles 韧带（腹股沟反转韧带）; **conoid l.,** the posteromedial portion of the coracoclavicular ligament, extending from the coracoid process to the inferior surface of the clavicle 锥状 韧 带; **conus l.,** a collagenous band connecting the posterior surface of the pulmonary annulus and the muscular infundibulum to the root of the aorta 圆锥韧带, 漏斗腱; **Cooper l.,** pectineal l. 库珀韧带; **coracoclavicular l.,** a band joining the coracoid process of the scapula and the acromial extremity of the clavicle, consisting of two ligaments, the conoid and trapezoid 喙锁

韧带; **cotyloid l.,** a ring of fibrocartilage connected with the rim of the acetabulum 髋臼韧带; **cruciate l's of knee,** more or less cross-shaped ligaments, one anterior and one posterior, arising from the femur and passing through the intercondylar space to attach to the tibia 膝交叉韧带; **cystoduodenal l.,** an anomalous fold of peritoneum extending between the gallbladder and the duodenum 胆囊十二指肠韧带; **diaphragmatic l.,** the involuting urogenital ridge that becomes the suspensory ligament of the ovary 膈韧带; **falciform l.,** a sickle-shaped sagittal fold of peritoneum that helps attach the liver to the diaphragm 镰突（骶结节韧带）, 镰状韧带; **flaval l's,** ligamenta flava 黄韧带; **glenohumeral l's,** bands, usually three, on the inner surface of the articular capsule of the humerus, extending from the glenoid lip to the anatomic neck of the humerus 盂肱韧带; **glenoid l.,** 1. *(in the pl.)* dense bands on the plantar surfaces of the metatarsophalangeal joints 跖趾关节足底韧带; 2. 见 *lip* 下词条; **Henle l.,** falx inguinalis 腹股沟镰; **Hey l.,** falciform process (1)Hey 韧 带; **iliofemoral l.,** a very strong triangular or inverted Y-shaped band covering the anterior and superior portions of the hip joint 髂股韧带; **iliotrochanteric l.,** a portion of the joint capsule of the hip joint 贝利尼韧带(髂转子韧带); **inguinal l.,** a fibrous band running from the anterior superior spine of the ilium to the spine of the pubis 腹股沟韧带; **lacunar l.,** a membrane with its base just medial to the femoral ring, one side attached to the inguinal ligament and the other to the pectineal line of the pubis 腔隙韧带; **Lisfranc l.,** a fibrous band extending from the medial cuneiform bone to the second metatarsal Lisfranc 韧带（楔趾韧带）; **Lockwood l.,** a suspensory sheath supporting the eyeball Lockwood 韧带（眼球悬韧带）; **medial l.,** 1. a large fan-shaped ligament on the medial side of the ankle 内侧韧带, 三角韧带; 2. the medial ligament of temporomandibular articulation 颞下颌关节内侧韧带; **meniscofemoral l's,** two small fibrous bands of the knee joint attached to the lateral meniscus, one (the anterior) extending to the anterior cruciate ligament and the other (the posterior) to the medial femoral condyle 半月板股骨韧带; **nephrocolic l.,** fasciculi from the fatty capsule of the kidney passing down on the right side to the mastoid wall of the ascending colon and on the left side to the mastoid wall of the descending colon 肾结肠韧带; **nuchal l.,** a broad, fibrous, roughly triangular sagittal septum in the back of the neck, separating the right and left sides 项韧带; **ovarian l.,** a musculofibrous cord in the broad ligament, joining the ovary to the upper part of the lateral margin of the uterus just below the attachment of the uterine tube 卵巢韧带；**patellar l.,** the continuation of the central portion of the tendon of the quadriceps femoris muscle distal to the patella, extending from the patella to the tuber of the tibia 髌韧带；**pectineal l.,** a strong aponeurotic lateral continuation of the lacunar ligament along the pectineal line of the pubis 耻骨梳韧带；**periodontal l.,** the fibrous connective tissue that surrounds the root of a tooth, separating it from and attaching it to the alveolar bone, and serving to hold the tooth in its socket. It extends from the base of the gingival mucosa to the fundus of the bony socket 牙周膜，牙周韧带；**phrenicocolic l.,** a peritoneal fold passing from the left colic flexure to the adjacent part of the respiratory diaphragm 膈结肠韧带；**Poupart l.,** inguinal l. 普帕尔韧带（腹股沟韧带）；**pulmonary l.,** a vertical fold extending from the hilus to the base of the lung 肺韧带；**rhomboid l. of clavicle,** a ligament connecting cartilage of the first rib to the undersurface of the clavicle 肋锁韧带；**Robert l.,** posterior meniscofemoral l. Robert 韧带（外侧半月板韧带）**round l.,** 1. *(of femur)* a broad ligament arising from the fatty cushion of the acetabulum and inserted on the head of the femur 股骨头韧带；2. *(of uterus)* a fibromuscular band attached to the uterus near the uterine tube, passing through the inguinal ring to the labium majus 子宫圆韧带；**Schlemm l's,** two ligamentous bands of the capsule of the glenohumeral joint Schlemm 韧带（盂肱韧带）；**subflaval l's,** ligamenta flava 黄韧带；**suspensory l.,** 1. *(of lens)* ciliary zonule 晶状体悬韧带；2. *(of axilla)* a layer ascending from the axillary fascia and ensheathing the pectoralis minor muscle 腋悬韧带；3. *(of ovary)* the portion of the broad ligament lateral to and above the ovary 卵巢悬韧带；4. *(of breast)* one of numerous fibrous processes extending from the body of the mammary gland to the dermis 乳房悬韧带；5. *(of clitoris)* a strong fibrous band attaching the root of the clitoris to the linea alba and pubic symphysis 阴蒂悬韧带；6. *(of penis)* a strong fibrous band that attaches the root of the penis to the linea alba and pubic symphysis 阴茎悬韧带；**synovial l.,** a large synovial fold 滑膜韧带；**tendinotrochanteric l.,** portion of the capsule of the hip joint 腱转子韧带；**tracheal l's,** circular horizontal ligaments that join the tracheal cartilages together 环状韧带，气管韧带；**transverse l.,** short fibers that connect the posterior surface of the neck of a rib with the anterior surface of the transverse process of the corresponding vertebra 横韧带；**tranverse carpal l.,** flexor retinaculum of hand 腕横韧带；**transverse humeral l.,** a band of fibers bridging the in-

tertubercular groove of the humerus and holding the tendon in the groove 肱横韧带；**trapezoid l.,** the anterolateral portion of the coracoclavicular ligament, extending from the upper surface of the coracoid process to the trapezoid line of the clavicle 斜方韧带；**umbilical l., median,** a fibrous cord, the remains of the obliterated umbilical artery, running cranialward beside the bladder to the umbilicus 脐正中韧带；**uteropelvic l's,** expansions of muscular tissue in the broad ligament, radiating from the fascia over the internal obturator to the side of the uterus and the vagina 子宫骨盆韧带；**ventricular l.,** 同 vestibular l.；**vesicoumbilical l., median** umbilical l. 膀胱脐韧带；**vesicouterine l.,** a ligament that extends from the anterior aspect of the uterus to the bladder 膀胱子宫韧带；**vestibular l.,** the membrane extending from the thyroid cartilage in front to the anterolateral surface of the arytenoid cartilage behind 前庭韧带；**vocal l.,** the elastic tissue membrane extending from the thyroid cartilage in front to the vocal process of the arytenoid cartilage behind 声带韧带；**Weitbrecht l.,** a small ligamentous band extending from the ulnar tuber to the radius Weitbrecht 韧带（前臂骨间膜斜索）；**Wrisberg l,** posterior meniscofemoral l. 里斯伯格韧带，板股后韧带；**Y l.,** iliofemoral l；**yellow l's,** ligamenta flava 黄韧带

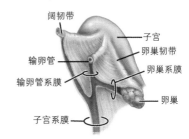

▲ 子宫阔韧带，包括卵巢系膜、子宫系膜和输卵管系膜；如侧视图所示，子宫体前表面朝向左

lig·a·men·to·pexy (lig″ə-men″to-pek′se) fixation of the uterus by shortening or suturing the round ligament 子宫圆韧带固定术

lig·a·men·tum (lig″ə-men′təm) pl. *ligamen′ta* [L.] ligament 韧带；**ligamen′ta fla′va,** yellow ligaments: a series of bands of yellow elastic tissue attached to and extending between the ventral portions of the laminae of two adjacent vertebrae, from the axis to the sacrum. They assist in maintaining or regaining the erect position and serve to close in the spaces between the arches 黄韧带

li·gand (li′gand) (lig′ənd) an organic molecule that

donates the necessary electrons to form coordinate covalent bonds with metallic ions. Also, an ion or molecule that reacts to form a complex with another molecule 配体

li·gase (li′gās) any of a class of enzymes that catalyze the joining together of two molecules coupled with the breakdown of a pyrophosphate bond in ATP or a similar triphosphate 连接酶

li·ga·tion (li-ga′shən) 1. the application of a ligature 结扎；2. the process of annealing or joining 退火和连接的过程；**tubal l.**, sterilization of the female by constricting, severing, or crushing the uterine tubes 输卵管结扎术

lig·a·ture (lig′ə-chər) any material, such as thread or wire, used for tying a vessel or to constrict a part 结扎线

light (līt) electromagnetic radiation with a range of wavelength between 3900 (violet) and 7700 (red) angstroms, capable of stimulating the subjective sensation of sight; sometimes considered to include ultraviolet and infrared radiation as well 光；**idioretinal l.**, the sensation of light in the complete absence of external stimuli 视网膜自发光感；**intrinsic l.**, the dim light always present in the visual field 固有光；**polarized l.**, light of which the vibrations are made over one plane or in circles or ellipses 偏振光；**ultraviolet l.**, 紫外线，见 *ray* 下词条；**Wood l.**, ultraviolet radiation from a mercury vapor source, transmitted through a filter that holds back all but a few violet rays and passes ultraviolet wavelengths of about 365 nm 伍德光

light·en·ing (līt′ən-ing) the sensation of decreased abdominal distention produced by the descent of the uterus into the pelvic cavity, 2 to 3 weeks before labor begins 胎儿下降感

lignoceric ac·id (lig″no-sēr′ik) a saturated 24-carbon fatty acid occurring in sphingomyelin and as a minor constituent of many plant fats 木蜡酸

limb (lim) 1. member or extremity; one of the paired appendages of the body used in locomotion or grasping 肢；2. a structure or part resembling such 分支；**anacrotic l.**, 同 ascending l. (2)；**ascending l.**, 1. the distal part of the loop of Henle（髓襻）升支；2. anacrotic l.; the ascending portion of an arterial pulse tracing 脉波升支；**catacrotic l.**, 同 descending l. (2)；**descending l.**, 1. the proximal part of the loop of Henle（髓襻）降支；2. catacrotic l.; the descending portion of an arterial pulse tracing 脉波降支；**lower l.**, the limb of the body extending from the gluteal region to the foot; it is specialized for weight bearing and locomotion 下肢，另见 *leg*；**phantom l.**, the sensation, after amputation of a limb, that the absent part is still present; there may

also be paresthesias, transient aches, and intermittent or continuous pain perceived as originating in the absent limb 幻肢；**upper l.**, the limb of the body extending from the descending part of the deltoid region to the hand; it is specialized for functions requiring great mobility 上肢，另见 *arm*

lim·bic (lim′bik) pertaining to a limbus, or margin 边缘的；另见 *system* 下词条

lim·bus (lim′bəs) pl. *lim′bi* [L.] an edge, fringe, or border 缘；**corneal l.**, the edge of the cornea where it joins the sclera 角膜缘；**spiral l.**, the thickened periosteum of the osseous spiral lamina of the cochlea 螺旋缘

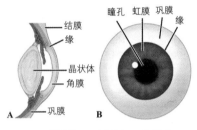

▲ 角膜缘 **A.** 水平面。**B.** 前视图

lime (līm) 1. calcium oxide, a corrosively alkaline and caustic earth, CaO; having various industrial uses and also a pharmaceutical necessity 氧化钙；2. the acid fruit of the tropical tree, *Citrus aurantifolia*; its juice contains ascorbic acid 酸柚；**soda l.**, 碱石灰，见 *soda* 下词条

li·men (li′mən) pl. *li′mina* [L.] a threshold or boundary 阈；**l. of insula, l. in′sulae**, the point at which the cortex of the insula is continuous with the cortex of the frontal lobe 岛 阈；**l. na′si**, the ridge marking the boundary between the vestibule of the nose and the nasal cavity proper 鼻阈

lim·i·nal (lim′ĭ-nəl) barely perceptible; pertaining to a threshold 阈限的，阈的

lim·i·nom·e·ter (lim″ĭ-nom′ə-tər) an instrument for measuring the strength of a stimulus that just induces a tendon reflex 反射阈计

lim·i·tans (lim′ĭ-tanz) [L.] limiting 界膜

lim·it dex·trin·ase (lim′it dek′strin-ās) α - dextrinase α - 糊精酶

limp (limp) any gait that avoids weight bearing by one leg 跛行

lin·a·glip·tin (si″tə-glip′tin) an agent that in response to elevated blood sugar slows the inactivation of incretins, thereby increasing insulin release and decreasing circulating glucagon levels; used in the treatment of type 2 diabetes mellitus 利格列汀

lin·co·my·cin (lin″ko-mi′sin) an antibiotic,

primarily a gram-positive specific antibacterial, produced by a variant of *Streptomyces lincolnensis;* used as the hydrochloride salt 林可霉素

lin·dane (lin'dān) the gamma isomer of benzene hexachloride, used as a topical pediculicide and scabicide 六氯化苯，林丹，γ-六六六

line (līn) 1. a stripe, streak, or narrow ridge 线；2. an imaginary line connecting different anatomic landmarks 连接不同解剖标志的假想线；**lin′ear** *adj.*；absorption l's, dark lines in the spectrum due to absorption of light by the substance through which the light has passed 吸收线；anocutaneous l., 同 pectinate l.；Beau l's transverse furrows on the fingernails, usually a sign of a systemic disease but also due to other causes 博氏线；bismuth l., a thin blue-black line along the gingival margin in bismuth poisoning 铋线；blood l., a line of direct descent through several generations 血统线；cement l., a line visible in microscopic examination of bone in cross section, marking the boundary of an osteon (haversian system) 黏合线；cervical l., anatomic designation for the cementoenamel junction, the dividing line between the crown and root portions of a tooth 牙颈线；cleavage l's, linear clefts in the skin indicative of the direction of the fibers 皮纹线；costoclavicular l., 同 parasternal l.；l. of Douglas, a crescentic line marking the termination of the posterior layer of the sheath of the rectus abdominis muscle 腹直肌鞘弓形线；epiphyseal l., 1. a plane or plate on a long bone, visible as a line, marking the junction of the epiphysis and diaphysis 骺线；2. a strip of lesser density on the radiograph of a long bone, representing that plane or plate 骨骺线；l's of expression, the natural skin lines and creases of the face and neck; the preferred lines of incision in facial and cervical surgery 表观线，头颈部手术首选线；gingival l., 1. a line determined by the level to which the gingiva extends on a tooth 牙龈线；2. any linear mark visible on the surface of the gingiva 牙龈表面可见的任何线性标记；gluteal l., any of the three rough curved lines (anterior, inferior, and posterior) on the gluteal surface of the ala of the ilium 臀线；Harris l's, lines of retarded growth seen radiographically at the epiphyses of long bones Harris 线；hot l., 热线，见 *H* 下词条；iliopectineal l., a ridge on the ilium and pubes showing the brim of the lesser pelvis 髂耻线；intertrochanteric l., a line running obliquely from the greater to the lesser trochanter on the anterior surface of the femur 转子间线；lead l., a gray or bluish black line at the gingival margin in lead poisoning 铅线；mammary l., 乳线，见 *ridge* 下

词条；mammillary l., an imaginary vertical line passing through the center of the nipple 乳头线；median l., an imaginary line dividing the body surface equally into right and left sides 正中线；milk l., mammary ridge 乳线，乳腺嵴；mylohyoid l., a ridge on the inner surface of the lower jaw from the base of the symphysis to the ascending rami behind the last molar tooth 下颌舌骨肌线；nasobasilar l., one through the basion and nasion 鼻基线；Nélaton l., one from the anterior superior spine of the ilium to the most prominent part of the tuber of the ischium Nélaton 线；nuchal l's, three lines (inferior, superior, highest) on the outer surface of the occipital bone 项线；另见 *external occipital crest*；parasternal l., an imaginary line midway between the mammillary line and the border of the sternum 胸骨旁线；pectinate l., one marking the junction of the zone of the anal canal lined with stratified squamous epithelium and the zone lined with columnar epithelium 齿状线；pectineal l., 1. a line running down the posterior surface of the shaft of the femur, giving attachment to the pectineus muscle 耻骨肌线；2. the anterior border of the superior ramus of the pubis 耻骨线；semilunar l., a curved line along the lateral border of each rectus abdominis muscle, marking the meeting of the aponeuroses of the internal abdominal oblique and transversus abdominis muscles 半月线；Shenton l., a curved line seen in radiographs of the normal hip, formed by the top of the obturator foramen Shenton 线；sternal l., an imaginary vertical line on the anterior body surface, corresponding to the lateral border of the sternum 骨线；subcostal l., a transverse line on the surface of the abdomen at the level f the lower edge of the tenth costal cartilage 肋下线；Sydney l., a palmar crease correlated with an increased risk for leukemia and other malignancies in childhood 西尼线；temporal l., 1. either of the curved ridges, inferior and superior, on the outside of the parietal bone, continuous with the temporal line of the frontal bone（顶骨）颞线；2. a ridge extending superiorly and posteriorly from the zygomatic process of the frontal bone（额骨）颞线；terminal l. of pelvis, one on the inner surface of each coxal bone, from the sacroiliac joint to the iliopubic eminence anteriorly, separating the greater from the lesser pelvis 骨盆分界线；trapezoid l., a ridge on the inferior surface of the clavicle for attachment of the trapezoid ligament 斜方线；Voigt l., a dorsoventral pigmented line of demarcation on the skin along the lateral edge of the biceps muscle; seen in 20 to 26 percent of blacks and rarely in whites Voigt 线

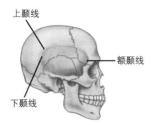

上颞线

额颞线

下颞线

li·nea (lin′e-ə) pl. *li′neae* [L.] line 线；l. al′ba, white line; the tendinous median line on the anterior abdominal wall between the two rectus muscles 腹白线；l. as′pera, a rough longitudinal line on the back of the femur for muscle attachments 肌骨嵴粗线；l. epiphysia′lis, epiphyseal line 骺线；l. glu′tea, gluteal line 臀线；l. ni′gra, the linea alba when it has become pigmented in pregnancy 黑线；l. splen′dens, the sheath for the anterior spinal artery formed by the pia mater in the anterior median fissure of the spinal cord 软脊膜前纤维索

lin·e·age (lin′e-əj) descent traced down from or back to a common ancestor 谱系；cell l., the developmental history of cells as traced from the first division of the original cell or cells 细胞谱系

lin·er (līn′ər) material applied to the inside of the walls of a cavity or container for protection or insulation of the surface 衬里

li·nez·o·lid (lĭ-nez′o-lid) a synthetic oxazolidinone antibacterial, effective against gram-positive organisms 利奈唑胺

lin·gua (ling′gwə) pl. *lin′guae* [L.] tongue 舌；**lin′gual** *adj.*; l. geogra′phica, benign migratory glossitis 地图样舌；l. ni′gra, black hairy tongue 黑舌；l. plica′ta, fissured tongue 裂纹舌

lin·gual (ling′gwəl) 1. pertaining to or near the tongue 舌的; 2. in dental anatomy, facing the tongue or oral cavity 牙的舌面

Lin·guat·u·la (ling-gwă′chə-lə) a genus of worm-like arthropods, the adults of which inhabit the respiratory tract of vertebrates; the larvae are found in the lungs and other internal organs. It includes *L. serra′ta* (*L. rhina′ria*), which parasitizes dogs and cats and sometimes humans 舌形虫属

lin·gu·la (ling′gu-lə) pl. *lin′gulae* [L.] a small tonguelike structure, such as the projection from the lower portion of the upper lobe of the left lung (*l. pulmo′nis sinis′tri*), the bony ridge between the body and greater wing of the sphenoid bone (*l. sphenoida′lis*), or the most anterior lobule of the anterior lobe of the cerebellum (*l. cerebel′li*) 小舌 **lin′gular** *adj.*

lin·gu·lec·to·my (ling″gu-lek′tə-me) excision of the lingula of the left lung 肺舌叶切除术

lin·guo·pap·il·li·tis (ling″gwo-pap″ĭ-li′tis) inflammation or ulceration of the papillae of the edges of the tongue 舌乳头炎

lin·guo·ver·sion (ling″gwo-vur′zhən) displacement of a tooth lingually from the line of occlusion 舌向错位

lin·i·ment (lin′ĭ-mənt) an oily liquid preparation to be used on the skin 搽剂，擦剂

li·ni·tis (lĭ-ni′tis) inflammation of gastric cellular tissue 胃蜂窝织炎；l. plas′tica, diffuse fibrous proliferation of the submucous connective tissue of the stomach, resulting in thickening and fibrosis so that the organ is constricted, inelastic, and rigid (like a leather bottle) 皮革样胃

link·age (lingk′əj) 1. the connection between different atoms in a chemical compound, or the symbol representing it in structural formulas 键；另见 *bond*; 2. in genetics, the association of genes having loci on the same chromosome, which results in the tendency of a group of such nonallelic genes to be associated in inheritance 连锁；sex l., the location of a gene responsible for a specific trait on a sex chromosome, resulting in sexually dependent inheritance and expression of the trait 性连锁

li·no·le·ate (lĭ-no′le-āt) a salt (soap), ester, or anionic form of linoleic acid 亚油酸盐（盐、酯或阴离子型）

lin·o·le·ic ac·id (lin″o-le′ik) a polyunsaturated fatty acid, occurring as a major constituent of many vegetable oils; it is used in the biosynthesis of prostaglandins and cell membranes 亚油酸

li·no·le·nate (lĭ-no′lə-nāt) a salt (soap), ester, or anionic form of linolenic acid 亚麻酸（盐、酯或阴离子型）

lin·o·len·ic ac·id (lin″o-len′ik) a polyunsaturated 18-carbon essential fatty acid occurring in some fish oils and many seed-derived oils 亚麻酸

lin·seed (lin′sēd) flaxseed; the dried ripe seed of *Linum usitatissimum,* the common flax plant, used as a laxative and a topic demulcent and emollient, and a source of α-linolenic acid 亚麻子

lint (lint) an absorbent surgical dressing material 布（外科用敷料）

li·o·thy·ro·nine (li″o-thi′ro-nēn) a synthetic pharmaceutical preparation of the levorotatory isomer of triiodothyronine, used as the sodium salt in the treatment of hypothyroidism and the treatment and prophylaxis of goiter and thyroid carcinoma 三碘甲状腺氨酸

li·o·trix (li′o-triks) a 1:4 mixture of liothyronine sodium and levothyroxine sodium by weight; used as the sodium salt in the treatment of hypothyroid-

L

ism and in the treatment and prophylaxis of goiter and thyroid carcinoma 复方甲状腺素

lip (lip) 1. the upper or lower fleshy margin of the mouth 唇；2. any liplike part; labium 边缘部分；**cleft l.**, a congenital cleft or defect in the upper lip 唇裂；**glenoid l.**, a ring of fibrocartilage joined to the rim of the glenoid fossa 盂缘；**Hapsburg l.**, a thick, overdeveloped lower lip that often accompanies Hapsburg jaw 哈布斯堡唇

lip·ac·i·du·ria (lip″as-ĭ-du′re-ə) fatty acids in the urine 脂酸尿

lip·ase (lip′ās) (li′pās) any enzyme that catalyzes the cleavage of a fatty acid anion from a triglyceride or phospholipid 脂肪酶

lip·ec·to·my (lĭ-pek′tə-me) excision of a localized area of subcutaneous adipose tissue 脂肪切除术；**suction l., suction-assisted l.**, liposuction; surgical removal of localized fat deposits via high-pressure vacuum, applied by means of a suction curet or cannula inserted subdermally through small incisions 脂肪抽吸术，辅助脂肪抽吸术

lip·ede·ma (lip″ə-de′mə) an accumulation of excess fat and fluid in the superficial fascia 脂肪水肿

lip·emia (lĭ-pe′me-ə) hyperlipidemia 脂血症；**lipe′mic** adj.；**alimentary l.**, that occurring after ingestion of food 饮食性脂血症；**l. retina′lis**, that manifested by a milky appearance of the veins and arteries of the retina 视网膜脂血症

lip·id (lip′id) any of a heterogeneous group of fats and fatlike substances, including fatty acids, neutral fats, waxes, and steroids, which are water-insoluble and soluble in nonpolar solvents. Lipids, which are easily stored in the body, serve as a source of fuel, are an important constituent of cell structure, and serve other biologic functions. Compound lipids comprise the glycolipids, lipoproteins, and phospholipids 脂质，类脂

lip·i·de·mia (lip″ĭ-de′me-ə) hyperlipidemia 脂血症

lip·i·do·sis (lip″ĭ-do′sis) pl. *lipido′ses*. 1. abnormal accumulations of lipids in the tissues 脂肪沉积；2. one of the lysosomal storage diseases in which there is abnormal accumulation of lipids in the reticuloendothelial cells 磷脂沉积病

lip·i·du·ria (lip″ĭ-du′re-ə) adiposuria; lipids in the urine 脂肪尿

lipo·am·ide (lip″o-am′īd) the functional form of lipoic acid, linked to the lysine side chain of any of several enzyme complexes that catalyze the oxidative decarboxylation of keto acids 硫辛酰胺

lipo·ar·thri·tis (lip″o-ahr-thri′tis) inflammation of fatty tissue of a joint 关节脂肪组织炎症

lipo·at·ro·phy (lip″o-at′ro-fe) atrophy of subcuta-

neous fatty tissues of the body 脂肪萎缩

lipo·blast (lip′o-blast) a connective tissue cell that develops into a fat cell 成脂肪细胞；**lipoblas′tic** adj.

lipo·blas·to·ma (lip″o-blas-to′mə) a benign fatty tumor composed of a mixture of embryonic lipoblastic cells in a myxoid stroma and mature fat cells, with the cells ar ranged in lobules 脂肪母细胞瘤

lipo·blas·to·ma·to·sis (lip″o-blas-to″mə-to′sis) the occurrence of multiple lipoblastomas locally diffused but without a tendency to metastasize 成脂肪细胞瘤病

lipo·car·di·ac (lip″o-kahr′de-ak) relating to a fatty heart 脂肪心的

lipo·chon·dro·ma (lip″o-kon-dro′mə) chondrolipoma 脂肪软骨瘤

lipo·chrome (lip′o-krōm) any of a group of fat-soluble hydrocarbon pigments, such as carotene, xanthophyll, lutein, chromophane, and the natural coloring material of butter, egg yolk, and yellow corn 脂色素

lipo·cyte (lip′o-sīt) 1. fat cell 脂肪细胞；2. a fat-storing cell of the liver（肝内的）储脂细胞

lipo·dys·tro·phy (lip″o-dis′trə-fe) any disturbance of fat metabolism 脂质营养不良，脂质营养不良；**congenital generalized l., congenital progressive l.**, 同 total l.；**generalized l.**, 同 total l.；**partial l., progressive l.**, progressive and symmetric loss of subcutaneous fat from the parts above the pelvis, beginning with facial emaciation and progressing downward, giving an apparent and possibly real accumulation of fat about the thighs and buttocks 进行性脂肪营养不良；**total l.**, a recessive condition marked by the virtual absence of subcutaneous adipose tissue, macrosomia, visceromegaly, hypertrichosis, acanthosis nigricans, and reduced glucose tolerance in the presence of high insulin levels 全身脂肪营养不良

lipo·fus·cin (lip″o-fu′sin) any of a class of fatty pigments formed by the solution of a pigment in fat 脂褐质

lipo·fus·cin·o·sis (lip″o-fu″sin-o′sis) any disorder due to abnormal storage of lipofuscins 脂褐质沉积症；**neuronal ceroid l.**, any of several genetic lipidoses characterized by progressive neurodegeneration, loss of vision, and a fatal course; included are *Haltia-Santavuori disease, Janský- Bielschowsky disease, Vogt-Spielmeyer disease,* and *Kufs disease* 神经元蜡样质脂褐质沉积症

lipo·gen·e·sis (lip″o-gen′ə-sis) the formation of fat; the transformation of nonfat food materials into body fat 脂肪生成；**lipogenet′ic** adj.

lip·o·gen·ic (lip″o-jen′ik) forming, producing, or caused by fat 脂肪生成的

lipo·gran·u·lo·ma (lip″o-gran″u-lo′mə) a foreign body inflammation of adipose tissue containing granulation tissue and oil cysts 脂肪肉芽肿

lipo·gran·u·lo·ma·to·sis (lip″o-gran″u-lomə-to′sis) a condition of faulty lipid metabolism in which yellow nodules of lipoid material are deposited in the skin and mucosae, giving rise to granulomatous reactions 脂肪肉芽肿病

lipo·hy·per·tro·phy (lip″o-hi-pur′trə-fe) hypertrophy of subcutaneous fat 脂肪增生；**insulin l.,** localized hypertrophy of subcutaneous fat at insulin injection sites caused by the lipogenic effect of insulin 胰岛素性脂肪增生

lipo·ic ac·id (lip-o′ik) a necessary cofactor for several enzyme complexes involved in the oxidative decarboxylation of keto acids, where it occurs in the form lipoamide. It is used as a dietary supplement for its antioxidant properties 硫辛酸

lip·oid (lip′oid) fatlike 类脂的

li·pol·y·sis (lĭ-pol′ə-sis) the splitting up or decomposition of fat 脂肪分解；**lipolyt′ic** *adj.*

lip·o·ma (lip-o′mə) a benign, soft, rubbery, encapsulated tumor of adipose tissue, usually composed of mature fat cells 脂肪瘤

lip·o·ma·to·sis (lip″o-mə-to′sis) abnormal localized or tumorlike accumulations of fat in the tissues 脂过多症；**multiple symmetric l.,** multiple lipomas that surround the neck 多发对称性脂肪瘤病；**renal l.,** fatty masses within the kidney 脂瘤性肾病

lipo·me·nin·go·cele (lip″o-mə-ning′go-sēl) meningocele associated with an overlying lipoma 脂性脑膜膨出

lipo·my·elo·me·nin·go·cele (lip″o-mi″ə-lo-mə-ning′go-sēl) myelomeningocele with an overlying lipoma 脂性脊髓脊膜突出

lipo·my·o·ma (lip″o-mi-o′mə) myolipoma 脂肌瘤

lipo·myx·o·ma (lip″o-mik-so′mə) myxolipoma 黏液脂瘤

lipo·pe·nia (lip″o-pe′ne-ə) deficiency of lipids in the body 脂肪减少

lipo·phage (lip′o-fāj) a cell that absorbs or ingests fat 噬脂细胞

lipo·pha·gia (lip″o-fa′je-ə) lipolysis 噬脂性；**lipopha′- gic** *adj.*

lipo·phil·ia (lip″o-fil′e-ə) 1. affinity for fat 亲脂性；2. solubility in lipids 脂溶性；**lipophil′ic** *adj.*

lipo·plas·ty (lip′o-plas″te) 同 liposuction

lipo·poly·sac·cha·ride (lip″o-pol″e-sak′ə-rīd) 1. a molecule in which lipids and polysaccharides are linked 脂多糖；2. a major component of the cell wall of gram-negative bacteria; lipopolysaccharides are endotoxins and important antigens 革兰阴

性菌细胞壁的主要成分

lipo·pro·tein (lip″o-) (li″po-pro′tēn) a complex of lipids and apolipoproteins, the form in which lipids are transported in the blood 脂蛋白；**α-l., alpha l.,** a lipoprotein belonging to the class of those having the most rapid electrophoretic mobility; the group comprises HDL$_2$ and HDL$_3$, the major high-density lipoproteins (q.v.) 高脂蛋白；**β-l., beta l.,** a lipoprotein belonging to the class of those having electrophoretic mobility slower than that of the pre-β lipoproteins but not remaining at the origin; the low-density and intermediate-density lipoproteins (q.v.)（低）脂蛋白；**floating beta l's,** β-VLDL β极低密度脂蛋白；**high-density l. (HDL),** a class of plasma lipoproteins that promote transport of cholesterol from extrahepatic tissue to the liver for excretion in the bile; serum levels have been negatively correlated with premature coronary heart disease 高密度脂蛋白；**intermediate-density l. (IDL),** a class of lipoproteins formed in the degradation of very-low-density lipoproteins; some are cleared rapidly into the liver and some are degraded to low-density lipoproteins 中密度脂蛋白；**lowden-sity l. (LDL),** a class of plasma lipoproteins that transport cholesterol to extrahepatic tissues; high serum levels have been correlated with premature coronary heart disease 低密度脂蛋白；**Lp(a) l.,** a lipoprotein particle containing apolipoprotein B-100 as well as an antigenically unique apolipoprotein; its occurrence at high levels in plasma has been correlated with an increased risk of heart disease Lp(a) 载脂蛋白，下沉前β-脂蛋白；**pre-β-l., pre-beta l.,** a lipoprotein belonging to the class of those having intermediate electrophoretic mobility between the α-lipoproteins and the β-lipoproteins, predominantly comprising the very-low-density lipoproteins (q.v.) 前β-脂蛋白；**sinking pre-β-l.,** 同 Lp(a) l.；**very-high-density l. (VHDL),** a class of lipoproteins composed predominantly of proteins and also containing a high concentration of free fatty acids 极高密度脂蛋白；**very-lowdensity l. (VLDL),** a class of lipoproteins that transport triglycerides from the intestine and liver to adipose and muscle tissues; they contain primarily triglycerides with some cholesteryl esters 极低密度脂蛋白

lipo·pro·tein li·pase (lip″o-pro′tēn li′pās) an enzyme that catalyzes the hydrolytic cleavage of fatty acids from triglycerides (or di- or monoglycerides) in chylomicrons, very-low-density lipoproteins, and low-density lipoproteins 脂蛋白脂肪酶

lipo·sar·co·ma (lip″o-sahr-ko′mə) a malignant mesenchymal tumor usually in the upper thigh, having primitive lipoblastic cells with lipoblastic or lipomatous differentiation, sometimes with foci of normal fat cells 脂肪肉瘤

li·po·sis (lī-po′sis) 同 lipomatosis

lipo·sol·u·ble (lip″o-sol′u-bəl) soluble in fats 脂溶性的

lipo·some (lip′o-sōm) a microscopic spherical particle formed by a lipid bilayer enclosing an aqueous compartment 脂质体

lipo·suc·tion (lip′o-suk″shən) suction-assisted lipectomy 抽脂术

li·pot·ro·phy (lī-pot′rə-fe) increase of bodily fat 脂肪增多；**lipotroph′ic** *adj.*

lipo·tro·pic (lip″o-tro′pik) acting on fat metabolism by hastening removal or decreasing the deposit of fat in the liver; also, an agent having such effects 抗脂肪肝的

lip·o·tro·pin (lip′o-tro″pin) any of several prohormones that promote lipolysis; the most important one in humans is *β-lipotropin* 促脂解素；β-l. a prohormone synthesized by cells of the anterior lobe of the pituitary; it promotes fat mobilization and skin darkening by stimulation of melanocytes and is the precursor of the endorphins β 促脂素

lipo·vac·cine (lip″o-vak′sēn) a vaccine in a vegetable oil vehicle 脂制菌苗

li·poxy·ge·nase (lī-pok′sī-jən-ās) an enzyme that catalyzes the oxidation of polyunsaturated fatty acids to form a peroxide of the acid 脂氧合酶，脂加氧酶，又称 *lipoxidase*

lip·ping (lip′ing) 1. a wedge-shaped shadow in the radiograph of chondrosarcoma between the cortex and the elevated periosteum 唇状阴影；2. bony overgrowth in osteoarthritis 骨关节炎骨质增生过度

liq·ue·fa·cient (lik″wə-fa′shənt) 1. producing or pertaining to liquefaction 液化的；2. an agent that causes liquefaction 液化剂

liq·ue·fac·tion (lik″wə-fak′shən) conversion into a liquid form 液化；**liquefac′tive** *adj.*

liq·ue·fy (lik′wə-fi) to become or cause to become liquid（使）液化

liq·uid (lik′wid) 1. a substance that flows readily in its natural state 液体；2. flowing readily; neither solid nor gaseous 液态

li·quor (lik′ər) (li′kwor) pl. *liquors, liquo′res* [L.] 1. a liquid, especially an aqueous solution containing a medicinal substance 溶液；2. a term applied to certain body fluids 某种体液；**l. am′nii,** amniotic fluid 羊水；**l. cerebrospina′lis,** cerebrospinal fluid 脑脊液；**l. folli′culi,** follicular fluid 滤泡液

li·sin·o·pril (li-sin′o-pril) an angiotensin-converting enzyme inhibitor used in the treatment of hypertension, congestive heart failure, and acute myocardial infarction 赖诺普利

lis·sen·ceph·a·ly (lis″ən-sef′ə-le) agyria 无脑回畸形；**lissencephal′ic** *adj.*

Lis·te·ria (lis-te′re-ə) a genus of small, grampositive, coccoid bacteria of the family Listeriaceae; *L. monocyto′genes* causes listeriosis 李斯特菌属

Lis·te·ri·a·ceae (lis-te″re-a′se-e) a family of gram-positive, non–spore-forming bacteria of the order Bacillales 李斯特菌科

lis·te·ri·o·sis (lis-te″re-o′sis) infection caused by *Listeria monocytogenes*. Infection in utero results in abortion, stillbirth, or prematurity; that during birth causes cardiorespiratory distress, diarrhea, vomiting, and meningitis; and in adults it causes meningitis, endocarditis, and disseminated granulomatous lesions 李斯特菌病

lis·ter·ism (lis′tər-iz″əm) the principles and practice of antiseptic and aseptic surgery 防腐无菌法

li·ter (L) (le′tər) a basic unit of volume used for liquids with the SI system, equal to 1000 cubic centimeters, or 1 cubic decimeter, or 1.0567 quarts liquid measure 升

li·thi·a·sis (lī-thi′ə-sis) the formation or presence of calculi or other concretions 结石

lith·i·um (Li) (lith′e-əm) a soft, light, silverwhite, alkali metal element; at. no. 3, at. wt. 6.94. Its salts, especially *l. carbonate* and *l. citrate,* are used to treat and prevent manic states in bipolar disorder 锂（化学元素）

litho·clast (lith′o-klast) lithotrite 碎石器

litho·gen·e·sis (lith″o-gen′ə-sis) formation of calculi. 结石形成 **lithogen′ic, lithog′enous** *adj.*

li·thol·a·paxy (lī-thol′ə-pak″se) 同 lithotripsy

li·thol·y·sis (lī-thol′ī-sis) 同 dissolution of calculi 结石溶解；**litholyt′ic** *adj.*

litho·ne·phri·tis (lith″o-nə-fri′tis) inflammation of the kidney due to irritation by calculi 结石性肾炎

li·thot·o·my (lī-thot′o-me) 1. incision of a duct or organ for removal of calculi 取石术；2. cystolithotomy 膀胱切开取石术

litho·trip·sy (lith′o-trip″se) the crushing of a calculus within the urinary system or gallbladder, followed at once by the washing out of the fragments; it may be performed surgically or by noninvasive methods, such as by laser or by shock waves 碎石术 **extracorporeal shock wave l.,** a procedure for treating upper urinary tract stones: the patient is immersed in a large tub of water and a high-energy shock wave generated by a high-voltage spark is focused on the stone by an ellipsoid reflector. The stone disintegrates into particles, which are passed in the urine 体外超声波碎石术；**pneumatic l.,** lithotripsy in which a rigid probe is inserted and pneumatic pressure is applied directly to the calculus 气压弹道碎石术

litho·trip·ter (lith′o-trip″tər) an instrument for crushing calculi in lithotripsy 碎石机

litho·trip·tic (lith′o-trip″tik) dissolving vesical calculi; also, an agent that so acts 碎石的

litho·trip·tor (lith′o-trip″tər) 同 lithotripter

litho·trite (lith′o-trīt) an instrument for crushing a urinary calculus 碎石器

li·thot·ri·ty (lĭ-thot′rĭ-te) 同 lithotripsy

lith·ure·sis (lith″u-re′sis) the passage of small calculi in the urine 石尿症

lit·mus (lit′məs) a pigment prepared from *Roccella tinctoria* and other lichens; used as an acidbase (pH) indicator 石蕊

lit·ter (lit′ər) stretcher 担架

lit·to·ral (lit′ə-rəl) pertaining to the shore of a large body of water 沿海的

li·ve·do (lĭ-ve′do) [L.] a discolored patch on the skin 青斑; **l. racemo′sa, l. reticula′ris,** a red to blue, netlike mottling of the skin on the limbs and trunk, which becomes more intense on exposure to cold. One type is normal, benign, and transient and other types are chronic, indicative of underlying conditions, and occasionally even ulcerative 网状青斑

liv·e·doid (liv′ə-doid) pertaining to livedo 青斑样的

liv·er (liv′ər) 1. the large, dark-red gland in the upper part of the abdomen on the right side, just beneath the respiratory diaphragm. Its functions include storage and filtration of blood, secretion of bile, conversion of sugars into glycogen, and many other metabolic activities 肝脏，见图 27; 2. the same gland of certain animals, sometimes used as food or from which pharmaceutical products are prepared 肝; **fatty l.,** one with fatty infiltration; the liver is enlarged but of normal consistency 脂肪肝; **hobnail l.,** one whose surface has naillike points from cirrhosis 结节性肝硬化

liv·er phos·phor·y·lase (liv′ər fos-for′ə-lās)the liver isozyme of glycogen phosphorylase; deficiency causes glycogen storage disease, type Ⅵ肝磷酸化酶

liv·er phos·phor·y·lase ki·nase (liv′ər fosfor′ə-lās ki′nās) the liver isozyme of phosphorylase kinase 肝磷酸化酶激酶

liv·id (liv′id) discolored, as from a contusion or bruise; black and blue 青紫的

li·vor (li′vor) pl. *livo′res* [L.] discoloration 青紫; **l. mor′tis,** discoloration of dependent parts of the body after death 尸斑

lix·iv·i·a·tion (lik-siv″e-a′shən) separation of soluble from insoluble material by use of an appropriate solvent, and drawing off the solution 浸滤

LMA left mentoanterior (position of fetus) 左颏前位（胎位）

LMF lymphocyte mitogenic factor 淋巴细胞有丝分裂因子

LMP last menstrual period 末次月经; left mentoposterior (position of fetus) 左颏后位（胎位）

LMT left mentotransverse (position of fetus) 左颏横位（胎位）

lncRNA long noncoding radionuclide angiography 长非编码放射性核素血管造影

LNMP last normal menstrual period 末次正常月经期

LNPF lymph node permeability factor 淋巴结通透性因子

LOA left occipitoanterior (position of fetus) 左枕前位（胎位）

Loa (lo′ə) a genus of filarial nematodes, including *L. lo′a,* a West African species that migrates freely throughout the subcutaneous connective tissue, seen especially about the orbit and even under the conjunctiva, and occasionally causing edematous swellings 罗阿（丝虫）属

load (l ō d) the quantity of something measurable carried by an object or organism 负荷; 负载; 装载; 充 填; **allostatic l.,** the physiologic consequences resulting from some combination of repeated or chronic exposure to adverse stimuli and inefficient management of allostasis 非稳态负荷; **viral l.** the number of copies of RNA of a given virus per milliliter of blood 病毒载量

load·ing (lōd′ing) 1. administering sufficient quantities of a substance to test a subject's ability to metabolize or absorb it 负荷试验; 2. exertion of lengthening force on a part such as a muscle or ligament 加荷

lo·bate (lo′bāt) divided into lobes 叶状的

lo·ba·tion (lo-ba′shən) the formation of lobes; the state of having lobes 叶状形成; **renal l.,** the appearance on x-ray films of small notches along the surface of the kidney, indicating the location of renal lobes 肾叶形成，X 线片上出现肾表面小切迹，表示肾叶的位置

lobe (lōb) 1. a more or less well-defined portion of an organ or gland 叶，器官的一部分; 2. one of the main divisions of a tooth crown 牙叶，牙冠主要分区之一; **lo′bar** *adj.*; **caudate l.,** a small lobe of the liver between the inferior vena cava and the left lobe 肝尾状叶; **ear l.,** earlobe 耳垂; **frontal l.,** the rostral (anterior) portion of the cerebral hemisphere 额叶; **hepatic l's,** the lobes of the liver, designated the right and left and the caudate and quadrate 肝叶; **insular l.,** insula (2) 岛叶; **occipital l.,** the most posterior portion of the cerebral hemisphere, forming a small part of its dorsolateral surface 枕叶; **parietal l.,** the upper central portion of the cerebral hemisphere, between the frontal and occipital lobes and above the temporal lobe 顶叶；**polyalveolar l.,** a congenital disorder characterized by early infancy by far more than the normal number of alveoli in the lung lobes; thereafter, normal multiplication of alveoli does not take place, and the alveoli become enlarged, i.e., emphysematous 多肺泡叶；**quadrate l.,** 1. precuneus 楔前叶；2. a small lobe of the liver, between the gallbladder on the right and the left lobe 肝方叶；**spigelian l.,** caudate l. of liver 肝尾状叶；**temporal l.,** the lower lateral lobe of the cerebral hemisphere 颞叶

lo·bec·to·my (lo-bek′tə-me) excision of a lobe, as of the lung, brain, or liver (脑、肺、肝等的) 叶切除术

lo·bo·my·co·sis (lo″bo-mi-ko′sis) 同 lacaziosis

lo·bot·o·my (lo-bot′ə-me) incision of a lobe; in psychosurgery, incision of all the fibers of a lobe of the brain 脑叶切断术；**frontal l., prefrontal l.,** incision of the white matter of the frontal lobe with a leukotome passed via a cannula through holes drilled in the skull 前脑叶白质切除术

lob·u·lat·ed (lob′u-lāt″əd) made up of lobules 分叶状

lob·ule (lob′ūl) a small segment or lobe, especially one of the smaller divisions making up a lobe 小叶；**lob′ular** adj.；**ansiform l.,** 同 semilunar l's；**anterior quadrangular l. of cerebellum,** the portion of the anterior lobe of the hemisphere of the cerebellum lying anterior to the primary fissure, continuous with the culmen 小脑方形小叶前部；**biventral l.,** a lobule of the cerebellar hemisphere, in the posterior lobe between the tonsil and the gracile lobule and continuous with the pyramid of the vermis 二腹小叶；**central l. of cerebellum,** the portion of the vermis of the cerebellum between the lingula and the culmen, in the anterior lobe, resting on the lingula and the anterior medullary velum 小脑中央小叶；**l's of epididymis,** the wedge-shaped parts of the head of the epididymis, each comprising an efferent ductule of the testis 附睾小叶；**gracile l.,** paramedian l.; a lobule of the posterior lobe of the hemisphere of the cerebellum between the semilunar and biventral lobules, lateral to the tuber vermis 正中旁小叶；**hepatic l's,** the small vascular units composing the substance of the liver 肝小叶；**paracentral l.,** a lobe on the medial surface of the cerebral hemisphere, continuous with the precentral and postcentral gyri, limited below by the cingulate sulcus; subdivided into anterior and posterior paracentral gyri 中央旁小叶；**paramedian l.,** 同 gracile l.；**parietal l.,** one of the two divisions, inferior and superior, of the parietal lobe of the cerebrum 顶小叶；**portal l.,** a polygonal mass of liver tissue containing portions of three adjacent hepatic lobules

and having a portal vein at its center and a central vein peripherally at each corner 门管小叶；**posterior quadrangular l. of cerebellum,** the portion of the posterior lobe of the hemisphere of the cerebellum between the primary and posterior superior fissures and continuous with the declive 小脑方形小叶后部；**primary l. of lung, respiratory l.,** terminal respiratory unit 初级肺小叶；**semilunar l's,** ansiform l.; the part of the posterior lobe of the hemisphere of the cerebellum between the posterior quadrangular lobule and the gracile lobule, continuous with the folium vermis and tuber vermis; subdivided into inferior and superior semilunar l's 襻状小叶；**simple l. of cerebellum,** the large anterior division of the posterior cerebellar lobe, comprising the posterior quadrangular lobule and declive 小脑单小叶；**l's of testis,** the pyramidal subdivisions of the testicular substance, each with its base against the tunica albuginea of the testis and its apex at the mediastinum, and composed largely of seminiferous tubules 睾丸小叶

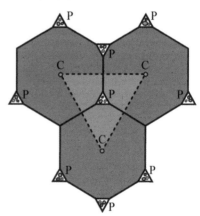

▲ 肝脏（实线）和门静脉（虚线）小叶图，显示门静脉区（**P**）和中央静脉（**C**）

lob·u·lus (lob′u-ləs) pl. lo′buli [L.] 同 lobule

lo·bus (lo′bəs) pl. lo′bi [L.] lobe 叶

lo·cal (lo′kəl) restricted to or pertaining to one spot or part; not general 局部的

lo·cal·iza·tion (lo″kəl-ĭ-za′shən) 1. the determination of the site or place of any process or lesion 定位；2. restriction to a circumscribed or limited area 局部化，局限；3. the localization in the oocyte or blastomere of materials that will develop into a particular tissue or organ 胚区定位；**cerebral l.,** determination of areas of the cortex involved in performance of certain functions 大脑皮质定位；**germinal l.,** the location on a blastoderm of prospective organs 胚区定位

lo·ca·tor (lo'ka-tər) a device for determining the site of foreign objects within the body 定位器；**electroacoustic l.,** a device that amplifies into an audible click the contact of the probe with a solid object in tissue 电声（异物）定位器

lo·chia (lo'ke-ə) a vaginal discharge occurring during the first week or two after childbirth 恶露；**lo'chial** *adj.* **l. al'ba,** the final vaginal discharge after childbirth, when the amount of blood is decreased and the leukocytes are increased 白色恶露；**l. ru'bra,** that occurring immediately after childbirth, consisting almost entirely of blood 血性恶露；**l. sanguinolen'ta,** 同 l. serosa；**l. sero'sa,** the serous vaginal discharge occurring 4 or 5 days after childbirth 浆液恶露

lock·jaw (lok'jaw) 1. tetanus 破伤风；2. trismus 牙关紧闭

lo·co·mo·tion (lo"kə-mo'shən) movement or the ability to move from one place to another 行进（运动）；**locomo'tive, locomo'tor** *adj.*

lo·co·re·gion·al (lo"ko-re'jən-əl) limited to a localized area, as contrasted with systemic or metastatic 局部区域的

loc·u·lus (lok'u-ləs) pl. *lo'culi* [L.] 1. a small space or cavity 小室；2. an enlargement in the uterus in some mammals, containing an embryo 子宫局部扩大部；**loc'ular** *adj.*

lo·cum (lo'kəm) [L.] place 部位；**l. te'nens, l. te'nent,** a practitioner who temporarily takes the place of another 代理医师

lo·cus (lo'kəs) pl. *lo'ci* [L.] 1. place; site 位置；轨迹；2. in genetics, the specific site of a gene on a chromosome 基因座；**l. coeru'leus,** a pigmented area in the pontine part of the fourth ventricle floor, extending through the rostral pons; its cells contain melanin 蓝斑

lo·dox·a·mide (lo-dok'sə-mīd) a mast cell stabilizer and antiallergic; applied topically to the eye as the tromethamine salt for the treatment of allergen-induced conjunctivitis, keratitis, and keratoconjunctivitis 洛度沙胺

log·a·dec·to·my (log"ə-dek'tə-me) excision of a portion of the conjunctiva 结膜部分切除术

log·am·ne·sia (log"am-ne'zhə) receptive aphasia 感觉性失语症

log·a·pha·sia (log"ə-fa'zhə) motor aphasia 运动性失语症

logo·clo·nia (log"o-klo'ne-ə) spasmodic repetition of words or parts of words, particularly the end syllables; often occurring in Alzheimer disease 词尾重复症。Cf. *stuttering*

logo·pe·dics (log-o-pe'diks) the study and treatment

of speech defects 言语矫正法

log·or·rhea (log"o-re'ə) pressured speech; excessive and rapid speech, seen in certain mental disorders 多语症

logo·spasm (log'o-spaz"əm) 1. logoclonia 言语痉挛；2. stuttering 口吃

lo·i·a·sis (lo-i'ə-sis) infection with nematodes of the genus *Loa* 罗阿丝虫病

loin (loin) that part of each side of the back between the thorax and pelvis 腰部

lo·me·flox·a·cin (lo"mə-flok'sə-sin) a broadspectrum antibiotic effective against a wide range of aerobic gram-negative and gram-positive organisms; used as the hydrochloride salt 洛美沙星

lo·mi·ta·pide (loh-mī'tə-pide) a microsomal triglyceride transfer protein inhibitor used as a lipid-lowering agent adjunct to other lipidlowering therapies to reduce total cholesterol, LDL-C, apolipoprotein B, and non–HDL-C levels in patients with homozygous familial hypercholesterolemia 洛美他派

lo·mus·tine (lo-mus'tēn) an alkylating agent of the nitrosourea group, used as an antineoplastic in the treatment of Hodgkin disease and brain tumors 洛莫司汀

lon·gis·si·mus (lon-jis'ĭ-məs) [L.] longest 最长的

lon·gi·tu·di·nal (lon"jĭ-too'di-nəl) lengthwise; parallel to the long axis of the body or an organ 纵向的

lon·gi·tu·di·na·lis (lon"ji-too"dĭ-na'lis) [L.] 同 longitudinal

lon·gus (long'gəs) [L.] long 长的

loop (loop) a turn or sharp curve in a cordlike structure 襻，环；**capillary l's,** minute endothelial tubes that carry blood in the papillae of the skin 毛细血管襻；**closed l.,** a type of feedback in which the input to one or more of the subsystems is affected by its own output 闭合循环；**Henle l.,** the long U-shaped part of the renal tubule, extending through the medulla from the end of the proximal convoluted tubule. It begins with a *descending limb* (comprising the *proximal straight tubule* and the *thin tubule*), followed by the *ascending limb* (the *distal straight tubule*), and ending at the *distal convoluted tubule* 细尿管襻；**open l.,** a system in which an input alters the output, but the output has no effect on the input 开环

loo·sen·ing (loo'sən-ing) freeing from restraint or strictness 松弛；**l. of associations,** in psychiatry, a disorder of thinking in which associations of ideas become so shortened, fragmented, and disturbed as to lack logical relationship 思维散漫

LOP left occipitoposterior (position of fetus) 左枕后位（胎位）

L

lo·per·amide (lo-per′ə-mīd) an antiperistaltic used as the hydrochloride salt as an antidiarrheal and to reduce the volume of discharge from ileostomies 洛哌丁胺

lo·phot·ri·chous (lo-fot′rī-kəs) having two or more flagella at one end (of a bacterial cell) 偏端丛毛的

lo·pin·a·vir (lo-pin′ə-vir) an antiviral HIV protease inhibitor, used with ritonavir in the treatment of HIV infection 洛匹那韦

lor·a·car·bef (lor″ə-kahr′bef) a carbacephem antibiotic closely related to cefaclor and having similar antibacterial actions and uses 氯碳头孢

lor·at·a·dine (lə-rat′ə-dēn) a nonsedating antihistamine used in the treatment of allergic rhinitis, chronic idiopathic urticaria, and asthma 氯雷他定

lor·a·ze·pam (lor-az′ə-pam) a benzodiazepine used as an antianxiety agent, sedative-hypnotic, preanesthetic medication, and anticonvulsant 劳拉西泮

lor·cas·er·in (lor-kayz′er-in) a serotonin 2C receptor agonist used to treat obesity and stimulate weight loss in combination with a lowcalorie diet and physical activity in adults 罗卡西林

lor·do·sis (lor-do′sis) 1. the anterior concavity in the curvature of the lumbar and cervical spine as viewed from the side 脊柱前凸；2. abnormal increase in this curvature 曲率异常增大

lo·sar·tan (lo-sahr′tan) an angiotensin Ⅱ receptor antagonist, used as an antihypertensive; used as the potassium salt 氯沙坦

LOT left occipitotransverse (position of fetus) 左枕横位（胎位）

lo·te·pred·nol (lo″tə-pred′nol) a corticosteroid applied topically to the conjunctiva in the treatment of seasonal allergic conjunctivitis, postoperative inflammation, and ocular inflammatory disorders 氯替泼诺

lo·tion (lo′shən) a liquid suspension, solution, or emulsion for external application to the body 洗剂

loupe (loop) [Fr.] a magnifying lens 放大镜

louse (lous) pl. lice. Any of various parasitic insects; species parasitic on humans are *Pediculus humanus capitis* (head l.), *P. humanus corporis* (body, or clothes, l.), and *Phthirus pubis* (crab, or pubic, l.). Lice are major vectors of typhus, relapsing fever, and trench fever 虱

lo·va·stat·in (lo′və-stat″in) an antihyperlipidemic agent that acts by inhibiting cholesterol synthesis, used in the treatment of hypercholesterolemia and other forms of dyslipidemia and to lower the risks associated with atherosclerosis and coronary heart disease 洛伐他汀

low-grade (lo′grād′) occurring near the low end of a range, as of a fever or malignancy 低级别

lox·a·pine (lok′sə-pēn) a tricyclic dibenzoxaze- pine derivative used as the succinate and hydrochloride salts as an antipsychotic 洛沙平

lox·os·ce·lism (lok-sos′ə-liz-əm) a morbid condition due to the bite of the spiders *Loxosceles laeta* and *L. reclusa*, beginning with a painful erythematous vesicle and progressing to a gangrenous slough of the affected area 棕花蛛中毒

lox·ot·o·my (lok-sot′ə-me) oval amputation 斜切断术，卵圆形切断术

loz·enge (loz′ənj) [Fr.] 1. troche; a discoidshaped, solid, medicinal preparation for solution in the mouth, consisting of an active ingredient incorporated in a suitably flavored base 锭剂；2. a triangular area of tissue marked for excision in plastic surgery 三角标记区

Lp (a) 脂蛋白（a）抗原，见 *lipoprotein* 下词条

LPN licensed practical nurse 执业护士

LPR laryngopharyngeal reflux 喉咽反流

LPV lymphotropic papovavirus 亲淋巴乳多空病毒

LSA left sacroanterior (position of fetus) 左骶前位（胎位）

LScA left scapuloanterior (position of fetus) 左肩前位（胎位）

LScP left scapuloposterior (position of fetus) 左肩后位（胎位）

LSD lysergic acid diethylamide 麦角酰二乙胺

LSP left sacroposterior (position of fetus) 左骶后位（胎位）

L-spine lumbar spine 腰椎

LST left sacrotransverse (position of fetus) 左骶横位（胎位）

LTF lymphocyte transforming factor 淋巴细胞转化因子

Lu utetium 元素镥的符号

lubb-dupp (ləb-dup′) syllables used to represent the first and second heart sounds 用来表示第一、第二心音音节

lu·bri·cant (loo′brī-kənt) a substance applied as a surface film to reduce friction between moving parts 润滑剂

lu·cid·i·ty (loo-sid′ĭ-te) clearness of mind 清醒度（神志）；**lu′cid** *adj.*

lu·es (loo′ēz) syphilis 梅毒；**luet′ic** *adj.*

lum·ba·go (ləm-ba′go) a nonmedical term for any pain in the lower back 腰痛

lum·bar (lum′bər) (-bahr) pertaining to the loins 腰的

lum·bar·iza·tion (lum″bər-ĭ-za′shən) nonfusion of the first and second segments of the sacrum so that there is one additional articulated vertebra, the sacrum consisting of only four segments 腰椎化

lum·bo·cos·tal (lum″bo-kos′təl) pertaining to the

lumbar vertebrae and ribs 腰肋三角

lum·bo·dyn·ia (lum″bo-din′e-ə) 同 lumbago

lum·bo·in·gui·nal (lum″bo-ing′gwĭ-nəl) pertaining to the lumbar and inguinal regions 腰腹股沟的

lum·bo·sa·cral (lum″bo-sa′krəl) pertaining to the lumbar vertebrae and sacrum, or to the lumbar and sacral regions 腰骶部

lum·bri·cide (lum′brĭ-sīd) ascaricide 驱蛔虫药

lum·bri·coid (lum′brĭ-koid) resembling an earthworm; said particularly of *Ascaris lumbricoides* 蚯蚓状的

lum·bri·cus (ləm-bri′kəs) pl. *lumbri′ci* [L.] any member of the genus *Lumbricus,* the earthworms 蚯蚓

lu·men (loo′mən) pl. *lu′mina* [L.] 1. the cavity or channel within a tube or tubular organ 管腔；2. the SI unit of luminous flux; it is the light emitted in a unit solid angle by a uniform point source with luminous intensity of 1 candela 流明（光通量的单位）；**residual l.,** the remains of the Rathke pouch, between the distal and intermediate parts of the pituitary gland 残留腔

lu·mi·nal (loo′mĭ-nəl) pertaining to or located in the lumen of a tubular structure 管腔的

lu·mi·nes·cence (loo″mĭ-nes′əns) the property of giving off light without a corresponding degree of heat 发光

lu·mi·no·phor (loo′mĭ-nə-for″) a chemical group that gives the property of luminescence to organic compounds 发光体

lu·mi·rho·dop·sin (loo″mĭ-ro-dop′sin) an intermediate product of exposure of rhodopsin to light 感光视紫红质

lum·pec·to·my (ləm-pek′tə-me) 1. surgical excision of only the palpable lesion in carcinoma of the breast 乳腺肿块切除术；2. surgical removal of a mass 肿块切除术

LUNA laparoscopic uterine nerve ablation 腹腔镜子宫神经消融术

lu·nate (loo′nāt) 1. moon-shaped or crescentic 新月形；2. lunate bone 月骨

lung (lung) the organ of respiration; either of the pair of organs that effect aeration of blood, lying on either side of the heart within the chest cavity 肺，见图 25 和图 26；**black l.,** pneumoconiosis of coal workers 尘肺；**brown l.,** byssinosis 棉尘肺；**farmer's l.,** hypersensitivity pneumonitis from inhalation of moldy hay dust 农民肺；**humidifier l.,** hypersensitivity pneumonitis caused by breathing air that has passed through humidifiers, dehumidifiers, or air conditioners contaminated by certain fungi, amebas, or thermophilic actinomycetes 加湿器肺；**iron l.,** popular name for *Drinker respirator* 铁肺；**pigeon breeder's l.,** hypersensitivity pneumonitis from inhalation of particles of bird feces by those who work closely with pigeons or other birds; it may eventually result in pulmonary fibrosis 饲鸽者肺；**white l.,** pneumonia alba 白肺

lung·worm (lung′wərm) any parasitic worm, such as *Paragonimus westermani,* that invades the lungs 肺蠕虫

lu·nu·la (loo′nu-lə) pl. *lu'nulae* [L.] a small, crescentic or moon-shaped area or structure, e.g., the white area at the base of the nail of a finger or toe, or one of the segments of the semilunar valves of the heart 甲弧影

lu·poid (loo′poid) pertaining to or resembling lupus 狼疮样的

lu·pus (loo′pəs) any of a group of skin diseases in which the lesions are characteristically eroded 狼疮；**chilblain l. erythematosus,** a form due to cold-induced microvascular injury, aggravated by cold; early lesions resemble chilblains, but later the condition resembles discoid lupus erythematosus 冻疮样红斑狼疮；**cutaneous l. erythematosus,** one of the two main forms of lupus erythematosus, in which the skin may be either the only or the first organ or system involved. It is usually classified as either *chronic, subacute,* or *acute* 皮肤红斑狼疮；**discoid l. erythematosus (DLE),** a chronic form of cutaneous lupus erythematosus, with red macules covered by scanty adherent scales that fall off and leave scars; lesions often form a butterfly pattern over the bridge of the nose and cheeks, but other areas may also be involved 盘状红斑狼疮；**drug-induced l.,** a syndrome similar to systemic lupus erythematosus, caused by prolonged use of certain drugs, such as hydralazine, isoniazid, various anticonvulsants, or procainamide 药物性狼疮；**l. erythemato′sus (LE),** a group of chronic connective tissue diseases, usually classified as either *cutaneous l. erythematosus* or *systemic l. erythematosus* 红斑狼疮；**l. erythemato′sus profun′dus,** cutaneous lupus erythematosus with deep brawny indurations or subcutaneous nodules on the skin; the overlying skin may be erythematous, atrophic, and ulcerated and on healing may leave a depressed scar 深部红斑狼疮；**l. erythemato′sus tu′midus,** a variant of the discoid or systemic type in which lesions are raised red, purple, or brown plaques 肿胀型红斑狼疮；**hypertrophic l. erythematosus,** a form of the discoid type having verrucous hyperkeratotic lesions 肥厚性红斑性狼疮；**l. milia′ris dissemina′tus fa′ciei,** a form marked by discrete, superficial nodules on the face, particularly the eyelids, upper lip, chin, and nostrils 颜面播散性粟粒性狼疮；**neonatal l.,** a rash resembling discoid lupus, sometimes with systemic abnormalities such as heart block or hepatosplenomegaly, in infants born to mothers with systemic lupus erythematosus; it is usually benign and selflimited 新生儿狼疮；l. per′nio, 1. a cutaneous manifestation of sarcoidosis consisting of smooth, shiny, purple plaques on the ears, forehead, nose, and digits, often with bone cysts 一种结节病的皮肤表现；2. chilblain l. erythematosus；systemic l. erythematosus (SLE), a chronic generalized connective tissue disorder, ranging from mild to fulminating, marked by skin eruptions, arthralgia, arthritis, leukopenia, anemia, visceral lesions, neurologic manifestations, lymphadenopathy, fever, and other constitutional symptoms. There may also be abnormal immunologic phenomena such as hypergammaglobulinemia, hypocomplementemia, antigen-antibody complexes, antinuclear antibodies, and LE cells 系统性红斑狼疮；l. vulga′ris, the most common, severe form of tuberculosis of the skin, usually on the face, with red-brown patches of nodules in the dermis that progressively spread peripherally, leaving central atrophy and later ulceration, scarring, and destruction of cartilage in involved sites 寻常狼疮

lu·ras·i·done (loo-rasˈĭ-dōn) an antipsychotic used as the hydrochloride salt in the treatment of schizophrenia 鲁拉西酮

lute (loot) 1. a substance such as cement, wax, or clay that coats a surface or joint area to make a tight seal 封泥；2. to coat or seal with such a substance 用封泥封

lu·te·al (looˈte-əl) pertaining to or having the properties of the corpus luteum or its active principle 黄体的

lu·te·in (looˈte-in) 1. a lipochrome from the corpus luteum, fat cells, and egg yolk 叶黄素；2. any lipochrome 脂色素

lu·te·in·ic (loo″te-inˈik) 1. pertaining to lutein 叶黄素的；2. 同 luteal；3. pertaining to luteinization 黄体化的

lu·te·in·iza·tion (loo″te-in″ĭ-za′shən) the process by which a postovulatory ovarian follicle transforms into a corpus luteum through vascularization, follicular cell hypertrophy, and lipid accumulation, the latter in some species giving the yellow color indicated by the term 黄体化

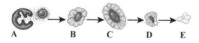

▲ 黄体化，以排卵期卵巢卵泡破裂起始（**A**），通过血管化和肥大进展为成熟的黄体（**B** 和 **C**），接下来是退化（**D**）形成白体（**E**）

lu·te·ol·y·sis (loo″te-olˈə-sis) degeneration of the corpus luteum 黄体溶解；**luteolyt′ic** *adj.*

lu·te·o·ma (loo″te-o′mə) 1. a luteinized granulosa-theca cell tumor 黄体瘤；2. nodular hyperplasia of ovarian lutein cells sometimes occurring in the last trimester of pregnancy 卵巢黄体细胞的结节状增生，常发生在妊娠的最后三个月

lu·teo·tro·pic (loo″te-o-tro′pik) stimulating formation of the corpus luteum 促黄体的

lu·te·ti·um (Lu) (loo-te′she-əm) a silvery white, heavy metal, rare earth element; at. no. 71, at. wt. 174.967 镥（化学元素）

Lut·zo·my·ia (loot-zo-mi′ə) a genus of sandflies of the family Psychodidae, the females of which suck blood. Various species are vectors of leishmaniasis in the New World 罗蛉属

lux (lx) (luks) the SI unit of illumination, being 1 lumen per square meter 勒（克斯），光照度的单位

lux·a·tion (lək-sa′shən) dislocation 脱位

lux·u·ri·ant (ləg-zhoor′e-ənt) growing freely or excessively 繁茂的

LV left ventricular 左心室；lupus vulgaris 寻常型狼疮

LVAD left ventricular assist device 左室辅助装置；见 *device* 下 *ventricular assist device*

LVN licensed vocational nurse 有执照的职业护士

ly·ase (li′ās) any of a class of enzymes that remove groups from their substrates (other than by hydrolysis or oxidation), leaving double bonds, or that conversely add groups to double bonds 裂解酶

ly·can·thro·py (li-kan′thrə-pe) a delusion in which the individual believes he or she is a wolf or other animal or that they can change into one 变兽妄想

ly·co·pene (li′ko-pēn) the red carotenoid pigment of tomatoes and various berries and fruits 番茄红素

ly·ing-in (li″ing-in′) 1. puerperal 产后；2. puerperium 产褥期

lymph (limf) a transparent, usually slightly yellow, often opalescent liquid found within the lymphatic vessels, collected from tissues in all parts of the body and returned to the blood via the lymphatic system. Its cellular component consists chiefly of lymphocytes 淋巴

lym·pha (lim′fə) [L.] 同 lymph

lym·phad·e·nec·to·my (lim-fad″ə-nek′tə-me) surgical excision of a lymph node or nodes 淋巴结切除术

lym·phad·e·ni·tis (lim-fad″ə-ni′tis) inflammation of one or more lymph nodes 淋巴结炎；**cervical l.**, 见 *lymphadenopathy* 下词条；**mesenteric l.**, inflammation of the mesenteric lymph nodes, causing pain and swelling resembling that of acute appendicitis 肠系膜淋巴结炎；**tuberculous l.**, tuberculosis of lymph nodes, usually either cervical or mediastinal 结核性淋巴结炎；**tuberculous cervical l.**, tuberculosis of the cervical lymph nodes; formerly called *scrofula* 颈淋巴结结核，曾称为瘰疬

lym·phad·e·nog·ra·phy (lim-fad″ə-nog′rə-fe) radiography of lymph nodes after injection of a contrast medium in a lymphatic vessel 淋巴结造影术

lym·phad·e·noid (lim-fad′ə-noid) resembling the tissue of lymph nodes 淋巴结样的

lym·phad·e·no·ma (lim-fad″ə-no′mə) 同 lymphoma

lym·phad·e·nop·a·thy (lim-fad″ə-nop′ə-the) disease of the lymph nodes, usually with swelling 淋巴结病；**angioimmunoblastic l., angioimmunoblastic l. with dysproteinemia (AILD)**, a systemic lymphoma-like disorder characterized by malaise, generalized lymphadenopathy, and constitutional symptoms; it is a nonmalignant hyperimmune reaction to chronic antigenic stimulation 血管免疫母细胞性淋巴结病；**cervical l.**, enlarged, inflamed, and tender cervical lymph nodes, seen in certain infectious diseases of children, such as acute infections of the throat 颈部淋巴结病；**dermatopathic l.**, regional lymph node enlargement associated with melanoderma and other dermatoses marked by chronic erythroderma 皮肤病性淋巴结病；**immunoblastic l.**, angioimmunoblastic l. 免疫母细胞性淋巴结病；**mediastinal l.**, inflammation and swelling of mediastinal lymph nodes, often caused by some underlying condition such as mediastinitis, a cyst, or a tumor that can be malignant 纵隔淋巴结病

lym·pha·gogue (lim′fə-gog) an agent promoting the production of lymph 利淋巴药

lym·phan·gi·ec·ta·sia (lim-fan″je-ək-ta′zhə) lymphangiectasis 淋巴管扩张

lym·phan·gi·ec·ta·sis (lim-fan″je-ek′tə-sis) dilatation of the lymphatic vessels 淋巴管扩张；**lymphangiectat′ic** *adj.*

lym·phan·gio·en·do·the·li·o·ma (lim-fan″je-o-en″do-the″le-o′mə) endothelioma of the lymphatic vessels 淋巴管内皮瘤

lym·phan·gi·og·ra·phy (lim-fan″je-og′rə-fe) angiography of lymphatic vessels 淋巴管造影术

lym·phan·gio·leio·myo·ma·to·sis (lim-fan″jeo-li″o-mi″o-mə-to′sis) lymphangiomyomatosis 淋巴管平滑肌瘤病

lym·phan·gi·o·ma (lim-fan″je-o′mə) a tumor composed of newly formed lymph spaces and channels 淋巴管瘤；**cavernous l.**, 1. a deeply seated lymphangioma composed of cavernous lymphatic spaces and occurring in the head or neck 海绵状淋巴管瘤；2. cystic hygroma 囊性水肿；**cystic l.**, cystic hygroma 囊性淋巴管瘤

lym·phan·gio·my·o·ma·to·sis (lim-fan″je-omi″o-mə-to′sis) a progressive disorder of women of child-bearing age, marked by nodular and diffuse interstitial proliferation of smooth muscle in the lungs, lymph nodes, and thoracic duct 淋巴管肌瘤病，又称 *lymphangioleiomyomatosis*

lym·phan·gio·phle·bi·tis (lim-fan″je-o-flə- bi′tis) inflammation of the lymphatic vessels and the veins 淋巴管静脉炎

lym·phan·gio·sar·co·ma (lim-fan″je-o-sahrko′mə) a malignant tumor of vascular endothelial cells arising from lymphatic vessels, usually in a limb that is the site of chronic lymphedema 淋巴管肉瘤

lym·phan·gi·tis (lim″fan-ji′tis) inflammation of a lymphatic vessel or vessels 淋巴管炎；**lymphangit′ic** *adj.*

lym·pha·phe·re·sis (lim″fə-fə-re′sis) 同 lymphocytapheresis

lym·phat·ic (lim-fat′ik) 1. pertaining to lymph or to a lymphatic vessel 淋巴；2. a lymphatic vessel 淋巴管

lym·pha·tism (lim′fə-tiz″əm) status lymphaticus 淋巴毒血症，淋巴体质

lym·phec·ta·sia (lim″fek-ta′zhə) distention with lymph 淋巴管扩张

lym·phe·de·ma (lim″fə-de′mə) chronic swelling of a part due to accumulation of interstitial fluid (edema) after obstruction of lymphatic vessels or lymph nodes 淋巴水肿；**l. prae′cox,** Meige disease; lymphedema of the lower limbs beginning at or near puberty, usually in young women 早发性淋巴水肿，原发性淋巴水肿；**l. tar′da,** primary lymphedema occurring after age 35 迟发性淋巴水肿

lymph·no·di·tis (limf″no-di′tis) 同 lymphadenitis

lym·pho·blast (lim′fo-blast) a morphologically immature lymphocyte, representing an activated lymphocyte that has been transformed in response to antigenic stimulation 成淋巴细胞；**lympho-blas′tic** *adj.*

lym·pho·blas·to·ma (lim″fo-blas-to′mə) lymphoblastic lymphoma 成淋巴细胞瘤

lym·pho·blas·to·sis (lim″fo-blas-to′sis) an excess of lymphoblasts in the blood 成淋巴细胞增多症

Lym·pho·cryp·to·vi·rus (lim″fo-krip′to-vi″rəs) a genus of viruses of the family Herpesviridae; it includes the species human herpesvirus 4 (Epstein-Barr virus) 淋巴隐病毒属，见 *herpesvirus* 下表

lym·pho·cy·ta·phe·re·sis (lim″fo-si″tə-fə- re′sis) the selective removal of lymphocytes from withdrawn blood, which is then retransfused into the donor 淋

巴细胞除血浆法

lym·pho·cyte (lim′fo-sīt) a mononuclear, non-granular leukocyte having a deeply staining nucleus containing dense chromatin and a pale-blue-staining cytoplasm. Chiefly a product of lymphoid tissue, it participates in immunity 淋巴细胞; **lymphocyt′ic** *adj.*; B l's, B cells, bursa-dependent lymphocytes; the precursors of antibody-producing cells (plasma cells) and the cells primarily responsible for humoral immunity B 淋巴细胞; **cytotoxic T l's (CTL)**, differentiated T lymphocytes that can recognize and lyse target cells bearing specific antigens; they are important in graft rejection and killing of tumor cells and virus-infected host cells 细胞毒性 T 淋巴细胞; **T l's**, cells, thymus-dependent lymphocytes; those derived from precursors that migrate to the thymus, where they differentiate under the influence of the thyroid hormones and acquire their characteristic cell-surface markers; they are responsible for cell-mediated immunity and delayed hypersensitivity T 淋巴细胞

lym·pho·cy·to·blast (lim″fo-si′to-blast) lymphoblast

lym·pho·cy·to·ma (lim″fo-si-to′mə) welldifferentiated lymphocytic malignant lymphoma 假淋巴瘤，淋巴细胞瘤; **l. cu′tis**, cutaneous lymphoid hyperplasia 皮肤淋巴细胞瘤

lym·pho·cy·to·pe·nia (lim″fo-si″to-pe′ne-ə) lymphopenia; reduction of the number of lymphocytes in the blood 淋巴细胞减少

lym·pho·cy·to·phe·re·sis (lim″fo-si″to-fə-re′sis) 同 lymphocytapheresis

lym·pho·cy·to·sis (lim″fo-si-to′sis) an excess of normal lymphocytes in the blood or an effusion 淋巴细胞增多

lym·pho·cy·to·tox·ic·i·ty (lim″fo-si″to-toksis′ĭ-te) the quality or capability of lysing lymphocytes, as in procedures in which lymphocytes having a specific cell surface antigen are lysed when incubated with antisera and complement 淋巴细胞毒性

lym·pho·epi·the·li·o·ma (lim″fo-ep″ĭ-the″leo′mə) a pleomorphic, poorly differentiated carcinoma arising from modified epithelium overlying lymphoid tissue of the nasopharynx 淋巴上皮瘤

lym·phog·e·nous (lim-foj′ə-nəs) 1. producing lymph 成淋巴的; 2. produced from lymph or in the lymphatics 淋巴原的

lym·pho·gran·u·lo·ma (lim″fo-gran″u-lo′mə) Hodgkin disease 淋巴肉芽肿，霍奇金病; **l. inguina′le**, **l. vene′reum**, a venereal infection due to strains of *Chlamydia trachomatis*, marked by a primary transient ulcerative lesion of the genitals, followed by acute lymphadenopathy. In men, primary infection on the penis usually leads to inguinal lymphadenitis; in women, primary infection of the labia, vagina, or cervix often leads to hemorrhagic proctocolitis, and may progress to ulcerations, rectal strictures, rectovaginal fistulas, and genital elephantiasis 腹股沟淋巴肉芽肿，性病（性）淋巴肉芽肿

lym·pho·gran·u·lo·ma·to·sis (lim″fo-gran″ulo-mə-to′sis) European synonym for *Hodgkin disease* 淋巴肉芽肿病，霍奇金病

lym·phog·ra·phy (lim-fog′rə-fe) radiography of the lymphatic channels and lymph nodes after injection of a radiopaque medium 淋巴造影

lym·pho·his·tio·cy·to·sis (lim″fo-his″te-o-sito′sis) lymphocytosis with histiocytosis 淋巴组织细胞增生; **hemophagocytic l.**, any of several closely related disorders with excessive hemophagocytosis in the lymphoreticular system or the central nervous system; it is usually secondary to infection but can also be secondary to rheumatologic or other conditions, or can be familial (*familial hemophagocytic l.*) 噬血性淋巴组织细胞增生症

lym·phoid (lim′foid) 1. resembling lymph or tissue of the lymphoid system 淋巴样的; 2. 同 lymphatic (1)

lym·pho·kine (lim′fo-kīn) a general term for soluble protein mediators postulated to be released by sensitized lymphocytes on contact with antigen, and believed to play a role in macrophage activation, lymphocyte transformation, and cell-mediated immunity 淋巴因子

lym·pho·lyt·ic (lim″fo-lit′ik) causing destruction of lymphocytes 溶淋巴细胞的

lym·pho·ma (lim-fo′mə) any neoplastic disorder of lymphoid tissue. Often used to denote *malignant l.*, classifications of which are based on predominant cell type and degree of differentiation; various categories may be subdivided into nodular and diffuse types depending on the predominant pattern of cell arrangement 淋巴瘤; **adult T-cell l.**, adult T-cell leukemia/l., 成人 T 细胞淋巴瘤，见 *leukemia* 下词条; **B-cell l.**, B any in a large group of non-Hodgkin lymphomas characterized by malignant transformation of the B lymphocytes B 细胞淋巴瘤; **B-cell monocytoid l.**, a low-grade lymphoma in which cells resemble those of hairy cell leukemia B 细胞单核细胞淋巴瘤; **Burkitt l.**, a form of small noncleaved cell lymphoma, usually occurring in Africa, manifested usually as a large osteolytic lesion in the jaw or as an abdominal mass; Epstein-Barr virus has been implicated as a cause 伯基特淋巴瘤; **centrocytic l.**, mantle cell l. 中心细胞性淋巴瘤; **convoluted T-cell l.**, lymphoblastic lymphoma with markedly convoluted nuclei 卷曲

核 T 细 胞 淋 巴 瘤; **cutaneous T-cell l.**, a group of lymphomas exhibiting both clonal expansion of malignant T lymphocytes and malignant infiltration of the skin. The lymphocytes are arrested at varying stages of differentiation into helper cells, and skin infiltration is often the chief or only manifestation of disease 皮肤 T 细胞淋巴瘤; **follicular l.**, any of several types of non-Hodgkin lymphoma in which the lymphomatous cells are clustered into nodules or follicles 滤泡性淋巴瘤; **follicular center cell l.**, B-cell lymphoma classified by the similarity of the cell size and nuclear characteristics to those of normal follicular center cells; the four previous subtypes are scattered among several types of follicular and diffuse lymphomas 滤泡中心细胞性淋巴瘤; **giant follicular l.**, 同 follicular l.; **histiocytic l.**, a rare type of non-Hodgkin lymphoma characterized by the presence of large tumor cells resembling histiocytes morphologically but considered to be of lymphoid origin 组织细胞性淋巴瘤; **Hodgkin l.**, 霍奇金淋巴瘤, 见 *disease* 下词条; **large cell l.**, non-Hodgkin lymphoma characterized by the formation of one or more types of malignant large lymphocytes in a diffuse pattern 大细胞淋巴瘤; **large cell immunoblastic l.**, a highly malignant type of non-Hodgkin lymphoma characterized by large lymphoblasts (B or T lymphoblasts or a mixture) resembling histiocytes and having a diffuse pattern of infiltration 成免疫细胞性大细胞淋巴瘤; **Lennert l.**, a type of non-Hodgkin lymphoma with a high content of epithelioid histiocytes and frequently with bone marrow involvement 伦纳特淋巴瘤; **lymphoblastic l.**, a highly malignant type of non-Hodgkin lymphoma composed of a diffuse, relatively uniform proliferation of cells with round or convoluted nuclei and scanty cytoplasm 淋巴母细胞性淋巴瘤; **malignant l.**, a group of malignancies characterized by the proliferation of cells native to the lymphoid tissues, i.e., lymphocytes, histiocytes, and their precursors and derivatives; the group is divided into two major clinicopathologic categories: *Hodgkin disease* and *nonHodgkin* 恶性淋巴瘤; **mantle cell l., mantle zone l.**, a rare form of non-Hodgkin lymphoma having a usually diffuse pattern with both small lymphocytes and small cleaved cells 套细胞淋巴瘤; **marginal zone l.**, a group of related B-cell neoplasms that involve the lymphoid tissues in the marginal zone 边缘区淋巴瘤; **mixed lymphocytic-histiocytic l.**, nonHodgkin lymphoma characterized by a mixed population of cells, the smaller cells resembling lymphocytes and the larger ones histiocytes 混合淋巴细胞 - 组织细胞性淋巴瘤; **nodular l.**, follicular l. 结节状

淋巴瘤 **non-Hodgkin l.**, a heterogeneous group of malignant lymphomas, the only common feature being an absence of the giant Reed-Sternberg cells characteristic of Hodgkin disease 非霍奇金淋巴瘤; **primary effusion l.**, a B-cell lymphoma associated with human herpesvirus 8 infection, characterized by the occurrence of lymphomatous effusions in body cavities without the presence of a solid tumor 原发性渗出性淋巴瘤; **small B-cell l.**, the usual type of small lymphocytic lymphoma, having predominantly B lymphocytes 小 B 细胞淋巴瘤; **small cleaved cell l.**, a group of non-Hodgkin lymphomas characterized by the formation of malignant small cleaved follicular center cells, with either a follicular or diffuse pattern 弥漫性小裂细胞淋巴瘤; **small lymphocytic l.**, a diffuse form of non-Hodgkin lymphoma representing the neoplastic proliferation of well-differentiated B lymphocytes, with focal lymph node enlargement or generalized lymphadenopathy and splenomegaly 小淋巴细胞性淋巴瘤; **small noncleaved cell l.**, a highly malignant type of non-Hodgkin lymphoma characterized by the formation of small noncleaved follicular center cells, usually in a diffuse pattern 小无裂细胞淋巴瘤; **T-cell l.**, any in a heterogeneous group of lymphoid neoplasms representing malignant transformation of T lymphocytes T 细胞淋巴瘤; **undifferentiated l.**, small noncleaved cell l. 未分化淋巴瘤

lym·pho·ma·to·sis (lim″fo-mə-to′sis) the formation of multiple lymphomas in the body 淋巴瘤病

lym·pho·myx·o·ma (lim″fo-mik-so′mə) any benign growth consisting of adenoid tissue 淋巴黏液瘤

lym·pho·no·dus (lim″fo-no′dəs) pl. *lymphono′di*. Lymph node 淋巴结

lym·phop·a·thy (lim-fop′ə-the) any disease of the lymphatic system 淋巴系统疾病

lym·pho·pe·nia (lim″fo-pe′ne-ə) 同 lymphocytopenia

lym·pho·plas·ma·phe·re·sis (lim″fo-plaz″ mə-fə-re′sis) selective separation and removal of plasma and lymphocytes from withdrawn blood, the remainder of the blood then being retransfused to the donor 淋巴血浆交换疗法

lym·pho·pro·lif·er·a·tive (lim″fo-pro-lif′ər-ə- tiv) pertaining to or characterized by proliferation of the cells of the lymphoreticular system 淋巴组织增生的

lym·pho·re·tic·u·lar (lim″fo-rə-tik′u-lər) pertaining to the cells or tissues of both the lymphoid and reticuloendothelial systems 淋巴网状内皮细胞的

lym·pho·re·tic·u·lo·sis (lim″fo-rə-tik″u-lo′sis) proliferation of the reticuloendothelial cells of the

L

lymph nodes 淋巴网状内皮细胞增生；benign l., cat-scratch disease 良性淋巴网状内皮细胞增生症，猫抓病

lym·phor·rhea (lim″fo-re′ə) flow of lymph from cut or ruptured lymph vessels 淋巴溢，又称 *lymphorrhagia*

lym·pho·sar·co·ma (lim″fo-sahr-ko′mə) a general term applied to malignant neoplastic disorders of lymphoid tissue, but not including Hodgkin disease 淋巴肉瘤；见 *lymphoma*

lym·pho·scin·tig·ra·phy (lim″fo-sin-tig′rə-fe) scintigraphic detection of metastatic tumor in radioactively labeled lymph nodes, particularly that using radioactively labeled technetium colloid *(radiocolloid l.)* 淋巴系闪烁造影（术）

lym·phos·ta·sis (lim-fos′tə-sis) stoppage of lymph flow 淋巴淤滞

lym·pho·tax·is (lim″fo-tak′sis) the property of attracting or repulsing lymphocytes 淋巴细胞趋向性

lym·pho·tox·in (lim″fo-tok″sin) tumor necrosis factor β; a lymphokine produced by activated T lymphocytes that inhibits growth of tumors and blocks transformation of cells 淋巴毒素

lym·pho·tro·pic (lim″fo-tro′pik) having an affinity for lymphatic tissue 嗜淋巴细胞的

ly·on·iza·tion (li′on-ī-za′shən) the process by which or the condition in which all X chromosomes of the somatic cells in excess of one are inactivated on a random basis 莱昂作用

lyo·phil·ic (li″o-fil′ik) having an affinity for, or stable in, solution 亲液的，又称 *lyotropic*

ly·oph·i·li·za·tion (li-of″ĭ-lĭ-za′shən) the creation of a stable preparation of a biologic substance by rapid freezing and dehydration of the frozen product under high vacuum 冷冻干燥

lyo·pho·bic (li″o-fo′bik) not having an affinity for, or unstable in, solution 疏液的

ly·pres·sin (li-pres′in) a synthetic preparation of lysine vasopressin, used as an antidiuretic and vasoconstrictor in the treatment of central diabetes insipidus 赖氨酸加压素

Lys 同 lysine

lyse (līz) 1. to cause or produce disintegration of a compound, substance, or cell 溶化；2. to undergo lysis 溶解

ly·ser·gic ac·id di·eth·yl·amide (LSD) (lisur′jik as′id di-eth′əl-ə-mīd) a widely abused psychomimetic derived from lysergic acid, with both sympathomimetic and serotoninergic blocking effects. Side effects can include ataxia, fever, hyperreflexia, mydriasis, piloerection, tremor, nausea and vomiting, visual perception disorders, and varying psychiatric disturbances. Anxiety may develop into acute panic

reactions, and a persistent toxic psychotic state may result 麦角酰二乙胺

ly·ser·gide (li-sur′jĭd) 同 lysergic acid diethylamide

ly·sin (li′sin) 1. an antibody that causes complement-dependent lysis of cells; often used with a prefix indicating the target cells, e.g., hemolysin（细胞）溶素；2. any substance that causes cytolysis 溶解素

ly·sine (**Lys, K**) (li′sēn) a naturally occurring, essential amino acid, necessary for optimal growth in human infants and for maintenance of nitrogen equilibrium in adults. The acetate and hydrochloride salts are used in dietary supplementation and the hydrochloride salt is used in the treatment of severe metabolic alkalosis refractory to treatment 赖氨酸

ly·sin·o·gen (li-sin′ə-jən) an antigenic substance capable of inducing the formation of lysins 溶素原

ly·sin·uria (li″sī-nu′re-ə) an aminoaciduria consisting of excessive lysine in the urine, as in hyperlysinemia 赖氨酸尿；**lysinu′ric** *adj.*

ly·sis (li′sis) 1. destruction or decomposition, as of a cell or other substance, under the influence of a specific agent 溶解分解；2. mobilization of an organ by division of restraining adhesions 松解术；3. gradual abatement of the symptoms of a disease 渐退，消散（指症状）

ly·so·gen (li′so-jən) 1. an agent that induces lysis 致溶解的药物；2. 同 lysinogen；3. a lysogenized bacterium 溶原菌

ly·so·gen·ic (li-so-jen′ik) 1. producing lysins or causing lysis 引起溶解的；2. pertaining to lysogeny 溶原性

ly·so·ge·nic·i·ty (li″so-jə-nis′ĭ-te) 1. the ability to produce lysins or cause lysis 溶原性；2. the potentiality of a bacterium to produce phage 产噬菌体；3. the specific association of the phage genome (prophage) with the bacterial genome in such a way that only a few, if any, phage genes are transcribed 与噬菌体共生性

ly·sog·e·ny (li-soj′ə-ne) the phenomenon in which a bacterium is infected by a temperate bacteriophage and the viral DNA is integrated in the chromosome of the host cell and replicated along with the host chromosome for many generations (the lysogenic cycle); production of virions and lysis of host cells (the lytic cycle) then begins again 溶源性

ly·so·phos·pha·ti·date (li″so-fos″fə-ti′dāt) the anionic form of lysophosphatidic acid 溶血磷脂酸（阴离子型）

ly·so·phos·pha·tid·ic ac·id (li″so-fos″fə-tid′ik) any phosphatidic acid–containing lysophospholipid; they are important in extracellular signaling, with their actions mediated through a set of G protein–

coupled receptors 溶血磷脂酸

ly·so·phos·pho·lip·id (li″so-fos″fo-lip′id) a phospholipid that lacks one of its fatty acyl chains; formed during phospholipid metabolism. Several (lysophosphatidic acid and sphingosine 1-phosphate) are important in extracellular signaling 溶血磷脂

ly·so·so·mal α-glu·co·si·dase (li″so-so′məl glooko′sī-dās) acid maltase 溶酶体 α - 葡糖苷酶

ly·so·some (li″so-sōm) a membrane-bound cytoplasmic organelle that contains hydrolytic enzymes and is involved in intracellular digestion. 溶 酶 体; **lysoso′mal** *adj.*; **secondary l.**, one that has fused with a phagosome or pinosome, bringing hydrolases in contact with the ingested material, which is then digested 次级溶酶体

ly·so·zyme (li′so-zīm) an enzyme present in saliva, tears, egg white, and many animal fluids, functioning as an antibacterial agent by catalyzing the hydrolysis of specific glycosidic linkages in peptidoglycans and chitin, breaking down some bacterial cell walls 溶菌酶

Lys·sa·vi·rus (lis′ə-vi″rəs) a genus of viruses of the family Rhabdoviridae that includes the rabies virus and related viruses 狂犬病病毒属

lys·so·pho·bia (lis″o-fo′be-ə) irrational fear of going insane 狂犬病恐怖症

lyt·ic (lit′ik) 1. pertaining to lysis or to a lysin 裂解的，溶解的; 2. producing lysis 引起溶解的

-lytic a word termination denoting lysis of the substance indicated by the stem to which it is affixed 溶解的后缀

lyze (līz) 同 lyse

M

M [符号] 同 mega- 百万，兆 (10⁶); methionine 蛋氨酸; molar¹ 摩尔浓度; molar² 磨牙; myopia 近视

M. [L.] [符号] mis′ce (mix) 混和; mistu′ra (a mixture) 合剂

M molar¹ 摩尔浓度的符号

M_r relative molecular mass 相对分子质量的符号，见 *weight* 下 *molecular weight*

m [符号] median 中位数; meter 米; milli- 毫

m. [L.] mus′culus (muscle) 肌的符号

m [符号] mass 质量; molal (重量)摩尔

m- meta- (2) 间(位)的化学符号

μ (mu, the twelfth letter of the Greek alphabet) (mu 希腊语的第 12 个字母) micro- 微的符号; the heavy chain of IgM (see *immunoglobulin*) 重链 IgM 的符号

MA Master of Arts 文学硕士; mental age 智力年龄，心理年龄

mA milliampere; one thousandth (10⁻³) of an ampere 毫安(培)的符号

MAC membrane attack complex 攻膜复合物; *Mycobacterium avium* complex 鸟分枝杆菌复合群 (见 *disease* 下词条)

mac·er·ate (mas′ər-āt) to soften by wetting or soaking 浸软

ma·chine (mə-shēn′) a mechanical contrivance for doing work or generating energy 机器，机械; **heart-lung m.**, a combination blood pump (artificial heart) and blood oxygenator (artificial lung) used in open-heart surgery 人工心肺机

MACRA Medicare Access and CHIP Re-author-ization Act 联邦医保可及性和儿童健康保险项目重新授权法案

Mac·ra·can·tho·rhyn·chus (mak″rə-kan″tho-ring′kəs) a genus of parasitic worms (phylum Acanthocephala), including *M. hirudina′ceus,* found in swine 巨吻棘头虫属

mac·ren·ceph·a·ly (mak″rən-sef′ə-le) hypertrophy of the brain 巨脑

mac·ro·ad·e·no·ma (mak″ro-ad″ə-no′mə) a pituitary adenoma over 10 mm in diameter 巨腺瘤

mac·ro·am·y·lase (mac″ro-am′ə-lās) a complex in which normal serum amylase is bound to a variety of specific binding proteins, forming a complex too large for renal excretion 巨淀粉酶

mac·ro·bi·o·ta (mak″ro-bi-o′tə) the macroscopic living organisms of a region 大 生 物 区 系; **macro-biot′ic** *adj.*

mac·ro·blast (mak′ro-blast″) an abnormally large immature erythrocyte; a large young erythroblast with megaloblastic features 巨成红细胞

mac·ro·ble·pha·ria (mak″ro-blə-far′e-ə) abnormal largeness of the eyelid 巨睑

mac·ro·ceph·a·ly (mak″ro-sef′ə-le) megalo-cephaly; unusually large size of the head 大头(畸形) **macrocephal′ic, macroceph′alous** *adj.*

mac·ro·chei·lia (mak″ro-ki′le-ə) excessive size of the lip 巨唇(症)

mac·ro·chei·ria (mak″ro-ki′re-ə) 同 mega-lochei-ria

mac·ro·co·lon (mak′ro-ko″lən) 同 megacolon

mac·ro·cra·nia (mak″ro-kra′ne-ə) abnormal increase in the size of the skull, the face appearing small in comparison 巨颅

mac·ro·cyte (mak′ro-sīt″) an abnormally large erythrocyte 巨红细胞

mac·ro·cy·the·mia (mak″ro-si-the′me-ə) the presence of macrocytes in the blood 巨红细胞血症

mac·ro·cyt·ic (mak″ro-sit′ik) pertaining to or characterized by macrocytes 大红细胞的

mac·ro·cy·to·sis (mak″ro-si-to′sis) 同 macro-cythemia

mac·ro·dac·ty·ly (mak″ro-dak′tə-le) 同 mega-lodactyly

mac·ro·el·e·ment (mak″ro-el′ə-mənt) any of the macronutrients that are chemical elements 常量元素，大量元素

mac·ro·fau·na (mak″ro-faw′nə) the macroscopic animal life present in or characteristic of a given location 大型动物区系

mac·ro·flo·ra (mak″ro-flor′ə) the macroscopic plant life present in or characteristic of a given location 大型植物区系

mac·ro·fol·lic·u·lar (mak″ro-fə-lik′u-lər) pertaining to or characterized by large follicles 巨滤泡腺瘤

mac·ro·gam·ete (mak″ro-gam′ēt) 1. the larger, less active female anisogamete 雌配子；2. the larger of two types of malarial parasites 大配子，见 gamete (2)

mac·ro·ga·me·to·cyte (mak″ro-gə-me′to-sīt)1. a cell that produces macrogametes 大配子母细胞；2. the female gametocyte of certain Sporozoa, such as malarial plasmodia, which matures into a macrogamete 大配子体

mac·ro·gen·i·to·so·mia (mak″ro-jen″ĭ-toso′me-ə) excessive bodily development, with unusual enlar-gement of the genital organs 巨生殖器；m. prae′-cox, macrogenitosomia occurring at an early age 生殖器巨大畸形

mac·rog·lia (mak-rog′le-ə) neuroglial cells of ectodermal origin, i.e., the astrocytes and oligodendrocytes considered together 大胶质

mac·ro·glob·u·lin (mak″ro-glob′u-lin) a globulin of unusually high molecular weight, in the range of 1,000,000 巨球蛋白；α₂-m., a plasma protein that inhibits a wide variety of proteolytic enzymes, including trypsin, plasmin, thrombin, kallikrein, and chymotrypsin, by entrapping and reducing the accessibility of their functional sites to large molecules α₂巨球蛋白

mac·ro·glob·u·lin·emia (mak″ro-glob″u-li-ne′me-ə) increased levels of macroglobulins in the blood 巨球蛋白血症；Waldenström m., a plasma cell dyscrasia resembling leukemia, with cells of lymphocytic, plasmacytic, or intermediate morphology that secrete an IgM M component, diffuse infiltration of bone marrow, weakness, fatigue, bleeding disorders, and visual disturbances 华氏巨球蛋白

血症

mac·ro·gna·thia (mak″ro-na′the-ə) enlargement of the jaw 巨颌；macrognath′ic adj.

mac·ro·gy·ria (mak″ro-ji′re-ə) moderate reduction in the number of sulci of the cerebrum, sometimes with increase in the brain substance, resulting in excessive size of the gyri 巨脑回畸形

mac·ro·lide (mak′ro-līd) 1. a compound characterized by a large lactone ring with multiple keto and hydroxyl groups 大环内酯类；2. any of a group of antibiotics containing this ring linked to one or more sugars, produced by certain species of Streptomyces 大环内酯类抗生素

mac·ro·mas·tia (mak″ro-mas′te-ə) excessive size of the breasts 巨乳房，乳房过大

mac·ro·me·lia (mak″ro-me′le-ə) abnormal largeness of one or more limbs 巨肢

mac·ro·mere (mak′ro-mēr″) one of the large blastomeres formed by unequal cleavage of a zygote as a result of asymmetric positioning of the mitotic spindle 大分裂球

mac·ro·meth·od (mak′ro-meth″əd) a chemical method using customary (not minute) quantities of the substance being analyzed 常量法

mac·ro·min·er·al (mak′ro-min″ər-əl) macro-element 常量矿物质

mac·ro·mol·e·cule (mak″ro-mol′ə-kūl) a very large molecule having a polymeric chain structure, as in proteins, polysaccharides, etc. 大分子，高分子；macromolec′ular adj.

mac·ro·mono·cyte (mak″ro-mon′o-sīt) an abnormally large monocyte 巨单核细胞

mac·ro·my·elo·blast (mak″ro-mi′ə-lo-blast) an abnormally large myeloblast 巨成髓细胞

mac·ro·nod·u·lar (mak″ro-nod′u-lər) characterized by large nodules 巨结的

mac·ro·nor·mo·blast (mak″ro-nor′mo-blast) 同 macroblast

mac·ro·nu·cle·us (mak″ro-noo′kle-əs) the larger of two types of nuclei when more than one is present in a cell 大核

mac·ro·nu·tri·ent (mak″ro-noo′tre-ənt) an essential nutrient required in relatively large amounts, such as carbohydrates, fats, proteins, or water; sometimes certain minerals are included, such as calcium, chloride, or sodium 常量营养素，宏量营养素

mac·ro·nych·ia (mak″ro-nik′e-ə) abnormal largeness of the nails 巨指甲

mac·ro·ovalo·cyte (mak″ro-o′və-lo-sīt) an enlarged, oval erythrocyte seen in megaloblastic anemia 巨卵性红细胞

mac·ro·pe·nis (mak″ro-pe′nis) excessive size of

the penis 巨阴茎

mac·ro·phage (mak′ro-fāj″) any of the large, mononuclear, highly phagocytic cells derived from monocytes that occur in the walls of blood vessels (adventitial cells) and in loose connective tissue (histiocytes, phagocytic reticular cells). They are components of the reticuloendothelial system. Macrophages are usually immobile but become actively mobile when stimulated by inflammation; they also interact with lymphocytes to facilitate antibody production 巨噬细胞；**alveolar m.**, one of the rounded granular, mononuclear phagocytes within the alveoli of the lungs that ingest inhaled particulate matter 肺泡巨噬细胞；**armed m′s**, those capable of inducing cytotoxicity as a consequence of antigen-binding by cytophilic antibodies on their surfaces or by factors derived from T lymphocytes 武装巨噬细胞

mac·roph·thal·mia (mak″rof-thal′me-ə) megalophthalmos; enlargement of the eyeball 大眼球

mac·ro·pino·cy·to·sis (mak″ro-pin″o-si-to′sis) (-pi″no-si-to′sis) pinocytosis in which large amounts of extracellular fluid are taken up by extension of the plasma membrane, with the formation of large vesicles 大型胞饮作用

mac·ro·poly·cyte (mak″ro-pol′e-sīt) a hypersegmented polymorphonuclear leukocyte of greater than normal size 大多核白细胞

mac·ro·pro·lac·ti·no·ma (mak″ro-pro-lak″tĭ-no′mə) a prolactinoma more than 10 mm in diameter, usually associated with serum prolactin levels above 500 ng per mL 巨催乳素瘤

ma·crop·sia (mə-krop′se-ə) a disorder of visual perception in which objects appear larger than their actual size 视物显大症

mac·ro·scop·ic (mak″ro-skop′ik) gross (2) 肉眼的

mac·ro·shock (mak′ro-shok″) in cardiology, a moderate to high level of electric current passing over two areas of intact skin, which can cause ventricular fibrillation 强震荡

mac·ro·so·ma·tia (mak″ro-so-ma′she-ə) great bodily size 巨体

mac·ro·sto·mia (mak″ro-sto′me-ə) greatly exagg-erated width of the mouth 巨口，大口畸形

mac·ro·tia (mak-ro′shə) abnormal enlargement of the pinna of the ear 巨耳畸形，大耳畸形

mac·u·la (mak′u-lə) pl. *ma′culae* [L.] 1. in anatomy, a stain, spot, or thickening; an area distinguishable by color or otherwise from its surroundings 斑；2. **m. lutea** 黄斑 黄体；3. 同 macule；4. a corneal scar, appreciated as a gray spot 灰 斑；**mac′ular, mac′ulate** *adj.*；**acoustic maculae**, the macula sacculi and macula utriculi considered together 听

斑；**ma′culae atro′phicae**, white scarlike patches formed on the skin by atrophy 萎缩斑；**cerebral m.**, tache cérébrale 脑膜性划痕；**ma′culae ceru′leae**, faint grayish blue spots sometimes found peripheral to the axilla or inguinal region in pediculosis 青斑；**ma′culae cribro′sae**, three perforated areas (inferior, medial, and superior) on the vestibular wall through which branches of the vestibulocochlear nerve pass to the saccule, utricle, and semicircular canals 筛斑；**m. den′sa**, a zone of heavily nucleated cells in the distal renal tubule 致密斑；**m. fla′va**, a yellow nodule at one end of a vocal cord 黄斑；**m. lu′tea, m. re′tinae**, an irregular yellowish depression on the retina, lateral to and slightly below the optic disk 视网膜黄斑；**m. sac′culi**, a thickening on the wall of the saccule where the epithelium contains hair cells that are stimulated by linear acceleration and deceleration and by gravity 球囊斑；**m. utri′culi**, a thickening in the wall of the utricle where the epithelium contains hair cells that are stimulated by linear acceleration and deceleration and by gravity 椭圆囊斑

mac·ule (mak′ūl) a discolored spot on the skin that is not raised above the surface 斑疹

mac·u·lo·cer·e·bral (mak″u-lo-ser′ə-brəl) cerebromacular 黄斑（与）脑的

mac·u·lop·a·thy (mak″u-lop′ə-the) any pathologic condition of the macula retinae 黄斑病变；**bull′s eye m.**, increase of pigment of a circular area of the macula retinae accompanying degeneration, occurring in various toxic states and diseases 牛眼样黄斑病

mad·a·ro·sis (mad″ə-ro′sis) loss of eyelashes or eyebrows 睫毛脱落，眉毛脱落

Mad·u·rel·la (mad″u-rel′ə) a genus of imperfect fungi. *M. gris′ea* and *M. myceto′mi* are etiologic agents of maduromycosis 马杜拉分枝菌属

ma·du·ro·my·co·sis (mə-du″ro-mi-ko′sis) mycetoma 足分枝菌病

maf·en·ide (maf′ən-īd) an antibacterial, used topically as the monoacetate salt in superficial infections 磺胺米隆（抗菌药）

mag·al·drate (mag′əl-drāt) a chemical combination of aluminum and magnesium hydroxides and sulfate; an antacid 镁加铝，氢氧化镁铝（抗酸药）

ma·gen·ta (mə-jen′tə) fuchsin or other salt of rosaniline 品红

mag·got (mag′ət) the soft-bodied larva of an insect, especially a form living in decaying flesh. Used in maggot debridement therapy 蛆

mag·ma (mag′mə) 1. a thick, viscous, aqueous suspension of finely divided, insoluble, inorganic material 晶浆；2. a thin, pastelike substance composed of organic material 岩浆

mag·ne·si·um (Mg) (mag-ne′ze-əm) a light, silvery, alkaline earth metal element; at. no. 12, at. wt. 24.305. Its salts are essential in nutrition, being required for the activity of many enzymes, especially those concerned with oxidative phosphorylation. Various salts, including *m. chloride, m. gluceptate, m. gluconate,* and *m. lactate* are used as electrolyte replenishers 镁；**m. carbonate,** an antacid 碳酸镁；**m. chloride,** an electrolyte replenisher and a pharmaceutical necessity for hemodialysis and peritoneal dialysis fluids 氯化镁；**m. citrate,** a saline laxative used for bowel evacuation before diagnostic procedures or surgery of the colon 柠檬酸镁；**m. hydroxide,** an antacid and laxative 氢氧化镁；**m. oxide,** an antacid and laxative; also used as a preventative for hypomagnesemia and as a sorbent in pharmaceutical preparations 氧化镁；**m. salicylate,** 水杨酸镁，见 *salicylate*；**m. silicate,** MgSiO₃, a silicate salt of magnesium; the most common hydrated forms found in nature are asbestos and talc 硅酸镁；**m. sulfate,** Epsom salt; an anticonvulsant and electrolyte replenisher, also used as a laxative and local antiinflammatory 硫酸镁；**m. trisilicate,** a compound of magnesium oxide and silicon dioxide with varying proportions of water; an antacid 三硅酸镁

mag·net (mag′nət) an object having polarity and capable of attracting iron 磁体；**magnet′ic** *adj.*

mag·net·ro·pism (mag-net′ro-piz-əm) a growth response in a nonmotile organism under the influence of a magnet 向磁性

mag·ni·fi·ca·tion (mag″nĭ-fĭ-ka′shən) 1. apparent increase in size, as under the microscope 增大；2. the process of making something appear larger, as by use of lenses 放大；3. the ratio of apparent (image) size to real size 放大率

MaHR major hematologic response 主要血液学反应

ma huang (mah hwahng′) [Chinese] any of various species of *Ephedra* used as herbs in Chinese medicine 麻黄

main·te·nance (mān′tə-nəns) providing a stable state over a long period, or the stable state so produced 维持

ma·jor (ma′jər) large; significant; great or greatest in scope, effect, number, size, extent, or importance 主要的

mal (mahl) [Fr.] disease 病；**grand m.,** (grahn) 大发作，见 *epilepsy* 下条条；**m. de mer,** (də mār′) seasickness 晕船；**petit m.,** (pə-te′) absence epilepsy 小发作

ma·la¹ (ma′lə) [L.] 1. cheek 脸 颊；2. zygomatic bone 颧骨

ma·la² (mū′lə) [Sanskrit] in ayurveda, waste products of the body formed during metabolism, including urine, feces, mucus, and sweat 在阿育吠陀中，在新陈代谢过程中形成的身体废物，包括尿液、粪便、黏液和汗液

mal·ab·sorp·tion (mal″əb-sorp′shən) impaired intestinal absorption of nutrients 吸收不良

ma·la·cia (mə-la′shə) morbid softening or softness of a part or tissue 软化

mal·a·co·pla·kia (mal″ə-ko-pla′ke-ə) the formation of soft patches of the mucous membrane of a hollow organ 软斑病；**m. vesi′cae,** a soft, yellowish, fungus-like growth on the mucosa of the bladder and ureters 膀胱软斑症

mal·a·co·sis (mal″ə-ko′sis) 同 malacia

mal·a·cos·te·on (mal″ə-kos′te-on) osteomalacia 骨软化

mal·ad·just·ment (mal″ə-just′mənt) in psychiatry, defective adaptation to the environment 失调

mal·a·dy (mal′ə-de) disease 疾病

mal·aise (mă-lāz′) a vague feeling of discomfort 乏力

mal·align·ment (mal″ə-līn′mənt) displacement, especially of teeth from their normal relation to the line of the dental arch 排列不齐

ma·lar (ma′lər) 1. buccal; pertaining to the cheek 颊的、脸颊的；2. zygomatic 颧骨的

ma·lar·ia (mə-lar′e-ə) an infectious febrile disease endemic in many warm regions of the world, caused by protozoa of the genus *Plasmodium,* which are parasitic in red blood cells; it is transmitted by *Anopheles* mosquitoes and marked by attacks of chills, fever, and sweating occurring at intervals that depend on the time required for development of a new generation of parasites in the body 疟疾；**malar′ial, malar′ious** *adj.*；**falciparum m.,** the most serious form, due to *Plasmodium falciparum,* with severe constitutional symptoms and sometimes causing death 恶性疟；**ovale m.,** a mild form due to *Plasmodium ovale,* with recurring tertian febrile paroxysms and a tendency to end in spontaneous recovery 卵型（疟原虫）疟；**quartan m.,** that in which the febrile paroxysms occur every 72 hours, or every fourth day counting the day of occurrence as the first day of each cycle; due to *Plasmodium malariae* 三日疟；**quotidian m.,** vivax malaria in which the febrile paroxysms occur daily 日发疟；**tertian m.,** vivax malaria in which the febrile paroxysms occur every 42 to 47 hours, or every third day counting the day of occurrence as the first day of the cycle 间日疟；**vivax m.,** that due to *Plasmodium vivax,* in which the febrile paroxysms commonly occur every other day *(tertian m.),* but may occur daily *(quotidian m.),* if there are two broods of parasites segmenting on alternate days 间日疟

Mal·as·se·zia (mal″ə-se′zhə) a genus of anamorphic fungi; various species, including *M. fur′fur* (and its cultural variant *M. ova′lis*) and *M. globo′sa* are part of the normal skin flora but can cause tinea versicolor in susceptible individuals 马拉色霉菌属

mal·as·sim·i·la·tion (mal″ə-sim″ĭ-la′shən) 1. imperfect, or disordered, assimilation 同化不良; 2. the inability of the gastrointestinal tract to take up ingested nutrients, due to faulty digestion (maldigestion) or to impaired intestinal mucosal transport (malabsorption) 消化吸收障碍

ma·late (ma′lāt) (mal′āt) any salt of malic acid 苹果酸盐

mal·a·thi·on (mal″ə-thi′on) an organophosphorus insecticide used as a topical pediculicide 马拉硫磷

mal·ax·a·tion (mal″ək-sa′shən) an act of kneading 揉捏法

mal·de·vel·op·ment (mal″də-vel′əp-mənt) abnormal growth or development 发育不良

male (māl) 1. the sex that produces spermatozoa 男性; 2. 同 masculine

mal·e·ate (mal′e-āt) any salt or ester of maleic acid 顺丁烯二酸阴离子

ma·le·ic ac·id (mə-le′ik) an unsaturated dibasic acid, the cis-isomer of fumaric acid 马来酸，顺丁烯二酸

mal·erup·tion (mal″ə-rup′shən) eruption of a tooth out of its normal position 错位长出

mal·for·ma·tion (mal″for-ma′shən) a morphologic defect resulting from an abnormal developmental process 畸形; **Arnold-Chiari m.,** Chiari m., usually specifically denoting the type II form 阿 - 基二氏畸形，小脑扁桃体下疝畸形; **cerebral arteriovenous m.,** a congenital anomaly of the brain vasculature composed of arterial and venous channels with many interconnecting shunts without a capillary bed; characteristics include hemorrhage, headache, and focal epileptic seizures 脑动静脉畸形; **Chiari m. (CM),** a group of related congenital anomalies in which the cerebellum and medulla oblongata, which is elongated and flattened, protrude into the spinal canal through the foramen magnum. It is classified into three or more types according to severity; type I is least severe 小脑扁桃体下疝畸形; **Dandy-Walker m.,** cystic dilatation of the fourth ventricle, absence or hypoplasia of the vermis, and enlargement of the posterior fossa, usually with hydrocephalus; due to failure of the roof of the fourth ventricle to develop during embryogenesis 先天性脑积水

mal·ic ac·id (ma′lik) (mal′ik) a crystalline acid from the juices of many fruits and plants and an intermediate in the tricarboxylic acid cycle 苹果酸

ma·lig·nan·cy (mə-lig′nən-se) 1. a tendency to progress in virulence 恶性，毒性; 2. the quality of being malignant 恶性程度; 3. a cancer, especially one with the potential to cause death 恶性肿瘤，癌

ma·lig·nant (mə-lig′nənt) 1. tending to become worse and end in death 致命的; 2. having the properties of anaplasia, invasiveness, and metastasis; said of tumors 恶性的（指肿瘤）

ma·lin·ger·ing (mə-ling′ər-ing) willful, fraudulent feigning or exaggeration of the symptoms of illness or injury to attain a consciously desired end 诈病

mal·le·a·ble (mal′e-ə-bəl) susceptible of being beaten out into a thin plate（金属）延展性的；易适应的

mal·leo·in·cu·dal (mal″e-o-ing′ku-dəl) pertaining to the malleus and incus 锤骨砧骨的

mal·le·o·lus (mə-le′o-ləs) pl. *malle′oli* [L.] a rounded process, such as the protuberance on either side of the ankle joint at the lower end of the fibula and the tibia 踝; **malle′olar** *adj.*

mal·le·ot·o·my (mal″e-ot′ə-me) 1. operative division of the malleus 锤骨切开术; 2. operative separation of the malleoli 踝切离术

mal·le·us (mal′e-əs) [L.] hammer; the outermost of the auditory ossicles, and the one attached to the tympanic membrane; its club-shaped head articulates with the incus 锤骨，见图 29

mal·nu·tri·tion (mal″noo-trish′ən) any disorder of nutrition 营养不良

mal·oc·clu·sion (mal″ə-kloo′zhən) improper relations of apposing teeth when the jaws are in contact 错殆

mal·po·si·tion (mal″pə-zish′ən) abnormal or anomalous placement 错位，异位

mal·prac·tice (mal-prak′tis) improper or injurious practice; unskillful and faulty medical or surgical treatment 过失行为，违法行为；治疗失当，医疗差错

mal·pres·en·ta·tion (mal″prez-ən-ta′shən) faulty fetal presentation 先露异常

mal·ro·ta·tion (mal″ro-ta′shən) 1. abnormal or pathologic rotation, as of the vertebral column 异常旋转; 2. failure of normal rotation of an organ, as of the gut, during embryonic development 旋转不良

MALT mucosa-associated lymphoid tissue 黏膜相关淋巴组织

mal·tase (mawl′tās) 1. α-glucosidase α 葡糖苷酶; 2. any enzyme with similar glycolytic activity, cleaving α -1,4 and sometimes α -1,6 linked glucose residues from nonreducing termini; in humans there are considered to be four such enzymes; two are the heat-stable enzymes, usually called maltases, constituting the glucoamylase complex; the other two are the heat-labile enzymes, usually called sucrase and isomaltase 麦芽糖酶

mal·ti·tol (mawl'tĭ-tol) a hydrogenated, partially hydrolyzed starch used as a bulk sweetener 麦芽糖醇

MALT·oma (mawl-to'mə) a form of extranodal marginal zone lymphoma originating in mucosaassociated lymphoid tissue, particularly that of the gastrointestinal tract 黏膜相关淋巴组织淋巴瘤

mal·tose (mawl'tōs) a disaccharide composed of two glucose residues, the fundamental structural unit of glycogen and starch 麦芽糖

mal·un·ion (mal-ūn'yən) faulty union of the fragments of a fractured bone 畸形愈合

mam·ba (mahm'bə) any member of the genus *Dendroaspis*, extremely venomous elapid snakes. Included are the black mamba (*D. polylepis*), a large black African tree snake, and the green mamba (*D. angusticeps*), a large green or black tree snake of eastern and southern Africa 窄头眼镜蛇

ma·mil·la (mə-mil'ə) [L.] 同 mammilla

mam·ma (mam'ə) pl. *mam'mae* [L.] the breast 乳房

mam·mal (mam'əl) an individual of the class Mammalia 哺乳动物; **mamma'lian** adj.

mam·mal·gia (mə-mal'jə) 同 mastalgia

mam·ma·lia (mə-mal'e-ə) a class of warm-blooded vertebrate animals, including all that have hair and suckle their young 哺乳动物类

mam·ma·plas·ty (mam'ə-plas''te) mammoplasty; plastic reconstruction of the breast, either to augment or reduce its size 乳房成形术

mam·ma·ry (mam'ər-e) pertaining to the mammary gland, or breast 乳房的

mam·mec·to·my (mə-mek'tə-me) 同 mastectomy

mam·mil·la (mə-mil'ə) pl. *mammil'lae* [L.] 1. a nipple 乳头; 2. any nipple-like structure 乳头状结构; **mam'millary** adj.

mam·mil·la·tion (mam''ĭ-la'shən) a nipple-like elevation or projection 乳头形成; **mam'millated** adj.

mam·mil·li·plas·ty (mə-mil'ĭ-plas''te) theleplasty 乳头成形术

mam·mil·li·tis (mam''ĭ-li'tis) thelitis 乳头炎

mam·mil·lo·tha·lam·ic (mam''ĭ-lo''thə-lam'ik) pertaining to or connecting the mammillary body and thalamus 乳头体丘脑的

mam·mi·tis (mə-mi'tis) 同 mastitis

mam·mo·gram (mam'ə-gram) a radiograph of the breast 乳房 X 线照片

mam·mog·ra·phy (mə-mog'rə-fe) radiography of the mammary gland 乳房 X 线照相术

mam·mo·pla·sia (mam''o-pla'zhə) development of breast tissue 乳腺生长

mam·mo·plas·ty (mam'o-plas''te) 同 mammaplasty

mam·mose (mam'ōs) 1. having large breasts 大乳房的; 2. mammillated 乳房状的

mam·mot·o·my (mə-mot'ə-me) 同 mastotomy

mam·mo·tro·phic (mam''o-tro'fik) 同 mammotropic

mam·mo·tro·pic (mam''o-tro'pik) having a stimu-lating effect on the mammary gland 促乳腺的

mam·mo·tro·pin (mam'o-tro''pin) prolactin 催乳素，促乳素

man·di·ble (man'dĭ-bəl) the horseshoe-shaped bone forming the lower jaw; the largest and strongest bone of the face, consisting of a body and a pair of rami, which articulate with the skull at the temporomandibular joints 下颌骨，见图 1; **mandib'ular** adj.

man·dib·u·la (man-dib'u-lə) pl. *mandib'ulae* [L.] 同 mandible

man·drel (man'drəl) the shaft on which a dental tool is held in the dental handpiece, for rotation by the dental engine 轴柄

man·drin (man'drin) a metal guide for a flexible catheter 导尿管导子

ma·neu·ver (mə-noo'vər) a skillful or dexterous method or procedure 手法，操作法; **Bracht m.,** a method of extraction of the aftercoming head in breech presentation Bracht 手法; **Brandt-Andrews m.,** a method of expressing the placenta from the uterus 布-安二氏手法; **forward-bending m.,** a method of detecting retraction signs in neoplastic changes in the mammae; the patient bends forward from the waist with chin held up and arms extended toward the examiner. If retraction is present, an asymmetry in the breast is seen 前弯手法; **Heimlich m.,** a method of dislodging food or other material from the throat of a choking victim: wrap one's arms around the victim, allowing the victim's upper torso to hang forward; with both hands against the victim's abdomen (slightly above the navel and below the rib cage), make a fist with one hand, grasp it with the other, and forcefully press into the abdomen with a quick upward thrust. Repeat several times if necessary 海姆利希手法，又称 *abdominal thrust*.; **Pajot m.,** a method of forceps delivery with traction along the axis of the superior pelvic aperture Pajot 法; **Pinard m.,** a method of bringing down the foot in breech extraction Pinard 手法; **Prague m.,** a method of extracting the aftercoming head in breech presentation 布拉格手法; **Scanzoni m.,** double application of forceps blades for delivery of a fetus in the occiput posterior position 斯坎佐尼手法；**Toynbee m.,** pinching the nostrils and swallowing; if the auditory tube is patent, the tympanic membrane will retract medially汤因比手法；**Valsalva m.,** 1. increase in intrathoracic pressure by forcible exhalation effort against the closed glottis 通过闭合声门强制呼气来增加胸内压；2. increase in the pressure in the eustachian tube and middle ear by forcible exhalation effort against occluded nostrils and closed mouth 瓦尔萨尔瓦动作，通过闭塞口鼻强制呼气来增加咽鼓管和中耳的压力

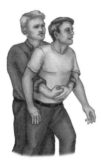

▲ 海姆利希手法

man·ga·fo·di·pir (mang″gə-fo′dī-pir) a contrast-enhancing agent used as the trisodium salt in magnetic resonance imaging (MRI) of hepatic lesions 锰福地吡

man·ga·nese (Mn) (mang′gə-nēs) a hard, brittle, silvery gray, heavy metallic element; at. no. 25, at. wt. 54.938. It is a trace element with roles in metabolic regulation, activation of numerous enzymes, and respiratory chain phosphorylation. Poisoning, usually due to inhalation of manganese dust, causes neurotoxicity with a syndrome resembling parkinsonism and inflammation throughout the respiratory system 锰

ma·nia (ma′ne-ə) [Gr.] a phase of bipolar disorders characterized by expansiveness, elation, agitation, hyperexcitability, hyperactivity, and increased speed of thought and ideas 躁狂（症）；**man′ic** *adj.*

man·ic-de·pres·sive (man′ik-de-pres′iv) al-ternating between attacks of mania and depression, as in bipolar disorders 躁狂抑郁的

man·i·kin (man′ĭ-kin) a model to illustrate anatomy or on which to practice surgical or other manipulations; used as patient simulation for a broad range of medical, nursing, and physical therapy training 人体模型

ma·nip·u·la·tion (mə-nip″u-la′shən) skillful or dexterous treatment 手法；手法治疗；推拿（术）

man·ni·tol (man′ĭ-tol) a sugar alcohol formed by reduction of mannose or fructose and widely distributed in plants and fungi; it is an osmotic diuretic used to prevent and treat acute renal failure, to promote excretion of toxic substances, and to reduce cerebral edema or elevated intracranial or intraocular pressure. It is used as an irrigating solution to prevent hemolysis during transurethral surgical procedures and is inhaled in a challenge test for bronchial hyperresponsiveness in the clinical evaluation of asthma 甘露醇

man·nose (man′ōs) a 6-carbon sugar epimeric with glucose and occurring in oligosaccharides of many glycoproteins and glycolipids 甘露糖

α-man·no·si·do·sis (man″o-sĭ-do′sis) a lysosomal storage disease due to a defect in α-mannosidase activity that results in lysosomal accumulation of mannose-rich substrates; it is characterized by coarse facies, upper respiratory problems, intellectual disability, hepatosplenomegaly, and cataracts α-甘露糖苷贮积症

ma·nom·e·ter (mə-nom′ə-tər) an instrument for measuring the pressure of liquids or gases 测压计，（液体）压力计；**manomet′ric** *adj.*

ma·nom·e·try (mə-nom′ə-tre) the measurement of pressure by means of a manometer 测压法；**anal m.,** the measurement of pressure generated by the anal sphincter; used in the evaluation of fecal incontinence 肛门测压

Man·son·el·la (man″sən-el′ə) a genus of filarial nematodes. *M. ozzar′di* is found in the mesentery and visceral fat of humans in Central and South America 曼森线虫属

Man·so·nia (mən-so′ne-ə) a genus of mosquitoes, several species of which transmit *Brugia malayi;* some may also transmit viruses, such as those of equine encephalomyelitis 曼蚊属

man·tle (man′təl) 1. an enveloping cover or layer 外套；2. cerebral cortex 大脑皮层，大脑皮质

man·u·al (man′u-əl) 1. of or pertaining to the hand; performed by the hand or hands 用手的；2. a small reference book, particularly one giving instructions or guidelines 手册；**Diagnostic and Statistical M. of Mental Disorders (DSM),** 精神疾病诊断与统计手册，见 *D.* 下词条

ma·nu·bri·um (mə-noo′bre-əm) pl. *manu′bria* [L.] a handle-like structure or part, such as the manubrium of the sternum 柄；**m. mal′lei, m. of malleus,** the longest process of the malleus; it is attached to the middle layer of the tympanic membrane and has the tensor tympani muscle attached to it 锤骨柄；**m. ster′ni, m. of sternum,** the cranial part of the sternum, articulating with the clavicles and first two pairs of ribs 胸骨柄

ma·nus (ma′nəs) pl. *ma′nus* [L.] hand 手

MAO monoamine oxidase 单胺氧化酶

MAOI monoamine oxidase inhibitor 单胺氧化酶抑制药

MAP mean arterial pressure 平均动脉压

map (map) a two-dimensional graphic representation of arrangement in space 图；**chromosome m.**, a map showing the position of genetic loci on a chromosome, such as a gene map or cytogenetic map 染色体图；**cytogenetic m.**, a map showing the position of gene loci relative to chromosome bands 细胞遗传学图；**gene m.**, one showing the linear arrangement of genetic loci on a DNA molecule and indicating the distance between them, either in relative or physical units 基因图（谱）；**genetic m.**, **linkage m.**, a gene map giving the positions of known genes and markers relative to each other, based on recombination frequencies, rather than as specific physical points 遗传图，连锁图；**physical m.**, a gene map showing the linear order of genes or markers in the genome, along with the physical distances between them, rather than the frequencies of recombination 物理图（谱）

ma·pro·ti·line (mə-pro′tĭ-lēn) a tetracyclic antidepressant with actions similar to those of the tricyclic antidepressants; used as the hydrochloride salt 马普替林（抗抑郁药）

ma·ras·mus (mə-raz′məs) a form of proteinenergy malnutrition predominantly due to prolonged severe caloric deficit, chiefly occurring in the first year of life, with growth retardation and wasting of subcutaneous fat and muscle 消瘦；**marasmat′ic**, **maras′mic** *adj.*

march (mahrch) the progression of electrical activity through the motor cortex 前进，进行；**jacksonian m.**, the spread of abnormal electrical activity from one area of the cerebral cortex to adjacent areas, characteristic of jacksonian epilepsy 杰克逊前进

mar·fa·noid (mahr′fən-oid) having the characteristic symptoms of Marfan syndrome 马方综合征的

mar·gin (mahr′jin) an edge or border 边缘；**margi′nal** *adj.*；**gingival m.**, **gum m.**, marginal gingiva 龈缘；**m. of safety**, a calculation estimating a maximum safe level of exposure for humans, now superseded by the reference dose 安全范围

mar·gi·na·tion (mahr″jĭ-na′shən) accumulation and adhesion of leukocytes to the endothelial cells of blood vessel walls at the site of injury in the early stages of inflammation 着边，壁立

mar·gino·plas·ty (mahr-jin′ə-plas″te) surgical restoration of a border, as of the eyelid 睑缘成形术

mar·go (mahr′go) pl. *mar′gines* [L.] 同 margin

mar·i·jua·na (mar″ĭ-hwah′nə) a preparation of the leaves and flowering tops of hemp plants *(Cannabis sativa)*, usually smoked in cigarettes for its euphoric properties 大麻。Spelled also *marihuana*

mar·i·tal (mar′ĭ-təl) of or pertaining to marriage 婚姻的

mark (mahrk) a spot, blemish, or other circumscribed area visible on a surface 痕迹，斑点；**birth m.**, 胎记，见 *birthmark*；**port-wine m.**, nevus flammeus 葡萄酒色痣；**strawberry m.**, 1. strawberry hemangioma (1) 草状血管瘤；2. cavernous hemangioma 海绵状血管瘤

mark·er (mahrk′ər) something that identifies or that is used to identify 标记，标志；**tumor m.**, a biochemical substance indicative of neoplasia, ideally specific, sensitive, and proportional to tumor load 肿瘤标志物

mar·row (mar′o) 1. 同 bone m.；2. any of various soft substances resembling bone marrow 髓；**bone m.**, the soft organic material filling the cavities of bones, made up of a fiber-rich meshwork of connective tissue, the meshes being filled with marrow cells, which consist variously of fat cells, large nucleated cells or myelocytes, and megakaryocytes. *Yellow bone m.* is that in which fat cells predominate; *red bone m.* is the site of production of erythrocytes and granular leukocytes and occurs in developing bone, as of the ribs and vertebrae 骨髓；**spinal m.**, spinal cord 脊髓

marsh·mal·low (mahrsh′mel″o) (-mal″o) a perennial Eurasian herb, *Althaea officinalis*, or preparations of its flowers, leaves, or roots, which are used in the treatment of cough and for irritation of the oral and pharyngeal mucosa; also used in folk medicine 药用蜀葵

Mar·su·pi·a·lia (mahr-soo″pe-a′le-ə) an order of mammals characterized by the possession of a marsupium, including opossums, kangaroos, wallabies, koala bears, and wombats 有袋目

mar·su·pi·al·iza·tion (mahr-soo″pe-al-ĭ-za′shən) conversion of a closed cavity into an open pouch, by incising it and suturing the edges of its wall to the edges of the wound 袋形缝术

mas·cu·line (mas′ku-lin″) pertaining to or having qualities normally associated with the male sex 男性的

mas·cu·lin·i·ty (mas″ku-lin′ĭ-te) virility; the possession of masculine qualities 男性

mas·cu·lin·iza·tion (mas″ku-lin-ĭ-za′shən) 1. normal development of male primary or secondary sex characters in a male 男性化；2. development of male secondary sex characters in a female or prepubescent male 女性男性化；3. the condition of having such sex characters 男性特征

ma·ser (ma′zər) a device that produces an extremely intense, small, and nearly nondivergent beam of monochromatic radiation in the microwave region, with all the waves in phase 微波激射器

mask (mask) 1. a covering or appliance for shading, protecting, or medicating the face 面罩；2. to cover or conceal 掩盖；3. in audiometry, to obscure or diminish a sound by the presence of another sound of different frequency 在听力测定时由于另外不同频率的声音存在，致所测声音模糊不清或减小；4. in dentistry, to camouflage metal parts of a prosthesis by covering them with opaque material 牙科用不透明物质涂布于金属假牙的表面

masked (maskt) 1. concealed from view; hidden 隐蔽的；2. not presenting or producing the usual symptoms 隐匿的；3. blind (2). 盲目的

maso·chism (mas′o-kiz-əm) the act or instance of gaining pleasure from physical or psychological pain; usually used to denote *sexual masochism* 受虐癖；**masochis′tic** *adj.*；**sexual m.**, a paraphilia in which sexual gratification is derived from being hurt, humiliated, or otherwise made to suffer physically or psychologically 性受虐癖

mass (mas) 1. a lump or collection of cohering particles 质，物质；2. a cohesive mixture to be made into pills 块，丸块，团；3. the characteristic of matter that gives it inertia. Symbol m 质量，符号 m；**atomic m.**, atomic weight; used particularly when describing a single isotope of a nuclide 原子质量；**inner cell m.**, embryoblast 内细胞团，内细胞群；**lean body m.**, the part of the body that comprises all its components except neutral storage lipid; in essence, the fat-free mass of the body 瘦体重；**molar m.** (*M*) the mass of a molecule in grams (or kilograms) per mole 摩尔质量；**molecular m.**, the mass of a molecule in daltons, derived by addition of the component atomic masses. Its dimensionless equivalent is molecular weight 分子质量；**relative molecular m.**, technically preferable term for *molecular weight*. Symbol M, 分子，符号 M,

mas·sa (mas′ə) pl. *mas′sae* [L.] 同 mass (1)

mas·sage (mə-sahzh′) [Fr.] systematic therapeutic friction, stroking, or kneading of the body 按摩，推拿；**cardiac m.**, intermittent compression of the heart by pressure applied over the sternum *(closed cardiac m.)* or directly to the heart through an opening in the chest wall *(open cardiac m.)* to reinstate and maintain circulation 心脏按压；**carotid sinus m.**, firm rotatory pressure applied to one side of the neck over the carotid sinus, causing

vagal stimulation and used to slow or terminate tachycardia 颈动脉窦按摩；**electrovibratory m., vibratory m.**, that performed with an electric vibrator 电除颤

mas·sa·sau·ga (mas″ə-saw′gə) *Sistrurus catenatus,* a small venomous rattlesnake in the United States and northern Mexico 侏响尾蛇

mas·se·ter (mə-se′tər) 咬肌，见 *muscle* 下词条；**masseter′ic** *adj.*

mas·seur (mə-soor′) [Fr.] 1. a man who performs massage 男按摩师；2. an instrument for performing massage 按摩器

mas·seuse (mə-sooz′) [Fr.] a woman who performs massage 女按摩师

MAST acronym for Military Anti-Shock Trousers, inflatable trousers used to induce autotransfusion of blood from the lower to the upper part of the body 军用抗休克裤

mas·tad·e·ni·tis (mas″tad-ə-ni′tis) 同 mastitis

Mas·tad·e·no·vi·rus (mast-ad′ə-no-vi″rəs) mammalian adenoviruses; a genus of viruses of the family Adenoviridae that infect mammals, causing disease of the gastrointestinal tract, conjunctiva, central nervous system, and urinary tract; many species induce malignancy 哺乳动物腺病毒属

mas·tal·gia (mas-tal′jə) pain in the breast 乳腺痛

mas·tat·ro·phy (mas-tat′rə-fe) atrophy of the breast 乳腺萎缩

mas·tec·to·my (mas-tek′tə-me) excision of the breast 乳房切除术；**extended radical m.**, radical mastectomy with removal of the ipsilateral half of the sternum and a portion of ribs two through five with the underlying pleura and the internal mammary lymph nodes 乳房扩大根治术；**modified radical m.**, simple mastectomy together with axillary lymphadenectomy, but with preservation of the pectoral muscles 乳房改良根治术；**partial m.**, removal of only enough breast tissue to ensure that the margins of the resected surgical specimen are free of tumor 乳腺区段切除术；**radical m.**, amputation of the breast with wide excision of the pectoral muscles and axillary lymph nodes 乳房根治术；**subcutaneous m.**, excision of breast tissue with preservation of the overlying skin, nipple, and areola so that the breast form may be reconstructed 皮下乳腺切除术

mas·ti·ca·tion (mas″tĭ-ka′shən) chewing; the biting and grinding of food 咀嚼

mas·ti·ca·to·ry (mas″tĭ-kə-tor″e) 1. subserving or pertaining to mastication; affecting the muscles of mastication 咀嚼的；2. a remedy to be chewed but not swallowed 咀嚼物

mas·ti·goph·o·ra (mas″tĭ-gof′ə-rə) a subphylum

of protozoa comprising those having one or more flagella throughout most of their life cycle and a simple, centrally located nucleus; many are parasitic in both invertebrates and vertebrates, including humans 鞭毛纲

mas·ti·goph·o·ran (mas″tĭ-gof′ə-rən) 1. a protozoan of the subphylum Mastigophora 鞭毛虫; 2. of or belonging to the subphylum Mastigophora 鞭毛虫亚门，又称 *flagellate* 和 *mastigote*

mas·ti·gote (mas′tĭ-gōt) 同 mastigophoran

mas·ti·tis (mas-ti′tis) inflammation of the breast 乳腺炎；**m. neonato′rum,** any abnormal condition of the breast in the newborn 新生儿乳腺炎；**periductal m.,** inflammation of the tissues about the ducts of the mammary gland 管周乳腺炎；**plasma cell m.,** infiltration of the breast stroma with plasma cells and proliferation of the cells lining the ducts 浆细胞性乳腺炎

mas·to·cyte (mas′to-sīt″) mast cell 肥大细胞

mas·to·cy·to·sis (mas″to-si-to′sis) an accumulation, local or systemic, of mast cells in the tissues; known as *urticaria pigmentosa* when widespread in the skin 肥大细胞增多症

mas·toid (mas′toid) 1. breast shaped 乳房状的；2. mastoid process 乳突；3. pertaining to the mastoid process 乳突的

mas·toid·al·gia (mas″toid-al′jə) pain in the mastoid region 乳突痛

mas·toid·ec·to·my (mas″toid-ek′tə-me) excision of the mastoid cells or the mastoid process 乳突切除术

mas·toi·deo·cen·te·sis (mas-toi″de-o-sente′sis) paracentesis of the mastoid cells 乳突穿刺术

mas·toid·itis (mas″toid-i′tis) inflammation of the mastoid antrum and cells 乳突炎

mas·top·a·thy (mas-top′ə-the) any disease of the mammary gland 乳腺病

mas·to·pexy (mas′to-pek″se) surgical fixation of a pendulous breast 乳房固定术

mas·to·plas·ty (mas′to-plas″te) 同 mammaplasty

mas·top·to·sis (mas″top-to′sis) pendulous breasts 乳房下垂

mas·to·squa·mous (mas-to-skwa′məs) pertaining to the mastoid and squama of the temporal bone 乳突鳞部的

mas·tot·o·my (mas-tot′ə-me) surgical incision of a breast 乳房切开术

mas·tur·ba·tion (mas″tər-ba′shən) selfstimulation of the genitals for sexual pleasure 手淫

MAT multifocal atrial tachycardia 多源性房性心动过速，见 *tachycardia* 下 *chaotic atrial tachycardia*

match·ing (mach′ing) 1. comparison and se-lec-tion of objects having similar or identical characteristics 匹配；2. selection of compatible donors and recipients for transfusion or transplantation 配型；3. selection of subjects for clinical trials or other studies so that the different groups are similar in selected characteristics 匹配的；**cross m.,** crossmatching 交叉配合

ma·te·ria (mə-tēr′e-ə) [L.] matter 物质；**m. al′ba,** whitish deposits on the teeth, composed of mucus and epithelial cells containing bacteria and filamentous organisms 白垢；**m. me′dica,** pharmacology 药物学

ma·ter·nal (mə-tur′nəl) pertaining to the mother 母体的

ma·ter·ni·ty (mə-tur′nĭ-te) 1. motherhood 母性；2. a lying-in hospital 产院

mat·ing (māt′ing) pairing of individuals of opposite sexes, especially for reproduction 交配；**assortative m.,** nonrandom mating in which the choice of a mate is influenced by phenotype; it is *positive* if phenotypically similar mates are chosen and *negative* if they are dissimilar 选型交配；**nonrandom m.,** mating in which partner selection is not independent of genotype, such as occurs with assortative mating, inbreeding, or stratification of populations into subgroups 非随机交配；**random m.,** mating in which partner selection is independent of genotype 随机交配

ma·trix (ma′triks) pl. *ma′trices* [L.] 1. the base or surrounding substance in which a thing develops, originates, or is contained 基质；2. an intergranular binding substance, such as resin in a dental resin composite filling 基体；3. a mold, form, or die for casting or shaping 铸造模型的模子；4. the principal metal in an alloy 合金中的主要金属；**bone m.,** the intercellular substance of bone, consisting of collagenous fibers, ground substance, and inorganic salts 骨基质；**cartilage m.,** the intercellular substance of cartilage, consisting of cells and extracellular fibers embedded in an amorphous ground substance 软骨基质；**extracellular m. (ECM),** any substance produced by cells and excreted to the extracellular space within the tissues, serving as a scaffolding to hold tissues together and helping to determine their characteristics 细胞外基质；**interterritorial m.,** a paler-staining region among the darker territorial matrices 区间基质；**nail m.,** m. unguis 甲母质；**territorial m.,** basophilic material around groups of cartilage cells 软骨区基质；**m. un′guis,** nail bed; also, the proximal part of the nail bed where growth occurs 甲床

mat·ter (mat′ər) 1. substance; anything that occupies space 物质；2. pus 脓；**gray m. of nervous**

system, substantia grisea 灰质；white m. of nervous system, substantia alba 白质

mat·u·ra·tion (mach″u-ra′shən) 1. the process of becoming mature 成熟；2. attainment of emotional and intellectual maturity 情感和智力成熟；3. in biology, a process of cell division during which the number of chromosomes in the germ cells is reduced to one-half the number characteristic of the species 减数分裂；4. suppuration 化脓

ma·ture (mə-choor′) 1. to develop to maturity; to ripen（使）成熟；2. fully developed; ripe 成熟的

max·il·la (mak-sil′ə) pl. *maxil′las, maxil′lae* [L.] the irregularly shaped bone that with its fellow forms the upper jaw; it assists in the formation of the orbit, the nasal cavity, and the palate, and lodges the upper teeth 上颌骨，见图 1；**max′illary** *adj.*

max·il·lo·eth·moi·dec·to·my (mak-sil″o-eth″-moi-dek′tə-me) excision of the portion of the maxilla surrounding the maxillary sinus and of the cribriform plate and anterior ethmoid cells 上颌筛骨切除术

max·il·lo·fa·cial (mak-sil″o-fa′shəl) pertaining to the maxilla and the face 上颌面的

max·il·lo·man·dib·u·lar (mak-sil″o-man-dib′ulər) pertaining to the upper and lower jaws 上下颌的

max·il·lot·o·my (mak″sĭ-lot′ə-me) surgical sectioning of the maxilla that allows movement of all or part of the maxilla into the desired position 上颌骨切开术

max·i·mum (mak′sĭ-məm) pl. *max′ima* [L.] 1. the greatest possible, or actual, effect or quantity 最大（量），最高（量），最大限度；2. largest, utmost 极限；**max′imal** *adj.*；**transport m., tubular m. (T_m),** the highest rate (milligrams per minute) at which the renal tubules can transfer a substance either from the tubular luminal fluid to the interstitial fluid or from the interstitial fluid to the tubular luminal fluid, beyond which it may be excreted in the urine（肾）小管最大转运率

maze (māz) a complicated system of intersecting paths used in intelligence tests and in demonstrating learning in experimental animals 迷宫，迷津

ma·zin·dol (ma′zin-dol) a sympathomimetic amine having amphetamine-like actions; used as an anorectic 氯苯咪吲哚

ma·zo·pexy (ma′zo-pek″se) 同 mastopexy

ma·zo·pla·sia (ma″zo-pla′zhə) degenerative epithelial hyperplasia of the mammary acini 乳房组织增生

MB [L.] Medici′nae Baccalau′reus (Bachelor of Medicine) 医学学士

MC¹ [L.] Magis′ter Chirur′giae (Master of Surgery) 外科硕士

MC² Medical Corps 军医队

MCFA medium-chain fatty acids 中链脂肪酸

mcg microgram 微克的符号

MCH mean corpuscular hemoglobin 平均红细胞血红蛋白

MCHC mean corpuscular hemoglobin concentration 平均红细胞血红蛋白浓度

mCi millicurie; one thousandth (10^{-3}) of a curie 毫居里的符号

μCi microcurie; one millionth (10^{-6}) of a curie 微居里的符号

MCP membrane cofactor protein 膜辅因子蛋白

MCPP microbiologically confirmed pneumococcal pneumonia 肺炎球菌性肺炎

mCPP meta-chlorophenylpiperazine 间氯苯哌嗪

mCRPC metastatic castration-resistant prostate cancer 转移性去势抵抗性前列腺癌

MCV mean corpuscular volume 平均红细胞容积；meningococcal conjugate vaccine 脑膜炎球菌结合疫苗

MCV4 meningococcal conjugate vaccine 流行性脑脊髓膜炎疫苗

MD [L.] Medici′nae Doc′tor (Doctor of Medicine) 医学博士

MDA methylenedioxyamphetamine 甲撑二氧苯丙胺

MDCT multidetector computed tomography 多排计算机体层摄影

MDF myocardial depressant factor 心肌抑制因子

MDMA 3,4-methylenedioxymethamphetamine 3,4- 亚甲二氧基甲基苯丙胺

meal (mēl) a portion of food or foods taken at some particular and usually stated or fixed time 膳食，餐；**test m.,** a meal containing material given to aid in diagnostic examination of the stomach 试餐，试（验）食

mean (mēn) an average; a numerical value that in some sense represents the central value of a set of numbers 平均数，均值；**arithmetic m.,** the sum of n numbers divided by n 算术平均数；**geometric m.,** the nth root of the product of n numbers 几何平均数

meas·ure (mezh′ər) 量，见 weight 处表

me·a·ti·tis (me″ə-ti′tis) inflammation of the urinary meatus 尿道炎

me·a·to·plas·ty (me-at′o-plas″te) plastic surgery of a meatus 外耳道成形术

me·a·tos·co·py (me″ə-tos′kə-pe) inspection of a meatus, especially the urinary meatus 尿道口镜检查

me·a·tot·o·my (me″ə-tot′ə-me) incision of an

acoustic or urinary meatus to enlarge it 尿道口切开术

me·a·tus (me-a'təs) pl. *mea'tus* [L.] an opening or passage 道；**mea'tal** *adj.*；**acoustic m.**, **auditory m.**, either of two passages in the ear, one leading to the tympanic membrane *(external acoustic m.)* and one for passage of nerves and blood vessels *(internal acoustic m.)* 耳道；**nasal m.**, one of the spaces (inferior, middle, and superior) below the corresponding nasal concha, on either side of the septum 鼻道；**urinary m.**, the opening of the urethra on the body surface through which urine is discharged 尿道口

me·ben·da·zole (mə-ben'də-zōl) an anthelmintic used against trichuriasis, enterobiasis, ascariasis, and hookworm disease 甲苯达唑，甲苯咪唑

mec·a·myl·amine (mek″ə-mil'ə-mēn) a ganglionic blocking agent used in the form of the hydrochloride salt as an antihypertensive 美加明，四甲双环庚胺

me·chan·ics (mə-kan'iks) the science dealing with the motions of bodies 力学；**body m.**, the application of kinesiology to prevent and correct problems related to posture 躯体力学

mech·a·nism (mek'ə-niz-əm) 1. a machine or machinelike structure 机械结构，机构；2. the manner of combination of parts, processes, etc., which subserve a common function 机理，机制；**defense m.**, a usually unconscious mental mechanism by which psychic tension is diminished, e.g., repression, rationalization 防御机制；**escape m.**, in the heart, the mechanism of impulse initiation by lower centers in response to lack of impulse propagation by the sinoatrial node 逃避机制；**mental m.**, 1. the organization of mental operations 心理机制；2. an unconscious and indirect manner of gratifying a repressed desire 一种无意识和间接的满足压抑欲望的方式

mech·a·no·re·cep·tor (mek″ə-no-re-sep'tər) a receptor that is excited by mechanical pressures or distortions, such as those responding to touch and muscular contractions 机械（性）感受器

me·cha·no·sen·so·ry (mek″ə-no-sen'sə-re) pertaining to sensory activation in response to mechanical pressures or distortions 机械感觉的

mech·lor·eth·amine (mek″lor-eth'ə-mēn) one of the nitrogen mustards, used in the form of the hydrochloride salt as an antineoplastic, particularly in disseminated Hodgkin disease 氮芥

mec·li·zine (mek'lĭ-zēn) an antihistamine used as the hydrochloride salt as an antinauseant in motion sickness and to manage vertigo associated with disease affecting the vestibular system 美其敏（抗组胺药）

mec·lo·cy·cline (mek″lo-si'klēn) a tetracycline antibiotic used topically as *m. sulfosalicylate* for the treatment of acne vulgaris 甲氯环素

mec·lo·fen·a·mate (mek″lo-fen'ə-māt) a nonsteroidal antiinflammatory drug used as the sodium salt in the treatment of rheumatic and nonrheumatic inflammatory disorders, pain, dysmenorrhea, hypermenorrhea, and vascular headaches 甲氯灭酸

me·co·ni·um (mə-ko'ne-əm) dark green mucilaginous material in the intestine of the full-term fetus 胎粪

MED minimal erythema dose 最小红斑量

me·dia (me'de-ə) 1. *medium* 的复数；2. middle 中间；3. tunica media vasorum 血管中膜

me·di·al (me'de-əl) 1. situated toward the median plane or midline of the body or a structure 内侧的，近中的；2. pertaining to the middle layer of structures 中层的

me·di·a·lis (me″de-a'lis) [L.] 同 medial

me·di·an (m) (me'de-ən) 1. situated in or near the midline of a body or structure 正中的；2. the value of the middle item of a series when the items are arranged in numerical order 中（位）数

me·di·a·nus (me″de-a'nəs) [L.] median 正中的

me·di·as·ti·nal (me″de-ə-sti'nəl) of or pertaining to the mediastinum 纵隔的

me·di·as·ti·ni·tis (me″de-as″tĭ-ni'tis) inflamma-tion of the mediastinum 纵隔炎；**fibrosing m.**, **fibrous m.**, mediastinal fibrosis 纤维性纵隔炎

me·di·as·ti·nog·ra·phy (me″de-as″tĭ-nog'rə-fe) radiography of the mediastinum 纵隔 X 线照像术

me·di·as·ti·no·peri·car·di·tis (me″de-as″tĭ- no-per″e-kahr-di'tis) pericarditis with adhesions extending from the pericardium to the mediastinum 纵隔心包炎

me·di·as·ti·nos·co·py (me″de-as″tĭ-nos'kə-pe) examination of the mediastinum by means of an endoscope inserted through an anterior midline incision just above the superior thoracic aperture 纵隔镜检查

me·di·as·ti·num (me″de-ə-sti'nəm) pl. *mediasti·na* [L.] 1. a median septum or partition 中隔；2. the mass of tissues and organs separating the two pleural sacs, between the sternum in front and the vertebral column behind, containing the heart and its large vessels, trachea, esophagus, thymus, lymph nodes, and other structures and tissues; it is divided into superior and inferior regions, the latter subdivided into anterior, middle, and posterior parts 纵隔；**m. tes'tis**, the partial septum of the testis, formed near its posterior border by a continuation of the tunica albuginea 睾丸纵隔

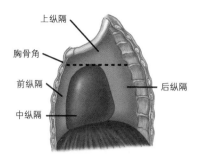

上纵隔
胸骨角
前纵隔
后纵隔
中纵隔

▲ 纵隔分区

me·di·ate[1] (me′de-ət) indirect; accomplished by means of an intervening medium 间接的；中介的
me·di·ate[2] (me′de-āt) to serve as an intermediate agent 介质
med·i·ca·ble (med′ĭ-kə-bəl) subject to treatment with reasonable expectation of cure 可治疗的
med·i·cal (med′ĭ-kəl) pertaining to medicine 医学的
med·i·care (med′ĭ-kār) a program of the Social Security Administration that provides medical care to the aged 医疗保险
med·i·cat·ed (med′ĭ-kāt″əd) imbued with a medicinal substance 含药的
med·i·ca·tion (med″ĭ-ka/shən) 1. 同 medicine (1)；2. impregnation with a medicine 药物疗法；3. administration of a medicine or other remedy 给药；**ionic m.,** iontophoresis 离子透药疗法
me·dic·i·nal (mə-dis′ĭ-nəl) having healing qualities; pertaining to a medicine 医治的，医药的，药用的
med·i·cine (med′ĭ-sin) 1. any drug or remedy 药物；2. the diagnosis and treatment of disease and the maintenance of health 医学；3. the treatment of disease by nonsurgical means 内科学；**alternative m.,** 见 *complementary* 和 *alternative medicine*；**aviation m.,** that dealing with the physiologic, medical, psychological, and epidemiologic problems involved in aviation 航空医学；**Chinese herbal m.,** a highly complex system of diagnosis and treatment using medicinal herbs, one of the branches of traditional Chinese medicine. Herbs range from the nontoxic and rejuvenating, used to support the body's healing system, to highly toxic ones, used to treat disease 中草药；**clinical m.,** 1. the study of disease by direct examination of the living patient 临床医学；2. the last 2 years of the usual curriculum in a medical college 医学院课程最后两年；**complementary m., complementary and alternative m. (CAM),** a large and diverse set of systems of diagnosis, treatment, and prevention based on philosophies and techniques other than those used in conventional Western medicine. Such practices may be described as *alternative,* existing as a body separate from and as a replacement for conventional Western medicine, or *complementary,* used in addition to conventional Western practice. CAM is characterized by its focus on the whole person as a unique individual, on the energy of the body and its influence on health and disease, on the healing power of nature and the mobilization of the body's own resources to heal itself, and on the treatment of the underlying causes, not symptoms, of disease. Many of the techniques used are controversial and have not been validated by controlled studies 辅助性医疗，补充和替代医疗；**emergency m.,** the medical specialty dealing with the acutely ill or injured who require immediate medical treatment 急救医学；**environmental m.,** that dealing with the effects of the environment on humans, including rapid population growth, water and air pollution, travel, etc. 环境医学；**evidence-based m.,** that in which the physician finds, assesses, and implements methods of diagnosis and treatment on the basis of the best available, current research, his or her clinical expertise, and the needs and preferences of the patient 循证医学，另见 *practice* 下词条；**experimental m.,** the study of diseases based on experimentation in animals 实验医学；**family m.,** 家庭医学，见 *practice* 下词条；**folk m.,** the use of home remedies and procedures as handed down by tradition 民间医学；**forensic m.,** the use of home remedies and procedures as handed down by tradition 法医学；**geographic m.,** 1. geomedicine 地理医学；2. 同 tropical m.；**group m.,** the practice of medicine by a group of physicians, usually representing various specialties, who are associated together for the cooperative diagnosis, treatment, and prevention of disease 联合医学；**herbal m.,** herbalism 草药；**holistic m.,** a system of medicine that considers the human being as an integrated whole or functioning unit 整体医学；**internal m.,** that dealing especially with diagnosis and medical treatment of diseases and disorders of internal structures of the body 内科学；**legal m.,** medical jurisprudence 法医学；**maternalfetal m.,** a subspecialty of obstetrics concerned with the obstetric, medical, genetic, and surgical complications of pregnancy and their effects on the mother and fetus 母胎医学；**mind-body m.,** a holistic approach to medicine that takes into account the effect of the mind on physical processes, including the effects of psychosocial stressors and conditioning, particularly as they affect the immune

M

system 心身医学；**naturopathic m.**, naturopathy 自然疗法；**nuclear m.**, the branch of medicine concerned with the use of radionuclides in the diagnosis and treatment of disease 核医学；**occupational m.**, the branch of medicine dealing with the study, prevention, and treatment of workplace-related injuries and occupational diseases 职业医学；**orthomolecular m.**, a system for the prevention and treatment of disease based on the theory that each person's biochemical environment is genetically determined and individually specific. Therapy involves supplementation with substances naturally present in the body (e.g., vitamins, minerals, trace elements, amino acids) in individually optimized amounts 正分子医学；**osteopathic m.**, an approach to medicine that emphasizes the unity of body, mind, and spirit, the interrelationship between structure and function, and an appreciation of the ability of the body to heal itself, combining these with the current practice of medicine, surgery, and obstetrics 整骨医学；**patent m.**, a drug or remedy protected by a trademark, available without a prescription; formerly used for quack remedies sold by peddlers 专卖药；**physical m.**, physiatry 物理医学；**preclinical m.**, 1. 同 preventive m.；2. the first 2 years of the usual curriculum in a medical college 医学院前两年的课程；**preventive m.**, science aimed at preventing disease 预防医学；**proprietary m.**, a remedy whose formula is owned exclusively by the manufacturer and which is marketed usually under a name registered as a trademark 成药；**psychosomatic m.**, the study of the interactions between psychological processes and physiological states 心身医学；**rehabilitation m.**, the branch of physiatry concerned with the restoration of form and function after injury or illness 康复医学；**socialized m.**, a system of medical care controlled by the government 公费医疗制度；**space m.**, the branch of aviation medicine concerned with conditions encountered by humans in space 航天医学；**sports m.**, the branch of medicine concerned with injuries sustained in athletics, including their prevention, diagnosis, and treatment 运动医学；**traditional Chinese m. (TCM)**, the diverse body of medical theory and practice that has evolved in China, comprising four branches: acupuncture and moxibustion, herbal medicine, qi gong, and tui na. In all of these, the body and mind are considered together as a dynamic system subject to cycles of change and affected by the environment, and emphasis is on supporting the body's self-healing ability. Fundamental to TCM are the yin/yang principle and the concept of basic substances that pervade the body: qi, jing, and shen, collectively

known as the three treasures, and the blood (a fluid and material manifestation of qi) and body fluids (which moisten and lubricate the body) 中医学；**travel m., travelers' m.**, the subspecialty of tropical medicine consisting of the diagnosis and treatment or prevention of diseases of travelers 旅行医学；**tropical m.**, the branch of medicine concerned with diseases of the tropics and subtropics 热带病学；**veterinary m.**, the diagnosis and treatment of diseases of animals other than humans 兽医学

med·i·co·le·gal (med″ĭ-ko-le′gəl) pertaining to medical jurisprudence 法医学

med·i·co·so·cial (med″ĭ-ko-so′shəl) having both medical and social aspects 医学社会的

me·dio·lat·er·al (me″de-o-lat′ər-əl) pertaining to the midline and one side 中间外侧的

me·dio·ne·cro·sis (me″de-o-nə-kro′sis) necrosis of the tunica media of a blood vessel 主动脉中层坏死

med·i·ta·tion (med″ĭ-ta′shən) an intentional and self-regulated focusing of attention intended to relax and calm the mind and body 冥想；**mindfulness m.**, a form in which distracting thoughts and feelings are not ignored but instead acknowledged and observed nonjudgmentally as they arise in order to detach from them and gain insight and awareness 正念冥想；**transcendental m.**, a technique for attaining a state of physical relaxation and psychological calm by the regular practice of a relaxation procedure that entails the repetition of a mantra to block distracting thoughts 超觉静坐

me·di·um (me′de-əm) pl. *mediums, me′dia* [L.] 1. a substance that transmits impulses 介质，媒质；2. 同 culture medium；3. a preparation used in treating histologic specimens 培养基；**active m.**, the aggregated atoms, ions, or molecules contained in a laser's optical cavity, in which stimulated emission will occur under the proper excitation 激活介质；**clearing m.**, a substance to render histologic specimens transparent 透明介质；**contrast m.**, a substance introduced into or around a structure or tissues, being different from the structure or tissues as to absorptivity of x-rays, allowing radiographic visualization 对比剂；**culture m.**, 培养基，见 C. 下词条；**dioptric media,** 同 refracting media；**disperse m., dispersion m., dispersive m.**, the continuous phase of a colloid system; the medium in which the particles of the disperse phase are distributed, analogous to the solvent in a true solution 分散介质；**nutrient m.**, a culture medium to which nutrient materials have been added 营养培养基；**radiolucent m.**, a contrast medium that permits passage of x-rays 射线穿透性造影剂；**radiopaque**

m., a contrast medium that blocks passage of x-rays 射线不透性造影剂; **refracting media,** the transparent tissues and fluid in the eye through which light rays pass and by which they are refracted and focused on the retina 屈光介质

me·di·us (me′de-əs) [L.] situated in the middle 中间的

med·roxy·pro·ges·ter·one (məd-rok″se-projes′tər-ōn) a progestin used as the acetate ester in treatment of menstrual disorders, in postmenopause hormone replacement therapy, as a test for endogenous estrogen production, as an antineoplastic in the treatment of metastatic endometrial, breast, and renal carcinoma, and as a long-acting contraceptive 甲羟孕酮

med·ry·sone (med′rə-sōn″) a synthetic glucocorticoid used topically in the treatment of corticosteroid-responsive allergic and inflammatory conditions of the eye 甲羟松

me·dul·la (mə-dul′ə) pl. *medul′lae* [L.] 1. the innermost part of an organ or structure 器官或结构最内部的组织; 2. 同 m. oblongata; 3. bone marrow 骨髓; **adrenal m., m. of suprarenal gland,** the inner, reddish brown, soft part of the suprarenal gland; it synthesizes, stores, and releases catecholamines 肾上腺髓质; **m. of bone,** bone marrow 骨髓; **m. oblonga′ta,** that part of the brainstem continuous with the pons above and the spinal cord below 延髓; **m. os′sium,** bone marrow 骨髓; **renal m.,** the inner part of the kidney substance, composed chiefly of collecting elements, Henle loops, and vasa recta, organized grossly into pyramids 肾髓质; **spinal m., m. spina′lis,** spinal cord 脊髓; **m. of thymus,** the central portion of each lobule of the thymus; it contains many more reticular cells and far fewer lymphocytes than does the surrounding cortex 胸腺髓质

med·ul·lary (med′ə-lar″e) (mə-dul′ə-re) 1. pertaining to a medulla 髓的; 2. pertaining to bone marrow 骨髓的; 3. pertaining to the spinal cord 脊髓的

med·ul·lat·ed (med′ə-lāt″əd) 同 myelinated

med·ul·li·za·tion (med″ə-lī-za′shən) enlargement of marrow spaces, as in rarefying osteitis 髓形成; 髓化

me·dul·lo·blast (mə-dul′o-blast) an undifferentiated cell of the embryonic neural tube that may develop into either a neuroblast or spongioblast 成神经管细胞

me·dul·lo·epi·the·li·o·ma (mə-dul″o-ep″ĭ-the″le-o′mə) a rare type of neuroepithelial tumor, usually in the brain or retina, composed of primitive neuroepithelial cells lining the tubular spaces 髓上皮瘤

me·fe·nam·ic ac·id (mef″ə-nam′ik) a nonsteroidal antiinflammatory drug used to treat or prevent pain, inflammation, dysmenorrhea, and vascular headache 甲灭酸

mef·lo·quine (mef′lo-kwin) an antimalarial effective against chloroquine-resistant strains of *Plasmodium falciparum* and *P. vivax;* used as the hydrochloride salt 甲氟喹

mega- word element [Gr.], large; also used in naming units of measurement (symbol M) to designate an amount one million (10^6) times the size of the unit to which it is joined [构词成分]巨，大；兆，百万(10^6)

mega·cal·y·co·sis (meg″ə-kal″ĭ-ko′sis) nonobstructive dilatation of the renal calices due to malformation of the renal papillae 巨肾盏

mega·caryo·cyte (meg″ə-kar′e-o-sīt″) 同 megakaryocyte

mega·co·lon (meg″ə-ko′lən) dilatation and hypertrophy of the colon 巨结肠; **acquired m.,** any type associated with chronic constipation but normal ganglion cell innervation 获得性巨结肠; **aganglionic m., congenital m.,** Hirschsprung disease; dilatation of one segment of the colon due to narrowing and loss of motor function in the next distal segment, which has a congenital lack of myenteric ganglion cells 无神经性巨结肠，先天性巨结肠; **idiopathic m., acquired m.** 特发性巨结肠; **toxic m.,** that associated with amebic or ulcerative colitis 中毒性巨结肠

mega·cys·tis (meg″ə-sis′tis) an abnormally enlarged urinary bladder 巨膀胱

mega·esoph·a·gus (meg″ə-ə-sof′ə-gəs) pathologic dilatation of the esophagus 巨食管，食管扩张；见 *achalasia*

mega·karyo·blast (meg″ə-kar′e-o-blast) the earliest cytologically identifiable precursor in the thrombocytic series, which matures to form the promegakaryocyte 原巨核细胞; **megakaryoblas′tic** *adj.*

mega·karyo·cyte (meg″ə-kar′e-o-sīt) the giant cell of bone marrow containing a greatly lobulated nucleus, from which mature blood platelets originate 巨核细胞; **megakaryocyt′ic** *adj.*

meg·al·gia (məg-al′jə) a severe pain 剧痛

meg·a·lo·blast (meg′ə-lo-blast″) a large, nucleated, immature progenitor of an abnormal erythrocytic series; the abnormal form corresponding to the normoblast 巨成红细胞; **megaloblas′tic** *adj.*

meg·a·lo·ceph·a·ly (meg″ə-lo-sef′ə-le) macrocephaly 巨头; **megalocephal′ic** *adj.*

meg·a·lo·chei·ria (meg″ə-lo-ki′re-ə) abnormal largeness of the hands 巨手

meg·a·lo·cyte (meg′ə-lo-sīt″) 同 macrocyte

meg·a·lo·dac·ty·ly (meg″ə-lo-dak′tə-le) excessive size of the fingers or toes 巨指（趾）；**megalo-dac′ty-lous** adj.

meg·a·lo·kary·o·cyte (meg″ə-lo-kar′e-o-sīt″) megakaryocyte 巨核细胞

meg·a·lo·ma·nia (meg″ə-lo-ma′ne-ə) unreasonable conviction of one's own extreme greatness, goodness, or power 夸大狂；**megaloma′niac** adj.

meg·a·lo·pe·nis (meg″ə-lo-pe′nis) 同 macropenis

meg·a·loph·thal·mos (meg″ə-lof-thal′mos) 同 macrophthalmia

meg·a·lo·pia (meg″ə-lo′pe-ə) 同 macropsia

meg·a·lo·po·dia (meg″ə-lo-po′de-ə) abnormal largeness of the feet 巨足

meg·a·lo·ure·ter (meg″ə-lo″u-re′tər) 同 megaureter 巨输尿管

meg·a·lo·ure·thra (meg″ə-lo″u-re′thrə) congenital dilation of the urethra, due usually to abnormal development of the corpus spongiosum but occasionally to some abnormality of the corpus cavernosum 巨尿道

mega·ure·ter (meg″ə-u-re′tər) congenital ureteral dilatation, which may be either primary or secondary to something else 巨输尿管

mega·vi·ta·min (meg″ə-vi″tə-min) a dose of vitamin(s) vastly exceeding the amount recommended for nutritional balance 大剂量维生素

mega·volt (MV) (meg′ə-vōlt″) one million (10⁶) volts 兆伏（特）

mega·vol·tage (meg′ə-vōl″təj) in radiotherapy, voltage greater than 1 megavolt, in contrast to orthovoltage and supervoltage 巨电压（在电离辐射治疗中电压超过 1 兆伏）

me·ges·trol (mə-jes′trol) a synthetic progestational agent, used as the acetate ester in the palliative treatment of some breast, endometrial, and prostate carcinomas and in the treatment of anorexia, cachexia, and weight loss associated with cancer or AIDS 甲地孕酮

meg·lu·mine (meg′loo-mēn) a crystalline base used in preparing salts of certain acids for use as a radiopaque medium, e.g., *diatrizoate m., iothalamate m.* 甲基葡胺

meg·ohm (meg′ōm) one million (10⁶) ohms 兆欧（姆）

mei·o·sis (mi-o′sis) a special type of cell division occurring in the maturation of germ cells, consisting of two successive cell divisions (meiosis I and meiosis II) without an interval of DNA replication, by means of which diploid germ cells give rise to haploid gametes 减数分裂；**meiot′ic** adj.

mel·ag·ra (məl-ag′rə) muscular pain in the limbs 肢痛，肢体肌痛

mel·al·gia (məl-al′jə) pain in the limbs 肢痛

mel·an·cho·lia (mel″an-ko′le-ə) former name for depression; currently used to denote severe forms of major depressive disorder 忧郁症；**melanchol′ic** adj.

mel·a·nin (mel′ə-nin) any of several closely related dark pigments of the skin, hair, choroid coat of the eye, substantia nigra, and various tumors, produced by polymerization of oxidation products of tyrosine and dihydroxyphenol compounds 黑（色）素

mel·a·nism (mel′ə-niz″əm) 同 melanosis

mel·a·no·a·melo·blas·to·ma (mel′ə-no″ə- mel″o-blas-to′mə) melanotic neuroectodermal tumor 黑素成釉细胞瘤

mel·a·no·blast (mel′ə-no-blast″) (mə-lan′oblast) a cell that originates from the neural crest and develops into a melanocyte 成黑（色）素细胞

mel·a·no·cyte (mel′ə-no-sīt″) (mə-lan′o-sīt″) a type of dendritic clear cell of the stratum basale of the epidermis that synthesizes the enzyme tyrosinase and contains melanosomes that produce melanin and can be later transferred from melanocytes to keratinocytes 黑（色）素细胞；**melanocyt′ic** adj.

mel·a·no·cy·to·ma (mel″ə-no″si-to′mə) a neoplasm or hamartoma composed of melanocytes 黑素细胞瘤

mel·a·no·der·ma (mel″ə-no-dur′mə) abnormally increased melanin in the skin 黑皮病

mel·a·no·der·ma·ti·tis (mel″ə-no-dur″mə- ti′tis) dermatitis with deposit of melanin in the skin 黑皮炎

me·lan·o·gen (mə-lan′o-jən) a colorless chromogen, convertible into melanin, which may occur in the urine in certain diseases 黑素原

mel·a·no·gen·e·sis (mel″ə-no-jen′ə-sis) the production of melanin 黑素生成

mel·a·no·glos·sia (mel″ə-no-glos′ē-ə) a condition in which the hypertrophied filiform papillae are brown or black 黑舌（病），又称 *black hairy tongue* 和 *black tongue*

mel·a·noid (mel′ə-noid″) 1. resembling melanin 黑素样的；2. a substance resembling melanin 类黑素

mel·a·no·ma (mel″ə-no′mə) a tumor arising from the melanocytic system of the skin and other organs; used alone, it denotes *malignant m.* 黑素瘤；**acral-lentiginous m.,** an irregular, enlarging black macule with a long noninvasive stage, seen chiefly on the palms and soles, the most common type of melanoma in nonwhite persons 肢端雀斑样

痣黑（色）素瘤；**amelanotic m.**, an unpigmented malignant melanoma 无黑（色）素性黑（色）素瘤；**juvenile m.**, Spitz nevus 幼年型黑素瘤；**lenti′go malig′na m.**, a cutaneous malignant melanoma arising in the site of a preexisting lentigo maligna, occurring on sun-exposed areas, particularly of the face 恶性雀斑样痣黑（色）素瘤；**malignant m.**, a malignant tumor usually developing from a nevus or lentigo maligna and consisting of black masses of cells with a marked tendency to metastasis 恶性黑（色）素瘤；**nodular m.**, a type of malignant melanoma without a perceptible radial growth phase, usually seen on the head, neck, or trunk as a uniformly pigmented, elevated, discolored, rapidly enlarging nodule that ulcerates 结节性黑（色）素瘤；**ocular m.**, malignant melanoma arising from the structures of the eye; it frequently metastasizes, which rapidly causes death 眼黑色素瘤；**subungual m.**, acral-lentiginous melanoma in the nail fold or bed 甲下黑（色）素瘤；**superficial spreading m.**, malignant melanoma with a period of radial growth atypical of epidermal melanocytes, which may be followed by invasive growth or may regress; it usually occurs as a small pigmented macule or papule with irregular outline on the lower leg or back 浅表扩散性黑（色）素瘤；**uveal m.**, ocular melanoma consisting of overgrowth of uveal melanocytes 葡萄膜黑素瘤

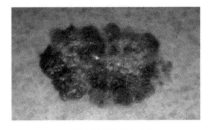

▲　浅表扩散性黑色素瘤

mel·a·no·nych·ia (mel″ə-no-nik′e-ə) blackening of the nails by melanin pigmentation 黑甲

mel·a·no·phage (mel′ə-no-fāj″) a histiocyte laden with phagocytosed melanin 噬黑素细胞

mel·a·no·pla·kia (mel″ə-no-pla′ke-ə) the formation of melanotic patches on the oral mucosa 黏膜黑斑

mel·a·no·sis (mel″ə-no′sis) melanism; disordered production of melanin, with darkening of the skin 黑变病；**m. co′li**, black or brown discoloration of the mucosa of the colon, due to pigment from cathartics that has leaked into the lamina propria 结肠黑色素

沉着病；**m. i′ridis, m. of iris**, abnormal pigmentation of the iris by infiltration of melanoblasts 虹膜黑变病；**neurocutaneous m.**, giant hairy nevus accompanied by malignant melanomas of the meninges 神经皮肤黑变病

mel·a·no·some (mel′ə-no-sōm″) any of the granules within the melanocytes that contain tyrosinase and synthesize melanin; they are transferred from the melanocytes to keratinocytes 黑素体

mel·a·not·ic (mel″ə-not′ik) 1. pertaining to or characterized by the presence of melanin 黑色素的；2. characterized by melanosis 黑变病的

mel·an·uria (mel″ə-nu′re-ə) excretion of urine that is darkly stained or turns dark on standing 黑尿；**melanu′ric** adj.

me·las·ma (mə-laz′mə) sharply demarcated, blotchy, brown macules, usually in a symmetrical distribution on the cheeks and forehead and sometimes the upper lip and neck, often associated with pregnancy or other altered hormonal state 黑斑病，黄褐斑

mel·a·to·nin (mel″ə-to′nin) a catecholamine hormone synthesized and released by the pineal body; in mammals it influences hormone production and in many species regulates seasonal changes such as reproductive pattern and fur color. In humans it is implicated in the regulation of sleep, mood, puberty, and ovarian cycles and it has been tried therapeutically for insomnia, jet lag, and other conditions 褪黑激素

me·le·na (mə-le′nə) the passage of dark stools stained with altered blood 黑粪症

me·li·oi·do·sis (me″li-oi-do′sis) a glanderslike disease of rodents, transmissible to humans, and caused by *Pseudomonas pseudomallei* 类鼻疽

melo·plas·ty (mel′o-plas″te) plastic surgery of the cheek 颊成形术

melo·rhe·os·to·sis (mel″o-re″os-to′sis) a form of osteosclerosis, with linear tracks extending through a long bone 肢骨纹状肥大。见 *rheostosis*

mel·ox·i·cam (mə-lok′sĭ-kam) a nonsteroidal anti-inflammatory drug used in the treatment of osteoarthritis 美洛昔康

mel·pha·lan (mel′fə-lan) a cytotoxic alkylating agent derived from mechlorethamine, used as an antineoplastic 美法仑，左旋溶肉瘤素

mem·ber (mem′bər) 1. a part of the body distinct from the rest in function or position 在功能和位置上不同于其他部位的肢体部分；2. limb 肢

mem·bra (mem′brə) [L.] *membrum* 的复数

mem·bra·na (mem-bra′nə) pl. *membra′nae* [L.] 同 membrane mem·brane (mem′brān) a thin layer of tissue that covers a surface, lines a cavity, or divides a space or organ 膜；alveolar-capillary m., alveolocapillary m., a thin tissue barrier through which gases are exchanged between the alveolar air and the blood in the pulmonary capillaries 肺泡毛细血管膜，又称 *blood-air barrier*, *blood-gas barrier*；alveolodental m., periodontium 牙周膜；arachnoid m., arachnoid (2) 蛛网膜；atlantooccipital m., either of two midline ligamentous structures, one (the *anterior*) passing from the anterior arch of the atlas to the anterior margin of the foramen magnum and the other (the *posterior*) connecting the posterior aspects of the same structures 寰枕前膜；basement m., a sheet of amorphous extracellular material upon which the basal surfaces of epithelial cells rest; it is also associated with muscle cells, Schwann cells, fat cells, and capillaries, interposed between the cellular elements and the underlying connective layer 基(底）膜；basilar m. of cochlear duct, lamina basilaris 蜗管基底层；Bichat m., 同 fenestrated m.；Bowman m., a thin layer of cornea between the outer layer of stratified epithelium and the substantia propria 鲍曼膜；Bruch m., the inner layer of the choroid, separating it from the pigmentary layer of the retina 布鲁赫膜，（脉络膜）玻璃膜；Brunn m., the epithelium of the olfactory part of the nose 鼻嗅区上皮；cloacal m., the thin temporary barrier between the embryonic hindgut and the exterior 泄殖腔膜；Corti m., a gelatinous mass resting on the organ of Corti, connected with the hairs of the hair cells 科蒂膜；croupous m., the false membrane of true croup 格鲁布膜；cytoplasmic m., 同 plasma m.；Descemet m., a thin hyaline membrane between the substantia propria and endothelial layer of the cornea 德塞梅膜，（角膜）后界层；diphtheritic m., a false membrane characteristic of diphtheria, formed by coagulation necrosis 白喉膜；elastic m., one made up largely of elastic fibers 弹性膜；enamel m., 1. dental cuticle 牙小皮；2. the inner layer of cells within the enamel organ of the fetal dental germ 釉膜；epiretinal m., a pathologic membrane partially covering the surface of the retina, probably originating chiefly from the retinal pigment epithelial and glial cells 视网膜前膜；extraembryonic m's, those that protect the embryo or fetus and provide for its nutrition, respiration, and excretion; the yolk sac (umbilical vesicle), allantois, amnion, chorion, decidua, and placenta 胎膜；false m., pseudomembrane 假膜；fenestrated m., one of the perforated elastic sheets of the tunica intima and tunica media of arteries 窗膜；fetal m's, 同 extraembryonic m's；fibroelastic m. of larynx, the fibroelastic layer beneath the mucous coat of the larynx 喉纤维弹性膜；glomerular m., the membrane covering a glomerular capillary 肾小球膜；hemodialyzer m., the semipermeable membrane that filters the blood in a hemodialyzer, commonly made of cuprophane, cellulose acetate, polyacrylonitrile, or polymethyl methacrylate 血液透析膜；hyaline m., 1. a membrane between the outer root sheath and inner fibrous layer of a hair follicle 透明膜（毛根），（毛囊）玻璃膜；2. a layer of eosinophilic hyaline material lining alveoli, alveolar ducts, and bronchioles, found at autopsy in infants who have died of respiratory distress syndrome of the newborn 透明膜；hyaloid m., 同 vitreous m. (1)；Jackson m., a web of adhesions sometimes covering the cecum and causing obstruction of the bowel Jackson 膜；limiting m., one that constitutes the border of some tissue or structure 界膜；medullary m., endosteum 骨内膜；mucous m., mucosa 黏膜；nuclear m., 1. either of the membranes, inner and outer, comprising the nuclear envelope 核膜；2. nuclear envelope 核被膜；olfactory m., the olfactory portion of the mucous membrane lining the nasal fossa 嗅膜；ovular m., 同 vitelline m.；peridental m., periodontal m., periodontal ligament 牙周膜；placental m., the membrane separating the fetal from the maternal blood in the placenta; sometimes inappropriately called the *placental barrier* 胎盘膜；plasma m., the structure, consisting of a lipid bilayer with embedded proteins, that encloses the cytoplasm of a cell, forming a selectively permeable barrier 质膜；pleuroperitoneal m's, a pair of partitions in the embryo that close off the passages connecting the primordial pericardial and peritoneal cavities, creating separate cavities and developing into the posterolateral portions of the respiratory diaphragm 胸腹隔膜；postsynaptic m., the area of plasma membrane of a postsynaptic cell that is within the synapse and has areas especially adapted for receiving neurotransmitters 突触后膜；presynaptic m., the area of plasma membrane of a presynaptic axon that is within the synapse and has sites especially adapted for the release of neurotransmitters 突触前膜；pupillary m., a mesodermal layer attached to the rim or front of the iris during embryonic development 瞳孔膜；Reissner m., the thin anterior wall of the cochlear duct, separating it from the scala vestibuli 赖斯纳膜，前庭膜；reticular m. of spiral organ, a netlike membrane over the spiral organ of the ear, through which pass the free ends of the outer hair cells 网状膜；m. of round window, secondary tympanic m. 圆窗膜；Ruysch m., ruyschian m., lamina choroidocapillaris 鲁伊施膜；Scarpa m., 同 secondary tympanic m.；schneiderian m., the mucous membrane lining the nose 施耐德膜；secondary tympanic m., the membrane enclosing the fenestra cochlearis 第二鼓膜；Shrapnell m., the thin upper part of the tympanic membrane Shrapnell 膜；suprapleural m., the strengthened portion of the endothoracic fascia attached to the inner part of the first rib and the transverse process of the seventh cervical vertebra 胸膜上膜；synaptic m., the part of the plasma membrane of a neuron that is within a synapse 突触膜；synovial m., the inner of the two layers of the joint capsule of a synovial joint, composed of loose connective tissue and having a free smooth surface that lines the joint cavity 滑膜；tectorial m., Corti m. 盖膜；tympanic m., the thin partition between the external acoustic meatus and the middle ear 鼓膜；undulating m., a protoplasmic membrane running like a fin along the bodies of certain protozoa 波动膜；vestibular m. of cochlear duct, the thin anterior wall of the cochlear duct, separating it from the scala tympani 蜗管前庭膜；vitelline m., the cytoplasmic, noncellular membrane surrounding an oocyte 卵黄膜；vitreous m., 1. a delicate boundary layer investing the vitreous body 玻璃体膜；2. 同 Bruch m.；3. 同 Descemet m.；4. hyaline m. (1) 透明膜（毛根）；yolk m., 同 vitelline m.；Zinn m., ciliary zonule 秦氏膜

mem·bra·no·car·ti·lag·i·nous (mem″brə-no-kahr″tĭ-laj′ĭ-nəs) 1. developed in both membrane and cartilage 在膜和软骨中均有发育；2. partly cartilaginous and partly membranous 膜（与）软骨性的

mem·bra·noid (mem′brə-noid) resembling a membrane 膜样的

mem·bran·ol·y·sis (mem″brān-ol′ĭ-sis) disruption of any membrane 细胞膜破裂

mem·bra·nous (mem′brə-nəs) pertaining to or of the nature of a membrane 膜的，膜性的，膜样的

mem·brum (mem′brəm) pl. *mem'bra* [L.] limb 肢，肢体

mem·o·ry (mem′ə-re) that faculty by which sensations, impressions, and ideas are stored and recalled 记忆；immunologic m., anamnesis; the capacity of the immune system to respond more rapidly and strongly to subsequent antigenic challenge than to the first exposure 免疫记忆；remote m., memory that is serviceable for events long past but is not able to make new recollections 远期记忆；replacement m., the replacing of one memory with another 替代记忆；screen m., a consciously tolerable memory serving to conceal another mem-

ory that might be disturbing or emotionally painful if recalled 筛选记忆；short-term m., memory that is lost within a brief period (from a few seconds to a maximum of about 30 minutes) unless reinforced 短期记忆

MEN multiple endocrine neoplasia 多发性内分泌腺瘤

me·nac·me (mə-nak′me) the period of a woman's life that is marked by menstrual activity 经潮期

men·a·di·ol (men″ə-di′ol) a vitamin K analogue; its sodium diphosphate salt is used as a prothrombinogenic vitamin 磷钠甲萘醌，甲萘二酚，甲萘氢醌

men·a·di·one (men″ə-di′ōn) vitamin K₃ 维生素 K₃ 1. a synthetic fat-soluble vitamin that can be converted in the body to active vitamin K 一种合成的脂溶性维生素；2. the basic double-ring quinone structure that is the parent structure of the related compounds with vitamin K activity, which can be formed by addition of long side chain substituents 甲萘醌

men·a·quin·one (men″ə-kwin′ōn) vitamin K₂; any of a series of compounds that have vitamin K activity and are structurally similar to phytonadione (vitamin K₁) but have a different side chain; synthesized by the intestinal flora 维生素 K₂，甲基萘醌类

me·nar·che (mə-nahr′ke) establishment or beginning of the menstrual function 月经初潮；**menar'chal, menar'cheal, menar'chial** *adj.*

me·nin·ges (mə-nin′jēz) sing. *me'ninx.* [Gr.] the three membranes covering the brain and spinal cord: dura mater, arachnoid mater, and pia mater 脑脊膜；**menin'geal** *adj.*

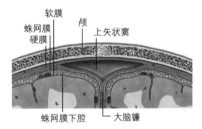

▲ 上冠状面视图中的颅脑膜，包括硬膜、蛛网膜和软膜

me·nin·gi·o·ma (mə-nin″je-o′mə) a benign, slow-growing tumor of the meninges, usually next to the dura mater, which may invade the skull or cause hyperostosis and often causes increased intracranial pressure; it is usually subclassified on the basis of anatomic location 脑（脊）膜瘤；angioblastic m., one containing many blood vessels of various sizes 成血管细胞型脑膜瘤; **convexity m's,** a diverse group of meningiomas located within the sulci of the brain, usually anterior to the central sulcus 凸面脑膜瘤; **psammomatous m.,** one containing many psammoma bodies 砂状性脑膜瘤

me·nin·gism (mə-nin′jiz-əm) the symptoms of meningitis with acute febrile illness or dehydration without infection of the meninges 假性脑（脊）膜炎

men·in·gis·mus (men″in-jis′məs) 同 meningism

men·in·gi·tis (men″in-ji′tis) pl. *meningi′tides* [Gr.] inflammation of the meninges 脑膜炎; **meningit′ic** *adj.*; **basilar m.,** that affecting the meninges at the base of the brain 基底性脑膜炎; **cerebral m.,** inflammation of the membranes of the brain 脑膜炎; **cerebrospinal m.,** inflammation of the membranes of the brain and spinal cord 脑脊膜炎; **chronic m.,** a variable syndrome of prolonged fever, headache, lethargy, stiff neck, confusion, nausea, and vomiting, with pleocytosis; due to a variety of infectious and noninfectious causes 慢性脑膜炎; **cryptococcal m.,** cryptococcosis in which the meninges are invaded by *Cryptococcus.* 隐球菌性脑膜炎; **eosinophilic m.,** meningitis characterized by an increase in lymphocytes and a high percentage of eosinophils in the cerebrospinal fluid, usually due to *Angiostrongylus cantonensis* infection 嗜酸性粒细胞增多性脑膜炎; **epidemic cerebrospinal m.,** meningococcal m. 流行性脑脊膜炎; **meningococcal m.,** an acute infectious, usually epidemic, disease attended by a seropurulent meningitis, due to *Neisseria meningitidis,* usually with an erythematous, herpetic, or hemorrhagic skin eruption 脑膜炎球菌性脑膜炎; **occlusive m.,** leptomeningitis of children, with closure of the lateral and median apertures of the fourth ventricle 闭塞性脑膜炎; **m. ossi′ficans,** ossification of the cerebral meninges 骨化性脑膜炎; **otitic m.,** that secondary to otitis media 耳炎性脑膜炎; **spinal m.,** inflammation of the membranes of the spinal cord 脊髓炎; **tubercular m., tuberculous m.,** severe meningitis due to *Mycobacterium tuberculosis* 结核性脑膜炎; **viral m.,** that due to a virus, e.g., coxsackieviruses, mumps virus, or the virus of lymphocytic choriomeningitis, marked by malaise, fever, headache and other aches, nausea, and cerebrospinal fluid pleocytosis (mainly lymphocytic); it usually runs a short uncomplicated course 病毒性脑膜炎

me·nin·go·cele (mə-ning′go-sēl″) hernial protrusion of the meninges through a defect in the cranium *(cranial m.)* or vertebral column *(spinal m.)* 脊膜膨出，脑（脊）膜膨出

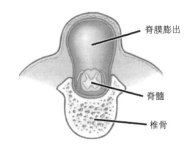

▲ **脊膜膨出的横截面**

me·nin·go·coc·ce·mia (mə-ning″go-kokse′me-ə) invasion of the blood by meningococci 脑膜炎球菌败血症

me·nin·go·coc·cus (mə-ning″go-kok′əs) pl. *meningococ′ci.* An individual organism of *Neisseria meningitidis* 脑膜炎双球菌; **meningococ′cal, meningococ′cic** *adj.*

me·nin·go·cyte (mə-ning′go-sīt″) a histiocyte of the meninges 脑膜细胞

me·nin·go·en·ceph·a·li·tis (mə-ning″go- ən-sef′ə-li′tis) inflammation of the brain and meninges 脑膜脑炎; **toxoplasmic m.,** meningoencephalitis occurring in toxoplasmosis, with seizures and mental confusion followed by coma; often fatal if untreated 弓形虫脑膜炎

me·nin·go·en·ceph·a·lo·cele (mə-ning″go- ən-sef′ə-lo-sēl″) encephalocele 脑膜脑膨出

me·nin·go·en·ceph·a·lop·a·thy (mə-ning″go-ən-sef′ə-lop′ə-the) noninflammatory disease of the cerebral meninges and brain 脑膜脑病

me·nin·go·gen·ic (mə-ning″go-jen′ik) arising in the meninges 脑膜源性

me·nin·go·ma·la·cia (mə-ning″go-mə- la′shə) softening of a membrane 脑膜软化

me·nin·go·my·eli·tis (mə-ning″go-mi″ə- li′tis) inflammation of the spinal cord and its membranes 脊髓脊膜炎

me·nin·go·my·elo·ra·dic·u·li·tis (mə- ning″go-mi″ə-lo″rə-dik″u-li′tis) inflammation of the meninges, spinal cord, and roots of the spinal nerves 脊膜脊髓神经根炎

me·nin·go-os·teo·phle·bi·tis (mə-ning″goos″te-o-flə-bi′tis) periostitis with inflammation of the veins of a bone 骨膜骨静脉炎

men·in·gop·a·thy (men″in-gop′ə-the) any disease of the meninges 脑膜病

me·nin·go·poly·neu·ri·tis (mə-ning″gopol″e-noo-ri′tis) the triad of radiculopathy, aseptic meningitis, and cranial neuritis 神经根病变、无菌性脑膜炎和颅神经炎的三联征

me·nin·go·ra·dic·u·lar (mə-ning″go-rə- dik′u-lər) pertaining to the meninges and the cranial or spinal nerve roots 脑脊膜神经根的

me·nin·gor·rha·gia (mə-ning″go-ra′jə) hemorrhage from cerebral or spinal membranes 脑膜出血

men·in·go·sis (men″in-go′sis) attachment of bones by membrane 膜性附着

me·ninx (me′ninks) pl. *menin′ges* [Gr.] *meninges* 的单数

men·is·ci·tis (men″ĭ-si′tis) inflammation of a meniscus of the knee joint 半月板炎

me·nis·co·fem·o·ral (mə-nis″ko-fem′ə-rəl) pertaining to or connecting the femur and a meniscus 半月板股骨间的

me·nis·co·syn·o·vi·al (mə-nis″ko-sə-no′ve-əl) pertaining to a meniscus and the synovial membrane 半月板滑膜的

me·nis·cus (mə-nis′kəs) pl. *menis′ci* [L.] some - thing of crescent shape, as the concave or convex surface of a column of liquid in a pipet or buret, or a crescent-shaped cartilage, particularly one in the knee joint 半月板；新月面，弯月面；**menis′cal** *adj.*; **tactile m.,** one of the small, cup-shaped nerve endings within the skin (deep epidermis, hair follicles, and hard palate); each is in contact with a single Merkel cell and they function as tactile receptors 触盘，触角半月板

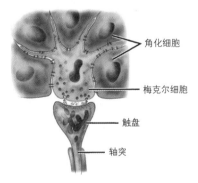

角化细胞

梅克尔细胞

触盘

轴突

▲ 与上皮梅克尔细胞接触的神经纤维的触盘

meno·met·ror·rha·gia (men″o-me″tro-ra′jə) excessive and prolonged uterine bleeding occurring at irregular, frequent intervals 月经频多

meno·pause (men′o-pawz″) cessation of menstruation 绝经（期）；**menopau′sal** *adj.*; **premature m.,** menopause before the age of 40; replaced by the broader term *primary ovarian insufficiency* 早期绝经

men·or·rha·gia (men″ə-ra′jə) hypermenorrhea 月经过多

men·or·rhea (men″ə-re′ə) 1. the normal discharge of the menses 行经，月经；2. profuse menstruation 月经过多；**menorrhe′al** *adj.*

me·nos·che·sis (mə-nos′kə-sis) retention of the menses 闭经，经闭

meno·stax·is (men″ə-stak′sis) excessively prolonged menstruation 经期延长

meno·tro·pins (men′o-tro″pinz) a purified preparation of gonadotropins extracted from the urine of postmenopausal women containing folliclestimulating hormone (FSH) and luteinizing hormone (LH); used to treat male hypogonadism, to induce ovulation and pregnancy in certain infertile, anovulatory women, and to stimulate oocyte development and maturation in patients using assisted reproductive technologies 尿促性素，促生育素，促月经素

men·ses (men′sēz) the monthly flow of blood from the female genital tract 月经

men·stru·al (men′stroo-əl) pertaining to the menses or to menstruation 月经的

men·stru·a·tion (men″stroo-a′shən) the cyclic, physiological discharge through the vagina of blood and muscosal tissues from the nonpregnant uterus; it is under hormonal control and normally recurs at approximately 4-week intervals, except during pregnancy and lactation, throughout the reproductive period (puberty through menopause) 月经；**anovular m., anovulatory m.,** periodic uterine bleeding without preceding ovulation 无排卵月经；**infrequent m.,** oligomenorrhea 月经稀少；**profuse m.,** hypermenorrhea 月经过多；**retrograde m.,** backflow of menstrual fluid, epithelial cells, and debris through the uterine tubes and into the peritoneal cavity 逆行月经；**scanty m.,** hypomenorrhea 月经过少；**vicarious m.,** discharge of blood from an extragenital source at the time menstruation is normally expected 代偿性月经

men·su·ra·tion (men″su-ra′shən) the act or process of measuring 测量

men·tal (men′təl) 1. pertaining to the mind 心理的，精神的；2. pertaining to the chin 颏的

men·thol (men′thol) an alcohol from various mint oils or produced synthetically; used topically to relieve itching and as an inhalation to treat upper respiratory tract disorders 薄荷醇

men·to·la·bi·al (men″to-la′be-əl) pertaining to the chin and lip 颏唇的

men·ton (men′ton) the most inferior point on the mandibular symphysis on a lateral jaw projection 颏下点

men·to·plas·ty (men′to-plas″te) plastic surgery of the chin; surgical correction of deformities and defects of the chin 颏成形术

men·tum (men′təm) [L.] chin 颏

MEP maximum expiratory pressure 最大呼气压

me·pen·zo·late (mə-pen′zo-lāt) a quaternary ammonium compound with anticholinergic and antimuscarinic effects, used in the form of the bromide salt in the treatment of peptic ulcers and disorders characterized by colon hypermotility 甲哌佐酯

me·per·i·dine (mə-per′ĭ-dēn) an opioid analgesic, used as the hydrochloride salt as an analgesic and an anesthesia adjunct 杜冷丁

me·phen·ter·mine (mə-fen′tər-mēn) an adrenergic used as the sulfate salt for its vasopressor effects in the treatment of certain hypotensive states 硫 酸甲苯丁胺（肾上腺素能药）

me·phen·y·to·in (mə-fen′ə-to-in) an anticonvulsant used for the control of a variety of epileptic seizures 美芬妥因（抗惊厥药）

me·phit·ic (mə-fit′ik) emitting a foul odor 臭气的

meph·o·bar·bi·tal (mef″o-bahr′bĭ-təl) a longacting barbiturate used as an anticonvulsant 甲基苯巴比妥（抗惊厥药）

me·piv·a·caine (mĕ-pi′və-kān) a lidocaine analogue used in the form of the hydrochloride salt as a local anesthetic 甲哌卡因（局部麻醉药）

me·pro·ba·mate (mə-pro′bə-māt) (mep″robam′āt) a carbamate derivative with tranquilizing and muscle relaxant actions 甲丙氨酯

mEq milliequivalent 毫（克）当量

mer·ad·i·mate (mer-ad′ĭ-māt) an absorber of ultraviolet A radiation, used topically as a sunscreen 美拉地酯（防晒药）

me·ral·gia (mə-ral′jə) pain in the thigh 股痛；**m. paresthe′tica,** paresthesia, pain, and numbness in the outer surface of the thigh due to entrapment of the lateral femoral cutaneous nerve at the inguinal ligament 感觉异常性股痛

mer·cap·tan (mər-kap′tan) thiol (2) 硫醇

mer·cap·to·pu·rine (6-MP) (mər-kap″to-pu′rēn) a sulfur-containing purine analogue, used as an antineoplastic and as an immunosuppressant 6-巯(基)嘌呤（抗肿瘤药）

mer·cu·ri·al (mər-kūr′e-əl) 1. pertaining to mercury 水银的，汞的；2. a preparation containing mercury 汞制剂

mer·cur·ic (mər-kūr′ik) pertaining to mercury as a bivalent element 汞的

mer·cu·rous (mur′kū-rəs) pertaining to mercury as a monovalent element 亚汞的

mer·cu·ry (Hg) (mur′kūr-e) a heavy, silvery white, liquid metallic element; at. no. 80; at. wt. 200.59. Acute poisoning, due to ingestion, is marked

by severe abdominal pain, metallic taste, vomiting, bloody diarrhea with watery stools, oliguria or anuria, and corrosion and ulceration of the digestive tract. Chronic poisoning, due to absorption through skin and mucous membranes, inhalation, or ingestion, is marked by stomatitis, metallic taste, sore bleeding gums with a blue line along the border, excessive salivation, excitability, memory loss, and nervous system damage 汞，水银

me·rid·i·an (mə-rid′e-ən) 1. an imaginary line on the surface of a spherical body, marking the intersection with the surface of a plane passing through its axis 子午线，经线；2. in acupuncture, a system of 20 lines connecting acupoints and regarded as channels through which qi flows 经络

me·rid·i·a·nus (mə-rid″e-a′nəs) pl. *meridia′ni* [L.] meridian 子午线，经线

mero·blas·tic (mer″o-blas′tik) partially dividing; undergoing cleavage in which only part of the zygote participates 部分分裂的，不全（卵）裂的

mero·crine (mer′o-krin) discharging only the secretory product and maintaining the secretory cell intact (e.g., salivary glands, pancreas) 部 分 分 泌（的），局（部分）泌的

mero·gen·e·sis (mer″o-jen′ə-sis) cleavage of a zygote 卵裂；**merogenet′ic, merogen′ic** *adj.*

mero·me·lia (mer″o-me′le-ə) congenital absence of any part of a limb 残肢畸形；cf. *amelia*

mero·myo·sin (mer″o-mi′o-sin) a fragment of the myosin molecule isolated by treatment with a proteolytic enzyme; there are two types, heavy *(H-meromyosin)* and light *(L-meromyosin)* 酶 解 肌球蛋白

mer·o·pen·em (mer″o-pen′əm) a broad-spectrum antibacterial effective against a wide variety of gram-positive and gram-negative organisms; used in the treatment of intra-abdominal infections and bacterial meningitis 美洛培南，广谱抗生素，用于治疗腹内感染和细菌性脑膜炎

mero·ra·chis·chi·sis (me″ro-rə-kis′kĭ-sis) fissure of a part of the vertebral column 部分脊柱裂，脊柱不全裂

mero·zo·ite (mer″o-zo′īt) one of the organisms formed by multiple fission (schizogony) of a sporozoite within the body of the host 裂殖子

MESA microsurgical epididymal sperm aspiration 显微附睾精子抽取术

me·sal·amine (mə-sal′ə-mēn) 5-aminosalicylic acid, an active metabolite of sulfasalazine, used in the prophylaxis and treatment of inflammatory bowel disease 氨基水杨酸，又称 *mesalazine*

mes·an·gio·cap·il·lary (mes-an″je-o-kap′ĭ- lar″e)

pertaining to or affecting the mesangium and the associated capillaries 肾小球膜毛细血管的
mes·an·gi·um (mes-an'je-əm) the thin membrane supporting the capillary loops in renal glomeruli 肾小球膜；**mesan'gial** *adj.*

mes·ax·on (mes-ak'son) a pair of parallel membranes marking the line of edge-to-edge contact of Schwann cells encircling an axon 轴突系膜

mes·ca·line (mes'kə-lēn) a poisonous alkaloid from the flowering heads (mescal buttons) of a Mexican cactus, *Lophophora williamsii*; it produces an intoxication with delusions of color and sound 麦司卡林，仙掌毒碱（一种致幻剂）

mes·ec·to·derm (mez-ek'to-dərm) embryonic migratory cells derived from the neural crest of the head that contribute to the formation of the meninges and become pigment cells 中外胚层

mes·en·ceph·a·lon (mez″en-sef'ə-lon) midbrain 中脑 1. the part of the brain developed from the middle of the three primary vesicles of the embryonic neural tube, comprising the tectum, midbrain tegmentum, and basis pedunculi; 2. the middle of the three primary brain vesicles in the embryo, lying between the prosencephalon and the rhombencephalon；**mesencephal'ic** *adj.*

mes·en·ceph·a·lot·o·my (mez″en-sef″ə-lot'ə- me) surgical production of lesions in the midbrain, especially for relief of intractable pain 中脑切开术

mes·en·chyme (mez'əng-kīm″) the meshwork of embryonic connective tissue in the mesoderm from which are formed the connective tissues of the body and the blood and lymphatic vessels 间充质，又称 *mesenchyma*；**mesen'chymal** *adj.*

mes·en·chy·mo·ma (mez″ən-ki-mo'mə) a mixed mesenchymal tumor composed of two or more cellular elements not commonly associated, exclusive of fibrous tissue 间叶瘤

mes·en·ter·ic (mez″ən-ter'ik) pertaining to the mesentery 肠系膜的

mes·en·ter·io·pexy (mez″ən-ter'e-o-pek″se) fixation or suspension of a torn mesentery 肠系膜固定术

mes·en·ter·i·pli·ca·tion (mez″ən-ter″ĭ-plĭ-ka'-shən) shortening of the mesentery by plication 肠系膜折术

mes·en·ter·i·um (mez″ən-ter'e-əm) [L.] 同 mes-en-tery (1)

mes·en·ter·on (mez-en'tər-on) the midgut 中肠

mes·en·tery (mez'ən-ter″e) 1. the peritoneal fold attaching the small intestine to the posterior body wall 肠系膜；2. a membranous fold attaching an organ to the body wall 隔（膜）

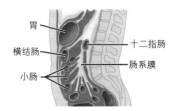

▲ 正中矢状面肠系膜

mesh·work (mesh'wərk) a network or reticulum 网；trabecular m., a trabecula of loose fibers found at the iridocorneal angle between the anterior chamber of the eye and the venous sinus of the sclera; the aqueous humor filters through the spaces between the fibers into the sinus and passes into the bloodstream. It is divided into a corneoscleral part and a uveal part 小梁网

me·si·ad (me'ze-ad) toward the middle or center 向中线，向中

me·si·al (me'ze-əl) nearer the center of the dental arch 正中的；近中的

me·si·al·ly (me'ze-al″e) toward the median line 向中线

me·sio·clu·sion (me″ze-o-kloo'zhən) anteroclusion; malrelation of the dental arches with the mandibular arch anterior to the maxillary arch (prognathism) 近中拾

me·sio·dens (me'ze-o-denz″) pl. *mesioden'tes.* A small supernumerary tooth, occurring singly or paired, generally palatally between the maxillary central incisors 额外牙，楔形牙，正中多生牙

me·sio·ver·sion (me″ze-o-vur'zhən) displacement of a tooth along the dental arch toward the midline of the face 近中向位，近中错位

mes·mer·ism (mez'mər-iz″əm) hypnotism 催眠术

mes·na (mez'nə) a sulfhydryl compound given with urotoxic antineoplastic agents because it inactivates some of their urotoxic metabolites 美司钠，巯乙磺酸钠

meso·ap·pen·dix (mez″o-) (me″zo-ə-pen'dix) the peritoneal fold connecting the appendix to the ileum 阑尾系膜

meso·bil·i·ru·bin·o·gen (mez″o-) (me″zobil″ĭ-roo-bin'o-jən) a reduced form of bilirubin, formed in the intestine, which on oxidation forms stercobilin 中胆红素原

meso·blast (mez'o-) (me'zo-blast″) mesoderm, especially in the early, undifferentiated stages 中胚层

meso·blas·te·ma (mez″o-) (me″zo-blas-te'mə) the cells composing the mesoblast 中胚层细胞

meso·blas·tic (mez'o-) (me″zo-blas'tik)pertaining to or derived from the mesoblast 中胚层的

meso·car·dia (mez″o-) (me″zo-kahr′de-ə) atypical location of the heart, with the apex in the midline of the thorax 中位心

meso·car·di·um (mez″o-) (me″zo-kahr′de-əm) that part of the embryonic mesentery connecting the heart with the body wall in front and the foregut behind 心系膜

meso·ce·cum (mez″o-) (me″zo-se′kəm) the occasionally occurring mesentery of the cecum 盲肠系膜

meso·co·lon (mez″o-) (me′zo-ko″lən) the peritoneal process attaching the colon to the posterior abdominal wall, and called ascending, descending, etc., according to the portion of colon to which it attaches 结肠系膜；**mesocol′ic** *adj.*

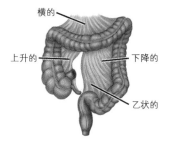

横的

上升的

下降的

乙状的

▲ 结肠系膜

meso·co·lo·pexy (mez″o-) (me″zo-ko′lopek″se) suspension or fixation of the mesocolon 结肠系膜固定术

meso·cor·tex (mez″o-) (me″zo-kor′teks) the cortex of the cingulate gyrus, intermediate in form between the allocortex and the isocortex and having five or six layers 中间皮质

meso·derm (mez′o-) (me′zo-dərm″) the middle of the three primary germ layers of the embryo, lying between the ectoderm and endoderm; from it are derived the connective tissue, bone, cartilage, muscle, blood and blood vessels, lymphatics, lymphoid organs, notochord, pleura, pericardium, peritoneum, kidneys, and gonads 中胚层；**mesoder′mal, mesoder′mic** *adj.*

meso·du·o·de·num (mez″o-) (me″zo-doo″ode′nəm) the mesenteric fold enclosing the duodenum of the early fetus 十二指肠系膜；**mesoduode′nal** *adj.*

meso·epi·did·y·mis (mez″o-) (me″zo-ep″ĭ-did′ĭ-mis) a fold of tunica vaginalis testis sometimes connecting the epididymis and testis 附睾系膜

meso·gas·tri·um (mez″o-) (me″zo-gas′tre-əm) the portion of the primitive mesentery that encloses the stomach and from which the greater omentum develops 胃系膜；**mesogas′tric** *adj.*

meso·ile·um (mez″o-) (me″zo-il′e-əm) the mesentery of the ileum 回肠系膜

meso·je·ju·num (mez″o-) (me″zo-jə-joo′nəm) the mesentery of the jejunum 空肠系膜

meso·mere (mez′o-) (me′zo-mēr) 1. a blastomere of size intermediate between a macromere and a micromere 中分裂球；2. a midzone of the mesoderm between the epimere and hypomere 中段（中胚层）

meso·me·tri·um (mez″o-) (me″zo-me′tre- əm) the portion of the broad ligament below the mesovarium 子宫系膜

meso·morph (mez′o-) (me′zo-morf″) an individual having the type of body build in which mesodermal tissues predominate: relative preponderance of muscle, bone, and connective tissue, usually with heavy, hard physique of rectangular outline 中胚层体型者

mes·on (mez′on) (me′zon) a subatomic particle having a rest mass intermediate between the mass of the electron and that of the proton, carrying either a positive, negative, or neutral electric charge 介子

meso·neph·ric (mez″o-) (me″zo-nef′rik) pertaining to the mesonephros 中肾的

mes·o·ne·phro·ma (mez″o-) (me″zo-nə- fro′mə) clear cell adenocarcinoma 中肾瘤

meso·neph·ros (mez″o-) (me″zo-nef′ros) pl. *mesoneph′roi* [Gr.] the excretory organ of the embryo, arising caudad to the pronephric rudiments or the pronephros and using its ducts 中肾

meso·phile (mez′o-) (me′zo-fīl″) an organism that grows best at 20℃ to 55℃ 中温（微）生物，嗜温菌；中温生物；**mesophil′ic** *adj.*

meso·phle·bi·tis (mez″o-) (me″zo-flə-bi′tis) inflammation of the middle coat of a vein 静脉中层炎

me·soph·ry·on (mə-sof′re-on) the glabella, or its central point 眉间

meso·pul·mo·num (mez″o-) (me″zo-pəlmo′nəm) the embryonic mesentery enclosing the laterally expanding lung 肺系膜

mes·or·chi·um (məz-or′ke-əm) the portion of the primordial mesentery enclosing the fetal testis, represented in the adult by a fold between the testis and epididymis 睾丸系膜；**mesor′chial** *adj.*

meso·rec·tum (mez″o-) (me″zo-rek′təm) the fold of peritoneum connecting the upper portion of the rectum with the sacrum 直肠系膜

meso·sal·pinx (mez″o-) (me″zo-sal′pinks) the portion of the broad ligament above the mesovarium 输卵管系膜

meso·sig·moid (mez″o-) (me″zo-sig′moid) the peritoneal fold attaching the sigmoid flexure to the posterior abdominal wall 乙状结肠系膜

meso·sig·moido·pexy (mez″o-) (me″zo-sigmoi′-do-pek″se) fixation of the mesosigmoid for prolapse of the rectum 乙状结肠系膜固定术

meso·some (mez′o-) (me′zo-sōm″) an invagination of the bacterial cell membrane, forming organelles thought to be the site of cytochrome enzymes and the enzymes of oxidative phosphorylation and the citric acid cycle 间体

meso·ten·din·e·um (mez″o-) (me″zo-təndin′e-əm) the connective tissue sheath attaching a tendon to its fibrous sheath 腱系膜

meso·the·li·o·ma (mez″o-) (me″zo-the″leo′mə) a tumor derived from mesothelial tissue (peritoneum, pleura, pericardium), occurring in both benign and malignant forms 间皮瘤

meso·the·li·um (mez″o-) (me″zo-the′le-əm) the layer of cells, derived from mesoderm, lining the body cavity of the embryo; in the adult, it forms the simple squamous epithelium that covers all true serous membranes (peritoneum, pericardium, pleura) 间皮; **mesothe′lial** *adj.*

meso·tym·pa·num (mez″o-) (me″zo-tim′pə- nəm) the portion of the middle ear medial to the tympanic membrane 中鼓室

meso·va·ri·um (mez″o-) (me″zo-var′e-əm) the portion of the broad ligament between the mesometrium and mesosalpinx, which encloses and holds the ovary in place 卵巢系膜

mes·sen·ger (mes′ən-jər) an information carrier 信使; **second m.,** any of several classes of intracellular signals acting at or situated within the plasma membrane and translating electrical or chemical messages from the environment into cellular responses 第二信使

mes·tra·nol (mes′trə-nol) an estrogen related to ethinyl estradiol; used in combination with a progestational agent as an oral contraceptive 美雌醇，炔雌醇甲醚

mes·y·late (mes′ə-lāt) USAN contraction for methanesulfonate 甲磺酸盐（methanesulfonate 的 USAN 的缩略词）

Met 同 methionine

met(a)- word element [Gr.], *(a) change; transformation; exchange; (b) after; next.* 更改，转换，交换；之后，下一步

meta- 1. symbol m-; in organic chemistry, a prefix indicating a 1,3-substituted benzene ring. 2. in inorganic chemistry, a prefix indicating a polymeric acid anhydride. 在有机化学中，表示 1，3- 取代苯环的前缀，在无机化学中，表示聚合酸酐的前缀

meta-anal·y·sis (met″ə-ə-nal′ə-sis) a systematic method that takes data from a number of independent studies and integrates them using statistical analysis 整合分析

me·tab·a·sis (mə-tab′ə-sis) a change in the manifestations or course of a disease 疾病转变；转移

meta·bi·o·sis (met″ə-bi-o′sis) dependence of one organism upon another for its existence; commensalism 共栖，共生

met·a·bol·ic (met″ə-bol′ik) pertaining to or of the nature of metabolism 代谢的

me·tab·o·lism (mə-tab′ə-liz″əm) 1. the sum of all the physical and chemical processes by which living organized substance is produced and maintained (anabolism) and also the transformation by which energy is made available for the uses of the organism (catabolism) 新陈代谢；2. biotransformation（生理）代谢作用；**metabol′ic** *adj.*; **basal m.,** the minimal energy expended to maintain respiration, circulation, peristalsis, muscle tonus, body temperature, glandular activity, and the other vegetative functions of the body 基础代谢

me·tab·o·lite (mə-tab′ə-līt) any substance produced by metabolism or by a metabolic process 代谢产物

meta·car·pal (met″ə-kahr′pəl) 1. pertaining to the metacarpus 掌骨的；2. a bone of the metacarpus 掌骨

meta·car·pus (met″ə-kahr′pəs) the part of the hand between the wrist and fingers, its skeleton being five bones (metacarpals) extending from the carpus to the phalanges 掌

meta·cen·tric (met″ə-sen′trik) having the centromere near the middle, so that the arms of the chromosome are approximately equal in length 中间着丝点的，具中间着丝粒的

meta·cer·ca·ria (met″ə-sər-kar′e-ə) pl. *metacerca′riae.* The encysted resting or maturing stage of a trematode parasite in the tissues of an intermediate host or on vegetation 后囊蚴

meta·chro·ma·sia (met″ə-kro-ma′zhə) 1. failure to stain true with a given stain 异染性；2. the different coloration of different tissues produced by the same stain 变色反应性；3. change of color produced by staining 变色现象

meta·chro·mat·ic (met″ə-kro-mat′ik) staining differently with the same dye; said of tissues in which a dye gives different colors to different elements 异染性的

meta·chro·mo·phil (met″ə-kro′mo-fil) not staining in the usual manner with a given stain 嗜异染的

meta·cone (met′ə-kōn) the distobuccal cusp of an upper molar tooth 后尖，上后尖（上磨牙的远中颊尖）

meta·con·id (met″ə-kon′id) the mesiolingual cusp of a lower molar tooth 下后尖(下磨牙的近中舌尖）

M

meta·gas·ter (met″ə-gas′tər) the permanent intestinal canal of the embryo 后肠管（胎）

Meta·gon·i·mus (met″ə-gon′ĭ-məs) a genus of flukes, including *M. yokoga'wai,* parasitic in the small intestine of humans and other mammals in Japan, China, Indonesia, the Balkans, and Israel 后殖吸虫属

met·al (met′əl) any element marked by luster, malleability, ductility, and conductivity of electricity and heat and which will ionize positively in solution 金属；**metal′lic** *adj.*；**alkali m.,** any of a group of monovalent metals, including lithium, sodium, potassium, rubidium, and cesium 碱土金属；**heavy m.,** one with a high specific gravity, usually defined as over 5.0 重金属

me·tal·lo·en·zyme (mə-tal″o-en′zīm) any enzyme containing tightly bound metal atoms, e.g., the cytochromes 金属酶

me·tal·lo·por·phy·rin (mə-tal″o-por′fə-rin) a combination of a metal with porphyrin, as in heme 金属卟啉

me·tal·lo·pro·tein (mĕ-tal″o-pro′tēn) a protein molecule with a bound metal ion, e.g., hemoglobin 金属蛋白

met·al·lur·gy (met′əl-ur″je) the science and art of using metals 冶金学，冶金术

meta·mere (met′ə-mēr) one of a series of homologous segments of the body of an animal 体节，节。Cf. *antimere*

meta·mor·pho·sis (met″ə-mor′fə-sis) change of structure or shape, particularly a transition from one developmental stage to another, as from larva to adult form 变态；**metamor′phic** *adj.*；**fatty m.,** fatty change 脂肪变态

meta·my·elo·cyte (met″ə-mi′ə-lo-sīt″) a precursor in the granulocytic series, being a cell intermediate in development between a promyelocyte and the mature, segmented (polymorphonuclear) granular leukocyte, and having a U-shaped nucleus 晚幼粒细胞

meta·neph·ric (met″ə-nef′rik) of or pertaining to the metanephros 后肾的

meta·neph·rine (met″ə-nef′rin) a metabolite of epinephrine excreted in urine and found in certain tissues 间甲肾上腺素，3-O-甲基肾上腺素

meta·neph·ros (met″ə-nef′ros) pl. *metaneph'roi* [Gr.] the primordium of the permanent kidney, developing later than and caudad to the mesonephros 后肾

meta·phase (met′ə-fāz″) the stage of cell division following prometaphase, during which the chromosomes move to the center of the cell and line up to form the equatorial plate 中期（细胞分裂）

meta·phos·phor·ic ac·id (met″ə-fos-for′ik) a polymer of phosphoric acid, used as a reagent for chemical analysis and as a test for albumin in the urine 偏磷酸

meta·phys·e·al (met″ə-fiz′e-əl) pertaining to or of the nature of a metaphysis 干骺端的。Spelled also *metaphysial*

me·taph·y·sis (mə-taf′ə-sis) pl. *metaph'yses* [Gr.] the wider part at the end of a long bone, adjacent to the epiphyseal disk 干骺端

meta·pla·sia (met″ə-pla′zhə) the change in the type of adult cells in a tissue to a form abnormal for that tissue 组织转化，化生；**metaplas′tic** *adj.*；**myeloid m.,** a syndrome characterized by myeloid tissue in extramedullary sites with nucleated erythrocytes and immature granulocytes in the circulating blood and extramedullary hematopoiesis in the liver and spleen, as well as anemia and splenomegaly. Both a primary form *(agnogenic myeloid m.)* and forms secondary to carcinoma, leukemia, leukoerythroblastosis, and tuberculosis are known 髓样化生

meta·pneu·mon·ic (met″ə-noo-mon′ik) succeeding or following pneumonia 肺炎后的

Meta·pneu·mo·vi·rus (met″ə-noo′mo-vi″rəs) a genus of viruses of the family Paramyxoviridae that cause respiratory infections in humans and other animals 偏肺病毒属

meta·pro·ter·e·nol (met″ə-pro-ter′ə-nol) a β_2-adrenergic receptor agonist with significant β_1-adrenergic activity, used in the form of the sulfate salt as a bronchodilator 硫酸异丙喘宁

meta·psy·chol·o·gy (met″ə-si-kol′ə-je) the branch of speculative psychology that deals with the significance of mental processes that are beyond empirical verification 心理玄学，心灵学

meta·ram·i·nol (met″ə-ram′ĭ-nol) a sympathomimetic agent acting mainly as an α-adrenergic agonist but also stimulating the β_1-adrenergic receptors of the heart and having potent vasopressor activity; used as the bitartrate salt in the treatment of certain hypotensive states 间羟胺，间羟基去甲麻黄碱

meta·ru·bri·cyte (met″ə-roo′bri-sīt) orthochromatic erythroblast 晚幼红细胞

me·tas·ta·sec·to·my (mə-tas″tə-sek′tə-me) excision of one or more metastases 转移瘤切除术

me·tas·ta·sis (mə-tas′tə-sis) pl. *metas'tases.* 1. transfer of disease from one organ or part of the body to another not directly connected with it, due either to transfer of pathogenic microorganisms or to transfer of cells; all malignant tumors are capable of metastasizing 转移；2. a growth of pathogenic microorganisms or of abnormal cells distant from the site primarily involved by the morbid process 转移瘤，转移灶；**metastat′ic** *adj.*

meta·tar·sal (met″ə-tahr′səl) 1. pertaining to the metatarsus 跖骨的；2. a bone of the metatarsus 跖骨

meta·tar·sal·gia (met″ə-tahr-sal′jə) pain and tenderness in the metatarsal region 跖骨痛

meta·tar·sus (met″ə-tahr′səs) the part of the foot between the ankle and the toes, its skeleton being the five bones (metatarsals) extending from the tarsus to the phalanges 跖

meta·thal·a·mus (met″ə-thal′ə-məs) the part of the diencephalon composed of the medial and lateral geniculate bodies; often considered to be part of the thalamus 丘脑后部，后丘脑

me·tath·e·sis (mə-tath′ə-sis) 1. artificial transfer of a morbid process 病变移植；2. a chemical reaction in which an element or radical in one compound exchanges places with another element or radical in another compound 复分解（作用），置换（作用），易位（作用）

meta·tro·phic (met″ə-tro′fik) utilizing organic matter for food 腐物寄生的，嗜有机质的

me·tax·a·lone (mə-taks′ə-lōn) a skeletal muscle relaxant used in the treatment of painful musculoskeletal conditions 美他沙酮，间噁酮

Meta·zoa (met″ə-zo′ə) that division of the animal kingdom embracing the multicellular animals whose cells differentiate to form tissues, i.e., all animals except the Protozoa 后生动物门；**metazo′al, metazo′an** *adj.*

meta·zo·on (met″ə-zo′on) pl. *metazo′a.* An individual organism of the Metazoa 后生动物

met·en·ceph·a·lon (met″en-sef′ə-lon) [Gr.] 1. the rostral part of the hindbrain, comprising the cerebellum and pons 后脑（头端部分，包括小脑和脑桥）；2. the anterior of two brain vesicles formed by specialization of the hindbrain in the developing embryo 前脑泡

me·te·orot·ro·pism (me″te-ə-rot′rə-piz″əm) response to influence by meteorologic factors noted in certain biologic events 气候影响反应（指受气候影响而产生的反应）；**meteorotrop′ic** *adj.*

me·ter (me′tər) 1. the base SI unit of linear measure, approximately equivalent to 39.37 inches. Symbol m 米，符号为 m；2. an apparatus to measure the quantity of anything passing through it 计，表，量器

met·for·min (mət-for′min) an antihyperglycemic agent that potentiates the action of insulin, used in the treatment of type 2 diabetes mellitus 甲福明，二甲双胍（口服降血糖药）

meth·ac·ry·late (meth-ak′rə-lāt) an ester of meth-acrylic acid, or the resin derived from polymerization of the ester 甲基丙烯酸树脂，另见 *resin* 下 *acrylic resins*

meth·a·cryl·ic ac·id (meth″ə-kril′ik) an organic acid that polymerizes easily to form a ceramic-like mass. Its esters, methyl and polymethyl methacrylate, are used in the manufacture of acrylic resins and plastics 甲基丙烯酸，异丁烯酸

meth·a·done (meth′ə-dōn) a synthetic opioid analgesic with actions similar to those of morphine and heroin, and almost equal in potential for addiction; the hydrochloride salt is used as an analgesic and in the management of heroin addiction 美沙酮（镇痛药）

meth·am·phet·amine (meth″am-fet′ə-mēn) a central nervous system stimulant and pressor substance with actions similar to amphetamine; used as the hydrochloride salt in the treatment of attention-deficit/hyperactivity disorder. Abuse may lead to dependence 去氧麻黄碱

meth·a·nal (meth′ə-nal) formaldehyde 甲醛

meth·ane (meth′ān) a flammable, explosive gas, CH_4, from decomposition of organic matter 甲烷

meth·a·no·gen (meth′ə-no-jen″) an anaerobic microorganism that grows in the presence of carbon dioxide and produces methane gas. Methanogens are found in the stomach of cows, in swamp mud, and in other environments in which oxygen is not present 产甲烷细菌

meth·a·nol (meth′ə-nol) methyl alcohol 甲醇

meth·a·zo·la·mide (meth″ə-zo′lə-mīd) a carbonic anhydrase inhibitor used as an adjunct to reduce intraocular pressure in the treatment of glaucoma 甲醋唑胺（碳酸酐酶抑制药）

meth·di·la·zine (məth-di′lə-zēn) an antihistamine with anticholinergic and sedative effects, used as the base or the hydrochloride salt as an antipruritic 甲地拉嗪，甲吡咯嗪

met·hem·al·bu·min (met″he-mal-bu′min) a brownish pigment formed in the blood by the binding of albumin with heme; indicative of intravascular hemolysis 正铁白蛋白，假正铁血红蛋白

met·he·mo·glo·bin (met-he′mo-glo″bin) a hematogenous pigment formed from hemoglobin by oxidation of the iron atom from the ferrous to the ferric state. A small amount is found in the blood normally, but injury or toxic agents convert a larger proportion of hemoglobin into methemoglobin, which does not function as an oxygen carrier 高铁血红蛋白

meth·en·amine (meth-en′ə-mēn) an antibacterial used in urinary tract infections; administered as the hippurate and mandelate salts 乌洛托品，环六亚甲基四胺（尿路抗菌药）

meth·i·cil·lin (meth″ĭ-sil′in) a semisynthetic penicillin highly resistant to inactivation by penicillinase; used as the sodium salt 甲氧西林，甲氧苯青霉素

meth·im·a·zole (meth-im′ə-zōl) a thyroid inhibitor used in the treatment of hyperthyroidism 甲巯咪唑（抗甲状腺药）

me·thi·o·nine (Met, M) (mə-thi′o-nēn) a naturally occurring, essential amino acid that furnishes both methyl groups and sulfur necessary for normal metabolism. Labeled with carbon 11, it is used in positron emission tomography for detection of neoplasms 甲硫氨酸，蛋氨酸

meth·o·car·ba·mol (meth″o-kahr′bə-mol) a skeletal muscle relaxant used in the treatment of painful musculoskeletal conditions 美索巴莫，氨甲酸愈甘醚酯

meth·od (meth′əd) the manner of performing any act or operation; a procedure or technique 方法；**dye dilution m.**, a type of indicator dilution method for assessing flow through the circulatory system, using a dye as an indicator 染剂稀释法；**fertility awareness m's,** methods of planning or preventing pregnancy based on prediction or identification of the timing of ovulation in a menstrual cycle 安全期避孕法；**indicator dilution m.**, any of several methods for assessing flow through the circulatory system by injecting a known quantity of an indicator and monitoring its concentration over time at a specific point in the system 指示剂稀释法；**Lamaze m.**, a method of preparing for delivery, involving education of the prospective mother in the physiology of pregnancy and parturition as well as in techniques such as breathing exercises and bearing down for the easing of delivery Lamaze 法；**Westergren m.**, the most common method for testing the erythrocyte sedimentation rate, measuring the timed fall of the level of red cells after mixing whole blood and sodium citrate anticoagulant-diluent solution Westergren 法；**Yuzpe m.**, a regimen for postcoital contraception, consisting of a combination of ethinyl estradiol and norgestrel taken twice, 12 hours apart Yuzpe 法

meth·od·ol·o·gy (meth″ə-dol′ə-je) the science of method; the science dealing with principles of procedure in research and study 方法论

meth·o·hex·i·tal (meth″o-hek′sĭ-təl) an ultrashort-acting barbiturate; its sodium salt is used as a general anesthetic, a general and local anesthesia adjunct, and a sedative for certain diagnostic procedures in children 美索比妥

meth·o·trex·ate (meth″o-trek′sāt) a folic acid antagonist used as the base or the sodium salt as an antineoplastic, antipsoriatic, and antiarthritic 甲氨蝶呤

me·thox·a·mine (mə-thok′sə-mēn) an α 1-adrenergic agonist, used as the hydrochloride salt as a vasopressor 甲氧氨

me·thox·sa·len (mə-thok′sə-lən) a psoralen that induces melanin production on exposure of the skin to ultraviolet light; used in the treatment of idiopathic vitiligo, mycosis fungoides, and psoriasis 甲氧沙林，甲氧补骨脂素

meth·oxy·flu·rane (mə-thok″se-floo′rān) a highly potent inhalational anesthetic agent 甲氧氟烷

meth·sux·i·mide (meth-suk′sĭ-mīd) an anticonvulsant used in the treatment of seizures in absence epilepsy 甲琥胺

meth·y·clo·thi·a·zide (meth″ĭ-klo-thi′ə-zīd) a thiazide diuretic used for treatment of hypertension and edema 甲氯噻嗪

meth·yl (meth′əl) the chemical group or radical CH₃– 甲基；**m. methacrylate,** a methyl ester of methacrylic acid, which polymerizes to form polymethyl methacrylate; used in the manufacture of acrylic resins and plastics 甲基丙烯酸甲酯；**m. salicylate,** a volatile oil with a characteristic wintergreen odor and taste; used as a flavoring agent and as a topical counterirritant for muscle pain 冬青油

meth·yl·amine (meth′əl-ə-mēn″) a flammable, explosive gas used in tanning and organic synthesis and produced naturally in some decaying fish, certain plants, and crude methanol; it is irritating to the eyes 甲胺

meth·yl·ate (meth′əl-āt) 1. a compound of methyl alcohol and a base 甲醇盐；2. to add a methyl group to a substance 甲基化，加甲基

meth·yl·a·tion (meth″əl-a′shən) addition of one or more methyl groups to a substance 甲基化（作用）；**DNA m.**, the postsynthetic addition of methyl groups to specific sites on DNA molecules; it is involved in gene expression and plays a role in a variety of epigenetic mechanisms DNA 甲基化

meth·yl·ben·ze·tho·ni·um (meth″əl-ben″zə-tho′ne-əm) a disinfectant quaternary compound; applied topically to skin coming in contact with urine, feces, or perspiration, and used in a rinse for diapers and linens of incontinent patients 甲基苄甲乙氧胺（消毒药）

meth·yl·cel·lu·lose (meth″əl-sel′u-lōs) a methyl ester of cellulose; used as a bulk laxative and as a suspending agent for drugs and applied topically to the conjunctiva to protect and lubricate the cornea during certain ophthalmic procedures 甲基纤维素

meth·yl·co·bal·a·min (meth″əl-ko-bal′ə-min) a metabolically active cobalamin derivative synthesized upon ingestion of vitamin B$_{12}$ 甲钴胺

meth·yl·do·pa (meth″əl-do′pə) a phenylalanine derivative used in the treatment of hypertension 甲基多巴（抗高血压药）

meth·yl·do·pate (meth″əl-do′pāt) the ethyl ester of methyldopa; its hydrochloride salt is used as an antihypertensive 甲基多巴乙酯

meth·y·lene (meth′ə-lēn) the bivalent hydrocarbon radical −CH$_2$− or CH$_2$= 甲叉，亚甲（基），甲撑

meth·y·lene·di·oxy·am·phet·amine (MDA) (meth″ə-lēn-di-ok″se-am-fet′ə-mēn) a hallucinogenic compound chemically related to amphetamine and mescaline; it is widely abused and causes dependence 甲撑二氧苯丙胺

3,4-meth·y·lene·di·oxy·meth·am·phet·amine (MDMA) (meth″ə-lēn″di-ok″se-meth″amfet′ə-mēn) a compound chemically related to amphetamine and having hallucinogenic properties; it is widely abused. Popularly called *Ecstasy* 3,4-亚甲基二氧甲基苯丙胺（俗称摇头丸）

meth·yl·er·go·no·vine (meth″əl-ur″go-no′vēn) an oxytocic, used as the maleate salt to prevent or combat postpartum or postabortion hemorrhage and atony 甲基麦角新碱

meth·yl·glu·ca·mine (meth″əl-gloo′kə-mēn) 同 meglumine

meth·yl·ma·lon·ic ac·id (meth″əl-mə-lon′ik) a carboxylic acid intermediate in fatty acid metabolism 甲基丙二酸

meth·yl·ma·lon·ic·ac·i·de·mia (meth″əlmə-lon″ik-as″ĭ-de′me-ə) 1. an aminoacidopathy characterized by an excess of methylmalonic acid in the blood and urine, with metabolic ketoacidosis, hyperglycinemia, hyperglycinuria, and hyperammonemia, resulting from any of several enzymatic defects 甲基丙二酸血症，由几种酶缺陷引起，伴有代谢性酮症酸中毒、高甘氨酸血症、高甘氨酸尿症和高氨血症等；2. excess of methylmalonic acid in the blood 血中甲基丙二酸过多

meth·yl·ma·lon·ic·ac·id·uria (meth″əl-mə-lon″ik-as″ĭ-du′re-ə) 1. excess of methylmalonic acid in the urine 甲基丙二酸尿；2. 同 methylmalonicacidemia (1)

meth·yl·meth·ac·ry·late (meth″əl-methak′rə-lāt) 见 *methyl* 下词条

meth·yl·phen·i·date (meth″əl-fen′ĭ-dāt) a central stimulant, used in the form of the hydrochloride salt in the treatment of attentiondeficit/hyperactivity disorder in children and narcolepsy 哌甲酯（中枢兴奋药）

meth·yl·pred·nis·o·lone (meth″əl-pred-nis′ə-lōn) a synthetic glucocorticoid derived from progester-

one, used in replacement therapy for adrenocortical insufficiency and as an antiinflammatory and immunosuppressant; also used as *m. acetate* and *m. sodium succinate* 甲泼尼龙

meth·yl·tes·tos·te·rone (meth″əl-tes-tos′tə- rōn) a synthetic androgenic hormone with actions and uses similar to those of testosterone 甲睾酮，甲基睾丸素

meth·yl·tet·ra·hy·dro·fo·late (meth″əltet″rə-hi″dro-fo′lāt) a derivative of folic acid that is the principal form of folic acid during transport and storage in the body and that also acts as a source of methyl groups for the regeneration of methionine 甲基四氢叶酸

meth·yl·trans·fer·ase (meth″əl-trans′fər- ās) any of a group of enzymes that catalyze the transfer of a methyl group from one compound to another 甲基转移酶

meth·y·ser·gide (meth″ĭ-sur′jīd) a potent serotonin antagonist with direct vasoconstrictor effects, used as the maleate salt in prophylaxis of migraine and cluster headaches 美西麦角，二甲麦角新碱

met·i·pran·o·lol (met″ĭ-pran′ə-lol) a betaadrenergic blocking agent, used as the hydrochloride salt in the treatment of glaucoma and ocular hypertension 一种β受体阻滞药，其盐酸盐用于治疗青光眼和高眼压

met·myo·glo·bin (mət-mi″o-glo′bin) a compound formed from myoglobin by oxidation of the ferrous to the ferric state 正铁肌红蛋白

met·o·clo·pra·mide (met″o-klo′prə-mīd) a dopamine receptor antagonist and prokinetic that stimulates gastric motility, used as the hydrochloride salt as an antiemetic, as an adjunct in gastrointestinal radiology and intestinal intubation, and in the treatment of gastroparesis and gastroesophageal reflux 胃复安，甲氧氯普胺

me·to·la·zone (mə-to′lə-zōn) a sulfonamide derivative with actions similar to the thiazide diuretics; used in the treatment of hypertension and edema 美托拉宗，甲苯喹唑酮

me·top·ic (me-top′ik) frontal (1) 额的

met·o·pro·lol (met″o-pro′lol) a cardioselective β$_1$-adrenergic blocking agent used in the form of the succinate and tartrate salts in the treatment of hypertension, chronic angina pectoris, and myocardial infarction 美托洛尔，甲氧乙心安，美多心安

me·tra (me′trə) the uterus 子宫

me·trec·to·pia (me″trek-to′pe-ə) uterine displacement 子宫异位，子宫移位

me·treu·ryn·ter (me″troo-rin′tər) an inflatable bag for dilating the cervical canal 子宫颈扩张袋

met·ric (met′rik) 1. pertaining to measures or

measurement（以米）测量的；2. having the meter as a basis 米（制）的

me·tri·tis (mə-tri′tis) inflammation of the uterus 子宫炎

me·triz·a·mide (mə-triz′ə-mīd) a nonionic, water-soluble, iodinated radiographic contrast medium used in myelography and cisternography 甲泛葡胺

met·ro·ni·da·zole (met″ro-ni′də-zōl) an antiprotozoal and antibacterial effective against obligate anaerobes; used as the base or the benzoate or hydrochloride salt. It is also used as a topical treatment for rosacea 甲硝唑

me·trop·a·thy (mə-trop′ə-the) hysteropathy 子宫病

me·tro·peri·to·ni·tis (me″tro-per″ĭ-to-ni′tis) inflammation of the peritoneum about the uterus 子宫腹膜炎

me·tro·phle·bi·tis (me″tro-flə-bi′tis) inflammation of the uterine veins 子宫静脉炎

me·tro·plas·ty (me′tro-plas″te) plastic surgery on the uterus 子宫成形术，子宫重建术

me·tror·rha·gia (me″tro-ra′jə) uterine bleeding occurring at irregular intervals and sometimes of prolonged duration 子宫出血

me·tror·rhea (me″tro-re′ə) a free or abnormal uterine discharge 子宫溢液

me·tror·rhex·is (me″tro-rek′sis) rupture of the uterus 子宫破裂

me·tro·stax·is (me″tro-stak′sis) slight but per-sistent uterine bleeding 子宫渗血

me·tro·ste·no·sis (me″tro-stə-no′sis) contraction or stenosis of the uterine cavity 子宫狭窄

me·tyr·a·pone (mə-tēr′ə-pōn) a synthetic compound that selectively inhibits an enzyme responsible for the biosynthesis of corticosteroids; it is used as a diagnostic aid for determination of hypothalamicopituitary-adrenocortical reserve 双甲吡丙酮，甲吡酮，美替拉酮

me·ty·ro·sine (mə-ti′ro-sēn) an inhibitor of the first step in catecholamine synthesis, used to control hypertensive attacks in pheochromocytoma 甲基酪氨酸（抗高血压药）

MeV megaelectron volt; one million (10^6) electron volts 兆电子伏（特）

mex·il·e·tine (mek′sĭ-lə-tēn) an antiarrhythmic agent used as the hydrochloride salt in the treatment of ventricular arrhythmias 美西律

mez·lo·cil·lin (mez″lo-sil′in) a semisynthetic broad-spectrum penicillin used as the sodium salt, particularly in the treatment of mixed infections 美洛西林（抗生素类药）

μF microfarad 微法（拉）的符号

Mg magnesium 元素镁的符号

mg milligram 毫克的符号

μg microgram (on The Joint Commission "Do Not Use" List) 微克的符号

MHC major histocompatibility complex 主要组织相容性复合体

MHz megahertz; one million (10^6) hertz 兆赫（兹）

MI myocardial infarction 心肌梗死

mi·ca·tion (mi-ka′shən) a quick motion, such as winking 急促动作

mi·con·a·zole (mi-kon′ə-zōl) an imidazole antifungal agent used as the base or the nitrate salt against tinea and cutaneous or vulvovaginal candidiasis 咪康唑

mi·cren·ceph·a·ly (mi″krən-sef′ə-le) abnormal smallness of the brain 脑过小；**micrenceph′alous** *adj.*

micr(o)- word element [Gr.] *small*; also used in naming units of measurement (symbol μ) to designate an amount one millionth (10^{-6}) the size of the unit to which it is joined, e.g., microgram [构词成分]小、细、微；百万分之一（10^{-6}）

mi·cro·ab·scess (mi″kro-ab′ses) a small, localized collection of pus 微脓疡；**Pautrier m.**, one of the intraepidermal nests of atypical mononuclear cells characteristic of T-cell lymphoma and mycosis fungoides 波特里耶小脓肿

mi·cro·ad·e·no·ma (mi″kro-ad″ə-no′mə) a pituitary adenoma less than 10 mm in diameter 微腺瘤

mi·cro·aero·phil·ic (mi″kro-ār′o-fil′ik) requiring oxygen for growth but at lower concentration than is present in the atmosphere; said of bacteria 微需氧的

mi·cro·ag·gre·gate (mi″kro-ag′rə-gət) a microscopic collection of particles, as of platelets, leukocytes, and fibrin, that occurs in stored blood 微聚集

mi·cro·al·bu·min·uria (mi″kro-al-bu″minu′re-ə) a very small increase in urinary albumin 微（白）蛋白尿

mi·cro·anal·y·sis (mi″kro-ə-nal′ə-sis) the chemical analysis of minute quantities of material 微量分析

mi·cro·anat·o·my (mi″kro-ə-nat′ə-me) histology 显微解剖学，组织学

mi·cro·an·eu·rysm (mi″kro-an′u-riz″əm) a microscopic aneurysm, a characteristic of thrombotic purpura 微动脉瘤

mi·cro·an·gi·op·a·thy (mi″kro-an″je-op′ə- the) angiopathy involving the small blood vessels 微血管病；**microangiopath′ic** *adj.*；**thrombotic m.**, thrombi in arterioles and capillaries, as in thrombotic thrombocytopenic purpura and hemolytic uremic syndrome 血栓性微血管病

Mi·cro·bac·te·ri·a·ceae (mi″kro-bak-tēr″ea′se-e)

a family of bacteria of the suborder Micrococcineae 微杆菌科

Mi·cro·bac·te·ri·um (mi″kro-bak-tēr′e-əm) a genus of small, gram-positive, aerobic, rodshaped bacteria of the family Microbacteriaceae, characterized by resistance to heat. It is an opportunistic pathogen, causing nosocomial infections 微杆菌属，小细菌属

mi·crobe (mi′krōb) a microorganism; sometimes restricted to ones that are disease-causing 微生物；**micro′bial, micro′bic** *adj.*

mi·cro·bi·cide (mi-kro′bĭ-sīd″) 1. a substance that destroys microbes; 2. a substance that destroys infectious agents, including also viruses; sometimes used specifically for that used to prevent transmission of sexually transmitted diseases 杀微生物剂；**microbici′dal** *adj.*

mi·cro·bi·ol·o·gy (mi″kro-bi-ol′ə-je) the science dealing with the study of microorganisms 微生物学；**microbiolog′ical** *adj.*

mi·cro·bio·pho·tom·e·ter (mi″kro-bi″o-fotom′ə-tər) an instrument for measuring the growth of bacterial cultures by the turbidity of the medium 微生物浊度计

mi·cro·bi·o·ta (mi″kro-bi-o′tə) the microscopic living organisms of a region 微生物区系；**microbiot′ic** *adj.*

mi·cro·blast (mi′kro-blast″) an erythroblast of 5 microns or less in diameter 小幼红血细胞

mi·cro·ble·pha·ria (mi″kro-blə-far′e-ə) abnormal shortness of the vertical dimensions of the eyelids 小（眼）睑

mi·cro·body (mi′kro-bod″e) any of a group of-related membrane-bound, ovoid or spherical, granular cytoplasmic organelles, containing numerous oxidative enzymes and other substances and occurring in virtually all eukaryotic cells 微体

mi·cro·bu·ret (mi″kro-bu-ret′) a buret with a capacity of the order of 0.1 to 10 mL, with graduated intervals of 0.001 to 0.02 mL 微量滴定管

mi·cro·ca·lix (mi″kro-ka′liks) a very small renal calix arising by caliceal branching, usually at the side of a calix of normal size 微肾盏

mi·cro·car·dia (mi″kro-kahr′de-ə) abnormal smallness of the heart 心过小，小心畸形

mi·cro·ceph·a·ly (mi″kro-sef′ə-le) abnormal smallness of the head 小头（畸形）；**microcephal′ic, microceph′alous** *adj.*

mi·cro·chei·lia (mi″kro-ki′le-ə) abnormal smallness of the lip 小唇（畸形）

mi·cro·chei·ria (mi″kro-ki′re-ə) abnormal smallness of the hands 小手畸形

mi·cro·chem·is·try (mi″kro-kem′is-tre) chemis-try concerned with exceedingly small quantities of chemical substances 微量化学

mi·cro·cin·e·ma·tog·ra·phy (mi″kro-sin″ə- mə- tog′rə-fe) moving picture photography of microscopic objects 显微电影术

mi·cro·cir·cu·la·tion (mi″kro-sur″ku-la′shən) the flow of blood through the fine vessels (arterioles, capillaries, and venules) 微循环；**microcirculato′ry** *adj.*

Mi·cro·coc·ca·ceae (mi″kro-kə-ka′se-e) a family of gram-positive, aerobic or facultatively anaerobic, spherical bacteria of the suborder Micrococcineae 微球菌科

Mi·cro·coc·ci·neae (mi″kro-kok-sin′e-e) a suborder of bacteria of the order Actinomycetales comprising a highly diverse group of organisms 微球菌亚目

Mi·cro·coc·cus (mi″kro-kok′əs) a genus of gram-positive, aerobic bacteria of the family Micrococcaceae found in soil, water, etc.; it occasionally causes infective endocarditis 微球菌属，微球菌科的革兰氏阳性需氧菌的一个属，存在于土壤、水等中，偶尔引起感染性心内膜炎

mi·cro·coc·cus (mi″kro-kok′əs) pl. *micrococ′ci*. 1. an organism of the genus *Micrococcus* 微球菌；2. a very small spherical microorganism 小球菌

mi·cro·co·lon (mi″kro-ko′lən) an abnormally small colon 小结肠

mi·cro·co·ria (mi″kro-ko′re-ə) smallness of the pupil 小瞳孔

mi·cro·crys·tal·line (mi″kro-kris′tə-lin) made up of minute crystals 微晶的，细晶质的

mi·cro·cyte (mi′kro-sīt) 1. an abnormally small erythrocyte, 5 microns or less in diameter 小红细胞；2. microglial cell 小胶质细胞

mi·cro·cyt·ic (mi″kro-sit′ik) pertaining to or characterized by microcytes 小红细胞的

mi·cro·cy·to·tox·ic·i·ty (mi″kro-si″to-toksis′ĭ-te) the capability of lysing or damaging cells as detected in procedures (e.g., lymphocytotoxicity procedures) using extremely minute amounts of material 微量细胞毒（性）

mi·cro·derm·abra·sion (mi″kro-dur″mə-bra′zhən) superficial dermabrasion done mainly to treat acne scars or other mild lesions or to stimulate and remodel skin collagen 微晶磨皮术

mi·cro·de·ter·mi·na·tion (mi″kro-de-tur″mī-na′shən) chemical examination of minute quantities of a substance 微量测定（法）

mi·cro·dis·kec·to·my (mi″kro-dis-kek′tə- me) debulking of a herniated nucleus pulposus using an operating microscope or loupe for magnification 显微椎间盘切除术

mi·cro·dis·sec·tion (mi″kro-dĭ-sek′shən) dissection

of tissue or cells under the microscope 显微解剖

mi·cro·drep·a·no·cyt·ic (mi″kro-drep″ə-nosit′ik) containing microcytic and drepanocytic elements 小镰状细胞的

mi·cro·en·vi·ron·ment (mi″kro-ən-vi′ronmənt) the environment at the microscopic or cellular level 微环境

mi·cro·eryth·ro·cyte (mi″kro-ə-rith′ro-sīt) microcyte 小红细胞

mi·cro·far·ad (μF) (mi″kro-far′əd) one millionth (10^{-6}) of a farad 微法（拉）（电容单位，等于 10^{-6}F，符号为 μF）

mi·cro·fau·na (mi″kro-faw′nə) the microscopic animal life present in or characteristic of a given location 微动物区系

mi·cro·fil·a·ment (mi″kro-fil′ə-mənt) 1. any of the submicroscopic filaments composed chiefly of actin, found in the cytoplasmic matrix of almost all cells, often with the microtubules 微丝; 2. a cytoplasmic structure, 5 to 7 nm in diameter, composed of two chains of G-actin coiled around each other to form an F-actin filament and acting as components of the cytoskeleton 微丝纤维

mi·cro·fi·la·ria (mi″kro-fī-lar′e-ə) pl. *microfila′riae.* The prelarval stage of Filarioidea in the blood of humans and in the tissues of the vector; sometimes incorrectly used as a genus name 微丝蚴

mi·cro·flo·ra (mi″kro-flor′ə) the population of microorganisms present in or characteristic of a given location 微植物区系

mi·cro·fol·lic·u·lar (mı″kro-fə-lik′u-lər) pertaining to or characterized by small follicles 微滤泡

mi·cro·frac·ture (mi″kro-frak′chər) a minute, incomplete break or small area of discontinuity in a bone 小骨折

mi·cro·gam·ete (mi″kro-gam′ēt) 1. the smaller, often flagellated, actively motile male anisogamete 小配子; 2. the smaller of two types of malarial parasites 雄配子，参见 *gamete* (2)

mi·cro·ga·me·to·cyte (mi″kro-gə-me′to-sīt) 1. a cell that produces microgametes 小配子母细胞; 2. the male gametocyte of certain Sporozoa, such as malarial plasmodia 雄配子体

mi·crog·lia (mi-krog′le-ə) small nonneural cells forming part of the supporting structure of the central nervous system. They are migratory and act as phagocytes to waste products of nerve tissue 小胶质细胞; **microg′lial** *adj.*

mi·cro·glio·cyte (mi-krog′le-o-sīt) microglial cell 小（神经）胶质细胞

mi·cro·glob·u·lin (mi″kro-glob′u-lin) any globulin, or any fragment of a globulin, of low molecular weight 微球蛋白; β₂-m., beta₂-m., a small (mol.

wt. 12,000), nonpolymorphic protein, homologous to the C3 domain of IgG, that is one subunit of class I major histocompatibility antigens β_2-微球蛋白

mi·cro·gna·thia (mi″kro-na′the-ə) unusual smallness of the jaws, especially the lower jaw 小颌，小颌畸形，小颌症; **micrognath′ic** *adj.*

mi·cro·go·nio·scope (mi″kro-go′ne-o-skōp) a gonioscope with a magnifying lens 前房角镜

mi·cro·gram (μg) (mi′kro-gram″) one millionth (10^{-6}) of a gram 微克

mi·cro·graph (mi′kro-graf″) 1. an instrument used to record very minute movements by making a greatly magnified photograph of the minute motions of a diaphragm 微动描记器; 2. a photograph of a minute object or specimen as seen through a microscope 显微照片

mi·cro·graph·ia (mi″kro-graf′e-ə) tiny handwriting, or handwriting that decreases in size from normal to minute, seen in parkinsonism 过小字体症

mi·cro·gy·ria (mi″kro-ji′re-ə) polymicrogyria 多小脑回畸形

mi·cro·gy·rus (mi″kro-ji′rəs) pl. *microgy′ri.* An abnormally small, malformed convolution of the brain 小脑回

mi·cro·in·farct (mi″kro-in′fahrkt) a very small infarct due to obstruction of circulation in capillaries, arterioles, or small arteries 微梗死

mi·cro·in·jec·tor (mi″kro-in-jek′tər) an instrument for infusion of very small amounts of fluids or drugs 微量注射器

mi·cro·in·va·sion (mi″kro-in-va′zhən) microscopic extension of malignant cells into adjacent tissue in carcinoma in situ 微观侵入; **microinva′sive** *adj.*

mi·cro·ker·a·tome (mi″kro-ker′ə-tōm) an instrument for removing a thin slice, or creating a thin hinged flap, on the surface of the cornea 显微角膜计

mi·cro·lec·i·thal (mi″kro-les′ĭ-thəl) containing little yolk, as do the eggs of mammals 卵黄过小的

mi·cro·li·ter (μL) (mi′kro-le″tər) one millionth (10^{-6}) of a liter 微升

mi·cro·li·thi·a·sis (mi″kro-lĭ-thi′ə-sis) the formation of minute concretions in an organ 小结石病，微石症; **m. alveola′ris pulmo′num, pulmonary alveolar m.,** deposition of minute, sandlike calculi in the pulmonary alveoli 肺泡小结石

mi·cro·ma·nip·u·la·tion (mi″kro-mə-nip″u-la′shən) surgery, injection, or other procedures done with a micromanipulator 显微操作

mi·cro·ma·nip·u·la·tor (mi″kro-mə-nip′ula″tər) an instrument for the moving, dissecting, etc., of minute specimens under the microscope 显微操作器

mi·cro·mere (mi′kro-mēr) one of the small blastomeres formed by unequal cleavage of a fertilized oocyte as the result of asymmetric positioning of the mitotic spindle 小分裂球

mi·cro·me·tas·ta·sis (mi″kro-mə-tas′tə-sis) the spread of cancer cells from the primary tumor to distant sites to form microscopic secondary tumors 微转移; **micrometastat′ic** *adj.*

mi·crom·e·ter[1] (mi-krom′ə-tər) an instrument for measuring objects seen through the microscope 测微计

mi·cro·me·ter[2] (μm) (mi′kro-me″tər) one millionth (10^{-6}) of a meter 微米

mi·cro·meth·od (mi″kro-meth′əd) any technique dealing with exceedingly small quantities of material 微量法，微量测定（法）

Mi·cro·mo·no·spo·ra (mi″kro-mon″o-spor′ə) a genus of gram-positive, spore-forming, generally aerobic soil and water bacteria of the family Micromonosporaceae. Various species, including *M. echinospo′ra* and *M. inyoen′sis,* are sources of aminoglycoside antibiotics 小单孢菌属

Mi·cro·mo·nos·po·ra·ceae (mi″kro-mon″o″spə-ra′se-e) a family of gram-positive, aerobic soil bacteria of the suborder Micromonosporineae. Some members produce antibiotics 小单孢菌科

Mi·cro·mo·no·spo·ri·neae (mi″kro-mon″ospə-rin′e-e) a phenotypically diverse suborder of gram-positive bacteria of the order Actinomycetales 小单孢亚目

mi·cro·my·elia (mi″kro-mi-e′le-ə) abnormal smallness of the spinal cord 小脊髓

mi·cro·my·elo·blast (mi″kro-mi′ə-lo-blast) a small, immature myelocyte 小原粒细胞; **micromyeloblas′tic** *adj.*

mi·cro·nee·dle (mi′kro-ne″dəl) a fine glass needle used in micromanipulation 显微操作针

mi·cro·neu·ro·sur·gery (mi″kro-noor″osur′jər-e) surgery conducted under high magnification with miniaturized instruments on microscopic vessels and structures of the nervous system 显微神经手术，显微神经外科（学）

mi·cro·nu·cle·us (mi″kro-noo′kle-əs) 1. in ciliate protozoa, the smaller of two types of nuclei in each cell, which functions in sexual reproduction 在纤毛虫细胞内两种细胞核中较小的一种，在有性生殖中起作用; cf. *macronucleus*; 2. a small nucleus 小核，微核; 3. nucleolus 核仁

mi·cro·or·gan·ism (mi″kro-or′gən-iz-əm) a microscopic organism; those of medical interest include bacteria, fungi, and protozoa. Viruses are often included but are sometimes excluded because they are not cellular and are unable to replicate without a host cell 微生物

mi·cro·pa·thol·o·gy (mi″kro-pə-thol′ə-je) 1. the sum of what is known about minute pathologic change 微生物病理学; 2. pathology of diseases caused by microorganisms 显微病理学

mi·cro·pe·nis (mi″kro-pe′nis) abnormal smallness of the penis 小阴茎

mi·cro·per·fu·sion (mi″kro-pər-fu′zhən) perfusion of a minute amount of a substance 微量灌注

mi·cro·phage (mi′kro-fāj″) a small phagocyte; an actively motile neutrophil capable of phagocytosis 小噬细胞

mi·cro·pha·kia (mi″kro-fa′ke-ə) abnormal smallness of the crystalline lens 小晶状体

mi·cro·phone (mi′kro-fōn) a device to pick up sound for amplification or transmission 扩音器

mi·cro·phon·ic (mi″kro-fon′ik) 1. serving to amplify sound 扩音的; 2. 同 cochlear m.; **cochlear m.,** the electrical potential generated in the hair cells of the organ of Corti in response to acoustic stimulation 耳蜗微音电位

mi·cro·pho·to·graph (mi″kro-fo′tə-graf) a photograph of small size 显微照片

mi·croph·thal·mos (mi″krof-thal′mos) moderate to severe reduction in size of one or both eyes 眼过小，小眼

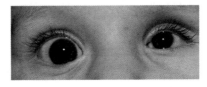

▲ 左眼小眼和左眼小角膜

mi·cro·pino·cy·to·sis (mi″kro-pin″o-si-to′sis) the taking up into a cell of specific macromolecules by invagination of the plasma membrane, which is then pinched off, resulting in small vesicles in the cytoplasm 微胞饮

mi·cro·pi·pet (mi′kro-pi-pet″) a pipet for handling small quantities of liquids (up to 1 mL) 微量吸移管

mi·cro·pleth·ys·mog·ra·phy (mi″kro-pleth″is-mog′rə-fe) the recording of minute changes in the size of a part as produced by circulation of blood 微差体积描记法

mi·cro·probe (mi′kro-prōb″) a minute probe, such as one used in microsurgery 微探子

mi·crop·sia (mi-krop′se-ə) a visual disorder in which objects appear smaller than their actual size 视物显小症

mi·cro·punc·ture (mi′kro-punk″chər) 1. the creation of minute openings by piercing 显微穿刺; 2. in renal physiology, the process by which nephron segments are pierced 肾单位穿刺

mi·cro·ra·di·og·ra·phy (mi″kro-ra″de-og′rə- fe) radiography under conditions that permit subsequent microscopic examination or enlargement of the radiograph up to several hundred linear magnifications 显微放射相术

mi·cro·re·frac·tom·e·ter (mi″kro-re″frak-tom′ə-tər) a refractometer for the discernment of variations in minute structures 显微折射计

mi·cro·res·pi·rom·e·ter (mi″kro-res″pī-rom′ə-tər) an apparatus to investigate oxygen usage in isolated tissues 微量呼吸计

micro·RNA (**miRNA**) (mi″kro-ahr′en-a) any of a number of very small RNA molecules that act as negative regulators of gene expression by binding to specific segments of messenger RNA, thus interfering with translation 微 RNA，小分子核糖核酸，一种非常小的 RNA 分子，通过结合信使 RNA 的特定片段，起到负调节基因表达的作用，从而干扰翻译

mi·cro·sat·el·lite (mi″kro-sat′ə-līt) a stretch of DNA consisting of tandem repeating units of two, three, or four nucleotides, occurring throughout the genome, and highly polymorphic, with codominant mendelian inheritance 微卫星

mi·cro·scope (mi′kro-skōp″) an instrument used to obtain an enlarged image of small objects and reveal details of structure not otherwise distinguishable 显微镜; **acoustic m.,** one using veryhigh-frequency ultrasound waves, which are focused on the object; the reflected beam is converted to an image by electronic processing 声学显微镜; **binocular m.,** one with two eyepieces, permitting use of both eyes 双目显微镜; **compound m.,** one consisting of two lens systems 复合式显微镜; **corneal m.,** one with a lens of high magnifying power, for observing minute changes in the cornea and iris 角膜显微镜; **darkfield m.,** a microscope made with illumination from the side of the field, so that details appear light against a dark background 暗视野显微镜; **electron m.,** one in which an electron beam, instead of light, forms an image for viewing on a fluorescent screen, or for photography 电子显微镜; **fluorescence m.,** a microscope used for the examination of specimens stained with fluorochromes or fluorochrome complexes, e.g., a fluorescein-labeled antibody, which fluoresces in ultraviolet light 荧光显微镜; **infrared m.,** one in which radiation of an 800-nm or longer wavelength is used as the image-forming energy 红外线显微镜; **light m.,** a microscope in

which the specimen is viewed under visible light 光学显微镜; **phase m., phase-contrast m.,** one altering the phase relationships of the light passing through and that passing around the object, the contrast permitting visualization without the necessity of staining or other special preparation 相差显微镜; **scanning m., scanning electron m.,** an electron microscope in which a beam of electrons scans over a specimen point by point and builds up an image on the fluorescent screen of a cathode ray tube 扫描显微镜; **simple m.,** one consisting of a single lens 单式显微镜; **slit lamp m.,** a corneal microscope with a special attachment that permits examination of the endothelium on the posterior surface of the cornea 裂隙灯显微镜; **stereoscopic m.,** a binocular microscope modified to give a three-dimensional view of the specimen 实体显微镜，体视显微镜; **ultraviolet m.,** one that utilizes reflecting optics or quartz and other ultraviolet-transmitting lenses 紫外线显微镜; **x-ray m.,** one in which x-rays are used instead of light, the image usually being reproduced on film X 光显微镜

mi·cro·scop·ic (mi″kro-skop′ik) 1. of extremely small size; visible only by the aid of the microscope 微观的; 2. pertaining or relating to a microscope or to microscopy 显微镜的

mi·cros·co·py (mi-kros′kə-pe) examination under or observation by means of the microscope 显微镜检查

mi·cro·shock (mi′kro-shok) in cardiology, a low level of electric current applied directly to myocardial tissue; as little as 0.1 mA causes ventricular fibrillation 微电击，微震荡

mi·cros·mat·ic (mi″kros-mat′ik) having a feebly developed sense of smell, as do humans 嗅觉不灵敏的

mi·cro·some (mi′kro-sōm″) any of the vesicular fragments of endoplasmic reticulum formed after disruption and centrifugation of cells 微粒体; **micro·so′mal** adj.

mi·cro·spec·tro·scope (mi″kro-spek′trə-skōp) a spectroscope and microscope combined 显微分光镜

mi·cro·sphe·ro·cyte (mi″kro-sfe′ro-sīt) spherocyte 小球形红细胞

mi·cro·sphero·cy·to·sis (mi″kro-sfe″ro-sito′sis) spherocytosis 小球形红细胞症

mi·cro·sphyg·mia (mi″kro-sfig′me-ə) a pulse that is difficult to perceive by the finger 微脉，细脉

mi·cro·sple·nia (mi″kro-sple′ne-ə) abnormal smallness of the spleen 小脾

Mi·cros·po·ron (mi-kros′pə-ron) 同 *Microsporum*

Mi·cros·po·rum (mi-kros′pə-rəm) a genus of

filamentous, dermatophytic, anamorphic fungi. It includes anthropophilic (*M. audoui'nii, M. ferrugi'neum*), zoophilic (*M. ca'nis, M. galli'nae, M. na'num, M. persi'color*), and geophilic (*M. coo'kei, M. ful'vum, M. gyp'seum*) species, which colonize keratinized tissues and may cause diseases of the skin, hair, and rarely nails. Teleomorphs are classified in the genus *Arthroderma* 小孢子癣菌属

mi·cro·sto·mia (mi″kro-sto'me-ə) unusually small size of the mouth 小口（畸形）

mi·cro·sur·gery (mi'kro-sur″jər-e) dissection of minute structures under the microscope by means of handheld instruments 显微手术，显微外科；**microsur′gical** *adj.*

mi·cro·syr·inge (mi″kro-sə-rinj') a syringe fitted with a screw-thread micrometer for accurate measurement of minute quantities 微量调节注射器

mi·cro·tia (mi-kro'shə) gross hypoplasia or aplasia of the auricle of the ear, with a blind or absent external acoustic meatus 小耳（畸形）

mi·cro·tome (mi'kro-tōm) an instrument for cutting thin sections for microscopic study 切片机

mi·cro·tu·bule (mi″kro-too'būl) a slender, tubular cytoplasmic structure composed of tubulin dimers; microtubules are involved in the maintenance of cell shape and in the movements of organelles and inclusions and form the spindle fibers of mitosis 微管

mi·cro·vas·cu·la·ture (mi″kro-vas″ku-lə-chər) the finer vessels of the body, such as the arterioles, capillaries, and venules 微脉管系统；**microvas′cular** *adj.*

mi·cro·ves·sel (mi'kro-ves″əl) any of the finer vessels of the body 微脉管

mi·cro·vil·lus (mi″kro-vil'əs) a minute process from the free surface of a cell, especially cells of the proximal convolution in renal tubules and of the intestinal epithelium 微绒毛

mi·cro·wave (mi'kro-wāv) a wave of electromagnetic radiation between far infrared and radio waves, regarded as extending from 300,000 to 100 megahertz (wavelength of 1 mm to 30 cm) 微波

mi·cro·zo·on (mi″kro-zo'on) pl. *microzo'a*. A microscopic animal organism 微（生）动物

Mi·cru·roi·des (mi″kroo-roi'dēz) a genus of venomous snakes of the family Elapidae. *M. euryxan'thus* is the Arizona or Sonoran coral snake of Mexico and the southwestern United States 类珊瑚毒蛇属

Mi·cru·rus (mi-kroo'rəs) a genus of venomous snakes of the family Elapidae. *M. ful'vius*, the Eastern or Texas coral snake, is found in the southern United States and tropical America; its body is marked with bright red, yellow, and black bands 珊瑚毒蛇属

mic·tu·rate (mik'tu-rāt) urinate 排尿

mic·tu·ri·tion (mik″tu-rĭ'shən) urination 排尿

mid·azo·lam (mid'a-zo-lam″) a benzodiazepine tranquilizer, used as the maleate ester for sedation and in the induction of anesthesia 咪达唑仑，咪唑安定

mid·brain (mid'brān″) 同 mesencephalon

mid·gut (mid'gut″) the region of the embryonic digestive tube into which the yolk sac opens and which gives rise to most of the intestines; ahead of it is the foregut and caudal to it is the hindgut 中肠

mi·do·drine (mi'do-drēn″) a vasopressor used as the hydrochloride salt in the treatment of orthostatic hypotension 一种血管加压药

mid·riff (mid'rif) the respiratory diaphragm; the region between the breast and waistline 隔

mid·wife (mid'wīf″) an individual who practices midwifery 助产士，参见 nurse-midwife

MIF macrophage migration inhibitory factor 巨噬细胞迁移抑制因子

mif·e·pris·tone (mif″ə-pris'tōn) RU-486; an antiprogestin used with misoprostol or other prostaglandin to terminate pregnancy in the first trimester 米非司酮

mig·li·tol (mig'lĭ-tol) an enzyme inhibitor that slows the absorption of glucose into the bloodstream and reduces postprandial hyperglycemia; used in the treatment of type 2 diabetes 降血糖药，用于治疗 2 型糖尿病

mi·graine (mi'grān) a symptom complex of periodic headaches, usually temporal and unilateral, often with irritability, nausea, vomiting, constipation or diarrhea, and photophobia, preceded by constriction of the cranial arteries, often with resultant prodromal sensory, especially ocular, symptoms (aura), and commencing with the vasodilation that follows 偏头痛；**mi′grainous** *adj.*；**abdominal m.**, that in which abdominal symptoms are predominant 腹型偏头痛；**basilar m., basilar artery m.**, a type of ophthalmic migraine with an aura that fills both visual fields and that may be accompanied by dysarthria and disturbances of equilibrium 基底型偏头痛；**ophthalmic m.**, migraine accompanied by amblyopia, teichopsia, or other visual disturbance 眼性偏头痛；**ophthalmoplegic m.**, periodic migraine accompanied by ophthalmoplegia 眼肌麻痹性偏头痛；**retinal m.**, a type of ophthalmic migraine with retinal symptoms, probably secondary to constriction of one or more retinal arteries 视网膜性偏头痛

mi·gra·tion (mi-gra'shən) 1. an apparently spontaneous change of place, as of symptoms 迁移，移动，移行，游走；2. diapedesis 血细胞渗出

mi·gra·to·ry (mi′grə-tor″e) 1. roving or wandering 流动的；移行的，游走的；2. of, pertaining to, or characterized by migration; undergoing periodic migration 迁徙的

mil·dew (mil′doo) colloquialism for any superficial fungus growth on plants or any organic material 霉菌病

mi·li·a·ria (mil″e-ar′e-ə) 1. a cutaneous condition with retention of sweat due to obstruction of sweat ducts, rupture of occluded ducts, and extravasation of sweat at different levels in the skin; when used alone, it refers to *m. rubra* 痱，汗疹，粟疹（单独使用时，指红痱）；2. 同 m. rubra；**m. crystalli′-na**, sudamina; miliaria in which the sweat escapes in or just beneath the stratum corneum, producing non-inflammatory vesicles with the appearance of clear droplets 白痱；**m. profun′da**, miliaria seen in hot humid climates, in which the occlusion of the sweat ducts is at the dermoepidermal junction; it follows severe, recurrent miliaria rubra and can lead to heat intolerance 深部痱；**m. ru′bra**, heat rash, prickly heat; miliaria in which the obstruction is deep in the epidermal layer, with rupture producing pruritic erythematous papulovesicles 红痱

mil·i·ary (mil′e-ar-e) 1. like millet seeds 粟粒状的；2. characterized by lesions resembling millet seeds 具粟粒状性质的

mil·i·um (mil′e-əm) pl. *mil′ia* [L.] a tiny spheroidal epithelial cyst lying superficially within the skin, usually of the face, containing lamellated keratin and often associated with vellus hair follicles 粟丘疹

milk (milk) 1. the fluid secretion of the mammary gland forming the natural food of young mammals 乳，奶；2. any whitish milklike substance, e.g., coconut milk or plant latex 乳状物；3. a liquid (emulsion or suspension) resembling the secretion of the mammary gland 乳剂；**m. of magnesia**, a suspension of magnesium hydroxide, used as an antacid and laxative 氧化镁混悬液；**modified m.**, cow's milk made to correspond to the composition of human milk 加工乳；**soy m.**, a liquid made from soybeans, used as a milk substitute and source of calcium 豆乳；**vitamin D m.**, cow's milk supplemented with 400 IU of vitamin D per quart 维生素 D 乳；**witch's m.**, milk secreted in the breast of the newborn infant 新生儿乳，婴乳

milk·ing (milk′ing) the pressing out of the contents of a tubular structure by running the finger along it 挤奶；挤出

milky (mil′ke) 1. having the appearance of milk; whitish, cloudy, and fluid 乳汁的；乳状的；乳色的；2. filled with or consisting of milk or a milklike fluid 牛奶的

milli- word element [L.], *one thousand;* also used in naming units of measurement (symbol m) to designate an amount 10^{-3} the size of the unit to which it is joined, e.g., milligram [构词成分] 千分之一；毫（符号 m）

mil·li·equiv·a·lent (mEq) (mil″e-e-kwiv′ə-lənt) one thousandth (10^{-3}) of the equivalent weight of an element, radical, or compound 毫（克）当量

mil·li·gram (mg) (mil′ĭ-gram) one thousandth (10^{-3}) of a gram 毫克

mil·li·li·ter (mL) (mil′ĭ-le″tər) one thousandth (10^{-3}) of a liter 毫升

mil·li·me·ter (mm) (mil′ĭ-me″tər) one thousandth (10^{-3}) of a meter 毫米

mil·li·mo·lar (mM) (mil′ĭ-mo″lər) denoting a concentration of 1 millimole per liter 毫摩尔的，每升 1 毫摩尔的浓度

mil·li·mole (mmol) (mil′ĭ-mōl) one thousandth (10^{-3}) of a mole 毫摩尔

mil·ri·none (mil′rĭ-nōn) a cardiotonic used in the treatment of congestive heart failure 米力农（强心药）

mi·me·sis (mĭ-me′sis) the simulation of one disease by another 模仿，模拟；拟态；疾病模仿

mi·met·ic (mĭ-met′ik) pertaining to or exhibiting imitation or simulation, as of one disease for another 模仿的，拟态的

mim·ic (mim′ik) 1. pertaining to imitation or simulation 模仿的；2. one who imitates, or that which imitates 模仿者或仿制品；3. to imitate or simulate 模仿

mind (mīnd) 1. the organ or seat of consciousness; the faculty, or brain function, by which one is aware of surroundings, and by which one experiences feelings, emotions, and desires, and is able to attend, remember, learn, reason, and make decisions 精神；2. the organized totality of an organism's mental and psychological processes, conscious and unconscious 智力；3. the characteristic thought process of a person or group 意志

min·er·al (min′ər-əl) any nonorganic homogeneous solid substance of the earth's crust 矿物；**trace m.**, a mineral that is a trace element 矿物质微量元素

min·er·alo·cor·ti·coid (min″ər-al″o-kor′tĭ-koid) 1. any of the group of corticosteroids, principally aldosterone, primarily involved in the regulation of electrolyte and water balance through its effect on ion transport in epithelial cells of the renal tubules, resulting in retention of sodium and loss of potassium 盐皮质激素. Cf. *glucocorticoid*；2. of, pertaining to, or resembling a mineralocorticoid 矿

质皮质激素

min·i·mal (min′ĭ-məl) smallest or least; the smallest possible 最低限度的，最小的

min·i·pill (min′e-pil) an oral contraceptive consisting of a small daily dose of a progestational agent 低剂量避孕丸

mini·plate (min′e-plāt) a small bone plate 小骨板

mini·sat·el·lite (min″e-sat′ə-līt) any of a series of short lengths of DNA comprising tandemly repeated nucleotide sequences, each repeating unit composed of approximately 10 to 60 base pairs. The number of repeating units in a given minisatellite varies between individuals 小卫星

mi·no·cy·cline (mĭ-no-si′klēn) a semisynthetic broad-spectrum tetracycline antibiotic, used as the hydrochloride salt 米诺环素

mi·nor (mi′nər) insignificant; small or least in scope, effect, number, size, extent, or importance 不重要的；次要的；较少的；少数的；未成年的

mi·nox·i·dil (mĭ-nok′sĭ-dil) a potent, long-acting vasodilator acting primarily on arterioles; used as an antihypertensive, also applied topically in androgenetic alopecia 米诺地尔（抗高血压药）

mi·nute (mi-no͞ot′) extremely small 微小的；微小体；**double m's,** acentric chromosomal fragments created by gene amplification and newly integrated into the chromosome; they are tumor markers indicative of solid neoplasms with a poor prognosis 双微体

mi·o·sis (mi-o′sis) contraction of the pupil 瞳孔缩小，缩瞳

mi·ot·ic (mi-ot′ik) 1. pertaining to, characterized by, or producing miosis 缩瞳的；2. an agent that causes contraction of the pupil 缩瞳药

MIP maximum inspiratory pressure 最大吸气压

mi·po·mer·sen (mih-poh″mir′sen) a lipid-lowering drug used to treat homozygous familial hypercholesterolemia 一种用于治疗纯合型家族性高胆固醇血症的降脂药物

mir·a·beg·ron (meer-ə-beg′ron) a β_3-adrenergic agonist that relaxes smooth muscle and is used as a urinary tract antispasmodic to treat symptoms of overactive bladder 一种 β_3 肾上腺素受体激动药，用作尿路解痉药

mi·ra·cid·i·um (mi-rə-sid′e-əm) pl. *miraci′dia*. The first-stage larva of a trematode, which undergoes further development in the body of a snail 毛蚴

mire (mēr) [Fr.] one of the figures on the arm of an ophthalmometer the images of which are reflected on the cornea; measurement of the variations determines the amount of corneal astigmatism 梯形目标（检眼计臂上的数字之一，其影像反射到角膜上，影像改变即可测量散光程度）

MIRL membrane inhibitor of reactive lysis 膜反应性溶解抑制物，见 *protectin*

miRNA microRNA. 微小 RNA

mir·ror (mir′ər) a polished surface that reflects sufficient light to yield images of objects in front of it. 镜子；**dental m.,** mouth m.；**frontal m., head m.,** a circular mirror strapped to the head of the examiner, used to reflect light into a cavity, especially the nose, pharynx, or larynx 额镜，头镜；**mouth m.,** a small mirror attached at an angle to a handle, for use in dentistry 口腔镜

mir·taz·a·pine (mir″taz-ə-pēn) an antidepressant structurally unrelated to any of the classes of antidepressants 一种抗抑郁药

mis·car·riage (mis′kar-əj) popular term for *spontaneous abortion* 流产

mis·ci·ble (mis′ĭ-bəl) able to be mixed 可混合的

mi·sog·a·my (mĭ-sog′ə-me) hatred of or aversion to marriage 厌婚症

mi·sog·y·ny (mĭ-soj′ĭ-ne) hatred of women 厌女症

mi·so·pro·stol (mi-so-pros′tol) a synthetic prostaglandin E_1 analogue used to treat gastric irritation resulting from long-term therapy with nonsteroidal antiinflammatory drugs; also used in conjunction with mifepristone (q.v.) for termination of pregnancy 米索前列醇（前列腺素 E_1 的衍生物）

mis·tle·toe (mis′əl-to) any of several related parasitic shrubs. *European m. (Viscum album)* contains small amounts of several toxins and is used for rheumatism and as an adjunct in cancer therapy; also used in traditional Chinese medicine and homeopathy 槲寄生

mite (mīt) any arthropod of the order Acarina except the ticks; they are minute animals, usually transparent or semitransparent, and may be parasitic on humans and domestic animals, causing various skin irritations 螨；**chigger m., harvest m.,** chigger 恙螨；**itch m., mange m.,** 疥癣虫，参见 *Notoedres* 和 *Sarcoptes*

mith·ra·my·cin (mith″rə-mi′sin) plicamycin 光神霉素

mi·ti·cide (mi′tĭ-sīd) an agent destructive to mites 杀螨剂

mi·to·chon·dria (mi″to-kon′dre-ə) sing. *mitochon′drion*. [Gr.] small spherical to rodshaped cytoplasmic organelles, enclosed by two membranes separated by an intermembranous space; the inner membrane is infolded, forming a series of projections (cristae). Mitochondria are the principal sites of ATP synthesis; they contain enzymes of the tricarboxylic acid cycle and for fatty acid oxidation, oxidative phosphorylation, and many other biochemical pathways. They contain their own nucleic acids and ribosomes, replicate independently, and code for the synthesis of some of their own proteins 线粒体; **mitochon'drial** *adj.*

mi·to·gen (mi'to-jən) a substance that induces mitosis and cell transformation, especially lymphocyte transformation 促分裂原; **mitogen'ic** *adj.*

mi·to·gen·e·sis (mi″to-jen'ə-sis) the production, or causation, of mitosis in or transformation of a cell 有丝分裂发生

mi·to·my·cin (mi″to-mi'sin) 1. any of a group of antitumor antibiotics (e.g., mitomycin A, B, C) produced by *Streptomyces caespitosus* 丝裂霉素（抗肿瘤抗生素）; 2. mitomycin C; used as a palliative antineoplastic 丝裂霉素 C

mi·to·sis (mi-to'sis) a complex of processes by which two daughter nuclei receive identical complements of the number of chromosomes characteristic of the somatic cells of the species 有丝分裂; **mitot'ic** *adj.*

mi·to·tane (mi'to-tān) an antineoplastic similar to the insecticide DDT; used for the treatment of inoperable adrenocortical carcinoma 米托坦, 邻氯苯对氯苯二氯乙烷（抗肿瘤药）

mi·to·xan·trone (mi″to-zan'trōn) a DNA-intercalating anthracenedione, used as the hydrochloride salt as an antineoplastic agent in the treatment of acute myelogenous leukemia and advanced, hormone-refractory prostate cancer; also used in the treatment of secondary multiple sclerosis 米托蒽醌（一种蒽二酮族抗肿瘤药）

mi·tral (mi'trəl) shaped like a miter; pertaining to the mitral valve 僧帽状的; 僧帽瓣的, 二尖瓣的, 左房室瓣的

mi·tral·iza·tion (mi″trəl-ĭ-za'shən) a straightening of the left border of the cardiac shadow, commonly seen radiographically in mitral stenosis 二尖瓣狭窄阴影

mit·tel·schmerz (mit'əl-shmɚrtz) pain associated with ovulation, usually occurring in the middle of the menstrual cycle 经间痛

mi·va·cu·rium (mi″və-ku're-əm) a nondepolarizing neuromuscular blocking agent of short duration, used as the chloride salt as an adjunct to anesthesia 美维库铵

mixed (mikst) affecting various parts at once; showing two or more different characteristics 混合的

mix·ture (miks'chər) a combination of different drugs or ingredients, such as a fluid with other fluids or solids or of a solid with a liquid 合剂, 混合物

mL ml milliliter 毫升的符号

μL microliter 微升的符号

MLD median lethal dose 半数致死量; minimum lethal dose 最小致死量

mM millimolar 毫摩尔的符号

mm millimeter 毫米的符号

μm micrometer 微米的符号

MMF mycophenolate mofetil 霉酚酸酯

MMIHS megacystis-microcolon–intestinal hypoperistalsis syndrome 巨膀胱 - 小结肠 - 肠蠕动迟缓综合征

mmol millimole 毫摩尔的符号

MMR measles-mumps-rubella (vaccine) 麻疹 - 腮腺炎 - 风疹（疫苗）, 见 *vaccine* 下 *measles, mumps, and rubella vaccine live*

MMRV measles, mumps, rubella, and varicella virus vaccine live 麻疹、腮腺炎、风疹和水痘病毒活疫苗

Mn manganese 元素锰的符号

MNCD mild neurocognitive disorder 轻度神经认知障碍

mne·mon·ics (ne-mon'iks) improvement of memory by special methods or techniques 记忆术; 记忆力培养法; **mnemon'ic** *adj.*

MO Medical Officer 医官

Mo molybdenum 元素钼的符号

mo·bi·li·za·tion (mo″bĭ-lĭ-za'shən) the rendering of a fixed part movable 活动法, 松动术; **stapes m.**, surgical correction of immobility of the stapes in treatment of deafness 镫骨松动术（治聋）

Mo·bi·lun·cus (mo″bĭ-lung'kəs) a genus of gram-negative, anaerobic, small, curved, rodshaped bacteria of the family Actinomycetaceae, frequently isolated from women with bacterial vaginosis 动弯杆菌属

mo·daf·i·nil (mo-daf'ĭ-nil″) a central nervous system stimulant used in the treatment of narcolepsy, obstructive sleep apnea, and shift work– associated sleep disorders 莫达非尼（中枢神经系统兴奋药）

mo·dal·i·ty (mo-dal'ĭ-te) 1. a method of application of, or the employment of, any therapeutic agent, especially a physical agent 药征; 2. in homeopathy, a condition that modifies drug action; a condition under which symptoms develop, becoming better or worse 用药程式; 3. a specific sensory entity, such as taste 感觉体（如味觉）

mode (mōd) 1. a manner, way, or method of acting; a particular condition of functioning 方式; 样式; 2. in statistics, the most frequently occurring value or item in a distribution 众数

mod·el (mod'əl) 1. something that represents or simulates something else 模型; 2. a reasonable facsimile of the body or any of its parts 型号, 特定模式; 3. cast (2). 样机, 样品; 4. to imitate another's behavior 使仿效, 仿仿; 5. a hypothesis or theory（用作分析与阐明）模型

mod·i·fi·ca·tion (mod″ĭ-fĭ-ka′shən) the process or result of changing the form or characteristics of an object or substance 矫正，改变；**behavior m.**, 行为矫正，参见 *therapy* 下词条

mod·i·fi·er (mod′ĭ-fi″ər) an agent that changes the form or characteristics of an object or substance 变更因子，变更基因，修饰因子，修饰基因；**biologic response m. (BRM)**, a method or agent that alters host-tumor interaction, usually by amplifying the antitumor mechanisms of the immune system or by some mechanism directly or indirectly affecting host or tumor cell characteristics 生物应答调节剂

mo·di·o·lus (mo-di′o-ləs) [L.] the central pillar or columella of the cochlea 蜗轴

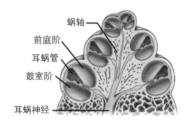

蜗轴
前庭阶
耳蜗管
鼓室阶
耳蜗神经

▲ 耳蜗轴的横截面

mod·u·la·tion (mod″u-la′shən) 1. the act of tempering 调整；2. the normal capacity of cell adaptability to its environment 适应（细胞适应环境的正常能力）；3. embryologic induction in a specific region 调变（胚胎学）；**antigenic m.**, the alteration of antigenic determinants in a living cell surface membrane following interaction with antibody 抗原调变；**biochemical m.**, in combination chemotherapy, the use of a substance to modulate the negative side effects of the primary agent, increasing its effectiveness or allowing a higher dose to be used 生化调整

mod·u·la·tor (mod′u-la″tər) a specific inductor that brings out characteristics peculiar to a definite region 调制器

mo·ex·i·pril (mo-ek′sĭ-pril″) an angiotensin-con-verting enzyme inhibitor used as the hydrochloride salt as an antihypertensive 莫尔普利，一种血管紧张素转化酶抑制药，其盐酸盐作为抗高血压药

moi·e·ty (moi′ə-te) any equal part; a half; also any part or portion, such as a portion of a molecule 等分，一半；一部分

mol (mol) 同 mole1

mo·lal (**m**) (mo′ləl) containing 1 mole of solute per kilogram of solvent. Note: *molal* refers to the weight of the solvent, *molar* to the volume of the solution（重量）摩尔的，（重量）克分子的（符号为 m）（注：molal 指溶剂的重量，molar 指溶液的体积）

mo·lal·i·ty (mo-lal′ĭ-te) the number of moles of a solute per kilogram of pure solvent 质量摩尔浓度，（重量）克分子浓度；Cf. *molarity*

mo·lar[1] (mo′lər) 1. pertaining to a mole of a substance（容积）摩尔的，（容积）克分子的；2. a measure of the concentration of a solute, expressed as the number of moles of solute per liter of solution. Symbol M, *M*, or mol/L 摩尔浓度，克分子浓度（符号为 M，*M* 或 mol/L）

mo·lar[2] (**M**) (mo′lər) 1. 磨牙，参见 *tooth* 和图 31；2. pertaining to a molar tooth 磨牙的

mo·lar·i·ty (mo-lar′ĭ-te) the number of moles of a solute per liter of solution 容积摩尔浓度，容积克分子浓度；Cf. *molality*

mold (mōld) 1. any of a group of parasitic and saprobic fungi causing a cottony growth on organic substances; also the deposit or growth produced by such fungi 霉菌；2. a form in which an object is shaped, or cast 模子；3. in dentistry, the shape of an artificial tooth 铸模

mold·ing (mōld′ing) the adjusting of the shape and size of the fetal head to the birth canal during labor（分娩时）胎头变形

mole[1] (mōl) the base SI unit of amount of matter, being that amount of substance that contains as many elementary entities as there are carbon atoms in 0.012 kg of carbon 12 (¹²C), Avogadro's number (6.023 × 10²³) 摩尔，克分子（量）

mole[2] (m ō l) 1. melanocytic nevus 黑素细胞痣；2. any pigmented skin lesion 色素沉着的皮损；**pigmented m.**, 色素痣，参见 *nevus* 下词条

mole[3] (mōl) a fleshy mass or tumor formed in the uterus by the degeneration or abnormal development of a zygote 胎块；**hydatid m., hydatidiform m.**, an abnormal pregnancy characterized by placental abnormality involving swollen chorionic villi, which form a large, grapelike mass of vesicles, by trophoblastic hyperplasia, and by loss of fetal blood vessels in the villi. It is *complete* when all villi are swollen and fetal tissues are absent, and it is *partial* when only some villi are swollen and fetal tissues are present. Complete moles usually possess only paternal chromosomes; partial moles are usually triploid and possess both maternal and paternal chromosomes 水泡状胎块，葡萄胎

mol·e·cule (mol′ə-kūl) a small mass of matter; the smallest amount of a substance that can exist alone; an aggregation of atoms, specifically a chemical combination of two or more atoms forming a specific chemical substance 分子; **molec′ular** *adj.*; **cell adhesion m's (CAM)**, cell surface glycoproteins that mediate intercell adhesions in vertebrates 细胞黏附分子

mo·lin·done hy·dro·chlo·ride (mo-lin′dōn) an antipsychotic agent, used as the hydrochloride salt 盐酸吗茚酮，盐酸吗啉吲酮（抗精神病药）

Mol·li·cu·tes (mol″ĭ-ku′tēz) a class of generally parasitic bacteria of the phylum Firmicutes, comprising the smallest and simplest microor-ganisms capable of self-replication 柔膜体纲

mol·lus·cum (mo-lus′kəm) 1. any of various skin diseases marked by the formation of soft rounded cutaneous tumors 软疣; 2. 同 m. contagiosum; **mollus′cous** *adj.*; **m. contagio′sum**, a common, benign, usually self-limited viral infection of the skin, caused by a poxvirus, with firm, round, trans-lucent, crateriform papules containing caseous mat-ter and pathognomonic intracytoplasmic inclusions in which replicating virions can be found 传染性软疣

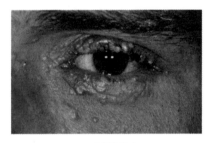

▲ 传染性软疣

Mol-wt mol wt molecular weight 分子量

mo·lyb·date (mə-lib′dāt) any salt of molybdic acid 钼酸盐

mo·lyb·den·um (Mo) (mə-lib′də-nəm) a hard, silvery white, metallic element; at. no. 42; at. wt. 95.96; a cofactor in numerous enzymes and an es-sential trace element for eukaryotes 钼（化学元素）

mo·lyb·do·pro·tein (mə-lib″do-pro′tēn) an en-zyme containing molybdenum 钼蛋白

mo·met·a·sone (mo-met′ə-sōn) a synthetic corti-costeroid used in the form of *m. furoate* for the relief of inflammation and pruritus in certain dermatoses and the treatment of allergic rhinitis and other in-flammatory nasal conditions 莫米松（合成皮质类固醇）

mon·ad (mon′əd) 1. a single-celled protozoan or coccus 单细胞（原）虫，单细胞（球）菌; 2. a univalent radical or element 一价基，一价物; 3. in meiosis, one member of a tetrad 单分体

mon·ar·thri·tis (mon″ahr-thri′tis) inflammation of a single joint 单关节炎

mon·ar·tic·u·lar (mon″ahr-tik′u-lər) pertaining to a single joint 单关节的

mon·ath·e·to·sis (mon″ath-ə-to′sis) athetosis of one limb 单肢（手足）徐动症

mon·atom·ic (mon″ə-tom′ik) 1. 同 monovalent (1); 2. 同 monobasic; 3. containing one atom 一原子的

mon·au·ral (mon-aw′rəl) pertaining to one ear 单耳的

mo·ne·cious (mo-ne′shəs) 同 monoecious

mon·es·thet·ic (mon″əs-thet′ik) pertaining to or affecting a single sense or sensation 单感觉的

mo·nil·e·thrix (mo-nil′ə-thriks) a hereditary con-dition in which the hairs have constrictions, giving a beading effect, and are brittle 念珠状发

Mo·nil·ia (mo-nil′e-ə) 1. former name for *Candida* 念珠菌属（旧名，现称 *Candida*）; 2. a genus of imperfect fungi of the family Moniliaceae 丛梗孢属

mo·nil·i·al (mo-nil′e-əl) pertaining to or caused by *Monilia (Candida)* 念珠菌的

mo·nil·i·form (mo-nil′ĭ-form) beaded. 念珠形的

mon·i·tor (mon′ĭ-tər) 1. to check constantly on a given condition or phenomenon, e.g., blood pressure or heart or respiratory rate 监护; 2. an apparatus by which such conditions can be constantly observed or recorded 监护仪; **ambulatory ECG m., Holter m.**, a portable continuous electrocardiographic recorder used to detect the frequency and duration of rhythm disturbances 动态心电监护仪

mon·key·pox (mung′ke-poks) a mild, epidemic, exanthematous disease occurring in monkeys and other mammals; when transmitted to humans, it causes a disease clinically similar to smallpox 猴痘

mono·am·ide (mon″o-am′īd) an amide compound with only one amide group 一酰胺

mono·amine (mon″o-ə-mēn′) an amine containing one amino group, e.g., serotonin, dopamine, epi-nephrine, and norepinephrine 单胺

mono·amine ox·i·dase (MAO) (mon″o-ə- mēn′ ok′sī-dās) a flavoprotein (FAD) enzyme that catalyz-es the oxidative deamination of primary amines to form aldehydes and hydrogen peroxide. Substrates include serotonin, norepinephrine, epinephrine, dopamine, and also some secondary and tertiary amines. It occurs in several isozymes 单胺氧化酶

mono·am·in·er·gic (mon″o-am″in-ur′jik) of or pertaining to neurons that secrete monoamine neu-rotransmitters (e.g., dopamine, serotonin) 单胺能的

mono·am·ni·ot·ic (mon″o-am″ne-ot′ik) having or developing within a single amniotic cavity, such as monozygotic twins 单羊膜的，一卵性的

mon·o·bac·tam (mon″o-bak′tam) a class of

synthetic antibiotics having a monocyclic β-lactam nucleus 单环 β- 内酰胺类（抗生素）

mono·ba·sic (mon″o-ba′sik) having but one atom of replaceable hydrogen 一价碱的

mono·ben·zone (mon″o-ben′zōn) a melanininhibiting agent used as a topical depigmenting agent in vitiligo 莫诺苯宗，双苄氧酚（黑素抑制药）

mono·blast (mon′o-blast) the earliest precursor in the monocytic series, which matures to develop into the promonocyte 原单核细胞

mono·blep·sia (mon″o-blep′se-ə) a condition in which vision is better when only one eye is used 单眼视症

mono·cho·rea (mon″o-kə-re′ə) chorea affecting only one limb 单肢舞蹈病

mono·cho·ri·on·ic (mon″o-kor″e-on′ik) having or developing in a common chorionic sac, such as monozygotic twins 单绒毛膜的（单卵双胎）

mono·chro·mat (mon″o-kro′mat) a person with monochromatic vision 全色盲者

mono·chro·mat·ic (mon″o-kro-mat′ik) 1. existing in or having only one color 单色的；2. pertaining to or affected by monochromatic vision 全色盲的；3. staining with only one dye at a time 单染色的

mono·chro·ma·tism (mon″o-kro′mə-tiz″əm) monochromatic vision 全色盲；cone m., that in which there is some cone function 锥体全色盲；rod m., that in which there is complete absence of cone function 杆体全色盲

mono·chro·mato·phil (mon″o-kro-mat′ə- fil) 1. stainable with only one kind of stain 单染色的；2. any cell or other element taking only one stain 单染性细胞或成分

mono·clo·nal (mon″o-klo′nəl) derived from or pertaining to a single clone 单克隆的

mon·oc·u·lar (mon-ok′u-lər) 1. pertaining to or having only one eye 单眼的；2. having only one eyepiece, as in a microscope 单目镜的（显微镜）

mono·cyte (mon′o-sīt) a mononuclear, phagocytic leukocyte, 13 to 25 μm in diameter, with an ovoid or kidney-shaped nucleus and azurophilic cytoplasmic granules. Formed in the bone marrow from promonocytes, monocytes are transported to tissues, such as the lung and liver, where they develop into macrophages 单核细胞，**monocyt′ic** adj.

mono·cy·toid (mon″o-si′toid) resembling a monocyte 单核细胞样的

mono·cy·to·pe·nia (mon″o-si″to-pe′ne-ə) deficiency of monocytes in the blood 单核细胞减少（症）

mono·der·mo·ma (mon″o-dər-mo′mə) a tumor developed from one germ layer 单胚叶瘤

mo·noe·cious (mo-ne′shəs) having reproductive organs typical of both sexes in a single individual 雌雄同体的，雌雄同株的

mono·eth·a·nol·amine (mon″o-eth″ə-nol′ə- mēn) an amino alcohol used as a pharmaceutical surfactant. The oleate salt is *ethanolamine oleate* 乙醇胺，氨基乙醇

mono·gen·ic (mon″o-jen′ik) pertaining to or influenced by a single gene 单基因的

mono·io·do·ty·ro·sine (mon″o-i-o″do-ti′rosēn) an iodinated amino acid intermediate in the synthesis of thyroxine and triiodothyronine 一碘酪氨酸

mono·kine (mon′o-kīn) a general term for soluble mediators of immune responses that are not antibodies or complement components and that are produced by mononuclear phagocytes (monocytes or macrophages) 单核因子

mono·loc·u·lar (mon″o-lok′u-lər) unilocular 单腔的，单房的

mono·ma·nia (mon″o-ma′ne-ə) a form of mental disorder characterized by preoccupation with one subject or idea 单狂，偏执（精神疾病）

mono·mer (mon′o-mər) 单体 1. a simple molecule of relatively low molecular weight, capable of reacting to form by repetition a dimer, trimer, or polymer 低分子量单分子化合物；2. some basic unit of a molecule, either the molecule itself or some structural or functional subunit of it 一个分子的基本单位

mono·mer·ic (mon″o-mer′ik) pertaining to, composed of, or affecting a single segment 单节的；单基因的

mono·mi·cro·bi·al (mon″o-mi-kro′be-əl) marked by the presence of a single species of microorganisms 单微生物的

mono·mo·lec·u·lar (mon″o-mo-lek′u-lər) pertaining to a single molecule or to a layer one molecule thick 单分子的

mono·mor·phic (mon″o-mor′fik) existing in only one form; maintaining the same form throughout all developmental stages 单形的

mono·neu·ri·tis (mon″o-noo-ri′tis) inflammation of a single nerve 单神经炎；m. mul′tiplex 多发性单神经炎，见 *mononeuropathy* 下词条

mono·neu·rop·a·thy (mon″o-noo-rop′ə-the) disease affecting a single nerve 单神经病；multiple m., m. multiplex, mononeuropathy of several different nerves simultaneously 多发性单神经病

mono·nu·cle·ar (mon″o-noo-kle-ər) 1. having but one nucleus 单核的；2. a cell having a single nucleus, especially a monocyte of the blood or tissues 单核细胞

mono·nu·cle·o·sis (mon″o-noo″kle-o′sis) excess of mononuclear leukocytes (monocytes) in the blood

单核细胞增多（症）；**cytomegalovirus m.**, an infectious disease caused by a cytomegalovirus and resembling infectious mononucleosis 巨细胞病毒性单核细胞增多症；**infectious m.**, an acute, usually self-limited, infectious disease caused by human herpesvirus 4; symptoms include fever, malaise, sore throat, lymphadenopathy, atypical lymphocytes (resembling monocytes) in the peripheral blood, and various immune reactions 传染性单核细胞增多症

mono·nu·cle·o·tide (mon″o-noo′kle-o-tīd) nucleotide 单核苷酸

mono·oc·ta·no·in (mon″o-ok′tə-no′in) a semisynthetic glycerol derivative used to dissolve cholesterol stones in the common and intrahepatic bile ducts 单辛精（半合成甘油衍生物）

mono·pha·sia (mon″o-fa′zhə) aphasia with ability to utter only one word or phrase 单语症；**mono-pha′sic** adj.

mono·phe·nol mono·oxy·gen·ase (mon″ofe′nol mon″o-ok′sĭ-jən-ās″) any of a group of oxidoreductases that catalyze a step in the formation of melanin pigments from tyrosine 单酚单（加）氧酶

mon·oph·thal·mus (mon″of-thal′məs) cyclops 独眼畸胎

mono·phy·let·ic (mon″o-fi-let′ik) descended from a common ancestor or stem cell 单源的（起源于单细胞型的）

mono·ple·gia (mon″o-ple′jə) paralysis of a single part 单（肢）瘫；**monople′gic** adj.

mono·pty·chi·al (mon″o-ti′ke-əl) arranged in a single layer; said of glands with cells arranged on the basement membrane in a single layer 单层的

mon·or·chid (mon-or′kid) 1. pertaining to or characterized by monorchism 单睾丸的；2. an individual with monorchism 单睾丸者

mon·or·chid·ism (mon-or′kid-iz-əm) 同 monorchism

mon·or·chism (mon′or-kiz″əm) the condition of having only one testis in the scrotum 单睾症，单侧睾丸缺如

mono·sac·cha·ride (mon″o-sak′ə-rīd) a simple sugar, having the general formula $C_nH_{2n}O_n$; a carbohydrate that cannot be decomposed by hydrolysis. The two main types are the aldoses and the ketoses 单糖

mono·so·di·um glu·ta·mate (mon″o-so′de-əm gloo′tə-māt) the monosodium salt of l-glutamic acid, used as a pharmaceutical necessity and to enhance the flavor of foods 谷氨酸钠

mono·so·my (mon″o-so″me) existence in a cell of only one instead of the normal diploid pair of a particular chromosome 单体性（染色体）；**monoso′mic** adj.

mono·spasm (mon′o-spaz″əm) spasm of a single limb or part 局部痉挛，单处痉挛

mono·spe·cif·ic (mon″o-spə-sif′ik) having an effect only on a particular kind of cell or tissue or reacting with a single antigen, as a monospecific antiserum might 单特异性的

mono·sper·my (mon″o-spur″me) fertilization in which only one spermatozoon enters the oocyte 单精受精

mono·stra·tal (mon″o-stra′təl) pertaining to a single layer or stratum 单层的

mono·syn·ap·tic (mon″o-sĭ-nap′tik) pertaining to or passing through a single synapse 单突触的

mono·ther·a·py (mon″o-ther′ə-pe) treatment of a condition by means of a single drug 单药治疗

mono·ther·mia (mon″o-thur′me-ə) maintenance of the same body temperature throughout the day 体温恒定

mon·ot·ri·chous (mə-not′rĭ-kəs) having a single polar flagellum 单鞭毛的

mono·un·sat·u·rat·ed (mon″o-ən-sach′ər- āt″əd) of a chemical compound, containing one double or triple bond 单不饱和的

mono·va·lent (mon″o-va′lənt) 1. having a valency of one 一价的；2. capable of combining with only one antigenic specificity or with only one antibody specificity 单特异性的

mon·ov·u·lar (mon-ov′u-lər) pertaining to or derived from a single oocyte, as monozygotic twins 单卵的

mono·xen·ic (mon″o-zen′ik) associated with a single known species of microorganisms; said of otherwise germ-free animals 单种菌（感染）的（实验动物）

mo·nox·e·nous (mə-nok′sə-nəs) requiring only one host to complete the life cycle 单栖的，单（宿主）寄生的

mon·ox·ide (mon-ok′sīd) an oxide with one oxygen atom in the molecule 一氧化物

mono·zy·got·ic (mon″o-zi-got′ik) pertaining to or derived from a single zygote, as are monozygotic twins 单合子的，单卵双生的

mons (monz) [L.] an elevation or eminence 山，阜，隆凸的统称；**m. pu′bis, m. ve′neris**, the rounded fleshy prominence over the symphysis pubis in the female 阴阜

mon·ster (mon′stər) a term formerly used to denote a fetus or infant with such pronounced developmental anomalies as to be grotesque and usually nonviable 畸胎

mon·te·lu·kast (mon″tə-loo′kast) a leukotriene antagonist used as the sodium salt in prophylaxis and chronic treatment of asthma 孟鲁司特（抗白

三烯类药物，抗过敏药）

mon·tic·u·lus (mon-tik′u-ləs) pl. *monti′culi* [L.] a small eminence 小山；m. cerebel′li, the projecting or central part of the vermis 小脑小山，小脑上蚓的中心突起

mood (mŏŏd) the emotional state or state of mind of an individual 心境，情绪

MOPP a cancer chemotherapy regimen consisting of mechlorethamine, Oncovin (vincristine), procarbazine, and prednisone 氮芥 - 长春新碱 - 甲基苄肼 - 泼尼松（联合化疗治癌）

Mo·rax·el·la (mo″rak-sel′ə) a genus of bacteria of the family Moraxellaceae, made up of gram-negative, short, aerobic, nonpigmented organisms found as parasites and pathogens on the mucous membranes of mammals; it includes two subgenera: *M. (Moraxella)* and *M. (Branhamella). M. (Branhamel′la) catarrha′lis* is a normal inhabitant of the human nasal cavity and nasopharynx, occasionally causing otitis media or respiratory disease. *M. (Moraxel′la) lacuna′ta* causes conjunctivitis and corneal infections 莫拉菌属

Mo·rax·el·la·ceae (mo″rak-sel-a′se-e) a family of gram-negative, rod-shaped, coccoid or coccal bacteria, of the order Pseudomonadales; organisms are nonmotile, chemo-organotrophic, and aerobic and are usually catalase-positive. Medically important organisms are contained in the genera *Acinetobacter* and *Moraxella* 莫拉菌科

mor·bid (mor′bid) 1. pertaining to, affected with, or inducing disease; diseased 疾病的；2. unhealthy or unwholesome 不健康的；3. characterized by preoccupation with gloomy or unwholesome feelings or thoughts 忧郁或令人不快的感觉

mor·bid·i·ty (mor-bid′ĭ-te) 1. a diseased condition or state 病态，成病，发病；2. the incidence or prevalence of a disease or of all diseases in a population 发病率

mor·bil·li·form (mor-bil′ĭ-form) measleslike; resembling the eruption of measles 麻疹样的

Mor·bil·li·vi·rus (mor-bil′ĭ-vi″rəs) measleslike viruses; a genus of viruses of the family Paramyxoviridae, including the agents of measles and canine distemper 麻疹病毒属

mor·cel·la·tion (mor″səl-a′shən) the division of solid tissue (such as a tumor) into pieces, which can then be removed 分碎术

mor·cel·la·tor (mor″səl-a′tor) a surgical instrument used for morcellation of bodily tissue or bodily organ parts during endoscopic surgical procedures 粉碎器

mor·dant (mor′dənt) 1. a substance capable of intensifying or deepening the reaction of a specimen

to a stain 媒染剂；2. to subject to the action of a mordant before staining 媒染

Mor·ga·nel·la (mor″gə-nel′ə) a genus of gramnegative, facultatively anaerobic, rod-shaped bacteria of the family Enterobacteriaceae. *M. morga′nii* is an opportunistic pathogen, causing secondary infections of blood, respiratory tract, and wounds 摩根菌属

morgue (morg) a place where dead bodies may be kept for identification or until claimed for burial 停尸室，太平间

mor·i·bund (mor′ĭ-bund″) in a dying state 濒死的

mor·i·ci·zine (mor-ĭ′sĭ-zēn) a phenothiazine derivative used as the hydrochloride salt as an antiarrhythmic in treatment of ventricular arrhythmias 莫雷西嗪，一种吩噻嗪衍生物，其盐酸盐作为抗心律失常药，用于治疗室性心律失常

mor·phea (mor-fe′ə) a localized type of scleroderma in which there is connective tissue replacement of skin and sometimes superficial fascia, with formation of firm white or pink patches, bands, or lines 硬斑病

mor·phine (mor′fēn) an opioid analgesic, the principal and most active alkaloid of opium; used as the sulfate or hydrochloride salt as an analgesic and antitussive and as an adjunct to anesthesia or to treatment of pulmonary edema secondary to left ventricular failure 吗啡（镇痛药）

mor·pho·gen (mor′fo-jən) a substance in embryonic tissue that forms a concentration gradient and influences morphogenesis 形态发生素

mor·pho·gen·e·sis (mor″fo-jen′ə-sis) the evolution and development of form, such as the development of the shape of a particular organ or part of the body or the development undergone by individuals who attain the type to which the majority of the individuals of the species approximate 形态发生

mor·pho·ge·net·ic (mor″fo-jə-net′ik) producing growth; producing form or shape 形态发生的

mor·phol·o·gy (mor-fol′ə-je) the science of the forms and structures of organisms; the form and structure of a particular organism, organ, or part 形态学；**morpholog′ic, morpholog′ical** *adj.*

mor·pho·sis (mor-fo′sis) the process of formation of a part or organ 形态形成；**morphot′ic** *adj.*

mor·rhu·ate (mor′u-āt) the fatty acids of cod liver oil; the sodium salt is used as a sclerosing agent, especially for the treatment of varicose veins and hemorrhoids 鱼肝油酸盐

mors (morz) [L.] death 死亡

mor·sus (mor′səs) [L.] bite 咬，螫

mor·tal (mor′təl) 1. subject to death, or destined to die 不能免死的，必死的；2. fatal 致命的

mor·tal·i·ty (mor-tal′ĭ-te) 1. the quality of being mortal 必死性; 2. death rate 死亡率; 3. the ratio of actual deaths to expected deaths 预期死亡率

mor·tar (mor′tər) a bell- or urn-shaped vessel in which drugs are beaten, crushed, or ground with a pestle 乳钵，研钵

mor·ti·fi·ca·tion (mor″tĭ-fĭ-ka′shən) gangrene 坏疽

mor·u·la (mor′u-lə) 1. the solid mass of blasto-meres formed by cleavage of a zygote 桑葚胚; 2. an inclusion body seen in circulating leukocytes in ehrlichiosis 桑葚胚（存在于埃立克体病患者血细胞中的包涵体）

mor·u·lar (mor′u-lər) 1. pertaining to a morula 桑葚胚的; 2. resembling a mulberry 桑葚状的

mo·sa·ic (mo-za′ik) 1. a pattern made of numerous small pieces fitted together 马赛克; 2. in genetics, an individual composed of two or more cell lines that are karyotypically or genotypically distinct but are derived from a single zygote 嵌合体

mo·sa·i·cism (mo-za′ĭ-siz″əm) the presence in an individual of two or more cell lines that are karyotypically or genotypically distinct and are derived from a single zygote 镶嵌现象，镶嵌现象

mOsm milliosmole; one thousandth (10⁻³) of an osmole 毫渗量，毫渗摩尔的符号

mos·qui·to (məs-ke′to) [Sp.] a bloodsucking and venomous insect of the family Culicidae, including the genera *Aedes, Anopheles, Culex,* and *Mansonia* 蚊

moth·er (muth′ər) 1. the female parent 母亲; 2. something from which another thing is derived 母体; surrogate m., a woman who carries a fetus for another; she may contribute the oocyte, or she may be impregnated with a donor oocyte via in vitro fertilization *(gestational surrogate m.)* 代孕母亲

mo·til·in (mo-til′in) a polypeptide hormone secreted by enterochromaffin cells of the gut; it causes increased motility of several portions of the gut and stimulates pepsin secretion. Its release is stimulated by the presence of acid and fat in the duodenum 促胃动素

mo·til·i·ty (mo-til′ĭ-te) the ability to move spontaneously 能动性，机动性，能动力; **mo′tile** *adj.*

mo·to·neu·ron (mo″to-noor′on) motor neuron; a neuron having a motor function; an efferent neuron conveying motor impulses 运动神经元; lower m., a peripheral neuron with a cell body that lies in the ventral gray columns of the spinal cord and whose termination is in a skeletal muscle 下运动神经元; peripheral m., in a reflex arc, a motoneuron that receives impulses from interneurons 外周运动神经元; upper m., a neuron in the cerebral cortex that conducts impulses from the motor cortex to a motor

nucleus of one of the cerebral nerves or to a ventral gray column of the spinal cord 上运动神经元

mo·tor (mo′tər) 1. a muscle, nerve, or center that effects or produces motion 指影响或产生运动的肌肉、运动神经或中枢; 2. producing or subserving motion 运动的

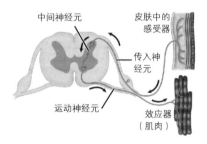

▲ 运动神经元在三神经元反射弧中作为传出神经元

mot·tled (mot′əld) marked by spots or blotches of different colors or shades 斑色的，花斑状的

mot·tling (mot′ling) a condition of spotting with patches of color 斑点状阴影，斑（状阴）影

mou·lage (moo-lahzh′) [Fr.] the making of molds or models in wax or plaster; also, a mold or model so produced 蜡模（型）

mound·ing (mound′ing) 同 myoedema (1)

mount (mount) 1. to fix in or on a support 安装; 2. a support on which something may be fixed 底座; 3. to prepare specimens and slides for study 制作标本或载片; 4. a specimen or slide for study 标本，载片

mourn·ing (mor′ning) 1. the normal psychological processes that follow the loss of a loved one; grief is the accompanying emotional state 悲伤; 2. social expressions of grief, such as funeral and burial services, prayers, or other rituals 哀悼

mouse (mous) 1. a small rodent, various species of which are used in laboratory experiments 小鼠; 2. a small weight or movable structure 游动小体; joint m., a movable fragment of cartilage or other body within a joint 关节内游动体，关节鼠; peritoneal m., a free body in the peritoneal cavity, probably a small detached mass of omentum, sometimes visible radiographically 腹膜腔游动体

mouth (mouth) 1. an opening 开口，小孔; 2. oral cavity 口腔; trench m., necrotizing ulcerative gingivitis 坏死性溃疡性齿龈炎，战壕口炎

mouth·wash (mouth′wahsh″) a solution for rinsing the mouth 漱口液

move·ment (moov′mənt) an act of changing position 运动; ameboid m., movement characteristic of amebae and leukocytes by extension of the plasma membrane to form pseudopodia into which the cytosol flows, moving the cell forward 阿米巴运动; **associated m.,** 1. movement of parts that act together, such as the eyes 联合运动（如眼）; 2. synkinesis 联带运动; **bowel m.,** defecation 肠蠕动; **brownian m.,** the random zigzag or dancing movement of minute solute particles suspended in a solvent, due to bombardment by rapidly moving solvent molecules 布朗运动; **rapid eye m. (REM),** the rapid conjugate movement of the eyes that occurs during REM sleep (see under *sleep*) 快速眼动，睡眠期间发生的眼睛快速共轭运动; **vermicular m.,** peristalsis 蠕动

mov·er (moov′ər) that which produces motion 行动者；原动力; **prime m.,** a muscle that acts directly to bring about a desired movement 原动肌

moxa (mok′sə) [Japanese] the dried leaves of *Artemisia vulgaris,* burned on or near acupoints in moxibustion 艾，灸料，灼烙剂

mox·i·bus·tion (mok″sĭ-bus′chən) the stimulation of an acupoint by the burning of a cone or cylinder of moxa placed at or near the point 灸术

mox·i·flox·a·cin (mok″sĭ-flok′sə-sin) a fluoroquinolone antibacterial effective against many gram-positive and gram-negative bacteria; used as the hydrochloride salt 莫西沙星（氟喹诺酮类抗菌药）

6-MP 同 mercaptopurine

MPD maximum permissible dose 最大容许剂量

MPH Master of Public Health 公共卫生硕士

MPO myeloperoxidase

MPSV meningococcal polysaccharide vaccine 脑膜炎球菌多糖疫苗

MR mitral regurgitation 二尖瓣反流

mR milliroentgen; one thousandth (10^{-3}) of a roentgen 毫伦琴的符号

MRA Medical Record Administrator 病案管理人员

mrad millirad; one thousandth (10^{-3}) of a rad 毫拉德的符号

MRC Medical Reserve Corps 军医预备队

MRCP Member of Royal College of Physicians 皇家内科医师学会会员

MRCS Member of Royal College of Surgeons 皇家外科医师学会会员

mrem millirem; one thousandth (10^{-3}) of a rem 毫雷姆

MRI magnetic resonance imaging 磁共振成像

MRL Medical Record Librarian 病案管理员，现称 Medical Record Administrator

mRNA messenger RNA 信使 RNA

MRSA methicillin-resistant *Staphylococcus aureus* 耐甲氧西林金黄色葡萄球菌

MS Master of Science 理科硕士; Master of Surgery 外科硕士; mitral stenosis 二尖瓣狭窄; multiple sclerosis 多发性硬化

ms millisecond; one thousandth (10^{-3}) of a second 毫秒的符号

μs microsecond; one millionth (10^{-6}) of a second 微秒的符号

MSA multiple system atrophy 多系统萎缩; **MSA-C,** multiple system atrophy with predominant cerebellar ataxia 小脑多系统萎缩; **MSA-P,** multiple system atrophy with predominant parkinsonism 帕金森多系统萎缩

MSD minimal systolic displacement 最小收缩位移

MSG monosodium glutamate 谷氨酸单钠

MSH melanocyte-stimulating hormone 促黑素细胞激素

MSUD maple syrup urine disease 枫糖尿病

MT Medical Technologist 医学技术员

mtDNA mitochondrial DNA 线粒体脱氧核糖核酸

mu·cif·er·ous (mu-sif′ər-əs) 同 muciparous

mu·ci·gen (mu′sĭ-jən) the substance from which mucin is derived 黏蛋白原

mu·ci·lage (mu′sĭ-ləj) an aqueous solution of a gummy substance, used as a vehicle or demulcent 胶浆剂; **mucilag′inous** *adj.*

mu·cil·loid (mu′sĭ-loid) a preparation of a mucilaginous substance 胶浆剂; **psyllium hydrophilic m.,** a powdered preparation of the mucilaginous portion of the seeds of blond psyllium *(Plantago ovata),* used as a bulk-forming laxative 车前子亲水胶浆（泻药）

mu·cin (mu′sin) 1. any of a group of proteincontaining glycoconjugates with high sialic acid or sulfated polysaccharide content that compose the chief constituent of mucus 黏蛋白; 2. any of a wide variety of glycoconjugates, including mucoproteins, glycoproteins, glycosaminoglycans, and glycolipids 含糖复合物的统称

mu·ci·noid (mu′sĭ-noid) resembling or pertaining to mucin 黏蛋白样的

mu·ci·no·sis (mu″sĭ-no′sis) a state with abnormal deposits of mucins in the skin 黏蛋白沉积症; **cutaneous focal m.,** a type of dermal mucinosis in which there is a solitary nodule on the skin 皮肤灶性黏蛋白沉积症; **dermal m.,** any of the types caused by deposition of mucin in the dermis, with nodules, papules, or plaques on the skin surface 皮肤黏蛋白沉积症; **follicular m.,** a disease of the pilosebaceous unit, characterized by plaques of follicular papules and alopecia 毛囊性黏蛋白沉积症; **reticular erythematous m.,** a type of dermal mucinosis characterized by papules or plaques in a reticular pattern on the back after sun exposure 网状红斑性黏蛋白沉积症

mu·ci·nous (mu'sĭ-nəs) resembling, or marked by formation of, mucin 黏蛋白的，黏蛋白状的

mu·cin·uria (mu″sin-u're-ə) the presence of mucin in the urine, suggesting vaginal contamination 黏蛋白尿

mu·cip·a·rous (mu-sip'ə-rəs) secreting mucus 分泌黏液的

mu·co·cele (mu'ko-sēl) 1. dilatation of a cavity with mucous secretion 黏液囊肿；2. mucus retention cyst 黏液潴留囊肿

mu·co·cil·i·ary (mu″ko-sil'e-ar-e) pertaining to mucus and to the cilia of the epithelial cells in the airways 黏膜纤毛的

mu·co·cu·ta·ne·ous (mu″ko-ku-ta'ne-əs) pertaining to or affecting the mucous membrane and the skin 皮肤黏膜的

mu·co·ep·i·der·moid (mu″ko-ep″ĭ-dur'moid) composed of mucus-producing epithelial cells 黏液表皮样的

mu·co·gin·gi·val (mu″ko-jin'jĭ-vəl) pertaining to the oral mucosa and gingiva, or to the line of demarcation between them 黏液龈的

mu·coid (mu'koid) 1. resembling mucus 黏液样的；2. 同 mucinoid

mu·co·lip·i·do·sis (mu″ko-lip″ĭ-do'sis) pl. *mucolipido'ses.* Any of a group of lysosomal storage diseases in which both glycosaminoglycans (mucopolysaccharides) and lipids accumulate in tissues but without excess of the former in the urine 黏脂贮积病；m. Ⅰ, sialidosis 黏脂贮积病Ⅰ型；m. Ⅱ, an autosomal recessive, rapidly progressing disease of young children, characterized by severe growth impairment, minimal hepatomegaly, extreme mental and motor retardation, and clear corneas; due to deficiency of an enzyme important for incorporation of lysosomal enzymes into lysosomes 黏脂贮积病Ⅱ型；m. Ⅲ, an autosomal recessive disorder similar to mucolipidosis Ⅱ but clinically less severe; there are two forms, each due to a different defect in the same enzyme affected in type Ⅱ 黏脂贮积病Ⅲ型；m. Ⅳ, an autosomal recessive disorder characterized by psychomotor retardation and severe visual impairment, initially manifest in infancy or childhood as corneal clouding; caused by a mutation affecting a membrane protein important in endocytosis and lysosomal transport 黏脂贮积病Ⅳ型

mu·co·lyt·ic (mu″ko-lit'ik) capable of reducing the viscosity of mucus, or an agent that so acts 溶解黏液的；黏液溶解药

mu·co·peri·chon·dri·um (mu″ko-per″e-kon'-dre-əm) perichondrium having a mucosal surface, such as that of the nasal septum 黏膜性软骨膜；**mucoperichon'drial** adj.

mu·co·peri·os·te·um (mu″ko-per″e-os'te-əm) periosteum having a mucous surface 黏膜骨膜；**mucoperios'teal** adj.

mu·co·poly·sac·cha·ride (mu″ko-pol″esak'ə-rīd) glycosaminoglycan 黏多糖，糖胺聚糖

mu·co·poly·sac·cha·ri·do·sis (mu″ko-pol″-e-sak″ə-ri-do'sis) pl. *mucopolysaccharido'ses.* Any of a group of lysosomal storage diseases due to defective metabolism of glycosaminoglycans, causing their accumulation and excretion and affecting the bony skeleton, joints, liver, spleen, eye, ear, skin, teeth, and cardiovascular, respiratory, and central nervous systems 黏多糖贮积病

mu·co·pro·tein (mu″ko-pro'tēn) a covalently linked conjugate of protein and polysaccharide, the latter containing many hexosamine residues and constituting 4 to 30 percent of the weight of the compound; they occur mainly in mucus secretions 黏蛋白

mu·co·pu·ru·lent (mu″ko-pu'roo-lənt) containing both mucus and pus 黏液脓性的

mu·co·pus (mu'ko-pus″) mucus blended with pus 黏液性脓

Mu·cor (mu'kor) a genus of fungi some species of which cause mucormycosis 毛霉菌属

Mu·co·ra·les (mu″kə-ra'lēz) an order of fungi, including bread molds and related fungi, most of which are saprobes. Species of genera *Absidia, Mucor,* and *Rhizopus* cause mucormycosis 毛霉菌目

mu·cor·my·co·sis (mu″kor-mi-ko'sis) infection by fungi of the order Mucorales, usually in debilitated or immunocompromised patients, the organisms are generally inhaled or enter via a cutaneous lesion, invade and spread via the blood vessels, and affect numerous systems, with clinical manifestations ranging from chronic to fulminant 毛霉菌病

mu·co·sa (mu-ko'sə) [L.] tunica mucosa; the mucous membrane lining of various tubular structures 黏膜；**muco'sal** adj.

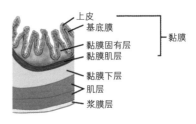

上皮
基底膜
黏膜固有层
黏膜肌层
黏膜
黏膜下层
肌层
浆膜层

▲ 小肠壁黏膜

mu·cous (mu′kəs) 1. pertaining to or resembling mucus 黏液或黏液样的；2. covered with mucus 被黏液覆盖的；3. secreting, producing, or containing mucus 分泌、产生或含有黏液的

mu·cus (mu′kəs) the free slime of the mucous membranes, composed of secretion of the glands, various salts, desquamated cells, and leukocytes 黏液

mug·wort (mug′wort) 1. any of several plants of the genus *Artemisia,* particularly *A. vulgaris* 蒿属植物；2. a preparation of *A. vulgaris,* used internally for gastrointestinal complaints and as a tonic; also used in homeopathy and traditional Chinese medicine 艾蒿

mul·ti·al·le·lic (mul″te-ə-le′lik) pertaining to or having many alleles at a single gene locus 多等位基因的

mul·ti·cen·tric (mul″te-sen′trik) polycentric 多中心的

mul·ti·fac·to·ri·al (mul″te-fak-tor′e-əl) 1. of or pertaining to, or arising through the action of, many factors 多因子的，多因素的；2. in genetics, arising as the result of the interaction of several genes and usually, to some extent, of nongenetic factors 多遗传因子的

mul·ti·fid (mul′tĭ-fid) cleft into many parts 多裂的

mul·ti·fo·cal (mul″te-fo′kəl) arising from or pertaining to many foci 多病灶的；由多病灶引起的；多疫源地的

mul·ti·grav·i·da (mul″te-grav′ĭ-də) a woman who is pregnant and has been pregnant at least twice before 经孕妇

mul·ti·loc·u·lar (mul″te-lok′u-lər) having many cells or compartments 多腔的，多房的

mul·ti·nod·u·lar (mul″te-nod′u-lər) composed of many nodules 多结节的

mul·ti·nu·cle·ate (mul″te-noo′kle-āt) 同 multinucleated

mul·ti·nu·cle·at·ed (mul″te-noo′kle-āt″əd) of cells, having more than one nucleus 多核的

mul·tip·a·ra (məl-tip′ə-rə) a woman who has had two or more pregnancies resulting in viable fetuses, whether or not the offspring were alive at birth 经产妇；**multip′arous** *adj.*；**grand m.,** a woman who has had six or more pregnancies resulting in viable fetuses 多产妇（妊娠 6 次或 6 次以上，而且胎儿都能存活）

mul·ti·par·i·ty (mul″te-par′ĭ-te) 1. the condition of being a multipara 经产；2. the production of several offspring in one gestation 多胎产

mul·ti·ple (mul′tĭ-pəl) manifold; occurring in or affecting various parts of the body at once 多数的；多发的

mul·ti·sen·so·ry (mul″te-sen′sə-re) capable of responding to more than one kind of sensory input, as certain neurons do in the central nervous system 多种感觉（并用）的

mul·ti·va·lent (mul″te-va′lənt) 多价体 1. having the power of combining with three or more univalent atoms 有两价或两价以上的；2. active against several strains of an organism 能抗多种抗原或微生物的

mum·mi·fi·ca·tion (mum″ĭ-fĭ-ka′shən) the shriveling up of a tissue, as in dry gangrene, or of a dead, retained fetus 干尸化，木乃伊化，干性坏疽

mumps (mumps) an acute contagious paramyxovirus disease seen mainly in childhood, involving chiefly the salivary glands, most often the parotids; other tissues such as meninges and testes are occasionally affected 流行性腮腺炎

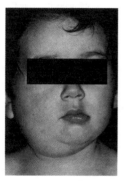

▲ 流行性腮腺炎

Mu·pap·il·lo·ma·vi·rus (mu-pap″ĭ-lo′mə-vi″rəs) a genus of the family Papillomaviridae that contains a few of the human papillomaviruses 乳头瘤病毒科中的一个属

mu·pir·o·cin (mu-pir′o-sin) an antibacterial derived from *Pseudomonas fluorescens,* effective against staphylococci and nonenteric streptococci; used topically in the treatment of impetigo and, intranasally as the calcium salt, in the treatment of nasal colonization by *Staphylococcus aureus* 莫匹罗星（抗生素）

mu·ral (mu′rəl) pertaining to or occurring in the wall of a body cavity 壁的，腔壁的

mu·ram·i·dase (mu-ram′ĭ-dās) lysozyme 胞壁质酶，溶菌酶

mu·rex·ine (mu-rek′sin) a neurotoxin from the hypobranchial gland of the snail *Murex*. It is called purpurine when derived from snails of the genus *Purpura* 骨螺毒素

mu·rine (mu′rin) pertaining to, derived from, or

characteristic of mice or rats 鼠的，鼠性的

mur·mur (mur′mər) [L.] an auscultatory sound, particularly a periodic sound of short duration of cardiac or vascular origin 杂音；**anemic m.,** a cardiac murmur heard in anemia 贫血性杂音；**aortic m.,** one generated by blood flowing through a diseased aorta or aortic valve 主动脉瓣杂音；**arterial m.,** one over an artery, sometimes aneurysmal and sometimes constricted 动脉杂音；**Austin Flint m.,** a presystolic murmur heard at the apex in aortic regurgitation 奥斯汀·弗林特杂音（主动脉瓣反流患者的心尖部舒张中、晚期杂音）；**cardiac m.,** one of finite length generated by turbulence of blood flow through the heart 心脏杂音；**Carey Coombs m.,** a rumbling mid-diastolic murmur occurring in the active phase of rheumatic fever 凯美库姆杂音（心尖部隆隆样舒张中期杂音，见于急性风湿热，愈后消失）；**continuous m.,** a humming cardiac murmur heard throughout systole and diastole 连续性杂音；**Cruveilhier-Baumgarten m.,** one heard at the abdominal wall over veins connecting the portal and caval systems Cruveilhier-Baumgarten 杂音（在腹壁闻及的连接门腔静脉系统的静脉杂音）；**diastolic m.,** cardiac murmurs heard during diastole, usually due to semilunar valve regurgitation or to altered blood flow through atrioventricular valves 舒张期杂音；**Duroziez m.,** a double murmur over the femoral or other large peripheral artery; due to aortic insufficiency Duroziez 杂音（股动脉双重杂音，发生于主动脉关闭不全时）；**ejection m.,** a type of systolic murmur usually heard in midsystole when ejection volume and velocity of blood flow are maximal, such as in aortic or pulmonary stenosis 喷射性杂音；**extracardiac m.,** one heard over the heart but originating from another structure 心外杂音；**friction m.,** 摩擦杂音，参见 *rub*；**functional m.,** a cardiac murmur generated in the absence of organic cardiac disease 功能性杂音；**Gibson m.,** a long, rumbling cardiac murmur heard for most of systole and diastole, usually in the second left interspace near the sternum, indicative of patent ductus arteriosus Gibson 杂音，机器样杂音（动脉导管未闭时，双期连续性杂音）；**Graham Steell m.,** one due to pulmonary regurgitation in patients with pulmonary hypertension and mitral stenosis 格雷厄姆·斯蒂尔杂音（肺动脉高压所致肺动脉瓣相对关闭不全时的舒张期杂音）；**heart m.,** 同 cardiac m.；**innocent m.,** 同 functional m.；**machinery m.,** 同 Gibson m.；**musical m.,** a cardiac murmur having a periodic harmonic pattern 音乐性杂音；**organic m.,** one due to a lesion in an organ, e.g., the heart, a vessel, or a lung 器质性杂音；**pansystolic m.,** a regurgitant murmur heard throughout systole 全收

缩期杂音；**pericardial m.,** 心包杂音，参见 *rub* 下词条；**prediastolic m.,** a cardiac murmur heard just before and with diastole; due to mitral obstruction or to aortic or pulmonary regurgitation 舒张前杂音；**presystolic m.,** a cardiac murmur heard just before ventricular ejection, usually associated with atrial contraction and the acceleration of blood flow through a narrowed atrioventricular valve 收缩期前杂音；**pulmonic m.,** a murmur due to disease of the pulmonary valve or artery 肺动脉杂音；**regurgitant m.,** one due to regurgitation of blood through an abnormal valvular orifice 反流杂音；**seagull m.,** a raucous murmur with musical qualities, such as that heard occasionally in aortic insufficiency 海鸥鸣样杂音；**Still m.,** a low-frequency, vibratory or buzzing, functional cardiac murmur of childhood, heard in midsystole Still 杂音（为儿童期的一种功能性收缩中期心脏杂音）；**systolic m.,** cardiac murmurs heard during systole; usually due to mitral or tricuspid regurgitation or to aortic or pulmonary obstruction 收缩期杂音；**to-and-fro m.,** a friction rub heard in both systole and diastole 往返性杂音；**vascular m.,** one heard over a blood vessel 血管杂音；**vesicular m.,** vesicular breath sounds 肺泡呼吸音

mu·ro·mo·nab-CD3 (mu″ro-mo′nab) a murine monoclonal antibody to the CD3 antigen of human T cells that functions as an immunosuppressant in the treatment of acute allograft rejection of renal, hepatic, and cardiac transplants 莫罗单抗 -CD3

Mus (mus) a genus of rodents, including *M. mus′culus,* the common house mouse 鼠属

Mus·ca (mus′kə) [L.] a genus of flies, including the common housefly, *M. domes′tica,* which may serve as a vector of various pathogens; its larvae may cause myiasis 蝇属

mus·ca (mus′kə) pl. *mus′cae.* A fly 蝇；**mus′cae volitan′tes** specks seen as floating before the eyes 飞蚊症

mus·ca·rine (mus′kə-rēn) a poisonous cholinomimetic alkaloid from various mushrooms, e.g., *Amanita muscaria;* its stimulatory effects cause salivation, lacrimation, urination, and diaphoresis in addition to gastrointestinal symptoms 毒蝇碱

mus·ca·rin·ic (mus″kə-rin′ik) denoting the cholinergic effects of muscarine on postganglionic parasympathetic neural impulses 毒蕈碱的

mus·cle (mus′əl) an organ that by contraction produces movement of an animal organism; see Plates 3 to 7. Note: the word "muscle" is often omitted from the names of individual muscles 肌，见图 3 至图 7；**abductor digiti minimi m. of foot,** abductor muscle of little toe: *origin,* medial and lateral tubercles of calcaneus, plantar fascia; *insertion,* lateral surface of base of proximal phalanx of little toe; *innervation,* superficial branch of lateral plantar; action, abducts little toe 小趾展肌，又称 *musculus abductor digiti minimi pedis*；**abductor digiti minimi m. of hand,** *origin,* pisiform bone, tendon of flexor carpi ulnaris muscle; *insertion,* medial surface of base of proximal phalanx of little finger; *innervation,* ulnar; *action,* abducts little finger 小指展肌，又称 *musculus abductor digiti minimi manus*；**abductor hallucis m.,** abductor muscle of great toe: *origin,* medial tubercle of calcaneus, plantar fascia; *insertion,* medial surface of base of proximal phalanx of great toe; *innervation,* medial plantar; *action,* abducts, flexes great toe 拇展肌，又称 *musculus abductor hallucis*；**abductor pollicis brevis m.,** short abductor muscle of thumb:*origin,*scaphoid, ridge of trapezium, flexor retinaculum of hand; *insertion,*lateral surface of base of proximal phalanx of thumb;*innervation,* median; *action,* abducts thumb 拇短展肌，又称 *musculus abductor pollicis brevis*；**abductor pollicis longus m.,** long abductor muscle of thumb: *origin,* posterior surfaces of radius and ulna; *insertion,* radial side of base of first metacarpal bone; *innervation,* posterior interosseous; *action,* abducts, extends thumb 拇长展肌，又称 *musculus abductor pollicis longus*；**adductor brevis m.,** short adductor muscle: *origin,* outer surface of body and inferior ramus of pubis; *insertion,* upper part of linea aspera of femur; *innervation,* obturator; *action,* adducts, rotates, flexes thigh 短收肌，又称 *musculus adductor brevis*；**adductor hallucis m.,** adductor muscle of great toe (2 heads): *origin,* OBLIQUE HEAD— bases of second through fourth metatarsals, and sheath of fibularis longus muscle, TRANSVERSE HEAD—capsules of metatarsophalangeal joints of three lateral toes; *insertion,* lateral side of base of proximal phalanx of great toe; *innervation,* lateral plantar; action, adducts great toe 拇收肌，又称 *musculus adductor hallucis*；**adductor longus m.,** long adductor muscle: *origin,* crest and symphysis of pubis; *insertion,* linea aspera of femur; innervation, obturator; *action,* adducts, rotates, flexes thigh 长收肌，又称 *musculus adductor longus*；**adductor magnus m.,** great adductor muscle (2 parts): *origin,* DEEP PART—inferior ramus of pubis, ramus of ischium, SUPERFICIAL PART—ischial tuber; *insertion,* DEEP PART—linea aspera of femur, SUPERFICIAL PART—adductor tubercle of femur; *innervation,* DEEP PART—obturator, SUPERFICIAL PART—sciatic; *action,* DEEP PART—adducts thigh, SUPERFICIAL PART—extends thigh 大收肌，又称 *musculus adductor magnus*；**adductor minimus m.,** smallest adductor muscle: a name given the anterior portion of the adductor magnus muscle; *insertion,* ischium, body and ramus of pubis; *innervation,* obturator and sciatic; *action,* adducts thigh 小收肌，又称 *musculus adductor minimus*；**adductor pollicis m.,** adductor muscle of thumb (2 heads): *origin,* OBLIQUE HEAD—sheath of flexor carpi radialis, palmar ligaments of carpus, capitate bone, and bases of second and third metacarpals, TRANSVERSE HEAD—anterior surface of third metacarpal; *insertion,* medial surface of base of proximal phalanx of thumb; *innervation,* ulnar; *action,* adducts, opposes thumb 拇收肌，又称 *musculus adductor pollicis*；**agonistic m.,** one opposed in action by another muscle (the antagonistic m.) 主动肌；**anconeus m.,** *origin,* back of lateral epicondyle of humerus; *insertion,* olecranon and posterior surface of ulna; *innervation,* radial; *action,* extends forearm 肘肌，又称 *musculus anconeus*；**anorectoperineal m's,** bands of smooth muscle fibers extending from the anorectal flexure of the rectum to the membranous urethra in the male 直肠尿道肌，又称 *musculi anorectoperineales*；**antagonistic m.,** one that counteracts the action of another muscle (the agonistic m.) 对抗肌，拮抗肌；**antigravity m's,** the muscles, mainly extensors of the knees, hips, and back, that by their tone resist the constant pull of gravity in the maintenance of normal posture 抗重力肌；**antitragicus m.,** *origin,* outer part of antitragus; *insertion,* caudate process of helix and anthelix; *innervation,* temporal and posterior auricular 对耳屏肌，又称 *musculus antitragicus*；**appendicular m's,** the muscles of a limb 附属肌，肢体肌；**arrector pili m.,** a type of tiny smooth muscle of the skin whose contraction causes the hair to stand erect with cutis anserina (goose flesh): *origin,* dermis; *insertion,* a hair follicle; *innervation,* sympathetic; *action,* elevates hair of skin 立毛肌，又称 *musculus arrector pili*；**articular m.,** one that has one end attached to a joint capsule 关节肌；**articularis cubiti m.,** articular muscle of elbow: a few fibers of the deep surface of the triceps brachii that insert into the posterior ligament and synovial membrane of the elbow joint 肘关节肌，又称 *musculus articularis cubiti*；**articularis genus m.,** articular muscle of knee: origin, distal anterior surface of femur; *insertion,* synovial membrane of knee joint; *innervation,* femoral; *action,* lifts capsule of knee joint 膝关节肌，又称 *musculus articularis genus*；**aryepiglottic m.,** an inconstant fascicle of the oblique arytenoid muscle, originating from the apex of the arytenoid cartilage and inserting on the lateral margin of the epiglottis 杓会厌肌；**arytenoid m., oblique,** one of the intrinsic muscles of the larynx:

M

origin, muscular process of arytenoid cartilage; *insertion,* apex of opposite arytenoid cartilage; *innervation,* recurrent laryngeal; *action,* closes inlet of larynx 杓斜肌, 又称 *musculus arytenoideus obliquus*；**arytenoid m., transverse,** one of the intrinsic muscles of the larynx: *origin,* lateral border of posterior surface of arytenoid cartilage; *insertion,* lateral border of posterior surface of opposite arytenoid cartilage; *innervation,* recurrent laryngeal; *action,* approximates arytenoid cartilages 杓横肌, 又称 *musculus arytenoideus transversus*；**m's of auditory ossicles,** the two muscles of the middle ear, the tensor tympani and the stapedius 听小骨肌；**auricular m's,** 1. the extrinsic auricular muscles, including the anterior, posterior, and superior auricular muscles 耳外肌；2. the intrinsic auricular muscles that extend from one part of the auricle to another, including the helicis major, helicis minor, tragicus, antitragicus, transverse auricular, and oblique auricular muscles 耳内肌；**auricular m., anterior,** *origin,* superficial temporal fascia; *insertion,* cartilage of ear; *innervation,* facial; *action,* draws the auricle forward 耳前肌, 又称 *musculus auricularis anterior*；**auricular m., oblique,** *origin,* cranial surface of concha; *insertion,* cranial surface of auricle above concha; *innervation,* temporal and posterior auricular 耳斜肌, 又称 *musculus obliquus auriculae*；**auricular m., posterior,** *origin,* mastoid process; *insertion,* cartilage of ear; *innervation,* facial; *action,* draws auricle backward 耳后肌, 又称 *musculus auricularis posterior*；**auricular m., superior,** *origin,* galea aponeurotica; *insertion,* cartilage of ear; *innervation,* facial; *action,* raises auricle 耳上肌, 又称 *musculus auricularis superior*；**auricular m., transverse,** *origin,* cranial surface of auricle; *insertion,* circumference of auricle; *innervation,* posterior auricular; *action,* retracts helix 耳横肌, 又称 *musculus transversus auriculae*；**Bell m.,** the muscular strands between the ureteric orifices and the uvula vesicae, bounding the trigone of the urinary bladder Bell 肌；**biceps brachii m.,** biceps muscle of arm (2 heads): *origin,* LONG HEAD— upper border of glenoid fossa, SHORT HEAD— apex of coracoid process; *insertion,* radial tuber and fascia of forearm; *innervation,* musculocutaneous; *action,* flexes forearm, supinates hand 肱二头肌, 又称 *musculus biceps brachii*；**biceps femoris m.,** biceps muscle of thigh (2 heads): *origin,* LONG HEAD— ischial tuberosity, SHORT HEAD— linea aspera of femur; *insertion,* head of fibula, lateral condyle of tibia; *innervation,* LONG HEAD— tibial, SHORT HEAD— peroneal, popliteal; *action,* flexes leg, extends thigh 股二头肌, 又称 *musculus biceps femoris*；**bipen-**nate m., 同 pennate m.；**brachialis m.,** brachial muscle: *origin,* anterior surface of humerus; *insertion,* coronoid process of ulna; *innervation,* radial, musculocutaneous; *action,* flexes forearm 肱肌, 又称 *musculus brachialis*；**brachioradialis m.,** brachioradial muscle: *origin,* lateral supracondylar ridge of humerus; *insertion,* lower end of radius; *innervation,* radial; *action,* flexes forearm 肱桡肌, 又称 *musculus brachioradialis*；**bronchoesophageus m.,** bronchoesophageal muscle: a name given muscular fasciculi that arise from the wall of the left bronchus and reinforce muscles of the esophagus 支气管食管肌, 又称 *musculus bronchooesophageus*；**Brücke m.,** the longitudinal fibers of the ciliary muscle Brücke 肌；**buccinator m.,** *origin,* buccinator ridge of mandible, alveolar process of maxilla, pterygomandibular ligament; *insertion,* orbicularis oris at angle of mouth; *innervation,* buccal branch of facial; *action,* compresses cheek and retracts angle of the mouth 颊肌, 又称 *musculus buccinator*；**bulbocavernosus m., bulbospongiosus m.,** *origin,* central point of perineum, median raphe of bulb; *insertion,* fascia of penis or clitoris; *innervation,* pudendal; *action,* constricts spongy urethra in males and vaginal orifice in females, contributes to erection of penis or clitoris 球海绵体肌, 又称 *musculus bulbospongiosus*；**cardiac m.,** the muscle of the heart, composed of striated but involuntary muscle fibers, comprising the chief component of the myocardium and lining the walls of the adjoining large vessels 心肌；**ceratocricoid m.,** a name given a muscular fasciculus arising from the cricoid cartilage and inserted on the inferior cornu of the thyroid cartilage, considered one of the intrinsic muscles of the larynx 角环肌, 又称 *musculus ceratocricoideus*；**cervical m's,** the muscles of the neck, including the sternocleidomastoid, longus colli, suprahyoid, infrahyoid, and scalene muscles 颈肌；**chondroglossus m.,** *origin,* medial side and base of lesser cornu of hyoid bone; *insertion,* substance of tongue; *innervation,* hypoglossal; *action,* depresses, retracts tongue 小角舌肌, 又称 *musculus chondroglossus*；**ciliary m.,** *origin,* scleral spur; *insertion,* outer layers of choroid and ciliary processes; *innervation,* oculomotor, parasympathetic; *action,* affects shape of lens in visual accommodation 睫状肌, 又称 *musculus ciliaris*；**coccygeus m.,** coccygeal muscle: *origin,* ischial spine; *insertion,* lateral border of lower part of sacrum, upper coccyx; *innervation,* third and fourth sacral; *action,* supports and raises coccyx 尾骨肌, 又称 *musculus ischiococcygeus*；**compressor urethrae m.,** compressor muscle of urethra (females): *origin,* ischiopubic ramus on each side; *insertion*, blends with its partner on the other side anterior to the urethra; *innervation*, perineal branches of pudendal nerve; *action*, accessory urethral sphincter 尿道膜部括约肌，又称 *musculus compressor urethrae*; **congenerous m's**, muscles having a common action or function 协同肌; **constrictor m. of pharynx, inferior**, *origin*, undersurfaces of cricoid and thyroid cartilages; *insertion*, median raphe of mastoid wall of pharynx; *innervation*, glossopharyngeal, pharyngeal plexus, branches of superior laryngeal and recurrent laryngeal; *action*, constricts pharynx. It is often described in two parts: cricopharyngeus and thyropharyngeus muscles 咽下缩肌，又称 *musculus constrictor pharyngis inferior*; **constrictor m. of pharynx, middle**, *origin*, horns of hyoid and stylohyoid ligament; *insertion*, median raphe of mastoid wall of pharynx; *innervation*, pharyngeal plexus of vagus and glossopharyngeal; *action*, constricts pharynx 咽中缩肌，又称 *musculus constrictor pharyngis medius*; **constrictor m. of pharynx, superior**, *origin*, medial pterygoid plate, pterygomandibular raphe, mylohyoid ridge of mandible, and mucous membrane of floor of mouth; *insertion*, median raphe of mastoid wall of pharynx; *innervation*, pharyngeal plexus of vagus; *action*, constricts pharynx 咽上缩肌，又称 *musculus constrictor pharyngis superior*; **coracobrachialis m.**, coracobrachial muscle: *origin*, coracoid process of scapula; *insertion*, medial surface of body of humerus; *innervation*, musculocutaneous; *action*, flexes, adducts arm 喙肱肌，又称 *musculus coracobrachialis*; **corrugator supercilii m.**, *origin*, medial end of superciliary arch; *insertion*, skin of eyebrow; *innervation*, facial; *action*, draws eyebrow downward and medially 皱眉肌，又称 *musculus corrugator supercilii*; **cremaster m.**, *origin*, inferior margin of internal oblique muscle of abdomen; *insertion*, pubic tubercle; *innervation*, genital branch of genitofemoral; *action*, elevates testis 提睾肌，又称 *musculus cremaster*; **cricoarytenoid m., lateral**, one of the intrinsic muscles of the larynx: *origin*, lateral surface of cricoid cartilage; *insertion*, muscular process of arytenoid cartilage; *innervation*, recurrent laryngeal; *action*, approximates vocal folds 环杓侧肌，又称 *musculus cricoarytenoideus lateralis*; **cricoarytenoid m., posterior**, one of the intrinsic muscles of the larynx: *origin*, lateral surface of cricoid cartilage; *insertion*, muscular process of arytenoid cartilage; *innervation*, recurrent laryngeal; *action*, approximates vocal folds 环杓后肌，又称 *musculus cricoarytenoideus lateralis*; **cricopharyngeus m.**, the part of the inferior pharyngeal constrictor muscle

arising from the cricoid cartilage 环咽肌；**cricothyroid m.**, one of the intrinsic muscles of the larynx: *origin*, front and side of cricoid cartilage; *insertion*, lamina of thyroid cartilage; *innervation*, external branch of superior laryngeal; *action*, tenses vocal folds 环甲肌，又称 *musculus cricothyroideus*; **cruciate m.**, a muscle in which the fiber bundles are arranged in the shape of an X 交叉肌；**cutaneous m.**, striated muscle that inserts into the skin 皮肌；**dartos m.**, dartos: the nonstriated muscle fibers of the tunica dartos, the deeper layers of which help to form the scrotal septum; the term may be used more broadly to denote the tunica dartos 肉膜肌，又称 *musculus dartos*; **deltoid m.**, *origin*, clavicle, acromion, spine of scapula; *insertion*, deltoid tuber of humerus; *innervation*, axillary; *action*, abducts, flexes, extends arm 三角肌，又称 *musculus deltoideus*; **depressor anguli oris m.**, depressor muscle of angle of mouth: *origin*, lower border of mandible; *insertion*, angle of mouth; *innervation*, facial; *action*, pulls down angle of mouth 降口角肌，又称 *musculus depressor anguli oris*; **depressor labii inferioris m.**, depressor muscle of lower lip: *origin*, anterior portion of lower border of mandible; *insertion*, orbicularis oris and skin of lower lip; *innervation*, facial; *action*, depresses lower lip 降下唇肌，又称 *musculus depressor labii inferioris*; **depressor septi nasi m.**, depressor muscle of nasal septum: *origin*, incisor fossa of maxilla; *insertion*, ala and septum of nose; *innervation*, facial; *action*, contracts nostril and depresses ala 降鼻中隔肌，又称 *musculus depressor septi nasi*; **depressor supercilii m.**, a name given a few fibers of the orbital part of the orbicularis oculi muscle that are inserted in the eyebrow, which they depress 降眉肌，又称 *musculus depressor supercilii*; **detrusor m.**, the bundles of smooth muscle fibers forming the muscular coat of the urinary bladder, which are arranged in a longitudinal and a circular layer and, on contraction, serve to expel urine 逼尿肌，又称 *musculus detrusor vesicae urinariae*; **digastric m.**, *origin*, ANTERIOR BELLY—digastric fossa on lower border of mandible near symphysis, POSTERIOR BELLY—mastoid notch of temporal bone; *insertion*, intermediate tendon on hyoid bone; *innervation*, ANTERIOR BELLY—mylohyoid, POSTERIOR BELLY—digastric branch of facial; *action*, elevates hyoid bone, lowers jaw 二腹肌，又称 *musculus digastricus*; **dilator m.**, a muscle that dilates 开大肌；**dilator pupillae m.**, a name applied to fibers extending radially from the sphincter of the pupil to the ciliary margin: *innervation*, sympathetic; *action*, dilates iris 瞳孔开大肌，又称 *musculus dilatator pupillae*; **epicranius m.**, epicranial muscle: a name given the muscular covering of the scalp, including the occipitofrontalis and temporoparietalis muscles, and the galea aponeurotica 颅顶肌，又称 *musculus epicranius*；**epimeric m.**, one derived from an epimere and innervated by a posterior ramus of a spinal nerve 上段（中胚层）肌；**erector spinae m.**, a name given the fibers of the more superficial of the deep muscles of the back, originating from the sacrum, spines of lumbar and eleventh and twelfth thoracic vertebrae, and iliac crest, which split and insert as the iliocostalis, longissimus, and spinalis muscles 竖脊肌，又称 *musculus erector spinae*；**m's of expression**, a group of cutaneous muscles of the facial structures, including the muscles of the scalp, ear, eyelids, nose, and mouth, and the platysma 表情肌；**extensor carpi radialis brevis m.**, short radial extensor muscle of wrist: *origin*, lateral epicondyle of humerus; *insertion*, base of third metacarpal bone; *innervation*, deep branch of radial; *action*, extends and abducts radiocarpal joint 桡侧腕短伸肌，又称 *musculus extensor carpi radialis brevis*；**extensor carpi radialis longus m.**, long radial extensor muscle of wrist: *origin*, lateral supracondylar ridge of humerus; *insertion*, base of second metacarpal bone; *innervation*, radial; *action*, extends and abducts radiocarpal joint 桡侧腕长伸肌，又称 *musculus extensor carpi radialis longus*；**extensor carpi ulnaris m.**, ulnar extensor muscle of wrist (2 heads): *origin*, SUPERFICIAL HEAD—lateral epicondyle of humerus, DEEP HEAD—posterior border of ulna; *insertion*, base of fifth metacarpal bone; *innervation*, deep branch of radial; *action*, extends and adducts radiocarpal joint 尺侧腕伸肌，又称 *musculus extensor carpi ulnaris*；**extensor digiti minimi m.**, extensor muscle of little finger: *origin*, common extensor tendon and adjacent intermuscular septa; *insertion*, extensor expansion of little finger; *innervation*, deep branch of radial; *action*, extends little finger 小指伸肌，又称 *musculus extensor digiti minimi*；**extensor digitorum m.**, extensor muscle of fingers: *origin*, lateral epicondyle of humerus; *insertion,* extensor expansion of each (nonthumb) finger; *innervation*, posterior interosseous; *action*, extends radiocarpal joint and phalanges 指伸肌，趾伸肌，又称 *musculus extensor digitorum*；**extensor digitorum brevis m.**, short extensor muscle of toes: *origin*, superior surface of calcaneus; *insertion*, tendons of extensor digitorum longus of first, second, third, and fourth toes; *innervation*, deep fibular; *action*, extends toes 趾短伸肌，又称 *musculus extensor digitorum brevis*；**extensor digitorum longus m.**, long extensor muscle of toes: *origin*, anterior surface of fibula, lateral condyle of tibia, interosseous membrane; *insertion*, extensor expansion of each of the four lateral toes; *innervation*, deep fibular; *action*, extends toes 趾长伸肌，又称 *musculus extensor digitorum longus*；**extensor hallucis brevis m.**, short extensor muscle of great toe: a name given the portion of the extensor digitorum brevis muscle that goes to the great toe 踇短伸肌，又称 *musculus extensor hallucis brevis*；**extensor hallucis longus m.**, long extensor muscle of great toe: *origin*, front of fibula and interosseous membrane; *insertion*, base of distal phalanx of great toe; *innervation*, deep fibular; *action*, dorsiflexes ankle joint, extends great toe 踇长伸肌，又 称 *musculus extensor hallucis longus*；**extensor indicis m.**, extensor muscle of index finger: *origin*, posterior surface of body of ulna, interosseous membrane; *insertion*, extensor expansion of index finger; *innervation*, posterior interosseous; *action*, extends index finger 示指伸肌，又称 *musculus extensor indicis*；**extensor pollicis brevis m.**, short extensor muscle of thumb: *origin*, posterior surface of radius and interosseous membrane; *insertion*, base of proximal phalanx of thumb; *innervation*, posterior interosseous; *action*, extends thumb 拇短伸肌，又称 *musculus extensor digitorum brevis*；**extensor pollicis longus m.**, long extensor muscle of thumb: *origin*, posterior surface of ulna and interosseous membrane; *insertion*, base of distal phalanx of thumb; *innervation*, posterior interosseous; *action*, extends thumb, adducts and rotates thumb laterally 拇长伸肌，又称 *musculus extensor pollicis longus*；**extraocular m's**, the six voluntary muscles that move the eyeball: superior, inferior, middle, and lateral recti, and superior and inferior oblique muscles 眼外肌；**extrinsic m.**, one not originating in the limb or part in which it is inserted 外部肌；**m's of eye**, 同 extraocular m's；**facial m's**, m's of expression 面肌；**fibularis brevis m.**, 同 peroneus brevis m.；**fibularis longus m.**, 同 peroneus longus m.；**fibularis tertius m.**, 同 peroneus tertius m.；**fixation m's**, **fixator m's**, accessory muscles that serve to steady a part. 固定肌群；**flexor accessorius m.**, *origin*, calcaneus and plantar fascia; *insertion*, tendons of flexor digitorum longus; *innervation*, lateral plantar; *action*, aids in flexing toes 副趾肌，足底方肌，又称 *musculus flexor accessorius* 和 *musculus quadratus plantae*；**flexor carpi radialis m.**, radial flexor muscle of wrist: *origin*, medial epicondyle of humerus; *insertion*, base of second metacarpal; *innervation*, median; *action*, flexes and abducts radiocarpal joint 桡侧腕屈肌，又 称 *musculus flexor carpi radialis*；**flexor carpi ulnaris m.**, ulnar flexor muscle of wrist (2 heads):

origin, SUPERFICIAL HEAD—medial epicondyle of humerus, DEEP HEAD—olecranon, ulna, intermuscular septum; *insertion*, pisiform, hook of hamate bone, proximal end of fifth metacarpal; *innervation*, ulnar; *action*, flexes and adducts radiocarpal joint 尺侧腕屈肌，又称 *musculus flexor carpi ulnaris*；**flexor digiti minimi brevis m.** of foot, short flexor muscle of little toe: *origin*, base of fifth metatarsal, sheath of fibularis longus muscle; *insertion*, lateral surface of base of proximal phalanx of little toe; *innervation*, lateral plantar; *action*, flexes little toe 小趾短屈肌，又称 *musculus flexor digiti minimi pedis*；**flexor digiti minimi brevis m.** of hand, short flexor muscle of little finger: *origin*, hook of hamate bone, palmar surface of flexor retinaculum; *insertion*, medial side of proximal phalanx of little finger; *innervation*, ulnar; *action*, flexes little finger 小指短屈肌，又称 *musculus flexor digiti minimi brevis manus*；**flexor digitorum brevis m.**, short flexor muscle of toes: *origin*, medial tuber of calcaneus, plantar fascia; *insertion*, middle phalanges of four lateral toes; *innervation*, medial plantar; *action*, flexes four lateral toes 趾短屈肌，又称 *musculus flexor digitorum brevis*；**flexor digitorum longus m.**, long flexor muscle of toes: *origin*, posterior surface of body of tibia; *insertion*, distal phalanges of four lateral toes; *innervation*, posterior tibial; *action*, flexes toes and plantarflexes foot 趾长屈肌，又称 *musculus flexor digitorum longus*；**flexor digitorum profundus m.**, deep flexor muscle of fingers: *origin*, body of ulna, coronoid process, interosseous membrane; *insertion*, bases of distal phalanges of fingers; *innervation*, ulnar and anterior interosseous; *action*, flexes distal phalanges 指深屈肌，又称 *musculus flexor digitorum profundus*；**flexor digitorum superficialis m.**, superficial flexor muscle of fingers (2 heads): *origin*, HUMEROULNAR HEAD—medial epicondyle of humerus, coronoid process of ulna, RADIAL HEAD—oblique line of radius, anterior border; *insertion*, sides of middle phalanges of four (nonthumb) fingers; *innervation*, median; *action*, primarily flexes middle phalanges 指浅屈肌，又称 *musculus flexor digitorum superficialis*；**flexor hallucis brevis m.**, short flexor muscle of great toe: *origin*, undersurface of cuboid, lateral cuneiform; *insertion* (2 heads): both sides of base of proximal phalanx of toe, one head on each side; *innervation*, medial plantar; *action*, flexes great toe 蹈短屈肌，又称 *musculus flexor hallucis brevis*；**flexor hallucis longus m.**, long flexor muscle of great toe: *origin*, posterior surface of fibula; *insertion*, base of distal phalanx of great toe; *innervation*, tibial; *action*, flexes great toe 蹈长屈肌，又称 *musculus*

flexor hallucis longus；**flexor pollicis brevis m.**, short flexor muscle of thumb: *origin*, SUPERFICIAL HEAD—flexor retinaculum, distal part of tubercle of trapezium bone; MEDIAL HEAD (when present)—trapezoid and capitate bones and palmar ligaments of distal row of carpal bones; *insertion*, radial side of base of proximal phalanx of thumb; *innervation*, median, ulnar; *action*, flexes and adducts thumb 拇短屈肌，又称 *musculus flexor pollicis brevis*；**flexor pollicis longus m.**, long flexor muscle of thumb: *origin*, anterior surface of radius, interosseous membrane, and medial epicondyle of humerus or coronoid process of ulna; *insertion*, base of distal phalanx of thumb; *innervation*, anterior interosseous; *action*, flexes thumb 拇长屈肌，又称 *musculus flexor pollicis longus*；**fusiform m.**, a spindle-shaped muscle in which the fibers are approximately parallel to the long axis of the muscle but converge upon a tendon at either end 梭形肌；**gastrocnemius m.**, *origin*, MEDIAL HEAD—popliteal surface of femur, upper part of medial condyle, and capsule of knee, LATERAL HEAD— lateral condyle and capsule of knee; *insertion*, aponeurosis unites with tendon of soleus to form Achilles tendon; *innervation*, tibial; *action*, plantarflexes ankle joint, flexes knee joint 腓肠肌，又称 *musculus gastrocnemius*；**gemellus m., inferior**, *origin*, tuber of ischium; *insertion*, greater trochanter of femur; *innervation*, nerve to quadratus femoris; *action*, rotates thigh laterally 下孖肌，又称 *musculus gemellus inferior*；**gemellus m., superior**, *origin*, spine of ischium; *insertion*, greater trochanter of femur; *innervation*, nerve to internal obturator; *action*, rotates thigh laterally 上孖肌，又称 *musculus gemellus superior*；**genioglossus m.**, *origin*, superior mental spine; *insertion*, hyoid bone and inferior surface of tongue; *innervation*, hypoglossal; *action*, protrudes and depresses tongue 颏舌肌，又称 *musculus genioglossus*；**geniohyoid m.**, *origin*, inferior mental spine; *insertion*, body of hyoid bone; *innervation*, a branch of first cervical nerve through hypoglossal; *action*, elevates and draws hyoid forward, or depresses mandible when hyoid is fixed by its depressors 颏舌骨肌，又称 *musculus geniohyoideus*；**gluteus maximus m.**, *origin*, posterior aspect of ilium, posterior surface of sacrum and coccyx, sacrotuberous ligament, fascia covering gluteus medius; *insertion*, iliotibial tract of fascia lata, gluteal tuber of femur; *innervation*, inferior gluteal; *action*, extends, abducts, and rotates thigh laterally 臀大肌，又称 *musculus gluteus maximus*；**gluteus medius m.**, *origin*, lateral surface of ilium between anterior and posterior gluteal lines; *insertion*, greater trochanter

M

of femur; *innervation*, superior gluteal; *action*, abducts and rotates thigh medially 臀中肌，又称 *musculus gluteus medius*；**gluteus minimus m.**，*origin*, lateral surface of ilium between anterior and inferior gluteal lines; *insertion*, greater trochanter of femur; *innervation*, superior gluteal; *action*, abducts, rotates thigh medially 臀小肌，又称 *musculus gluteus minimus*；**gracilis m.** *origin*, body and inferior ramus of pubis; *insertion*, medial surface of body of tibia; *innervation*, obturator; *action*, adducts thigh, flexes knee joint 股薄肌，又称 *musculus gracilis*；**hamstring m's**, the muscles of the back of the thigh: biceps femoris, semitendinosus, and semimembranosus muscles 腘绳肌；**helicis major m.**, *origin*, spine of helix; *insertion*, anterior border of helix; *innervation*, auriculotemporal and posterior auricular; *action*, tenses skin of auditory canal 耳轮大肌，又称 *musculus helicis major*；**helicis minor m.**, *origin*, anterior rim of helix; *insertion*, concha; *innervation*, temporal, posterior auricular 耳轮小肌，又称 *musculus helicis minor*；**Horner m.**, the lacrimal part of the orbicularis oculi muscle 霍纳肌，眼轮匝肌泪道部；**Houston m.**, fibers of the bulbocavernosus muscle compressing the dorsal vein of the penis Houston 肌，豪斯顿肌，即阴茎背静脉压肌；**hyoglossus m.**, hyoglossal muscle: *origin*, body and greater horn of hyoid bone; *insertion*, side of tongue; *innervation*, hypoglossal; *action*, depresses and retracts tongue 舌骨舌肌，又称 *musculus hyoglossus*；**m's of hyoid bone**, the infrahyoid and suprahyoid muscles 舌骨肌群；**hypomeric m.**, one derived from a hypomere and innervated by an anterior ramus of a spinal nerve 下段（中胚层）肌；**hypothenar m's**, the intrinsic muscles of the little finger, flexing, abducting, and opposing it: they comprise the palmaris brevis, abductor digiti minimi, flexor digiti minimi brevis, and opponens digiti minimi muscles 小鱼际肌；**iliacus m.**, iliac muscle: *origin*, iliac fossa and base of sacrum; *insertion*, greater psoas tendon and lesser trochanter of femur; *innervation*, femoral; *action*, flexes thigh, trunk on limb 髂肌，又称 *musculus iliacus*；**iliococcygeus m.**, iliococcygeal muscle: the posterior portion of the levator ani, which originates as far anteriorly as the obturator canal and inserts on the side of the coccyx and the anococcygeal ligament: *innervation*, third and fourth sacral; *action*, helps to support pelvic viscera and resist increases in intra-abdominal pressure 髂尾肌，又称 *musculus iliococcygeus*；**iliocostalis m.**, iliocostal muscle: the lateral division of the erector spinae, which includes the *iliocostalis cervicis, iliocostalis thoracis*, and *iliocostalis lumborum muscles* 髂肋肌，又称 *musculus iliococcy-*

geus；**iliocostalis cervicis m.**, *origin*, angles of third, fourth, fifth, and sixth ribs; *insertion*, transverse processes of fourth, fifth, and sixth cervical vertebrae; *innervation*, branches of cervical; *action*, extends cervical spine 颈髂肋肌，又称 *musculus iliocostalis cervicis*；**iliocostalis lumborum m.**, *origin*, iliac crest; *insertion*, angles of lower six or seven ribs; *innervation*, branches of thoracic and lumbar; *action*, extends lumbar spine. The term is sometimes used to denote the combination of both the lumbar and thoracic (iliocostalis thoracis) parts, not just the lumbar 腰髂肋肌，又称 *musculus iliocostalis lumborum*；**iliocostalis thoracis m.**, *origin*, upper borders of angles of six lower ribs; *insertion*, angles of six upper ribs and transverse process of seventh cervical vertebra; *innervation*, branches of thoracic; *action*, keeps thoracic spine erect 胸髂肋肌。Cf. *iliocostalis lumborum m.*；**iliopsoas m.**, a compound muscle consisting of the iliacus and the psoas major 髂腰肌，又称 *musculus iliopsoas*；**incisive m's of inferior lip**, small bundles of muscle fibers, one arising from the incisive fossa of the mandible on each side and passing laterally to the angle of the mouth: *innervation*, facial; *action*, closely apply lower lip to teeth and alveolar arch 下唇切牙肌，又称 *musculi incisivi labii inferioris*；**incisive m's of superior lip**, small bundles of muscle fibers, one arising from the incisive fossa of the maxilla on each side and passing laterally to the angle of the mouth: *innervation*, facial; *action*, closely apply upper lip to teeth and alveolar arch 上唇切牙肌，又称 *musculi incisivi labii superioris*；**infrahyoid m's**, the muscles that anchor the hyoid bone to the sternum, clavicle, and scapula, including the sternohyoid, omohyoid, sternothyroid, and thyrohyoid muscles 舌骨下肌群；**infraspinatus m.**, *origin*, infraspinous fossa of scapula; *insertion*, greater tubercle of humerus; *innervation*, suprascapular; *action*, rotates humerus laterally 冈下肌，又称 *musculus infraspinatus*；**inspiratory m's**, those acting during inhalation, such as the respiratory diaphragm and the intercostal and pectoralis muscles 吸气肌；**intercostal m's, external**, *origin*, inferior border of rib (11 on each side); *insertion*, superior border of rib below; *innervation*, intercostal; *action*, primarily elevate ribs in inspiration, also active in expiration 肋间外肌，又称 *musculi intercostales externi*；**intercostal m's, innermost**, the layer of muscle fibers separated from the internal intercostal muscles by the intercostal nerves 肋间最内肌，又称 *musculi intercostales intimi*；**intercostal m's, internal**, *origin*, inferior border of rib and costal cartilage (11 on each side); *insertion*, superior border of rib and costal cartilage below; *innervation*, intercostal; *action*, draw ribs together in respiration and expulsive movements, also act in inspiration 肋间内肌，又称 *musculi intercostales interni*；**interossei m's, palmar**, palmar interosseous muscles (3): *origin*, sides of second, fourth, and fifth metacarpal bones; *insertion*, bases of proximal phalanges and corresponding extensor expansions of second, fourth, and fifth fingers; *innervation*, ulnar; *action*, adduct fingers, flex proximal phalanges, extend middle and distal phalanges 骨间掌侧肌，又称 *musculi interossei palmares*；**interossei m's, plantar**, plantar interosseous muscles (3): *origin*, medial surfaces of third, fourth, and fifth metatarsal bones; *insertion*, medial side of base of proximal phalanges of third, fourth, and fifth toes and their extensor expansions; *innervation*, lateral plantar; *action*, adduct, flex toes 骨间足底肌，又称 *musculi interossei plantares*；**interossei m's of foot,dorsal**, dorsal interosseous muscles of foot (4): *origin*, adjacent surfaces of metatarsal bones; *insertion*, base of proximal phalanges of second, third, and fourth toes and their extensor expansions; *innervation*, lateral plantar; *action*, abduct, flex toes 足骨间背侧肌，又称 *musculi interossei dorsales pedis*；**interossei m's of hand, dorsal**, dorsal interosseous muscles of hand (4): *origin*, by two heads from adjacent sides of metacarpal bones; *insertion*, bases of proximal phalanges and corresponding extensor expansions of second, third, and fourth fingers; *innervation*, ulnar; *action*, abduct fingers, flex proximal phalanges, extend middle and distal phalanges 手骨间背侧肌，又称 *musculi interossei dorsales manus*；**interspinales m's**, short bands of muscle fibers between spinous processes of contiguous vertebrae, including the *interspinales cervicis, thoracis*, and *lumborum muscles* 棘间肌，包括颈棘间肌、腰棘间肌和胸棘间肌，又称 *musculi interspinales*；**interspinales cervics m's**, paired bands of muscle fibers extending between spinous processes of contiguous cervical vertebrae, innervated by spinal nerves, and acting to extend the vertebral column 颈棘间肌，又称 *musculi interspinales cervicis*；**interspinales lumborum m's**, paired bands of muscle fibers extending between spinous processes of contiguous lumbar vertebrae, innervated by spinal nerves, and acting to extend the vertebral column 腰棘间肌，又称 *musculi interspinales lumborum*；**interspinales thoracis m's**, paired bands of muscle fibers extending between spinous processes of contiguous thoracic vertebrae, innervated by spinal nerves, and acting to extend the vertebral column 胸棘间肌，又称 *musculi interspinales thoracis*；**intertransversarii m's**, small mus-

cles passing between the transverse processes of contiguous vertebrae, including the lateral and medial lumbar, thoracic, and anterior, lateral posterior, and medial posterior cervical intertransversarii muscles 横突间肌，又称 *musculi intertransversarii*；**intertransversarii m's, anterior cervical**, small muscles passing between the anterior tubercles of adjacent cervical vertebrae, innervated by anterior primary rami of spinal nerves and acting to bend the vertebral column laterally 颈横突间前肌，又称 *musculi intertransversarii anteriores cervicis*；**intertransversarii m's, lateral lumbar**, small muscles passing between the transverse processes of adjacent lumbar vertebrae, innervated by anterior primary rami of spinal nerves, and acting to bend the vertebral column laterally 腰横突间外侧肌，又称 *musculi intertransversarii laterales lumborum*；**intertransversarii m's, lateral posterior cervical**, small muscles passing between the posterior tubercles of adjacent cervical vertebrae, lateral to the medial posterior intertransversarii, innervated by anterior primary rami of spinal nerves, and acting to bend the vertebral column laterally 颈横突间后外侧肌，又称 *musculi intertransversarii posteriores laterales cervicis*；**intertransversarii m's, medial lumbar**, small muscles passing from the accessory process of one lumbar vertebra to the mammillary process of the contiguous lumbar vertebra, innervated by posterior primary rami of spinal nerves, and acting to bend the vertebral column laterally 腰横突间内侧肌，又称 *musculi intertransversarii mediales lumborum*；**intertransversarii m's, medial posterior cervical**, small muscles passing between the posterior tubercles of adjacent cervical vertebrae, close to the vertebral body, innervated by posterior primary rami of spinal nerves, and acting to bend the vertebral column laterally 颈横突间后内侧肌，又称 *musculi intertransversarii posteriores mediales cervicis*；**intertransversarii m's,thoracic**, poorly developed muscle bundles extending between the anterior tubercles of adjacent thoracic vertebrae, innervated by posterior primary rami of spinal nerves and acting to bend the vertebral column laterally 胸横突间肌，又称 *intertransversarii thoracis*；**intra-auricular m's**, the stapedius and tensor tympani muscles 耳内肌；**intraocular m's**, the intrinsic muscles of the eyeball 眼内肌；**intrinsic m.**, one that is contained (origin, belly, and insertion) in the same limb or structure 内在肌；**involuntary m.**, one that is not under the control of the will, including both smooth and cardiac muscle 不随意肌；**iridic m's**, those controlling the iris 虹膜肌；**ischiocavernosus m.**, ischiocavernous muscle:

origin, ramus of ischium; *insertion*, crus of penis (or of clitoris); *innervation*, perineal; *action*, maintains erection of penis (clitoris) 坐骨海绵体肌，又称 *musculus ischiocavernosus*；**ischiococcygeus m.**，同 coccygeus m.；**Landström m.**，minute muscle fibers in the fascia around and behind the eyeball, attached in front to the anterior orbital fascia and eyelids Landström 肌，眼球后方及周围筋膜内的细小肌纤维，附着于眼眶前筋膜和眼睑上；**m's of larynx**, the intrinsic and extrinsic muscles of the larynx, including the oblique and transverse arytenoid, ceratocricoid, lateral and posterior cricoarytenoid, cricothyroid, thyroarytenoid, and vocalis muscles 喉肌；**latissimus dorsi m.**，*origin*, spines of lower thoracic vertebrae, lumbar and sacral vertebrae through attachment to thoracolumbar fascia, iliac crest, lower ribs, inferior angle of scapula; *insertion*, floor of intertubercular sulcus of humerus; *innervation*, thoracodorsal; *action*, adducts, extends, and rotates humerus medially 背阔肌，又称 *musculus latissimus dorsi*；**levator anguli oris m.**，*origin*, canine fossa of maxilla; *insertion*, orbicularis oris and skin at angle of mouth; *innervation*, facial; *action*, raises angle of mouth 提口角肌，又称 *musculus levator anguli oris*；**levator ani m.**，a name applied collectively to important muscular components of the pelvic diaphragm, including the pubococcygeus, puborectalis, and iliococcygeus muscles 肛提肌，又称 *musculus levator ani*；**levatores costarum m's**, levator muscles of ribs (12 on each side): originating from the transverse processes of the seventh cervical and first to eleventh thoracic vertebrae and inserting medial to the angle of a lower rib; innervated by intercostal nerves and aiding in elevation of the ribs in respiration 肋提肌，又称 *musculi levatores costarum*；**levatores costarum breves m's**, short levator muscles of ribs: the levatores costarum muscles of each side that insert medial to the angle of the rib next below the vertebra of origin 肋短提肌，又称 *musculi levatores costarum breves*；**levatores costarum longi m's**, long levator muscles of ribs: the lower levatores costarum muscles of each side, which have fascicles extending down to the second rib below the vertebra of origin 肋长提肌，又称 *musculi levatores costarum longi*；**levator glandulae thyroideae m.**, levator muscle of thyroid gland: an inconstant muscle originating on the isthmus or pyramid of the thyroid gland and inserting on the body of the hyoid bone 甲状腺提肌，又称 *musculus levator glandulae thyroideae*；**levator labii superioris m.**, levator muscle of upper lip: *origin*, lower orbital margin; *insertion*, muscle of upper lip; *innervation*, facial nerve; *ac-*

tion, raises upper lip 提上唇肌，又称 *musculus levator labii superioris*；**levator labii superioris alaeque nasi m.**, levator muscle of upper lip and ala of nose: *origin*, upper part of frontal process of maxilla; *insertion*, cartilage and skin of ala nasi, and upper lip; *innervation*, infraorbital branch of facial; *action*, raises upper lip and dilates nostril 提上唇鼻翼肌，又称 *musculus levator labii superioris alaeque nasi*；**levator palpebrae superioris m.**, levator muscle of upper eyelid: *origin*, sphenoid bone above optic canal; *insertion*, tarsal plate and skin of upper eyelid; *innervation*, oculomotor; *action*, raises upper lid 上睑提肌，又称 *musculus levator palpebrae superioris*；**levator prostatae m.**, puboprostaticus m. 前列腺提肌即耻骨前列腺肌；**levator scapulae m.**, levator muscle of scapula: *origin*, transverse processes of four upper cervical vertebrae; *insertion*, medial border of scapula; *innervation*, third and fourth cervical; *action*, raises scapula 肩胛提肌，又称 *musculus levator scapulae*；**levator veli palatini m.**, *origin*, apex of petrous portion of temporal bone and cartilaginous part of auditory tube; *insertion*, aponeurosis of soft palate; *innervation*, pharyngeal plexus of vagus; *action*, raises and draws back soft palate 腭帆提肌，又称 *musculus levator veli palatini*；**lingual m's**, the extrinsic and intrinsic muscles that move the tongue 舌肌；**longissimus m.**, the largest element of the erector spinae, which includes the *longissimus capitis, cervicis*, and *thoracis muscles* 最长肌，包括头最长肌、颈最长肌和胸最长肌，又称 *musculus longissimus*；**longissimus capitis m.**, *origin*, transverse processes of four or five upper thoracic vertebrae, articular processes of three or four lower cervical vertebrae; *insertion*, mastoid process of temporal bone; *innervation*, branches of cervical; *action*, draws head backward, rotates head 头最长肌，又称 *musculus longissimus capitis*；**longissimus cervicis m.**, *origin*, transverse processes of four or five upper thoracic vertebrae; *insertion*, transverse processes of second to sixth cervical vertebrae; *innervation*, lower cervical and upper thoracic; *action*, extends cervical vertebrae 颈最长肌，又称 *musculus longissimus cervicis*；**longissimus thoracis m.**, *origin*, transverse and articular processes of lumbar vertebrae and thoracolumbar fascia; *insertion*, transverse processes of all thoracic vertebrae, nine or ten lower ribs; *innervation*, lumbar and thoracic; *action*, extends thoracic vertebrae 胸最长肌，又称 *musculus longissimus thoracis*；**longitudinal m. of tongue, inferior**, *origin*, inferior surface of tongue at base; *insertion*, apex of tongue; *innervation*, hypoglossal; *action*, changes shape of tongue in mastication and deglutition 舌下纵肌，又称 *musculus longitudinalis inferior linguae*；**longitudinal m. of tongue, superior**, *origin*, submucosa and septum of tongue; *insertion*, margins of tongue; *innervation*, hypoglossal; *action*, changes shape of tongue in mastication and deglutition 舌上纵肌，又称 *musculus longitudinalis superior linguae*；**longus capitis m.**, *origin*, transverse processes of third to sixth cervical vertebrae; *insertion*, basilar part of occipital bone; *innervation*, branches from first, second, and third cervical; *action*, flexes head 头长肌，又称 *musculus longus capitis*；**longus colli m.**, *origin*, SUPERIOR OBLIQUE PORTION— transverse processes of third to fifth cervical vertebrae, INFERIOR OBLIQUE PORTION— bodies of first to third thoracic vertebrae, VERTICAL PORTION—bodies of three upper thoracic and three lower cervical vertebrae; *insertion*, SUPERIOR OBLIQUE PORTION—tubercle of anterior arch of atlas, INFERIOR OBLIQUE PORTION—transverse processes of fifth and sixth cervical vertebrae, VERTICAL PORTION—bodies of second to fourth cervical vertebrae; *innervation*, anterior cervical; *action*, flexes and supports cervical vertebrae 颈长肌，又称 *musculus longus colli*；**m's of lower limb**, the muscles acting on the thigh, leg, and foot 下肢肌；**lumbrical m's of foot**, *origin*, tendons of flexor digitorum longus; *insertion*, extensor expansions of four lateral toes; *innervation*, medial and lateral plantar; *action*, flex metatarsophalangeal joints, extend distal phalanges 足蚓状肌，又称 *musculi lumbricales pedis*；**lumbrical m's of hand**, *origin*, tendons of flexor digitorum profundus; *insertion*, extensor expansions of the four nonthumb fingers; *innervation*, median and ulnar; *action*, flex metacarpophalangeal joint and extend middle and distal phalanges 手蚓状肌，又称 *musculi lumbricales manus*；**masseter m.**, *origin*, SUPERFICIAL PART—zygomatic process of maxilla and inferior border of zygomatic arch, DEEP PART—inferior border and medial surface of zygomatic arch; *insertion*, SUPERFICIAL PART— angle and ramus of mandible, DEEP PART— superior half of ramus and lateral surface of coronoid process of mandible; *innervation*, masseteric, from mandibular division of trigeminal; *action*, raises mandible, closes jaws 咬肌，又称 *musculus masseter*；**masticatory m's**, a group of muscles responsible for the movement of the jaws during mastication, including the masseter, temporalis, and medial and lateral pterygoid muscles 咀嚼肌；**mentalis m.**, *origin*, incisive fossa of mandible; *insertion*, skin of chin; *innervation*, facial; *action*, wrinkles skin of chin 颏肌，又称 *musculus mentalis*；**Müller m.**, 1. the circular fibers of the ciliary muscle 米勒肌，睫状肌的环形纤维；2. 同 orbit-

alis m.；**multifidus m's, *origin***, sacrum, sacroiliac ligament, mammillary processes of lumbar, transverse processes of thoracic, and articular processes of cervical vertebrae; *insertion*, spines of contiguous vertebrae above; *innervation*, posterior ramus of spinal nerves; *action*, extend, rotate vertebral column 多裂肌，又称 *musculi multifidi*；**multipennate m.**, one in which the fiber bundles converge to several tendons 多羽肌；**mylohyoid m.**, *origin*, mylohyoid line of mandible; *insertion*, body of hyoid bone and median raphe; *innervation*, mylohyoid branch of inferior alveolar; *action*, elevates hyoid bone, supports floor of mouth 下颌舌骨肌，又称 *musculus mylohyoideus*；**nasalis m.**, *origin*, maxilla; *insertion*, ALAR PART—ala nasi, HORIZONTAL PART—by aponeurotic expansion with fellow of opposite side; *innervation*, facial; *action*, ALAR PART—aids in widening nostril, HORIZONTAL PART—depresses cartilage of nose 鼻肌，又称 *musculus nasalis*；**m's of neck,** 同 cervical m's；**nonstriated m., nonstriated involuntary m.,** 同 smooth m.；**oblique m. of abdomen，external**, *origin*, lower eight ribs at costal cartilages; *insertion*, crest of ilium, linea alba through rectus sheath; *innervation*, seventh to twelfth intercostal; *action*, flexes and rotates vertebral column, increases intra-abdominal pressure, acts as accessory respiratory muscle 腹外斜肌，又称 *musculus obliquus externus abdominis*；**oblique m. of abdomen, internal**, *origin*, inguinal ligament, iliac crest, thoracolumbar fascia; *insertion*, inferior three or four costal cartilages, linea alba, conjoined tendon to pubis; *innervation*, seventh to twelfth intercostal, first lumbar; *action*, flexes and rotates vertebral column, increases intraabdominal pressure, acts as accessory respiratory muscle 腹内斜肌，又称 *musculus obliquus internus abdominis*；**oblique m. of auricle**, *origin*, cranial surface of concha; *insertion*, cranial surface of auricle above concha; *innervation*, temporal and posterior auricular (branches of facial) 耳廓斜肌，又称 *musculus obliquus auriculae*；**oblique m. of eyeball, inferior**, *origin*, orbital surface of maxilla; *insertion*, sclera; *innervation*, oculomotor; *action*, rotates eyeball upward and outward 眼球下斜肌，又称 *musculus obliquus inferior bulbi*；**oblique m. of eyeball, superior**, *origin*, lesser wing of sphenoid bone above optic canal; *insertion*, sclera; *innervation*, trochlear; *action*, rotates eyeball downward and outward 眼球上斜肌，又称 *musculus obliquus superior bulbi*；**obliquus capitis inferior m.**, *origin*, spinous process of axis; *insertion*, transverse process of atlas; *innervation*, posterior ramus of spinal nerves; *action*, rotates atlas and head 头下斜肌，又称 *musculus obliquus capi-*

tis inferior; **obliquus capitis superior m.**, *origin*, transverse process of atlas; *insertion*, occipital bone; *innervation*, posterior ramus of spinal nerves; *action*, extends and moves head laterally 头上斜肌，又称 *musculus obliquus capitis superior*; **obturator externus m.**, external obturator muscle: *origin*, pubis, ischium, and external surface of obturator membrane; *insertion*, trochanteric fossa of femur; *innervation*, obturator; *action*, rotates thigh laterally 闭孔外肌，又称 *musculus obturatorius externus*; **obturator internus m.**, internal obturator muscle: *origin*, pelvic surface of coxal bone and obturator membrane, margin of obturator foramen, ramus of ischium, inferior ramus of pubis; *insertion*, greater trochanter of femur; *innervation*, fifth lumbar, first and second sacral; *action*, rotates thigh laterally 闭孔内肌，又称 *musculus obturatorius internus*; **occipitofrontalis m.**, occipitofrontal muscle: *origin*, FRONTAL BELLY—galea aponeurotica, OCCIPITAL BELLY— supreme nuchal line of occipital bone; *insertion*, FRONTAL BELLY—skin of eyebrows and root of nose, OCCIPITAL BELLY—galea aponeurotica; *innervation*, FRONTAL BELLY—temporal branch of facial, OCCIPITAL BELLY—posterior auricular branch of facial; *action*, FRONTAL BELLY—raises eyebrows, OCCIPITAL BELLY—draws scalp posteriorly 枕额肌，又称 *musculus occipitofrontalis*; **ocular m's**, 同 extraocular m's; **omohyoid m.**, *origin*, superior border of scapula; *insertion*, lateral border of hyoid bone; *innervation*, upper cervical through ansa cervicalis; *action*, depresses hyoid bone. It comprises two bellies (superior and inferior) connected by a central tendon that is bound to the clavicle by a fibrous expansion of the cervical fascia 肩胛舌骨肌，又称 *musculus omohyoideus*; **opponens digiti minimi m.**, *origin*, hook of hamate bone, flexor retinaculum; *insertion*, ulnar margin of fifth metacarpal; *innervation*, eighth cervical through ulnar; *action*, rotates, abducts, and flexes fifth metacarpal 小指对掌肌，又称 *musculus opponens digiti minimi*; **opponens pollicis m.**, *origin*, tubercle of trapezium bone, flexor retinaculum; *insertion*, radial side of first metacarpal; *innervation*, sixth and seventh cervical through median; *action*, flexes and opposes thumb 拇对掌肌，又称 *musculus opponens pollicis*; **orbicular m.**, one that encircles a body opening, e.g., the eye or mouth 轮匝肌; **orbicularis oculi m.**, the oval sphincter muscle surrounding the eyelids, consisting of three parts: *origin*, ORBITAL PART—medial margin of orbit, including frontal process of maxilla, PALPEBRAL PART—medial palpebral ligament, LACRIMAL PART—posterior lacrimal crest; *insertion*, ORBITAL PART—near origin after encircling orbit, PALPEBRAL PART—

fibers intertwine to form lateral palpebral raphe, LACRIMAL PART—lateral palpebral raphe, upper and lower tarsi; *innervation*, facial; *action*, closes eyelids, wrinkles forehead, compresses lacrimal sac 眼轮匝肌，又称 *musculus orbicularis oculi*; **orbicularis oris m.**, a name applied to a complicated sphincter muscle of the mouth, comprising a *labial part*, fibers restricted to the lips, and a *marginal part*, fibers blending with those of adjacent muscles: *innervation*, facial; *action*, closes and protrudes lips 口轮匝肌，又称 *musculus orbicularis oris*; **orbitalis m.**, orbital muscle: a thin layer of nonstriated muscle that bridges the inferior orbital fissure: *innervation*, sympathetic branches 眶肌，又称 *musculus orbitalis*; **palatine m's**, the intrinsic and extrinsic muscles that act upon the soft palate and the adjacent pharyngeal wall 腭肌; **palatoglossus m.**, *origin*, undersurface of soft palate; *insertion*, side of tongue; *innervation*, pharyngeal plexus of vagus; *action*, elevates tongue, constricts fauces 腭舌肌，又称 *musculus palatoglossus*; **palatopharyngeus m.**, palatopharyngeal muscle: one of the intrinsic muscles of the larynx; *origin*, soft palate; *insertion*, aponeurosis of pharynx, posterior border of thyroid cartilage; *innervation*, pharyngeal plexus of vagus; *action*, aids in deglutition 腭咽肌，又称 *musculus palatopharyngeus*; **palmaris brevis m.**, *origin*, palmar aponeurosis; *insertion*, skin of medial border of hand; *innervation*, ulnar; *action*, assists in deepening hollow of palm 掌短肌，又称 *musculus palmaris brevis*; **palmaris longus m.**, *origin*, medial epicondyle of humerus; *insertion*, flexor retinaculum, palmar aponeurosis; *innervation*, median; *action*, flexes radiocarpal joint, anchors skin and fascia of hand 掌长肌，又称 *musculus palmaris longus*; **papillary m's**, conical muscular projections from the walls of the cardiac ventricles, attached to the leaflets of the atrioventricular valves by the chordae tendineae. There is an anterior and an inferior papillary muscle in each ventricle, as well as a group of small papillary muscles on the septum in the right ventricle 乳头肌，又称 *musculi papillares*; **pectinate m's of left atrium**, small ridges of muscle fibers projecting from the inner walls of the left auricle of the heart 左心房梳状肌，又称 *musculi pectinati atrii sinistri*; **pectinate m's of right atrium**, small ridges of muscle fibers projecting from the inner walls of the right auricle of the heart and extending in the right atrium to the crista terminalis 右心房梳状肌，又称 *musculi pectinati atrii dextri*; **pectineus m.**, pectineal muscle: *origin*, pectineal line of pubis; *insertion*, pectineal line of femur; *innervation*, obturator and femoral; *action*, flexes,

adducts thigh 耻骨肌，又称 *musculus pectineus*；
pectoralis major m., greater pectoral muscle: *origin*, clavicle, sternum, six upper costal cartilages, aponeurosis of external abdominal oblique muscle; the origins are reflected in the subdivision of the muscle into clavicular, sternocostal, and abdominal plexuses; *insertion*, crest of intertubercular groove of humerus; *innervation*, medial and lateral pectoral; *action*, adducts, flexes, rotates arm medially 胸大肌，又 称 *musculus pectoralis major*；**pectoralis minor m.**, smaller pectoral muscle: *origin*, third, fourth, and fifth ribs; *insertion*, coracoid process of scapula; *innervation*, lateral and medial pectoral; *action*, draws shoulder forward and downward, raises third, fourth, and fifth ribs in forced inspiration 胸小肌，又 称 *musculus pectoralis minor*；**pennate m., penniform m.**, a muscle in which the fibers approach the tendon of insertion from a wide area and are inserted through a large segment of its circumference 羽状肌；**peroneus brevis m.**, short fibular muscle: *origin*, lateral surface of fibula; *insertion*, tuber on base of fifth metatarsal bone; *innervation*, superficial fibular; *action*, everts, abducts, plantarflexes foot 腓骨短肌，又称 *musculus peroneus brevis* 和 *musculus fibularis brevi*；**peroneus longus m.**, long fibular muscle: *origin*, lateral condyle of tibia, head and lateral surface of fibula; *insertion*, medial cuneiform, first metatarsal; *innervation*, superficial fibular; *action*, abducts, everts, plantarflexes foot 腓 骨 长肌，又称 *musculus peroneus longus* 和 *musculus fibularis longus*；**peroneus tertius m.**, third fibular muscle: *origin*, anterior surface of fibula, interosseous membrane; *insertion*, base of fifth metatarsal; *innervation*, deep fibular; *action*, everts, dorsiflexes foot 第三腓骨肌，又称 *musculus peroneus tertius* 和 *musculus fibularis tertius*；**pharyngeal m's**, the muscular coat of the pharynx, comprising the three constrictor muscles and the stylopharyngeus, salpingopharyngeus, and palatopharyngeus muscles 咽肌；**piriformis m.**, piriform muscle: *origin*, ilium, second to fourth sacral vertebrae; *insertion*, greater trochanter of femur; *innervation*, first and second sacral; *action*, rotates thigh laterally 梨状肌，又称 *musculus piriformis*；**plantaris m.**, plantar muscle: *origin*, oblique popliteal ligament, lateral supracondylar line of femur; *insertion*, posterior part of calcaneus; *innervation*, tibial; *action*, plantarflexes foot, flexes knee 跖肌，又称 *musculus plantaris*；**pleuroesophageus m.**, pleuroesophageal muscle: a bundle of smooth muscle fibers usually connecting the esophagus with the left mediastinal pleura 胸膜食管肌，又称 *musculus pleurooesophageus*；**popliteus m.**, popliteal muscle: *origin*, lateral condyle

of femur, lateral meniscus; *insertion*, posterior surface of tibia; *innervation*, tibial; *action*, flexes leg, rotates leg medially 腘肌，又称 *musculus popliteus*；**procerus m.**, *origin*, fascia over nasal bone; *insertion*, skin of forehead; *innervation*, facial; *action*, draws medial angle of eyebrows down 降眉间肌，又称 *musculus procerus*；**pronator quadratus m.**, *origin*, anterior surface and border of distal third or fourth of body of ulna; *insertion*, anterior surface and border of distal fourth of body of radius; *innervation*, anterior interosseous; *action*, pronates forearm 旋前方肌，又称 *musculus pronator quadratus*；**pronator teres m.**, (2 heads): *origin*, SUPERFICIAL HEAD—medial epicondyle of humerus, DEEP HEAD—coronoid process of ulna; *insertion*, lateral surface of radius; *innervation*, median; *action*, flexes elbow and pronates forearm 旋前圆肌，又称 *musculus pronator teres*；**psoas major m.**, *origin*, lumbar vertebrae; *insertion*, lesser trochanter of femur; *innervation*, second and third lumbar; *action*, flexes thigh or trunk 腰大肌，又称 *musculus psoas major*；**psoas minor m.**, *origin*, last thoracic and first lumbar vertebrae; *insertion*, pecten pubis, iliopectineal eminence, iliac fascia; *innervation*, first lumbar; *action*, flexes trunk 腰小肌，又称 *musculus psoas minor*；**pterygoid m., lateral**, *origin*, SUPERIOR HEAD—infratemporal surface of greater wing of sphenoid bone and infratemporal crest, INFERIOR HEAD—lateral surface of lateral pterygoid plate; *insertion*, neck of condyle of mandible, temporomandibular joint capsule; *innervation*, mandibular; *action*, protrudes mandible, opens jaws, moves mandible from side to side 翼外肌，又称 *musculus pterygoideus lateralis*；**pterygoid m., medial**, *origin*, medial surface of lateral pterygoid plate, tuberosity of maxilla; *insertion*, medial surface of ramus and angle of mandible; *innervation*, mandibular; *action*, closes jaws 翼内肌，又称 *musculus pterygoideus medialis*；**puboanalis m.**, puboanal muscle: fibers from the medial part of the pubococcygeus muscle that decussate and blend with the longitudinal muscle layer and fascia of the rectum 耻骨肛门肌，又称 *musculus puboanalis*；**pubococcygeus m.**, pubococcygeal muscle: the anterior portion of the levator ani, originating anterior to the obturator canal: *insertion*, anococcygeal body and side of coccyx; *innervation*, pudendal; *action*, helps support pelvic viscera and resist increases in intraabdominal pressure 耻尾肌，又称 *musculus pubococcygeus*；**puboperinealis m.**, puboperineal muscle: fibers from the medial part of the pubococcygeus muscle that insert into the perineal body 耻骨会阴肌，又称 *musculus puboperinealis*；**puboprostaticus m.**,

M

puboprostatic muscle: a part of the anterior portion of the pubococcygeus muscle, inserted in the prostate and the tendinous center of the perineum; innervated by the pudendal nerve, it supports and compresses the prostate and is involved in control of urination 耻骨前列腺肌，又称 *musculus puboprostaticus*；**puborectalis m.**, puborectal muscle: a portion of the levator ani having a more lateral origin from the pubic bone, and continuous posteriorly with the corresponding muscle of the opposite side: *innervation*, third and fourth sacral; *action*, helps support pelvic viscera and resist increases in intra-abdominal pressure, maintains anorectal flexure at anorectal junction 耻骨直肠肌，又称 *musculus puborectalis*；**pubovaginalis m.**, pubovaginal muscle: a part of the anterior portion of the pubococcygeus muscle, which is inserted into the urethra and vagina; innervated by the pudendal nerve, it is involved in control of urination 耻骨阴道肌，又称 *musculus pubovaginalis*；**pubovesicalis m.**, pubovesical muscle: smooth muscle fibers extending from the neck of the urinary bladder to the pubis 耻骨膀胱肌，又称 *musculus pubovesicalis*；**pyramidal m. of auricle**, a prolongation of the fibers of the tragicus to the spine of helix 耳廓锥状肌，又称 *musculus pyramidalis auriculae*；**pyramidalis m.**, pyramidal muscle: *origin*, anterior aspect of pubis, anterior pubic ligament; *insertion*, linea alba; *innervation*, last thoracic; *action*, tenses abdominal wall 锥状肌，又称 *musculus pyramidalis*；**quadrate m.**, a square-shaped muscle 方形肌；**quadratus femoris m.**, *origin*, upper part of lateral border of tuber of ischium; *insertion*, quadrate tubercle of femur, intertrochanteric crest; *innervation*, fourth and fifth lumbar and first sacral; *action*, adducts, rotates thigh laterally 股方肌，又称 *musculus quadratus femoris*；**quadratus lumborum m.**, *origin*, iliac crest, thoracolumbar fascia; *insertion*, twelfth rib, transverse processes of four upper lumbar vertebrae; *innervation*, first and second lumbar and twelfth thoracic; *action*, flexes lumbar vertebrae laterally, fixes last rib 腰方肌，又称 *musculus quadratus lumborum*；**quadratus plantae m.**, *origin*, calcaneus and plantar fascia; *insertion*, tendons of flexor digitorum longus; *innervation*, lateral plantar; *action*, aids in flexing toes 足底方肌，又称 *musculus flexor accessorius* 和 *musculus quadratus plantae*；**quadriceps femoris m.**, a name applied collectively to the rectus femoris, vastus intermedius, vastus lateralis, and vastus medialis, inserting by a common tendon that surrounds the patella and ends on the tuber of the tibia, and acting to extend the leg upon the thigh 股四头肌，又称 *musculus quadriceps femoris*；

rectococcygeus m., rectococcygeal muscle: smooth muscle fibers originating on the anterior surface of the second and third coccygeal vertebrae and inserting on the posterior surface of the rectum, innervated by autonomic nerves, and acting to retract and elevate the rectum 直肠尾骨肌，又称 *musculus rectococcygeus*；**rectourethral m's**, 同 anorectoperineal m's；**rectouterinus m.**, rectouterine muscle: a band of fibers running between the cervix of the uterus and the rectum, in the rectouterine fold 直肠子宫肌，又称 *musculus rectouterinus*；**rectovesicalis m.**, rectovesical muscle: a band of fibers in the male, connecting the longitudinal musculature of the rectum with the external muscular coat of the bladder 直肠膀胱肌，又称 *musculus rectovesicalis*；**rectus abdominis m.**, *origin*, pubic crest and symphysis; *insertion*, xiphoid process, cartilages of fifth, sixth, and seventh ribs; *innervation*, branches of lower thoracic; *action*, flexes lumbar vertebrae, supports abdomen 腹直肌，又称 *musculus rectus abdominis*；**rectus capitis anterior m.**, *origin*, lateral mass of atlas; *insertion*, basilar part of occipital bone; *innervation*, first and second cervical; *action*, flexes, supports head 头前直肌，又称 *musculus rectus capitis anterior*；**rectus capitis lateralis m.**, *origin*, upper surface of transverse process of atlas; *insertion*, jugular process of occipital bone; *innervation*, first and second cervical; *action*, flexes, supports head 头外侧直肌，又称 *musculus rectus capitis lateralis*；**rectus capitis posterior major m.**, *origin*, spinous process of axis; *insertion*, occipital bone; *innervation*, suboccipital and greater occipital; *action*, extends head 头后大直肌，又称 *musculus rectus capitis posterior major*；**rectus capitis posterior minor m.**, *origin*, posterior tubercle of atlas; *insertion*, occipital bone; *innervation*, suboccipital and greater occipital; *action*, extends head 头后小直肌，又称 *musculus rectus capitis posterior minor*；**rectus m. of eye ball, inferior**, *origin*, common tendinous ring; *insertion*, underside of sclera; *innervation*, oculomotor; *action*, adducts, rotates eyeball downward and medially 眼下直肌，又称 *musculus rectus inferior bulbi*；**rectus m. of eyeball, lateral**, *origin*, common tendinous ring; *insertion*, lateral side of sclera; *innervation*, abducens; *action*, abducts eyeball 眼外直肌，又称 *musculus rectus lateralis bulbi*；**rectus m. of eyeball, medial**, *origin*, common tendinous ring; *insertion*, medial side of sclera; *innervation*, oculomotor; *action*, adducts eyeball 眼内直肌，又称 *musculus rectus medialis bulbi*；**rectus m. of eyeball, superior**, *origin*, common tendinous ring; *insertion*, upper aspect of sclera; *innervation*, oculomotor; *action*, adducts, rotates eyeball upward and medially 眼上直肌，又称 *musculus rectus superior bulbi*； **rectus femoris m.,** *origin*, anterior inferior iliac spine, rim of acetabulum; *insertion*, base of patella, tuber of tibia; *innervation*, femoral; *action*, extends knee, flexes thigh at hip 股直肌，又称 *musculus rectus femoris*； **Reisseisen m's,** the smooth muscle fibers of the smallest bronchi Reisseisen 肌，最小支气管的平滑肌纤维； **rhomboid major m.,** *origin*, spinous processes of second, third, fourth, and fifth thoracic vertebrae; *insertion*, medial margin of scapula; *innervation*, dorsal scapular; *action*, retracts, elevates scapula 大菱形肌，又称 *musculus rhomboideus major*； **rhomboid minor m.,** *origin*, spinous processes of seventh cervical to first thoracic vertebrae, lower part of nuchal ligament; *insertion*, medial margin of scapula at root of the spine; *innervation*, dorsal scapular; *action*, adducts, elevates scapula 小菱形肌，又称 *musculus rhomboideus minor*； **risorius m.,** *origin*, fascia over masseter; *insertion*, skin at angle of mouth; *innervation*, buccal branch of facial; *action*, draws angle of mouth laterally 笑肌，又称 *musculus risorius*； **rotatores m's,** rotator muscles: a series of small muscles deep in the groove between the spinous and transverse processes of the vertebrae; each connects a vertebra with the vertebra one or two above it. They are subdivided by region into *rotatores cervicis, thoracis,* and *lumborum* 回旋肌，又称 *musculi rotatores*； **Ruysch m.,** the muscular tissue of the fundus of the uterus Ruysch 肌，子宫底肌组织； **salpingopharyngeus m.,** salpingopharyngeal muscle: *origin*, auditory tube near its orifice; *insertion*, posterior part of palatopharyngeus; *innervation*, pharyngeal plexus of vagus; *action*, elevates upper lateral wall of pharynx 咽鼓管咽肌，又称 *musculus salpingopharyngeus*； **sartorius m.,** *origin*, anterior superior iliac spine; *insertion*, proximal part of medial surface of tibia; *innervation*, femoral; *action*, flexes leg at knee and thigh at pelvis 缝匠肌，又称 *musculus sartorius*； **scalene m., anterior,** *origin*, transverse processes of third to sixth cervical vertebrae; *insertion*, scalene tubercle of first rib; *innervation*, fourth to sixth cervical; *action*, raises first rib, flexes cervical vertebrae forward and laterally and rotates to opposite side 前斜角肌，又称 *musculus scalenus anterior*； **scalene m., middle,** *origin*, transverse processes of second to seventh cervical vertebrae and often atlas; *insertion*, upper surface of first rib; *innervation*, third to eighth cervical; *action*, raises first rib, flexes cervical vertebrae forward and laterally and rotates to opposite side 中斜角肌，又称 *musculus scalenus medius*； **scalene m., posterior,** *origin*, posterior tubercles of transverse processes of fourth to sixth cervical vertebrae; *insertion*, second rib; *innervation*, sixth to eighth cervical; *action*, raises second rib, flexes cervical vertebrae laterally 后斜角肌，又称 *musculus scalenus posterior*； **scalene m., smallest,** a band occasionally found between the anterior and middle scalene muscles; *origin*, transverse process of seventh cervical vertebra; *insertion*, first rib, suprapleural membrane; *innervation*, seventh cervical; *action*, raises first rib, flexes and rotates cervical vertebrae, supports suprapleural membrane 小斜角肌，又称 *musculus scalenus minimus*； **semimembranosus m.,** semimembranous muscle: *origin*, tuber of ischium; *insertion*, medial condyle and border of tibia, lateral condyle of femur; *innervation*, tibial; *action*, flexes and rotates leg medially, extends thigh at hip 半膜肌，又称 *musculus semimembranosus*； **semipennate m.,** a muscle in which the fiber bundles approach the tendon of insertion from only one direction and are inserted through only a small segment of its circumference 半羽肌； **semispinalis capitis m.,** *origin*, transverse processes of five or six upper thoracic and four lower cervical vertebrae; *insertion*, between superior and inferior nuchal lines of occipital bone; *innervation*, suboccipital, greater occipital, and other branches of cervical; *action*, extends head and rotates to opposite side 头半棘肌，又称 *musculus semispinalis capitis*； **semispinalis cervicis m.,** *origin*, transverse processes of five or six upper thoracic vertebrae; *insertion*, spinous processes of second to fifth cervical vertebrae; *innervation*, branches of cervical; *action*, extends, rotates vertebral column 颈半棘肌，又称 *musculus semispinalis cervicis*； **semispinalis thoracis m.,** *origin*, transverse processes of sixth to tenth thoracic vertebrae; *insertion*, spinous processes of two lower cervical and four upper thoracic vertebrae; *innervation*, spinal nerves; *action*, extends, rotates vertebral column 胸半棘肌，又称 *musculus semispinalis thoracis*； **semitendinosus m.,** semitendinous muscle: *origin*, tuber of ischium; *insertion*, upper part of medial surface of tibia; *innervation*, tibial; *action*, flexes and rotates leg medially, extends thigh 半腱肌，又称 *musculus semitendinosus*； **serratus anterior m.,** *origin*, eight or nine upper ribs; *insertion*, medial border of scapula; *innervation*, long thoracic; *action*, draws scapula forward; rotates scapula to raise shoulder in abduction of arm 前锯肌，又称 *musculus serratus anterior*； **serratus posterior inferior m.,** *origin*, spines of two lower thoracic and two or three upper lumbar vertebrae; *insertion*, inferior border of four lower ribs; *innervation*, ninth to twelfth thoracic; *action*, lowers ribs in expiration 下后锯肌，又称

musculus serratus posterior inferior; **serratus posterior superior m.**, *origin*, nuchal ligament, spinous processes of upper thoracic vertebrae; *insertion*, second, third, fourth, and fifth ribs; *innervation*, first four thoracic; *action*, raises ribs in inspiration 上后锯肌，又称 *musculus serratus posterior superior*; **skeletal m.**, any of the striated muscles attached to bones, typically crossing at least one joint; under voluntary control 骨骼肌；**smooth m., smooth involuntary m.**, a type without transverse striations in its constituent fibers; not under voluntary control 平滑肌；**soleus m.**, *origin*, fibula, tibia, muscular trochlea between tibia and fibula and passing over popliteal vessels; *insertion*, calcaneus by Achilles tendon; *innervation*, tibial; *action*, plantarflexes foot 比目鱼肌，又称 *musculus soleus*；**sphincter m.**, sphincter. For specific sphincter muscles, see entries under *sphincter* 括约肌；**spinalis m.**, the medial division of the erector spinae, including the *spinalis capitis, spinalis cervicis,* and *spinalis thoracis muscles* 棘肌，包括头棘肌、颈棘肌和胸棘肌，又称 *musculus spinalis*；**spinalis capitis m.**, *origin*, spines of upper thoracic and lower cervical vertebrae; *insertion*, occipital bone; *innervation*, branches of cervical; *action*, extends head 头棘肌，又称 *musculus spinalis capitis*；**spinalis cervicis m.**, *origin*, lower part of nuchal ligament, spinous processes of seventh cervical and sometimes two upper thoracic vertebrae; *insertion*, spinous processes of axis and sometimes of second to fourth cervical vertebrae; *innervation*, branches of cervical; *action*, extends vertebral column 颈棘肌，又称 *musculus spinalis cervicis*；**spinalis thoracis m.**, *origin*, spinous processes of two upper lumbar and two lower thoracic vertebrae; *insertion*, spines of upper thoracic vertebrae; *innervation*, branches of thoracic and lumbar; *action*, extends vertebral column 胸棘肌，又称 *musculus spinalis thoracis*；**splenius capitis m.**, *origin*, lower half of nuchal ligament, spinous processes of seventh cervical and three or four upper thoracic vertebrae; *insertion*, mastoid part of temporal bone, occipital bone; *innervation*, middle and lower cervical; *action*, extends, rotates head 头夹肌，又称 *musculus splenius capitis*；**splenius cervicis m.**, *origin*, spinous processes of third to sixth thoracic vertebrae; *insertion*, transverse processes of two or three upper cervical vertebrae; *innervation*, posterior ramus of lower cervical; *action*, extends, rotates head and neck 颈夹肌，又称 *musculus splenius cervicis*；**stapedius m.**, *origin*, interior of pyramidal eminence of tympanic cavity; *insertion*, posterior surface of neck of stapes; *innervation*, stapedial branch of facial; *action*, dampens stapedial

movement 镫骨肌，又称 *musculus stapedius*；**sternalis m.**, sternal muscle: a band occasionally found parallel to the sternum on the sternocostal origin of the pectoralis major 胸骨肌，又称 *musculus sternalis*；**sternocleidomastoid m.**, (2 heads): *origin*, STERNAL HEAD—manubrium sterni, CLAVICULAR HEAD—superior surface of medial third of clavicle; *insertion*, mastoid process and superior nuchal line of occipital bone; *innervation*, accessory nerve and cervical plexus; *action*, flexes vertebral column, rotates head upward and to opposite side 胸锁乳突肌，又称 *musculus sternocleidomastoideus*；**sternohyoid m.**, *origin*, manubrium sterni, posterior sternoclavicular ligament, clavicle; *insertion*, body of hyoid bone; *innervation*, upper ansa cervicalis; *action*, depresses hyoid bone and larynx 胸骨舌骨肌，又称 *musculus sternohyoideus*；**sternothyroid m.**, *origin*, manubrium sterni; *insertion*, lamina of thyroid cartilage; *innervation*, ansa cervicalis; *action*, depresses thyroid cartilage 胸骨甲状肌，又称 *musculus sternothyroideus*；**striated m.**, one whose fibers are divided by transverse bands into striations, including cardiac *(striated involuntary m.)* and skeletal *(striated voluntary m.)* muscles; often used synonymously with the latter 横纹肌；**styloglossus m.**, *origin*, styloid process; *insertion*, margin of tongue; *innervation*, hypoglossal; *action*, raises and retracts tongue 茎突舌肌，又称 *musculus styloglossus*；**stylohyoid m.**, *origin*, styloid process; *insertion*, body of hyoid bone; *innervation*, facial; *action*, draws hyoid and tongue superiorly and posteriorly 茎突舌骨肌，又称 *musculus stylohyoideus*；**stylopharyngeus m.**, stylopharyngeal muscle: one of the intrinsic muscles of the larynx: *origin*, styloid process; *insertion*, thyroid cartilage and pharyngeal constrictors; *innervation*, pharyngeal plexus, glossopharyngeal; *action*, raises and dilates pharynx 茎突咽肌，又称 *musculus stylopharyngeus*；**subclavius m.**, *origin*, first rib and its cartilage; *insertion*, lower surface of clavicle; *innervation*, fifth and sixth cervical; *action*, depresses lateral end of clavicle 锁骨下肌，又称 *musculus subclavius*；**subcostales m's**, subcostal muscles: *origin*, inner surface of ribs: *insertion*, inner surface of first, second, and third ribs below; *innervation*, intercostal; *action*, draw adjacent ribs together, depress ribs 肋下肌，又称 *musculus subclavius*；**suboccipital m's**, those situated just below the occipital bone, including the rectus capitis, obliquus capitis, splenius capitis, and longus capitis muscles 枕下肌，又称 *musculi subcostales*；**subscapularis m.**, subscapular muscle: *origin*, subscapular fossa of scapula; *insertion*, lesser tubercle of humerus; *innervation*, subscapular; *ac-*

tion, rotates humerus medially 肩胛下肌，又称 *musculus subscapularis*；**supinator m.**, *origin*, lateral epicondyle of humerus, ulna, elbow joint fascia; *insertion*, radius; *innervation*, deep radial; *action*, supinates forearm 旋后肌，又称 *musculus supinator*；**suprahyoid m's**, the muscles that attach the hyoid bone to the skull, including the digastric, stylohyoid, mylohyoid, and geniohyoid muscles 舌骨上肌；**supraspinatus m.**, supraspinous muscle: *origin*, supraspinous fossa of scapula; *insertion*, greater tubercle of humerus; *innervation*, suprascapular; *action*, abducts humerus 冈上肌，又称 *musculus supraspinatus*；**suspensory m. of duodenum**, a flat band of smooth muscle originating from the left crus of the respiratory diaphragm, and continuous with the muscular coat of the duodenum at its junction with the jejunum 十二指肠旋肌，又称 *musculus suspensorius duodeni*；**synergic m's, synergistic m's**, those that assist one another in action 协同肌；**tarsal m., inferior**, *origin*, inferior rectus muscle of eyeball; *insertion*, tarsal plate of lower eyelid; *innervation*, sympathetic; *action*, widens palpebral fissure 下睑板肌，又称 *musculus tarsalis inferior*；**tarsal m., superior**, *origin*, levator palpebrae superioris muscle; *insertion*, tarsal plate of upper eyelid; *innervation*, sympathetic; *action*, widens palpebral fissure 上睑板肌，又称 *musculus tarsalis superior*；**temporalis m.**, temporal muscle: *origin*, temporal fossa and fascia; *insertion*, coronoid process of mandible; *innervation*, mandibular; *action*, closes jaws 颞肌，又称 *musculus temporalis*；**temporoparietalis m.**, temporoparietal muscle: *origin*, temporal fascia above ear; *insertion*, galea aponeurotica; *innervation*, temporal branches of facial; *action*, tightens scalp 颞顶肌，又称 *musculus temporoparietalis*；**tensor fasciae latae m.**, *origin*, iliac crest; *insertion*, iliotibial tract of fascia lata; *innervation*, superior gluteal; *action*, flexes, rotates thigh medially 阔筋膜张肌，又称 *musculus tensor fasciae latae*；**tensor tympani m.**, *origin*, cartilaginous portion of auditory tube; *insertion*, manubrium of malleus; *innervation*, mandibular; *action*, tenses tympanic membrane 鼓膜张肌，又称 *musculus tensor tympani*；**tensor veli palatini m.**, *origin*, scaphoid fossa at base of medial pterygoid plate, wall of auditory tube, spine of sphenoid bone; *insertion*, aponeurosis of soft palate, horizontal part of palatine bone; *innervation*, mandibular; *action*, tenses soft palate, opens auditory tube 腭帆张肌，又称 *musculus tensor veli palatini*；**teres major m.**, *origin*, inferior angle of scapula; *insertion*, lip of intertubercular sulcus of humerus; *innervation*, lower subscapular; *action*, adducts, extends, rotates arm medially 大圆肌；**teres minor m.**, *origin*, lateral margin of scapula; *insertion*, greater tubercle of humerus; *innervation*, axillary; *action*, rotates arm laterally 小圆肌，又称 *musculus teres minor*；**m. of terminal notch**, an inconstant muscular slip continuing forward from the tragicus muscle to bridge the incisure of the cartilaginous meatus 耳界切迹肌，从耳屏肌向前延续，连接软骨性耳道切迹的肌肉，非普遍存在，易发生变异；Called also *musculus incisurae terminalis*；**thenar m's**, the abductor and flexor muscles of the thumb 鱼际肌；**thyroarytenoid m.**, one of the intrinsic muscles of the larynx: *origin*, lamina of thyroid cartilage; *insertion*, muscular process of arytenoid cartilage; *innervation*, recurrent laryngeal; *action*, relaxes, shortens vocal folds 甲杓肌，又称 *musculus thyroarytenoideus*；**thyroepiglottic m.**, the thyroepiglottic part of the thyroarytenoid muscle: fibers of the thyroarytenoid muscle that continue to the margin of the epiglottis, closing the inlet to the larynx 甲状会厌肌；**thyrohyoid m.**, *origin*, lamina of thyroid cartilage; *insertion*, greater cornu of hyoid bone; *innervation*, first cervical; *action*, raises and changes form of larynx 甲状舌骨肌，又称 *musculus thyrohyoideus*；**thyropharyngeus m.**, the part of the inferior pharyngeal constrictor muscle arising from the thyroid cartilage 甲咽肌；**tibialis anterior m.**, anterior tibial muscle: *origin*, lateral condyle and lateral surface of tibia, interosseous membrane; *insertion*, medial cuneiform and base of first metatarsal; *innervation*, deep fibular; *action*, dorsiflexes and inverts foot 胫骨前肌，又称 *musculus tibialis anterior*；**tibialis posterior m.**, posterior tibial muscle: *origin*, tibia, fibula, interosseous membrane; *insertion*, bases of second to fourth metatarsals and tarsals, except talus; *innervation*, tibial; *action*, plantarflexes and inverts foot 胫骨后肌，又称 *musculus tibialis posterior*；**m's of tongue**, 同 lingual m's；**trachealis m.**, tracheal muscle: a transverse layer of smooth fibers in the dorsal portion of the trachea; *insertion*, tracheal cartilages; *innervation*, autonomic fibers; *action*, lessens caliber of trachea 气管肌，又称 *musculus trachealis*；**tragicus m.**, muscle of tragus: a short, flattened vertical band on the lateral surface of the tragus, innervated by the auriculotemporal and posterior auricular nerves 耳屏肌，又称 *musculus tragicus*；**transverse m. of auricle**, *origin*, cranial surface of auricle; *insertion*, circumference of auricle; *innervation*, posterior auricular; *action*, retracts helix 耳廓横肌，又称 *musculus transversus auriculae*；**transverse perineal m., deep**, *origin*, ramus of ischium; *insertion*, tendinous center of perineum; *innervation*, perineal; *action*, fixes tendinous center of

652

perineum 会阴深横肌，又称 *musculus transversus perinei profundus*；**transverse perineal m.**, superficial, *origin*, ramus of ischium; *insertion*, tendinous center of perineum; *innervation*, perineal; *action*, fixes tendinous center of perineum 会阴浅横肌，又称 *musculus transversus perinei superficialis*；**transverse m. of tongue**, *origin*, median septum of tongue; *insertion*, dorsum and margins of tongue; *innervation*, hypoglossal; *action*, changes shape of tongue in mastication and deglutition 舌横肌，又称 *musculus transversus linguae*；**transversospinales m's**, a general term including the semispinalis, multifidus, and rotatores muscles 横突棘肌，又称 *musculi transversospinales*；**transversus abdominis m.**, *origin*, cartilages of six lower ribs, thoracolumbar fascia, iliac crest, inguinal ligament; *insertion*, linea alba through rectus sheath, conjoined tendon to pubis; *innervation*, lower intercostals, iliohypogastric, ilioinguinal; *action*, increases intra-abdominal pressure, acts as accessory respiratory muscle 腹横肌，又称 *musculus transversus abdominis*；**transversus menti m.**, superficial fibers of the depressor anguli oris that turn back and cross to the opposite side 颏横肌，又称 *musculus transversus menti*；**transversus nuchae m.**, a small muscle often present, passing from the occipital protuberance to the posterior auricular muscle; it may be either superficial or deep to the trapezius 项横肌，又 称 *musculus transversus nuchae*；**transversus thoracis m.**, *origin*, mediastinal surface of sternum and of xiphoid process; *insertion*, cartilages of second to sixth ribs; *innervation*, intercostal; *action*, draws ribs downward 胸横肌，又称 *musculus transversus thoracis*；**trapezius m.**, *origin*, occipital bone, nuchal ligament, spinous processes of seventh cervical and all thoracic vertebrae; *insertion*, clavicle, acromion, spine of scapula; *innervation*, accessory nerve and cervical plexus; *action*, elevates shoulder, rotates scapula to raise shoulder in abduction of arm, draws scapula backward 斜方肌，又称 *musculus trapezius*；**triangular m.**, 1. a muscle that is triangular in shape 三角肌；2. depressor anguli oris m. 降口角肌；**triceps brachii m.**, triceps muscle of arm (3 heads): *origin*, LONG HEAD— infraglenoid tubercle of scapula, LATERAL HEAD—posterior surface of humerus, lateral border of humerus, lateral intermuscular septum, MEDIAL HEAD—posterior surface of humerus below radial groove, medial border of humerus, medial intermuscular septum; *insertion*, olecranon of ulna; *innervation*, radial; *action*, extends forearm, long head adducts and extends arm 肱三头肌，又称 *musculus triceps brachii*；**triceps surae m.**, the gastrocnemius and soleus considered

together 小腿三头肌，又称 *musculus triceps surae*；**trigonal m's**, a submucous sheet of smooth muscle at the vesical trigone, continuous with ureteral muscles above and with those of the proximal urethra below; divided into morphologically distinct superficial and deep layers 膀胱三角肌，又称 *musculi trigoni vesicae urinariae*；**trigonal m., deep**, the deep layer of trigonal muscles, which is continuous with the detrusor muscle of bladder 深膀 胱三角肌，又称 *musculus trigoni vesicae urinariae profundus*；**trigonal m., superficial**, the superficial layer of the trigonal muscles, continuous proximally with the muscles of the ureteral wall 浅膀胱 三角肌，又称 *musculus trigoni vesicae urinariae superficialis*；**unipennate m.**, 同 semipennate m.；**m's of upper limb**, the muscles acting on the arm, forearm, and hand 上肢肌；**m. of uvula**, *origin*, posterior nasal spine of palatine bone and aponeurosis of soft palate; *insertion*, uvula; *innervation*, pharyngeal plexus of vagus; *action*, raises uvula 腭垂 肌，又称 *musculus uvulae*；**vastus intermedius m.**, *origin*, anterior and lateral surfaces of femur; *insertion*, patella, common tendon of quadriceps femoris; *innervation*, femoral; *action*, extends leg 股中间肌，又称 *musculus vastus intermedius*；**vastus lateralis m.**, *origin*, lateral aspect of femur; *insertion*, patella, common tendon of quadriceps femoris; *innervation*, femoral; *action*, extends leg 股外侧肌，又称 *musculus vastus lateralis*；**vastus medialis m.**, *origin*, medial aspect of femur; *insertion*, patella, common tendon of quadriceps femoris; *innervation*, femoral; *action*, extends leg 股内侧肌，又称 *musculus vastus medialis*；**vertical m. of tongue**, *origin*, dorsal fascia of tongue; *insertion*, sides and base of tongue; *innervation*, hypoglossal; *action*, changes shape of tongue in mastication and deglutition 舌垂直肌，又 称 *musculus verticalis linguae*；**vestigial m.**, a muscle that was once well developed but through evolution has become rudimentary 遗迹肌；**visceral m.**, muscle fibers associated chiefly with the hollow viscera; except for the striated fibers in the heart, they are smooth muscle fibers bound together by reticular fibers 内脏肌；**vocalis m.**, vocal muscle: one of the intrinsic muscles of the larynx: *origin*, angle between laminae of thyroid cartilage; *insertion*, vocal process of arytenoid cartilage; *innervation*, recurrent laryngeal; *action*, shortens and relaxes vocal folds 声带肌，又称 *musculus vocalis*；**voluntary m.**, skeletal m. 随意肌（正常时 受意志控制的肌肉，几乎均由横纹肌纤维构成）；**yoked m's**, those that normally act simultaneously and equally, as in moving the eyes 共轭肌，同时产 生相同动作的肌肉，如动眼时涉及的相关肌肉；

zygomaticus major m., greater zygomatic muscle: *origin*, zygomatic bone in front of temporal process; *insertion*, angle of mouth; *innervation*, facial; *action*, draws angle of mouth backward and upward 颧大肌，又 称 *musculus zygomaticus major*；**zygomaticus minor m.**, lesser zygomatic muscle: *origin*, zygomatic bone near maxillary suture; *insertion*, orbicularis oris and levator labii superioris; *innervation*, facial; *action*, draws upper lip upward and laterally 颧小肌，又称 *musculus zygomaticus minor*

mus·cle phos·pho·fruc·to·ki·nase (mus′əl fos-″fo-frook″to-ki′nās) the muscle isozyme of 6-phosphofructokinase 肌磷酸果糖激酶

mus·cle phos·phor·y·lase (mus′əl fos-for′ə- lās) the muscle isozyme of glycogen phosphorylase; deficiency causes glycogen storage disease, type V 肌磷酸化酶

mus·cu·lar (mus′ku-lər) 1. pertaining to, composed of, or composing muscle 肌肉的；2. having a well-developed musculature 壮健的，肌肉发达的

mus·cu·la·ris (mus″ku-lar′is) [L.] 1. muscular 肌的；2.pertaining to a muscular layer or coat肌层的；**m. exter′na**, tunica muscularis 肌层；**m. muco′sae**, the thin layer of smooth muscle fibers usually found as part of the mucosa deep to the lamina propria 黏膜肌层

mus·cu·la·ture (mus′ku-lə-chər) the muscular apparatus of the body or of a part 肌肉系统

mus·cu·lo·apo·neu·rot·ic (mus″ku-lo-ap′onōo-rot′ik) pertaining to a muscle and its aponeurosis 肌腱膜的

mus·cu·lo·cu·ta·ne·ous (mus″ku-lo″ku-ta′- ne-əs) myocutaneous; pertaining to, composed of, or supplying both muscles and skin 肌皮的

mus·cu·lo·phren·ic (mus″ku-lo-fren′ik) pertaining to or supplying the respiratory diaphragm and adjoining muscles 肌膈的

mus·cu·lo·skel·e·tal (mus″ku-lo-skel′ə-təl) pertaining to or comprising the skeleton and muscles 肌（与）骨骼的

mus·cu·lo·spi·ral (mus″ku-lo-spi′rəl) pertaining to muscles and having a spiral direction, as does the radial nerve 肌螺旋的，与肌肉有关，具有螺旋方向，如桡神经螺旋

mus·cu·lo·ten·di·nous (mus″ku-lo-ten′dī-nəs) pertaining to or composed of muscle and tendon 肌腱的

mus·cu·lus (mus′ku-ləs) pl. *mus′culi* [L.] 同 muscle

mush·room (mush′room) the fleshy fruiting body of any of a variety of fungi, especially one that is edible; most are in the order Agaricales 蕈菌，蘑菇

mus·tard (mus′tərd) 1. a plant of the genus *Bras-* *sica* 芥属植物；2. the ripe seeds of *Brassica alba* (white mustard) and *B. nigra* (black mustard), whose oils have irritant, stimulant, and emetic properties 芥子，白芥和黑芥的成熟种子，其油具有刺激性和催吐性；3. resembling, or something resembling, mustard in one or more of its properties 在一种或多种性质上类似于芥末的东西；**nitrogen m.**, 1. 同 mechlorethamine；2. any of a group of cytotoxic, blistering alkylating agents homologous to the vesicant war gas dichlorodiethyl sulfide (mustard gas), some of which have been used as antineoplastics and immunosuppressants 任何一种与糜烂性毒气二氯二乙基硫醚（芥子气）同源的细胞毒性起泡烷基化剂，其中一些已被用作抗肿瘤药和免疫抑制药

mu·ta·gen (mu′tə-jən) an agent that induces genetic mutation 诱变剂，致突变原

mu·ta·gen·e·sis (mu″tə-jen′ə-sis) the induction of genetic mutation 诱变，遗传突变的诱导

mu·ta·gen·ic (mu″tə-jen′ik) inducing genetic mutation 诱变的

mu·ta·ge·nic·i·ty (mu″tə-jə-nis′ĭ-te) the ability to induce genetic mutation 诱变性

mu·tant (mu′tənt) 1. something, as an organism, cell, virus, or gene, that has undergone genetic mutation 突变体，突变型；2. produced by mutation 变异的

mu·ta·ro·tase (mu″tə-ro′tās) an isomerase that catalyzes the interconversion of the α- and β-forms of d-glucose, l-arabinose, d-galactose, d-xylose, lactose, and maltose 变旋酶

mu·ta·ro·ta·tion (mu″tə-ro-ta′shən) a change in optical activity of a freshly prepared solution of a pure compound, occurring because of the formation of diastereoisomers having different optical activity 变旋（现象）

mu·tase (mu′tās) a group of enzymes (transferases) that catalyze the intramolecular shifting of a chemical group from one position to another 变位酶

mu·ta·tion (mu-ta′shən) 1. a permanent transmissible change in the genetic material 突变；2. a cell, virus, or organism exhibiting such a change 表现出这种变化的细胞、病毒或有机体；**germline m.**, one in a germ cell, altering the gametes and thus transmitted to progeny 生殖细胞突变；**missense m.**, one that changes a codon so that it codes for a different amino acid 错义突变；**nonsense m.**, one in which a codon signaling chain termination appears in the middle of an mRNA, causing premature transcription termination and production of an incomplete, usually nonfunctional, polypeptide 无义突变；**point m.**, a mutation resulting from a change in a single base pair in the DNA molecule 点突变；

M

reverse m., 回复突变，反突变，参见 *reversion* (2)；**silent m.**, one that does not affect function or production of the gene product; sometimes more specifically a change in the DNA sequence of a coding region that does not change the amino acid sequence of the polypeptide product 沉默突变，同义突变；**somatic m.**, one occurring in a somatic cell, and thus not transmitted to progeny 体细胞突变；**suppressor m.**, one that partially or completely masks phenotypic expression of another mutation but occurs at a different site from it (i.e., causes suppression); used particularly to describe a secondary mutation that suppresses a nonsense codon created by a primary mutation 抑制（基因）突变

mute (mūt) 1. unable to speak 哑的；2. to muffle or soften a sound 消减（噪声）

mu·ti·la·tion (mu″tī-la′shən) the act of depriving an individual of a limb, member, or other important part. Also, the condition resulting therefrom 残毁，残缺；阉割

mu·tism (mu′tiz-əm) inability or refusal to speak 缄默症；**akinetic m.**, a state in which the person appears to be alert but can make no spontaneous movement or sound 无动性缄默，运动不能性缄默症，个体处于无自发运动及失声的状态；**selective m.**, a mental disorder of childhood characterized by continuous refusal to speak in social situations by a child who is able and willing to speak to selected persons 选择性缄默症，一种儿童性精神疾病，其特征为在公共场合下一直不说话，但他有说话的能力，并且愿意和他喜欢的人讲话

mu·tu·al·ism (mu′choo-əl-iz-əm) the biologic association of two individuals or populations of different species, both of which are benefited by the relationship and sometimes unable to exist without it 互惠共生，互利共生

MV¹ [L.] Med′icus Veterina′rius (veterinary physician) 兽医师

MV² megavolt 兆伏（特）；minute volume 每分输出量

mV millivolt; one thousandth (10⁻³) of a volt 毫伏（特）

μV microvolt; one millionth (10⁻⁶) of a volt 微伏（特）

MVP mitral valve prolapse 二尖瓣脱垂，见 syndrome 下词条

MW molecular weight 分子量

MWIA Medical Women's International Association 国际女医务工作者协会

my·al·gia (mi-al′jə) muscular pain 肌痛；**myal′gic** *adj.*；**epidemic m.**, 流行性肌痛；流行性胸肌痛，见 *pleurodynia* 下词条

my·as·the·nia (mi″əs-the′ne-ə) muscular debility

or weakness 肌无力；**myasthen′ic** *adj.*；**familial infantile m. gravis**, choline acetyltransferase deficiency 家族性婴儿重症肌无力；**m. gra′vis**, an autoimmune disease of neuromuscular function, possibly due to presence of antibodies to acetylcholine receptors at the neuromuscular junction, marked by fatigue and exhaustion of the muscular system, often with fluctuating severity, without sensory disturbance or atrophy 重症肌无力；**neonatal m.**, a transient myasthenia affecting offspring of myasthenic women 新生儿肌无力

my·a·to·nia (mi″ə-to′ne-ə) amyotonia 肌张力缺乏，肌迟缓

my·at·ro·phy (mi-at′rə-fe) atrophy of a muscle 肌萎缩

my·ce·li·um (mi-se′le-əm) pl. *myce′lia*. The mass of threadlike processes (hyphae) constituting the fungal thallus 菌丝体；**myce′lial, myce′lian** *adj.*

my·cete (mi′sēt) a fungus 霉菌，真菌

my·ce·to·ma (mi″sə-to′mə) a chronic, progressive, destructive infection of the cutaneous and subcutaneous tissues, fascia, and bone caused by traumatic implantation of certain actinomycetes (*actinomycotic m.*), true fungi (*eumycotic m.*), or other organisms; it usually involves the foot (*Madura foot*) or leg 足菌肿，足分枝菌病

My·co·bac·te·ri·a·ceae (mi″ko-bak-tēr″e′a′se-e) a family of gram-positive, aerobic, rodshaped bacteria of the order Actinomycetales 分枝杆菌科

My·co·bac·te·ri·um (mi″ko-bak-tēr′e-əm) a genus of gram-positive, aerobic, acid-fast, rodshaped bacteria of the family Mycobacteriaceae 结核分枝杆菌属；**M. a′vium**, the avian type of tubercle bacillus, which causes pulmonary disease in humans 鸟分枝杆菌，另参见 *complex* 下 *Mycobacterium avium-intracellulare complex*；**M. bo′vis**, a virulent species that causes tuberculosis in cattle and can be acquired by humans from infected milk. An attenuated strain is used to prepare BCG vaccine 牛分枝杆菌；**M. chelo′nae**, a species that is an opportunistic pathogen, causing soft tissue abscesses throughout the body 龟分枝杆菌；**M. intracellula′re**, a species associated with chronic pulmonary infection in humans 胞内分枝杆菌，另参见 *complex* 下 *Mycobacterium avium-intra- cellulare complex*；**M. kansa′sii**, a slow-growing species that causes tuberculosislike disease in humans, particularly among immunocompromised persons 堪萨斯分枝杆菌；**M. lep′rae**, the species that causes leprosy 麻风（分枝）杆菌；**M. mari′num**, a species that causes cutaneous lesions and granulomas (swimming pool granuloma) 海分枝杆菌；**M. tuberculo′sis**, the tubercle bacillus; a slow-growing species that causes tuberculosis, most commonly in the lungs 结核（分枝杆）菌

my·co·bac·te·ri·um (mi″ko-bak-tēr′e-əm) pl. *mycobacte′ria.* An individual organism of the genus *Mycobacterium* 分 枝 杆 菌；**anonymous myco-bacteria, atypical mycobacteria,** nontuberculous mycobacteria 无名分枝杆菌，非典型分枝杆菌；**Group Ⅰ to Ⅳ mycobacteria,** 参见 *nontuberculous mycobacteria*；**nontuberculous mycobacteria,** mycobacteria other than *Mycobacterium tuberculosis* or *M. bovis;* they are divided into four groups, Ⅰ to Ⅳ, on the basis of several physical characteristics 非结核性分枝杆菌，Ⅰ～Ⅳ类分枝杆类

my·col·o·gy (mi-kol′ə-je) the science and study of fungi 真菌学

my·co·pheno·late (mi″ko-fen′ə-lāt) an immuno-suppressant used as *m. mofetil* to prevent rejection of allogeneic cardiac, hepatic, and renal transplants 霉酚酸酯

My·co·plas·ma (mi′ko-plaz″mə) a genus of gram-negative, aerobic to facultatively anaerobic bacteria of the family Mycoplasmataceae, including the pleuropneumonia-like organisms; species include *M. ho′minis,* which is associated with non-gonococcal urethritis and mild pharyngitis, and *M. pneumo′niae,* a cause of primary atypical pneumonia 支原体属

my·co·plas·mal (mi″ko-plaz′məl) of, pertaining to, or caused by *Mycoplasma* 支原体的

My·co·plas·ma·ta·ceae (mi″ko-plaz″mə-ta′- se-e) a family of schizomycetes of the class Mollicutes, comprising organisms that require sterol for growth 支原体科

my·co·sis (mi-ko′sis) any disease caused by fungi 真菌病；**m. fungoi′des,** a chronic or rapidly progressive form of cutaneous T-cell lymphoma, characterized by Sézary cells and later painful, ulcerating tumors 蕈样肉芽肿病

my·cot·ic (mi-kot′ik) 1. pertaining to mycosis 真菌病的；2. caused by a fungus 由真菌引起的；3. pertaining to or caused by any microorganism; obsolete except in the phrase *mycotic aneurysm* 由微生物引起或与之相关的；如今除真菌性动脉瘤，已不再使用

my·co·tox·i·co·sis (mi″ko-tok″sī-ko′sis) poisoning caused by a mycotoxin 真菌（毒素）中毒症

my·co·tox·in (mi′ko-tok″sin) a toxic secondary metabolite produced by a microscopic fungus 真菌毒素

my·dri·a·sis (mĭ-dri′ə-sis) [Gr.] dilatation of the pupil 瞳孔散大

myd·ri·at·ic (mid″re-at′ik) dilating the pupil, or an agent that so acts 散瞳的；散瞳药

my·ec·to·my (mi-ek′tə-me) excision of a muscle 肌（部分）切除术

my·ec·to·pia (mi-ek-to′pe-ə) displacement of a muscle 肌异位

my·el·at·ro·phy (mi″əl-at′rə-fe) atrophy of the spinal cord 脊髓萎缩

my·el·emia (mi″ə-le′me-ə) 同 myelocytosis

my·el·en·ceph·a·lon (mi″əl-en-sef′ə-lon) 1. medulla oblongata 延髓；2. the posterior of two brain vesicles formed by specialization of the hindbrain in embryonic development 末脑

my·elin (mi′ə-lin) the lipid-rich substance of the cell membrane of Schwann cells that coils to form the myelin sheath surrounding the axon of myelinated nerve fibers 髓磷脂，髓鞘质；**myelin′ic** adj.

my·eli·nat·ed (mi′ə-lĭ-nāt′əd) having a myelin sheath 有髓（鞘）的

my·elin·i·za·tion (mi″ə-lin″ĭ-za′shən) the act of adding myelin; formation of a myelin sheath 髓鞘形成，又称 myelination

my·elin·ol·y·sis (mi″ə-lin-ol′ə-sis) demyelination 脱髓鞘，髓鞘破坏；**central pontine m.,** symmetric demye - lination affecting the central pons, possibly caused by rapid correction of hyponatremia, and characterized by rapidly progressing paraparesis or quadriparesis, dysarthria, dysphagia, and impaired consciousness 中心性脑桥髓鞘破坏

my·eli·no·sis (mi″ə-lĭ-no′sis) fatty degeneration, with formation of myelin 脂肪坏死性髓磷脂生成

my·elino·tox·ic (mi″ə-lin-o-tok″sik) having a deleterious effect on myelin; causing demyelination 对髓鞘有毒性的；致脱髓鞘的

my·eli·tis (mi″ə-li′tis) 1. inflammation of the spinal cord; often expanded to include noninflammatory spinal cord lesions 脊髓炎；2. inflammation of the bone marrow (osteomyelitis) 骨髓炎；**myelit′ic** adj.

my·elo·ab·la·tion (mi″ə-lo-ab-la′shən) the severe or complete depletion of bone marrow cells, as with the administration of high doses of chemotherapy or radiation therapy prior to stem cell transplantation 脊髓抑制；**myeloab′lative** adj.

my·elo·blast (mi′ə-lo-blast) an immature cell found in the bone marrow and not normally in the peripheral blood; it is the most primitive precursor in the granulocytic series, which matures to develop into the promyelocyte and eventually the granular leukocyte 原粒细胞，成髓细胞；**myeloblas′tic** adj.

my·elo·blas·te·mia (mi″ə-lo-blas-te′me-ə) the presence of myeloblasts in the blood 成髓细胞血症

my·elo·blas·to·ma (mi″ə-lo-blas-to′mə) a focal malignant tumor composed of myeloblasts or early myeloid precursors occurring outside the bone marrow 成髓细胞瘤

my·elo·cele (mi′ə-lo-sēl) protrusion of the spinal cord through a defect in the vertebral arch 脊髓膨出

my·elo·cyst (mi′ə-lo-sist) a benign cyst developed from rudimentary medullary canals 脊髓囊肿

my·elo·cys·to·cele (mi″ə-lo-sis′to-sēl) my - elo - meningocele 脊髓囊肿状突出，脊髓脊膜膨出

my·elo·cys·to·me·nin·go·cele (mi″ə-lo-sis″tomə-ning′go-sēl) 同 myelomeningocele

my·elo·cyte (mi′ə-lo-sīt) a precursor in the granulocyte series, being a cell intermediate in development between a promyelocyte and a metamyelocyte 中幼粒细胞；**myelocyt′ic** adj.

my·elo·cy·to·sis (mi″ə-lo-si-to′sis) excessive number of myelocytes in the blood 髓细胞血症，髓细胞增多症

myelodysplasia (mi″ə-lo-dis-pla′zhə) 1. a neural tube defect causing defective development of any part of the spinal cord 脊髓发育不良；2. dysplasia of myelocytes and other elements of the bone marrow 骨髓增生异常；**myelodysplas′tic** adj.

my·elo·en·ceph·a·li·tis (mi″ə-lo-en-sef″ə- li′tis) inflammation of the spinal cord and brain 脑脊髓炎

my·elo·fi·bro·sis (mi″ə-lo-fi-bro′sis) replacement of bone marrow by fibrous tissue 骨髓纤维化(症)

my·elo·gen·e·sis (mi″ə-lo-jen′ə-sis) 同 myelinization

my·elog·e·nous (mi″ə-loj′ə-nəs) produced in bone marrow 骨髓性的

my·elog·ra·phy (mi″ə-log′rə-fe) radiography of the spinal cord after injection of a contrast medium into the subarachnoid space 脊髓造影(术)

my·eloid (mi′ə-loid) 1. medullary; pertaining to, derived from, or resembling bone marrow or the spinal cord 骨髓的；脊髓的；2. having the appearance of myelocytes, but not derived from bone marrow 髓细胞样的

my·eloi·do·sis (mi″ə-loi-do′sis) formation of myeloid tissue, especially hyperplastic development of such tissue 骨髓组织增生

my·elo·li·po·ma (mi″ə-lo-lǐ-po′mə) a rare benign tumor of the suprarenal gland composed of adipose tissue, lymphocytes, and primitive myeloid cells 髓脂瘤

my·elo·ma (mi″ə-lo′mə) 1. a tumor composed of cells of the type normally found in the bone marrow 骨髓瘤；2. 同 multiple m.；**giant cell m.**, 巨细胞性骨髓瘤，参见 tumor (1) 下词条；**multiple m.**, a disseminated type of plasma cell dyscrasia characterized by multiple bone marrow tumor foci and secretion of an M component, manifested by skeletal destruction, pathologic fractures, bone pain,

the presence of anomalous circulating immunoglobulins, Bence Jones proteinuria, and anemia 多发性骨髓瘤；**plasma cell m.**, multiple m. 浆细胞性骨髓瘤；**sclerosing m.**, myeloma associated with osteosclerosis, most often manifested by peripheral neuropathy 硬化性骨髓瘤；**solitary m.**, a variant of multiple myeloma in which there is a single localized tumor focus 孤立性骨髓瘤

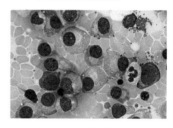

▲ 骨髓内多发性骨髓瘤，可见大的伴核仁的浆细胞

my·elo·ma·la·cia (mi″ə-lo-mə-la′shə) morbid softening of the spinal cord 脊髓软化

my·elo·ma·to·sis (mi″ə-lo-mə-to′sis) multiple myeloma 骨髓瘤，多发性骨髓瘤

my·elo·men·in·gi·tis (mi″ə-lo-men″in-ji′tis) 同 meningomyelitis

my·elo·men·in·go·cele (mi″ə-lo-mə-nin′gosēl″) hernial protrusion of the spinal cord and its meninges through a defect in the vertebral arch 脊髓脊膜膨出

my·elo·mere (mi′ə-lo-mēr) one of the segments of the embryonic brain or spinal cord 髓节，胚胎大脑或脊髓的一部分

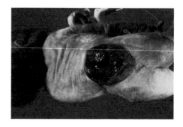

▲ 髓节

my·elo·mono·cyt·ic (mi″ə-lo-mon″o-sit′ik) characterized by both myelocytes and monocytes 髓单核细胞的

my·elop·a·thy (mi″ə-lop′ə-the) 1. any functional disturbance and/or pathologic change in the spinal cord; often used to denote nonspecific lesions, as opposed to myelitis 脊髓病；2. pathologic bone marrow changes 骨髓病；**myelopath′ic** adj.；

carcinomatous m., rapidly progressive degeneration or necrosis of the spinal cord associated with a carcinoma 癌（性）脊髓病；**chronic progressive m.,** gradually progressive spastic paraparesis associated with infection by human T-lymphotropic virus 1 慢性进行性脊髓病；**HTLV-1–associated m.,** chronic progressive m. HTLV-1 相关脊髓病；**paracarcinomatous m., paraneoplastic m.,** carcinomatous m. 副癌脊髓病；**spondylotic cervical m.,** that secondary to encroachment of cervical spondylosis upon a congenitally small cervical spinal canal 颈椎硬化性脊髓病；**transverse m.,** that extending across the spinal cord 横贯性脊髓病；**vacuolar m.,** loss of myelin and spongy degeneration of the spinal cord with microscopic vacuolization, caused by infection with human immunodeficiency virus 空泡性脊髓病

my·elo·per·ox·i·dase (MPO) (mi″ə-lo-pər-ok′sĭ- dās) a green hemoprotein in neutrophils and monocytes that catalyzes the reaction of hydrogen peroxide and halide ions to form cytotoxic acids and other intermediates; these play a role in the oxygen-dependent killing of tumor cells and microorganisms 髓过氧化物酶

my·elop·e·tal (mi″ə-lop′ə-təl) moving toward the spinal cord 向脊髓的

my·e·loph·thi·sis (mi″ə-lof′thĭ-sis) 1. wasting of the spinal cord 脊髓痨；2. bone marrow suppression secondary to marrow infiltration by tumor with local production of myelosuppressive cytokines 骨髓痨，全骨髓萎缩

my·elo·plast (mi′ə-lo-plast″) any leukocyte of the bone marrow 骨髓白细胞

my·elo·poi·e·sis (mi″ə-lo-poi-e′sis) the formation of marrow or the cells arising from it 骨髓组织生成，骨髓细胞生成；**myelopoiet′ic** adj.

my·elo·pro·lif·er·a·tive (mi″ə-lo-pro-lif′ər-ə- tiv) pertaining to or characterized by medullary and extramedullary proliferation of bone marrow constituents 骨髓增生的，骨髓增殖的；参见 disorder 下词条

my·elo·ra·dic·u·li·tis (mi″ə-lo-rə-dik″u-li′tis) inflammation of the spinal cord and posterior nerve roots 脊髓神经根炎

my·elo·ra·dic·u·lo·dys·pla·sia (mi″ə-lo-rə-dik″u-lo-dis-pla′zhə) developmental abnormality of the spinal cord and spinal nerve roots 脊髓神经根发育异常

my·elo·ra·dic·u·lop·a·thy (mi″ə-lo-rə-dik″u-lop′ə-the) disease of the spinal cord and spinal nerve roots 脊髓神经根病

my·elor·rha·gia (mi″ə-lo-ra′jə) hematomyelia 脊髓出血

my·elo·sar·co·ma (mi″ə-lo-sahr-ko′mə) a sarcomatous growth made up of myeloid tissue or bone marrow cells 骨髓肉瘤

my·elos·chi·sis (mi″ə-los′kĭ-sis) a developmental anomaly characterized by a cleft spinal cord 脊髓裂

my·elo·scle·ro·sis (mi″ə-lo-sklə-ro′sis) 1. sclerosis of the spinal cord 脊骨髓硬化；2. obliteration of the medullary cavity by small spicules of bone 骨髓硬化症；3. 同 myelofibrosis

my·elo·sis (mi″ə-lo′sis) 1. 同 myelocytosis；2. formation of a tumor of the spinal cord 脊髓瘤形成；**erythremic m.,** erythroleukemia 红细胞增多性骨髓增殖

my·elo·spon·gi·um (mi″ə-lo-spun′je-əm) a network developing into the neuroglia 髓管网

my·elo·sup·pres·sion (mi″ə-lo-sə-presh′ən) bone marrow suppression 骨髓抑制

my·elo·sup·pres·sive (mi″ə-lo-sə-pres′iv) 1. causing bone marrow suppression 骨髓抑制的；2. an agent that so acts 骨髓抑制药

my·elo·tox·ic (mi″ə-lo-tok″sik) 1. destructive to bone marrow 骨髓毒性的；2. myelosuppressive 骨髓抑制的；3. arising from diseased bone marrow 骨髓病性的

my·en·ter·on (mi-en′tər-on) the muscular coat of the intestine 肠肌层；**myenter′ic** adj.

my·es·the·sia (mi″es-the′zhə) muscle sense (1) 肌觉

my·i·a·sis (mi-i′ə-sis) invasion of the body by the larvae of flies, characterized as cutaneous (subdermal tissue), gastrointestinal, nasopharyngeal, ocular, or urinary, depending on the region invaded 蝇蛆病，苍蝇幼虫侵入身体，其特征症状取决于被侵入的区域，如皮肤（皮下组织）、胃肠道、鼻咽、眼或尿

my·lo·hy·oid (mi″lo-hi′oid) pertaining to molar teeth and the hyoid bone 下颌舌骨的

myo·ar·chi·tec·ton·ic (mi″o-ahr″kĭ-tek-ton′- ik) pertaining to structural arrangement of muscle fibers 肌结构的

myo·at·ro·phy (mi″o-at′rə-fe) muscular atrophy 肌萎缩

myo·blast (mi′o-blast) an embryonic cell that becomes a muscle cell or fiber 成肌细胞；**myoblas′tic** adj.

myo·blas·to·ma (mi″o-blas-to′mə) a benign circumscribed tumor-like lesion of soft tissue, possibly composed of myoblasts 成肌细胞瘤；**granular cell m.,** 颗粒细胞成肌细胞瘤，参见 tumor 下词条

myo·car·di·al (mi″o-kahr′de-əl) pertaining to the muscular tissue of the heart 心肌的

myo·car·di·op·a·thy (mi″o-kahr″de-op′ə-the)

cardiomyopathy 心肌病

myo·car·di·tis (mi″o-kahr-di′tis) inflammation of the muscular walls of the heart 心肌炎；**acute isolated m.**, a frequently fatal, idiopathic, acute myocarditis affecting chiefly the interstitial fibrous tissue 急性孤立性心肌炎；**Fiedler m.**, acute isolated myocarditis 菲德勒心肌炎；**giant cell m.**, a subtype of acute isolated myocarditis characterized by the presence of multinucleate giant cells and other inflammatory cells, and by ventricular dilatation, mural thrombi, and wide areas of necrosis 巨细胞性心肌炎；**granulomatous m.**, giant cell myocarditis, including also granuloma formation 粒细胞性心肌炎；**hypersensitivity m.**, that due to allergic reactions caused by hypersensitivity to various agents, particularly sulfonamides, penicillins, and methyldopa 过敏性心肌炎；**interstitial m.**, that affecting chiefly the interstitial fibrous tissue 间质性心肌炎

myo·car·di·um (mi″o-kahr′de-əm) the middle and thickest layer of the heart wall, composed of cardiac muscle 心肌；**hibernating m.**, 冬眠心肌，参见 *hibernation* 下 *myocardial hibernation*; **stunned m.**, 顿抑心肌，参见 *stunning* 下 *myocardial stunning*

myo·cele (mi′o-sēl) protrusion of a muscle through its ruptured sheath 肌突出

my·oc·lo·nus (mi-ok′lo-nəs) shocklike contractions of a muscle or a group of muscles 肌阵挛；**myoclon′ic** *adj.*; **essential m.**, myoclonus of unknown etiology, involving one or more muscles and elicited by excitement or an attempt at voluntary movement 原发性肌阵挛，病因不明的肌阵挛，累及一块或多块肌肉，由兴奋或自主运动引起；**intention m.**, that occurring when voluntary muscle movement is initiated 行为性肌阵挛，自发的肌肉运动时发生的；**nocturnal m.**, nonpathologic myoclonic jerks occurring as a person is falling asleep or is asleep 夜间肌阵挛，非病理性肌阵挛，发生于人入睡或睡着时；**palatal m.**, rapid rhythmic, up-and-down movement of one or both sides of the palate, often with ipsilateral synchronous clonic movements of the tongue, pharynx, and respiratory diaphragm muscles 腭肌阵挛，上腭一侧或两侧的快速有节奏的上下运动，通常伴有面部、舌头、咽和呼吸隔膜肌肉的同侧同步阵挛运动

myo·coele (mi′o-sēl) the cavity within a myotome (2) 肌节腔

my·o·cu·ta·ne·ous (mi″o-ku-ta′ne-əs) 同 musculocutaneous

myo·cyte (mi′o-sīt) a muscle cell 肌细胞；**Anichkov (Anitschkow) m.**, Anichkov 肌细胞，参见 *cell* 下词条

myo·cy·tol·y·sis (mi″o-si-tol′ĭ-sis) disintegration

of muscle fibers 肌细胞崩溃，肌纤维崩溃

myo·dys·to·nia (mi″o-dis-to′ne-ə) disorder of muscular tone 肌张力障碍

myo·dys·tro·phy (mi″o-dis′trə-fe) 1. muscular dystrophy 肌营养不良；2. myotonic dystrophy 肌强直性营养不良

myo·ede·ma (mi″o-ə-de′mə) 1. the rising in a lump by a wasting muscle when struck 肌耸起；2. edema of a muscle 肌水肿

myo·epi·the·li·o·ma (mi″o-ep″ĭ-the″le-o′mə) a tumor composed of outgrowths of myoepithelial cells from a sweat gland 肌上皮（细胞）瘤

myo·epi·the·li·um (mi″o-ep″ĭ-the″le-əm) tissue made up of contractile epithelial cells 肌上皮；**myoepithe′lial** *adj.*

myo·fas·ci·al (mi″o-fash′e-əl) pertaining to or involving the fascia surrounding and associated with muscle tissue 肌筋膜的

myo·fas·ci·tis (mi″o-fə-si′tis) inflammation of a muscle and its fascia 肌筋膜炎

myo·fi·ber (mi′o-fi″bər) muscle fiber 肌纤维

myo·fi·bril (mi″o-fi′bril) muscle fibril; one of the slender threads of a muscle fiber, composed of numerous myofilaments 肌原纤维，见图 7；**myo·ofi′brillar** *adj.*

myo·fi·bro·blast (mi″o-fi′bro-blast) an atypical fibroblast combining the ultrastructural features of a fibroblast and a smooth muscle cell 肌成纤维细胞

myo·fi·bro·ma (mi″o-fi-bro′mə) leiomyoma 肌纤维瘤

myo·fi·bro·sis (mi″o-fi-bro′sis) replacement of muscle tissue by fibrous tissue 肌纤维化，肌纤维变性

myo·fila·ment (mi″o-fil′ə-mənt) any of the ultramicroscopic threadlike structures composing the myofibrils of striated muscle fibers; thick ones contain myosin, thin ones contain actin, and intermediate ones contain desmin and vimentin 肌丝，见图 7

myo·gen·e·sis (mi″o-jen′ə-sis) the development of muscle tissue, especially its embryonic development 肌生成；**myogenet′ic** *adj.*

my·o·gen·ic (mi″o-jen′ik) 1. pertaining to myogenesis 生肌的；2. originating in myocytes or muscle tissue 肌（源）性的

my·og·e·nous (mi-oj′ə-nəs) originating in muscular tissue 生肌的，肌（源）性的

myo·glo·bin (mi′o-glo′bin) the oxygen-transporting pigment of muscle, a hemoprotein that resembles a single subunit of hemoglobin, being composed of one globin polypeptide chain and one heme group 肌红蛋白

myo·glob·u·lin (mi″o-glob′u-lin) a globulin from muscle serum 肌球蛋白

myo·graph (mi′o-graf) apparatus for recording effects of muscular contraction 肌动描记器，记录肌肉收缩效应的仪器

my·og·ra·phy (mi-og′rə-fe) 1. the use of a myograph 肌动描记（法）；2. description of muscles 肌 学；3. radiography of muscle tissue after injection of a radiopaque medium 肌组织 X 线摄影（术）；**myograph′ic** *adj.*

my·oid (mi′oid) resembling muscle 肌样的；肌样质，肌样体

myo·ki·nase (mi″o-ki′nās) adenylate kinase; an enzyme of muscle that catalyzes the phosphorylation of ADP to molecules of ATP and AMP 肌激酶

myo·ki·ne·sis (mi″o-kĭ-ne′sis) movement of muscles, especially displacement of muscle fibers in operation 肌运动，肌移位（尤指肌纤维的位移）；**myokinet′ic** *adj.*

myo·kym·ia (mi″o-ki′me-ə) a benign condition marked by brief spontaneous tetanic contractions of motor units or groups of muscle fibers, usually adjacent groups of fibers contracting alternately 肌纤维颤搐；**myoky′mic** *adj.*

myo·li·po·ma (mi″o-lĭ-po′mə) a benign mesenchymoma containing fatty or lipomatous elements 肌脂瘤

my·ol·o·gy (mi-ol′ə-je) the scientific study or description of the muscles and accessory structures (bursae and synovial sheath) 肌学

my·ol·y·sis (mi-ol′ĭ-sis) disintegration or de - generation of muscle tissue 肌溶解

my·o·ma (mi-o′mə) pl. *myomas, myo′mata.* A benign tumor formed of muscle elements 肌 瘤；**myo′matous** *adj.*；**uterine m.,** leiomyoma uteri 子宫肌瘤

my·o·ma·to·sis (mi″o-mə-to′sis) the formation of multiple myomas 肌瘤病，多发性肌瘤形成

my·o·mec·to·my (mi″o-mek′tə-me) 1. surgical removal of a myoma, particularly of the uterus (leiomyoma) 子宫肌瘤切除术；2. 同 myectomy

myo·mel·a·no·sis (mi″o-mel′ə-no′sis) melanosis of muscle tissue 肌黑变病

myo·mere (mi′o-mēr) 同 myotome (2)

my·om·e·ter (mi-om′ə-tər) an apparatus for measuring muscle contraction 肌收缩计，肌力计

myo·me·tri·tis (mi″o-me-tri′tis) inflammation of the myometrium 子宫肌（层）炎

myo·me·tri·um (mi-o-me′tre-əm) the tunica muscularis of the uterus 子宫肌层；**myome′trial** *adj.*

myo·neme (mi′o-nēm) a fine contractile fiber found in the cytoplasm of certain protozoa 肌线

myo·neu·ral (mi″o-noor′əl) pertaining to nerve terminations in muscles 肌神经的

myo·pal·mus (mi″o-pal′məs) muscle twitching 肌颤搐

myo·par·e·sis (mi″o-pə-re′sis) slight muscle paralysis 肌瘫痪，肌麻痹

my·op·a·thy (mi-op′ə-the) any disease of muscle 肌 病；**myopath′ic** *adj.*；**centronuclear m.,** myotubular m. 中心核肌病；**mitochondrial m.,** any of a group of myopathies associated with an increased number of large, often abnormal, mitochondria in muscle fibers and manifested by exercise intolerance, weakness, lactic acidosis, infantile quadriparesis, ophthalmoplegia, and cardiac abnormalities 线粒体肌病；**myotubular m.,** an often fatal congenital myopathy marked by myofibers resembling the myotubules of early fetal muscle; inheritance may be X-linked, dominant, or recessive 肌管性肌病；**nemaline m.,** a congenital abnormality of myofibrils in which small threadlike fibers are scattered through the muscle fibers; marked by hypotonia and proximal muscle weakness 线状体肌病，杆状体肌病；**ocular m.,** progressive external ophthalmoplegia 眼 肌 病；**thyrotoxic m.,** weakness and wasting of skeletal muscles, especially of the pelvic and pectoral girdles, accompanying hyperthyroidism 甲状腺毒性肌病

myo·peri·car·di·tis (mi″o-per″ĭ-kahr-di′tis) myocarditis combined with pericarditis 心肌心包炎

myo·phos·phor·y·lase (mi″o-fos-for′ə-lās) the muscle isozyme of glycogen phosphorylase; deficiency causes glycogen storage disease, type Ⅴ 肌磷酸化酶

my·o·pia (M) (mi-o′pe-ə) nearsightedness; an error of refraction in which rays of light entering the eye parallel to the optic axis are brought to a focus in front of the retina 近视；**myop′ic** *adj.*；**curvature m.,** myopia due to changes in curvature of the refracting surfaces of the eye 曲率性近视，屈光面曲率变化引起的近视；**index m.,** myopia due to abnormal refractivity of the media of the eye 指 数 性近视；**malignant m., pernicious m.,** progressive myopia with disease of the choroid, leading to retinal detachment and blindness 恶性近视，进行性近视伴脉络膜疾病，导致视网膜脱离和失明；**progressive m.,** myopia increasing in adult life 进行性近视

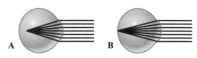

▲ 近视　**A.** 近视眼的屈光度误差；**B.** 正视眼的正常折射

myo·plasm (mi′o-plaz″əm) the contractile part of a muscle cell, or myofibril 肌质，肌浆

myo·plas·ty (mi′o-plas″te) plastic surgery on muscle 肌成形术；**myoplas′tic** *adj.*

my·or·rhex·is (mi″o-rek′sis) rupture of a muscle 肌断裂

myo·sar·co·ma (mi″o-sahr-ko′mə) a malignant tumor derived from muscle tissue 肌肉瘤

myo·scle·ro·sis (mi″o-sklə-ro′sis) hardening of muscle tissue 肌硬化

my·o·sin (mi′o-sin) any of a family of ATPsplitting proteins that move along actin filaments (F-actin). Myosin is involved in the transport of vesicles and organelles and is responsible for the contraction and relaxation of muscle; it also is the motor that drives cytokinesis 肌球蛋白。Cf. *actomyosin*

myo·si·tis (mi″o-si′tis) inflammation of a voluntary muscle 肌炎。**m. fibro′sa,** a type in which connective tissue forms within the muscle 纤维性肌炎；**inclusion body m.,** a progressive type that primarily involves muscles of the pelvic region and legs 包涵体肌炎，主要累及骨盆和腿部肌肉的渐进式肌炎；**m. ossi′ficans,** myositis marked by bony deposits or by ossification of muscle 骨化性肌炎；**proliferative m.,** a benign, rapidly growing, reactive, nodular lesion similar to nodular fasciitis, but characterized by fibroblast proliferation within skeletal muscle 增生性肌炎

myo·tac·tic (mi″o-tak′tik) pertaining to the proprioceptive sense of muscles 肌触觉的，肌本体感觉的

my·ot·a·sis (mi-ot′ə-sis) stretching of muscle 肌伸张；**myotat′ic** *adj.*

myo·teno·si·tis (mi″o-ten″o-si′tis) inflammation of a muscle and tendon 肌腱炎

myo·tome (mi′o-tōm) 1. an instrument for performing myotomy 肌刀；2. the muscle plate or portion of a somite that develops into noncardiac striated muscle 肌节；3. a group of muscles innervated from a single spinal segment 同神经肌丛。**myotom′ic** *adj.*

my·ot·o·my (mi-ot′ə-me) the cutting or dissection of a muscle or of muscular tissue 肌切开术

myo·to·nia (mi″o-to′ne-ə) dystonia involving increased muscular irritability and contractility with decreased power of relaxation 肌强直；**myoton′ic** *adj.*；**m. conge′nita,** tonic spasm and rigidity of certain muscles when attempts are made to move them after rest, improving with sustained motion; there are autosomal dominant and autosomal recessive forms, both due to mutation in a gene encoding a muscle chloride channel; the recessive form is more severe and is also characterized by muscle weakness 先天性肌强直

my·ot·o·noid (mi-ot′ə-noid) denoting muscle reactions marked by slow contraction or relaxation 肌强直样的

my·ot·o·nus (mi-ot′ə-nəs) tonic spasm of a muscle or a group of muscles 肌强直，肌强直性痉挛

myo·tro·phic (mi″o-tro′fik) 1. increasing the weight of muscle 增加肌重量的；2. pertaining to myotrophy 肌营养的

my·ot·ro·phy (mi-ot′rə-fe) nutrition of muscle 肌营养

myo·tu·bule (mi″o-too′būl) a developing muscle cell or fiber with a centrally located nucleus 肌管；**myotu′bular** *adj.*

Myr·i·ap·o·da (mir″e-ap′ə-də) a superclass of arthropods, including centipedes and millipedes 多足纲

my·rin·ga (mĭ-ring′gə) the tympanic membrane 鼓膜

my·rin·gec·to·my (mir″in-jek′tə-me) tympa-nectomy 鼓膜切除术

my·rin·gi·tis (mir″in-ji′tis) inflammation of the tympanic membrane 鼓膜炎；**m. bullo′sa, bullous m.,** a form of viral otitis media in which serous or hemorrhagic blebs appear on the tympanic membrane and often on the adjacent wall of the auditory meatus 大疱性鼓膜炎

my·rin·got·o·my (mir″ing-got′o-me) tympa-notomy; creation of a hole in the tympanic mem-brane, as for tympanocentesis 鼓膜切开术

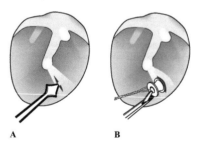

A   B

▲ A. 鼓膜切开术；B. 鼓膜置管术

my·ris·tic ac·id (mĭ-ris′tik) a saturated 14-carbon fatty acid occurring in most animal and vegetable fats, particularly butterfat and coconut, palm, and nutmeg oils 肉豆蔻酸，十四（烷）酸

My·roi·da·ceae (mi″roi-da′se-e) in some systems of classification, a family of bacteria of the phylum Bacteroidetes 类香味菌科

My·roi·des (mi-roi′dēz) a genus of gramnegative, non–spore-forming, rod-shaped bacteria of the family Myroidaceae. *M. odoratimi′mus* and *M. odora′tus*

cause nosocomial infections 类香味菌属

myrrh (mər) the oleo-gum-resin obtained from species of *Commiphora;* applied topically in mild inflammations of the oral and pharyngeal mucosa 没药树脂（局部用于口腔和咽黏膜的轻度炎症）

myr·ti·form (mir′tĭ-form) shaped like myrtle or myrtle berries 桃金娘形的

my·so·pho·bia (mi″so-fo′be-ə) irrational fear of dirt and contamination 洁癖，污秽恐怖

myx·ad·e·ni·tis (miks″ad-ə-ni′tis) inflammation of a mucous gland 黏液腺炎

myx·as·the·nia (miks″əs-the′ne-ə) deficient secretion of mucus 黏液分泌功能衰弱，黏液（分泌）不足

myx·ede·ma (miks″ə-de′mə) a dry, waxy type of swelling (nonpitting edema) with abnormal deposits of mucin in the skin (mucinosis) and other tissues, associated with hypothyroidism; the facial changes are distinctive, with swollen lips and thickened nose 黏液（性）水肿; **myxedem′atous** *adj.*; **congenital m.**, cretinism 呆小病，先天性黏液水肿，克汀病; **papular m.**, lichen myxedematosus 黏液水肿性苔藓，丘疹性黏液水肿; **pituitary m.**, that due to deficient secretion of the pituitary hormone thyrotropin 垂体性黏液水肿; **pretibial m.**, localized edema associated with preceding hyperthyroidism and exophthalmos, occurring typically on the anterior (pretibial) surface of the legs, the mucin deposits appearing as both plaques and papules 胫前黏液（性）水肿

myxo·chon·dro·ma (mik″so-kon-dro′mə) chondroma with stroma resembling primitive mesenchymal tissue 黏液软骨瘤

myxo·fi·bro·ma (mik″so-fi-bro′mə) a fibroma containing myxomatous tissue 黏液纤维瘤

myxo·fi·bro·sar·co·ma (mik″so-fi″bro-sahrko′mə) the myxoid subtype of malignant fibrous histiocytoma 黏液纤维肉瘤

myx·oid (mik′soid) mucoid 黏液样的

myxo·li·po·ma (mik″so-lĭ-po′mə) lipoma with foci of myxomatous degeneration 黏液脂瘤

myx·o·ma (mik-so′mə) pl. *myxomas, myxo′-mata.* A benign tumor composed of primitive connective tissue cells and stroma resembling mesenchyme 黏液瘤

myx·o·ma·to·sis (mik″so-mə-to′sis) 1. the development of multiple myxomas 多发（性）黏液瘤病; 2. myxomatous degeneration 黏液瘤变性

myx·o·ma·tous (mik-so′mə-təs) of the nature of a myxoma 黏液瘤的

myxo·sar·co·ma (mik″so-sahr-ko′mə) a sarcoma with myxomatous tissue 黏液肉瘤

myxo·vi·rus (mik′so-vi″rəs) any of a group of RNA viruses, including the viruses of influenza, parainfluenza, mumps, and Newcastle disease, characterically causing agglutination of erythrocytes 黏病毒

N

N [符号] newton 牛顿; nitrogen 氮; normal (2a) 当量（溶液）

N [符号] Avogadro's number 阿伏伽德罗常数; normal (2a) 当量（溶液）; number 数

*N*ᴀ [符号] Avogadro's number 阿伏伽德罗常数

n [符号] nano- 纳（诺）; neutron 中子; refractive index 折射率

n. [符号] [L.] ner′vus (nerve) 神经

n [符号] haploid chromosome number 单倍体染色体数; refractive index 折射率; sample size (statistics) 样本量（统计学）

n- [符号] normal (2b) 正（链）

ν (nu, the thirteenth letter of the Greek alphabet) （nu, 希腊字母的第 13 个字母）frequency (1) 频率的符号

NA *Nomina Anatomica,* a former official body of anatomic nomenclature, superseded by the *Terminologia Anatomica* [TA] (1998) Nomina Anatomica, 前解剖学命名法官方机构, 后被 Terminologia Anatomica [TA]（1998）取代

Na [符号] sodium ([L.] *na′trium*) 元素钠

NAACLS National Accrediting Agency for Clinical Laboratory Sciences 国家临床实验学科认证机构

na·bu·me·tone (nə-bu″mə-tōn″) a nonsteroidal antiinflammatory drug used in the treatment of osteoarthritis and rheumatoid arthritis 萘丁美酮，一种非甾体抗炎药，用于治疗骨关节炎和类风湿关节炎

na·cre·ous (na′kre-əs) having a pearllike luster 珍珠色的，具珠光的

NACT National Alliance of Cardiovascular Technologists 全国心血管技术专家联盟

NAD nicotinamide adenine dinucleotide 烟酰胺腺嘌呤二核苷酸，辅酶 I

NAD⁺ the oxidized form of NAD 烟酰胺腺嘌呤二核苷酸的氧化型

NADH the reduced form of NAD 烟酰胺腺嘌呤二核苷酸的还原型

na·di (nah′de) in ayurveda, any of the channels

that carry vital energy through the body 在阿育吠陀中，在身体内传递生命能量的任何通道

NADL National Association of Dental Laboratories 全国牙科技工室协会

na·do·lol (na-do′lol) a nonselective β-adrenergic blocking agent used for the treatment of angina pectoris and hypertension 纳多洛尔，一种非选择性β受体阻滞药，用于治疗心绞痛和高血压

NADP nicotinamide adenine dinucleotide phosphate 烟酰胺腺嘌呤二核苷酸磷酸，辅酶Ⅱ

NADP⁺ the oxidized form of NADP 烟酰胺腺嘌呤二核苷酸磷酸的氧化型

NADPH the reduced form of NADP 烟酰胺腺嘌呤二核苷酸磷酸的还原型

NAEMD National Academy of Emergency Medical Dispatch 全国紧急医疗调度研究院

NAEMT National Association of Emergency Medical Technicians 全国紧急医疗技术员协会

naf·a·rel·in (naf′ə-rel″in) a synthetic preparation of gonadotropin-releasing hormone, used as the acetate ester in the treatment of central precocious puberty and endometriosis 那法瑞林，促性腺激素释放激素的合成制剂，其醋酸酯用于治疗中枢性早熟和子宫内膜异位症

naf·cil·lin (naf-sil′in) a semisynthetic, acidand penicillinase-resistant penicillin that is effective against staphylococcal infections; used as the sodium salt 乙氧萘青霉素，一种半合成的、耐酸和耐青霉素酶的青霉素，对葡萄球菌感染有效；用作钠盐形式

naf·ti·fine (naf′tĭ-fēn) a broad-spectrum antifungal agent, used topically as the hydrochloride salt 桂奈甲胺，萘替芬，一种广谱抗真菌药，其盐酸盐常作为局部用药

NAHC National Association for Home Care and Hospice 全国家庭护理和临终关怀协会

nail (nāl) 1. the horny cutaneous plate on the dorsal surface of the distal end of a finger or toe. 指甲，趾甲；2. a rod of metal, bone, or other material for fixation of fragments of fractured bones 骨钉；**ingrown n.**, aberrant growth of a toenail, with one or both lateral margins pushing deeply into adjacent soft tissue 内长甲，嵌甲，趾甲的异常生长，其中一个或两侧缘嵌入邻近的软组织；**pincer n.**, a nail that curves outward at the end and pinches the nailbed 钳甲，在末端向外弯曲并挤压甲床；**pitted n.**, one with surface pits, seen most often in psoriasis 点状凹陷甲，有表面凹陷的一种指甲，最常见于银屑病；**racket n.**, a short broad thumbnail or fingernail 球拍状甲；**spoon n.**, koilonychia 反甲，匙状甲；**Terry n's,** 1. opaque, whitish discoloration affecting the entire nail except for 1–2 mm at the distal margin; commonly seen in

cirrhosis, congestive heart failure, and certain other conditions Terry甲，除远端边缘1～2mm外，整个指甲的不透明白色变色；常见于肝硬化、充血性心力衰竭和某些其他情况；2. A type of apparent leukonychia 白甲

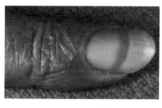

▲ **Terry 甲**

Nai·ro·vi·rus (ni′ro-vi″rəs) a genus of viruses of the family Bunyaviridae, including CrimeanCongo hemorrhagic fever virus 内罗毕病毒属

Na·ja (na′jə) the cobras, a genus of venomous snakes (family Elapidae) found in Asia and Africa 眼镜蛇属

Na⁺,K⁺-ATP·ase (a-te-pe′ās) an enzyme that spans the plasma membrane and hydrolyzes ATP to drive the active transport mechanism by which sodium (Na⁺) is extruded from a cell and potassium (K⁺) is brought in, so as to maintain gradients of these ions across the cell membrane Na⁺, K⁺-腺苷三磷酸酶，又称 *sodium pump*

nal·bu·phine (nal′bu-fēn) an opioid analgesic, used as the hydrochloride salt in the treatment of moderate to severe pain and as an anesthesia adjunct 纳布啡，环丁甲羟氢吗啡，一种阿片类镇痛药，其盐酸盐用于治疗中重度疼痛和作为麻醉辅助剂

nal·i·dix·ic ac·id (nal″ĭ-dik′sik) a synthetic antibacterial agent used in the treatment of genitourinary infections caused by gram-negative organisms 萘啶酸，萘啶酮酸，一种合成抗菌药，用于治疗革兰阴性菌引起的泌尿生殖道感染

nal·me·fene (nal′mə-fēn″) an opioid antagonist, used as the hydrochloride salt in the treatment of opioid overdose and postoperative opioid depression 纳美芬，阿片类拮抗药

nal·or·phine (nal′or-fēn) a semisynthetic congener of morphine; the hydrochloride salt is used as an antagonist to morphine and related opioids and in the diagnosis of narcotic addiction 烯丙吗啡，纳洛芬，吗啡的半合成同系物；其盐酸盐作为吗啡和相关阿片类药物的拮抗药，并用于麻醉成瘾的诊断

nal·ox·one (nal-ok′sōn) an opioid antagonist, used as the hydrochloride salt in opioid toxicity, opioid-induced respiratory depression, and hypotension associated with septic shock 纳洛酮，一种阿片类

拮抗药，其盐酸盐用于治疗阿片类药物毒性、阿片类药物引起的呼吸抑制和败血症性休克相关的低血压

nal·trex·one (nal-trek′sōn) an opioid antagonist used in the treatment of opioid or alcohol addiction 纳曲酮，一种用于治疗阿片类或酒精成瘾的阿片类拮抗药

name (nām) a word or words used to designate a unique entity and distinguish it from others 名字，名称；**generic n.**, 1. in chemistry, a name applied to a class of compounds, e.g., alkane（化学）类名；2. 同 nonproprietary n.; 3. in biology, the name applied to a genus（生物学）属名；**International Nonproprietary N. (INN)**, the nonproprietary designation recommended by the World Health Organization for any pharmaceutical preparation 国际非专利药名；**nonproprietary n.**, a short name coined for a drug or chemical not subject to proprietary (trademark) rights and recommended or recognized by an official body 非专利名称；**pharmacy equivalent n. (PEN)**, a shortened name for a drug or combination of drugs; when used for a combination of drugs, the term usually consists of the prefix co- plus an abbreviation for each drug in the combination 药剂对应名称，药物或药物组合的简称；当用于药物组合时，该术语通常由前缀 co- 加上组合中每种药物的缩写组成；**proprietary n.**, a brand name or trademark under which a proprietary product is marketed 专利药名，参见 *proprietary*; **systematic n.**, in chemical nomenclature, a name of a substance based on the chemical structure of a compound 系统名（称），学名（根据化合物的化学结构而定的物质的名称）；**trivial n.**, in chemical nomenclature, a name of a substance that does not reflect its chemical structure; many trivial names are semisystematic, e.g., the -ol in glycerol indicates that it is an alcohol 通用名（在化学命名法中不反映化学结构的物质的名称，许多通用名都是半系统名）；**United States Adopted N. (USAN)**, a nonproprietary designation for any compound used as a drug, established by negotiation between their manufacturers and a council sponsored jointly by the American Medical Association, American Pharmaceutical Association, and United States Pharmacopeial Convention 美国采用药名（美国药物命名委员会采用的非专利商标名称）

NANDA North American Nursing Diagnosis Association 北美护理诊断协会

nan·dro·lone (nan′dro-lōn) an anabolic steroid with lesser androgenic effects; used as *n. decanoate* and *n. phenpropionate* in the treatment of severe growth retardation in children and of metastatic breast cancer and as an adjunct in the treatment of chronic wasting diseases and anemia associated with renal insufficiency 诺龙，19- 去甲睾酮，一种具有较小雄激素作用的合成类固醇；常以癸酸诺龙和苯丙酸诺龙治疗儿童严重生长迟缓和转移性乳腺癌；也作为辅助手段用于治疗慢性消耗性疾病和肾功能不全引起的贫血

na·nism (na′niz-əm) former name for *dwarfism* 矮小，侏儒症的曾用名；**mulibrey n.**, a rare autosomal recessive disorder due to mutation of a peroxisomal protein; marked by dwarfism, constrictive pericarditis, craniofacial abnormalities including triangular face and scaphocephaly, muscular hypotonia, high-pitched voice, and abnormalities of the ocular fundus 肌肝脑眼侏儒

nan(o)- word element [Gr.], *dwarf; small size;* also used in naming units of measurement (symbol n) to designate an amount one billionth (10^{-9}) the size of the unit to which it is joined, e.g., nanocurie [构词成分] 矮小；小尺寸；纳（诺），毫微，在命名测量单位（符号 n）中也用于表示与其连接的单位的十亿分之一（10^{-9}）

nano·ceph·a·ly (nan″o-sef′ə-le) microcephaly 小头畸形；**nanoceph′alous** *adj.*

nano·gram (ng) (nan′o-gram) one billionth (10^{-9}) of a gram 纳克，毫微克

nano·me·ter (nm) (nan′o-me″tər) one billionth (10^{-9}) of a meter 纳米，毫微米

nan·oph·thal·mia (nan″of-thal′me-ə) 同 nanoph-thalmos

nan·oph·thal·mos (nan″of-thal′məs) abnormal smallness in all dimensions of one or both eyes in the absence of other ocular defects; pure microphthalmos 小眼，眼小

NANT National Association of Nephrology Technicians/Technologists 全国肾脏病学技术员 / 技师协会

na·nu·ka·ya·mi (nah″noo-kah-yah′me) a leptospirosis marked by fever and jaundice, first reported in Japan, due to *Leptospira hebdomadis* 七日热，一种以发热和黄疸为特征的钩端螺旋体病，首次在日本报告，由希伯来钩端螺旋体引起

nape (nāp) the back of the neck 项，（后）颈

naph·az·o·line (naf-az′o-lēn) an adrenergic used in the form of the hydrochloride salt as a vasoconstrictor to decongest nasal and ocular mucosae 萘甲唑啉，一种 α 受体激动药，其盐酸盐用作血管收缩药，以减轻鼻和眼黏膜的充血

naph·tha (naf′thə) any of various volatile liquid hydrocarbon mixtures from petroleum, natural gas, or coal tar, sometimes specifically petroleum benzoin or ligroin; used as solvents, dry cleaning fluids, in synthesis, in varnishes, or as fuels 石脑油

NAPNAP National Association of Pediatric Nurse Associates and Practitioners 全国儿科护士和执业医师协会

NAPNES National Association for Practical Nurse Education and Services 全国实用护理教育和服务协会

na·prap·a·thy (nə-prap′ə-the) a system of therapy employing manipulation of connective tissue (ligaments, muscles, and joints) and dietary measures to facilitate the recuperative and regenerative processes of the body 推拿疗法

na·prox·en (nə-prok′sən) a nonsteroidal antiinflammatory drug used as the base or the sodium salt in the treatment of pain, inflammation, arthritis, gout, calcium pyrophosphate deposition disease, fever, and dysmenorrhea and in the prophylaxis and suppression of vascular headache 萘普生，一种非甾体抗炎药，常用其碱或钠盐，用于治疗疼痛、炎症、关节炎、痛风、焦磷酸钙沉积症、发热和痛经以及预防和抑制血管性头痛

nap·sy·late (nap′sə-lāt) USAN contraction for 2-naphthalenesulfonate 萘磺酸盐，2- 萘磺酸盐的 USAN 缩约词

NAPT National Association for Poetry Therapy 全国诗歌治疗协会

nar·a·trip·tan (narʺə-trip′tan) a selective serotonin receptor agonist used as the hydrochloride salt in the acute treatment of migraine 那拉曲坦，一种选择性 5- 羟色胺受体激动药，其盐酸盐用于偏头痛的急性治疗

Nar·can (nahr′kan) trademark for a preparation of naloxone hydrochloride 盐酸纳洛酮制剂的商品名

nar·cis·sism (nahr′sĭ-siz-əm) dominant interest in one's self; the state in which the ego is invested in oneself rather than in another person; self-love 自恋；**narcissis′tic** adj.

nar·co·hyp·no·sis (nahrʺko-hip-no′sis) hypnotic suggestions made while the patient is narcotized 麻醉（药）催眠

nar·co·lep·sy (nahr′ko-lepʺse) recurrent, uncontrollable, brief episodes of sleep, often with hypnagogic or hypnopompic hallucinations, cataplexy, and sleep paralysis 发作性睡病；**narcolep′tic** adj.

nar·co·sis (nahr-ko′sis) reversible depression of the central nervous system produced by drugs, marked by stupor or insensibility 麻醉

nar·cot·ic (nahr-kot′ik) 1. pertaining to or producing narcosis 麻醉的；2. an agent that produces insensibility or stupor, especially an opioid 麻醉药

nar·co·tize (nahr′ko-tīz) to put under the influence of a narcotic 使麻醉

na·res (na′rēz) sing. *na′ris*. [L.] the nostrils; the external openings of the nasal cavity 鼻孔

na·sal (na′zəl) pertaining to the nose 鼻的；鼻音的

na·sa·lis (na-za′lis) [L.] nasal 鼻的

nas·cent (nas′ənt) (na′sənt) 1. being born; just coming into existence 新 生 的；2. just liberated from a chemical combination, and hence more reactive because uncombined（化）初生的，刚从化学结合中解放出来，因未结合而更具反应活性

na·si·on (na′ze-on) the middle point of the frontonasal suture 鼻根点

na·so·an·tral (naʺzo-an′trəl) pertaining to the nose and maxillary antrum 鼻上颌窦的

na·so·an·tros·to·my (naʺzo-an-tros′tə-me) surgical formation of a nasoantral window for drainage of an obstructed maxillary sinus 鼻上颌窦造口术

na·so·cil·i·ary (naʺzo-sil′e-arʺe) pertaining to the eyes, brow, and root of the nose 鼻睫（状）的

na·so·fron·tal (naʺzo-fron′təl) pertaining to the nose and forehead or to nasal and frontal bones 鼻额骨的

na·so·gas·tric (naʺzo-gas′trik) pertaining to the nose and stomach 鼻胃的

na·so·la·bi·al (naʺzo-la′be-əl) pertaining to the nose and lip 鼻唇的

na·so·lac·ri·mal (naʺzo-lak′rĭ-məl) pertaining to the nose and lacrimal apparatus 鼻泪的

na·so·pal·a·tine (naʺzo-pal′ə-tīn) pertaining to the nose and palate 鼻腭的

na·so·phar·yn·gi·tis (naʺzo-farʺin-ji′tis) inflammation of the nasopharynx 鼻咽炎

na·so·pha·ryn·go·la·ryn·go·scope (naʺzo-fə-ringʺgo-lə-ring′go-skōp) a flexible fiberoptic endoscope for examining the nasopharynx and larynx 鼻咽喉镜

na·so·phar·ynx (naʺzo-far′inks) the part of the pharynx above the soft palate 鼻咽；**nasopharyn′geal** adj.

na·so·si·nus·itis (naʺzo-siʺnə-si′tis) rhinosinusitis 鼻鼻窦炎

na·so·tra·che·al (naʺzo-tra′ke-əl) pertaining to the nose and the trachea 鼻支气管的

NASS North American Spine Society 北美脊柱学会

na·sus (na′səs) 同 nose

NASW National Association of Social Workers 全国社会工作者协会

na·tal (na′təl) 1. pertaining to birth 分娩的，生产的；2. gluteal 臀的

nat·al·iz·u·mab (natʺə-liz′u-mab) a recombinant monoclonal antibody that binds to α_4- integrin; used in the treatment of patients with relapsing forms of multiple sclerosis, administered intravenously 那他珠单抗，一种与 α_4 整合素结合的重组单克隆抗体；经静脉注射用于治疗复发型多发性硬化症

nat·a·my·cin (nat″ə-mi′sin) a polyene antibiotic used in topical treatment of fungal keratitis, blepharitis, and conjunctivitis 纳他霉素，一种多烯类抗生素，用于真菌性角膜炎、眼睑炎和结膜炎的局部治疗

na·teg·li·nide (nə-teg′lĭ-nīd) an agent that stimulates release of insulin from pancreatic islet beta cells, used in the treatment of type 2 diabetes 那格列奈，一种刺激胰岛 β 细胞释放胰岛素的药物，用于治疗 2 型糖尿病

Na·tion·al For·mu·lary (NF) a book of standards for certain pharmaceuticals and preparations that are not included in the USP *(United States Pharmacopeia)* 美国国家处方集

na·tri·ure·sis (na″tre-u-re′sis) excretion of sodium in the urine, particularly in excessive amounts 尿钠症；**pressure n.**, increased urinary excretion of sodium along with water when arterial pressure increases; a compensatory mechanism to maintain blood pressure within the normal range 压力性尿钠尿症

na·tri·uret·ic (na″tre-u-ret′ik) 1. pertaining to, characterized by, or promoting natriuresis 促钠尿排泄的，利钠的；2. an agent that promotes natriuresis 促钠尿排泄剂，利钠剂

nat·u·ral (nach′ə-rəl) neither artificial nor pathologic 自然的，天然的

na·tur·op·a·thy (na″chər-op′ə-the) a drugless system of health care, using a wide variety of therapies, including hydrotherapy, heat, massage, and herbal medicine, intended to treat the whole person to stimulate and support the person's own innate healing capacity 自然疗法；**naturopath′ic** *adj.*

nau·sea (naw′ze-ə) an unpleasant sensation vaguely referred to the epigastrium and abdomen, with a tendency to vomit 恶心；**n. gravida′rum**, the morning sickness of pregnancy 妊娠期恶心

nau·se·ant (naw′ze-ənt) 1. inducing nausea 使恶心的；2. an agent causing nausea 恶心药

nau·se·ate (naw′ze-āt) to affect with nausea 使恶心，作呕

nau·seous (naw′shəs) pertaining to or producing nausea 恶心的，致恶心的

na·vel (na′vəl) the umbilicus 脐

na·vic·u·la (nə-vĭ′ku-lə) frenulum of pudendal labia 舟状窝

na·vic·u·lar (nə-vik′u-lər) scaphoid 舟状的

Nb niobium 元素铌的符号

NBNA National Black Nurses Association 全国黑人护士协会

NBTE nonbacterial thrombotic endocarditis 非细菌性血栓性心内膜炎

NCI National Cancer Institute 全国癌症研究所

nCi nanocurie; one billionth (10⁻⁹) of a curie 纳居里

NCIL National Council on Independent Living 全国独立生活理事会

NCN National Council of Nurses 全国护士理事会

NCoV novel coronavirus 新型冠状病毒

NCPDP National Council for Prescription Drug Programs 处方药物计划全国理事会

ND Doctor of Naturopathy 自然疗法医学博士

Nd neodymium 元素钕的符号

NDA National Dental Association 全国牙科协会

NDHA National Dental Hygienists' Association 全国牙齿卫生员协会

nDNA nuclear DNA 核 DNA，核脱氧核糖核酸

Nd:YAG neodymium:yttrium-aluminum-garnet 钕：钇-铝-石榴石，参见 *laser* 下词条

Ne neon 元素氖的符号

near·sight·ed·ness (nēr′sīt″əd-nis) myopia 近视

ne·ar·thro·sis (ne″ahr-thro′sis) a false or artificial joint 假关节；人工关节

neb·u·la (neb′u-lə) pl. *ne′bulae* [L.] 1. a slight corneal opacity 角膜薄翳；2. a preparation, particularly an oily preparation, for use in a nebulizer 喷雾剂

neb·u·li·za·tion (neb″u-li-za′shən) 1. conversion into an aerosol or spray 雾化；2. treatment by an aerosol 喷雾治疗

neb·u·liz·er (neb′u-li″zər) atomizer; a device for throwing a spray 雾化器，喷雾器

Ne·ca·tor (ne-ka′tor) a genus of hookworms. *N. america′nus* (American or New World hookworm) causes hookworm disease 板口线虫属

ne·ca·to·ri·a·sis (ne-ka″to-ri′ə-sis) hookworm disease caused by species of *Necator* 钩虫病，板口线虫病

ne·ces·si·ty (nə-ses′ĭ-te) something necessary or indispensable 必需的，必要的；**pharmaceutical n.**, a substance having slight or no value therapeutically but used in the preparation of various pharmaceuticals, including preservatives, solvents, ointment bases, and flavoring, coloring, diluting, emulsifying, and suspending agents 佐剂

neck (nek) 1. cervix or collum; the constricted part connecting the head and trunk 颈；2. the constricted part of an organ or other structure 颈状部位，细长部分；**anatomic n. of humerus**, a constriction of the humerus just below its proximal articular surface. 肱骨解剖颈；**bladder n.**, a constricted portion of the urinary bladder, formed by the meeting of its inferolateral surfaces proximal to the opening of the urethra 膀胱颈；**n. of femur**, the heavy column of bone connecting the head of the femur and the shaft 股骨颈；**surgical n. of humerus,** the constricted part of the humerus just below the tuberosities 肱骨外科颈；**n. of tooth,** the narrowed part of a tooth between the crown and the root 牙颈；**webbed n.,** pterygium colli 蹼（状）颈；**wry n.,** torticollis (1) 斜颈

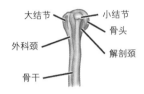

大结节 小结节
骨头
外科颈
解剖颈
骨干

▲ **右肱骨前部，显示解剖和外科颈部**

neck·lace (nek'ləs) a structure encircling the neck 项环，环绕颈部的结构；**Casal n.,** an eruption in pellagra, encircling the lower part of the neck 颈蜀黍红疹，围绕脖子下部的暴发性糙皮病

nec·rec·to·my (nek-rek'tə-me) excision of necrotic tissue 坏死（组织）切除术

nec·ro·bac·il·lo·sis (nek″ro-bas′ĭ-lo′sis) infection of animals with *Fusobacterium necrophorum* 坏死杆菌病

nec·ro·bi·o·sis (nek″ro-bi-o′sis) swelling, bas-ophilia, and distortion of collagen bundles in the dermis, sometimes with obliteration of normal structure but short of actual necrosis 渐进性坏死；**necrobiot′ic** *adj.*

nec·ro·cy·to·sis (nek″ro-si-to′sis) death and decay of cells 细胞坏死

nec·ro·gen·ic (nek″ro-jen′ik) productive of necrosis or death 死质性的，坏死源的

ne·crog·e·nous (nə-kroj′ə-nəs) originating or arising from dead matter 死质性的，坏死源的

ne·crol·o·gy (nə-krol′ə-je) statistics or records of death 死亡统计；**necrolog′ic** *adj.*

ne·crol·y·sis (nə-krol′ĭ-sis) separation or exfoliation of necrotic tissue 坏死松解；**toxic epidermal n.,** an exfoliative skin disease, primarily a reaction to drugs; characterized by full-thickness epidermal necrosis resulting in bulla formation, subepidermal separation, and inflammatory dermal changes, with the widespread loss of skin leaving raw denuded areas 毒性表皮坏死松解

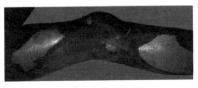

▲ **毒性表皮坏死松解**

nec·ro·phil·ia (nek″ro-fil′e-ə) sexual attraction to or sexual contact with dead bodies 恋尸癖

nec·ro·phil·ic (nek″ro-fil′ik) 1. pertaining to necrophilia 恋尸癖的；2. showing preference for dead tissue, as necrophilic bacteria 对坏死组织偏好的，如腐败菌

ne·croph·i·lous (nə-krof′ĭ-ləs) 同 necrophilic

nec·ro·pho·bia (nek″ro-fo′be-ə) irrational fear of death or of dead bodies 死亡恐怖，尸体恐怖

nec·rop·sy (nek′rop-se) examination of a body after death; autopsy 尸体剖检，验尸

nec·rose (nek′rōs) to become necrotic or to undergo necrosis（使）发生坏死

ne·cro·sis (nə-kro′sis) pl. *necro′ses* [Gr.] the morphologic changes indicative of cell death caused by progressive enzymatic degradation; it may affect groups of cells or part of a structure or an organ 坏死；**acute retinal n. (ARN),** necrotizing retinitis with uveitis and other retinal pathology, severe loss of vision, and often retinal detachment; caused by herpesvirus infection 急性视网膜坏死；**aseptic n.,** necrosis without infection, usually in the head of the femur after traumatic hip dislocation 无菌性坏死；**caseous n.,** cheesy n. 干酪性坏死；**central n.,** that affecting the central portion of an affected bone, cell, or lobule of the liver 中心性坏死；**cheesy n.,** that in which the tissue is soft, dry, and cottage cheese-like; most often seen in tuberculosis and syphilis 干酪样坏死；**coagulation n.,** necrosis of a portion of some organ or tissue, with formation of fibrous infarcts, the protoplasm of the cells becoming fixed and opaque by coagulation of the protein elements, the cellular outline persisting for a long time 凝固性坏死；**colliquative n.,** 同 liquefactive n.；**contraction band n.,** a cardiac lesion characterized by hypercontracted myofibrils and contraction bands and mitochondrial damage, caused by calcium influx into dying cells resulting in arrest of the cells in the contracted state 萎缩带坏死；**fat n.,** that in which the neutral fats in adipose tissue are split into fatty acids and glycerol, usually affecting the pancreas and peripancreatic fat in acute hemorrhagic pancreatitis 脂肪坏死；**liquefaction n.,** liquefactive n.,** necrosis in which the necrotic material becomes softened and liquefied 液化性坏死；**phosphorus n.,** necrosis of the jaw bone due to exposure to phosphorus 磷中毒性坏死；**postpartum pituitary n.,** necrosis of the pituitary during the postpartum period, often associated with shock and excessive uterine bleeding during delivery, and leading to variable patterns of hypopituitarism 产后垂体坏死；**subcutaneous fat n.,** induration of the subcutaneous fat in newborn and young infants 新生儿皮下脂肪

坏死；*n. ustilagi′nea,* dry gangrene due to ergotism 麦角中毒性坏死；**Zenker n.,** Zenker 坏死，参见 *degeneration* 下词条

nec·ro·sper·mia (nek″ro-spur′me-ə) a condition in which the spermatozoa of the semen are either motionless or dead 死精症；**necrosper′mic** *adj.*

ne·crot·ic (nə-krot′ik) pertaining to or characterized by necrosis 坏死的

nec·ro·tiz·ing (nek′ro-tīz″ing) causing necrosis 引起坏死的

ne·crot·o·my (nə-krot′ə-me) 1. dissection of a dead body 尸体解剖；2. sequestrectomy 死骨摘除术

ned·o·cro·mil (ned″o-kro′mil) a nonsteroidal antiinflammatory drug used by inhalation in the treatment of bronchial asthma and topically as the sodium salt in the treatment of allergic conjunctivitis 一种非甾体抗炎药，用于吸入治疗支气管哮喘，局部以钠盐形式治疗过敏性结膜炎

nee·dle (ne′dəl) 1. a sharp instrument for suturing or puncturing 针；2. to puncture or separate with a needle 用针刺穿或分离；**aneurysm n.,** a needle with a handle, used in ligating blood vessels 动脉瘤针；**aspirating n.,** a long, hollow needle for removing fluid from a cavity 吸液针；**cataract n.,** a needle used in removing a cataract 白内障针；**discission n.,** a special form of cataract needle 晶状体刺开针；**hypodermic n.,** a short, slender, hollow needle, used in injecting drugs beneath the skin 皮下注射针；**stop n.,** one with a shoulder that prevents too-deep penetration 有档针；**transseptal n.,** one used to puncture the interatrial septum in transseptal catheterization 经间隔穿刺针

neem (nēm) *Azadirachta indica,* a large evergreen tree having antifungal, antibacterial, antiviral, and antimalarial activity; long used medicinally for a wide variety of indications 印楝，一种有抗真菌、抗菌、抗病毒和疟症疾活性的常青树；因具有广泛的适应证而长期使用

NEFA nonesterified fatty acids 非酯化脂肪酸

ne·fa·zo·done (nə-fa′zo-dōn) an antidepressant, used as the hydrochloride salt 奈法唑酮，一种抗抑郁药，常用其盐酸盐

neg·a·tive (neg′ə-tiv) 1. having a value less than zero 负的；2. indicating absence, as of a condition or organism 隐性的；3. characterized by refusal, denial, resistance, or opposition 消极的

neg·a·tiv·ism (neg′ə-tĭ-viz″əm) opposition to suggestion or advice; behavior opposite to that appropriate to a specific situation or against the wishes of others, including direct resistance to efforts to be moved 否定态度；违拗症；抗拒症

ne·glect (nə-glekt′) disregard of or failure to perform some task or function 忽视；忽略；疏忽；**unilateral n.,** hemiapraxia with failure to pay attention to bodily grooming and stimuli on one side but not the other, usually due to a lesion in the central nervous system 单侧忽略

Neis·se·ria (ni-se′re-ə) a genus of gramnegative, aerobic or facultatively anaerobic bacteria of the family Neisseriaceae, including *N. gonorrhoe′ae,* the cause of gonorrhea, and *N. meningi′tidis,* which causes meningococcal meningitis 奈瑟菌属

Neis·se·ri·a·ceae (ni-se″re-a′se-e) a family of gram-negative, aerobic cocci and rod-shaped bacteria of the order Neisseriales 奈瑟菌科

Neis·se·ri·a·les (ni-se″re-a′lēz) an order of aerobic, coccal to rod-shaped bacteria of the class Betaproteobacteria 奈瑟菌目

nel·fin·a·vir (nel-fin′ə-vir) an HIV protease inhibitor that causes formation of immature, noninfectious viral particles; used as the mesylate salt in the treatment of HIV infection 一种 HIV 蛋白酶抑制药，能形成不成熟的非感染性病毒颗粒；其甲磺酸盐用于治疗 HIV 感染

nem·a·line (nem′ə-lēn) threadlike or rodshaped 线样的，杆状的

Nem·a·thel·min·thes (nem″ə-thəl-min′thēz) in some classifications, a phylum including the Acanthocephala and Nematoda 线形动物门

nem·a·to·cide (nem′ə-to-sīd″) 1. destroying nematodes 杀线虫的；2. an agent that so acts 杀线虫剂

Nem·a·to·da (nem″ə-to′də) a class of helminths (phylum Aschelminthes), the roundworms, many of which are parasites; in some classifications, considered to be a phylum, and sometimes known as Nemathelminthes, or a class of that phylum 线虫纲

nem·a·tode (nem′ə-tōd) a roundworm; any individual of the class Nematoda 线虫

neo·ad·ju·vant (ne″o-aj′oo-vənt) referring to preliminary cancer therapy, usually chemotherapy or radiation therapy, that precedes a necessary second modality of treatment 新辅助治疗

neo·an·ti·gen (ne″o-an′tī-jən) tumor-associated antigen 新抗原，肿瘤抗原

neo·blad·der (ne″o-blad′ər) a continent urinary reservoir constructed from a detubularized bowel segment or from a segment of the stomach, with implantation of the ureters and urethra; used to replace the bladder following cystectomy 人工新膀胱

neo·blas·tic (ne″o-blas′tik) originating in or of the nature of new tissue 新组织的

neo·cer·e·bel·lum (ne″o-ser″ə-bel′əm) phylogenetically, the newer parts of the cerebellum, consisting of those parts predominantly supplied by corticopontocerebellar fibers 新小脑，小脑的较新部分，主要由皮质桥小脑纤维供应的部分组成

neo·cor·tex (ne″o-kor′teks) the newer, sixlayered portion of the cerebral cortex, showing the most highly evolved stratification and organization 新皮质。Cf. *archicortex and paleocortex*

neo·dym·i·um (Nd) (ne″o-dim′e-əm) a silvery white, heavy, rare earth element; at. no. 60, at. wt. 144.242 钕（化学元素）

neo·glot·tis (ne″o-glot′is) a glottis created by suturing the pharyngeal mucosa over the superior end of the transected trachea above the primary tracheostoma and making a permanent stoma in the mucosa; done to permit phonation after laryngectomy 新声门；**neoglot′tic** *adj*.

ne·ol·o·gism (ne-ol′ə-jiz″əm) a newly coined word; in psychiatry, a new word whose meaning may be known only to the patient using it 新词语；新语；语词新作

neo·mem·brane (ne″o-mem′brān) pseudomembrane 假膜

neo·my·cin (ne″o-mi′sin) a broad-spectrum aminoglycoside antibiotic produced by *Streptomyces fradiae*, effective against a wide range of gramnegative bacilli and some gram-positive bacteria; used as the sulfate salt 新霉素

ne·on (Ne) (ne′on) a colorless, odorless, tasteless, inert noble gas element; at. no. 10, at. wt. 20.180. In a high-voltage electrical field, it exhibits an orange-red glow 氖（化学元素）

neo·na·tal (ne″o-na′təl) pertaining to the first 4 weeks after birth 新生（期）的

neo·nate (ne′o-nāt) newborn infant 新生儿

neo·na·tol·o·gy (ne″o-na-tol′ə-je) the diagnosis and treatment of disorders of the newborn 新生儿学

neo·pal·li·um (ne″o-pal′e-əm) 同 neocortex

neo·pla·sia (ne″o-pla′zhə) the formation of a neoplasm 瘤形成；**cervical intraepithelial n. (CIN)**, dysplasia of the cervical epithelium, often premalignant, characterized by various degrees of hyperplasia, abnormal keratinization, and the presence of condylomata 宫颈上皮内瘤变；**gestational trophoblastic n. (GTN)**, a group of neoplastic disorders that originate in the placenta, including hydatidiform mole, chorioadenoma destruens, and choriocarcinoma 妊娠滋养细胞肿瘤；**multiple endocrine n. (MEN)**, a group of autosomal dominant disorders characterized by hyperplasia and hyperfunction of two or more components of the endocrine system; *type 1* is characterized by tumors of the pituitary, parathyroid glands, and pancreatic islet cells, with peptic ulcers and sometimes ZollingerEllison syndrome; *type 2A* is characterized

by thyroid medullary carcinoma, pheochromocytoma, and parathyroid hyperplasia; *type 2B* is similar to type 2A but includes neuromas of the oral region, neurofibromas, ganglioneuromas of the gastrointestinal tract, and café-au-lait spots 多发性内分泌腺瘤形成；**penile intraepithelial n.**, erythroplasia of Queyrat; a form of epithelial dysplasia, ranging from mild to forms of carcinoma, manifested as a circumscribed, velvety, erythematous lesion on the penis 阴茎上皮内瘤变

neo·plasm (ne′o-plaz″əm) tumor; any new and abnormal growth, specifically one in which cell multiplication is uncontrolled and progressive. Neoplasms may be benign or malignant 新生物，赘生物，（肿）瘤，任何新生的和异常的生长，特别是细胞增殖不受控制和进行的生长。肿瘤可为良性或恶性

neo·plas·tic (ne″o-plas′tik) 1. pertaining to a neoplasm 新生物的，赘生物的，（肿）瘤的；2. pertaining to neoplasia 瘤形成的

ne·op·ter·in (ne-op′tər-in) 1. a pteridine derivative excreted at elevated levels in the urine in some disorders of tetrahydrobiopterin synthesis, certain malignant diseases, viral infection, and graft rejection 新蝶呤；2. any of a class of related compounds 任何与新蝶呤相关的同类化合物

Neo·rick·ett·sia (ne″o-rĭ-ket′se-ə) a genus of gram-negative bacteria of the family Anaplasmataceae, transmitted by flukes and occurring in cytoplasmic vacuoles. *N. helmin′thoeca* is a parasite of various fish, especially salmon and trout, and causes hemorrhagic enteritis in those ingesting raw infected fish 新立克次体

neo·stig·mine (ne″o-stig′mēn) a cholinergic (cholinesterase inhibitor), used as the bromide or methylsulfate salt in the treatment of myasthenia gravis, in the prevention and treatment of postoperative stasis and atony of the gastrointestinal tract or urinary bladder, and for postsurgical reversal of the effects of nondepolarizing neuromuscular blocking agents 新斯的明

neo·thal·a·mus (ne″o-thal′ə-məs) the part of the thalamus connected to the neocortex 新丘脑，丘脑与新皮质相连的部分

neo·u·re·thra (ne″o-u-re′thrə) a surgically created urethra 新尿道，手术形成的尿道

neo·vas·cu·lar·iza·tion (ne″o-vas″ku-lər-ĭ-za′shən) 1. new blood vessel formation in abnormal tissue or in abnormal positions 新血管形成；2. revascularization 血管再生

neph·e·lom·e·ter (nef″ə-lom′ə-tər) an instrument for measuring the concentration of substances in suspension by means of light scattering by the suspended particles 比浊计，浊度计，通过悬浮粒子的光散射测量悬浮物质浓度的仪器

ne·phral·gia (nə-fral′jə) pain in a kidney 肾痛

neph·rec·ta·sia (nef″rek-ta′zhə) distention of the kidney 肾扩张，囊状肾

ne·phrec·to·my (nə-frek′tə-me) excision of a kidney 肾切除术

neph·ric (nef′rik) renal 肾的

ne·phrit·ic (nə-frit′ik) pertaining to or affected with nephritis 肾炎的

ne·phri·tis (nə-fri′tis) pl. *nephri′tides* [Gr.] inflammation of the kidney; a focal or diffuse proliferative or destructive disease that may involve the glomerulus, tubule, or interstitial renal tissue 肾炎; **glomerular n.**, glomerulonephritis 肾小球肾炎; **interstitial n.**, primary or secondary disease of the renal interstitial tissue 间质性肾炎; **lupus n.**, glomerulonephritis associated with systemic lupus erythematosus 狼疮（性）肾炎; **potassium-losing n.**, 失钾性肾炎, 参见 *uropathy* 下词条; **radiation n.**, kidney damage caused by ionizing radiation; symptoms include glomerular and tubular damage, hypertension, and proteinuria, sometimes leading to renal failure. It may be acute or chronic, and some varieties do not manifest until years after the radiation exposure 放射性肾炎; **salt-losing n.**, 失盐性肾炎, 参见 *nephropathy* 下词条; **transfusion n.**, nephropathy following transfusion from an incompatible donor 输血性肾炎; **tubulointerstitial n.**, nephritis of the renal tubules and interstitial tissues, usually secondary to drug sensitization, systemic infection, graft rejection, or autoimmune disease. An acute type and a chronic type have been distinguished 肾小管间质性肾炎

ne·phrit·o·gen·ic (nə-frit″o-jen′ik) causing nephritis 致肾炎的

neph·ro·blas·to·ma·to·sis (nef″ro-blas-to″mə-to′sis) clusters of microscopic blastema cells, tubules, and stromal cells at the periphery of the renal lobes in an infant; believed to be a precursor of Wilms tumor 肾母细胞瘤病

neph·ro·cal·ci·no·sis (nef″ro-kal″si-no′sis) precipitation of calcium phosphate in the renal tubules, with resultant renal insufficiency 肾钙质沉着

neph·ro·cele (nef′ro-sēl) hernia of a kidney 肾突出

neph·ro·col·ic (nef″ro-kol′ik) pertaining to or connecting the kidney and colon 肾结肠的

neph·ro·gen·ic (nef″ro-jen′ik) producing kidney tissue 肾原性的

ne·phrog·e·nous (nə-froj′ə-nəs) arising in a kidney 肾原性的，肾发生的

ne·phrog·ra·phy (nə-frog′rə-fe) radiography of the kidney 肾造影术

neph·ro·lith (nef′ro-lith) renal calculus 肾石

neph·ro·li·thi·a·sis (nef″ro-lĭ-thi′ə-sis) presence of renal calculi 肾石病

neph·ro·li·thot·o·my (nef″ro-lĭ-thot′o-me) incision of the kidney for removal of calculi 肾石切除术

ne·phrol·o·gy (nə-frol′o-je) the branch of medical science that deals with the kidneys 肾病学

ne·phrol·y·sis (nə-frol′ə-sis) 1. freeing of a kidney from adhesions 肾松解术; 2. destruction of kidney substance 肾溶解; **nephrolyt′ic** *adj.*

ne·phro·ma (nə-fro′mə) a tumor of the kidney or of kidney tissue 肾瘤; **congenital mesoblastic n.**, a renal tumor similar to Wilms tumor but appearing earlier and infiltrating more surrounding tissue 先天性中胚层细胞肾瘤

neph·ro·meg·a·ly (nef″ro-meg′ə-le) enlargement of the kidney 肾肥大, 巨肾

neph·ron (nef′ron) the structural and functional unit of the kidney, numbering about a million in the renal parenchyma, each being capable of forming urine 肾单位, 另参见 *tubule* 下 *renal tubules*

neph·ron·oph·thi·sis (nef″ron-of′thĭ-sis) an autosomal recessive kidney disorder characterized by chronic renal tubule dysfunction resulting in end-stage renal disease. It often occurs as part of a multisystem disorder, such as SeniorLoken syndrome 肾消耗病, 一种常染色体隐性肾脏疾病, 以慢性肾小管功能障碍为特征, 导致终末期肾病。其经常作为多系统疾病的一部分发生, 如 SeniorLoken 综合征; **familial juvenile n.**, a progressive, autosomal recessive kidney disorder marked by anemia, polyuria, renal loss of sodium, tubular atrophy, interstitial fibrosis, glomerular sclerosis, and medullary cysts, and progressing to end-stage renal disease 家族性青年性肾消耗病

ne·phrop·a·thy (nə-frop′ə-the) disease of the kidneys 肾病; **nephropath′ic** *adj.*; **analgesic n.**, interstitial nephritis with renal papillary necrosis, seen with abuse of analgesics such as aspirin or acetaminophen 镇痛药性肾病; **diabetic n.**, the nephropathy seen in later stages of diabetes mellitus, with first hyperfiltration, renal hypertrophy, microalbuminuria, and hypertension, and later proteinuria and end-stage renal disease 糖尿病肾病; **gouty n.**, any of a group of chronic kidney diseases associated with the abnormal production and excretion of uric acid 痛风肾病; **HIV-associated n.**, renal pathology in patients infected with the human immunodeficiency virus, a condition resembling focal segmental glomerulosclerosis 人类免疫缺陷病毒相关性肾病; **IgA n.**, IgA 肾病, 参见 *glomerulonephritis* 下词条; **ischemic n.**, nephropathy resulting from partial or complete

N

obstruction of a renal artery and the accompanying ischemia; there is a significant reduction in the glomerular filtration rate 缺血性肾病；**membranous n.**, 膜性肾病，参见 *glomerulonephritis* 下词条；**minimal change n.**, 微小病变性肾小球病，参见 *disease* 下词条；**obstructive n.**, nephropathy from obstruction of the urinary tract with hydronephrosis and a slowed glomerular filtration rate 梗阻性肾病；**potassium-losing n.**, persistent urinary potassium losses in the presence of hypokalemia, such as in metabolic alkalosis or intrinsic renal disease 失钾性肾病；**reflux n.**, childhood pyelonephritis in which the renal scarring results from vesicoureteric reflux, with radiologic appearance of intrarenal reflux 反流性肾病；**salt-losing n.**, any intrinsic renal disease causing abnormal urinary sodium loss to the point of hypotension 失盐性肾病；**sickle cell n.**, chronic kidney disease in sickle cell disease, including vascular abnormalities, fibrosis, and an increased glomerular filtration rate 镰状细胞肾病；**urate n.**, **uric acid n.**, any of a group of kidney diseases with hyperuricemia, including an acute form, a chronic form *(gouty n.)*, and nephrolithiasis with uric acid calculi 尿酸盐肾病

neph·ro·pexy (nefʹro-pek″se) fixation or suspension of a hypermobile kidney 肾固定术

neph·rop·to·sis (nef″rop-toʹsis) floating or hypermobile kidney; downward displacement of a kidney 肾下垂

neph·ro·py·elog·ra·phy (nef″ro-pi″ə-logʹrə-fe) radiography of the kidney and its pelvis 肾盂造影（术）

neph·ror·rha·gia (nef″ro-raʹjə) hemorrhage from the kidney 肾出血

neph·ror·rha·phy (nef-rorʹə-fe) suture of the kidney 肾缝术

neph·ro·scle·ro·sis (nef″ro-sklə-roʹsis) hardening of the kidney due to renovascular disease 肾硬化，肾硬变（病）；**arteriolar n.**, that involving mainly arterioles, with degeneration of renal tubules and fibrotic thickening of glomeruli; there are both benign and malignant forms 小动脉性肾硬化症，细动脉性肾硬化

neph·ro·scope (nefʹro-skōp) an instrument inserted into an incision in the renal pelvis for viewing the inside of the kidney 肾镜

ne·phro·sis (nə-froʹsis) [Gr.] 1. 同 nephropathy；2. any kidney disease characterized by purely degenerative lesions of the renal tubules 任何一种以肾小管的纯致变性病变为特征的肾病；**amyloid n.**, renal amyloidosis 淀粉样肾病变；**lipid n.**, minimal change disease 脂性肾病

neph·ro·so·ne·phri·tis (nə-fro″so-nə-friʹtis) renal disease with nephrotic and nephritic components 肾病性肾炎

ne·phros·to·my (nə-frosʹtə-me) creation of a permanent fistula leading into the renal pelvis 肾造口术

ne·phrot·ic (nə-frotʹik) pertaining to, resembling, or caused by nephrosis 肾病的

neph·ro·tome (nefʹro-tōm) one of the segmented divisions of the mesoderm connecting the somite with the lateral plates of unsegmented mesoderm; the source of much of the urogenital system 生肾节

neph·ro·to·mog·ra·phy (nefʹro-to-mogʹrə- fe) radiologic visualization of the kidney by tomography 肾断层造影（术）；**nephrotomograph′ic** *adj.*

ne·phrot·o·my (nə-frotʹə-me) incision of a kidney 肾切开术

neph·ro·tox·ic (nefʹro-tok″sik) destructive to kidney cells 肾中毒的

neph·ro·tox·in (nefʹro-tok″sin) a toxin having a specific destructive effect on kidney cells 肾毒素，溶肾素

neph·ro·tro·pic (nefʹro-troʹpik) having a special affinity for kidney tissue 向肾性的

neph·ro·tu·ber·cu·lo·sis (nef″ro-too-bur″kuloʹsis) renal tuberculosis 肾结核

neph·ro·ure·ter·ec·to·my (nef″ro-u-re″tərekʹtə-me) excision of a kidney and all or part of the ureter 肾输尿管切除术

nep·tu·ni·um (Np) (nep-tooʹne-əm) a silvery white, ductile, reactive transuranium element; at. no. 93, at. wt. 237 镎（化学元素）

nerve (nurv) a cordlike structure comprising a collection of nerve fibers that convey impulses between a part of the central nervous system and some other body region 神经，见图 8 至图 14；**abducent n.**, sixth cranial nerve: *origin*, a nucleus in the pons, immediately internal to the facial colliculus in the floor of the fourth ventricle, emerging from the brainstem anteriorly between the pons and medulla oblongata; *distribution*, lateral rectus muscle of eye; *modality*, motor（外）展神经，又称 *nervus abducens*；**accelerator n's**, the cardiac sympathetic nerves, which, when stimulated, accelerate the action of the heart 加速神经，心脏交感神经，当受到刺激时，加速心脏的活动；**accessory n.**, eleventh cranial nerve: *origin*, by spinal roots from the cervical spinal cord; the roots unite briefly with socalled cranial roots of the nerve (actually part of the vagus nerve) to form the trunk of the accessory nerve; upon exiting the jugular foramen, the cranial roots split off and join the vagus nerve; *distribution* (spinal roots), sternocleidomastoid and trapezius muscles; *modality*, motor 副神经，又称 *nervus ac-*

cessorius; **acoustic n.**, 同 vestibulocochlear n.; **afferent n.**, any nerve that transmits impulses from the periphery toward the central nervous system 传入神经, 参见 *sensory n.*; **alveolar n.**, **inferior**, *origin*, mandibular nerve; *branches*, inferior dental plexus, mylohyoid and mental nerves; *distribution*, teeth and gums of lower jaw, skin of chin and lower lip, mylohyoid muscle and anterior belly of digastric muscle; *modality*, motor and general sensory 下牙槽神经, 又称 *nervus alveolaris inferior*; **alveolar n's, superior**, a collective name for the superior alveolar branches (anterior, middle, and posterior) arising from the maxillary and infraorbital nerves, innervating the teeth and gums of the upper jaw and the maxillary sinus, and forming the superior dental plexus 上牙槽神经, 又称 *nervi alveolares superiores*; **ampullary n., anterior**, the branch of the vestibular nerve that innervates the ampulla of the anterior semicircular duct, ending around the hair cells of the ampullary crest 前壶腹神经, 又称 *nervus ampullaris anterior*; **ampullary n., inferior**, 同 ampullary n., posterior; **ampullary n., lateral**, the branch of the vestibular nerve that innervates the ampulla of the lateral semicircular duct, ending around the hair cells of the ampullary crest 外壶腹神经, 又称 *nervus ampullaris lateralis*; **ampullary n., posterior**, the branch of the vestibular nerve that innervates the ampulla of the posterior semicircular duct, ending around the hair cells of the ampullary crest 后壶腹神经, 又称 *nervus ampullaris posterior*; **ampullary n., superior**, 同 ampullary n., anterior; **anal n's, inferior**, *origin*, pudendal nerve, or independently from the sacral plexus; *distribution*, external anal sphincter, skin around anus, and lining of anal canal up to pectinate line; *modality*, general sensory and motor 肛门下神经, 又称 *nervi anales inferiores*; **anococcygeal n.**, *origin*, coccygeal plexus; *distribution*, sacrococcygeal joint, coccyx, skin over the coccyx; *modality*, general sensory 肛尾神经, 又称 *nervus anococcygeus*; **antebrachial cutaneous n's**, cutaneous n's of forearm 前臂皮神经; **articular n.**, any mixed peripheral nerve that supplies a joint and its associated structures 关节神经; **auricular n's, anterior**, *origin*, auriculotemporal nerve; *distribution*, skin of anterosuperior part of external ear; *modality*, general sensory 耳前神经, 又称 *nervi auriculares anteriores*; **auricular n., great**, *origin*, cervical plexus—C2-C3; *branches*, anterior and posterior branches; *distribution*, skin over parotid gland and mastoid process, and both surfaces of auricle; *modality*, general sensory 耳大神经, 又称 *nervus auricularis magnus*; **auricular n., posterior**, *origin*, facial nerve; *branches*, occipital branch; *distribution*, posterior auricular and occipitofrontalis muscles and skin of external acoustic meatus; *modality*, motor and general sensory 耳后神经, 又称 *nervus auricularis posterior*; **auriculotemporal n.**, *origin*, by two roots from the mandibular nerve; *branches*, anterior auricular nerve, nerve of external acoustic meatus, parotid branches, branch to tympanic membrane, and branches communicating with facial nerve; its terminal branches are superficial temporal to the scalp; *distribution*, parotid gland, scalp in temporal region, tympanic membrane (see also *anterior auricular n's* and *n. of external acoustic meatus*); *modality*, general sensory 耳颞神经, 又称 *nervus auriculotemporalis*; **autonomic n.**, any of the parasympathetic or sympathetic nerves of the autonomic nervous system 自主神经; **axillary n.**, *origin*, posterior cord of brachial plexus (C5-C6); *branches*, lateral superior cutaneous nerve of arm and muscular branches; *distribution*, deltoid and teres minor muscles, skin on back of arm; *modality*, motor and general sensory 腋神经, 又称 *nervus axillaris*; **brachial cutaneous n's**, cutaneous n's of arm 臂皮神经; **buccal n.**, *origin*, mandibular nerve; *distribution*, skin and mucous membrane of cheeks, gums, and perhaps the first two molars and the premolars; *modality*, general sensory 颊神经, 又称 *nervus buccalis*; **cardiac n., inferior**, cardiac n., inferior cervical, *origin*, cervicothoracic ganglion; *distribution*, heart via cardiac plexus; *modality*, sympathetic (accelerator) and visceral afferent (chiefly pain) 颈下心神经, 又称 *nervus cardiacus cervicalis inferior*; **cardiac n., middle**, cardiac n., middle cervical, *origin*, middle cervical ganglion; *distribution*, heart; *modality*, sympathetic (accelerator) and visceral afferent (chiefly pain) 颈中心神经, 又称 *nervus cardiacus cervicalis medius*; **cardiac n., superior**, cardiac n., superior cervical, *origin*, superior cervical ganglion; *distribution*, heart; *modality*, sympathetic (accelerator) 颈上心神经, 又称 *nervus cardiacus cervicalis superior*; **cardiac n's, thoracic**, thoracic cardiac branches: branches of the second through fourth or fifth thoracic ganglia of the sympathetic trunk, supplying the heart and having a sympathetic (accelerator) modality as well as a visceral afferent one (chiefly for pain) 胸心神经; **caroticotympanic n's**, *origin*, internal carotid plexus; together with tympanic nerve, these nerves form the tympanic plexus; *distribution*, tympanic region and parotid gland; *modality*, sympathetic 颈鼓神经, 又称 *nervi caroticotympanici*; **carotid n's, external**, *origin*, superior cervical ganglion; *distribution*, cranial blood vessels and glands via the external carotid

N

plexus; *modality*, sympathetic 颈外动脉神经，又称 *nervi carotici externi*；**carotid n., internal,** *origin*, superior cervical ganglion; *distribution*, cranial blood vessels and glands via internal carotid plexus; *modality*, sympathetic 颈内动脉神经，又称 *nervus caroticus internus*；**cavernous n's of clitoris,** *origin*, uterovaginal plexus; *distribution*, erectile tissue of clitoris; *modality*, parasympathetic, sympathetic, and visceral afferent 阴蒂海绵体神经，又称 *nervi cavernosi clitoridis*；**cavernous n's of penis,** *origin*, prostatic plexus; *distribution*, erectile tissue of penis; *modality*, sympathetic, parasympathetic, and visceral afferent 阴茎海绵体神经，又称 *nervi cavernosi penis*；**centrifugal n.,** 同 efferent n.；**centripetal n.,** 同 afferent n.；**cerebral n's,** 同 cranial n's；**cervical n's,** the eight pairs of nerves (C1–C8) that arise from the cervical segments of the spinal cord and, except for the last pair, leave the vertebral column above the correspondingly numbered vertebra. The anterior rami of the upper four, on either side, unite to form the cervical plexus, and those of the lower four, together with the anterior branch of the first thoracic nerve, form most of the brachial plexus 颈神经，又称 *nervi cervicales*；**cervical n., transverse,** *origin*, cervical plexus (C2–C3); *branches*, superior and inferior branches; *distribution*, skin on side and front of neck; *modality*, general sensory 颈横神经，又称 *nervus transversus colli*；**cervical cardiac n's,** 颈心神经，参见 *cardiac n., inferior cervical, cardiac n., middle cervical,* 和 *cardiac n., superior cervical*；**ciliary n's, long,** *origin*, nasociliary nerve, from ophthalmic nerve; *distribution*, dilator pupillae, uvea, cornea; *modality*, sympathetic and general sensory 睫状长神经，又称 *nervi ciliares longi*；**ciliary n's, short,** *origin*, ciliary ganglion; *distribution*, smooth muscle and tunics of eye; *modality*, parasympathetic, sympathetic, and general sensory 睫状短神经，又称 *nervi ciliares breves*；**cluneal n's, inferior,** general sensory nerve branches of the posterior femoral cutaneous nerve, innervating the skin of the lower part of the buttocks 臀下皮神经，又称 *nervi clunium inferiores*；**cluneal n's, middle,** general sensory nerve branches of the plexus formed by the diagonal branches of the posterior rami of the first four sacral nerves, innervating ligaments of the sacrum and the skin over the posterior buttocks 臀中皮神经，又称 *nervi clunium medii*；**cluneal n's, superior,** general sensory nerve branches of the posterior branches of the upper lumbar nerves, innervating the skin of the upper part of the buttocks 臀上皮神经，又称 *nervi clunium superiores*；**coccygeal n.,** either of the thirty-first pair of spinal nerves, arising from the coccy-geal segment of the spinal cord 尾神经，又称 *nervus coccygeus*；**cochlear n.,** the part of the vestibulocochlear nerve concerned with hearing, consisting of fibers that arise from the bipolar cells in the spiral ganglion and have their receptors in the spiral organ of the cochlea 蜗神经，又称 *nervus cochlearis*；**cranial n's,** the twelve pairs of nerves that are connected with the brain, including the olfactory（Ⅰ）, optic（Ⅱ）, oculomotor（Ⅲ）, trochlear（Ⅳ）, trigeminal（Ⅴ）, abducent（Ⅵ）, facial（Ⅶ）, vestibulocochlear（Ⅷ）, glossopharyngeal（Ⅸ）, vagus（Ⅹ）, accessory（Ⅺ）, and hypoglossal（Ⅻ）nerves 脑神经，又称 *nervi craniales*，见图 8；**crural interosseous n.,** 同 interosseous n. of leg；**cubital n.,** 同 ulnar n.；**cutaneous n.,** any mixed peripheral nerve that supplies a region of the skin 皮神经；**cutaneous n., perforating,** one arising from the posterior surface of the second and third sacral nerves, piercing the sacrotuberous ligament, and supplying the skin over the inferomedial gluteus maximus; it is absent in one-third of the population 穿皮神经，又称 *nervus cutaneus perforans*；**cutaneous n. of arm, inferior lateral,** *origin*, radial nerve; *distribution*, skin of lateral surface of lower part of arm; *modality*, general sensory 臂外侧下皮神经，又称 *nervus cutaneus brachii lateralis inferior*；**cutaneous n. of arm, medial,** *origin*, medial cord of brachial plexus (T1); *distribution*, skin on medial and posterior aspects of arm; *modality*, general sensory 臂内侧皮神经，又称 *nervus cutaneus brachii medialis*；**cutaneous n. of arm, posterior,** *origin*, radial nerve in the axilla; *distribution*, skin on back of arm; *modality*, general sensory 臂后侧皮神经，又称 *nervus cutaneus brachii posterior*；**cutaneous n. of arm, superior lateral,** *origin*, axillary nerve; *distribution*, skin of back of arm; *modality*, general sensory 臂外侧上皮神经，又称 *nervus cutaneus brachii lateralis superior*；**cutaneous n's of calf,** sural cutaneous n's 腓肠皮神经；**cutaneous n. of foot, intermediate dorsal,** *origin*, superficial fibular nerve; *branches*, dorsal digital nerves of foot; *distribution*, skin of front of lower third of leg and dorsal region of foot, and skin and joints of adjacent sides of third and fourth, and of fourth and fifth toes; *modality*, general sensory 足背中间皮神经，又称 *nervus cutaneus dorsalis intermedius*；**cutaneous n. of foot, lateral dorsal,** *origin*, continuation of sural nerve; *distribution*, skin and joints of lateral side of foot and fifth toe; *modality*, general sensory 足背外侧皮神经，又称 *nervus cutaneus dorsalis lateralis*；**cutaneous n. of foot, medial dorsal,** *origin*, superficial fibular nerve; *distribution*, skin and joints of medial side of foot and big toe, and adjacent sides of second and third toes; *modality*, general sensory 足背内侧皮神经, 又称 *nervus cutaneus dorsalis medialis*; **cutaneous n. of forearm, lateral**, *origin*, continuation of musculocutaneous nerve; *distribution*, skin over radial side of forearm and sometimes an area of skin of back of hand; *modality*, general sensory 前臂外侧皮神经, 又称 *nervus cutaneus antebrachii lateralis*; **cutaneous n. of forearm, medial**, *origin*, medial cord of brachial plexus (C8, T1); *branches*, anterior and posterior; *distribution*, skin of front, medial, and posteromedial aspects of forearm; *modality*, general sensory 前臂内侧皮神经, 又称 *nervus cutaneus antebrachii medialis*; **cutaneous n. of forearm, posterior**, *origin*, radial nerve; *distribution*, skin of dorsal aspect of forearm; *modality*, general sensory 前臂后皮神经, 又称 *nervus cutaneus antebrachii posterior*; **cutaneous n. of neck, transverse**, transverse cervical n. 颈横神经; **cutaneous n. of thigh, intermediate**, a branch of the anterior cutaneous branch of the femoral nerve; it supplies the skin on the anterior side of the thigh and knee and ends as part of the patellar plexus 股内中皮神经; **cutaneous n. of thigh, lateral**, *origin*, lumbar plexus—L2–L3; *distribution*, skin of lateral and anterior aspects of thigh; *modality*, general sensory 股外侧皮神经, 又称 *nervus cutaneus femoris lateralis*; **cutaneous n. of thigh, medial**, a branch of the anterior cutaneous branch of the femoral nerve; it supplies the skin on the medial side of the thigh and knee and has a branch that forms part of the patellar plexus 股中皮神经; **cutaneous n. of thigh, posterior**, *origin*, sacral plexus—S1– S3; *branches*, inferior cluneal nerves and perineal branches; *distribution*, skin of buttock, external genitalia, and back of thigh and calf; *modality*, general sensory 股后皮神经, 又称 *nervus cutaneus femoris posterior*; **depressor n.**, 1. a nerve that lessens the activity of an organ 抑制神经; 2. an afferent nerve whose stimulation causes a fall in blood pressure 降压神经; **digital n's, radial dorsal**, dorsal digital n's of radial nerve (桡神经) 指背神经; **digital n's, ulnar dorsal**, dorsal digital n's of ulnar nerve (尺神经) 指背神经; **digital n's of foot, dorsal**, 1. nerves supplying the third, fourth, and fifth toes: *origin*, intermediate dorsal cutaneous nerve; *distribution*, skin and joints of adjacent sides of third and fourth, and of fourth and fifth toes; *modality*, general sensory 足背内侧皮神经; 2. nerves supplying the first and second toes: *origin*, medial terminal division of deep fibular nerve; *distribution*,skin and joints of adjacent sides of great and second toes; *modality*, general sensory(腓深神经) 趾背神经, 又称 *nervi digitales dorsales pedis*;

digital n's of lateral plantar n., common plantar, *number*, two; *origin*, superficial branch of lateral plantar nerve; *branches*, the medial nerve gives rise to two proper plantar digital nerves; *distribution*, the lateral one to the flexor digiti minimi brevis muscle of foot and to skin and joints of lateral side of sole and little toe; the medial one to adjacent sides of fourth and fifth toes and see individual nerve branches; *modality*, motor and general sensory（足底外侧神经）趾足底总神经, 又称 *nervi digitales plantares communes nervi plantaris lateralis*; **digital n's of lateral plantar n., proper plantar**, *origin*, common plantar digital nerves; *distribution*, flexor digiti minimi brevis muscle of foot, skin and joints of lateral side of sole and little toe, and adjacent sides of fourth and fifth toes; *modality*, motor and general sensory(足底外侧神经)趾足底固有神经, 又称 *nervi digitales plantares proprii nervi plantaris lateralis*; **digital n's of medial plantar n., common plantar**, *number*, four; *origin*, medial plantar nerve; *branches*, muscular branches and proper plantar digital nerves; *distribution*, flexor hallucis brevis muscle and first lumbrical muscles, skin and joints of medial side of foot and great toe, and adjacent sides of great and second, second and third, and third and fourth toes; *modality*, motor and general sensory（足底内侧神经）趾足底总神经, 又称 *nervi digitales plantares communes nervi plantaris medialis*; **digital n's of medial plantar n., proper plantar**, *origin*, common plantar digital nerves; *distribution*, skin and joints of medial side of great toe, and adjacent sides of great and second, second and third, and third and fourth toes; the nerves extend to the dorsum to supply nail beds and tips of toes; *modality*, general sensory（趾足底总神经）趾足底固有神经, 又称 *nervi digitales plantares proprii nervi plantaris medialis*; **digital n's of median n., common palmar**, *number*, four; *origin*, lateral and medial divisions of median nerve; *branches*, proper palmar digital nerves; *distribution*, thumb, index, middle, and ring fingers and first two lumbrical muscles; *modality*, motor and general sensory（正中神经）指掌侧总神经, 又称 *nervi digitales palmares communes nervi mediani*; **digital n's of median n., proper palmar**, *origin*, common palmar digital nerves; *distribution*, first two lumbrical muscles, skin and joints of both sides and palmar aspect of thumb, index, and middle fingers, radial side of ring finger, and back of distal aspect of these digits; *modality*, general sensory and motor（正中神经）指掌侧固有神经, 又称 *nervi digitales palmares proprii nervi mediani*; **digital n's of radial n., dorsal**, *origin*, superficial branch of radial nerve; *distri-*

bution, skin and joints of back of thumb, index finger, middle finger, and medial aspect of ring finger, as far distally as the distal phalanx; *modality*, general sensory（桡神经）指背神经，又称 *nervi digitales dorsales nervi radi alis*; **digital n's of ulnar n.**, **common palmar**, *number*, two; *origin*, superficial branch of ulnar nerve; *branches*, proper palmar digital nerves; *distribution*, little and ring fingers; *modality*, general sensory（尺神经）指掌侧总神经，又 称 *nervi digitales palmares communes nervi ulnaris*; **digital n's of ulnar n., dorsal**, *origin*, dorsal branch of ulnar nerve; *distribution*, skin and joints of medial side of little finger, dorsal aspects of adjacent sides of little and ring fingers; *modality*, general sensory（尺神经）指背神经，又称 *nervi digitales dorsales nervi ulnaris*; **digital n's of ulnar n., proper palmar**, *origin*, the lateral of the two common palmar digital nerves from the superficial branch of the ulnar nerve; *distribution*, skin and joints of adjacent sides of fourth and fifth fingers; *modality*, general sensory（尺神经）指掌侧固有 神经，又称 *nervi digitales palmares proprii nervi ulnaris*; **dorsal n. of clitoris**, *origin*, pudendal nerve; *distribution*, deep transverse perineal and urethral sphincter muscles; corpus cavernosum clitoridis; and skin, prepuce, and glans of clitoris; *modality*, general sensory and motor 阴蒂背神经，又 称 *nervus dorsalis clitoridis*; **dorsal n. of penis**, *origin*, pudendal nerve; *distribution*, deep transverse perineal and urethral sphincter muscles; corpus cavernosum penis; and skin, prepuce, and glans of penis; *modality*, general sensory and motor 阴茎背神 经，又称 *nervus dorsalis penis*; **dorsal scapular n.**, *origin*, brachial plexus—anterior ramus of C5; *distribution*, rhomboid muscles and occasionally the levator scapulae muscle; *modality*, motor 肩胛背神 经，又 称 *nervus dorsalis scapulae*; **efferent n.**, any nerve that carries impulses from the central nervous system to the periphery, e.g., a motor nerve 传 出神经; **ethmoidal n., anterior**, *origin*, continuation of nasociliary nerve, from ophthalmic nerve; *branches*, internal, external, lateral, and medial nasal branches; *distribution*, mucosa of upper and anterior nasal septum, lateral wall of nasal cavity, skin of lower bridge and tip of nose; *modality*, general sensory 筛前神经，又称 *nervus ethmoidalis anterior*; **ethmoidal n., posterior**, *origin*, nasociliary nerve, from ophthalmic nerve; *distribution*, mucosa of posterior ethmoid cells and of sphenoidal sinus; *modality*, general sensory 筛后神经，又称 *nervus ethmoidalis posterior*; **excitor n.**, one that transmits impulses resulting in an increase in functional activity 兴奋神经; **excitoreflex n.**, an autonomic nerve that produces reflex action 兴奋反射性神经; **n. of external acoustic meatus**, *origin*, auriculotemporal nerve; *distribution*, skin lining external acoustic meatus, and tympanic membrane; *modality*, general sensory. Called also *nervus meatus acustici externi* 外耳道神经; **facial n.**, the seventh cranial nerve, consisting of two roots: a large motor root, which supplies the muscles of facial expression, and a smaller root, the intermediate nerve (q.v.). *Origin*, inferior border of pons, between olive and inferior cerebellar peduncle; *branches* (of motor root), stapedius and posterior auricular nerves, parotid plexus, digastric, stylohyoid, temporal, zygomatic, buccal, lingual, marginal mandibular, and cervical branches, and a communicating branch with the tympanic plexus; *distribution*, various structures of face, head, and neck; *modality*, motor, parasympathetic, general sensory, special sensory 面神经，又 称 *nervus facialis*; **femoral n.**, *origin*, lumbar plexus (L2–L4); descending behind the inguinal ligament to the femoral triangle; *branches*, saphenous nerve, muscular and anterior cutaneous branches; *distribution*, skin of thigh and leg, muscles of front of thigh, and hip and knee joints; *modality*, general sensory and motor 股神经，又称 *nervus femoralis*; **femoral cutaneous n's**, cutaneous n's of thigh 股皮 神经; **fibular n's**, peroneal n's 腓神经; **fibular n., common**, *origin*, sciatic nerve in lower part of thigh; *branches and distribution*, supplies short head of biceps femoris muscle (while still incorporated in sciatic nerve), gives off lateral sural cutaneous nerve and sural communicating branch as it descends in popliteal fossa, supplies knee and superior tibiofibular joints and tibialis anterior muscle, and divides into superficial and deep fibular nerves; *modality*, general sensory and motor 腓总神经，又称 *nervus fibularis communis and nervus peronaeus communis*; **fibular n., deep**, *origin*, a terminal branch of common fibular nerve; *branches and distribution*, winds around the neck of the fibula and descends on the interosseous membrane to the front of the ankle; gives off muscular branches to tibialis anterior, extensor hallucis longus, extensor digitorum longus, and fibularis tertius muscles, and a twig to the ankle joint; and an articular branch; and divides into lateral and medial terminal branches, the former supplying the extensor digitorum brevis muscle and tarsal joints and the latter dividing into dorsal digital nerves for skin and joints of adjacent sides of first and second toes; *modality*, general sensory and motor 腓深神经，又称 *nervus fibularis profundus and nervus peronaeus profundus*; **fibular n., superficial**, *origin*, a terminal branch of common peroneal nerve; *branches and distribution,* descends in front of the fibula, supplies fibularis longus and brevis muscles and, in the lower part of the leg, divides into the muscular branches, and medial and intermediate dorsal cutaneous nerves; *modality,* general sensory and motor 腓浅神经，又称 *nervus fibularis superficialis and nervus peronaeus superficialis*; **frontal n.**, *origin,* ophthalmic division of trigeminal nerve; enters the orbit through the superior orbital fissure; *branches,* supraorbital and supratrochlear nerves; *distribution,* chiefly to the forehead and scalp; *modality,* general sensory 额神经，又称 *nervus frontalis*; **fusimotor n's,** nerves with a special type of ending that innervates intrafusal fibers of the muscle spindle 肌梭运动神经；**gangliated n.**, any nerve of the sympathetic nervous system 有节神经，交感神经；**genitofemoral n.**, *origin,* lumbar plexus (L1–L2); *branches,* genital and femoral branches; *distribution,* cremaster muscle, skin of scrotum or labia majora and of adjacent area of thigh and femoral triangle; *modality,* general sensory and motor 生殖股神经，又称 *nervus genitofemoralis*; **glossopharyngeal n.**, the ninth cranial nerve: *origin,* several rootlets from lateral side of upper part of medulla oblongata, between the olive and the inferior cerebellar peduncle; *branches,* tympanic nerve, pharyngeal, stylopharyngeal, carotid, tonsillar, and lingual branches, and communicating branches with the auricular and meningeal branches of the vagus nerve, with the chorda tympani, and with the auriculotemporal nerve; *distribution,* it has two enlargements (superior and inferior ganglia) and supplies the tongue, pharynx, and parotid gland; *modality,* motor, parasympathetic, and general, special, and visceral sensory 舌咽神经，又称 *nervus glossopharyngeus*; **gluteal n's,** 1. the superior and inferior gluteal nerves 臀上神经和臀下神经；2. the cluneal nerves (superior, middle, and inferior) in the lumbar and sacral regions 腰骶部的臀（上、中、下）皮神经；**gluteal n., inferior,** *origin,* sacral plexus (L5–S2); *distribution,* gluteus maximus muscle; *modality,* motor 臀下神经，又称 *nervus gluteus inferior*; **gluteal n., superior,** *origin,* sacral plexus (L4–S1); *distribution,* gluteus medius and minimus muscles, tensor fasciae latae muscle, and hip joint; *modality,* motor and general sensory 臀上神经，又称 *nervus gluteus superior*; **gustatory n's,** sensory nerve fibers innervating the taste buds and associated with taste, including branches from the lingual and glossopharyngeal nerves 味觉神经；**hemorrhoidal n's, inferior,** 同 anal n's, inferior；**hypogastric n.**, a nerve trunk situated on either side (right and left), interconnecting the superior and inferior

hypogastric plexuses 腹下神经（左及右），又称 *nervus hypogastricus*；**hypoglossal n.,** the twelfth cranial nerve: *origin,* several rootlets in the anterolateral sulcus between the olive and the pyramid of the medulla oblongata; it passes through the hypoglossal canal to the tongue; *branches,* lingual branches; *distribution,* styloglossus, hyoglossus, and genioglossus muscles and intrinsic muscles of the tongue; *modality,* motor 舌下神经，又称 *nervus hypoglossus*；**iliohypogastric n.**, *origin,* lumbar plexus—L1 (sometimes T12); *branches,* lateral and anterior cutaneous branches; *distribution,* the skin above the pubis and over the lateral side of the buttock, and occasionally the pyramidalis muscle; *modality,* motor and general sensory 髂腹下神经，又称 *nervus iliohypogastricus*；**ilioinguinal n.**, *origin,* lumbar plexus—L1 (sometimes T12); accompanies the spermatic cord through the inguinal canal; *branches,* anterior scrotal or labial branches; *distribution,* skin of scrotum or labia majora, and adjacent part of thigh; *modality,* general sensory 髂腹股沟神经，又称 *nervus ilioinguinalis*；**infraorbital n.**, *origin,* continuation of the maxillary nerve, entering the orbit through the inferior orbital fissure, and occupying in succession the infraorbital groove, canal, and foramen; *branches,* middle and anterior superior alveolar, inferior palpebral, internal and external nasal, and superior labial arteries; *distribution,* incisor, cuspid, and premolar teeth of upper jaw, skin and conjunctiva of lower eyelid, mobile septum and skin of side of nose, mucous membrane of mouth, skin of upper lip; *modality,* general sensory 眶下神经，又称 *nervus infraorbitalis*；**infratrochlear n.**, *origin,* nasociliary nerve from ophthalmic nerve; *branches,* palpebral branches; *distribution,* skin of root and upper bridge of nose and lower eyelid, conjunctiva, lacrimal duct; *modality,* general sensory 滑车下神经，又称 *nervus infratrochlearis*；**inhibitory n.,** one that transmits impulses resulting in a decrease in functional activity 抑制神经；**intercostal n's,** anterior ramus of the first eleven thoracic spinal nerves, situated between the ribs. The first three send branches to the brachial plexus as well as to the thoracic wall; the fourth, fifth, and sixth supply only the thoracic wall; and the seventh through eleventh are thoracoabdominal in distribution 肋间神经，又称 *nervi intercostales*，另参见 *subcostal n.*；**intercostobrachial n's,** two nerves arising from the intercostal nerves. The first is constant: *origin,* second intercostal nerve; *distribution,* skin on back and medial aspect of arm; *modality,* general sensory. A second is often present: *origin,* third intercostal nerve; *distribution,* skin of axilla and medial aspect of arm;

N

modality, general sensory 肋间臂神经，又称 *nervi intercostobrachiales*；**intermediate n.**, the smaller root of the facial nerve, lying between the main root and the vestibulocochlear nerve; *branches*, chorda tympani and greater petrosal nerve; *distribution*, lacrimal, nasal, palatine, submandibular, and sublingual glands, and anterior two-thirds of tongue; *modality*, parasympathetic and special sensory 中间神经，又称 *nervus intermedius*；**interosseous n. of forearm, anterior**, *origin*, median nerve; *distribution*, flexor pollicis longus, flexor digitorum profundus, and pronator quadratus muscles, wrist and intercarpal joints; *modality*, motor and general sensory 前臂骨间前神经，又称 *nervus interosseus antebrachii anterior*；**interosseous n. of forearm, posterior**, *origin*, continuation of deep branch of radial nerve; *distribution*, abductor pollicis longus, extensors of the thumb and second finger, and wrist and intercarpal joints; *modality*, motor and general sensory 前臂骨间后神经，又称 *nervus interosseus antebrachii posterior*；**interosseous n. of leg**, *origin*, tibial nerve; *distribution*, interosseous membrane and tibiofibular syndesmosis; *modality*, general sensory 小腿骨间神经，又称 *nervus interosseus cruris*；**ischiadic n.**, 同 sciatic n.；**jugular n.**, a branch of the superior cervical ganglion that communicates with the vagus and glossopharyngeal nerves 颈静脉神经，又称 *nervus jugularis*；**labial n's, anterior**, *origin*, ilioinguinal nerve; *distribution*, skin of anterior labial region of labia majora, and adjacent part of thigh; *modality*, general sensory 阴唇前神经，又称 *nervi labiales anteriores*；**labial n's, posterior**, *origin*, perineal nerve; *distribution*, labia majora; *modality*, general sensory 阴唇后神经，又称 *nervi labiales posteriores*；**lacrimal n.**, *origin*, ophthalmic division of trigeminal nerve, entering the orbit through the superior orbital fissure; *distribution*, lacrimal gland, conjunctiva, lateral commissure of eye, and skin of upper eyelid; *modality*, general sensory 泪腺神经，又称 *nervus lacrimalis*；**laryngeal n., external**, external branch of superior laryngeal nerve: the smaller of the two branches into which the superior laryngeal nerve divides, descending under cover of the sternothyroid muscle and innervating the cricothyroid and the inferior pharyngeal constrictor muscle of the pharynx; *modality*, motor 喉上神经外支；**laryngeal n., inferior**, a name sometimes given to the anterior branch of the recurrent laryngeal nerve 喉返神经前支；**laryngeal n., internal**, internal branch of superior laryngeal nerve: the larger of the two branches of the superior laryngeal nerve, which innervates the mucosa of the epiglottis, base of the tongue, and larynx; *modality*,

general sensory 喉上神经内支；**laryngeal n., recurrent**, *origin*, vagus nerve (chiefly the cranial part of the accessory nerve); *branches*, inferior laryngeal nerve and tracheal, esophageal, pharyngeal, and inferior cardiac branches; *distribution*, tracheal mucosa, esophagus, inferior pharyngeal constrictor muscle of pharynx, cardiac plexus; *modality*, parasympathetic, visceral afferent, and motor 喉返神经，又称 *nervus laryngeus recurrens*；**laryngeal n., superior**, *origin*, inferior ganglion of vagus nerve; *branches*, external, internal, and communicating branches; *distribution*, inferior pharyngeal constrictor muscle of pharynx and cricothyroid muscles, and mucosa of epiglottis, base of tongue, and larynx; *modality*, motor, general sensory, visceral afferent, and parasympathetic 喉上神经，又称 *nervus laryngeus superior*；**n. to lateral pterygoid**, *origin*, mandibular nerve; *distribution*, lateral pterygoid muscle; *modality*, motor 翼外肌神经，又称 *nervus pterygoideus lateralis*；**n. to levator ani**, a branch of the sacral plexus that innervates the levator ani muscle 肛提肌神经，骶神经丛的一个分支，支配着肛提肌；**lingual n.**, *origin*, mandibular nerve, descending to the tongue, first medial to the mandible and then under cover of the mucosa of mouth; *branches*, sublingual nerve, lingual branches, branches to isthmus of fauces, and branches communicating with the hypoglossal nerve and chorda tympani; *distribution*, anterior two-thirds of tongue, adjacent areas of mouth, gums, isthmus of fauces, sublingual gland and overlying mucosa; *modality*, general sensory 舌神经，又称 *nervus lingualis*；**lumbar n's**, the five pairs of nerves (L1–L5) that arise from the lumbar segments of the spinal cord, each pair leaving the vertebral column below the correspondingly numbered vertebra. The anterior rami of these nerves participate in the formation of the lumbosacral plexus 腰神经，又称 *nervi lumbales*；**mandibular n.**, one of three terminal divisions of the trigeminal nerve, passing through the foramen ovale to the infratemporal fossa. *Origin*, trigeminal ganglion; *branches*, meningeal branch, masseteric, deep temporal, lateral and medial pterygoid, buccal, auriculotemporal, lingual, and inferior alveolar nerves; *distribution*, extensive distribution to muscles of mastication, skin of face, mucous membrane of mouth, teeth, dura mater, mucous membrane of mastoid air cells; *modality*, general sensory and motor 下颌神经，又称 *nervus mandibularis*；**masseteric n.**, *origin*, mandibular division of trigeminal nerve; *distribution*, masseter muscle and temporomandibular joint; *modality*, motor and general sensory 咬肌神经，又称 *nervus* *massetericus*; **maxillary n.**, one of the three terminal divisions of the trigeminal nerve, passing through the foramen rotundum, and entering the pterygopalatine fossa. *Origin*, trigeminal ganglion; *branches*, meningeal branch, zygomatic, superior alveolar, and infraorbital nerves, branches to pterygopalatine ganglion, and, indirectly, the branches of the pterygopalatine ganglion; *distribution*, dura mater, extensive distribution to skin of face and scalp, mucous membrane of maxillary sinus and nasal cavity, and teeth; *modality*, general sensory 上颌神经，又称 *nervus maxillaris*; **n. to medial pterygoid**, *origin*, mandibular nerve; *branches*, nerve to tensor tympani, nerve to tensor veli palatini; *distribution*, medial pterygoid, tensor tympani, and tensor veli palatini muscles; *modality*, motor 翼内肌神经，又称 *nervus pterygoideus medialis*; **median n.**, *origin*, lateral and medial cords of brachial plexus (C6–T1); *branches*, anterior interosseous nerve of forearm, common palmar digital nerves, muscular and palmar branches, and a communicating branch with the ulnar nerve; *distribution*, the elbow, wrist, and intercarpal joints, anterior muscles of the forearm, muscles of the digits, skin of the palm, thenar eminence, and digits; *modality*, general sensory 正中神经，又称 *nervus medianus*; **mental n.**, *origin*, inferior alveolar nerve; *branches*, mental, gingival, and inferior labial arteries; *distribution*, skin of chin, and lower lip; *modality*, general sensory 颏神经，又称 *nervus mentalis*; **mixed n.**, one composed of both sensory and motor fibers 混合神经; **motor n.**, an efferent nerve that stimulates muscle contraction 运动神经; **musculocutaneous n.**, *origin*, lateral cord of brachial plexus—C5–C7; *branches*, lateral antebrachial cutaneous nerve and muscular branches; *distribution*, coracobrachialis, biceps brachii, and brachialis muscles, the elbow joint, and skin of radial side of forearm; *modality*, general sensory and motor 肌皮神经，又称 *nervus musculocutaneus*; **myelinated n.**, a nerve, especially a peripheral nerve, whose fibers (axons) are encased in a myelin sheath, which in turn is enclosed by a neurilemma 有髓神经; **n. to mylohyoid**, *origin*, inferior alveolar nerve; *distribution*, mylohyoid muscle, anterior belly of digastric muscle; *modality*, motor 下颌舌骨肌神经，又称 *nervus mylohyoideus*; **nasociliary n.**, *origin*, ophthalmic division of trigeminal nerve; *branches*, long ciliary, posterior ethmoidal, anterior ethmoidal, and infratrochlear nerves, and a communicating branch to the ciliary ganglion; *distribution*—see individual nerve branches; *modality*, general sensory 鼻睫神经，又称 *nervus nasociliaris*; **nasopalatine n.**, *origin*, pterygopalatine ganglion;

distribution, mucosa and glands of most of nasal septum and anterior part of hard palate; *modality*, parasympathetic and general sensory 鼻腭神经，又称 *nervus nasopalatinus*; **obturator n.**, *origin*, lumbar plexus (L3– L4); *branches*, anterior, posterior, and muscular branches; *distribution*, adductor muscles and gracilis muscle, skin of medial part of thigh, and hip and knee joints; *modality*, general sensory and motor 闭孔神经，又称 *nervus obturatorius*; **obturator n., accessory**, *origin*, anterior branches of anterior ramus of L3–L4; *distribution*, pectineus muscle, hip joint, communicates with obturator nerve; *modality*, general sensory and motor 副闭孔神经，又称 *nervus obturatorius accessorius*; **n. to obturator internus**, *origin*, anterior branches of anterior rami of L5, S1–S2; *distribution*, superior gemellus and obturator internus muscles; *modality*, general sensory and motor 闭孔内肌神经，又称 *nervus musculi obturatorii interni*; **occipital n., greater**, *origin*, medial branch of posterior ramus of C2; *distribution*, semispinalis capitis muscle and skin of scalp as far forward as the vertex; *modality*, general sensory and motor 枕大神经，又称 *nervus occipitalis major*; **occipital n., lesser**, *origin*, superficial cervical plexus (C2–C3); *distribution*, ascends behind the auricle and supplies some of the skin on the side of the head and on the cranial surface of the auricle; *modality*, general sensory 枕小神经，又称 *nervus occipitalis minor*; **occipital n., third**, *origin*, medial branch of posterior ramus of C3; *distribution*, skin of upper part of back of neck and head; *modality*, general sensory 第三枕神经，又称 *nervus occipitalis tertius*; **oculomotor n.**, third cranial nerve: *origin*, brainstem, emerging medial to cerebral peduncles and running forward in the cavernous sinus; *branches*, superior and inferior branches; *distribution*, entering the orbit through the superior orbital fissure, the branches supply the levator palpebrae superioris muscle and all of the extrinsic eye muscles except the lateral rectus and superior oblique, and carry parasympathetic fibers for the ciliaris and sphincter pupillae muscles; *modality*, motor and parasympathetic 动眼神经，又称 *nervus oculomotorius*; **olfactory n.**, first cranial nerve; the nerve of smell, consisting of about 20 bundles (sometimes called olfactory nerves) arising in the olfactory epithelium and passing through the cribriform plate of the ethmoid bone to the olfactory bulb 嗅神经，又称 *nervus olfactorius*; **ophthalmic n.**, one of the three terminal divisions of the trigeminal nerve: *origin*, trigeminal ganglion; *branches*, recurrent meningeal (tentorial) branch, frontal, lacrimal, and nasociliary nerves; *distribution*, eyeball and

N

678

conjunctiva, lacrimal gland and sac, nasal mucosa and frontal sinus, external nose, upper eyelid, forehead, and scalp; *modality*, general sensory 眼神经, 又称 *nervus ophthalmicus*; **optic n.**, second cranial nerve, the nerve of sight; misnamed as a nerve because of its cordlike appearance, it is actually part of the central nervous system. It consists chiefly of axons and central processes of cells of the ganglionic layer of the retina that leave each orbit through the optic canal, joining with those of the opposite side to form the optic chiasm (the medial fibers of each nerve crossing over to the opposite side), then continuing on each side as the optic tract 视神经, 又称 *nervus opticus*; **pain n.**, a sensory nerve that conducts stimuli producing the sensation of pain 痛觉神经; **palatine n.**, **greater**, *origin*, pterygopalatine ganglion; *branches*, posterior inferior (lateral) nasal branches; *distribution*, emerges through the greater palatine foramen and supplies the palate; *modality*, parasympathetic, sympathetic, and general sensory 腭大神经, 又称 *nervus palatinus major*; **palatine n's, lesser**, *origin*, pterygopalatine ganglion; *distribution*, emerge through the lesser palatine foramen and supply the soft palate and tonsil; *modality*, parasympathetic, sympathetic, and general sensory 腭小神经, 又称 *nervi palatini minores*; **parasympathetic n.**, any of the nerves of the parasympathetic nervous system 副交感神经; **pectoral n., lateral**, *origin*, lateral cord of brachial plexus or anterior division of upper and middle trunks (C5–C7); *distribution*, usually several nerves supplying the pectoralis minor muscle and acromioclavicular and glenohumeral joints; *modality*, motor and general sensory 胸外侧神经, 又称 *nervus pectoralis lateralis*; **pectoral n., medial**, *origin*, medial cord or lower trunk of brachial plexus (C8, T1); *distribution*, usually several nerves supplying the pectoralis major and pectoralis minor muscles; *modality*, motor 胸内侧神经, 又称 *nervus pectoralis medialis*; **perforating cutaneous n.**, 同 cutaneous n., perforating; **perineal n's**, *origin*, pudendal nerve in the pudendal canal; *branches*, muscular branches and posterior scrotal or labial nerves; *distribution*, muscular branches supply the bulbospongiosus, ischiocavernosus, and superficial transverse perineal muscles and bulb of the penis and, in part, the external anal sphincter and levator ani muscles; the scrotal or labial nerves supply the scrotum or labia majora; *modality*, general sensory and motor 会阴神经, 又称 *nervi perineales*; **peripheral n.**, any nerve outside the central nervous system 周围神经; **petrosal n., deep**, *origin*, internal carotid plexus; *distribution*, joins greater petrosal nerve to form

nerve of pterygoid canal, and supplies lacrimal, nasal, and palatine glands via pterygopalatine ganglion and its branches; *modality*, sympathetic 岩深神经, 又称 *nervus petrosus profundus*; **petrosal n., greater**, *origin*, intermediate nerve via geniculate ganglion; *distribution*, running forward from the geniculate ganglion, it joins the deep petrosal nerve of the pterygoid canal, and reaches lacrimal, nasal, and palatine glands and nasopharynx, via pterygopalatine ganglion and its branches; *modality*, parasympathetic and general sensory 岩大神经, 又称 *nervus petrosus major*; **petrosal n., lesser**, *origin*, tympanic plexus; *distribution*, parotid gland via otic ganglion and auriculotemporal nerve; *modality*, parasympathetic and general sensory 岩小神经, 又称 *nervus petrosus minor*; **pharyngeal n.**, a nerve running from the posterior part of the pterygopalatine ganglion, through the pharyngeal canal with the pharyngeal branch of the maxillary artery, to the mucous membrane of the nasal part of the pharynx posterior to the auditory tube 咽神经, 又称 *nervus pharyngeus*; **phrenic n.**, *origin*, cervical plexus (C4–C5); *branches*, pericardial and phrenicoabdominal branches; *distribution*, pleura, pericardium, respiratory diaphragm, peritoneum, and sympathetic plexuses; *modality*, general sensory and motor 膈神经, 又称 *nervus phrenicus*; **phrenic n's, accessory**, inconstant contributions of the fifth cervical nerve to the phrenic nerve; when present, they run a separate course to the root of the neck or into the thorax before joining the phrenic nerve 膈副神经, 又称 *nervi phrenici accessorii*; **n. to piriformis**, *origin*, posterior branches of anterior rami of S1–S2; *distribution*, piriformis muscle; *modality*, general sensory and motor 梨状肌神经, 又称 *nervus musculi piriformis*; **plantar n., lateral**, *origin*, the smaller of terminal branches of tibial nerve; *branches*, muscular, superficial, and deep branches; *distribution*, lying between first and second layers of muscles of sole, the nerve supplies the quadratus plantae, abductor digiti minimi, flexor digiti minimi brevis, adductor hallucis, interossei, and second, third, and fourth lumbrical muscles, and gives off cutaneous and articular twigs to lateral side of sole and fourth and fifth toes; *modality*, general sensory and motor 足底外侧神经, 又称 *nervus plantaris lateralis*; **plantar n., medial**, *origin*, the larger of the terminal branches of tibial nerve; *branches*, common plantar digital nerves and muscular branches; *distribution*, abductor hallucis, flexor digitorum brevis, flexor hallucis brevis, and first lumbrical muscles, and cutaneous and articular twigs to the medial side of the sole, and to the first to fourth toes; *modality*, general sensory and motor 足底内侧神经，又称 *nervus plantaris medialis*；**popliteal n., lateral, common fibular n.** 腓总神经；**popliteal n., medial,** 同 tibial n.；**pressor n.,** any afferent nerve whose irritation stimulates a vasomotor center and increases intravascular tension 加压神经；**pterygoid n., lateral,** 同 n. to lateral pterygoid；**pterygoid n., medial, n.** to medial pterygoid 翼内肌神经；**n. of pterygoid canal,** *origin,* union of deep and greater petrosal nerves; *distribution,* pterygopalatine ganglion and branches; *modality,* parasympathetic and sympathetic 翼管神经，又称 *nervus canalis pterygoidei*；**pudendal n.,** *origin,* sacral plexus (S2–S4); *branches,* enters the pudendal canal, gives off the inferior anal nerve, and then divides into the perineal nerve and dorsal nerve of the penis (clitoris); *distribution,* muscles, skin, and erectile tissue of perineum; *modality,* general sensory, motor, and parasympathetic 阴部神经，又称 *nervus pudendus*；**n. to quadratus femoris,** *origin,* anterior branches of anterior ramus of L4–L5; *distribution,* gemellus inferior, anterior quadratus femoris muscle, hip joint; *modality,* general sensory and motor. Called also *nervus musculi quadrati femoris* 股方肌神经；**radial n.,** *origin,* posterior cord of brachial plexus (C6–C8, and sometimes C5 and T1); *branches,* posterior cutaneous and inferior lateral cutaneous nerves of arm, posterior cutaneous nerve of forearm, muscular, deep, and superficial branches; *distribution,* descending in the back of arm and forearm, it is ultimately distributed to skin on back of arm, forearm, and hand, extensor muscles on back of arm and forearm, and elbow joint and many joints of hand; *modality,* general sensory and motor 桡神经，又称 *nervus radialis*；**rectal n's, inferior,** inferior anal n's 直肠下神经；**recurrent n.,** recurrent laryngeal n. 喉返神经；**saccular n.,** the branch of the vestibular nerve that innervates the macula of the saccule 球囊神经，又称 *nervus saccularis*；**sacral n's,** the five pairs of nerves (S1–S5) that arise from the sacral segments of the spinal cord; the anterior ramus of the first four pairs participates in the formation of the sacral plexus 骶神经，又称 *nervi sacrales*；**saphenous n.,** *origin,* termination of femoral nerve, descending first with femoral vessels and then on medial side of leg and foot; *branches,* infrapatellar and medial crural cutaneous branches; *distribution,* knee joint, subsartorial and patellar plexuses, skin on medial side of leg and foot; *modality,* general sensory 隐神经，又称 *nervus saphenus*；**sciatic n.,** the largest nerve of the body: *origin,* sacral plexus (L4–S3); it leaves the pelvis through the greater sciatic foramen; *branches,* divides into the tibial and common fibular nerves, usually in lower third of thigh; *distribution*—see individual nerve branches; *modality,* general sensory and motor 坐骨神经，又称 *nervus ischiadicus*；**scrotal n's, anterior,** *origin,* ilioinguinal nerve; *distribution,* skin of anterior scrotal region; *modality,* general sensory 阴囊前神经，又称 *nervi scrotales anteriores*；**scrotal n's, posterior,** *origin,* perineal nerve; *distribution,* skin of scrotum; *modality,* general sensory 阴囊后神经，又称 *nervi scrotales posteriores*；**secretory n.,** any efferent nerve whose stimulation increases glandular activity 分泌神经；**sensory n.,** a peripheral nerve that conducts impulses from a sense organ to the spinal cord or brain 感觉神经；**somatic n's,** the motor and sensory nerves that supply skeletal muscle and somatic tissues 体神经；**spinal n's,** the 31 pairs of nerves that arise from the spinal cord and pass out between the vertebrae, including the eight pairs of cervical, twelve of thoracic, five of lumbar, five of sacral, and one pair of coccygeal nerves 脊神经，又称 *nervi spinales*；**splanchnic n's,** those of the blood vessels and viscera, especially the visceral branches of the thoracic, lumbar, and pelvic parts of the sympathetic trunks 内脏神经；**splanchnic n., greater,** *origin,* thoracic sympathetic trunk and fifth through tenth thoracic ganglia; *distribution,* descending through the respiratory diaphragm or its aortic openings, it ends in the celiac ganglia and plexuses, with a splanchnic ganglion commonly occurring near the respiratory diaphragm; *modality,* preganglionic sympathetic and visceral afferent 内脏大神经，又称 *nervus splanchnicus major*；**splanchnic n., least,** *origin,* last ganglion of sympathetic trunk or lesser splanchnic nerve; *distribution,* aorticorenal ganglion and adjacent plexus; *modality,* sympathetic and visceral afferent 内脏最小神经，又称 *nervus splanchnicus imus*；**splanchnic n., lesser,** *origin,* ninth and tenth thoracic ganglia of sympathetic trunk; *branches,* renal branch; *distribution,* pierces the respiratory diaphragm, joins the aorticorenal ganglion and celiac plexus, and communicates with the renal and superior mesenteric plexuses; *modality,* preganglionic sympathetic and visceral afferent 内脏小神经，又称 *nervus splanchnicus minor*；**splanchnic n., lowest, least** splanchnic n. 内脏最下神经；**splanchnic n's, lumbar,** *origin,* lumbar ganglia or sympathetic trunk; *distribution,* upper nerves join celiac and adjacent plexuses, middle ones go to intermesenteric and adjacent plexuses, and lower ones descend to superior hypogastric plexus; *modality,* preganglionic sympathetic and visceral afferent 腰内脏神经，又称 *nervi splanchnici lumbales*；**splanchnic n's, pelvic,**

N

parasympathetic root of pelvic ganglia: *origin*, sacral plexus (S3–S4); *distribution*, leaving the sacral plexus, the nerves enter the inferior hypogastric plexus and supply the pelvic organs; *modality*, preganglionic parasympathetic and visceral afferent 骨盆内脏神经; **splanchnic n's, sacral**, *origin*, sacral part of sympathetic trunk; *distribution*, pelvic organs and blood vessels via inferior hypogastric plexus; *modality*, preganglionic sympathetic and visceral afferent 骶内脏神经, 又称 *nervi splanchnici sacrales*; **n. to stapedius**, *origin*, facial nerve; *distribution*, stapedius muscle; *modality*, motor 镫骨肌神经, 又称 *nervus stapedius*; **n. to subclavius**, *origin*, upper trunk of brachial plexus (C5); *distribution*, subclavius muscle and sternoclavicular joint; *modality*, motor and general sensory 锁骨下神经, 又称 *nervus subclavius*; **subcostal n.**, *origin*, anterior ramus of twelfth thoracic nerve; *distribution*, skin of lower abdomen and lateral side of gluteal region, parts of transversus, oblique, and rectus muscles, and usually the pyramidalis muscle, and adjacent peritoneum; *modality*, general sensory and motor 肋下神经, 又称 *nervus subcostalis*; **sublingual n.**, *origin*, lingual nerve; *distribution*, sublingual gland and overlying mucous membrane; *modality*, parasympathetic and general sensory 舌下神经, 又称 *nervus sublingualis*; **suboccipital n.**, *origin*, posterior ramus of first cervical nerve; *distribution*, emerges above posterior arch of atlas and supplies muscles of suboccipital triangle and semispinalis capitis muscle; *modality*, motor 枕下神经, 又称 *nervus suboccipitalis*; **subscapular n's**, *origin*, posterior cord of brachial plexus (C5); *distribution*, usually two or more nerves, upper and lower, supplying subscapularis and teres major muscles; *modality*, motor 肩胛下神经, 又称 *nervi subscapulares*; **sudomotor n's**, the nerves that innervate the sweat glands 泌汗神经; **supraclavicular n's**, a term denoting collectively the common trunk, which is a branch of the cervical plexus (C3–C4) and which emerges under cover of the posterior border of the sternocleidomastoid muscle and divides into the intermediate, lateral, and medial supraclavicular nerves 锁骨上神经, 又称 *nervi supraclaviculares*; **supraclavicular n's, anterior**, medial supraclavicular n's 锁骨上神经前支; **supraclavicular n's, intermediate**, *origin*, cervical plexus (C3–C4); *distribution*, descend in the posterior triangle, cross the clavicle, and supply the skin over pectoral and deltoid regions; *modality*, general sensory 锁骨上中间支, 又称 *nervi supraclaviculares intermedii*; **supraclavicular n's, lateral**, *origin*, cervical plexus (C3–C4); *distribution*, descend in the posterior tri-angle, cross the clavicle, and supply the skin of superior and posterior parts of shoulder; *modality*, general sensory 锁骨上外侧神经, 又称 *nervi supraclaviculares laterales*; **supraclavicular n's, medial**, *origin*, cervical plexus (C3–C4); *distribution*, descend in posterior triangle, cross the clavicle, and supply the skin of medial infraclavicular region; *modality*, general sensory 锁骨上内侧神经, 又称 *nervi supraclaviculares mediales*; **supraclavicular n's, middle**, intermediate supraclavicular n's 锁骨上神经中间支; **supraclavicular n's, posterior**, lateral supraclavicular n's 锁骨上神经后支; **supraorbital n.**, *origin*, continuation of frontal nerve, from ophthalmic nerve; *branches*, lateral and medial branches; *distribution*, leaves orbit through supraorbital notch or foramen, and supplies the skin of upper eyelid, forehead, anterior scalp (to vertex), mucosa of frontal sinus; *modality*, general sensory 眶上神经, 又称 *nervus supraorbitalis*; **suprascapular n.**, *origin*, brachial plexus (C5–C6); *distribution*, descends through suprascapular and spinoglenoid notches and supplies acromioclavicular and glenohumeral joints, and supraspinatus and infraspinatus muscles; *modality*, motor and general sensory 肩胛上神经, 又称 *nervus suprascapularis*; **supratrochlear n.**, *origin*, frontal nerve, from ophthalmic nerve; *distribution*, leaves orbit at medial end of supraorbital margin and supplies the forehead and upper eyelid; *modality*, general sensory 滑车上神经, 又称 *nervus supratrochlearis*; **sural n.**, *origin*, medial sural cutaneous nerve and communicating branch of common fibular nerve; *branches*, lateral dorsal cutaneous nerve and lateral calcaneal branches; *distribution*, skin on back of leg, and skin and joints on lateral side of heel and foot; *modality*, general sensory 腓肠神经, 又称 *nervus suralis*; **sural cutaneous n., lateral**, *origin*, common fibular nerve; *distribution*, skin of lateral side of back of leg, rarely may continue as the sural nerve; *modality*, general sensory 腓肠外侧皮神经, 又称 *nervus cutaneus surae lateralis*; **sural cutaneous n., medial**, *origin*, tibial nerve; usually joins sural communicating branch of common fibular nerve to form the sural nerve; *distribution*, may continue as the sural nerve; *modality*, general sensory 腓肠内侧皮神经, 又称 *nervus cutaneus surae medialis*; **sympathetic n.**, 1. 交感干, 参见 *trunk* 下词条; 2. any nerve of the sympathetic nervous system 交感神经; **temporal n's, deep**, *number*, usually two, anterior and posterior, with a third middle one often seen; *origin*, mandibular nerve; *distribution*, temporalis muscle; *modality*, motor 颞深神经, 又称 *nervi temporales profundi*; **n. to tensor tympani**, *origin*, nerve to medial pterygoid; *distribution*, tensor tympani muscle; *modality*, motor 鼓膜张肌神经，又称 *nervus musculi tensoris tympani*；n. to tensor veli palatini, *origin*, nerve to medial pterygoid; *distribution*, tensor veli palatini muscle; *modality*, motor 腭帆张肌神经，又称 *nervus musculi tensoris veli palatini*；tentorial n., tentorial branch of ophthalmic nerve: a branch that arises from the ophthalmic nerve close to its origin from the trigeminal ganglion, turning back to innervate the dura mater of the tentorium cerebelli and falx cerebri; *modality*, general sensory 幕神经；terminal n., the collection of nerve filaments found in the pia mater between the olfactory bulb and the crista galli, and passing through the cribriform plate to the nasal mucosa; ganglion cells occur along their course 终神经，又称 *nervus terminalis*；thoracic n's, the twelve pairs of spinal nerves (T1–T12) that arise from the thoracic segments of the spinal cord, each pair leaving the vertebral column below the correspondingly numbered vertebra. They innervate the body wall of the thorax and upper abdomen 胸神经，又称 *nervi thoracici*；thoracic n., long, *origin*, brachial plexus (anterior rami of C5–C7); *distribution*, descends behind the brachial plexus to the serratus anterior muscle; *modality*, motor 胸长神经，又称 *nervus thoracicus longus*；thoracodorsal n., *origin*, posterior cord of brachial plexus (C7–C8); *distribution*, latissimus dorsi muscle; *modality*, motor 胸背神经，又称 *nervus thoracodorsalis*；tibial n., *origin*, sciatic nerve in lower part of thigh; *branches*, crural interosseous nerve, medial sural cutaneous and sural nerves, medial and lateral plantar nerves, and muscular and medial calcaneal branches; *distribution*, while still incorporated in the sciatic nerve, it supplies the semimembranosus and semitendinosus muscles, long head of biceps, and adductor magnus muscle; it supplies the knee joint as it descends in the popliteal fossa and, continuing into the leg, supplies the muscles and skin of the calf and sole of the foot, and the toes; *modality*, general sensory and motor 胫神经，又称 *nervus tibialis*；trigeminal n., fifth cranial nerve, which emerges from the lateral surface of the pons as a motor and a dorsal root, together with some intermediate fibers. The dorsal root expands into the trigeminal ganglion, which contains the cells of origin of most of the sensory fibers, and from which the three divisions of the nerve arise. See *mandibular n., maxillary n.,* and *ophthalmic n.* The trigeminal nerve is sensory in supplying the face, teeth, mouth, and nasal cavity, and motor in supplying the muscles of mastication 三叉神经，又称 *nervus trigeminus*；trochlear n., fourth cranial nerve; *origin*, the fibers of the trochlear nerve on each side decussate across the median plane and emerge from the back of the brainstem below the corresponding inferior colliculus; *distribution*, runs forward in lateral wall of cavernous sinus, traverses the superior orbital fissure, and supplies superior oblique muscle of eyeball; *modality*, motor 滑车神经，又称 *nervus trochlearis*；tympanic n., *origin*, inferior ganglion of glossopharyngeal nerve; *branches*, helps form tympanic plexus; *distribution*, mucous membrane of tympanic cavity, mastoid air cells, auditory tube, and, via lesser petrosal nerve and otic ganglion, the parotid gland; *modality*, general sensory and parasympathetic 鼓室神经，又称 *nervus tympanicus*；ulnar n., *origin*, medial and lateral cords of brachial plexus (C7–T1); *branches*, muscular, dorsal, palmar, superficial, and deep branches; *distribution*, ultimately to skin on front and back of medial part of hand, some flexor muscles on front of forearm, many short muscles of hand, elbow joint, many joints of hand; *modality*, general sensory and motor 尺神经，又称 *nervus ulnaris*；unmyelinated n's, one whose fibers (axons) are not encased in a myelin sheath 无髓鞘神经；utricular n., the branch of the vestibular nerve that innervates the macula of the utricle 椭圆囊神经，又称 *nervus utricularis*；utriculoampullary n., a nerve that arises by peripheral division of the vestibular nerve, and supplies the utricle and ampullae of the semicircular ducts 椭圆囊壶腹神经，又称 *nervus utriculoampullaris*；vaginal n's, *origin*, uterovaginal plexus; *distribution*, vagina; *modality*, sympathetic and parasympathetic 阴道神经，又称 *nervi vaginales*；vagus n., tenth cranial nerve: *origin*, by numerous rootlets from lateral side of medulla oblongata in the groove between the olive and the inferior cerebellar peduncle; *branches*, superior and recurrent laryngeal nerves, meningeal, auricular, pharyngeal, cardiac, bronchial, gastric, hepatic, celiac, and renal branches, pharyngeal, pulmonary, and esophageal plexuses, and anterior and posterior trunks; *distribution*, descending through the jugular foramen, it presents as a superior and an inferior ganglion, and continues through the neck and thorax into the abdomen. It supplies sensory fibers to the ear, tongue, pharynx, and larynx, motor fibers to the pharynx, larynx, and esophagus, and parasympathetic and visceral afferent fibers to thoracic and abdominal viscera; *modality*, parasympathetic, visceral afferent, motor, general sensory 迷走神经，又称 *nervus vagus*；vascular n's, the nerve branches that supply the adventitia of the blood vessels 血管神经；vasoconstrictor n., one whose stimulation causes contraction of the blood vessels 缩血管神经; **vasodilator** n., one whose stimulation causes dilation of the blood vessels 舒血管神经; **vasomotor** n., one concerned in controlling the caliber of vessels, whether as a vasodilator or a vasoconstrictor 血管运动神经; **vertebral** n., *origin*, cervicothoracic and vertebral ganglia; *distribution*, ascends with vertebral artery and gives fibers to spinal meninges, cervical nerves, and posterior cranial fossa; *modality*, sympathetic 椎神经，又称 *nervus vertebralis*; **vestibular** n., the posterior part of the vestibulocochlear nerve, which is concerned with the sense of equilibrium. It consists of fibers arising from bipolar cells in the vestibular ganglion, and divides peripherally into a superior and an inferior part, with receptors in the ampullae of the semicircular canals, the utricle, and the saccule 前庭神经，又称 *nervus vestibularis*; **vestibulocochlear** n., eighth cranial nerve; it emerges from the brain between the pons and the medulla oblongata, at the cerebellopontine angle and behind the facial nerve. It divides near the lateral end of the internal acoustic meatus into two functionally distinct and incompletely united components, the vestibular nerve and the cochlear nerve, and is connected with the brain by corresponding roots, the vestibular and the cochlear roots 前庭蜗神经，听神经，又称 *nervus vestibulocochlearis*; **vidian** n., n. of pterygoid canal 翼管神经; **visceral** n., autonomic n. 内脏神经; **zygomatic** n., *origin*, maxillary nerve, entering the orbit through the inferior orbital fissure; *branches*, zygomaticofacial and zygomaticotemporal branches; *distribution*, communicates with the lacrimal nerve and supplies the skin of the temple and adjacent part of the face; *modality*, general sensory 颧神经，又称 *nervus zygomaticus*

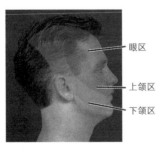

▲ 三叉神经的一般分布。眼部、上颌和下颌这三个区域分别由眼神经、上颌神经和下颌神经这三个主要分支支配

ner·vi·mo·tor (nur″vĭ-mo′tər) pertaining to a motor nerve 运动神经的

ner·vous (nur′vəs) 1. 同 neural (1); 2. unduly excitable 焦虑的

ner·vus (nur′vəs) pl. *ner′vi* [L.] 同 nerve

ne·sid·i·ec·to·my (ne-sid″e-ek′tə-me) excision of the islet cells of the pancreas 胰岛切除术

ne·sid·io·blast (ne-sid′e-o-blast″) any of the cells giving rise to islet cells of the pancreas 成胰岛细胞

nest (nest) a small mass of cells, usually foreign to the area in which they are found 巢; **junctional** n., a nest of dysplastic cells seen at the dermoepidermal junction as part of a junctional nevus 接合处巢，皮毛接合处的一个发育不良细胞巢，作为交界痣的一部分

net·il·mi·cin (net″il-mi′sin) a semisynthetic aminoglycoside antibiotic having a wide range of activity; used as the sulfate salt in the treatment of infection caused by severe systemic gramnegative infection 奈替霉素，一种具有广泛活性的半合成氨基糖苷类抗生素；其硫酸盐用于治疗由革兰阴性菌引起的感染

net·tle (net′əl) any plant of the genus *Urtica*, characterized by stinging hairs and secretion of a poisonous fluid. *U. dioica* is a type of *stinging nettle* that grows in temperate regions; its root is used to treat urinary problems associated with benign prostatic hyperplasia. The flowering plant is used for urinary tract infections, kidney and bladder stones, and rheumatism and is also widely used in folk medicine 荨麻

neu·ral (noor′əl) 1. pertaining to a nerve or to the nerves 神经的; 2. situated in the region of the spinal axis, as is the neural arch 位于脊髓轴包括椎弓的区域

neu·ral·gia (noo-ral′jə) paroxysmal pain extending along the course of one or more nerves 神经痛; **neural′gic** *adj.*; **geniculate** n., Ramsay Hunt syndrome (1) 膝状节神经痛; **glossopharyngeal** n., that affecting the petrosal and jugular ganglion of the glossopharyngeal nerve, marked by severe paroxysmal pain originating on the side of the throat and extending to the ear 舌咽神经痛; **Hunt** n., Ramsay Hunt syndrome (1) 亨特神经痛，膝状节神经痛; **intercostal** n., neuralgia of the intercostal nerves 肋间神经痛; **migrainous** n., cluster headache 偏头痛性神经痛; **Morton** n., Morton toe: a form of foot pain, metatarsalgia due to compression of a branch of the plantar nerve by the metatarsal heads; it may lead to formation of a neuroma. 跖痛症，莫顿趾，脚痛的一种形式，由于跖骨头压迫足底神经的一个分支而引起的跖骨痛；它可能导致神经瘤的形成; **postherpetic** n., persistent burning pain and hyperesthesia along the distribution of a cutaneous nerve following an attack of herpes zoster 带状疱疹（后）神经痛；**triafacial n., trifocal n., trigeminal n.,** severe episodic pain in the area of the trigeminal nerve, often precipitated by stimulation of trigger points 三叉神经痛

neu·ra·min·ic   ac·id (noor″ə-min′ik) a 9-carbon amino sugar whose *N*-acyl derivatives are the sialic acids 神经氨（糖）酸，甘露糖胺丙酮酸

neu·ra·min·i·dase (noor″ə-min′ ĭ-dās) sialidase; an enzyme that catalyzes the cleavage of sialic acid residues from the nonreducing terminal of oligosaccharides in glycoproteins, glycolipids, and proteoglycans. Deficiency of the lysosomal form of the enzyme causes sialidosis. Viral neuraminidase is important in influenza 神经氨酸酶，唾液酸酶

neu·rana·gen·e·sis (noor″an-ə-jen′ə-sis) re - generation of nerve tissue 神经再生

neu·ra·poph·y·sis (noor″ə-pof′ə-sis) the structure forming either side of the neural arch 神经突，神经弓的任意一侧

neu·ra·prax·ia (noor″ə-prak′se-ə) usually temporary failure of nerve conduction in the absence of structural changes, due to blunt injury, compression, or ischemia 神经失用症，功能性麻痹

neu·ras·the·nia (noor″əs-the′ne-ə) a term virtually obsolete in Western medicine but still used in traditional Chinese medicine, denoting a mental disorder marked by chronic weakness and easy fatigability 神经衰弱，该术语在西医中已不再使用，中医里表示一种长期疲乏的神经症状

neu·rec·ta·sia (noor″ək-ta′zhə) 同 neurotony

neu·rec·to·my (noo-rek′tə-me) excision of a part of a nerve 神经（部分）切除术

neu·rec·to·pia (noor″ək-to′pe-ə) displacement of or abnormal situation of a nerve 神经异位

neu·ren·ter·ic (noor″ən-ter′ik) pertaining to the neural tube and archenteron of the embryo 神经管（与）原肠的（胚胎中神经管和原肠的附属物）

neu·rer·gic (noo-rur′jik) pertaining to or dependent on nerve action 神经作用的，由神经活动产生的

neu·ri·lem·ma (noor″ĭ-lem′ə) the thin membrane spirally enwrapping the myelin layers of certain fibers, especially of the peripheral nerves, or the axons of some unmyelinated nerve fibers 神 经 鞘，神经膜

neu·ri·lem·mi·tis (noor″ĭ-lem-i′tis) inflammation of the neurilemma 神经鞘膜炎

neu·ri·lem·o·ma (noor″ĭ-lem-o′mə) a tumor of a peripheral nerve sheath (neurilemma), the most common type of neurogenic tumor, usually benign 神经鞘瘤

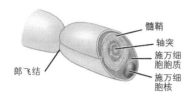

▲ **外周神经纤维的神经鞘包绕轴突**

neu·ri·tis (noo-ri′tis) inflammation of a nerve 神经炎；**neurit′ic** *adj.*；**hereditary optic n.,** Leber hereditary optic neuropathy 遗传性视神经炎；**multiple n.,** polyneuritis 多 神 经 炎；**optic n.,** inflammation of the optic nerve, affecting part of the nerve within the eyeball *(papillitis)* or the part behind the eyeball *(retrobulbar n.)* 视神经炎，包括视神经乳头炎和球后视神经炎；**retrobulbar n.,** 参见 *optic n.*；**toxic n.,** 见 *neuropathy* 下词条

neu·ro·anas·to·mo·sis (noor″o-ə-nas″tə-mo′- sis) surgical anastomosis of one nerve to another 神经吻合术

neu·ro·anat·o·my (noor″o-ə-nat′ə-me) anatomy of the nervous system 神经解剖学

neu·ro·ar·throp·a·thy (noor″o-ahr-throp′ə- the) any disease of joint structures associated with disease of the central or peripheral nervous system 神经性关节病

neu·ro·as·tro·cy·to·ma (noor″o-as″tro-sito′mə) a glioma composed mainly of astrocytes, found mostly in the floor of the third ventricle and the temporal lobes 神经星形细胞瘤

neu·ro·be·hav·ior·al (noor″o-be-hāv′u-rəl) relating to neurologic status as assessed by observation of behavior 神经行为的

neu·ro·bi·ol·o·gy (noor″o-bi-ol′ə-je) biology of the nervous system 神经生物学

neu·ro·blast (noor′o-blast) an embryonic cell that develops into a nerve cell or neuron 神经母细胞，成神经细胞

neu·ro·blas·to·ma (noor″o-blas-to′mə) sarcoma of nervous system origin, composed chiefly of neuroblasts, affecting mostly infants and young children, usually arising in the autonomic nervous system (sympathicoblastoma) or in the adrenal medulla 神经母细胞瘤，成神经细胞瘤

neu·ro·car·di·ac (noor″o-kahr′de-ak) pertaining to the nervous system and the heart 神经心脏的

neu·ro·cen·tral (noor″o-sen′trəl) pertaining to the body (centrum) of a vertebra and the pedicles of the

N

vertebral arch 髓椎体的

neu·ro·cen·trum (noor″o-sen′trəm) one of the embryonic vertebral elements from which the spinous processes of the vertebrae develop 髓椎体（胚胎）; **neurocen′tral** *adj.*

neu·ro·chem·is·try (noor″o-kem′is-tre) the branch of neurology dealing with the chemistry of the nervous system 神经化学

neu·ro·chon·drite (noor″o-kon′drīt) one of the embryonic cartilaginous elements that develop into the vertebral arch of a vertebra 胚神经弓，胚胎软骨成分之一，最终形成椎体的椎弓

neu·ro·cho·rio·ret·i·ni·tis (noor″o-kor″e-oret″ī-ni′tis) inflammation of the optic nerve, choroid, and retina 视神经脉络膜视网膜炎

neu·ro·cho·roi·di·tis (noor″o-kor″oi-di′tis) inflammation of the optic nerve and choroid 视神经脉络膜炎

neu·ro·cir·cu·la·to·ry (noor″o-sur′ku-lə-tor″e) pertaining to the nervous and circulatory systems 神经（与）循环系统的

neu·roc·la·dism (noo-rok′lə-diz″əm) the formation of new branches by the process of a neuron 神经分支

neu·ro·cog·ni·tive (noor″o-kog′nĭ-tiv) said of those aspects of cognition that are most closely connected to specific areas of the brain 神经认知; cf. *neuropsychology*

neu·ro·com·mu·ni·ca·tions (noor″o-kə- mu″nĭ-ka′shənz) the branch of neurology dealing with the transfer and integration of information within the nervous system 神经信息学，神经学的分支，研究神经系统中信息的传递与整合

neu·ro·cra·ni·um (noor″o-kra′ne-əm) the part of the cranium enclosing the brain 脑颅; **neurocra′nial** *adj.*

neu·ro·cris·top·a·thy (noor″o-kris-top′ə-the) any disease arising from maldevelopment of the neural crest 神经嵴病

neu·ro·cu·ta·ne·ous (noor″o-ku-ta′ne-əs) pertaining to the nerves and skin, or the cutaneous nerves 神经（与）皮肤的; 皮神经的

neu·ro·cys·ti·cer·co·sis (noor″o-sis″tĭ-sərko′sis) infection of the central nervous system with the larval forms (cysticerci) of *Taenia solium*; variable manifestations include seizures, hydrocephalus, and other neurologic dysfunctions 神经囊尾蚴病，中枢神经系统感染猪肉绦虫的蚴型（囊尾蚴），临床表现十分多变，包括癫痫发作、脑积水以及许多其他神经功能障碍

neu·ro·cy·tol·y·sin (noor″o-si-tol′ ĭ-sin) a constituent of certain snake venoms which lyses nerve cells 溶神经细胞素

neu·ro·cy·to·ma (noor″o-si-to′mə) 1. medulloepithelioma 髓上皮瘤; 2. ganglioneuroma 神经节瘤，节细胞神经瘤

neu·ro·de·gen·er·a·tion (noor″o-de-jen″əra′shən) degeneration of nerve tissue 神经退行性变; 见 *degeneration* 下类型; **neurodegen′erative** *adj.*; **pantothenate kinase–associated n.**, an autosomal recessive disorder of acyl coenzyme A metabolism characterized by a marked reduction in the number of myelin sheaths of the globus pallidus and substantia nigra, with accumulation of iron pigment, progressive rigidity beginning in the legs, choreoathetoid movements, dysarthria, and progressive mental deterioration 泛酸盐激酶依赖性神经退化症

neu·ro·der·ma·ti·tis (noor″o-dur″mə-ti′tis) [Gr.] a general term for an eczematous dermatosis presumed to be a cutaneous response to prolonged vigorous scratching, rubbing, or pinching to relieve severe pruritus; believed by some to be a psychogenic disorder 神经性皮炎

neu·ro·dyn·ia (noor″o-din′e-ə) 同 neuralgia

neu·ro·ec·to·derm (noor″o-ek′to-dərm) the portion of the ectoderm of the early embryo that gives rise to the central and peripheral nervous systems, including some glial cells 神经外胚层; **neuroectoder′mal** *adj.*

neu·ro·ef·fec·tor (noor″o-ə-fek′tər) of or relating to the junction between a neuron and the effector organ it innervates 神经效应器

neu·ro·en·ceph·a·lo·my·elop·a·thy (noor″oensef″ə-lo-mi″ə-lop′ə-the) disease involving the nerves, brain, and spinal cord 神经脑脊髓病

neu·ro·en·do·crine (noor″o-en′do-krin) pertaining to neural and endocrine influence, and particularly to the interaction between the nervous and endocrine systems 神经内分泌的

neu·ro·en·do·cri·nol·o·gy (noor″o-en″dokrī-nol′ə-je) the study of the interactions of the nervous and endocrine systems 神经内分泌学

neu·ro·en·do·scope (noor″o-en′do-skōp″) an endoscope for examining and performing various interventions in the central nervous system 神经内镜

neu·ro·epi·the·li·o·ma (noor″o-ep″ī-the″leo′mə) medulloepithelioma 神经上皮瘤

neu·ro·epi·the·li·um (noor″o-ep″ī-the′le- əm) 神经上皮 1. epithelium made up of cells specialized to serve as sensory cells for reception of external stimuli 由感知细胞组成的上皮，能够感受外界刺激; 2. the ectodermal epithelium, from which the central nervous system is derived 外胚层上皮，发生为神经系统; **neuroepithe′lial** *adj.*

neu·ro·eth·ics (noor″o-eth′ĭks) the study of how developments in neuroscience impact human self-understanding, ethics, and policy decisions 神经伦理学

neu·ro·f·bril (noor″o-fi′brĭl) one of the delicate threads running in every direction through the cytoplasm of a nerve cell and extending into the axon and dendrites in a silver-stained preparation; believed to be neurofilament bundles, and perhaps neurotubules, coated with silver 神经原纤维

neu·ro·f·bro·ma (noor″o-fi-bro′mə) a tumor of peripheral nerves due to abnormal proliferation of Schwann cells 神经纤维瘤

neu·ro·f·bro·ma·to·sis (noor″o-fi-bro″mə- to′sis) either of two autosomal dominant disorders affecting the bones, nervous system, soft tissue, and skin, with formation of neurofibromas. Neurofibromatosis 1 is marked by numerous neurofibromas with café-au-lait spots, intertriginous freckling, and Lisch nodules; neurofibromatosis 2 is marked also by acoustic neuromas, central and peripheral nerve tumors, and presenile lens opacities 常染色体显性遗传病的一种，累及骨质、神经、软组织和皮肤，并伴有神经纤维瘤的形成。Ⅰ型神经纤维瘤伴咖啡斑，原发性雀斑和 Lisch 结节；Ⅱ型神经纤维瘤表现为听神经瘤，中枢或外周神经肿瘤和早发性晶状体浑浊

neu·ro·f·bro·sar·co·ma (noor″o-fi″bro-sahrko′mə) a malignant type of schwannoma superficially resembling a fibrosarcoma, sometimes occurring in association with neurofibromatosis that is undergoing malignant transformation 神经纤维肉瘤

neu·ro·fil·a·ment (noor″o-fil′ə-ment) an intermediate filament occurring with neurotubules in the neurons and having cytoskeletal, and perhaps transport, functions 神经（微）丝

neu·ro·gen·e·sis (noor″o-jen′ə-sis) the development of nervous tissue 神经发生

neu·ro·ge·net·ic (noor″o-jə-net′ik) 1. pertaining to neurogenesis 神经发生的；2. neurogenic 神经原（性）的

neu·ro·gen·ic (noor″o-jen′ik) 1. forming nervous tissue 神经发生的；2. originating in the nervous system or from a lesion in the nervous system 神经原（性）的

neu·rog·e·nous (noo-roj′ə-nəs) neurogenic 神经原（性）的

neu·rog·lia (noo-rog′le-ə) the supporting structure of nervous tissue, consisting of a fine web of tissue enclosing neuroglial cells, which is of three types: astrocytes, oligodendrocytes, and microglial cells 神经胶质；**neurog′lial** *adj.*

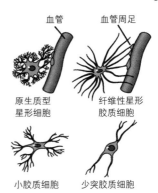

血管　血管周足

原生质型星形细胞　纤维性星形胶质细胞

小胶质细胞　少突胶质细胞

▲ 神经胶质，不同类型的神经胶质细胞

neu·rog·lio·cyte (noo-rog′le-o-sīt″) one of the cells composing the neuroglia 神经胶质细胞

neu·rog·li·o·ma (noo-rog″le′o-mə) glioma 神经胶质瘤；n. gangliona′re, ganglioglioma 神经节神经胶质瘤

neu·rog·li·o·sis (noo-rog″le-o′sis) gliomatosis 神经胶质瘤病

neu·ro·gly·co·pe·nia (noor″o-gli″ko-pe′ne-ə) chronic hypoglycemia of a degree sufficient to impair brain function, resulting in personality changes and intellectual deterioration 神经性低血糖症

neu·ro·his·tol·o·gy (noor″o-his-tol′ə-je)histology of the nervous system 神经组织学

neu·ro·hor·mone (noor′o-hor″mōn) a hormone secreted by a specialized neuron into the bloodstream, the cerebrospinal fluid, or the intercellular spaces of the nervous system 神经激素

neu·ro·hy·poph·y·sis (noor″o-hi-pof′ə-sis) the posterior (or neural) lobe of the pituitary gland, which stores oxytocin and vasopressin 神经垂体，垂体后部；**neurohypophys′ial** *adj.*

neu·ro·im·mu·nol·o·gy (noor″o-im″u-nol′ə- je) the study of the interaction between the nervous and immune systems 神经免疫学；**neuroimmunolog′ic** *adj.*

neu·ro·ker·a·tin (noor″o-ker′ə-tin) a protein network seen in histologic specimens of the myelin sheath after the myelin has been removed, probably not existing in vivo 神经角蛋白

neu·ro·lep·tan·al·ge·sia (noor″o-lep″tan-əl-je′ze-ə) a state of quiescence, altered awareness, and analgesia produced by a combination of an opioid analgesic and a neuroleptic 神经安定镇痛术

neu·ro·lep·tic (noor″o-lep′tik) originally, referring to the effects on cognition and behavior of the first antipsychotic agents: a state of apathy, lack of initiative, and limited range of emotion, and in psychotic patients, reduction in confusion and agitation and normalization of psychomotor activity. It is still used for agents (e.g., droperidol) producing such effects as part of anesthesia or analgesia, but is outdated as a synonym for antipsychotic agents because newer agents do not necessarily have such effects 神经安定药，精神安定药

neu·ro·log·ic (noor″o-loj′ik) pertaining to neurology or to the nervous system 神经学的，神经病学的，神经系统的

neu·rol·o·gy (noo-rol′ə-je) the branch of medicine that deals with the nervous system, both when normal and in disease 神经学，神经病学；**clinical n.**, that especially concerned with the diagnosis and treatment of disorders of the nervous system 临床神经病学

neu·rol·y·sin (noo-rol′ĭ-sin) a cytolysin with a specific destructive action on neurons 溶神经素

neu·rol·y·sis (noo-rol′ĭ-sis) 1. release of a nerve sheath by cutting it longitudinally 神经鞘纵向切开；2. operative breaking up of perineural adhesions 手术分离神经周围粘连；3. relief of tension upon a nerve obtained by stretching 神经减压术；4. destruction or dissolution of nerve tissue 神经组织崩解；**neurolyt′ic** adj.

neu·ro·ma (noo-ro′mə) a tumor growing from a nerve or made up largely of nerve cells and nerve fibers 神经瘤；**neuro′matous** adj.; **acoustic n.**, a benign tumor within the internal auditory canal arising from Schwann cells of the eighth cranial (acoustic) nerve 听神经瘤；**amputation n.**, traumatic n. 截断性神经瘤；**n. cu′tis,** neuroma in the skin 皮肤神经瘤；**false n.,** 1. something that looks like a neuroma but does not contain nerve cells 假神经瘤；2. 同 traumatic n.；**Morton n., Morton,** the neuroma that results from Morton neuralgia 莫顿神经瘤；**plexiform n.,** one made up of contorted nerve trunks 丛状神经瘤；**n. telangiecto′des,** one containing an excess of blood vessels 血管扩张性神经瘤；**traumatic n.,** a nonneoplastic, unorganized, bulbous or nodular mass of nerve fibers and Schwann cells produced by hyperplasia of nerve fibers and their supporting tissues after accidental or purposeful sectioning of the nerve 创伤性神经瘤

neu·ro·ma·la·cia (noor″o-mə-la′shə) morbid softening of the nerves 神经软化

neu·ro·ma·to·sis (noo-ro″mə-to′sis) 1. any disease marked by the presence of many neuromas 多发性神经纤维瘤；2. neurofibromatosis 神经纤维瘤病

neu·ro·mere (noor′o-mēr) any of a series of transitory segmental elevations in the wall of the neural tube in the developing embryo 菱脑节

neu·ro·mi·met·ic (noor″o-mĭ-met′ik) 1. eliciting a response in effector organs that simulates that elicited by nervous impulses 模仿神经冲动的；2. an agent that elicits such a response 神经冲动模仿物

neu·ro·mod·u·la·tion (noor″o-mod″u-la′shən) 1. electrical stimulation of a peripheral nerve, the spinal cord, or the brain for relief of pain 神经调镇痛术；2. the effect of a neuromodulator on another neuron 神经调质作用

neu·ro·mod·u·la·tor (noor″o-mod″u-la″tər) a substance, other than a neurotransmitter, released by a neuron and transmitting information to other neurons, altering their activities 神经调质

neu·ro·mus·cu·lar (noor″o-mus′ku-lər) pertaining to nerves and muscles, or to the relationship between them 神经肌肉的

neu·ro·my·eli·tis (noor″o-mi″ə-li′tis) inflammation of nervous and medullary substance; myelitis attended with neuritis 神经脊髓炎

neu·ro·my·op·a·thy (noor″o-mi-op′ə-the) any disease of both muscles and nerves, especially a muscular disease of nervous origin 神经肌病，尤指神经起源导致的肌肉疾病；**neu-romyopath′ic** adj.

neu·ro·myo·si·tis (noor″o-mi″o-si′tis) neuritis blended with myositis 神经肌炎

neu·ro·myo·to·nia (noor″o-mi″o-to′ne-ə) myotonia caused by electrical activity of a peripheral nerve; characterized by stiffness, delayed relaxation, fasciculations, and myokymia 神经肌强直

neu·ron (noor′on) nerve cell; any of the conducting cells of the nervous system, consisting of a cell body, containing the nucleus and its surrounding cytoplasm, and the axon and dendrites 神经元，参见图14；**neuro′nal** adj.; **afferent n.,** one that conducts a nervous impulse from a receptor to a center 传入神经元；**efferent n.,** one that conducts a nervous impulse from a center to an organ of response 传出神经元；**Golgi n's,** (type I): pyramidal cells with long axons, which leave the gray matter of the central nervous system, traverse the white matter, and terminate in the periphery 高尔基Ⅰ型神经元；2. (type II): stellate neurons with short axons that are particularly numerous in the cerebral and cerebellar cortices and in the retina 高尔基Ⅱ型神经元；**motor n.,** motoneuron 运动神经元；**multisensory n.,** a neuron in the cerebral cortex or subcortical regions that can receive input from more than one sensory modality 多感觉神经元；**postganglionic n's,** neurons whose cell bodies lie in the autonomic ganglia and whose purpose is to

relay impulses beyond the ganglia 节后神经元；
preganglionic n's, neurons whose cell bodies lie in the central nervous system and whose efferent fibers terminate in the autonomic ganglia 节前神经元；
sensory n., any neuron having a sensory function; an afferent neuron conveying sensory impulses. The first in an afferent pathway is the *primary sensory n.* and the second is the *secondary sensory n.* 感觉神经元

neu·ro·ne·vus (noor″o-ne′vəs) an intradermal nevus whose cells differentiate toward nervelike structures; it may resemble a neurofibroma or a giant pigmented nevus 真皮内痣

neu·ro·ni·tis (noor″o-ni′tis) inflammation of one or more neurons 神经元炎；**vestibular n.,** a disturbance of vestibular function consisting of a single attack of severe vertigo with nausea and vomiting but without auditory symptoms 前庭神经元炎

neu·ro·nop·a·thy (noor″on-op′ə-the) polyneuropathy involving destruction of the cell bodies of neurons 神经元病

neu·ro·oph·thal·mol·o·gy (noor″o-of″thəlmol′ə-je) the specialty dealing with the portions of the nervous system related to the eye 神经眼科学，眼神经学

neu·ro·pap·il·li·tis (noor″o-pap″ĭ-li′tis) papillitis (2) 视神经乳头炎，视神经炎

neu·ro·par·a·lyt·ic (noor″o-par″ə-lit′ik) affected with or pertaining to paralysis of a nerve or nerves 神经性麻痹的

neu·ro·path·ic (noor″o-path′ik) pertaining to or characterized by neuropathy 神经病的

neu·ro·patho·ge·nic·i·ty (noor″o-path″ojə-nis′ĭ-te) the quality of producing or the ability to produce pathologic changes in nerve tissue 致神经病性，神经发病性

neu·ro·pa·thol·o·gy (noor″o-pə-thol′ə-je) pathology of diseases of the nervous system 神经病理学

neu·rop·a·thy (noo-rop′ə-the) a functional disturbance or pathologic change in the peripheral nervous system, sometimes limited to noninflammatory lesions as opposed to those of neuritis 神经病；**alcoholic n.,** neuropathy due to thiamine deficiency in chronic alcoholism 酒精性神经病变；**angiopathic n.,** that caused by arteritis of the blood vessels supplying the nerves, usually a systemic complication of disease 血管性神经病变；**axonal n.,** axonopathy 轴突神经病；**diabetic n.,** any of several clinical types of peripheral neuropathy (sensory, motor, autonomic, and mixed) occurring with diabetes mellitus; the most common is a chronic, symmetrical sensory polyneuropathy affecting first the nerves of the lower limbs and often affecting autonomic nerves 糖尿病性神经病，糖尿病神经病变；**entrapment n.,** any of a group of neuropathies, often overuse injuries such as carpal tunnel syndrome, due to mechanical pressure on a peripheral nerve 受压性神经病变；**giant axonal n.,** an autosomal recessive disorder affecting the central and peripheral nervous systems, due to mutation of a protein involved in targeting damaged proteins for destruction; characterized by enlarged axons made up of masses of tightly woven neurofilaments 巨轴突神经病（常染色体隐性遗传病）；**hereditary n. with liability to pressure palsies (HNPP),** an autosomal dominant neuropathy due to deletion of a gene encoding a specific myelin protein; characterized by pain, weakness, and pressure palsy in the arms and hands, with swelling of the myelin sheaths 遗传性压迫易感性神经病；**hereditary motor and sensory n. (HMSN),** a general term for the group of hereditary polyneuropathies encompassing Charcot-MarieTooth disease and Dejerine-Sottas disease 遗传性运动感觉神经病；**hereditary optic n.,** 同 Leber hereditary optic n.；**hereditary sensory and autonomic n. (HSAN),** any of several inherited neuropathies that involve slow ascendance of lesions of the sensory nerves, resulting in pain, distal trophic ulcers, and variable autonomic disturbances without significant motor involvement 遗传性感觉和自主神经病；**ischemic n.,** an injury to a peripheral nerve caused by a reduction in blood supply 缺血性神经病；**Leber hereditary optic n.,** an inherited disorder of ATP manufacture, usually in males, usually as bilateral progressive optic atrophy and loss of central vision, which may remit spontaneously Leber 遗传性视神经病变；**multiple n.,** 1. polyneuropathy 多（发性）神经病；2. multiple mononeuropathy 多发性单神经病；**peripheral n.,** polyneuropathy 周围神经病；**progressive hypertrophic n.,** Dejerine-Sottas disease 进行性肥大性神经病，德热里纳－索塔斯病；**radial n.,** any type of entrapment neuropathy of part of the radial nerve, usually in the axilla or cubital region, causing sensory deficits and paralysis of muscles in the wrist and hand 桡神经病；**sarcoid n.,** a polyneuropathy sometimes seen in sarcoidosis, characterized by either cranial polyneuritis or spinal nerve deficits 肉瘤样神经病变；**toxic n.,** that due to ingestion of a toxin 中毒性神经病变；**vasculitic n.,** 同 angiopathic n.

neu·ro·pep·tide (noor″o-pep′tīd) any of the molecules composed of short chains of amino acids (endorphins, enkephalins, vasopressin, etc.) found in brain tissue 神经肽

neu·ro·phar·ma·col·o·gy (noor″o-fahr″mə-kol′ə-je) the scientific study of the effects of drugs on the nervous system 神经药理学

neu·ro·phy·sin (noor″o-fi′sin) any of a group of soluble proteins secreted in the hypothalamus that serve as binding proteins for vasopressin and oxytocin, playing a role in their transport in the neurohypophyseal tract and their storage in the posterior pituitary 后叶激素运载蛋白，神经垂体素运载蛋白

neu·ro·phys·i·ol·o·gy (noor″o-fiz″e-ol′ə-je) physiology of the nervous system 神经生理学

neu·ro·pil (noor′o-pil) a feltwork of interwoven dendrites and axons and of neuroglial cells in the gray matter of the central nervous system 神经毡

neu·ro·plasm (noor′o-plaz″əm) the protoplasm of a nerve cell 神经胞质，神经浆．**neuroplas′mic** *adj.*

neu·ro·plas·ty (noor′o-plas″te) plastic repair of a nerve 神经成形术

neu·ro·pore (noor′o-por) the open anterior *(rostral n.)* or posterior *(caudal n.)* end of the neural tube of the early embryo, which closes as the embryo develops 神经孔（胚胎）

neu·ro·psy·chi·a·try (noor″o-si-ki′ə-tre) the combined specialties of neurology and psychiatry 神经精神病学

neu·ro·psy·chol·o·gy (noor″o-si-kol′ə-je) a discipline combining neurology and psychology to study the relationship between the functioning of the brain and cognitive processes or behavior 神经心理学；**neuropsycholog′ical** *adj.*

neu·ro·ra·di·ol·o·gy (noor″o-ra″de-ol′o-je) radiology of the nervous system 神经放射学

neu·ro·ret·i·ni·tis (noor″o-ret″ĭ-ni′tis) inflammation of the optic nerve and retina 视神经视网膜炎

neu·ro·ret·i·nop·a·thy (noor″o-ret″ĭ-nop′ə- the) pathologic involvement of the optic disk and retina 视神经视网膜病

neu·ror·rha·phy (noo-ror′ə-fe) suture of a divided nerve 神经缝合术

neu·ro·sar·co·ma (noor″o-sahr-ko′mə) a sarcoma with neural elements 神经肉瘤

neu·ro·se·cre·tion (noor″o-sə-kre′shən) 1. secretory activities of nerve cells 神经分泌；2. the product of such activities; a neurosecretory substance 神经分泌物；**neurosecre′tory** *adj.*

neu·ro·sis (noo-ro′sis) pl. *neuro′ses*. 1. former name for a category of mental disorders characterized by anxiety and avoidance behavior, with symptoms distressing to the patient, intact reality testing, no violations of gross social norms, and no apparent organic etiology 神经官能症的旧称；2. in psychoanalytic theory, the process that gives rise to these disorders as well as personality disorders and some

psychotic disorders, being triggering of unconscious defense mechanisms by unresolved conflicts 神经症；**character n.**, a type of high-level personality disorder with some neurotic characteristics 性格神经症；**hysterical n.**, former name for a group of conditions now divided between *conversion disorder* and *dissociative disorders* 癔病性神经症

neu·ro·spasm (noor″o-spaz″əm) a spasm caused by a disorder in the motor nerve supplying the muscle 神经性痉挛

neu·ro·splanch·nic (noor″o-splangk′nik) pertaining to the cerebrospinal and sympathetic nervous systems 脑脊髓（与）交感神经系统的

neu·ro·sur·gery (noor″o-sur′jər-e) surgery of the nervous system 神经外科学

neu·ro·su·ture (noor″o-soo′chər) 同 neurorrhaphy

neu·ro·syph·i·lis (noor″o-sif′ĭ-lis) syphilis of the central nervous system 神经梅毒

neu·ro·ten·di·nous (noor″o-ten′dĭ-nəs) pertaining to both nerve and tendon 神经（与）腱的

neu·ro·ten·sin (noor″o-ten′sin) a tridecapeptide found in small intestine and brain tissue; it induces vasodilation and hypotension, and in the brain it is a neurotransmitter 神经降压素，神经降压肽

neu·rot·ic (noo-rot′ik) 1. pertaining to or characterized by a neurosis 神经功能病的，神经（官能）症的；神经过敏的，神经质的；2. a person affected with a neurosis 神经过敏者，神经质者

neu·rot·iza·tion (noo-rot″ĭ-za′shən) regeneration of a nerve after its division 神经植入术

neu·rot·me·sis (noor″ot-me′sis) partial or complete severance of a nerve, with disruption of the axon and its myelin sheath and the connective tissue elements 神经断伤

neu·ro·tome (noor′o-tōm) 1. a needlelike knife for dissecting nerves 神经刀；2. 同 neuromere

neu·ro·to·mog·ra·phy (noor″o-to-mog′rə-fe) tomography of the central nervous system 神经 X 线断层照像术

neu·rot·o·my (noo-rot′ə-me) dissection or cutting of nerves 神经切断术

neu·rot·o·ny (noo-rot′ə-ne) stretching of a nerve 神经牵伸术

neu·ro·tox·ic·i·ty (noor″o-tok-sis′ ĭ-te) the quality of exerting a destructive or poisonous effect upon nerve tissue 神经毒性；**neurotox′ic** *adj.*

neu·ro·tox·in (noor′o-tok″sin) a substance that is poisonous or destructive to nerve tissue 神经毒素

neu·ro·trans·duc·er (noor″o-trans-doos′ər) a neuron that synthesizes and releases hormones that serve as the functional link between the nervous system and the pituitary gland 介导神经元

neu·ro·trans·mit·ter (noor″o-trans′mit-ər) a

substance released from the axon terminal of a presynaptic neuron on excitation, which diffuses across the synaptic cleft to either excite or inhibit the target cell 神经递质；**false n.,** an amine that can be stored in and released from presynaptic vesicles but that has little effect on postsynaptic receptors 假性神经递质

neu·ro·trau·ma (noor″o-traw′mə) mechanical injury to a nerve 神经外伤

neu·rot·ro·pism (noo-rot′ro-piz″əm) 1. the quality of having a special affinity for nervous tissue 嗜神经性；2. the alleged tendency of regenerating nerve fibers to grow toward specific portions of the periphery 神经趋向性；**neurotro′pic** adj.

neu·ro·tu·bule (noor″o-too′būl) a microtubule occurring in a neuron 神经微管

neu·ro·vac·cine (noor″o-vak-sēn′) vaccine virus prepared by growing the virus in a rabbit's brain 兔脑疫苗

neu·ro·vas·cu·lar (noor″o-vas′ku-lər) pertaining to both nervous and vascular elements, or to nerves controlling the caliber of blood vessels 神经血管的

neu·ro·vis·cer·al (noor″o-vis′ər-əl) neurosplanchnic 脑脊髓（与）交感神经系统的

neu·ru·la (noor′u-lə) the early embryonic stage following the gastrula, marked by the first appearance of the nervous system 神经胚

neu·ru·la·tion (noor″u-la′shən) formation in the early embryo of the neural plate, followed by its closure with development of the neural tube 神经胚形成

neu·tral (noo′trəl) neither basic nor acidic 中性的

neu·tro·cyte (noo′tro-sīt) 同 neutrophil (1)；**neutrocyt′ic** adj.

neu·tron (n) (noo′tron) an electrically neutral or uncharged particle of matter existing along with protons in the nucleus of atoms of all elements except the mass 1 isotope of hydrogen 中微子

neu·tro·pe·nia (noo″tro-pe′ne-ə) diminished number of neutrophils in the blood 中性粒细胞减少（症）

neu·tro·phil (noo′tro-fil) 1. a granular leukocyte having a nucleus with three to five lobes connected by threads of chromatin, and cytoplasm containing very fine granules（嗜）中性粒细胞；cf. *heterophil*；2. any cell, structure, or histologic element readily stainable with neutral dyes 嗜中性的；**rod n., stab n.,** one whose nucleus is not divided into segments 杆状核中性粒细胞

neu·tro·phil·ia (noo″tro-fil′e-ə) increase in the number of neutrophils in the blood 中性粒细胞增多

neu·tro·phil·ic (noo″tro-fil′ik) 1. pertaining to neutrophils 中性粒细胞的；2. stainable by neutral dyes 嗜中性染色的

ne·vir·a·pine (nə-vir′ə-pēn) a nonnucleoside inhibitor of HIV-1 reverse transcriptase, used in combination with other antiretroviral agents in the treatment of HIV infection 奈韦拉平，HIV-1 的非核苷类逆转录酶抑制药

ne·void (ne′void) resembling a nevus 痣样的

ne·vo·li·po·ma (ne″vo-lĭ-po′mə) a nevus containing a large amount of fibrofatty tissue 痣脂瘤，脂瘤痣

ne·vus (ne′vəs) pl. *ne′vi* [L.] 1. any congenital skin lesion; a birthmark 痣；2. a type of hamartoma representing a circumscribed stable malformation of the skin and occasionally of the oral mucosa, which is not due to external causes; the excess (or deficiency) of tissue may involve epidermal, connective tissue, adnexal, nervous, or vascular elements 色素痣，**balloon cell n.,** an intradermal nevus consisting of balloon cells with pale cytoplasm that contains large vacuoles formed of altered melanosomes 气球状细胞痣；**Becker n.,** a usually acquired type, seen mostly in males on the shoulder or upper trunk, consisting of epidermal melanosis with light hyperpigmentation and later growth of long dark hairs from the lesions 贝克痣；**blue n.,** a dark blue nodular lesion composed of closely grouped melanocytes and melanophages situated in the mid-dermis 蓝痣；**blue rubber bleb n.,** a hereditary condition marked by multiple bluish cutaneous hemangiomas with soft raised centers, frequently associated with hemangiomas of the gastrointestinal tract 蓝色橡皮疱样痣；**cellular blue n.,** a large blue to blue-black, lobulated, circumscribed, nodular tumor composed of melanocytes and spindle cells, found on the buttocks or sacrococcygeal region, with a slight incidence of transformation to melanoma 细胞性蓝痣；**comedo n., n. comedo′nicus,** a rare type of epidermal nevus having small patches in which there are collections of large comedones or comedolike lesions 黑头粉刺痣；**compound n.,** a melanocytic nevus composed of fully formed nests of nevus cells in the epidermis and newly forming ones in the dermis 混合痣；**connective tissue n.,** any of a group of hamartomas involving various components of the connective tissue, usually present at birth or soon after 结缔组织痣；**dysplastic n.,** an acquired atypical melanocytic nevus with an irregular border and mixed coloring, characterized by intraepidermal melanocytic dysplasia; it may be a precursor of malignant melanoma 发育不良痣；**epidermal n.,** any of various types of hamartoma of the epidermis representing developmental anomalies with faulty cutaneous structures; many patients also have involvement of other organ systems 表皮痣；**n. flam′meus,** a common congenital vascular malformation involving mature capillaries, ranging from pink *(salmon patch)* to dark-colored *(port-wine stain),* usually found on the face or neck 表皮鲜红斑痣，焰色痣，毛细血管扩张痣；**giant hairy n., giant pigmented n.,** any of a group of large, darkly pigmented, hairy nevi, present at birth; they are associated with other cutaneous and subcutaneous lesions, neurofibromatosis, and leptomeningeal melanocytosis and tend to development of malignant melanoma 巨大色素痣；**halo n.,** a melanocytic nevus surrounded by a halo of depigmentation, occasionally related to development of melanoma 晕痣；**intradermal n.,** a melanocytic nevus, clinically identical to a compound nevus, in which the nests of nevus cells lie exclusively within the dermis 皮内痣；**n. of Ito,** a type similar to nevus of Ota but found in areas of distribution of the posterior supraclavicular and lateral cutaneous brachial nerves 伊藤痣；**junction n., junctional n.,** a melanocytic nevus in which the nests of nevus cells are confined to the dermal-epidermal junction 交界痣；**n. lipomato'sus, lipomatous n.,** 同lipoma；**melanocytic n.,** 黑素细胞痣；**nevocellular n., nevus cell n.,** any of numerous acquired or inherited nevi composed of nests of nevus cells, usually tan or brown macules or papules with well-defined, rounded borders 痣细胞痣；**n. of Ota,** a type resembling a mongolian spot, usually present at birth, involving the conjunctiva, eyelids, and adjacent facial skin, sclera, ocular muscles, periosteum, and buccal mucosa, usually unilaterally 太田痣，眼上腭部褐青色痣；**pigmented n.,** any nevus containing pigment, especially melanin 色素痣；**sebaceous n., n. seba'ceus,** a circumscribed, tan, epidermal nevus, present at birth, containing hyperplastic sebaceous glands and hair follicles, found on the scalp, face, or neck; there may also be neurologic or ophthalmic abnormalities. In time, some lesions become nodular and may develop benign or malignant adnexal tumors or basal cell carcinoma 皮脂腺痣；**spider n.,** 蜘蛛痣，参见 *angioma*；**n. spi'lus,** a smooth, tan to brown, macular nevus composed of melanocytes, and speckled with smaller, darker macules 斑痣；**Spitz n.,** a benign compound nevus, seen usually in children, composed of dermal spindle and epithelioid cells; it resembles malignant melanoma histologically and appears as a smooth, raised, firm, pink to purple nodule or papule 斯皮茨痣；**n. uni'us la'teris,** a verrucous epidermal nevus occurring as a linear band or patch, usually along the margin between two neuromeres 单侧痣；**vascular n., n. vascula'ris,** any nevus caused by a vascular malformation 血管痣；**white sponge n.,** a benign, congenital,

inherited disorder characterized by extensive spongy whiteness and gray-white, soft, fissured lesions of the mucous membranes, especially of the oral mucosa 白色海绵状斑痣

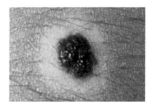

▲ 晕痣

new·born (noo'born) 1. recently born 新生的；2. newborn infant 新生儿

new·ton (N) (noo'tən) the SI unit of force; that when applied in a vacuum to a body having a mass of 1 kilogram accelerates it at the rate of 1 meter per second squared 牛（顿），力的单位

nex·us (nek'səs) pl. *nex'us* [L.] 1. a bond, especially one between members of a series or group 结合，接合；2. gap junction 融合膜（缝隙连接）

NF *National Formulary* 国家处方集

NFLPN National Federation of Licensed Practical Nurses 全国执业护士联合会

ng nanogram 纳克

NHSC National Health Service Corps 国家卫生服务队

Ni nickel 元素镍的符号

ni·a·cin (ni'ə-sin) nicotinic acid; a water-soluble vitamin of the B complex required by the body for the formation of the coenzymes NAD and NADP, important in biochemical oxidations; used to prevent and treat pellagra and to treat hyperlipidemia 烟酸尼克酸

ni·a·cin·a·mide (ni″ə-sin'ə-mīd) nicotinamide, a B complex vitamin used in the prophylaxis and treatment of pellagra 烟酰胺，尼克酰胺

NIAID National Institute of Allergy and Infectious Diseases 国立变态反应和传染病研究所

ni·car·di·pine (ni-kahr'dĭ-pēn) a calcium channel blocker that acts as a vasodilator; used as the hydrochloride salt in the treatment of angina pectoris and hypertension 尼卡地平

NICHD National Institute of Child Health and Human Development 美国国立儿童健康与人类发展研究所

niche (nich) a defect in an otherwise even surface, especially a depression or recess in the wall of a hollow organ, as seen in a radiograph, or such a depression in an organ visible to the naked eye 壁龛，龛影（如 X 线片所见或肉眼所见的器官上

的凹陷）；**enamel n.**, either of two depressions between the dental lamina and the developing tooth germ, one pointing distally *(distal enamel n.)* and the other mesially *(mesial enamel n.)* 釉隙

nick·el (Ni) (nik′əl) a shiny, silver-white, ductile metallic element; at. no. 28, at. wt. 58.693. Long-term exposure to metallic nickel, as in jewelry, can cause contact (nickel) dermatitis; nickel fumes can be toxic and carcinogenic 镍

nick·ing (nik′ing) localized constriction of the retinal blood vessels 血管局部缩窄

nic·o·tin·a·mide (nik″o-tin′ə-mīd) 同 niacinamide; **n. adenine dinucleotide (NAD)**, a coenzyme composed of nicotinamide mononucleotide in pyrophosphate linkage with adenosine monophosphate; it is involved in numerous enzymatic reactions, in which it serves as an electron carrier by being alternately oxidized (NAD$^+$) and reduced (NADH) 烟酰胺腺嘌呤二核苷酸; **n. adenine dinucleotide phosphate (NADP)**, a coenzyme composed of nicotinamide mononucleotide coupled by pyrophosphate linkage to adenosine 2′, 5′-bisphosphate; it serves as an electron carrier in numerous reactions, being alternately oxidized (NADP+) and reduced (NADPH) 烟酰胺腺嘌呤二核苷酸磷酸

nic·o·tine (nik′o-tēn) a very poisonous alkaloid, obtained from tobacco or produced synthetically; used as an agricultural insecticide and as an aid to smoking cessation 尼古丁，烟碱; **n. polacrilex**, nicotine bound to a cation exchange resin; used in nicotine chewing gum as an aid to smoking cessation 烟碱结合物

nic·o·tin·ic (nik″o-tin′ik) denoting the effect of nicotine and other drugs in initially stimulating and subsequently, in high doses, inhibiting neural impulses at autonomic ganglia and the neuromuscular junction 尼古丁的，烟碱的

nic·o·tin·ic ac·id (nik″o-tin′ik) 同 niacin

nic·o·tin·ism (nik′o-tin-iz″əm) nicotine poisoning 烟碱中毒

nic·ti·ta·tion (nik″tī-ta′shən) winking 眨眼

ni·dal (ni′dəl) pertaining to a nidus 巢的

ni·da·tion (ni-da′shən) implantation (1) 着床（受精卵在子宫内）

NIDCR National Institute of Dental and Craniofacial Research 美国国立口腔与颅面研究所

NIDD, NIDDM non–insulin-dependent diabetes mellitus 非胰岛素依赖型糖尿病; 参见 diabetes 下 *type 2 diabetes mellitus*

ni·dus (ni′dəs) pl. *ni′di* [L.] 1. the point of origin or focus of a morbid process 病灶; 2. nucleus (2) 核; **n. a′vis**, a depression in the cerebellum between the posterior velum and uvula 小脑禽巢

ni·fed·i·pine (ni-fed′ĭ-pēn) a calcium channel blocking agent used as a coronary vasodilator in the treatment of coronary insufficiency and angina pectoris; also used in the treatment of hypertension 硝苯地平

night·mare (nīt′mār″) a terrifying dream, usually awakening the dreamer 梦魇

night·shade (nīt′shād″) a plant of the genus *Solanum* 茄属植物; **deadly n.**, belladonna 颠茄叶

ni·gra (ni′grə) [L.] substantia nigra 黑质; **ni′gral** *adj.*

ni·gro·sin (ni′gro-sin) an aniline dye having a special affinity for ganglion cells 苯胺黑

ni·gro·stri·a·tal (ni″gro-stri-a′təl) projecting from the substantia nigra to the corpus striatum; said of a bundle of nerve fibers 黑质纹状体的，指一束神经纤维

NIH National Institutes of Health 国立卫生研究院

ni·hil·ism (ni′il-iz″əm) 1. an attitude of skepticism regarding traditional values and beliefs or their frank rejection 虚无主义; 2. a delusion of nonexistence of part or all of the self or the world 虚无妄想; **nihilis′tic** *adj.*

ni·lo·ti·nib (ni-lo′tĭ-nib) a tyrosine kinase inhibitor with actions similar to those of imatinib; used as the hydrochloride salt in the treatment of Philadelphia chromosome–positive chronic myelogenous leukemia 一种酪氨酸激酶抑制药，作用类似伊马替尼，其盐酸盐用于治疗费城染色体阳性慢性髓细胞性白血病

ni·lu·ta·mide (ni-loo′tə-mīd) a nonsteroidal antiandrogen used as an antineoplastic in the treatment of prostatic carcinoma 尼鲁米特

NIMH National Institute of Mental Health 美国国立精神卫生研究所

ni·mo·di·pine (ni-mo′dī-pēn) a calcium channel blocker used as a vasodilator in the treatment of neurologic deficits associated with subarachnoid hemorrhage from a ruptured intracranial aneurysm 尼莫地平

NINR National Institute of Nursing Research 美国国立护理研究所

ni·o·bi·um (Nb) (ni-o′be-əm) a silvery white, soft, ductile, metallic element; at. no. 41, at. wt. 92.906 铌（化学元素）

NIOSH National Institute for Occupational Safety and Health 美国国立职业安全与卫生研究所

nip·ple (nip′əl) 1. mammary papilla; the pigmented projection on the anterior surface of the breast, surrounded by the areola; in women it gives outlet to the lactiferous ducts 乳头; 2. any similarly shaped structure 乳头样结构

ni·sol·di·pine (ni-sol′dī-pēn) a calcium channel blocker used in the treatment of hypertension 尼索

N

地平

nit (nit) the egg of a louse 虮，虱卵

ni·trate (niʹtrāt) any salt of nitric acid; organic nitrates are used in the treatment of angina pectoris 硝酸盐

ni·tric (niʹtrik) pertaining to or containing nitrogen in one of its higher valences 含氮的; n. oxide, endothelium-derived relaxing factor; a naturally occurring gas that in the body is a short-lived dilator substance released from vascular endothelial cells in response to the binding of vasodilators; it inhibits muscular contraction and produces relaxation and is toxic in the central nervous system. A preparation is used in the treatment of persistent fetal circulation in term and near-term neonates 一氧化氮

ni·tric ac·id (niʹtrik) a colorless liquid, HNO_3, which fumes in moist air and has a characteristic choking odor; used as a cauterizing agent. Its potassium salt *(potassium nitrate)* is used in potassium deficiencies and as a diuretic; its sodium salt *(sodium nitrate)* as a reagent 硝酸

ni·tri·fi·ca·tion (niʺtrī-fĭ-kaʹshən) the bacterial oxidation of ammonia to nitrite and then to nitrate in the soil 硝化（作用）

ni·trite (niʹtrīt) any salt or ester of nitrous acid 亚硝酸盐

ni·tro·cel·lu·lose (niʺtro-selʹu-lōs) pyroxylin 硝酸纤维素，火棉

ni·tro·fu·ran (niʺtro-fuʹran) any of a group of antibacterials, including nitrofurantoin, nitrofurazone, etc., that are effective against a wide range of bacteria 硝基呋喃

ni·tro·fu·ran·to·in (niʺtro-fu-ranʹto-in) an antibacterial effective against many gram-negative and gram-positive organisms; used in urinary tract infections 呋喃妥因

ni·tro·fu·ra·zone (niʺtro-fuʹrə-zōn) an antibacterial effective against a wide variety of gramnegative and gram-positive organisms; used topically as a local antiinfective 呋喃西林

ni·tro·gen (N) (niʹtro-jən) a colorless, odorless, tasteless, inert gaseous element; at. no. 7, at. wt. 14.007. It forms about 79 percent by volume of the earth's atmosphere and is a constituent of all proteins and nucleic acids. Release of nitrogen from the blood and body tissues as bubbles of gas upon overly rapid reduction of ambient pressure can cause decompression sickness 氮; n. 13, a radioactive isotope of nitrogen having a half-life of 9.97 minutes and decaying by positron emission (1.190 MeV); used as a tracer in positron emission tomography 氮 13; n. mustard, 氮芥, 参见 *mustard* 下词条; **nonprotein n.**, the nitrogenous constituents of the blood exclusive of the protein bodies, consisting of the nitrogen of urea, uric acid, creatine, creatinine, amino acids, polypeptides, and an undetermined part known as *rest nitrogen* 非蛋白氮

ni·trog·e·nous (ni-trojʹə-nəs) containing nitrogen 含氮的

ni·tro·glyc·er·in (niʺtro-glisʹər-in) an antianginal, antihypertensive, and vasodilator used for the prophylaxis and treatment of angina pectoris, the treatment of congestive heart failure and myocardial infarction, and blood pressure control or controlled hypotension during surgery 硝酸甘油

ni·tro·prus·side (niʺtro-prusʹīd) the anion $[Fe(CN)_5NO]^{2-}$ 硝普盐，硝基氢氰酸盐; 参见 *sodium nitroprusside*

Ni·tro·so·mo·na·da·les (ni-troʺso-moʹnə- daʹlēz) a morphologically, metabolically, and ecologically diverse order of bacteria of the class Betaproteobacteria 亚硝化单胞菌目

ni·tro·so·urea (ni-troʺso-uʹre-ə) any of a group of lipid-soluble biologic alkylating agents, including carmustine and lomustine, which cross the blood-brain barrier and are used as antineoplastic agents 亚硝脲

ni·trous (niʹtrəs) pertaining to nitrogen in its lowest valency 亚硝的; n. oxide, a gas, N_2O, used as a general anesthetic, usually in combination with another agent 一氧化二氮氧化亚氮，笑气（麻醉药）

ni·trous ac·id (niʹtrəs) a weak acid, HNO_2, existing only in aqueous solution 亚硝酸

ni·za·ti·dine (nĭ-za·tĭ-dēn) a histamine H_2 receptor antagonist, used to inhibit gastric acid secretion in the treatment of gastric and duodenal ulcer, gastroesophageal reflux disease, and conditions that cause gastric hypersecretion 尼扎替丁（组胺 H_2 受体拮抗药）

NLDO nasolacrimal duct obstruction 鼻泪管阻塞

NLN National League for Nursing 全国护理联合会

NLNAC National League for Nursing Accrediting Commission 美国护理联盟护理教育评估委员会

nm nanometer 纳米

NMIBC non–muscle-invasive bladder cancer 非肌层浸润性膀胱癌

NMR nuclear magnetic resonance 核磁共振

nn. [L.] nervi (nerves) 神经

NNBA National Nurses in Business Association, Inc 全国商业护士协会

No·car·dia (no-kahrʹde-ə) a genus of grampositive, mainly saprophytic bacteria of the family Nocardiaceae. Pathogenic species include *N. asteroiʹdes*, which produces a tuberculosis-like infection, *N. brasilienʹsis*, which causes nocardiosis and actinomycotic mycetoma, and *N. farciʹnica*, which produces a tuberculosis-like infection in cattle and causes actinomycotic mycetoma 诺卡菌属

No·car·di·a·ceae (no-kahr″de-a′se-e) a family of gram-positive, aerobic, nonmotile bacteria of the order Actinomycetales, consisting of microorganisms that form branching hyphae that fragment into rod-shaped to coccoid elements 诺卡菌科

no·car·di·al (no-kahr′de-əl) pertaining to or caused by *Nocardia* 诺卡菌的

No·car·di·op·sa·ceae (no-kahr″de-op-sa′se-e) a family of gram-positive, aerobic, filamentforming bacteria of the order Actinomycetales 拟诺卡菌科

No·car·di·op·sis (no-kahr″de-op′sis) a genus of gram-positive, aerobic soil bacteria of the family Nocardiopsaceae. *N. dassonvil′lei* causes mycetoma, conjunctivitis, skin infections, and hypersensitivity pneumonitis 拟诺卡菌属

no·car·di·o·sis (no-kahr″de-o′sis) infection with *Nocardia* 诺卡菌病

no·ce·bo (no-se′bo) [L.] an adverse, nonspecific side effect occurring in conjunction with a medication but not directly resulting from the pharmacologic action of the medication 反安慰剂效应

no·ci·as·so·ci·a·tion (no″se-ə-so″se-a′shən) unconscious discharge of nervous energy under the stimulus of trauma 伤害性联合反应

no·ci·cep·tion (no″sĭ-sep′shən) pain sense 伤害性感受

no·ci·cep·tor (no″sĭ-sep′tər) a receptor for pain caused by injury, physical or chemical, to body tissues 伤害性感受器；**nocicep′tive** *adj.*

no·ci·per·cep·tion (no″sĭ-pər-sep′shən) pain sense 疼痛性知觉

noc·tu·ria (nok-tu′re-ə) excessive urination at night 夜尿（症），又称 nycturia

noc·tur·nal (nok-tur′nəl) pertaining to, occurring at, or active at night 夜间的，夜发的，夜间活动的

NOD nucleotide oligomerization domain 核苷酸寡聚域

node (nōd) a small mass of tissue in the form of a swelling, knot, or protuberance, either normal or pathologic 结，结节；**no′dal** *adj.*；**atrioventricular n., AV n. (AVN),** a collection of Purkinje fibers beneath the endocardium of the right atrium, continuous with the atrial muscle fibers and atrioventricular bundle; it receives the cardiac impulses from the sinoatrial node and passes them on to the ventricles 房室结；**Bouchard n's,** cartilaginous and bony enlargements of the proximal interphalangeal joints of the fingers in degenerative joint disease 布夏尔结节；**Flack n.,** 同 sinoatrial n.；**Heberden n's,** small hard nodules, usually at the distal interphalangeal joints of the fingers, formed by calcific spurs of the articular cartilage and associated with osteoarthritis 赫伯登结节；**Hensen n.,** primitive node 亨森结；**Keith n., Keith Flack n.,** 同 sinoatrial n.；**lymph n.,** any of the accumulations of lymphoid tissue organized as definite lymphoid organs along the course of lymphatic vessels, consisting of an outer cortical and an inner medullary part; they are the main source of lymphocytes of the peripheral blood and, as part of the reticuloendothelial system, serve as a defense mechanism by removing noxious agents, e.g., bacteria and toxins, and probably play a role in antibody formation 淋巴结；**Osler n's,** small, raised, swollen, tender areas, bluish or sometimes pink or red, occurring commonly in the pads of the fingers or toes, the thenar or hypothenar eminences, or the soles of the feet; they are practically pathognomonic of subacute bacterial endocarditis 奥斯勒结节；**primitive n.,** a mass of cells at the cranial end of the primitive streak in the early embryo 原结；**n's of Ranvier,** constrictions of myelinated nerve fibers at regular intervals at which the myelin sheath is absent and the axon is enclosed only by Schwann cell processes 郎飞结，见图 14；**Schmorl n.,** an irregular or hemispherical bone defect in the upper or lower margin of the body of a vertebra Schmorl 结节；**sentinel n.,** 1. the first lymph node to receive drainage from a tumor; if it is free from mestastasis, other regional lymph nodes are also free from metastasis 前哨淋巴结；2. 同 signal n.；**signal n.,** an enlarged supraclavicular lymph node; often the first sign of a malignant abdominal tumor 信号淋巴结；**singer's n's,** vocal cord nodules 声带小结；**sinoatrial n., sinuatrial n., sinus n.,** a microscopic collection of atypical cardiac muscle fibers (Purkinje fibers) at the junction of the superior vena cava and right atrium, in which the cardiac rhythm normally originates and which is therefore called the cardiac pacemaker 窦房结；**teacher's n's,** vocal cord nodules 声带小结；**Troisier n., Virchow n.,** 同 signal n.

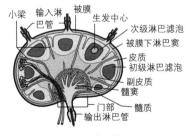

小梁　输入淋巴管　被膜　生发中心
次级淋巴滤泡
被膜下淋巴窦
皮质
初级淋巴滤泡
副皮质
髓窦
门部
髓质
输出淋巴管

▲ 淋巴结

N

no·di (no′di) [L.] *nodus* 的复数
no·dose (no′dōs) having nodes or projections 有结节的，结节状的

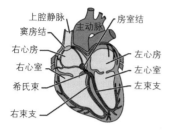

▲ 心脏搏动通过窦房结和房室结传导

no·dos·i·ty (no-dos′ĭ-te) 1. a node 结节；2. the quality of being nodose 结节性
no·do·ven·tric·u·lar (no″do-ven-trik′u-lər) connecting the atrioventricular node to the ventricle 房室结
nod·ule (nod′ūl) a small knot or node, a comparatively minute collection of tissue 结，小结节；**nod′ular** *adj.*；**Albini n's,** gray nodules of the size of small grains, sometimes seen on the free edges of the atrioventricular valves of infants; they are remains of fetal structures Albini 结节；**apple jelly n's,** minute, yellowish or reddish brown, translucent nodules, seen on the lesions of lupus vulgaris 苹果酱状结节；**n's of Arantius,** 阿朗希乌斯小结，参见 *body* 下词条；**Aschoff n's,** 阿绍夫小体，参见 *body* 下词条；**Brenner n's,** nodular masses of tumor in the cyst wall in cases of Brenner tumor 博拉纳尔结；**Jeanselme n's, juxtaarticular n's,** gummata of tertiary syphilis and of nonvenereal treponemal diseases, located on joint capsules, bursae, or tendon sheaths 近关节结节；**Lisch n's,** hamartomas of the iris occurring in neurofibromatosis 里斯克节；**lymphatic n., lymphoid n.,** a small, dense accumulation of lymphocytes expressing tissue cytogenetic and defense functions; some are encapsulated within lymph nodes. *Primary lymphoid n's* have not been exposed to antigen; exposure causes development to *secondary lymphoid n's*, which contain germinal centers 淋巴小结，初级淋巴小结是未经受抗原暴露的，刺激淋巴小结受到抗原刺激，产生生发中心；**milker's n's,** paravaccinia 副痘，挤乳者结节；**pulp n.,** denticle (2) 髓石；**rheumatic n's,** small, round or oval, mostly subcutaneous nodules similar to Aschoff bodies; seen in rheumatic fever 风湿性结节；**rheumatoid n's,** subcutaneous nodules consisting of central foci of necrosis surrounded by palisade-like coronas of fibroblasts,

seen in rheumatoid arthritis 类风湿结节；**Schmorl n.,** an irregular or hemispherical bone defect in the upper or lower margin of the body of the vertebra 施莫尔结节；**solitary lymphoid n's,** small concentrations of lymphoid tissue scattered throughout the mucosa and submucosa of the small and large intestines 孤立淋巴小结；**triticeous n.,** 麦粒软骨，参见 *cartilage*；**typhus n's,** minute nodules, originally described in typhus, produced by perivascular infiltration of polymorphonuclear leukocytes and mononuclear cells in typhus 斑疹伤寒小结；**n. of vermis,** the most anterior lobule on the inferior surface of the vermis of the cerebellum, where the inferior medullary velum attaches 蚓部小结；**vocal cord n's,** singer's or teacher's nodes; small white nodules on the vocal cords in those who use their voice excessively 声带小结
nod·u·lus (nod′u-ləs) pl. *no′duli* [L.] 同 nodule
no·dus (no′dəs) pl. *no′di* [L.] 同 node
no·ma (no′mə) gangrenous process of the mouth or genitalia. In the mouth *(cancrum oris, gangrenous stomatitis)*, it begins as a small gingival ulcer and results in gangrenous necrosis of surrounding facial tissues; on the genitalia, the appearance is similar, affecting the penis in males and the labia majora, one after the other, in females 坏疽性口炎
no·men·cla·ture (no′mən-kla″chər) a classified system of names, as of anatomic structures, organisms, etc. 命名法；**binomial n.,** the system of designating plants and animals by two latinized words signifying the genus and species 双名法，二名法
nom·i·nal (nom′ĭ-nəl) pertaining to a name or names 命名的，称名的
nom·o·gram (nom′o-gram) a graph with several scales arranged so that a straightedge laid on the graph intersects the scales at related values of the variables; the values of any two variables can be used to find the values of the others 列线图
non com·pos men·tis (non kom′pos men′tis) [L.] not of sound mind, and so not legally responsible 精神不健全
non·con·duc·tor (non″kən-duk′tər) a substance that does not readily transmit electricity, light, or heat 不传导
non·di·a·bet·ic (non″di-ə-bet′ik) not caused by or affected with diabetes 非糖尿病的
non·dis·junc·tion (non″dis-junk′shən) failure either of two homologous chromosomes to pass to separate cells during the first meiotic division, or of the two chromatids of a chromosome to pass to separate cells during mitosis or during the second meiotic division. As a result, one daughter cell has two chromosomes or two chromatids and the other

has none 不分离

non·elec·tro·lyte (non″e-lek′tro-līt) a substance that does not dissociate into ions; in solution it is a nonconductor of electricity 非电解质

non·heme (non′hēm) not bound within a porphyrin ring; said of iron so contained within a protein 非血红素的（指蛋白质内的铁）

non·neu·ro·nal (non″noo-ro′nəl) pertaining to or composed of nonconducting cells of the nervous system, e.g., neuroglial cells 非神经元的

non·ox·y·nol 9 (non-ok′sĭ-nol) a spermaticide used in contraceptive agents 壬苯醇醚 9，一种用于避孕的杀精剂

NONPF The National Organization of Nurse Practitioner Faculties 美国护士执业联盟

non·re·spond·er (non″re-spon′dər) a person or animal that after vaccination against a given virus does not show any immune response when challenged with the virus 无应答者，指人或动物接种某一病毒疫苗后，在受到该病毒攻击时未显示免疫应答

non·se·cre·tor (non″se-kre′tər) a person with A or B type blood whose body secretions do not contain the particular (A or B) substance 非分泌者，指 A 型血或 B 型血的人，其体液中并不含有特殊的（A 或 B）物质

non·self (non′self″) in immunology, pertaining to foreign antigens 非自身的，在免疫学中指外来的抗原

non·spe·cif·ic (non″spə-sif′ik) 1. not due to any single known cause 原因不明的；2. not specific or definite; not having a specific cause or target 非特异性的

non·union (non-ūn′yən) failure of the ends of a fractured bone to unite 骨折不愈合，骨不连接

non·vi·a·ble (non-vi′ə-bəl) not capable of living 不能存活的，不能生活的

NOPHN National Organization for Public Health Nursing 国家公共卫生护理组织

nor- chemical prefix denoting (a) a compound of normal structure (having an unbranched chain of carbon atoms) that is isomeric with one having a branched chain, or (b) a compound whose chain or ring contains one less methylene (CH_2) group than does that of its homologue 化学前缀，（a）化合物的无分支的碳链结构与有分支的为同分异构体；（b）化合物的链或环比同系物少一个亚甲基

nor·adren·a·line (nor″ə-dren′ə-lin) 同 norepine-phrine

nor·ad·ren·er·gic (nor″ad-rən-ur′jik) activated by or secreting norepinephrine 去甲肾上腺素能的

nor·cloz·a·pine (nor-clŏz′uh-peen) the major metabolite of clozapine; used in the treatment of

schizophrenia 去甲氯氮平

nor·epi·neph·rine (nor″ep-ĭ-nef′rin) a catecholamine, which is the principal neurotransmitter of postganglionic adrenergic neurons, having predominant α -adrenergic activity; also secreted by the adrenal medulla in response to splanchnic stimulation, being released predominantly in response to hypotension. It is a powerful vasopressor and is used, in the form of the bitartrate salt, to restore the blood pressure in certain cases of acute hypotension and to improve cardiac function during decompensation associated with congestive heart failure or cardiovascular surgery 去甲肾上腺素

nor·eth·in·drone (nor-eth′in-drōn) a progestational agent having some anabolic, estrogenic, and androgenic properties; used as the base or the acetate ester in the treatment of amenorrhea, dysfunctional uterine bleeding, and endometriosis, and as an oral contraceptive 炔诺酮

nor·ethy·no·drel (nor″ə-thi′no-drəl) a progestin, used in combination with an estrogen as an oral contraceptive, to control endometriosis, for the treatment of hypermenorrhea, and to produce cyclic withdrawal bleeding 异炔诺酮

nor·flox·a·cin (nor-flok′sə-sin) a broad-spectrum antibacterial effective against a wide range of aerobic gram-negative and gram-positive organisms 诺氟沙星

nor·ges·ti·mate (nor-jes′tĭ-māt) a synthetic progestational agent with little androgenic activity, used in combination with an estrogen component as an oral contraceptive 诺孕酯，肟炔诺酮

nor·ges·trel (nor-jes′trəl) a synthetic progestational agent used as an oral contraceptive 甲基炔诺酮

norm (norm) a fixed or ideal standard 标准，规格，准则；定额；范数；常模

nor·mal (nor′məl) 1. agreeing with the regular and established type. 正规的；2. in chemistry, (a) denoting a solution containing, in each 1000 ml, 1 g equivalent weight of the active substance, symbol N or N; (b) denoting aliphatic hydrocarbons in which no carbon atom is combined with more than two other carbon atoms, symbol n-; (c) denoting salts not containing replaceable hydrogen or hydroxide ions 在化学中，（a）指 1000ml 溶液中含有 1g 当量的活性物质，符号为 N 或 N；（b）脂肪烃，符号 n-；（c）指不包含可置换氢或氢氧离子的盐

nor·meta·neph·rine (nor-met″ə-nef′rin) a metabolite of norepinephrine excreted in the urine and found in certain tissues 去甲变肾上腺素

nor·mo·blast (nor′mo-blast) 1. orthochromatic erythroblast 晚幼红细胞，正成红细胞；2. term

N

now often used as a synonym of *erythroblast*; sometimes more specifically, a nucleated cell in the normal course of erythrocyte maturation, as opposed to a megaloblast. When used in the latter sense, the four developmental stages of the nucleated cells of the erythrocytic series are usually named pronormoblasts *(proerythroblasts)* and basophilic, polychromatophilic, and orthochromatic normoblasts (see under *erythroblast*) 红细胞或有核红细胞；**normoblas′tic** *adj.*

nor·mo·blas·to·sis (nor″mo-blas-to′sis) excessive production of normoblasts by the bone marrow 正成红细胞过多（症）

nor·mo·cal·ce·mia (nor″mo-kal-se′me-ə) a normal level of calcium in the blood 血钙正常；**normocalce′mic** *adj.*

nor·mo·chro·mia (nor″mo-kro′me-ə) normal color; indicating the color of erythrocytes having a normal hemoglobin content 血（细胞）色正常；**normochro′mic** *adj.*

nor·mo·cyte (nor′mo-sīt) an erythrocyte that is normal in size, shape, and color（正常）红细胞；**normocyt′ic** *adj.*

nor·mo·cy·to·sis (nor″mo-si-to′sis) a normal state of the blood in respect to erythrocytes 血细胞正常

nor·mo·gly·ce·mia (nor″mo-gli-se′me-ə) euglycemia 血糖量正常；**normoglyce′mic** *adj.*

nor·mo·ka·le·mia (nor″mo-kə-le′me-ə) a normal level of potassium in the blood 血钾正常；**normo-kale′mic** *adj.*

nor·mo·sper·mia (nor″mo-spur′me-ə) production of spermatozoa normal in number and motility 精子正常；**normosperm′ic** *adj.*

nor·mo·ten·sive (nor″mo-ten′siv) 1. characterized by normal tone, tension, or pressure, as by normal blood pressure 血压正常的；2. a person with normal blood pressure 血压正常者

nor·mo·ther·mia (nor″mo-thur′me-ə) a normal state of temperature 体温正常，温度正常；**normother′mic** *adj.*

nor·mo·vo·le·mia (nor″mo-vo-le′me-ə) normal blood volume 血量正常

Nor·o·vi·rus (nor′o-vi″rəs) a genus of viruses of the family Caliciviridae, including Norwalk virus, that cause self-limited acute gastroenteritis 诺如病毒

nor·trip·ty·line (nor-trip′tə-lēn) a tricyclic antidepressant, used as the hydrochloride salt to treat depression and panic disorder and to relieve chronic severe pain 去甲替林

nose (nōz) the specialized facial structure serving as an organ of the sense of smell and as part of the respiratory apparatus 鼻，见图 25；**saddle n., swayback n.,** a nose with a sunken bridge 鞍（状）鼻

nose·bleed (nōz′blēd″) epistaxis 鼻出血，鼻衄

No·se·ma (no-se′mə) a genus of intracellular protozoa, including *N. ocula′rum,* which causes corneal infections 微孢子虫属

nose·piece (nōz′pēs″) the portion of a microscope nearest to the stage, which bears the objective or objectives（显微镜的）物镜旋座

noso·co·mi·al (nos″o-ko′me-əl) pertaining to or originating in a hospital 医院的

no·sog·e·ny (no-soj′ə-ne) pathogenesis 发病机制

no·sol·o·gy (no-sol′ə-je) the science of the classification of diseases 疾病分类学；**nosolog′ic** *adj.*

Noso·psyl·lus (nos″o-sil′əs) a genus of fleas, including *N. fascia′tus,* the common rat flea of North America and Europe, a vector of murine typhus and probably of plague 病蚤属

nos·tril (nos′tril) either of the nares 鼻孔

nos·trum (nos′trəm) a quack, patent, or secret remedy 秘方

no·tal·gia (no-tal′jə) pain in the back 背痛

notch (noch) incisure; an indentation on the edge of a bone or other organ 切迹；**aortic n.,** 同dicrotic n.；**cardiac n.,** 1. *(of stomach)* a notch at the junction of the esophagus and the greater curvature of the stomach 食管和胃大弯连接处的切迹；2. *(of left lung)* a notch in the anterior border of the left lung 左肺心切迹；**dicrotic n.,** a small downward deflection in the arterial pulse or pressure contour immediately following the closure of the semilunar valves and preceding the dicrotic wave, sometimes used as a marker for the end of systole or the ejection period 降中峡，重搏波切迹；**frontal n.,** a notch in the supraorbital margin of the frontal bone medial to the supraorbital notch (or foramen), for transmission of the supraorbital nerve and vessels; frequently converted into a foramen by a bridge of osseous tissue 额切迹；**jugular n.** suprasternal n.; the notch in the midline on the upper border of the manubrium of the sternum 颈静脉切迹；**mastoid n. of temporal bone,** a deep groove on the medial surface of the mastoid process of the temporal bone, giving attachment to the posterior belly of the digastric muscle 颞骨乳突切迹；**Rivinus n.,** tympanic n. 里维努斯切迹；**supraorbital n.,** a passage in the frontal bone for the supraorbital artery and nerve. It is bridged by fibrous tissue, which is sometimes ossified, forming a bony aperture *(supraorbital foramen)* 眶上切迹；**suprasternal n.,** jugular n. 胸骨上切迹；**tentorial n.,** an opening at the anterior part of the cerebellum, formed by the internal border of the tentorium cerebelli and the dorsum of the sella turcica, and containing the midbrain 小脑幕切

迹；**trochlear n.**, a large concavity on the anterior surface at the proximal end of the ulna, formed by the olecranon and coronoid processes, for articulation with the trochlea of the humerus 滑车切迹；**tympanic n.**, a defect in the upper tympanic ring of the temporal bone, filled by the upper portion of the tympanic membrane 鼓切迹；**vertebral n.**, the indentation found below (*inferior vertebral n.*) and above (*superior vertebral n.*) each pedicle of a vertebra. The inferior notch of one vertebra together with the superior notch of the next-lower vertebra form the intervertebral foramen 椎切迹

No·tech·is (no-tek′is) a genus of extremely venomous Australian snakes of the family Elapidae. *N. scuta′tus* is the tiger snake, whose body is brown with dark bands 澳大利亚的一属剧毒蛇。*N. scutatus* 虎蛇

no·ti·fi·a·ble (no″tĭ-fi′ə-bəl) necessary to be reported to a government health agency 须报告卫生当局的，应具报的，应报告的

no·to·chord (no′to-kord) a rod-shaped cord of cells on the dorsal aspect of an embryo, defining the primitive axis of the body and serving as the center of development of the axial skeleton; it is the common factor of all chordates 脊索

No·to·ed·res (no″to-ed′rēz) a genus of mites, including *N. ca′ti*, an itch mite causing a persistent, often fatal, mange in cats; it also infests domestic animals and sometimes temporarily humans 耳螨属

No·vo·cain (no′və-kān) trademark for preparations of procaine 普鲁卡因

NOWS neonatal opioid withdrawal syndrome 新生儿阿片戒断综合征

nox·ious (nok′shəs) hurtful; injurious; pernicious 有害的

Np neptunium 元素镎的符号

NPDS National Poison Data System 国家毒物控制中心系统

NPN nonprotein nitrogen 非蛋白质氮

NPO [L.] nil per os (nothing by mouth) 禁食

NPWH National Association of Nurse Practitioners in Women's Health 全国妇女保健护士执业协会

NRCA National Rehabilitation Counseling Association 国家康复咨询协会

NREM non-rapid eye movement (see under *sleep*) 非快速眼动（睡眠）

NREMT National Registry of Emergency Medical Technicians 紧急医疗技术人员国家登记处

NRI selective norepinephrine reuptake inhibitor 选择性肾上腺素再吸收抑制药

ns nanosecond; one billionth (10^{-9}) of a second 纳秒 (10^{-9}s)

NSAIA nonsteroidal antiinflammatory analgesic (or agent) 非甾体抗炎镇痛药；参见 *drug* 下词条

NSAID nonsteroidal antiinflammatory drug 非甾体抗炎药

NSCLC non-small cell lung carcinoma (or cancer) 非小细胞肺癌

NSH National Society for Histotechnology 美国国家病理组织技术协会

NSIAD nephrogenic syndrome of inappropriate antidiuresis 抗利尿药不适当肾病综合征

NSNA National Student Nurses' Association 全国护士生协会

NST nonstress test 无应激试验

NTDB National Trauma Data Bank 国家创伤数据库

NTRS National Therapeutic Recreation Society 国家治疗性娱乐协会

NTSS National Tuberculosis Surveillance System 国家结核病监测系统

nu·cha (noo′kə) 同 nape; **nu′chal** *adj.*

nu·cle·ar (noo′kle-ər) pertaining to a nucleus（原子）核的，核心的

nu·cle·ase (noo′kle-ās) any of a group of enzymes that split nucleic acids into nucleotides and other products 核酸酶

nu·cle·at·ed (noo′kle-āt″əd) having a nucleus or nuclei 有核的

nu·clei (noo′kle-i) [L.] *nucleus* 复数

nu·cle·ic ac·id (noo-kle′ik) a high-molecular-weight nucleotide polymer. There are two types: *deoxyribonucleic acid* (DNA) and *ribonucleic acid* (RNA) 核酸

nu·cleo·cap·sid (noo″kle-o-kap′sid) a unit of viral structure, consisting of a capsid with the enclosed nucleic acid 核（衣）壳

nu·cle·of·u·gal (noo″kle-of′u-gəl) moving away from a nucleus 离核的

nu·cle·oid (noo′kle-oid) 1. resembling a nucleus 拟核的，核样的；2. a DNA-containing region lacking a surrounding nuclear membrane, occurring in prokaryotes, mitochondria, and chloroplasts; analogous to the eukaryotic cell nucleus 拟核，类核；3. the core of nucleic acid surrounded by the protein capsid in some viruses 病毒核心

nu·cleo·lo·ne·ma (noo″kle-o″lo-ne′mə) a network of strands formed by organization of fine ribonucleoprotein granules in the nucleolus of a cell 核仁线

nu·cle·o·lus (noo-kle′ə-ləs″) pl. *nucle′oli* [L.] a rounded refractile body in the nucleus of most cells, which is the site of synthesis of ribosomal RNA 核仁

nu·cle·op·e·tal (noo″kle-op′ə-təl) moving toward a nucleus 入核

N

nu·cleo·phago·cy·to·sis (noo″kle-o-fa″go-sito′sis) the engulfing of the nuclei of other cells by phagocytes. 噬核现象

nu·cleo·phile (noo′kle-o-fīl″) an electron donor in chemical reactions involving covalent catalysis in which the donated electrons bond other chemical groups (electrophiles) 亲核体，亲核试剂；**nucleophil′ic** *adj.*

nu·cleo·plasm (noo′kle-o-plaz″əm) the protoplasm of the nucleus of a cell, comprising the contents of the nucleus other than the nucleolus and chromatin and containing macromolecules and particles necessary for maintenance of the cell 核质。 Cf. *cytoplasm*；**nucleoplas′mic** *adj.*

nu·cleo·pro·tein (noo″kle-o-pro′tēn) a substance composed of a simple basic protein (e.g., a histone) combined with a nucleic acid 核蛋白

nu·cleo·si·dase (noo″kle-o-si′dās) an enzyme that catalyzes the splitting of a nucleoside to form a purine or pyrimidine base and a sugar 核苷酶

nu·cleo·side (noo′kle-o-sīd″) one of the compounds into which a nucleotide is split by the action of nucleotidase or by chemical means; it consists of a sugar (a pentose) with a purine or pyrimidine base 核苷

nu·cleo·some (noo′kle-o-sōm) the primary structural unit of eukaryotic chromatin, seen with the electron microscope as one of the characteristic "beads on a string"; it comprises a segment of DNA wrapped twice around an octamer core of histones and is connected to each adjacent nucleosome by a short DNA segment 核小体

nu·cleo·ti·dase (noo″kle-o-ti′dās) an enzyme that catalyzes the cleavage of a nucleotide into a nucleoside and an orthophosphate 核苷酸酶

nu·cleo·tide (noo′kle-o-tīd) one of the compounds into which nucleic acid is split by the action of nuclease; nucleotides are composed of a base (purine or pyrimidine), a sugar (ribose or deoxyribose), and a phosphate group 核苷酸；**cyclic n's,** those in which the phosphate group bonds to two atoms of the sugar, forming a ring, as in cyclic AMP and cyclic GMP, which act as intracellular second messengers 环核苷酸

nu·cleo·tid·yl (noo″kle-o-tid′əl) a nucleotide residue 核苷酸基

nu·cleo·tox·in (noo′kle-o-tok″sin) 1. a toxin from cell nuclei 核毒素；2. any toxin affecting cell nuclei 有损害细胞核作用的任何毒素

nu·cle·us (noo′kle-əs) pl. *nu′clei* [L.] 1. the central core of a body or object 中 心；2. cell nucleus: a spheroid body within a eukaryotic cell, separated from the cytoplasm by the nuclear envelope, and containing chromatin, a nucleolus or nucleoli, and nucleoplasm 细 胞 核；3. a group of nerve cells, usually within the central nervous system, bearing a direct relationship to the fibers of a particular tract or system 中枢神经系统内的核团；4. in organic chemistry, the combination of atoms forming the central element or basic framework of the molecule of a specific compound or class of compounds 核 基，环核；5. 参见 *atomic n.*；**nu′clear** *adj.*；n. **ambi′guus,** the nucleus of origin of motor fibers of the vagus and glossopharyngeal nerves in the medulla oblongata 疑 核；**anterior olfactory n.,** scattered groups of neurons intermingled with the olfactory tract that run caudally from the end of the olfactory bulb, some receiving synaptic stimuli from the fibers of the olfactory tract 前嗅觉核；**arcuate n.,** 1. a nucleus of nerve cells in the posterior hypothalamic region, extending into the median eminence and almost entirely surrounding the base of the infundibulum 弓状核；2. one of the small irregular areas of gray substance on the ventromedial aspect of the pyramid of the medulla oblongata 延 髓 椎体腹内侧的灰质中不规则的小区域；**atomic n.,** the central core of an atom, composed of protons and neutrons, constituting most of its mass but only a small part of its volume 原 子 核；**basal nuclei, nu′clei basa′les,** specific interconnected groups of masses of gray substance deep in the cerebral hemispheres, constituting the corpus striatum 基底核；n. **caeru′leus,** a compact aggregation of pigmented neurons subjacent to the locus caeruleus, sometimes considered one of the medial reticular nuclei 蓝 斑核；n. **cauda′tus,** an elongated, arched gray mass closely related to the lateral ventricle throughout its entire extent, which, together with the putamen, forms the neostriatum 尾 状 核；**central nuclei of thalamus,** two small intralaminar nuclei, medial and lateral, situated in the internal medullary lamina 丘脑中央核；**centromedian n. of thalamus,** the largest and most caudal of the intralaminar nuclei of the dorsal thalamus 丘脑中央核；**cochlear nuclei,** the nuclei, anterior and posterior, of termination of sensory fibers of the cochlear part of the vestibulocochlear nerve, which partly encircle the restiform body at the junction of the medulla oblongata and pons 蜗神经核；**cuneate n., n. cunea′tus,** a nucleus in the medulla oblongata, in which the fibers of the fasciculus cuneatus synapse 楔 束 核；**Deiters n.,** lateral vestibular nucleus 前庭外侧 核，参见 *vestibular nuclei*；**dentate n., n. denta′tus,** the largest and most lateral of the deep cerebellar nuclei, lying in the white matter of the cerebellum just lateral to the emboliform nucleus（小脑）

齿 状 核；**droplet nuclei,** dried particles of pathogencontaining material expelled from the respiratory tract and capable of causing droplet infections 微滴核；**emboliform n., n. embolifor′mis,** a small cerebellar nucleus that lies between the dentate nucleus and globose nucleus and contributes to the superior cerebellar peduncles 栓 状 核；**n. endopeduncula′ris,** a small nucleus in the internal capsule of the hypothalamus, adjacent to the medial edge of the globus pallidus 脚 内 核；**fastigial n., n. fasti′gii,** the most medial of the cerebellar nuclei, near the midline in the roof of the fourth ventricle 顶核；**n. gra′cilis,** a nucleus in the medulla oblongata, in which the fibers of the fasciculus gracilis of the spinal cord synapse 薄束核；**hypoglossal n., n. of hypoglossal nerve,** the nucleus of origin of the hypoglossal nerve, forming a column in the central gray matter from below the level of the inferior olive to the upper part of the medulla oblongata 舌 下 神经核；**interpeduncular n., n. interpeduncula′ris,** a nucleus between the cerebral peduncles immediately dorsal to the interpeduncular fossa 脚间核；**lenticular n., lentiform n.,** the part of the corpus striatum just lateral to the internal capsule, comprising the putamen and globus pallidus 豆状核；**Meynert n.,** a group of neurons in the basal forebrain that has wide projections to the neocortex and is rich in acetylcholine and choline acetyltransferase; it undergoes degeneration in paralysis agitans and Alzheimer disease 迈 纳 特 基 底 核；**motor n.,** any collection of cells in the central nervous system giving origin to a motor nerve 运动核；**oculomotor n.,** the origin of the fibers of the oculomotor nerve, situated in the tegmentum of the midbrain immediately ventral to the central gray matter, between the medial longitudinal fasciculi. Innervation of the superior rectus of one eye originates in the contralateral oculomotor nucleus; the other elements of the nucleus supply ipsilateral eye muscles via the oculomotor nerve 动眼神经核；**olivary n.,** 1. a folded band of gray substance enclosing a white core and producing the elevation (olive) of the medulla oblongata （ 延 髓切面 ） 橄榄核；2. olive (2) 橄榄体；**n. of origin,** any of the groups of nerve cells in the central nervous system from which arise the motor, or efferent, fibers of the cranial nerves 起始核；**paraventricular n. of hypothalamus,** a band of cells in the wall of the third ventricle in the anterior hypothalamic region; many of its cells are neurosecretory in function (secreting oxytocin) and project to the posterior lobe of the pituitary 下丘脑室旁核；**pontine nuclei, nu′clei pon′tis,** masses of nerve cells scattered throughout the ventral part of the pons, in which the longitudinal fibers of the pons terminate; the majority of the axons arising from these cells cross to the opposite side and form the middle cerebellar peduncle 脑 桥 核；**posterior thoracic n.,** a well-defined column of cells in the medial part of the intermediate zone of the spinal gray matter, usually extending from the eighth cervical segment to the second or third lumbar segment 胸 后 核；**n. pro′prius,** a column of large neurons that extends throughout the posterior column of the spinal cord, ventral to the gelatinous substance 固有核；**n. pulpo′sus,** a semifluid mass of fine white and elastic fibers forming the center of an intervertebral disk 髓核；**raphe nuclei,** a subgroup of the reticular nuclei of the brainstem, found in narrow longitudinal sheets along the raphae of the medulla oblongata, pons, and midbrain; they include many neurons that synthesize serotonin 中缝核；**red n.,** a distinctive oval nucleus centrally placed in the upper mesencephalic reticular formation 红核；**reticular nuclei,** nuclei found in the reticular formation of the brainstem, occurring primarily in longitudinal columns in three groups: median column reticular nuclei (raphe nuclei), medial column reticular nuclei, and lateral column reticular nuclei 网状核；**n. ru′ber,** 同 red n.；**salivatory nuclei,** cells in the posterolateral part of the reticular formation of the pons, subdivided into inferior and superior nuclei, together comprising the parasympathetic outflow for the supply of the salivary glands 泌涎核；**sensory n.,** the nucleus of termination of the afferent (sensory) fibers of a peripheral nerve 感觉核；**solitary nuclei,** any of various nuclei of termination of the visceral afferent fibers of the facial, glossopharyngeal, and vagus nerves, which enter the solitary tract 孤立核；**subthalamic n., n. subthala′micus,** a nucleus on the medial side of the junction of the internal capsule and crus cerebri 底 丘 脑核；**supraoptic n.,** a nucleus of nerve cells just above the lateral part of the optic chiasm; many of its cells are neurosecretory in function (secreting vasopressin) and project to the posterior lobe of the pituitary; other cells are osmoreceptors, which respond to increased osmotic pressure to signal the release of vasopressin by the posterior lobe of the pituitary 视 上 核；**tegmental n., laterodorsal,** a nucleus of nerve cells in the mesencephalic tegmentum, situated dorsal to the nucleus of the trochlear nerve 背侧被盖核；**terminal n.,** groups of nerve cells within the central nervous system on which the axons of primary afferent neurons of various cranial nerves synapse 终止核；**nuclei of trapezoid body,** groups of nerve cell bodies lying within the fibers of the trapezoid body 斜方体核；**trigeminal nuclei,** four nuclei associated with the trigeminal nerve, located in the midbrain, pons, and medulla oblongata, and extending as far caudally as the upper cervical spinal cord 三叉神经核；**vestibular nuclei,** the four (superior, lateral, medial, and inferior) cellular masses in the floor of the fourth ventricle in which the branches of the vestibular nerve terminate and in which cerebellar projections are received. The nuclei give rise to widely dispersed projections to motor nuclei in the brainstem and cervical cord and to motor cells throughout the spinal cord. Additional connections provide for conscious perception of, and autonomic reactions to, labyrinthine stimulation 前庭神经核

nu·clide (noo′klīd) a species of atom characterized by the charge, mass, number, and quantum state of its nucleus, and capable of existing for a measurable lifetime (usually more than 10^{-10} seconds)（原子）核素

null (nul) 1. insignificant; having no consequence or value 无结果，无意义；2. absent or nonexistent 不存在的；3. zero; nothing 零位的；空的

nul·lip·a·ra (nə-lip′ə-rə) para 0; a woman who has never borne a viable child 未产妇，参见 *para*；**nullip′arous** *adj.*

nul·li·par·i·ty (nul″ĭ-par′ĭ-te) the state of being a nullipara 未经产

numb (num) anesthetic (1) 麻木的，感觉缺失的

num·ber (num′bər) a symbol, such as a figure or word, expressive of a certain value or a specified quantity determined by count 数字符号；**atomic n.** (Z), a number expressive of the number of protons in an atomic nucleus 原子序数；**Avogadro's n.** (N) (NA), the number of molecules in 1 mole of a substance: 6.023×10^{23} 阿伏伽德罗常数；**mass n.** (A), the number expressive of the mass of a nucleus, being the total number of protons and neutrons in the nucleus of an atom or nuclide 质量数；**oxidation n.,** a number assigned to each atom in a molecule or ion that represents the number of electrons theoretically lost (negative numbers) or gained (positive numbers) in converting the atom to the elemental form (which has an oxidation number of zero). The sum of the oxidation numbers for all atoms in a neutral compound is zero; for polyatomic ions, it is equal to the ionic charge 氧化数；**tooth n.,** a number or letter assigned to each of the permanent or primary teeth to denote its place in the dentition 牙号；**turnover n.,** the number of molecules of substrate acted upon by one molecule of enzyme per minute 催化常数

numb·ness (num′nis) anesthesia (1) 麻木，感觉缺失

num·mu·lar (num′u-lər) 1. coin-sized and coin-shaped 钱币形的；2. made up of round, flat disks 圆串状的；3. arranged like a stack of coins 钱串排列的

nurse (nurs) 1. one who is especially prepared in the scientific basis of nursing and who meets certain prescribed standards of education and clinical competence 护士；2. to provide services essential to or helpful in the promotion, maintenance, and restoration of health and well-being 照料，护理；3. to breast-feed an infant 喂奶；**clinical n. specialist,** a registered nurse with a high degree of knowledge, skill, and competence in a specialized area of nursing, and usually having a master's degree in nursing 临床护理专家；**community n.,** in Great Britain, a public health nurse 地段护士（英国）；**community health n.,** public health n. 社区保健护士；**district n.,** 同 community n.；**general duty n.,** a registered nurse, usually one who has not undergone training beyond the basic nursing program, who sees to the general nursing care of patients in a hospital or other health agency 普通护士；**graduate n.,** a graduate of a school of nursing; often used to designate one who has not been registered or licensed 毕业护士；**licensed practical n.,** a graduate of a school of practical nursing whose qualifications have been examined by a state board of nursing and who has been legally authorized to practice as a licensed practical or vocational nurse (LPN or LVN), under supervision of a physician or registered nurse 执照护士；**licensed vocational n.,** 同 licensed practical n.；**n. practitioner,** a registered nurse with advanced education and clinical training within a specialty area 从业护士；**private n., private duty n.,** a nurse who attends an individual patient, usually on a fee-for-service basis, and who may specialize in a specific class of diseases 私人护士；**probationer n.,** a person who has entered a school of nursing and is under observation to determine fitness for the nursing profession; applied principally to nursing students enrolled in hospital schools of nursing 护士生；**public health n.,** an especially prepared registered nurse employed in a community agency to safeguard the health of persons in the community, giving care to the sick in their homes, promoting health and wellbeing by teaching families how to keep well, and assisting in programs for the prevention of disease 公共卫生护士；**Queen's N.,** in Great Britain, a district nurse who has been trained at or in accordance with the regulations of the Queen Victoria Jubilee Institute for Nurses 地段护士（英国）；**registered n.,** a graduate nurse who has been legally authorized (registered) to practice after examination by a state board of nurse examiners or similar regulatory authority, and who is legally entitled to use the designation RN 注册护士；**scrub n.**, a nurse who directly assists the surgeon in the operating room 手术室护士；**n. specialist**, clinical n. specialist. 专科护理师；**visiting n.**, 同 public health n. 访视护士；**wet n.**, a woman who breastfeeds the infant of another 乳母，奶妈

nurse-mid·wife (nurs-mid′wīf) an individual educated in the two disciplines of nursing and midwifery, who possesses evidence of certification according to the requirements of the American College of Nurse-Midwives. Abbreviated CNM (Certified Nurse-Midwife) 助产士

nurse-mid·wi·fery (nurs-mid′wi-fər-e) the independent management of care of essentially normal newborns and women, antepartally, intrapartally, postpartally, and/or gynecologically, occurring within a health care system that provides for medical consultation, collaborative management, or referral, and is in accord with the functions, standards, and qualifications as defined by the American College of Nurse-Midwives 助产护士学

nur·se·ry (nur′sə-re) the department in a hospital providing care for newborn infants 婴儿室

nurs·ing (nurs′ing) 1. the provision, at various levels of preparation, of services essential to or helpful in the promotion, maintenance, and restoration of health and well-being or in the prevention of illness, as of infants, of the sick and injured, or of others for any reason unable to provide such services for themselves 照料、护理（婴儿、病人和伤员）；2. breastfeeding 哺乳

nu·ta·tion (noo-ta′shən) the act of nodding, especially involuntary nodding 点头（尤指不随意性点头）

nu·tri·ent (noo′tre-ənt) 1. nourishing; providing nutrition 滋养的，营养的；2. a food or other substance that provides energy or building material for the survival and growth of a living organism 营养素，营养物，又称 *nutriment*

nu·tri·tion (noo-tri′shən) the taking in and metabolism of nutrients (food and other nourishing material) by an organism so that life is maintained and growth can take place 营养，养分；**nutri′tional**, **nu′tritive** *adj.*；**enteral n.**, the delivery of nutrients in liquid form directly into the stomach, duodenum, or jejunum 肠道营养；**parenteral n.**, administration of nutriment intravenously 肠外营养；**total parenteral n. (TPN)**, intravenous administration, via a central venous catheter, of the total nutrient requirements of a patient with gastrointestinal dysfunction 全静脉营养

nu·tri·tious (noo-tri′shəs) affording nourishment 有营养的，滋养的

nu·tri·tive (noo′trĭ-tiv″) 1. nutritional 营养的；2. 同 nutritious

nu·tri·ture (noo′trĭ-chur″) the status of the body in relation to nutrition 营养状况

nyc·ta·lo·pia (nik″tə-lo′pe-ə) 1. night blindness 夜盲；2. in French (and incorrectly in English), day blindness 昼盲症（法语）

nyc·to·hem·er·al (nik″to-hem′ər-əl) pertaining to both day and night 昼夜的

nyc·to·pho·bia (nik″to-fo′be-ə) irrational fear of darkness 黑夜恐怖，黑暗恐怖，恐夜症

nymph (nimf) a developmental stage in certain arthropods, e.g., ticks, between the larval form and the adult, and resembling the latter in appearance 若虫（与成虫相似的昆虫幼体）

nym·pha (nim′fə) pl. *nym′phae* [Gr.] one of the labia minora pudendi 小阴唇

nym·phec·to·my (nim-fek′tə-me) excision of the nymphae (labia minora) 小阴唇切除术

nym·phi·tis (nim-fi′tis) inflammation of the nymphae (labia minora) 小阴唇炎

nym·pho·ma·nia (nim″fo-ma′ne-ə) excessive sexual desire in a female 慕男狂；**nymphoman′iac** *adj.*

nym·phot·o·my (nim-fot′ə-me) surgical incision of the nymphae (labia minora) or clitoris 小阴唇切开术，阴蒂切开术

nys·tag·mi·form (nis-tag′mĭ-form) 同 nystagmoid

nys·tag·mo·graph (nis-tag′mo-graf) an instrument for recording the movements of the eyeball in nystagmus 眼球震颤描记器

nys·tag·moid (nis-tag′moid) resembling nystagmus 眼球震颤样的

nys·tag·mus (nis-tag′məs) involuntary rapid movement (horizontal, vertical, rotatory, or mixed, i.e., of two types) of the eyeball 眼球震颤，眼震；**nystag′mic** *adj.*；**aural n.**, vestibular n. 耳源性眼球震颤；**caloric n.**, rotatory nystagmus induced by irrigating the ears with warm or cold water or air 温热性眼球震颤，参见 *test* 下 *caloric test*；**dissociated n.**, that in which the movements in the two eyes are dissimilar 分离性眼球震颤；**endposition n.**, that occurring in normal individuals only at extremes of gaze 终位性眼球震颤；**fixation n.**, that occurring only on gazing fixedly at an object 凝视性眼球震颤；**gaze n.**, nystagmus made apparent by looking to the right or to the left 注视性眼震；**gaze paretic n.**, a form of gaze nystagmus seen in patients recovering from central nervous system lesions; the eyes fail to stay fixed to the affected side with a cerebral or pontine lesion 注视不全麻痹性

眼 球 震 颤；**labyrinthine** n., **vestibular** n. 迷路性眼球震颤；**latent** n., that occurring only when one eye is covered 隐性眼球震颤；**lateral** n., involuntary horizontal movement of the eyes 摆动性眼球震颤；**opticokinetic** n., **optokinetic** n., the normal nystagmus occurring when looking at objects passing across the field of vision, as in viewing from a moving vehicle 视动性眼球震颤；**pendular** n., that which consists of to-and-fro movements of equal velocity 钟摆型眼球震颤（曾称为摆动性眼球震颤）；**positional** n., that which occurs, or is altered in form or intensity, on assumption of certain positions of the head 位置性眼震；**retraction** n., n. **retracto′rius**, a spasmodic backward movement of the eyeball occurring on attempts to move the eye; a sign of midbrain disease 退缩性眼球震颤；**rotatory** n., involuntary rotation of eyes about the visual axis 旋转性眼球震颤；**spontaneous** n., that occurring without specific stimulation of the vestibular system 自发性眼球震颤；**undulatory** n., pendular n. 振动性眼球震颤；**vertical** n., involuntary up-and-down movement of the eyes 垂直性眼球震颤；**vestibular** n., that due to disturbance of the vestibular system; eye movements are rhythmic, with slow and fast components 前庭性眼球震

ny·sta·tin (ni-stat′in) an antifungal produced by growth of *Streptomyces noursei*; used in treatment of infections caused by *Candida albicans* and other *Candida* species 制霉菌素

nyx·is (nik′sis) puncture, or paracentesis 穿刺术

O

O oxygen 元素氧的符号

O. [L.] o′culus (eye) 眼的符号

o- ortho- (2) 正，邻的化学符号

Ω ohm 欧姆的符号

ω- (omega, the twenty-fourth letter of the Greek alphabet)（omega，希腊语第 24 个字母）1. the carbon atom farthest from the principal functional group in a molecule 末位的（离主要功能基最远的碳原子的符号）；2. last in a series of related entities or chemical compounds 最后位的

OA ocular albinism 眼白化病

OAF osteoclast-activating factor 破骨细胞激活因子

OB obstetrics 产科学

obes·i·ty (o-bēs′ĭ-te) an increase in body weight beyond the limitation of skeletal and physical requirements as the result of excessive accumulation of body fat 肥胖（症）；**obese′** adj.；**adultonset o.**, obesity that begins in adulthood and is characterized by increase in size (hypertrophy) of adipose cells with no increase in their number 成年型肥胖症；**android o.**, obesity in which fat is localized around the waist and in the upper body, most frequently seen in men 男性肥胖；**gynecoid o., gynoid o.**, obesity in which fat is localized in the lower half of the body, most frequently seen in women 女性肥胖；**lifelong o.**, that beginning in childhood and characterized by an increase both in number (hyperplasia) and in size (hypertrophy) of adipose cells 终身性肥胖症；**morbid o.**, obesity in which a person is 45 kg (100 pounds) or more over ideal weight or has a body mass index of 40 or more 病态肥胖症

obex (o′beks) the ependyma-lined junction of the taeniae of the fourth ventricle of the brain at the inferior angle 闩（菱形窝下角处，两侧外下界之间的圆弧形移行部）

ob·jec·tive (ob-jek′tiv) 1. perceptible by the external senses 客观的；2. a result achieved by an effort 目标；3. the lens or system of lenses of a microscope (or telescope) nearest the object that is being examined 物镜

ob·li·gate (ob′lĭ-gāt) pertaining to or characterized by the ability to survive only in a particular environment or to assume only a particular role, such as an obligate anaerobe 专性的（如专性厌氧菌）；有义务的

ob·lig·a·to·ry (ob-lig′ə-tor″e) 同 obligate

obliq·ui·ty (o-blik′wĭ-te) the state of being inclined or slanting 倾斜，斜度；**oblique′** adj.；**Litzmann o.**, inclination of the fetal head so that the posterior parietal bone presents to the birth canal 利次曼倾斜；**Nägele o.**, presentation of the anterior parietal bone to the birth canal, the biparietal diameter being oblique to the brim of the pelvis Nägele 斜度，前顶骨朝向产道，双顶径倾向于骨盆口

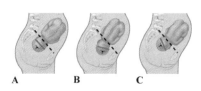

▲ 斜度

oblit·er·a·tion (ob-lit″ər-a′shən) complete removal by disease, degeneration, surgical procedure, irradiation, etc. 消灭，消失（因疾病、变性、外科手术、照射法等使之完全消除）

ob·lon·ga·ta (ob″long-gah′tə) medulla oblongata 延髓；**oblonga′tal** *adj.*

ob·ses·sion (ob-sesh′ən) a persistent unwanted idea or impulse that cannot be eliminated by reasoning 强迫症，强迫观念；**obses′sive** *adj.*

ob·ses·sive-com·pul·sive (əb-ses′iv-kəmpul′siv) pertaining to obsessions and compulsions, to obsessive-compulsive disorder, or to obsessive-compulsive personality disorder 强迫观念与行为的

ob·ste·tri·cian (ob″stə-trĭ′shən) one who practices obstetrics 产科医生

ob·stet·rics (ob-stet′riks) the branch of medicine dealing with pregnancy, labor, and the puerperium 产科学；**obstet′ric, obstet′rical** *adj.*

ob·sti·pa·tion (ob″stĭ-pa′shən) intractable constipation 顽固便秘

ob·struc·tion (ob-struk′shən) 1. the act of blocking or clogging 阻塞；2. block; occlusion; the state or condition of being clogged 梗阻；**obstruc′tive** *adj.*

ob·tund (ob-tund′) to render dull, blunt, or less acute, or to reduce alertness 变钝；缓和，抑制（疼痛等）

ob·tun·da·tion (ob″tən-da′shən) mental blunting with mild to moderate reduction in alertness and a diminished sensation of pain 意识混浊不清

ob·tun·dent (ob-tun′dənt) 1. pertaining to or causing obtundation 使感觉迟钝的；2. having the power to soothe pain 止痛的；3. an agent that blunts irritation or soothes pain 缓和药，安抚药

ob·tu·ra·tor (ob′tə-ra′tər) a disk or plate, natural or artificial, that closes an opening 闭塞器

ob·tu·sion (ob-too′zhən) a deadening or blunting of sensitivity 感觉迟钝

OCA 1. Oculocutaneous albinism 眼皮肤白化病；2. Obeticholic acid 奥贝胆酸

Oc·a·liv·a (oh-ca′liv-ə) trademark for a preparation of obeticholic acid 奥贝胆酸

oc·cip·i·tal (ok-sip′ĭ-təl) pertaining to or near the occiput or the occipital bone 枕部的，枕骨的

oc·cip·i·ta·lis (ok-sip″ĭ-ta′lis) [L.] 1. 同 occipital; 2. the occipital belly of the occipitofrontalis muscle 枕额肌的枕腹

oc·cip·i·tal·iza·tion (ok-sip″ĭ-təl-ĭ-za′shən) synostosis of the atlas with the occipital bone 寰椎骨性接合，寰（椎）枕骨化

oc·cip·i·to·cer·vi·cal (ok-sip″ĭ-to-sur′vĭ-kəl) pertaining to the occiput and neck 枕颈的

oc·cip·i·to·fron·tal (ok-sip″ĭ-to-frun′təl) pertaining to the occiput and the forehead 枕额的

oc·cip·i·to·mas·toid (ok-sip″ĭ-to-mas′toid) pertaining to the occipital bone and mastoid process 枕乳突的

oc·cip·i·to·men·tal (ok-sip″ĭ-to-men′təl) pertaining to the occiput and chin 枕颏的

oc·cip·i·to·pa·ri·e·tal (ok-sip″ĭ-to-pə-ri′ə-təl) pertaining to the occipital and parietal bones or lobes of the brain 枕顶的

oc·cip·i·to·tem·po·ral (ok-sip″ĭ-to-tem′pə-rəl) pertaining to the occipital and temporal bones 枕颞的

oc·cip·i·to·tha·lam·ic (ok-sip″ĭ-to-thə-lam′ik) pertaining to the occipital lobe and thalamus 枕叶丘脑的

oc·ci·put (ok′sĭ-pət) the posterior part of the head 枕（骨）部；**occip′ital** *adj.*

oc·clude (ə-klood′) to fit close together; to close tight; to obstruct or close off 殆，咬合；闭塞，闭合

oc·clu·sal (ə-kloo′zəl) 1. pertaining to the masticating surfaces of the premolar and molar teeth（上下齿）咬合（面）的；2. 同 occlusive

oc·clu·sion (ə-kloo′zhən) 1. obstruction; 2. the trapping of a liquid or gas within cavities in a solid or on its surface 液体或气体栓塞；3. the relation of the teeth of both jaws when in functional contact during activity of the mandible 殆，咬合；4. momentary complete closure of some area in the vocal tract, causing the breath to stop and pressure to accumulate 声道闭塞；**abnormal o.,** malocclusion 异常殆；**balanced o.,** occlusion in which the teeth are in harmonious working relation 平衡咬合；**centric o.,** that in the vertical and horizontal position of the mandible in which the cusps of the mandibular and maxillary teeth interdigitate maximally 正中殆；**coronary o.,** complete obstruction of an artery of the heart 冠状动脉闭塞；**eccentric o.,** occlusion of the teeth when the lower jaw has moved from the centric position. 偏心咬合；**habitual o.,** the consistent relationship of the teeth in the maxilla to those of the mandible when the teeth in both jaws are brought into maximum contact 习惯性咬合；**lateral o.,** occlusion of the teeth when the lower jaw is moved to the right or left of centric occlusion 侧向殆；**lingual o.,** malocclusion in which the tooth is lingual to the line of the normal dental arch 舌侧集中殆；**mesial o.,** the position of a lower tooth when it is mesial to its opposite number in the maxilla 近中殆；**normal o.,** the contact of the upper and lower teeth in the centric relationship 正常殆；**protrusive o.,** anteroclusion 前伸殆；**retrusive o.,** distoclusion. 后退殆；**venous o.,** the blocking of venous return 静脉闭塞

oc·clu·sive (ə-kloo′siv) pertaining to or causing occlusion 闭塞的，闭合的；咬合的

oc·cult (ə-kult′) obscure or hidden from view 隐

的，隐伏的，潜隐的；难懂的

OCD obsessive-compulsive disorder 强迫症

Ochro·bac·trum (o″kro-bak′trəm) a widely distributed genus of gram-negative, aerobic, motile, rod-shaped bacteria that is a cause of nosocomial infections 苍白杆菌属

Ochro·co·nis (o″krə-co′nis) a genus of dematiaceous anamorphic fungi that has been found in opportunistic infections. *O. gallopa′va* causes infections of the central nervous system, particularly brain abscesses, and respiratory tracts 赭霉属

ochrom·e·ter (o-krom′ə-tər) an instrument for measuring capillary blood pressure 毛细管血压计

ochro·no·sis (o″krə-no′sis) deposition of dark pigment in the connective tissues, usually secondary to alkaptonuria, characterized by urine that darkens on standing and dusky discoloration of the sclerae and ears 褐黄病；**ochronot′ic** *adj.*

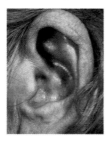

▲ 褐黄病

OCRD obsessive-compulsive and related disorders 强迫观念与行为及相关疾病

oc·ri·plas·min (awk-ri-plaz′min) a recombinant proteolytic enzyme that inhibits vitreous proteins such as laminin, fibronectin, and collagen to dissolve the protein matrix and treat the symptoms of vitreomacular adhesion 奥克纤溶酶

OCT optical coherence tomography 光学相干断层成像；ornithine carbamoyltransferase 鸟氨酸氨基甲酰转移酶；oxytocin challenge test 催产素激惹试验

oc·tin·ox·ate (ok-tin′ok-sāt) an absorber of ultraviolet B radiation, used topically as a sunscreen 桂皮酸盐，甲氧基肉桂酸辛酯，一种防晒成分

oc·ti·sal·ate (ok″tĭ-sal′āt) a substituted salicylate that absorbs ultraviolet light in the UVB range, used as a sunscreen 水杨酸盐

oc·to·cryl·ene (ok′to-kril″ēn) a sunscreen that absorbs ultraviolet B radiation 氰双苯丙烯酸辛酯（遮光剂）

oc·to·pam·ine (ok″to-pam′ēn) a sympathomimetic amine thought to result from inability of the diseased liver to metabolize tyrosine; it is called a false neurotransmitter because it can be stored in presynaptic vesicles, replacing norepinephrine, but has little effect on postsynaptic receptors 章胺，羟基苯乙醇胺

oc·tre·o·tide (ok-tre′o-tīd) a synthetic analogue of somatostatin, used as the acetate ester in the palliative treatment of the symptoms of gastrointestinal endocrine tumors and in the treatment of acromegaly 奥曲肽

oc·tyl meth·oxy·cin·na·mate (ok′təl mə- thok″se-sin′ə-māt) 同 octinoxate

oc·u·lar (ok′u-lər) 1. of, pertaining to, or affecting the eye 眼的；2. eyepiece 目镜

oc·u·lo·cu·ta·ne·ous (ok″u-lo-ku-ta′ne-əs) pertaining to or affecting the eyes and the skin 眼（与）皮的

oc·u·lo·fa·cial (ok″u-lo-fa′shəl) pertaining to the eyes and the face 眼面的

oc·u·lo·gy·ra·tion (ok″u-lo-ji-ra′shən) movement of the eye about the anteroposterior axis 眼球转动；**oculogy′ric** *adj.*

oc·u·lo·mo·tor (ok″u-lo-mo′tər) 1. pertaining to or affecting eye movements 眼球运动的；2. pertaining to the oculomotor nerve 动眼神经的

oc·u·lo·my·co·sis (ok″u-lo-mi-ko′sis) a fungal disease of the eye 眼真菌病

oc·u·lo·na·sal (ok″u-lo-na′səl) pertaining to the eye and the nose 眼鼻的

oc·u·lo·zy·go·mat·ic (ok″u-lo-zi″go-mat′ik) pertaining to the eye and the zygoma 眼颧的

oc·u·lus (ok′u-ləs) pl. *o′culi* [L.] eye 眼

OD[1] [L.] o′culus dex′ter (right eye) 右眼

OD[2] Doctor of Optometry 视力测定术博士；overdose 过量

odon·tal·gia (o-don-tal′jə) toothache 牙痛

odon·tec·to·my (o″don-tek′tə-me) excision of a tooth 牙切除术，拔牙

odon·tic (o-don′tik) pertaining to the teeth 牙的

odon·to·blast (o-don′to-blast) one of the connective tissue cells that deposit dentin and form the outer surface of the dental pulp 成牙质细胞；**odontoblas′tic** *adj.*

odon·to·blas·to·ma (o-don″to-blas-to′mə) a tumor made up of odontoblasts 成牙质细胞瘤

odon·to·clast (o-don′to-klast) an osteoclast associated with absorption of the roots of deciduous teeth 破牙质细胞

odon·to·gen·e·sis (o-don″to-jen′ə-sis) the origin and histogenesis of the teeth 牙发生，牙生成；**odontogenet′ic** *adj.*；*o. imperfec′ta*, dentinogenesis imperfecta 牙生长不全

odon·to·gen·ic (o-don″to-jen′ik) 1. forming teeth

生牙的；2. arising in tissues that give origin to the teeth 牙源性的

odon·toid (o-don'toid) like a tooth 牙样，牙形的

odon·tol·o·gy (o″don-tol'ə-je) 1. scientific study of the teeth 针对牙齿的科学研究；2. dentistry 牙科学

odon·tol·y·sis (o-don-tol'ĭ-sis) the resorption of dental tissue 牙质溶解

odon·to·ma (o-don-to'mə) 1. odontogenic tumor 牙源性肿瘤；2. a specific type of mixed odontogenic tumor, in which both the epithelial and mesenchymal cells exhibit complete differentiation, resulting in formation of tooth structures 复合牙瘤；**composite o.,** one consisting of both enamel and dentin in an abnormal pattern 复质牙瘤；**radicular o.,** one associated with a tooth root, or formed when the root was developing 连根牙瘤

odon·top·a·thy (o″don-top'ə-the) any disease of the teeth 牙病；**odontopath'ic** adj.

odon·tot·o·my (o″don-tot'ə-me) incision of a tooth 牙切开术，牙体洞术

odor (o'dər) a volatile emanation perceived by the sense of smell 气味

odor·ant (o'dər-ənt) any substance capable of stimulating the sense of smell 臭气物质

odyn·om·e·ter (o″din-om'ə-tər) algesimeter 痛觉计

od·y·no·pha·gia (od″ĭ-no-fa'jə) a dysphagia in which swallowing causes pain 吞咽痛

Oer·sko·via (er-sko've-ə) a genus of grampositive bacteria, consisting of branching hyphae that break up into motile flagellate rods; it is an opportunistic pathogen 厄氏菌属

oesoph·a·go·sto·mi·a·sis (ə-sof″ə-go-stomi'ə-sis) infection with *Oesophagostomum* 结节线虫病

Oesoph·a·gos·to·mum (ə-sof″ə-gos'to-məm) a genus of nematode worms found in the intestines of various animals 结节线虫属

Oes·trus (es'trəs) a genus of botflies. *O. o'vis* deposits its larvae in nasal passages of sheep and goats, and may cause ocular myiasis in humans 狂蝇属

OFC orbitofrontal cortex 眶额皮质

of·fi·cial (ə-fish'əl) authorized by a current pharmacopeia or recognized formulary 官方的，法定的，正式的

of·fic·i·nal (o-fis'ĭ-nəl) denoting pharmaceutical preparations that are regularly kept at pharmacies 药房常备有售的

oflox·a·cin (o-flok'sə-sin) an antibacterial agent effective against a wide variety of gram-negative and gram-positive aerobic organisms 氧氟沙星

ohm (Ω) (ōm) the SI unit of electrical resistance, being that of a resistor in which a current of 1 ampere is produced by a potential difference of 1 volt 欧（姆），电阻单位

ohm·me·ter (ōm'me-tər) an instrument that measures electrical resistance in ohms 欧姆计

OI osteogenesis imperfecta 成骨不全

OIC opioid-induced constipation 阿片类药物相关性便秘

oil (oil) 1. an unctuous, combustible substance that is liquid, or easily liquefiable, on warming, and is soluble in ether but not in water. Oils may be animal, vegetable, or mineral in origin, and volatile or nonvolatile (fixed). A number of oils are used as flavoring or perfuming agents in pharmaceutical preparations 油；2. a fat that is liquid at room temperature 油脂，室温下为液体；**borage o.,** that extracted from the seeds of borage; used for the treatment of neurodermatitis and as a food supplement 琉璃苣油；**cajeput o.,** a volatile oil from the fresh leaves and twigs of cajeput; used as a stimulant and rubefacient in rheumatism and other muscle and joint pain 玉树油；**canola o.,** rapeseed oil, specifically that prepared from plants bred to be low in erucic acid 油菜籽油；**castor o.,** a fixed oil obtained from the seed of *Ricinus communis;* used as a bland topical emollient and also occasionally as a strong cathartic 蓖麻油；**clove o.,** a volatile oil from cloves; used externally in the treatment of colds and headache and as a dental antiseptic and analgesic; it also has various uses in Indian medicine 丁香油；**cod liver o.,** partially desteararated, fixed oil from fresh livers of *Gadus morrhua* and other fish of the family Gadidae; used as a source of vitamins A and D 鱼肝油；**corn o.,** a refined fixed oil obtained from the embryo of *Zea mays;* used as a solvent and vehicle for various medicinal agents and as a vehicle for injections. It has also been promoted as a source of polyunsaturated fatty acids in special diets 玉米油；**cottonseed o.,** a fixed oil from seeds of cultivated varieties of the cotton plant *(Gossypium);* used as a solvent and vehicle for drugs 棉籽油；**essential o.,** 同 volatile o.；**ethiodized o.,** an iodine addition product of the ethyl ester of fatty acids of poppyseed oil; used as a diagnostic radiopaque medium 乙碘油；**eucalyptus o.,** a volatile oil from the fresh leaf of species of *Eucalyptus;* used as a pharmaceutical flavoring agent, as an expectorant and local antiseptic, for rheumatism, and in folk medicine 桉树油；**evening primrose o.,** that produced from the ripe seeds of evening primrose *(Oenothera biennis);* used in the treatment of mastalgia, premenstrual syndrome, and atopic eczema 月见草油；**expressed o., fatty o., fixed o.,** a nonvolatile oil, i.e., one that does not evaporate on warming; such oils consist of a mixture of fatty acids and their esters, and are classified as solid, semisolid, and liquid or as drying, semidrying, and nondrying as a function of their tendency to solidify on exposure to air 压榨油；**fennel o.,** a volatile oil distilled from fennel (the seeds of *Foeniculum vulgare*); used for cough, bronchitis, and dyspepsia and as a pharmaceutical flavoring agent 茴香油；**iodized o.,** an iodine addition product of vegetable oil; used as a diagnostic radiopaque medium 碘油；**lavender o.,** a volatile oil distilled from the flowering tops of lavender or prepared synthetically; used for loss of appetite, dyspepsia, nervousness, and insomnia; also widely used in folk medicine 薰衣草油；**mineral o.,** a mixture of liquid hydrocarbons from petroleum; used as a lubricant laxative, drug vehicle, and skin emollient and cleanser. *Light mineral o.,* of lesser density, is used similarly 矿物油；**olive o.,** a fixed oil obtained from ripe fruit of *Olea europaea;* used as a setting retardant for dental cements, topical emollient, pharmaceutical necessity, and sometimes as a laxative 橄榄油；**peanut o.,** the refined fixed oil from peanuts (*Arachis hypogaea);* used as a solvent and vehicle for drugs 花生油；**peppermint o.,** a volatile oil from fresh overground parts of the flowering plant of peppermint (*Mentha piperita);* used as a flavoring agent for drugs, and as a gastric stimulant and carminative 薄荷油；**rapeseed o.,** the oil expressed from the seeds of the rapeseed plant; used in the manufacture of soaps, margarines, and lubricants 菜籽油，另参见 *canola o.*；**safflower o.,** an oily liquid extracted from the seeds of the safflower, *Carthamus tinctorius,* containing predominantly linoleic acid; used as a pharmaceutical aid, as a component of total parenteral nutrition solutions, and in the management of hypercholesterolemia 红花油；**silicone o.,** any of various longchain fluid silicone polymers, some of which are injected into the vitreous to serve as a vitreous substitute during or after vitreoretinal surgery 硅油；**tea tree o.,** an essential oil from the leaves and branch tips of the tea tree; it has bacteriostatic and weak antiviral and antimycotic properties, is used topically for skin infections and internally and externally in folk medicine for various indications 茶树油；**thyme o.,** the volatile oil extracted from fresh, flowering thyme; used as an antitussive and expectorant 麝香草油；**volatile o.,** one that evaporates readily, usually found in aromatic plants; most are a mixture of two or more terpenes 精油，挥发油；**volatile o. of mustard,** a volatile oil distilled from the seeds of black mustard (*Brassica nigra);* used as a strong counterirritant and rubefacient 挥发性芥子油

oint·ment (oint′mənt) a semisolid preparation for external application to the skin or mucous membranes, usually containing a medicinal substance 软膏（剂），油膏

oja (o′jə) in ayurveda, the imprint of self in the physical body, which arises from the strength of the metabolism and balance a body maintains in knowing itself, thus governing the immune system 营养要素

OL [L.] o′culus lae′vus (left eye) 左眼

-ol word termination indicating a hydroxyl derivative of a hydrocarbon, e.g., an alcohol or a phenol [后缀] 醇，酚

ol·amine (ol′ə-mēn) USAN contraction for ethanolamine 乙醇胺（ethanolamine 的 USAN 缩约词）

olan·za·pine (o-lan′zə-pēn) a monoaminergic antagonist used as an antipsychotic 奥氮平

ole·ag·i·nous (o″le-aj′ĭ-nəs) oily; greasy 油脂性的，油状的

ole·ate (o′le-āt) 1. a salt, ester, or anion of oleic acid 油酸盐，油酸酯，油酸根；2. a solution of a substance in oleic acid; used as an ointment 油酸制剂

olec·ran·ar·thri·tis (o-lek″rə-nahr-thri′tis) anconitis 肘关节炎

olec·ra·non (o-lek′rə-non) bony projection of the ulna at the elbow 鹰嘴；**olec′ranal** *adj.*

ole·ic ac·id (o-le′ik) a monounsaturated 18- carbon fatty acid found in most animal fats and vegetable oils; used in pharmacy as an emulsifier and to assist absorption of some drugs by the skin 油酸

ole·in (o′le-in) the triglyceride formed from oleic acid, occurring in most fats and oils 油酸甘油酯，油酰甘油

oleo·res·in (o″le-o-rez′in) 1. a natural combination of a resin and a volatile oil, such as exudes from pines 松脂；2. a compound extracted from a drug, containing both volatile oil and resin, by percolation with a volatile solvent, such as acetone, alcohol, or ether, and removal of the solvent 油树脂

oleo·vi·ta·min (o″le-o-vi′tə-min) a preparation of fish liver oil or edible vegetable oil containing one or more fat-soluble vitamins or their derivatives 维生素油剂

ole·um (o′le-əm) pl. *o′lea* [L.] 同 oil

ol·fact (ol′fakt) a unit of odor, the minimum perceptible odor, being the minimum concentration of a substance in solution that can be perceived by a large number of normal individuals; expressed in grams per liter 嗅阈值，嗅觉系数

ol·fac·tion (ol-fak′shən) 1. smell; the ability to perceive and distinguish odors 嗅觉；2. the act of perceiving and distinguishing odors 嗅（动作）

ol·fac·tol·o·gy (ol″fak-tol′ə-je) the science of the sense of smell 嗅觉学

ol·fac·tom·e·ter (ol″fak-tom′ə-tər) an instrument for testing the sense of smell 嗅觉计

ol·fac·to·ry (ol-fak′tə-re) pertaining to the sense of smell 嗅觉的

Oli·gel·la (ol″ĭ-gel′ə) a genus of gram-negative, aerobic, rod-shaped bacteria that includes species that cause urinary tract infections and septicemia 寡源杆菌属

ol·i·go·as·then·o·sper·mia (ol″ĭ-go-as″thə-no-spur′me-ə) oligospermia with decreased sperm motility 少精症，弱精症

ol·i·go·clo·nal (ol″ĭ-go-klo′nəl) pertaining to or derived from a few clones 寡克隆的

ol·i·go·cys·tic (ol″ĭ-go-sis′tik) containing few cysts 少囊的

ol·i·go·dac·ty·ly (ol″ĭ-go-dak′tə-le) the presence of less than the usual number of fingers or toes 少指（畸形），少趾（畸形）

ol·i·go·den·dro·cyte (ol″ĭ-go-den′dro-sīt) a cell of the oligodendroglia 少突胶质细胞

ol·i·go·den·drog·lia (ol″ĭ-go-den-drog′le-ə) 1. the nonneural cells of ectodermal origin forming part of the adventitial structure (neuroglia) of the central nervous system 少突胶质细胞；2. the tissue composed of such cells 少突胶质

ol·i·go·den·dro·gli·o·ma (ol″ĭ-go-den″drogli-o′mə) a neoplasm derived from and composed of oligodendrocytes in varying stages of differentiation 少突神经胶质瘤，少突胶质（细胞）瘤

ol·i·go·dip·sia (ol″ĭ-go-dip′se-ə) hypodipsia 渴感过少

ol·i·go·don·tia (ol″ĭ-go-don′shə) the presence of fewer than the normal number of teeth 少牙（畸形）

ol·i·go·ga·lac·tia (ol″ĭ-go-gə-lak′she-ə) hypogalactia 乳汁分泌过少

ol·i·go·gen·ic (ol″ĭ-go-jen′ik) produced or influenced by the action of a few different genes 寡基因的

ol·i·go·hy·dram·ni·os (ol″ĭ-go-hi-dram′ne-os) deficiency in the amount of amniotic fluid 羊水过少

ol·i·go·meg·a·ne·phro·nia (ol″ĭ-go-meg″ə- nə-fro′ne-ə) congenital renal hypoplasia in which there is a reduced number of lobes and nephrons, with hypertrophy of the nephrons 先天性肾单位减少代偿肥大; **oligomeganephron′ic** adj.

ol·i·go·men·or·rhea (ol″ĭ-go-men″ə-re′ə) abnormally infrequent menstruation 月经稀少

ol·i·go·mer (ol″ĭ-go-mər) a polymer formed by the combination of relatively few monomers 寡聚体

ol·i·go·nu·cle·o·tide (ol″ĭ-go-noo′kle-o-tīd) a sin-gle-stranded nucleic acid segment of a few (usually fewer than 20) nucleotides 寡核苷酸

ol·i·go·sac·cha·ride (ol″ĭ-go-sak′ə-rīd) a carbohydrate which on hydrolysis yields a small number of monosaccharides 寡糖，低聚糖

ol·i·go·sper·mia (ol″ĭ-go-spur′me-ə) decreased number of spermatozoa in the semen 精子减少（症），少精液症

ol·i·go·syn·ap·tic (ol″ĭ-go-sin-ap′tik) involving a few synapses in series and therefore a sequence of only a few neurons 少突触的

ol·i·go·zo·o·sper·mia (ol″ĭ-go-zo″o-spur′me-ə) 同 oligospermia

ol·i·gu·ria (ol″ĭ-gu′re-ə) diminished urine production and excretion in relation to fluid intake 少尿; **oligu′ric** adj.

oli·va (o-li′və) pl. *oli′vae* [L.] 同 olive (2)

ol·i·vary (ol′ĭ-var″e) 1. shaped like an olive 橄榄状的；2. pertaining to the olive 橄榄的

ol·ive (ol′iv) 1. the tree *Olea europaea* and its fruit 橄榄；2. olivary body; a rounded elevation lateral to the upper part of each pyramid of the medulla oblongata 橄榄体

ol·i·vif·u·gal (ol″ĭ-vif′u-gəl) moving or conducting away from the olive 离橄榄体的

ol·i·vip·e·tal (ol″ĭ-vip′ə-təl) moving or conducting toward the olive 向橄榄体的

ol·i·vo·pon·to·cer·e·bel·lar (ol″ĭ-vo-pon″toser″ə-bel′ər) pertaining to the olive, the middle peduncles, and the cerebellar cortex 橄榄体脑桥小脑的

ol·me·sar·tan **me·dox·o·mil** (ol″mə-sahr′tan mə-dok′sə-mil) an angiotensin II receptor antagonist, used in the treatment of hypertension 奥美沙坦

olo·pa·ta·dine (o″lo-pat′ə-dēn) an antihistamine used as the hydrochloride salt in the topical treatment of allergic conjunctivitis 奥洛他定

ol·sal·a·zine (ol-sal′ə-zēn) a derivative of mesalamine used as the sodium salt as an antiinflammatory in ulcerative colitis 奥沙拉秦

OMD Doctor of Oriental Medicine 东方医学博士

omen·tal (o-men′təl) pertaining to the omentum 网膜的

omen·tec·to·my (o″mən-tek′tə-me) excision of all or part of the omentum 网膜切除术

omen·ti·tis (o″mən-ti′tis) inflammation of the omentum 网膜炎

omen·to·pexy (o-men′to-pek″se) fixation of the omentum, especially to establish collateral circulation in portal obstruction 网膜固定术

omen·tor·rha·phy (o″mən-tor′ə-fe) suture or repair of the omentum 网膜缝合术

omen·tum (o-men′təm) pl. *omen′ta* [L.] a fold of

peritoneum extending from the stomach to adjacent abdominal organs 网膜；**colic o., gastrocolic o.,** 同 greater o.；**gastrohepatic o.,** 同 lesser o.；**greater o.,** a peritoneal fold suspended from the greater curvature of the stomach and attached to the anterior surface of the transverse colon 大网膜；**lesser o.,** a peritoneal fold joining the lesser curvature of the stomach and the first part of the duodenum to the porta hepatis 小网膜；**o. ma′jus,** 同 greater o.；**o. mi′nus,** 同 lesser o.

omep·ra·zole (o-mep′rə-zōl) an inhibitor of gastric acid secretion used in the treatment of dyspepsia, gastroesophageal reflux disease, disorders of gastric hypersecretion, and peptic ulcer, including that associated with *Helicobacter pylori* infection 奥美拉唑

omo·cla·vic·u·lar (o″mo-klə-vik′u-lər) pertaining to the shoulder and clavicle 肩锁的

omo·hy·oid (o″mo-hi′oid) pertaining to the shoulder and the hyoid bone 肩胛舌骨的

om·pha·lec·to·my (om″fə-lek′tə-me) excision of the umbilicus 脐切除术

om·phal·ic (om-fal′ik) umbilical 脐的

om·pha·li·tis (om″fə-li′tis) inflammation of the umbilicus 脐炎

om·pha·lo·cele (om′fə-lo-sēl″) protrusion, at birth, of part of the intestine through a defect in the abdominal wall at the umbilicus 脐膨出

om·pha·lo·mes·en·ter·ic (om″fə-lo-mes″ənter′ik) pertaining to the umbilicus and mesentery 脐肠系膜的

om·pha·lo·phle·bi·tis (om″fə-lo-flə-bi′tis) inflammation of the umbilical veins 脐静脉炎

om·pha·lor·rha·gia (om″fə-lo-ra′jə) hemorrhage from the umbilicus 脐出血

om·pha·lor·rhea (om″fə-lo-re′ə) effusion of lymph at the umbilicus 脐溢液

om·pha·lor·rhex·is (om″fə-lo-rek′sis) rupture of the umbilicus 脐破裂

om·pha·lot·o·my (om″fə-lot′ə-me) the cutting of the umbilical cord 断脐术

Om·pha·lo·tus (om″fə-lo′təs) a genus of mushrooms including several species, *O. olea′rius* and *O. oliva′scens* (jack-o-lantern mushrooms), that cause severe gastrointestinal irritation 类脐菇属

ona·bot·u·li·num·tox·in A (on″ə-boch″u-li′-nəm-tok″sin) a preparation of botulinum toxin type A, used to prevent migraine and to treat cervical dystonia, upper limb spasticity, strabismus, blepharospasm, primary axillary hyperhidrosis, and glabellar lines 肉毒毒素 A 制剂，可用于预防偏头痛，治疗颈部肌张力障碍、上肢痉挛、斜视、眼睑痉挛、原发性腋窝多汗症和眉间纹

On·cho·cer·ca (ong″ko-sur′kə) a genus of nematode parasites of the superfamily Filarioidea, including *O. vol′vulus,* which causes onchocerciasis 盘尾（丝虫）属

on·cho·cer·ci·a·sis (ong″ko-sər-ki′ə-sis) infection by nematodes of the genus *Onchocerca.* Parasites invade the skin, superficial fascia, and other parts of the body, producing fibrous nodules; blindness occurs after ocular invasion 盘尾丝虫病

on·cho·cer·co·ma (ong″ko-sər-ko′mə) one of the dermal or subcutaneous nodules containing *Onchocerca volvulus* in human onchocerciasis 盘尾丝虫瘤

on·co·cyte (ong′ko-sīt) a large epithelial cell with an extremely acidophilic and granular cytoplasm, containing vast numbers of mitochondria; such cells may undergo neoplastic transformation 嗜酸瘤细胞；**oncocyt′ic** adj.

on·co·cy·to·ma (ong″ko-si-to′mə) 1. a usually benign adenoma composed of oncocytes with granular, eosinophilic cytoplasm 大嗜酸粒细胞瘤，一种常见的良性腺瘤，由颗粒状大嗜酸粒细胞组成；2. a benign Hürthle cell tumor 良性 Hürthle 细胞瘤；**renal o.,** a benign neoplasm of the kidney resembling a renal cell carcinoma but encapsulated and not invasive 肾嗜酸细胞瘤

on·co·cy·to·sis (on″ko-si-to′sis) metaplasia of oncocytes 嗜酸瘤细胞化生

on·co·fe·tal (ong″ko-fe′təl) carcinoembryonic 癌胚的

on·co·gen·e·sis (ong″ko-jen′ə-sis) tumorigenesis 瘤形成，瘤发生；**oncogenet′ic** adj.

on·co·gen·ic (ong″ko-jen′ik) giving rise to tumors or causing tumor formation; said especially of tumor-inducing viruses 致瘤的

on·cog·e·nous (ong-koj′ə-nəs) arising in or originating from a tumor 肿瘤源的

on·col·o·gy (ong-kol′ə-je) the sum of knowledge regarding tumors; the study of tumors 肿瘤学

on·col·y·sate (ong-kol′ĭ-sāt) any agent that lyses or destroys tumor cells 肿瘤溶解剂

on·col·y·sis (ong-kol′ĭ-sis) destruction or dissolution of a neoplasm 癌细胞溶解，溶癌作用；**oncolyt′ic** adj.

on·co·sis (ong-ko′sis) a morbid condition marked by the development of tumors 肿瘤病

on·co·sphere (ong′ko-sfēr) the larva of the tapeworm contained within the external embryonic envelope and armed with six hooks 六钩蚴

on·cot·ic (ong-kot′ik) 1. pertaining to swelling 肿胀的；2. 参见 *pressure* 下词条

on·cot·o·my (ong-kot′ə-me) the incision of a tumor or swelling 肿块切开术

on·co·tro·pic (ong″ko-tro′pik) having special affinity for tumor cells 亲肿瘤的

On·co·vin (on′ko-vin) trademark for a preparation of vincristine sulfate 硫酸长春新碱制剂的商品名

on·co·vi·rus (ong′ko-vi″rəs) any of various tumor-producing RNA viruses 肿瘤病毒

on·dan·se·tron (on-dan′sə-tron) a serotonin receptor antagonist used as the base or the hydrochloride salt as an antiemetic 昂丹司琼

onei·ric (o-ni′rik) pertaining to or characterized by dreaming or oneirism 梦样的，梦的

onei·rism (o-ni′riz-əm) a waking dream state 梦幻症，梦样状态，醒梦状态

on·lay (on′la″) 高嵌体 1. a graft applied or laid on the surface of an organ or structure 放在器官或组织表面上的移植物；2. a cast metal restoration that overlays cusps and lends strength to the restored tooth 覆盖牙尖的铸造金属修复体

on·o·mato·ma·nia (on″ə-mat″ə-ma′ne-ə) irresistible preoccupation with specific words or names 强迫性观念插入症，称名癖

ONS Oncology Nursing Society 肿瘤护理学会

on·to·gen·e·sis (on″to-jen′ə-sis) 同 ontogeny

on·tog·e·ny (on-toj′ə-ne) the complete developmental history of an individual organism 个体发育，个体发生；**ontogenet′ic, ontogen′ic** adj.

ony·al·ai (on′ne-al′a-e) a form of thrombocytopenic purpura due to a nutritional disorder occurring in blacks in Africa 奥尼赖病（血小板减少性紫癜的一型，见于非洲）

on·y·cha·tro·phia (on″ī-kə-tro′fe-ə) atrophy of a nail or the nails 甲萎缩

on·y·chaux·is (on″ī-kawk′sis) hypertrophy of the nails 甲肥厚

on·y·chec·to·my (on″ī-kek′tə-me) excision of a nail or nail bed 甲切除术

onych·ia (o-nik′e-ə) inflammation of the nail bed, resulting in loss of the nail 甲床炎

on·y·chi·tis (on″ī-ki′tis) 同 onychia

on·y·cho·dys·tro·phy (on″ī-ko-dis′trə-fe) malformation of a nail 指甲营养不良

on·y·cho·graph (o-nik′o-graf″) an instrument for observing and recording the nail pulse and capillary circulation 指甲毛细管搏动描记器

on·y·cho·gry·pho·sis (on″ī-ko-grə-fo′sis) hypertrophy and curving of the nails, giving them a claw-like appearance 甲弯曲

on·y·cho·gry·po·sis (on″ī-ko-grə-po′sis) 同 onychogryphosis

on·y·cho·het·ero·to·pia (on″ī-ko-het″ər-oto′pe-ə) abnormal location of the nails 指甲异位

on·y·chol·y·sis (on″ī-kol′ī-sis) loosening or separation of a nail from its bed 甲剥离

on·y·cho·ma·de·sis (on″ī-ko-mə-de′sis) complete loss of the nails 脱甲病

on·y·cho·ma·la·cia (on″ī-ko-mə-la′shə) softening of a nail or nails 甲软化，软甲

on·y·cho·my·co·sis (on″ī-ko-mi-ko′sis) fungal infection of the nails, often with thickening, opacification, crumbling, and onycholysis; often used interchangeably with *tinea unguium* because most infections are caused by dermatophytes 甲癣

on·y·chop·a·thy (on″ī-kop′ə-the) any disease of the nails 甲病；**onychopath′ic** adj.

on·y·cho·pha·gia (on″ī-ko-fa′jə) biting of the nails 咬甲癣

on·y·choph·a·gy (on″ī-kof′ə-je) 同 onychophagia

on·y·chor·rhex·is (on″ī-ko-rek′sis) spontaneous splitting or breaking of the nails 脆甲症

on·y·cho·schi·zia (on″ī-ko-skiz′e-ə) splitting of a nail in layers, usually at the free edge 甲分裂

on·y·cho·til·lo·ma·nia (on″ī-ko-til″o-ma′ne-ə) compulsive picking or tearing at the nails 剔甲癣

on·y·chot·o·my (on″ī-kot′ə-me) incision into a fingernail or toenail 甲切开术

on·yx (on′iks) nail (1) 甲

oo·blast (o′o-blast) a primordial cell from which an oocyte ultimately develops 成卵细胞

oo·cyst (o′o-sist) the encysted or encapsulated ookinete in the wall of a mosquito's stomach; also, the analogous stage in the development of any sporozoan 卵囊

oo·cyte (o′o-sīt) the immature female reproductive cell prior to fertilization; derived from an oogonium. It is a *primary o.* prior to completion of the first maturation division, and a *secondary o.* in the period between the first and second maturation divisions 卵母细胞

oog·a·my (o-og′ə-me) in the most restrictive sense, fertilization of a large nonmotile female gamete by a small motile male gamete, as in certain algae; often used more generally to mean the sexual union of two dissimilar gametes (heterogamy) 卵式生殖；**oog′amous** adj.

oo·gen·e·sis (o″o-jen′ə-sis) the process of formation of female gametes (oocytes) 卵子发生；**ooge-net′ic** adj.

oo·go·ni·um (o″o-go′ne-əm) pl. *oogo′nia* [Gr.] 1. a primordial oocyte during fetal development; it is derived from a primordial germ cell and before birth becomes a primary oocyte 卵原细胞；2. the female reproductive structure in certain fungi and algae 藏卵器，某些藻类和真菌中包含一个或多个配子的性结构

oo·ki·ne·sis (o″o-kī-ne′sis) the mitotic movements of the oocyte during maturation and fertilization 卵核分裂

oo·ki·nete (o″o-ki′nēt) (o″o-kī-net′) the fertilized

form of the malarial parasite in a mosquito's body, formed by fertilization of a macrogamete by a microgamete and developing into an oocyst 动合子（蚊体内疟原虫的授精型）

oo·lem·ma (o″o-lem′ə) zona pellucida 卵膜

ooph·o·rec·to·my (o″of-ə-rek′tə-me) excision of one or both ovaries 卵巢切除术

ooph·o·ri·tis (o″of-ə-ri′tis) inflammation of an ovary 卵巢炎

ooph·o·ro·cys·tec·to·my (o-of″ə-ro-sis-tek′tə-me) excision of an ovarian cyst 卵巢囊肿切除术

ooph·o·ro·cys·to·sis (o-of″ə-ro-sis-to′sis) the formation of ovarian cysts 卵巢囊肿形成

ooph·o·ro·hys·ter·ec·to·my (o-of″ə-ro-his″tərek′tə-me) excision of the ovaries and uterus 卵巢子宫切除术

ooph·o·ron (o-of′ə-ron) 同 ovary

ooph·o·ro·pexy (o-of′ə-ro-pek″se) the operation of elevating and fixing an ovary to the abdominal wall 卵巢固定术

ooph·o·ro·plas·ty (o-of′ə-ro-plas″te) plastic surgery of an ovary 卵巢成形术

ooph·o·ros·to·my (o-of″ə-ro-ros′tə-me) the creation of an opening into an ovarian cyst 卵巢（囊肿）造口（引流）术

ooph·o·rot·o·my (o-of″ə-rot′ə-me) incision of an ovary 卵巢切除术

oo·plasm (o′o-plaz″əm) the cytoplasm of an oocyte 卵质

oo·tid (o′o-tid) a mature oocyte; one of four cells derived from the two consecutive divisions of the primary oocyte. In mammals, the second maturation division is not completed unless fertilization occurs 卵（细胞）

opac·i·fi·ca·tion (o-pas″ĭ-fĭ-ka′shən) 1. the development of an opacity 浑浊化；2. the rendering opaque to x-rays of a tissue or organ by introduction of a contrast medium 造影

opac·i·ty (o-pas′ĭ-te) 1. the condition of being opaque 浑浊，不透明；2. an opaque area 不透明区

opal·es·cent (o″pəl-es′ənt) showing a milky iridescence, like an opal 乳色的，乳光的

opaque (o-pāk′) impervious to light rays or, by extension, to x-rays or other electromagnetic radiation （光束、X线或其他电磁辐射）不可穿透的

Op·di·vo (op-dee′voh) trademark for a preparation of nivolumab 纳武单抗

OPDM oculopharyngodistal myopathy 眼咽型远端肌病

open (o′pən) 1. not obstructed or closed 通畅的，开放的；2. exposed to the air; not covered by unbroken skin 敞开，暴露；3. pertaining to a study in which both subjects and experimenters know which treatment is administered to each subject 公开研究中每个受试者接受的治疗信息

open·ing (o′pən-ing) an aperture or open space; an anatomic opening may be called an *aditus, foramen, fossa, hiatus, orifice*, or *ostium* 开口或开放空间，解剖学开口可被称为 aditus, foramen, fossa, hiatus, orifice, ostium；**aortic o.**, 1. the aperture in the respiratory diaphragm for passage of the descending aorta 呼吸膈降主动脉的开口；2. see under *orifice*. 参见 orifice；**cardiac o.**, the opening from the esophagus into the stomach 贲门口；**caval o.**, foramen venae cavae 腔静脉裂口；**pyloric o.**, the opening between the stomach and duodenum 幽门口；**saphenous o.**, 隐静脉裂孔，参见 *hiatus* 下词条

op·er·a·ble (op′ər-ə-bəl) subject to being operated upon with a reasonable degree of safety; appropriate for surgical removal 可行手术的

op·er·ant (op′ər-ənt) in psychology, any response that is not elicited by specific external stimuli but that recurs at a given rate in a particular set of circumstances 操作性反应

op·er·a·tion (op″ər-a′shən) 1. any action performed with instruments or by the hands of a surgeon; a surgical procedure 操作，手术；2. any effect produced by a therapeutic agent 作用；**op′erative** *adj.*；**Albee o.**, an operation for ankylosis of the hip Albee 手术（股骨头髋臼融合术）；**Bassini o.**, plastic repair of inguinal hernia Bassini 手术（腹股沟疝修补术）；**Belsey Mark IV o.**, an operation for gastroesophageal reflux performed through a thoracic incision; the fundus ıs wrapped 270 degrees around the circumference of the esophagus, leaving its mastoid wall free Belsey Mark IV 手术，通过胸腔切口做的一种治疗胃食管反流病的手术；**Billroth o.**, partial resection of the stomach with anastomosis to the duodenum (Billroth I) or to the jejunum (Billroth II) 毕式手术；**Blalock-Taussig o.**, sideto-side anastomosis of the left subclavian artery to the left pulmonary artery to shunt some of the systemic circulation into the pulmonary circulation; performed as palliative treatment of tetralogy of Fallot or other congenital anomalies associated with insufficient pulmonary arterial flow 布 - 陶二式手术（锁骨下动脉肺动脉吻合术）；**Browne o.**, a type of urethroplasty for hypospadias repair, in which an intact strip of epithelium is left on the ventral surface of the penis to form the roof of the urethra, and the floor of the urethra is formed by epithelialization from the lateral wound margins 布朗手术（尿道成形术）；**Brunschwig o.**, pancreatoduodenectomy performed in two stages Brunschwig 手术（胰十二指肠切除术）；**Caldwell-Luc o.**, 1. antrostomy in which an opening is made into the maxillary sinus via an incision through the roof of the mouth opposite the premolar teeth 上颌窦造口术；2. in compound fractures of the zygomatic bone and maxilla, a method of packing of the maxillary sinus to allow reduction of displaced fragments of the zygoma by upward and outward pressure 上颌窦根治手术；**Cotte o.,** removal of the presacral nerve Cotte 手术（骶前神经切除术）；**Denis Browne o.,** 同 Browne o.；**Dührssen o.,** vaginal fixation of the uterus Dührssen 手术；**Dupuy-Dutemps o.,** blepharoplasty of the lower lid with tissue from the upper lid 经阴道子宫固定术；**Elliot o.,** sclerectomy by trephine 埃利奥特手术（环形巩膜切除术）；**equilibrating o.,** tenotomy of the direct antagonist of a paralyzed eye muscle 平衡手术（麻痹性斜视矫正术）；**exploratory o.,** incision into a body area to determine the cause of unexplained symptoms 探查术；**flap o.,** 1. any operation involving the raising of a flap of tissue 翻瓣术；2. in periodontics, an operation to secure greater access to granulation tissue and osseous defects, consisting of detachment of the gingivae and/or all or a portion of the alveolar mucosa 牙周翻瓣术；**Fothergill o.,** an operation for uterine prolapse by fixation of the cardinal ligaments Fothergill 手术（子宫主韧带固定术）；**Frazier-Spiller o.,** trigeminal rhizotomy using an approach through the middle cranial fossa 弗-斯二氏手术（经颅中窝三叉神经切断术）；**Fredet-Ramstedt o.,** pyloromyotomy 弗-腊二氏手术（先天幽门狭窄环状肌切断术）；**Hartmann o.,** resection of a diseased portion of the colon, with the proximal end of the colon brought out as a colostomy and the distal stump or rectum being closed by suture Hartmann 手术，手术切除憩室或病变肠道；**Kelly o.,** 凯利手术，参见 *plication* 下词条；**King o.,** arytenoidopexy 杓状软骨固定术；**Kraske o.,** removal of the coccyx and part of the sacrum for access to a rectal carcinoma 经骶尾部入路的肛门直肠手术；**Le Fort o., Le Fort-Neugebauer o.,** uniting the anterior and posterior vaginal walls at the middle line to repair or prevent uterine prolapse 阴道纵隔形成术，阴道闭合术；**Lorenz o.,** an operation for congenital dislocation of the hip Lorenz 手术（治先天性髋脱位）；**McDonald o.,** an operation for incompetent cervix, in which the cervical os is closed with a purse-string suture 宫颈环扎术；**McGill o.,** suprapubic transvesical prostatectomy McGill 手术（耻骨上前列腺切除术）；**McVay o.,** McVay 法手术，参见 *repair* 下词条；**Manchester o.,** Fothergill o. 曼彻斯特手术（经阴道手术治子宫脱垂）；**Marshall-Marchetti-Krantz o.,** suture of the anterior portion of the urethra, vesical neck, and bladder to the posterior surface of the pubic bone for correction of stress incontinence 马-马-克手术，治疗压迫性尿失禁的一种手术；**Motais o.,** transplantation of a portion of the tendon of the superior rectus muscle of the eyeball into the upper lid, for ptosis 莫泰手术，将眼球上直肌的部分肌腱移植到上睑，治疗上睑下垂；**Partsch o.,** a technique for marsupialization of a dental cyst 帕尔奇手术；**radical o.,** one involving extensive resection of tissue for complete extirpation of disease 根治手术；**Ramstedt o.,** pyloromyotomy Ramstedt 手术（先天幽门狭窄环状肌切断术）；**Shirodkar o.,** an operation for incompetent cervix in which the cervical os is closed with a surrounding purse-string suture 宫颈环扎缩窄术；**Wertheim o.,** radical hysterectomy 根治性子宫切除术

op·er·a·tor (op′ər-a-tər) a DNA sequence preceding the coding sequence of a structural gene in an operon, to which a regulator protein binds to control expression of the structural genes 操纵基因

oper·cu·lum (o-pur′ku-ləm) pl. *oper′cula* [L.] 1. a lid or covering 盖；2. the folds of pallium from the frontal, parietal, and temporal lobes of the cerebrum overlying the insula 前额和顶部大脑皮质皱褶，小脑覆盖小脑岛的颞叶；**oper′cular** *adj.*；**dental o.,** the hood of gingival tissue overlying the crown of an erupting tooth 牙盖；**trophoblastic o.,** the plug of trophoblast that helps close the gap in the endometrium made by the implanting blastocyst 滋养层盖，滋养细胞闭合由胚囊引起的子宫内膜缺损

op·er·on (op′ər-on) a prokaryotic chromosomal segment constituting a functional unit of transcription, comprising one or more structural genes, their promoter, and an operator region 操纵子

ophi·a·sis (o-fi′ə-sis) a form of alopecia areata involving the temporal and occipital margins of the scalp in a continuous band 匐行性脱发

ophi·dism (o′fi-diz-əm) poisoning by snake venom 蛇咬中毒

oph·ry·on (of′re-on) the middle point of the transverse supraorbital line 印堂，眉间中点

oph·ry·o·sis (of″re-o′sis) spasm of the eyebrow 眉痉挛

oph·thal·mag·ra (of″thəl-mag′rə) sudden pain in the eye 眼骤痛

oph·thal·mal·gia (of″thəl-mal′jə) pain in the eye 眼痛

oph·thal·mec·to·my (of″thəl-mek′tə-me) excision of an eye; enucleation of the eyeball 眼球摘除术

oph·thal·men·ceph·a·lon (of″thəl-men-sef′ə-lon) the retina, optic nerve, and visual apparatus of the brain 视脑（视网膜、视神经及脑内视器的总称）

oph·thal·mia (of-thal′me-ə) severe inflammation of the eye 眼炎；**Egyptian o.,** trachoma 沙眼；

O

gonorrheal o., gonorrheal conjunctivitis 淋病性眼炎；o. neonato′rum, any hyperacute purulent conjunctivitis occurring during the first 10 days of life, usually contracted during birth from infected vaginal discharge of the mother 新生儿眼炎；**phlyctenular o.**, 泡性眼炎，参见 *keratoconjunctivitis* 下词条；**purulent o.**, ophthalmia with purulent discharge, commonly due to gonorrheal infection 脓性眼炎；**sympathetic o.**, granulomatous inflammation of the uveal tract of the uninjured eye following a wound involving the uveal tract of the other eye, resulting in bilateral granulomatous inflammation of the entire uveal tract 交感性眼炎

oph·thal·mic (of-thal′mik) 同 ocular (1)

oph·thal·mi·tis (of″thəl-mi′tis) inflammation of the eye 眼炎；**ophthalmit′ic** *adj.*

oph·thal·mo·blen·nor·rhea (of-thal″mo-blen″o-re′ə) gonorrheal conjunctivitis 脓性眼炎

oph·thal·mo·cele (of-thal′mo-sēl) exophthalmos 眼球突出

oph·thal·mo·dy·na·mom·e·try (of-thal″modi″nə-mom′ə-tre) determination of the blood pressure in the retinal artery 视网膜血管血压测量（法）

oph·thal·mo·dyn·ia (of-thal″mo-din′e-ə) pain in the eye 眼痛

oph·thal·mo·ei·ko·nom·e·ter (of-thal″moi″kə-nom′ə-tər) an instrument for determining both the refraction of the eye and the relative size and shape of the ocular images 眼影像计

oph·thal·mog·ra·phy (of″thəl-mog′rə-fe) description of the eye and its diseases 眼球运动照相术；眼科专著

oph·thal·mo·gy·ric (of-thal″mo-ji′rik) oculogyric 眼球旋动的

oph·thal·mol·o·gist (of″thəl-mol′ə-jist) a physician who specializes in ophthalmology 眼科医生，眼科学家

oph·thal·mol·o·gy (of″thəl-mol′ə-je) the branch of medicine dealing with the eye, including its anatomy, physiology, and pathology 眼科学；**ophthalmolog′ic** *adj.*

oph·thal·mo·ma·la·cia (of-thal″mo-mə-la′-shə) abnormal softness of the eyeball 眼球软化

oph·thal·mo·my·ot·o·my (of-thal″mo-miot′ə-me) surgical division of the muscles of the eyes 眼肌切开术

oph·thal·mo·neu·ri·tis (of-thal″mo-noori′tis) optic neuritis 眼神经炎

oph·thal·mop·a·thy (of″thəl-mop′ə-the) any disease of the eye 眼病

oph·thal·mo·plas·ty (of-thal′mo-plas″te) plastic surgery of the eye or its appendages 眼成形术

oph·thal·mo·ple·gia (of-thal″mo-ple′jə) paral-

ysis of the eye muscles 眼肌麻痹，眼肌瘫痪；**ophthalmople′gic** *adj.*；**external o.**, paralysis of the external ocular muscles 眼外肌麻痹；**internal o.**, paralysis of the iris and ciliary apparatus 眼内肌麻痹；**nuclear o.**, that due to a lesion of nuclei of motor nerves of the eye 核性眼肌麻痹；**partial o.**, that affecting some of the eye muscles 部分眼肌麻痹；**progressive external o.**, gradual paralysis affecting the extraocular muscles and sometimes also the orbicularis oculi, leading to ptosis and progressive total ocular paresis 进行性眼外肌麻痹；**total o.**, paralysis of all the eye muscles, both intraocular and extraocular 全部眼肌麻痹

oph·thal·mor·rha·gia (of-thal″mo-ra′jə) hemorrhage from the eye 眼出血

oph·thal·mor·rhea (of-thal″mo-re′ə) oozing of blood from the eye 眼渗血

oph·thal·mor·rhex·is (of-thal″mo-rek′sis) rupture of an eyeball 眼球破裂

oph·thal·mo·scope (of-thal′mo-skōp) an instrument containing a perforated mirror and lenses used to examine the interior of the eye 眼底镜，检眼镜；**direct o.**, an ophthalmoscope that produces an upright, or unreversed, image of approximately 15 times magnification 直接检眼镜；**indirect o.**, one that produces an inverted, or reversed, direct image of two to five times magnification 间接检眼镜；**scanning laser o.**, an instrument for retinal imaging in which the retina is scanned by a low-power laser and the reflected light is used to create a digital image 激光扫描检眼镜

oph·thal·mos·co·py (of″thəl-mos′kə-pe) examination of the eye by means of the ophthalmoscope 检眼镜检查（法）；**medical o.**, that performed for diagnostic purposes 医用检眼镜诊断法；**metric o.**, that performed for measurement of refraction 检眼镜屈光测量法

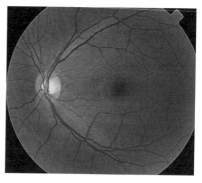

▲ 检眼镜下的正常眼底

oph·thal·mos·ta·sis (of″thəl-mos′tə-sis) fixation of the eye with the ophthalmostat 眼球固定法

oph·thal·mo·stat (of-thal′mo-stat″) an instrument for holding the eye steady during operation 眼球固定器

oph·thal·mot·o·my (of″thəl-mot′ə-me) incision of the eye 眼球切开术

oph·thal·mo·trope (of-thal′mo-trōp) a mechanical eye that moves like a real eye 眼肌模型

opi·ate (o′pe-ət) 1. any drug derived from opium 阿片类药物；2. hypnotic (2) 安眠药

opi·oid (o′pe-oid) 阿片类（物质）1. any synthetic narcotic that has opiate-like activities but is not derived from opium 类阿片样活性合成麻醉药；2. more broadly, any compound with opiate-like activity, including the opiates, synthetic agents not derived from opium, and naturally occurring peptides that bind at or otherwise influence the opiate receptors of cell membranes 所有有阿片样活性的化合物，包括阿片类药物、非阿片来源的合成药剂和天然存在的能结合或影响阿片受体的肽；**abuse-deterrent o.**, opioid formulations that are made taking into account and intending to prevent known or expected routes of abuse, such as crushing in order to inhale or dissolving in order to inject 滥用阿片类药物

opis·thi·on (o-pis′the-on) the midpoint of the lower border of the foramen magnum 颅后点（枕骨大孔后缘的中点）

opis·thor·chi·a·sis (o″pis-thor-ki′ə-sis) infection of the biliary tract by *Opisthorchis* 后睾吸虫病

Opis·thor·chis (o″pis-thor′kis) a genus of flukes parasitic in the liver and biliary tract of various birds and mammals; *O. feli′neus* and *O. viver′rini* cause opisthorchiasis and *O. sinen′sis* causes clonorchiasis in humans 后睾（吸虫）属

opis·thot·o·nos (o″pis-thot′ə-nəs) a form of extreme hyperextension of the body in which the head and heels are bent backward and the body bowed forward 角弓反张；**opisthoton′ic** *adj.*

opi·um (o′pe-əm) [L.] air-dried milky exudation from incised unripe capsules of *Papaver somniferum* or its variety *album*, containing some 20 alkaloids, the more important being morphine, codeine, and thebaine; the alkaloids are used for their narcotic and analgesic effects. Because it is highly addictive, opium production is restricted and cultivation of the plants from which it is obtained is prohibited by most nations under an international agreement 阿片，鸦片

op·por·tu·nis·tic (op″ər-too-nis′tik) 1. denoting a microorganism that does not ordinarily cause disease but becomes pathogenic under certain circumstances 机会致病菌；2. denoting a disease or infection caused by such an organism 机会致病

oprel·ve·kin (o-prel′və-kin″) recombinant interleukin-11, used as a hematopoietic stimulator to prevent thrombocytopenia following myelo-suppressive chemotherapy 重组白细胞介素 -11

op·sin (op′sin) a protein of the retinal rods (scotopsin) and cones (photopsin) that combines with 11-cis-retinal to form visual pigments 视蛋白

op·so·clo·nus (op″so-klo′nəs) involuntary, non-rhythmic horizontal and vertical oscillations of the eyes. 视性眼阵挛

op·so·nin (op′sə-nin) an antibody that renders bacteria and other cells susceptible to phagocytosis 调理素；**opson′ic** *adj.*；**immune o.**, an antibody that sensitizes a particulate antigen to phagocytosis, after combination with the homologous antigen in vivo or in vitro 免疫调理素

op·so·ni·za·tion (op″sə-nĭ-za′shən) the rendering of bacteria and other cells subject to phagocytosis 调理作用

op·so·no·cy·to·phag·ic (op″sə-no-si″to-faj′ik) denoting the phagocytic activity of blood in the presence of serum opsonins and homologous leukocytes 调理素细胞吞噬的

op·tic (op′tik) 同 ocular (1)

op·ti·cal (op′tĭ-kəl) visual 眼的；视力的；视觉的；光学的

op·ti·cian (op-tish′ən) a specialist in opticianry 眼镜师

op·ti·cian·ry (op-tish′ən-re) the translation, filling, and adapting of ophthalmic prescriptions, products, and accessories 眼科光学

op·ti·co·chi·as·mat·ic (op″tĭ-ko-ki″az-mat′ik) pertaining to the optic nerves and chiasma 视交叉的

op·ti·co·cil·i·ary (op″tĭ-ko-sil′e-ar-e) pertaining to the optic and ciliary nerves 视（神经）睫状神经的

op·ti·co·pu·pil·lary (op″tĭ-ko-pu″pĭ-lar-e) pertaining to the optic nerve and pupil 视神经瞳孔的

op·tics (op′tiks) the science of light and vision 光学

op·to·gram (op′to-gram) the retinal image formed by the bleaching of visual purple under the influence of light 视网膜象

op·to·ki·net·ic (op″to-kĭ-net′ik) pertaining to movement of the eyes, as in nystagmus 视运动的，视动性

op·tom·e·ter (op-tom′ə-tər) refractometer 视力计

op·tom·e·trist (op-tom′ə-trist) a specialist in optometry 验光师

op·tom·e·try (op-tom′ə-tre) the professional practice consisting of examination of the eyes to evaluate health and visual abilities, diagnosis of eye diseases and conditions of the eye and visual system, and provision of necessary treatment by the use of eyeglasses, contact lenses, and other functional, optical, surgical, and pharmaceutical means as regulated by state law 验光（法），视力测定法

op·to·my·om·e·ter (op″to-mi-om′ə-tər) a device for measuring the power of ocular muscles 眼肌力计

OPV poliovirus vaccine live oral 口服脊髓灰质炎病毒活疫苗

OR operating room 手术室

ora[1] (o′rə) pl. *o′rae* [L.] an edge or margin 缘；*o. serra′ta re′tinae,* the zigzag margin of the retina of the eye 视网膜锯齿缘

ora[2] (o′rə) *os* (1) 的复数

orad (o′rad) toward the mouth 向口

oral (or′əl) 1. pertaining to the mouth; taken through or applied in the mouth 口腔的；2. lingual (2) 舌的

oral·i·ty (o-ral′ĭ-te) the psychic organization of all the sensations, impulses, and personality traits derived from the oral stage of psychosexual development 口欲性欲，口欲色情

or·ange (or′ənj) 1. the trees *Citrus aurantium* and *Citrus sinensis* or their fruits; the flowers and peels are used in pharmaceutical preparations 枳实树、柑橘树或它们的果实；其花和果皮被用于药物制剂；2. a color between red and yellow, produced by energy of wavelengths between 590 and 630 nm 橙色；3. a dye or stain with this color 橙色染料

or·bic·u·lar (or-bik′u-lər) circular; rounded 环状的，圆的

or·bic·u·la·re (or-bik″u-la′re) a small oval knob on the long limb of the incus, articulating with or ossified to the head of the stapes 豆状突（砧骨）

or·bic·u·lus (or-bik′u-ləs) pl. *orbi′culi* [L.] a small disk 小环，盘

or·bit (or′bit) the bony cavity containing the eyeball and its associated muscles, vessels, and nerves 眶，眶腔；**or′bital** *adj.*

or·bi·ta (or′bĭ-tə) pl. *or′bitae* [L.] 同 orbit

or·bi·ta·le (or″bĭ-ta′le) the lowest point on the inferior edge of the orbit 眶下缘点，眶下点

or·bi·ta·lis (or″bĭ-ta′lis) [L.] pertaining to the orbit 眶的

or·bi·tog·ra·phy (or″bĭ-tog′rə-fe) visualization of the orbit and its contents using radiography or computed tomography 眶造影（术）

or·bi·to·na·sal (or″bĭ-to-na′zəl) pertaining to the orbit and nose 眶（和）鼻的

or·bi·to·nom·e·ter (or″bĭ-to-nom′ə-tər) an instrument for measuring backward displacement of the eyeball produced by a given pressure on its anterior aspect 眶压计

or·bi·top·a·thy (or″bĭ-top′ə-the) disease affecting the orbit and its contents 眶病

or·bi·tot·o·my (or″bĭ-tot′ə-me) incision into the orbit 眶切开术

Or·bi·vi·rus (or′bĭ-vi″rəs) orbiviruses; a genus of viruses of the family Reoviridae that infect a variety of vertebrates and cause fever in humans 环状病毒属

or·bi·vi·rus (or′bĭ-vi″rəs) any virus of the genus *Orbivirus* 环状病毒

or·ce·in (or-se′in) a brownish-red coloring substance obtained from orcinol; used as a stain for elastic tissue 地衣红

or·chi·al·gia (or″ke-al′jə) pain in a testis 睾丸痛

or·chi·dec·to·my (or″kĭ-dek′tə-me) 同 orchiectomy

or·chi·ec·to·my (or″ke-ek′tə-me) excision of one or both testes. If bilateral it is called also *castration* 睾丸切除术

or·chi·epi·did·y·mi·tis (or″ke-ep″ĭ-did″ə-mi′tis) epididymo-orchitis 睾丸附睾炎

or·chi·op·a·thy (or″ke-op′ə-the) any disease of the testis 睾丸病

or·chio·pexy (or′ke-o-pek″se) fixation in the scrotum of an undescended testis 睾丸固定术

or·chio·plas·ty (or′ke-o-plas″te) plastic surgery of a testis 睾丸成形术

or·chi·ot·o·my (or″ke-ot′ə-me) incision into a testis 睾丸切开术

or·chi·tis (or-ki′tis) inflammation of a testis 睾丸炎；**orchit′ic** *adj.*

or·ci·nol (or′sĭ-nol) an antiseptic principle, mainly derived from lichens, used as a reagent in various tests 苔黑素，地衣酚，5- 甲基间苯二酚

or·der (or′dər) a taxonomic category subordinate to a class and superior to a family (or suborder) 目（生物分类）

or·der·ly (or′dər-le) an attendant in a hospital who works under the direction of a nurse 男护理员

or·di·nate (y) (or′dĭ-nət) the vertical line in a graph along which is plotted one of two sets of factors considered in the study 纵坐标

orel·la·nine (o-rel′ə-nēn) a heat-stable nephrotoxin found in some *Cortinarius* mushrooms; ingestion causes delayed gastrointestinal symptoms followed by renal toxicity that may progress to renal failure 联吡啶四醇

orex·i·gen·ic (o-rek″sĭ-jen′ik) increasing or stimulating the appetite 促进食欲的，开胃的

orf (orf) contagious ecthyma 羊痘

or·gan (or′gən) a somewhat independent body part that performs a special function 器官；*o. of Corti,* the organ lying against the basilar membrane in the cochlear duct, containing special sensory receptors for hearing and consisting of neuroepithelial hair cells and several types of supporting cells 螺旋器，科尔蒂器；**effector o.**, effector (2) 效应器；**enamel o.**, a process of epithelium forming a cap over a dental papilla and developing into the enamel 成釉器，造釉器；**end o.**, end-organ 终末器官；**genital o's**, 同 reproductive o's；**Golgi tendon o.**, any of the mechanoreceptors arranged in series with muscle in the tendons of mammalian muscles, being the receptors for stimuli responsible for the lengthening reaction 高尔基腱器；**Jacobson o.**, 同 vomeronasal o.；**reproductive o's**, the various internal and external organs that are concerned with reproduction 生殖器官；**rudimentary o.**, 1. a primordium 原基；2. an imperfectly or incompletely developed organ 残余器官；**sense o's, sensory o's**, organs that receive stimuli that give rise to sensations, i.e., organs that translate certain forms of energy into nerve impulses that are perceived as special sensations 感觉器官；**spiral o.**, 同 o. of Corti；**vestigial o.**, an undeveloped organ that, in the embryo or in some ancestor, was well developed and functional 退化器官；**vomeronasal o.**, a short rudimentary canal just above the vomeronasal cartilage, opening in the side of the nasal septum and passing from there blindly upward and backward 犁鼻器；**Weber o.**, prostatic utricle 韦伯器（官），前列腺囊；**o's of Zuckerkandl**, para-aortic bodies 主动脉旁体

or·ga·nelle (or″gə-nel′) a specialized structure of a cell, such as a mitochondrion, Golgi complex, lysosome, endoplasmic reticulum, ribosome, centriole, chloroplast, cilium, or flagellum 细胞器

or·gan·ic (or-gan′ik) 1. pertaining to or arising from an organ or organs 器官的；2. having an organized structure 有组织结构的；3. arising from an organism 有机体的；4. pertaining to substances derived from living organisms 来源于生物体物质的；5. denoting chemical substances containing covalently bonded carbon atoms. 由共价碳原子结合的化学物的；6. pertaining to or cultivated by use of animal or vegetable fertilizers, rather than synthetic chemicals 利用动植物肥料，而不是化肥培育的

or·gan·ism (or′gə-niz″əm) an individual living thing, whether animal or plant 生物，有机体；**pleuro-pneumonialike o's**, any of various bacteria of the genus *Mycoplasma*, originally found causing pleuropneumonia in cattle and later found in other animals, including humans 类胸膜肺炎菌

or·ga·ni·za·tion (or″gə-nī-za′shən) 1. the process of organizing or of becoming organized 组织；2. an organized body, group, or structure 有组织的机体，团体或结构；3. the replacement of blood clots by fibrous tissue 机化（血栓或坏死组织）；**health maintenance o. (HMO)**, a broad term encompassing a variety of health care delivery systems utilizing group practice and providing alternatives to the fee-for-service private practice of medicine and allied health professions 健康维护组织；**Peer Review O., Professional Review O. (PRO)**, a regional organization of health care professionals established to monitor health care services paid for by Medicare, Medicaid, and Maternal and Child Health programs 同行审查组织；**Professional Standards Review O. (PSRO)**, former name for *Professional Review O.* 专业标准审查组织

or·ga·nize (or′gə-nīz″) 1. to provide with an organic structure 使有机化，使成有机体；2. to form into organs 构成器官

or·ga·niz·er (or′gə-nīz″ər) a region of the embryo that is capable of determining the differentiation of other regions 组织者

or·ga·no·gen·e·sis (or″gə-no-jen′ə-sis) the origin and development of organs 器官发生；**organogenet′ic** *adj.*

or·ga·nog·e·ny (or″gə-noj′ə-ne) 同 organogenesis

or·ga·noid (or′gə-noid) 1. resembling an organ 器官样的；2. a structure that resembles an organ 类器官

or·ga·no·meg·a·ly (or″gə-no-meg′ə-le) enlargement of an internal organ or organs 器官巨大症

or·ga·no·mer·cu·ri·al (or″gə-no-mər-ku′re-əl) any mercury-containing organic compound 有机汞的

or·ga·no·me·tal·lic (or″gə-no-mə-tal′ik) consisting of a metal combined with an organic radical, used particularly for a compound in which the metal is linked directly to a carbon atom 有机金属的

or·ga·no·phos·phate (or″gə-no-fos′fāt) an organic ester of phosphoric or thiophosphoric acid; such compounds are powerful acetylcholinesterase inhibitors and are used as insecticides and nerve gases 有机磷酸酯；**organophos′phorous** *adj.*

or·ga·no·sil·ane (or″gə-no-sil′ān) any of the class of silanes containing at least one direct carbon–silicon bond 有机硅烷

or·ga·no·tro·phic (or″gə-no-tro′fik) heterotrophic 器官营养的；有机营养的（指细菌）

or·ga·not·ro·pism (or″gə-not′rə-piz″əm) the special affinity of chemical compounds or pathogenic agents for particular tissues or organs of the body 亲器官性；**organotrop′ic** *adj.*

or·gasm (or′gaz-əm) the apex and culmination of sexual excitement 性快感；**orgas′mic** *adj.*

O

ori·en·ta·tion (or″e-ən-ta′shən) 1. awareness of one's environment with reference to time, place, and people（根据时间，地点，人物）定位（环境）; 2. the relative positions of atoms or groups in a chemical compound 化合物中原子（组合）的相对位置

Ori·en·tia (or″e-en′she-ə) a genus of gramnegative bacteria of the family Rickettsiaceae that includes organisms formerly classified in the genus *Rickettsia. O. tsutsugamu'shi* is the cause of scrub typhus 东方体属

or·i·fice (or′ ĭ-fis) 1. the entrance or outlet of any body cavity 体腔出入口; 2. any opening or meatus 口; 道; **orific'ial** *adj.*; **aortic o.,** the opening of the left ventricle into the aorta 主动脉口; **cardiac o.,** 贲门, 参见 *opening* 下词条; **ileal o., ileocecal o.,** the opening between the small and large intestines (ileum and cecum); the ileum forms the cone-shaped ileal papilla 回盲口; **left atrioventricular o., mitral o.,** the opening between the left atrium and ventricle of the heart 左房室口; **pulmonary o., o. of pulmonary trunk,** the opening between the pulmonary trunk and the right ventricle 肺动脉口; **right atrioventricular o., tricuspid o.,** the opening between the right atrium and ventricle of the heart 右房室口

or·i·gin (or′ĭ-jin) the source or beginning of anything, especially the more fixed end or attachment of a muscle (as distinguished from its insertion) or the site of emergence of a peripheral nerve from the central nervous system 起源; 起因, 起端

Or·ip·ro A trademark preparation of progesterone 一种黄体酮制剂的商品名

or·li·stat (or′lĭ-stat) an inhibitor of gastrointestinal lipases that prevents the digestion, and therefore absorption, of dietary fat; used in the treatment of obesity 奥利司他

or·ni·thine (or′nĭ-thēn) an amino acid obtained from arginine by splitting of urea; it is an intermediate in urea biosynthesis 鸟氨酸

or·ni·thine car·ba·mo·yl·trans·fer·ase (or′nĭ-thēn kahr-bam″o-əl-trans′fər-ās) an enzyme that catalyzes the carbamoylation of ornithine to form citrulline, a step in the urea cycle; deficiency of the enzyme is an X-linked aminoacidopathy causing hyperammonemia, neurologic abnormalities, and oroticaciduria and is usually fatal in the neonatal period in males 鸟氨酸氨甲酰转移酶

or·ni·thin·emia (or″nĭ-thī-ne′me-ə) hyperornithinemia 高鸟氨酸血症

Or·ni·thod·o·ros (or″nĭ-thod′ə-rəs) a genus of soft-bodied ticks, many species of which are reservoirs and vectors of species of *Borrelia* 纯缘蜱属

or·ni·tho·sis (or″nĭ-tho′sis) psittacosis 鹦鹉热

oro·lin·gual (or″o-ling′gwəl) pertaining to the mouth and tongue 口舌的

oro·na·sal (or″o-na′zəl) pertaining to the mouth and nose 口鼻的

oro·pha·ryn·ge·al (or″o-fə-rin′je-əl) 1. pertaining to the mouth and pharynx 口腔和咽部的; 2. pertaining to the oropharynx 口咽部的

oro·phar·ynx (or″o-far′inks) the part of the pharynx between the soft palate and the upper edge of the epiglottis 口咽

oro·tra·che·al (or″o-tra′ke-əl) pertaining to the mouth and trachea 口腔气管的

or·phen·a·drine (or-fen′ə-drēn) an analogue of diphenhydramine having anticholinergic, antihistaminic, and antispasmodic actions; its citrate salt is used as a skeletal muscle relaxant 奥芬那君（邻甲苯海拉明）

ORS oral rehydration salts 口服补液盐

ORT oral rehydration therapy 口服补液疗法

ortho- 1. symbol *o-*; in organic chemistry, a prefix indicating a 1,2-substituted benzene ring 符号 *o-*; 有机化学中表示 1,2- 代苯环; 2. in inorganic chemistry, the common form of an acid 无机化学中表示一种 "- 酸"

Or·tho·bun·ya·vi·rus (or″tho-bun′yə-vi″rəs) a genus of viruses of the family Bunyaviridae. It is transmitted most often by the bite of an infected mosquito and causes fever and encephalitis. Important disease-causing species include California encephalitis, Jamestown Canyon, La Crosse, and Oropouche viruses 正布尼亚病毒属

or·tho·cho·rea (or″tho-kə-re′ə) choreic movements in the erect posture 立位舞蹈病

or·tho·chro·mat·ic (or″tho-kro-mat′ik) staining normally 正染的

or·tho·de·ox·ia (or″tho-de-ok′se-ə) accentuation of arterial hypoxemia in the erect position 直立低氧血症

or·tho·don·tia (or″tho-don′shə) 同 orthodontics

or·tho·don·tics (or″tho-don′tiks) the branch of dentistry concerned with irregularities of teeth and malocclusion, and associated facial abnormalities 口腔正畸学; **orthodon'tic** *adj.*

or·tho·don·tist (or″tho-don′tist) a dentist who specializes in orthodontics 正牙学家

or·tho·dro·mic (or″tho-dro′mik) conducting impulses in the normal direction; said of nerve fibers 顺行的，顺向传导的（神经纤维）

or·thog·nath·ia (or″thog-nath′e-ə) the branch of oral medicine dealing with the cause and treatment of malposition of the bones of the jaw 正颌学

or·thog·na·thic (or″thog-nath′ik) 1. pertaining to

orthognathia 正颌的；2. 同 orthognathous

or·thog·na·thous (or-thog′nə-thəs″) pertaining to or characterized by minimal protrusion of the mandible or minimal prognathism 直颌的

or·tho·grade (or′tho-grād″) walking with the body upright 直体步行的

Or·tho·hep·ad·na·vi·rus (or″tho-hep-ad′nə- vi″rəs) hepatitis B viruses that infect mammals; a genus of the family Hepadnaviridae that includes hepatitis B virus 正去氧核糖核酸病毒属

or·tho·ker·a·to·sis (or″tho-ker′ə-to′sis) thickening of the stratum corneum without parakeratosis, i.e., without the abnormal retention of keratinocyte nuclei 正角化

or·thom·e·ter (or-thom′ə-tər) instrument for determining relative protrusion of the eyeballs 突眼比较计

or·tho·mo·lec·u·lar (or″tho-mo-lek′u-lər) relating to or aimed at restoring the optimal concentrations and functions at the molecular level of the substances (e.g., vitamins) normally present in the body 正分子的

Or·tho·myxo·vi·ri·dae (or″tho-mik″so-vir′ĭ-de) a family of RNA viruses that cause influenza; genera include *Influenzavirus A, Influenzavirus B,* and *Influenzavirus C* 正粘病毒科

or·tho·myxo·vi·rus (or″tho-mik″so-vi″rəs) any virus of the family Orthomyxoviridae 正粘病毒

or·tho·pe·dic (or″tho-pe′dik) pertaining to the correction of deformities of the musculoskeletal system; pertaining to orthopedics 矫形外科的，矫形的

or·tho·pe·dics (or″tho-pe′diks) the branch of surgery dealing with the preservation and restoration of the function of the skeletal system, its articulations, and associated structures 矫形外科学，矫形学

or·tho·pe·dist (or″tho-pe′dist) an orthopedic surgeon 矫形外科医师

or·tho·per·cus·sion (or″tho-pər-kush′ən) percussion with the distal phalanx of the finger held perpendicularly to the body wall 直指叩诊法

or·tho·pho·ria (or″tho-fo′re-ə) normal equilibrium of the eye muscles, or muscular balance 位置正常，正位；视轴正常，直视；**orthophor′ic** *adj.*

or·tho·phos·phor·ic ac·id (or″tho-fos-for′ik) phosphoric acid 正磷酸

or·thop·nea (or″thop-ne′ə) dyspnea that is relieved in the upright position 端坐呼吸；**orthopne′ic** *adj.*

Or·tho·pox·vi·rus (or′tho-poks-vi″rəs) a genus of viruses of the family Poxviridae, which causes generalized infections with a rash in mammals. It includes cowpox, monkeypox, and variola viruses

正痘病毒属

or·tho·pox·vi·rus (or′tho-poks-vi″rəs) a virus of the genus *Orthopoxvirus* 正痘病毒

or·tho·prax·is (or″tho-prak′sis) 同 orthopraxy

or·tho·praxy (or′tho-prak″se) mechanical correction of deformities 机械矫形术

or·thop·tic (or-thop′tik) correcting obliquity of one or both visual axes 视轴矫正的

or·thop·tics (or-thop′tiks) treatment of strabismus by exercise of the ocular muscles 视轴矫正法

Or·tho·reo·vi·rus (or″tho-re′o-vi″rəs) a genus of viruses of the family Reoviridae; no causative relationship to any disease has been proved in humans, but in other mammals they have been associated with respiratory and enteric disease, and in chickens and turkeys with arthritis 正呼肠病毒属

or·tho·scope (or′tho-skōp) an apparatus that neutralizes corneal refraction by means of a layer of water 水检眼镜

or·tho·scop·ic (or″tho-skop′ik) 1. affording a correct and undistorted view 正常无畸变的；2. pertaining to an orthoscope 水检眼镜的

or·tho·sis (or-tho′sis) pl. *ortho′ses* [Gr.] an orthopedic appliance or apparatus used to support, align, prevent, or correct deformities or to improve function of movable parts of the body 矫形器；**cervical o.,** one that encircles the neck and supports the chin for treatment of injuries of the cervical spine 颈椎矫形器；**dynamic o., functional o.,** a support or protective apparatus for the hand or other body part that also aids in initiating, performing, and reacting to motion 动力支具，功能性矫形器；**halo o.,** a cervical orthosis consisting of a stiff halo attached to the upper skull and to a rigid jacket on the chest, providing maximal rigidity 颈部支具；**spinal o.,** one that surrounds the trunk to support or align the vertebral column or to prevent movement after trauma 脊柱支架；**static o.,** one that does not allow motion of the part and is primarily for support only 静态矫正器

or·tho·stat·ic (or″tho-stat′ik) pertaining to or caused by standing erect 直立的，直体的

or·tho·stat·ism (or′tho-stat″iz-əm) an erect standing position of the body 直立位，直立姿势

or·thot·ics (or-thot′iks) the field of knowledge relating to orthoses and their use 整直学，矫正学，矫形器修配学

or·thot·ist (or-thot′ist) a person skilled in orthotics and practicing its application in individual cases 整直师，矫形师，矫正器修配者

or·thot·o·nos (or-thot′ə-nəs) tetanic spasm that fixes the head, body, and limbs in a rigid straight line 挺直性痉挛，身体强直

or·thot·o·nus (or-thot′ə-nəs) 同 orthotonos

or·tho·top·ic (or″tho-top′ik) occurring at the normal place 正位的，常位的

or·tho·vol·tage (or′tho-vōl″təj) in radiotherapy, voltage in the range of 140 to 400 kilovolts, as contrasted to supervoltage and megavoltage 正电压

OS [L.] o′culus sinis′ter (left eye) 左眼

Os osmium 元素锇的符号

os^1 (os) pl. *o′ra* [L.] 1. any body orifice 孔，口；2. oral cavity (mouth) 口腔；**external o. of uterus,** ostium uteri; the external opening of the uterine cervix into the vagina 子宫外口；**internal o. of uterus,** the internal orifice of the uterine cervix, opening into the cavity of the uterus 子宫内口

os^2 (os) pl. *os′sa* [L.] bone 骨

OSA Optical Society of America 美国光学学会

os·cil·la·tion (os″ĭ-la′shən) a backward-andforward motion, like that of a pendulum 振动，振荡，摆动

os·cil·lom·e·ter (os″ĭ-lom′ə-tər) an instrument for measuring oscillations 示波计

os·cil·lop·sia (os″ĭ-lop′se-ə) a visual sensation that stationary objects are swaying back and forth 振动幻视

os·cil·lo·scope (ə-sil′ə-skōp) an instrument that displays a visual representation of electrical variations on the fluorescent screen of a cathoderay tube 示波器

-ose a suffix indicating that the substance is a carbohydrate（糖类）碳水化合物的后缀

osel·tam·i·vir (o″səl-tam′ĭ-vir) an inhibitor of viral neuraminidase, used as the phosphate salt in the treatment of influenza 奥司他韦

os·mate (oz′māt) a salt containing the osmium tetroxide anion 锇酸盐

os·mic ac·id (oz′mik) osmium tetroxide 四氧化锇

os·mi·um (Os) (oz′me-əm) a very hard, brittle, blue-gray, metallic element; at. no. 76, at. wt. 190.23 锇（化学元素），**o. tetroxide,** a fixative used in preparing histologic specimens, OsO_4 四氧化锇（制组织标本时用作固定液）

os·mo·lal·i·ty (oz″mo-lal′ĭ-te) the concentration of a solution in terms of osmoles of solute per kilogram of solvent 渗量，渗透摩尔量

os·mo·lar (oz-mo′lər) pertaining to the concentration of osmotically active particles in solution 摩尔渗透压的

os·mo·lar·i·ty (oz″mo-lar′ĭ-te) the concentration of a solution in terms of osmoles of solutes per liter of solution 渗量

os·mole (Osm) (oz′mōl) a unit of osmotic pressure equivalent to the amount of solute that dissociates in solution to form 1 mole (Avogadro's number) of particles (molecules and ions) 渗摩，渗模，渗量（用摩尔表示渗透压单位）

os·mom·e·ter (oz-mom′ə-tər) an instrument for measuring osmotic concentration or pressure 渗（透）压计

os·mo·phil·ic (oz″mo-fil′ik) having an affinity for solutions of high osmotic pressure 嗜高渗的

os·mo·phore (oz′mo-for″) the group of atoms responsible for the odor of a compound 生臭基，生臭团

os·mo·re·cep·tor (oz″mo-re-sep′tər) 1. any of a group of specialized neurons in the hypothalamus that are stimulated by increased osmolality (chiefly, increased sodium concentration) of the extracellular fluid; their excitation promotes the release of antidiuretic hormone by the posterior pituitary 渗透压感受器；2. olfactory receptor 嗅觉感受器

os·mo·reg·u·la·tion (oz″mo-reg″u-la′shən) maintenance of osmolarity by a simple organism or body cell relative to the surrounding medium 渗透（压）调节；**osmoreg′ulatory** *adj.*

os·mo·sis (oz-mo′sis) (os-mo′sis) the diffusion of pure solvent across a membrane in response to a concentration gradient, usually from a solution of lesser to one of greater solute concentration 渗透（作用）；**osmot′ic** *adj.*

os·mo·stat (oz′mo-stat″) the regulatory centers that control the osmolality of the extracellular fluid 渗（透）压控制器

os·sa (os′ə) [L.] *os* 的复数（见 *os*^{2}）

os·se·in (os′e-in) the collagen of bone 骨胶原

os·seo·car·ti·lag·i·nous (os″e-o-kahr″tĭ-laj′ĭ-nəs) composed of bone and cartilage 骨软骨的

os·seo·fi·brous (os″e-o-fi′brəs) made up of fibrous tissue and bone 骨（与）纤维组织的

os·seo·mu·cin (os″e-o-mu′sin) the ground substance that binds together the collagen and elastic fibrils of bone 骨黏素

os·se·ous (os′e-əs) of the nature or quality of bone; bony 骨性的，骨的

os·si·cle (os′ĭ-kəl) a small bone, especially one of those in the middle ear 小骨；**ossic′ular** *adj.*；**Andernach o's,** sutural bones 缝间骨；**auditory o's,** the small bones of the middle ear: incus, malleus, and stapes 听小骨，见图 29

os·sic·u·lec·to·my (os″ĭ-ku-lek′tə-me) excision of one or more ossicles of the middle ear 听小骨切除术

os·sic·u·lot·o·my (os″ĭ-ku-lot′ə-me) incision of the auditory ossicles 听小骨切开术

os·sic·u·lum (ə-sik′u-ləm) pl. *ossi′cula* [L.] 同 ossicle

os·sif·er·ous (ə-sif′ər-əs) producing bone 生骨的

os·sif·ic (ə-sif′ik) forming or becoming bone 骨化的，成骨的

os·si·fi·ca·tion (os″ĭ-fĭ-ka′shən) formation of or conversion into bone or a bony substance 骨化，成骨；**ectopic o.**, a pathologic condition in which bone arises in tissues not in the osseous system and in connective tissues usually not manifesting osteogenic properties 异位骨化；**endochondral o.**, ossification that occurs in and replaces cartilage 软骨内成骨；**heterotopic o.**, the formation of bone in abnormal locations, secondary to pathology 异位骨化；**intramembranous o.**, ossification that occurs in and replaces connective tissue 膜内成骨

os·si·fy·ing (os′ĭ-fi″ing) changing or developing into bone 骨化的

os·te·al·gia (os″te-al′jə) pain in the bones 骨痛

os·te·ar·throt·o·my (os″te-ahr-throt′ə-me) excision of an articular end of a bone 骨关节端切除术

os·tec·to·my (os-tek′tə-me) excision of a bone or part of a bone 骨切除术

os·te·ec·to·pia (os″te-ek-to′pe-ə) displacement of a bone 骨异位

os·te·itis (os″te-i′tis) inflammation of bone 骨炎；**o. conden′sans**, 同 condensing o.；**condensing o.**, a focal inflammatory reaction of bone marked by the formation of radiopaque sclerotic lesions; it occurs in the jaw as a reaction to infection and in the clavicle, ilium, or pubis, probably as the result of repeated mechanical stress 致密性骨炎；**o. defor′mans**, rarefying osteitis resulting in weakened, deformed bones of increased mass, which may lead to bowing of long bones and deformation of flat bones; when the bones of the skull are affected, deafness may result 畸形性骨炎，又称 *Paget disease of bone*；**o. fbro′sa cys′tica**, rarefying osteitis with fibrous degeneration and formation of cysts and with the presence of fibrous nodules on the affected bones, due to marked osteoclastic activity secondary to hyperparathyroidism 纤维囊性骨炎，囊性纤维性骨炎；**o. fungo′sa**, chronic osteitis in which the haversian canals are dilated and filled with granulation tissue 肉芽性骨炎；**parathyroid o.**, 同 o. fibrosa cystica；**sclerosing o.**, sclerosing nonsuppurative osteomyelitis 硬化性骨炎

os·tem·py·e·sis (os″təm-pi-e′sis) suppuration within a bone 骨化脓

os·te·o·ana·gen·e·sis (os″te-o-an′ə-jen′ə-sis) regeneration of bone 骨重建

os·te·o·ar·thri·tis (os″te-o-ahr-thri′tis) noninflammatory degenerative joint disease marked by degeneration of the articular cartilage, hypertrophy of bone at the margins, and changes in the synovial membrane, accompanied by pain and stiffness 骨（性）关节炎；**osteoarthrit′ic** *adj.*

os·teo·ar·throp·a·thy (os″te-o-ahr-throp′ə-the) any disease of the joints and bones 骨关节病；**hypertrophic pulmonary o.**, **secondary hypertrophic o.**, symmetrical osteitis of the four limbs, chiefly localized to the phalanges and terminal epiphyses of the long bones of the forearm and leg; it is often secondary to chronic lung and heart conditions 肥大性肺性骨关节病

os·teo·ar·thro·sis (os″te-o-ahr-thro′sis) 同 osteo-arthritis

os·teo·ar·throt·o·my (os″te-o-ahr-throt′ə-me) 同 ostearthrotomy

os·teo·blast (os′te-o-blast″) a cell arising from a fibroblast, which, as it matures, is associated with bone production 成骨细胞

os·teo·blas·to·ma (os″te-o-blas-to′mə) a benign, painful, vascular tumor of bone marked by formation of osteoid tissue and primitive bone 成骨细胞瘤

os·teo·camp·sia (os″te-o-kamp′se-ə) curvature of a bone 骨屈曲

os·teo·chon·dral (os″te-o-kon′drəl) pertaining to bone and cartilage 骨软骨的

os·teo·chon·dri·tis (os″te-o-kon-dri′tis) inflammation of bone and cartilage 骨软骨炎；**o. defor′mans juveni′lis**, osteochondrosis of the capitular epiphysis of the femur 幼年变形性骨软骨炎；**o. defor′mans juveni′lis dor′si**, osteochondrosis of vertebrae 幼年脊柱变形性骨软骨炎；**o. dis′secans**, that resulting in splitting of pieces of cartilage into the affected joint 剥脱性骨软骨炎

os·teo·chon·dro·dys·pla·sia (os″te-o-kon″drodis-pla′zhə) any of a large group of inherited disorders of cartilage and bone growth 骨软骨发育不良

os·teo·chon·dro·dys·tro·phy (os″te-o-kon″dro-dis′trə-fe) Morquio syndrome 骨软骨营养不良

os·teo·chon·drol·y·sis (os″te-o-kon-drol′ə-sis) osteochondritis dissecans 骨软骨脱离，分离性骨软骨炎

os·teo·chon·dro·ma (os″te-o-kon-dro′mə) a benign bone tumor consisting of projecting adult bone capped by cartilage projecting from the lateral contours of endochondral bones 骨软骨瘤

os·teo·chon·dro·ma·to·sis (os″te-o-kon-dro″mə-to′sis) occurrence of multiple osteochondromas, as in multiple cartilaginous exostoses or enchondromatoses; sometimes specifically denoting one of these disorders 骨软骨瘤病

os·teo·chon·dro·myx·o·ma (os″te-o-kon″dro-mik-so′mə) osteochondroma containing myxoid elements 骨软骨黏液瘤

os·teo·chon·dro·sis (os″te-o-kon-dro′sis) a disease of the growth ossification centers in children, beginning as a degeneration or necrosis followed by regeneration or recalcification; known by various names, depending on the bone involved 骨软骨病

os·te·oc·la·sis (os″te-ok′lə-sis) surgical fracture or refracture of bones 折骨术（外科的骨折或再骨折）

os·te·o·clast (os′te-o-klast″) 1. a large multinuclear cell associated with absorption and removal of bone 破骨细胞；2. an instrument used for osteoclasis 折骨器；**osteoclas′tic** adj.

os·teo·clas·to·ma (os″te-o-klas-to′mə) giant cell tumor of bone 破骨细胞瘤

os·teo·cra·ni·um (os″te-o-kra′ne-əm) the fetal skull during its stage of ossification 骨颅（在骨化期的胎儿头颅）

os·teo·cys·to·ma (os″te-o-sis-to′mə) a bone cyst 骨囊瘤

os·teo·cyte (os′te-o-sīt″) an osteoblast that has become embedded within the bone matrix, occupying a bone lacuna and sending, through the canaliculi, slender cytoplasmic processes that make contact with processes of other osteocytes 骨细胞

os·teo·di·as·ta·sis (os″te-o-di-as′tə-sis) the separation of two adjacent bones 骨分离

os·te·odyn·ia (os″te-o-din′e-ə) 同 ostealgia

os·teo·dys·tro·phy (os″te-o-dis′trə-fe) abnormal development of bone 骨营养不良；**Albright hereditary o.**, a constellation of physical features, including short stature, round facies, brachydactyly, obesity, and ectopic soft tissue or dermal ossification; associated with resistance to parathyroid hormone Albright 遗传性骨营养不良；**renal o.**, a condition due to chronic kidney disease and renal failure, with elevated serum phosphorus levels, low or normal serum calcium levels, and stimulation of parathyroid function, resulting in a variable admixture of bone disease 肾性骨营养不良（症）

os·teo·epiph·y·sis (os″te-o-ə-pif′ə-sis) any bony epiphysis 骨骺

os·teo·fi·bro·ma (os″te-o-fi-bro′mə) a benign tumor combining both osseous and fibrous elements 骨纤维瘤，纤维骨瘤

os·teo·fluo·ro·sis (os″te-o-floo-ro′sis) skeletal changes, usually consisting of osteomalacia and osteosclerosis, caused by the chronic intake of excessive quantities of fluorides 氟骨病

os·teo·gen (os′te-o-jen″) the substance composing the inner layer of the periosteum, from which bone is formed 成骨质

os·teo·gen·e·sis (os″te-o-ə-sis) the formation of bone; the development of the bones 骨发生，骨形成；**osteogenet′ic** adj.；**o. imperfec′ta (OI)**, a group of connective tissue disorders, of variable inheritance, due to a variety of mutations causing defects in biosynthesis of type I collagen and characterized by brittle, easily fractured bones; other defects may include blue sclerae, muscle weakness, joint laxity, shortened limbs and limb defects, hearing loss, and dentinogenesis imperfecta 成骨不全

os·teo·gen·ic (os″te-o-jen′ik) derived from or composed of any tissue concerned in bone growth or repair 成骨的

os·teo·ha·lis·ter·e·sis (os″te-o-hə-lis″tər-e′sis) deficiency in mineral elements of bone 骨质缺乏

os·te·oid (os′te-oid) 1. resembling bone 类骨的；2. the organic matrix of bone; young bone that has not undergone calcification 类骨质，尚未钙化的幼骨

os·teo·in·duc·tion (os″te-o-in-duk′shən) the act or process of stimulating osteogenesis 骨诱导

os·teo·lipo·chon·dro·ma (os″te-o-lip″o-kon-dro′mə) a benign cartilaginous tumor with osseous and fatty elements 骨脂软骨瘤

os·te·ol·o·gy (os″te-ol′ə-je) scientific study of the bones 骨学

os·te·ol·y·sis (os″te-ol′ə-sis) dissolution of bone; applied especially to the removal or loss of the calcium of bone 溶骨性反应，骨质溶解；**osteolyt′ic** adj.

os·te·o·ma (os″te-o′mə) a benign, slow-growing tumor composed of well-differentiated, densely sclerotic, compact bone, occurring particularly in the skull and facial bones 骨瘤；**compact o.**, a small, dense, compact tumor of mature lamellar bone with little medullary space, usually in the craniofacial or nasal bones 致密骨瘤；**o. cu′tis**, the formation of bone tissue in the dermis or subcutis; it may be sporadic, inherited, metastatic, or secondary to a preexisting lesion or inflammatory process 皮肤骨瘤；**o. du′rum, ivory o.**, compact o. 密质骨瘤；**osteoid o.**, a small, benign but painful, circumscribed tumor of spongy bone, usually in the bones of the limbs or vertebrae of young persons 骨样骨瘤

os·teo·ma·la·cia (os″te-o-mə-la′shə) inadequate or delayed mineralization of osteoid in mature cortical and spongy bone; it is the adult equivalent of rickets and accompanies that disorder in children 骨软化（症）；**osteomala′cic** adj.；**hepatic o.**, osteomalacia as a complication of cholestatic liver disease, which may lead to severe bone pain and multiple fractures 肝性骨软化；**oncogenic o., tumor-induced o.**, osteomalacia occurring in association with mesenchymal neoplasms, which are usually benign 肿瘤源性骨软化病

os·te·o·mere (os'te-o-mēr″) one of a series of similar bony structures, such as the vertebrae 单骨，骨件

os·te·om·e·try (os″te-om'ə-tre) measurement of the bones 骨测量法

os·te·o·my·eli·tis (os″te-o-mi'ə-li'tis) inflammation of bone, localized or generalized, due to infection, usually by pyogenic organisms 骨髓炎；**osteomyelit'ic** adj.; **Garré o., sclerosing non-suppurative o.,** a chronic form involving the long bones, especially the tibia and femur, marked by a diffuse inflammatory reaction, increased density and spindle-shaped sclerotic thickening of the cortex, and an absence of suppuration Garré 骨髓炎，硬化性非化脓性骨髓炎

os·te·o·my·elo·dys·pla·sia (os″te-o-mi'ə-lodis-pla'zhə) a condition characterized by thinning of the osseous tissue of bones and increase in size of the marrow cavities, attended by leukopenia and fever 骨髓发育不良

os·te·on (os'te-on) [Gr.] the basic unit of structure of compact bone, comprising a haversian canal and its concentrically arranged lamellae 骨单位

os·te·o·ne·cro·sis (os″te-o-nə-kro'sis) necrosis of a bone 骨坏死

os·te·o·neu·ral·gia (os″te-o-noo-ral'jə) neuralgia of a bone 骨神经痛

os·te·o·path (os'te-o-path″) a health care practitioner who practices based on the principles of osteopathic philosophy 按摩术医士，疗骨术医士

os·te·o·path·ia (os″te-o-path'e-ə) 同 osteopathy (1); **o. conden'sans dissemina'ta,** 同 osteopoikilosis; **o. stria'ta,** an asymptomatic condition characterized radiographically by multiple condensations of cancellous bone tissue, giving a striated appearance 条纹状骨病

os·te·op·a·thy (os″te-op'ə-the) 1. any disease of a bone 骨病；2. a system of therapy founded on the theory that the body is capable of making the remedies necessary to protect itself against disease and other toxic conditions when it is in normal structural relationship and has favorable environmental conditions and adequate nutrition. It considers the person as a unit combining body, mind, and spirit and emphasizes maintenance of normal body mechanics and manipulative methods of detecting and correcting faulty structure 整骨疗法；**osteopath'ic** adj.

os·te·o·pe·nia (os″te-o-pe'ne-ə) 1. reduced bone mass due to a decrease in the rate of osteoid synthesis to a level insufficient to compensate for normal bone lysis 骨量减少；2. any decrease in bone mass

below the normal 骨量缺乏；**osteopen'ic** adj.

os·te·o·peri·os·te·al (os″te-o-per″e-os'te-əl) pertaining to bone and its periosteum 骨骨膜的

os·te·o·peri·os·ti·tis (os″te-o-per″e-os-ti'tis) inflammation of a bone and its periosteum 骨骨膜炎

os·te·o·pe·tro·sis (os″te-o-pe-tro'sis) a hereditary disease marked by abnormally dense bone, and by the common occurrence of fractures of affected bone 骨硬化病

os·te·o·phle·bi·tis (os″te-o-flə-bi'tis) inflammation of the veins of a bone 骨静脉炎

os·te·o·phy·ma (os″te-o-fi'mə) a tumor or outgrowth of bone 骨赘

os·te·o·phyte (os'te-o-fit″) a bony excrescence or outgrowth of bone 骨赘

os·te·o·plas·ty (os'te-o-plas″te) plastic surgery of the bones 骨成形术

os·te·o·poi·ki·lo·sis (os″te-o-poi″kī-lo'sis) an autosomal dominant trait in which there are multiple sclerotic foci in the ends of long bones and scattered stippling in round and flat bones, usually without symptoms 全身脆弱性骨硬化；**osteopoikilot'ic** adj.

os·te·o·po·ro·sis (os″te-o-pə-ro'sis) abnormal rarefaction of bone; it may be idiopathic or occur secondary to other diseases 骨质疏松（症）；**osteoporot'ic** adj.; **postmenopausal o.,** osteoporosis in women after menopause, usually affecting trabecular bone and manifested by vertebral fractures, hip fractures, Colles fractures, and increased tooth loss 绝经妇女骨质疏松症；**posttraumatic o.,** loss of bone substance following a nerve-damaging injury, sometimes due to an increased blood supply caused by the neurogenic insult, or to disuse secondary to pain; a component of complex regional pain syndrome type 1 创伤后骨质疏松

os·te·o·ra·dio·ne·cro·sis (os″te-o-ra″de-o-nə-kro'sis) necrosis of bone as a result of exposure to radiation 放射性骨坏死

os·te·or·rha·gia (os″te-o-ra'jə) hemorrhage from bone 骨出血

os·te·or·rha·phy (os″te-or'ə-fe) fixation of fragments of bone with sutures or wires 骨缝术

os·te·o·sar·co·ma (os″te-o-sahr-ko'mə) a malignant primary neoplasm of bone composed of a malignant connective tissue stroma with evidence of malignant osteoid, bone, or cartilage formation; it is subclassified as osteoblastic, chondroblastic, or fibroblastic 骨肉瘤；**osteosarco'matous** adj.; **parosteal o.,** a variant consisting of a slowly growing tumor resembling cancellous bone but arising from the cortex of the bone and slowly growing outward to surround the bone 骨 旁 骨 肉 瘤；**periosteal o.**, a variant of osteochondroma consisting of a soft, lobulated tumor arising from the periosteum of a long bone and growing outward 骨 膜 骨 肉 瘤；**small-cell o.**, a variant of osteosarcoma resembling Ewing sarcoma, with areas of osteoid and sometimes chondroid formation 小细胞骨肉瘤

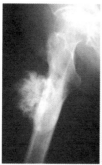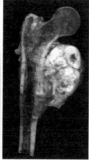

▲ 67 岁老年女性股骨近端骨膜骨肉瘤。病变发生在骨表面，尚未侵犯骨髓腔

os·teo·sar·co·ma·to·sis (os″te-o-sahr-ko″mə- to′-sis) the simultaneous occurrence of multiple osteosarcomas; synchronous multicentric osteosarcoma 多发性骨肉瘤

os·teo·scle·ro·sis (os″te o sklə-ro′sis) the hardening or abnormal density of bone 骨硬化；**osteosclerot′ic** adj.；**o. conge′nita**, achondroplasia 软 骨 发育不全；**o. fra′gilis**, 同 osteopetrosis

os·te·o·sis (os″te-o′sis) the formation of bony tissue 骨质生成，骨化（病）

os·teo·su·ture (os′te-o-soo″chər) 同 osteorrhaphy

os·teo·syn·o·vi·tis (os″te-o-sin″o-vi′tis) synovitis with osteitis of neighboring bones 骨滑膜炎

os·teo·syn·the·sis (os″te-o-sin′thə-sis) surgical fastening of the ends of a fractured bone 骨缝术，骨接合术

os·teo·ta·bes (os″te-o-ta′bēz) a disease, chiefly of infants, in which bone marrow cells are destroyed and the marrow disappears 骨髓痨，骨耗病

os·teo·throm·bo·sis (os″te-o-throm-bo′sis) thrombosis of the veins of a bone 骨内静脉血栓形成

os·teo·tome (os′te-o-tōm″) a chisel-like knife for cutting bone 骨凿

os·te·ot·o·my (os″te-ot′ə-me) incision or transection of a bone 截骨术；**cuneiform o.**, removal of a wedge of bone 楔形切骨术；**displacement o.**, surgical division of a bone and shifting of the divided ends to change the alignment of the bone or

to alter weight-bearing stresses 骨切断错位术；**Le Fort o.**, transverse sectioning and repositioning of the maxilla; the incision for each of the three types (*Le Fort I, II, and III o's*) is placed along the line defined by the corresponding Le Fort fracture 勒福型截骨术；**linear o.**, the sawing or linear cutting of a bone 线状截骨术，线性缝骨术；**sandwich o.**, a surgical procedure for augmenting an atrophic mandible, resembling a visor osteotomy but having a horizontal split confined between the mental foramina 三明治切骨术；**visor o.**, a surgical technique for augmenting an atrophic mandible, in which the mandible is split sagitally and the cranial fragment is slid upward and supported with grafts 盔式截骨术

os·ti·tis (os-ti′tis) 同 osteitis

os·ti·um (os′te-əm) pl. *os′tia* [L.] an opening or orifice. 孔，口；**os′tial** adj.；**o. abdomina′le tu′bae uteri′nae**, the funnel-shaped opening where the uterine tube meets the abdominal cavity 输卵管腹腔口；**coronary o.**, either of the two openings in the aortic sinus that mark the origin of the (left and right) coronary arteries 冠 状 口；**o. pharyn′geum tu′bae auditi′vae**, the pharyngeal opening of the auditory tube 咽鼓管咽口；**o. pri′mum**, an opening in the lower portion of the membrane dividing the embryonic heart into right and left sides 原中隔孔；**o. secun′dum**, an opening high in the septum of the embryonic heart, approximately where the foramen ovale will later appear 第二房间孔；**tympanic o., o. tympa′nicum tu′bae auditi′vae**, the opening of the auditory tube on the carotid wall of the tympanic cavity 咽鼓管鼓口；**o. u′teri**, external os of uterus 子宫颈管外口；**o. vagi′nae**, the external orifice of the vagina 阴道口

os·to·mate (os′tə-māt) one who has undergone enterostomy or ureterostomy 造口者

os·to·my (os′tə-me) general term for an operation in which an artificial opening is formed 吻合术，造口术

OT old tuberculin 旧结核菌素；参见 *tuberculin*

otal·gia (o-tal′jə) pain in the ear; earache 耳痛

OTC over the counter; said of drugs not required by law to be sold on prescription only 柜台有售非处方药

otic (o′tik) auditory (1) 耳的

oti·tis (o-ti′tis) inflammation of the ear 耳 炎；**otit′ic** adj.；**aviation o.**, barotitis media 航空中耳炎；**o. exter′na**, inflammation of the external ear, usually caused by a bacterial or fungal infection; it may be either circumscribed, with formation of a furuncle, or *diffuse* 外 耳 炎；**furuncular o.**, otitis externa with formation of a furuncle 外耳道疖；**o.**

inter′na, labyrinthitis 内耳炎；o. me′dia, inflammation of the middle ear, classified as either *serous (secretory)*, due to obstruction of the eustachian tube, or *suppurative (purulent)*, due to bacterial infection. Both types may involve hearing loss 中耳炎

Oto·bi·us (o-to′be-əs) a genus of soft-bodied ticks parasitic in the ears of various animals, including humans 耳蜱属，残喙蜱属

oto·ceph·a·ly (o″to-sef′ə-le) a congenital anomaly characterized by lack of a lower jaw and by ears that are united below the face 无下颌并耳畸形

oto·cra·ni·um (o″to-kra′ne-əm) the area of the petrous part of the temporal bone surrounding the osseous labyrinth 耳颅；otocra′nial adj.

oto·cyst (o′to-sist″) the auditory vesicle of the embryo 听泡（胚胎）

Oto·dec·tes (o″to-dek′tēz) a genus of mites 耳螨属

oto·en·ceph·a·li·tis (o″to-ən-sef″ə-li′tis) inflammation of the brain due to extension from an inflamed middle ear 中耳性脑炎

oto·gen·ic (o″to-jen′ik) 同 otogenous

otog·e·nous (o-toj′ə-nəs) originating within the ear 耳源性的

oto·lar·yn·gol·o·gy (o″to-lar″ing-gol′ə-je) the branch of medicine dealing with disease of the ear, nose, and throat 耳鼻咽喉（科）学

oto·lith (o′to-lith″) statolith 耳石，位砂

otol·o·gy (o-tol′ə-je) the branch of medicine dealing with the ear, its anatomy, physiology, and pathology 耳科学；otolog′ic adj.

oto·my·co·sis (o″to-mi-ko′sis) otitis externa caused by a fungal infection 耳真菌病，耳癣

oto·neu·rol·o·gy (o″to-noo-rol′ə-je) the branch of otology dealing especially with those portions of the nervous system related to the ear 耳神经科学；otoneurolog′ic adj.

oto·pha·ryn·ge·al (o″to-fə-rin′je-əl) pertaining to the ear and pharynx 耳咽的

oto·plas·ty (o′to-plas″te) plastic surgery of the ear 耳成形术

oto·py·or·rhea (o″to-pi″o-re′ə) otorrhea that is purulent 耳脓溢

oto·rhi·no·lar·yn·gol·o·gy (o″to-ri″no-lar″ing-gol′ə-je) the branch of medicine dealing with the ear, nose, and throat 耳鼻咽喉（科）学

oto·rhi·nol·o·gy (o″to-ri-nol′ə-je) the branch of medicine dealing with the ear and nose 耳鼻科学

otor·rhea (o″to-re′ə) a discharge from the ear 耳漏

oto·scle·ro·sis (o″to-sklə-ro′sis) a condition in which otospongiosis may cause bony ankylosis of the stapes, resulting in conductive hearing loss 耳硬化（症）；otosclerot′ic adj.

oto·scope (o′to-skōp″) an instrument for inspecting or auscultating the ear 耳镜

oto·spon·gi·o·sis (o″to-spun″je-o′sis) the formation of spongy bone in the bony labyrinth of the ear 耳绵化，耳硬化症

oto·tox·ic (o″to-tok″sik) having a deleterious effect upon the eighth nerve or on the organs of hearing and balance 耳毒性的（对第八脑神经或听觉及平衡器官有毒性作用的）

OU [L.] o′culus uter′que (each eye) 每眼

ounce (oz) (ouns) a measure of weight. In the avoirdupois system, 1/16 lb, 28.3495 g, or 437.5 grains; in the apothecaries' system, 1/12 lb, 31.03 g, or 480 grains 盎司，英两（常衡＝1/16磅，或28.3495g；药衡＝1/12磅，或31.03g）；fluid o. (fl oz), a unit of liquid measure of the apothecaries' system; in the United States it is one-sixteenth of a pint, or 29.57 ml. In Great Britain *(imperial ounce)*, it is one-twentieth of an (imperial) pint, or 28.41 ml 流质英两

out·breed·ing (out′brēd-ing) the mating of genetically unrelated individuals 杂交繁殖，远交

out·let (out′lət) a means or route of exit or egress 出口，pelvic o., the inferior opening of the pelvis 骨盆下口；thoracic o., the irregular opening at the inferior part of the thorax, bounded by the twelfth thoracic vertebra, the twelfth ribs, and the lower edge of the costal cartilages. Note: In clinical usage, the term "thoracic outlet syndrome" refers not to this but to the thoracic inlet (q.v.) 胸腔下口

out·li·er (out′li-ər) an observation so distant from the central mass of the data that it noticeably influences results 离群值

out·pa·tient (out′pa-shənt) a patient who comes to the hospital, clinic, or dispensary for diagnosis and/or treatment but does not occupy a bed 门诊病人

out·pock·et·ing (out-pok′ət-ing) evagination 外包缝合法

out·pouch·ing (out′pouch-ing) evagination 突出，外突

out·put (out′poot″) the yield or total of anything produced by any functional system of the body 排出量，输出量；排泄物；cardiac o. (CO), the effective volume of blood expelled by either ventricle of the heart per unit of time (usually per minute) 心排血量，心输出量；stroke o., 心搏排出量，参见 *volume* 下的词条；urinary o., the amount of urine excreted by the kidneys 尿量

ova (o′və) *ovum* 的复数

ovar·i·an (o-var′e-ən) pertaining to an ovary or ovaries 卵巢的，卵巢性的

ovar·i·ec·to·my (o-var″e-ek′tə-me) 同 oopho-rec-tomy

ovar·io·cen·te·sis (o-var″e-o-sen-te′sis) surgical puncture of an ovary 卵巢穿刺术

ovar·io·pexy (o-var″e-o-pek′se) 同 oophoropexy

ovar·i·or·rhex·is (o-var″re-o-rek′sis) rupture of an ovary 卵巢破裂

ovar·i·os·to·my (o-var″e-os′tə-me) 同 oopho-ro-stomy

ovar·i·ot·o·my (o-var″e-ot′ə-me) 1. 同 oopho-rec-tomy; 2. removal of an ovarian tumor 卵巢肿瘤切除术

ovar·io·tu·bal (o-var″e-o-too′bəl) tuboovarian 输卵管卵巢的

ova·ri·tis (o″və-ri′tis) 同 oophoritis

ova·ri·um (o-var′e-əm) pl. *ova′ria* [L.] ovary 卵巢

ova·ry (o′və-re) the female gonad: either of the paired female sexual glands in which oocytes are formed 卵巢; **ova′rian** *adj.*; **polycystic o's,** ova-ries containing multiple small follicular cysts filled with yellow or blood-stained thin serous fluid, as in polycystic ovary syndrome 多囊性卵巢

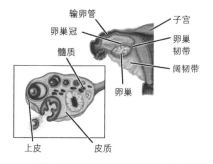

▲ 卵巢，插图展示卵巢的微观结构：右上方逆时针方向表示卵泡发育的不同阶段，表明卵泡逐渐从成熟到排卵之后，最终黄体成熟后退化

over·bite (o′vər-bīt″) the extension of the upper incisor teeth over the lower ones vertically when the opposing posterior teeth are in contact 覆𬌗

over·com·pen·sa·tion (o″vər-kom″pən-sa′-shən) exaggerated correction of a real or imagined physi-cal or psychological defect 过度补偿

over·den·ture (o″vər-den′chər) a complete den-ture supported both by mucosa and by a few remain-ing natural teeth that have been altered to permit the denture to fit over them 覆盖义齿

over·de·ter·mi·na·tion (o″vər-de-ter″mĭ-na′-shən) the concept that every dream, disorder, aspect of behavior, or other emotional reaction or symptom

has multiple causative factors 多因素决定

over·do·sage (o″vər-do′səj) 1. the administration of an excessive dose 超剂量; 2. the condition re-sulting from an excessive dose 超剂量反应

over·dose (o′vər-dōs″) 1. to administer an exces-sive dose 使……服药过量; 2. an excessive dose 用量（用药）

over·drive (o′vər-drīv″) a more rapid heart rate produced in the correction of an underlying patho-logic rhythm 超律（法）; 另参见 *pacing* 下词条

over·hy·dra·tion (o″vər-hi-dra′shən) hyperhydra-tion 水中毒

over·jet (o′vər-jet″) extension of the incisal or buccal cusp ridges of the upper teeth labially or buc-cally to the incisal margins and ridges of the lower teeth when the jaws are closed normally 覆盖

over·rid·ing (o″vər-rīd′ing) 1. the slipping of either part of a fractured bone past the other 骨折断端滑动; 2. extending beyond the usual position 异常突起

over·ven·ti·la·tion (o″vər-ven″tĭ-la′shən) hyper-ventilation 换气过度

ovi·cide (o′vĭ-sīd) an agent destructive to the eggs of certain organisms 杀卵剂

ovi·duct (o′vĭ-dukt″) 1. uterine tube 输卵管; 2. in nonmammals, a passage through which ova leave the female or pass to an organ that communi-cates with the exterior of the body 非哺乳动物体内卵子排出体外的通道; **ovidu′cal, oviduct′al** *adj.*

ovif·er·ous (o-vif′ər-əs) producing ova 产卵的

ovi·gen·e·sis (o″vĭ-jen′ə-sis) 同 oogenesis

ovip·a·rous (o-vip′ə-rəs) producing eggs in which the embryo develops outside the maternal body, as do birds 卵生的

ovi·pos·i·tor (o″vĭ-poz′ĭ-tər) a specialized organ by which many female insects deposit their eggs 产卵器

ovo·lac·to·veg·e·tar·i·an (o″vo-lak″to-vej″ə-tar′e-ən) 1. one whose diet is restricted to vege-tables, dairy products, and eggs, eschewing other foods of animal origin 乳蛋素食者; 2. pertaining to ovolac-tovegetarianism 乳蛋素食主义的; 3. one who practices ovolactovegetarianism 乳蛋素食主义者

ovo·lac·to·veg·e·tar·i·an·ism (o″vo-lak″tovej″ə-tar′e-ən-iz″əm) restriction of the diet to vegetables, dairy products, and eggs, eschewing other foods of animal origin 乳蛋素食主义

ovo·plasm (o′vo-plaz″əm) 同 ooplasm

ovo·tes·tis (o″vo-tes′tis) a gonad containing both testicular and ovarian tissue 两性生殖腺，卵睾体

ovo·veg·e·tar·i·an (o″vo-vej″ə-tar′e-ən) 1. per-taining to ovovegetarianism 蛋素食主义的; 2. one who practices ovovegetarianism 蛋素食主义者

ovo·veg·e·tar·i·an·ism (o″vo-vej″ə-tar′e- ən-iz″əm) restriction of the diet to vegetables and eggs, eschewing other foods of animal origin 蛋素食主义

ovu·lar (ov′u-lər) 1. pertaining to an ovule 原卵的；2. pertaining to an oocyte 卵母细胞的

ovu·la·tion (ov″u-la′shən) the discharge of a secondary oocyte from a graafian follicle 排卵；**ov′ulatory** adj.

ovule (o′vūl) 1. the oocyte within the graafian follicle 原卵，卵泡内卵；2. any small, egglike structure 卵状小体，小卵

ovum (o′vəm) pl. o′va [L.] 1. the female reproductive cell which, after fertilization, becomes a zygote that develops into a new member of the same species 卵子；2. imprecise term for oocyte 卵母细胞（的不精确术语）；3. formerly, any of various stages from the primary oocyte to the implanting blastocyst 之前指代从初级卵母细胞到着床囊胚的任何阶段；4. in some species, any stage from the unfertilized female reproductive cell, through the developing embryo surrounded by nutrient material and protective covering, up to the point when the young emerge 卵

ox·a·cil·lin (ok″sə-sil′in) a semisynthetic penicillinase-resistant penicillin used as the sodium salt in infections due to penicillin-resistant, gram-positive organisms 苯唑西林，苯唑青霉素

ox·a·late (ok′sə-lāt) any salt of oxalic acid 草酸盐

ox·a·le·mia (ok″sə-le′me-ə) excess of oxalates in the blood 草酸盐血

ox·al·ic ac·id (ok-sal′ik) a dicarboxylic acid occurring in various fruits and vegetables and as a metabolic product of glyoxylic or ascorbic acid; it is not metabolized but is excreted in the urine. Excess may lead to formation of calcium oxalate calculi in the kidney 草酸

ox·al·ism (ok′səl-iz″əm) poisoning by oxalic acid or by an oxalate 草酸中毒

ox·a·lo·ac·e·tate (ok″sə-lo-as′ə-tāt) a salt or ester of oxaloacetic acid 草酰乙酸盐（或酯）

ox·a·lo·ace·tic ac·id (ok″sə-lo-ə-se′tik) a metabolic intermediate in the tricarboxylic acid cycle; it is convertible to aspartic acid by aspartate transaminase 草酰乙酸

ox·a·lo·sis (ok″sə-lo′sis) generalized deposition of calcium oxalate in renal and extrarenal tissues, as may occur in primary hyperoxaluria 草酸盐沉着症

ox·al·uria (ok″səl-u′re-ə) hyperoxaluria 草酸尿

ox·an·dro·lone (ok-san′dro-lōn) an androgenic and anabolic steroid that is used in the treatment of catabolic or tissue-wasting diseases or states 氧甲氢龙

ox·a·pro·zin (ok″sə-pro′zin) a nonsteroidal anti-inflammatory drug, used in the treatment of rheumatoid arthritis and osteoarthritis 噁丙嗪

ox·az·e·pam (ok-saz′ə-pam) a benzodiazepine tranquilizer, used as an antianxiety agent and as an adjunct in the treatment of acute alcohol withdrawal symptoms 去甲羟基安定

oxa·zo·lid·in·one (ok″sə-zo-lid′ĭ-nōn) any of a class of synthetic antibacterial agents effective against gram-positive organisms 噁唑烷酮

ox·car·baz·e·pine (oks″kahr-baz′ə-pēn) an anticonvulsant used in the treatment of partial seizures 奥卡西平

ox·i·con·a·zole (ok″sĭ-kon′ə-zōl) an imidazole antifungal used topically as the nitrate salt in the treatment of various forms of tinea 奥昔康唑

ox·i·dant (ok′sĭ-dənt) the electron acceptor in an oxidation-reduction (redox) reaction 氧化剂

ox·i·dase (ok′sĭ-dās) any enzyme of the class of oxidoreductases in which molecular oxygen is the hydrogen acceptor 氧化酶

ox·i·da·tion (ok″sĭ-da′shən) the act of oxidizing or state of being oxidized 氧化（作用）；**ox′idative** adj.

ox·i·da·tion-re·duc·tion (ok″sĭ-da′shən re-duk′shən) the chemical reaction whereby electrons are removed (oxidation) from atoms of the substance being oxidized and transferred to those being reduced (reduction) 氧化还原（作用）

ox·ide (ok′sīd) a compound of oxygen with an element or radical 氧化物

ox·i·dize (ok′sĭ-dīz″) to cause to combine with oxygen or to remove hydrogen（使）氧化

ox·i·do·re·duc·tase (ok″sĭ-do-re-duk′tās) any of a class of enzymes that catalyze the reversible transfer of electrons from a substrate that becomes oxidized to one that becomes reduced (oxidation-reduction, or redox reaction) 氧化还原酶

ox·ime (ok′sēm) any of a series of compounds containing the CH(=NOH) group, formed by the action of hydroxylamine upon an aldehyde or a ketone 肟。Spelled also oxim

ox·im·e·ter (ok-sim′ə-tər) a photoelectric device for determining the oxygen saturation of the blood 血氧计

ox·im·e·try (ok-sim′ə-tre) determination of the oxygen saturation of arterial blood using an oximeter 血氧定量法

5-ox·o·pro·line (ok″so-pro′lēn) an acidic lactam of glutamic acid occurring at the N-terminus of several peptides and proteins 5-羟脯氨酸

5-ox·o·pro·lin·u·ria (ok″so-pro″lin-u′re-ə) 1. excess of 5-oxoproline in the urine 尿中 5-羟脯

氨酸过多；2. generalized deficiency of glutathione synthetase 全身性谷胱甘肽合成酶缺乏症

ox·triph·yl·line (oks-trif'ə-lēn) the choline salt of theophylline, used chiefly as a bronchodilator 胆茶碱

oxy·ben·zone (ok″se-ben′zōn) a topical sunscreen that absorbs UVB rays and some UVA rays 氧苯酮

oxy·bu·ty·nin (ok″se-bu′tĭ-nin) an anticholinergic having a direct antispasmodic effect on smooth muscle; used as the chloride salt in the treatment of uninhibited or reflex neurogenic bladder 奥昔布宁，羟丁宁

oxy·ceph·a·ly (ok″se-sef′ə-le) increased skull height owing to premature closure of multiple sutures, with the skull high and narrow and shallow orbits; however, sometimes used interchangeably with acrocephaly for any abnormally tall skull 尖头（畸形）；**oxycephal′ic** *adj.*

oxy·co·done (ok″se-ko′dōn) an opioid analgesic derived from morphine; used in the form of the hydrochloride and terephthalate salts 羟考酮

ox·y·gen (O) (ok′sĭ-jən) a colorless, odorless, tasteless gaseous element; at. no. 8, at. wt. 15.999. Diatomic oxygen gas (O$_2$) constitutes about 21 percent of the volume of air, is the essential agent in the respiration of plants and animals, and is necessary to support combustion 氧；**o. 15,** an artificial radioactive isotope of oxygen having a half-life of 2.04 minutes and decaying by positron emission; used as a tracer in positron emission tomography 氧^{15}；**hyperbaric o.,** oxygen under greater than atmospheric pressure 高压氧

ox·y·gen·ase (ok′sĭ-jən-ās) any oxidoreductase that catalyzes the incorporation of both atoms of molecular oxygen into a single substrate 加氧酶，氧合酶

ox·y·gen·ate (ok′sĭ-jə-nāt) to saturate with oxygen 氧合，充氧

ox·y·gen·a·tion (ok″sĭ-jə-na′shən) 1. the act or process of adding oxygen 充氧；2. the result of having oxygen added 氧合；**extracorporeal membrane o. (ECMO),** extracorporeal life support 体外膜氧合；**hyperbaric o.,** exposure to oxygen under pressure greater than normal atmospheric pressure, done for those needing more oxygen than they can take in through breathing or use of an oxygen mask 高压氧治疗

oxy·hem·a·to·por·phy·rin (ok″se-hem″ə-topor′fĭ-rin) a pigment sometimes found in the urine, closely allied to hematoporphyrin 血氧卟啉

oxy·he·mo·glo·bin (ok″se-he′mo-glo″bin) hemoglobin that contains bound O$_2$, a compound formed from hemoglobin on exposure to alveolar gas in the lungs 氧合血红蛋白

oxy·met·az·o·line (ok″se-mət-az′o-lēn) an adrenergic used as the hydrochloride salt as a vasoconstrictor to reduce nasal or conjunctival congestion 羟甲唑啉

oxy·meth·o·lone (ok″se-meth′ə-lōn) an anabolic steroid used in the treatment of anemia and for the prophylaxis and treatment of hereditary angioedema 羟甲烯龙

oxy·mor·phone (ok″se-mor′fōn) an opioid analgesic, used as the hydrochloride salt as an analgesic and anesthesia adjunct 羟吗啡酮

oxy·myo·glo·bin (ok″se-mi′o-glo″bin) myoglobin charged with oxygen 氧合肌红蛋白

ox·yn·tic (ok-sin′tik) secreting acid, as the parietal (oxyntic) cells 泌酸的

oxy·phil (ok′se-fil) 1. *(in the pl.)* oxyphil cells 嗜酸性细胞；2. *(in the pl.)* Askanazy cells Askanazy 细胞；3. acidophilic (1) 嗜酸（性）的

oxy·phil·ic (ok″se-fil′ik) acidophilic (1) 嗜酸的

oxy·quin·o·line (ok″se-kwin′o-lēn) a dicyclic aromatic compound used as a chelating agent; also used in the form of the base or the sulfate salt as a bacteriostatic, fungistatic, antiseptic, and disinfectant 羟喹啉

oxy·tet·ra·cy·cline (ok″se-tet″rə-si′klēn) a broad-spectrum tetracycline antibiotic produced by *Streptomyces rimosus,* used as the base or the hydrochloride salt 氧四环素

oxy·to·cia (ok-se-to′se-ə) rapid labor 快速分娩

oxy·to·cic (ok-se-to′sik) 1. pertaining to, marked by, or promoting oxytocia 催产的；2. an agent that promotes rapid labor by stimulating contractions of the myometrium 催产药

oxy·to·cin (ok″se-to′sin) a hypothalamic hormone stored in the posterior pituitary, which has uterine-contracting and milk-releasing actions; it may also be prepared synthetically or obtained from the posterior pituitary of domestic animals; used to induce active labor, increase the force of contractions in labor, contract uterine muscle after delivery of the placenta, control postpartum hemorrhage, and stimulate milk ejection 催产素，缩宫素

oxy·uri·a·sis (ok″se-u-ri′ə-sis) 1. infection with an oxyurid such as *Enterobius vermicularis* 蛲虫感染；2. enterobiasis 蛲虫病

oxy·urid (ok-se-u′rid) a pinworm, seatworm, or threadworm; any individual of the superfamily Oxyuroidea 蛲虫

Oxy·uris (ok″se-u′ris) a genus of intestinal nematodes (superfamily Oxyuroidea) 尖尾线虫属，蛲虫属

Oxy·uroi·dea (ok″se-u″roi-de′ə) a superfamily

of small nematodes—the pinworms, seatworms, or threadworms—parasitic in the cecum and colon of vertebrates and sometimes infecting invertebrates 尖尾总科，蛲虫总科

oz ounce 盎司

oze·na (o-ze′nə) an atrophic rhinitis marked by a thick mucopurulent discharge, mucosal crusting, and fetor 臭鼻（症）

ozone (o′zōn) a bluish explosive gas or blue liquid, being an allotropic form of oxygen, O_3; it is antiseptic and disinfectant, and irritating and toxic to the pulmonary system 臭氧

P

P [符号] para 产次; peta- 称; phosphate (group) 磷酸基; phosphorus 磷; posterior 后的; premolar 前磨牙; proline 脯氨酸; pupil 瞳孔

P [符号] power 功率; pressure 压力

P₁ parental generation 亲代的符号

P₂ pulmonic second sound 肺动脉第二心音的符号

p [符号] pico- 皮（可）; proton 质子; the short arm of a chromosome 染色体短臂

p- para; beside, beyond 对（位）

PA physician assistant 医师助理; posteroanterior 后前位的; pulmonary artery 肺动脉

Pa [符号] pascal 帕（斯卡）; protactinium 元素镤

PAB, PABA p-aminobenzoic acid 对氨基苯甲酸

pace·mak·er (pās′ma-kər) 1. that which sets the pace at which a phenomenon occurs 起步点，起搏点; 2. the natural cardiac pacemaker or an artificial cardiac pacemaker 起搏器; 3. in biochemistry, a substance whose rate of reaction sets the pace for a series of related reactions（生化反应中）关键酶; **artificial cardiac p.,** a device designed to reproduce or regulate the rhythm of the heart. It is worn by or implanted in the body of the patient, is battery-driven, is usually triggered or inhibited to modify output by sensing the intracardiac potential in one or more cardiac chambers, and may also have antitachycardia functions. Many are designated by a three- to five-letter code used to categorize them functionally 人工心脏起搏器; **cardiac p.,** a group of cells rhythmically initiating the heartbeat, characterized physiologically by a slow loss of membrane potential during diastole; usually it is the sinoatrial node 心脏起搏点，心脏起步点; **demand p.,** an implanted cardiac pacemaker in which the generator stimulus is inhibited by a signal derived from the heart's electrical activation (depolarization), thus minimizing the risk of pacemakerinduced fibrillation 按需型起搏器; **dual-chamber p.,** an artificial pacemaker with two leads, one in the atrium and one in the ventricle, so that electromechanical synchrony can be approximated 双室起搏器; **ectopic p.,** any biologic cardiac pacemaker other than the sinoatrial node; it is normally inactive 异位起搏点，异位起步点; **escape p.,** an ectopic pacemaker that assumes control of cardiac impulse propagation because of failure of the sinoatrial node to initiate one or more impulses 脱逸起搏器; **fixed-rate p.,** an artificial cardiac pacemaker set to pace at only a single rate 固定频率起搏器; **rate-responsive p.,** an artificial cardiac pacemaker that can deliver stimuli at a rate adjustable to some parameter independent of atrial activity 频率适应性起搏器; **runaway p.,** a malfunctioning artificial cardiac pacemaker that abruptly accelerates its pacing rate, inducing tachycardia 失速起搏器; **secondary p.,** ectopic p. 异位起搏点; **single-chamber p.,** an implanted cardiac pacemaker with only one lead, placed in either the atrium or the ventricle 单室起搏器; **wandering atrial p.,** a condition in which the site of origin of the impulses controlling the heart rate shifts from one point to another within the atria, almost with every beat 移动性起搏点

pachy·bleph·a·ron (pak″e-blef′ə-ron) thickening of the eyelids 睑缘肥厚

pachy·ceph·a·ly (pak″e-sef′ə-le) abnormal thickness of the bones of the skull 颅骨肥厚; **pachycephal′ic, pachyceph′alous** adj.

pachy·chei·lia (pak″e-ki′le-ə) thickening of the lips 唇肥厚

pachy·der·ma (pak″e-dur′mə) abnormal thickening of the skin 皮肥厚，厚皮; **pachyder′matous, pachyder′mic** adj.

pachy·der·mo·peri·os·to·sis (pak″e-dur″moper″e-os-to′sis) pachyderma of the face and scalp, thickening of the bones of the distal limbs, and acropachy 厚皮性骨膜病

pachy·glos·sia (pak″e-glos′e-ə) abnormal thickness of the tongue 舌肥厚，厚舌

pachy·gy·ria (pak″e-ji′re-ə) macrogyria 巨脑回畸形

pachy·lep·to·men·in·gi·tis (pak″e-lep″-tomen″in-ji′tis) inflammation of the dura mater and pia mater 硬软脑膜炎

pachy·men·in·gi·tis (pak″e-men″in-ji′tis) inflammation of the dura mater 硬脑膜炎

pachy·men·in·gop·a·thy (pak″e-men″ingo-p′ə-the) noninflammatory disease of the dura mater 硬脑脊膜病

pachy·me·ninx (pak″e-me′ninks) pl. *pachy-menin'ges.* Dura mater 硬脑（脊）膜

pa·chyn·sis (pə-kin′sis) an abnormal thickening 肥厚; **pachyn′tic** *adj.*

pachy·onych·ia (pak″e-o-nik′e-ə) abnormal thickening of the nails 甲肥厚，厚甲; **p. conge′nita**, an autosomal dominant disorder due to mutation in any of several genes encoding keratins, marked by dystrophic, thickened nails, palmoplantar hyperkeratosis, hyperhidrosis of the palms and soles, and bullae following trauma. Oral leukoplakia is also common 先天性甲肥厚

pachy·peri·os·ti·tis (pak″e-per″e-os-ti′tis) periostitis of the long bones resulting in abnormal thickness of affected bones 肥厚性骨膜炎

pachy·pleu·ri·tis (pak″e-ploo-ri′tis) 1. fibrothorax 纤维胸; 2. pleural fibrosis 肥厚性胸膜炎

pachy·sal·pin·gi·tis (pak″e-sal″pin-ji′tis) chronic salpingitis with thickening 肥厚性输卵管炎，实质性输卵管炎

pachy·sal·pin·go·ova·ri·tis (pak″e-sal-ping″-goo″və-ri′tis) chronic inflammation of the ovary and uterine tube, with thickening 肥厚性输卵管卵巢炎

pachy·tene (pak′e-tēn) the third stage of prophase in meiosis I, during which synapsis is complete and genetic material may be exchanged by crossing over 粗线期

pach·y·vag·i·ni·tis (pak″e-vaj″ĭ-ni′tis) chronic vaginitis with thickening of the vaginal walls 肥厚性阴道炎

pac·ing (pās′ing) setting of the pace 定速，调速，起搏; **asynchronous p.**, cardiac pacing in which impulse generation by the pacemaker occurs at a fixed rate, independent of underlying cardiac activity 非同步起搏; **burst p.**, overdrive p. 短阵快速起搏; **cardiac p.**, regulation of the rate of contraction of the heart muscle by an artificial cardiac pacemaker 心脏起搏; **coupled p.**, a variation of paired pacing in which the patient's natural depolarization serves as the first of the two stimuli, with the second induced by an artificial cardiac pacemaker 双重调节; **diaphragm p., diaphragmatic p.**, electrophrenic respiration 膈肌起搏; **overdrive p.**, the process of increasing the heart rate by means of an artificial cardiac pacemaker in order to suppress certain arrhythmias 超速起搏; **paired p.**, cardiac pacing in which two impulses are delivered to the heart in close succession, to slow tachyarrhythmias and to improve cardiac performance 双脉冲心

律调节; **ramp p.**, cardiac pacing in which stimuli are delivered at a rapid but continually altering rate, either from faster to slower *(rate decremental or tune down)*, from fast to faster *(cycle length decremental or ramp up)*, or in some cyclic combination of increasing and decreasing rates; used to control tachyarrhythmias 斜坡心律调节; **synchronous p.**, cardiac pacing in which information about sensed activity in one or more cardiac chambers is used to determine the timing of impulse generation by the pacemaker 同步起搏; **underdrive p.**, a method for terminating certain tachycardias by means of slow asynchronous pacing at a rate not an even fraction of the tachycardia rate 亚速起搏

pack (pak) 1. treatment by wrapping a patient in blankets or sheets or a limb in towels, either wet or dry and hot or cold; also, the blankets or towels used for this purpose 包扎; 2. a tampon 棉塞

pack·er (pak′ər) an instrument for introducing a dressing into a cavity or a wound 填塞器

pack·ing (pak′ing) the filling of a wound or cavity with gauze, sponges, pads, or other material; also, the material used for this purpose（用纱布、棉花等）填塞（伤口或腔）；填料，填塞物

pac·li·tax·el (pak″lĭ-tak′səl) an antineoplastic that promotes and stabilizes polymerization of microtubules, isolated from the Pacific yew tree *(Taxus brevifolia)*; used in the treatment of advanced ovarian or breast carcinoma, non– small-cell lung carcinoma, and AIDS-related Kaposi sarcoma 紫杉醇

PACU postanesthesia care unit 术后麻醉恢复室; 参见 *unit* 下词条

pad (pad) a cushionlike mass of soft material 垫，托; 纱布垫; **abdominal p.**, a pad for the absorption of discharges from abdominal wounds or for packing off abdominal viscera to improve exposure during surgery 腹垫; **buccal fat p.**, 同 sucking p.; **dinner p.**, a pad placed over the stomach before a plaster jacket is applied; the pad is then removed, leaving space under the jacket to accommodate expansion of the stomach after eating 胃托; **infrapatellar fat p.**, a large pad of fat lying behind and below the patella 髌下脂体; **knuckle p's**, nodular thickenings of the skin on the dorsal surface of the interphalangeal joints 指节垫; **retromolar p.**, a cushionlike mass of tissue situated at the distal termination of the mandibular residual ridge 磨牙后垫; **sucking p., suctorial p.**, a lobulated mass of fat that occupies the space between the masseter and the external surface of the buccinator; it is well developed in infants 吸垫，颊脂体，颊脂垫

pad·i·mate O (pad′ĭ-māt) a substituted aminobenzoate used as a sunscreen, absorbing UVB rays 二

甲氨苯酸辛酯（遮光剂）

PAF platelet-activating factor 血小板激活因子

PAH, PAHA *p*-aminohippuric acid 对氨基马尿酸

PAI plasminogen activator inhibitor 纤溶酶原激活物抑制物

pain (pān) a feeling of distress, suffering, or agony, caused by stimulation of specialized nerve endings（疼）痛; **bearing-down p.,** pain accompanying uterine contractions during the second stage of labor 坠痛（分娩第二期）; **false p's,** ineffective pains resembling labor pains, not accompanied by cervical dilatation 假阵痛; **growing p's,** recurrent quasirheumatic limb pains peculiar to early youth 发育期痛; **hunger p.,** pain coming on at the time for feeling hunger for a meal; a symptom of gastric disorder 饥饿痛; **intermenstrual p.,** pain accompanying ovulation, occurring during the period between the menses, usually about midway 经间期疼痛; **labor p's,** the rhythmic pains of increasing severity and frequency due to contraction of the uterus at childbirth 阵痛, 分娩痛; **phantom limb p.,** pain felt as though arising in an absent (amputated) limb 幻肢痛; **psychogenic p.,** symptoms of physical pain having psychological origin 精神性疼痛; **referred p.,** pain felt in a part other than that in which the cause that produced it is situated 牵涉痛; **rest p.,** a continuous burning pain due to ischemia of the lower leg, which begins or is aggravated after reclining and is relieved by sitting or standing 静息痛

paint (pānt) 1. a liquid designed for application to a surface, as of the body or a tooth 涂层; 2. to apply a liquid to a specific area as a remedial or protective measure 涂抹

pair (pār) 1. a combination of two related, similar, or identical entities or objects 配对; 2. in cardiology, two successive premature beats, particularly two ventricular premature complexes 偶联; **base p.,** a pair of hydrogen-bonded bases, a pyrimidine with a purine base, that bind together two strands, or two parts of a strand, of nucleic acid 碱基对

pal·ate (pal′ət) roof of the mouth; the partition separating the nasal and oral cavities 腭; **pal′atal, pal′atine** *adj.*; **cleft p.,** congenital fissure of median line of palate 腭裂; **hard p.,** the anterior portion of the palate, separating the oral and nasal cavities, consisting of the bony framework and covering membranes 硬腭; **soft p.,** the fleshy part of the palate, extending from the posterior edge of the hard palate; the uvula projects from its free inferior border 软腭

pal·a·ti·tis (pal″ə-ti′tis) inflammation of the palate 腭炎

pal·a·to·glos·sal (pal″ə-to-glos′əl) pertaining to the palate and tongue 舌腭的

pal·a·tog·na·thous (pal″ə-tog′nə-thəs) having a cleft palate 腭裂的

pal·a·to·pha·ryn·ge·al (pal″ə-to-fə-rin′je-əl) pertaining to the palate and pharynx 腭咽的

pal·a·to·plas·ty (pal′ə-to-plas″te) plastic reconstruction of the palate 腭成形术

pal·a·to·ple·gia (pal″ə-to-ple′jə) paralysis of the palate 腭麻痹

pal·a·tor·rha·phy (pal″ə-tor′ə-fe) surgical correction of a cleft palate 腭裂修复术

pa·la·tum (pə-la′təm) pl. *pala′ta* [L.] 同 palate

pa·leo·cer·e·bel·lum (pa″le-o-ser″ə-bel′əm) the phylogenetically second oldest part of the cerebellum, namely the vermis of the anterior lobe and the pyramis, uvula, and paraflocculus of the posterior lobe. Because this corresponds roughly to the primary site of termination of the major spinocerebellar afferents, the term is sometimes equated with *spinocerebellum* 旧小脑。Spelled also *palaeocerebellum*; **paleocerebel′lar** *adj.*

pa·leo·cor·tex (pa″le-o-kor′teks) that portion of the cerebral cortex that, with the archicortex, develops in association with the olfactory system and is phylogenetically older and less stratified than the neocortex. It is composed chiefly of the piriform cortex and the parahippocampal gyrus 旧皮质。Spelled also *palaeocortex*; **paleocor′tical** *adj.*

pa·le·o·on·col·o·gy (pa′le-ō-ong-kol″ə-je) study of the history of cancer and other neoplastic diseases using archaeologic, historical, clinical, and biomolecular analysis 古肿瘤学

pa·leo·pa·thol·o·gy (pa″le-o-pə-thol′ə-je) study of disease in bodies that have been preserved from ancient times 古生物病理学

pa·leo·stri·a·tum (pa″le-o-stri-a′təm) the phylogenetically older portion of the corpus striatum, represented by the globus pallidus 旧纹状体, 原纹状体; **paleostria′tal** *adj.*

pal·in·dro·mia (pal″in-dro′me-ə) [Gr.] a recurrence or relapse（病的）复发, 再发; **palindro′mic** *adj.*

pali·nop·sia (pal″ĭ-nop′se-ə) the continuance of a visual sensation after the stimulus is gone 持续后像

pal·i·viz·u·mab (pal″ĭ-viz′u-mab) a monoclonal antibody against respiratory syncytial virus (RSV); used as a passive immunizing agent in susceptible infants and children 帕立珠单抗

pal·la·di·um (Pd) (pə-la′de-əm) a rare, hard, silvery white, metallic element; at. no. 46, at. wt. 106.42 钯（化学元素）

pall·an·es·the·sia (pal″ən-es-the′zhə) loss or absence of pallesthesia 振动（感）觉缺失

pall·es·the·sia (pal″es-the′zhə) the ability to feel mechanical vibrations on or near the body, such as when a vibrating tuning fork is placed over a bony prominence 振动觉；**pallesthet′ic** *adj.*

pal·li·a·tive (pal′e-ə-tiv) affording relief; also, a drug that so acts 减轻的；缓和剂

pal·li·dec·to·my (pal″ĭ-dek′tə-me) extirpation of the globus pallidus 苍白球切除术

pal·li·do·an·sot·o·my (pal″ĭ-do-ən-sot′ə-me) production of lesions in the globus pallidus and ansa lenticularis 苍白球豆状核袢切开术

pal·li·dot·o·my (pal″ĭ-dot′ə-me) a stereotaxic surgical technique for the production of lesions in the globus pallidus for treatment of extrapyramidal disorders 苍白球切开术

pal·li·dum (pal′ĭ-dəm) globus pallidus 苍白球；**pal′lidal** *adj.*

pal·li·um (pal′e-əm) [L.] 1. cerebral cortex 大脑皮质，大脑皮层；2. the cerebral cortex during its period of development 大脑皮质发育；**pal′lial** *adj.*

pal·lor (pal′ər) paleness, as of the skin 苍白

palm (pahm) (pahlm) the hollow or flexor surface of the hand 掌

pal·ma (pahl′mə) pl. *pal′mae* [L.] 同 palm

pal·mar (pahl′mər) pertaining to the palm of the hand 掌的

pal·mar·is (pahl-mar′is) 同 palmar

pal·mate (pahl′māt) having a shape resembling that of a hand with the fingers spread 掌状的

pal·mit·ic ac·id (pal-mit′ik) a 16-carbon saturated fatty acid found in most fats and oils, particularly associated with stearic acid; one of the most prevalent saturated fatty acids in body lipids 棕榈酸，软脂酸，十六（烷）酸

pal·mi·tin (pal′mĭ-tin) glyceryl tripalmitate; a crystallizable and saponifiable fat from various fats and oils（三）棕榈酸甘油酯

pal·mi·to·le·ate (pal″mĭ-to′le-āt) a salt (soap), ester, or anionic form of palmitoleic acid 棕榈油酸盐（酯或阴离子型）

pal·mi·to·le·ic ac·id (pal″mĭ-to-le′ik) a mono-unsaturated 16-carbon fatty acid occurring in many oils, particularly those derived from marine animals 棕榈油酸，十六（碳）烯 - 9 - 酸

pal·pa·tion (pal-pa′shən) the act of feeling with the hand; the application of the fingers with light pressure to the surface of the body for the purpose of determining the condition of the parts beneath in physical diagnosis 触诊；**pal′patory** *adj.*

pal·pe·bra (pal′pə-brə) pl. *pal′pebrae* [L.] eyelid 眼睑；**pal′pebral** *adj.*

pal·pe·bri·tis (pal″pə-bri′tis) blepharitis 眼睑炎

pal·pi·ta·tion (pal″pĭ-ta′shən) a subjective sensation of an unduly rapid or irregular heartbeat 心悸

PALS periarteriolar lymphoid sheath 动脉周围淋巴鞘

pal·sy (pawl′ze) 同 paralysis；Bell p., unilateral facial paralysis of sudden onset due to a lesion of the facial nerve, resulting in characteristic facial distortion 贝尔麻痹，特发性面神经麻痹；cerebral p., any of a group of persisting qualitative motor disorders appearing in young children, resulting from brain damage caused by birth trauma or intrauterine pathology 大脑性瘫痪，脑瘫；Erb p., Erb-Duchenne p., Erb-Duchenne paralysis 臂麻痹上丛型；facial p., Bell p. 面瘫；progressive bulbar p., chronic, progressive, generally fatal paralysis and atrophy of the muscles of the lips, tongue, mouth, pharynx, and larynx due to lesions of the motor nuclei of the lower brainstem, usually occurring in late adult years 慢性延髓麻痹；pseudobulbar p., spastic weakness of the muscles innervated by the cranial nerves, i.e., the facial muscles, pharynx, and tongue, due to bilateral lesions of the corticospinal tract, often accompanied by uncontrolled weeping or laughing 假延髓性麻痹；wasting p., spinal muscular atrophy 消瘦性麻痹

pam·a·brom (pam′ə-brom) a mild diuretic used in preparations for the relief of premenstrual symptoms 柏马溴

pam·i·dro·nate (pam″ĭ-dro′nāt) an inhibitor of bone resorption used to treat malignancyassociated hypercalcemia, osteitis deformans, and osteolytic metastasis secondary to breast cancer or myeloma; used as the disodium salt. Complexed with technetium 99m, it is used in bone imaging 帕米膦酸二钠

pam·pin·i·form (pam-pin′ĭ-form) shaped like a tendril 蔓状的，卷须状的

PAN polyarteritis nodosa 结节性多动脉炎

Pan·ae·o·lus (pan″e-o′lus) a genus of mushrooms, several species of which contain the hallucinogens psilocybin and psilocin 斑褶菇属

pan·ag·glu·ti·nin (pan″ə-gloo′tĭ-nin) an agglutinin that agglutinates the erythrocytes of all human blood groups 泛凝集素，全凝集素

pan·ar·ter·i·tis (pan″ahr-tə-ri′tis) 同 polyarteritis

pan·at·ro·phy (pan-at′rə-fe) atrophy of several parts; diffuse atrophy 全身萎缩

pan·au·to·nom·ic (pan″aw-tə-nom′ik) pertaining to or affecting the entire autonomic (sympathetic and parasympathetic) nervous system 全自主神经系统的

pan·car·di·tis (pan″kahr-di′tis) diffuse inflammation of the heart 全心炎

pan·cha·kar·ma (pahn″chə-kahr′mə) [Sanskrit]

a fivefold purification treatment used in ayurveda, usually including a purgative to eliminate kapha, a laxative to eliminate pitta, an enema to eliminate vata, inhalation treatment to clear doshas from the head, and bloodletting to purify the blood 排毒治疗

pan·co·lec·to·my (pan″ko-lek′tə-me) excision of the entire colon, with creation of an ileostomy 全结肠切除术

pan·cre·as (pan′kre-əs) pl. *pancre′ata* [Gr.] a large, elongated, racemose gland lying transversely behind the stomach, between the spleen and duodenum. Its external secretion contains digestive enzymes. One internal secretion, insulin, is produced by the beta cells, and another, glucagon, is produced by the alpha cells. The alpha, beta, and delta cells form aggregates, called *islets of Langerhans* 胰（腺），见图 27；**endocrine p.**, that part of the pancreas that acts as an endocrine gland, consisting of the islets of Langerhans, which secrete insulin and other hormones 胰腺内分泌；**exocrine p.**, that part of the pancreas that acts as an exocrine gland, consisting of the pancreatic acini, which produce pancreatic juice and secrete it into the duodenum to aid in protein digestion 胰腺外分泌

pan·cre·a·tec·to·my (pan″kre-ə-tek′tə-me) excision of the pancreas 胰切除术

pan·cre·at·ic (pan″kre-at′ik) pertaining to the pancreas 胰（腺）的

pan·cre·at·ic elas·tase (pan″kre-at′ik e-las′tās) an endopeptidase catalyzing the cleavage of specific peptide bonds in protein digestion; it is activated in the duodenum by trypsin-induced cleavage of its inactive precursor proelastase. In humans the form expressed is *p. e. II* 胰脏弹性蛋白酶

pan·cre·at·i·co·du·o·de·nal (pan″kre-at″ĭ- ko-doo″o-de′nəl) pertaining to or connecting the pancreas and duodenum 胰十二指肠的

pan·cre·at·i·co·du·o·de·nos·to·my (pan″ kre-at″ĭ-ko-doo″o-də-nos′tə-me) pancreaticoenterostomy with the duct or pancreas anastomosed to the duodenum 胰管十二指肠吻合术

pan·cre·at·i·co·en·ter·os·to·my (pan″kreat″ĭ-ko-en″tər-os′tə-me) anastomosis of the pancreatic duct to the intestine 胰管小肠吻合术

pan·cre·at·i·co·gas·tros·to·my (pan″kreat″ĭ-ko-gas-tros′tə-me) anastomosis of the pancreatic duct to the stomach 胰管胃吻合术

pan·cre·at·i·co·je·ju·nos·to·my (pan″kreat″ĭ-ko-jə-joo-nos′tə-me) pancreaticoenterostomy with the duct or pancreas anastomosed to the jejunum 胰管空肠吻合术

pan·cre·a·tin (pan′kre-ə-tin) a substance from the pancreas of the hog or ox containing enzymes, principally amylase, protease, and lipase; used as a digestive aid 胰酶（助消化药）

pan·cre·a·ti·tis (pan″kre-ə-ti′tis) inflammation of the pancreas 胰腺炎；**acute hemorrhagic p.**, a condition due to autolysis of pancreatic tissue caused by escape of enzymes into the substance, resulting in hemorrhage into the parenchyma and surrounding tissues 急性出血性胰腺炎

pan·cre·a·to·du·o·de·nec·to·my (pan″kre- ə-to-doo″o-də-nek′tə-me) excision of the head of the pancreas along with the encircling loop of the duodenum 胰头十二指肠切除术

pan·cre·a·to·gen·ic (pan″kre-ə-to-jen′ik) arising in the pancreas 胰发生的，胰源性的

pan·cre·a·tog·ra·phy (pan″kre-ə-tog′rə-fe) radiography of the pancreas 胰造影术

pan·cre·a·to·li·thec·to·my (pan″kre-ə-tolĭ-thek′tə-me) excision of a calculus from the pancreas 胰石切除术

pan·cre·a·to·li·thi·a·sis (pan″kre-ə-to-lĭ- thi′ə-sis) presence of calculi in the ductal system or parenchyma of the pancreas 胰石病

pan·cre·a·to·li·thot·o·my (pan″kre-ə-to-lĭ- thot′ə-me) incision of the pancreas for the removal of calculi 胰切开取石术

pan·cre·a·tol·y·sis (pan″kre-ə-tol′ĭ-sis) destruction of pancreatic tissue 胰组织破坏；**pancreatolyt′ic** *adj.*

pan·cre·a·tot·o·my (pan″kre-ə-tot′ə-me) incision of the pancreas 胰切开术

pan·cre·a·to·tro·pic (pan″kre-ə-to-tro′pik) having an affinity for the pancreas 促胰腺的

pan·cre·li·pase (pan″kre-li′pās) a preparation of hog pancreas containing enzymes, principally lipase with amylase and protease; used as a digestive aid in pancreatic insufficiency 胰脂肪酶

pan·creo·zy·min (pan′kre-o-zi″min) cholecystokinin 肠促胰酶素

pan·cu·ro·ni·um (pan″ku-ro′ne-um) a neuromuscular blocking agent used as the bromide salt as an adjunct to anesthesia 泮库溴铵

pan·cys·ti·tis (pan″sis-ti′tis) cystitis involving the entire thickness of the wall of the urinary bladder, as occurs in interstitial cystitis 全膀胱炎

pan·cy·to·pe·nia (pan″si-to-pe′ne-ə) abnormal depression of all the cellular elements of the blood 全血细胞减少症

pan·dem·ic (pan-dem′ik) 1. a widespread epidemic of a disease 大流行病；2. widely epidemic 大流行的，泛流行的

pan·en·ceph·a·li·tis (pan″ən-sef″ə-li′tis) encephalitis, probably of viral origin, which produces intranuclear or intracytoplasmic inclusion bodies that result in parenchymatous lesions of both the gray and white matter of the brain 全脑炎

pan·en·do·scope (pan-en′do-skōp) 1. an endoscope that permits wide-angle viewing广视野内镜 2. a cystoscope that permits wide-angle viewing of the bladder and urethra 广角膀胱镜

pan·hy·po·pi·tu·i·ta·rism (pan-hi″po-pī-too′ĭ- tə-riz-əm) generalized hypopituitarism due to absence or damage of the pituitary gland, which, in its complete form, leads to absence of gonadal function and insufficiency of thyroid and adrenal function. When cachexia is a prominent feature, it is called *Simmonds disease* or *pituitary cachexia* 全垂体功能减退（症）

pan·hys·tero·sal·pin·gec·to·my (pan-his″tər-o-sal″pin-jek′tə-me) excision of the body of the uterus, cervix, and uterine tubes 全子宫输卵管切除术

pan·hys·tero·sal·pin·go-ooph·o·rec·to·my (pan-his″tər-o-sal″ping-go-o″of-ə-rek′tə-me) excision of the uterus, cervix, uterine tubes, and ovaries 全子宫输卵管卵巢切除术

pan·ic (pan′ik) acute, extreme, and unreasoning fear and anxiety 恐慌，惊恐；极度焦虑；**homosexual p.**, an acute, extreme anxiety reaction brought on by circumstances that induce the unconscious fear of being homosexual or of succumbing to homosexual impulses 同性恋恐慌

pan·my·eloph·thi·sis (pan-mi″ə-lof′thĭ-sis) aplastic anemia 再生障碍性贫血

pan·nic·u·lec·to·my (pə-nik″u-lek′tə-me) surgical excision of the abdominal apron of superficial fat in the obese 脂膜切除术

pan·nic·u·li·tis (pə-nik″u-li′tis) inflammation of the panniculus adiposus, especially of the abdomen 脂膜炎；**lobular p.**, any of the types affecting mainly the lobules of adipose tissue,often with necrosis or other types of degeneration 小叶脂膜炎；**nodular nonsuppurative p., relapsing febrile nodular nonsuppurative p.**, a type of predominantly lobular panniculitis of the lower legs, with fever and formation of tender nodules 结节性非化脓性脂膜炎；**septal p.**, any of the types affecting mainly the septa between the lobules of adipose tissue, usually with formation of nodules 间隔性脂膜炎

pan·nic·u·lus (pə-nik′u-ləs) pl. *panni′culi* [L.] a layer of membrane 膜；**p. adipo′sus**, the subcutaneous fat: a layer of fat underlying the dermis 脂膜

pan·nus (pan′əs) [L.] 1. superficial vascularization of the cornea with infiltration of granulation tissue 角膜翳；2. an inflammatory exudate overlying the synovial cells on the inside of a joint 关节翳；3. panniculus adiposus 脂膜；**p. trachomato′sus**, pannus of the cornea secondary to trachoma 沙眼血

管翳

pan·oph·thal·mi·tis (pan″of-thəl-mi′tis) inflammation of all the eye structures or tissues 全眼球炎

pan·oti·tis (pan″o-ti′tis) inflammation of all the parts or structures of the ear 全耳炎

pan·pho·bia (pan-fo′be-ə) fear of everything; vague and persistent dread of an unknown evil 广泛性恐怖症

pan·ret·i·nal (pan-ret′ĭ-nəl) pertaining to or encompassing the entire retina 全视网膜的

Pan·stron·gy·lus (pan-stron′jə-ləs) a genus of hemipterous insects, species of which transmit trypanosomes 锥蝽属

pan·sys·tol·ic (pan″sis-tol′ik) pertaining to or affecting all of, or occurring throughout, systole 全收缩的

pan·te·the·ine (pan-tə-the′in) an amide of pantothenic acid, an intermediate in the biosynthesis of CoA, a growth factor for *Lactobacillus bulgaricus*, and a cofactor in certain enzyme complexes 泛酰巯基乙胺

Pan·toea (pan-te′ə) a widely distributed genus of gram-negative, usually motile, rod-shaped bacteria, including *P. agglo′merans*, which causes nosocomial infections 泛生菌属

pan·to·pra·zole (pan-to′prə-zōl) a gastric acid pump inhibitor similar to omeprazole, used as the sodium salt in the treatment of erosive esophagitis associated with gastroesophageal reflux disease and of pathologic hypersecretion associated with Zollinger-Ellison syndrome or other neoplastic condition 泮托拉唑

pan·to·then·ate (pan″to-then′āt) any salt of pantothenic acid; *calcium p.* is used as a dietary source of pantothenic acid 泛酸盐

pan·to·then·ic ac·id (pan″to-then′ik) a component of coenzyme A and a member of the vitamin B complex; necessary for nutrition in some animal species but of uncertain importance for humans 泛酸

pan·tro·pic (pan-tro′pik) having an affinity for or affecting many tissues or cells 泛向的（对许多组织或细胞有亲和力的）

pa·pa·in (pə-pa′in) (pə-pi′in) a proteolytic enzyme from the latex of papaw, *Carica papaya*, which catalyzes the hydrolysis of proteins and polypeptides to amino acids; used as a protein digestant and as a topical application for enzymatic débridement 木瓜蛋白酶

pa·pav·er·ine (pə-pav′ər-in) a smooth muscle relaxant and vasodilator used as the hydrochloride salt to relieve arterial spasms causing cerebral, peripheral, or myocardial ischemia and also injected into the penis in the diagnosis and treatment of erectile dysfunction 罂粟碱

pa·per (pa′pər) a material manufactured in thin sheets from fibrous substances that have first been reduced to a pulp 纸；**litmus p.**, moistureabsorbing paper impregnated with a solution of litmus: if slightly acid, it is red and alkalis turn it blue; if slightly alkaline, it is blue and acid turns it red 石蕊（试）纸；**test p.**, paper stained with a compound that changes visibly on occurrence of a chemical reaction 试纸

pa·pil·la (pə-pil′ə) pl. *papil′lae* [L.] a small nipple-shaped projection or elevation 乳突，乳头状突起；**circumvallate papillae**, vallate papillae 轮廓乳头；**conical papillae**, sparsely scattered elevations on the tongue, often considered to be modified filiform papillae 圆锥乳头；**dental p., dentinal p.**, a small mass of condensed mesenchyme in the enamel organ; it differentiates into the dentin and dental pulp 牙乳头；**dermal p.**, any of the conical extensions of the fibers, capillary blood vessels, and sometimes nerves of the dermis into corresponding spaces among downward- or inwardprojecting rete ridges on the undersurface of the epidermis 真皮乳头；**duodenal p.**, either of two small elevations on the mucosa of the duodenum, the *major* at the entrance of the conjoined pancreatic and common bile ducts and the *minor* at the entrance of the accessory pancreatic duct 十二指肠乳头；**filiform papillae**, threadlike elevations covering most of the tongue surface 丝状乳头；**foliate papillae**, parallel mucosal folds on the tongue margin at the junction of its body and root 叶状乳头；**fungiform papillae**, knoblike projections of the tongue scattered among the filiform papillae 菌状乳头；**gingival p.**, the cone-shaped pad of gingiva filling the space between the teeth up to the contact area（牙）龈乳头；**hair p.**, a fibrovascular dermal papilla enclosed within the hair bulb 毛乳头；**ileal p., ileocecal p.**, the conical projection formed by the terminal ileum at its junction with the cecum, corresponding to the *ileocecal valve* in the cadaver 回盲乳头；**incisive p.**, an elevation at the anterior end of the raphe of the palate 切牙乳头；**interdental p.**, gingival p. 牙间乳头；**lacrimal p.**, one in the conjunctiva near the medial angle of the eye 泪乳头；**mammary p.**, nipple (1) 乳房乳头；**optic p.**, optic disk 视神经乳头；**palatine p.**, incisive p. 腭乳头；**renal papillae**, the blunted apices of the renal pyramids 肾乳头；**p. of tongue**, 舌乳头，参见 *conical, filiform, foliate, fungiform* 和 *vallate papillae*；**vallate papillae**, eight to twelve large papillae arranged in a V near the base of the tongue 轮廓乳头

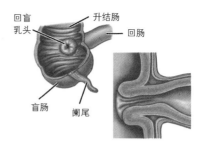

回盲乳头　升结肠　回肠　盲肠　阑尾

pap·il·lary (pap′ĭ-lar″e) pertaining to or resembling a papilla, or nipple 乳头的，乳头状的

pa·pil·le·de·ma (pap″il-ə-de′mə) edema of the optic disk 视神经乳头水肿

pa·pil·li·tis (pap″ĭ-li′tis) 1. inflammation of a papilla 乳头炎；2. a form of optic neuritis involving the optic papilla (disk) 视神经乳头炎波

pap·il·lo·ma (pap″ĭ-lo′mə) a benign tumor derived from epithelium 乳头状瘤；**papillo′matous** *adj.*；**fibroepithelial p.**, a type containing extensive fibrous tissue 纤维上皮乳头状瘤；**intracanalicular p.**, an arborizing nonmalignant growth within the ducts of certain glands, particularly the breast 小管内乳头状瘤；**intraductal p.**, a tumor in a lactiferous duct, usually attached to the wall by a stalk; it may be solitary, often with a serous or bloody nipple discharge, or multiple 导管内乳头状瘤；**inverted p.**, one in which the proliferating epithelial cells invaginate into the underlying stroma 内翻性乳头状瘤

pap·il·lo·ma·to·sis (pap″ĭ-lo-mə-to′sis) development of multiple papillomas 乳头（状）瘤病

Pap·il·lo·ma·vi·ri·dae (pap″ĭ-lo″mə-vir′ ĭ-de) the papillomaviruses, a family of viruses formerly grouped with the polyomaviruses in a family called Papovaviridae; many species cause tumors or other types of cancer. Genera that infect humans include *Alphapapillomavirus, Betapapillomavirus, Gammapapillomavirus,* and *Mupapillomavirus* 乳头瘤病毒科

pap·il·lo·ma·vi·rus (pap″ĭ-lo′mə-vi″rəs) any virus of the family Papillomaviridae 乳头瘤病毒；**human p. (HPV)**, any of a number of species that cause warts, particularly plantar warts and genital warts, on the skin and mucous membranes in humans; some are associated with malignancies of the genital tract 人乳头瘤病毒

pap·il·lo·ret·i·ni·tis (pap″ĭ-lo-ret″ĭ-ni′tis) inflammation of the optic disk and retina 乳头视网膜炎

pap·il·lot·o·my (pap″ĭ-lot′ə-me) incision of a papilla, as of a duodenal papilla 乳头括约肌切开

（术）

Pa·po·va·vi·ri·dae (pə-po″və-vir′ĭ-de) a former family of DNA viruses now subdivided into the two families Papillomaviridae and Polyomaviridae 乳多空病毒科，乳头多瘤空泡病毒科

pa·po·va·vi·rus (pə-po′və-vi″rəs) any of the viruses of the former family Papovaviridae 乳多空病毒，乳头多瘤空泡病毒；**lymphotropic p. (LPV),** a polyomavirus originally isolated from a B-lymphoblastic cell line of an African green monkey; antigenically related viruses are widespread in primates and may infect humans 亲淋巴乳多空病毒

pap·u·la·tion (pap″u-la′shən) the formation of papules 丘疹形成

pap·ule (pap′ūl) a small, circumscribed, solid, elevated lesion of the skin 丘疹；**pap′ular** *adj.*; **piezogenic p's,** soft, sometimes painful, large papules above the heel on the side of one or both feet, caused by weight bearing associated with prolonged standing or running 压力性丘疹

pap·u·lo·ne·crot·ic (pap″u-lo-nə-krot′ik) characterized by both papules and necrosis 丘疹坏死性的

pap·u·lo·sis (pap-u-lo′sis) the presence of multiple papules 丘疹病；**bowenoid p.,** benign reddish brown papules, usually on the genitalia, particularly the penis, in young adults; believed to have a viral etiology Bowe 样丘疹病

pap·y·ra·ceous (pap″ĭ-ra′shəs) like paper 纸状的

para (P) (par′ə) a woman who has produced one or more viable offspring, regardless of whether the child or children were living at birth. Used with Roman numerals to designate the number of such pregnancies, as *para 0 (none—nullipara), para I (one—primipara), para II (two—secundipara),* etc. 产次，指产过能存活的婴儿者称之，用数字表示分娩之存活婴儿的妊娠次数，如 para 0（0 产），para 1（1 产），para 2（2 产）等

para-ami·no·ben·zo·ic ac·id (par″ə-ə-me″nobenzo′ik) *p*-aminobenzoic acid 对氨苯甲酸

para-ami·no·hip·pu·ric ac·id (par″ə-ə-me″nohĭpūr′ik) *p*-aminohippuric acid 对氨马尿酸

para-ami·no·sal·i·cyl·ic ac·id (par″ə-ə-me″nosal-ĭ-sil′ik) *p*-aminosalicylic acid 对氨水杨酸

para-an·es·the·sia (par″ə-an-es-the′zhə) anesthesia of the lower part of the body 下身痛觉缺失

para-aor·tic (par″ə-a-or′tik) near or next to the aorta 主动脉旁的

para·bio·sis (par″ə-bi-o′sis) the union of two individuals, as conjoined twins, or of experimental animals by surgical operation 异种共生；**parabiot′ic** *adj.*

para·ca·sein (par″ə-ka′sēn) the chemical product of the action of rennin on casein 衍酪蛋白，副酪蛋白

para·cen·te·sis (par″ə-sen-te′sis) surgical puncture of a cavity for the aspiration of fluid（放液）穿刺术；**paracentet′ic** *adj.*

para·cen·tral (par″ə-sen′trəl) near a center 旁中央的，近中心的

para·cer·vi·cal (par″ə-sur′vĭ-kəl) near a neck or cervix, particularly the uterine cervix 宫颈旁的

Para·chla·my·dia (par″ə-klə-mid′e-ə) a genus of gram-variable coccoid bacteria of the family Parachlamydiaceae that are naturally parasites of free-living amebae and cause respiratory infections in humans 副衣原体属

Para·chla·my·di·a·ceae (par″ə-klə-mid″ea′se-e) a family of bacteria of the order Chlamydiales that are natural parasites of freeliving amebae 副衣原体科

para·chol·era (par″ə-kol′ər-ə) a disease resembling Asiatic cholera but not caused by *Vibrio cholerae* 类霍乱病

para·chor·dal (par″ə-kor′dəl) situated beside the notochord 脊索旁的

para·clin·i·cal (par″ə-klin′ĭ-kəl) pertaining to abnormalities (e.g., morphologic or biochemical) underlying clinical manifestations (e.g., chest pain or fever) 近似临床的

para·coc·cid·i·oi·dal (par″ə-kok-sid″e-oi′dəl) pertaining to or caused by fungi of the genus *Paracoccidioides* 副球孢子菌的

Para·coc·cid·i·oi·des (par″ə-kok-sid″e-oi′dēz) a genus of anamorphic fungi comprising the single species *P. brasilien′sis*, which is thermally dimorphic, growing in yeast form in tissues and causing paracoccidioidomycosis 副球孢子菌属

para·coc·cid·i·oi·do·my·co·sis (par″ə-koksid″e-oi″do-mi-ko′sis) an often fatal, chronic granulomatous disease caused by *Paracoccidioides brasiliensis*, primarily involving the lungs but spreading to the skin, mucous membranes, lymph nodes, and internal organs 副球孢子菌病

para·crine (par′ə-krin) 1. denoting a type of hormone function in which a hormone synthesized in and released from endocrine cells binds to its receptor in nearby cells and affects their function 旁分泌；2. denoting the secretion of a hormone by an organ other than an endocrine gland（非内分泌腺）分泌

par·acu·sia (par″ə-ku′zhə) 1. any deficiency in the sense of hearing 误听，又称 *paracusis*；2. auditory hallucination 幻听

para·did·y·mis (par″ə-did′ĭ-mis) a group of several convoluted tubules in the anterior part of the spermatic cord; probably a remnant of the mesonephros

旁睾

para·dox (par′ə-doks) a seemingly contradictory occurrence 悖论；**paradox′ic, paradox′ical** *adj.*；**Weber p.,** elongation of a muscle that has been so stretched that it cannot contract Weber 悖论，肌肉足够拉紧以至无法收缩而延长

para·du·o·de·nal (par″ə-doo″o-de′nəl) (-doood′ə-nəl) alongside, near, or around the duodenum 十二指肠旁的

para·esoph·a·ge·al (par″ə-e-sof″ə-je′əl) near or beside the esophagus 食管周围的

par·af·fin (par′ə-fin) 1. a purified hydrocarbon wax used for embedding histologic specimens and as a stiffening agent in pharmaceutical preparations 石蜡；2. alkane 烷烃；**liquid p.,** mineral oil 液体石蜡

par·af·fin·o·ma (par″ə-fin-o′mə) a chronic granuloma produced by prolonged exposure to paraffin 石蜡瘤

para·floc·cu·lus (par″ə-flok′u-ləs) a small lobe of the cerebellar hemisphere, immediately cranial to the flocculus 旁绒球，副绒球

para·gan·gli·o·ma (par″ə-gang′gle-o′mə) a tumor of the tissue composing the paraganglia 副神经节瘤，神经节细胞瘤；**nonchromaffin p.,** chemodectoma 非嗜铬性副神经节瘤

para·gan·gli·on (par″ə-gang′gle-on) pl. *paragan′glia.* A collection of chromaffin cells derived from neural ectoderm, occurring outside the adrenal medulla, usually near the sympathetic ganglia and in relation to the aorta and its branches 副神经节，嗜铬体

para·geu·sia (par″ə-goo′zhə) 1. perversion of the sense of taste 味觉倒错；2. a bad taste in the mouth 味觉异常

par·a·gon·i·mi·a·sis (par″ə-gon″ĭ-mi′ə-sis) infection with flukes of the genus *Paragonimus* 肺吸虫病，肺并殖吸虫病

Par·a·gon·i·mus (par″ə-gon′ĭ-məs) a genus of parasitic flukes that have two invertebrate hosts, the first a snail, the second a crab or crayfish. *P. westerma′ni* is the lung fluke of southern and eastern Asia, found in cysts in the lungs and sometimes elsewhere in humans and other animals that have eaten infected freshwater crayfish and crabs 并殖吸虫属

para·gran·u·lo·ma (par″ə-gran″u-lo′mə) the most benign form of Hodgkin disease, largely confined to the lymph nodes 副肉芽肿

para·he·mo·phil·ia (par″ə-he″mo-fil′e-ə) a hereditary hemorrhagic tendency due to deficiency of coagulation factor 副血友病

para·hip·po·cam·pal (par″ə-hip″o-kam′pəl) near or next to the hippocampus 海马旁的

para·hor·mone (par″ə-hor′mōn) a substance, not a true hormone, which has a hormone-like action in controlling the functioning of some distant organ 副激素

para·in·fec·tious (par″ə-in-fek′shəs) pertaining to manifestations of infectious disease that are caused by the immune response to the infectious agent 副感染的

para·ker·a·to·sis (par″ə-ker″ə-to′sis) persistence of the nuclei of keratinocytes as they rise into the stratum corneum of the epidermis. It is normal in the epithelium of the true mucous membrane of the mouth and vagina 角化不全

para·ki·ne·sia (par″ə-kĭ-ne′zhə) perversion of motor function; in ophthalmology, irregular action of an individual ocular muscle 运动倒错

para·la·lia (par″ə-la′le-ə) a disorder of speech, especially the production of a vocal sound different from the one desired 言语障碍，构音倒错，错语症

par·al·lag·ma (par″ə-lag′mə) displacement of a bone or of the fragments of a broken bone 骨移位

par·al·ler·gy (par-al′ər-je) a condition in which an allergic state, produced by specific sensitization, predisposes the body to react to other allergens with clinical manifestations that differ from the original reaction 副变态反应；**paraller′gic** *adj.*

pa·ral·y·sis (pə-ral′ĭ-sis) pl. *paral′yses.* Loss or impairment of motor function in a part due to a lesion of the neural or muscular mechanism; also, by analogy, impairment of sensory function *(sensory p.).* 麻痹，瘫痪；**p. of accommodation,** cycloplegia 调节麻痹；**p. a′gitans,** Parkinson disease 震颤麻痹，帕金森病病；**ascending p.,** spinal paralysis that progresses cephalad 上行性麻痹；**brachial p.,** paralysis of an upper limb from a lesion of the brachial plexus 臂丛麻痹；**bulbar p.,** progressive bulbar palsy 延髓麻痹；**central p.,** any paralysis due to a lesion of the brain or spinal cord 中枢性麻痹；**compression p.,** that caused by pressure on a nerve 压迫性麻痹；**conjugate p.,** loss of ability to perform some parallel ocular movements 共向性麻痹；**crossed p., cruciate p.,** that affecting one side of the face and the other side of the body 交叉麻痹；**crutch p.,** a type of radial neuropathy caused by pressure of the crutch in the axilla 腋杖麻痹；**decubitus p.,** that due to pressure on a nerve from lying for a long time in one position 久卧性麻痹；**Duchenne p.,** 1. 同 ErbDuchenne p.；2. progressive bulbar palsy 进展性球麻痹；**ErbDuchenne p.,** paralysis of the upper roots of the brachial plexus, caused by birth injury 上臂丛麻痹（产伤所致）；**facial p.,** weakening or paralysis of the facial nerve, as in Bell palsy 口眼歪斜，面

瘫；**familial periodic p.**, any of several autosomal dominant conditions marked by recurring attacks of rapidly progressive flaccid paralysis, subclassified on the basis of serum potassium levels *(hypokalemic periodic p., hyperkalemic periodic p.)* 家族性周期性麻痹；**flaccid p.**, any paralysis accompanied by loss of muscle tone and absence of tendon reflexes in the paralyzed part 松弛性瘫痪，弛缓性瘫痪；**hyperkalemic periodic p.**, familial periodic paralysis with high serum potassium levels; due to mutation in a skeletal muscle sodium channel 高钾性周期性麻痹；**hypokalemic periodic p.**, familial periodic paralysis with low serum potassium levels. Several types have been distinguished: type 1 is due to mutation in a skeletal muscle calcium channel; type 2 is due to mutation in a skeletal muscle sodium channel 低钾性周期性麻痹；**hysterical p.**, paralysis in a part owing to a conversion disorder, without any organic neurologic cause 癔症性瘫痪；**juvenile p. agitans**, increased muscle tonus with the characteristic attitude and facies of paralysis agitans, occurring in infants because of progressive degeneration of the globus pallidus 幼年型震颤麻痹；**Klumpke p., Klumpke-Dejerine p.**, lower brachial plexus paralysis caused by birth injury, particularly during a breech delivery 下臂丛麻痹；**Landry p.**, Guillain-Barré syndrome 兰德里麻痹；**mixed p.**, combined motor and sensory paralysis 混合性麻痹；**motor p.**, paralysis of voluntary muscles 运动麻痹；**obstetric p.**, paralysis caused by injury received at birth 产伤麻痹；**periodic p.**, any of various diseases characterized by episodic flaccid paralysis or muscular weakness 周期性麻痹；**postepileptic p.**, Todd p. 癫痫后麻痹；**progressive bulbar p.**, 进行性延髓麻痹，参见 *palsy* 下词条；**radial p.**, 桡神经麻痹，参见 *neuropathy* 下词条；**sensory p.**, loss of sensation due to a morbid process 感觉麻痹；**sleep p.**, paralysis upon awakening or sleep onset because of extension of the atonia of REM sleep into the waking state, often seen in those suffering from narcolepsy or sleep apnea 睡眠麻痹；**spastic p.**, paralysis marked by spasticity of the muscles of the paralyzed part and increased tendon reflexes, due to upper motor neuron lesions 痉挛麻痹；**thyrotoxic periodic p.**, recurrent episodes of generalized or local paralysis accompanied by hypokalemia occurring in association with Graves disease, especially after exercise or a high-carbohydrate or high-sodium meal 甲状腺毒性周期性麻痹；**tick p.**, a progressive ascending type of flaccid paralysis seen in children and domestic animals following the bite of certain ticks, usually the result of toxins from the tick's saliva that enter the central nervous system of the host 蜱麻痹；**Todd p.**, transient hemiplegia or monoplegia after an epileptic seizure 癫痫后麻痹；**vasomotor p.**, cessation of vasomotor control 血管运动性麻痹

par·a·lyt·ic (par″ə-lit′ik) 1. affected with or pertaining to paralysis 麻痹的，瘫痪的；2. a person affected with paralysis 麻痹者，瘫痪病人

par·a·lyz·ant (par′ə-līz″ənt) 1. causing paralysis 致瘫痪的；2. a drug that causes paralysis 瘫痪药

para·mag·net·ic (par″ə-mag-net′ik) being attracted by a magnet and assuming a position parallel to that of a magnetic force, but not becoming permanently magnetized 顺磁的

para·mas·ti·tis (par″ə-mas-ti′tis) inflammation of tissues around the mammary gland 乳腺周炎

Par·a·me·ci·um (par″ə-me′se-əm) a genus of ciliate protozoa 草履虫属

par·a·me·ci·um (par″ə-me′se-əm) pl. *parame′cia*. An organism of the genus *Paramecium* 草履虫

pa·ram·e·ter (pə-ram′ə-tər) 1. a constant that distinguishes specific cases, having a definite fixed value in one case but different values in other cases 参数；2. in statistics, a value that specifies one of the members of a family of probability distributions, such as the mean or standard deviation 参数；3. a variable whose measure is indicative of a quantity or function that cannot itself be directly determined precisely 系数

para·me·tric (par″ə-me′trik) situated near the uterus; parametrial 子宫旁的

para·met·ric (par″ə-met′rik) pertaining to or defined in terms of a parameter 参数的

para·me·tri·tis (par″ə-mə-tri′tis) inflammation of the parametrium 子宫旁（组织）炎

para·me·tri·um (par″ə-me′tre-əm) the extension of the subserous coat of the portion of the uterus just above the cervix, out laterally between the layers of the broad ligament 子宫旁组织；**parame′trial** *adj.*

par·am·ne·sia (par″am-ne′zhə) a disturbance of memory in which reality and fantasy are confused 记忆倒错，记忆错构，错构症

Par·amoe·ba (par″ə-me′bə) a genus of parasitic or free-living ameboid protozoa 副变形虫属

par·am·y·loi·do·sis (par-am″ə-loi-do′sis) accumulation of an atypical form of amyloid in tissues 副淀粉样变性

para·my·oc·lo·nus (par″ə-mi-ok′lə-nəs) myoclonus in several unrelated muscles 肌阵挛（状态）；**p. mul′tiplex**, a form of myoclonus of unknown etiology starting in the muscles of the upper arms and shoulders and spreading to other parts of the upper body 多发性肌阵挛

para·myo·to·nia (par″ə-mi″o-to′ne-ə) tonic

spasms caused by a disorder of muscular tonicity 副肌强直; **p. conge′nita,** an autosomal dominant disorder clinically similar to myotonia congenita, except that it is precipitated by cold exposure and is aggravated by activity; due to a defect in a voltage-gated sodium channel 先天性副肌强直症

Para·myxo·vi·ri·dae (par″ə-mik″so-vir′ĭ-de) the paramyxoviruses, a family of RNA viruses that includes the viruses causing measles and mumps; genera that infect humans include *Metapneumovirus, Morbillivirus, Respirovirus,* and *Pneumovirus* 副粘病毒科

Para·myxo·vi·ri·nae (par″ə-mik″so-vir-i′ne) a subfamily of the family Paramyxoviridae, containing the genera *Avulavirus, Henipavirus, Morbillivirus, Respirovirus,* and *Rubulavirus* 副粘病毒亚科

Para·myxo·vi·rus (par″ə-mik′so-vi′rəs) former name for *Respirovirus* 副粘病毒属

para·myxo·vi·rus (par″ə-mik′so-vi″rəs) any virus of the family Paramyxoviridae 副粘病毒

para·na·sal (par″ə-na′zəl) alongside or near the nose 鼻旁的

para·neo·plas·tic (par″ə-ne″o-plas′tik) pertaining to changes produced in tissue remote from a tumor or its metastases 癌旁的

para·neph·ric (par″ə-nef′rik) near the kidney 肾旁的

para·ne·phri·tis (par″ə-nə-fri′tis) 1. inflammation of the suprarenal gland 肾上腺炎; 2. inflammation of the connective tissue around the kidney 肾周炎

par·an·es·the·sia (par″an-es-the′zhə) 同 paraanes-thesia

para·noia (par″ə-noi′ah) 1. behavior characterized by well-systematized delusions of grandeur or persecution or a combination 偏执狂; 2. former name for *delusional disorder* 妄想性障碍的曾用名; **paranoi′ac, par′anoid** *adj.*

par·a·no·mia (par″ə-no′me-ə) amnestic aphasia 命名错乱

para·oral (par″ə-or′əl) 1. near or adjacent to the mouth 口腔旁的; 2. administered by some route other than by the mouth; said of medication 非经口（给药）的

para·pa·re·sis (par″ə-pə-re′sis) partial paralysis of the lower limbs 轻截瘫; **tropical spastic p.,** chronic progressive myelopathy 热带痉挛性截瘫

para·per·tus·sis (par″ə-pər-tus′is) an acute respiratory disease clinically indistinguishable from mild or moderate pertussis, caused by *Bordetella parapertussis* 副百日咳

para·pha·sia (par″ə-fa′zhə) partial aphasia in which the patient employs wrong words, or uses words in wrong and senseless combinations *(choreic*

p.) 语言错乱，错语

pa·ra·phia (pə-ra′fe-ə) perversion of the sense of touch 触觉倒错

para·phil·ia (par″ə-fil′e-ə) a psychosexual disorder marked by sexual urges, fantasies, and behavior involving objects, suffering or humiliation, or children or other nonconsenting partners 性欲倒错; **paraphil′iac** *adj.*

para·phi·mo·sis (par″ə-fi-mo′sis) retraction of phimotic prepuce, causing a painful swelling of the glans, sometimes progressing to dry gangrene 包皮嵌顿，嵌顿包茎

para·plec·tic (par″ə-plek′tik) 同 paraplegic

para·ple·gia (par″ə-ple′jə) paralysis of the lower part of the body, including the legs 截瘫

para·ple·gic (par″ə-ple′jik) 1. pertaining to or of the nature of paraplegia 截瘫的; 2. an individual with paraplegia 截瘫病人

Para·pox·vi·rus (par″ə-poks′vi-rəs) a genus of viruses of the family Poxviridae, including paravaccinia virus 副痘病毒属

para·prax·is (par″ə-prak′sis) pl. *paraprax′es.* A faulty action, such as a slip of the tongue or misplacement of an object, which in psychoanalytic theory is due to unconscious associations and motives 动作倒错

para·pro·tein (par″ə-pro′tēn) M component 副蛋白

para·pro·tein·emia (par″ə-pro″tēn-e′me-ə) plasma cell dyscrasia 副蛋白血症

para·pso·ri·a·sis (par″ə-sə-ri′ə-sis) any of a group of slowly developing, persistent, maculopapular scaly erythrodermas, without subjective symptoms and resistant to treatment 类银屑病

para·quat (par′ə-kwaht) a poisonous compound, some of whose salts are used as contact herbicides. Contact with concentrated solutions causes irritation of the skin, cracking and shedding of the nails, and delayed healing of cuts and wounds. After ingestion of large doses, renal and hepatic failure may develop, followed by pulmonary insufficiency 百草枯

para·ro·san·i·line (par″ə-ro-zan′ĭ-lin) a basic dye; a triphenylmethane derivative, one of the components of basic fuchsin 碱性副品红

par·ar·rhyth·mia (par″ə-rith′me-ə) 同 parasystole

para·sa·cral (par″ə-sa′krəl) beside or near the sacrum 骶骨旁的

para·sex·u·al (par″ə-sek′shoo-əl) accomplished by other than sexual means, as by genetic study of in vitro somatic cell hybrids 拟有性的，准性的，超性的

para·si·noi·dal (par″ə-si-noi′dəl) situated along the course of a sinus 窦旁的

par·a·site (par′ə-sīt) 1. a plant or animal that lives upon or within another living organism at whose expense it obtains some advantage 寄生物，寄生虫；参见 *symbiosis*；2. the smaller, less complete member of asymmetrical conjoined twins, attached to and dependent upon the autosite 寄生胎；**parasit′ic** *adj.*；**malarial p.**, *Plasmodium* 疟原虫；**obligatory p.**, one that is entirely dependent on a host for its survival 专性寄生物

par·a·si·te·mia (par″ə-si-te′me-ə) the presence of parasites, especially malarial forms, in the blood 寄生物血症

par·a·sit·ism (par″ə-si′tiz-əm) 1. symbiosis in which one population (or individual) adversely affects another but cannot live without it 寄生；2. infection or infestation with parasites 寄生物感染

par·a·si·to·gen·ic (par″ə-si″to-jen′ik) due to parasites 寄生物原的，寄生物所致的

par·a·si·tol·o·gy (par″ə-si-tol′ə-je) the scientific study of parasites and parasitism 寄生虫学

par·a·si·to·tro·pic (par″ə-si″to-tro′pik) having an affinity for parasites 亲寄生物的

para·som·nia (par″ə-som′ne-ə) a category of sleep disorders in which abnormal events occur during sleep, such as sleepwalking or talking; due to inappropriately timed activation of physiologic systems 睡眠异态，深眠状态

para·spa·di·as (par″ə-spa′de-əs) a congenital condition in which the urethra opens on one side of the penis 尿道旁裂

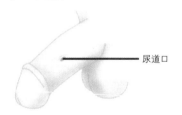

————— 尿道口

▲ 尿道旁裂

par·a·spi·nal (par″ə-spi′nəl) near the spine; pertaining to a plane along the spine 脊柱旁的

para·ster·nal (par″ə-stur′nəl) beside the sternum 胸骨旁的

para·sui·cide (par″ə-soo′ ĭ-sīd) attempted suicide, emphasizing that in most such attempts death is not the desired outcome 准自杀

para·sym·pa·thet·ic (par″ə-sim″pə-thet′ik) 副交感（神经）的，参见 *system* 下词条

para·sym·pa·tho·lyt·ic (par″ə-sim″pə-tho-lit′ik) anticholinergic 副交感神经阻滞药

para·sym·pa·tho·mi·met·ic (par″ə-sim″pə- tho-mĭ-met′ik) cholinergic 拟副交感神经药

para·sys·to·le (par″ə-sis′tə-le) a cardiac irregularity attributed to the interaction of two foci independently initiating cardiac impulses at different rates 并行收缩

para·ten·on (par″ə-ten′on) the fatty areolar tissue filling the interstices of the fascial compartment in which a tendon is situated 腱旁组织

para·thi·on (par″ə-thi′on) a highly toxic agricultural insecticide 对硫磷

para·thor·mone (par″ə-thor′mōn) parathyroid hormone 甲状旁腺激素

para·thy·mia (par″ə-thi′me-ə) a perverted, contrary, or inappropriate mood 情感倒错

par·a·thy·roid (par″ə-thi′roid) 1. situated beside the thyroid gland 甲状腺旁的；2. 甲状旁腺，参见 *gland* 下词条

para·thy·ro·pri·val (par″ə-thi″ro-pri′vəl) hypoparathyroid 无甲状旁腺的，甲状旁腺缺失的

para·thy·ro·tro·pic (par″ə-thi″ro-tro′pik) having an affinity for the parathyroid glands 促甲状旁腺的

para·tope (par′ə-tōp) the site on the antibody molecule that attaches to an antigen 抗原结合部位，互补位

para·tu·ber·cu·lo·sis (par″ə-too-bur″ku-lo′sis) a tuberculosis-like disease not due to *Mycobacterium tuberculosis* 副结核

para·ty·phoid (par″ə-ti′foid) infection due to *Salmonella* of all groups except *S. typhi* 副伤寒

para·ure·thral (par″ə-u-re′thrəl) near the urethra 尿道旁的

para·vac·cin·ia (par″ə-vak-sin′e-ə) an infection due to the paravaccinia virus, producing papular, and later vesicular, pustular, and scabular, lesions on the udders and teats of milk cows, the oral mucosa of suckling calves, and the hands of humans milking infected cows 副痘

para·vag·i·ni·tis (par″ə-vaj″ĭ-ni′tis) inflammation of the tissues alongside the vagina 阴道旁炎，阴道周炎

para·ver·te·bral (par″ə-vur′tə-brəl) beside the vertebral column 椎旁的

para·ves·i·cal (par″ə-ves′ĭ-kəl) perivesical 膀胱旁的

para·zone (par′ə-zōn) one of the white bands alternating with dark bands (diazones) seen in cross-section of a tooth 明带（在釉柱层内，见于牙的横切面）

Par·echo·vi·rus (par-ek′o-vi″rəs) a genus of viruses of the family Picornaviridae; two species called *parechovirus 1* and *parechovirus 2* infect humans 副肠孤病毒属

par·ei·do·lia (per-ī-dō′hlēə) an imagined visual,

or auditory, perception of a representational pattern or meaning where such interpretation does not actually exist 空想性错视；**face p.**, the tendency to see faces in certain shapes, patterns, or inanimate objects 人脸空想性错视

pa·ren·chy·ma (pə-reng′kĭ-mə) [Gr.] the essential or functional elements of an organ, as distinguished from its stroma or framework 实质；**paren′chymal**, **parenchym′atous** adj.；**renal p.**, the functional tissue of the kidney, consisting of the nephrons 肾实质

pa·ren·ter·al (pə-ren′tər-əl) not through the alimentary canal, but rather by injection through some other route, such as subcutaneous, intramuscular, etc. 肠胃外的，不经肠的非肠道的（采取消化道以外的其他途径，如皮下、肌内注射）

pa·re·sis (pə-re′sis) slight or incomplete paralysis 轻瘫；**general p.**, paralytic dementia; a form of neurosyphilis in which chronic meningoencephalitis causes gradual loss of cortical function, progressive dementia, and generalized paralysis 麻痹性痴呆

par·es·the·sia (par″es-the′zhə) morbid or perverted sensation; an abnormal sensation, such as burning, prickling, formication, etc. 感觉异常

pa·ret·ic (pə-ret′ik) pertaining to or affected with paresis 轻瘫的

par·i·cal·ci·tol (par″ĭ-kal′sĭ-tol) a synthetic vitamin D analogue, used for the prevention and treatment of hyperparathyroidism secondary to chronic renal failure 帕立骨化醇

par·i·es (par′e-ēz) pl. pari′etes [L.] a wall, as of an organ or cavity 壁

pa·ri·e·tal (pə-ri′ə-təl) 1. of or pertaining to the walls of a cavity 壁 的；2. pertaining to or located near the parietal bone 顶骨的

pa·ri·e·to·fron·tal (pə-ri″ə-to-frun′təl) pertaining to the parietal and frontal bones, gyri, or fissures 顶额的

pa·ri·e·to·oc·cip·i·tal (pə-ri″ə-to-ok-sip′ĭ-təl) pertaining to the parietal and occipital bones or lobes 顶枕的

par·i·ty (par′ĭ-te) 同 para; the condition of a woman with respect to having borne viable offspring 经产状况（指妇女产过存活婴儿的状况）

par·kin·son·ism (pahr′kin-sən-iz″əm) a group of neurologic disorders marked by hypokinesia, tremor, and muscular rigidity, including the parkinsonian syndrome and Parkinson disease 帕金森综合征；**parkinson′ian** adj.

par·oc·cip·i·tal (par″ok-sip′ĭ-təl) near the occipital bone 枕骨旁部

par·o·mo·my·cin (par′ə-mo-mi″sin) a broadspectrum antibiotic derived from *Streptomyces rimosus*

var. *paromomycinus*; the sulfate salt is used as an antiamebic 巴龙霉素

par·onych·ia (par″o-nik′e-ə) inflammation involving the folds of tissue around the fingernail 甲沟炎

par·o·nych·i·al (par″o-nik′e-əl) pertaining to paronychia or to the nail folds 甲沟炎的

par·oöph·o·ron (par″o-of′ə-ron) an inconstantly present small group of coiled tubules between the layers of the mesosalpinx, being a remnant of the excretory part of the mesonephros 卵巢旁体

par·oph·thal·mia (par″of-thal′me-ə) inflammation of the connective tissue around the eye 眼周炎

par·os·te·al (par-os′te-əl) pertaining to the outer surface of the periosteum 骨膜外面的

par·os·to·sis (par″os-to′sis) ossification of tissues outside the periosteum 骨膜外组织骨化

pa·rot·id (pə-rot′id) 1. near the ear 耳旁的；2. pertaining to a parotid gland 腮腺的

par·oti·tis (par″o-ti′tis) inflammation of the parotid gland 腮腺炎；**epidemic p., infectious p.**, 1. parotitis caused by an infectious agent, usually bacteria or viruses 由传染源引起的腮腺炎；2. mumps 流行性腮腺炎

par·ovar·i·an (par″o-var′e-ən) 1. beside the ovary 卵巢旁的；2. pertaining to the epoöphoron 卵巢冠的

par·ox·e·tine (pah-rok′sĕ-tēn) a selective serotonin uptake inhibitor used as the hydrochloride salt to treat depression and obsessive-compulsive, panic, and social anxiety disorders 帕罗西汀，氟苯哌苯醚

par·ox·ysm (par′ok-siz-əm) 1. a sudden recurrence or intensification of symptoms 发作，突发；2. a spasm or seizure 痉挛或癫痫；**paroxys′mal** adj.

pars (pahrz) pl. par′tes [L.] 同 part；**p. pla′na**, ciliary disk; the thin part of the ciliary body 睫状体扁平部

pars pla·ni·tis (pahrz pla-ni′tis) granulomatous uveitis of the pars plana of the ciliary body 睫状体平坦部炎

part (pahrt) a division of a larger structure 部分；（身体的）部位；**mastoid p. of temporal bone**, mastoid bone; the irregular, posterior part of the temporal bone 颞骨乳突部；**petromastoid p. of temporal bone**, 颞骨岩部乳突部，参见 *petrous p. of temporal bone*；**petrous p. of temporal bone**, petrous bone; the part of the temporal bone at the base of the cranium, containing the inner ear. Some divide it into two subparts, calling the posterior section the *mastoid part*, reserving the term *petrous part* for the anterior section only, and calling the entire area the *petromastoid part* 颞骨岩部；**squamous p. of temporal bone**, squamous bone; the flat, scalelike, anterior superior portion of the temporal bone 颞骨鳞部；**tympanic p. of temporal bone,** tympanic bone; the part of the temporal bone forming the anterior and inferior walls and part of the mastoid wall of the external acoustic meatus 颞骨鼓室部

par·ti·cle (pahr′tĭ-kəl) a tiny mass of material 颗粒，粒子，微粒，质点；**Dane p.,** an intact hepatitis B viral particle Dane 颗粒，乙型肝炎病毒颗粒；**viral p., virus p.,** virion 病毒粒子

par·ti·tion·ing (pahr-tĭ′shən-ing) dividing into parts 分隔；**gastric p.,** any of various gastroplasty procedures for morbid obesity in which a small stomach pouch is walled off, and when filled signals satiety 分胃术

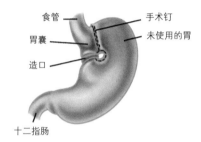

食管　　　手术钉
胃囊　　　未使用的胃
造口
十二指肠

▲ 垂直袖带胃成形术

par·tu·ri·ent (pahr-tu′re-ənt) giving birth or pertaining to birth; by extension, a woman in labor 分娩的，临产的；产妇

par·tu·ri·om·e·ter (pahr″tu-re-om′ə-tər) a device used in measuring the expulsive power of the uterus 分娩力计

par·tu·ri·tion (pahr″tu-rĭ′shən) childbirth 分娩，生产

pa·ru·lis (pə-roo′lis) a subperiosteal abscess of the gum 龈脓肿

par·vi·cel·lu·lar (pahr″vĭ-sel′u-lər) composed of small cells 小细胞性的

Par·vo·vi·ri·dae (pahr″vo-vir′ĭ-de) the parvoviruses, a family of DNA viruses that includes the genera *Parvovirus* and *Dependovirus* 细小病毒科

Par·vo·vi·rus (pahr′vo-vi″rəs) a genus of viruses of the family Parvoviridae that infect mammals and birds; those infecting humans can cause aplastic crisis, erythema infectiosum, hydrops fetalis, spontaneous abortion, and fetal death 细小病毒属

par·vo·vi·rus (pahr′vo-vi″rəs) any virus of the family Parvoviridae 细小病毒

PAS, PASA *p*-aminosalicylic acid 对氨（基）水杨酸；Pediatric Academic Societies 儿科学术协会

pas·cal (Pa) (pas-kal′) the SI unit of pressure, which corresponds to a force of 1 newton per square

meter 帕斯卡（压强单位，1Pa = 1N/m²)

pas·sive (pas′iv) neither spontaneous nor active; not produced by active efforts 被动的；消极的

PASSOR Physiatric Association of Spine, Sports, and Occupational Rehabilitation 脊柱、运动和职业康复物理治疗协会

paste (pāst) a semisolid preparation containing one or more drug substances, for topical application 糊剂，膏剂

Pas·teur·el·la (pas″tər-el′ə) a genus of gramnegative bacteria of the family Pasteurellaceae, including *P. multo′cida,* the etiologic agent of the hemorrhagic septicemias 巴氏杆菌属

Pas·teur·el·la·ceae (pas″tər-el-a′se-e) a family of facultatively anaerobic, nonmotile, gramnegative, coccoid to rod-shaped bacteria of the order Pasteurellales, occurring as parasites in mammals and birds 巴斯德菌科

Pas·teu·rel·la·les (pas″tər-el-a′lēz) an order of bacteria of the class Gammaproteobacteria 巴斯德菌目

pas·teu·rel·lo·sis (pas″tər-ə-lo′sis) infection with organisms of the genus *Pasteurella* 巴斯德菌病

patch (pach) 1. a small area differing from the rest of a surface 斑；2. a small piece of cloth or other material that covers part of another surface 补片；3. a macule more than 1 cm in diameter 斑疹（直径小于 1cm）；**Peyer p's,** oval elevated patches of closely packed lymph follicles on the mucosa of the small intestines 派尔集合淋巴结；**salmon p.,** a common type of pink or skincolored nevus flammeus seen on the forehead or nape of the neck in neonates 粉黄色斑；**transdermal p.,** a drug delivery system in which a patch with medication is placed on the skin so that the medication is gradually absorbed over time 皮肤药贴

pa·tel·la (pə-tel′ə) [L.] knee cap; a triangular sesamoid bone situated at the front of the knee in the tendon of insertion of the quadriceps femoris muscle 髌骨，见图 1；**patel′lar** adj.

pat·el·lec·to·my (pat″ə-lek′tə-me) excision of the patella 髌骨切除术

pat·ent (pa′tənt) 1. open, unobstructed, or not closed 开放的，不闭的；2. apparent, evident 明显的

path·er·gy (path′ər-je) 1. a condition in which the application of a stimulus leaves the organism unduly susceptible to subsequent stimuli of a different kind 过应性；2. a condition of being allergic to numerous antigens 过敏反应性；**pather′gic** adj.

path·find·er (path′find-ər) 1. an instrument for locating urethral strictures 尿道狭窄探针；2. a dental instrument for tracing the course of root canals 牙根

管探针

patho·an·a·tom·i·cal (path″o-an″ə-tom′ ĭ-kəl) pertaining to anatomic pathology 病理解剖的

patho·bi·ol·o·gy (path″o-bi-ol′ə-je) a branch of pathology that focuses on biologic aspects such as structural and functional changes of organs 病理生物学

patho·cli·sis (path″o-klis′is) a specific sensitivity to specific toxins, or a specific affinity of certain toxins for certain systems or organs 特异感受性

patho·gen (path′o-jən) any disease-producing agent or microorganism 病原体; **pathogen′ic** adj.

patho·gen·e·sis (path″o-jen′ə-sis) the development of morbid conditions or of disease; more specifically the cellular events and reactions and other pathologic mechanisms occurring in the development of disease 发病机制; **pathogenet′ic** adj.

pa·thog·no·mon·ic (path″og-no-mon′ik) specifically distinctive or characteristic of a disease or pathologic condition; denoting a sign or symptom on which a diagnosis can be made 特殊（病征）的，能确定诊断的（病征）

patho·log·ic (path″o-loj′ik) 1. indicative of or caused by some morbid condition 病态的；2. pertaining to pathology 病理的

patho·log·i·cal (path″o-loj′ĭ-kəl) pathologic 病理的

pa·thol·o·gy (pə-thol′ə-je) 1. the branch of medicine dealing with the essential nature of disease, especially changes in body tissues and organs that cause or are caused by disease 病理学；2. the structural and functional manifestations of disease 病理; **anatomic p.**, the anatomic study of changes in the function, structure, or appearance of organs or tissues, including postmortem examinations and the study of biopsy specimens 解剖病理学; **cellular p.**, cytopathology 细胞病理学; **clinical p.**, pathology applied to the solution of clinical problems, especially the use of laboratory methods in clinical diagnosis 临床病理学; **comparative p.**, that which considers human disease processes in comparison with those of other animals 比较病理学; **oral p.**, that treating of conditions causing or resulting from morbid anatomic or functional changes in the structures of the mouth 口腔病理学; **surgical p.**, the pathology of disease processes that are surgically accessible for diagnosis or treatment 外科病理学

patho·mi·me·sis (path″o-mi-me′sis) mimicry of a disease or disorder, particularly malingering 疾病模仿

patho·mor·phism (path″o-mor′fiz-əm) perverted or abnormal morphology 病理形态学

patho·phys·i·ol·o·gy (path″o-fiz″e-ol′ə-je) the physiology of disordered function 病理生理学

patho·psy·chol·o·gy (path″o-si-kol′o-je) the psychology of mental disease 病理心理学

patho·var (path′o-vahr) (path′o-var) a variant strain of a bacterial species, differentiated by reactions in one or more hosts 致病型

path·way (path′wa) 1. a course usually followed 途径；2. the nerve structures through which an impulse passes between groups of nerve cells or between the central nervous system and an organ or muscle 神经通路；3. 同 metabolic p.；**accessory conducting p.**, myocardial fibers that propagate the atrial contraction impulse to the ventricles but are not a part of the normal atrioventricular conducting system 副传导途径; **afferent p.**, the nerve structures through which an impulse, especially a sensory impression, is conducted to the cerebral cortex 传入通路; **alternative complement p.**, a pathway of complement activation initiated by a variety of factors other than those initiating the classical pathway, including IgA immune complexes, bacterial endotoxins, microbial polysaccharides, and cell walls. It does not include factors C1, C2, and C4 of the classical complement pathway but does include factors B and D and properdin 补体旁路途径; **amphibolic p.**, a group of metabolic reactions providing small metabolites for further metabolism to end products or for use as precursors in synthetic, anabolic reactions 两用代谢途径; **circus p.**, a ring or circuit traversed by an abnormal excitatory wavefront, as in reentry 环形途径; **classical complement p.**, a pathway of complement activation,comprising nine components (C1 to C9), initiated by antigen-antibody complexes containing immunoglobulins IgG or IgM 经典补体途径; **common p. of coagulation**, the steps in the mechanism of coagulation from the activation of factor X through the conversion of fibrinogen to fibrin 共同凝血途径; **efferent p.**, the nerve structures through which an impulse passes away from the brain, especially for the innervation of muscles, effector organs, or glands 传出通路; **EmbdenMeyerhof p.**, the series of enzymatic reactions in the anaerobic conversion of glucose to lactic acid, resulting in energy in the form of adenosine triphosphate (ATP) 糖酵解途径; **extrinsic p. of coagulation**, the mechanism that produces fibrin following tissue injury, beginning with formation of an activated complex between tissue factor and factor VII and leading to activation of factor X, inducing the reactions of the common pathway of coagulation 外在凝血途径; **final common p.**, a motor pathway consisting of the motor neurons by which nerve impulses from

P

many central sources pass to a muscle or gland in the periphery 最终共同通路; **intrinsic p. of co-agulation,** a sequence of reactions leading to fibrin formation, beginning with the contact activation of factor XII and resulting in the activation of factor X to initiate the common pathway of coagulation 内源性凝血途径; **lipoxygenase p.,** a pathway for the formation of leukotrienes and hydroxyeicosatetraenoic acid from arachidonic acid 脂肪氧合酶途径; **metabolic p.,** a series of enzymatic reactions that convert one biologic material to another 代谢途径; **motor p.,** an efferent pathway conducting impulses from the central nervous system to a muscle 运动通路; **pentose phosphate p.,** a major branching of the Embden-Meyerhof pathway of carbohydrate metabolism, successively oxidizing hexoses to form pentose phosphates 磷酸戊糖途径; **reentrant p.,** that over which the impulse is conducted in reentry 折返途径

pa·tri·lin·e·al (pat″rĭ-lin′e-əl) descended through the male line 父系的

pat·u·lous (pat′u-ləs) spread widely apart; open; distended 扩展的，开放的，膨胀的

pau·ci·syn·ap·tic (paw″se-sin-ap′tik) oligosynaptic 少突触的

pause (pawz) an interruption or rest 中止，暂停，间歇; **compensatory p.,** the pause in impulse generation after an extrasystole, either *full* if the sinus node is not reset or *incomplete* or *noncompensatory* if the node is reset and the cycle length is disrupted 代偿（性）间歇; **sinus p.,** a transient interruption in the sinus rhythm, of a duration that is not a simple multiple of the normal cardiac cycle 窦性收缩间歇

pa·vor (pa′vor) [L.] terror 惊，惊悸; **p. noc-tur′nus,** a sleep disturbance of children causing them to cry out in fright and awake in panic, with poor recall of a nightmare. Repeated occurrences are called *sleep terror disorder* 夜惊，梦惊（反复出现的症状称为睡惊症）

PAWP pulmonary artery wedge pressure 肺动脉楔压

Pax·il·lus (pak-sil′əs) a genus of mushrooms including many toxic species; *P. involu′tus* causes gastroenteritis and sometimes causes an immune-mediated hemolytic anemia with syncope, oliguria, hemoglobinuria, back pain, and hemolysis 桩菇属

Pb lead[1] (L. *plum′bum*) 元素铅的符号

PBI protein-bound iodine 蛋白结合碘

PC phosphocreatine 磷酸肌酸

p.c. [L.] post ci′bum (after meals) 饭后，食后

PCB polychlorinated biphenyl 多氯化联（二）苯

PCC prothrombin complex concentrate 凝血酶原复合物

PCE pseudocholinesterase 假胆碱酯酶; 参见 *cholinesterase*

PCEC PCECV purified chick embryo cell (vaccine) 纯化鸡胚细胞（疫苗）; 参见 *rabies vaccine*

PCI percutaneous coronary intervention 经皮冠状动脉介入治疗

PCL posterior cruciate ligament 后交叉韧带; pubococcygeal line 耻尾线

P_{CO_2} the partial pressure of carbon dioxide in the blood; also written P_{CO_2}, pCO_2, or pCO_2 血二氧化碳分压

PCOS polycystic ovary syndrome 多囊卵巢综合征

PCR polymerase chain reaction 聚合酶链（式）反应

PCT porphyria cutanea tarda 迟发性皮肤卟啉症

PCV packed-cell volume 血细胞压积

PCV7 pneumococcal 7-valent conjugate vaccine 七价肺炎球菌结合疫苗

PCWP pulmonary capillary wedge pressure 肺毛细（血）管楔压

Pd palladium 元素钯的符号

PDA patent ductus arteriosus 动脉导管未闭

peak (p ē k) the top or upper limit of a graphic tracing or of any variable 峰; **kilovolts p. (kVp),** the highest kilovoltage used in producing a radiograph kV 峰值

pearl (purl) 1. a small rounded mass or body 珠，珍珠，小珠（药），珠剂; 2. a rounded mass of tough sputum as seen in the early stages of an attack of bronchial asthma 痰珠，早期支气管哮喘发作所见的圆形硬块痰; **epidermic p's, epithelial p's,** rounded concentric masses of epithelial cells found in squamous cell carcinomas 上皮珠; **Laënnec p's,** soft casts of the smaller bronchial tubes expectorated in bronchial asthma Laënnec 珠，支气管哮喘病人痰液中的小圆形透明小体

pec·ten (pek′tən) pl. *pec′tines* [L.] 1. a comb; in anatomy, any of certain comblike structures 梳，栉; 2. p. analis 肛梳; **p. of anal canal, p. ana′lis,** the zone in the lower half of the anal canal between the pectinate line and the anal verge 肛门梳; **p. os′sis pu′bis,** pectineal line (2) 耻骨梳

pec·te·no·sis (pek″tə-no′sis) stenosis of the anal canal due to an inelastic ring of tissue between the anal groove and anal crypts 肛门梳硬结

pec·tin (pek′tin) a polymer of sugar acids of fruit that forms gels with sugar at the proper pH; a purified form obtained from the acid extract of the rind of citrus fruits or from apple pomace is used as an antidiarrheal and as a pharmaceutical aid 果胶; **pec′tic** *adj.*

pec·ti·nate (pek′tĭ-nāt) comb-shaped 梳状的，栉状的

pec·tin·e·al (pek-tin′e-əl) (pek″tĭ-ne′əl) pertaining to the os pubis 耻骨的

pec·tin·i·form (pek-tin′ĭ-form) comb-shaped 梳状的，栉状的

pec·to·ral (pek′tər-əl) thoracic 胸的

pec·to·ra·lis (pek″tə-ra′lis) (-ral′is) [L.] thoracic 胸的

pec·to·ril·o·quy (pek″tə-ril′ə-kwe) voice sounds of increased resonance heard through the chest wall 胸语音

pec·tus (pek′təs) pl. *pec′tora* [L.] thorax 胸；
p. carina′tum, pigeon breast or chest; a group of deformities of the anterior chest wall marked by protrusion of the sternum and costal cartilages鸡胸；
p. excava′tum, funnel breast or chest; a congenital deformity in which the sternum is depressed 漏斗胸

ped·al (ped′əl) pertaining to the foot or feet 足的，脚的

ped·er·as·ty (ped′ər-as″te) anal intercourse between a man and a boy 鸡奸

pe·di·at·ric (pe″de-at′rik) pertaining to the health of children 儿科的

pe·di·at·rics (pe″de-at′riks) the branch of medicine dealing with children, their development and care, and with the nature and treatment of diseases of children 儿科学

ped·i·cel (ped′ĭ-sel) a footlike part, especially any of the secondary processes of a podocyte 蒂

ped·i·cle (ped′ĭ-kəl) a footlike, stemlike, or narrow basal part or structure 蒂

pe·dic·u·lar (pə-dik′u-lər) pertaining to or caused by lice 虱的

pe·dic·u·li·cide (pə-dik′u-lĭ-sīd) 1. destroying lice 灭虱的；2. an agent that destroys lice 灭虱药；**pediculici′dal** adj.

pe·dic·u·lo·sis (pə-dik″u-lo′sis) infestation with lice of the family Pediculidae, especially *Pediculus humanus* 虱病；**p. pu′bis,** phthiriasis; infestation with the pubic louse *Phthirus pubis* 阴虱病

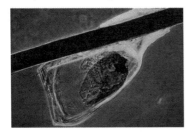

▲ 虱病：虱卵黏附在毛干上

pe·dic·u·lous (pə-dik′u-ləs) infested with lice 有虱的

Pe·dic·u·lus (pə-dik′u-ləs) a genus of lice. *P. huma′nus,* a species feeding on human blood, is a major vector of typhus, trench fever, and relapsing fever; it has two subspecies: *P. huma′nus cap′itis* (head louse), found on the scalp hair, and *P. huma′nus huma′nus* (body, or clothes, louse), found on the body 虱属

pe·dic·u·lus (pə-dik′u-ləs) pl. *pedic′uli* [L.] 1. louse 虱；2. pedicle 蒂

ped·i·gree (ped′ĭ-gre) 1. lineage 普系，系普；2. a list of ancestors 家谱；3. a chart or diagram of an individual's ancestors used in genetics in the analysis of inheritance of specific traits 纯种系普

pe·do·don·tics (pe-do-don′tiks) the branch of dentistry dealing with the teeth and mouth conditions of children 儿童牙科学

pe·do·phil·ia (pe″do-fil′e-ə) a paraphilia in which an adult has recurrent, intense sexual urges or sexually arousing fantasies of engaging or repeatedly engages in sexual activity with a prepubertal child 恋童癖；**pedophil′ic** adj.

pe·dor·thics (pə-dor′thiks) the design, manufacture, fitting, and modification of shoes and related foot appliances as prescribed for the amelioration of painful or disabling conditions of the foot and leg 脚病鞋制造业；**pedor′thic** adj.

pe·dun·cle (pə-dung′kəl) a stemlike connecting part, especially *(a)* a collection of nerve fibers cours ing between different areas in the central nervous system, or *(b)* the stalk by which a nonsessile tumor is attached to normal tissue 脚，蒂，茎；**pedun′cular** adj.; **cerebellar p′s,** three sets of paired bundles of the hindbrain *(superior, middle,* and *inferior),* connecting the cerebellum to the midbrain, pons, and medulla oblongata, respectively 小脑脚；**cerebral p.,** either of the two large paired portions of the midbrain; divisible into an anterior part *(crus cerebri)* and a posterior part *(tegmentum),* which are separated by the substantia nigra 大脑脚；**pineal p.,** habenula (2) 松果体脚；**p′s of thalamus,** thalamic radiations 丘脑辐射

pe·dun·cu·lus (pə-dung′ku-ləs) pl. *pedun′culi* [L.] 同 peduncle

PEEP positive end-expiratory pressure 呼气末正压；参见 *pressure* 下词条

PEF peak expiratory flow 呼气流量峰值

PEG pneumoencephalography 气脑造影术；polyethylene glycol 聚乙二醇

peg (peg) a projecting structure 钉；**rete p′s,** 表皮突，钉突；参见 *ridge* 下词条

peg·ad·e·mase (peg-ad′ə-mās) adenosine deam-

P

inase derived from bovine intestine and attached covalently to polyethylene glycol, used in replacement therapy for adenosine deaminase deficiency in immunocompromised patients 腺苷脱氨酶

peg·as·par·gase (peg-as′pahr-jās) l-asparaginase covalently linked to polyethylene glycol, used as an antineoplastic in the treatment of acute lymphoblastic leukemia 培门冬酶

peg·i·nes·a·tide (peg″ĭ-nes′ə-tīd) a synthetic erythropoiesis-stimulating agent, used as the acetate salt in the treatment of anemia associated with chronic kidney disease 聚乙二醇肽

peg·in·ter·fer·on (peg″in″tər-fēr′on) a covalent conjugate of recombinant interferon and polyethylene glycol (PEG); used in the treatment of chronic hepatitis C infection (interferon alfa-2a or alfa-2b) and chronic hepatitis B infection (interferon alfa-2a) 聚乙二醇干扰素 α

peg·lo·ti·case (peg-lo′tĭ-kās) a recombinant urate oxidase linked to polyethylene glycol, which catalyzes the conversion of urate to allantoin, reducing plasma uric acid levels; used for the treatment of severe, treatment-refractory, chronic gout 聚乙二醇重组尿酸酶

pel·i·o·sis (pel″e-o′sis) purpura 紫癜; **p. he′pa-tis**, a mottled blue liver, due to blood-filled lacunae in the parenchyma 肝紫癜症

pel·lag·ra (pə-lag′rə) a syndrome due to niacin deficiency (or failure to convert tryptophan to niacin), marked by dermatitis on parts of the body exposed to light or trauma, inflammation of the mucous membranes, diarrhea, and psychic disturbances 糙皮病, 烟酸缺乏症; **pellag′ral, pellag′rous** adj.

pel·la·groid (pə-lag′roid) resembling pellagra 类糙皮病

pel·li·cle (pel′ĭ-kəl) a thin scum forming on the surface of liquids 表膜, 菌膜

pel·lu·cid (pə-loo′sid) translucent 透明的, 清澈的

pel·vic (pel′vik) pertaining to the pelvis 骨盆的

pel·vi·cal·y·ce·al (pel″vĭ-kal′ə-se′əl) 同 pyelo-cal-yceal

pel·vi·ceph·a·lom·e·try (pel″vĭ-sef′ə-lom′ə-tre) measurement of the fetal head in relation to the maternal pelvis 骨盆胎头测量法

pel·vi·fix·a·tion (pel″vĭ-fik-sa′shən) surgical fixation of a displaced pelvic organ 盆腔器官固定术

pel·vim·e·try (pel-vim′ə-tre) measurement of the capacity and diameter of the pelvis 骨盆测量（法）

pel·vi·ot·o·my (pel″ve-ot′ə-me) 1. incision or transection of a coxal bone 骨盆切开术; 2. 同 py-elotomy

pel·vis (pel′vis) pl. **pel′ves** [L.] the lower (caudal) portion of the trunk, bounded anteriorly and later-

ally by the two coxal bones and posteriorly by the sacrum and coccyx. Also applied to any basinlike structure (e.g., the renal pelvis) 骨盆, 盂, 肾盂; **pel′vic** adj.; **android p.**, one with a wedge-shaped inlet and narrow anterior segment; used to describe a female pelvis with characteristics usually found in the male 男子型骨盆; **anthropoid p.**, a female pelvis in which the anteroposterior diameter of the inlet equals or exceeds the transverse diameter 类人猿型骨盆; **assimilation p.**, one in which the ilia articulate with the vertebral column higher (high-assimilation p.) or lower (lowassimilation p.) than normal, the number of lumbar vertebrae being correspondingly decreased or increased 混化骨盆; **beaked p.**, one with the coxal bones laterally compressed and their anterior junction pushed forward 喙状骨盆; **brachypellic p.**, one in which the transverse diameter exceeds the anteroposterior diameter by 1 to 3 cm 短状骨盆; **contracted p.**, one showing a decrease of 1.5 to 2 cm in any important diameter; when all dimensions are proportionately diminished it is a generally contracted p. (p. justo minor) 骨盆狭窄; **dolichopellic p.**, an elongated pelvis, the anteroposterior diameter being greater than the transverse diameter 长型骨盆; **extrarenal p.**, 肾外型肾盂, 参见 renal p.; **false p.**, the part of the pelvis superior to a plane passing through the iliopectineal lines 假骨盆; **flat p.**, a pelvis whose anteroposterior dimension is abnormally reduced 扁平骨盆; **funnel-shaped p.**, one with a normal inlet but a greatly narrowed outlet 漏斗型骨盆; **gynecoid p.**, the normal female pelvis: a rounded oval pelvis with well-rounded anterior and posterior segments 女性骨盆; **infantile p.**, a generally contracted pelvis with an oval shape, high sacrum, and marked inclination of the walls 婴儿样骨盆; **p. jus′to ma′jor**, an unusually large gynecoid pelvis, with all dimensions increased 均大骨盆; **p. jus′to mi′nor**, a small gynecoid pelvis, with all dimensions symmetrically reduced 均小骨盆; 另参见 contracted p.; **juvenile p.**, 同 infantile p.; **p. ma′jor**, 同 false p.; **mesatipellic p.**, one in which the transverse diameter is equal to the anteroposterior diameter or exceeds it by no more than 1 cm 中型骨盆; **p. mi′nor**, 同 true p.; **platypellic p., platypelloid p.**, one shortened in the anteroposterior aspect, with a flattened transverse oval shape 扁骨盆; **rachitic p.**, a pelvis that is distorted as a result of rickets 佝偻病性骨盆; **renal p.**, the funnel-shaped expansion of the upper end of the ureter into which the renal calices open; it is usually within the renal sinus, but under certain conditions a large part of it may be outside the kidney (extrarenal p.) 肾盂

scoliotic p., a pelvis that is deformed as a result of scoliosis 脊柱侧凸性骨盆；**split p.**, one with a congenital separation at the pubic symphysis 分裂骨盆；**spondylolisthetic p.**, one in which the last, or rarely the fourth or third, lumbar vertebra is dislocated in front of the sacrum, more or less occluding the pelvic brim 脊柱滑出性骨盆；**true p.**, the part of the pelvis inferior to a plane passing through the iliopectineal lines 真骨盆

pe·mir·o·last (pə-mir′o-last″) a mast cell stabilizer that inhibits type Ⅰ hypersensitivity reactions; administered topically as the potassium salt to prevent pruritus associated with allergic conjunctivitis 吡嘧司特

pem·o·line (pem′o-lēn) a central nervous system stimulant used in the treatment of attentiondeficit/hyperactivity disorder 匹莫林，苯异妥英（中枢神经系统兴奋药）

pem·phi·goid (pem′fǐ-goid) 1. resembling pemphigus 天疱疮样的；2. any of a group of dermatologic syndromes similar to but clearly distinguishable from the pemphigus group 类天疱疮

pen·bu·to·lol (pen-bu′tə-lol) a beta-adrenergic blocking agent with intrinsic sympathomimetic activity; used as the sulfate salt in the treatment of hypertension 喷布洛尔，硫酸环戊丁心安（β受体阻滞药）

pen·ci·clo·vir (pen-si′klo-vir) a compound that inhibits viral DNA synthesis in herpesviruses 1 and 2, used in the treatment of recurrent herpes labialis 喷昔洛韦

pen·del·luft (pen′də-looft″) the movement of air back and forth between the lungs, resulting in increased dead space ventilation 摆动呼吸，空气在肺内来回流动，结果造成死腔通气增加

pen·du·lar (pen′du-lər) having a pendulumlike movement 摆动的

pen·du·lous (pen′du-ləs) hanging loosely; dependent 悬垂的，下垂的

pe·nec·to·my (pe-nek′tə-me) surgical removal of the penis 阴茎切除术

pen·e·trance (pen′ə-trəns) in genetics, the frequency of expression of a genotype under defined conditions 外显率（在遗传学上指基因与其相应有关遗传性状的表现的个体的比率）

pen·e·trom·e·ter (pen′ə-trom′ə-tər) an instrument for measuring the penetrating power of x-rays（X线）硬度计，（X线）透度计

pen·i·cil·la·mine (pen′ĭ-sil′ə-mēn) a degradation product of penicillin that chelates certain heavy metals and also binds cystine and promotes its excretion; used in the treatment of Wilson disease, cystinuria, recurrent cystine renal calculi, and rheumatoid arthritis 青霉胺

pen·i·cil·lin (pen′ĭ-sil′in) any of a large group of natural *(p. G, p. V)* or semisynthetic antibacterial antibiotics derived directly or indirectly from strains of fungi of the genus *Penicillium* and other soil-inhabiting fungi, which exert a bactericidal as well as a bacteriostatic effect on susceptible bacteria by interfering with the final stages of the synthesis of peptidoglycan, a substance in the bacterial cell wall. The penicillins, despite their relatively low toxicity for the host, are active against many bacteria, especially gram-positive pathogens (streptococci, staphylococci, pneumococci); clostridia; some gram-negative forms (gonococci, meningococci); some spirochetes (*Treponema pallidum* and *T. pertenue*); and some fungi. Certain strains of some target species, e.g., staphylococci, secrete the enzyme penicillinase, which inactivates penicillin and confers resistance to the antibiotic 青霉素

pen·i·cil·lin·ase (pen″ĭ-sil′ĭ-nās) a β-lactamase preferentially cleaving penicillin 青霉素酶

Pen·i·cil·li·um (pen″ĭ-sil′e-əm) a genus of fungi 青霉（菌）属

pen·i·cil·lo·yl pol·y·ly·sine (pen″ĭ-sil′o-əl pol″eli′sēn) benzylpenicilloyl polylysine 青霉噻唑酰 - 聚赖氨酸

pen·i·cil·lus (pen″ĭ-sil′əs) pl. *penicil′li* [L.] a brushlike structure, particularly any of the brushlike groups of arterial branches in the lobules of the spleen 笔毛（状）动脉丛，脾内微动脉丛

pe·nile (pe′nīl) of or pertaining to the penis 阴茎的

pe·nis (pe′nis) the male organ of urination and copulation 阴茎；**concealed p.**, a small penis hidden by a skin abnormality or the suprapubic fat pad 隐匿阴茎；**webbed p.**, a penis that is enclosed by the skin of the scrotum, which extends onto its shaft 蹼状阴茎

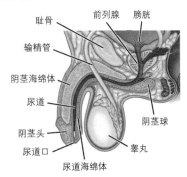

▲ 阴茎

pe·ni·tis (pe-ni′tis) inflammation of the penis 阴茎炎

pen·ni·form (pen′ĭ-form) shaped like a feather 羽状的

pe·no·plas·ty (pe′no-plas″te) 同 phalloplasty

pen·ta·gas·trin (pen″tə-gas′trin) a synthetic pentapeptide consisting of β-alanine and the C-terminal tetrapeptide of gastrin; used as a test of gastric secretory function 五肽胃泌素

pen·tam·i·dine (pen-tam′ĭ-dēn) an antiinfective used as the isethionate salt in the treatment of pneumocystis pneumonia, leishmaniasis, and early African trypanosomiasis 戊烷脒, 喷他脒 (抗感染药)

pen·ta·starch (pen″tə-stahrch″) an artificial colloid derived from a waxy starch and used as an adjunct in leukapheresis to increase the erythrocyte sedimentation rate 五羟淀粉, 一种源自蜡质淀粉的人造胶体, 用作白细胞分离术中的辅助剂, 以提高红细胞沉降率

pen·taz·o·cine (pen-taz′o-sēn) a synthetic opioid analgesic, used in the form of the hydrochloride and lactate salts as an analgesic and anesthesia adjunct 喷他佐辛 (代替吗啡的合成阿片类镇痛药, 其盐酸盐和乳酸盐用作镇痛和麻醉辅助剂, 不易成瘾)

pen·te·tate (pen′te-tāt) a salt, anion, ester, or complex of pentetic acid 三胺五乙酸

pen·te·tic ac·id (pen-tet′ik) diethylenetriamine pentaacetic acid, DTPA; a chelating agent (iron) with the general properties of the edetates; used in preparing radiopharmaceuticals 二乙撑三胺五乙酸, DTPA; 螯合剂 (铁) 具有乙二胺四乙酸盐的一般性质; 用于制备放射性药物

pen·to·bar·bi·tal (pen″to-bahr′bĭ-təl) a shortto intermediate-acting barbiturate; the sodium salt is used as a hypnotic and sedative, usually presurgery, and as an anticonvulsant 戊巴比妥

pen·to·san (pen′to-san) a carbohydrate derivative used in the form of *p. polysulfate sodium* as an anti-inflammatory in the treatment of interstitial cystitis 戊聚糖

pen·tose (pen′tōs) a monosaccharide containing five carbon atoms in a molecule 戊糖

pen·to·stat·in (pen″to-stat′in) an antineoplastic used in the treatment of hairy cell leukemia 喷司他丁, 用于治疗毛细胞白血病的抗肿瘤药

pen·tos·uria (pen″to-su′re-ə) excretion of pentoses in the urine 戊糖尿; **alimentary p.,** that occurring as a normal consequence of excessive ingestion of some fruits or their juices 营养性戊糖尿; **essential p.,** a benign autosomal recessive deficiency of the enzyme l-xylulose reductase, resulting in excessive urinary excretion of l-xylulose 左旋木酮糖尿

pen·tox·i·fyl·line (pen″tok-sif′ə-lin) a xanthine derivative that reduces blood viscosity; used for the symptomatic relief of intermittent claudication 己酮可可碱

pep·lo·mer (pep′lo-mər) a subunit of a peplos 包膜体; 外包膜突起

pep·los (pep′ləs) envelope (2) 包膜

pep·per (pep′ər) 1. any of various plants of the genus *Piper*, or their fruits, particularly the black pepper *(P. nigrum)*, the common spice 胡椒; 2. any of various plants of the genus *Capsicum*, or their fruits 辣椒; **cayenne p., red p.,** capsicum 辣椒

pep·per·mint (pep′ər-mint) the perennial herb *Mentha piperita,* or a preparation of its dried leaves and flowering tops, which have carminative, gastric stimulant, and counterirritant properties; used for gastrointestinal, liver, and gallbladder disturbances; also used in folk medicine and in homeopathy 薄荷

pep·sin (pep′sin) the proteolytic enzyme of gastric juice that catalyzes the hydrolysis of native or denatured proteins to form a mixture of polypeptides; it is formed from pepsinogen in the presence of acid or, autocatalytically, in the presence of pepsin 胃蛋白酶

pep·sin·o·gen (pep-sin′ə-jən) a zymogen secreted by the chief cells of the gastric glands and converted into pepsin in the presence of gastric acid or of pepsin itself 胃蛋白酶原

pep·tic (pep′tik) pertaining to pepsin or to digestion or to the action of gastric juices 胃蛋白酶的

pep·ti·dase (pep′tĭ-dās) any of a subclass of proteolytic enzymes that catalyze the hydrolysis of peptide linkages; it comprises the exopeptidases and endopeptidases 肽酶

pep·tide (pep′tīd) any of a class of compounds of low molecular weight that yield two or more amino acids on hydrolysis; known as di-, tri-, tetra-, (etc.) peptides, depending on the number of amino acids in the molecule. Peptides form the constituent parts of proteins 肽; **atrial natriuretic p. (ANP),** a hormone involved in natriuresis and the regulation of renal and cardiovascular homeostasis 心房钠尿肽; **glucagon-like p. (GLP),** either of two intestinal peptide hormones (GLP-1 and GLP-2) secreted by the L cells in response to ingestion of nutrients, especially carbohydrates and fat-rich meals. GLP-1 inhibits gastric emptying and food intake and has several antidiabetic effects, including stimulation of insulin secretion and pancreatic islet proliferation; GLP-2 inhibits antral motility and gastric acid secretion and induces crypt cell proliferation 胰高血糖素样肽; **opioid p.,** opioid (2) 鸦片肽

pep·ti·der·gic (pep″tĭ-dur′jĭk) of or pertaining to

neurons that secrete peptide hormones 肽能的

pep·ti·do·gly·can (pep″tĭ-do-gli′kən) a glycan (polysaccharide) attached to short cross-linked peptides; found in bacterial cell walls 肽聚糖

pep·ti·dyl-di·pep·ti·dase A (pep′tĭ-dəl di-pep′tĭ-dās) an enzyme that catalyzes the cleavage of a dipeptide from the C-terminal end of oligopeptides; when catalyzing the cleavage of angiotensin Ⅰ to form the activated angiotensin Ⅱ, it is also called *angiotensinconverting enzyme;* when catalyzing the cleavage and inactivation of kinins, it is also called *kininase Ⅱ* 血管紧张肽Ⅰ转化酶

pep·to·gen·ic (pep″to-jen′ik) 1. producing pepsin or peptones 生胃蛋白酶的；生胨的；2. promoting digestion 助消化的

pep·tol·y·sis (pep-tol′ĭ-sis) the splitting up of peptones 胨分解；**peptolyt′ic** *adj.*

pep·tone (pep′tōn) a derived protein, or a mixture of cleavage products produced by partial hydrolysis of native protein（蛋白）胨；**pepton′ic** *adj.*

Pep·to·strep·to·coc·ca·ceae (pep″to-strep″-to-kok-a′se-e) a family of gram-positive, coccoid bacteria of the order Clostridiales 消化链球菌科

per·ac·id (per-as′id) an acid containing more than the usual quantity of oxygen 过酸

per·acute (per″ə-kūt′) excessively acute or sharp 极急性的

per·am·pa·nel (per-am′pə-nel) a noncompetitive antagonist of the glutamate receptor AMPA, used as an anticonvulsant in combination to treat partial-onset seizures 吡仑帕奈

per anum (pər a′nəm) [L.] through the anus 经肛门

per·cept (pur′sept) the object perceived; the mental image of an object in space perceived by the senses 知觉对象

per·cep·tion (pər-sep′shən) the conscious mental registration of a sensory stimulus 知觉，感知；**percep′tive** *adj.*

per·cep·tiv·i·ty (pur″sep-tiv′ĭ-te) ability to receive sense impressions 知觉，感知力

per·chlor·ic acid (pər-klor′ik) a colorless volatile liquid, HClO₄, which can cause powerful explosions in the presence of organic matter or anything reducible 高氯酸，过氯酸

per·co·late (pur′kə-lāt) 1. to strain; to submit to percolation 过滤；2. to trickle slowly through a substance 渗滤；3. a liquid that has been submitted to percolation 渗滤液，渗出液，滤出液

per·co·la·tion (pur″kə-la′shən) the extraction of soluble parts of a drug by passing a solvent liquid through it 渗滤法，渗滤

per·cus·sion (pər-kush′ən) the act of striking a part with short, sharp blows as an aid in diagnosing the condition of the underlying parts by the sound obtained 叩诊；**auscultatory p.,** auscultation of the sound produced by percussion 听叩诊；**immediate p.,** that in which the blow is struck directly against the body surface 直接叩诊；**mediate p.,** that in which a pleximeter is used 间接叩诊；**palpatory p.,** a combination of palpation and percussion, affording tactile rather than auditory impressions 触叩诊

per·cus·sor (pər-kus′ər) 1. a vibrator that produces relatively coarse movements 振动器，产生相对粗糙的运动；2. percussion hammer 叩诊锤

per·cu·ta·ne·ous (pur″ku-ta′ne-əs) performed through the skin 经皮的

per·en·ni·al (pə-ren′e-əl) lasting through the year or for several years 多年生的，常年性的

per·fect (pur′fəkt) of a fungus, capable of reproducing sexually (with sexual spores) 一种真菌，有性繁殖力（有性孢子）

per·fo·rans (pur′fə-ranz) pl. *perforan′tes* [L.] penetrating; applied to various muscles, nerves, arteries, and veins 穿通的，用于各种肌肉、神经、动脉和静脉

per·fu·sate (pər-fu′zāt) a liquid that has been subjected to perfusion 灌注液

per·fu·sion (pər-fu′zhən) 1. the act of pouring over or through, especially the passage of a fluid through the vessels of a specific organ 灌注；2. a liquid poured over or through an organ or tissue 灌注液；**luxury p.** abnormally increased flow of blood to an area of the brain, leading to swelling 过度灌注

per·go·lide (pur′go-līd) a long-acting ergot derivative with dopaminergic properties; formerly used as the mesylate salt in the treatment of parkinsonism 培高利特，硫丙麦角林，具有多巴胺能特性的长效麦角衍生物；其甲磺酸盐曾用于治疗帕金森病

peri·ac·i·nal (per″e-as′ĭ-nəl) around an acinus 腺泡周的

peri·ac·i·nous (per″e-as′ĭ-nəs) periacinal 同 periacinal

peri·ad·e·ni·tis (per″e-ad″ə-ni′tis) inflammation of tissues around a gland 腺周炎；**p. muco′san-ecro′tica recur′rens,** the more severe form of aphthous stomatitis, marked by recurrent attacks of aphtha-like lesions that begin as small firm nodules and enlarge, ulcerate, and heal to leave numerous atrophied scars on the oral mucosa 复发性坏死性黏膜腺周炎

peri·am·pul·lary (per″e-am′pu-lar″e) around an ampulla 壶腹周围的

peri·ap·i·cal (per″e-ap′ĭ-kəl) around the apex of

P

the root of a tooth 根尖周的

peri·ap·pen·di·ci·tis (per″e-ə-pen″dĭ-si′tis) inflammation of the tissues around the vermiform appendix 阑尾周围炎

peri·ar·ter·i·tis (per″e-ahr″tə-ri′tis) inflammation of the external coats of an artery and of the tissues around the artery 动脉周围炎，动脉外膜炎；**p. nodo′sa**, 1. polyarteritis nodosa 结节性多动脉炎；2. a group comprising polyarteritis nodosa, allergic granulomatous angiitis, and many systemic necrotizing vasculitides with clinicopathologic characteristics overlapping these two 一组包括结节性多动脉炎、过敏性肉芽肿性血管炎和许多临床病理学特征与这两者重叠的系统性坏死性血管炎（结节性动脉周围炎）

peri·ar·thri·tis (per″e-ahr-thri′tis) inflammation of tissues around a joint 关节周围炎

peri·ar·tic·u·lar (per″e-ahr-tik′u-lər) around a joint 关节周的

peri·ax·i·al (per″e-ak′se-əl) near or around an axis 轴周的

peri·bron·chio·li·tis (per″e-brong″ke-o-li′tis) inflammation of tissues around the bronchioles 细支气管周炎

peri·bron·chi·tis (per″e-brong-ki′tis) bronchitis with inflammation and thickening of tissues around the bronchi 支气管周炎

peri·cal·lo·sal (per″e-kə-lo′səl) around the corpus callosum 胼胝体周的

peri·ca·lyc·e·al (per″e-kal″ĭ-se′əl) near or around a renal calyx 肾盏周的

peri·car·di·al (per″e-kahr′de-əl) 1. pertaining to the pericardium 心包的；2. surrounding the heart 心脏周围的

peri·car·di·ec·to·my (per″e-kahr″de-ek′tə-me) removal of all or part of the pericardium 心包切除术

peri·car·dio·cen·te·sis (per″e-kahr″de-o-sente′-sis) surgical puncture of the pericardial cavity for the aspiration of fluid 心包穿刺术

peri·car·di·ol·y·sis (per″e-kahr″de-ol′ĭ-sis) the operative freeing of adhesions between the visceral and parietal pericardium 心包松解术

peri·car·dio·phren·ic (per″e-kahr″de-o-fren′ik) pertaining to the pericardium and respiratory diaphragm 心包膈的

peri·car·di·or·rha·phy (per″e-kahr″de-or′ə-fe) suture of the pericardium 心包缝合术

peri·car·di·os·to·my (per″e-kahr″de-os′tə-me) creation of an opening into the pericardium, usually for the drainage of effusions 心包造口术

peri·car·di·ot·o·my (per″e-kahr″de-ot′ə-me) incision of the pericardium 心包切开术

peri·car·di·tis (per″e-kahr-di′tis) inflammation of the pericardium 心包炎；**pericardit′ic** *adj.*；**adhesive p.**, a condition due to the presence of dense fibrous tissue between the parietal and visceral layers of the pericardium 粘连性心包炎；**constrictive p.**, a chronic form in which a fibrotic, thickened, adherent pericardium restricts diastolic filling and cardiac output, usually resulting from a series of events beginning with fibrin deposition on the pericardial surface followed by fibrotic thickening and scarring and obliteration of the pericardial space 缩窄性心包炎；**fibrinous p.**, **fibrous p.**, that characterized by a fibrinous exudate, sometimes accompanied by a serous effusion; usually manifested as a pericardial friction rub 纤维性心包炎；**p. obli′terans**, **obliterating p.**, adhesive pericarditis that leads to obliteration of the pericardial cavity 闭塞性心包炎

peri·car·di·um (per″ĭ-kahr′de-əm) the fibroserous sac enclosing the heart and the roots of the great vessels 心包；**pericar′dial** *adj.*；**adherent p.**, one abnormally connected with the heart by dense fibrous tissue 粘连性心包

peri·ce·ci·tis (per″e-se-si′tis) inflammation of the tissues around the cecum 盲肠周围炎

peri·ce·men·ti·tis (per″e-se″mən-ti′tis) periodontitis 牙周膜炎

peri·cho·lan·gi·tis (per″e-ko″lan-ji′tis) inflammation of the tissues around the bile ducts 胆管周围炎

peri·cho·le·cys·ti·tis (per″e-ko″lə-sis-ti′tis) inflammation of tissues around the gallbladder 胆囊周炎

peri·chon·dri·um (per″ĭ-kon′dre-əm) the layer of fibrous connective tissue investing all cartilage except the articular cartilage of synovial joints 软骨膜，**perichon′drial** *adj.*

peri·chor·dal (per″e-kor′dəl) around the notochord 脊索膜的

peri·cho·roi·dal (per″e-kor-oi′dəl) surrounding the choroid coat 脉络膜周的，脉络膜外的

peri·co·li·tis (per″e-ko-li′tis) inflammation around the colon, especially of its peritoneal coat 结肠周炎，又称 *pericolonitis*

peri·col·pi·tis (per″e-kol-pi′tis) inflammation of tissues around the vagina 阴道周炎

peri·cor·o·nal (per″e-kor′ə-nəl) around the crown of a tooth（牙）冠周的

peri·cra·ni·tis (per″e-kra-ni′tis) inflammation of the pericranium 颅骨膜炎

peri·cra·ni·um (per″e-kra′ne-əm) the periosteum of the skull 颅骨膜，**pericra′nial** *adj.*

peri·cyte (per′e-sīt) a type of elongated cell having the power of contraction, found wrapped about the outside of precapillary arterioles, postcapillary venules, and capillaries 周皮细胞，外膜细胞

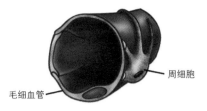

毛细血管　周细胞

▲　周细胞。包裹在毛细血管上皮周围

peri·cy·ti·al (per″e-si′te-əl) around a cell 细胞周的

peri·den·tal (per″e-den′təl) 同 periodontal

peri·derm (per′ĭ-durm″) 1. the outer layer of the bilaminar fetal epidermis, generally disappearing before birth 胎儿表皮；2. the cuticle (eponychium) and hyponychium considered together 周皮；**periderm′al** *adj.*

peri·des·mi·um (per″e-dez′me-əm) the areolar membrane that covers the ligaments 韧带膜

peri·di·ver·tic·u·li·tis (per″e-di″vər-tik″u-li′tis) inflammation of the structures around a diverticulum of the intestine 憩室周围炎

peri·duc·tal (per″e-duk′təl) surrounding a duct, particularly of the mammary gland 导管周的

peri·du·o·de·ni·tis (per″e-doo″o-də-ni′tis) inflammation around the duodenum 十二指肠周炎

peri·en·ceph·a·li·tis (per″e-en-sef″ə-li′tis) meningoencephalitis 脑表层炎

peri·en·ter·itis (per″e-en″tər-i′tis) inflammation of the peritoneal coat of the intestines 肠周炎，肠腹膜炎

peri·esoph·a·gi·tis (per″e-ə-sof′ə-ji′tis) inflammation of tissues around the esophagus 食管周炎

peri·fol·lic·u·lar (per″e-fə-lik′u-lər) surrounding a follicle, particularly a hair follicle 滤泡周的（一般指毛囊周的）

peri·fol·lic·u·li·tis (per″e-fə-lik″u-li′tis) inflammation around the hair follicles 毛囊周炎

peri·gan·gli·itis (per″e-gang″gle-i′tis) inflammation of tissues around a ganglion 神经节周炎

peri·gas·tri·tis (per″e-gas-tri′tis) inflammation of the peritoneal coat of the stomach 胃周炎，胃腹膜炎

peri·hep·a·ti·tis (per″e-hep″ə-ti′tis) inflammation of the peritoneal capsule of the liver and the surrounding tissue 肝周炎

peri·is·let (per″e-i′let) around the islets of Langerhans 胰岛周围的

peri·je·ju·ni·tis (per″e-jĕ″joo-ni′tis) inflammation around the jejunum 空肠周炎

peri·kary·on (per″e-kar′e-on) the cell body as distinguished from the nucleus and the processes; applied particularly to neurons 核周体

peri·lab·y·rin·thi·tis (per″e-lab″ə-rin-thi′tis) circumscribed labyrinthitis 迷路周炎

peri·lymph (per′e-limf) the fluid within the space separating the membranous and osseous labyrinths of the ear 外淋巴（内耳迷路与膜迷路之间的液体）

peri·lym·phan·gi·tis (per″e-lim″fan-ji′tis) inflammation around a lymphatic vessel 淋巴管周炎

peri·lym·phat·ic (per″e-lim-fat′ik) 1. pertaining to the perilymph 外淋巴的；2. around a lymphatic vessel 淋巴管周的

peri·men·in·gi·tis (per″e-men″in-ji′tis) pachymeningitis 硬脑膜炎，硬脊膜炎

peri·meno·pause (per″e-men′o-pawz) the time just before and after menopause 围绝经期；**perimenopau′sal** *adj.*

peri·me·tri·um (per″ĭ-me′tre-əm) the tunica serosa surrounding the uterus 子宫外膜

per·i·mor·tem (pair′ē-mohr-tem) at or near the time of death 濒死期

peri·myo·si·tis (per″e-mi″o-si′tis) inflammation of connective tissue around a muscle 肌周炎

peri·mys·i·um (per″ĭ-mis′e-əm) pl. *perimys′ia*. The connective tissue demarcating a fascicle of skeletal muscle fibers 肌束膜，参见图7；**perimys′ial** *adj.*

peri·na·tal (per″e-na′təl) relating to the period shortly before and after birth; from the twentieth to twenty-ninth week of gestation to 1 to 4 weeks after birth 围生期的

peri·na·tol·o·gy (per″e-na-tol′ə-je) the branch of medicine (obstetrics and pediatrics) dealing with the fetus and infant during the perinatal period 围生医学

peri·ne·al (per″ĭ-ne′əl) pertaining to the perineum 会阴的

peri·neo·plas·ty (per″ĭ-ne′o-plas″te) plastic repair of the perineum 会阴成形术

peri·ne·or·rha·phy (per″ĭ-ne-or′ə-fe) suture of the perineum 会阴修复术

peri·ne·ot·o·my (per″ĭ-ne-ot′ə-me) incision of the perineum 会阴切开术

peri·neo·vag·i·nal (per″ĭ-ne″o-vaj′ ĭ-nəl) pertaining to or communicating with the perineum and vagina 会阴阴道的

peri·neph·ric (per″e-nef′rik) perirenal; surrounding the kidney 肾周的

peri·ne·phri·tis (per″e-nə-fri′tis) inflammation of the perinephrium 肾周（围）炎

peri·neph·ri·um (per″ĭ-nef′re-əm) the peritoneal envelope and other tissues around the kidney 肾周膜，肾外膜；**perineph′rial** *adj.*

peri·ne·um (per″ĭ-ne′əm) 1. the region and associated structures occupying the pelvic outlet and beneath the pelvic diaphragm; bounded anteriorly by the pubic symphysis, anterolaterally by the ischiopubic rami and the ischial tuberosities, posterolaterally by the sacrotuberous ligaments, and posteriorly by the coccyx 会阴（广义）; 2. the region between the thighs, bounded in the male by the scrotum and anus and in the female by the vulva and anus, and containing the roots of the external genitalia 会阴（狭义）

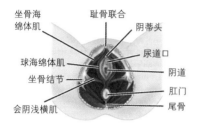

坐骨海绵体肌　　　耻骨联合
　　　　　　　　　阴蒂头
球海绵体肌　　　　尿道口
坐骨结节　　　　　阴道
　　　　　　　　　肛门
会阴浅横肌　　　　尾骨

▲ 会阴（女性）

peri·neu·ri·tis (per″e-noo-ri′tis) inflammation of the perineurium 神经束膜炎

peri·neu·ri·um (per″e-noor′e-əm) an intermediate layer of connective tissue in a peripheral nerve, surrounding each bundle of nerve fibers 神经束膜，参见图 14; **perineu′rial** *adj.*

peri·nu·cle·ar (per″e-noo′kle-ər) near or around a nucleus 核周的

pe·ri·od (pēr′e-əd) an interval or division of time 期，时期; **ejection p.,** the second phase of ventricular systole, being the interval between the opening and closing of the semilunar valves, during which the blood is discharged into the aortic and pulmonary arteries; it is divided into a *p. of rapid ejection* followed by a *p. of reduced ejection* 射血期; **gestation p.,** the duration of pregnancy, in humans being about 266 days (38 weeks) from the time of fertilization until birth. In obstetrics, it is instead considered to begin on the first day of the woman's last normal menstrual period prior to fertilization, thus being about 280 days (40 weeks) 妊娠期; **incubation p.,** 1. the interval of time required for development 孵化期; 2. the interval between the receipt of infection and the onset of the consequent illness or the first symptoms of the illness 潜伏期; 3. the interval between the entrance into a vector of an infectious agent and the time at which the vector is capable of transmitting the infection 潜伏期; **latency p.,** 1. 同 latent p.; 2. 性成熟前期，参见 *stage* 下词条; **latent p.,** a seemingly inactive period, as that between exposure to an infection and subsequent illness, or that between the instant of stimulation and the beginning of response 潜伏期; **menstrual p.,** the time of menstruation 月经期; **pacemaker refractory p.,** the period immediately following either pacemaker sensing or pacing, during which improper inhibition of the pacemaker by inappropriate signals is prevented by inactivation of pacemaker sensing 起搏器不应期; **quarantine p.,** 1. the length of time that must elapse before a person exposed to contagion is regarded as incapable of transmitting or acquiring the disease (see also *quarantine*) 检疫期; 2. a period of detention of vessels, vehicles, or travelers coming from infected or suspected ports or places 留验期; **refractory p.,** the period of depolarization and repolarization of the cell membrane after excitation; during the first portion *(absolute refractory p.),* the nerve or muscle fiber cannot respond to a second stimulus, whereas during the *relative refractory period,* it can respond only to a strong stimulus 不应期; **sphygmic p.,** 同 ejection p.; **Wenckebach p.,** the steadily lengthening P–R interval occurring in successive cardiac cycles in Wenckebach block 文克巴赫周期，在文氏阻滞连续的心脏周期中，P-R 间期持续延长

pe·ri·od·ic (pēr″e-od′ik) 1. recurring at regular intervals of time 周期性的; 2. recurring intermittently or occasionally 间发性的，定期的

pe·ri·o·dic·i·ty (pēr″e-o-dis′ĭ-te) recurrence at regular intervals of time 周期性，间发性

peri·odon·tal (per″e-o-don′təl) 1. pertaining to the periodontal ligament or periodontium 牙周膜的; 2. near or around a tooth 牙周的

peri·odon·tics (per″e-o-don′tiks) the branch of dentistry dealing with the study and treatment of diseases of the periodontium 牙周病学

peri·odon·ti·tis (per″e-o-don-ti′tis) inflammatory reaction of the periodontium 牙周炎; **marginal p.,** a chronic destructive inflammatory periodontal disease that begins as a simple marginal gingivitis and may migrate along the tooth toward the apex, producing periodontal pockets, usually with pus formation, and destruction of the periodontal and alveolar structures, causing the teeth to become loose 边缘性牙周炎

peri·odon·ti·um (per″e-o-don′she-əm) pl. *periodon′tia*. The tissues investing and supporting the teeth, including the cement, periodontal ligament, alveolar bone, and gingiva 牙周组织，牙周膜

peri·odon·to·sis (per″e-o-don-to′sis) a degenerative disorder of the periodontal structures, marked by tissue destruction 牙周变性

peri·onych·i·um (per″e-o-nik′e-əm) eponychium (1) 甲周膜

peri·ooph·o·ri·tis (per″e-o-of″o-ri′tis) inflammation of tissues around the ovary 卵巢周炎

peri·ooph·o·ro·sal·pin·gi·tis (per″e-o-of″oro-sal″pin-ji′tis) inflammation of tissues around an ovary and uterine tube 卵巢输卵管周炎

peri·op·er·a·tive (per″e-op′ər-ə-tiv) pertaining to the period extending from the time of hospitalization for surgery to the time of discharge 手术期间的

peri·oph·thal·mic (per″e-of-thal′mik) around the eye 眼周的

peri·op·tom·e·try (per″e-op-tom′ə-tre) measurement of acuity of peripheral vision or of limits of the visual field 视野检查法

peri·or·bi·ta (per″e-or″bĭ-tə) periosteum of the bones of the orbit, or eye socket 眶骨膜; **peri·or′bital** adj.

peri·or·bi·ti·tis (per″e-or″bĭ-ti′tis) inflammation of the periorbita 眶骨膜炎

peri·or·chi·tis (per″e-or-ki′tis) inflammation of the tunica vaginalis testis 睾丸鞘膜炎

peri·os·te·al (per″e-os′te-əl) pertaining to the periosteum 骨膜的

peri·os·te·itis (per″e-os″te-i′tis) 同 periostitis

peri·os·te·o·ma (per″e-os-te-o′mə) a morbid bony growth surrounding a bone 骨膜瘤

peri·os·teo·my·eli·tis (per″e-os″te-o-mi″ə-li′tis) inflammation of the entire bone, including periosteum and marrow 骨膜脊髓炎

peri·os·teo·phyte (per″e-os′te-o-fīt″) a bony growth on the periosteum 骨膜骨赘

peri·os·te·ot·o·my (per″e-os″te-ot′ə-me) incision of the periosteum 骨膜切开术

peri·os·te·um (per″e-os′te-əm) a specialized connective tissue covering all bones and having bone-forming potentialities 骨膜

peri·os·ti·tis (per″e-os-ti′tis) inflammation of the periosteum 骨膜炎

peri·os·to·sis (per″e-os-to′sis) abnormal deposition of periosteal bone; the condition manifested by development of periosteomas 骨膜骨赘形成

peri·otic (per″e-o′tik) 1. situated about the ear, especially the internal ear 耳周的(尤指内耳周的); 2. the petrous and mastoid portions of the temporal bone, at one stage a distinct bone 耳周骨

peri·ovu·lar (per″e-ov′u-lər) 1. surrounding an ovum 卵周的; 2. around the time of ovulation 排卵期前后

peri·pap·il·lary (per″e-pap′ ĭ-lar″e) around the optic papilla 视乳头周围的

peri·par·tum (per″e-pahr′təm) occurring during the last month of gestation or the first few months after delivery, with reference to the mother 围生期

pe·riph·er·ad (pə-rif′ər-əd) toward the periphery 向外周, 向周围, 向末梢

pe·riph·er·al (pə-rif′ər-əl) pertaining to or situated at or near the periphery; situated away from a center or central structure 外周的, 周围的; 末梢的

peri·phe·ra·lis (pə-rif″ə-ra′lis) 同 peripheral

peri·phe·ri·cus (per″ĭ-fer′ĭ-kəs) [L.] 同 peripheral

pe·riph·ery (pə-rif′ə-re) an outward surface or structure; the portion of a system outside the central region 外周(部), 周围(部)

peri·phle·bi·tis (per″e-flə-bi′tis) inflammation of tissues around a vein, or of the external coat of a vein 静脉周围炎

Per·i·pla·ne·ta (per″ĭ-plə-ne′tə) a genus of roaches, including *P. america′na,* the American cockroach, and *P. australa′siae,* the Australian cockroach 大蠊属

peri·plas·mic (per″e-plas′mik) around the plasma membrane; between the plasma membrane and the cell wall of a bacterium 周质的, 胞质的

peri·proc·ti·tis (per″e-prok-ti′tis) inflammation of tissues around the rectum and anus 直肠周围炎

peri·pros·ta·ti·tis (per″e-pros″tə-ti′tis) inflammation of tissues around the prostate 前列腺周围炎

peri·py·le·phle·bi·tis (per″e-pi″le-flə-bi′tis) inflammation of tissues around the portal vein 门静脉周围炎

peri·rec·ti·tis (per″e-rek-ti′tis) 同 periproctitis

peri·re·nal (per″e-re′nəl) 同 perinephric

peri·sal·pin·gi·tis (per″e-sal″pin-ji′tis) inflammation of the tissues and peritoneum around a uterine tube 输卵管腹膜炎

peri·sig·moid·itis (per″e-sig″moid-i′tis) inflammation of the peritoneum of the sigmoid flexure 乙状结肠周围炎

peri·si·nus·itis (per″e-si″nəs-i′tis) inflammation of tissues about a sinus 窦周炎

peri·splanch·ni·tis (per″e-splank-ni′tis) inflammation of tissues around the viscera 内脏周围炎

peri·sple·ni·tis (per″e-splə-ni′tis) inflammation of the peritoneal surface of the spleen 脾周围炎

peri·spon·dy·li·tis (per″e-spon″də-li′tis) inflammation of tissues around a vertebra 椎骨周围炎

peri·stal·sis (per″ĭ-stawl′sis) the wormlike movement by which the alimentary canal or other tubular organs having both longitudinal and circular muscle fibers propel their contents, consisting of a wave of contraction passing along the tube for variable distances 蠕动; **peri·stal′tic** adj.

peri·staph·y·line (per″e-staf′ə-līn) around the uvula 悬雍垂周的

peri·tec·to·my (per″ĭ-tek′tə-me) excision of a ring of conjunctiva around the cornea in treatment of pannus 球结膜环状切除术

peri·ten·din·e·um (per″ĭ-tən-din′e-əm) connective tissue investing larger tendons and extending between the fibers composing them 腱鞘

peri·ten·di·ni·tis (per″e-ten″dĭ-ni′tis) tenosynovitis 腱鞘炎

peri·ten·o·ni·tis (per″e-ten′ə-ni′tis) tenosynovitis 腱鞘炎

peri·the·li·o·ma (per″ĭ-the″le-o′mə) hemangiopericytoma 血管外皮细胞瘤

peri·the·li·um (per″e-the′le-əm) the connective tissue layer surrounding the capillaries and smaller vessels 周皮

peri·thy·roi·di·tis (per″e-thi″roi-di′tis) inflammation of the capsule of the thyroid gland 甲状腺囊炎

pe·rit·o·my (pə-rit′ə-me) incision of the conjunctiva and subconjunctival tissue about the entire circumference of the cornea 球结膜环状切开术

peri·to·ne·al (per″ĭ-to-ne′əl) pertaining to the peritoneum 腹膜的

peri·to·ne·al·gia (per″ĭ-to″ne-al′jə) pain in the peritoneum 腹膜痛

peri·to·neo·cen·te·sis (per″ĭ-to″ne-o-sen-te′sis) paracentesis of the abdominal cavity 腹腔穿刺（术）

peri·to·ne·os·co·py (per″ĭ-to″ne-os′kə-pe) laparoscopy 腹腔镜检查

peri·to·neo·ve·nous (per″ĭ-to-ne″o-ve′nəs) communicating with the peritoneal cavity and the venous system 腹腔静脉短路

peri·to·ne·um (per″ĭ-to-ne′əm) the serous membrane lining the walls of the abdominal and pelvic cavities *(parietal p.)* and investing the contained viscera *(visceral p.),* the two layers enclosing a potential space, the peritoneal cavity 腹膜；**peritone′al** *adj.*

peri·to·ni·tis (per″ĭ-to-ni′tis) inflammation of the peritoneum, which may be due to chemical irritation or bacterial invasion 腹膜炎

peri·ton·sil·lar (per″e-ton′sĭ-lər) around a tonsil 扁桃体周的

peri·ton·sil·li·tis (per″e-ton″sĭ-li′tis) inflammation of peritonsillar tissues 扁桃体周炎

pe·rit·ri·chous (pə-rit′rĭ-kəs) 1. having flagella around the entire surface; said of bacteria; sometimes used to describe the flagella themselves 周毛的；2. having flagella around the cytostome only; said of Ciliophora 围口纤毛的（指纤毛虫）

peri·tu·bu·lar (per″e-too′bu-lər) situated around or near tubules 小管周

peri·um·bil·i·cal (per″e-əm-bil′ĭ-kəl) around the umbilicus 脐周的

peri·un·gual (per″e-ung′gwəl) around the nail 甲周的

peri·ure·ter·itis (per″e-u-re″tər-i′tis) inflammation of tissues around a ureter 输尿管周围炎

peri·ure·thri·tis (per″e-u″rə-thri′tis) inflammation of the tissues around the urethra 尿道周围炎

peri·vag·i·ni·tis (per″e-vaj″ĭ-ni′tis) 同 pericolpitis

peri·vas·cu·lar (per″e-vas′ku-lər) near or around a vessel 血管周的

peri·vas·cu·li·tis (per″e-vas″ku-li′tis) inflammation of the tissue surrounding a blood or lymph vessel 血管周围炎

peri·ves·i·cal (per″e-ves′ĭ-kəl) near the urinary bladder 膀胱周的

peri·ve·sic·u·li·tis (per″e-və-sik″u-li′tis) inflammation of tissue around the seminal vesicle 精囊周围炎

per·lèche (per-lesh′) inflammation with exudation, maceration, and fissuring at the labial commissures 传染性口角炎，念珠菌性口角炎

per·man·ga·nate (pər-mang′gə-nāt) a salt containing the MnO_4^- ion 高锰酸盐

per·me·a·bil·i·ty (pur″me-ə-bil′ĭ-te) the property or state of being permeable 渗透性；通透性

per·me·a·ble (pur′me-ə-bəl) allowing passage of a substance 可渗透的，可透过的

per·me·ase (pur′me-ās) former name for *transport protein* 通透酶

per·me·ate (pur′me-āt″) 1. to penetrate or pass through, as through a filter 渗透，透过；2. the constituents of a solution or suspension that pass through a filter 渗透液，滤过液

per·meth·rin (pər-meth′rin) a topical insecticide used in the treatment of infestations by *Pediculus humanus capitis, Sarcoptes scabiei,* or any of various ticks; also applied to objects such as furniture and bedding 扑灭司林，氯菊酯，一种局部杀虫剂，用于治疗头足虱、疥螨或任何一种蜱虫的侵扰；也适用于家具和床上用品等物体

perm·se·lec·tiv·i·ty (pərm″sə-lek-tiv′ĭ-te) restriction of permeation of macromolecules across a glomerular capillary wall on the basis of molecular size, charge, and physical configuration 通透选择

per·ni·cious (pər-nish′əs) tending toward a fatal issue 有害的，恶性的

per·nio (pur′ne-o) pl. *pernio′nes* [L.] chilblain 冻疮

pe·ro·me·lia (pe″ro-me′le-ə) severe dysmelia 四肢不全（畸形）

per·o·ne·al (per″o-ne′əl) pertaining to the fibula or to the lateral aspect of the leg; fibular 腓骨的，腓侧的

pe·ro·ne·a·lis (pə-ro″ne-a′lis) [L.] fibular 腓骨

per·oral (pər-or′əl) performed or administered

through the mouth 经口的，由口的，口服的

per os (pər os) [L.] by mouth 口服，经口

per·ox·i·dase (pər-ok′sĭ-dās) any of a group of iron-porphyrin enzymes that catalyze the oxidation of some organic substrates in the presence of hydrogen peroxide 过氧化物酶

per·ox·ide (pər-ok′sīd) that oxide of any element containing more oxygen than any other; more correctly applied to compounds having such linkage as —O—O— 过氧化物

per·ox·i·some (pər-ok′sĭ-sōm) a microbody (q.v.), present in all animal cells except erythrocytes and many plant cells, containing enzymes that participate in a variety of oxidative processes, including reactions involving hydrogen peroxide, purine metabolism, cellular lipid metabolism, and gluconeogenesis 过氧化物酶体，微体

per·phen·a·zine (pər-fen′ə-zēn) a phenothiazine used as an antipsychotic and as an antiemetic 奋乃静羟哌氯丙嗪，用作抗精神病药和止吐药

per pri·mam in·ten·ti·o·nem (pər pri′məm in-ten″she-o′nəm) [L.] by first intention 第一期愈合；见 *healing* 下词条。又写作 *per primam*

per rec·tum (pər rek′təm) [L.] by way of the rectum 经直肠

per se·cun·dam in·ten·ti·o·nem (pər se-kun′dəm in-ten″she-o′nəm) [L.] by second intention 第二期愈合；见 *healing* 下词条。又写作 *per secundam*

per·sev·er·a·tion (pər-sev″ər-a′shən) persistent repetition of the same verbal or motor response to varied stimuli; continuance of activity after cessation of the causative stimulus 持续症，持续动作

per·so·na (pər-so′nə) [L.] in jungian psychology, the personality mask or facade presented by a person to the outside world, as opposed to the anima, the inner being 人格面具，伪装人格

per·so·nal·i·ty (pur″sə-nal′ĭ-te) the characteristic, relatively stable, and predictable way a person thinks, feels, and behaves, including conscious attitudes, values, and styles, and also unconscious conflicts and defense mechanisms 人格，个性；**cyclothymic p.,** a temperament characterized by rapid, frequent swings between sad and cheerful moods 循环型人格；**split p.,** a colloquial term used for either schizophrenia or dissociative identity disorder 人格分裂

per·spi·ra·tion (pur″spī-ra′shən) 1. sweating 出汗；2. sweat 汗

per·sul·fate (pər-sul′fāt) a salt of persulfuric acid 过硫酸盐

per tu·bam (pər too′bəm) [L.] through a tube 经管

per·tus·sis (pər-tus′is) whooping cough; an infectious disease caused by *Bordetella pertussis,* marked by inflammation of the respiratory tract and peculiar paroxysms of cough, ending in a prolonged crowing or whooping respiration 百日咳

per·tus·soid (pər-tus′oid) 1. resembling whooping cough 百日咳样的；2. an influenzal cough resembling that of whooping cough 百日咳样咳嗽

per va·gi·nam (pər və-ji′nəm) [L.] through the vagina 经阴道

per·ver·sion (pər-vur′zhən) 1. deviation from the normal course 倒错，反常；2. sexual perversion 性反常行为；参见 *deviation* 下词条

pes (pes) pl. *pe′des* [L.] 1. foot 足，脚；2. any footlike part 足状部分，足样的部分

pes·sa·ry (pes′ə-re) 1. an instrument placed in the vagina to support the uterus or rectum or as a contraceptive device 子宫托，阴道环；2. a medicated vaginal suppository 医用阴道栓剂

pes·ti·lence (pes′tĭ-ləns) a virulent contagious epidemic or infectious epidemic disease 疫病；疫病流行；**pestilen′tial** *adj.*

pes·tle (pes′əl) an implement for pounding drugs in a mortar 杵，研棒

PET positron emission tomography 正电子发射体层摄影（术）

peta- (P), a word element used in naming units of measurement to designate a quantity 10^{15} (a quadrillion) times the unit to which it is joined [构词成分] 秤（10^{15}）

pe·te·chia (pə-te′ke-ə) pl. *pete′chiae* [L.] a pinpoint, nonraised, round, purplish red spot caused by intradermal or submucous hemorrhage 瘀点，瘀斑；**pete′chial** *adj.*

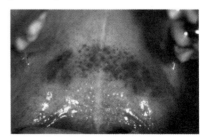

▲ 由咳嗽引起的软腭瘀点

pet·i·ole (pet′e-ōl) a stalk or pedicle 柄，茎，又称 *petiolus*；**epiglottic p.,** the pointed lower end of the epiglottic cartilage, attached to the thyroid cartilage 会厌软骨柄

pe·tit mal (pə-te′ mahl) [Fr.]（癫痫）小发作，参见 *epilepsy* 下词条

pet·ro·la·tum (pet″ro-la′təm) a purified mixture of semisolid hydrocarbons obtained from petroleum; used as an ointment base, protective dressing, and soothing application to the skin 矿脂，凡士林；
liquid p., mineral oil 液体石蜡

pe·tro·le·um (pə-tro′le-əm) a thick natural mixture of gaseous, liquid, and solid hydrocarbons obtained from beneath the surface of the earth 石油；**p. benzin**, a colorless, volatile, flammable fraction from petroleum distillation, containing largely hydrocarbons of the methane series; it has been variously described as a special grade of ligroin or as a separate but similar fraction with a lower boiling range. It is used chiefly as an extractive solvent 石油醚

pet·ro·mas·toid (pet″ro-mas′toid) 1. pertaining to the petrous portion of the temporal bone and its mastoid process 岩部乳突的；2. otocranium (2) 耳外骨

pet·ro·oc·cip·i·tal (pet″ro-ok-sip′ĭ-təl) pertaining to the petrous portion of the temporal bone and to the occipital bone 岩枕的

pe·tro·sal (pə-tro′səl) pertaining to the petrous part of the temporal bone 岩部的（颞骨）

pet·ro·si·tis (pet″ro-si′tis) inflammation of the petrous part of the temporal bone 岩锥炎，（颞骨）岩部炎

pet·ro·sphe·noid (pet″ro-sfe′noid) pertaining to the petrous portion of the temporal bone and to the sphenoid bone 岩部蝶骨的

pet·ro·squa·mous (pet″ro-skwa′məs) pertaining to the petrous and squamous parts of the temporal bone 岩鳞（部）的

pet·rous (pet′rəs) resembling a rock; hard; stony 岩石样的，石状的

PETS percutaneous epiphysiodesis using transphyseal screws 经皮椎体螺钉外固定术；经皮松质骨螺钉骺板阻滞术

PEXG pseudoexfoliative glaucoma 假性表皮脱落性青光眼

pex·is (pek′sis) 1. the fixation of matter by a tissue 固定；2. surgical fixation 固定术；**pex′ic** adj.

pey·o·te (pa-yo′ta) a stimulant drug from mescal buttons, whose active principle is mescaline; used by North American Indians in certain ceremonies to produce an intoxication marked by feelings of ecstasy 拍约他，仙人球膏（制自墨西哥仙人球的一种兴奋剂）

PFS progression-free survival 无进展生存期，无进展生存

pg picogram 皮克

pH the symbol relating the hydrogen ion (H^+) concentration or activity of a solution to that of a given standard solution. Numerically the pH is approximately equal to the negative logarithm of H^+ concentration expressed in molarity. pH 7 is neutral; above it alkalinity increases and below it acidity increases 氢离子指数，pH 值

phaco·ana·phy·lax·is (fak″o-an″ə-fə-lak′sis) hypersensitivity to the protein of the crystalline lens of the eye, induced by escape of material from the lens capsule 晶状体蛋白过敏性

phaco·cele (fak′o-sēl) herniation of the lens of the eye 晶状体突出

phaco·cys·tec·to·my (fak″o-sis-tek′tə-me) excision of part of the lens capsule for cataract 晶状体囊（部分）切除术（治疗白内障）

phaco·cys·ti·tis (fak″o-sis-ti′tis) inflammation of the lens capsule 晶状体囊炎

phaco·emul·si·fi·ca·tion (fak″o-e-mul″sī-fĭ-ka′shən) a method of cataract extraction in which the lens is fragmented by ultrasonic vibrations and simultaneously irrigated and aspirated 超声乳化白内障吸出术（一种白内障摘除方法）

phaco·ery·sis (fak″o-ə-re′sis) removal of the lens of the eye by suction, for cataract 晶状体吸出术

phac·oid (fak′oid) shaped like a lens 透镜状的

phac·oid·itis (fak″oi-di′tis) 同 phakitis

pha·col·y·sis (fə-kol′ĭ-sis) dissolution or discission of the lens of the eye 晶状体溶解；**phaco·lyt′ic** adj.

phaco·ma·la·cia (fak″o-mə-la′shə) softening of the lens 晶状体软化

phaco·meta·cho·re·sis (fak″o-met″ə-ko-re′sis) displacement of the lens of the eye 晶状体移位

phaco·scle·ro·sis (fak″o-sklə-ro′sis) hardening of the crystalline lens, or a cataract that has become hard 晶状体硬化，硬白内障

phaco·scope (fak′o-skōp) an instrument for viewing accommodative changes of the lens of the eye 晶状体镜

phaco·tox·ic (fak′o-tok″sik) exerting a deleterious effect upon the crystalline lens 晶状体毒性的

phaeo·hy·pho·my·co·sis (fe″o-hi″fo-mi-ko′sis) any of a wide variety of infections, ranging from localized cutaneous infectious disease to systemic disease, caused by dematiaceous fungi that form hyphae or yeast-like cells, or both, in tissue 暗色丝孢霉病

phage (fāj) bacteriophage 噬菌体

phag·e·de·na (faj″ə-de′nə) ulceration that spreads rapidly and causes sloughing 崩蚀性溃疡，蚀疮；**phagede′nic** adj.

phag·e·den·ic (faj″ə-den′ik) pertaining to or characterized by phagedena 崩蚀性溃疡的

phago·cyte (fa′go-sīt) any cell that ingests microorganisms or other cells and foreign particles, such as a microphage, macrophage, or monocyte 吞噬细胞；**phagocyt′ic** adj.

phago·cy·tol·y·sis (fa″go-si-tol′ĭ-sis) destruction of phagocytes 吞噬细胞溶解；**phagocytolyt′ic** adj.

phago·cy·to·sis (fa″go-si-to′sis) the engulfing of microorganisms or other cells and foreign particles by phagocytes 吞噬作用；**phagocytot′ic** adj.

phago·some (fag′o-sōm) a membrane-bound vesicle in a phagocyte containing the phagocytized material 吞噬体

phago·type (fag′o-tīp) phage type 吞噬体型，参见 type 下词条

pha·ki·tis (fa-ki′tis) inflammation of the crystalline lens 晶状体炎

pha·ko·ma (fə-ko′mə) any of the hamartomas found in the phakomatoses, such as the herald lesions of tuberous sclerosis 晶状体瘤；另参见 tuber (2)

phak·o·ma·to·sis (fak″o-mə-to′sis) pl. phakomato′ses. Any of a group of congenital hereditary developmental anomalies having selective involvement of tissues of ectodermal origin, primarily the skin and central nervous system 斑痣性错构瘤病

pha·lan·ge·al (fə-lan′je-əl) pertaining to a phalanx 指（趾）骨的

phal·an·gec·to·my (fal″ən-jek′tə-me) excision of a phalanx 指（趾）骨切除术

phal·an·gi·tis (fal″ən-ji′tis) inflammation of one or more phalanges 指（趾）骨炎

pha·lanx (fa′lanks) pl. phalan′ges [Gr.] 1. any bone of a finger or toe; there are two for the thumb and great toe and three for each of the other fingers and toes 指骨，趾骨，见图 1；2. any one of a set of plates that are disposed in rows and make up the reticular membrane of the organ of Corti 指状板；**phalan′geal** adj.

phal·lec·to·my (fə-lek′tə-me) 同 penectomy

phal·li (fal′i) phallus 的复数

phal·lic (fal′ik) pertaining to or resembling a phallus 阴茎的

phal·li·tis (fə-li′tis) 同 penitis

phal·lo·plas·ty (fal′o-plas″te) plastic surgery of the penis 阴茎成形术

phal·lus (fal′əs) pl. phal′li. 1. 同 penis；2. a representation of the penis 代表阴茎；3. the primordium of the penis or clitoris that develops from the genital tubercle 阴茎或阴蒂的原基

phan·tasm (fan′taz-əm) an impression or image not evoked by actual stimuli, and usually recognized as false by the observer 幻象，幻觉

phan·tom (fan′tom) 1. 同 phantasm；2. a model of the body or a body part 人体模型；3. a device

for simulating the in vivo effect of radiation on tissues 体内放射模拟器，一种模拟体内辐射对组织影响的装置

phan·tos·mia (fant-oz′me-ə) a parosmia consisting of a sensation of smell in the absence of any external stimulus 嗅幻觉

phar pharm pharmaceutical 药的，制药的；药学的；pharmacopeia 药典；pharmacy 药学，药剂学，药房

phar·ma·ceu·tic (fahr″mə-soo′tik) 同 pharmaceu-tical (1)

phar·ma·ceu·ti·cal (fahr″mə-soo′tĭ-kəl) 1. pertaining to pharmacy or drugs 药的，制药的；药学的；2. a medicinal drug 药品，药剂

phar·ma·cist (fahr″mə-sist) one who is licensed to prepare and sell or dispense drugs and compounds, and to make up prescriptions 药剂师，调剂员；药商

pharmaco- word element [Gr.], drug; medicine [构词成分] 药，药学

phar·ma·co·an·gi·og·ra·phy (fahr″mə-koan″je-og′rə-fe) angiography in which visualization is enhanced by manipulating the flow of blood by the administration of vasodilating and vasoconstricting agents 药物性血管造影

phar·ma·co·dy·nam·ics (fahr″mə-ko-dinam′iks) the study of the biochemical and physiologic effects of drugs and the mechanisms of their actions, including the correlation of their actions and effects with their chemical structure 药物效应动力学，药效学；**pharmacodynam′ic** adj.

phar·ma·co·ge·net·ics (fahr″mə-ko-jə-net′-iks) the clinical study of inherited variation in the nature of responses to drugs, focusing on single genes. In practice, often used interchangeably with pharmacogenomics 药物遗传学

phar·ma·co·ge·no·mics (fahr″mə-ko-jə-no′-miks) the study of the inherited variations in many genes that dictate a drug response and the way these variations can be used to predict individual responses to drugs. In practice, often used interchangeably with pharmacogenetics 药物基因组学

phar·ma·cog·no·sy (fahr″mə-kog′nə-se) the branch of pharmacology dealing with natural drugs and their constituents 生药学

phar·ma·co·ki·net·ics (fahr″mə-ko-kĭ-net′-iks) the action of drugs in the body over a period of time, including the processes of absorption, distribution, localization in tissues, biotransformation, and excretion 药代动力学，药动学；**pharmacokinet′ic** adj.

phar·ma·co·log·ic (fahr″mə-kə-loj′ik) pertaining to pharmacology or to the properties and actions of drugs 药理学的

P

phar·ma·col·o·gist (fahr″mə-kol′ə-jist) a specialist in the study of the actions of drugs 药理学家

phar·ma·col·o·gy (fahr″mə-kol′ə-je) the science that deals with the origin, nature, chemistry, effects, and uses of drugs; it includes pharmacognosy, pharmacokinetics, pharmacodynamics, pharmacotherapeutics, and toxicology 药理学

phar·ma·co·pe·ia (fahr″mə-ko-pe′ə) an authoritative treatise on drugs and their preparations 药典，另参见 *USP*; **pharmacopei′al** *adj.*; **United States P.**, 美国药典，参见 *U* 下词条

phar·ma·co·ther·a·py (fahr″mə-ko-ther′ə-pe) treatment of disease with medicines 药物治疗，药物疗法

phar·ma·cy (fahr′mə-se) 1. the branch of the health sciences dealing with the preparation, dispensing, and proper utilization of drugs 药学，药剂学; 2. a place where drugs are compounded or dispensed 药房

Pharm D [L.] Pharma′ciae Doc′tor (Doctor of Pharmacy) 药学博士

phar·yn·gal·gia (far″in-gal′jə) 同 pharyngodynia

pha·ryn·ge·al (fə-rin′je-əl) pertaining to the pharynx 咽的

phar·yn·gec·to·my (far″in-jek′tə-me) excision of part of the pharynx 咽（部分）切除术

phar·yn·gis·mus (far″in-jiz′məs) muscular spasm of the pharynx 咽痉挛

phar·yn·gi·tis (far″in-ji′tis) sore throat; inflammation of the pharynx 咽炎; **pharyngit′ic** *adj.*

pha·ryn·go·cele (fə-ring′go-sēl) herniation or cystic deformity of the pharynx 咽突出

pha·ryn·go·dyn·ia (fə-ring″go-din′e-ə) pain in the pharynx 咽痛

pha·ryn·go·esoph·a·ge·al (fə-ring″go-ə- sof′ə-je″əl) pertaining to the pharynx and esophagus 咽食管的

pha·ryn·go·my·co·sis (fə-ring″go-mi-ko′sis) any fungal infection of the pharynx 咽真菌病

pha·ryn·go·pa·ral·y·sis (fə-ring″go-pə-ral′ ĭ- sis) paralysis of the pharyngeal muscles 咽麻痹

pha·ryn·go·ple·gia (fə-ring″go-ple′jə) pharyngoparalysis 咽麻痹

phar·yn·gos·co·py (far″ing-gos′kə-pe) direct visual examination of the pharynx 咽镜检查

pha·ryn·go·ste·no·sis (fə-ring″go-stə-no′sis) narrowing of the pharynx 咽狭窄

phar·yn·got·o·my (far″ing-got′ə-me) incision of the pharynx 咽切开术

phar·ynx (far′inks) the throat; the musculomembranous cavity behind the nasal cavities, mouth, and larynx, communicating with them and with the esophagus 咽

phase (fāz) 1. one of the aspects or stages through which a varying entity may pass 阶段; 期; 2. in physical chemistry, any physically or chemically distinct, homogeneous, and mechanically separable part of a system 相; **pha′sic** *adj.*; **erythrocytic p.**, that phase in the life cycle of a malarial plasmodium in which the parasites multiply in the red blood cells 红细胞内期（疟原虫）; **five p's**, in traditional Chinese medicine, a set of dynamic relations (designated earth, metal, water, wood, and fire) that can be used to categorize relationships among phenomena 五行，五相; **follicular p.**, the first part of the ovarian cycle, lasting from the end of the menstrual phase until ovulation and corresponding to the proliferative phase of the uterine cycle; it is characterized by the development of a dominant ovarian follicle 卵泡期增殖期; G_0 **p.**, a special subtype of the G_1 phase, in which cells carry out their normal physiologic functions but do not proliferate G_0 期, G_1 期的一种特殊亚型, 细胞执行正常的生理功能, 但不增殖; G_1 **p.**, the part of the cell cycle lasting from the end of cell division (the M phase) until the start of DNA synthesis (the S phase) G_1 期, 细胞周期的一部分, 从细胞分裂结束（M 期）到 DNA 合成开始（S 期）; G_2 **p.**, a relatively quiescent part of the cell cycle, lasting from the end of the S phase until the start of cell division, during which the accuracy of DNA replication is checked and faulty sections repaired G_2 期, 细胞周期中相对静止的部分, 从 S 期结束一直持续到细胞分裂开始, 在此期间检查 DNA 复制的准确性并修复有缺陷的部分; **luteal p.**, the phase of the ovarian cycle, lasting from ovulation to menstruation, during which the ovarian follicle transforms into the corpus luteum; it corresponds to the secretory phase in the uterus 黄体期; **M p.**, the part of the cell cycle during which mitosis occurs; subdivided into prophase, metaphase, anaphase, and telophase M 期, 有丝分裂期; **menstrual p.**, the phase of the human menstrual cycle, following the luteal phase and occurring only if fertilization has not taken place. The corpus luteum regresses and is shed through menstruation and growth begins for the ovarian follicle, leading to the follicular phase 月经期; **proliferative p.**, the phase of the uterine cycle, corresponding to the follicular phase of the ovarian cycle, during which the functional layer of the endometrium is repaired and proliferates following menstruation（子宫内膜）增生期; **S p.**, the part of the cell cycle between the G_1 and G_2 phases, during which DNA is synthesized and chromosomes are replicated S 期, 细胞周期在 G_1 和 G_2 阶段之间的一部分, 在此期间 DNA 被合成, 染色体被

复制；**secretory p.**, the phase of the uterine cycle, corresponding to the luteal phase of the ovarian cycle, characterized by thickening and increased vascularity of the endometrium 分泌期

phas·mid (faz′mid) 1. either of the two caudal chemoreceptors occurring in certain nematodes (Phasmidia) 尾感器；2. any nematode containing phasmids 尾感器线虫

phe·nac·e·tin (fə-nas′ə-tin) an analgesic and antipyretic, whose major metabolite is acetaminophen, now little used because of its toxicity 非那西丁，一种止痛药和退热药，其主要代谢产物为对乙酰氨基酚，由于其毒性，现在很少使用

phe·nan·threne (fə-nan′thrēn) a tricyclic aromatic hydrocarbon occurring in coal tar; toxic and carcinogenic 菲，一种存在于煤焦油中的三环芳香烃；具有毒性和致癌性

phen·ar·sa·zine chlor·ide (fen-ahr′sə-zēn) a toxic, irritant compound used as a war gas and, with tear gas, in riot control, as well as in some wood-preserving solutions 氯化吩砒嗪，一种有毒、刺激性的化合物，用作战争气体，与催泪瓦斯一起用于防暴，也用于一些木材保存溶液中

phen·a·zone (fen′ə-zōn) antipyrine 非那宗，安替比林

phen·a·zo·pyr·i·dine (fen″ə-zo-pir′ĭ-dēn) a urinary tract analgesic, used as the hydrochloride salt 苯偶氮吡啶，非那吡啶，其盐酸盐用作泌尿道镇痛药

phen·cy·cli·dine (PCP) (fen-si′klĭ-dēn) a potent veterinary analgesic and anesthetic, used as a drug of abuse in the form of the hydrochloride salt; its abuse by humans may lead to serious psychological disturbances 苯环己哌啶（兽医用镇痛药和麻醉药）

phen·di·met·ra·zine (fen″di-met′rə-zēn) a sympathomimetic amine used as an anorectic in the form of the tartrate salt 苯双甲吗啉，苯甲曲秦（食欲抑制药）

phen·el·zine (fen′əl-zēn) a monoamine oxidase inhibitor used as the sulfate salt as an antidepressant and in the prophylaxis of migraine 苯乙肼，单胺氧化酶抑制药，其硫酸盐用作抗抑郁药和治疗偏头痛

phe·nin·da·mine (fə-nin′də-mēn) an antihistamine with anticholinergic and sedative effects, used as the tartrate salt 苯茚胺（抗组胺药）

phen·ir·amine (fen-ir′ə-mēn) an antihistamine with anticholinergic and sedative effects, used as the maleate salt 非尼拉敏（抗组胺药）

phen·met·ra·zine (fen-met′rə-zēn) a central nervous system stimulant formerly used as an anorectic in the form of the hydrochloride salt 芬美曲秦，苯甲吗啉，中枢神经兴奋药，其盐酸盐曾作为食欲抑制药

phe·no·bar·bi·tal (fe″no-bahr′bĭ-təl) a longacting barbiturate, used as the base or sodium salt as a sedative, hypnotic, and anticonvulsant 苯巴比妥

phe·no·copy (fe′no-kop″e) 1. an environmentally induced phenotype mimicking one usually produced by a specific genotype 表型模拟，拟表型；2. an individual exhibiting such a phenotype 表型模拟者

phe·nol (fe′nol) 1. an extremely poisonous compound, C_6H_5OH, which is caustic and disinfectant; used as a pharmaceutical preservative and in dilution as an antimicrobial and topical anesthetic and antipruritic. Poisoning, due to ingestion or transdermal absorption, causes symptoms including colic, local irritation, corrosion, seizures, cardiac arrhythmias, shock, and respiratory arrest 苯酚，碳酸；2. any organic compound containing one or more hydroxyl groups attached to an aromatic carbon ring 酚

phe·no·late (fe′nə-lāt) 1. to treat with phenol for purposes of sterilization 用酚消毒；2. a salt formed by union of a base with phenol, in which a monovalent metal, such as sodium or potassium, replaces the hydrogen of the hydroxyl group 酚盐，一种碱与苯酚结合形成的盐，其中单价金属，如钠或钾，取代羟基的氢

phe·nol·phthal·ein (fe″nol-thal′ēn) a cathartic and pH indicator, with a range of 8.5 to 9.0 酚酞

phe·nom·e·non (fə-nom′ə-non) pl. *phenom′ena*. Any sign or objective symptom; an observable occurrence or fact 迹象，症状，现象；**booster p.**, on a tuberculin test, an initial false-negative result due to a diminished amnestic response, becoming positive on subsequent testing 复强现象，助强效应；**dawn p.**, the early-morning increase in plasma glucose concentration and thus insulin requirement in patients with type 1 diabetes mellitus 黎明现象；**Koebner p.**, a cutaneous response seen in certain dermatoses, manifested by the appearance on uninvolved skin of lesions typical of the skin disease at the site of trauma, on scars, or at points where articles of clothing produce pressure 同形反应，科布内现象；**Marcus Gunn pupillary p.**, with unilateral optic nerve or retinal disease, a difference between the pupillary reflexes of the two eyes; on the affected side there is abnormally slight contraction or even dilatation of the pupil when a light is shone in the eye Marcus Gunn 瞳孔现象；**no-reflow p.**, when cerebral blood flow is restored following prolonged global cerebral ischemia, there is initial hyperemia followed by a gradual decline in perfusion until there is almost no blood flow 无复流现象；**Somogyi p.**, a rebound phenomenon occurring in diabetes: overtreatment with insulin

抑制药

induces hypoglycemia, thus initiating hormone release; this stimulates lipolysis, gluconeogenesis, and glycogenolysis, which in turn cause rebound hyperglycemia and ketosis 索莫奇现象

phe·no·thi·a·zine (fe″no-thi′ə-zēn) any of a group of antipsychotic agents having a similar tricyclic structure and acting as potent alphaadrenergic and dopaminergic blocking agents, as well as having hypotensive, antispasmodic, antihistaminic, analgesic, sedative, and antiemetic activity 吩噻嗪

phe·no·type (fe′no-tīp) the observable characteristics of an individual, either in whole or with respect to a single or a few traits, as determined by a combination of the genotype and the environment 表型; **phenotyp′ic** *adj.*

phe·noxy·benz·amine (fə-nok″se-ben′zə- mēn) an irreversible α-adrenergic blocking agent; the hydrochloride salt is used to control hypertension in pheochromocytoma and to treat urinary symptoms in benign prostatic hyperplasia 苯氧苄胺, 酚苄明（α- 肾上腺素受体阻滞药）

phen·pro·pi·o·nate (fen-pro′pe-ə-nāt″) USAN contraction for 3-phenylpropionate 苯丙酸盐；苯丙酸酯（3-phenylpropionate 的 USAN 缩约词）

phen·ter·mine (fen′tər-mēn) a sympathomimetic amine related to amphetamine, used as an anorectic either as the hydrochloride salt or as the base complexed with an ion exchange resin 芬特明，苯丁胺

phen·yl (fen′əl) (fe′nəl) the monovalent radical C_6H_5, derived from benzene by removal of a hydrogen 苯基; **phenyl′ic** *adj.*

phen·yl·a·ce·tic ac·id (fen″əl-ə-se′tik) a catabolite of phenylalanine, excessively formed and excreted in the urine in phenylketonuria 苯乙酸

phen·yl·al·a·nine (Phe, F) (fen″əl-al′ə-nēn) an aromatic essential amino acid necessary for optimal growth in infants and for nitrogen equilibrium in human adults 苯丙氨酸

phen·yl·bu·ta·zone (fen″əl-bu′tə-zōn) a nonsteroidal antiinflammatory drug used in the short-term treatment of severe rheumatoid disorders unresponsive to less toxic agents 保泰松，布他酮，二苯丁唑酮

***p*-phen·yl·ene·di·amine** (par″ə-fen″əl-ēndi′ə- mēn) a derivative of benzene used as a dye for hair, garments, and textiles, as a photographic developing agent, and in a variety of other processes; it is a strong allergen, causing contact dermatitis and bronchial asthma 对苯二胺苯的一种衍生物，用作染发、服装和织品的染料，用作摄影的显影剂，本品为强变应原，可致接触性皮炎和支气管哮喘

phen·yl·eph·rine (fen″əl-ef′rin) an adrenergic

used as the hydrochloride salt for its potent vasoconstrictor properties 苯福林，去氧肾上腺素

phen·yl·ke·ton·uria (PKU, PKU1) (fen″əlke″- to-nu′re-ə) an autosomal recessive disorder due to deficiency of the enzyme necessary to convert phenylalanine into tyrosine so that phenylalanine and related compounds accumulate; characterized by severe intellectual disability, tumors, seizures, hypopigmentation of hair and skin, eczema, and mousy odor, all preventable by early restriction of dietary phenylalanine 苯丙酮尿症; **phenylketonu′ric** *adj.*

phen·yl·mer·cu·ric (fen″əl-mər-ku′rik) denoting a compound containing the radical C_6H_5Hg—, forming various antiseptic, antibacterial, and fungicidal salts; compounds of the acetate and nitrate salts are used as bacteriostatic pharmaceutical preservatives, and the former is used as a herbicide 苯汞基

phen·yl·pro·pa·nol·amine (fen″əl-pro″pə- nol′ə- mēn) an adrenergic, used in the form of the hydrochloride salt as nasal and sinus decongestant, as an appetite suppressant, and in the treatment of stress incontinence 去甲麻黄碱，苯丙醇胺

phen·yl·py·ru·vic ac·id (fen″əl-pi-roo′vik) an intermediary product produced when the normal pathway of phenylalanine catabolism is blocked, and excreted in the urine in phenylketonuria 苯丙酮酸

phen·yl·thio·urea (fen″əl-thi″o-u-re′ə) a compound used in genetics research; the ability to taste it is inherited as a dominant trait. It is intensely bitter to about 70 percent of the population and nearly tasteless to the rest 苯基硫脲，苯硫脲，一种用于遗传学研究的化合物，人们对这种化合物的味觉的显性性状是遗传的，约 70% 的人能尝出它的苦味，其余的人则尝不出

phen·yl·tol·ox·amine (fen″əl-tol-ok′sə-mēn) a sedating antihistamine, used as the citrate salt 苄苯醇胺，苯托沙敏（抗组胺药）

phen·y·to·in (fen′ĭ-toin) an anticonvulsant used in the control of various kinds of epilepsy and of seizures associated with neurosurgery 苯妥英，二苯乙内酰脲（抗惊厥药）

pheo·chrome (fe′o-krōm″) chromaffin 嗜铬的

pheo·chro·mo·blast (fe′o-kro′mo-blast) any of the embryonic structures that develop into chromaffin (pheochrome) cells 成嗜铬细胞

pheo·chro·mo·cyte (fe″o-kro′mo-sīt) chromaffin cell 嗜铬细胞

pheo·chro·mo·cy·to·ma (fe″o-kro″mo-si-to′mə) a tumor of chromaffin tissue of the adrenal medulla or prevertebral ganglia; symptoms, notably hypertension, reflect the increased secretion of epinephrine and norepinephrine 嗜铬细胞瘤

phe·re·sis (fə-re′sis) apheresis 除去法，提取法

pher·o·mone (fer′ə-mōn) a substance secreted to the outside of the body and perceived (as by smell) by other individuals of the same species, releasing specific behavior in the percipient 外激素，信息素

PhG Graduate in Pharmacy 药学毕业生

Phi·al·e·mo·ni·um (fi″əl-ə-mo′ne-əm) a genus of dematiaceous anamorphic fungi; *P. curva′tum* and *P. obova′tum* are opportunistic human pathogens 单胞瓶霉属，属于暗色变形真菌属

Phi·a·loph·o·ra (fi″ə-lof′ə-rə) a genus of dematiaceous anamorphic fungi; *P. verruco′sa* and other species cause chromoblastomycosis, eumycotic mycetoma, and phaeohyphomycosis 瓶霉菌属

phil·trum (fil′trəm) the vertical groove in the median portion of the upper lip 人中

phi·mo·sis (fi-mo′sis) constriction of the orifice of the prepuce so that it cannot be drawn back over the glans 包茎；**phimot′ic** adj.

phleb·an·gi·o·ma (fleb″an-je-o′mə) a venous aneurysm 静脉瘤

phleb·ar·te·ri·ec·ta·sia (fleb″ahr-tēr″e-ekta′zhə) general dilatation of veins and arteries 动静脉扩张

phleb·ec·ta·sia (fleb″ek-ta′zhə) a varicosity of a vein 静脉扩张

phle·bec·to·my (flə-bek′tə-me) excision of a vein, or a segment of a vein 静脉切除术

phleb·em·phrax·is (fleb″əm-frak′sis) stoppage of a vein by a plug or clot 静脉梗阻

phle·bi·tis (flə-bi′tis) inflammation of a vein 静脉炎；**phlebit′ic** adj.; **sinus p.,** inflammation of a cerebral sinus 静脉窦炎

phle·boc·ly·sis (flə-bok′lī-sis) injection of fluid into a vein 静脉输液法

phle·bog·ra·phy (flə-bog′rə-fe) 1. venography; angiography of a vein 静脉造影术；2. the graphic recording of the venous pulse 静脉搏动描记法

phlebo·li·thi·a·sis (fleb″o-lī-thi′ə-sis) the development of calculi in veins 静脉石病

phlebo·ma·nom·e·ter (fleb″o-mə-nom′ə-tər) an instrument for the direct measurement of venous blood pressure 静脉血压计

phlebo·phle·bos·to·my (fleb″o-flə-bos′tə-me) operative anastomosis of vein to vein 静脉 - 静脉吻合术

phlebo·rhe·og·ra·phy (fleb″o-re-og′rə-fe) a technique employing a plethysmograph with cuffs applied to the abdomen, thigh, calf, and foot, for measuring venous volume changes in response to respiration and to compression of the foot or calf 静脉血流摄术

phle·bor·rha·phy (flə-bor′ə-fe) suture of a vein

静脉缝术

phlebo·scle·ro·sis (fleb″o-sklə-ro′sis) fibrous thickening of the walls of veins 静脉硬化

phle·bos·ta·sis (flə-bos′tə-sis) 1. venous stasis 静脉淤滞法；2. temporary sequestration of a portion of blood from the general circulation by compressing the veins of a limb 静脉止血法

phlebo·throm·bo·sis (fleb″o-throm-bo′sis) the development of venous thrombi in the absence of associated inflammation 静脉血栓形成

Phle·bot·o·mus (flə-bot′ə-məs) a genus of biting sandflies, the females of which suck blood. They are vectors of various diseases, including cutaneous and visceral leishmaniasis, Carrión disease, and phlebotomus fever 白蛉属

phle·bot·o·my (flə-bot′ə-me) venotomy; incision of a vein 静脉切开术

Phle·bo·vi·rus (fleb′o-vi″rəs) the sandfly fever viruses, a genus of the family Bunyaviridae, including the virus that causes phlebotomus fever 白蛉热病毒属；白蛉热病毒

phlegm (flem) viscid mucus excreted in abnormally large quantities from the respiratory tract 痰，黏痰

phleg·ma·sia (fleg-ma′zhə) [Gr.] inflammation 炎（症），热；**p. al′ba do′lens,** phlebitis of the femoral vein with swelling of the leg, occasionally following parturition or an acute febrile illness 股白肿；**p. ceru′lea do′lens,** an acute fulminating form of deep venous thrombosis, with pronounced edema and severe cyanosis of the limb 股蓝肿

phleg·mon (fleg′mon) diffuse inflammation of the soft or connective tissue due to infection 蜂窝织炎；**phleg′monous** adj.

phlo·go·gen·ic (flo″go-jen′ik) producing inflammation 致炎的

phlo·rhi·zin hy·dro·lase (flo-ri′zin hi′dro-lās) glycosylceramidase 根皮苷水解酶

phlyc·te·na (flik-te′nə) pl. *phlycte′nae* [Gr.] 1. a small blister made by a burn 水疱（烧伤所致）；2. a small vesicle containing lymph seen on the conjunctiva in certain conditions 小（水）疱（内含淋巴，见于结膜）；**phlyc′tenar** adj.

phlyc·ten·u·lar (flik-ten′u-lər) associated with the formation of phlyctenules, or of vesiclelike prominences 小疱（形成）的

phlyc·ten·ule (flik′tən-ūl) a minute vesicle; an ulcerated nodule of cornea or conjunctiva 小（水）疱；角膜或结膜的溃烂小结

pho·bia (fo′be-ə) a persistent, irrational, intense fear of a specific object, activity, or situation (the phobic stimulus), fear that is recognized as being excessive or unreasonable by the individual himself.

When a phobia is a significant source of distress or interferes with social functioning, it is considered a mental disorder (sometimes called a *phobic disorder*); in DSM-Ⅳ phobias are classified with the anxiety disorders and are subclassified as agoraphobia, specific phobias, and social phobias 恐惧症，恐怖症；**pho′bic** *adj.*；**simple p.**, specific p. 单纯恐怖症；**social p.**, an anxiety disorder characterized by fear and avoidance of social or performance situations in which the individual fears possible embarrassment and humiliation 社交恐怖症；**specific p.**, persistent and excessive or unreasonable fear of a circumscribed, welldefined object or situation 特定恐怖症

pho·co·me·lia (fo″ko-me′le-ə) congenital absence of the proximal portion of a limb or limbs, the hands or feet being attached to the trunk by a small, irregularly shaped bone 海豹肢畸形，短肢畸形；**phocome′lic** *adj.*

pho·com·e·lus (fo-kom′ə-ləs) a person with phocomelia 海豹肢畸胎，短肢畸胎

phon·as·the·nia (fo″nəs-the′ne-ə) weakness of the voice; difficult phonation from fatigue 发声无力

phon·en·do·scope (fōn-en′do-skōp) a stethoscopic device that intensifies auscultatory sounds 扩音听诊器

pho·no·car·di·og·ra·phy (fo″no-kahr″de-og′rə-fe) the graphic representation of heart sounds or murmurs; by extension, the term also includes pulse tracings (carotid, apex, and jugular pulses) 心音描记法；**phonocardiograph′ic** *adj.*

pho·no·cath·e·ter (fo″no-kath′ə-tər) a device similar to a conventional catheter, with a microphone at the tip 检音导管

pho·nol·o·gy (fə-nol′ə-je) the science of vocal sounds 音系学；**phonolog′ical** *adj.*

pho·no·my·oc·lo·nus (fo″no-mi-ok′lə-nəs) myoclonus in which a sound is heard on auscultation of an affected muscle, indicating fibrillar contractions 有声肌阵挛

pho·no·my·og·ra·phy (fo″no-mi-og′rə-fe) the recording of sounds produced by muscle contraction 肌音描记法

pho·no·stetho·graph (fo″no-steth′o-graf) an instrument by which chest sounds are amplified, filtered, and recorded 听诊录音机

pho·no·sur·gery (fo′no-sur′jər-e) a group of surgical procedures whose purpose is to restore, maintain, or enhance the voice 嗓音外科学

phor·bol (for′bol) a polycyclic alcohol occurring in croton oil; it is the parent compound of the phorbol esters 佛波醇（使用于生化研究中）；**p. ester**, any of several esters of phorbol that are potent

cocarcinogens, activating a cellular protein kinase; used in research to enhance the induction of mutagenesis or tumors by carcinogens 佛波酯，大戟二萜醇酯

pho·ria (for′e-ə) heterophoria 隐斜，隐斜视

phor·op·ter (for-op′tər) an instrument for retinoscopic evaluation of vision, with lenses placed on dials in a unit that is positioned in front of the patient 综合屈光检查仪

phose (fōz) any subjective visual sensation, as of light or color 光幻视

phos·gene (fos′jēn) a suffocating and highly poisonous gas, carbonyl chloride, $COCl_2$, which causes rapidly fatal pulmonary edema or pneumonia on inhalation; used in the synthesis of organic compounds and formerly as a war gas 光气，碳酰氯

phos·pha·gen (fos′fə-jən) any of a group of high-energy compounds, including phosphocreatine, that act as reservoirs of phosphate bond energy, donating phosphoryl groups for ATP synthesis when supplies are low 磷酸肌酸，磷酸原

phos·pha·tase (fos′fə-tās) any of a group of enzymes that catalyze the hydrolytic cleavage of inorganic phosphate from esters 磷酸（酯）酶

phos·phate (fos′fāt) any salt or ester of phosphoric acid 磷酸盐；**phosphat′ic** *adj.*

phos·pha·te·mia (fos″fə-te′me-ə) an excess of phosphates in the blood 磷酸盐血，磷酸血症

phos·pha·ti·dic ac·id (fos″fə-ti′dik) any of a group of compounds formed by esterification of three hydroxyl groups of glycerol with two fatty acid groups and one phosphoric acid group; from it are derived the phosphoglycerides 磷脂酸

phos·pha·ti·dyl·cho·line (fos″fə-ti″dəl-ko′- lēn) a phospholipid comprising choline linked to phosphatidic acid; it is a major component of cell membranes and is localized preferentially in the outer surface of the plasma membrane 磷脂酰胆碱，卵磷脂

phos·pha·tu·ria (fos″fə-tu′re-ə) 1. excretion of phosphates in the urine 尿（内）磷酸盐过多；2. hyperphosphaturia 高磷酸盐尿

phos·phene (fos′fēn) a sensation of light due to a stimulus other than light rays, e.g., a mechanical stimulus 压眼闪光，光幻视

phos·pho·cre·a·tine (PC) (fos″fo-kre′ə-tin) the phosphagen of vertebrates, a creatine–phosphoric acid compound occurring in muscle, being an important storage form of high-energy phosphate, the energy source in muscle contraction 磷酸肌酸

phos·pho·di·es·ter·ase (fos″fo-di-es′tər-ās) any of a group of enzymes that catalyze the hydrolytic cleavage of an ester linkage in a phosphoric acid compound containing two such ester linkages 磷酸二酯酶

phos·pho·enol·py·ru·vate (fos″fo-e″nolpi′roo-vāt) a high-energy derivative of pyruvate occurring as an intermediate in the EmbdenMeyerhof pathway of glucose metabolism, in gluconeogenesis, and in the biosynthesis of some amino acids 磷酸烯醇丙酮酸

6-phos·pho·fruc·to·ki·nase (fos″fo-frook″toki′nās) an enzyme catalyzing the phosphorylation of fructose 6-phosphate, a site of regulation in the Embden-Meyerhof pathway of glucose metabolism; deficiency of the muscle isozyme causes glycogen storage disease, type Ⅶ 6- 磷酸果糖激酶

phos·pho·glyc·er·ate (fos″fo-glis′ər-āt) an anionic form of phosphoglyceric acid; *2-p.* and *3-p.* are interconvertible intermediates in the Embden-Meyerhof pathway of glucose metabolism 磷酸甘油酸

phos·pho·glyc·er·ide (fos″fo-glis′ər-īd) a class of phospholipids whose parent compound is phosphatidic acid; they consist of a glycerol backbone, two fatty acids, and a phosphorylated alcohol (e.g., choline, ethanolamine, serine, or inositol) and are major components of cell membranes 磷酸甘油酯

phos·pho·ino·si·tide (fos″fo-in-o′sī-tīd) any of a number of phosphorylated inositol-containing compounds that play roles in cell activation and calcium mobilization in response to hormones 磷酸肌醇

phos·pho·lip·ase (fos″fo-lip′ās) any of four enzymes (phospholipase A to D) that catalyze the hydrolysis of specific ester bonds in phospholipids 磷脂酶

phos·pho·lip·id (fos″fo-lip′id) any lipid that contains phosphorus, including those with a glycerol backbone (phosphoglycerides and plasmalogens) or a backbone of sphingosine or a related substance (sphingomyelins). They are the major lipids in cell membranes 磷脂

phos·pho·ne·cro·sis (fos″fo-nə-kro′sis) phosphorus necrosis 磷毒性颌骨坏死

phos·pho·pro·tein (fos″fo-pro′tēn) a conjugated protein in which phosphoric acid is esterified with a hydroxy amino acid 磷蛋白

phos·phor·ic ac·id (fos-for′ik) 1. orthophosphoric acid, the monomeric form H_3PO_4 正磷酸; 2. a general term encompassing the monomeric (orthophosphoric acid), dimeric (pyrophosphoric acid), and polymeric (metaphosphoric acid) forms of the acid. *Diluted p. a.* is used as a pharmaceutical solvent and a gastric acidifier 泛指单体（正磷酸）、二聚体（焦磷酸）和聚合（偏磷酸）形式的酸。稀磷酸用作药物制剂的溶剂和口服胃酸化药

phos·pho·rism (fos′fə-riz″əm) chronic phosphorus

poisoning 慢性磷中毒；参见 *phosphorus*

phos·pho·rol·y·sis (fos″fə-rol′ ī-sis) cleavage of a chemical bond with simultaneous addition of the elements of phosphoric acid to the residues 磷酸分解（作用）

phos·pho·rous ac·id (fos-for′əs) H_3PO_3; its salts are the phosphites 亚磷酸

phos·pho·rus (P) (fos′fə-rəs) a poisonous, highly inflammable, nonmetallic element; at. no. 15, at. wt. 30.974. It occurs in several allotropic forms, the two most common of which are *white* (or yellow) and *red p.* It is an essential trace element; it is a major component of the mineral phase of bone and occurs in all tissues, being involved in almost all metabolic processes. Ingestion or inhalation of free phosphorus causes toothache, phosphorus necrosis, anorexia, weakness, and anemia, and contact with white phosphorus causes severe burns 磷（化学元素）; **phosphor′ic, phos′phorous** *adj.*; **p. 32**, a radioisotope of phosphorus having a half-life of 14.28 days and emitting beta particles (1.71 MeV); therapeutic uses include treatment of polycythemia vera, chronic myelogenous leukemia, chronic lymphocytic leukemia, and certain ovarian and prostate carcinomas, palliation of metastatic skeletal disease, and treatment of intraperitoneal and intrapleural malignant effusions 磷[32]，磷的一种放射性同位素，半衰期为 14.28 天，可释放 β 粒子（1.71 MeV）；治疗用途包括治疗真性红细胞增多症、慢性粒细胞白血病、慢性淋巴细胞白血病、某些卵巢和前列腺癌、缓解转移性骨骼疾病、腹腔和胸腔恶性积液

phos·phor·y·lase (fos-for′ə-lās) 1. any of a group of enzymes that catalyze the phosphorolysis of glycosides, transferring the cleaved glycosyl group to inorganic phosphate. When not qualified with the substrate name, the term usually denotes *glycogen phosphorylase* (animals) or *starch phosphorylase* (plants). 2. any of a group of enzymes that catalyze the transfer of a phosphate group to an organic acceptor 磷酸化酶

phos·phor·y·lase ki·nase (fos-for′ə-lās ki′nās) phosphorylase *b* kinase; an enzyme that catalyzes the phosphorylation and activation of glycogen phosphorylase, a step in the cascade of reactions regulating glycogenolysis. Deficiency causes glycogen storage disease, type IX 磷酸化酶激酶

phos·phor·y·la·tion (fos-for″ə-la′shən) the metabolic process of introducing a phosphate group into an organic molecule 磷酸化（作用）; **oxidative p.**, the formation of high-energy phosphate bonds by phosphorylation of ADP to ATP coupled to the transfer of electrons from reduced coenzymes to molecular oxygen via the electron trans-

P

port chain; it occurs in the mitochondria 氧化磷酸化（作用）；**substrate-level p.**, the formation of high-energy phosphate bonds by phosphorylation of ADP to ATP (or GDP to GTP) coupled to cleavage of a high-energy metabolic intermediate 底物水平磷酸化（作用）

phos·pho·trans·fer·ase (fos″fo-trans′fər-ās) any of a subclass of enzymes that catalyze the transfer of a phosphate group 磷酸转移酶，转磷酸酶

pho·tal·gia (fo-tal′jə) pain, as in the eye, caused by light 光痛（如眼）

pho·tic (fo′tik) pertaining to light 光的，感光的

pho·to·abla·tion (fo″to-ab-la′shən) volatilization of tissue by ultraviolet radiation emitted by a laser 光切除术，光挥发（作用）

pho·to·ac·tive (fo″to-ak′tiv) reacting chemically to sunlight or ultraviolet radiation 光敏的

pho·to·ag·ing (fo″to-āj′ing) photodamage with premature aging of the skin 光照性皮肤老化

pho·to·al·ler·gen (fo″to-al′ər-jən) an agent that elicits an allergic response to light 光过敏原

pho·to·al·ler·gy (fo″to-al′ər-je) a delayed immunologic type of photosensitivity involving a chemical substance to which the individual has previously become sensitized, combined with radiant energy 光过敏，光变态反应；**photoaller′gic** adj.

pho·to·bi·ol·o·gy (fo″to-bi-ol′ə-je) the branch of biology dealing with the effect of light on organisms 光生物学；**photobiolog′ic, photobiolog′ical** adj.

pho·to·bi·ot·ic (fo″to-bi-ot′ik) living only in the light 需光生存的，感光生存的

pho·to·ca·tal·y·sis (fo″to-kə-tal′ ĭ-sis) promotion or stimulation of a chemical reaction by light 光催化（作用）；**photocatalyt′ic** adj.

pho·to·cat·a·lyst (fo″to-kat′ə-list) a substance, e.g., chlorophyll, that brings about a chemical reaction to light 光催化剂

pho·to·chem·is·try (fo″to-kem′is-tre) the branch of chemistry dealing with the chemical properties or effects of light rays or other radiation 光化学；**photochem′ical** adj.

pho·to·che·mother·a·py (fo″to-ke″mother′ə-pe) treatment by means of drugs (e.g., methoxsalen) that react to ultraviolet radiation or sunlight 光化学疗法

pho·to·co·ag·u·la·tion (fo″to-ko-ag″ula′shən) condensation of protein material by the controlled use of an intense beam of light (e.g., argon laser) used especially in the treatment of retinal detachment and destruction of abnormal retinal vessels or intraocular tumor masses 光凝固（术）

pho·to·dam·age (fo′to-dam″əj) damage to the skin from prolonged exposure to ultraviolet radiation 光损害

pho·to·der·ma·ti·tis (fo″to-dur″mə-ti′tis) 1. phototoxic dermatitis 光毒性皮炎；2. any of the types of dermatitis caused by exposure to ultraviolet radiation, such as that in sunlight 光照性皮炎

pho·to·dy·nam·ic (fo″to-di-nam′ik) powerful in the light; used particularly for the action exerted by fluorescent substances in the light 光动力（作用）的

pho·to·flu·o·rog·ra·phy (fo″to-floor-og′rə-fe) the photographic recording of fluoroscopic images on small films, using a fast lens 荧光屏图像摄影

pho·to·gen·ic (fo″to-jen′ik) 1. produced by light, as photogenic epilepsy 光所致的，光源性的；2. producing or emitting light 发光的

pho·to·lu·mi·nes·cence (fo″to-loo″mĭ-nes′əns) the quality of being luminescent after exposure to light or other electromagnetic radiation 光致发光

pho·tol·y·sis (fo-tol′ĭ-sis) chemical decomposition or cleavage of a bond by the action of light or other radiant energy 光解（作用）；**photolyt′ic** adj.

pho·to·med·i·cine (fo″to-med′ĭ-sin) the medical specialty dealing with interactions between light and living systems, such as therapeutic uses such as phototherapy and pathologic effects such as photodermatitis 光医学

pho·tom·e·try (fo-tom′ə-tre) measurement of the intensity of light 光度测量，光度学

pho·to·mi·cro·graph (fo″to-mi′kro-graf) a photograph of an object as seen through an ordinary light microscope 显微照片

pho·ton (fo′ton) a particle (quantum) of radiant energy 光子，光量子

pho·to·par·ox·ys·mal (fo″to-par″ok-siz′məl) photoconvulsive; denoting an abnormal electroencephalographic response to photic stimulation (brief flashes of light), marked by diffuse paroxysmal discharge recorded as spike-wave complexes; the response may be accompanied by minor seizures 光致发作的

pho·to·pe·ri·od (fo′to-pēr″e-əd) the period of time per day that an organism is exposed to daylight (or to artificial light) 光周期；**photoperiod′ic** adj.

pho·to·pe·ri·od·ism (fo″to-pēr′e-əd-iz-əm) the physiologic and behavioral reactions brought about in organisms by changes in the duration of daylight and darkness 光周期现象，光周期性

pho·to·phe·re·sis (fo″to-fə-re′sis) a technique for treating cutaneous T-cell lymphoma, in which a photoactive chemical is administered, the blood is removed and circulated through a source of ultraviolet radiation, then returned to the patient; it is believed to stimulate the immune system 光免疫化学疗法，光敏治疗

pho·to·phil·ic (fo″to-fil′ik) thriving in light 嗜光的

pho·to·pho·bia (fo″to-fo′be-ə) abnormal visual intolerance to light 畏光; **photopho′bic** adj.

pho·toph·thal·mia (fo″tof-thal′me-ə) ophthalmia due to exposure to intense light, as in snow blindness 光照性眼炎

pho·to·pia (fo-to′pe-ə) day vision 光适应; **photop′ic** adj.

pho·to·pig·ment (fo″to-pig′mənt) a pigment that is unstable in the presence of light 感光色素

pho·top·sia (fo-top′se-ə) appearance as of sparks or flashes in retinal irritation 闪光感

pho·top·sin (fo-top′sin) the opsin of the cones of the retina that combines with retinal to form photochemical pigments 光视蛋白

pho·top·tar·mo·sis (fo″to-tahr-mo′sis) sneezing caused by the influence of light 感光喷嚏

pho·top·tom·e·ter (fo″top-tom′ə-tər) an instrument for measuring visual acuity by determining the smallest amount of light that will render an object just visible 光觉计

pho·to·re·ac·ti·va·tion (fo″to-re-ak″tĭ-va′-shən) reversal of the biologic effects of ultraviolet radiation on cells by subsequent exposure to visible light 光致复活（作用）

pho·to·re·cep·tor (fo″to-re-sep′tər) a nerve end-organ or receptor sensitive to light 光受体

pho·to·re·frac·tive (fo″to-re-frak′tiv) pertaining to the refraction of light 光折变的

pho·to·ret·i·ni·tis (fo″to-ret″ĭ-ni′tis) retinitis due to exposure to intense light 光照性视网膜炎

Pho·to·rhab·dus (fo″to-rab′dəs) a genus of gram-negative, non–spore-forming, luminescent, motile, rod-shaped bacteria; organisms occur as symbionts of nematodes and as parasites of insects and are opportunistic pathogens for humans 发光杆菌属

pho·to·scan (fo′to-skan) a two-dimensional representation of gamma rays emitted by a radioactive isotope in body tissue, produced by a printout mechanism utilizing a light source to expose a photographic film 光扫描图

pho·to·sen·si·tiv·i·ty (fo″to-sen″sĭ-tiv′ĭ-te) 1. ability of a cell, organ, or organism to react to light 感光性，光感性; 2. an abnormal response of the skin or eyes to sunlight 光过敏; **photosen′sitive** adj.

pho·to·sen·si·ti·za·tion (fo″to-sen″sĭ-tĭ-za′-shən) development of abnormally increased reactivity of the skin or eyes to sunlight 光敏化（作用）

pho·to·sta·ble (fo′to-sta′bəl) unchanged by the influence of light 不感光的，耐光的

pho·to·syn·the·sis (fo″to-sin′thə-sis) a chemical combination caused by the action of light; specifically, the formation of carbohydrates from carbon dioxide and water in the chlorophyll tissue of plants under the influence of light 光合作用; **photosynthet′ic** adj.

pho·to·tax·is (fo″to-tak′sis) the movement of cells and microorganisms in response to light 趋光性，指细胞和微生物在光影响下的活动; **phototac′tic** adj.

pho·to·ther·a·py (fo″to-ther′ə-pe) 1. treatment of disease by exposure to light 光疗法，光疗; 2. photodynamic therapy 光动力（学）疗法

pho·to·tox·ic (fo′to-tok″sik) pertaining to, characterized by, or producing phototoxicity 光毒性的，光线损害的

pho·to·tox·ic·i·ty (fo″to-tok-sis′ĭ-te) a type of photosensitivity that is induced by a toxic substance, as opposed to a photoallergy 光毒性; **phototox′ic** adj.

pho·to·tro·phic (fo″to-tro′fik) capable of deriving energy from light 光营养的

pho·tot·ro·pism (fo-tot′rə-piz-əm) 1. the tendency of an organism to turn or move toward or away from light 向光性; 2. color change produced in a substance by the action of light 光色互变（现象）; **phototrop′ic** adj.

phren·ic (fren′ik) 1. diaphragmatic 膈的; 2. mental (1) 精神上的

phren·i·co·col·ic (fren″ĭ-ko-kol′ik) pertaining to or connecting the respiratory diaphragm and colon 膈结肠的

phre·ni·tis (frə-ni′tis) diaphragmitis; inflammation of the respiratory diaphragm 膈炎

phreno·gas·tric (fren″o-gas′trik) pertaining to the respiratory diaphragm and stomach 膈胃的

phreno·he·pat·ic (fren″o-hə-pat′ik) pertaining to the respiratory diaphragm and liver 膈肝的

phreno·ple·gia (fren″o-ple′jə) paralysis of the respiratory diaphragm 膈瘫痪

phren·o·tro·pic (fren″o-tro′pik) exerting its principal effect upon the mind 作用于精神的，向精神的

phryno·der·ma (frin″o-dur′mə) a follicular hyperkeratosis probably due to deficiency of vitamin A or of essential fatty acids 蟾皮病

phthal·ein (thal′ēn) any one of a series of coloring matters formed by the condensation of phthalic anhydride with the phenols 酞

phthir·i·a·sis (thir-i′ə-sis) pediculosis pubis 虱病

Phthir·us (thir′əs) a genus of lice. P. *pu′bis* is the pubic, or crab, louse, which infests the hair of the hypogastric region and sometimes the eyebrows and eyelashes 阴虱属

phthi·sis (thi′sis) (ti′sis) a wasting of the body 肺结核

phy·co·my·co·sis (fi″ko-mi-ko′sis) zygomycosis 藻菌病

phy·log·e·ny (fi-loj′ə-ne) the complete developmental history of a group of organisms 系统发育，系统发生，种系发生；**phylogenet′ic, phylogen′ic** *adj.*

phy·lum (fi′ləm) pl. *phy′la* [L.] a primary division of a kingdom, composed of a group of related classes; in the taxonomy of plants and fungi, the term *division* is used instead. Mycologists sometimes use the word to denote any important group of organisms（生物分类学的）门

phy·ma (fi′mə) pl. *phy′mata* [Gr.] a skin swelling or tumor larger than a tubercle（皮肤）肿块，（皮肤）结块，肿瘤

phys·iat·rics (fiz″e-at′riks) 同 physiatry

phys·iat·rist (fiz″e-at′rist) a physician who specializes in physiatry 理疗医师，理疗学家

phys·iat·ry (fiz″e-at′re) the branch of medicine that deals with the prevention, diagnosis, and treatment of disease or injury, and the rehabilitation from resultant impairments and disabilities, using physical and sometimes pharmaceutical agents 理疗学

phys·i·cal (fiz′ĭ-kəl) pertaining to the body, to material things, or to physics 物理的；身体的；物质的

phy·si·cian (fĭ-zish′ən) 1. an authorized practitioner of medicine, as one graduated from a college of medicine or osteopathy and licensed by the appropriate board 医师；另参见 *doctor*；2. one who practices medicine as distinct from surgery 内科医师；**p. assistant (PA),** one who has been trained in an accredited program and certified by an appropriate board to perform certain of a physician's duties, including history taking, physical examination, diagnostic tests, treatment, and certain minor surgical procedures, all under the responsible supervision of a licensed physician 助理医师；**attending p.,** 主治医师 1. a physician who has admitting privileges at a hospital 在医院有办理住院特权的医生；2. the physician with primary responsibility for the care of a patient in a particular case 在特定病例中，对患者负有主要责任的医生；**emergency p.,** a specialist in emergency medicine 急诊医师；**family p.,** a medical specialist who plans and provides the comprehensive primary health care of all members of a family, regardless of age or sex, on a continuous basis 家庭医师；**resident p.,** a graduate and licensed physician receiving training in a specialty, usually in a hospital 住院

医师

phys·i·co·chem·i·cal (fiz″ĭ-ko-kem′ ĭ-kəl) pertaining to both physics and chemistry 物理化学的

phys·ics (fiz′iks) the study of the laws and phenomena of nature, especially of forces and general properties of matter and energy 物理学

phys·io·chem·i·cal (fiz″e-o-kem′ ĭ-kəl) pertaining to both physiology and chemistry 生理化学的

phys·i·og·no·my (fiz″e-og′nə-me) 1. determination of mental or moral character and qualities by the face 面相法；2. the countenance, or face 面部表情，面容；3. the facial expression and appearance as a means of diagnosis 面容诊断

phys·i·o·log·ic (fiz″e-o-loj′ik) 同 physiological

phys·i·o·log·i·cal (fiz″e-o-loj′ĭ-kəl) pertaining to physiology; normal; not pathologic 生理的，生理学的

phys·i·ol·o·gist (fiz″e-ol′ə-jist) a specialist in physiology 生理学家

phys·i·ol·o·gy (fiz″e-ol′ə-je) 1. the science of the functions of the living organism and its parts, and of the physical and chemical factors and processes involved 生理学；2. the basic processes underlying the functioning of a species or class of organism, or any of its parts or processes 生理功能；**morbid p., pathologic p.,** the study of disordered function or of function in diseased tissues 病理生理学

phys·io·patho·log·ic (fiz″e-o-path″ə-loj′ik) pertaining to pathologic physiology 病理生理的

phys·io·ther·a·pist (fiz″e-o-ther′ə-pist) physical therapist 物理治疗师，理疗师

phys·io·ther·a·py (fiz″e-o-ther′ə-pe) physical therapy 物理疗法，理疗

phy·sique (fĭ-zēk′) the body organization, development, and structure 体格，体形

phy·so·hem·a·to·me·tra (fi″so-he″mə-tome′trə) gas and blood in the uterine cavity 子宫积血气

phy·so·hy·dro·me·tra (fi″so-hi″dro-me′trə) gas and serum in the uterine cavity 子宫积水气

phy·so·me·tra (fi″so-me′trə) gas in the uterine cavity 子宫积气

phy·so·stig·mine (fi″zo-stig′mēn) a cholinergic alkaloid usually obtained from the dried ripe seed of *Physostigma venenosum* (Calabar bean), used as a topical miotic and to reverse the central nervous system effects of an overdosage of anticholinergic drugs; used in the form of the salicylate and sulfate salts 毒扁豆碱

phy·tan·ic ac·id (fi-tan′ik) a 20-carbon branched-chain fatty acid occurring at high levels in dairy products and the fat of ruminants and accumulated in the tissues in Refsum disease 植烷酸

phy·tic ac·id (fi′tik) the hexaphosphoric acid ester

of inositol, found in many plants and microorganisms and in animal tissues 植酸，肌醇六磷酸

phy·to·be·zoar (fi″to-be′zor) a bezoar composed of vegetable fibers 植物石

phy·to·es·tro·gen (fi″to-es′tro-jən) any of a roup of weakly estrogenic, nonsteroidal compounds widely occurring in plants 植物雌激素

phy·to·he·mag·glu·ti·nin (fi″to-he″mə-gloo′tĭ-nin) a hemagglutinin of plant origin 植物血凝素，植物凝集素

phy·to·med·i·cine (fi″to-med′ĭ-sin) 1. a preparation of a medicinal herb 植物药；2. herbalism 本草学

phy·to·na·di·one (fi-to″nə-di′ōn) vitamin K₁: a vitamin found in green plants or prepared synthetically, used as a prothrombinogenic agent 植物甲萘醌，维生素 K₁（止血药）

phy·to·par·a·site (fi″to-par′ə-sīt) any parasitic plant organism or species 寄生植物

phy·to·path·o·gen·ic (fi″to-path″o-jen′ik) producing disease in plants 致植物病的

phy·to·pa·thol·o·gy (fi″to-pə-thol′ə-je) the pathology of plants 植物病理学

phy·to·pho·to·der·ma·ti·tis (fi″to-fo″to-dur″mə-ti′tis) phototoxic dermatitis induced by exposure to certain plants and then to sunlight 植物光皮炎，植物日光性皮炎

phy·to·pre·cip·i·tin (fi″to-pre-sip′ĭ-tin) a precipitin formed in response to vegetable antigen 植物沉淀素

phy·to·sis (fi-to′sis) any disease caused by a phytoparasite 植物病，植物原病，植物寄生病

phy·to·ther·a·py (fi″to-ther′ə-pe) treatment by use of plants 植物（药）疗法

phy·to·tox·ic (fi′to-tok″sik) 1. pertaining to phytotoxin 植物毒性的；2. poisonous to plants 对植物有毒的

phy·to·tox·in (fi′to-tok″sin) an exotoxin produced by certain species of higher plants; any toxin of plant origin 植物毒素

pia-ar·ach·ni·tis (pi″ə-ar″ak-ni′tis) leptomeningitis 软脑膜炎，软膜蛛网膜炎

pia-arach·noid (pi″ə-ə-rak′noid) the pia mater and arachnoid considered together as one functional unit; the leptomeninges 软膜蛛网膜，柔脑膜

pia-glia (pi″ə-gli′ə) a membrane constituting one of the layers of the pia-arachnoid 软膜神经胶（质）层

pi·al (pi′əl) (pe′əl) pertaining to the pia mater 软膜的

pia ma·ter (pi′ə ma′tər) (pe′ə mah′tər) [L.] the innermost of the three meninges covering the brain and spinal cord 软膜

pi·arach·noid (pi″ə-rak′noid) 同 pia-arachnoid

pi·ca (pi′kə) [L.] compulsive eating of nonnutritive substances, such as ice, dirt, flaking paint, clay, hair, or laundry starch 异食癖

pi·co·gram (pg) (pi′ko-gram) one-trillionth (10⁻¹²) of a gram 皮克，微微克（10⁻¹²g）

Pi·cor·na·vi·ri·dae (pi-kor″nə-vir′ĭ-de) a family of extremely small RNA viruses; genera that infect humans include *Aphthovirus, Cardiovirus, Enterovirus, Hepatovirus, Parechovirus,* and *Rhinovirus* 微小 RNA 病毒科

pi·cor·na·vi·rus (pi-kor′nə-vi″rəs) any virus of the family Picornaviridae 小 RNA 病毒

pic·rate (pik′rāt) any salt of picric acid 苦味酸盐

pic·ric ac·id (pik′rik) trinitrophenol 苦味酸，三硝基酚

pic·ro·car·mine (pik″ro-kahr′min) a histologic stain consisting of a mixture of carmine, ammonia, distilled water, and aqueous solution of picric acid 苦味酸卡红，苦胭脂红

PID pelvic inflammatory disease 盆腔炎症性疾病

pie·bald·ism (pi′bawld-iz-əm) a congenital, autosomal dominant pigmentary disorder characterized by patchy areas of lightened or white skin lacking melanocytes, usually associated with a white forelock 斑驳病

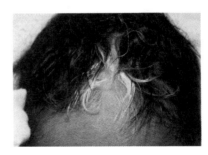

▲ 色素沉着不足的表皮斑块和斑驳病的白色额发

pie·dra (pya′drə) a fungal disease of the hair in which fungi form white *(white p.)* or black *(black p.)* nodules on the hair shafts 毛结节菌病

Pi·e·draia (pi″ə-dri′ə) a genus of keratolytic, dematiaceous, filamentous fungi found in soil, particularly in tropical areas; *P. hor′tae* causes black piedra 毛结节菌属

pi·es·es·the·sia (pi-e″zes-the′zhə) the sense by which pressure stimuli are felt 压觉

pi·esim·e·ter (pi″ə-sim′ə-tər) instrument for testing the sensitiveness of the skin to pressure 压力计（测皮肤对压力的敏感度）

PIGF phosphatidylinositol-glycan biosynthesis class F protein 磷脂酰肌醇聚糖生物合成 F 类蛋白

pig·ment (pig′mənt) 1. any coloring matter of the body 色素；2. a stain or dye 颜料；**pig′mentary** *adj.*；**bile p.**, any of the coloring matters of the bile, including bilirubin, biliverdin, etc. 胆色素；**blood p.,hematogenous p.**, any of the pigments derived from hemoglobin 血色素；**respiratory p′s**, substances, e.g., hemoglobin, myoglobin, or cytochromes, which take part in the oxidative processes of the animal body 呼吸色素；**retinal p′s, visual p′s**, the photopigments in retinal rods and cones that respond to certain colors of light and initiate the process of vision 视网膜色素

pig·men·ta·tion (pig″mən-ta′shən) the deposition of coloring matter; the coloration or discoloration of a part by a pigment 色素沉着，着色

pig·ment·ed (pig′mən-təd) colored by deposit of pigment 色素沉着的，着色的

PIGO phosphatidylinositol glycan anchor biosynthesis class O 磷脂酰肌醇聚糖锚生物合成 O 类蛋白

pi·lar (pi′lər) pertaining to the hair 毛发的

pile (pīl) 1. hemorrhoid 痔；2. an aggregation of similar elements for generating electricity 痔；**sentinel p.**, a hemorrhoid-like thickening of the mucous membrane at the lower end of an anal fissure 前哨痔

pi·li (pi′li) [L.] *pilus* 的属格和复数

pi·lif·er·ous (pi-lif′ər-əs) bearing or producing hair 有毛的

pill (pil) tablet 丸剂

pil·lar (pil′ər) a supporting column, usually occurring in pairs 柱；**articular p′s**, columnlike structures formed by the articulation of the superior and inferior articular processes of the vertebrae 关节柱；**p′s of fauces**, the palatoglossal arch and palatopharyngeal arch considered together 腭弓

pi·lo·car·pine (pi″lo-kahr′pēn) a cholinergic alkaloid, used as the base or the hydrochloride or nitrate salt as an antiglaucoma agent and miotic and, as the hydrochloride salt in the treatment of xerostomia associated with radiotherapy or Sjögren syndrome 毛果芸香碱

pi·lo·cys·tic (pi″lo-sis′tik) hollow or cystlike, and containing hair; said of dermoid cysts 囊样含毛的（指某些皮样瘤）

pi·lo·erec·tion (pi″lo-e-rek′shən) horripilation 竖毛

pi·lo·leio·myo·ma (pi″lo-li″o-mi-o′mə) a cutaneous leiomyoma that arises from the arrectores pilo-

rum muscles 毛平滑肌瘤

pi·lo·ma·tri·co·ma (pi″lo-ma″trī-ko′mə) a solitary, benign, calcifying adnexal tumor of hair follicle origin, appearing as a circumscribed, firm, intracutaneous nodule, usually on the face or upper body 毛母质瘤

pi·lo·ma·trix·o·ma (pi″lo-ma″trik-so′mə) 同 pilomatricoma

pi·lo·mo·tor (pi″lo-mo′tər) pertaining to the arrector pili muscles and horripilation 毛发运动的（指竖毛）

pi·lo·ni·dal (pi″lo-ni′dəl) having a nidus of hairs 藏毛的

pi·lo·se·ba·ceous (pi″lo-sə-ba′shəs) pertaining to the hair follicles and the sebaceous glands 毛囊皮脂腺的

pi·lus (pi′ləs) pl. *pi′li* [L.] 1. a hair 毛；2. one of the minute filamentous appendages of certain bacteria, associated with antigenic properties and sex functions of the cell（细胞、微生物等表面的）毛，纤毛，菌毛；**pi′lial, pi′liate** *adj.*；**pi′li incarna′ti**, a condition characterized by ingrown hairs 内嵌毛；**pi′li tor′ti**, a condition characterized by twisted hairs 卷毛

pim·e·cro·li·mus (pim″ə-kro-li′məs) a calcineurin inhibitor immunosuppressant produced by a variant of *Streptomyces hygroscopicus;* applied topically to treat moderate to severe atopic dermatitis 吡美莫司

pim·e·lop·ter·yg·i·um (pim″ə-lo-tər-ij′e-əm) a fatty outgrowth on the conjunctiva 脂肪性翼状胬肉

pi·mo·zide (pi′mə-zīd) an antipsychotic and antidyskinetic agent used in the treatment of Gilles de la Tourette syndrome 哌迷清

pim·ple (pim′pəl) a papule or pustule 丘疹小脓疱

pin (pin) a slender, elongated piece of metal used for securing fixation of parts 针；**Steinmann p.**, a metal rod for the internal fixation of fractures 施氏针，骨圆针

pin·do·lol (pin′də-lol) a nonselective betaadrenergic blocking agent with intrinsic sympathomimetic activity; used in the treatment of hypertension 吲哚洛尔

pin·e·al (pin′e-əl) 1. pertaining to the pineal body 松果体的；2. shaped like a pine cone 松果状的

pin·e·al·ec·to·my (pin″e-əl-ek′tə-me) excision of the pineal body 松果体切除术

pin·e·al·ism (pin′e-əl-iz″əm) the condition due to deranged secretion of the pineal body 松果体功能障碍

pin·e·a·lo·blas·to·ma (pin″e-ə-lo-blas-to′mə) pinealoma in which the pineal cells are not well differentiated 成松果体细胞瘤

pin·e·a·lo·cyte (pin′e-ə-lo-sīt″) an epithelioid cell of the pineal body 松果体细胞

pin·e·a·lo·ma (pin″e-ə-lo′mə) a tumor of the pineal body composed of neoplastic nests of large epithelial cells; it may cause hydrocephalus, precocious puberty, and gait disturbances 松果体瘤

pin·gue·cu·la (ping-gwek′u-lah) pl. *pingue′- culae* [L.] a benign yellowish spot on the bulbar conjunctiva 结膜黄斑

pin·i·form (pin′ī-form) conical or cone shaped 圆锥形的

pink·eye (pink′i) acute contagious conjunctivitis 红眼（急性触染性结膜炎）

pin·na (pin′ə) auricle (1) 耳廓; **pin′nal** *adj.*

pino·cyte (pin′o-) (pi′no-sīt) a cell that exhibits pinocytosis 胞饮细胞; **pinocyt′ic** *adj.*

pino·cy·to·sis (pin″o-) (pi′no-si-to′sis) the cellular uptake of extracellular fluid and its contents by the formation of invaginations by the cell membrane, which pinch off to form fluidfilled vesicles in the cytoplasm 胞饮作用; **pinocytot′ic** *adj.*

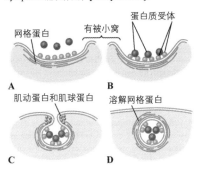

▲ 胞外蛋白胞饮作用机制

pino·some (pin′o-) (pi′no-sōm) the intracellular vacuole formed by pinocytosis 胞饮体，吞饮体

pint (pīnt) a unit of liquid measure; in the United States it is 16 fluid ounces (0.473 liter). In Great Britain, it is the *imperial pint,* equal to 20 fluid ounces (0.568 liter) 品脱（归糖量单位）

pin·ta (pēn′tah) a treponemal infection of tropical America, characterized by bizarre pigmentary changes in the skin 品他病

pin·worm (pin′wurm″) oxyurid 蛲虫

pi·o·glit·a·zone (pi″o-glit′ə-zōn) an antidiabetic agent that decreases insulin resistance in the peripheral tissues and liver; used as the hydrochloride salt in the treatment of type 2 diabetes mellitus 吡格列酮（降糖药）

pip·ecol·ic **ac·id** (pip″ə-kol′ik) a cyclic amino acid occurring as an intermediate in a minor pathway of lysine degradation and at elevated levels in the blood in cerebrohepatorenal syndrome and in hyperlysinemia 哌可酸

pip·e·cu·ro·ni·um (pip″ə-ku-ro′ne-əm) a nondepolarizing neuromuscular blocking agent used as the bromide salt as an adjunct to anesthesia, inducing skeletal muscle relaxation 哌库溴铵（非神经肌肉松弛药）

pi·per·a·cil·lin (pi-per′ə-sil″in) a semisynthetic broad-spectrum penicillin effective against a wide variety of gram-positive and gram-negative bacteria; used as the sodium salt 哌拉西林

pi·per·a·zine (pi-per′ə-zēn) an anthelmintic used against *Ascaris lumbricoides* and *Enterobius vermicularis;* used as the citrate salt 哌嗪（抗蛔虫药）

pi·pette (pi-pet′) [Fr.] 1. a glass or transparent plastic tube used in measuring or transferring small quantities of liquid or gas. Spelled also *pipet* 吸管; 2. to dispense by means of a pipette 用移液管吸移

pir·bu·ter·ol (pir-bu′tər-ol) a β_2-adrenergic receptor agonist, used in the form of the acetate ester as a bronchodilator 吡丁醇（支气管扩张药）

pir·i·form (pir′ī-form) pear-shaped 梨状的，梨形的

Pir·mel·la (pur″meh′luh) 1. trademark for a combination preparation of norethindrone and ethinyl estradiol 炔诺酮和炔雌醇联合制剂的商品名; 2. trademark for a combination preparation of progestin and estrogen 孕激素和雌激素联合制剂的商品名

Pi·ro·plas·ma (pi″ro-plaz′mə) *Babesia* 梨浆虫属（现名巴贝虫属 Babesia）

pi·ro·plas·mo·sis (pi″ro-plaz-mo′sis) babesiasis 梨浆虫病

pir·ox·i·cam (pir-ok′sī-kam) a nonsteroidal anti-inflammatory drug used in the treatment of various rheumatic disorders and dysmenorrhea 吡罗昔康，吡氧噻嗪，炎痛喜康（非甾体抗炎药）

pi·si·form (pi′sī-form) (piz′ ī-form) resembling a pea in shape and size 豌豆状的

PIT plasma iron turnover 血浆铁周转率

pit (pit) 1. a fovea or indentation, either normal or abnormal 窝，凹; 2. pockmark 痘凹; 3. to indent, or to become and remain for a few minutes indented, by pressure 使成凹; **anal p.,** proctodeum 肛道，肛窝; **auditory p.,** a depression on the auditory placode, marking the beginning of embryonic development of the internal ear 听窝; **coated p's,** small proteincoated pits in the plasma membrane of many cells, involved in receptor-mediated endocytosis 有被小窝；**ear p.**, 同 preauricular p.；**lens p.**, a pitlike depression in the ectoderm of the lens placode where the primordial lens is developing 晶状体窝；**olfactory p.**, the primordium of a nasal cavity 鼻窝；**otic p.**, 同 auditory p.；**preauricular p.**, a small depression anterior to the helix of the ear, sometimes leading to a fistula or congenital preauricular cyst 耳前凹；**p. of stomach**, epigastrium 胃窝

pitch (pich) 1. a dark viscous residue from distillation of tar and other substances 沥青；2. any of various bituminous substances such as natural asphalt 人造沥青；3. a resin from the sap of some coniferous trees（针叶树的）树脂，松脂；4. the quality of sound dependent principally on its frequency 音调，音高

pith·e·coid (pith′ə-koid) apelike 猿样的

pit·ta (pit′ə) [Sanskrit] in ayurveda, one of the three doshas, condensed from the elements fire and water. It is the principle of transformation energy and governs heat and metabolism in the body, is concerned with the digestive, enzymatic, and endocrine systems, and is eliminated from the body through sweat 在阿育吠陀中，三种 doshas 的一种，由火和水元素浓缩而成。它是转换能量的原理，控制着体内的热量和新陈代谢，与消化、酶和内分泌系统有关，通过汗液排出体外

pit·ting (pit′ing) 1. the formation, usually by scarring, of a small depression 凹陷；2. the removal from erythrocytes, by the spleen, of such structures as iron granules, without destruction of the cells 脾从红细胞中清除铁颗粒等结构而不破坏细胞；3. remaining indented for a few minutes after removal of firm finger pressure, distinguishing fluid edema from myxedema 指凹性水肿

pi·tu·i·cyte (pĭ-too′ĭ-sīt) the distinctive fusiform cell composing most of the posterior lobe of the pituitary 垂体细胞

pi·tu·i·ta·rism (pĭ-too′ĭ-tə-riz″əm) disorder of pituitary function 垂体功能障碍；参见 *hyper-* and *hypopituitarism*

pi·tu·i·tary (pĭ-too′ĭ-tar″e) 1. hypophysial 垂体的；2. pituitary gland 垂体；参见 *gland* 下条条；**anterior p.**, adenohypophysis 垂体前叶；**posterior p.**, neurohypophysis 垂体后叶

pit·y·ri·a·sis (pit″ĭ-ri′ə-sis) any of various skin diseases characterized by fine, branny scales 糠疹；**p. al′ba**, a chronic type with patchy scaling and hypopigmentation of the skin of the face 白糠疹；**p. lichenoi′des**, a rare self-limited type with discolored papular lesions and sometimes ulceration; there are both acute and chronic forms 苔藓样糠疹；**p. ro′sea**, a type marked by scaling, pink, oval macules

arranged with the long axes parallel to the cleavage lines of the skin 玫瑰糠疹；**p. ru′bra pila′ris**, a chronic inflammatory type marked by pink scaling macules and horny follicular papules; it usually begins with seborrhea of the scalp and face and then progresses to keratoderma of palms and soles 毛发红糠疹；**p. versi′color**, tinea versicolor 花斑癣

pit·y·roid (pit′ĭ-roid) furfuraceous; branny 糠状的

Pit·y·ros·po·rum (pit″ĭ-ros′pə-rəm) former name for *Malassezia* 糠疹癣菌属

piv·a·late (piv′ə-lāt) USAN contraction for trimethylacetate 特戊酸盐、三甲基醋酸（或酯）（trimethylacetate 的 USAN 缩约词）

PJIA polyarticular juvenile idiopathic arthritis 多关节幼年特发性关节炎

pK_a the negative logarithm of the ionization constant (K) of an acid, the pH of a solution in which half of the acid molecules are ionized 酸的电离常数（Ka）的负对数

PKU, PKU1 phenylketonuria 苯丙酮酸尿症

pla·ce·bo (plə-se′bo) [L.] any dummy medical treatment; originally, a medicinal preparation having no specific pharmacologic activity against the patient's illness or complaint given solely for the psychophysiologic effects of the treatment; more recently, a dummy treatment administered to the control group in a controlled clinical trial in order that the specific and nonspecific effects of the experimental treatment can be distinguished 安慰治疗；安慰剂，无剂（对照）剂

pla·cen·ta (plə-sen′tə) pl. *placentas, placen′tae* [L.] an organ characteristic of true mammals during pregnancy, joining mother and fetus, providing endocrine secretion and selective exchange of soluble blood-borne substances through apposition of uterine and trophoblastic vascularized parts 胎盘；**placen′tal** *adj.*；**p. accre′ta**, one abnormally adherent to the myometrium, with partial or complete absence of the decidua basalis 侵入性胎盘；**circumvallate p.**, one in which a dense peripheral ring is raised from the surface and the attached membranes are doubled back over the placental edge 轮廓胎盘；**deciduate p., deciduous p.**, a placenta or type of placentation in which the decidua or maternal parts of the placenta separate from the uterus and are cast off together with the trophoblastic parts 蜕膜胎盘；**fetal p.**, the part of the placenta derived from the chorionic sac that encloses the embryo, consisting of a chorionic plate and villi 胎盘胎儿部；**hemochorial p.**, one in which maternal blood comes in direct contact with the chorion, as in humans 血性绒毛膜胎盘；**p. incre′ta**, placenta accreta with penetration of the myometrium 植入性胎盘；**maternal p.,** the maternally contributed part of the placenta, derived from the decidua basalis 胎盘母体部；**p. membrana′cea,** one that is abnormally thin and spread out over an unusually large area of the uterine wall 膜状胎盘；**p. percre′ta,** placenta accreta with invasion of the myometrium to its peritoneal covering, sometimes causing rupture of the uterus 穿透性胎盘；**p. pre′via,** one located in the lower uterine segment, so that it partially or completely covers or adjoins the internal os 前置胎盘；**p. spu′ria,** an accessory portion having no blood vessel attachment to the main placenta 假胎盘；**p. succenturia′ta, succenturiate p.,** an accessory portion attached to the main placenta by an artery or vein 副胎盘；**villous p.,** a placenta having villi that are outgrowths of the chorion, such as that in humans 绒毛胎盘

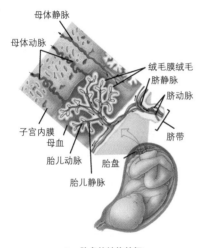

▲ 胎盘的结构特征

plac·en·ta·tion (plas″ən-ta′shən) the series of events following implantation of the embryo and leading to development of the placenta 胎盘形成

plac·en·ti·tis (plas″ən-ti′tis) inflammation of the placenta 胎盘炎

plac·en·tog·ra·phy (plas″ən-tog′rə-fe) radiologic visualization of the placenta after injection of a contrast medium 胎盘造影术

pla·cen·toid (plə-sen′toid) resembling the placenta 胎盘样的

plac·ode (plak′ōd) a platelike structure, especially a thickened plate of ectoderm in the early embryo, from which a sense organ develops, e.g., *otic p.* (ear), *lens p.* (eye), and *nasal p.* (nose) 基板

pla·gio·ceph·a·ly (pla″je-o-sef′ə-le) an asymmetric condition of the head, due to irregular closure of the cranial sutures 斜形头；**plagiocephal′ic** *adj.*

plague (plāg) a severe acute or chronic infectious disease due to *Yersinia pestis,* beginning with chills and fever, quickly followed by prostration, often with delirium, headache, vomiting, and diarrhea; primarily a disease of rats and other rodents, it is transmitted to humans by flea bites or communicated from patient to patient 鼠疫；**bubonic p.,** plague with swelling of the lymph nodes, which form buboes in the femoral, inguinal, axillary, and cervical regions; there is also fever, headache, chills, and weakness. It is transmitted by the bite of infected fleas and may progress to pneumonic or septicemic plague 腺鼠疫；**pneumonic p.,** a rapidly progressive, highly contagious, and often fatal form of plague occurring when *Y. pestis* infects the lungs; it is characterized by pneumonia and productive cough with mucoid, blood-stained, foamy, plague bacillus-laden sputum. It may be a primary infection due to inhalation of aerosolized bacteria, can be a secondary complication of bubonic plague, via hematogenous spread of infection to the lungs 肺鼠疫；**septicemic p.,** an acute fulminating form of plague with high-density bacteremia. It can occur as a complication of bubonic or pneumonic plague, or can be a primary infection transmitted by fleas that may present and result in death before the appearance of buboes 败血症鼠疫；**sylvatic p.,** plague in wild rodents, such as the ground squirrel, which serve as a reservoir from which humans may be infected 野生啮齿动物鼠疫

pla·nar (pla′nər) 1. flat 平面；2. of or pertaining to a plane 平面的

plane (plān) 1. a flat surface determined by the position of three points in space 平面；2. a specified level, as the plane of anesthesia 麻醉平面；3. to rub away or abrade 刨平；参见 *planing*；4. a superficial incision in the wall of a cavity or between tissue layers, especially in plastic surgery, made so that the precise point of entry into the cavity or between the layers can be determined 平面切口；**axial p.,** a plane parallel with the long axis of a structure 轴平面；**base p.,** an imaginary plane upon which is estimated the retention of an artificial denture 基底平面；**coronal p's,** 同 frontal p's；**Frankfort horizontal p.,** a horizontal plane represented in profile by a line between the lowest point on the margin of the orbit and the highest point on the margin of the auditory meatus 法兰克福平面，眼耳平面；**frontal p's,** those passing longitudinally through the body from side to side, at right angles to the median plane, dividing the body into front and back parts

冠状面，额状面；**horizontal p.**, 1. one passing through the body, at right angles to both the frontal and median planes, dividing the body into upper and lower parts 水平面；2. one passing through a tooth at right angles to its long axis 横剖面；**median p.**, one passing longitudinally through the middle of the body from front to back, dividing it into right and left halves 正中矢状面；**nuchal p.**, the outer surface of the occipital bone between the foramen magnum and the superior nuchal line 项平面；**occipital p.**, the outer surface of the occipital bone above the superior nuchal line 枕平面；**orbital p.**, 1. the orbital surface of the maxilla 眶平面；2. 同 visual p.；**sagittal p's**, vertical planes passing through the body parallel to the median plane (or to the sagittal suture), dividing the body into left and right portions 矢状平面；**temporal p.**, the depressed area on the side of the skull below the inferior temporal line 颞平面；**transverse p.**, one passing horizontally through the body, at right angles to the sagittal and coronal planes, and dividing the body into upper and lower portions 横剖面；**vertical p.**, one perpendicular to a horizontal plane, dividing the body into left and right, or front and back portions 矢状面；**visual p.**, one passing through the visual axes of the two eyes 视平面

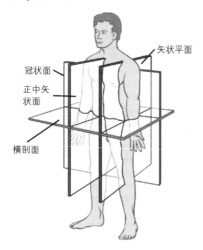

▲ 身体平面及解剖位置

pla·nig·ra·phy (plə-nig′rə-fe) tomography 层析 X 射线照相术；**planigraph′ic** adj.

plan·ing (plān′ing) abrasion of disfigured skin to promote epithelialization with minimal scarring; it may be done mechanically *(dermabrasion)* or by means of caustic substances *(chemabrasion)*（皮肤）

整平法

pla·no·cel·lu·lar (pla″no-sel′u-lər) composed of flat cells 扁平细胞的

pla·no·con·cave (pla″no-kon-kāv′) flat on one side and concave on the other 平凹的

pla·no·con·vex (pla″no-kon-veks′) flat on one side and convex on the other 平凸的

plant (plant) any multicellular eukaryotic organism that performs photosynthesis to obtain its nutrition; plants comprise one of the six kingdoms in the most widely used classification of living organisms 植物

plan·ta (plan′tə) the sole of the foot 足底，又称 *plantar region*

Plan·ta·go (plan-ta′go) a genus of herbs, including *P. in'dica, P. psyl'lium* (Spanish psyllium), and *P. ova'ta* (blond psyllium) 车前属，另参见 *psyllium*

plan·tal·gia (plan-tal′jə) pain in the sole of the foot 足底痛

plan·tar (plan′tər) pertaining to the sole of the foot 足底的，跖的

plan·ta·ris (plan-ta′ris) [L.] 同 plantar

plan·ti·grade (plan′tĭ-grād) walking on the full sole of the foot 跖行的

plan·u·la (plan′u-lə) 1. a larval coelenterate 浮浪幼体（腔肠动物）；2. something resembling such an animal 类浮浪幼体

pla·num (pla′nəm) pl. *pla′na* [L.] 同 plane

plaque (plak) 1. any patch or flat area 斑；2. a superficial, solid, elevated skin lesion 蚀斑，空斑；**attachment p's**, small regions of increased density along the sarcolemma of skeletal muscles to which myofilaments seem to attach 附着斑；**bacterial p., dental p.**, a soft thin film of food debris, mucin, and dead epithelial cells on the teeth, providing the medium for bacterial growth. It contains calcium, phosphorus, and other salts, polysaccharides, proteins, carbohydrates, and lipids, and plays a role in the development of caries, dental calculus, and periodontal and gingival diseases 牙菌斑；**fibrous p.**, the lesion of atherosclerosis, a pearly white area within an artery that causes the intimal surface to bulge into the lumen; it is composed mainly of collagen and, often, calcium, together with lipid, cell debris, and smooth muscle cells 纤维斑块；**Hollenhorst p's**, atheromatous emboli containing cholesterol crystals in the retinal arterioles, a sign of impending serious cardiovascular disease 视网膜淤肿栓塞；**neuritic p's, senile p's**, microscopic argyrophilic masses composed of fragmented axon terminals and dendrites surrounding a core of amyloid, seen in small amounts in the cerebral cortex of healthy elderly people and in larger amounts in those with Alzheimer disease 神经斑炎，老年斑

plasm (plaz′əm) 1. 同 plasma；2. formative substance (cytoplasm, hyaloplasm, etc.) 形成物质

plas·ma (plaz′mə) 1. blood plasma; the fluid portion of the blood in which the particulate components are suspended 血浆；2. the fluid portion of the lymph 原生质，原浆；**plasmat′ic** *adj.*；**antihemophilic human p.**, human plasma that has been processed promptly to preserve the antihemophilic properties of the original blood; used for temporary correction of a bleeding tendency in hemophilia 抗血友病性人血浆；**blood p.**, 同 plasma (1)；**citrated p.**, blood plasma treated with sodium citrate, which prevents clotting 枸橼酸钠血浆；**seminal p.**, the fluid portion of the semen, in which the spermatozoa are suspended 精液浆

plas·ma·blast (plaz′mə-blast) the immature precursor of a plasma cell 浆母细胞，成浆细胞

plas·ma·cyte (plaz′mə-sīt) plasma cell 浆细胞；**plasmacyt′ic** *adj.*

plas·ma·cy·to·ma (plaz″mə-si-to′mə) 1. plasma cell dyscrasias 浆细胞瘤；2. solitary myeloma 孤立性骨髓瘤

plas·ma·cy·to·sis (plaz″mə-si-to′sis) an excess of plasma cells in the blood 浆细胞增多（症）

plas·ma·lem·ma (plaz″mə-lem′ə) 1. plasma membrane 质膜；2. a thin peripheral layer of the ectoplasm in a fertilized egg 卵细胞膜

plas·ma·lo·gen (plaz-mal′ə-jən) any of various phospholipids in which the group at one C1 of glycerol is an ether-linked alcohol in place of an ester-linked fatty acid, found in myelin sheaths of nerve fibers, cell membranes of muscle, and platelets 缩醛磷脂

plas·ma·phe·re·sis (plaz″mə-fə-re′sis) the removal of plasma from withdrawn blood, with retransfusion of the formed elements into the donor; generally, type-specific fresh frozen plasma or albumin is used to replace the withdrawn plasma. The procedure may be done for purposes of collecting plasma components or for therapeutic purposes 血浆除去术，血浆置换

plas·mid (plaz′mid) an extrachromosomal self-replicating structure of bacterial cells that carries genes for a variety of functions not essential for cell growth and that can be transferred to other cells by conjugation or transduction 质粒，另参见 *episome*；**F p.**, a conjugative plasmid found in F⁺ (male) bacterial cells that leads with high frequency to its transfer, and much less often to transfer of the bacterial chromosome, to an F⁻ (female) cell lacking such a plasmid 生殖质粒；**R p., resistance p.**, a conjugative factor in bacterial cells that promotes

resistance to agents such as antibiotics, metal ions, ultraviolet radiation, and bacteriophages 抗药质粒，R 质粒

plas·min (plaz′min) an endopeptidase occurring in plasma as plasminogen, which is activated via cleavage by plasminogen activators; it solubilizes fibrin clots, degrades other coagulationrelated proteins, and can be activated for use in therapeutic thrombolysis 纤溶酶

plas·min·o·gen (plaz-min′ə-jən) the inactive precursor of plasmin, occurring in plasma and converted to plasmin by the action of urokinase 纤维蛋白溶酶原，纤溶酶原

plas·min·o·gen ac·ti·va·tor (plaz-min′ə-jən ak′tĭ-va″tər) 纤维蛋白溶酶原激活剂，参见 *activator* 下词条

plas·mo·cyte (plaz′mo-sīt) plasma cell 浆细胞

plas·mo·di·ci·dal (plaz″mo-dĭ-si′dəl) destructive to plasmodia 杀疟原虫的

Plas·mo·di·um (plaz-mo′de-əm) a genus of sporozoa parasitic in the red blood cells of humans and other animals. Four species, *P. falci′parum*, *P. mala′riae*, *P. ova′le*, and *P. vi′vax*, cause the four specific types of malaria in humans 疟原虫属

plas·mo·di·um (plaz-mo′de-əm) pl. *plasmo′dia*. 1. a protozoan of the genus *Plasmodium* 疟原虫；2. a multinucleate continuous mass of protoplasm formed by aggregation and fusion of myxamebae 原形体，原质团；合胞体；**plasmo′dial** *adj.*

plas·mol·y·sis (plaz-mol′ĭ-sis) contraction of cell protoplasm due to loss of water by osmosis 质壁分离；**plasmolyt′ic** *adj.*

plas·ter (plas′tər) 1. a gypsum material that hardens when mixed with water, used for immobilizing or making impressions of body parts 石膏，灰泥；2. a pastelike mixture that can be spread over the skin and that is adhesive at body temperature; varied uses include skin protectant and counterirritant 硬膏（剂）；**p. of Paris**, calcined calcium sulfate; on addition of water it forms a porous mass that is used in making casts and bandages to support or immobilize body parts, and in dentistry for making study models 煅石膏，干燥硫酸钙

plas·tic (plas′tik) 1. tending to build up tissues to restore a lost part 成形的；2. capable of being molded 可塑的；3. a high-molecular-weight polymeric material, usually organic, capable of being molded, extruded, drawn, or otherwise shaped and hardened into a form 塑料；4. material that can be molded 可塑材料

plate (plāt) 1. a flat structure or layer, as a thin layer of bone 板；2. 同 dental p.；3. to apply a culture medium to a Petri dish 基片；4. to inoculate such a plate with bacteria 培养皿；**bite p.**, biteplate 咬托；**bone p.**, a metal bar with perforations for the insertion of screws, used to immobilize fractured segments 骨板；**cribriform p.**, fascia cribrosa 筛板；**dental p.**, a plate of acrylic resin, metal, or other material, which is fitted to the shape of the mouth and serves to support artificial teeth 牙板；**dorsal p.**, 同 roof p.；**epiphyseal p.**, 骺板, 参见 disk 下词条；**equatorial p.**, the collection of chromosomes at the equator of the cell during metaphase 赤道板；**floor p.**, the unpaired ventral longitudinal zone of the neural tube 底板；**foot p.**, 1. 足板, 参见 footplate；2. the embryonic precursor of a foot 足的胚胎先质；**growth p.**, epiphyseal disk 生长板；**hand p.**, a flattened expansion at the end of the embryonic limb; the precursor of the hand 手板；**medullary p.**, 同 neural p.；**motor end p.**, end plate 终板；**muscle p.**, myotome (2) 肌板；**nail p.**, nail (1) 甲板；**neural p.**, the thickened plate of ectoderm in the embryo that develops into the neural tube 神经板；**roof p.**, the unpaired dorsal longitudinal zone of the neural tube 顶板；**tarsal p.**, tarsus (2) 睑板；**tympanic p.**, the bony plate forming the floor and sides of the meatus auditorius 鼓板；**ventral p.**, 同 floor p.

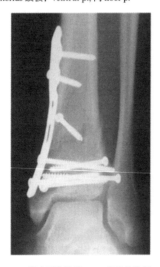

▲ 经皮固定治疗 **Pilon** 骨折的骨板

plate·let (plāt′lət) thrombocyte; a disk-shaped structure, 2 to 4 μm in diameter, found in the blood of mammals and important for its role in blood coagulation; platelets, which are formed by detachment of part of the cytoplasm of a megakaryocyte, lack a nucleus and DNA but contain active enzymes and mitochondria 血小板

plate·let·phe·re·sis (plāt″lət-fə-re′sis) thrombocytapheresis 血小板去除法

plat·i·num (Pt) (plat′ĭ-nəm) a heavy, soft, malleable, ductile, gray-white, metallic element; at. no. 78, at. wt. 195.084 铂（化学元素）

platy·ba·sia (plat″ĭ-ba′se-ə) 1. basilar impression 扁颅底, 扁后脑；2. malformation of the base of the skull due to softening of skull bones or a developmental anomaly, with bulging upwards of the floor of the posterior cranial fossa, upward displacement of the upper cervical vertebrae, and bony impingement on the brainstem 后颅（骨）凹陷症

platy·co·ria (plat″ĭ-kor′e-ə) a dilated condition of the pupil of the eye 瞳孔开大

platy·hel·minth (plat″ĭ-hel′minth) one of the Platyhelminthes; a flatworm 扁形动物

Platy·hel·min·thes (plat″ĭ-həl-min′thēz) a phylum of acoelomate, dorsoventrally flattened, bilaterally symmetrical animals, commonly known as flatworms; it includes the classes Cestoidea (tapeworms) and Trematoda (flukes) 扁形动物门

platy·hi·er·ic (plat″e-hi-er′ik) having a sacral index above 100 阔骶（骨）的

platy·pel·lic (plat″ĭ-pel′ik) having a wide, flat pelvis 骨盆扁型, 阔骨盆的

platy·pel·loid (plat″ĭ-pel′oid) 同 platypellic

pla·tys·ma (plə-tiz′mə) [Gr.] a platelike muscle that originates from the fascia of the cervical region and inserts in the mandible and the skin around the mouth. It is innervated by the cervical branch of the facial nerve, and acts to wrinkle the skin of the neck and to depress the jaw 颈阔肌

pledge (plej) a solemn statement of intention 誓言，保证；**Nightingale p.**, a statement of principles for the nursing profession, formulated by a committee in 1893 and subscribed to by student nurses at the time of the capping ceremonies 南丁格尔誓言（护理专业的道德准则誓言）

pled·get (plej′ət) a small compress or tuft 小拭子

plei·ot·ro·pism (pli-ot′rə-piz-əm) 同 pleiotropy

plei·ot·ro·py (pli-ot′rə-pe) the production by a single gene of multiple phenotypic effects 多效性（一个基因对多种遗传性状产生影响的现象）；**pleiotrop′ic** adj.

pleo·cy·to·sis (ple″o-si-to′sis) presence of a greater than normal number of cells in cerebrospinal fluid 脑脊液细胞增多

pleo·mor·phism (ple″o-mor′fiz-əm) the occurrence of various distinct forms by a single organism or within a species 多形性；**pleomor′phic, pleomor′phous** adj.

ple·on·os·te·o·sis (ple″on-os″te-o′sis) abnormally increased ossification 骨化过早, 骨化过度；**Léri**

p., a hereditary syndrome of premature and excessive ossification, with short stature, limitation of movement, broadening and deformity of digits, and mongolian facies Léri 骨化过早

ples·ses·the·sia (ples″es-the′zhə) palpatory percussion 触叩诊

pleth·ys·mo·graph (plə-thiz′mo-graf) an instrument for recording variations in volume of an organ, part, or limb 体积描记器

pleth·ys·mog·ra·phy (pleth″iz-mog′rə-fe) the determination of changes in volume by means of a plethysmograph 体积描记（术）

pleu·ra (ploor′ə) pl. *pleu′rae* [Gr.] the serous membrane investing the lungs *(visceral p.)* and lining the walls of the thoracic cavity *(parietal p.);* the two layers enclose a potential space, the *pleural cavity.* The two pleurae, right and left, are entirely distinct from each other 胸膜; **pleu′ral** *adj.*

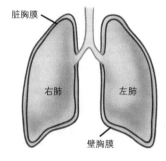

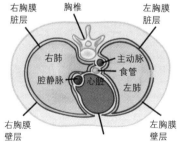

▲ 胸膜。为便于说明，胸膜腔显示为一个实际的空间

pleu·ra·cot·o·my (ploor″ə-kot′ə-me) thoracotomy 胸膜切开术，胸膜腔切开术

pleu·ral·gia (ploo-ral′jə) 1. 同 pleurodynia (1); 2. costalgia (2) 肋痛; **pleural′gic** *adj.*

pleu·rec·to·my (ploo-rek′tə-me) excision of part of the pleura 胸膜（部分）切除术

pleu·ri·sy (ploor′ĭ-se) inflammation of the pleura

胸膜炎; **pleurit′ic** *adj.*; **adhesive p.**, fibrinous p. 粘连性胸膜炎; **dry p.**, 同 fibrinous p.; **p. with effusion**, that marked by serous exudation 渗出性胸膜炎; **fibrinous p.**, a type with fibrinous adhesions between the visceral and parietal pleurae, obliterating part or all of the pleural space 纤维蛋白性胸膜炎，干性胸膜炎; **interlobular p.**, a form enclosed between the lobes of the lung 小叶间胸膜炎; **plastic p.**, fibrinous p. 成形性胸膜炎; **purulent p.**, empyema (2) 化脓性胸膜炎，脓胸; **serous p.**, that marked by free exudation of fluid 浆液性胸膜炎; **suppurative p.**, empyema (2) 化脓性胸膜炎; **wet p.**, 同 p. with effusion 湿性胸膜炎

pleu·ri·tis (ploo-ri′tis) 同 pleurisy; **pleurit′ic** *adj.*

pleu·ro·cele (ploor′o-sēl) pneumonocele (1) 胸膜疝; 胸膜突出

pleu·ro·cen·te·sis (ploor″o-sen-te′sis) thoracentesis 胸腔穿刺术

pleu·ro·dyn·ia (ploor″o-din′e-ə) 1. pain in the pleural cavity 胸膜痛; 2. costalgia (2) 肋痛; **epidemic p.**, an epidemic disease usually due to coxsackievirus B, marked by sudden violent pain in the chest, fever, and a tendency toward recrudescence on the third day 流行性胸痛

pleu·ro·gen·ic (ploor″o-jen′ik) 同 pleurogenous

pleu·rog·e·nous (ploo-roj′ə-nəs) originating in the pleura 胸膜原（性）的

pleu·rog·ra·phy (ploo-rog′rə-fe) radiography of the pleural cavity 胸膜射线摄影术

pleu·ro·hep·a·ti·tis (ploor″o-hep″ə-ti′tis) hepatitis with inflammation of a portion of the pleura near the liver 胸膜肝炎

pleu·rol·y·sis (ploo-rol′ĭ-sis) surgical separation of pleural adhesions 胸膜松解术

pleu·ro·pa·ri·e·to·pexy (ploor″o-pə-ri′ə-topek″se) fixation of the lung to the chest wall by adhesion of the visceral and parietal pleura 胸膜胸壁固定术

pleu·ro·peri·car·di·tis (ploor″o-per″ĭ-kahrdi′tis) inflammation of the pleura and pericardium 胸膜心包炎

pleu·ro·peri·to·ne·al (ploor″o-per″ĭ-to-ne′əl) pertaining to the pleura and peritoneum 胸膜腹膜的

pleu·ro·pneu·mo·nia (ploor″o-noo-mo′ne-ə) pleurisy complicated by pneumonia 胸膜肺炎

pleu·ro·thot·o·nos (ploor″o-thot′ə-nəs) tetanic bending of the body to one side 侧弓反张

pleu·rot·o·my (ploo-rot′ə-me) thoracotomy 胸膜切开术

plex·ec·to·my (plek-sek′tə-me) surgical excision of a plexus 神经丛切除术

plex·i·form (plek′sĭ-form) resembling a plexus or

P

network 丛状的

plex·i·tis (plek-si′tis) inflammation of a nerve plexus 神经丛炎

plex·o·gen·ic (plek′so-jen″ik) giving rise to a plexus or plexiform structure 丛原的

plex·op·a·thy (plek-sop′ə-the) any disorder of a plexus, especially of nerves 神经丛（神经）病；**lumbar p.**, neuropathy of the lumbar plexus 腰丛病

plex·us (plek′səs) pl. *plex′us, plexuses* [L.] a network or tangle, chiefly of vessels or nerves（血管、淋巴管、神经等的）丛；**plex′al** *adj.*; **abdominal aortic p.**, one composed of fibers that arise from the celiac and superior mesenteric plexuses and descend along the aorta. Receiving branches from the lumbar splanchnic nerves, it becomes the superior hypogastric plexus below the bifurcation of the aorta. Branches are distributed along the adjacent branches of the aorta 腹主动脉丛；**autonomic p.**, any of the extensive networks of nerve fibers and cell bodies associated with the autonomic nervous system; found particularly in the thorax, abdomen, and pelvis, and containing sympathetic, parasympathetic, and visceral afferent fibers 自主神经丛；**Batson p.**, the vertebral plexus (1) considered as a whole system 巴特森丛，视为一个整体系统的椎丛；**brachial p.**, a nerve plexus originating from the anterior branches of the last four cervical and the first thoracic spinal nerves, giving off many of the principal nerves of the shoulder, chest, and arms 臂丛；**cardiac p.**, the plexus around the base of the heart, chiefly in the epicardium, formed by cardiac branches from the vagus nerves and the sympathetic trunks and ganglia 心丛；**carotid p.**, any of three nerve plexuses surrounding the common, external, and internal carotid arteries, particularly the last 颈动脉神经丛；**cavernous p.**, a plexus of sympathetic nerve fibers related to the cavernous sinus of the dura mater 海绵窦丛；**celiac p.**, 1. a network of ganglia and nerves lying in front of the aorta behind the stomach, supplying the abdominal viscera 腹腔丛；2. a network of lymphatic vessels, the superior mesenteric lymph nodes, and the celiac lymph nodes 肠系膜上淋巴结和腹腔淋巴结丛；**cervical p.**, a nerve plexus formed by the anterior branches of the first four cervical nerves, supplying structures in the neck region 颈丛；**choroid p's**, infoldings of blood vessels of the pia mater covered by a thin coat of ependymal cells that form tufted projections into the third, fourth, and lateral ventricles of the brain; they secrete the cerebrospinal fluid 脉络丛；**coccygeal p.**, a nerve plexus formed by the anterior branches of the coccygeal and fifth sacral nerves and by a communication from the fourth sacral nerve, giving off the anococcygeal nerve 尾丛；**cystic p.**, a nerve plexus near the gallbladder. 胆囊丛；**dental p.**, either of two plexuses (inferior and superior) of nerve fibers, one from the inferior alveolar nerve situated around the roots of the lower teeth and the other from the superior alveolar nerve situated around the roots of the upper teeth 牙丛；**enteric p.**, a plexus of autonomic nerve fibers within the wall of the digestive tube, made up of the submucosal, myenteric, and subserosal plexuses 肠丛；**esophageal p.**, a plexus surrounding the esophagus, formed by branches of the left and right vagi and sympathetic trunks and containing also visceral afferent fibers from the esophagus 食管丛；**Exner p.**, superficial tangential fibers in the molecular layer of the cerebral cortex 埃克斯内神经丛，大脑皮层分子层的浅切向神经纤维；**gastric p's**, subdivisions of the celiac portions of the prevertebral plexuses, accompanying the gastric arteries and branches and supplying nerve fibers to the stomach 胃（神经）丛；**Heller p.**, an arterial network in the submucosa of the intestine 海勒丛，肠黏膜下层的动脉网；**hemorrhoidal p.**, rectal p. 痔静脉丛；**hypogastric p., inferior**, the plexus formed on each side anterior to the lower part of the sacrum, formed by the junction of the hypogastric and pelvic splanchnic nerves; branches are given off to the pelvic organs 下腹下丛；**hypogastric p., superior**, the downward continuation of the abdominal aortic plexus; it lies in front of the upper part of the sacrum, just below the bifurcation of the aorta, receives fibers from the lower lumbar splanchnic nerves, and divides into right and left hypogastric nerves 腹下上丛；**lumbar p.**, 1. one formed by the anterior branches of the second to fifth lumbar nerves in the psoas major muscle (the branches of the first lumbar nerve often are included) 腰丛；2. a lymphatic plexus in the lumbar region 腰部淋巴丛；**lumbosacral p.**, the lumbar and sacral plexuses considered together, because of their continuous nature 腰骶丛；**lymphatic p.**, an interconnecting network of lymph vessels, i.e., the lymphocapillary vessels, collecting vessels, and trunks, which provides drainage of lymph in a one-way flow 淋巴管丛；**Meissner p.**, submucosal p. 迈斯纳神经丛；**mesenteric p., inferior**, a subdivision of the abdominal aortic plexus accompanying the inferior mesenteric artery 肠系膜下丛；**mesenteric p., superior**, a subdivision of the celiac plexus accompanying the superior mesenteric artery 肠系膜上丛；**myenteric p.**, that part of the enteric plexus within the tunica muscularis 肠肌丛；**pampiniform p.**, 1. a plexus of veins from the testicle and epididymis, constituting part of the spermatic cord 蔓状静脉丛；2. a plexus of ovarian veins in the broad ligament 卵巢宽韧带静脉丛；**pelvic p.,** inferior hypogastric p. 盆丛；**pharyngeal p.,** 1. a venous plexus posterolateral to the pharynx, formed by the pharyngeal veins, communicating with the pterygoid venous plexus, and draining into the internal jugular vein. 咽静脉丛；2. a nerve plexus formed chiefly by fibers from branches of the vagus nerves, but also by fibers from the glossopharyngeal nerves and sympathetic trunks, and supplying most of the muscles and mucosa of the pharynx and soft palate 咽（神经）丛；**phrenic p.,** a nerve plexus accompanying the inferior phrenic artery to the respiratory diaphragm and suprarenal glands 膈丛；**prevertebral p's,** autonomic nerve plexuses situated in the thorax, abdomen, and pelvis, anterior to the vertebral column; they consist of visceral afferent fibers, preganglionic parasympathetic fibers, preganglionic and postganglionic sympathetic fibers, and ganglia containing sympathetic ganglion cells, and they give rise to postganglionic fibers 椎前丛；**prostatic p.,** 1. a subdivision of the inferior hypogastric plexus that supplies nerve fibers to the prostate and adjacent organs 前列腺（神经）丛；2. a venous plexus around the prostate gland, receiving the deep dorsal vein of the penis and draining through the vesical plexus and the prostatic veins 前列腺（静脉）丛；**pterygoid p.,** a network of veins corresponding to the second and third parts of the maxillary artery; situated on the medial and lateral pterygoid muscles and draining into the facial vein 翼丛；**pulmonary p.,** one formed by several strong trunks of the vagus nerve that are joined at the root of the lung by branches from the sympathetic trunk and cardiac plexus; it is often divided into anterior and posterior parts 肺丛；**rectal p.,** 1. a venous plexus that surrounds the lower part of the rectum and drains into the rectal veins 直肠（静脉）丛；2. any of the rectal nerve plexuses (inferior, middle, or superior) 直肠（神经）丛（上，中，下）；**rectal p., external,** inferior rectal p. (1) 直肠外静脉丛；**rectal p., inferior,** 1. the subcutaneous portion of the rectal venous plexus, below the pectinate line 直肠下静脉丛；2. a nerve plexus accompanying the inferior rectal artery, derived chiefly from the inferior rectal nerve 直肠下（神经）丛；**rectal p., internal,** superior rectal p. (1) 直肠内静脉丛；**rectal p., middle,** a subdivision of the inferior hypogastric plexus, in proximity with and supplying nerve fibers to the rectum 直肠中丛；**rectal p., superior,** 1. the submucosal portion of the rectal venous plexus, above the pectinate line 直肠上静脉丛；2. a nerve plexus

accompanying the superior rectal artery to the rectum, derived from the inferior mesenteric and hypogastric plexuses 直肠上丛（神经）；**sacral p.,** 1. a nerve plexus arising from the anterior branches of the last two lumbar and the first four sacral nerves 骶丛（神经）；2. a venous plexus on the pelvic surface of the sacrum, receiving the sacral intervertebral veins 骶丛（静脉）；**solar p.,** 同celiac p. (1)；**submucosal p.,** the part of the enteric plexus that is situated in the submucosa 黏膜下神经丛；**subserosal p.,** the part of the enteric plexus situated deep to the serosal surface of the tunica serosa 浆膜下丛，肠神经丛的一部分，位于浆膜表面深处；**thoracic aortic p.,** one around the descending thoracic aorta formed by filaments from the sympathetic trunks and vagus nerves, and from which fine twigs accompany branches of the aorta; continuous below with the celiac plexus and the abdominal aortic plexus 胸主动脉丛；**tympanic p.,** a network of nerve fibers supplying the mucous lining of the tympanum, mastoid air cells, and auditory tube 鼓室丛；**uterine p.,** 1. the part of the uterovaginal plexus that supplies nerve fibers to the cervix and lower part of the uterus 子宫丛（神经），子宫阴道丛的一部分，供应宫颈和子宫下部神经纤维；2. the venous plexus around the uterus, draining into the internal iliac veins by way of the uterine veins 子宫丛（血管），子宫周围的静脉丛，通过子宫静脉流入髂内静脉；**uterovaginal p.,** 1. the subdivision of the inferior hypogastric plexus that supplies nerve fibers to the uterus, ovary, vagina, urethra, and erectile tissue of the vestibule 子宫阴道丛（神经），下腹神经丛的一个分支，支配前庭的子宫、卵巢、阴道、尿道和勃起组织；2. the uterine and vaginal venous plexuses considered together 子宫阴道丛（血管），子宫和阴道静脉丛；**vaginal p.,** 1. a nerve plexus that is part of the uterovaginal plexus and innervates the walls of the vagina 阴道丛（神经）；2. a venous plexus in the walls of the vagina, which drains into the internal iliac veins by way of the internal pudendal veins 阴道丛（血管）；**vascular p.,** 1. a network of intercommunicating blood vessels 血管丛；2. a plexus of peripheral nerves through which blood vessels receive innervation 支配血管的外周神经丛；**venous p.,** a network of interconnecting veins 静脉丛；**vertebral p.,** 1. a plexus of veins related to the vertebral column 椎动脉丛；2. a nerve plexus accompanying the vertebral artery, carrying sympathetic fibers to the posterior cranial fossa via cranial nerves 椎丛，伴随椎动脉的神经丛，通过颅神经将交感神经纤维输送到颅后窝；**vesical p.,** 1. the subdivision of the inferior hypogastric plexus that supplies sympathetic nerve fibers to the urinary bladder and parts of the ureter, ductus deferens, and seminal vesicle 膀胱（神经）丛；2. a venous plexus surrounding the upper part of the urethra and the neck of the bladder, communicating with the vaginal plexus in the female and with the prostatic plexus in the male 膀胱（静脉）丛

pli·ca (pli′kə) pl. *pli′cae* [L.] a ridge or fold 皱襞，褶

pli·ca·my·cin (pli″kə-mi′sin) an antineoplastic antibiotic produced by *Streptomyces plicatus*; used in the treatment of advanced testicular carcinoma. It also has an inhibiting effect on osteoclasts and is used to treat hypercalcemia and hypercalciuria associated with malignancy 光神霉素

pli·cate (pli′kāt) plaited or folded 有襞的，折襞的，具褶的

pli·ca·tion (pli-ka′shən) the operation of taking tucks in a structure to shorten it 折襞，折术；**Kelly p.**, suture of the connective tissue between the vagina and the urethra and the floor of the bladder for correction of stress incontinence in women　Kelly 折叠术，缝合阴道、尿道和膀胱底部之间的结缔组织，以矫正女性压力性尿失禁

pli·cot·o·my (pli-kot′ə-me) surgical division of the posterior fold of the tympanic membrane（鼓膜）襞切断术

plug (plug) an obstructing mass 塞子，栓；充填剂，填料；**closing p.**, a fibrinous coagulum of blood that fills the defect in the endometrial epithelium created by implantation of the blastocyst 封闭塞，一种血纤维蛋白凝结物，填充胚胎植入造成的子宫内膜上皮缺损；**Dittrich p's**, masses of fat globules, fatty acid crystals, and bacteria sometimes seen in the bronchi in bronchitis and bronchiectasis Dittrich 塞，在支气管炎和支气管扩张时，支气管内有时可见的大量脂肪球、脂肪酸晶体和细菌；**epithelial p.**, 1. a mass of ectodermal cells that temporarily closes an opening in the fetus, particularly in the external nares 上皮栓，暂时阻塞胎儿开口，尤其是外鼻孔的大量上皮细胞；2. a mass of epithelium clogging or obstructing an opening 阻塞开口的上皮团；**mucous p.**, 1. a plug formed by secretions of the mucous glands of the cervix uteri and closing the cervical canal during pregnancy 黏液栓，子宫颈黏液腺分泌物在怀孕期间关闭宫颈管形成的塞子；2. abnormally thick mucus occluding the bronchi and bronchioles 阻塞支气管和细支气管的厚黏液栓

plug·ger (plug′ər) an instrument for compacting filling material in a tooth cavity 充填器，在齿腔中压实填充材料的仪器

plum·bic (plum′bik) pertaining to lead 铅的

plum·bism (plum′biz-əm) chronic lead poisoning

慢性铅中毒，参见 *lead*¹

pluri- word element [L.], *more* [构词成分] 多数，多

plu·ri·glan·du·lar (ploor″ī-glan′du-lər) pertaining to or affecting several glands 多腺性的

plu·ri·hor·mo·nal (ploor″ī-hor-mo′nəl) of or pertaining to several hormones 多激素的

plu·rip·o·tent (ploo-rip′ə-tənt) able to develop or act in any one of several possible ways 多能的；**pluripotency** *n.*

plu·ri·po·ten·tial (ploor″ī-po-ten′shal) 同 pluripotent

plu·to·ni·um (Pu) (ploo-to′ne-əm) a heavy, silvery white, reactive transuranium element; at. no. 94, at. wt. 244 钚（化学元素）

Pm promethium 元素钷的符号

PMDD premenstrual dysphoric disorder 月经前焦虑障碍

PMFC posterior medial frontal cortex 后内侧额叶皮质

PMI point of maximal impulse (of the heart) 最强心尖搏动点

PMMA polymethyl methacrylate 聚甲基丙烯酸甲酯

PNET primitive neuroectodermal tumor 原发性神经外胚层瘤

pneu·mar·throg·ra·phy (noo″mahr-throg′-rə-fe) radiography of a joint after injection of air or gas as a contrast medium 关节充气造影术

pneu·mar·thro·sis (noo″mahr-thro′sis) 1. gas or air in a joint 关节气肿；2. inflation of a joint with air or gas for radiographic examination 充气以进行射线照相检查关节

pneu·mat·ic (noo-mat′ik) 1. pertaining to air 空气的，气体的；2. respiratory 呼吸的

pneu·ma·ti·za·tion (noo″mə-tī-za′shən) the formation of air cells or cavities in tissue, especially in the temporal bone 气腔形成

pneu·ma·to·cele (noo-mat′o-sēl) 1. aerocele; a tumor or cyst formed by air or other gas filling an adventitious pouch, such as a laryngocele, tracheocele, or gaseous swelling of the scrotum 气瘤，气囊，由空气或其他气体形成的囊肿，如喉囊肿、气管囊肿或阴囊气肿；2. a usually benign, thin-walled, air-containing cyst of the lung, as in staphylococcal pneumonia 肺膨出

pneu·ma·to·graph (noo-mat′o-graf″) spirograph 呼吸描记器

pneu·ma·to·sis (noo″mə-to′sis) [Gr.] air or gas in an abnormal location in the body 气肿，积气症；**p. cystoi′des intestina′lis**, presence of thin-walled, gas-containing cysts in the wall of the intestines 肠壁囊样积气

pneu·ma·tu·ria (noo″mə-tu′re-ə) gas or air in the urine 气尿，尿中有气体或空气

pneu·mo·ar·throg·ra·phy (noo″mo-ahr-throg′-rə-fe) pneumarthrography 关节充气造影术

pneu·mo·bil·ia (noo″mo-bil′e-ə) gas in the biliary system 胆道积气，气性胆汁

pneu·mo·cele (noo″mo-sēl″) 1. 同 pneumonocele (1); 2. 同 pneumatocele (1); 3. 同 pneumatocele (2)

pneu·mo·ceph·a·lus (noo″mo-sef′ə-ləs) air in the cranial cavity 颅腔积气

pneu·mo·coc·cal (noo″mo-kok′əl) pertaining to or caused by pneumococci 肺炎球菌的

pneu·mo·coc·ce·mia (noo″mo-kok-se′me-ə) pneumococci in the blood 肺炎球菌血症

pneu·mo·coc·co·su·ria (noo″mo-kok″o-su′re-ə) pneumococci in the urine 肺炎球菌尿

pneu·mo·coc·cus (noo″mo-kok′əs) pl. pneumococ′ci. A member of the species Streptococcus pneumoniae 肺炎球菌

pneu·mo·co·ni·o·sis (noo″mo-ko″ne-o′sis) deposition of large amounts of dust or other particulate matter in the lungs, causing a tissue reaction, usually in workers in certain occupations and in residents of areas with excessive particulates in the air; there are many types, including anthracosis, asbestosis, bituminosis, and silicosis 肺尘埃沉着病，尘肺病；coal workers'p., black lung; a form caused by deposition of coal dust in the lungs, usually characterized by centrilobular emphysema. Different varieties of coal have different risks; bituminosis is usually more severe than anthracosis 煤矿工尘肺；talc p., talcosis; a type of silicatosis caused by the inhalation of talc; prolonged exposure may result in pulmonary fibrosis 肺滑石沉着病，滑石肺

pneu·mo·ceph·a·lus (noo″mo-kra′ne-əm) pneumocephalus 颅腔积气

pneu·mo·cys·ti·a·sis (noo″mo-sis-ti′ə-sis) pneumocystis pneumonia 肺囊虫病

Pneu·mo·cys·tis (noo″mo-sis′tis) a genus of yeast-like fungi. P. jirove′ci causes pneumocystis pneumonia; it was formerly called P. carinii, now reserved for the species infecting rats 肺囊虫属

pneu·mo·cys·tog·ra·phy (noo″mo-sis-tog′-rə-fe) cystography after injection of air or gas into the bladder 膀胱充气造影术

pneu·mo·en·ceph·a·lo·cele (noo″mo-ensef′ə-lo-sēl) pneumocephalus 颅腔积气

pneu·mo·en·ceph·a·log·ra·phy (PEG) (noo″mo-ən-sef″ə-log′rə-fe) radiography of fluidcontaining structures of the brain after cerebrospinal fluid is intermittently withdrawn by lumbar puncture and replaced by a gas 气脑造影术

pneu·mo·en·ter·itis (noo″mo-en″tər-i′tis) inflam-mation of the lungs and intestine 肺肠炎

pneu·mog·ra·phy (noo″mo-mog′rə-fe) 1. spirography 呼吸描记法；2. radiography of a part after injection of a gas 充气造影术

pneu·mo·he·mo·peri·car·di·um (noo″mohe″mo-per″ĭ-kahr′de-əm) air or gas and blood in the pericardium 气血心包，心包积气血

pneu·mo·he·mo·tho·rax (noo″mo-he″mothor′aks) hemopneumothorax 气血胸

pneu·mo·hy·dro·me·tra (noo″mo-hi″drome′trə) gas and fluid in the uterus 子宫积气水

pneu·mo·hy·dro·peri·car·di·um (noo″mohi″dro-per″ĭ-kahr′de-əm) air or gas and fluid in the pericardium 气水心包，心包积水气

pneu·mo·hy·dro·tho·rax (noo″mo-hi″drothor′aks) hydropneumothorax 气水胸

pneu·mo·li·thi·a·sis (noo″mo-lĭ-thi′ə-sis) the presence of concretions in the lungs 肺石病

pneu·mo·me·di·as·ti·num (noo″mo-me″de-ə-sti′nəm) air or gas in the mediastinum, which may be pathologic or introduced intentionally 纵隔积气

pneu·mo·my·co·sis (noo″mo-mi-ko′sis) any fungal disease of the lungs 肺真菌病，肺霉菌病

pneu·mo·my·elog·ra·phy (noo″mo-mi″ə-log′rə-fe) radiography of the spinal canal after withdrawal of cerebrospinal fluid and injection of air or gas 气脊髓造影术

pneu·mo·nec·to·my (noo″mo-nek′tə-me) excision of lung tissue; it may be total, partial, or of a single lobe (lobectomy) 肺切除术

pneu·mo·nia (noo-mōn′yə) inflammation of the lungs with exudation and consolidation 肺炎；p. al′ba., a fatal desquamative pneumonia of the newborn due to congenital syphilis, with fatty degeneration of the lungs 白色肺炎；aspiration p., that due to aspiration of foreign material into the lungs. 吸入性肺炎；atypical p., 同 primary atypical p.；bacterial p., that due to bacteria, usually species of Streptococcus, Staphylococcus, Klebsiella, and Mycoplasma 细菌性肺炎；bronchial p., bronchopneumonia 支气管肺炎；desquamative interstitial p., chronic pneumonia with desquamation of large alveolar cells and thickening of the walls of distal air passages; marked by dyspnea and nonproductive cough 脱屑性间质性肺炎；double p., that affecting both lungs 双侧肺炎；Friedländer p., 同 Klebsiella p.；hypostatic p., a type seen in the weak or elderly, due to excessive lying on the back 坠积性肺炎；influenzal p., influenza virus p., an acute, usually fatal type due to influenza virus, with high fever, prostration, sore throat, aching pains, dyspnea, massive edema, and consolidation. It may be complicated by bacterial pneumonia 流感（病

毒）性肺炎；**inhalation p.**, 1. 同 aspiration p.；2. bronchopneumonia due to inhalation of irritating vapors 吸入性支气管肺炎；**interstitial p.**, 1. any of various types of pneumonia characterized by thickening of the interstitial tissue 间质性肺炎；2. idiopathic pulmonary fibrosis 特发性肺纤维化；**interstitial plasma cell p.**, pneumocystis pneumonia 间质性浆细胞肺炎；*Klebsiella p.*, Friedländer p.；a form with massive mucoid inflammatory exudates in a lobe of the lung, due to *Klebsiella pneumoniae* 肺炎克雷伯菌肺炎；**lipid p., lipoid p.**, aspiration pneumonia due to aspiration of oil 类脂性肺炎；**lobar p.**, 1. acute bacterial pneumonia with edema, usually in one lung; the most common type is pneumococcal p. 大叶性肺炎；2. 同 pneumococcal p.；**lobular p.**, bronchopneumonia 小叶性肺炎；**mycoplasmal p.**, primary atypical pneumonia caused by *Mycoplasma pneumoniae* 支原体肺炎；**Pittsburgh p.**, a type resembling legionnaires' disease, caused by *Legionella micdadei*, seen in immunocompromised patients 匹兹堡肺炎；**pneumococcal p.**, the most common type of lobar pneumonia, caused by *Streptococcus pneumoniae.* 肺炎球菌性肺炎；**pneumocystis p.**, a form caused by *Pneumocystis jiroveci*, seen in infants and debilitated or immunocompromised persons; cellular detritus containing plasma cells appears in lung tissue 肺孢子虫性肺炎；*Pneumocystis carinii* p., former name for pneumocystis p. 肺孢子菌肺炎，肺孢子虫病；**primary atypical p.**, any of numerous types of acute pneumonia, caused by bacteria such as species of *Mycoplasma, Rickettsia,* or *Chlamydophila,* or viruses such as adenoviruses or parainfluenza virus 原发性非典型病原体肺炎；**rheumatic p.**, a rare, usually fatal complication of acute rheumatic fever, with extensive pulmonary consolidation and rapidly progressive functional deterioration, alveolar exudate, interstitial infiltrates, and necrotizing arteritis 风湿性肺炎；**varicella p.**, that developing after the skin eruption in varicella (chickenpox), apparently due to the same virus; symptoms may be severe, with violent cough, hemoptysis, and severe chest pain 水痘性肺炎；**ventilator-associated p.**, the most common type of nosocomial pneumonia seen in patients breathing with a ventilator; it is usually caused by aspiration of contaminated secretions or stomach contents; it may be bacterial, viral, or fungal and is frequently fatal 呼吸机相关性肺炎；**viral p.**, that due to a virus, e.g., adenovirus, influenza virus, parainfluenza virus, or varicella virus 病毒性肺炎；**white p.**, 同 p. alba

pneu·mon·ic (noo-mon′ik) 1. 同 pulmonary (1)；2. pertaining to pneumonia 肺炎的

pneu·mo·ni·tis (noo″mo-ni′tis) inflammation of the lung 肺炎，另参见 *pneumonia*；**hyper-sensitivity p.**, extrinsic allergic alveolitis; a hypersensitivity reaction to repeated inhalation of organic particles, usually on the job, with onset a few hours after exposure to the allergen 过敏性肺炎

pneu·mo·no·cele (noo-mon′o-sēl) 1. pleurocele; pneumocele; hernial protrusion of lung tissue, as through a fissure in the chest wall 胸膜疝；气瘤；2. 同 pneumatocele (2)

pneu·mo·no·cen·te·sis (noo-mo″no-sente′sis) paracentesis of a lung 肺穿刺术

pneu·mo·no·cyte (noo-mon′o-sīt) alveolar cell 肺细胞

pneu·mo·nop·a·thy (noo″mo-nop′ə-the) pneumonosis; any lung disease 肺病

pneu·mo·no·pexy (noo-mo′no-pek″se) surgical fixation of the lung to the thoracic wall 肺固定术

pneu·mo·nor·rha·phy (noo″mo-nor′ə-fe) suture of the lung 肺缝合术（肺修补术）

pneu·mo·no·sis (noo″mo-no′sis) 同 pneumopathy

pneu·mo·not·o·my (noo″mo-not′ə-me) incision of the lung 肺切开术

pneu·mo·peri·car·di·um (noo″mo-per″ĭ-kahr′de-əm) air or gas in the pericardial cavity 心气包，心包积气

pneu·mo·peri·to·ne·um (noo″mo-per″ĭ-tone′əm) air or gas in the peritoneal cavity 气腹

pneu·mo·peri·to·ni·tis (noo″mo-per″ĭ-toni′tis) peritonitis with air or gas in the peritoneal cavity 气性腹膜炎

pneu·mo·pleu·ri·tis (noo″mo-ploo-ri′tis) 同 pleuropneumonia (1)

pneu·mo·py·elog·ra·phy (noo″mo-pi″ə-log′rə-fe) radiography after injection of oxygen or air into the renal pelvis 肾盂充气造影术

pneu·mo·pyo·peri·car·di·um (noo″mo-pi″oper″ĭ-kahr′de-əm) pyopneumopericardium 气脓心包，心包积脓气

pneu·mo·pyo·tho·rax (noo″mo-pi″o-thor′aks) pyopneumothorax 气脓胸

pneu·mo·ra·di·og·ra·phy (noo″mo-ra″deog′rə-fe) radiography after injection of air or oxygen X线充气造影术

pneu·mo·ret·ro·peri·to·ne·um (noo″moret″ro-per″ĭ-to-ne′əm) air in the retroperitoneal space 腹膜后腔积气，腹膜后气肿

pneu·mo·ta·chom·e·ter (noo″mo-tə-kom′ə- tər) a transducer for measuring exhaled air flow 呼吸速度计

pneu·mo·tach·y·graph (noo″mo-tak′ĭ-graf) an instrument for recording the velocity of respired air

呼吸速度描记器

pneu·mo·tax·ic (noo″mo-tak′sik) regulating the respiratory rate 调节呼吸的

pneu·mo·tho·rax (noo″mo-thor′aks) air or gas in the pleural space, usually as a result of trauma *(traumatic* or *open p.)* or some pathologic process 气胸;

tension p., a type in which the pressure within the pleural space is greater than atmospheric pressure; the positive pressure in the cavity displaces the mediastinum to the opposite side, with consequent interference with respiration 张力性气胸

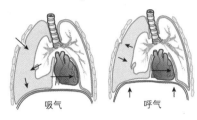

吸气　　呼气

▲ 张力性气胸致右侧肺不张，纵隔结构向左侧移位。吸气时空气被迫进入胸膜腔内，呼气时气体不能排出

pneu·mot·o·my (noo-mot′o-me) 同 pneumonotomy

pneu·mo·ven·tric·u·log·ra·phy (noo″ movən-trik″u-log′rə-fe) radiography of the cerebral ventricles after injection of air or gas 脑室充气造影术

Pneu·mo·vi·rus (noo″mo-vi″rəs) the respiratory syncytial viruses, a genus of the family Paramyxoviridae that causes respiratory infections in humans and other animals 呼吸道合胞病毒属

PNH paroxysmal nocturnal hemoglobinuria 阵发性睡眠性血红蛋白尿

PNS peripheral nervous system 周围神经系统

PO [L.] per os (by mouth, orally) 经口，口服

Po₂ oxygen partial pressure (tension); also written P_{O_2}, pO_2, and pO_2 氧分压

Po polonium 元素钋的符号

POAG primary open-angle glaucoma 原发性开角型青光眼

pock (pok) a pustule, especially of smallpox 痘疱（尤指天花）

pock·et (pok′ət) a bag or pouch 袋，囊; **endocardial p’s**, sclerotic thickenings of the mural endocardium, occurring most often on the left ventricular septum below an insufficient aortic valve. 心 内膜 袋; **gingival p.**, a gingival sulcus deepened by pathologic conditions, caused by gingival enlargement without destruction of the periodontal tissue 龈袋; **pacemaker p.**, the subcutaneous area in which the pulse generator and pacing leads of an internal pacemaker are implanted, usually developed in the prepectoral fascia or the retromammary area 起 搏器 袋; **periodontal p.**, a gingival sulcus deepened into the periodontal ligament apically to the original level of the resorbed alveolar crest 牙周袋

pock·mark (pok′mahrk) a depressed scar left by a pustule 痘痕

po·dag·ra (pə-dag′rə) gouty pain in the great toe 足痛风

po·dal·gia (pə-dal′jə) pain in the foot 足痛

po·dal·ic (pə-dal′ik) accomplished by means of the feet 足的，脚的; 参见 *version* 下词条

pod·ar·thri·tis (pod″ahr-thri′tis) inflammation of the joints of the feet 足关节炎

po·di·a·try (pə-di′ə-tre) chiropody; the specialized field dealing with the study and care of the foot, including its anatomy, pathology, medicinal and surgical treatment, etc. 足医术；足病学; **podiat′ric adj.**

podo·cyte (pod′o-sīt) an epithelial cell of the visceral layer of a renal glomerulus, having a number of footlike radiating processes (pedicels) 足细胞

podo·dy·na·mom·e·ter (pod″o-di″nə-mom′ə-tər) a device for determining the strength of leg muscles 腿肌力计，足力计

podo·dyn·ia (pod″o-din′e-ə) 同 podalgia

po·dof·i·lox (po-dof′ĭ-loks) an agent that inhibits cell mitosis and is used for topical treatment of condyloma acuminatum 普达非洛，一种抑制细胞分裂的制剂，主要用于尖锐湿疣的局部外涂治疗

po·dol·o·gy (po-dol′ə-je) 同 podiatry

podo·phyl·lin (pod″o-fil′in) podophyllum resin 鬼臼树脂

podo·phyl·lum (pod″o-fil′əm) the dried rhizome and roots of *Podophyllum peltatum* 鬼臼根，参见 *resin* 下词条

po·go·ni·a·sis (po″go-ni′ə-sis) excessive growth of the beard, or growth of a beard on a woman 多须，妇女多须

po·go·ni·on (po-go′ne-on) the most anterior point in the midline of the chin 颏点

poi·ki·lo·blast (poi′kĭ-lo-blast″) an abnormally shaped erythroblast 异形成红细胞

poi·ki·lo·cyte (poi′kĭ-lo-sīt″) an abnormally shaped erythrocyte, such as a burr cell, sickle cell, target cell, acanthocyte, elliptocyte, schistocyte, spherocyte, or stomatocyte 异形红细胞

poi·ki·lo·cy·to·sis (poi″kĭ-lo-si-to′sis) presence in the blood of erythrocytes showing abnormal variation in shape 异形红细胞症

poi·ki·lo·der·ma (poi″kĭ-lo-dur′mə) pigmentary and atrophic changes in the skin, giving it a mottled appearance 皮肤异色病

point (point) 1. a small area or spot; the sharp end of an object 点，尖（端）; 2. to approach the surface, like the pus of an abscess, at a definite spot or place（脓肿等）出现脓头; **p. A,** subspinale 上颌牙槽座点, **acupuncture p.,** acupoint 穴位; **p. B,** a radiographic cephalometric landmark, determined on the lateral head film; it is the most posterior midline point in the concavity between the infradentale and pogonium 下颌牙槽座点, **boiling p.,** the temperature at which a liquid will boil; at sea level, water boils at 100℃ (212 ℉) 沸点; **cardinal p's,** 1. the points on the different refracting media of the eye that determine the direction of the entering or emerging light rays 基点; 2. four points within the pelvic inlet—the two sacroiliac articulations and the two iliopectineal eminences 骨盆主点; **craniometric p.,** one of the established points of reference for measurement of the skull 测颅点; **far p.,** the remotest point at which an object is clearly seen when the eye is at rest 远点; **p. of fixation,** 1. the point on which the vision is fixed 凝视点; 2. the point on the retina on which are focused the rays coming from an object directly regarded 注视点; **freezing p.,** the temperature at which a liquid begins to freeze; for water, 0℃, or 32 ℉冰点; **isoelectric p.,** the pH of a solution at which a charged molecule does not migrate in an electric field 等电点; **jugal p.,** the point at the angle formed by the masseteric and maxillary edges of the zygomatic bone 颧点; **lacrimal p.,** the opening on the lacrimal papilla of an eyelid, near the medial angle of the eye, into which tears from the lacrimal lake drain to enter the lacrimal canaliculi 泪点; **p. of maximal impulse (PMI),** the point on the chest where the impulse of the left ventricle is felt most strongly, normally in the fifth costal interspace inside the mammillary line 最强心尖搏动点; **McBurney p.,** a point about one-third the distance between the right anterior superior iliac spine and the umbilicus; it is especially tender upon pressure in a patient with appendicitis 麦克伯尼点（麦氏点）; **melting p. (mp),** the minimum temperature at which a solid begins to liquefy 熔点; **near p.,** the nearest point of clear vision, the *absolute near p.* being that for either eye alone with accommodation relaxed, and the *relative near p.* that for both eyes with the employment of accommodation 近点; **nodal p's,** two points on the axis of an optical system situated so that a ray falling on one will produce a parallel ray emerging through the other 节点; **pressure p.,** 1. a point that is particularly sensitive to pressure 压觉点; 2. one of various locations on the body at which digital pressure may be applied for the control of hemorrhage 压迫

止血点; **subnasal p.,** the central point at the base of the nasal spine 鼻下点; **trigger p.,** a spot on the body at which pressure or other stimulus gives rise to specific sensations or symptoms. 扳机点; **triple p.,** the temperature and pressure at which the solid, liquid, and gas phases of a substance are in equilibrium 三相点

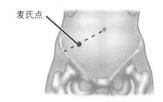

麦氏点

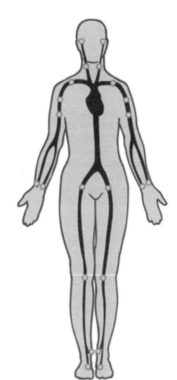

▲ 全身压迫止血点

point·er (point′ər) contusion at a bony eminence（骨隆突）挫伤; **hip p.,** a contusion of the bone of the iliac crest, or avulsion of muscle attachments at the iliac crest 髂嵴挫伤

poi·son (poi′zən) a substance that, on ingestion,

inhalation, absorption, application, injection, or development within the body, in relatively small amounts, may cause structural damage or functional disturbance 毒药，毒物; **poi′sonous** *adj.*

poi·son·ing (poi′zən-ing) the damaging physiologic effects resulting from exposure to poison 中毒; **blood p.,** septicemia 败血症; **food p.,** a group of illnesses caused by ingestion of food that is contaminated, as by pathogenic bacteria or their toxins, or that is inherently poisonous; characterized by gastroenteritis and sometimes affecting other systems, and varying in severity 食物中毒; **nicotine p.,** poisoning by exposure to excessive levels of nicotine; marked by stimulation and then depression of the central and autonomic nervous systems, and occasionally death from respiratory paralysis 尼古丁中毒; **scombroid p.,** epigastric pain, nausea, vomiting, headache, dysphagia, thirst, urticaria, and pruritus, usually lasting for less than 24 hours, caused by the ingestion of a toxic histamine-like substance produced by bacterial action on histidine in fish flesh; occurring when inadequately preserved scombroid fish (tuna, bonito, mackerel, etc.) are eaten 鲭鱼肉中毒; **shellfish p.,** poisoning from eating bivalve mollusks contaminated with a neurotoxin secreted by protozoa 贝类中毒

poi·son ivy (poi′zən i′ve) *Rhus radicans* 毒漆藤

poi·son oak (poi′zən ōk) *Rhus diversiloba* or *R. toxicodendron* 槲叶毒葛

poi·son su·mac (poi′zən soo′mak) *Rhus vernix* 美国毒漆树

po·lar (po′lər) 1. of or pertaining to a pole 极的; 2. being at opposite ends of a spectrum of manifestations 处于一系列表现形式的两端（相反的两端）

po·la·rim·e·try (po″lə-rim′ə-tre) measurement of the rotation of plane polarized light 旋光法，测偏振术

po·lar·i·ty (po-lar′ĭ-te) the condition of having poles or of exhibiting opposite effects at the two extremities 极性

po·lar·iza·tion (po″lər-ĭ-za′shən) 1. the presence or establishment of polarity 极性化; 2. the production of that condition in light in which its vibrations take place all in one plane, or in circles and ellipses 偏振; 3. the process of producing a relative separation of positive and negative charges, such as in a body, cell, molecule, or atom 极化

po·lar·og·ra·phy (po″lər-og′rə-fe) an electrochemical technique for identifying and estimating the concentration of reducible elements in an electrochemical cell by means of the dual measurement of the current flowing through the cell and the electrical potential at which each element is reduced 极

谱法; **polarograph′ic** *adj.*

pole (pōl) 1. either extremity of any axis, as of the fetal ellipse or a body organ 极; 2. either one of two points that have opposite physical qualities 具有相反物理性质的两点之一（电极，磁极，轴极）; **po′lar** *adj.*; **animal p.,** 动物极 1. the site of an oocyte to which the nucleus is approximated, and from which the polar bodies pinch off 卵母细胞中细胞核偏向的一端; 2. in nonmammalian species, the pole of an egg less heavily laden with yolk than the vegetal pole and exhibiting faster cell division 在非哺乳动物种中，成熟卵子含卵黄较少的一端，卵裂进行比较迅速; **cephalic p.,** the end of the fetal ellipse at which the head of the fetus is situated 头极; **frontal p. of cerebral hemisphere,** the most prominent part of the anterior end of each hemisphere 大脑半球额极; **germinal p.,** 同 animal p.; **occipital p. of cerebral hemisphere,** the posterior end of the occipital lobe 大脑半球枕极; **pelvic p.,** the end of the fetal ellipse at which the breech of the fetus is situated 骨盆极; **temporal p. of cerebral hemisphere,** the prominent anterior end of the temporal lobe 大脑半球颞极; **vegetal p.,** that pole of an oocyte at which the greater amount of food yolk is deposited 植物极

po·lice·man (pə-lēs′mən) a glass rod with a piece of rubber tubing on one end, used as a stirring rod and transfer tool in chemical analysis 淀帚，一端包有橡皮的玻璃棒，在化学分析时用作搅拌棒

poli·clin·ic (pol″e-klin′ik) a city hospital, infirmary, or clinic 市立（医院）门诊部; 综合门诊部 cf. *polyclinic*

po·lio (po′le-o) 同 poliomyelitis

po·lio·clas·tic (po″le-o-klas′tik) destroying the gray matter of the nervous system 破坏神经系统灰质的

po·lio·dys·tro·phia (po″le-o-dis-tro′fe-ə) 同 poliodystrophy

po·lio·dys·tro·phy (po″le-o-dis′trə-fe) atrophy of the cerebral gray matter 灰质营养不良，灰质营养障碍

po·lio·en·ceph·a·li·tis (po″le-o-ən-sef′ə-li′-tis) inflammatory disease of the gray matter of the brain 脑灰质炎; **inferior p.,** progressive bulbar palsy 脑下部灰质炎; 延髓性麻痹

po·lio·en·ceph·a·lo·me·nin·go·my·eli·tis (po″le-o-ən-sef″ə-lo-mə-ning″go-mi′ə- li′tis) inflammation of the gray matter of the brain and spinal cord and of the meninges 脑脊髓灰质脑脊膜炎

po·lio·en·ceph·a·lop·a·thy (po″le-o-ensef″ə-lop′ə-the) disease of the gray matter of the brain 脑灰质病

po·lio·my·eli·tis (po″le-o-mi″ə-li′tis) an acute

viral disease usually caused by a poliovirus and marked clinically by fever, sore throat, headache, vomiting, and often stiffness of the neck and back; in the *minor illness*, these may be the only symptoms. In the *major illness*, which may or may not be preceded by the minor illness, there is central nervous system involvement, stiff neck, pleocytosis in spinal fluid, and sometimes paralysis *(paralytic p.)*; there may be subsequent atrophy of muscle groups, ending in contraction and permanent deformity 脊髓灰质炎；**abortive p.**, the minor illness of poliomyelitis 轻型脊髓灰质炎；**acute anterior p.**, the major illness of poliomyelitis 急性脊髓前角灰质炎；**bulbar p.**, a serious form of paralytic poliomyelitis in which the medulla oblongata is affected, so that there is often dysfunction of the swallowing mechanism, breathing, and circulation 延髓型脊髓灰质炎；**nonparalytic p.**, the major illness of poliomyelitis when it does not involve paralysis 非麻痹性脊髓灰质炎；**paralytic p.**, the major illness of poliomyelitis when it involves paralysis 麻痹性脊髓灰质炎；**spinal p., spinal paralytic p.**, the classic form of the major illness, a type of paralytic poliomyelitis affecting the spinal cord and characterized primarily by flaccid paralysis in a limb or limbs 脊髓型脊髓灰质炎

po·lio·my·elop·a·thy (po″le-o-mi″ə-lop′ə-the) any disease of the gray matter of the spinal cord 脊髓灰质病

po·li·o·sis (po″le-o′sis) circumscribed loss of pigment of the hair, especially following some pathologic process 白发（症），灰发（症）

po·lio·vi·rus (po′le-o-vi″rəs) a virus that causes poliomyelitis, separable into three serotypes designated types 1, 2, and 3 脊髓灰质炎病毒；**poliovi′ral** *adj.*

pol·len (pol′ən) the male fertilizing element of flowering plants 花粉

pol·lex (pol′əks) pl. *pol′lices* [L.] the thumb 拇指，拇；**p. val′gus**, deviation of the thumb toward the ulnar side 拇外翻；**p. va′rus**, deviation of the thumb toward the radial side 拇内翻

pol·lic·i·za·tion (pol″is-ĭ-za′shən) surgical construction of a thumb from a finger 拇指整复

pol·li·no·sis (pol″ĭ-no′sis) an allergic reaction to pollen; hay fever 花粉症，季节性变应性鼻炎

po·lo·cytes (po′lo-sīts) polar bodies (1) 极体

po·lo·ni·um (Po) (pə-lo′ne-əm) a very rare, highly reactive, radioactive, metalloid element; at. no. 84, at. wt. 209 钋（化学元素）

pol·ox·a·mer (pol-ok′sə-mər) any of a series of nonionic surfactants of the polyoxypropylene-polyoxyethylene copolymer type, used as surfactants, emulsifiers, stabilizers, and food additives 泊洛沙姆，聚羟亚烃（聚羟乙烯聚羟丙烯共聚物），可以作表面活性剂、乳化剂、稳定剂和食品添加剂）

po·lus (po′ləs) pl. *po′li* [L.] 同 pole 极

poly·ad·e·ni·tis (pol″e-ad″ə-ni′tis) inflammation of several glands 多腺炎

poly·ad·e·no·sis (pol″e-ad″ə-no′sis) disorder of several glands, particularly endocrine glands 多腺病（尤指内分泌腺体的）

poly·al·ve·o·lar (pol″e-al-ve′ə-lər) having more than the usual number of alveoli, as a polyalveolar pulmonary lobe 多肺泡的

poly·am·ine (pol″e-am′ēn) any compound of a group of compounds containing two or more amino groups joined by a short hydrocarbon chain; they are important for many cellular growth processes 多胺

poly·an·dry (pol″e-an′dre) 1. polygamy in which a woman is concurrently married to multiple men （一妻）多夫配合；2. animal mating in which the female mates with more than one male （一雌）多雄配合；3. union of two or more male pronuclei with one female pronucleus, resulting in polyploidy of the zygote 多雄配合

poly·an·gi·itis (pol″e-an″je-i′tis) inflammation involving multiple blood or lymph vessels 多血管炎，多淋巴管炎

poly·ar·cu·ate (pol″e-ahr′ku-ət) characterized by multiple arch-shaped curves 多弧（拱／弓）形的

poly·ar·ter·i·tis (pol″e-ahr″tə-ri′tis) 1. multiple inflammatory and destructive arterial lesions 多发性大动脉炎；2. polyarteritis nodosa 结节性多动脉炎；**p. nodo′sa (PAN)**, classically, a form of systemic necrotizing vasculitis involving small to medium-sized arteries with signs and symptoms resulting from infarction and scarring of the affected organ system 结节性多动脉炎

poly·ar·thric (pol″e-ahr′thrik) polyarticular 多关节的

poly·ar·thri·tis (pol″e-ahr-thri′tis) inflammation of several joints 多关节炎；**chronic villous p.**, chronic inflammation of the synovial membrane of several joints 慢性多关节滑膜炎

poly·ar·tic·u·lar (pol″e-ahr-tik′u-lər) affecting many joints 多关节的

poly·atom·ic (pol″e-ə-tom′ik) made up of several atoms 多原子的

poly·ba·sic (pol″e-ba′sik) having several replaceable hydrogen atoms 多碱（价）的多元的

poly·car·bo·phil (pol″e-kahr′bo-fil) a hydrophilic resin that is a bulk-forming laxative and also a gastrointestinal absorbent in the treatment of diarrhea; usually used as *calcium p.* 聚卡波非（较强亲水性，导泻药，也用作治疗腹泻的胃肠吸附剂）

poly·cen·tric (pol″e-sen′trik) having many centers 多中心的；具有多着丝点的，具多着丝粒的

poly·chon·dri·tis (pol″e-kon-dri′tis) inflammation of many cartilages of the body 多软骨炎；**chronic atrophic p., p. chro′nica atro′phicans,** relapsing p. 慢性萎缩性多软骨炎；**relapsing p.,** an acquired idiopathic chronic disease with a tendency to recurrence, marked by inflammatory and degenerative lesions of various cartilaginous structures 复发性多软骨炎

poly·chro·ma·sia (pol″e-kro-ma′zhə) 1. variation in the hemoglobin content of erythrocytes 多染（色）性；2. 同 polychromatophilia

poly·chro·mat·ic (pol″e-kro-mat′ik) manycolored 多色的

poly·chro·mato·cyte (pol″e-kro-mat′o-sīt) a cell stainable with various kinds of stain 多染（性）细胞

poly·chro·mato·phil (pol″e-kro-mat′o-fil) a structure stainable with many kinds of stain 多染（性）细胞

poly·chro·ma·to·phil·ia (pol″e-kro″mə-tofil′e-ə) 1. the property of being stainable with various stains; affinity for all sorts of stains 多染（色）性；2. a condition in which the erythrocytes, on staining, show various shades of blue combined with tinges of pink 多染（性）细胞增多；**polychromatophil′ic** *adj.*

poly·clin·ic (pol″e-klin′ik) a hospital and school where diseases and injuries of all kinds are studied and treated 综合医院

poly·clo·nal (pol″e-klo′nəl) 1. derived from different cells 多细胞系的，多细胞株的；2. of or pertaining to multiple clones 多克隆的

poly·co·ria (pol″e-kor′e-ə) 1. more than one pupil in an eye 多瞳；2. the deposit of reserve material in an organ or tissue so as to produce enlargement 储备质过多

pol·y·cro·tism (pol-ik′rə-tiz-əm) the quality of having several secondary waves to each beat of the pulse 多波脉（现象）；**polycrot′ic** *adj.*

poly·cy·e·sis (pol″e-si-e′sis) multiple pregnancy 多胎妊娠

poly·cys·tic (pol″e-sis′tik) containing many cysts 多囊的

poly·cy·the·mia (pol″e-si-the′me-ə) an increase in the total cell mass of the blood 红细胞增多（症）；**absolute p.,** an increase in red cell mass caused by increased erythropoiesis, which may occur as a compensatory physiologic response to tissue hypoxia or as the principal manifestation of polycythemia vera 绝对红细胞增多；**hypertonic p.,** 同 stress p.；**relative p.,** a decrease in plasma

volume without change in red blood cell mass so that the erythrocytes become more concentrated (elevated hematocrit), which may be an acute transient or a chronic condition 相对性红细胞增多；**p. ru′bra,** 同 p. vera；**secondary p.,** any absolute increase in the total red cell mass other than polycythemia vera, occurring as a physiologic response to tissue hypoxia 继发性红细胞增多（症）；**stress p.,** chronic relative polycythemia usually affecting white, middle-aged, mildly obese males who are active, anxiety-prone, and hypertensive 应激性红细胞增多（症）；**p. ve′ra,** a myeloproliferative disorder of unknown etiology, characterized by abnormal proliferation of all hematopoietic bone marrow elements and an absolute increase in red cell mass and total blood volume, associated frequently with splenomegaly, leukocytosis, and thrombocythemia 真性红细胞增多症

poly·dac·tyl·ism (pol″e-dak′təl-iz-əm) 同 polydactyly

poly·dac·ty·ly (pol″e-dak′tə-le) the presence of more than the usual number of fingers or toes 多指趾（畸形）

poly·di·meth·yl·si·lox·ane (pol″ī-di-meth″əlsilok′sān) a polymeric siloxane in which the substituents are methyl groups; it is the most common form of silicone 聚二甲硅氧烷

poly·dip·sia (pol″e-dip′se-ə) chronic excessive thirst and fluid intake 烦渴，多饮

poly·dys·pla·sia (pol″e-dis-pla′zhə) faulty development in several types of tissue or several organs or systems 多种发育障碍

poly·dys·tro·phy (pol″e-dis′trə-fe) dystrophy of several tissues or structures at the same time 多发性营养不良；**polydystroph′ic** *adj.*；**pseudo-Hurler p.,** mucolipidosis Ⅲ 黏脂贮积症Ⅲ型

poly·em·bry·o·ny (pol″e-em-bri′o-ne) the production of two or more embryos from the same oocyte or seed 多胚性

pol·y·ene (pol′e-ēn) 1. a chemical compound with a carbon chain of four or more atoms and several conjugated double bonds 多烯（烃）；2. any of a group of antifungal antibiotics with such a structure (e.g., amphotericin and nystatin) produced by species of *Streptomyces* that damage cell membranes by forming complexes with sterols 聚烯

poly·es·the·sia (pol″e-es-the′zhə) a sensation as if several points were touched on application of a stimulus to a single point 多处感觉，一物多感（症），复觉

poly·es·tra·di·ol phos·phate (pol″e-es″trə- di′ol) a polymer of estradiol phosphate having estrogenic activity similar to that of estradiol; used in the palliative therapy of prostatic carcinoma 聚磷酸雌二醇（雌激素，用于治疗前列腺癌）

poly·eth·y·lene (pol″e-eth′ə-lēn) polymerized ethylene (−CH$_2$−CH$_2$−)n, a synthetic plastic material, forms of which have been used in reparative surgery 聚乙烯；**p. glycol (PEG)**, a generic name for mixtures of condensation polymers of ethylene oxide and water, available in liquid form (polymers with average molecular weights between 200 and 700) or as waxy solids (average molecular weights above 1000); some are used as pharmaceutical aids, and *p. glycol 3350* is used as a laxative 聚乙二醇

poly·ga·lac·tia (pol″e-gə-lak′she-ə) excessive secretion of milk 泌乳过多

po·lyg·a·my (pə-lig′ə-me) 1. the concurrent marriage of a woman or man to more than one spouse 多婚（多配偶的性关系，一夫多妻或一妻多夫）；2. animal mating in which the individual mates with more than one partner 多配性（一雌多雄或一雄多雌）

poly·gene (pol′e-jēn) a member of a group of non-allelic genes whose interaction has an additive effect on a quantitative character, each one having a small effect individually 多基因

poly·gen·ic (pol″e-jen′ik) pertaining to or determined by multiple different genes 多基因的

poly·glac·tin 910 (pol″e-glak′tin) a filamentous material that is braided and used for absorbable sutures 聚糖乳酸复合物910，一种编织的丝状材料，用于可吸收缝线

poly·glan·du·lar (pol″e-glan′du-lər) 同 pluriglan-dular

poly·glu·ta·mine (pol″e-gloo′tə-mēn) a stretch of glutamine residues in a protein; expanded numbers of such residues are associated with several triplet repeat disorders 多聚谷氨酰胺

poly·graph (pol′e-graf) an apparatus for simultaneously recording blood pressure, pulse, and respiration, and variations in electrical resistance of the skin; popularly known as a lie detector 多种（生理）记录仪（俗称测谎仪）

po·lyg·y·ny (pə-lij′ĭ-ne) 1. polygamy in which a man is married concurrently to more than one woman 一夫多妻（配合）；2. animal mating in which the male mates with more than one female 一雄多雌（配合）；3. union of two or more female pronuclei with one male pronucleus, resulting in polyploidy of the zygote 多配性

poly·gy·ria (pol″e-ji′re-ə) 同 polymicrogyria

poly·he·dral (pol″e-he′drəl) having many sides or surfaces 多面体的

poly·hi·dro·sis (pol″e-hĭ-dro′sis) hyperhidrosis 多汗（症）

poly·hy·dram·ni·os (pol″e-hi-dram′ne-os) excess of amniotic fluid, usually exceeding 2000ml 羊水过多

poly·hy·dric (pol″e-hi′drik) containing more than two hydroxyl groups 多羟（基）的

poly·ion·ic (pol″e-i-on′ik) containing several different ions (e.g., potassium, sodium), as does a polyionic solution 多离子的

poly·iso·pre·noid (pol″e-i″so-pre′noid) any isoprenoid that contains multiple isoprene units, such as rubber 类聚异戊二烯

poly·lac·tic ac·id (pol″e-lak′tik) a hydrophobic hydroxy acid polymer that is formed into granules and used as a surgical dressing for dental extraction sites 聚乳酸（用作牙拔除部位的外科敷料）

poly·lep·tic (pol″e-lep′tik) having many remissions and exacerbations 多次复发的

poly·mas·tia (pol″e-mas′te-ə) the presence of supernumerary mammary glands 多乳房

poly·me·lia (pol″e-me′le-ə) a developmental anomaly characterized by the presence of supernumerary limbs 多肢（畸形）

poly·men·or·rhea (pol″e-men″o-re′ə) abnormally frequent menstruation 月经频繁

poly·mer (pol′ĭ-mər) a compound, usually of high molecular weight, formed by the combination of simpler molecules (monomers); it may be formed without formation of any other product (*addition p.*) or with simultaneous elimination of water or other simple compound (*condensation p.*) 聚合物；**polyme′ric** adj.

po·lym·er·ase (pə-lim′ər-ās) an enzyme that catalyzes polymerization 聚合酶

po·lym·er·iza·tion (pə-lim″ər-ĭ-za′shən) the combining of several simpler molecules (monomers) to form a polymer 聚合作用

po·lym·er·ize (pə-lim′ər-īz) to subject to or to undergo polymerization 聚合

poly·meth·yl meth·ac·ryl·ate (PMMA) (pol″emeth″əl meth-ak′rəl-āt) a thermoplastic acrylic resin formed by polymerization of methyl methacrylate 聚甲基丙烯酸甲酯；另写为 *polymethylmethacrylate*

poly·mi·cro·bi·al (pol″e-mi-kro′be-əl) marked by the presence of several species of microorganisms 多种微生物的

poly·mi·cro·gy·ria (pol″e-mi″kro-ji′re-ə) a developmental anomaly of the brain marked by development of numerous small convolutions (microgyri), causing intellectual disability 多小脑回

poly·morph (pol′e-morf) colloquial term for polymorphonuclear leukocyte 多形核白细胞

poly·mor·phic (pol″e-mor′fik) occurring in several or many forms; appearing in different forms in different developmental stages 多形的，多型的，多形态的

pol·y·mor·phism (pol″e-mor′fiz-əm) 1. the existence within a population or species of several different forms of individuals, or the occurrence of different forms or stages in an individual over time 多态性，多态现象；2. genetic p.; the long-term occurrence in a population of multiple alternative alleles at a locus 遗传多态性；**balanced p.**, a state of equilibrium in which a genetic polymorphism is maintained by a balance between mutation and selection 平衡多态性，平衡多态现象；**restriction fragment length p. (RFLP)**, a genetic polymorphism in DNA sequence that can be detected on the basis of differences in DNA fragment lengths produced by digestion with a specific restriction endonuclease 限制性（内切酶）片段长度多态性；**single nucleotide p. (SNP)**, a genetic polymorphism between two genomes that is based on deletion, insertion, or exchange of a single nucleotide 单核苷酸多态性

pol·y·mor·pho·cel·lu·lar (pol″e-mor″fo-sel′ulər) having cells of many forms 多形细胞的

pol·y·mor·pho·nu·cle·ar (pol″e-mor″fo-noo′-kle-ər) having a nucleus so deeply lobed or so divided as to appear to be multiple 多形核的

pol·y·mor·phous (pol″e-mor′fəs) 同 polymorphic

pol·y·my·al·gia (pol″e-mi-al′jə) pain involving many muscles 多肌痛

pol·y·my·oc·lo·nus (pol″e-mi-ok′lə-nəs) myoclonus in several muscles or groups simultaneously or in rapid succession 多肌阵挛

pol·y·my·op·a·thy (pol″e-mi-op′ə-the) disease affecting several muscles simultaneously 多肌病

pol·y·myo·si·tis (pol″e-mi″o-si′tis) inflammation of several or many muscles at once, along with degenerative and regenerative changes marked by muscle weakness out of proportion to the loss of muscle bulk 多发性肌炎，多肌炎

pol·y·myx·in (pol″e-mik′sin) generic term for antibiotics derived from *Bacillus polymyxa;* they are differentiated by affixing different letters of the alphabet 多黏菌素；**p. B,** the least toxic of the polymyxins; its sulfate is used in the treatment of various gram-negative infections 硫酸多黏菌素 B

pol·y·ne·sic (pol″e-ne′sik) occurring in many foci 多灶性的

pol·y·neu·ral (pol″e-noor′əl) pertaining to or supplied by many nerves 多神经的

pol·y·neu·ral·gia (pol″e-noo-ral′jə) neuralgia of several nerves 多神经痛

pol·y·neu·ri·tis (pol″e-noo-ri′tis) inflammation of

several peripheral nerves simultaneously 多神经炎；**acute febrile p., acute idiopathic p.,** Guillain-Barré syndrome 急性热病性多神经炎

pol·y·neu·ro·myo·si·tis (pol″e-noor″o-mi″osi′tis) polyneuritis with polymyositis 多神经肌炎

pol·y·neu·rop·a·thy (pol″e-noo-rop′ə-the) neuropathy of several peripheral nerves simultaneously 多发性（周围）神经病；**amyloid p.,** polyneuropathy associated with amyloidosis, of either the primary or the familial type; symptoms may include dysfunction of the autonomic nervous system, carpal tunnel syndrome, and sensory disturbances in the limbs 淀粉样多神经病；**chronic inflammatory demyelinating p. (CIDP),** a slowly progressive autoimmune neurologic disorder with demyelination of the peripheral nerves and nerve roots; characterized by progressive weakness and impaired sensory function in the limbs and enlargement of the peripheral nerves and usually by elevated protein in the cerebrospinal fluid 慢性炎性脱髓鞘性多发性神经病；**erythredema p.,** acrodynia 红皮水肿性多（发性）神经病；**familial amyloid p.,** autosomal dominant amyloid polyneuropathy, associated with familial amyloidosis and most commonly involving a mutant form of the protein transthyretin; it may be subclassified on the basis of symptoms and the biochemical composition of the affected fibrils, or on the basis of affected kinships 家族性淀粉样多神经病变

pol·y·neu·ro·ra·dic·u·li·tis (pol″e-noor″o-rə-dik″u-li′tis) Guillain-Barré syndrome 多神经根炎（吉兰-巴雷综合征）

pol·y·nu·cle·ar (pol″e-noo′kle-ər) having several nuclei, multinucleated; said of cells 多核的，多形核的

pol·y·nu·cle·ate (pol″e-noo′kle-āt) 同 polynuclear

pol·y·nu·cleo·tide (pol″e-noo′kle-o-tīd) a linear polymer of mononucleotides 多核苷酸；参见 *nucleic acid*

Pol·y·o·ma·vir·i·dae (pol″e-o″mə-vir″ĭ-de) the polyomaviruses, a family of DNA viruses formerly grouped with the papillomaviruses in the family Papovaviridae. The family contains the single genus *Polyomavirus* 多瘤病毒科

Pol·y·o·ma·vi·rus (pol″e-o′mə-vi″rəs) a genus of the family Papovaviridae that induces tumors in experimental animals. Two species, BK polyomavirus and JC polyomavirus, infect humans 多瘤病毒属

pol·y·o·ma·vi·rus (pol″e-o′mə-vi″rəs) any virus of the family Polyomaviridae 多瘤病毒；**BK p.,** a species of the genus *Polyomavirus* that causes widespread infection in childhood and remains latent in the host; it is believed to cause hemorrhagic cystitis and nephritis in immunocompromised patients BK 多瘤病毒，多瘤病毒属的一种，在儿童期可引起广泛感染，并在宿主中保持潜伏状态；在免疫功能低下的患者中可引起出血性膀胱炎和肾炎；**JC p.**, a species of the genus *Polyomavirus* that causes widespread infection in childhood and remains latent in the host; it can cause progressive multifocal leukoencephalopathy JC 多瘤病毒，多瘤病毒属的一种，在儿童期可引起广泛感染，并在宿主中保持潜伏状态；可引起进行性多灶性白质脑病

poly·opia (pol″e-o′pe-ə) visual perception of several images of a single object 视物是多症

poly·or·chi·dism (pol″e-or′kĭ-diz-əm) the presence of more than two testes 多睾（畸形）

poly·os·tot·ic (pol″e-os-tot′ik) affecting several bones 多骨的

poly·ov·u·lar (pol″e-ov′u-lər) pertaining to or produced from more than one oocyte, as in dizygotic twins 多卵的

poly·ov·u·la·to·ry (pol″e-ov′u-lə-tor″e) discharging several oocytes in one ovarian cycle 多排卵的

poly·ox·yl (pol″e-oks′əl) a group of surfactants consisting of a mixture of mono- and diesters of stearate and polyoxyethylene diols; they are numbered according to the average polymer length of oxyethylene units, e.g., polyoxyl 40 stearate, and many are used in pharmaceutical preparations 聚乙二醇

pol·yp (pol′ip) an abnormal protruding growth from a mucous membrane; originally, but not currently, restricted to those on the nasal mucous membrane 息肉；**adenomatous p.**, a benign neoplastic growth with variable malignant potential, representing proliferation of epithelial tissue in the lumen of the sigmoid colon, rectum, or stomach 腺瘤性息肉；**cervical p.**, a common, innocuous tumor of the cervix uteri that often produces irregular vaginal bleeding 宫颈息肉；**juvenile p's**, small, benign, hemispheric hamartomas of the large intestine sometimes found in children 幼年性息肉；**nasal p's**, focal accumulations of edema fluid in the mucous membrane of the nose, with hyperplasia of the associated submucosal connective tissue 鼻息肉；**retention p's**, juvenile p's 潴留性息肉

pol·yp·ec·to·my (pol″ĭ-pek′tə-me) excision of a polyp 息肉切除术

poly·pep·tide (pol″e-pep′tīd) a peptide containing more than two amino acids linked by peptide bonds 多肽；**vasoactive intestinal p.**, a hormone that has vasoactive properties, stimulates intestinal secretion of water and electrolytes, inhibits gastric secretion, promotes glycogenolysis, causes hyperglycemia,

and stimulates production of pancreatic juice 血管活性肠肽

poly·pep·ti·de·mia (pol″e-pep″tī-de′me-ə) the presence of polypeptides in the blood 多肽血（症）

poly·pha·gia (pol″e-fa′jə) excessive eating 多食；另参见 *bulimia*

poly·pha·lan·gia (pol″e-fə-lan′jə) side-by-side duplication of one or more phalanges in a digit 多指（趾）骨（畸形）

poly·pha·lan·gism (pol″e-fə-lan′jiz-əm) 同 polyphalangia

poly·phar·ma·cy (pol″e-fahr′mə-se) 1. administration of many drugs together 复方药剂；2. administration of excessive medication 给药过多

poly·pho·bia (pol″e-fo′be-ə) irrational fear of many things 多样恐怖

poly·plas·tic (pol″e-plas′tik) 1. containing many structural or constituent elements 多种构造的；2. undergoing many changes of form 多种变形的，多塑性的

poly·ploid (pol′e-ploid) 1. characterized by polyploidy of 多倍体；2. an individual or cell characterized by polyploidy 多倍体生物，多倍体细胞

poly·ploi·dy (pol′e-ploi′de) possession of more than two sets of homologous chromosomes 多倍性

pol·yp·nea (pol″ip-ne′ə) hyperpnea 呼吸过速，呼吸急促，呼吸加快

pol·yp·oid (pol′ĭ-poid) resembling a polyp 息肉状的

poly·po·rous (pol′e-por″əs) having many pores 多孔的

pol·yp·osis (pol″ĭ-po′sis) the formation of numerous polyps 息肉病；**familial adenomatous p.**, an autosomal dominant disorder in which multiple adenomatous polyps with high malignant potential line the intestinal mucosa, especially that of the colon, beginning at about puberty 家族性腺瘤性息肉病；**juvenile p.**, the occurrence of multiple juvenile polyps in the gastrointestinal tract; it can be sporadic or can be an autosomal dominant disorder 幼年性息肉病

pol·yp·ous (pol′ĭ-pəs) polyp-like 息肉的，息肉样的

poly·pro·py·lene (pol″e-pro′pə-lēn) a synthetic, crystalline, thermoplastic polymer with a molecular weight of 40,000 or more and the general formula $(C_3H_5)_n$; uses include nonabsorbable sutures, surgical casts, and the membranes for membrane oxygenators 聚丙烯

poly·pty·chi·al (pol″e-ti′ke-əl) arranged in several layers 多层的，复层的

poly·pus (pol′ĭ-pəs) pl. *pol′ypi* [L.] 同 polyp

poly·ra·dic·u·li·tis (pol″e-rə-dik″u-li′tis) inflammation of the nerve roots 多神经根炎

poly·ra·dic·u·lo·neu·ri·tis (pol″e-rə-dik″u-lonoo-ri′tis) Guillain-Barré syndrome 多神经根神经炎

poly·ra·dic·u·lo·neu·rop·a·thy (pol″e-rə-dik″u-lo-noo-rop′ə-the) 1. any disease of the peripheral nerves and spinal nerve roots 多神经根神经病; 2. acute idiopathic polyneuritis 急性特发性多神经炎

poly·ri·bo·some (pol″e-ri′bo-sōm) a cluster of ribosomes connected with messenger RNA; they play a role in peptide synthesis 多核糖体

poly·sac·cha·ride (pol″e-sak′ə-rīd) a carbohydrate that on hydrolysis yields many monosaccharides 多糖

poly·se·ro·si·tis (pol″e-sēr″o-si′tis) general inflammation of serous membranes, with effusion 多浆膜炎

poly·si·lox·ane (pol″e-si′lok-sān) any of various polymeric siloxanes, particularly the silicones 聚硅氧烷

poly·some (pol′e-sōm) 同 polyribosome

poly·som·nog·ra·phy (pol″e-som-nog′rə-fe) the polygraphic recording during sleep of multiple physiologic variables related to the state and stages of sleep to assess possible biologic causes of sleep disorders 多导睡眠图

poly·so·my (pol″e-so′me) an excess of a particular chromosome 多体性

poly·sor·bate (pol″e-sor′bāt) any of various oleate esters of sorbitol and its anhydrides condensed with polymers of ethylene oxide, numbered to indicate chemical composition and used as surfactant agents 聚山梨酯, 聚山梨醇酯 (表面活性剂)

poly·sper·my (pol″e-spur′me) fertilization of an oocyte by more than one spermatozoon; occurring normally in certain species *(physiologic p.)* and sometimes abnormally in others *(pathologic p.)* 多精入卵, 又称 *polyspermia*

poly·sty·rene (pol″e-sti′rēn) the resin produced by polymerization of styrol, a clear resin of the thermoplastic type, used in the construction of denture bases 聚苯乙烯

poly·syn·ap·tic (pol″e-sĭ-nap′tik) pertaining to or relayed through two or more synapses 多突触的

poly·syn·dac·ty·ly (pol″e-sin-dak′tə-le) association of polydactyly and syndactyly of varying degrees of the hand and foot 多指 (趾) 并指 (趾) 畸形

poly·tef (pol′ĭ-tef) a polymer of tetrafluoroethylene, used as a surgical implant material for many prostheses, such as artificial vessels and orbital floor implants and for many applications in skeletal augmentation and skeletal fixation 聚四氟乙烯

poly·teno·syn·o·vi·tis (pol″e-ten″o-sin″o-vi′tis)

inflammation of several or many tendon sheaths at the same time 多腱鞘炎

poly·the·lia (pol″e-the′le-ə) the presence of supernumerary nipples 多乳头 (畸形)

poly·thi·a·zide (pol″ĭ-thi′ə-zīd) a thiazide diuretic used in the treatment of hypertension and edema 多噻嗪

poly·to·mo·gram (pol″e-to′mo-gram) the record produced by polytomography 多 X 线断层照片

poly·to·mog·ra·phy (pol″e-to-mog′rə-fe) tomography of tissue at several predetermined planes 多 X 线断层照相术

poly·trau·ma (pol″e-traw′mə) the occurrence of injuries to more than one body system 多发性损伤

poly·trich·ia (pol″e-trik′e-ə) hypertrichosis 多毛 (症)

poly·un·sat·u·rat·ed (pol″e-ən-sach″ər-āt″əd) denoting a chemical compound, particularly a fatty acid, having two or more double or triple bonds in its hydrocarbon chain 多不饱和的

poly·uria (pol″e-u′re-ə) excessive secretion of urine 多尿

poly·va·lent (pol″e-va′lənt) multivalent 多价的

poly·vi·nyl (pol″e-vi′nəl) a polymerization product of a monomeric vinyl compound 聚乙烯, 乙烯聚合体; p. alcohol, 聚乙烯醇, 参见 *alcohol* 下词条; p. chloride, a tasteless, odorless, clear, hard resin formed by the polymerization of vinyl chloride; its uses include packaging, clothing, and insulating pipes and wires. Workers in its manufacture are at risk because of the toxicity of vinyl chloride 聚氯乙烯

poly·vi·nyl·pyr·rol·i·done (pol″e-vi″nəl-pī-rōl′ĭ-dōn) povidone 聚乙烯吡咯酮, 聚烯吡酮

poly·zo·o·sper·mia (pol″e-zo″o-spur′me-ə) excessive numbers of highly motile sperm in the semen 多精子症

po·ma·lid·o·mide (poe″ma-lid′o-mide) a thalidomide analog immunomodulator used to treat multiple myeloma; administered with dexamethasone as third-line treatment 泊马度胺

Pom·a·lyst (pom′uh-list) trademark for a preparation of pomalidomide 泊马度胺制剂的商品名

pom·pho·lyx (pom′fo-liks) [Gr.] an intensely pruritic skin eruption on the sides of the digits or on the palms and soles, consisting of small, discrete, round vesicles, typically occurring in repeated self-limited attacks 汗疱疹

po·na·ti·nib (poe-na′tih-nib) a targeted tyrosine kinase inhibitor that blocks native or mutant Bcr-Abl activity to treat chronic myelocytic leukemia or Philadelphia chromosome–positive acute lymphoblastic leukemia in adults who are resistant or intolerant to other tyrosine kinase inhibitors 帕纳替尼（一种靶向酪氨酸激酶抑制药）

pons (ponz) pl. *pon′tes* [L.] 1. any slip of tissue connecting two parts of an organ 桥；2. that part of the central nervous system lying between the medulla oblongata and the midbrain, ventral to the cerebellum 脑桥；参见 *brainstem*；**p. he′patis,** an occasional projection partially bridging the longitudinal fissure of the liver 肝桥

pon·tic (pon′tik) the portion of a dental bridge that substitutes for an absent tooth 桥体（牙）

pon·tic·u·lus (pon-tik′u-ləs) pl. *ponti′culi* [L.] a small ridge or bridgelike structure 小桥，前桥；**pontic′ular** *adj.*

pon·tine (pon′tīn) (pon′tēn) pertaining to the pons 脑桥的

pon·to·bul·bar (pon″to-bul′bər) pertaining to the pons and the region of the medulla oblongata inferior to it 脑桥延髓的

pon·to·cer·e·bel·lar (pon″to-ser′ə-bel′ər) pertaining to the pons and cerebellum 脑桥小脑的

pon·to·mes·en·ce·phal·ic (pon″to-mes′ənsə-fal′ik) pertaining to or involving the pons and the midbrain 脑桥中脑的

PONV postoperative nausea and vomiting 术后恶心呕吐

pool (pool) 1. a common reservoir on which to draw; a supply available to be used by a group 池（集中起来供集体使用）；2. to create such a reservoir or supply, as when mixing plasma from several donors 库（储存多个供体的血浆）；3. an accumulation, as of blood in a part of the body due to retardation of the venous circulation 淤积（由于静脉循环受阻，身体某一部位积累了血液）

POP pelvic organ prolapse 盆腔器官脱垂

pop·lit·e·al (pop-lit′e-əl) pertaining to the area behind the knee 腘的

POR problem-oriented record 针对问题的记录

por·ac·tant al·fa (por-ak′tant al′fə) an extract of porcine lung surfactant used in the treatment of neonatal respiratory distress syndrome 猪肺磷脂，猪肺表面活性物质，用于治疗新生儿呼吸窘迫综合征

por·cine (por′sīn) pertaining to swine 猪的

pore (por) a small opening or empty space 孔，门；**alveolar p's,** openings between adjacent pulmonary alveoli that permit passage of air from one to another 肺泡孔；**nuclear p's,** small octagonal openings in the nuclear envelope at sites where the two nuclear membranes are in contact; together with their associated structures, they form the nuclear pore complex 核孔；**slit p's,** small slitlike spaces between the pedicels of the podocytes of the renal glomerulus 裂孔；**sweat p.,** the pore connecting a sweat duct to the surface of the skin 汗孔

por·en·ceph·a·li·tis (por″en-sef′ə-li′tis) porencephaly associated with an inflammatory process 穿通性脑炎；孔洞脑炎

por·en·ceph·a·ly (por″en-sef′ə-le) development or presence of abnormal cysts or cavities in the brain tissue, usually communicating with a lateral ventricle 脑穿通畸形；**porencephal′ic, porenceph′alous** *adj.*

por·fi·mer (por′fi-mer″) a light-activated antineoplastic related to porphyrin; used as the sodium salt in the treatment of esophageal and non–small-cell lung carcinomas 卟菲尔钠

po·ro·ker·a·to·sis (por″o-ker′ə-to′sis) a hereditary dermatosis marked by a centrifugally spreading hypertrophy of the stratum corneum around the sweat pores followed by atrophy 汗孔角化病，另写为 *p. of Mibelli*；**porokeratot′ic** *adj.*

po·ro·ma (pə-ro′mə) a type of benign adnexal tumor arising in a sweat pore; there are both apocrine and eccrine types 汗孔瘤

po·ro·sis (pə-ro′sis) 1. the formation of the callus in repair of a fractured bone 骨痂形成；2. cavity formation 空洞形成

po·ros·i·ty (pə-ros′ĭ-te) the condition of being porous; a pore 多孔性；孔

por·ous (por′əs) penetrated by pores and open spaces 多孔的；能渗透的

por·phin (por′fin) the fundamental ring structure of four linked pyrrole nuclei around which porphyrins, hemin, cytochromes, and chlorophyll are built 卟吩

por·pho·bi·lin·o·gen (por″fo-bĭ-lin′ə-jən) an intermediary product in the biosynthesis of heme; it is produced in excess and excreted in the urine in acute intermittent porphyria 胆色素原

por·phy·ria (por-fēr′e-ə) any of a group of disturbances of porphyrin metabolism characterized by an increase in formation and excretion of porphyrins or their precursors 卟啉病；**acute intermittent p. (AIP),** an autosomal dominant hepatic porphyria due to a defect of pyrrole metabolism, with recurrent attacks of abdominal pain, gastrointestinal and neurologic disturbances, and excessive amounts of δ-aminolevulinic acid and porphobilinogen in the urine 急性间歇性卟啉病；**congenital erythropoietic p. (CEP),** an autosomal recessive erythropoietic porphyria, with cutaneous photosensitivity leading to mutilating lesions, hemolytic anemia, splenomegaly, excessive urinary excretion of uroporphyrin and coproporphyrin and invariably erythrodontia and hypertrichosis 先天性红细胞生成性卟啉病；

p. cuta′nea tar′da (PCT), porphyria characterized by cutaneous sensitivity that causes scarring bullae, hyperpigmentation, facial hypertrichosis, and sometimes sclerodermatous thickenings and alopecia; it is associated with reduced activity of the enzyme catalyzing the conversion of uroporphyrinogen to coproporphyrinogen in heme biosynthesis, with symptom onset in adulthood precipitated by environmental factors or disease. Type I, the most common, is sporadic; type Ⅱ results from an inherited systemic defect in the enzyme 迟发性皮肤卟啉病；**erythropoietic p.**, that in which excessive formation of porphyrin or its precursors occurs in bone marrow normoblasts, including congenital erythropoietic porphyria and erythropoietic protoporphyria 红细胞生成性卟啉病；**hepatic p.**, that in which the excess formation of porphyrin or its precursors occurs in the liver 肝卟啉病；**hepatoerythropoietic p. (HEP)**, a homozygous form of porphyria cutanea tarda (PCT) type Ⅱ, clincally identical to PCT but with onset in childhood and virtual systemic absence of the affected enzyme activity 肝性红细胞生成性卟啉病；**p. variega′ta, variegate p. (VP)**, an autosomal dominant hepatic porphyria, with various combinations of chronic cutaneous photosensitivity with lesions and extreme skin fragility, attacks of abdominal pain, neuropathy, and gastrointestinal dysfunction, and typically an excess of coproporphyrin and protoporphyrin in bile and feces 复杂性卟啉病

por·phy·rin (por′fə-rin) any of a group of compounds containing the porphin structure to which a variety of side chains are attached, the nature of the side chain indicated by a prefix; they occur in the prosthetic groups of hemoglobins, myoglobin, and cytochromes, complexed with metal ions, and occur free in tissues in porphyrias. The term is sometimes used to include or to denote porphin specifically 卟啉

por·phy·rin·o·gen (por″fə-rin′ə-jən) the reduced form of any porphyrin; they are the functional intermediates in the biosynthesis of heme 卟啉原

por·phy·rin·uria (por″fə-rĭ-nu′re-ə) excess of one or more porphyrins in the urine 卟啉尿

Por·phy·ro·mo·na·da·ceae (por″fĭ-ro-mo″na-da′se-e) a family of gram-negative, rod-shaped bacteria of the phylum Bacteroidetes 卟啉单胞菌科

Por·phy·ro·mo·nas (por″fĭ-ro-mo′nəs) a genus of gram-negative, anaerobic, nonmotile, non–spore-forming, rod-shaped bacteria of the family Porphyromonadaceae that are normal inhabitants of the oral mucous membranes of the oral cavity and have been isolated from oral infections. *P. asaccharoly′ticus* is an important pathogen, causing infections of the head, neck, and other parts of the body 卟啉单胞菌属

por·ta (por′tə) pl. *por′tae* [L.] an entrance, especially the site of entrance to an organ of the blood vessels and other structures supplying or draining it 入口，门；**p. he′patis**, the transverse fissure on the visceral surface of the liver where the portal vein and hepatic artery enter and the hepatic ducts leave 肝门

por·ta·ca·val (por″tə-ka′vəl) pertaining to the portal vein and inferior vena cava 门（静脉与）腔静脉的

por·tal (por′təl) 1. 同 porta；2. pertaining to a porta, especially the porta hepatis 门的（尤指肝门的）

por·tio (por′she-o) pl. *portio′nes* [L.] a part or division 部，部分；**p. supravagina′lis cer′vicis**, the part of the cervix uteri that does not protrude into the vagina 子宫颈阴道上部；**p. vagina′lis cer′vicis**, the portion of the cervix uteri that projects into the vagina 阴道部子宫颈

por·to·en·ter·os·to·my (por″to-en″tər-os′tə-me) surgical anastomosis of the jejunum to a decapsulated area of liver in the porta hepatis region and to the duodenum; done to establish a conduit from the intrahepatic bile ducts to the intestine in biliary atresia 肝门肠造口术

por·tog·ra·phy (por-tog′rə-fe) radiography of the portal vein after injection of opaque material into the superior mesenteric vein or one of its branches during operation *(portal p.)*, or percutaneously into the spleen *(splenic p.)* 门静脉造影术

por·to·sys·tem·ic (por″to-sis-tem′ik) connecting the portal and systemic venous circulations 门体循环的（连接门静脉和体静脉循环的）

po·rus (por′əs) pl. *po′ri* [L.] an opening or pore 孔，门；**p. acus′ticus exter′nus**, the outer end of the external acoustic meatus 外耳门；**p. acus′ticus inter′nus**, the opening of the internal acoustic meatus 内耳门；**p. op′ticus**, the opening in the sclera for passage of the optic nerve 视神经盘中心动脉孔

po·si·tion (pə-zish′ən) 1. a bodily posture or attitude 位置；姿势；2. the relationship of a given point on the presenting part of the fetus to a designated point of the maternal pelvis; see accompanying table 胎位，参见附表。Cf. *presentation* and *lie*；**anatomic p.**, that of the human body standing erect with face and feet pointed anteriorly, and upper limbs at the sides with palms turned forward; used as the position of reference in designating the site or direction of structures of the body 解剖位置；**Bozeman p.**, the knee-elbow position with straps used for support Bozeman 位置；**decubitus p.**, 卧位，参见 *decubitus*；**Fowler p.**, a position in which the patient is sitting straight upright or leaning back slightly; the legs can be straight or bent at the knees 斜坡卧位; **knee-chest p.**, the patient resting on knees and upper chest 膝胸卧位; **knee-elbow p.**, the patient resting on knees and elbows with the chest elevated 膝肘卧位; **lithotomy p.**, the patient supine with hips and knees flexed and thighs abducted and externally rotated 截石位; **Mayer p.**, a radiographic position that gives a unilateral superoinferior view of the temporomandibular joint, external auditory canal, and mastoid and petrous processes 梅耶位置; **Rose p.**, a supine position with the head over the table edge in full extension, to prevent aspiration or swallowing of blood 罗斯卧位; **semi-Fowler p.**, one similar to the Fowler position but with the head less elevated 半坐卧位; **Sims p.**, the patient on the left side and chest, the right knee and thigh drawn up, the left arm along the back 俯卧位; **Trendelenburg p.**, the patient is supine on a surface inclined 45 degrees, head at the lower end and legs flexed over the upper end 头低足高位; **verticosubmental p.**, a radiographic position that gives an axial projection of the mandible, including the coronoid and condyloid processes of the rami, the base of the skull and its foramina, the petrous pyramids, the sphenoidal, posterior ethmoidal, and maxillary sinuses, and the nasal septum 顶颏下位置; **Waters p.**, a radiographic position that gives a posteroanterior view of the maxillary sinus, maxilla, orbits, and zygomatic arches Waters 位

pos·i·tive (poz'ĭ-tiv) 1. having a value greater than zero 正的（数值）; 2. indicating existence or presence, as chromatin-positive 阳性的; 3. characterized by affirmation or cooperation 肯定的。

pos·i·tron (poz'ĭ-tron) the antiparticle of an electron; a positively charged electron 阳电子，正电子

po·sol·o·gy (po-sol'ə-je) the science or a system of dosage 剂量学; **posolog′ic** adj.

post·anal (pōst-a'nəl) behind or beyond the anus 肛门后的

post·au·ric·u·lar (pōst″aw-rik'u-lər) located or performed behind the auricle of the ear 耳后的

post·ax·i·al (pōst-ak'se-əl) behind an axis; in anatomy, referring to the medial (ulnar) aspect of the upper arm and the lateral (fibular) aspect of the lower leg 轴后的

post·bra·chi·al (pōst-bra'ke-əl) on the posterior part of the upper arm 臂后部的

post·cap·il·lary (pōst-kap'ĭ-lar'e) 1. located just to the venous side of a capillary 后毛细血管（毛细血管静脉侧）; 2. venous capillary 静脉性毛细血管

post·ca·va (pōst-ka'və) the inferior vena cava 下腔静脉; **postca′val** adj.

post·cen·tral (pōst-sen'trəl) posterior to a center,

as is the postcentral gyrus 中央后的，中枢后的

post·ci·bal (pōst-si'bəl) 同 postprandial

post·coi·tal (post-koi'təl) after coitus 性交后的

post·di·as·tol·ic (pōst″di-əs-tol'ik) after diastole 舒张期后的

post·di·crot·ic (pōst″di-krot'ik) after the dicrotic elevation of the sphygmogram 重脉（波）后的

pos·te·ri·or (pos-tēr'e-ər) directed toward or situated at the back; opposite of anterior 后的；后面的

pos·tero·an·te·ri·or (pos″tər-o-an-tēr'e-ər) directed from the back toward the front 后前位的

pos·tero·clu·sion (pos″tər-o-kloo'zhən) distocclusion 后拾，远中拾

pos·tero·ex·ter·nal (pos″tər-o-ek-stur'nəl) situated on the outside of a posterior aspect 后外的

pos·tero·in·fe·ri·or (pos″tər-o-in-fēr'e-ər) posterior and inferior 后下的

pos·tero·lat·er·al (pos″tər-o-lat'ər-əl) situated on the side and toward the posterior aspect 后外侧的

pos·tero·me·di·an (pos″tər-o-me'de-ən) situated on the middle of a posterior aspect 后正中的

pos·tero·su·pe·ri·or (pos″tər-o-soo-pēr'e-ər) posterior and superior 后上的

post·gan·gli·on·ic (pōst″gang-gle-on'ik) distal to a ganglion（神经）节后的

post·glo·mer·u·lar (pōst″glo-mer'u-lər) located or occurring distal to a renal glomerulus 肾小球后的

pos·thi·tis (pos-thi'tis) inflammation of the prepuce 包皮炎

post·hyp·not·ic (pōst″hip-not'ik) following the hypnotic state 催眠后的

post·ic·tal (pōst-ik'təl) following a seizure 发作后的

post·in·fec·tious (pōst″in-fek'shəs) occurring after infection 感染后的

post·in·flam·ma·to·ry (pōst″in-flam'ə-tor″e) occurring after or secondary to inflammation 炎症后的

post·ma·tur·i·ty (pōst″mə-choor'ĭ-te) the condition of an infant after a prolonged gestation period 过度成熟（指婴儿）; **postmature′** adj.

post mor·tem (pōst mor'təm) [L.] after death 死后

post·mor·tem (pōst-mor'təm) performed or occurring after death 死后的；事后的

post·na·sal (pōst-na'zəl) posterior to the nose 鼻后的

post·na·tal (pōst-na'təl) occurring after birth, with reference to the newborn 出生后的，生后的，产后的

post·op·er·a·tive (pōst-op-ər-ə'tive) occurring after a surgical operation 手术后的

post par·tum (pōst pahr'təm) [L.] after parturition

产后

post·par·tum (pōst-pahr′təm) occurring after childbirth, with reference to the mother 产后的

post·pran·di·al (pōst-pran′de-əl) occurring after a meal 饭后的，食后的

post·pu·ber·tal (pōst-pu′bər-təl) after puberty 青春期后的，又称 *postpuberal*

post·pu·bes·cent (pōst″pu-bes′ənt) 同 postpubertal

post·re·nal (pōst-re′nəl) 1. located behind a kidney 肾后的；2. occurring after leaving a kidney 肾切除后的

post·si·nu·soi·dal (pōst″si-nə-soi′dəl) located behind a sinusoid or affecting the circulation beyond a sinusoid 窦状隙后的

post·sphe·noid (pōst-sfe′noid) pertaining to the posterior portion of the body of the sphenoid bone 后蝶骨

post·ste·not·ic (pōst″stə-not′ik) located or occurring distal to or beyond a stenosed segment 狭窄后的

post·sy·nap·tic (pōst″sī-nap′tik) distal to or occurring beyond a synapse 突触后的

post·term (pōst-tərm′) extending beyond term; said of a pregnancy or of an infant 过期的（指妊娠或新生儿）

post·trau·mat·ic (pōst″traw-mat′ik) occurring as a result of or after injury 外伤后的

pos·tu·late (pos′tu-lāt) a proposition that is assumed or taken for granted 假定，原则

pos·ture (pos′choor) a position of the body 姿势，体位；**pos′tural** *adj.*

post·vac·ci·nal (pōst-vak′sī-nəl) occurring after vaccination for smallpox 接种后的

pot·a·ble (po′tə-bəl) fit to drink 可饮的

pot·as·se·mia (pot″ə-se′me-ə) hyperkalemia 高钾血症

po·tas·si·um (K) (pə-tas′e-əm) a soft, silvery white, alkali metal element; at. no. 19, at. wt. 39.098. Potassium is the chief cation of intracellular fluid, and many of its salts are used as electrolyte replenishers and systemic and urinary alkalizers, including *p. acetate, p. bicarbonate, p. citrate,* and *p. gluconate* 钾；**p. bitartrate,** a compound administered rectally with sodium bicarbonate to produce carbon dioxide; used for relief of constipation, evacuation of the colon before surgical or diagnostic procedures, and pre- and postpartum bowel emptying 酒石酸氢钾；**p. chloride,** an electrolyte replenisher, KCl 氯化钾；**p. citrate,** a systemic and urinary alkalizer, electrolyte replenisher, and diuretic 枸橼酸钾；**dibasic p. phosphate,** the dipotassium salt, K_2HPO_4; used alone or in combination with other phosphate compounds as an electrolyte replenisher

磷酸氢二钾；**p. hydroxide,** an alkalizer used in pharmaceutical preparations 氢氧化钾；**p. iodide,** a thyroid inhibitor used in the treatment of hyperthyroidism, as a radiation protectant to the thyroid, as an iodine replenisher, and as an antifungal 碘化钾；**monobasic p. phosphate,** the monopotassium salt, KH_2PO_4; used as a buffering agent in pharmaceutical preparations and, alone or in combination with other phosphate compounds, as an electrolyte replenisher, urinary acidifier, and antiurolithic 磷酸二氢钾；**p. permanganate,** the potassium salt of permanganic acid, used as a topical anti-infective, an oxidizing agent, and an antidote for certain poisons 高锰酸钾；**p. phosphate,** a compound combining potassium and phosphoric acid, usually dibasic potassium phosphate 磷酸钾

po·ten·cy (po′tən-se) 1. the ability of the male to perform coitus（男性）性交能力；2. the relationship between the therapeutic effect of a drug and the dose necessary to achieve that effect 药物的效能和效力；3. the ability of an embryonic part to develop and complete its destiny 胚胎的发育能力；**po′tent** *adj.*

po·ten·tial (po-ten′shəl) 1. existing and ready for action, but not active 潜在的，有可能性的；2. the work per unit charge necessary to move a charged body in an electric field from a reference point to another point, measured in volts 电位，电势；**action p. (AP),** the electrical activity developed in a muscle or nerve cell during activity 动作电位；**after-p.,** afterpotential 后电位；**electric p., electrical p.,** 同 potential (2)；**evoked p. (EP),** the electrical signal recorded from a sensory receptor, nerve, muscle, or area of the central nervous system that has been stimulated, usually by electricity 诱发电位；**membrane p.,** the electrical potential across a plasma membrane 膜电位；**resting p.,** the potential difference across the membrane of a normal cell at rest 静息电位；**spike p.,** the initial, very large change in potential of an excitable cell membrane during excitation 峰电位

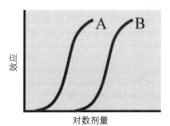

▲ 两种不同效能药物的剂量－效能曲线。药物 A 的效能强于药物 B

po·ten·tial·iza·tion (po-ten″shəl-ĭ-za′shən) 同 potentiation (1)

po·ten·ti·a·tion (po-ten″she-a′shən) 1. increase of the activity of one agent by another so that their combined effect is greater than the sum of the effects they each have alone 增强; 2. 同 posttetanic p.; **posttetanic p.,** an incrementing response without change of action potential amplitude, occurring with repetitive nerve stimulation 强直刺激后增强

po·ten·ti·za·tion (po-ten″tĭ-za′shən) in homeopathy, the process of making a remedy more potent by serial dilution (even to the extent that it is unlikely to contain a single molecule of the original substance) and succussion 药效强化

pouch (pouch) a pocket or sac 囊，窝，凹陷; **abdominovesical p.,** one formed by reflection of the peritoneum from the abdominal wall to the anterior surface of the bladder 腹壁膀胱凹陷; **branchial p.,** pharyngeal p. 鳃囊; **p. of Douglas,** rectouterine p. 道格拉斯腔; **ileoanal p.,** 回肠肛门，参见 *reservoir*; **Kock p.,** 1. a continent ileal reservoir with a capacity of 500 to 1000 ml and a valve made by intussusception of the terminal ileum 可控性回肠膀胱术; 2. a modification of this pouch, used as a neobladder 改良版科克膀胱; **pharyngeal p.,** a lateral endodermal diverticulum of the pharynx that meets a corresponding pharyngeal groove in the embryonic ectoderm, forming a closing membrane 咽囊; **Prussak p.,** a recess in the tympanic membrane between the flaccid part of the membrane and the neck of the malleus 普鲁萨克间隙; **Rathke p.,** a diverticulum from the embryonic buccal cavity from which the anterior lobe of the pituitary is developed 拉特克囊; **rectouterine p., rectovaginal p.,** a sac or recess formed by a fold of the peritoneum dipping down between the rectum and the uterus 直肠子宫陷凹; **rectovesical p.,** the space between the rectum and bladder in the male peritoneal cavity 直肠膀胱陷凹; **Seessel p.,** an outpouching of the embryonic pharynx rostral to the pharyngobasilar fascia and caudal to the Rathke pouch 西赛耳憩室; **vesicouterine p.,** the space between the bladder and the uterus in the female peritoneal cavity 膀胱子宫陷凹

pouch·itis (pouch-i′tis) inflammation of the mucosa, or of the full thickness, of the intestinal wall of an ileal or ileoanal reservoir 囊炎

poul·tice (pōl′tis) a soft, moist mass about the consistency of cooked cereal, spread between layers of muslin, linen, gauze, or towels and applied hot to a given area in order to create moist local heat or counterirritation 泥罨剂，泥敷剂

pound (lb) (pound) a unit of weight in the avoirdupois (453.6 grams, or 16 ounces) or apothecaries' (373.2 grams, or 12 ounces) system 磅

po·vi·done (po′vĭ-dōn) a synthetic polymer used as a dispersing and suspending agent 聚维酮; **p.-iodine,** a complex produced by reacting iodine with povidone; used as a topical antiinfective 聚维酮碘

POW Powassan (virus) 波瓦生病毒

pow·er (pou′ər) 1. capability; potency; the ability to act 力，能力; 2. a measure of magnification, as of a microscope 放大率; 3. the rate at which work is done; symbol P 功率; 符号 P; 4. of a statistical test: the probability of correctly rejecting the null hypothesis when a specified alternative holds true 检验力; **defining p.,** the ability of a lens to make an object clearly visible 清晰度; **resolving p.,** the ability of the eye or of a lens to make small objects that are close together separately visible, thus revealing the structure of an object 分辨力

pox (poks) any eruptive or pustular disease, especially one caused by a virus, such as chickenpox or smallpox 痘

Pox·vi·ri·dae (poks″vir′ĭ-de) the poxviruses, a family of DNA viruses, including the viruses that cause smallpox, cowpox, and paravaccinia. Genera that infect humans are *Orthopoxvirus* and *Parapoxvirus* 痘病毒科

pox·vi·rus (poks′vi-rəs) any virus of the family Poxviridae 痘病毒

PPD pigmented purpuric dermatoses 色素性紫癜性皮肤病; purified protein derivative 纯蛋白衍生物; 参见 *tuberculin*

ppm parts per million 兆比率，百万分之几

PPSV pneumococcal polysaccharide vaccine 肺炎球菌多糖疫苗

PR prosthion（上）牙槽中点; pulmonic regurgitation 肺动脉瓣反流

Pr [符号] praseodymium 镨; presbyopia 老视; prism 棱镜，棱晶

PRA panel-reactive antibody 群反应性抗体

prac·tice (prak′tis) the use of one's knowledge in a particular profession; the practice of medicine is the exercise of one's knowledge for recognition and treatment of disease 实践; **evidence-based p.,** that in which the practitioner systematically finds, appraises, and uses the most current and valid research findings as the basis for clinical decisions. The term is sometimes used to denote evidence-based medicine specifically, but can also include other specialties 循证实践; **family p.,** the medical specialty concerned with the planning and provision of the comprehensive primary health care of all members of a family on a continuing basis 家庭医疗；**general p.,** the provision of comprehensive medical care regardless of age of the patient or presence of a condition that may temporarily require the services of a specialist 综合医疗；**group p.,** 集体医疗，参见 *medicine* 下词条

prac·ti·tion·er (prak-tish′ən-ər) one who has met the requirements of and is engaged in the practice of medicine, dentistry, or nursing 行医者，医师；**nurse p.,** 从业护士，参见 *nurse* 下词条

prag·mat·ag·no·sia (prag″mat-ag-no′zhə) agnosia 物体认识不能，物体失认

prag·mat·am·ne·sia (prag″mat-am-ne′zhə) visual agnosia 物体记忆不能，物体遗忘

praj·na·pa·ra·dha (pruj″nə-pah-rə-thah′) [Sanskrit] in ayurveda, deliberate, willful indulgence in unhealthy practices that leads to unbalanced body functions and disease 在阿育吠陀中，故意放纵不健康的行为，导致身体功能不平衡和疾病

pra·kri·ti (prŭ′kre-the) [Sanskrit] according to ayurveda, a person's underlying characteristic physical and mental constitution and tendencies of expression 依据根据阿育吠陀的说法，一个人的潜在特征，由机体和精神构成，具有表达倾向

pral·i·dox·ime (pral″ĭ-doks′ēm) a cholinesterase reactivator, used as the chloride salt as an antidote in the treatment of organophosphate poisoning and to counteract the effects of overdosage by anticholinesterases used in treating myasthenia gravis 解磷定

pram·i·pex·ole (pram″ĭ-pek′sōl) a dopamine agonist used in the form of the dihydrochloride salt as an antidyskinetic in the treatment of Parkinson disease 普拉克索

pra·mox·ine (prə-mok′sēn) a local anesthetic applied topically as the hydrochloride salt for temporary relief of pain and pruritus associated with skin and anorectal disorders 普莫卡因

pra·na (prah′nə) [Sanskrit] in ayurvedic tradition, the life force or vital energy, which permeates the body and is especially concentrated along the midline in the chakras 生命素；生命能

pra·na·ya·ma (prah″nə-yah′mə) according to ayurveda, breath control, occurring as one of the eight limbs of yoga; used for controlling the energy within the body and the mind and acting as a vitalizing and regenerating force to increase oxygen exchange that can be used for physical healing 调息；控制呼吸；瑜珈修炼的一种呼吸术

pran·di·al (pran′de-əl) pertaining to a meal 膳食的

pra·seo·dym·i·um (Pr) (pra″ze-o-dim′e-əm) a soft, malleable, ductile, silvery white, rare earth element; at. no. 59, at. wt. 140.908 镨（化学元素）

prav·a·stat·in (prav′ə-stat″in) an antihyperlipidemic agent that acts by inhibiting cholesterol synthesis, used as the sodium salt in the treatment of hypercholesterolemia and other forms of dyslipidemia and to lower the risks associated with atherosclerosis and coronary heart disease 普伐他汀（一种胆固醇生物合成抑制药）

prax·i·ol·o·gy (prak″se-ol′ə-je) the science or study of conduct 实践学

pra·zi·quan·tel (pra″zĭ-kwahn′təl) a broadspectrum anthelmintic used for the treatment of a wide variety of fluke and tapeworm infections 吡喹酮

pra·zo·sin (pra′zə-sin) an alpha-adrenergic blocking agent with vasodilator properties, used as the hydrochloride salt in the treatment of hypertension 哌唑嗪

pre·ag·o·nal (pre-ag′ə-nəl) immediately before the death agony 濒死前的

pre·an·es·thet·ic (pre″an-əs-thet′ik) occurring before administration of an anesthetic 前驱麻醉的

pre·au·ric·u·lar (pre″aw-rik′u-lər) in front of the auricle of the ear 耳前的

pre·ax·i·al (pre-ak′se-əl) situated before an axis; in anatomy, referring to the lateral (radial) aspect of the upper arm and the medial (tibial) aspect of the lower leg 轴前的

pre·be·ta·lipo·pro·tein·emia (pre-ba″tə-lip″o-pro″te-ne′me-ə) hyperprebetalipoproteinemia 前 β 脂蛋白血症

pre·can·cer·ous (pre-kan′sər-əs) pertaining to a pathologic process that tends to become malignant 癌前期的

pre·cap·il·lary (pre-kap′ĭ-lar″e) 1. located just to the arterial side of a capillary 前毛细血管；2. arterial capillary 后小动脉

pre·car·di·ac (pre-kahr′de-ak) situated anterior to the heart 心前区的

pre·ca·va (pre-ka′və) the superior vena cava 上腔静脉；**preca′val** adj.

pre·cen·tral (pre-sen′trəl) anterior to a center, as is the precentral gyrus 中央前的，中枢前的

pre·chor·dal (pre-kor′dəl) situated cranial to the notochord 脊索前的

pre·cip·i·tant (pre-sip′ĭ-tənt) a substance that causes precipitation 沉淀剂

pre·cip·i·tate (pre-sip′ĭ-tāt) 1. to cause settling in solid particles of a substance in a solution 使沉淀；2. a deposit of solid particles settled out of a solution 沉淀物；3. occurring with undue rapidity 使突然发生

pre·cip·i·tin (pre-sip′ĭ-tin) an antibody to a soluble antigen that specifically aggregates the macromolecular antigen in vivo or in vitro to give a visible precipitate 沉淀素

pre·cip·i·tin·o·gen (pre-sip″ĭ-tin′o-jən) a soluble antigen that stimulates the formation of and reacts with a precipitin 沉淀原

pre·clin·i·cal (pre-klin′ĭ-kəl) before a disease becomes clinically recognizable 临床前的

pre·clot·ting (pre-klot′ing) the forcing of a patient's blood through the interstices of a knitted vascular prosthesis prior to implantation to render the graft temporarily impervious to blood by short-term deposition of fibrin and platelets in the interstices 预凝血

pre·coc·i·ty (pre-kos′ĭ-te) unusually early development of mental or physical traits 早熟，过早发育；**preco′cious** adj.; **sexual p.**, precocious puberty 性早熟

pre·cog·ni·tion (pre″kog-nish′ən) extrasensory perception of a future event 早知，预见，预知

pre·co·ma (pre-ko′mə) the neuropsychiatric state preceding coma, as in hepatic encephalopathy 前驱昏迷；**precom′atose** adj.

pre·con·scious (pre-kon′shəs) the part of the mind not present in consciousness but readily recalled into it 前意识的

pre·cor·di·um (pre-kor′de-əm) pl. *precor′dia*. The region of the anterior surface of the body covering the heart and lower thorax 心口，心前区；**pre·cor′dial** adj.

pre·cos·tal (pre-kos′təl) in front of the ribs 肋骨前的

pre·cu·ne·us (pre-kos′təl) in front of the ribs 楔前叶

pre·cur·sor (pre′kər-sər) something that precedes. In biologic processes, a substance from which another, usually more active or mature, substance is formed. In clinical medicine, a sign or symptom that heralds another 先兆，预兆；先质，前体；**precur′sory** adj.

pre·di·a·be·tes (pre-di′ə-be′tēz) a state of latent impairment of carbohydrate metabolism in which the criteria for diabetes mellitus are not all satisfied 糖尿病前期

pre·di·as·to·le (pre″di-as′tə-le) the interval immediately preceding diastole 舒张前期；**predi·astol′ic** adj.

pre·di·crot·ic (pre″di-krot′ik) occurring before the dicrotic wave of the sphygmogram 重波前的

pre·di·ges·tion (pre″di-jes′chən) partial artificial digestion of food before its ingestion 预消化

pre·dis·po·si·tion (pre″dis-pə-zish′ən) a latent susceptibility to disease that may be activated under certain conditions 因素

pre·di·ver·tic·u·lar (pre-di″vər-tik′u-lər) denoting a condition of thickening of the muscular wall of the colon and increased intraluminal pressure without evidence of diverticulosis 憩室前的

pred·ni·car·bate (pred″nĭ-kahr′bāt) a synthetic corticosteroid used topically for the relief of inflammation and pruritus in certain dermatoses 泼尼卡酯

pred·nis·o·lone (pred-nis′ə-lōn″) a synthetic glucocorticoid derived from cortisol, used in the form of the base or the acetate, sodium phosphate, or tebutate ester in replacement therapy for adrenocortical insufficiency, as an antiinflammatory, and as an immunosuppressant 泼尼松龙

pred·ni·sone (pred′nĭ-sōn) a synthetic glucocorticoid derived from cortisone, used as an antiinflammatory and immunosuppressant 泼尼松

pre·eclamp·sia (pre″ə-klamp′se-ə) a toxemia of late pregnancy, characterized by hypertension, proteinuria, and edema 先兆子痫

pre·ejec·tion (pre″e-jek′shən) occurring prior to ejection 排泄前期

pre·ex·ci·ta·tion (pre-ek″si-ta′shən) premature activation of a portion of the ventricles due to transmission of cardiac impulses along an accessory pathway not subject to the physiologic delay of the atrioventricular node; sometimes used as a synonym of Wolff-Parkinson-White syndrome 预激（心室部分过早兴奋）；预激综合征

pre·fron·tal (pre-fron′təl) situated in the anterior part of the frontal lobe or region 额叶前部的

pre·gab·a·lin (pre-gab′ə-lin) a derivative of γ-aminobutyric acid (GABA), used for the relief of pain in diabetic neuropathy and postherpetic neuralgia γ-氨基丁酸（GABA）的一种衍生物，用于减轻糖尿病神经经病变和疱疹后神经痛

pre·gan·gli·on·ic (pre″gang-gle-on′ik) proximal to a ganglion（神经）节前的

pre·gen·i·tal (pre-jen′ĭ-təl) antedating the emergence of genital interests 性前期的（生殖器发育前的）

pre·glo·mer·u·lar (pre″glo-mer′u-lər) located or occurring proximal to a renal glomerulus 肾小球前的

preg·nan·cy (preg′nən-se) 1. the condition of having a developing embryo or fetus in the body, after union of an oocyte and spermatozoon 妊娠；2. the period during which one is pregnant 妊娠期，参见 *period* 下 *gestation period*；**preg′nant** adj.; **abdominal p.**, ectopic pregnancy within the abdominal cavity 腹腔妊娠；**ampullar p.**, ectopic pregnancy in the ampulla of the uterine tube 壶腹妊娠；**cervical p.**, ectopic pregnancy within the cervical canal 宫颈妊娠；**combined p.**, simultaneous intrauterine and extrauterine pregnancies 联合妊娠；**cornual p.**, pregnancy in one of the horns of a bicornuate uterus 子宫角妊娠；**ectopic p.**, **extrauterine p.**, development of the embryo outside the uterine cavity 宫外孕；**false p.**, development of the signs of pregnancy without the presence of an embryo 假妊娠；**heterotopic p.**, combined p. 异位妊娠；**interstitial p.**, ectopic pregnancy in the part of the uterine tube within the uterine wall 输卵管间质部妊娠；**intraligamentary p.**, **intraligamentous p.**, ectopic pregnancy within the broad ligament 阔韧带内妊娠；**molar p.**, conversion of the early embryo into a mole 葡萄胎妊娠；**multiple p.**, presence of more than one fetus in the uterus at the same time 多胎妊娠；**mural p.**, 同 interstitial p.；**ovarian p.**, ectopic pregnancy occurring in an ovary 卵巢妊娠；**phantom p.**, false pregnancy due to psychogenic factors 精神性假妊娠；**postterm p.**, one that has extended beyond 42 weeks from the onset of the last menstrual period or 40 completed weeks from conception 过期妊娠；**tubal p.**, ectopic pregnancy within a uterine tube 输卵管妊娠；**tuboabdominal p.**, ectopic pregnancy partly in the fimbriated end of a uterine tube and partly in the abdominal cavity 输卵管腹腔妊娠；**tubo-ovarian p.**, ectopic pregnancy occurring partly in the ovary and partly in a uterine tube 输卵管卵巢妊娠

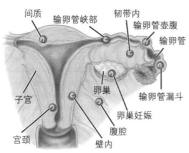

间质　输卵管峡部　韧带内　输卵管壶腹　输卵管　子宫　卵巢　输卵管漏斗　卵巢妊娠　腹腔　宫颈　壁内

▲ 异位妊娠的不同部位

preg·nane (preg′nān) a crystalline saturated steroid hydrocarbon, $C_{21}H_{36}$; β-*pregnane* is the form from which several hormones, including progesterone, are derived; α-*pregnane* is the form excreted in the urine 孕甾烷

preg·nane·di·ol (preg″nān-di′ol) a crystalline, biologically inactive dihydroxy derivative of pregnane, formed by reduction of progesterone and found especially in urine of pregnant women 孕二醇

preg·nane·tri·ol (preg″nān-tri′ol) a metabolite of 17-hydroxyprogesterone; its excretion in the urine is greatly increased in certain disorders of the adrenal cortex 孕三醇

preg·ne·no·lone (preg-nēn′ə-lōn) an intermediate in steroid hormone synthesis 孕烯醇酮

pre·hal·lux (pre-hal′əks) a supernumerary bone of the foot growing from the medial border of the scaphoid bone 踻前骨

pre·hen·sile (pre-hen′sil) adapted for grasping or seizing（适于）抓握的，捕捉的

pre·hen·sion (pre-hen′shən) the act of grasping 抓握，捕捉

pre·hor·mone (pre-hor′mōn) 同 prohormone

pre·hy·oid (pre-hi′oid) in front of the hyoid bone 舌骨前的

pre·ic·tal (pre-ik′təl) occurring before a stroke, seizure, or attack 发作前的

pre·in·va·sive (pre″in-va′siv) not yet invading tissues outside the site of origin 侵袭前的，蔓延前的

pre·kal·li·kre·in (pre″kal-ĭ-kre′in) the proenzyme of plasma kallikrein; it is cleaved and activated by coagulation factor XII 前激肽释放酶

pre·leu·ke·mia (pre-loo-ke′me-ə) myelodysplastic syndrome 白血病前期；**preleuke′mic** *adj.*

pre·lim·bic (pre-lim′bik) in front of a limbus 缘前的

pre-β-lipo·pro·tein (pre″ba-tə-lip″o-pro′tēn) very-low-density lipoprotein 前 β- 脂蛋白

pre·load (pre′lōd) the mechanical state of the heart at the end of diastole, the magnitude of the maximal (end-diastolic) ventricular volume or the end-diastolic pressure stretching the ventricles 前负荷（舒张末期心脏的机械性状态）

pre·ma·lig·nant (pre″mə-lig′nənt) precancerous 恶化前的，癌前期的

pre·ma·tur·i·ty (pre″mə-choor′ĭ-te) underdevelopment; the condition of a premature infant 早熟；早产儿；**premature′** *adj.*

pre·max·il·la (pre″mak-sil′ə) 1. incisive bone 切牙骨；2. the embryonic bone that later fuses with the maxilla to form the incisive bone 前颌

pre·max·il·lary (pre-mak′sĭ-lar′e) 1. in front of the maxilla 颌骨前的；2. pertaining to the premaxilla (incisive bone) 切牙骨的

pre·med·i·ca·tion (pre″med-ĭ-ka′shən) 1. preliminary administration of a drug preceding a diagnostic, therapeutic, or surgical procedure, such as an antibiotic or antianxiety agent 前驱给药法；2. a drug administered for such a purpose 术前用药

pre·me·nar·che·al (pre″mə-nahr′ke-əl) pertaining to the period before menarche（月）经前期的

P

pre·meno·pau·sal (pre″men-o-paw′zəl) preceding menopause 绝经前期的

pre·men·stru·al (pre-men′stroo-əl) occurring before menstruation 经前的

pre·men·stru·um (pre-men′stroo-əm) pl. *premen′strua* [L.] the interval immediately preceding a menstrual period 经前期

pre·mo·lar (P) (pre-mo′lər) 1. 前磨牙，参见 *tooth* 下词条；2. situated in front of the molar teeth 磨牙前的

pre·mor·bid (pre-mor′bid) occurring before development of disease 发病前的

pre·my·elo·blast (pre-mi′ə-lo-blast″) precursor of a myeloblast 前成髓细胞

pre·na·tal (pre-na′təl) preceding birth 产前的，出生前的

pre·neo·plas·tic (pre″ne-o-plas′tik) preceding the development of a tumor 肿瘤（发生）前的

pre·op·tic (pre-op′tik) in front of the optic chiasm 视交叉前的

pre·pa·tel·lar (pre″pə-tel′ər) in front of the patella 髌前的

pre·peri·to·ne·al (pre″per-ī-to-ne′əl) 1. situated between the parietal peritoneum and the anterior abdominal wall 腹膜外的（壁腹膜与前腹壁之间）；2. occurring anterior to the peritoneum 腹膜前的

pre·pro·in·su·lin (pre″pro-in′sə-lin) the precursor of proinsulin, containing an additional polypeptide sequence at the N-terminal 前胰岛素原

pre·pro·pro·tein (pre″pro-pro′tēn) any precursor of a proprotein 前蛋白质

pre·pros·thet·ic (pre″pros-thet′ik) performed or occurring before insertion of a prosthesis 前假体的，修复前的

pre·pu·ber·al (pre-pu′bər-əl) 同 prepubertal

pre·pu·ber·tal (pre-pu′bər-təl) before puberty; pertaining to the period of accelerated growth preceding gonadal maturity 青春期前的

pre·pu·bes·cent (pre″pu-bes′ənt) 同 prepubertal

pre·puce (pre′pūs) 1. a covering fold of skin 包皮；2. 同 p. of penis; **prepu′tial** *adj.*; **p. of clitoris**, a fold capping the clitoris, formed by union of the labia minora and the clitoris 阴蒂包皮; **p. of penis**, foreskin; the fold of skin covering the glans penis 阴茎包皮

pre·pu·ti·o·plas·ty (pre-pu′she-o-plas″te) plastic surgery of the prepuce 包皮背切术

pre·pu·ti·ot·o·my (pre-pu″she-ot′ə-me) incision of the prepuce to relieve phimosis 包皮切开术

pre·pu·ti·um (pre-pu′she-əm) 同 prepuce

pre·py·lor·ic (pre″pi-lor′ik) just proximal to the pylorus 幽门前的

pre·re·nal (pre-re′nəl) 1. located in front of a kidney 肾前的；2. occurring before the kidney is reached 肾前区的

pre·sa·cral (pre-sa′krəl) anterior to or preceding the sacrum 骶骨前的

pres·by·car·dia (pres″be-kahr′de-ə) impaired cardiac function attributed to aging, with senescent changes in the body and no evidence of other cause of heart disease 老年心脏病

pres·by·cu·sis (pres″bĭ-ku′sis) progressive, bilaterally symmetric sensorineural hearing loss occurring with age 老年（性）聋

pres·by·opia (Pr) (pres″be-o′pe-ə) diminution of accommodation of the lens of the eye occurring normally with aging 老视; **presbyop′ic** *adj.*

pre·scrip·tion (prĕ-skrip′shən) a written directive for the preparation and administration of a remedy 命令，指示，规定；另参见 *inscription, signature, subscription, superscription*

pre·se·nile (pre-se′nīl) pertaining to a condition resembling senility but occurring in early or middle life 早老的

pre·sen·ta·tion (pre″zən-ta′shən) 1. the act or process of presenting 表达，呈现；2. that part of the fetus lying over the pelvic inlet; the presenting body part of the fetus 胎先露. Cf. *position* and *lie*; **antigen p.**, the display of antigens bound by major histocompatibility molecules on the surface of specific (antigen-presenting) cells, allowing recognition by T-cell receptors and activation of T cells 抗原表达; **breech p.**, presentation of the fetal buttocks or feet in labor; the feet may be alongside the buttocks *(complete breech p.)*; the legs may be extended against the trunk and the feet lying against the face *(frank breech p.)*; or one or both feet or knees may be prolapsed into the maternal vagina *(incomplete breech p.)* 臀先露; **brow p.**, presentation of the fetal brow in labor 额先露; **cephalic p.**, presentation of any part of the fetal head in labor, whether the vertex, face, or brow 头先露; **compound p.**, prolapse of a limb of the fetus alongside the head in a cephalic presentation or of one or both arms in a breech presentation 复合先露; **footling p.**, presentation of the fetus with one (single footling) or both (double footling) feet prolapsed into the maternal vagina 足先露; **funic p., funis p.**, presentation of the umbilical cord in labor 脐带先露; **placental p.**, placenta previa 前置胎盘; **shoulder p.**, presentation of the fetal shoulder in labor 肩先露，参见 *oblique lie, transverse lie*; **transverse p.**, 横产位，参见 *lie* 下词条; **vertex p.**, that in which the vertex of the fetal head is the presenting part 顶先露

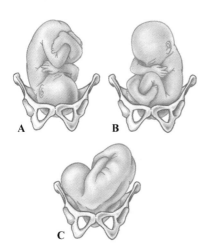

▲ A. 顶先露；B. 臀先露；C. 肩先露

pre·ser·va·tive (prə-zur′və-tiv) a substance or preparation added to a product to destroy or inhibit the multiplication of microorganisms 防腐剂，保护剂

pre·si·nu·soi·dal (pre″si-nə-soi′dəl) located in front of a sinusoid or affecting the circulation before the sinusoids 窦状隙前的

pre·so·mite (pre-so′mīt) referring to embryos before the appearance of somites 体节前胚胎

pre·sphe·noid (pre-sfe′noid) pertaining to the anterior portion of the body of the sphenoid bone 蝶骨前部

pres·sor (pres′or) tending to increase blood pressure 升压的，增压的

pres·so·re·cep·tive (pres″o-re-sep′tiv) sensitive to stimuli due to vasomotor activity 压力感受的

pres·so·re·cep·tor (pres″o-re-sep′tər) baroreceptor 压力感受器

pres·so·sen·si·tive (pres″o-sen′sĭ-tiv) pressoreceptive 压力感受的

pres·sure (*P*) (presh′ər) force per unit area 压力；**arterial p.,** 同 blood p. (2)；**blood p.,** 1. the pressure of blood against the walls of any blood vessel 血压；2. the pressure of blood on the walls of the arteries, dependent on the energy of the heart action, elasticity of the arterial walls, and volume and viscosity of the blood; the *maximum* or *systolic* pressure occurs near the end of the stroke output of the left ventricle, and the *minimum* or *diastolic* late in ventricular diastole 动脉血压；**central venous p. (CVP),** the venous pressure as measured at the right atrium, done by means of a catheter introduced through the median cubital vein to the superior vena cava 中心静脉压；**cerebrospinal p.,** the pressure or tension of the cerebrospinal fluid, normally 100 to 150 mm as measured by the manometer 脑脊液压；**detrusor p.,** the pressure exerted inwards by the detrusor urinae muscles of the bladder wall 逼尿肌压力；**diastolic p., diastolic blood p.,** 舒张压，参见 *blood p.*；**end-diastolic p.,** the pressure in the ventricles at the end of diastole, usually measured in the left ventricle as an approximation of the end-diastolic volume, or preload 舒张末期压力；**intracranial p. (ICP),** pressure of the subarachnoidal fluid 颅内压；**intraocular p.,** the pressure exerted against the outer coats by the contents of the eyeball 眼内压；**intravesical p.,** the pressure exerted on the contents of the urinary bladder; the sum of the intraabdominal pressure from outside the bladder and the detrusor pressure 膀胱内压；**maximum expiratory p. (MEP),** a measure of the strength of respiratory muscles, obtained by having the patient exhale as strongly as possible against a mouthpiece; the maximum value is near total lung capacity 最大呼气压；**maximum inspiratory p. (MIP),** a measure of the strength of respiratory muscles, obtained by having the patient inhale as strongly as possible with the mouth against a mouthpiece; the maximum value is near the residual volume 最大吸气压；**mean arterial p. (MAP),** the average pressure within an artery over a complete cycle of one heartbeat 平均动脉压；**mean circulatory filling p.,** a measure of the average (arterial and venous) pressure necessary to cause filling of the circulation with blood; it varies with blood volume and is directly proportional to the rate of venous return and thus to cardiac output 循环系统平均血充盈压；**negative p.,** pressure less than that of the atmosphere 负压；**oncotic p.,** the osmotic pressure due to the presence of colloids in solution 胶体渗透压；**osmotic p. (ϖ),** the pressure required to prevent osmosis through a semipermeable membrane between a solution and pure solvent; it is proportional to the osmolality of the solution 渗透压；**partial p.,** the pressure exerted by each of the constituents of a mixture of gases 分压；**positive p.,** pressure greater than that of the atmosphere 正压；**positive end-expiratory p. (PEEP),** a method of mechanical ventilation in which pressure is maintained to increase the volume of gas left in the lungs at the end of exhalation, reducing shunting of blood through the lungs and improving gas exchange 呼气末正压；**pulmonary artery wedge p. (PAWP), pulmonary capillary wedge p. (PCWP),** intravascular pressure as measured by a catheter wedged into the distal pulmonary artery; used to measure indirectly the

P

mean left atrial pressure 肺动脉楔压；**pulse p.**, the difference between systolic and diastolic pressures 脉搏压；**systolic p., systolic blood p.**, 收缩压，参见 *blood p.*；**Valsalva leak point p.**, the amount of pressure on the bladder by a Valsalva maneuver at which leakage of urine occurs; a measure of strength of the urethral sphincters 屏气漏尿点压；**venous p.**, the pressure of blood in the veins 静脉压；**wedge p.**, blood pressure measured by a small catheter wedged into a vessel, occluding it, e.g., pulmonary capillary wedge p. 契压；**wedged hepatic vein p.**, the venous pressure measured with a catheter wedged into the hepatic vein; used to locate the site of obstruction in portal hypertension 肝静脉楔压

pre·su·bic·u·lum (pre″soo-bik′u-ləm) a modified six-layered cortex between the subiculum and the main part of the parahippocampal gyrus 海马回沟前部，海马回下脚前部

pre·syn·ap·tic (pre″sĭ-nap′tik) situated or occurring proximal to a synapse 突触前的

pre·sys·to·le (pre-sis′to-le) the interval just before systole 收缩前期

pre·sys·tol·ic (pre″sis-tol′ik) 1. pertaining to the beginning of systole 收缩期期的；2. occurring just before systole 收缩前的

pre·tec·tal (pre-tek′təl) located anterior to the tectum mesencephali 顶盖前的

pre·term (pre-turm′) before completion of the full term; said of pregnancy or of an infant 早产儿

pre·thy·roid (pre-thi′roid) anterior to the thyroid gland or thyroid cartilage 甲状腺前的，甲状软骨前的

pre·tib·i·al (pre-tib′e-əl) in front of the tibia 胫骨前的，胫前的

prev·a·lence (prev′ə-ləns) the number of cases of a specific disease present in a given population at a certain time 患病率

pre·ven·tive (pre-ven′tiv) 1. serving to avert the occurrence of something 预防措施；2. 同 prophylactic (1)

pre·ver·te·bral (pre-vur′tə-brəl) anterior to a vertebra or vertebrae 椎骨前的

pre·ves·i·cal (pre-ves′ĭ-kəl) anterior to the bladder 膀胱前的

Pre·vo·tel·la (pre″vo-tel′ə) a genus of gramnegative, anaerobic, rod-shaped bacteria of the family Prevotellaceae. They are normal inhabitants of the mucous membranes and are found especially in the oral cavity, colon, and vagina; some species cause infection 普雷沃菌属

Pre·vo·tel·la·ceae (pre″vo-tel-a′se-e) a family of gram-negative, rod-shaped bacteria of the phylum Bacteroidetes 普雷沃菌科

pre·zy·got·ic (pre-zi-got′ik) occurring before

completion of fertilization 合子形成前的

PRFM platelet-rich fibrin matrix 富含血小板的纤维蛋白基质

pri·a·pism (pri′ə-piz″əm) persistent abnormal erection of penis, accompanied by pain and tenderness 阴茎异常勃起

prick·le (prik′əl) 1. a small, sharp spine or point 刺；2. a tingling or smarting sensation 刺痛（感）；**prick′ly** *adj.*

pril·o·caine (pril′o-kān) a local anesthetic, used parenterally as the hydrochloride salt or topically, together with lidocaine, as the base 丙胺卡因（局部麻醉药）

prim·a·quine (prim′ah-kwēn) an 8-aminoquinoline compound used as an antimalarial in the form of the phosphate salt 伯氨喹（抗疟药）

pri·ma·ry (pri′mar-e) first in order or in time of development; principal 最初的；主要的

Pri·ma·tes (pri-ma′tēz) the highest order of mammals, including humans, apes, monkeys, and lemurs 灵长目

prim·i·done (prim′ĭ-dōn) an anticonvulsant used in the treatment of generalized tonic-clonic, nocturnal myoclonic, and partial seizures 扑米酮, 扑痫酮, 去氧苯比妥

pri·mi·grav·i·da (pri″mĭ-grav′ĭ-də) a woman pregnant for the first time; gravida I 初孕妇

pri·mip·a·ra (pri-mip′ə-rə) pl. *primip′arae*. Para I; a woman who has had one pregnancy that resulted in one or more viable young 初产妇，参见 *para*；**primip′arous** *adj.*

prim·i·tive (prim′ĭ-tiv) first in point of time; existing in a simple or early form that shows little complexity 初级的，原始的

pri·mor·di·al (pri-mor′de-əl) 同 primitive

pri·mor·di·um (pri-mor′de-əm) pl. *primor′dia* [L.] the earliest indication of an organ or part during embryonic development 原基（器官）

prim·rose (prim′rōz) 1. a plant of the genus *Primula; P. obco′nica* (the cultivated primrose plant) is a common cause of allergic contact dermatitis 报春花（樱草）；2. 同 evening p.；**evening p.**, the herb *Oenothera biennis,* or a preparation of oil from its seeds 月见草，参见 *oil* 下词条

prin·ceps (prin′seps) [L.] principal; chief 主要的，首要的

prin·ci·ple (prin′sĭ-pəl) 1. a chemical component 成分；2. a substance on which certain of the properties of a drug depend 确定药物特性的物质；3. a law of conduct 原则；**p. of infinitesimal dose**, a fundamental principle of homeopathy: the more a remedy is diluted (even to the point that none of the medicinal substance is likely to be present), the more powerful and longer lasting will be its effect 无限小剂量原理; **yin/yang p.**, in Chinese philosophy, the concept of polar complements existing in dynamic equilibrium and always present simultaneously. In traditional Chinese medicine, a disturbance of the proper balance of yin and yang causes disease, and the goal is to maintain or to restore this balance 阴阳规律

pri·on (pri′on) (pre′on) any of several transmissible forms of the core of prion protein that cause a group of neurodegenerative diseases (prion diseases). Prions differ in structure from normal prion protein, lack detectable nucleic acid, and do not elicit an immune response 朊病毒

prism (priz′əm) a solid with a triangular or polygonal cross-section; used to correct deviations of the eyes 棱晶; 棱镜; **adamantine p's, enamel p's**, the structural units of the tooth enamel, consisting of parallel rods or prisms composed mainly of hydroxyapatite crystals and organic substance 釉柱

pris·mo·sphere (priz′mo-sfĕr) a prism combined with a spherical lens 棱球镜

PRK photorefractive keratectomy 屈光性角膜切削术

PRL Prl prolactin 催乳素

p.r.n. [L.] pro re na′ta (according to circumstances) 需要时，必要时

PRO Professional (or Peer) Review Organization 专业（或同行）评审机构

Pro proline 脯氨酸

pro·ac·cel·er·in (pro″ak-sel′ər-in) coagulation factor V 前加速因子，凝血因子V

pro·ac·ti·va·tor (pro-ak′tĭ-va″tər) a precursor of an activator; a factor that reacts with an enzyme to form an activator 激活剂前体

pro·ar·rhyth·mia (pro″ə-rith′me-ə) cardiac arrhythmia that is either drug-induced or drugaggravated 药物性心律失常; **proarrhyth′mic** adj.

pro·at·las (pro-at′ləs) a rudimentary vertebra which in some animals lies in front of the atlas; sometimes seen in humans as an anomaly 前寰椎

prob·a·bil·i·ty (prob″ə-bil′ĭ-te) the likelihood of occurrence of a specified event, often represented as a number between 0 (never) and 1 (always) corresponding to the long-run frequency at which an event occurs in a sequence of random independent trials as the number of trials approaches infinity 概率

pro·band (pro′band) an affected person ascertained independently of relatives in a genetic study 先证者

pro·bang (pro′bang) a flexible rod with a ball, tuft, or sponge at one end; used to apply medications

to or remove matter from the esophagus or larynx 食管探子，除鲠器

probe (prōb) 1. a long, slender instrument for exploring wounds or body cavities or passages 探针; 2. a labeled DNA or RNA sequence used to detect the presence of a complementary nucleic acid sequence by nucleic acid hybridization 核酸（DNA或RNA）探针

pro·ben·e·cid (pro-ben′ə-sid) a uricosuric agent used in the treatment of gout; also used to increase serum concentration of certain antibiotics and other drugs 丙磺舒，羧苯磺胺

pro·bi·ot·ic (pro″bi-ot′ik) a preparation of nonpathogenic microorganisms introduced into the body for their health benefits, such as *Lactobacillus acidophilus* ingested to modify the intestinal microflora 益生菌

pro·cain·amide (pro-kān′ə-mīd) a cardiac depressant used as the hydrochloride salt in the treatment of arrhythmias 普鲁卡因胺

pro·caine (pro′kān) a local anesthetic; the hydrochloride salt is used for infiltration and spinal anesthesia and peripheral nerve block 普鲁卡因

pro·car·ba·zine (pro-kahr′bə-zēn) an alkylating agent used as the hydrochloride salt as an antineoplastic, primarily in the treatment of Hodgkin disease 甲基苄肼

pro·car·boxy·pep·ti·dase (pro″kahr-bok″sepep′tĭ-dās) the inactive precursor of carboxypeptidase, which is converted to the active enzyme by the action of trypsin 羧（基）肽酶原

pro·car·cin·o·gen (pro″kahr-sin′ə-jən) a chemical substance that becomes carcinogenic only after it is altered by metabolic processes 前致癌物

pro·ce·dure (pro-se′jər) the manner of performing something; a method or technique 操作，步骤; **arterial switch p.**, a one-step method for correction of transposition of the great arteries 动脉转位术; **Burch p.**, a type of bladder neck suspension 膀胱颈cooper韧带悬吊术; **endocardial resection p. (ERP)**, surgical removal of a portion of left ventricular endocardium and underlying myocardium containing an arrhythmogenic area from the base of an aneurysm or infarction in order to relieve ventricular tachycardia associated with ischemic heart disease 心内膜切除术; **Fontan p.**, functional correction of tricuspid atresia by anastomosis of, or insertion of a nonvalved prosthesis between, the right atrium and pulmonary artery with closure of the interatrial communication 福沃坦手术; **Pereyra p.**, a type of bladder neck suspension 尿道旁悬吊术

pro·ce·phal·ic (pro″sə-fal′ik) pertaining to the anterior part of the head 头前部的

P

pro·cer·coid (pro-sur′koid) a larval stage of fish tapeworms 前尾蚴

proc·ess (pros′əs) (pro′səs) 1. a prominence or projection, as from a bone 突，突起; 2. a series of operations, events, or steps leading to achievement of a specific result; also, to subject to such a series to produce desired changes 过 程; **acromial p.**, acromion 肩峰; **alveolar p.**, the part of the bone in either the maxilla or mandible surrounding and supporting the teeth 牙槽突; **caudate p.**, the right of the two processes on the caudate lobe of the liver 尾状突; **ciliary p's**, meridionally arranged ridges or folds projecting from the crown of the ciliary body 睫状突; **clinoid p.**, any of three (anterior, medial, and posterior) processes of the sphenoid bone 床状突; **coracoid p.**, a curved process arising from the upper neck of the scapula and overhanging the glenohumeral joint 喙突（肩胛骨）; **coronoid p.**, 1. the anterior part of the upper end of the ramus of the mandible 喙突（下颌骨）; 2. a projection at the proximal end of the ulna 冠突; **ethmoidal p.**, a bony projection above and behind the maxillary process of the inferior nasal concha 筛突; **falciform p.**, 1. (of fascia lata) the lateral margin of the saphenous hiatus 阔筋膜镰状突; 2. (of pelvic fascia) thickening of the superior fascia, from the ischial spine to the pubis 盆筋膜镰状突; 3. Henle ligament Henle 韧带; **frontonasal p.**, 额鼻突，参见 *prominence* 下词条; **funicular p.**, the portion of the tunica vaginalis surrounding the spermatic cord 精索突; **lacrimal p.**, a process of the inferior nasal concha that articulates with the lacrimal bone 泪突; **malar p.**, zygomatic p. of maxilla 颧突（上颌骨）; **mammillary p.**, a tubercle on the superior articular process of each lumbar vertebra（腰椎）乳突; **mandibular p.**, 下颌突，参见 *prominence* 下词条; **mastoid p.**, the conical projection at the base of the mastoid portion of the temporal bone 乳突; **maxillary p.**, 1. 上颌突，参见 *prominence* 下词条; 2. (of inferior nasal concha) a bony process descending from the ethmoid process of the inferior nasal concha 下鼻甲上颌突; **nasal p.**, lateral, 鼻侧突，参见 *prominence* 下词条; **nasal p.**, medial, 鼻中突，参见 *prominence* 下词条; **odontoid p. of axis**, a toothlike projection of the axis that articulates with the atlas 齿突; **pterygoid p.**, one of the wing-shaped processes of the sphenoid bone 翼状突; **spinous p.**, 1. spine (1) 脊柱; 2. a part of a vertebra projecting backward from the arches, giving attachment to the back muscles 棘突; **styloid p.**, a long, pointed projection, especially a long spine projecting downward from the inferior surface of the temporal bone 茎突; **uncinate p.**, any hooklike process, as of a vertebra, the lacrimal bone, or the pancreas 钩突; **xiphoid p.**, the pointed process of cartilage, supported by a core of bone, connected with the lower end of the sternum 剑突; **zygomatic p.**, a projection in three parts, from the frontal bone, temporal bone, and maxilla, by which each articulates with the zygomatic bone 颧突

pro·ces·sus (pro-ses′əs) pl. *proces′sus* [L.] process; used in official names of various anatomic structures 突

pro·chlor·per·a·zine (pro″klor-per′ə-zēn) a phenothiazine derivative, used as the base or the edisylate or maleate salts as an antiemetic and antipsychotic 甲哌氯丙嗪

pro·chon·dral (pro-kon′drəl) occurring before the formation of cartilage 软骨生成前的

pro·ci·den·tia (pro″sĭ-den′shə) prolapse (1) 脱垂

pro·co·ag·u·lant (pro″ko-ag′u-lənt) 1. tending to promote coagulation 促凝血的; 2. a precursor of a natural substance necessary to coagulation of the blood 前凝血质

pro·col·la·gen (pro-kol′ə-jən) the precursor molecule of collagen, synthesized in the fibroblast, osteoblast, etc., and cleaved to form collagen extracellularly 原胶原

pro·con·ver·tin (pro″kən-vur′tin) coagulation factor Ⅶ 凝血因子Ⅶ

pro·cre·a·tion (pro″kre-a′shən) reproduction (1) 生殖; **pro′creative** adj.

proc·tal·gia (prok-tal′jə) pain in the rectum 肛部 痛; **p. fu′gax**, sudden, severe anorectal pain, up to a few minutes in duration, chiefly affecting young men; episodes are infrequent and separated by symptom-free intervals 痉挛性肛部痛，另参见 *syndrome* 下 *levator ani syndrome*

proc·tec·ta·sia (prok″tek-ta′zhə) dilatation of the rectum or anus 直肠扩张

proc·tec·to·my (prok-tek′tə-me) excision of the rectum 直肠切除术

proc·ti·tis (prok-ti′tis) inflammation of the rectum 直肠炎

proc·to·cele (prok′to-sēl″) rectocele 直肠膨出

proc·to·co·li·tis (prok″to-ko-li′tis) inflammation of the colon and rectum 直肠结肠炎

proc·to·de·um (prok″to-de′əm) the ectodermal depression of the caudal end of the embryo, where later the anus is formed 原肛，肛凹

proc·tol·o·gy (prok-tol′ə-je) the branch of medicine concerned with disorders of the rectum and anus 直肠病学; **proctolog′ic** adj.

proc·to·pa·ral·y·sis (prok″to-pə-ral′ĭ-sis) paralysis of the anal and rectal muscles 直肠（肛门）麻痹

proc·to·pexy (prok′to-pek″se) surgical fixation of the rectum 直肠固定术

proc·to·plas·ty (prok′to-plas″te) plastic repair of the rectum 直肠成形术

proc·to·ple·gia (prok″to-ple′jə) 同 proctoparalysis

proc·top·to·sis (prok″top-to′sis) prolapse of the rectum 脱肛，直肠脱垂

proc·tor·rha·phy (prok-tor′ə-fe) surgical repair of the rectum 直肠修补术

proc·to·scope (prok′to-skōp) a speculum or tubular instrument with illumination for inspecting the rectum 直肠镜

proc·to·sig·moi·di·tis (prok″to-sig″moi-di′tis) inflammation of the rectum and sigmoid colon 直肠乙状结肠炎

proc·to·sig·moi·dos·co·py (prok″to-sig″moidos′kə-pe) examination of the rectum and sigmoid colon with the sigmoidoscope 直肠乙状结肠镜检查

proc·to·ste·no·sis (prok″to-stə-no′sis) stricture of the rectum 直肠狭窄

proc·tos·to·my (prok-tos′tə-me) creation of a permanent artificial opening from the body surface into the rectum 直肠造口术

proc·tot·o·my (prok-tot′ə-me) incision of the rectum 直肠切开术

pro·cur·sive (pro-kur′siv) tending to run forward 前奔的

pro·cy·cli·dine (pro-si′klī-dēn) an antidyskinetic used as the hydrochloride salt in the treatment of parkinsonism and for the control of drug-induced extrapyramidal reactions 丙环啶

pro·drome (pro′drōm) a premonitory symptom; a symptom indicating the onset of a disease 前驱症状；**prodro′mal, prodro′mic adj.**

pro·drug (pro′drug′) a compound that, on administration, must undergo chemical conversion by metabolic processes before becoming an active pharmacologic agent; a precursor of a drug 前体药物，前药，潜药

prod·uct (prod′əkt) something produced 产品，产物；**cleavage p.**, a substance formed by splitting of a compound molecule into a simpler one 分裂产物，分解产物；**fibrin degradation p's, fibrinogen degradation p's,fibrin split p's,** the protein fragments produced after digestion of fibrinogen or fibrin by plasmin 纤维蛋白降解产物，纤维蛋白裂解产物；**fission p.**, an isotope, usually radioactive, of an element in the middle of the periodic table, produced by fission of a heavy element under bombardment with high-energy particles 核裂产物；**spallation p's,** the isotopes of many different chemical elements produced in small amounts in nuclear

fission 散裂产物；**substitution p.**, a substance formed by substitution of one atom or radical in a molecule by another atom or radical 取代产物

pro·duc·tive (pro-duk′tiv) producing or forming; said especially of an inflammation that produces new tissue or of a cough that brings forth sputum or mucus 生产的；形成的；产生新组织的（炎症）；生痰的（咳嗽）

pro·en·zyme (pro-en′zīm) an inactive precursor that can be converted to active enzyme 酶原

pro·eryth·ro·blast (pro″ə-rith′ro-blast) the earliest erythrocyte precursor in the *erythrocytic series*, having a large nucleus containing several nucleoli, surrounded by a small amount of cytoplasm 原红细胞

pro·es·tro·gen (pro-es′tro-jən) a substance without estrogenic activity but able to be metabolized in the body to active estrogen 前雌激素

pro·fes·sion·al (pro-fesh′ə-nəl) 1. pertaining to one's profession or occupation 职业的，专业的；2. one who is a specialist in a particular field or occupation 专家；**allied health p.**, a person with special training and licensed when necessary, who works under the supervision of a health professional with responsibilities bearing on patient care 助理卫生人员

pro·file (pro′fīl) 1. a simple outline, as of the side view of the head or face 侧影，轮廓，外形；2. a graph, table, or other summary representing quantitatively a set of characteristics determined by tests 量变曲线，图表

pro·fun·dus (pro-fun′dəs) [L.] deep 深的

pro·gas·trin (pro-gas′trin) an inactive precursor of gastrin 前（促）胃液素，前胃泌素

pro·ger·ia (pro-jēr′e-ə) Hutchinson-Gilford syndrome: an autosomal dominant syndrome characterized by precocious senility, with growth retardation, thinning skin, atherosclerosis, fragile bones, and death in childhood from stroke or coronary artery disease. It is caused by a mutation in the gene encoding the nuclear membrane protein lamin A（儿童的）早老症

pro·ges·ta·tion·al (pro″jəs-ta′shən-əl) 1. referring to that phase of the menstrual cycle just before menstruation, when the corpus luteum is active and the endometrium secreting 促孕的，孕前的；2. having effects similar to those of progesterone 促孕用药的，类黄体酮的，另参见 agent 下词条

pro·ges·te·rone (pro-jes′tə-rōn) the principal progestational hormone liberated by the corpus luteum, adrenal cortex, and placenta, whose function is to prepare the uterus for the reception and development of the fertilized oocyte by inducing

P

transformation of the endometrium from the proliferative to the secretory stage; used as a progestational agent in the treatment of dysfunctional uterine bleeding and abnormalities of the menstrual cycle, as part of postmenopausal hormone replacement therapy, as a test for endogenous estrogen production, and as an adjunct in infertility therapy 孕酮，黄体酮

pro·ges·tin (pro-jes′tin) progestational agent 黄体制剂

pro·ges·to·gen (pro-jes′to-jən) progestational agent 孕激素

pro·glos·sis (pro-glos′is) the tip of the tongue 舌尖

pro·glot·tid (pro-glot′id) one of the segments making up the body of a tapeworm 节片（绦虫），参见 *strobila*

pro·glot·tis (pro-glot′is) pl. *proglot′tides*. Proglottid 节片

prog·na·thism (prog′nə-thiz″əm) abnormal protrusion of one or both jaws, particularly the mandible 凸颌畸形，下颌前突；**prognath′ic, prog′na-thous** *adj.*

prog·no·sis (prog-no′sis) a forecast of the probable course and outcome of a disorder 预后；**prog-nos′tic** *adj.*

pro·grav·id (pro-grav′id) denoting the phase of the endometrium in which it is prepared for pregnancy 孕前的，黄体期的

pro·gres·sion (pro-gresh′ən) 1. the act of moving or walking forward 进行，促进；2. the process of spreading or becoming more severe 进展，发展；**progres′sive** *adj.*

pro·hor·mone (pro-hor′mōn) a hormone preprotein; a biosynthetic, usually intraglandular, hormone precursor, such as proinsulin 激素原

pro·in·su·lin (pro-in′sə-lin) a precursor of insulin, having low biologic activity 胰岛素原

pro·jec·tion (pro-jek′shən) 1. a throwing forward, especially the reference of impressions made on the sense organs to their proper source, so as to locate correctly the objects producing them 投影，投射；2. a connection between the cerebral cortex and other parts of the nervous system or organs of special sense（神经系统的其他部位或特殊感官与大脑皮质间的）神经连接，投射；3. the act of extending or jutting out, or a part that juts out 突出，突出物；4. an unconscious defense mechanism by which a person attributes to someone else unacknowledged ideas, thoughts, feelings, and impulses that they cannot accept as their own 投射（一种下意识的自我防卫机制，指人们把自己也不能接受的，也未被大家公认的观念、思想、

感觉和冲动归咎于他人）；5. the orientation of a radiographic machine in relation to the body or a body part 影像定位

pro·kary·ote (pro-kar′e-ōt) an organism lacking a true nucleus and nuclear membrane, having genetic material composed of a single molecule of naked double-stranded DNA. It lacks a cytoskeleton, and organelles are rare. Most have a true cell wall, and all reproduce by cell fission. They are predominantly unicellular but may have multicellular forms. Prokaryotes are classified into Archaea and Bacteria 原核生物。Cf. *eukaryote*；**prokaryot′ic** *adj.*

pro·ki·net·ic (pro″kī-net′ik) stimulating movement or motility 促动力，原动力

pro·la·bi·um (pro-la′be-əm) the prominent central part of the upper lip 前唇

pro·lac·tin (pro-lak′tin) a hormone of the anterior pituitary that stimulates and sustains lactation in postpartum mammals and shows luteotropic activity in certain mammals 催乳素，促乳素

pro·lac·ti·no·ma (pro-lak″tī-no′mə) a pituitary adenoma that secretes prolactin 催乳素瘤

pro·lapse (pro-laps′) 1. ptosis; the falling down, or downward displacement, of a part or viscus 上睑下垂；脱垂；2. to undergo such displacement 脱出；**anal p.**, protrusion of modified anal skin through the anal orifice 脱肛；**p. of cord**, protrusion of the umbilical cord ahead of the presentingpart of the fetus in labor（分娩时）脐脱垂；**p. of iris**, protrusion of the iris through a wound in the cornea 虹膜脱出；**Morgagni p.**, chronic inflammatory hyperplasia of the mucosa and submucosa of the sacculus laryngis 莫尔加尼脱垂（喉室前脱）；**rectal p.**, protrusion of the rectal mucous membrane through the anus 直肠脱垂；**uterine p., p. of uterus**, downward displacement of the uterus so that the cervix is within the vaginal orifice (*first-degree p.*), the cervix is outside the orifice (*second-degree p.*), or the entire uterus is outside the orifice (*third-degree p.*) 子宫脱垂

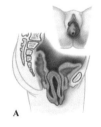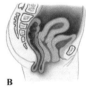

▲ **A. 子宫脱垂；B. 直肠脱垂**

pro·lap·sus (pro-lap′səs) [L.] 同 prolapse

pro·lep·sis (pro-lep′sis) recurrence of a paroxysm before the expected time（疾病的）提早发作；**prolep′tic** adj.

pro·li·dase (pro′lĭ-dās) an enzyme that catalyzes the cleavage of imidodipeptides. In prolidase deficiency, an autosomal recessive aminoacidopathy, imidodipeptides are excreted in urine; other manifestations include chronic skin lesions, impaired motor or cognitive development, frequent infections, and skeletal abnormalities 氨酰（基）脯氨酸二肽酶

pro·lif·er·a·tion (pro-lif″ə-ra′shən) the reproduction or multiplication of similar forms, especially of cells 增殖，增生；**prolif′erative, prolif′erous** adj.

pro·lig·er·ous (pro-lij′ər-əs) producing offspring 繁殖的，多育的

pro·line (Pro, P) (pro′lēn) a cyclic, nonessential amino acid occurring in proteins; it is a major constituent of collagen 脯氨酸

pro·lym·pho·cyte (pro-lim′fo-sīt) a developmental form in the lymphocytic series, intermediate between the lymphoblast and lymphocyte 幼淋巴细胞

pro·mas·ti·gote (pro-mas′tĭ-gōt) a morphologic stage in the life cycle of certain trypanosomatid protozoa, characterized by an anteriorly located kinetoplast and basal body giving rise to a free-flowing flagellum, and no undulating membrane 前鞭毛体

pro·mega·karyo·cyte (pro-meg″ə-kar′e-o-sīt) a precursor in the thrombocytic series, being a cell intermediate between the megakaryoblast and the megakaryocyte 幼巨核细胞，前巨核细胞

pro·meg·a·lo·blast (pro-meg′ə-lo-blast) the earliest form in the abnormal erythrocyte maturation sequence occurring in vitamin B_{12} and folic acid deficiencies; it corresponds to the pronormoblast and develops into a megaloblast 原巨红细胞

pro·meta·phase (pro-met′ə-fās) the phase of cell division that follows prophase, during which the nuclear membrane disintegrates and the chromosomes, attached to the spindle, begin moving toward the cell equator 前中期（指有丝分裂时期，一般自细胞核膜解体时起）

pro·meth·a·zine (pro-meth′ə-zēn) a phenothiazine derivative, used in the form of the hydrochloride salt as an antihistaminic, antiemetic, antivertigo agent, as a sedative, and in the prevention and treatment of motion sickness 异丙嗪

pro·me·thi·um (Pm) (pro-me′the-əm) a radioactive metallic element; at. no. 61, at. wt. 145 钷，（化学元素）

prom·i·nence (prom′ĭ-nəns) a protrusion or projection 隆凸，凸；突出，显著；**frontonasal p.**, frontonasal process; an expansive facial process in the embryo that develops into the forehead and bridge of the nose 额鼻突；**laryngeal p.**, Adam's apple; a subcutaneous prominence on the front of the neck produced by the thyroid cartilage of the larynx 喉结；**mandibular p.**, mandibular process; the ventral prominence formed by bifurcation of the mandibular (first pharyngeal) arch in the embryo, which unites ventrally with its fellow to form the lower jaw 下颌隆起，下颌突；**maxillary p.**, maxillary process; the dorsal prominence formed by bifurcation of the mandibular (first pharyngeal) arch in the embryo, which joins with the ipsilateral medial nasal prominence in the formation of the upper jaw 上颌隆起，上颌突；**nasal p., lateral**, the more lateral of the two limbs of a horseshoe-shaped elevation in the future nasal region of the embryo; it participates in formation of the side and wing of the nose 外侧鼻突；**nasal p., medial**, the more central of the two limbs of a horseshoe-shaped elevation in the future nasal region of the embryo; it joins with the ipsilateral maxillary prominence in the formation of half of the upper jaw 内侧鼻突

PROMM proximal myotonic myopathy 近端肌强直性肌病

pro·mono·cyte (pro-mon′o-sīt) a cell of the monocytic series intermediate between the monoblast and monocyte, with a coarse chromatin structure and one or two nucleoli 幼单核细胞，前单核细胞

prom·on·to·ry (prom′on-tor″e) a projecting process or eminence 岬

pro·mo·ter (prə-mo′tər) 1. a segment of DNA usually occurring upstream from a gene-coding region and acting as a controlling element in the expression of that gene 启动子；2. a substance in a catalyst that increases its rate of activity 促进剂，助催化剂；3. a type of epigenetic carcinogen that promotes neoplastic growth only after initiation by another substance 促癌物

pro·mo·til·i·ty (pro″mo-til′ĭ-te) serving to stimulate motility in the gastrointestinal tract; said of medications 促胃肠动力；促胃肠动力药

pro·my·elo·cyte (pro-mi′ə-lo-sīt) a precursor in the granulocytic series, intermediate between myeloblast and myelocyte, containing a few, as yet undifferentiated, cytoplasmic granules 早幼粒细胞；**promyelocyt′ic** adj.

pro·na·tion (pro-na′shən) the act of assuming the prone position, or the state of being prone. Applied to the hand, the act of turning the palm backward (posteriorly) or downward, performed by medial rotation of the forearm. Applied to the foot, rotation of the front of the foot laterally relative to the back of the foot, resulting in lowering of the medial margin of the foot and hence of the longitudinal arch 俯卧；前旋

prone (prōn) lying face downward 俯卧的

pro·neph·ros (pro-nef′ros) pl. *proneph′roi*. 1. a vestigial excretory structure developing in the embryo before the mesonephros; its duct is later used by the mesonephros, which arises caudal to it 前肾，原肾；2. the definitive excretory organ of primitive fishes 原始鱼类的最终排泄器官；**proneph′ric** *adj.*

pro·nor·mo·blast (pro-nor′mo-blast) term often considered a synonym of *proerythroblast*, but sometimes limited to one in a normal course of erythrocyte maturation, as opposed to a promegaloblast 原正成红细胞，原（始）红细胞

pro·nu·cle·us (pro-noo′kle-əs) the haploid nucleus occurring after meiosis in a germ cell 原核，前核

pro·ot·ic (pro-ot′ik) 同 preauricular

pro·pa·fe·none (pro″pə-fe′nōn) a sodium channel blocking agent acting on the Purkinje fibers and the myocardium; used as the hydrochloride salt as an antiarrhythmic 普罗帕酮（一种钠通道阻滞药，作用于浦肯野纤维和心肌，用于治疗危及生命的心律失常）

prop·a·ga·tion (prop″ə-ga′shən) reproduction (1) 繁殖，增殖；**prop′agative** *adj.*

pro·pa·no·ic ac·id (pro″pə-no′ik) systematic name for propionic acid 丙酸（propionic acid 的系统名）

pro·pan·the·line (pro-pan′thə-lēn) an anticholinergic, used as the bromide salt in the treatment of peptic ulcer and other gastrointestinal disorders 普鲁本辛，丙胺太林（抗胆碱药）

pro·par·a·caine (pro-par′ə-kān) a topical ophthalmic anesthetic; used as the hydrochloride salt 丙美卡因（服用局部麻醉药）

pro·per·din (pro′pər-din) factor P; a nonimmunoglobulin gamma globulin component of the alternative pathway of complement activation 备解素，P因子

pro·peri·to·ne·al (pro″pər-ĭ-to-ne′əl) 同 preperitoneal

pro·phage (pro′fāj) the latent stage of a phage in a lysogenic bacterium, in which the viral genome becomes inserted into a specific portion of the host chromosome and is duplicated in each cell generation 前噬菌体

pro·phase (pro′fāz) the first stage in cell reduplication in either meiosis or mitosis 前期（指ami丝分

裂和减数分裂过程的最早一个时期）

pro·phy·lac·tic (pro″fə-lak′tik) 1. tending to ward off disease; pertaining to prophylaxis 预防性的；2. an agent that tends to ward off disease 预防药，预防剂

pro·phy·lax·is (pro″fə-lak′sis) prevention of disease; preventive treatment（疾病的）预防，预防法

pro·pi·o·nate (pro′pe-ə-nāt) any salt of propionic acid 丙酸盐

Pro·pi·on·i·bac·te·ri·a·ceae (pro″pe-on″ĭ-bak-tēr′e-a′se-e) a family of gram-positive rodshaped or filamentous bacteria of the order Actinomycetales; organisms are inhabitants of the skin and respiratory and intestinal tracts and sometimes cause soft tissue infections 丙酸杆菌科

Pro·pi·on·i·bac·te·ri·um (pro″pe-on″ĭ-baktēr′e-əm) a genus of gram-positive bacteria of the family Propionibacteriaceae; they are found as saprophytes in humans, animals, and dairy products and sometimes cause soft tissue infections 丙酸杆菌属

pro·pi·on·ic ac·id (pro″pe-on′ik) a 3-carbon saturated fatty acid produced as a fermentation product by several species of bacteria; its salts, calcium and sodium propionate, are used as preservatives for food and pharmaceuticals 丙酸

pro·pi·on·ic·ac·i·de·mia (pro″pe-on″ik-as″ĭ-de′me-ə) 1. an autosomal recessive aminoacidopathy characterized by an excess of propionic acid in the blood and urine, with ketosis, acidosis, hyperglycinemia, hyperglycinuria, and often neurologic complicis due to deficiency of an enzyme involved in amino acid and fatty acid catabolism 丙酸血症；2. excess of propionic acid in the blood 血液内丙酸过多

pro·po·fol (pro′po-fol) a short-acting sedative and hypnotic used as a general anesthetic and adjunct to anesthesia 丙泊酚，异丙酚

pro·pos·i·tus (pro-poz′ĭ-təs) pl. *propo′siti* [L.] proband; often specifically the first proband to be ascertained（遗传病史研究中的）渊源者；（常特指第一个遗传疾病的）先证者

pro·poxy·phene (pro-pok′sĭ-fēn) an opioid analgesic structurally related to methadone, used as the hydrochloride and napsylate salts 丙氧芬

pro·pran·o·lol (pro-pran′ə-lol) a β -adrenergic blocking agent, used as the hydrochloride salt in the treatment and prophylaxis of certain cardiac disorders, the treatment of tremors and of inoperable pheochromocytomas, and the prophylaxis of migraine 普萘洛尔，心得安（一种 β-受体阻滞药，用于治疗和预防心律不齐和偏头痛，治疗心颤及不宜手术的嗜铬细胞瘤亦

有效）

pro·pri·e·tary (pro-pri′ə-tar-e) protected against free competition as to name, composition, or manufacturing process by patent, trademark, copyright, or other means 专有的，专卖的

pro·prio·cep·tion (pro″pre-o-sep′shən) perception mediated by proprioceptors or proprioceptive tissues 本体感受

pro·prio·cep·tor (pro″pre-o-sep′tər) any of the sensory nerve endings that give information concerning movements and position of the body; they occur chiefly in muscles, tendons, and joint capsules; receptors in the labyrinth may be included 本体感受器; **propriocep′tive** adj.

pro·pro·tein (pro-pro′tēn) a protein that is cleaved to form a smaller protein, e.g., proinsulin, the precursor of insulin 蛋白质原

prop·tom·e·ter (prop-tom′ə-tər) an instrument for measuring the degree of exophthalmos 突眼计

prop·to·sis (prop-to′sis) forward displacement or bulging, especially of the eye 突出，前垂（尤指眼）

pro·pul·sion (pro-pul′shən) 1. a tendency to fall forward in walking（走路时）前倾，前趋; 2. festination 慌张步态

pro·pyl (pro′pəl) the univalent radical $CH_3CH_2CH_2-$, from propane 丙基

pro·pyl·ene (pro′pə-lēn) a gaseous hydrocarbon, $CH_3CH=CH_2$ 丙烯; **p. glycol**, a colorless viscous liquid used as a humectant and solvent in pharmaceutical preparations 丙二醇

pro·pyl·thio·ura·cil (pro″pəl-thi″o-u′rə-sil) a thyroid inhibitor used in the treatment of hyperthyroidism 丙硫氧嘧啶

pro re na·ta (p.r.n.) (pro re na′tə) [L.] according to circumstances（处方用语）需要时，必要时

pro·ren·nin (pro-ren′in) the zymogen (proenzyme) in the gastric glands that is converted to rennin 原肾素，高血压蛋白酶原（胃腺中转化为肾素的酶原）

pro·ru·bri·cyte (pro-roo′brĭ-sīt) basophilic erythroblast 早幼红细胞，嗜碱性成红细胞

pro·se·cre·tin (pro″se-kre′tin) the precursor of secretin 前分泌素，原促胰液素

pro·sec·tion (pro-sek′shən) carefully programmed dissection for demonstration of anatomic structure（示教）解剖

pro·sec·tor (pro-sek′tər) [L.] one who dissects anatomic subjects for demonstration（示教）解剖员

pros·en·ceph·a·lon (pros″ən-sef′ə-lon) forebrain. 1. the part of the brain developed from the anterior of the three primary brain vesicles, comprising the diencephalon and cerebrum 前脑; 2. the most anterior of the primary brain vesicles, later dividing into the cerebrum and diencephalon 脑前部

proso·de·mic (pros″o-dem′ik) passing directly from one person to another; said of disease（以个人接触的方式）缓渐流行的（指疾病）

proso·pag·no·sia (pros″o-pag-no′zhə) inability to recognize faces due to damage to the underside of both occipital lobes 面部失认，指由于双侧枕叶下部受损而丧失辨认面貌的能力

proso·pla·sia (pros″o-pla′zhə) 1. abnormal differentiation of tissue（组织）分化异常; 2. development into a higher level of organization or function 进行性分化

pros·o·po·ple·gia (pros″o-po-ple′jə) facial paralysis 面瘫，面神经麻痹; **prosopople′gic** adj.

pros·o·pos·chi·sis (pros″o-pos′kĭ-sis) facial cleft (2) 面裂畸形

pros·ta·cy·clin (pros″tə-si′klin) a prostaglandin, PGI_2, synthesized by endothelial cells lining the cardiovascular system; it is a potent vasodilator and inhibitor of platelet aggregation. It is used pharmaceutically as *epoprostenol* 前列环素

pros·ta·glan·din (pros″tə-glan′din) any of a group of naturally occurring, chemically related fatty acids that stimulate contractility of the uterine and other smooth muscle and have the ability to lower blood pressure, regulate acid secretion of the stomach, regulate body temperature and platelet aggregation, and control inflammation and vascular permeability; they also affect the action of certain hormones. Nine primary types are labeled A through I, the degree of saturation of the side chain of each being designated by subscripts 1, 2, and 3. The types of prostaglandins are abbreviated PGE_2, $PGF_{2\alpha}$, and so on 前列腺素

pros·ta·glan·din syn·thase (pros″tə-glan′din sin′thās) an enzyme catalyzing the initial steps in the synthesis of prostaglandins from arachidonic acid; it comprises the component activities of cyclooxygenase, catalyzing cyclization and oxidation reactions, and peroxidase, catalyzing a reduction reaction 前列腺素合成酶

pros·ta·noid (pros′tə-noid) any of a group of complex fatty acids derived from arachidonic acid, including the prostaglandins, prostanoic acid, and the thromboxanes 前列腺素类（化合物）

pros·tate (pros′tāt) a gland surrounding the bladder neck and urethra in the male; it contributes a secretion to the semen 前列腺; **prostat′ic** adj.; **female p.,** paraurethral glands 尿道旁腺

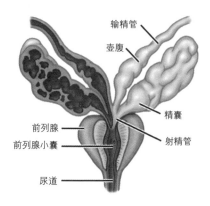

输精管

壶腹

精囊

前列腺

前列腺小囊

射精管

尿道

▲ 前列腺和精囊

pros·ta·tec·to·my (pros″tə-tek′tə-me) excision of all or part of the prostate 前列腺切除术；**radical p.**, removal of the prostate with its capsule, seminal vesicles, ductus deferens, some pelvic fasciae, and sometimes pelvic lymph nodes; performed via either the retropubic or the perineal route 根治性前列腺切除术；**radical retropubic p.**, radical prostatectomy through the retropubic space via a suprapubic incision 耻骨后根治性前列腺切除术；**suprapubic transvesical p.**, removal of the prostate through a suprapubic incision and an incision in the urinary bladder 耻骨后经膀胱前列腺切除术

pros·ta·tism (pros′tə-tiz″əm) a symptom complex resulting from compression or obstruction of the urethra, due most commonly to nodular hyperplasia of the prostate 前列腺病态

pros·ta·ti·tis (pros″tə-ti′tis) inflammation of the prostate 前列腺炎；**prostatit′ic** adj.；**allergic p.**, **eosinophilic p.**, a condition seen in certain allergies, characterized by diffuse infiltration of the prostate by eosinophils, with small foci of fibrinoid necrosis 过敏性前列腺炎，嗜酸性前列腺炎；**nonspecific granulomatous p.**, prostatitis characterized by focal or diffuse tissue infiltration by peculiar, large, pale macrophages 非特异性肉芽肿性前列腺炎

pros·ta·to·cys·ti·tis (pros″tə-to-sis-ti′tis) inflammation of the bladder, bladder neck, and prostatic urethra 前列腺膀胱炎

pros·ta·to·cys·tot·o·my (pros″tə-to-sis-tot′ə-me) incision of the bladder and prostate 前列腺膀胱切开术

pros·ta·to·dyn·ia (pros″tə-to-din′e-ə) pain in the prostate 前列腺痛（症）

pros·ta·to·li·thot·o·my (pros″tə-to-lī-thot′ə-me) incision of the prostate for removal of a calculus 前列腺石切除术

pros·ta·to·meg·a·ly (pros″tə-to-meg′ə-le) enlargement of the prostate 前列腺肥大

pros·ta·tor·rhea (pros″tə-to-re′ə) a discharge from the prostate 前列腺液溢

pros·ta·tot·o·my (pros″tə-tot′ə-me) surgical incision of the prostate 前列腺切开术

pros·ta·to·ve·sic·u·lec·to·my (pros″tə-to-və-sik″u-lek′tə-me) excision of the prostate and seminal vesicles 前列腺精囊切除术

pros·ta·to·ve·sic·u·li·tis (pros″tə-to-və-sik″uli′tis) inflammation of the prostate and seminal vesicles 前列腺及精囊炎

pros·the·sis (pros-the′sis) pl. *prosthe′ses* [Gr.] an artificial substitute for a missing body part, such as an arm, leg, eye, or tooth; used for functional or cosmetic reasons, or both 假体；赝复体；**prosthet′ic** adj.；**penile p.**, a semirigid rod or inflatable device implanted in the penis to provide an erection for men with organic impotence 阴茎假体，人工阴茎

pros·thi·on (PR) (pros′the-on) the point on the maxillary alveolar process that projects most anteriorly in the midline（上）牙槽中点

pros·tho·don·tics (pros″tho-don′tiks) the branch of dentistry dealing with construction of artificial appliances designed to restore and maintain oral function by replacing missing teeth and sometimes other oral structures or parts of the face 假牙修复学，假牙修复术

pros·tra·tion (pros-tra′shən) extreme exhaustion or lack of energy or power 衰竭，虚脱；**heat p.**, 热虚脱，中暑虚脱，参见 *exhaustion* 下词条

pro·tac·tin·i·um (Pa) (pro″tak-tin′e-əm) a dense, silvery gray, radioactive, metallic element; at. no. 91, at. wt. 231.036 镤（化学元素）

pro·ta·mine (pro′tə-mēn) one of a class of basic proteins occurring in the sperm of certain fish, having the property of neutralizing heparin; the sulfate salt is used as an antidote to heparin overdosage 鱼精蛋白

pro·ta·nom·a·ly (pro″tə-nom′ə-le) anomalous trichromatic vision with defective perception of red 红色觉变常

pro·ta·no·pia (pro″tə-no′pe-ə) dichromatic vision with perception of two hues only (blue and yellow) of the normal four primaries, lacking that for red and green and their derivatives 甲型色盲，红绿色盲；**protanop′ic** adj.

pro·te·ase (pro′te-ās) endopeptidase 蛋白酶

pro·te·a·some (pro′te-ə-sōm) a large, cylindrical protease complex that degrades intracellular proteins that have been marked by the attachment of ubiquitin 蛋白酶体

pro·tec·tant (pro-tek′tənt) 同 protective

pro·tec·tin (pro-tek′tin) a membrane-bound protein that prevents insertion of the membrane attack complex into the membrane, thereby protecting normal bystander cells from complement-induced lysis 保护素，保护蛋白

pro·tec·tive (pro-tek′tiv) 1. affording defense or immunity 保护的，免疫的；2. an agent affording defense or immunity 保护剂，免疫（物）

pro·tein (pro′tēn) any of a group of complex organic compounds containing carbon, hydrogen, oxygen, nitrogen, and sulfur. Proteins, the principal constituents of the protoplasm of all cells, are of high molecular weight and consist of α-amino acids joined by peptide linkages. Twenty different amino acids are commonly found in proteins, each protein having a unique, genetically defined amino acid sequence that determines its specific shape and function. Their roles include enzymatic catalysis, transport and storage, coordinated motion, nerve impulse generation and transmission, control of growth and differentiation, immunity, and mechanical support 蛋白质；AA p., 淀精样 A 蛋白，AA 蛋白，参见 amyloid 下词条；acute-phase p., any of the nonantibody proteins found in increased amounts in serum during the acutephase response, including C-reactive protein and fibrinogen 急性期蛋白；AL p., 淀粉样轻链蛋白，参见 amyloid 下词条；amyloid A p., AA amyloid 淀粉样 A 蛋白；amyloid light-chain p., AL amyloid 淀粉样轻链蛋白；amyloid precursor p. (APP), a large transmembrane glycoprotein expressed on the cell surface and of uncertain function; endocytosis and cleavage can produce abnormal 40- to 43-amino acid peptides, which aggregate to form Aβ amyloid, associated with Alzheimer disease 淀粉样前体蛋白；Bence Jones p., a low-molecular-weight, heatsensitive urinary protein found in multiple myeloma, which coagulates when heated to 45° to 55℃ and redissolves partially or wholly on boiling 本周蛋白；binding p., 1. any protein able to specifically and reversibly bind other substances, such as ions, sugars, nucleic acids, or amino acids; they are believed to function in transport 结合蛋白；2. 同 transport p.; bone morphogenetic p. (BMP), any of a group of related proteins involved in induction of bone and cartilage formation and important in embryonic patterning and early skeleton formation 骨形态发生蛋白，骨形成蛋白；p. C, a vitamin K–dependent plasma protein that, when activated by thrombin, inhibits the clotting cascade by enzymatic cleavage of factors Ⅴ and Ⅷ and also enhances fibrinolysis. Deficiency results in recurrent venous thrombosis 蛋白 C；C4-binding p., a complement system regulatory protein that inhibits activation of the classical pathway C4 结合蛋白；complete p., one containing the essential amino acids in the proportion required in the human diet 完全蛋白；compound p., conjugated p., any of those in which the protein is combined with nonprotein molecules or prosthetic groups other than as a salt; e.g., nucleoproteins, glycoproteins, lipoproteins, and metalloproteins 复合蛋白，结合蛋白；C-reactive p., a globulin that forms a precipitate with the C-polysaccharide of the pneumococcus; the most predominant of the acutephase proteins C 反应蛋白；fibrillar p., any of the generally insoluble proteins that comprise the principal structural proteins of the body, e.g., collagens, elastins, keratin, actin, and myosin 纤维蛋白；G p., any of a family of proteins of the intracellular portion of the plasma membrane that bind activated receptor complexes and, through conformational changes and cyclic binding and hydrolysis of GTP, effect alterations in channel gating and so couple cell surface receptors to intracellular responses 鸟苷酸结合蛋白，G 蛋白；glial fibrillary acidic p. (GFAP), the protein forming the glial filaments of the astrocytes and used as an immunohistochemical marker of these cells 胶质细胞原纤维酸性蛋白，胶质纤维酸性蛋白；globular p., any of the water-soluble proteins yielding only α-amino acids on hydrolysis, including most of the proteins of the body, e.g., albumins and globulins 球蛋白；guanyl-nucleotide–binding p., 同 G p.；heat shock p., any of a group of proteins first identified as synthesized in response to hyperthermia, hypoxia, or other stresses and believed to enable cells to recover from these stresses. Many have been found to be molecular chaperones and are synthesized abundantly regardless of stress 热休克蛋白；HIV p's, proteins specific to the human immunodeficiency virus; the presence of certain specific HIV proteins together with certain HIV glycoproteins constitutes a serologic diagnosis of HIV infection HIV 蛋白；incomplete p., one having a ratio of essential amino acids different from that of the average body protein 不完全蛋白；membrane cofactor p. (MCP), an inhibitor of complement activation found in most blood cells, endothelial and epithelial cells, and fibroblasts 细胞膜辅助蛋白；microtubule-associated p. (MAP), any of a large family of proteins that regulate microtubule assembly and structure 微管相关蛋白；myeloma p., any of the abnormal immunoglobulins or fragments, such as Bence Jones proteins, secreted by myeloma cells 骨髓瘤蛋白；partial p., 同 incomplete p.；plasma p's, all the proteins present in the blood plasma, including the

P

immunoglobulins 血浆蛋白; **prion p. (PrP)**, a constitutively expressed cell surface glycoprotein, 33 to 35 kD, of uncertain function. The protease-resistant core is the functional, and perhaps only, component of prions; several abnormal forms have been identified and are responsible for prion disease 朊病毒蛋白; **p. S**, a vitamin K–dependent plasma protein that inhibits blood clotting by serving as a cofactor for activated protein C 蛋白 S; **S p.**, S 蛋白, 玻连蛋白, 参见 *vitronectin*; **SAA p.**, 同 serum amyloid A p.; **serum p.'s**, proteins in the blood serum, including immunoglobulins, albumin, complement, coagulation factors, and enzymes 血清蛋白; **serum amyloid A p., SAA p.**; a high-molecular-weight protein synthesized in the liver; it is an acutephase protein and circulates in association with HDL lipoprotein. It is the precursor to AA amyloid and accumulates in inflammation 血清淀粉样蛋白 A; **sphingolipid activator p. (SAP)**, any of a group of nonenzyme lysosomal proteins that stimulate the actions of specific lysosomal hydrolases by binding and solubilizing their sphingolipid substrates 鞘脂激活蛋白; **transport p.**, a protein that binds to a substance and provides a transport system for it, either in the plasma or across a plasma membrane 运载蛋白, 转运蛋白

pro·tein·a·ceous (pro″tēn-a′shəs) pertaining to or of the nature of protein 蛋白质的, 蛋白性质的

pro·tein·ase (pro′tēn-ās) endopeptidase 蛋白酶

pro·tein·emia (pro″tēn-e′me-ə) excess of protein in the blood 蛋白血症

pro·tein ki·nase (pro′tēn ki′nās) an enzyme that catalyzes the phosphorylation of serine, threonine, or tyrosine groups in enzymes or other proteins, using ATP as a phosphate donor 蛋白激酶

pro·tein·o·sis (pro″tēn-o′sis) the accumulation of excess protein in the tissues 蛋白沉积（症）; **lipoid p.**, an autosomal recessive disorder of lipid metabolism marked by hyaline deposits in the skin and mucosa of the mouth, pharynx, laryngopharynx, and larynx, resulting in hoarseness due to infiltration of the vocal cords. Skin lesions occur mainly on the face and limbs 类脂质蛋白沉积症; **pulmonary alveolar p.**, a chronic lung disease in which the distal alveoli become filled with eosinophilic, probably endogenous, proteinaceous material that prevents ventilation of affected areas 肺泡蛋白沉积症, 肺泡蛋白沉着症

pro·tein-ty·ro·sine ki·nase (pro′tēn ti′ro-sēn ki′nās) a group comprising the protein kinases that catalyze the phosphorylation of tyrosine residues in specific proteins. The enzymes play a variety of roles in the control of cell growth and differen-tiation. Many of the known oncogenes and proto-oncogenes encode protein-tyrosine kinases, and unregulated activation of these enzymes can lead to oncogenesis as well as to benign proliferative conditions 蛋白 - 酪氨酸激酶

pro·tein·uria (pro″te-nu′re-ə) an excess of serum proteins in the urine, as in renal disease or after strenuous exercise 蛋白尿（症）; **proteinu′ric** *adj.*

Pro·teo·bac·te·ria (pro″te-o-bak-tēr′e-ə) a large, diverse phylum of gram-negative bacteria, comprising over 1300 species 变形菌门

pro·teo·gly·can (pro″te-o-gli′kan) any of a group of polysaccharide-protein conjugates present in connective tissue and cartilage, consisting of a polypeptide backbone to which many glycosaminoglycan chains are covalently linked; they form the ground substance in the extracellular matrix of connective tissue and also have lubricant and support functions 蛋白聚糖, 蛋白多糖

pro·te·ol·y·sis (pro″te-ol′ĭ-sis) the splitting of proteins by hydrolysis of the peptide bonds with formation of smaller polypeptides 蛋白酶解; **proteolyt′ic** *adj.*

pro·te·ome (pro′te-ōm) the complete set of proteins produced from the information encoded in a genome 蛋白质组

pro·teo·me·tab·o·lism (pro″te-o-mə-tab′ə-liz-əm) the metabolism of protein 蛋白质代谢

pro·teo·pep·tic (pro″te-o-pep′tik) digesting protein 蛋白消化的

Pro·te·us (pro′te-əs) a genus of gram-negative, motile bacteria of the family Enterobacteriaceae, usually found in fecal and other putrefying matter; members, including *P. vulga′ris*, are associated with urinary tract infections, bacteremia, and abdominal and wound infections 变形杆菌属

pro·throm·bin (pro-throm′bin) coagulation factor Ⅱ 凝血酶原, 凝血因子 Ⅱ

pro·throm·bin·ase (pro-throm′bin-ās) 1. the complex of activated coagulation factor Ⅹ and calcium, phospholipid, and modified factor Ⅴ; it can cleave and activate prothrombin to thrombin 凝血酶原酶; 2. sometimes specifically the active enzyme center of the complex, activated factor Ⅹ 凝血因子 Ⅱ a, 在其活性酶中心, 可激活凝血酶原 Ⅹ

pro·throm·bi·no·gen·ic (pro-throm″bĭ-nojen′ik) promoting the production of prothrombin 促凝血酶原的, 凝血因子 Ⅱ 的

pro·ti·re·lin (pro-ti′rə-lin) a synthetic preparation of thyrotropin-releasing hormone (q.v.), used diagnostically 普罗瑞林, 一种用于诊断的促甲状腺

素释放激素 (q.v.) 的合成制剂

pro·tist (pro′tist) 1. a single-celled eukaryote 单细胞原生生物; 2. any member of the kingdom Protista 任何一种原生生物

Pro·tis·ta (pro-tis′tə) in some systems of classification, a kingdom comprising a diverse group of phylogenetically distinct, unicellular eukaryotes, including protozoa, algae, and certain intermediate forms 原生生物的统称，指在某些分类中，原生生物包含多种系统发育上不同的单细胞真核生物，包括原生动物、藻类和某些中间形式

pro·ti·um (pro′te-əm) 氕，参见 *hydrogen*

pro·to·col (pro′tə-kol) 1. an explicit, detailed plan of an experiment, procedure, or test 科学实验报告; 2. the original notes made on a necropsy, an experiment, or a case of disease 原始记录（尸体剖检、实验或病案时用）

pro·to·di·a·stol·ic (pro″to-di″ə-stol′ik) pertaining to early diastole, i.e., immediately following the second heart sound 舒张初期的

pro·to·du·o·de·num (pro″to-doo″o-de′nəm) the first or proximal portion of the duodenum, extending from the pylorus to the duodenal papilla 前十二指肠，十二指肠头

pro·ton (p) (pro′ton) an elementary particle that is the core or nucleus of an ordinary hydrogen atom of mass 1; the unit of positive electricity, being equivalent to the electron in charge and approximately to the hydrogen ion in mass 质子

pro·to·on·co·gene (pro″to-ong′ko-jēn) a normal gene that with slight alteration by mutation or other mechanism becomes an oncogene; most are believed to normally function in cell growth and differentiation 原致癌基因，指一种由正常基因通过轻微基因突变或其他机制改变而变成的致癌基因，大多数被认为在细胞的生长和分化过程中起正常作用

pro·to·path·ic (pro″to-path′ik) affected first; pertaining to sensing of stimuli in a nonspecific, usually nonlocalized, manner 粗觉的，原始感觉的

pro·to·plasm (pro′to-plaz″əm) the viscid, translucent colloid material, the essential constituent of the living cell, including cytoplasm and nucleoplasm 原生质，指黏质半透明的胶体物质，是活细胞的基本成分，包括细胞质和核质; **protoplasmat′ic, protoplas′mic** *adj.*

pro·to·plast (pro′to-plast″) a bacterial or plant cell deprived of its rigid wall but with its plasma membrane intact; the cell is dependent for its integrity on an isotonic or hypertonic medium 原生质体，指无坚硬的细胞壁但质膜完整的细菌或

植物细胞，细胞的完整性依赖于等渗或高渗介质

pro·to·por·phyr·ia (pro″to-por-fir′e-ə) erythropoietic p. 原卟啉症; **erythropoietic p. (EPP),** a form of erythropoietic porphyria marked by excessive protoporphyrin in erythrocytes, plasma, liver, and feces, and by widely varying photosensitive skin changes ranging from a burning or pruritic sensation to erythema, plaquelike edema, and wheals; caused by mutation in the gene encoding ferrochelatase 红细胞生成性原卟啉病

pro·to·por·phy·rin (pro″to-por′fə-rin) any of several porphyrin isomers, one of which is an intermediate in heme biosynthesis; it is accumulated and excreted excessively in feces in erythropoietic protoporphyria and variegate porphyria 原卟啉

pro·to·por·phy·rin·o·gen (pro″to-por″fə-rin′ə-jən) any of fifteen isomers of a porphyrinogen derivative, one of which is an intermediate produced from coproporphyrinogen in heme synthesis 原卟啉原

Pro·to·the·ca (pro″to-the′kə) a genus of ubiquitous yeastlike organisms generally considered to be algae; *P. wickerha′mii* and *P. zop′fii* are pathogenic 原壁菌属，指普遍存在的一类酵母样的有机体，通常是指藻类

pro·to·troph (pro′to-trōf) an organism with the same growth factor requirements as the ancestral strain; said of microbial mutants 原养型，指具有与原始菌株相同的生长因子需求的有机体，指微生物突变体; **prototroph′ic** *adj.*

pro·to·ver·te·bra (pro″to-vur′tə-brə) 1. somite 体节; 2. the caudal half of a somite that forms most of a vertebra 原脊椎

Pro·to·zoa (pro″to-zo′ə) a group comprising the simplest organisms of the eukaryotes, consisting of unicellular organisms that are usually motile and heterotrophic 原生动物门，指真核生物中包含的具有最简单生物体的一组，由可游动的和异养的单细胞有机体组成

pro·to·zo·a·cide (pro″to-zo′ə-sīd) an agent that kills protozoa 杀原生动物药

pro·to·zo·al (pro″to-zo′əl) 同 protozoan (2)

pro·to·zo·an (pro″to-zo′ən) 1. any individual of the Protozoa 原生动物; 2. of or pertaining to the Protozoa 原生动物的

pro·to·zo·ia·sis (pro″to-zo-i′ə-sis) any disease caused by protozoa 原虫病

pro·to·zo·ol·o·gy (pro″to-zo-ol′ə-je) the study of protozoa 原生动物学

pro·to·zo·on (pro″to-zo′on) pl. *protozo′a.* Any individual of the Protozoa 原虫，属于原生动物门的任何个体

pro·to·zo·o·phage (pro″to-zo′o-fāj) a cell having a phagocytic action on protozoa 噬原虫细胞

pro·trac·tion (pro-trak′shən) 1. drawing out or lengthening 拉出，延长；2. extension or protrusion 伸长，突出；3. a condition in which the teeth or other maxillary or mandibular structures are situated anterior to their normal position 前伸，指牙齿或其他上颌骨或下颌结构位于正常位置之前的状态；**mandibular p.**, 1. the protrusive movement of the mandible initiated by the lateral and medial pterygoid muscles acting simultaneously 下颌关节的前突活动）；2. a facial anomaly in which the gnathion lies anterior to the orbital plane 下颌关节前脱位；**maxillary p.**, a facial anomaly in which the subnasion is anterior to the orbital plane 上颌关节前脱位

pro·trac·tor (pro-trak′tər) an instrument for extracting foreign bodies from wounds 钳取器，一种从伤口中取出异物的工具

pro·trans·glu·tam·i·nase (pro-tranz″gloota-m′ĭ-nās) the inactive precursor of transglutaminase; it is the inactive form of coagulation factor XIII 转谷氨酰胺酶原, 转谷氨酰胺酶的非活性前体, 是凝血因子XIII的非活性形式

pro·trip·ty·line (pro-trip′tə-lēn) a tricyclic antidepressant, also used in the treatment of attentiondeficit/hyperactivity disorder, and narcolepsy; used as the hydrochloride salt 普罗替林，一种三环类抗抑郁药，也用于治疗注意力缺陷／多动障碍和发作性睡病；常用其盐酸盐

pro·tru·sion (pro-troo′zhən) 1. extension beyond the usual limits, or above a plane surface 突起；2. the state of being thrust forward or laterally, as in masticatory movements of the mandible 伸出，前突；**protrus′ive** adj.

pro·tu·ber·ance (pro-too′bər-əns) a projecting part, or prominence 隆凸；**mental p.**, a triangular prominence on the anterior surface of the body of the mandible, on or near the median line 颏隆凸

pro·tu·ber·an·tia (pro-too″bər-an′shə) [L.] 同 protuberance

pro·uro·ki·nase (pro-UK) (pro″u-ro-ki′nās) the single-chain proenzyme cleaved by plasmin to form u-plasminogen activator (urokinase); it is slowly activated in the presence of fibrin clots and is used for therapeutic thrombolysis 尿激酶原

pro·ver·te·bra (pro-vur′tə-brə) 同 protovertebra

Pro·vi·den·cia (prov″ĭ-den′shə) a genus of gram-negative, facultatively anaerobic, rodshaped bacteria of the family Enterobacteriaceae, occurring in normal urine and feces and sometimes causing infections. *P. alcalifa′ciens* is associated with diarrhea in children, and *P. rett′geri* and *P. stuar′tii* cause nosocomial infections 普罗威登菌属，属肠杆菌科细菌，兼性厌氧的革兰阴性小杆菌，存在于正常的尿液和粪便中，有时可引起感染。儿童腹泻与埃氏普罗威登菌有关，雷氏普罗威登菌和斯氏普罗威登菌可引起院内感染

prov·ing (proov′ing) in homeopathy, the administration of a medicinal substance to healthy persons in doses large enough to elicit a symptomatic response without causing irreversible toxicity in order to determine its therapeutic properties 验证

pro·vi·rus (pro-vi′rəs) the genome of an animal virus integrated (by crossing over) into the chromosome of the host cell, and thus replicated in all of its daughter cells. It can be activated to produce a complete virus; it can also cause transformation of the host cell 原病毒

pro·vi·sion·al (pro-vizh′ən-əl) formed or performed for temporary purposes; temporary 临时的，暂时性的

pro·vi·ta·min (pro-vi′tə-min) a precursor of a vitamin 维生素原，维生素的前体；**p. A,** usually β-carotene, including any of the provitamin A carotenoids 维生素 A 原；**p. D2,** ergosterol 麦角固醇；**p. D3,** 7-dehydrocholesterol 维生素 D_3 原，7- 脱氢胆固醇

prox·i·mad (prok′sĭ-mad) in a proximal direction 在近侧，向近端

prox·i·mal (prok′sĭ-məl) nearest; closer to a point of reference 接近的，邻近的，近端的

prox·i·ma·lis (prok″sĭ-ma′lis) [L.] 同 proximal

prox·i·mate (prok′sĭ-mət) immediate or nearest 邻近的，近似的

prox·i·mo·buc·cal (prok″sĭ-mo-buk′əl) pertaining to the proximal and buccal surfaces of a posterior tooth 邻颊的

pro·zone (pro′zōn) the phenomenon exhibited by some sera, in which agglutination or precipitation occurs at higher dilution ranges but is not visible at lower dilutions or when undiluted 前带，指在某些血清所表现出的现象，即凝集或沉淀发生在较高的稀释度范围内，但在较低的稀释度或未稀释时不可见

PRRT peptide receptor radionuclide therapy 肽受体放射性核素治疗

pru·ri·go (proo-ri′go) [L.] any of several itchy skin eruptions in which the characteristic lesion is dome-shaped with a small transient vesicle on top, followed by crusting or lichenification 痒疹；**pru·rig′inous** adj.; **p. mi′tis,** a mild type that begins in childhood, is intensely pruritic, and is progressive 脓疱疮，是儿童时期多发的一种的痒疹类型，有强烈的瘙痒并且是进行性的；**nodular p.,** a form of neurodermatitis, usually on the limbs, with discrete, firm, rough-surfaced, dark brown to gray, itchy nodules 结节性痒疹；p. sim′plex, a type with crops of papules at various stages of development on the trunk and extensor surfaces of the limbs 单纯痒疹

pru·rit·o·gen·ic (proo″rit-o-jen′ik) causing pruritus, or itching 引起瘙痒的

pru·ri·tus (proo-ri′təs) itching 瘙　痒；**prurit′ic** *adj.*；p. a′ni, intense chronic itching in the anal region 肛门瘙痒症；senile p., p. seni′lis, itching in the aged, possibly due to dryness of the skin 老年性皮肤瘙痒症；uremic p., generalized itching associated with chronic renal failure and not attributable to other internal or skin disease 尿毒性瘙痒症；p. vul′vae, intense itching of the female external genitals 外阴瘙痒症

prus·sic ac·id (prus′ik) hydrogen cyanide 氢氰酸；参见 *hydrogen* 下词条

PS pulmonary stenosis 肺动脉瓣狭窄

PSA prostate-specific antigen 前列腺特异性抗原

psal·te·ri·um (sal-tēr′e-əm) commissure of the fornix 海马连合

psam·mo·ma (sam-o′mə) 1. any tumor containing psammoma bodies 砂样瘤；2. psammomatous meningioma 砂样脑膜瘤

psam·mo·ma·tous (sam-o′mə-təs) characterized by the presence of or containment of psammoma bodies 砂粒体型, 指以含有砂粒小体为特征的

Pseud·al·les·che·ria (sood″al-əs-kēr′e-ə) a genus of fungi of the family Microascaceae; *P. boy′dii* (anamorph *Scedosporium angiospermum*) causes mycetoma and other fungal infections 假性阿利什利菌属

pseud·dal·les·che·ri·a·sis (sood-al″əs-kə-ri′ə-sis) infection by *Pseudallescheria boydii* other than mycetoma, without production of grains, most commonly affecting the lungs, bones, joints, or central nervous system and varying from localized to invasive to disseminated disease 假性阿利什利菌病, 指由波氏假性阿利什利菌引起的感染, 无颗粒产生, 最常影响肺、骨、关节或中枢神经系统, 从局限性疾病到侵袭性疾病到播散性疾病不等

pseud·ar·thro·sis (sood″ahr-thro′sis) a pathologic condition in which failure of callus formation following pathologic fracture through an area of deossification in a weight-bearing long bone results in formation of a false joint 假关节, 指病理性骨折后, 骨痂形成失败, 骨痂通过负重长骨脱骨化区域而导致假关节形成的一种病理状态

Pseud·ech·is (soo-dek′is) a genus of venomous Australian snakes of the family Elapidae. *P. por-*

phyria′cus is the Australian blacksnake 拟蝮蛇属

pseud·es·the·sia (sood″es-the′zhə) 1. synesthesia 联觉，牵连感觉；2. a sensation felt in the absence of any external stimulus 假感觉，幻觉

pseu·do·ac·an·tho·sis (soo″do-ak″an-tho′sis) a condition clinically resembling acanthosis 假性棘皮症；p. ni′gricans, a benign form of acanthosis nigricans associated with obesity; the obesity is sometimes associated with endocrine disturbance 假性黑（色）棘皮症

pseu·do·achon·dro·pla·sia (soo″do-a-kon″-dro-pla′zhə) an autosomal dominant disorder causing a form of dwarfism in which limbs are short but head size and facial features are normal, with knee and other skeletal deformities, joint hypermobility, and precocious osteoarthritis; caused by a mutation affecting assembly of collagen fibers 假性软骨发育不全

pseu·do·agraph·ia (soo″do-ə-graf′e-ə) echographia 假性失写症

pseu·do·ain·hum (soo″do-īn′yoom) annular constrictions around the digits, limbs, or trunk, occurring congenitally (sometimes causing intrauterine autoamputation) and also associated with a wide variety of disorders 假性箍趾病, 假性自发性断趾病, 假阿洪病

pseu·do·al·leles (soo″do-ə-lēlz′) genes that behave functionally as if they were alleles at the same locus but that can be shown to be at distinct loci, separable by recombination 拟等位基因；**pseudoallel′ic** *adj.*

pseu·do·ane·mia (soo″do-ə-ne′me-ə) marked pallor with no evidence of anemia 假贫血

pseu·do·an·eu·rysm (soo″do-an′u-riz″əm) false aneurysm; dilatation or tortuosity of a vessel, giving the appearance of an aneurysm 假动脉瘤

pseu·do·an·gi·na (soo″do-an-ji′nə) a nervous disorder resembling angina 假性心绞痛

pseu·do·ap·o·plexy (soo″do-ap′o-plek″se) a condition resembling apoplexy, but without hemorrhage 假卒中（似中风，但无脑出血情况）

pseu·do·bul·bar (soo″do-bul′bər) apparently, but not really, due to a bulbar lesion 假延髓的

pseu·do·cast (soo′do-kast″) a formation of urinary sediment that by chance resembles a true cast 假管型

pseu·do·cho·lin·es·ter·ase (PCE) (soo″-doko″lin-es′tər-ās) cholinesterase 拟胆碱酯酶

pseu·do·chrom·hi·dro·sis (soo″do-kro″mī- dro′sis) the presence of pigment on the skin caused by the action of pigment-producing bacteria 假色汗症（产色素细菌作用所致）

pseu·do·co·arc·ta·tion (soo″do-ko″ahrk-ta′-

812

shən) a condition radiographically resembling coarctation but without compromise of the lumen, as occurs in a congenital anomaly of the aortic arch 假缩窄

pseu·do·col·loid (soo″do-kol′oid) a mucoid substance sometimes found in ovarian cysts 假性胶体（一种黏液样物质，有时见于卵巢囊内）

pseu·do·cow·pox (soo″do-kou′poks) 同 paravaccinia

pseu·do·cox·al·gia (soo″do-kok-sal′jə) osteochondrosis of the capitular epiphysis of the femur 假性髋关节痛（股骨小头骨骺骨软骨病）

pseu·do·cri·sis (soo″do-kri″sis) sudden but temporary abatement of febrile symptoms 假极期，假（热度）骤退

pseu·do·croup (soo″do-kroop′) laryngismus stridulus 假格鲁布（喘鸣性喉痉挛；胸腺性气喘）

pseu·do·cy·e·sis (soo″do-si-e′sis) false pregnancy 假孕

pseu·do·cy·lin·droid (soo″do-sə-lin′droid) a shred of mucin in the urine resembling a cylindroid 假圆柱状体

pseu·do·cyst (soo′do-sist″) 1. an abnormal or dilated space resembling a cyst but not lined with epithelium 假性囊肿；2. a cluster of small, comma-shaped forms of *Toxoplasma gondii* found particularly in muscle and brain tissue in toxoplasmosis 伪包囊；**pancreatic p.,** a complication of acute pancreatitis, characterized by a cystic collection of fluid and necrotic debris whose walls are formed by the pancreas and nearby organs 胰腺假囊肿

pseu·do·de·men·tia (soo″do-də-men′shə) a state of general apathy resembling dementia but due to a psychiatric disorder rather than organic brain disease and potentially reversible 假性痴呆

pseu·do·diph·the·ria (soo″do-dif-thēr′e-ə) diphtheroid; any of a group of infections resembling diphtheria but not caused by *Corynebacterium diphtheriae* 假性白喉

pseu·do·dom·i·nance (soo″do-dom′ĭ-nəns) 1. appearance of a recessive phenotype in a pedigree, the recessive allele being expressed due to loss of the dominant allele, as by a chromosomal deletion 假显性；2. quasidominance 类显性，准显性

pseu·do·dom·i·nant (soo″do-dom′ĭ-nənt) 1. pertaining to pseudodominance (1) 假显性的；2. quasidominant 类显性的，准显性的，参见 *quasidominance*

pseu·do·ephed·rine (soo″do-ə-fed′rin) one of the optical isomers of ephedrine; used as the hydrochloride or sulfate salt as a nasal decongestant 伪麻黄碱

pseu·do·epi·lepsy (soo″do-ep′ĭ-lep″se) 同 pseu-

doseizure

pseu·do·ex·stro·phy (soo″do-eks′trə-fe) a developmental anomaly marked by the characteristic musculoskeletal defects of bladder exstrophy but with no other major defect of the urinary tract 假性膀胱外翻

pseu·do·fol·lic·u·li·tis (soo″do-fə-lik″u-li′tis) a condition resembling folliculitis 假性毛囊炎；**p. bar′bae,** "razor bumps;" a chronic disorder of the shaved beard region of the neck, seen primarily in black men, consisting of erythematous papules containing buried hairs 须部假性毛囊炎

pseu·do·frac·ture (soo″do-frak′chər) a condition seen in the radiograph of a bone as a thickening of the periosteum and formation of new bone over what looks like an incomplete fracture 假性骨折，指在 X 线片上表现为骨膜增厚和新骨形成的状态，看起来像是不完全骨折

pseu·do·gene (soo′do-jēn″) a DNA sequence that is similar in sequence to an active gene at another locus but that has been inactivated by mutation and is not expressed 假基因，指基因组中存在的一段与正常基因非常相似但不能表达的 DNA 序列

pseu·do·gli·o·ma (soo″do-gli-o′mə) any condition mimicking retinoblastoma, e.g., retrolental fibroplasia or exudative retinopathy 假性胶质瘤

pseu·do·glot·tis (soo″do-glot′is) 1. the aperture between the false vocal cords 假声门；2. neoglottis 人工声门；**pseudoglot′tic** *adj.*

pseu·do·gout (soo′do-gout″) 假（性）痛风，参见 *disease* 词条下 *calcium pyrophosphate deposition disease*

pseu·do·he·ma·tu·ria (soo″do-he″mə-tu′re-ə) presence in urine of pigments that make it pink or red with no detectable hemoglobin or blood cells 假性血尿

pseu·do·he·mo·phil·ia (soo″do-he″mo-fil′e-ə) von Willebrand disease 假性血友病

pseu·do·her·maph·ro·dite (soo″do-hər-maf′ro-dīt) an individual with pseudohermaphroditism 假两性体，假半阴阳体

pseu·do·her·maph·ro·dit·ism (soo″do-hər-maf″ro-dit-iz″əm) incongruence between some combination of the genetic, gonadal, and anatomic sex of an organism; it has been subsumed into disorders of sex development (q.v.) 假两性畸形，假半阴阳；**female p.,** former name for *46, XX disorder of sex development* 女性假两性畸形，XX 性染色体异常导致的性发育异常；**male p.,** former name for *46, XY disorder of sex development* 男性假两性畸形，XY 性染色体异常导致的性发育异常

pseu·do·her·nia (soo″do-hur′ne-ə) an inflamed

sac or gland simulating strangulated hernia 假疝

pseu·do·hy·per·ten·sion (soo″do- hi″pərten′shən) falsely elevated blood pressure reading by sphygmomanometry, caused by loss of compliance of arterial walls 假性高血压

pseu·do·hy·per·tro·phy (soo″do-hi-pur′trə- fe) increase in size without true hypertrophy 假性肥大；**pseudohypertro′phic** adj.

pseu·do·hy·po·al·dos·ter·on·ism (soo″dohi″po-al-dos′tər-ōn-iz″əm) elevated levels of aldosterone and increased plasma renin activity together with signs and symptoms of mineralocorticoid deficiency, caused by resistance of target tissues to mineralocorticoids 假性醛固酮减少症；p. type 1, a hereditary disorder of infancy characterized by severe salt wasting, failure to thrive in association with normal or elevated aldosterone levels, caused by defects in the mineralocorticoid receptor 假性醛固酮减少症Ⅰ型，是一种婴儿期遗传性疾病，其特点是严重的钠丢失，血钠不能在正常或升高的醛固酮水平下升高，这是由盐皮质激素受体缺陷引起的；p. type 2, a familial endocrine abnormality, seen primarily in adults, characterized by hyperkalemia without salt wasting and caused by resistance to the mineralocorticoid effects of aldosterone 假性醛固酮减少症Ⅱ型，是一种家族性内分泌异常，主要见于成人，以无盐耗的高钾血症为特征，是由于对醛固酮的盐皮质激素代谢产生抵抗而引起的

pseu·do·hy·po·para·thy·roi·dism (soo″dohi″po-par″ə-thi′roi-diz″əm) a heterogeneous group of hereditary disorders resembling hypoparathyroidism but caused by failure of response to parathyroid hormone (PTH), marked by hypocalcemia and hyperphosphatemia; associated with defects in the signal transduction pathway linking receptor–ligand interactions with the activation of adenylate cyclase. The most common form, type 1A, is characterized by multihormone resistance and Albright hereditary osteodystrophy; type 1B shows PTH resistance only, confined to the kidney 假性甲状旁腺功能减退症

pseu·do·iso·chro·mat·ic (soo″do-i″so-kromat′ik) seemingly of the same color throughout; applied to a solution for testing color vision deficiency, having two pigments that can be distinguished by the normal eye 假等色的，指整个看似相同的颜色，用于测试色觉缺陷，有两种可以被正常眼睛区分的颜色

pseu·do·jaun·dice (soo″do-jawn′dis) skin discoloration due to blood changes and not to liver disease 假黄疸

pseu·do·mel·a·no·sis (soo″do-mel″ə-no′sis) discoloration of tissue after death by blood pigments 假黑变病

pseu·do·mem·brane (soo″do-mem′brān) false membrane; a membranous exudate, such as the diphtheritic membrane 假膜，伪膜；**pseudomem′-branous** adj.

pseudomeningocele abnormal collection of cerebrospinal fluid (CSF) that communicates with the CSF space around the brain or spinal cord 假性脑膜膨出

Pseu·do·mo·na·da·ceae (soo″do-mo″nə-da′see) a family of aerobic, mostly motile bacteria of the order Pseudomonadales 假单胞菌科

Pseu·do·mo·na·da·les (soo″do-mo″nə-da′lēz) an order of motile, aerobic bacteria of the class Gammaproteobacteria 假单胞菌目

Pseu·do·mo·nas (soo″do-mo′nəs) a genus of gramnegative, aerobic, rod-shaped, motile bacteria of the family Pseudomonadaceae, some species of which are pathogenic. *P. aerugino′sa* produces the blue-green pigment pyocyanin, which gives the color to "blue pus" and causes various human diseases; *P. alcali′genes, P. fluores′cens, P. pseudoalcali′- genes, P. pu′tida,* and *P. stut′zeri* are opportunistic pathogens 假单胞菌属

pseu·do·myx·o·ma (soo″do-mik-so′mə) 1. a mass of epithelial mucus resembling a myxoma 假黏液瘤；2. 同 p. peritonei；**p. peritone′i,** the presence in the peritoneal cavity of mucoid matter from a ruptured ovarian cyst or a ruptured mucocele of the appendix 腹膜假黏液瘤

pseu·do·neu·ri·tis (soo″do-noo-ri′tis) a congenital hyperemic condition of the optic papilla 假性视神经炎

Pseu·do·no·car·di·a·ceae (soo″do-no-kahr″dea′se-e) a phenotypically diverse family of gram-positive, aerobic bacteria of the order Actinomycetales 假诺卡氏菌科

pseu·do·pap·il·le·de·ma (soo″do-pap″ĭ-lə-de′mə) anomalous elevation of the optic disk 假视神经乳头水肿

pseu·do·pa·ral·y·sis (soo″do-pə-ral′ĭ-sis) 1. apparent loss of muscular power because of pain that is not neurologic in origin 假瘫；2. hysterical paralysis 癔症性瘫痪；**Parrot p., syphilitic p.,** apparent paralysis of a limb of an infant because of osteochondritis of an epiphysis in congenital syphilis 梅毒性假性麻痹，指先天性梅毒骨骺骨软骨炎引起的婴儿肢体明显瘫痪

pseu·do·pe·lade (soo″do-pə-lahd′) patchy alopecia roughly simulating alopecia areata; it may be due to various diseases of the hair follicles, some of which are associated with scarring 假性斑秃

pseu·do·po·di·um (soo″do-po′de-əm) pl. *pseudo-po′dia*. A temporary protrusion of the cytoplasm of an ameba, serving for locomotion or the engulfment of food 伪足

pseu·do·poly·me·lia (soo″do-pol″e-me′le-ə) an illusory sensation that may be referred to many extreme portions of the body, including the hands, feet, nose, nipples, and glans penis 多肢幻觉, 是一种虚幻的感觉, 可能涉及身体的许多极端部位, 包括手、脚、鼻子、乳头和龟头

pseu·do·pol·yp (soo″do-pol′ip) a hypertrophied tab of mucous membrane resembling a polyp 假息肉

pseu·do·pol·yp·osis (soo″do-pol″ĭ-po′sis) numerous pseudopolyps in the colon and rectum, due to long-standing inflammation 假息肉病

pseu·do·preg·nan·cy (soo″do-preg′nən-se) 1. false pregnancy 假孕, 假妊娠; 2. the premenstrual stage of the endometrium; so called because it resembles the endometrium just before implantation of the blastocyst 子宫内膜经前期

pseu·do·hy·po·para·thy·roid·ism (soo″do-soo″do-hi″po-par″ə-thi′roi-diz″əm) an autosomal dominant disorder clinically resembling pseudohypoparathyroidism but not showing resistance to parathyroid hormone (PTH) or other hormones and having normal serum levels of calcium and phosphorus. Clinical features of Albright hereditary osteodystrophy are present 假性甲状旁腺功能减退症

pseu·do·pter·yg·i·um (soo″do-tər-ij′e-əm) an adhesion of the conjunctiva to the cornea following a burn or other injury 假性翼状胬肉

pseu·do·pto·sis (soo″dop-to′sis) decrease in the size of the palpebral aperture 假性上睑下垂

pseu·do·pu·ber·ty (soo″do-pu′bər-te) development of secondary sex characters and reproductive organs that is not associated with pubertal levels of gonadotropins and gonadotropin-releasing hormone; it may be either heterosexual or isosexual 假青春期; **precocious p.**, the appearance of some of the secondary sex characters without maturation of the gonads, before the normal age of onset of puberty 假性性早熟

pseu·do·re·ac·tion (soo″do-re-ak′shən) a false or deceptive reaction; a skin reaction in intradermal tests that is not due to the specific test substance but to protein in the medium employed in producing the toxin 假反应, 是一种虚假的反应; 皮内反应试验中的皮肤反应, 不是由特定的试验物质引起, 而是由能产生毒素的介质中提取出来的蛋白质引起的

pseu·do·rick·ets (soo″do-rik′əts) renal osteodys-trophy 假佝偻病, 肾病性骨营养不良

pseu·do·sar·co·ma·tous (soo″do-sahr-ko′-mə-təs) mimicking sarcoma; used of both benign and malignant lesions that histologically resemble sarcoma 假性肉瘤

pseu·do·scle·ro·sis (soo″do-sklə-ro′sis) a condition with the symptoms but without the lesions of multiple sclerosis 假硬化症; **Strümpell-Westphal p.**, Westphal-Strümpell p., Wilson disease 肝豆状核变性

pseu·do·sei·zure (soo″do-se′zhər) an attack resembling an epileptic seizure but having purely psychological causes, lacking the electroencephalographic changes of epilepsy and sometimes able to be stopped by an act of will 假癫痫发作

pseu·do·sto·ma (soo″do-sto′mə) an apparent communication between silver-stained epithelial cells 假孔, 指银染上皮细胞间明显的细胞交流

pseu·do·syn·dac·ty·ly (soo″do-sin-dak′tə-le) fusion of one or more web spaces between the digits secondary to a pathologic process 假性并指

pseu·do·ta·bes (soo″do-ta′bēz) any neuropathy with symptoms like those of tabes dorsalis 假性脊髓痨

pseu·do·tet·a·nus (soo″do-tet′ə-nəs) persistent muscular contractions resembling tetanus but unassociated with *Clostridium tetani* 假破伤风

pseu·do·trun·cus ar·te·ri·o·sus (soo″-do-trung′kəs ahr-tēr″e-o′səs) the most severe form of tetralogy of Fallot 假性动脉干

pseu·do·tu·mor (soo″do-too′mər) an enlargement that resembles a tumor, resulting from inflammation, fluid accumulation, or other causes 假性肿瘤; **p. ce′rebri**, cerebral edema and raised intracranial pressure without neurologic signs except occasional sixth nerve palsy 假性脑瘤; **inflammatory p.**, a tumorlike mass representing an inflammatory reaction 炎性假瘤

pseu·do·uri·dine (ψ) (soo′do-ūr′ĭ-dēn) a nucleotide derived from uridine by isomerization and occurring in transfer RNA 假尿苷

pseu·do·ver·ti·go (soo″do-vur′tĭ-go) any dizziness or other form of light-headedness that resembles vertigo but does not involve a sense of rotation 假性眩晕

pseu·do·xan·tho·ma elas·ti·cum (soo″do-zan-tho′mə e-las′tĭ-kəm) a progressive, inherited disorder with skin, eye, and cardiovascular manifestations, most resulting from basophilic degeneration of elastic tissues, including small yellowish macules and papules; lax, inelastic, and redundant skin; premature arterial calcification; symptoms of coronary insufficiency; hypertension; left atrioventricular valve prolapse; angioid streaks in the retina; and gastrointestinal and other hemorrhages 弹 性 假 黄 色瘤

psi　pounds per square inch 每平方英寸磅数

psi·lo·cin　(si′lo-sin) a hallucinogenic, euphoria-producing metabolite of psilocybin, found in certain mushrooms; it affects the central nervous system via stimulation of serotonin receptors 二甲 - 4 - 羟色胺，脱磷酸裸盖菇素

Psi·lo·cy·be　(si″lo-si′be) a genus of mushrooms; *P. cuben'sis, P. mexica'na,* and other species contain the hallucinogens psilocybin and psilocin 裸盖菇

psi·lo·cy·bin　(si″lo-si′bin) a prodrug occurring in certain mushrooms and metabolized to the hallucinogen psilocin 二甲 - 4 - 羟色胺磷酸，裸头草碱

psit·ta·co·sis　(sit″ə-ko′sis) a disease due to infection with *Chlamydophila psittaci,* seen first in parrots and later in other wild and domestic birds; it is transmissible to humans, usually characterized by fever, cough, splenomegaly, and sometimes pneumonia 鹦鹉热

psor·a·len　(sor′ə-lən) any of the constituents of certain plants (e.g., *Psoralea corylifolia*) that have the ability to produce phototoxic dermatitis on subsequent exposure of the individual to sunlight; certain perfumes and drugs (e.g., methoxsalen) contain psoralens 补骨脂素

pso·ri·a·sis　(sə-ri′ə-sis) a chronic, hereditary, recurrent dermatosis marked by discrete vivid red macules, papules, or plaques covered with silvery lamellated scales 银屑病，白疕；**psoriat'ic** *adj.*; **erythrodermic p.,** a severe, generalized erythrodermic condition seen in chronic forms of psoriasis, characterized by massive exfoliation of skin and serious systemic illness 红皮病性银屑病；**guttate p.,** a form seen mainly in children and young adults after streptococcal infections, with abrupt appearance of small droplike lesions over much of the body 滴状银屑病；**inverse p.,** a type with moist, erythematous lesions, usually found in flexures such as the axillae and the inguinal region, or in skinfolds 反向银屑病，屈侧银屑病；**pustular p.,** a chronic, relapsing type with vesicles or pustules, generally occurring in association with a focal infection elsewhere in the body. Two types are recognized: a less severe *localized pustular* type, usually found on the palms and soles, and a more severe *generalized pustular* type, often accompanied by fever, which can be fatal 脓疱性银屑病

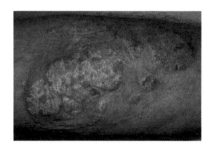

▲　银屑病

PSRO　Professional Standards Review Organization 职业标准评定组织

PSVT　paroxysmal supraventricular tachycardia 阵发性室上性心动过速

psy·chal·gia　(si-kal′jə) 1. pain, usually in the head and perceived as being of emotional origin, that may accompany intolerable ideas, obsessions, or hallucinations 精神痛苦；2. psychogenic pain 精神性疼痛，心因性疼痛；**psychal'gic** *adj.*

psy·cha·tax·ia　(si″kə-tak′se-ə) a disordered mental condition marked by confusion and inability to concentrate 精神失调

psy·che　(si′ke) 1. the human faculty for thought, judgment, and emotion; the mental life, including both conscious and unconscious processes; the mind in its totality, as distinguished from the body 心灵，心理，精神；2. the soul or self 灵魂；**psy'chic** *adj.*

psy·che·del·ic　(si″kə-del′ik) 1. pertaining to or characterized by hallucinations, distortions of perception and awareness, and sometimes psychotic-like behavior 致幻觉的；2. a drug that produces such effects 致幻药

psy·chi·a·trist　(si-ki′ə-trist) a physician who specializes in psychiatry 精神病学家

psy·chi·a·try　(si-ki′ə-tre) the branch of medicine dealing with the study, treatment, and prevention of mental disorders 精神病学；**psychiat'ric** *adj.*; **biologic p.,** that which emphasizes physical, chemical, and neurologic causes and treatment approaches 生物精神病学；**community p.,** that concerned with the detection, prevention, and treatment of mental disorders as they develop within designated psychosocial, cultural, or geographic areas 社区精神病学；**descriptive p.,** that based on the study of observable symptoms and behavioral phenomena, rather than underlying psychodynamic processes 描述性精神病学；**dynamic p.,** that based on the study of emotional processes, their origins, and the mental mechanisms underlying them, rather than

P

observable behavioral phenomena.that based on the study of emotional processes, their origins, and the mental mechanisms underlying them, rather than observable behavioral phenomena 动力精神病学；**forensic p.**, that dealing with the legal aspects of mental disorders 司法精神病学；**geriatric p.**, geropsychiatry 老年精神病学；**preventive p.**, that broadly concerned with the amelioration, control, and limitation of psychiatric disability 预防精神病学；**social p.**, that concerned with the cultural and social factors that engender, precipitate, intensify, or prolong maladaptive patterns of behavior and complicate treatment 社会精神病学

psy·chic (si′kik) 1. pertaining to the psyche 心理的；2. mental (1) 精神的

psy·cho·acous·tics (si″ko-ə-koos′tiks) a branch of psychophysics studying the relationship between acoustic stimuli and behavior 心理声学

psy·cho·ac·tive (si″ko-ak′tiv) 同 psychotropic

psy·cho·an·a·lep·tic (si″ko-an″ə-lep′tik) exerting a stimulating effect upon the mind（促）精神兴奋药的；精神兴奋药

psy·cho·anal·y·sis (si″ko-ə-nal′ĭ-sis) 1. a theory of human mental phenomena and behavior focusing on the influence of unconscious forces on the mental state (Freud) 精神分析；2. a method of investigation into the contents of the mind 精神分析学；3. a therapeutic technique based on Freud's theory, diagnosing and treating mental and emotional disorders through ascertaining and analyzing the facts of the patient's present and past mental life and emotional experiences 心理分析；**psychoanalyt′ic** *adj.*

psy·cho·bi·ol·o·gy (si″ko-bi-ol′ə-je) 1. biopsychology; a field of study examining the relationship between brain and mind, studying the effect of biologic influences on psychological functioning or mental processes 生物心理学；2. a psychiatric theory in which the human being is viewed as an integrated unit, incorporating psychological, social, and biologic functions, with behavior a function of the total organism 精神生物学；**psychobiolog′ical** *adj.*

psy·cho·dra·ma (si′ko-drah″mə) a form of group psychotherapy in which patients dramatize emotional problems and life situations in order to achieve insight and to alter faulty behavior patterns 心理剧

psy·cho·dy·nam·ics (si″ko-di-nam′iks) the interplay of motivational forces that gives rise to the expression of mental processes, as in attitudes, behavior, or symptoms 心理动力学，精神动力学

psy·cho·gen·e·sis (si″ko-jen′ə-sis) 1. mental development 心理发生；2. production of a symptom or illness by psychic factors 由精神因素造成症状

或疾患的

psy·cho·gen·ic (si″ko-jen′ik) having an emotional or psychological origin 心理性的，精神性的

psy·cho·graph (si″ko-graf) 1. a chart for recording graphically a person's personality traits 心理记录表；2. a written description of a person's mental functioning 心理记录

psy·chol·o·gy (si-kol′ə-je) the science dealing with the mind and mental processes, especially in relation to human and animal behavior 心理学；**psycholog′ic, psycholog′ical** *adj.*；**analytic p.**, psychology based on the concept of the collective unconscious and the complex 分析心理学；**child p.**, the study of the development of the mind of the child 儿童心理学；**clinical p.**, the use of psychological knowledge and techniques in the treatment of persons with emotional difficulties 临床心理学；**community p.**, a broad term referring to the organization of community resources for the prevention of mental disorders 社区心理学；**criminal p.**, the study of the mentality, motivation, and social behavior of criminals 犯罪心理学；**depth p.**, psychoanalysis 心理分析学；**developmental p.**, the study of behavioral change through the life span 发展心理学；**dynamic p.**, that stressing the element of energy in mental processes 动力心理学；**environmental p.**, the study of the effects of the physical and social environment on behavior 环境心理学；**experimental p.**, the study of the mind and mental operations by the use of experimental methods 实验心理学；**gestalt p.**, gestaltism 完形心理学，格式塔心理学；**physiologic p., physiological p.**, the branch of psychology that studies the relationship between physiologic and psychological processes 生理心理学；**social p.**, that treating of the social aspects of mental life 社会心理学

psy·chom·e·try (si-kom′ə-tre) the testing and measuring of mental and psychological ability, efficiency, potentials, and functioning 心理测量；**psychomet′ric** *adj.*

psy·cho·mo·tor (si″ko-mo′tər) pertaining to motor effects of cerebral or psychic activity 心理运动

psy·cho·neu·ral (si″ko-noor′əl) relating to the totality of neural events initiated by a sensory input and leading to storage, discrimination, or an output of any kind 精神神经的

psy·cho·neu·ro·im·mu·nol·o·gy (si″ko-noor″o-im″u-nol′ə-je) the study of the interactions between psychological factors, the central nervous system, and immune function as modulated by the neuroendocrine system 心理神经免疫学

psy·cho·neu·ro·sis (si″ko-noo-ro′sis) neurosis 神经官能症；**psychoneurot′ic** *adj.*

psy·cho·path·ic (si″ko-path′ik) pertaining to psychopathy, particularly to antisocial behavior or antisocial personality disorder 精神病态的，变态人格的

psy·cho·pa·thol·o·gy (si″ko-pə-thol′ə-je) 1. the branch of medicine dealing with the causes and processes of mental disorders 心理病理学，精神病理学; 2. abnormal, maladaptive behavior or mental activity 精神功能障碍

psy·chop·a·thy (si-kop′ə-the) broadly, a mental disorder; sometimes used specifically for *antisocial personality disorder* 精神病态，心理病态

psy·cho·phar·ma·col·o·gy (si″ko-fahr″mə- kol′ə-je) 1. the study of the action of drugs on psychological functions and mental states 精神药理学; 2. the use of drugs to modify psychological functions and mental states 使用药物来改变心理功能和精神状态; **psychopharmacolog′ic** *adj.*

psy·cho·phys·i·cal (si″ko-fiz′ ĭ-kəl) pertaining to the mind and its relation to physical manifestations 心理物理的

psy·cho·phys·ics (si″ko-fiz′iks) scientific study of quantitative relations between characteristics or patterns of physical stimuli and the sensations induced by them 心理物理学

psy·cho·phys·i·ol·o·gy (si″ko-fiz″e-ol′ə-je) physiologic psychology 心理生理学

psy·cho·ple·gic (si″ko-ple′jik) an agent lessening cerebral activity or excitability 精神抑制药

psy·cho·sen·so·ry (si″ko-sen′sə-re) perceiving and interpreting sensory stimuli 心理感觉的

psy·cho·sex·u·al (si″ko-sek′shoo-əl) pertaining to the mental or emotional aspects of sex 性心理的

psy·cho·sis (si-ko′sis) pl. *psycho′ses.* Any major mental disorder of organic or emotional origin marked by derangement of personality and loss of contact with reality, with delusions and hallucinations and often with incoherent speech, disorganized and agitated behavior, or illusions 精 神 病。Cf. *neurosis*; **alcoholic p's,** those associated with excessive use of alcohol and involving organic brain damage 酒精中毒性精神病; **bipolar p.,** 双相情感障碍，参见 *disorder* 下词条; **brief reactive p.,** an episode of a brief psychotic disorder that is a reaction to a recognizable, distressing life event 突发反应性精神病; **Korsakoff p.,** Korsakoff 精神病，参见 *syndrome* 下词条; **reactive p.,** brief reactive p.反应性精神病,应激相关障碍; **senile p.,** depressive or paranoid delusions or hallucinations or other mental disorders associated with degeneration of the brain in old age, as in senile dementia 老年性精神病; **symbiotic p., symbiotic infantile p.,** a condition seen in 2- to 4-yearold children having

an abnormal relationship to the mothering figure, characterized by intense separation anxiety, severe regression, giving up of useful speech, and autism 共生性精神病; **toxic p.,** one due to the ingestion of toxic agents or to the presence of toxins within the body 中毒性精神病

psy·cho·so·cial (si″ko-so′shəl) pertaining to or involving both psychic and social aspects 社 会 心 理的

psy·cho·so·mat·ic (si″ko-so-mat′ik) pertaining to the mind-body relationship; having bodily symptoms of psychic, emotional, or mental origin 心身的

psy·cho·stim·u·lant (si″ko-stim′u-lənt) 1. producing a transient increase in psychomotor activity 精神刺激的; 2. a drug that produces such effects 精神兴奋药

psy·cho·sur·gery (si″ko-sur′jər-e) brain surgery performed for treatment of psychiatric disorders 精神外科，为治疗精神疾病而进行的脑外科手术; **psychosur′gical** *adj.*

psy·cho·ther·a·py (si″ko-ther′ə-pe) treatment of mental disorders and behavioral disturbances using verbal and nonverbal communication, as opposed to agents such as drugs or electric shock, to alter maladaptive patterns of coping, relieve emotional disturbance, and encourage personality growth 心理疗法; **psychoanalytic p.,** psychoanalysis (3) 精神分析性心理治疗

psy·chot·ic (si-kot′ik) 1. pertaining to, characterized by, or caused by psychosis（患）精神病的; 2. a person exhibiting psychosis 精神病患者

psy·chot·o·gen·ic (si-kot″o-jen′ik) 同 psychotomimetic

psy·chot·o·mi·met·ic (si-kot″o-mĭ-met′ik) pertaining to, characterized by, or producing symptoms similar to those of a psychosis 拟 精 神 病 的; 致幻药

psy·cho·tro·pic (si″ko-tro′pik) exerting an effect on the mind; capable of modifying mental activity; said especially of drugs 亲精神的（尤指影响精神状态的药物）

psy·chro·al·gia (si″kro-al′jə) a painful sensation of cold 冷痛

psy·chro·phil·ic (si″kro-fil′ik) fond of cold; said of bacteria growing best in the cold (15° to 20°C) 嗜冷的（指细菌）

psyl·li·um (sil′e-əm) 1. a plant of the genus *Plantago* 车前草; 2. the husk *(psyllium husk)* or seed *(plantago* or *psyllium seed)* of various species of *Plantago;* used as a bulk-forming laxative 车前子壳，车前子

PT prothrombin time 凝血酶原时间

Pt platinum 元素铂的符号

PTA plasma thromboplastin antecedent (coagulation factor Ⅺ) 血浆凝血酶原前体（凝血因子Ⅺ）

ptar·mic (tahr'mik) causing sneezing 引嚏的

ptar·mus (tahr'məs) spasmodic sneezing 痉挛性喷嚏

PTC plasma thromboplastin component (coagulation factor Ⅸ) 血浆促凝血酶原激酶组分（凝血因子Ⅸ）

pte·ri·on (tēr'e-on) a point of junction of frontal, parietal, temporal, and sphenoid bones 翼点

pter·o·yl·glu·tam·ic ac·id (ter″o-əl-glootam'ik) folic acid 蝶酰谷氨酸，叶酸

pte·ryg·i·um (tə-rij'e-əm) pl. *ptery'gia* [Gr.] a winglike structure, especially an abnormal triangular fold of membrane in the interpalpebral fissure, extending from the conjunctiva to the cornea 翼状胬肉，胬肉攀睛。**p. col'li,** webbed neck; a thick skin fold on the side of the neck from the mastoid region to the acromion 翼状颈皮

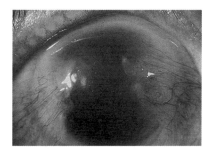

▲ 眼外眦与眼内眦的翼状胬肉

pter·y·goid (ter'ĭ-goid) shaped like a wing 翼状的

pter·y·go·man·dib·u·lar (ter″ĭ-go-man-dib'-u-lər) pertaining to the pterygoid process and the mandible 翼突下颌的

pter·y·go·max·il·lary (ter″ĭ-go-mak'sĭ-lar-e) pertaining to the pterygoid process and the maxilla 翼突上颌的

pter·y·go·pal·a·tine (ter″ĭ-go-pal'ə-tīn) pertaining to the pterygoid process and the palate bone 翼突腭的

PTMA percutaneous transvenous mitral annuloplasty 经皮经静脉二尖瓣成形术；posttransplantation thrombotic microangiopathy 移植后血栓性微血管病变

ptosed (tōst) affected with ptosis 上睑下垂的

pto·sis (to'sis) 1. 同 prolapse (1); 2. paralytic drooping of the upper eyelid 上睑麻痹性下垂，**ptot'ic** *adj.*

PTSD posttraumatic stress disorder 创伤后应激障碍

pty·al·a·gogue (ti-al'ə-gog) sialagogue 催涎药

pty·a·lec·ta·sis (ti″ə-lek'tə-sis) 1. a state of dilatation of a salivary duct 涎管扩张；2. surgical dilation of a salivary duct 涎腺导管扩张术

pty·a·lin (ti'ə-lin) α -amylase occurring in saliva 唾液淀粉酶

pty·a·lism (ti'ə-liz″əm) excessive secretion of saliva 多涎

pty·alo·cele (ti-al'o-sēl) a cystic tumor containing saliva 涎（液）囊肿

pty·al·o·gen·ic (ti″ə-lo-jen'ik) formed from or by the action of saliva 涎原的，涎性的

pty·a·lor·rhea (ti″ə-lo-re'ə) 同 ptyalism

Pu plutonium 元素钚的符号

pu·bar·che (pu-bahr'ke) the first appearance of pubic hair 阴毛初现

pu·ber·tas (pu-bur'təs) 同 puberty；**p. prae'cox,** precocious puberty 性早熟

pu·ber·ty (pu'bər-te) the period during which the secondary sex characters begin to develop and the capability of sexual reproduction is attained 青春期；**pu'beral, pu'bertal** *adj.*；**central precocious p.,** precocious puberty due to premature hypothalamic-pituitary-gonadal maturation; it is always isosexual and involves not only development of secondary sex characters but also development of the gonads. Increases in height and weight and osseous maturation are accelerated, and early closing of the epiphyses leads to short stature 中枢性性早熟；**precocious p.,** the onset of puberty at an earlier age than normal, defined as before age 8 in girls and 9 in boys; it is usually hormonal but occasionally occurs in otherwise normal children 性早熟

pu·bes (pu'bēz) [L.] 1. the hairs growing over the hypogastric region 阴毛；2. the hypogastric region 耻骨区；**pu'bic** *adj.*

pu·bes·cent (pu-bes'ənt) 1. arriving at the age of puberty 青春期的；2. covered with down or lanugo 有毛的

pu·bic (pu'bik) pertaining to or situated near the pubes, the pubic bone, or the hypogastric region 耻骨的

pu·bi·ot·o·my (pu″be-ot'ə-me) surgical separation of the pubic bone lateral to the symphysis 耻骨切开术

pu·bis (pu'bis) [L.] pubic bone 耻骨

pu·bo·ves·i·cal (pu″bo-ves'ĭ-kəl) vesicopubic 膀胱耻骨的

PUBS percutaneous umbilical blood sampling 经皮脐血抽样；参见 *cordocentesis*

pu·den·dum (pu-den'dəm) pl. *puden'da* [L.] the external genitalia of humans, especially of the female 阴部；参见 *vulva*；**puden'dal, pu'dic** *adj.*；**p. femininum,** the female pudendum 女阴

pu·er·ile (pu′ər-il) pertaining to childhood or to children; childish 童年的，儿童的；幼稚的

pu·er·pera (pu-ur′pər-ə) a woman who has just given birth to a child 产妇

pu·er·per·al (pu-ur′pər-əl) pertaining to a puerpera or to the puerperium 产褥期的

pu·er·pe·ri·um (pu″ər-pēr′e-əm) the period or state of confinement after childbirth 产褥期

PUFA polyunsaturated fatty acid 多不饱和脂肪酸，多烯酸

Pu·lex (pu′leks) a genus of fleas, including *P. ir′ri-tans,* the common flea or human flea, which attacks humans and domestic animals and may act as an intermediate host of certain helminths 蚤属，包括人蚤，可攻击人类和家畜，并可能作为某些蠕虫的中间宿主

pu·lic·i·cide (pu-lis′ĭ-sīd) an agent destructive to fleas 灭蚤药

pull (pool) 1. to strain a muscle 拉伤肌肉；2. the injury sustained in a muscle strain 牵拉伤

pul·lu·la·tion (pul″u-la′shən) development by sprouting or budding 出芽，生芽，发芽

pul·mo (pool′mo) pl. *pulmo′nes* [L.] lung 肺

pul·mo·nary (pool′mo-nar″e) 1. pertaining to the lungs 肺部的；2. pertaining to the pulmonary artery 肺动脉的

pul·mon·ic (pool-mon′ik) 同 pulmonary

pul·mo·ni·tis (pool″mo-ni′tis) 同 pneumonitis

pulp (pulp) any soft, juicy tissue 髓；**pul′pal** *adj.*；coronal p., the part of the dental pulp contained in the crown portion of the pulp cavity 牙冠髓；dental p., richly vascularized and innervated connective tissue inside the pulp cavity of a tooth 牙髓，齿髓；devitalized p., 同 necrotic p.；digital p., a cushion of soft tissue on the palmar or plantar surface of the distal phalanx of a finger or toe. 指腹；necrotic p., nonvital p., dental pulp that has been deprived of its blood and nerve supply and is no longer composed of living tissue; there may be bacterial invasion 坏死性牙髓，失活髓；red p., the dark, reddish brown substance filling the interspaces of the splenic sinuses and acting as a filter for the blood 红 髓；splenic p., the parenchyma of the spleen, composed of red p. and white p. 脾髓；vital p., dental pulp that has both vascularity and sensation, i.e., is not necrotic 活 髓；white p., the portion of the spleen involved in the immune response, comprising the T lymphocyte–rich periarteriolar lymphoid sheaths in which are interspersed the B lymphocyte–containing malpighian corpuscles 白髓

pul·pa (pul′pə) pl. *pul′pae* [L.] 同 pulp

pul·pec·to·my (pəl-pek′tə-me) removal of dental pulp 牙髓摘除术

pul·pi·tis (pəl-pi′tis) pl. *pulpi′tides.* Inflammation of dental pulp 牙髓炎

pul·pot·o·my (pəl-pot′ə-me) excision of the coronal pulp 牙髓切断术

pul·py (pul′pe) soft or pulteaceous 软的，髓样的

pul·sa·tile (pul′sə-tīl) characterized by a rhythmic pulsation 搏动的

pul·sa·tion (pəl-sa′shən) a throb, or rhythmic beat, as of the heart 搏动（如心脏）

pulse (puls) the rhythmic expansion of an artery that may be felt with the finger 脉搏；**alternating p.,** one with regular alternation of weak and strong beats without changes in cycle length 交 替 脉；**anacrotic p.,** one in which the ascending limb of the tracing shows a transient drop in amplitude 升线一波脉；**bigeminal p.,** one in which two beats occur in rapid succession, the groups of two being separated by a longer interval 二联脉；**cannonball p.,** 同 Corrigan p.；**capillary p.,** 同 Quincke p.；**catadicrotic p.,** one in which the descending limb of the tracing shows two small notches 降线二波脉；**Corrigan p.,** jerky pulse with full expansion and sudden collapse 水冲脉；**dicrotic p.,** a pulse characterized by two peaks, the second peak occurring in diastole and being an exaggeration of the dicrotic wave 二波脉；**entoptic p.,** a phose occurring with each pulse beat 闪光感性心搏；**hard p.,** one characterized by high tension 硬 脉；**jerky p.,** one in which the artery is suddenly and markedly distended 急 冲 脉；**paradoxical p.,** one that markedly decreases in size during inhalation, as often occurs in constrictive pericarditis 奇 脉；**pistol-shot p.,** Corrigan p. 射击脉；**plateau p.,** a pulse that is slowly rising and sustained 丘状脉；**quadrigeminal p.,** a pulse with a pause after every fourth beat 四联脉；**Quincke p.,** alternate blanching and flushing of the nail bed due to pulsation of subpapillary arteriolar and venous plexuses; seen in aortic insufficiency and other conditions and occasionally in normal persons 毛细管脉搏；**Riegel p.,** one that is smaller during respiration Riegel 脉搏（呼气时脉搏变小）；**thready p.,** one that is very fine and scarcely perceptible 细 脉；**tricrotic p.,** one in which the tracing shows three marked expansions in one beat of the artery 三重搏脉；**trigeminal p.,** a pulse with a pause after every third beat 三联脉；**vagus p.,** a slow pulse 迷走神经性脉搏；**venous p.,** the pulsation over a vein, especially over the right jugular vein 静脉脉搏；**water-hammer p.,** 同 Corrigan p.；**wiry p.,** a small, tense pulse 弦脉

pulse·less (puls′ləs) lacking a pulse 无脉的

pul·sion (pul′shən) a pushing forward or outward

推出，压出

pul·sus (pul′səs) pl. *pul′sus* [L.] 同 pulse；p. al·ter′nans, alternating pulse 交替脉；p. bisfe′riens, a pulse characterized by two strong systolic peaks separated by a midsystolic dip, most commonly occurring in pure aortic regurgitation and in aortic regurgitation with stenosis 双峰脉；p. dif′ferens, inequality of the pulse observable at corresponding sites on the two sides of the body 不对称脉

pul·ta·ceous (pəl-ta′shəs) like a poultice; pulpy 软糊状的，髓样的

pul·vi·nar (pəl-vi′nər) the prominent medial part of the posterior end of the thalamus 丘脑枕

pum·ice (pum′is) a very light, hard, rough, porous, grayish powder consisting of silicates of aluminum, potassium, and sodium; used in dentistry as an abrasive 浮石（牙科用作研磨剂）

pump 1. an apparatus for drawing or forcing liquids or gases 泵；2. to draw or force liquids or gases 压出，抽吸（液体或气体）；breast p., a manual or electric pump for abstracting breast milk 吸乳器；calcium p., the mechanism of active transport of calcium (Ca^{2+}) across a membrane, as of the sarcoplasmic reticulum of muscle cells, against a concentration gradient; the mechanism is driven by enzymatic hydrolysis of ATP 钙泵；intra-aor·tic balloon p. (IABP), a pump used in intra-aortic balloon counterpulsation 主动脉内球囊反搏；proton p., a system for transporting protons across cell membranes, often exchanging them for other positively charged ions 质子泵；sodium p., sodium-potassium p., Na^+, K^+-ATPase 钠泵，钠钾泵，钠钾 ATP 酶

pump-oxy·gen·a·tor (pump′ok″sĭ-jə-na′tər) an apparatus consisting of a blood pump and oxygenator, plus filters and traps, for saturating the blood with oxygen during heart surgery 泵式充氧器

punch drunk (punch′drunk″) showing symptoms of chronic traumatic encephalopathy 拳击手酩酊醉的（脑病），指表现出慢性创伤性脑病的症状

punc·tate (pungk′tāt) spotted; marked with points or punctures 点状的

punc·ti·form (pungk′tĭ-form) like a point 点状的

punc·tum (pungk′təm) pl. *punc′ta* [L.] a point or small spot 点，尖，p. cae′cum, blind spot 盲点；p. lacrima′le, lacrimal point 泪点；p. prox′imum, near point 近点；p. remo′tum, far point 远点

punc·ture (pungk′chər) the act of piercing or penetrating with a pointed object or instrument; a wound so made 穿刺（术）；刺伤；cisternal p., puncture of the cisterna cerebellomedullaris through the posterior atlanto-occipital membrane to obtain cerebrospinal fluid 小脑延髓池穿刺；lumbar p.,

spinal p., the withdrawal of fluid from the subarachnoid space in the lumbar region, usually between the third and fourth lumbar vertebrae 腰椎穿刺；sternal p., removal of bone marrow from the manubrium of the sternum through an appropriate needle 胸骨穿刺；ventricular p., puncture of a cerebral ventricle for the withdrawal of fluid 脑室穿刺

pu·pa (pu′pə) [L.] the second stage in the development of an insect, between the larva and the imago 蛹；pu′pal *adj.*

pu·pil (P) (pu′pil) the opening in the center of the iris through which light enters the eye 瞳孔，见图 30；pu′pillary *adj.*；Adie p., tonic p. 阿迪瞳孔；Argyll Robertson p., a pupil that is miotic and responds to accommodation effort, but not to light, usually a sign of neurosyphilis 阿·罗瞳孔；fixed p., a pupil that does not react either to light or on convergence, or in accommodation 固定性瞳孔；Hutchinson p., one that is dilated while the other is not 哈钦森瞳孔；tonic p., a usually unilateral condition of the eye in which the affected pupil is larger than the other; responds to accommodation and convergence in a slow, delayed fashion; and reacts to light only after prolonged exposure to dark or light 强直性瞳孔

pu·pil·la (pu-pil′ə) [L.] 同 pupil

pu·pil·lom·e·try (pu″pĭ-lom′ə-tre) measurement of the diameter or width of the pupil of the eye 瞳孔测量（法）

pu·pil·lo·ple·gia (pu″pĭ-lo-ple′jə) tonic pupil 强直性瞳孔

pu·pil·lo·sta·tom·e·ter (pu-pil″o-stə-tom′ə-tər) an instrument for measuring the distance between the pupils 瞳孔距离计

pure (pūr) free from mixture with or contamination by other materials 纯的，纯净的

pur·ga·tion (pər-ga′shən) evacuation (2) 净化

pur·ga·tive (pur′gə-tiv) cathartic (1, 2) 净化的，催泻的

purge (purj) 1. to cleanse or purify; to remove undesirable substances from something（使）净化；2. to cause evacuation of feces 催泻

pu·ri·fi·ca·tion (pūr″ĭ-fĭ-ka′shən) the separating of foreign or contaminating elements from a substance of interest 纯化，提纯

pu·rine (pu′rēn) a compound, $C_5H_4N_4$, not found in nature, but variously substituted to produce a group of compounds, *purines* or *purine bases,* which include adenine and guanine found in nucleic acids and xanthine and hypoxanthine 嘌呤

pur·ple (pur′pəl) 1. a color between blue and red 紫色；2. a substance of this color used as a dye or indicator 用作染料或指示剂的紫色的物质；visual p., rhodopsin 视紫红质

pur·pu·ra (pur′pu-rə) 1. a small hemorrhage in the skin, mucous membrane, or serosal surface 紫斑；2. a group of disorders characterized by the presence of purpuric lesions, ecchymoses, and a tendency to bruise easily 紫癜；**purpu′ric** *adj.*；
p. annula′ris telangiecto′des, a rare form in which punctate erythematous lesions coalesce to form an annular or serpiginous pattern 毛细血管扩张性环状紫癜；**chronic pigmented p.,** any of a group of benign dermatoses of unknown etiology, consisting of minimal inflammation with cayenne pepper spots on the skin 慢性色素性紫癜；**fibrinolytic p.,** purpura associated with increased fibrinolytic activity of the blood 纤维蛋白溶解性紫癜；**p. ful′minans,** nonthrombocytopenic purpura seen mainly in children, usually after an infectious disease, marked by fever, shock, anemia, and sudden, rapidly spreading symmetric skin hemorrhages of the lower limbs, often associated with extensive intravascular thromboses and gangrene 暴发性紫癜；**p. hemorrha′gica,** idiopathic thrombocytopenic p. 出血性紫癜；**Henoch p.,** Henoch-Schönlein purpura in which abdominal symptoms predominate 腹型过敏性紫癜；**Henoch-Schönlein p.,** nonthrombocytopenic purpura of unknown cause, usually in children; associated with symptoms such as urticaria, erythema, arthropathy and arthritis, gastrointestinal disorder, and renal involvement 过敏性紫癜；**idiopathic thrombocytopenic p.,** thrombocytopenic purpura not directly associated with a systemic disease, although often following a systemic infection; believed to be due to an IgG immunoglobulin that acts as an antibody against platelets 特发性血小板减少性紫癜；**nonthrombocytopenic p.,** purpura without any decrease in the platelet count of the blood 非血小板减少性紫癜；**Schönlein p.,** Henoch-Schönlein purpura with articular symptoms and without gastrointestinal symptoms 不伴有关节症状和无胃肠症状的过敏性紫癜；**Schönlein-Henoch p.,** 同 Henoch-Schönlein p.；**p. seni′lis,** dark purplish red ecchymoses on the forearms and backs of the hands in the elderly 老年性紫癜；**thrombocytopenic p.,** any form in which the platelet count is decreased, either as a primary disease *(idiopathic thrombocytopenic p.)* or resulting from a primary hematologic disorder *(secondary thrombocytopenic p.)* 血小板减少性紫癜；**thrombotic thrombocytopenic p.,** a form of thrombotic microangiopathy marked by thrombocytopenia, hemolytic anemia, neurologic manifestations, azotemia, fever, and thromboses in terminal arterioles and capillaries 血栓性血小板减少性紫癜
pu·ru·lence (pu′roo-ləns) suppuration 脓；**pur′u-**lent *adj.*

pus (pus) a protein-rich liquid inflammation product made up of leukocytes, cellular debris, and a thin fluid (liquor puris) 脓
pus·tu·la (pus′tu-lə) pl. *pus′tulae* [L.] 同 pustule
pus·tule (pus′tūl) a small, elevated, circumscribed, pus-containing lesion of the skin 脓疱；**pus′tular** *adj.*
pus·tu·lo·sis (pus″tu-lo′sis) a condition marked by an eruption of pustules 脓疱病
pu·ta·men (pu-ta′mən) the larger and more lateral part of the lentiform nucleus 壳、硬膜；**puta′minal** *adj.*
pu·tre·fac·tion (pu″trə-fak′shən) enzymatic decomposition, especially of proteins, with the production of foul-smelling compounds, such as hydrogen sulfide, ammonia, and mercaptans 腐败；**putrefac′tive, pu′trid** *adj.*
pu·tres·cence (pu-tres′əns) the condition of undergoing putrefaction 腐败，正在腐烂的东西；**putres′cent** *adj.*
pu·tres·cine (pu-tres′ēn) a polyamine precursor of spermidine occurring in most tissues and believed to be a growth factor necessary for cell division; first found in decaying animal tissues 腐胺
pu·trid (pu′trid) rotten; putrefied 腐烂的，恶臭的
PVC polyvinyl chloride 聚氯乙烯
PVP polyvinylpyrrolidone 聚乙烯吡咯酮（参见 *povidone*）
PVP-I povidone-iodine 聚维酮碘，聚烯吡咯碘，聚乙烯吡咯酮碘
PWI perfusion-weighted imaging 灌注加权像
py·ar·thro·sis (pi″ahr-thro′sis) suppuration within a joint cavity; acute suppurative arthritis 关节积脓；急性化脓性关节炎
py·elec·ta·sis (pi″ə-lek′tə-sis) dilatation of the renal pelvis 肾盂扩张
py·eli·tis (pi″ə-li′tis) inflammation of the renal pelvis 肾盂炎；**pyelit′ic** *adj.*
py·elo·cali·ec·ta·sis (pi″ə-lo-kal″e-ek′tə-sis) hydronephrosis 肾盂肾盏扩张
py·elo·cal·y·ce·al (pi″ə-lo-kal″ĭ-se′əl) pertaining to the renal pelvis and calices 肾盂肾盏的
py·elo·cys·ti·tis (pi″ə-lo-sis-ti′tis) inflammation of the renal pelvis and bladder 肾盂膀胱炎
py·elog·ra·phy (pi″ə-log′rə-fe) radiography of the renal pelvis and ureter after injection of contrast material 肾盂造影（术）；**antegrade p.,** pyelography in which the contrast medium is introduced by percutaneous needle puncture into the renal pelvis 顺行肾盂造影；**retrograde p.,** pyelography after introduction of contrast material through the ureter

逆行肾盂造影

py·elo·in·ter·sti·tial (pi″ə-lo-in″tər-stish′əl) pertaining to the interstitial tissue of the renal pelvis 肾盂间质的

py·elo·li·thot·o·my (pi″ə-lo-lĭ-thot′ə-me) incision of the renal pelvis for removal of calculi 肾盂切开取石术

py·elo·ne·phri·tis (pi″ə-lo-nə-fri′tis) inflammation of the kidney and its pelvis due to bacterial infection 肾盂肾炎

py·elo·ne·phro·sis (pi″ə-lo-nə-fro′sis) any disease of the kidney and its pelvis 肾盂肾病

py·e·lo·plas·ty (pi′ə-lo-plas″te) plastic operation on the renal pelvis 肾盂成形术

py·elos·to·my (pi″ə-los′tə-me) surgical formation of an opening into the renal pelvis 肾盂造瘘术

py·elot·o·my (pi″ə-lot′ə-me) incision of the renal pelvis 肾盂切开术

py·elo·ure·ter·i·tis (pi″ə-lo-u-re″tər-i′tis) inflammation of a ureter and the renal pelvis 肾盂输尿管炎

py·elo·ve·nous (pi″ə-lo-ve′nəs) pertaining to the renal pelvis and renal veins 肾盂肾静脉的

py·e·mia (pi-e′me-ə) septicemia in which secondary foci of suppuration occur and multiple abscesses are formed 脓血症，脓毒血症；**pye′mic** adj.；**arterial p.**, that due to dissemination of septic emboli from the heart 动脉性脓毒症；**cryptogenic p.**, that in which the source of infection is in an unidentified tissue 隐原性脓血症

Py·e·mo·tes (pi″ə-mo′tēz) a genus of parasitic mites. *P. ventrico′sus* attacks certain insect larvae found on straw, grain, and other plants, and causes grain itch in humans 蒲螨属

py·en·ceph·a·lus (pi″en-səf′ə-ləs) brain abscess 脑脓肿

py·gal (pi′gəl) gluteal 臀的

py·gal·gia (pi-gal′jə) pain in the buttocks 臀痛

pyk·nic (pik′nik) having a short, thick, stocky build 矮胖型的

pyk·no·cyte (pik′no-sīt″) a distorted and contracted, occasionally spiculed erythrocyte 固缩红细胞

pyk·no·dys·os·to·sis (pik″no-dis″os-to′sis) a hereditary syndrome of dwarfism, osteopetrosis, and skeletal anomalies of the cranium, digits, and mandible 致密性成骨不全症

pyk·nom·e·ter (pik-nom′ə-tər) an instrument for determining the specific gravity of fluids 比重计，比重管

pyk·no·mor·phous (pik″no-mor′fəs) having the stained portions of the cell body compactly arranged 致密排列的，密形的

pyk·no·sis (pik-no′sis) a thickening, especially degeneration of a cell in which the nucleus shrinks

in size and the chromatin condenses to a solid, structureless mass or masses 固缩；**pyknot′ic** adj.

py·le·phle·bi·tis (pi″le-flə-bi′tis) inflammation of the portal vein 门静脉炎

py·lo·rec·to·my (pi″lo-rek′tə-me) excision of the pylorus 幽门切除术

py·lo·ric (pi-lor′ik) pertaining to the pylorus or to the pyloric part of the stomach 幽门（部）的

py·lo·ri·ste·no·sis (pi-lor″ĭ-stə-no′sis) pyloric stenosis 幽门狭窄

py·lo·ro·du·od·e·ni·tis (pi-lor″o-doo-od″ə-ni′tis) inflammation of the pyloric and duodenal mucosa 幽门十二指肠炎

py·lo·ro·gas·trec·to·my (pi-lor″o-gas-trek′-tə-me) excision of the pylorus and adjacent portion of the stomach 幽门（及邻近部分胃）切除术

py·lo·ro·my·ot·o·my (pi-lor″o-mi-ot′ə-me) incision of the longitudinal and circular muscles of the pylorus 幽门肌切开术

py·lo·ro·plas·ty (pi-lor′o-plas″te) plastic surgery of the pylorus 幽门成形术；**double p.**, posterior pyloromyotomy combined with the HeinekeMikulicz pyloroplasty 双重幽门成形术；**Finney p.**, enlargement of the pyloric canal by establishment of an inverted U-shaped anastomosis between the stomach and duodenum after longitudinal incision 芬尼幽门成形术，指通过在胃和十二指肠之间建立一个纵向切开后的倒 U 形吻合口来扩大幽门管；**Heineke-Mikulicz p.**, enlargement of a pyloric stricture by incising the pylorus longitudinally and suturing the incision transversely 海 - 米二氏纵切横缝法幽门成形术，指通过纵向切开幽门并横向缝合切口来扩大幽门狭窄

py·lo·ros·to·my (pi″lor-os′tə-me) surgical formation of an opening through the abdominal wall into the stomach near the pylorus 幽门造口术

py·lo·rot·o·my (pi″lor-ot′ə-me) incision of the pylorus 幽门切开术

py·lo·rus (pi-lor′əs) the distal aperture of the stomach, opening into the duodenum; variously used to mean the pyloric part of the stomach, and pyloric antrum, canal, opening, or sphincter 幽门；**pylor′ic** adj.

pyo·cele (pi′o-sēl″) a collection of pus, as in the scrotum 鞘膜积脓

pyo·coc·cus (pi″o-kok′əs) any pus-forming coccus（化）脓球菌

pyo·cyst (pi′o-sist) a cyst containing pus 脓囊肿

pyo·der·ma (pi″o-dur′mə) any purulent skin disease 脓皮病；**p. gangreno′sum**, a rapidly evolving, irregular, boggy, blue-red cutaneous ulcer with an undermined border, seen with ulcerative colitis and other conditions 坏疽性脓皮病

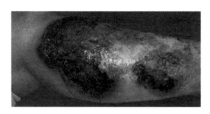

▲ 慢性溃疡性结肠炎患者的坏疽性脓皮病

pyo·gen·e·sis (pi″o-jen′ə-sis) suppuration; the formation of pus 化脓，生脓，脓生成

pyo·gen·ic (pi″o-jen′ik) suppurative 生脓的

pyo·he·mo·tho·rax (pi″o-he″mo-thor′aks) pus and blood in the pleural space 脓血胸

pyo·hy·dro·ne·phro·sis (pi″o-hi″dro-nə-fro′sis) accumulation of pus and urine in the kidney 脓性肾积水

pyo·me·tri·tis (pi″o-mə-tri′tis) purulent inflammation of the uterus 脓性子宫炎

pyo·myo·si·tis (pi″o-mi″o-si′tis) an acute bacterial infection of skeletal muscle, usually seen in the tropics, most commonly caused by *Staphylococcus aureus* 脓性肌炎

pyo·ne·phri·tis (pi″o-nə-fri′tis) purulent inflammation of the kidney 脓性肾炎

pyo·neph·ro·sis (pi″o-nə-fro′sis) suppurative destruction of the renal parenchyma, with total or almost complete loss of kidney function 肾盂积脓，脓肾

pyo-ova·ri·um (pi″o-o-var′e-əm) abscess of an ovary 卵巢积脓

pyo·peri·car·di·um (pi″o-per″ĭ-kahr′- de-əm) pus in the pericardium 心包积脓

pyo·peri·to·ne·um (pi″o-per″ĭ-to-ne′əm) pus in the peritoneal cavity 腹（膜）腔积脓

py·oph·thal·mi·tis (pi″of-thəl-mi′tis) purulent inflammation of the eye 脓性眼炎

pyo·phy·so·me·tra (pi″o-fi″so-me′trə) pus and gas in the uterus 子宫积脓气

pyo·pneu·mo·hep·a·ti·tis (pi″o-noo″mohep″ə-ti′tis) abscess of the liver with pus and gas 脓气性肝炎

pyo·pneu·mo·peri·car·di·um (pi″o-noo″moper″ĭ-kahr′de-əm) pus and gas or air in the pericardium 脓气心包

pyo·pneu·mo·peri·to·ni·tis (pi″o-noo″ moper″ĭ-to-ni′tis) peritonitis with pus and gas 脓气性腹膜炎

pyo·pneu·mo·tho·rax (pi″o-noo″mo-thor′aks) pus and air or gas in the pleural cavity 脓气胸

pyo·poi·e·sis (pi″o-poi-e′sis) 同 pyogenesis

pyo·py·elec·ta·sis (pi″o-pi″ə-lek′tə-sis) dilatation of the renal pelvis with pus 脓性肾盂扩张

py·or·rhea (pi″o-re′ə) a copious discharge of pus 溢脓；**pyorrhe′al** *adj.*；p. alveola′ris, marginal periodontitis 齿槽脓溢

pyo·sal·pin·gi·tis (pi″o-sal″pin-ji′tis) uterine salpingitis with suppuration 脓性输卵管炎

pyo·sal·pin·go-ooph·o·ri·tis (pi″o-sal-ping″- go-o″of-ə-ri′tis) purulent inflammation of a uterine tube and ovary 脓性输卵管卵巢炎

pyo·sal·pinx (pi″o-sal′pinks) a collection of pus in a uterine tube 输卵管积脓

pyo·sper·mia (pi″o-spur′me-ə) pus in the semen 脓性精液（症），精液含脓

pyo·stat·ic (pi″o-stat′ik) stopping or hindering pus formation; an agent that does this 抑制（化）脓的；制（化）脓的

pyo·tho·rax (pi″o-tho′raks) empyema (2) 脓胸

pyo·ure·ter (pi″o-u-re′tər) pus in a ureter 输尿管积脓

pyr·a·mid (pir′ə-mid) a pointed or coneshaped structure or part; often used to indicate the pyramid of the medulla oblongata 锥体；p. of cerebellum, 同 p. of vermis; Lalouette p., 同 p. of thyroid；p. of light, 光锥，参见 *cone* 下词条；p. of medulla oblongata, either of two rounded masses, one on either side of the median fissure of the medulla oblongata 延髓锥体；renal p's, the conical masses composing the medullary substance of the kidney 肾锥体；p. of thyroid, an occasional third lobe of the thyroid gland, extending upward from the isthmus 甲状腺锥体叶；p. of tympanum, the hollow elevation in the inner wall of the middle ear containing the stapedius muscle（鼓室）锥隆起；p. of vermis, the part of the vermis cerebelli between the tuber vermis and the uvula 蚓锥体

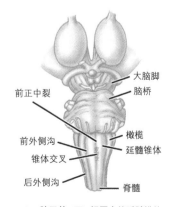

▲ 脑干前（下）视图中的延髓锥体

py·ram·i·dal (pĭ-ram′ĭ-dəl) 1. shaped like a pyr-

P

amid 金字塔型的，锥形的；2. pertaining to the pyramidal tract 椎体的

pyr·a·mis (pir'ə-mis) pl. *pyra'mides* [Gr.] 同 pyramid

py·ran (pi'ran) a cyclic compound in which the ring consists of five carbon atoms and one oxygen atom 吡喃

pyr·a·nose (pir'ə-nōs) any sugar containing the 5-carbon pyran ring structure; it is a cyclic form that ketoses and aldoses may take in solution 吡喃糖

py·ran·tel (pĭ-ran'təl) a broad-spectrum anthelmintic effective against roundworms and pinworms, used as the pamoate and tartrate salts 噻嘧啶，一种对蛔虫和蛲虫有效的广谱驱虫剂

pyr·a·zin·a·mide (pir'ə-zin'ə-mīd) an antibacterial derived from nicotinic acid, used as a tuberculostatic 吡嗪酰胺，一种从烟酸中提取的抗菌药物，用于治疗结核

py·reth·rin (pi-reth'rin) either of two esters, *p. I* and *p. II*, found in the flowers of certain species of *Chrysanthemum*; used as an insecticide and as a topical pediculicide 除虫菊酯

py·ret·ic (pi-ret'ik) 1. febrile 发热的（参见 fever）；2. 同 pyrogenic；3. 同 pyrogen

py·re·to·gen·e·sis (pi'rə-to-jen'ə-sis) the origin and causation of fever 发热，热发生

py·rex·ia (pi-rek'se-ə) fever 发热；**pyrex'ial** *adj.*

pyr·i·dine (pir'ĭ-dēn) 1. a coal tar derivative, C_5H_5N, derived also from tobacco and various organic matter 吡啶；2. any of a group of substances homologous with normal pyridine 与正常吡啶类似物质中的任一种

pyr·i·do·stig·mine (pir″ĭ-do-stig'mēn) a cholinesterase inhibitor, used as the bromide salt in the treatment of myasthenia gravis and as an antidote to nondepolarizing neuromuscular blocking agents 吡斯的明，一种胆碱酯酶抑制药，用于治疗重症肌无力和神经肌肉阻滞

pyr·i·dox·al (pir″ĭ-dok'səl) a form of vitamin B_6 吡哆醛；**p. phosphate**, the prosthetic group of many enzymes involved in amino acid transformations 磷酸吡哆醛

pyr·i·dox·amine (pir″ĭ-dok'sə-mēn) one of the three active forms of vitamin B_6 吡哆胺

pyr·i·dox·ine (pēr″ĭ-dok'sēn) one of the forms of vitamin B_6, used as the hydrochloride salt in the prophylaxis and treatment of vitamin B_6 deficiency and as an antidote in cycloserine and isoniazid poisoning 吡哆醇

py·ril·amine (pə-ril'ə-mēn) an antihistamine with anticholinergic and sedative effects, used as the maleate and tannate salts 吡拉明，一种具有抗胆碱能和镇静作用的抗组胺药

pyr·i·meth·amine (pir″ĭ-meth'ə-mēn) a folic acid antagonist, used in the treatment of malaria and of toxoplasmosis 乙胺嘧啶，一种叶酸拮抗药，用于治疗疟疾和弓形虫病

py·rim·i·dine (pə-rim'ĭ-dēn) an organic compound, $C_4H_4N_2$, the fundamental form of the pyrimidine bases, including uracil, cytosine, and thymine 嘧啶

py·ro·cat·e·chol (pi″ro-kat'ə-kol) a compound comprising the aromatic portion in the synthesis of endogenous catecholamines; it has been used as a topical antiseptic and as a reagent 邻苯二酚，焦儿茶酚

py·ro·gen (pi'ro-jən) a fever-producing substance 致热原，热原

py·ro·gen·ic (pi″ro-jen'ik) causing fever 致热的

py·ro·glob·u·lin·emia (pi″ro-glob″u-lin-e′-mə) presence in the blood of an abnormal globulin constituent that is precipitated by heat 热球蛋白血（症）

py·ro·ma·nia (pi″ro-ma'ne-ə) the compulsion to set or watch fires in the absence of monetary or other gain, the act being preceded by tension or arousal and resulting in pleasure or relief 纵火狂

py·ro·nin (pi'ro-nin) a red aniline histologic stain 派若宁，是一种红色的苯胺组织染色

py·ro·pho·bia (pi″ro-fo'be-ə) irrational fear of fire 恐火症，火（焰）恐怖

py·ro·phos·pha·tase (pi″ro-fos'fə-tās) any enzyme that catalyzes the hydrolysis of a pyrophosphate bond, cleaving between the two phosphate groups 焦磷酸酶

py·ro·phos·phate (pi″ro-fos'fāt) a salt of pyrophosphoric acid 焦磷酸盐

py·ro·phos·pho·ric ac·id (pi″ro-fos-for'ik) a dimer of phosphoric acid, $H_4P_2O_7$; its esters are important in energy metabolism and biosynthesis, e.g., ATP 焦磷酸

py·ro·sis (pi-ro'sis) heartburn 胃灼热；**pyrot'ic** *adj.*

py·roxy·lin (pir-ok'sə-lin) a product of the action of a mixture of nitric and sulfuric acids on cotton; used to make collodion 焦木素

pyr·role (pir-ōl′) 1. a toxic, basic, heterocyclic compound; obtained by destructive distillation of various animal substances and used in the manufacture of pharmaceuticals 吡咯；2. a substituted derivative of this structure 吡咯衍生物

pyr·rol·i·dine (pir-ol'ĭ-dēn) a simple base, $(CH_2)_4NH$, obtained from tobacco or prepared from pyrrole 四氢吡咯

py·ru·vate (pi'roo-vāt) a salt, ester, or anion of

pyruvic acid. Pyruvate is the end product of glycolysis and may be metabolized to lactate or to acetyl CoA 丙酮酸盐、酯、阴离子

py·ru·vate ki·nase (PK) (pi′roo-vāt ki′nās) an enzyme that catalyzes the transfer of highenergy phosphate from phospho*enol*pyruvate to ADP to yield ATP and pyruvate; it is one of two reactions generating ATP in the Embden-Meyerhof pathway and a key regulatory site in the pathway. The enzyme has three isozymes; deficiency of the erythrocyte isozyme, an autosomal recessive trait, causes hemolytic anemia 丙酮酸激酶

py·ru·vic ac·id (pi-roo′vik) CH₃COCOOH, an intermediate in carbohydrate, lipid, and protein metabolism 丙酮酸

py·uria (pi-u′re-ə) pus in the urine 脓尿

Q

Q ubiquinone 泛醌的符号

Q₁₀ ubiquinone 泛醌的符号

q the long arm of a chromosome 染色体长臂

q.d. [L.] qua′que di′e (every day) (on The Joint Commission "Do Not Use" List) 每日

q.h. [L.] qua′que ho′ra (every hour) 每小时

qi (che) [Chinese] chi or ch′i; one of the basic substances that according to traditional Chinese medicine pervade the body; a subtle influence or vital energy that is the cause of most physiologic processes and whose proper balance is necessary for maintaining health 气，属中医学范畴

q.i.d. [L.] qua′ter in di′e (four times a day) 每日 4 次

qi gong (che′ kung′) [Chinese] qi cultivation, a broad range of practices, incorporating meditation, movement exercises, and breath control, whose purpose is to manipulate and develop qi, and ranging in application from the meditative systems of spiritual practitioners to the martial arts 气功，属中医学范畴

QNS quantity not sufficient 量不足；Queen's Nursing Sister (of Queen's Institute of District Nursing) 女王护士长（皇家地区护理学会）

q.s. [L.] quan′tum sa′tis (sufficient quantity) 适量，足量

q-sort (ku′sort) a technique of personality assessment in which the subject (or an observer) indicates the degree to which a standardized set of descriptive statements applies to the subject q 分类，q 选择，一种人格鉴定法，其中受试者（或实验者）对一套标准化描述的符合程度

quack (kwak) one who misrepresents their ability and experience in diagnosis and treatment of disease or effects to be achieved by their treatment 庸医，江湖医

quack·ery (kwak′ər-e) the practice or methods of a quack 江湖医术

quad·rant (kwod′rənt) 1. one-fourth of the circumference of a circle 四分之一圆；2. one of four corresponding parts, or quarters, as of the surface of the abdomen or of the field of vision 四分体象限

quad·rant·an·o·pia (kwod″rənt-ə-no′pe-ə) defective vision or blindness in one-fourth of the visual field 象限盲

quad·ran·tec·to·my (kwod″rən-tek′tə-me) a form of partial mastectomy involving en bloc excision of tumor in one quadrant of breast tissue, as well as the pectoralis major muscle fascia and overlying skin 象限切除术

quad·rate (kwod′rāt) square or squared 正方形；方形的

quad·ri·ceps (kwod′rĭ-seps) having four heads 四头肌

quad·ri·gem·i·nal (kwod″rĭ-jem′ĭ-nəl) 1. fourfold; in four parts; forming a group of four 四倍的，四叠的，四联的；2. pertaining to the corpora quadrigemina 四叠体的

quad·ri·gem·i·ny (kwod″rĭ-jem′ĭ-ne) 1. occurrence in fours 四次出现；2. the occurrence of four beats of the pulse followed by a pause 四联脉

quad·rip·a·ra (kwod-rip′ə-rə) a woman who has had four pregnancies that resulted in viable offspring; para IV 四产妇

quad·ri·ple·gia (kwod″rĭ-ple′jə) paralysis of all four limbs 四肢麻痹，四肢瘫痪

quad·ri·ple·gic (kwod″rĭ-ple′jik) 1. of, pertaining to, or characterized by quadriplegia 四肢瘫痪者的；2. an individual with quadriplegia 四肢瘫痪者

quad·ri·tu·ber·cu·lar (kwod″rĭ-too-bur′kulər) having four tubercles or cusps 四结节的；四尖的

quad·ri·va·lent (kwod″rĭ-va′lənt) 1. effective against four different entities, as diseases or strains of a pathogen 四价体；2. tetravalent 四价的

quad·ru·ped (kwod′roo-ped″) 1. four-footed 四足的；2. an animal having four feet 四足动物；**quadru′pedal** *adj.*

quad·rup·let (kwod-roop′lət) one of four offspring produced at one birth 一胎四儿，四胎

qual·i·ta·tive (kwahl′ĭ-ta″tiv) pertaining to quality 性质的，定性的；品质的。Cf. *quantitative*

quan·ti·ta·tive (kwahn″tĭ-ta″tiv) 1. denoting or

expressing a quantity 量的，数量的；2. relating to the proportionate quantities or to the amount of the constituents of a compound 定量的

quan·tum (kwahn′təm) pl. *quan′ta* [L.] a unit of measure under the quantum theory (q.v.) 量子

quar·an·tine (kwor′ən-tēn) (kwahr′ən-tēn) 1. restriction of freedom of movement of apparently well individuals who have been exposed to infectious disease, which is imposed for the maximal incubation period of the disease 隔离检疫期；2. quarantine period 检疫期；3. the place where persons are detained for inspection 隔离区；4. to detain or isolate on account of suspected contagion 隔离

quart (kwort) one-fourth of a gallon; in the United States it is 0.946 liter, and in Great Britain *(imperial quart)* it is 1.14 liters 夸脱（1/4加仑）

quar·tan (kwor′tən) recurring in 4-day cycles 每第四日（复发）的；三日疟

quartz (kworts) a crystalline form of silica (silicon dioxide) 石英

qua·si·dom·i·nance (kwah″ze-dom′ĭ-nəns) the mimicking of dominance in inheritance, caused by mating of a carrier of a recessive gene with an individual homozygous for the gene 类显性，准显性；**quasidom′inant** *adj.*

qua·ter·nary (kwah′tər-nar″e) (kwah-tur′nər-e) 1. fourth in order 第四的；2. containing four elements or groups 四元的，四价的

qua·ze·pam (kwah′zə-pam) a benzodiazepine used as a sedative and hypnotic in the treatment of insomnia 夸西泮，四氟硫草安定，苯二氮䓬类药物，用于治疗失眠的镇静催眠药

quench·ing (kwench′ing) 1. suppressing or diminishing a physical property, as of heat in a metal by immersion in cold liquid（金属的）淬火；2. decrease of fluorescence from an excited molecule by other molecules that absorb some emission energy that would otherwise occur as light（光化学的）猝灭；3. in liquid scintillation counting, interference with fluorescence generation or propagation, decreasing the counting efficiency（液体闪烁的）淬灭；4. the termination of secondary and subsequent ionizations in a detector to give it time to become sensitive again（电离的）淬灭

que·ti·a·pine (kwə-ti′ə-pēn) a serotonin and dopamine antagonist used as the fumarate salt as an antipsychotic 喹硫平，一种血清素和多巴胺拮抗药，用抗精神病药物

quick·en·ing (kwik′ən-ing) the first perceptible movement of the fetus in the uterus 胎动感

quin·a·crine (kwin′ə-krin) an antimalarial, antiprotozoal, and anthelmintic, used as the hydrochloride salt, especially for suppressive therapy of ma-

laria and in the treatment of giardiasis and tapeworm infestations 阿的平，一种抗疟药，抗原生动物和驱虫药，尤指用于疟疾治疗和治疗贾第虫和绦虫感染

quin·a·pril (kwin′ə-pril) an angiotensin-converting enzyme inhibitor used as the hydrochloride salt in the treatment of hypertension and congestive heart failure 喹那普利，一种血管紧张素转换酶抑制药，用于治疗高血压和充血性心力衰竭

quin·eth·a·zone (kwin-eth′ə-zōn) a diuretic used in the treatment of edema and hypertension 喹噻酮，用于治疗水肿和高血压的利尿药

quin·i·dine (kwin′ĭ-dēn) the dextrorotatory isomer of quinine, used in the form of the gluconate, polygalacturonate, and sulfate salts in the treatment of cardiac arrhythmias; also used in the treatment of severe falciparum malaria 奎尼丁，奎宁的右旋异构体，用于治疗心律失常和恶性疟疾

qui·nine (kwin′in) (kwin-ēn′) (kwi′nīn) an alkaloid of cinchona that was once widely used to control and prevent malaria; also has analgesic, antipyretic, mild oxytocic, cardiac depressant, and sclerosing properties, and it decreases the excitability of the motor end plate. It is used as the dihydrochloride, hydrochloride, or sulfate salt in the treatment of resistant falciparum malaria 奎宁

quin·in·ism (kwin′ĭ-niz″əm) cinchonism 奎宁中毒，金鸡纳中毒

quin·o·lone (kwin′o-lōn) any of a group of synthetic antibacterial agents that includes nalidixic acid and the fluoroquinolones 喹诺酮

qui·none (kwi′nōn) any of a group of highly aromatic compounds derived from benzene or from multiple-ring hydrocarbons and containing two ketone group substitutions; they are subclassified on the basis of ring structure (i.e., anthraquinone, benzoquinone) and are mild oxidizing agents. Often used specifically to denote benzoquinone, particularly 1,4-benzoquinone 醌

quin·sy (kwin′ze) peritonsillar abscess 扁桃体周脓肿

quin·tan (kwin′tən) recurring every fifth day, as a fever 每第五日（复发）的（如五日热）

quin·tip·a·ra (kwin-tip′ə-rə) a woman who has had five pregnancies that resulted in viable offspring; para V 五产妇

quin·tup·let (kwin-tup′lət) one of five offspring produced at one birth 一胎五儿，五胎

quin·u·pris·tin (kwin-u′pris-tin) a semisynthetic antibacterial used in conjunction with dalfopristin against various gram-positive organisms, including vancomycin-resistant *Enterococcus faecium* 奎奴普汀，一种半成成抗生素，可抗各种革兰阳性菌

quo·tid·i·an　(kwo-tid'e-ən) recurring every day 每日的，日发的；参见 *malaria*
quo·tient　(kwo'shənt) a number obtained by division 商；**achievement q.**, the achievement age divided by the mental age, indicating progress in learning 能力商，成绩商；**caloric q.**, the heat evolved (in calories) divided by the oxygen consumed (in milligrams) in a metabolic process 热量商；**intelligence q.**, a measure of intelligence obtained by dividing the mental age by the chronological age and multiplying the result by 100 智商；**respiratory q. (RQ)**, the ratio of the volume of carbon dioxide given off by the body tissues to the volume of oxygen absorbed by them; usually equal to the corresponding volumes given off and taken up by the lungs 呼吸商

R

R　[符号] arginine 精氨酸；electrical resistance 电阻；organic radical 有机基；rate 率；respiration 呼吸；rhythm 节律；right 右（侧）的；roentgen 伦琴
R　resistance (3) 电阻的符号
R-　a stereodescriptor used to specify the absolute configuration of compounds having asymmetric carbon atoms; opposed to *S*- 右的，与 *S*- 相反
R$_A$, R$_{AW}$　airway resistance 气道阻力
R　[L.] re'cipe (take) 取的符号（用于处方）；参见 *prescription*
r　ring chromosome 环形染色体的符号
Ra　radium 元素镭的符号
ra·bep·ra·zole　(rə-bep'rə-zōl) a proton pump inhibitor used as the sodium salt to inhibit gastric acid secretion in the treatment of gastroesophageal reflux disease and conditions marked by excessive secretion of gastric acid 雷贝拉唑，一种质子泵抑制药，可抑制胃酸分泌，治疗胃食管反流病和胃酸分泌过多的病症
rab·id　(rab'id) affected with rabies; pertaining to rabies 患狂犬病的
ra·bies　(ra'bēz) (ra'be-ēz) an acute, usually fatal, infectious viral disease of the central nervous system of mammals, human infection resulting from the bite of a rabid animal (bats, dogs, etc.). In the later stages, it is marked by paralysis of the muscles of deglutition and glottal spasm provoked by the drinking or the sight of liquids, and by maniacal behavior, convulsions, tetany, and respiratory paralysis 狂犬病；**rab'id** *adj.*
ra·ce·mase　(ra'sə-mās) an enzyme that catalyzes inversion around the asymmetric carbon atom in a substrate having only one center of asymmetry 消旋酶
ra·ce·mate　(ra'sə-māt) a racemic mixture or compound 外消旋体
ra·ce·mic　(ra-se'mik) optically inactive, being composed of equal amounts of dextrorotatory and levorotatory isomers 外消旋的
ra·ce·mi·za·tion　(ra"sə-mī-za'shən) the transfor-

mation of one-half of the molecules of an optically active compound into molecules having exactly the opposite configuration, with complete loss of rotatory power because of the statistical balance between the equal numbers of dextrorotatory and levorotatory molecules（外消旋化）
rac·e·mose　(ras'ə-mōs) shaped like grapes on their stem 葡萄状的
ra·ceph·e·drine　(ra-sef'ĕ-drēn) the racemic form of ephedrine, having the same actions and uses; used as the hydrochloride salt 消旋麻黄碱
ra·chi·al·gia　(ra"ke-al'jə) 同 rachiodynia
ra·chi·cen·te·sis　(ra"ke-sen-te'sis) lumbar puncture 腰椎穿刺，椎管穿刺
ra·chid·i·al　(ra-kid'e-əl) spinal (1) 脊柱的
ra·chid·i·an　(ra-kid'e-ən) spinal (1) 脊柱的
ra·chil·y·sis　(ra-kil'ĭ-sis) correction of lateral curvature of the spine by combined traction and pressure 弯脊矫正术
ra·chi·odyn·ia　(ra"ke-o-din'e-ə) pain in the vertebral column 脊柱痛
ra·chi·om·e·ter　(ra"ke-om'ə-tər) an apparatus for measuring spinal curvature 脊柱弯度计
ra·chi·ot·o·my　(ra"ke-ot'ə-me) incision of a vertebra or the vertebral column 脊柱切开术
ra·chis　(ra'kis) vertebral column 脊柱，脊椎
ra·chis·chi·sis　(ra-kis'kĭ-sis) congenital fissure of the vertebral column 脊柱裂畸形；**r. poste'rior,** spina bifida 脊柱后裂
ra·chit·ic　(ra-kit'ik) pertaining to rickets 佝偻病的
ra·chi·tis　(ra-ki'tis) 同 rickets
ra·chit·o·gen·ic　(rə-kit"o-jen'ik) causing rickets 致佝偻病的
rad　(rad) *radiation absorbed dose:* a unit of measurement of the absorbed dose of ionizing radiation, corresponding to an energy transfer of 100 ergs per gram of any absorbing material 拉德（已废除的辐射吸收剂量单位，每克组织中吸收 100 erg 的能量为 1rad，1rad = 0.01Gy）
rad.　[L.] ra'dix (root) 根
ra·dec·to·my　(ra-dek'tə-me) excision of the root

of a tooth 牙根切除术

ra·di·ad (ra′de-ad) toward the radius or radial side 向桡侧

ra·di·al (ra′de-əl) 1. pertaining to a radius 桡骨的; 2. pertaining to the radius of the forearm or to the lateral aspect of the forearm as opposed to the medial (ulnar) aspect 桡侧的; 3. radiating; spreading outward from a common center 放射状的

ra·di·a·lis (ra′de-a′lis) [L.] radial (2) 桡侧的

ra·di·a·tio (ra-de-a′she-o) pl. *radiatio'nes* [L.] a radiation or radiating structure 辐射线

ra·di·a·tion (ra′de-a′shən) 1. divergence from a common center 辐射; 2. a structure made up of divergent elements, such as one of the fiber tracts in the brain 辐射线（解剖）; 3. energy transmitted by waves through space or through some medium; usually referring to electromagnetic radiation, when used without a modifier. By extension, a stream of particles, such as electrons or alpha particles 辐射能，放射能; **acoustic r.,** a fiber tract arising in the medial geniculate nucleus and passing laterally to terminate in the transverse temporal gyri of the temporal lobe 听辐射; **r. of corpus callosum,** the fibers of the corpus callosum radiating to all parts of the neopallium 胼胝体辐射; **corpuscular r's,** streams of subatomic particles emitted in nuclear disintegration, such as protons, neutrons, positrons, and deuterons 粒子辐射; **electromagnetic r.,** 电磁辐射，参见 *wave* 下词条; **ionizing r.,** corpuscular or electromagnetic radiation capable of producing ionization, directly or indirectly, in its passage through matter 电离辐射; **occipitothalamic r., optic r.,** a fiber tract starting at the lateral geniculate body, passing through the pars retrolentiformis of the internal capsule, and terminating in the striate area on the medial surface of the occipital lobe, on either side of the calcarine sulcus 视辐射; **pyramidal r.,** fibers extending from the pyramidal tract to the cortex 锥形辐射; **tegmental r.,** fibers radiating laterally from the red nucleus 被盖辐射; **thalamic r's,** fibers that reciprocally connect the thalamus and cerebral cortex by way of the internal capsule, usually grouped into four subradiations): anterior, central, inferior, and posterior 丘脑辐射; **ultraviolet r.,** 紫外（线）辐射，参见 *ray* 下词条

rad·i·cal (rad′i-kəl) 1. directed to the root or cause; designed to eliminate all possible extensions of a morbid process 根本的，基本的; 2. a group of atoms that enters and goes out of chemical combination without change 基，根，基团（化学上主要指原子团）; **free r.,** a radical that carries an unpaired electron; such radicals are extremely reactive, with a very short half-life 自由基

rad·i·cle (rad′i-kəl) ramulus; one of the smallest branches of a vessel or nerve 小根，细根，指血管或神经的最小分支

rad·i·cot·o·my (rad″ĭ-kot′ə-me) 同 rhizotomy

ra·dic·u·lal·gia (rə-dik″u-lal′jə) pain due to a disorder of the spinal nerve roots 神经根痛

ra·dic·u·lar (rə-dik′u-lər) of or pertaining to a root or radicle 根的

ra·dic·u·li·tis (rə-dik″u-li′tis) inflammation of the spinal nerve roots 脊神经根炎

ra·dic·u·lo·gan·gli·o·ni·tis (rə-dik″u-logang″gle-o-ni′tis) inflammation of the posterior spinal nerve roots and their ganglia 脊神经根神经节炎

ra·dic·u·lo·me·nin·go·my·eli·tis (rə-dik″ulo-mə-ning″go-mi′ə-li′tis) meningomyeloradiculitis 脊髓脊膜脊神经根炎

ra·dic·u·lo·my·elop·a·thy (rə-dik″u-lo-mi′ə-lop′ə-the) myeloradiculopathy 脊髓脊神经根病

ra·dic·u·lo·neu·rop·a·thy (rə-dik″u-lo-noorop′ə-the) disease of the nerve roots and spinal nerves 神经根神经病

ra·dic·u·lop·a·thy (rə-dik″u-lop′ə-the) disorder of the nerve roots, such as from inflammation of or impingement on a nerve root by a tumor or a bony spur 神经根病变; **spondylotic caudal r.,** compression of the cauda equina due to encroachment upon a congenitally small spinal canal by spondylosis, resulting in neural disorders of the lower limbs 尾椎关节强硬性神经根病

ra·dio·ac·tiv·i·ty (ra′de-o-ak-tiv′ĭ-te) emission of corpuscular or electromagnetic radiation consequent to nuclear disintegration; it is a natural property of all chemical elements of atomic number above 83 and can be induced in all other known elements 放射性; **radioac′tive** *adj.*; **artificial r., induced r.,** that produced by bombarding an element with high-velocity particles 人工放射性；人工放射现象

ra·dio·al·ler·go·sor·bent (ra′de-o-al″ər-gosor′bənt) denoting a radioimmunoassay technique for the measurement of specific IgE antibody to a variety of allergens 放射变应原吸附法

ra·dio·bi·cip·i·tal (ra′de-o-bi-sip′ĭ-təl) pertaining to the radius and the biceps muscle 桡骨（与）肱二头肌的

ra·dio·bi·ol·o·gy (ra″de-o-bi-ol′ə-je) the branch of science concerned with effects of light and of ultraviolet and ionizing radiations on living tissues or organisms 放射生物学; **radiobiolog′ical** *adj.*

ra·dio·car·di·og·ra·phy (ra″de-o-kahr″ deog′rəfe) graphic recording of variation with time of the concentration, in a selected chamber of the heart, of a radioactive isotope, usually injected intravenously

放射能心电图测定

ra·dio·car·pal (ra″de-o-kahr′pəl) pertaining to the radius and carpus 桡腕的

ra·dio·chem·is·try (ra″de-o-kem′is-tre) the branch of chemistry dealing with radioactive materials 放射化学

ra·dio·col·loids (ra″de-o-kol′oids) radioisotopes in pure form in solution; they often behave more like colloids than solutes 放射胶质

ra·dio·cys·ti·tis (ra″de-o-sis-ti′tis) radiation cystitis 放射性膀胱炎

ra·dio·den·si·ty (ra″de-o-den′sĭ-te) 同 radiopacity

ra·dio·der·ma·ti·tis (ra″de-o-dur″mə-ti′tis) a cutaneous inflammatory reaction to exposure to biologically effective levels of ionizing radiation 放射性皮炎

ra·dio·di·ag·no·sis (ra″de-o-di″əg-no′sis) diagnosis by means of x-rays and radiographs 放射诊断，X 线诊断

ra·di·odon·tics (ra″de-o-don′tiks) dental radiology 牙放射学

ra·di·odon·tist (ra″de-o-don′tist) a dentist who specializes in dental radiology 牙放射学家

ra·dio·gold (ra′de-o-gōld″) one of the radioactive isotopes of gold, particularly ^{198}Au 放射性金；参见 *gold 198*

ra·dio·gram (ra′de-o-gram″) 同 radiograph

ra·dio·graph (ra′de-o-graf″) the film produced by radiography 射线照片

ra·di·og·ra·phy (ra″de-og′rə-fe) the making of film records (radiographs) of internal structures of the body by passing x-rays or gamma rays through the body to act on specially sensitized film X 线射摄影；**radiograph′ic** *adj.*; **body section r.**, tomography 体层放射照相术; **digital r.**, a technique in which x-ray absorption is quantified by assignment of a number to the amount of x-rays reaching the detector; the information is manipulated by a computer to produce an optimal image 数字 X 线摄影; **electron r.**, a technique in which a latent electron image is produced on clear plastic by passing x-ray photons through a gas with a high atomic number; this image is then developed into a black-and-white picture 电子放射摄影; **mucosal relief r.**, two-stage radiography of the gastrointestinal mucosa, in which a suspension of barium is injected into and evacuated from the organ to be studied, followed by inflation of the organ with air to leave a light coating of contrast medium on the mucosa 双对比造影术; **serial r.**, the making of several exposures of a particular area at arbitrary intervals 系列放射照相术; **spot-film r.**, the making of localized instantaneous radiographic exposures during fluoroscopy 局部瞬时放射照

相术

ra·dio·hu·mer·al (ra″de-o-hu′mər-əl) pertaining to the radius and humerus 桡（骨）肱（骨）的

ra·dio·im·mu·ni·ty (ra″de-o-ĭ-mu′nĭ-te) diminished sensitivity to radiation 放射免疫性

ra·dio·im·mu·no·as·say (ra″de-o-im″u-noas′a) a highly sensitive and specific assay method that uses the competition between radiolabeled and unlabeled substances in an antigen-antibody reaction to determine the concentration of the unlabeled substance, which may be an antibody or a substance against which specific antibodies can be produced 放射免疫测定（法）

ra·dio·im·mu·no·dif·fu·sion (ra″de-oim″u-no-dĭ-fu′zhən) immunodiffusion conducted with radioisotope-labeled antibodies or antigens 放射免疫扩散（法）

ra·dio·im·mu·no·scin·tig·ra·phy (ra″de-oim″u-no-sin-tig′rə-fe) immunoscintigraphy 放射免疫闪烁显象

ra·dio·im·mu·no·sor·bent (ra″de-o-im″u-no-sor′bənt) denoting a radioimmunoassay technique for measuring IgE in samples of serum 放射免疫吸附的

ra·dio·io·dine (ra″de-o-i′o-dīn) any radioactive isotope of iodine, particularly ^{123}I, ^{125}I, and ^{131}I; used in the diagnosis and treatment of thyroid disease and in scintiscanning 放射性碘，又称 *radioactive iodine*

ra·dio·iso·tope (ra″de-o-i′sə-tōp) a radioactive isotope; one having an unstable nucleus and emitting characteristic radiation during its decay to a stable form 放射性同位素

ra·dio·la·bel (ra′de-o-la″bəl) 1. radioactive label 放射性标志物；2. to incorporate such a radioactive label into a compound 放射性示踪（标记）

ra·dio·li·gand (ra″de-o-li′gand) (rad″e-oli-g′ənd) a radioisotope-labeled substance, e.g., an antigen, used in the quantitative measurement of an unlabeled substance by its binding reaction to a specific antibody or other receptor site 放射性配体

ra·di·ol·o·gist (ra″de-ol′ə-jist) a physician specializing in radiology 放射科医生，放射学家

ra·di·ol·o·gy (ra″de-ol′ə-je) the branch of the health sciences concerned with radioactive substances and radiant energy and with the diagnosis and treatment of disease by means of both ionizing (e.g., x-rays) and nonionizing (e.g., ultrasound) radiation 放射学；**radiolog′ic, radiolog′ical** *adj.*

ra·dio·lu·cent (ra″de-o-loo′sənt) permitting the passage of radiant energy, such as x-rays, with little attenuation, the representative areas appearing dark on the exposed film 射线透射的，X 线可透的的

ra·di·om·e·ter (ra″de-om′ə-tər) an instrument for detecting and measuring radiant energy 辐射计

ra·dio·ne·cro·sis (ra″de-o-nə-kro′sis) tissue destruction due to radiant energy 放射性坏死

ra·dio·neu·ri·tis (ra″de-o-noo-ri′tis) neuritis from exposure to radiant energy 放射性神经炎

ra·dio·nu·clide (ra″de-o-noo′klīd) a nuclide that disintegrates with the emission of corpuscular or electromagnetic radiations 放射性核素

ra·di·opac·i·ty (ra″de-o-pas′ĭ-te) the quality or property of obstructing the passage of radiant energy, such as x-rays, the representative areas appearing light or white on the exposed film 射线不透性; **radiopaque′** adj.

ra·dio·pa·thol·o·gy (ra″de-o-pə-thol′ə-je) the pathology of the effects of radiation on tissues 放射病理学

ra·dio·phar·ma·ceu·ti·cal (ra″de-o-fahr″mə-soo′tĭ-kəl) a radioactive pharmaceutical, nuclide, or other chemical used for diagnostic or therapeutic purposes 放射性药品

ra·dio·pro·tec·tor (ra″de-o-pro-tek′tər) an agent that provides protection against the toxic effects of ionizing radiation 防辐射药，辐射防护剂

ra·dio·re·cep·tor (ra″de-o-re-sep′tər) 1. a receptor for the stimuli that are excited by radiant energy, such as light or heat 放射感受器; 2. a receptor to which a radioligand can bind 放射受体

ra·dio·re·sis·tance (ra″de-o-re-zis′təns) resistance, as of tissue or cells, to irradiation 辐射抗性; **radioresist′ant** adj.

ra·di·os·co·py (ra″de-os′kə-pe) fluoroscopy X 射线透视，荧光透视法

ra·dio·sen·si·tiv·i·ty (ra″de-o-sen″sĭ-tiv′ĭ-te) sensitivity, as of the skin, tumor tissue, etc., to radiant energy, such as x-rays or other radiation 辐射敏感性; **radiosen′sitive** adj.

ra·dio·sur·gery (ra″de-o-sur′jər-e) surgery in which tissue destruction is performed by means of ionizing radiation rather than by surgical incision 放射外科学; **stereotactic r., stereotaxic r.,** stereotactic surgery in which lesions are produced by ionizing radiation 立体定位放射手术，立体定向放射外科

ra·dio·ther·a·py (ra″de-o-ther′ə-pe) treatment of disease by means of ionizing radiation; tissue may be exposed to a beam of radiation, or a radioactive element may be contained in devices (e.g., needles or wire) and inserted directly into the tissues (*interstitial r.*), or it may be introduced into a natural body cavity (*intracavitary r.*) 放射治疗

ra·dio·tox·emia (ra″de-o-tok-se′me-ə) toxemia produced by radiant energy 放射性毒血症

ra·dio·tra·cer (ra″de-o-tra′sər) radioactive tracer 放射示踪物

ra·dio·trans·par·ent (ra″de-o-trans-par′ənt) 同 radiolucent

ra·di·o·tro·pic (ra″de-o-tro′pik) influenced by radiation 放射影响的

ra·dio·ul·nar (ra″de-o-ul′nər) pertaining to the radius and ulna 桡骨尺骨的

ra·di·um (Ra) (ra′de-əm) a rare, silvery white, radioactive, alkaline earth metal element, formed as a decay product of uranium; at. no. 88, at. wt. 226. All of its isotopes are radioactive, variously emitting α - or β -rays; all emit γ -rays. Its most stable isotope, ^{226}Ra, has a half-life of 1600 years and decays to radon 镭（化学元素）

ra·di·us (ra′de-əs) pl. *ra′dii* [L.] 1. a line from the center of a circle to a point on its circumference 半径; 2. the bone on the outer side of the forearm, articulating proximally with the humerus and ulna and distally with the ulna and carpus 桡骨，见图 1

ra·dix (ra′diks) pl. *ra′dices* [L.] root 根

ra·don (Rn) (ra′don) a heavy, colorless, odorless, tasteless, radioactive, noble gas element; at. no. 86, at. wt. 222; produced as an intermediate in the decay of radium, thorium, and actinium. Its most stable isotope, ^{222}Rn, has a half-life of 3.8 days. Natural radon gas is considered a significant public health hazard 氡（化学元素）

rag·o·cyte (rag′o-sīt) a polymorphonuclear phagocyte, found in the joints in rheumatoid arthritis, with cytoplasmic inclusions of aggregated IgG, rheumatoid factor, fibrin, and complement 类风湿细胞

ra·jas (rah-jus′) [Sanskrit] according to ayurveda, one of the three gunas, characterized by activity, stimulation, and movement 激性

rale (rahl) crackle; a discontinuous sound consisting of a series of short sounds, heard during inhalation 啰音; **amphoric r.,** a coarse musical rale due to splashing of fluid in a cavity connected with a bronchus 空瓮音; **clicking r.,** a small sound heard when inhaled air passes through secretions in smaller bronchi 喀喇音; **crackling r.,** 同 subcrepitant r.; **crepitant r.,** a sound like that made by rubbing hairs between the fingers, heard at the end of inhalation 捻发音; **dry r.,** a fine sound heard in interstitial lung diseases such as idiopathic pulmonary fibrosis 干啰音; **moist r.,** a sound heard over fluid in the bronchial tubes 湿啰音; **subcrepitant r.,** a fine moist rale heard over liquid in the smaller tubes 细捻发音

ral·ox·i·fene (ral-ok′sĭ-fēn) a selective activator of estrogen receptors that increases bone mineral density and decreases total and LDL cholesterol without affecting breast and uterine tissue; used as the hydrochloride salt for the prevention of postmenopausal osteoporosis 一种选择性的雌激素受体激活药，可增加骨密度，降低总胆固醇和低密度脂蛋白，而不影响乳腺和子宫组织，可用作预防绝经后骨质疏松症

Ral·sto·nia (rawl-sto′ne-ə) a genus of gramnegative, aerobic, rod-shaped bacteria of the family Burkholderiaceae; several species, including *R. picket'tii*, are associated with human infections 青枯菌属

ra·mal (ra′məl) pertaining to a ramus 支的，分支的

ra·mel·te·on (rə-mel′te-ən) a melatonin receptor agonist used in the treatment of insomnia 一种用于治疗失眠的褪黑素受体激活药

Ra·mi·chlo·rid·i·um (ra″mī-klor-id′e-əm) a genus of dematiaceous anamorphic fungi; *R. macken'ziei* causes brain abscesses and sometimes meningitis 枝氯霉属

ram·i·fi·ca·tion (ram″ĭ-fĭ-ka′shən) 1. distribution in branches 支状分布；2. a branching 分支

ram·i·fy (ram′ĭ-fi) 1. to branch; to diverge in different directions 使分支，使分叉；2. to traverse in branches 支状横越

ra·mi·pril (rə-mi′pril) an angiotensin-converting enzyme inhibitor used in treatment of hypertension and congestive heart failure and the prevention of a major cardiovascular event in highrisk patients 雷米普利，一种血管紧张素转换酶抑制药，用于治疗高血压和充血性心力衰竭，以及预防高危患者的主要心血管疾病

rami·sec·tion (ram″ĭ-sek′shən) section of one or more rami communicantes of the sympathetic nervous system 神经支切断术

ram·itis (ram-i′tis) inflammation of a ramus 神经根炎

ra·mose (ra′mōs) branching; having many branches 分支的

ra·mu·lus (ra′mu-ləs) pl. *ra'muli* [L.] 同 radicle

ra·mus (ra′məs) pl. *ra'mi* [L.] a branch, as of a nerve, vein, or artery 支；r. articula'ris, a branch of a mixed (afferent or efferent) peripheral nerve supplying a joint and its associated structures 关节神经分支；r. autono'micus, any of the branches of the parasympathetic or sympathetic nerves of the autonomic nervous system 自主神经系统分支；r. commu'nicans, a branch connecting two nerves or two arteries 神经交通支；动脉交通支；r. cuta'neus, a branch of a mixed (afferent or efferent) peripheral nerve innervating a region of the skin 皮支

ran·dom (ran′dəm) pertaining to a chancedependent process, particularly one that occurs according to a known probability distribution 随机的

range (r ā nj) 1. the difference between the upper and lower limits of a variable or of a series of values 极差；2. an interval in which values sampled from a population, or the values in the population itself, are known to lie 值域，r. of motion, the range, measured in degrees of a circle, through which a joint can be extended and flexed 关节活动度，关节活动范围

ra·nine (ra′nīn) 1. pertaining to a frog 蛙的；2. ranular 舌下囊肿的；3. sublingual 舌下的

ra·ni·ti·dine (rah-nĭ′tĭ-dēn) a histamine H_2 receptor antagonist, used as the hydrochloride salt to inhibit gastric acid secretion in the treatment of gastric and duodenal ulcer, gastroesophageal reflux disease, and conditions that cause gastric hypersecretion 雷尼替丁，一种组胺 H_2 受体拮抗药，在治疗胃和十二指肠溃疡、胃食管反流病以及引起胃高分泌的情况中可抑制胃酸分泌

ran·u·la (ran′u-lə) a cystic tumor beneath the tongue 舌下囊肿；ran'ular *adj.*

rape (rāp) nonconsensual sexual penetration of an individual, obtained by force or threat, or when the victim is not capable of consent 强奸

ra·phe (ra′fe) pl. *ra'phae.* A seam; the line of union of the halves of various symmetric parts 缝（际）；r. of penis, a narrow dark streak or ridge continuous posteriorly with the raphe of scrotum and extending forward along the midline on the underside of the penis 阴茎缝；perineal r., a ridge along the median line of the perineum that runs forward from the anus; in the male, it is continuous with the raphe of scrotum 会阴缝；r. of scrotum, a ridge along the surface of the scrotum in the median line, continuous with the perineal raphe and the raphe of penis 阴囊缝

rap·port (rah-por′) a relation of harmony and accord, as between patient and physician 关系（融洽）（病人与医师间）

rar·e·fac·tion (rar″ə-fak′shən) condition of being or becoming less dense 稀疏

ra·sa·ya·na (rah″sah-yah′nə) any of a group of herbal remedies with antioxidant properties used in ayurveda to promote health, provide defense against disease, and promote longevity 阿育吠陀使用的一类具有抗氧化特性的草药中的任何一种，可促进健康，防御疾病，并促进长寿

rash (rash) a temporary eruption on the skin 疹；butterfly r., a skin eruption across the nose and adjacent areas of the cheeks in the pattern of a butterfly, as in lupus erythematosus and seborrheic

R

dermatitis 蝶形皮疹；**diaper r.**, irritant dermatitis in infants on the areas covered by the diaper, usually due to soiling or fungal contamination 尿布疹；**drug r.**, 药疹，参见 *eruption* 下词条；**heat r.**, miliaria rubra 热疹

rasp (rasp) 1. raspatory; a coarse file used in surgery 骨锉，刮器，刮骨刀；2. to file with a rasp 用锉刀锉

ras·pa·to·ry (ras′pə-to-re) 同 rasp (1)

RAST radioallergosorbent test 放射变应原吸附试验

rate (rāt) the speed or frequency with which an event or circumstance occurs per unit of time, population, or other standard of comparison 率；**basal metabolic r. (BMR)**, an expression of the rate at which oxygen is used by body cells, or the calculated equivalent heat production by the body, in a fasting subject at complete rest 基础代谢率；**birth r.**, the number of births in a specified area during a defined period for the total population, often further qualified as to which portion of the population is being examined 出生率；**case fatality r.**, the ratio of the number of deaths caused by a specified disease to the number of diagnosed cases of that disease 病死率；**circulation r.**, the amount of blood pumped through the body by the heart per unit time 循环率；**death r.**, an expression of the number of deaths in a population at risk during 1 year. The *crude death r.* is the ratio of the number of deaths to the total population of an area; the *age-specific death r.* is the ratio of the number of deaths in a specific age group to the number of persons in that age group; the *cause-specific death r.* is the ratio of the number of deaths due to a specified cause to the total population 死亡率；**dose r.**, the amount of any agent administered per unit of time 剂量率；**erythrocyte sedimentation r. (ESR)**, the rate at which erythrocytes sediment from a well-mixed specimen of venous blood, as measured by the distance that the top of a column of erythrocytes falls in a specified time interval under specified conditions 红细胞沉降率；**fatality r.**, 同 case fatality r.；**fertility r.**, a measure of fertility in a specified population over a specified period of time, particularly the *general fertility r.*, the number of live births in a geographic area in a year per 1000 women of childbearing age 生育率；**fetal death r.**, the ratio of the number of fetal deaths in 1 year to the total number of both live births and fetal deaths in that year 胎儿死亡率；**five-year survival r.**, an expression of the number of survivors with no trace of disease 5 years after each has been diagnosed or treated for the same disease 五年存活率；**glomerular filtration r. (GFR)**, an expression of the quantity of glomerular filtrate formed each minute in the nephrons of both kidneys, usually measured by the rate of clearance of creatinine 肾小球滤过率；**growth r.**, an expression of the increase in size of an organic object per unit of time 增长率；**heart r.**, the number of contractions of the cardiac ventricles per unit of time 心率；**incidence r.**, the probability of developing a particular disease during a given period of time; the numerator is the number of new cases during the specified time period and the denominator is the population at risk during the period 发病率；**morbidity r.**, an inexact term that can mean either the *incidence rate* or the *prevalence rate* 患病率；**mortality r.**, 同 death r.；**prevalence r.**, the number of people in a population who have a disease at a given time: the numerator is the number of existing cases of disease at a specified time and the denominator is the total population 流行率；**pulse r.**, the number of pulsations noted in a peripheral artery per unit of time 脉率；**respiration r.**, the number of movements of the chest wall per unit of time, indicative of inhalation and exhalation 呼吸频率；**sedimentation r.**, the rate at which a sediment is deposited in a given volume of solution, especially when subjected to the action of a centrifuge 沉降速率；**stillbirth r.**, 同 fetal death r.

ra·tio (ra′she-o) [L.] an expression of the quantity of one substance or entity in relation to that of another; the relationship between two quantities expressed as the quotient of one divided by the other 比（率）；**A-G r., albumin-globulin r.**, the ratio of albumin to globulin in blood serum, plasma, or urine in various renal diseases 白蛋白球蛋白比率；**cardiothoracic r.**, on a radiograph, the ratio of the transverse diameter of the heart to the internal diameter of the chest at its widest point just above the dome of the respiratory diaphragm 心胸比；**lecithin/sphingomyelin r., L/S r.**, the ratio of lecithin to sphingomyelin concentration in the amniotic fluid, used to predict the degree of pulmonary maturity of the fetus and thus the risk of respiratory distress syndrome (RDS) if the fetus is delivered prematurely 卵磷脂与鞘磷脂比值；**sex r.**, the proportion of one sex to another, traditionally the number of males in a population per number of females 性别比；**ventilation-perfusion r.**, the ratio of oxygen received in the pulmonary alveoli to the flow of blood through the alveolar capillaries 通气-灌注比

ra·tion·al (rā′shən-əl) based upon reason; characterized by possession of one's reason 合理的；有理性的

ra·tion·al·iza·tion (ră″shən-əl-ī-za′shən) an unconscious defense mechanism by which one justifies attitudes and behavior that would otherwise be unacceptable 合理化

rat·tle·snake (rat′əl-snāk) any of the New World pit vipers of the genera *Crotalus* and *Sistrurus*, having a series of cornified interlocking segments at the tip of the tail; when disturbed they vibrate the tail to produce the characteristic rattling or buzzing sound. Included are the massasauga, the *eastern diamondback r. (C. adamanteus)*, the *Mojave r. (C. scutulatus scutulatus)*, the *prairie r. (C. viridis viridis)*, the *pygmy r. (S. miliarius)*, the *timber r. (C. horridus)*, and the *western diamondback r. (C. atrox)* 响尾蛇

Rau·wol·fia (rou-wool′fe-ə) a genus of tropical trees and shrubs, including *R. serpentina* and over 100 other species, that provide numerous alkaloids, notably reserpine, of medical interest 萝芙木属

rau·wol·fia (rou-wool′fe-ə) 1. any member of the genus *Rauwolfia* 萝芙木; 2. the dried root of *Rauwolfia*, or an extract of it 萝芙木的干燥根或其提取物; *r. serpenti′na*, the dried root of *Rauwolfia serpentina*; used as an antihypertensive; also used in folk medicine and Indian medicine 萝芙木干根（可作抗高血压药）

RAV Rous-associated virus 鲁斯相关病毒

rax·i·bac·u·mab (rak-see″bak′ū-mab) a recombinant human IgG monoclonal antibody that blocks the activity of the *Bacillus anthracis* toxin; used in adults and children to treat and prevent inhalational anthrax 一种重组人 IgG 单克隆抗体，阻断炭疽芽孢杆菌毒素的活性，可用于成人和儿童治疗和预防吸入性炭疽

ray (ra) 1. a line emanating from a center 射线，指从中心发出的一条线; 2. a more or less distinct portion of radiant energy (light or heat), proceeding in a specific direction 射线，指沿特定方向传播的光或热辐射; 3. a distinct portion of electromagnetic radiation that proceeds in a specific direction 射线，指沿特定方向传播的电磁辐射; α-r′s, high-speed helium nuclei ejected from radioactive substances; they have less penetrating power than beta rays α 射线; **actinic r′s**, light rays that produce chemical action, especially those beyond the violet end of the spectrum 光化射线; **alpha r′s**, 同 α-r′s; **β-r′s/beta r′s**, electrons ejected from radioactive substances with velocities as high as 0.98 of the velocity of light; they have more penetrating power than alpha rays, but less than gamma rays β 射线; **digital r.**, 1. a digit of the hand or foot and the corresponding portion of the metacarpus or metatarsus, considered as a continuous structural unit 指骨线，趾骨线; 2. in the embryo, a mesenchymal condensation of the hand or foot plate that outlines the pattern of a future digit 胎儿的指线或趾线; γ-r′s/gamma r′s, electromagnetic radiation of short wavelengths emitted by an atomic nucleus during a nuclear reaction, consisting of high-energy photons, having no mass and no electric charge, and traveling with the speed of light and with great penetrating power γ 射线; **grenz r′s**, very soft x-rays having wavelengths about 20 nm, lying between x-rays and ultraviolet rays 跨界射线; **infrared r′s**, radiations just beyond the red end of the visible spectrum, having wavelengths of 0.75 to 1000 μm 红外线; 另参见 *infrared*; **medullary r′s**, the intracortical prolongations of the renal pyramids 髓射线; **roentgen r′s**, x-r′s 伦琴射线; **ultraviolet r′s**, invisible rays that are just beyond the violet end of the visible spectrum; their wavelengths range between 4 and 400 nm 紫外线; 参见 *ultraviolet*; **x-r′s**, electromagnetic vibrations of short wavelengths (about 0.01 to 10 nm), or corresponding quanta produced when electrons moving at high velocity impinge on various substances; they are able to penetrate most substances to some extent, to affect a photographic plate, to cause certain substances to fluoresce, and to strongly ionize tissue X 射线

Rb rubidium 元素铷的符号

RBBB right bundle branch block 右束支传导阻滞, 参见 *bundle* 下 *branch block*

RBC red blood cell 红细胞

RBE relative biological effectiveness 相对生物效应

rcp reciprocal translocation 相互易位

RDI respiratory disturbance index 呼吸紊乱指数

Re rhenium 元素铼的符号

re·ab·sorp·tion (re″ab-sorp′shən) 1. the act or process of absorbing again, such as the absorption by the kidneys of substances (glucose, proteins, sodium, etc.) already secreted into the renal tubules 重吸收; 2. 同 resorption

re·ac·tant (re-ak′tənt) a substance entering into a chemical reaction 反应物

re·ac·tion (re-ak′shən) 1. opposite action, or counterreaction; the response to stimuli 反作用; 2. a phenomenon caused by the action of chemical agents; a chemical process in which one substance is transformed into another substance or other substances 化学反应; 3. the mental and/or emotional state that develops in any particular situation 回应; **acrosome r.**, structural changes and liberation of acrosomal enzymes occurring in spermatozoa in the vicinity of an oocyte, facilitating entry into the oocyte 顶体反应; **acute situational r., acute stress r.,** a transient, self-limiting acute emotional reaction to severe psychological stress; it is variably defined as comprising one or more of the following categories: *adjustment disorder, brief reactive psychosis, acute stress disorder,* and *posttraumatic stress disorder* 急性应激反应；**agglutination r.,** a positive result on an agglutination test (q.v.) 凝集反应；**alarm r.,** the physiologic effects (increase in blood pressure, cardiac output, blood flow to skeletal muscles, rate of glycolysis, and blood glucose concentration; decrease in blood flow to viscera) mediated by sympathetic nervous system discharge and release of adrenal medullary hormones in response to stress, fright, or rage 惊恐反应；**allergic r.,** hypersensitivity r., sometimes specifically a type Ⅰ hypersensitivity reaction 变态反应；**allograft r.,** homograft r.; the rejection of an allogeneic graft by a normal host 同种移植物反应；**anaphylactic r.,** anaphylaxis. 过敏反应；**anaphylactoid r.,** one resembling generalized anaphylaxis but not caused by an IgE-mediated allergic reaction 类过敏反应；**antibody-mediated hypersensitivity r.,** 1. type Ⅱ hypersensitivity r. Ⅱ型超敏反应，参见 *Gell* 和 *classification* 下 *Coombs classification*；2. occasionally, any hypersensitivity reaction in which antibodies are the primary mediators, i.e., types Ⅰ to Ⅲ 抗体介导的超敏反应，包括Ⅰ～Ⅲ型超敏反应；**antigen-antibody r.,** the reversible binding of antigen to homologous antibody by the formation of weak bonds between antigenic determinants on antigen molecules and antigen binding sites on immunoglobulin molecules 抗原-抗体反应；**anxiety r.,** a reaction characterized by abnormal apprehension or uneasiness; see also *anxiety disorders,* under *disorder* 焦虑反应；**Arias-Stella r.,** nuclear and cellular hypertrophy of the endometrial epithelium, associated with ectopic pregnancy A-S 反应；**Arthus r.,** the development of an inflammatory lesion, with induration, erythema, edema, hemorrhage, and necrosis, a few hours after intradermal injection of antigen into a previously sensitized animal producing precipitating antibody; it is classed as a type Ⅲ hypersensitivity reaction 阿蒂斯反应，实验性局部过敏反应；**associative r.,** a reaction in which the response is withheld until the idea presented has suggested an associated idea 联想反应；**biuret r.,** formation of a chelate having a violet-red color when biuret or compounds having two or more adjacent peptide bonds (e.g., proteins) are reacted with copper sulfate in alkaline solution; used as the basis of a colorimetric method for detection of protein 双缩脲反应；**cell-mediated hypersensitivity r.,** 细胞介导的超敏反应，指Ⅳ型超敏反应；参见 *Gell* 和 *classification* 下 *Coombs classifica-*

tion；**conversion r.,** 转化反应，参见 *disorder* 下词条；**cross r.,** the interaction of an antigen with an antibody formed against a different antigen with which the first antigen shares identical or closely related antigenic determinants 交叉反应；**cytotoxic hypersensitivity r.,** type Ⅱ hypersensitivity r. 细胞毒型超敏反应，指Ⅱ型超敏反应；参见 *Gell* 和 *classification* 下 *Coombs classification*；**defense r.,** 防御反应，参见 *mechanism* 下词条；**r. of degeneration,** the reaction to electrical stimulation of muscles whose nerves have degenerated, consisting of loss of response to a faradic stimulation in a muscle, and to galvanic and faradic stimulation in the nerve 变性反应；**delayed hypersensitivity r., delayed-type hypersensitivity r.,** a hypersensitivity reaction that takes 24 to 72 hours to develop and is mediated by T lymphocytes rather than by antibodies; usually denoting the subset of type Ⅳ hypersensitivity reactions involving cytokine release and macrophage activation, as opposed to direct cytolysis, but sometimes used more broadly, even as a synonym for *type IV hypersensitivity r.* (see *Gell and Coombs classification,* under *classification*) 迟发型超敏反应；**fight-or-flight r.,** 同 alarm r.；**foreign body r.,** a granulomatous inflammatory reaction evoked by the presence of exogenous material in the tissues, characterized by the formation of foreign body giant cells 异物反应；**hemianopic pupillary r.,** in certain cases of hemianopia, light thrown upon one side of the retina causes the iris to contract, while light thrown upon the other side arouses no response 偏盲性瞳孔反应；**homograft r.,** 同 allograft r.；**hypersensitivity r.,** one in which the body mounts an exaggerated or inappropriate immune response to a substance perceived as foreign, resulting in local or general tissue damage. Such reactions are usually classified as *types I to IV* on the basis of the Gell and Coombs classification (q.v.) 超敏反应；**id r.,** a secondary skin eruption occurring in sensitized patients as a result of circulation of allergenic products from a primary site of infection 附发疹反应；**immediate hypersensitivity r.,** 1. type Ⅰ hypersensitivity r.; see *Gell and Coombs classification,* under *classification.* 2. occasionally, any hypersensitivity reaction mediated by antibodies and developing rapidly, generally in minutes to hours (i.e., *types I to III*), as distinguished from those mediated by T lymphocytes and macrophages and requiring days to develop (*type IV,* or *delayed hypersensitivity r.*) 速发型超敏反应；**immune r.,** 免疫反应，参见 *response* 下词条；**immune complex-mediated hypersensitivity r.,** type Ⅲ hypersensitivity r. 免疫复合物介导的超敏反应；参见 *classifi-*

cation 下 *Gell and Coombs classification*; **Jarisch-Herxheimer r.,** a transient immunologic reaction following antibiotic treatment of syphilis and certain other diseases, marked by fever, chills, headache, myalgia, and exacerbation of cutaneous lesions, probably due to release of toxic or antigenic substances by the infecting microorganisms Jarisch-Herxheimer 反应; **Jones-Mote r.,** a mild skin reaction of the delayed (type Ⅳ) hypersensitivity type occurring after challenge with protein antigens 嗜碱性粒细胞聚集反应; **late-phase r.,** an IgE-mediated immune reaction occurring 5 to 8 hours after exposure to an antigen, after the wheal-and-flare reactions of immediate hypersensitivity have diminished, with inflammation peaking around 24 hours and then subsiding 迟发相反应; **lengthening r.,** reflex elongation of the extensor muscles that permits flexion of a limb 伸长反应; **lepra r.,** an acute or subacute hypersensitivity reaction occurring either during the course of antileprosy treatment or in untreated cases of leprosy 麻风反应; **leukemoid r.,** a peripheral blood picture resembling that of leukemia or indistinguishable from it on the basis of morphologic appearance alone; seen in certain infectious diseases, inflammatory conditions, and intoxications 类白血病反应; **Mazzotti r.,** the set of adverse reactions that accompany the administration of diethylcarbamazine in onchocerciasis, most commonly an intensely pruritic rash but sometimes also systemic manifestations such as fever, malaise, lymph node swelling, eosinophilia, arthralgias, tachycardia, and hypotension; if numerous microfilariae are present in the eyes, blindness may occur Mazzotti 反应, 指乙胺嗪治疗盘尾丝虫病时伴随的一系列不良反应, 最常见的是强烈瘙痒的皮疹, 有时也会出现系统性表现, 如发热、不适、淋巴结肿大、嗜酸性粒细胞增多、关节痛、心动过速和低血压; 如果眼睛中存在大量微丝虫, 可能会发生失明; **Neufeld r.,** swelling of the capsules of pneumococci, seen under the microscope, on mixture with a specific immune serum, owing to the binding of antibody with the capsular polysaccharide Neufeld 反应或溶菌现象, 指在显微镜下, 由于抗体与荚膜多糖的结合, 在与特定免疫血清的混合物中可见肺炎球菌肿胀; **oxidation-reduction r.,** 同 redox r.; **Pirquet r.,** appearance of a papule with a red areola 24 to 48 hours after introduction of two small drops of Old tuberculin by slight scarification of the skin; a positive test indicates previous infection 划痕反应, 指皮肤轻微擦伤后, 引入两小滴灭活结核菌素后 24～48h 出现带有红色乳晕的丘疹, 阳性检测表明以前有过感染; **polymerase chain r. (PCR),** a rapid technique for in vitro amplification of specific DNA or RNA sequences, allowing small quantities of short sequences to be analyzed without cloning 聚合酶链式反应; **precipitin r.,** the formation of an insoluble precipitate by reaction of antigen and antibody 沉淀反应; **redox r.,** a reaction oxidizing one substrate while reducing another 氧化还原反应; **righting r's,** responses of the head and eyes that occur as the body processes sensory input from the visual and vestibular systems 翻正反应; **serum r.,** seroreaction 血清反应; **startle r.,** the various psychophysiologic phenomena, including involuntary motor and autonomic reactions, evidenced by an individual in reaction to a sudden, unexpected stimulus, such as a loud noise 惊跳反应; **stress r.,** any physiologic or psychological reaction to physical, mental, or emotional stress that disturbs the organism's homeostasis 应激反应; **substitution r.,** a chemical reaction in which one atom or functional group replaces another in a molecule 取代反应; **T cell-mediated hypersensitivity r.,** type Ⅳ hypersensitivity r. T 细胞介导的超敏反应; 参见 *Gell* 和 *classification* 下 *Coombs classification*; **transfusion r.,** any symptoms due to agglutination or hemolysis of the recipient's blood cells when blood for transfusion is incorrectly matched or when the recipient has a hypersensitivity reaction to some element of the donor blood 输血反应; **Weil-Felix r.,** agglutination by blood serum of typhus patients of a bacillus of the proteus group from the urine and feces 外-斐反应; **Wernicke r.,** 同 hemianopic pupillary r.; **wheal-and-erythema r., wheal-and-flare r.,** a cutaneous sensitivity reaction to skin injury or administration of antigen, due to histamine production and marked by edematous elevation and erythematous flare 风团与红斑反应, 风团潮红反应; **white-graft r.,** an immune reaction to a tissue graft as a result of which the grafted tissue does not become vascularized due to rapid rejection 苍白移植物反应

re·ac·tion-for·ma·tion (re-ak′shən for-ma′shən) an unconscious defense mechanism in which a person assumes an attitude that is the reverse of the wish or impulse actually harbored 心理反应形成, 反向形成, 指一种无意识的防御机制, 在这种机制中, 一个人采取了一种与实际所怀有的欲望或动机相反的态度

re·ac·tive (re-ak′tiv) characterized by reaction; readily responsive to a stimulus 反应的

read·ing (rēd′ing) understanding of written or printed symbols representing words 解读; **lip r., speech r.,** understanding of speech through observation of the speaker's lip movements 读唇

R

re·a·gent (re-a′jənt) a substance used to produce a chemical reaction so as to detect, measure, produce, etc., other substances 试剂

re·a·gin (re′ə-jin) the antibody that mediates immediate hypersensitivity reactions; in humans, IgE 反应素；**reagin′ic** *adj.*

ream·er (rēm′ər) an instrument used in dentistry for enlarging root canals 根管扩孔钻

re·bound (re′bound) a reversed response occurring upon withdrawal of a stimulus 弹回，回缩，反跳；**acid r.**, an increased rate of stomach acid secretion occurring soon after eating 应激性胃酸再增加；**heparin r.**, the return of anticoagulant activity following neutralization of heparin in a patient's blood by protamine 肝素反跳；**urea r.**, a sudden increase in release of urea into the bloodstream by cells and organs that normally store it, seen in the first 15 minutes to an hour after urea has been removed by dialysis 尿素反弹

re·can·a·li·za·tion (re-kan″ə-lĭ-za′shən) formation of new canals or paths, especially blood vessels, through an obstruction such as a clot 再通，重通

re·cep·tac·u·lum (re″səp-tak′u-ləm) pl. *receptac′-ula* [L.] a vessel or receptacle 容器，（接）受器；**r. chy′li**, cisterna chyli 乳糜池

re·cep·tive (re-cep′tiv) capable of receiving or of responding to a stimulus 接受的，感受的

re·cep·tor (re-sep′tər) 1. a molecule on the surface or within a cell that recognizes and binds with specific molecules, producing a specific effect in the cell; e.g., the cell-surface receptors for antigens or cytoplasmic receptors for steroid hormones 受体；2. a sensory nerve ending that responds to various stimuli 感受器；**α-adrenergic r's**, adrenergic receptors that respond to norepinephrine and to such blocking agents as phenoxybenzamine. They are subdivided into two types: α_1, found in smooth muscle, heart, and liver, with effects including vasoconstriction, intestinal relaxation, uterine contraction, and pupillary dilation, and α_2, found in platelets, vascular smooth muscle, nerve termini, and pancreatic islets, with effects including platelet aggregation, vasoconstriction, and inhibition of norepinephrine release and of insulin secretion α-肾上腺素受体；**adrenergic r's**, receptors for epinephrine or norepinephrine, such as those on effector organs innervated by postganglionic adrenergic fibers of the sympathetic nervous system. Classified as α-*adrenergic r's* and β-*adrenergic r's* 肾上腺素受体；**alpha-adrenergic r's**, 同 α-adrenergic r's；**β-adrenergic r's/beta-adrenergic r's**, adrenergic receptors that respond particularly to epinephrine and to such blocking agents as propran-

olol. They are subdivided into two basic types: β_1, in myocardium and causing lipolysis and cardiac stimulation, and β_2, in smooth and skeletal muscle and liver and causing bronchodilation and vasodilation. The atypical type β_3 may be involved in lipolysis regulation in adipose tissue β-肾上腺素受体；**cholinergic r's**, cell-surface receptor molecules that bind the neurotransmitter acetylcholine and mediate its action on postjunctional cells 胆碱（能）受体；**complement r's**, cell-surface receptors for products of complement reactions, playing roles including recognition of pathogens, phagocytosis, adhesion, and clearance of immune complexes. The best characterized are C1 to C4, which bind C3 fragments already bound to a surface 补体受体；**cutaneous r.**, any of the various types of sense organs found in the dermis or epidermis, usually a mechanoreceptor, thermoreceptor, or nociceptor 皮肤感受器；**cytokine r's**, membrane-spanning proteins that bind cytokines via extracellular domains, acting to convert an extracellular signal to an intracellular one 细胞因子受体；**G protein–coupled r's**, a large superfamily of membrane receptors, specific for a wide range of signals, whose intracellular effects are mediated by G proteins G 蛋白耦联受体；**H₁ r's, H₂ r's**, H_1 受体，H_2 受体，参见 *histamine*；**joint r.**, any of several mechanoreceptors that occur in joint capsules and respond to deep pressure and to other stimuli such as stress or change in position 关节感受器；**muscarinic r.**, cholinergic receptors that are stimulated by the alkaloid muscarine and blocked by atropine; they are found on automatic effector cells and on central neurons in the thalamus and cerebral cortex 毒蕈碱受体；**muscle r.**, a mechanoreceptor found in a muscle or tendon 肌肉受体；**nicotinic r.**, cholinergic receptors that are stimulated initially and blocked at high doses by the alkaloid nicotine and blocked by tubocurarine; they are found on automatic ganglion cells, striated muscle cells, and spinal central neurons 烟碱受体；**nonadapting r.**, a mechanoreceptor, such as a nociceptor, that responds to stimulation with a continual steady discharge and little or no accommodation over time 非适应性感受器；**olfactory r.**, a chemoreceptor in the nasal epithelium that is sensitive to stimulation, giving rise to the sensation of odors 嗅觉感受器；**opiate r., opioid r.**, any of a number of receptors for opiates and opioids, grouped into at least seven types on the basis of their substrates and physiologic effects 阿片受体；**orphan r.**, a protein identified as a putative receptor on the basis of its structure but without identification of possible ligands or evidence of function 孤儿受体；**pain r.**, nociceptor

疼痛觉受体；**purinergic r's,** membrane receptors widely expressed in the brain, peripheral tissues, and circulating blood cells that bind purine bases or nucleotides. Most mediate their responses by G proteins 嘌呤受体；**rapidly adapting r.,** a mechanoreceptor that responds quickly to stimulation but that rapidly accommodates and stops firing if the stimulus remains constant 快适应感受器；**sensory r.,** receptor (2) 感 受 器；**slowly adapting r.,** a mechanoreceptor that responds slowly to stimulation and continues firing as long as the stimulus continues 慢适应感受器；**stretch r.,** a sense organ in a muscle or tendon that responds to elongation 牵 张 感受器；**tactile r.,** a mechanoreceptor for the sense of touch 触觉感受器；**thermal r.,** thermoreceptor 温度感受器

re·cess (re′ses) a small empty space, hollow, or cavity 隐窝；**epitympanic r.,** attic or epitympanum; the upper part of the tympanic cavity, above the level of the tympanic membrane, containing part of the incus and malleus 鼓室上隐窝；**infundibuliform r.,** 同 pharyngeal r.；**laryngopharyngeal r.,** piriform r. 喉咽隐窝；**pharyngeal r.,** a wide, slitlike lateral extension in the wall of the nasopharynx, cranial and dorsal to the pharyngeal orifice of the auditory tube 咽 隐 窝；**piriform r.,** a pear-shaped fossa in the wall of the laryngeal pharynx 梨状隐窝；**pleural r's,** the spaces where the different portions of the pleura join at an angle and which are never completely filled by lung tissue 胸膜隐窝；**r. of Rosenmüller,** 同 pharyngeal r.；**sphenoethmoidal r.,** the most superior and posterior part of nasal cavity, above the superior nasal concha, into which the sphenoidal sinus opens 蝶筛隐窝；**subpopliteal r.,** a prolongation of the synovial tendon sheath of the popliteus muscle outside the knee joint into the popliteal space 腘肌下隐窝；**superior r. of tympanic membrane,** Prussak pouch 鼓膜上隐窝；**utricular r.,** utricle (2) 椭圆囊隐窝

re·ces·sive (re-ses′iv) 1. tending to recede退缩的；2. in genetics, pertaining to phenotypic expression of an allele only in homozygotes (or hemizygotes, for X-linked traits) 隐性的

re·ces·sus (re-ses′əs) pl. *reces′sus* [L.] a recess 隐窝

re·cid·i·va·tion (re-sid′ĭ-va′shən) relapse, recurrence, or repetition, as of a disease or condition or of a pattern of behavior, particularly a criminal act 复发，再犯

re·cid·i·vism (re-sid′ĭ-viz-əm) a tendency to relapse, particularly a return to criminal behavior （疾病）复发，再发；（罪犯）累犯

rec·i·pe (res′ĭ-pe) [L.] 1. take; used at the head of a prescription, indicated by the symbol ℞ 取（处方头语），用符号℞表示；2. a formula for the preparation of a specific combination of ingredients 处方

re·cip·i·ent (re-sip′e-ənt) one who receives, e.g., a blood transfusion or a tissue or organ graft 受者，受体（接受移植的个体）；受血者，接受者；**universal r.,** a person thought to be able to receive blood of any group without agglutination of the donor cells 万能受血者

re·cip·ro·cal (re-sip′rə-kəl″) 1. being equivalent or complementary 等同的，互补的；2. inversely related; opposing 反向相关的；相反的

re·cip·ro·ca·tion (re-sip″ro-ka′shən) 1. the act of giving and receiving in exchange; the complementary interaction of two distinct entities 交互作用；2. an alternating back-and-forth movement 往复运动

RECIST Response Evaluation Criteria in Solid Tumors 实体瘤疗效反应评价标准

re·cog·ni·tion (rek″əg-nĭ′shən) in immunology, the interaction of immunologically competent cells with antigen, involving antigen binding to a specific receptor on the cell surface and resulting in an immune response 识别

re·coil (re′koil) a quick pulling back 反 冲；**elastic r.,** the ability of a stretched object or organ, such as the bladder or lung, to return to its resting position 弹性回缩

re·com·bi·nant (re-kom′bĭ-nənt) 1. the new entity (e.g., gene, protein, cell, individual) that results from genetic recombination 重组体；2. pertaining to or relating to such an entity 重组体的

re·com·bi·na·tion (re″kom-bĭ-na′shən) 1. the reunion, in the same or different arrangement, of formerly united elements that have been separated 再化合；2. in genetics, the process that creates new combinations of genes by shuffling the linear order of the DNA 重组（遗传学上指基因重组）

re·com·pres·sion (re″kəm-presh′ən) return to normal environmental pressure after exposure to greatly diminished pressure 再压缩（作用）

re·con·struc·tion (re″kən-struk′shən) 1. the reassembling or re-forming of something from constituent parts 重构；2. surgical restoration of function of a body part 功能重建

rec·ord (rek′ord) 1. a permanent or long-lasting account of something (as on film, in writing, etc.) 记录；2. in dentistry, a registration 牙科的注册；**problemoriented r. (POR),** a method of patient care record keeping that focuses on specific health care problems and a cooperative health care plan designed to cope with the identified problems. The

R

components of the POR are *database*, which contains information required for each patient regardless of diagnosis or presenting problems; *problem list,* which contains the major problems currently needing attention; *plan*, which specifies what is to be done with regard to each problem; *progress notes,* which document the observations, assessments, nursing care plans, physician's orders, etc., of all health care personnel directly involved in the care of the patient 面向问题记录（主要内容为数据库，问题一览表，保障计划和病程记录），另见 *SOAP*

re·cru·des·cence (re″kroo-des′əns) recurrence of symptoms after temporary abatement 复发，再燃；**recrudes′cent** *adj.*

re·cruit·ment (re-kroot′mənt) 1. the gradual increase to a maximum in a reflex when a stimulus of unaltered intensity is prolonged 募集反应，当强度不变的刺激延长时，反射中逐渐增加到最大值；2. in audiology, an abnormally rapid increase in the loudness of a sound caused by a slight increase in its intensity 声音的增益补偿；3. the orderly increase in number of activated motor units with increasing strength of voluntary muscle contractions 募集，随着肌肉自主收缩的强度的增加，兴奋的运动单位数目也进一步增加；4. the process by which certain primordial ovarian follicles begin growing in a particular menstrual cycle 卵泡的募集

rec·tal (rek′təl) pertaining to the rectum 直肠的

rec·tec·to·my (rek-tek′tə-me) proctectomy 直肠切除术

rec·ti·fi·ca·tion (rek″tĭ-fĭ-ka′shən) 1. the act of making straight, pure, or correct 矫正调整；2. redistillation of a liquid to purify it 精馏

rec·ti·tis (rek-ti′tis) proctitis 直肠炎

rec·to·ab·dom·i·nal (rek″to-ab-dom′ĭ-nəl) pertaining to the rectum and abdomen 直肠腹（部）的

rec·to·cele (rek′to-sēl) hernial protrusion of part of the rectum into the vagina 直肠膨出

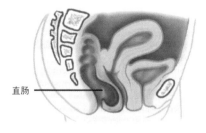

▲ 直肠膨出

rec·to·co·li·tis (rek″to-ko-li′tis) proctocolitis 直肠结肠炎

rec·to·cu·ta·ne·ous (rek″to-ku-ta′ne-əs) pertaining to the rectum and the skin 直肠皮肤的

rec·to·la·bi·al (rek″to-la′be-əl) relating to the rectum and a labium majus 直肠阴唇的

rec·to·pexy (rek′to-pek″se) proctopexy 直肠固定术

rec·to·plas·ty (rek′to-plas″te) proctoplasty 直肠成形术

rec·to·scope (rek′to-skōp) proctoscope 直肠镜

rec·to·sig·moid (rek″to-sig′moid) the terminal portion of the sigmoid colon and the proximal portion of the rectum 直肠乙状结肠的

rec·to·sig·moi·dec·to·my (rek″to-sig″ moidek′tə-me) excision of the rectosigmoid 直肠乙状结肠切除术

rec·tos·to·my (rek-tos′tə-me) proctostomy 直肠造口术

rec·to·ure·thral (rek″to-u-re′thrəl) pertaining to or communicating with the rectum and urethra 直肠尿道的

rec·to·uter·ine (rek″to-u′tər-in) pertaining to the rectum and uterus 直肠子宫的

rec·to·vag·i·nal (rek″to-vaj′ĭ-nəl) pertaining to or communicating with the rectum and vagina 直肠阴道的

rec·to·ves·i·cal (rek″to-ves′ĭ-kəl) pertaining to or communicating with the rectum and bladder 直肠膀胱的

rec·tum (rek′təm) the distal portion of the large intestine 直肠

rec·tus (rek′təs) [L.] straight 直的

re·cum·bent (re-kum′bənt) lying down 躺着的

re·cu·per·a·tion (re-koo″pər-a′shən) recovery of health and strength 恢复健康或力量

re·cur·rence (re-kur′əns) the return of symptoms after a remission 复发；**recur′rent** *adj.*

re·cur·rent (re-kur′ənt) 1. running back, or toward the source 回归的；2. returning after remissions 复发的

re·cur·va·tion (re″kər-va′shən) a backward bending or curvature 反弯，反屈

red (red) 1. the color produced by the longest waves of the visible spectrum, approximately 630 to 750 nm 红色；2. a dye or stain with this color 红色染料；**scarlet r.,** an azo dye used as a biologic stain for fats 猩红

re·dia (re′de-ə) pl. *re′diae.* A larval stage of certain trematode parasites, which develops in the body of a snail host and gives rise to daughter rediae or to the cercariae 雷蚴

red·in·te·gra·tion (red-in″tə-gra′shən) 1. the res-

直肠

toration or repair of a lost or damaged part 复原，恢复；2. a psychic process in which part of a complex stimulus provokes the complete reaction that was previously made only to the complex stimulus as a whole 重整作用（指一种心理过程）；3. 同 reintegration (2)

re·dox (re′doks) oxidation-reduction 氧化还原反应

re·duce (re-doos′) 1. to restore to the normal place or relation of parts, e.g., to reduce a fracture 使（骨折等）复位；2. to undergo reduction 使还原；3. to decrease in weight or size 减轻重量或减少尺寸

re·du·ci·ble (re-doo′sĭ-bəl) capable of being reduced 可还原的

re·duc·tant (re-duk′tənt) the electron donor in an oxidation-reduction (redox) reaction 还原剂

re·duc·tase (re-duk′tās) a term used in the names of some of the oxidoreductases, usually specifically those catalyzing reactions important solely for reduction of a metabolite 还原酶；5α-r., an enzyme that catalyzes the irreversible reduction of testosterone to dihydrotestosterone; enzyme deficiency causes ambiguous genitalia in males at birth, with some masculinization at puberty 5α- 还原酶，一种催化睾酮不可逆地还原为二氢睾酮的酶，酶缺乏将导致男性出生时生殖器不明确，并在青春期有一些男性化

re·duc·tion (re-duk′shən) 1. the correction of a fracture, luxation, or hernia（骨折、脱位、疝气的）复位术；2. the addition of hydrogen to a substance, or more generally, the gain of electrons 还原（作用）；closed r., the manipulative reduction of a fracture without incision 闭合复位术；open r., reduction of a fracture after incision into the fracture site 切开复位术

re·du·pli·ca·tion (re″doo-plĭ-ka′shən) 1. a doubling back 双背；2. the recurrence of paroxysms of a double type 双发型阵发性复发；3. duplication (3) 重复

re·en·try (re-en′tre) reexcitation of a region of cardiac tissue by a single impulse, continuing for one or more cycles and sometimes resulting in ectopic beats or tachyarrhythmias; it also requires refractoriness of the tissue to stimulation and an area of unidirectional block to conduction 折返（过早心搏时）；**reen′trant** *adj.*

re·feed·ing (re-fēd′ing) restoration of normal nutrition after a period of fasting or starvation 再补给

re·ferred (re-furd′) of sensory phenomena, perceived at a site other than the one being stimulated 牵涉的

re·flec·tion (re-flek′shən) 1. a turning or bending back upon a course 反映；2. an image produced by reflection 镜射，指反射产生的图像；3. in physics, the turning back of a ray of light, sound, or heat when it strikes against a surface that it does not penetrate 指光、声音或热量的反射；4. a special form of reentry in which an impulse crosses an area of diminished responsiveness to excite distal tissue and then returns, retracing its path rather than traversing a circuit, to seesaw back and forth 指组织的反射作用。

re·flex (re′fleks) a reflected action or movement; the sum total of any particular automatic response mediated by the nervous system 反射，指神经系统介导的任何特定的自动反应；**abdominal r's,** contractions of the abdominal muscles on stimulation of the abdominal skin 腹壁反射；**accommodation r.,** the coordinated changes that occur when the eye adapts itself to near vision; constriction of the pupil, convergence of the eyes, and increased convexity of the lens 调节反射（视）；**Achilles tendon r.,** triceps surae r. 跟腱反射；**acoustic r.,** contraction of the stapedius muscle in response to intense sound 听觉反射；**anal r.,** contraction of the anal sphincter on irritation of the anal skin 肛门反射；**ankle r.,** triceps surae r 踝反射；**auditory r.,** any reflex caused by stimulation of the vestibulocochlear nerve, especially momentary closure of both eyes produced by a sudden sound 听觉反射；**Babinski r.,** dorsiflexion of the big toe on stimulation of the sole, occurring in lesions of the pyramidal tract, although a normal reflex in infants 巴宾斯基反射，指刺激脚底时大脚趾的背屈，发生在锥体束的病变中，但在婴儿中是正常的反射；**Babkin r.,** pressure by the examiner's thumbs on the palms of both hands of the infant results in opening of the infant's mouth 巴布肯反射，指检查者的拇指对婴儿双手手掌施加的压力导致婴儿的嘴巴张开；**baroreceptor r.,** the reflex response to stimulation of baroreceptors of the carotid sinus and aortic arch, regulating blood pressure by controlling heart rate, strength of heart contractions, and diameter of blood vessels 压力感受器反射，指对颈动脉窦和主动脉弓压力感受器刺激的反射，可通过控制心率、心脏收缩力和血管直径来调节血压；**Bezold r., Bezold-Jarisch r.,** reflex bradycardia and hypotension resulting from stimulation of cardiac chemoreceptors by antihypertensive alkaloids and similar substances 贝（措尔德）-雅（里施）反射（迷走反射），指用抗高血压生物碱和类似物质刺激心脏化学感受器引起的反射性心动过缓和低血压；**biceps r.,** contraction of the biceps muscle when its tendon is tapped 肱二头肌反射；**Brain r.,** extension of a hemiplegic flexed arm on assumption of a quadrupedal posture 四肢伸直反射；**brain-stem r's**, those regulated at the level of the brainstem, such as pupillary, pharyngeal, and cough reflexes, and the control of respiration; their absence is one criterion of brain death 脑干反射；**bulbospongiosus r.**, contraction of the bulbospongiosus muscle in response to a tap on the dorsum of the penis 球海绵体肌反射；**carotid sinus r.**, slowing of the heartbeat on pressure on the carotid artery at the level of the cricoid cartilage 颈动脉窦反射；**Chaddock r.**, in lesions of the pyramidal tract, stimulation below the external malleolus causes extension of the great toe 查多克征，指在锥体束的病变中，外踝下方的刺激会导致大脚趾的伸展；**chain r.**, a series of reflexes, each serving as a stimulus to the next one, representing a complete activity 连锁反应；**ciliary r.**, the movement of the pupil in accommodation 睫状体反射；**ciliospinal r.**, dilation of the ipsilateral pupil on painful stimulation of the skin at the side of the neck 睫状肌脊髓反射；**closed loop r.**, a reflex, such as a stretch reflex, in which the stimulus decreases when it receives feedback from the response mechanism 闭合式环反射，指当刺激从响应机制接收反馈时，刺激减少的一种反射，如伸展反射；**conditioned r.**, 条件反射，参见 *response* 下词条；**conjunctival r.**, closure of the eyelid when the conjunctiva is touched 结膜反射；**corneal r.**, closure of the lids on irritation of the cornea 角膜反射；**cough r.**, the events initiated by the sensitivity of the lining of the airways and mediated by the medulla as a consequence of impulses transmitted by the vagus nerve, resulting in coughing 咳嗽反射；**cremasteric r.**, stimulation of the skin on the front and inner thigh retracts the testis on the same side 提睾反射；**deep r.**, tendon r. 深反射；**digital r.**, Hoffmann sign (2) 指反射（霍夫曼征）；**diving r.**, a reflex involving cardiovascular and metabolic adaptations to conserve oxygen occurring in animals during diving into water; observed in reptiles, birds, and mammals, including humans 潜水反射；**doll's eye r.**, oculocephalic r. 玩偶眼反射；**elbow r.**, triceps r. 肘反射；**embrace r.**, 同 Moro r.；**finger-thumb r.**, opposition and adduction of the thumb combined with flexion at the metacarpophalangeal joint and extension at the interphalangeal joint on downward pressure of the index finger 指拇反射；**gag r.**, 同 pharyngeal r.；**gastrocolic r.**, increase in intestinal peristalsis after food enters the empty stomach 胃结肠反射；**gastroileal r.**, increase in ileal motility and opening of the ileocecal orifice when food enters the empty stomach 胃小肠反射；**grasp r.**, flexion or clench-

ing of the fingers or toes on stimulation of the palm or sole, normal only in infancy 握持反射；**Hering-Breuer r.**, the reflex that limits excessive expansion and contraction of the chest during respiration prior to sending impulses to the brain via the vagus nerve 黑-伯反射，指在通过迷走神经向大脑输送冲动之前，在呼吸期间限制胸部过度膨胀和收缩的反射；**Hoffmann r.**, H 反射，霍夫曼反射，*sign* (2)；**hypogastric r.**, contraction of the muscles of the lower abdomen on stroking the skin on the inner surface of the thigh 下腹反射；**jaw r., jaw jerk r.**, closure of the mouth caused by a downward blow on the passively hanging chin; rarely seen in health but very noticeable in corticospinal tract lesions 下颌反射；**knee jerk r.**, 同 patellar r.；**light r.**, 1. cone of light 光锥反射；2. contraction of the pupil when light falls on the eye 瞳孔对光反射；3. a spot of light seen reflected from the retina with the retinoscopic mirror 视网膜对光反射；**Magnus and de Kleijn neck r's**, extension of both ipsilateral limbs, or one, or part of a limb; increase of tonus on the side to which the chin is turned when the head is rotated to the side; and flexion with loss of tonus on the side to which the occiput points; sign of decerebrate rigidity except in infants 马-德反射（视丘障碍时的颈-肢体运动反射），指双侧肢体或一侧或部分肢体的伸展，当头部向一侧旋转时，下巴转向一侧的张力增加，枕骨指向的一侧的屈曲而失去张力，是去脑强直的征兆，婴儿除外；**Mayer r.**, finger-thumb r. 基底关节反射；**Mendel-Bekhterev r.**, dorsal flexion of the second to fifth toes on percussion of the dorsum of the foot; in certain organic nervous disorders, plantarflexion occurs 足背反射，指足背敲击时第二至第五个脚趾的背部屈曲，在某些器质性神经疾病中，会发生足底屈曲；**micturition r.**, any of the reflexes necessary for effortless urination and subconscious maintenance of continence 排尿反射；**Moro r.**, flexion of an infant's thighs and knees, fanning and then clenching of fingers, with arms first thrown outward and then brought together as though embracing something; produced by a sudden stimulus and seen normally in the newborn 莫罗反射，拥抱反射；**myotatic r.**, 同 stretch r.；**neck r's**, reflex adjustments in trunk posture and limb position caused by stimulation of proprioceptors in the neck joints and muscles when the head is turned, tending to maintain a constant orientation between the head and body 颈反射；**neck righting r.**, rotation of the trunk in the direction in which the head of the supine infant is turned; absent or decreased in infants with spasticity 颈翻正反射；**nociceptive r's**, reflexes initiated by painful stimuli 伤害性反射；**oculocardiac r.**, a slowing of the rhythm of the heart following compression of the eyes; slowing of from 5 to 13 beats per minute is normal 眼心反射；**oculocephalic r.**, when the head is rotated laterally, the eyes deviate synergistically in the opposite direction; assessed in premature infants and coma to test oculomotor nerve and brainstem function 眼脑反射；**open loop r.**, a reflex in which the stimulus causes activity that it does not further control and from which it does not receive feedback 开环反应；**Oppenheim r.**, dorsiflexion of the big toe on stroking downward along the medial side of the tibia, seen in pyramidal tract disease 奥本海姆反射，指沿胫骨内侧向下划动，出现踇趾背屈，见于锥体束病变；**orbicularis oculi r.**, normal contraction of the orbicularis oculi muscle, with resultant closing of the eye, on percussion at the outer aspect of the supraorbital ridge, over the glabella, or around the margin of the orbit 眼轮匝肌反射；**orbicularis pupillary r.**, unilateral contraction of the pupil followed by dilatation after closure or attempted closure of eyelids that are forcibly held apart 眼轮匝肌瞳孔反射；**palatal r., palatine r.**, stimulation of the palate causes swallowing 吞咽反射；**patellar r.**, contraction of the quadriceps and extension of the leg when the patellar ligament is tapped 膝反射；**peristaltic r.**, when a portion of the intestine is distended or irritated, the area just proximal contracts and the area just distal relaxes 蠕动反射，指当肠道的一部分膨胀或受到刺激时，该区域近端收缩，而远端区域松弛；**pharyngeal r.**, contraction of the pharyngeal constrictor muscle elicited by touching the back of the pharynx 呕吐反射；**pilomotor r.**, the production of goose flesh on stroking the skin 竖毛反射；**placing r.**, flexion followed by extension of the leg when the infant is held erect and the dorsum of the foot is drawn along the under edge of a table top; it is obtainable in the normal infant up to the age of 6 weeks 放置反射；**plantar r.**, irritation of the sole contracts the toes 足趾反射；**primitive r.**, any of a group of stereotypical reflexes, such as the Moro reflex, that are normal in newborns but disappear in infancy in most individuals 原始反射；**proprioceptive r.**, one initiated by a stimulus to a proprioceptor 本体感受反射；**pupillary r.**, 1. contraction of the pupil on exposure of the retina to light 瞳孔对光反射；2. any reflex involving the iris, resulting in change in the size of the pupil, occurring in response to various stimuli, e.g., change in illumination or point of fixation, sudden loud noise, or emotional stimulation 瞳孔反射；**quadriceps r.**, 同 patellar r.；**quadrupedal extensor r.**, 同 Brain r.；**red r.**, a luminous red appearance seen upon the retina in retinoscopy 视网膜红反射；**righting r.**, the ability to assume an optimal position when there has been a departure from it 翻正反射；**Rossolimo r.**, in pyramidal tract lesions, plantarflexion of the toes when their plantar surface is tapped Rossolimo 反射，指在锥体束病变中，当脚趾的足底表面被敲击时，脚趾的足底屈曲；**scratch r.**, a spinal reflex by which an itch or other irritation of the skin causes a nearby body part to move over and briskly rub the affected area 搔反射；**spinal r.**, any reflex action mediated through a center of the spinal cord 脊髓反射；**startle r.**, 同 Moro r.；**stepping r.**, movements of progression elicited when the infant is held upright and inclined forward with the soles of the feet touching a flat surface 跨步反射；**stretch r.**, reflex contraction of a muscle in response to passive longitudinal stretching 牵张反射；**sucking r.**, sucking movements of the lips of an infant elicited by touching the lips or the skin near the mouth 吸吮反射；**superficial r.**, any withdrawal reflex elicited by noxious or tactile stimulation of the skin, cornea, or mucous membrane, including the corneal reflex, pharyngeal reflex, cremasteric reflex, etc. 浅反射；**swallowing r.**, 同 palatal r.；**tendon r.**, one elicited by a sharp tap on the appropriate tendon or muscle to induce brief stretch of the muscle, followed by contraction 腱反射；**tonic neck r.**, extensions of the arm and sometimes of the leg on the side to which the head is forcibly turned, with flexion of the contralateral limbs; seen normally in the newborn 颈部强直反射；**triceps r.**, contraction of the belly of the triceps muscle and slight extension of the arm when the tendon of the muscle is tapped directly, with the arm flexed and fully supported and relaxed 肱三头肌反射；**triceps surae r.**, plantarflexion caused by a twitchlike contraction of the triceps surae muscle, elicited by a tap on the Achilles tendon, preferably while the patient kneels on a bed or chair, the feet hanging free over the edge 小腿三头肌反射；**vestibular r's**, the reflexes for maintaining the position of the eyes and body in relation to changes in orientation of the head 前庭反射；**vestibuloocular r.**, nystagmus or deviation of the eyes in response to stimulation of the vestibular system by angular acceleration or deceleration or when the caloric test is performed 前庭眼球反射；**withdrawal r.**, a nociceptive reflex in which a body part is quickly moved away from a painful stimulus 退避反射

R

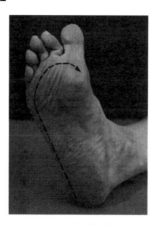

▲ 巴宾斯基反射

re·flex·o·gen·ic (re-flek″so-jen′ik) producing or increasing reflex action 发生反射的，促反射的

re·flex·og·e·nous (re″flek-soj′ə-nəs) 同 reflexogenic

re·flexo·graph (re-flek′so-graf) an instrument for recording a reflex 反射描记器

re·flex·ol·o·gy (re″flek-sol′ə-je) 1. the science or study of reflexes 反射学；2. a therapeutic technique based on the premise that areas in the hands or feet correspond to the organs and systems of the body and stimulation of these areas by pressure can affect the corresponding organ or system 反射疗法

re·flex·om·e·ter (re″flek-som′ə-tər) an instrument for measuring the force required to produce myotatic contraction 反射计

re·flux (re′fləks) a backward or return flow 回流反流；**duodenogastric r.**, reflux of the contents of the duodenum into the stomach; it may occur normally, especially during fasting 十二指肠胃反流；**gastroesophageal r.**, reflux of the stomach and duodenal contents into the esophagus 胃食管反流；**hepatojugular r.**, distention of the jugular vein induced by applying manual pressure over the liver; it suggests insufficiency of the right heart 肝颈静脉反流；**intrarenal r.**, reflux of urine into the renal parenchymal tissue 肾内反流；**laryngopharyngeal r. (LPR)**, a complication of gastroesophageal reflux caused by reflux from the esophagus into the pharynx, characterized by a variety of intermittent chronic symptoms, including hoarseness, cough, throat clearing, globus pharyngeus, and dysphagia 喉咽反流；**valvular r.**, backflow of blood past a venous valve in the lower limb due to venous insufficiency 瓣膜反流，由于静脉功能不全，血液通过下肢的静脉瓣回流；**vesicoureteral r., vesicoureteric**

r., backward flow of urine from the bladder into a ureter 膀胱输尿管反流

re·fract (re-frakt′) 1. to cause to deviate 使折射；2. to ascertain errors of ocular refraction 验光

re·frac·tion (re-frak′shən) 1. the act or process of refracting; specifically, the determination of the refractive errors of the eye and their correction with lenses 屈光；2. the deviation of light in passing obliquely from one medium to another of different density 折射；**refrac′tive** *adj.*；**double r.**, refraction in which incident rays are divided into two refracted rays, so as to produce a double image 双折射，其中入射光线被分成两个折射光线，从而产生双重图像；**dynamic r.**, the normal accommodation of the eye that is continually exerted without conscious effort 动态屈光，在无意识下不断进行的眼睛的正常调节

re·frac·tion·ist (re-frak′shən-ist) one skilled in determining the refracting power of the eyes and correcting refracting defects 验光师

re·frac·tom·e·ter (re″frak-tom′ə-tər) 1. an instrument for measuring the refractive power of the eye 屈光计；2. an instrument for determining the indexes of refraction of various substances, particularly for determining the strength of lenses for spectacles 折射计

re·frac·to·ry (re-frak′tə-re) 1. resistant to treatment 难治的，顽固性的；2. not responding to a stimulus 不感受的

re·fran·gi·ble (re-fran′jĭ-bəl) susceptible to being refracted 可折射的

re·fresh (re-fresh′) to denude an epithelial wound to enhance tissue repair 使复新，指去除上皮伤口以增强组织修复

re·frig·er·a·tion (re-frij″ər-a′shən) therapeutic application of low temperature 冷冻，一种低温治疗

re·fu·sion (re-fu′zhən) the return of blood to the circulation after temporary removal or stoppage of flow 血回输法

re·gen·er·a·tion (re-jen″ər-a′shən) the natural renewal of a structure, as of a lost tissue or part 再生；**guided tissue r.**, treatment of wound tissue using microporous membranes as barriers, so that only specific, desired types of cells can enter the wound and regenerate 引导性组织再生术，使用微孔膜作为屏障处理伤口组织，使得只有特定的所需类型的细胞才能进入伤口并再生

reg·i·men (rej′ĭ-mən) a strictly regulated scheme of diet, exercise, or other activity designed to achieve certain ends 制度，生活制度，为达到某种目的而进行的严格控制饮食、锻炼及其他活动的方法

re·gio (re′je-o) pl. *regio′nes* [L.] 同 region

re·gion (re′jən) a plane area with more or less definite boundaries 区，部（位）；**re′gional** *adj.*；**r's of back,** the areas into which the back is divided, including the *vertebral, sacral, scapular, infrascapular,* and *lumbar* 背区，包括椎体区、骶区、肩胛区、肩胛下区和腰椎区；**facial r.,** that comprising the various anatomic regions of the face: *buccal* (side of oral cavity), *infraorbital* (below eye), *mental* (chin), *nasal* (nose), *oral* (lips), *orbital* (eye), *parotid* (angle of jaw), and *zygomatic* (cheek bone) regions 面部区域，包括面部的各种解剖区域：颊区（口腔侧）、眶下区（眼睛下方）、颏区（下巴）、鼻区（鼻）、口区（嘴唇）、眶区（眼）、腮腺区（下颌角）和颧骨区（颧骨）；**homogeneously staining r's (HSR),** long unbanded regions of chromosomes created by gene amplification; they are tumor markers indicative of solid neoplasms with poor prognosis 均染区，通过基因扩增产生的染色体长的未折叠区域；它们是标志着实体肿瘤预后不良的肿瘤标志物；**pectoral r.,** the aspect of the chest bounded by the pectoralis major muscle, and including the lateral pectoral, mammary, and inframammary regions 胸肌区，由胸大肌包围的胸部，包括胸外侧区、乳房和乳房下区域；**perineal r.,** the region overlying the pelvic outlet, including the *anal* and *genitourinary* regions 会阴部，覆盖骨盆出口的区域，包括肛门和泌尿生殖区；**precordial r.,** the part of the anterior surface of the body covering the heart and the pit of the stomach 心前区，身体前表面覆盖心脏和胃的凹陷的部分

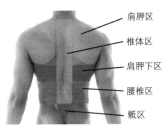

▲ 背区

reg·is·trant (rej′is-trənt) a nurse listed on the books of a registry as available for duty 登记护士

reg·is·trar (rej′is-trahr) 1. an official keeper of records 登记员，挂号员；2. in British hospitals, a resident specialist who acts as assistant to the chief or attending specialist（英国医院的）专科住院医师

reg·is·tra·tion (rej″is-tra′shən) in dentistry, the making of a record of the jaw relations present or desired, or the record so produced 记录（牙科中指颌位关系记录）

reg·is·try (rej′is-tre) 1. an office where a nurse's name may be listed as being available for duty（值班护士）登记处；2. a central agency for the collection of pathologic material and related data in a specified field of pathology 集中登记

re·go·raf·e·nib (ree″goh-raf′ə-nib) an antineoplastic multikinase inhibitor used to treat advanced gastrointestinal stromal tumors and previously treated metastatic colorectal cancer 一种抗肿瘤的多激酶抑制药，用于治疗晚期胃肠道间质瘤和既往经治疗的转移性结直肠癌

re·gres·sion (re-gresh′ən) 1. return to a former or earlier state 消退；2. subsidence of symptoms or of a disease process（疾病）恢复；3. the statistical tendency in successive generations to exhibit values closer and closer to the mean 回归，指连续世代的统计趋势越来越接近平均值的现象；4. defensive retreat to an earlier, often infantile, pattern of behavior or thought（心理学）退行，防御性地退回到早期的、且通常是幼稚的行为或思想模式；5. a functional relationship between a random variable and the corresponding values of one or more independent variables（统计学）回归，随机变量与一个或多个自变量的对应值之间的函数关系；**regres′sive** *adj.*

reg·u·lar (reg′u-lər) normal or conforming to rule; occurring at proper or fixed intervals 规律的，有规律的；定期的

reg·u·la·tion (reg″u-la′shən) 1. the act of adjusting or state of being adjusted to a certain standard 调控，调整或调整到一定标准的行为；2. in biology, the adaptation of form or behavior of an organism to changed conditions（生物学）调节，生物体为适应外界条件变化而改变自身的形态或行为；3. the power to form a whole embryo from stages before the gastrula（胚胎学）调整，指在原肠胚前，胚胎的各个形成阶段演化成完整胚胎的能力；**reg′ulatory** *adj.*

reg·u·la·tor (reg′u-lə-tər) a mechanism or process that controls another mechanism or process 调节因子；**cystic fibrosis transmembrane r. (CFTR),** a transmembrane protein primarily functioning as a cAMP-regulated chloride channel that also regulates other ion channels, and found in cell membranes of the respiratory epithelium, pancreas, salivary glands, sweat glands, intestines, and reproductive tract. Mutations have been associated with cystic fibrosis 囊性纤维化跨膜调节因子

re·gur·gi·tant (re-gur′jĭ-tənt) flowing backward 反流的

re·gur·gi·ta·tion (re-gur″jĭ-ta′shən) 1. flow in the

opposite direction from normal 反流；2. movement of undigested or partially digested food upward through the esophagus, as in vomiting or rumination 反胃；**aortic r. (AR)**, backflow of blood from the aorta into the left ventricle due to aortic valve insufficiency 主动脉瓣反流；**mitral r. (MR)**, backflow of blood from the left ventricle into the left atrium due to left atrioventricular valve insufficiency 二尖瓣反流；**pulmonic r. (PR)**, backflow of blood from the pulmonary artery into the right ventricle due to pulmonary valve insufficiency 肺动脉瓣反流；**tricuspid r. (TR)**, backflow of blood from the right ventricle into the right atrium due to right atrioventricular valve insufficiency 三尖瓣反流；**valvular r.**, backflow of blood through the orifices of the heart valves due to imperfect closing of the valves 瓣膜反流

re·ha·bil·i·ta·tion (re″hə-bil″ĭ-ta′shən) 1. the restoration of normal form and function after illness or injury 恢复；2. the restoration of the ill or injured patient to an optimal functional level in all areas of activity 康复

re·hy·dra·tion (re″hi-dra′shən) the restoration of water or fluid content to a patient or to a substance that has become dehydrated 补液

rei·ki (ra′ke) [Japanese] a healing tradition of Eastern origin whose purpose is to rebalance the complex energy systems that compose the body when they have become out of balance, using channeling of energy from an unlimited universal energy source through the hands of the practitioner 灵气疗法，一种东方的传统治疗，其目的是当构成身体的复杂能量系统失去平衡时，通过医生的手触摸患者向其体内输送来自外界的无限能量，使其重新恢复平衡

re·im·plan·ta·tion (re″im-plan-ta′shən) replacement of tissue or a structure in the site from which it was previously lost or removed 再植术；**ureteral r.**, ureteroneocystostomy 输尿管再植术

re·in·fec·tion (re″in-fek′shən) a second infection by the same agent or a second infection of an organ with a different agent 再感染

re·in·force·ment (re″in-fors′mənt) in behavioral science, the presentation of a stimulus following a response that increases the frequency of subsequent responses, whether *positive* to desirable events or *negative* to undesirable events, which are reinforced in their removal（行为学）强化

re·in·forc·er (re″in-for′sər) any stimulus that produces reinforcement, a *positive r.* being a desirable event strengthening responses preceding its occurrence and a *negative r.* being an undesirable event strengthening responses leading to its termination（心理学）强化物，指任何可以导致强化的刺激

re·in·fu·sate (re″in-fu′zāt) fluid for reinfusion into the body, usually after being subjected to a treatment process 再输注液

re·in·fu·sion (re″in-fu′zhən) infusion of body fluid that has previously been withdrawn from the same individual, e.g., reinfusion of ascitic fluid after ultrafiltration 再输注

re·in·ner·va·tion (re″in-ər-va′shən) restoration of nerve supply to a part from which it has been lost; it may occur spontaneously or by nerve grafting 神经移植术

re·in·te·gra·tion (re″in-tə-gra′shən) 1. biologic integration after a state of disruption 再整合（作用）；2. restoration of harmonious mental function after disintegration of the personality in mental illness 重整（作用）（指精神活动）

re·jec·tion (re-jek′shən) an immune reaction against grafted tissue that results in failure of the graft to survive 排斥（反应）

re·lapse (re′laps) (rə-laps′) 1. the return of a disease after its apparent cessation 复发；2. to fall back into an illness after a period of remission 再发

re·laps·ing (rə-lap′sing) (re′lap-sing) recurrent; likely to have periods of remission alternating with attacks of symptomatic disease 复发的

re·la·tion (re-la′shən) the condition or state of one object or entity when considered in connection with another 关系联系；**rel′ative** *adj.*；**object r's**, the emotional bonds formed between one person and another, as contrasted with love for and interest in oneself 对象关系，一个人与另一个人之间形成的情感纽带，与一个人对自己的爱和兴趣相对

re·lax·ant (re-lak′sənt) 1. lessening or reducing tension 松弛的，舒张的；2. an agent that so acts 松弛药，松弛剂；**muscle r.**, an agent that specifically aids in reducing muscle tension 肌肉松弛药

re·line (re-lin′) to resurface the tissue side of a denture with new base material in order to achieve a more accurate fit 重衬，为实现更精确的贴合而用新的基础材料重新塑造的义齿的组织侧面

REM rapid eye movements 快速眼动睡眠（参见 *sleep* 下词条）

rem (rem) *r*oentgen-*e*quivalent–*m*an: the amount of any ionizing radiation that has the same biological effectiveness as 1 rad of x-rays; 1 rem = 1 rad × RBE (relative biological effectiveness) 雷姆，人体伦琴当量

rem·e·dy (rem′ə-de) anything that cures, palliates, or prevents disease 治疗，药物，疗法；**reme′dial** *adj.*；**concordant r's**, in homeopathy, remedies of similar action but of dissimilar origin 协同药，指在顺势疗法中，来源不同但作用相似的药物；**in-**

imic r's, in homeopathy, remedies whose actions are antagonistic 拮抗药, 指在顺势疗法中, 作用相反的药物; **tissue r's,** the twelve remedies which, according to the biochemical school of homeopathy, form the mineral bases of the body 组织药, 指在顺势疗法中, 构成身体的矿物质基础的十二种药物

rem·i·fen·ta·nil (rem″ĭ-fen′tə-nil) an opioid analgesic used as the hydrochloride salt as an anesthesia adjunct 瑞芬太尼, 一种阿片类镇痛药, 其盐酸盐可用作麻醉辅助剂

re·min·er·al·i·za·tion (re-min″ər-əl-ĭ-za′shən) restoration of mineral elements, as of calcium salts to bone 再矿化

re·mis·sion (re-mish′ən) diminution or abatement of the symptoms of a disease; the period during which such diminution occurs 缓解

re·mit·tent (re-mit′ənt) having periods of abatement and of exacerbation 弛张的, 忽轻忽重的

re·mod·el·ing (re-mod′əl-ing) reorganization or renovation of an old structure 重塑; **bone r.,** absorption of bone tissue and simultaneous deposition of new bone; in normal bone the two processes are in dynamic equilibrium 骨重塑

re·mo·ti·va·tion (re-mo″tĭ-va′shən) any of various group therapy techniques used with longterm, withdrawn patients in mental hospitals to stimulate their communication, vocational, and social skills and interest in their environment 再激发, 一种集体治疗技术, 用于治疗长期住在精神病院的患者, 以激发他们的沟通、职业和社交技能以及对环境的兴趣

ren (ren) pl. *re′nes* [L.] kidney 肾

re·nal (re′nəl) pertaining to the kidney 肾脏的

ren·i·form (ren′ĭ-form) kidney-shaped 肾形的

re·nin (re′nin) a proteolytic enzyme synthesized, stored, and secreted by the juxtaglomerular cells of the kidney; it plays a role in regulation of blood pressure by catalyzing the conversion of angiotensinogen to angiotensin Ⅰ 肾素

re·nin·ism (re′nin-iz″əm) a condition marked by overproduction of renin 肾素产生过多; **primary r.,** a syndrome of hypertension, hypokalemia, hyperaldosteronism, and elevated plasma renin activity, due to proliferation of juxtaglomerular cells 原发性肾素增多症, 一种由于肾小球旁细胞增殖引起的以高血压、低钾血症、醛固酮增多症和血浆肾素活性升高为特征的综合征

reni·pel·vic (ren″ĭ-pel′vik) pertaining to the pelvis of the kidney 肾盂的

ren·nin (ren′in) chymosin 凝乳酶

re·no·gas·tric (re″no-gas′trik) pertaining to the kidney and stomach 肾胃的

re·nog·ra·phy (re-nog′rə-fe) radiography of the kidney 肾造影术

re·no·in·tes·ti·nal (re″no-in-tes′tĭ-nəl) pertaining to the kidney and intestine 肾肠的

re·no·pri·val (re″no-pri′vəl) pertaining to or caused by lack of kidney function 肾功能缺乏的, 肾无能的

re·no·vas·cu·lar (re″no-vas′ku-lər) pertaining to or affecting the blood vessels of the kidney 肾血管性的

ren·ule (ren′ūl) an area of kidney supplied by a branch of the renal artery, usually consisting of three or four medullary pyramids and their corresponding cortical substance 肾段, 由肾动脉分支供应的肾脏区域, 通常由三个或四个髓质三角及其相应的皮质组成

Reo·vi·ri·dae (re″o-vir′ĭ-de) the reoviruses: a family of RNA viruses that includes the genera *Orbivirus, Orthoreovirus, Rotavirus,* and *Coltivirus* 呼肠孤病毒科

reo·vi·rus (re′o-vi″rəs) 1. any virus belonging to the family Reoviridae 任何一种属于呼肠孤病毒科的病毒; 2. any virus belonging to the genus *Orthoreovirus* 正呼肠孤病毒

re·ox·y·gen·a·tion (re-ok″sĭ-jə-na′shən) in radiobiology, the phenomenon in which hypoxic (and thus radioresistant) tumor cells become more exposed to oxygen (and thus more radiosensitive) by coming into closer proximity to capillaries after death and loss of other tumor cells due to previous irradiation 再氧合（作用）, 在放射生物学中, 由于肿瘤细胞死亡后更接近毛细血管以及其他肿瘤细胞因先前的照射而损失, 低氧（对放射抵抗）的肿瘤细胞变得更多地暴露于氧（对放射敏感）的现象

re·pag·li·nide (rĕ-pag′lĭ-nīd) an oral hypoglycemic agent used in the treatment of type 2 diabetes mellitus 一种口服降糖药, 用于治疗 2 型糖尿病

re·pair (re-pār′) the physical or mechanical restoration of damaged or diseased tissues by the growth of healthy new cells or by surgical apposition 修复; **repar′ative** adj.; **Cooper ligament r., McVay r.,** repair of an inguinal hernia by suturing the inguinal falx to the pectineal (Cooper) and inguinal ligaments Cooper 韧带修复术, McVay 修复术, 一种通过将腹股沟镰缝合到耻骨梳状韧带（Cooper 韧带）和腹股沟韧带来修复腹股沟疝的手术

re·peat (re-pēt′) something done or occurring more than once, particularly over and over 重复; **long terminal r's (LTR),** identical DNA sequences, usually several hundred base pairs long, occurring at each end of an integrated retrovirus and essential for integration of the molecule into host DNA 长末端

R

重复（序列）；**short tandem r. (STR)**, microsatellite 短串联重复；**tandem r.**, 串联重复（序列）1. arrangement of two or more copies of a nucleotide sequence adjacent to each other within a segment of DNA 两个或多个彼此相邻的核苷酸序列的拷贝在 DNA 片段内排列；2. arrangement of two or more copies of a gene or two or more copies of a segment of a chromosome adjacent to each other on a chromosome 两个或多个彼此相邻的基因的拷贝或两个或多个彼此相邻的染色体片段的拷贝在染色体上排列；**triplet r.**, an unstable DNA sequence of three nucleotides, occurring in some human genes and normally repeated in tandem 5 to 50 times 三联重复序列，发生在一些人类基因中的三个核苷酸的不稳定 DNA 序列，通常串联重复 5 到 50 次；**variable number tandem r's (VNTR)**, different numbers of tandemly repeated oligonucleotide sequences in the alleles of a gene; such a polymorphism can be useful in genetic mapping 可变数目串联重复序列，参见 *minisatellite*

re·place·ment (re-plās′ment) 1. substitution 替换，参见 *therapy* 下 *replacement therapy*；2. arthroplasty 置换术；**joint r.**, arthroplasty 关节置换术

re·plan·ta·tion (re″plan-ta′shən) 同 reimplantation

rep·li·case (rep′lĭ-kās) 1. a polymerase synthesizing RNA from an RNA template RNA 复制酶，一种以 RNA 为模板合成 RNA 的聚合酶；2. more generically, any enzyme that replicates nucleic acids, i.e., a DNA or RNA polymerase 复制酶，广义上指任何可以复制核酸的酶，即 DNA 或 RNA 聚合酶

rep·li·ca·tion (rep″lĭ-ka′shən) 1. a turning back of a part so as to form a duplication 折转；2. repetition of an experiment to ensure accuracy 再试验；3. the process of duplicating or reproducing, as in the replication of an exact copy of a strand of DNA or RNA（DNA 或 RNA 的）复制；**rep′licative** *adj.*

re·po·lar·iza·tion (re-po″lər-ĭ-za′shən) the reestablishment of polarity, especially the return of cell membrane potential to resting potential after depolarization 复极化

re·pos·i·tor (re-poz′ĭ-tər) an instrument used in returning a displaced organ or tissue to the normal position 复位器

re·pos·i·to·ry (re-poz′ĭ-tor-e) a place where something is stored, in pharmacology referring to the injection, usually intramuscularly, of a long-acting drug, which is slowly absorbed and is therefore prolonged in its action 贮藏处（一般指长效药物的肌肉注射部位）

re·pres·si·ble (re-pres′ĭ-bəl) capable of undergoing repression 可抑制的

re·pres·sion (re-presh′ən) 1. the act of restraining, inhibiting, or suppressing 抑制；2. in psychiatry, an unconscious defense mechanism in which unacceptable ideas, fears, and impulses are thrust out or kept out of consciousness（心理学）压抑；3. 同 gene r.；**enzyme r.**, interference, usually by the end product of a pathway, with synthesis of the enzymes of that pathway 酶阻遏；**gene r.**, the inhibition of gene transcription of an operon; in prokaryotes repressor binding to the operon is involved 基因阻遏

re·pres·sor (re-pres′ər) in genetics, a protein produced by a regulator gene that binds to the operator region of a structural gene to block initiation of transcription of the gene or operon 阻遏蛋白，阻遏物

re·pro·duc·tion (re″pro-duk′shən) 1. the production of offspring by organized bodies 生殖，繁殖；2. the creation of a similar object or situation; duplication; replication 复制；**reproduc′tive** *adj.*；**asexual r.**, reproduction without the fusion of gametes 无性生殖；**cytogenic r.**, production of a new individual from a single germ cell or zygote 细胞性生殖；**sexual r.**, reproduction by the fusion of a female gamete and a male gamete *(bisexual r.)* or by development of an unfertilized egg *(unisexual r.)* 有性生殖；**somatic r.**, production of a new individual from a multicellular fragment by fission or budding 分体生殖

rep·til·ase (rep′til-ās) an enzyme from Russell's viper venom used in determining blood clotting time 蛇毒血凝酶（立止血）（用于测定凝血时间）

re·pul·sion (re-pul′shən) 1. the act of driving apart or away; a force that tends to drive two bodies apart 排斥，斥力；2. in genetics, the occurrence on opposite chromosomes in a double heterozygote of the two mutant alleles of interest（遗传学）相斥，在双杂合子中的两个相反染色体上发生的等位基因突变

RES reticuloendothelial system 网状内皮系统

re·scin·na·mine (re-sin′ə-min) an alkaloid from various species of *Rauwolfia;* used as an antihypertensive 瑞西那明（抗高血压药）

re·sect (re-sekt′) to excise part or all of an organ or other structure 切除

re·sec·tion (re-sek′shən) excision. **root r.**, apicoectomy 切除；**root r.**,（牙）根尖切除术；**transurethral r. of the prostate (TURP)**, resection of the prostate by means of an instrument passed through the urethra 经尿道前列腺切除术；**wedge r.**, removal of a triangular mass of tissue 楔形切除术

re·sec·to·scope (re-sek′to-skōp) an instrument with a wide-angle telescope and an electrically activated wire loop for transurethral removal or biopsy of lesions of the bladder, prostate, or urethra 电切镜

re·ser·pine (rə-sur′pēn) an alkaloid from various

species of *Rauwolfia*; used as an antihypertensive 利血平（抗高血压药）

re·serve (re-zurv′) 1. to hold back for future use 保留；2. a supply, beyond that ordinarily used, which may be utilized in emergency 储备；**alkali r., alkaline r.,** the amount of conjugate base components of the blood buffers, the most important being bicarbonate 碱储备；**cardiac r.,** potential ability of the heart to perform work beyond that necessary under basal conditions 心脏储备；**ovarian r.,** the number and quality of oocytes in the ovaries of a woman of childbearing age 卵巢储备

re·ser·voir (rez′ər-vwahr) 1. a storage place or cavity 储器；2. an alternate host or passive carrier of a pathogenic organism or parasite（寄生物或病菌的）贮主；**continent ileal r.,** 1. a valved intra-abdominal pouch that maintains continence of the feces and is emptied by a catheter when full 可控性回肠贮器，一种带瓣膜的腹内袋，可保持对粪便的控制，并可在充满时用导管清空；2. a neobladder made from a section of ileum 可控性回肠膀胱；**continent urinary r.,** neobladder 可控性膀胱术；**ileoanal r.,** a pouch for the retention of feces, formed by suturing together multiple limbs of ileum and connected to the anus by a short conduit of ileum; used with colectomy and ileoanal anastomosis to maintain continence in the treatment of ulcerative colitis 回肠肛门腔，一个用于保留粪便的小袋，通过将多段回肠的分支缝合在一起并通过回肠的短导管连接到肛门而形成；与结肠切除术和回肠吻合术一起使用，以维持治疗溃疡性结肠炎后患者对粪便的自主控制

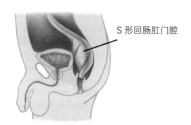

S 形回肠肛门腔

res·i·dent (rez′ĭ-dənt) 1. resident physician 住院医师；2. being or pertaining to such a physician 住院医师的

res·i·due (rez′ĭ-doo) 1. a remainder; that remaining after removal of other substances 残余物；2. in biochemistry, that portion of a monomer that is incorporated in a polymer（生物化学）残基，并入聚合物中的单体；**resid′ual** adj.

res·in (rez′in) 1. a solid or semisolid organic substance exuded by plants or by insects feeding on plants, or produced synthetically; they are insoluble in water but mostly soluble in alcohol or ether 树脂；2. a compound made by condensation or polymerization of low-molecular-weight organic compounds 合成树脂；**res′inous** adj.；**acrylic r's,** a class of thermoplastic resins produced by polymerization of acrylic or methacrylic acid or their derivatives; used in a variety of medical and dental applications 丙烯酸树脂；**anion exchange r.,** 阴离子交换树脂，参见 *ion exchange r.*；**cation exchange r.,** 阳离子交换树脂，参见 *ion exchange r.*；**cholestyramine r.,** a synthetic, strongly basic anion exchange resin in the chloride form that chelates bile acids in the intestine, thus preventing their reabsorption; used as an adjunctive therapy to diet in management of certain hypercholesterolemias and in the symptomatic relief of pruritus associated with bile stasis 消胆胺；**epoxy r.,** a heat-set resin with toughness, adhesibility, chemical resistance, dielectric properties, and dimensional stability; several modified types are used as denture base material 环氧树脂；**ion exchange r.,** a high-molecular-weight insoluble polymer of simple organic compounds capable of exchanging its attached ions for other ions in the surrounding medium; classified as *(a) cation* or *anion exchange r's,* depending on which ions the resin exchanges; and *(b)* carboxylic, sulfonic, etc., depending on the nature of the active groups 离子交换树脂，一种由简单有机化合物聚合而成的高分子量不溶性聚合物，能够将其附着的离子交换为周围介质中的其他离子；分类为（a）阳离子或阴离子交换树脂，取决于树脂交换的离子；（b）羧酸树脂、磺酸树脂等，取决于活性基团的性质；**podophyllum r.,** podophyllin; a mixture of resins from podophyllum, used as a topical caustic in the treatment of certain papillomas, condylomata acuminata, keratoses, and other epitheliomas 鬼臼树脂

re·sis·tance (re-zis′təns) 1. opposition, or counteracting force 阻力；2. the natural ability of an organism to resist microorganisms or toxins produced in disease（机体对病原微生物或毒物的）抵抗力；3. the opposition to the flow of electrical current between two points of a circuit 电阻，符号 R 或 *R*；4. in psychiatry, conscious or unconscious defenses that prevent material in the unconscious from coming into awareness（心理学）潜抑，一种心理防御机制；**airway r. (R_A) (R_{AW}),** the opposition of the tracheobronchial tree to air flow 气道阻力；**drug r.,** the ability of a microorganism to withstand the effects of a drug that are lethal to most members of its species 耐药性；**electri-**

848

cal r., 同 resistance (3)；**multidrug r., multiple drug r.,** in some malignant cell lines, resistance to many structurally unrelated chemotherapy agents in cells that have developed natural resistance to a single cytotoxic compound 多重耐药性；**vascular r.,** the opposition to blood flow in a vascular bed 血管阻力

re·sis·tin (re-zis′tin) an adipocytokine that has been implicated in the development of insulin resistance; it has been suggested that it may be the link between obesity and insulin resistance, but its role remains unclear 抵抗素

re·sis·tive (re-zis′tiv) pertaining to or characterized by resistance 抵抗的，有抵抗力的

res·o·lu·tion (rez″o-loo′shən) 1. subsidence of a pathologic state（疾病的）消退；2. perception as separate of two adjacent points; in microscopy, the smallest distance at which two adjacent objects can be distinguished as separate 分辨率，指对两个相邻点的感知，即能清楚区分被检物体细微结构最小间隔的能力；指在显微镜中，两个相邻物体可以被独立区分的最小距离；3. a measure of the fineness of detail that can be discerned in an image 分辨率

re·sol·vent (re-zol′vənt) 1. promoting resolution or the dissipation of a pathologic growth 使分解的；消散的；2. an agent that promotes resolution 消散药

Re·so·ma·tion (rē″sō-mā′shun) trademark for a process of disposing of dead bodies using primarily water and the process of alkaline hydrolysis Resomation 公司，该公司生产主要应用水和碱水解过程处理尸体的尸体液化机

res·o·nance (rez′o-nəns) 1. the prolongation and intensification of sound produced by transmission of its vibrations to a cavity, especially such a sound elicited by percussion 共振；2. a vocal sound heard on auscultation 清音；3. the existence of organic chemical structures that cannot be accurately represented by a single structural formula, the actual formula lying intermediate between several possible representations differing only in electron position（有机化学）共振结构；**amphoric r.,** an auscultatory sound like that produced by blowing over the mouth of an empty bottle 空瓮音，一种类似空气吹过空瓶口产生的声音；**nuclear magnetic r.,** a measure, by means of applying an external magnetic field to a solution in a constant radiofrequency field, of the magnetic moment of atomic nuclei to determine the structure of organic compounds; the technique is used in magnetic resonance imaging 核磁共振；**skodaic r.,** increased percussion resonance at the upper part of the chest, with flatness below it

skodaic 叩响，胸上部叩响增强而胸下部呈实音；**tympanitic r.,** 1. the percussion sound heard on an abdomen with tympanites 叩诊时在腹部听到叩响；2. the drumlike reverberation of a cavity full of air 鼓音，充满空气的空腔的鼓状混响；**vocal r. (VR),** the sound of ordinary speech as heard through the chest wall 语音共振，听觉语音

res·o·na·tor (rez′o-na″tər) 1. an instrument used to intensify sounds 共鸣箱；2. an electric circuit in which oscillations of a certain frequency are set up by oscillations of the same frequency in another circuit 谐振器

re·sorb (re-sorb′) (re-zorb′) to take up or absorb again 重吸收，再吸收

re·sor·ci·nol (rə-sor′sĭ-nol) a bactericidal, fungicidal, keratolytic, exfoliative, and antipruritic agent, used especially as a topical keratolytic in the treatment of acne and other dermatoses 间苯二酚，一种可杀细菌、真菌，溶解角质层，去角质和止痒的局部角质层分离剂，尤其用于治疗痤疮和其他皮肤病

re·sorp·tion (re-sorp′shən) 1. the lysis and assimilation of a substance, as of bone 吸收，如骨吸收；2. 同 reabsorption

res·pi·ra·ble (res′spər-ə-bəl) 1. suitable for respiration 可呼吸的；2. small enough to be inhaled 吸入性的

res·pi·ra·tion (res″pĭ-ra′shən) 1. the exchange of oxygen and carbon dioxide between the atmosphere and the body cells, including ventilation (inhalation and exhalation); diffusion of oxygen from alveoli to blood and of carbon dioxide from blood to alveoli; and transport of oxygen to and carbon dioxide from body cells 呼吸；2. ventilation (1) 通气；3. the metabolic processes by which cells generate energy, chiefly in the form of ATP, by the oxidation of organic molecules such as glucose, with the release of carbon dioxide, water, and other oxidized products 细胞呼吸；**abdominal r.,** breathing accomplished mainly by the abdominal muscles and respiratory diaphragm 腹式呼吸；**aerobic r.,** the oxidative transformation of certain substrates into secretory products, the released energy being used in the process of assimilation 有氧呼吸；**anaerobic r.,** respiration in which energy is released from chemical reactions in which free oxygen takes no part 无氧呼吸；**artificial r.,** any artificial method of ventilation in which air is forced into and out of the lungs of a person who has stopped breathing. It may be mechanical (see *mechanical ventilation*) or nonmechanical, e.g., mouth-to-mouth resuscitation 人工呼吸；**Biot r.,** rapid, short breathing with pauses of several seconds, indicating increased intracranial pressure 比奥

呼 吸；**Cheyne-Stokes r.**, breathing with rhythmic waxing and waning of depth of breaths and regularly recurring apneic periods 陈 - 施氏呼吸；**cogwheel r.**, breathing with jerky inhalation 齿 轮 状 呼 吸；**electrophrenic r.**, diaphragmatic pacing; induction of respiration by electric stimulation of the phrenic nerve 膈神经电刺激呼吸；**external r.**, exchange of gases between the lungs and blood 外呼吸；**internal r.**, exchange of gases between the body cells and blood 内呼吸；**Kussmaul r., Kussmaul-Kien r.**, air hunger; deep rapid breathing as seen in respiratory acidosis 库斯莫尔呼吸；**paradoxical r.**, that in which all or part of a lung is deflated during inhalation and inflated during exhalation, such as in flail chest or paralysis of the respiratory diaphragm 反常呼吸；**tissue r.**, internal r. 组织呼吸

res·pi·ra·tor (res′pĭ-ra″tər) ventilator (2) 呼吸机；**cuirass r.**, 胸甲式呼吸机，参见 *ventilator* 下词条；**Drinker r.**, popularly, "iron lung": an apparatus formerly in wide use for producing artificial respiration over long periods of time, consisting of a metal tank, enclosing the patient's body, with the head outside, and within which artificial respiration is maintained by alternating negative and positive pressure 德 林克人工呼吸器（铁肺）

res·pi·ra·to·ry (res′pər-ə-tor″e) pertaining to respiration 呼吸的

res·pi·rom·e·ter (res″pĭ-rom′ə-tər) an instrument for determining the nature of respiration 呼吸计

Res·pi·ro·vi·rus (res″pĭ-ro-vi″rəs) a genus of viruses of the family Paramyxoviridae that cause respiratory infections; included are mumps virus and several human parainfluenza viruses 呼吸道病毒属

re·sponse (re-spons′) any action or change of condition evoked by a stimulus 反应，应答；**respon′sive** *adj.*；**acute-phase r.**, a group of physiologic processes occurring soon after the onset of infection, trauma, inflammatory processes, and some malignant conditions; it includes an increase in acute-phase proteins in serum, fever, increased vascular permeability, and metabolic and pathologic changes 急 性 期 反 应；**anamnestic r.**, secondary immune r. 回忆应答；**autoimmune r.**, the immune response against an autoantigen 自身免疫应答；**conditioned r.**, a response evoked by a conditioned stimulus; a response to a stimulus that was incapable of evoking it before conditioning 条 件 反 应；**galvanic skin r.**, the alteration in the electrical resistance of the skin associated with sympathetic nerve discharge 皮 肤 电 反 应；**immune r.**, any response of the immune system to an antigenic stimulus, including antibody production, cell-mediated immunity, and

immunologic tolerance 免疫应答；**inflammatory r.**, the various changes that tissue undergoes when it becomes inflamed 炎性反应，参见 *inflammation*；**primary immune r.**, the immune response occurring on the first exposure to an antigen, with specific antibodies appearing in the blood after a multiple-day latent period 初次免疫应答；**relaxation r.**, a group of physiologic changes that cause decreased activity of the sympathetic nervous system and consequent relaxation after stimulation of certain regions of the hypothalamus. They may be self-induced through techniques such as meditation and biofeedback 迟缓反应；**secondary immune r.**, the immune response occurring on second and subsequent exposures to an antigen, with a stronger response to a lesser amount of antigen and a shorter lag time compared with the primary immune response 再次免疫应答；**triple r.**, a triphasic skin reaction to being stroked with a blunt instrument: first a red line develops at the site due to histamine release, then a flare develops around the red line, and lastly a wheal is formed as a result of local edema 三 重 反 应，钝器敲击皮肤产生的三相反应：首先由于组胺释放而在该部位出现红线，然后在红线周围形成一个红斑，最后由于局部水肿而形成风团；**unconditioned r.**, an unlearned response, i.e., one that occurs naturally to an unconditioned stimulus 无条件反应

rest (rest) 1. repose after exertion 休息；2. a fragment of embryonic tissue retained within the adult organism 胎性剩余；3. an extension that helps support a removable partial denture 支托，用于支撑可摘局部义齿的延伸部分；**adrenal r's,** accessory suprarenal glands 肾上腺剩余；**incisal r., lingual r., occlusal r.**, a metallic part or extension from a removable partial denture to aid in supporting the prosthesis 切支托，舌面支托，𬌗支托；**suprarenal r's,** accessory suprarenal glands 肾上腺剩余

re·ste·no·sis (re″stə-no′sis) recurrent stenosis, especially of a cardiac valve after surgical correction of the primary condition 再狭窄；**restenot′ic** *adj.*

res·ti·form (res′tĭ-form) shaped like a rope 绳 状的，索状的

res·ti·tu·tion (res″tĭ-too′shən) the spontaneous realignment of the fetal head with the fetal body, after delivery of the head 转回（胎头）

res·to·ra·tion (res″tə-ra′shən) 1. induction of a return to a previous state, as a return to health or replacement of a part to normal position 恢复；2. partial or complete reconstruction of a body part, or the device used in its place 修 重；**restor′ative** *adj.*

re·straint (re-strānt′) the forcible confinement or

control of a subject 限制，约束

re·stric·tion (re-strik'shən) 1. a limitation 限制；2. a thing or process that limits 限制物，限制步骤；**restric'tive** *adj.*；**intrauterine growth r. (IUGR),** 宫内发育迟缓，参见 *retardation* 下词条

re·sus·ci·ta·tion (re-sus'ĭ-ta'shən) restoration to life of one apparently dead 复 苏；**cardiopulmonary r. (CPR),** the reestablishing of heart and lung action after cardiac arrest or apparent sudden death resulting from electric shock, drowning, respiratory arrest, and other causes. The two major components of CPR are rescue breathing and closed chest cardiac massage 心肺复苏术；**mouth-to-mouth r.,** a rescue breathing technique: with the victim supine, the rescuer places a hand under the nape of the victim's neck and a hand on the victim's forehead, also pressing the victim's nostrils closed; the rescuer takes a deep breath and exhales between the victim's lips. This is repeated quickly four times to inflate the victim's lungs before allowing the first exhalation 口对口复苏

re·sus·ci·ta·tor (re-sus'ĭ-ta″tər) an apparatus for initiating respiration in persons whose breathing has stopped 人工呼吸器

re·tain·er (re-ta'nər) an appliance or device that keeps a tooth or partial denture in proper position 固位体（牙）；保持器

re·tar·da·tion (re″tahr-da'shən) delay; hindrance; delayed development 阻滞，迟缓，延滞发育；**fetal growth r., intrauterine growth r. (IUGR),** birth weight below the tenth percentile for gestational age for infants born in a given population, defined as *symmetric* (both weight and length below normal) or *asymmetric* (weight below normal, length normal) 胎儿发育迟缓，宫内发育迟缓；**mental r.,** a mental disorder characterized by significantly subaverage general intellectual functioning associated with impairment in adaptive behavior and manifested in the developmental period; classified according to IQ as *mild* (50 to 70), *moderate* (35 to 50), *severe* (20 to 35), and *profound* (less than 20) 精神发育迟缓；**psychomotor r.,** generalized slowing of mental and physical activity 精神运动性抑制

retch·ing (rech'ing) strong involuntary effort to vomit 干呕

re·te (re'te) pl. *re'tia* [L.] a network or meshwork, especially of blood vessels 网，尤指血管网；**r. arterio'sum,** an anastomotic network of minute arteries, just before they become arterioles or capillaries 动脉网；**articular r.,** a network of anastomosing blood vessels in or around a joint 关节血管网；**r. mira'bile,** 1. a vascular network formed by division of an artery or vein into many smaller vessels that reunite into a single vessel 细脉网；2. arterial anastomosis of the brain occurring between the external and internal carotid arteries due to long-standing thrombosis of the latter 颅底微血管网，由于颈内动脉的长期血栓形成，在颈外动脉和颈内动脉之间发生的动脉吻合；**r. ova'rii,** a homologue of the rete testis, developed in the early female fetus but vestigial in the adult 卵巢网；**r. subpapilla're,** the network of arteries at the boundary between the papillary and reticular layers of the dermis 乳头下动脉网；**r. tes'tis,** a network formed in the mediastinum testis by the seminiferous tubules 睾丸网；**r. veno'sum,** an anastomotic network of small veins 静脉网

re·ten·tion (re-ten'shən) the process of holding back or keeping in position, as persistence in the body of material normally excreted or maintenance of a dental prosthesis in proper position in the mouth 潴留，停滞；保留，保持；固位

ret·e·plase (ret'ə-plās) a recombinant form of tissue plasminogen activator; used as a thrombolytic agent in the treatment of myocardial infarction 瑞替普酶，一种重组形式的组织纤溶酶原激活物，用作血栓溶解剂治疗心肌梗死

re·tic·u·la (rə-tik'u-lə) [L.] *reticulum* 的复数

re·tic·u·lar (rə-tik'u-lər) resembling a net 网状的

re·tic·u·lat·ed (rə-tik'u-lāt″əd) 同 reticular

re·tic·u·la·tion (rə-tik″u-la'shən) the formation or presence of a network 网状形成

re·tic·u·lin (rə-tik'u-lin) a scleroprotein from the connective fibers of reticular tissue 网硬蛋白

re·tic·u·lo·cyte (rə-tik'u-lo-sīt″) a young erythrocyte showing a basophilic reticulum under vital staining 网织红细胞

re·tic·u·lo·cy·to·pe·nia (rə-tik″u-lo-si″tope'ne-ə) deficiency of reticulocytes in the blood 网状细胞减少

re·tic·u·lo·cy·to·sis (rə-tik″u-lo-si-to'sis) an excess of reticulocytes in the peripheral blood 网状细胞增多

re·tic·u·lo·en·do·the·li·al (rə-tik″u-lo-en″dothe'le-əl) pertaining to the reticuloendothelium or to the reticuloendothelial system 网状内皮的

re·tic·u·lo·en·do·the·li·o·sis (rə-tik″u-loen″do-the-le-o'sis) hyperplasia of reticuloendothelial tissue 网状内皮组织增殖

re·tic·u·lo·en·do·the·li·um (rə-tik″u-loen″do-the'le-əm) the tissue of the reticuloendothelial system 网状内皮组织

re·tic·u·lo·his·tio·cyt·ic (rə-tik″u-lo-his″teo-sit'ik) pertaining to or of the nature of a reticulohistiocytoma 网状组织细胞的，参见 *granuloma* 下词条

re·tic·u·lo·his·tio·cy·to·ma (re-tik″u-lohis″te-o-si-to'mə) a granulomatous aggregation of lipid-laden histiocytes and multinucleated giant cells with pale eosinophilic cytoplasm having a ground glass appearance. It occurs in two forms, *reticulohistiocytic granuloma* and *multicentric reticulohistiocytosis* 网状组织细胞瘤

re·tic·u·lo·his·tio·cy·to·sis (rə-tik″u-lo-his″teo-si-to'sis) the formation of multiple reticulohistiocytomas 网状组织细胞增多症; **multicentric r.,** a systemic disease of polyarthritis of the hands and large joints with nodular reticulohistiocytomas in the skin, bone, and mucous and synovial membranes; it may progress to polyvisceral involvement and death 多中心网状组织细胞增多症

re·tic·u·lo·pe·nia (rə-tik″u-lo-pe'ne-ə) 同 reticulocytopenia

re·tic·u·lo·sis (rə-tik″u-lo'sis) an abnormal increase in cells derived from or related to the reticuloendothelial cells 网状细胞增多（症）; **histiocytic medullary r.,** hemophagocytic lymphohistiocytosis 组织细胞性髓性网状细胞增多; **malignant midline r., polymorphic r.,** a form of angiocentric immunoproliferative lesion involving midline structures of the nose and face 恶性中线网状细胞增多，多形性网状细胞增多

re·tic·u·lo·spi·nal (rə-tik″u-lo-spi'nəl) pertaining to a reticular formation and the spinal cord 网状脊髓（束）的

re·tic·u·lum (rə-tik'u-ləm) pl. *retic'ula* [L.] 1. a small network, especially a protoplasmic network in cells 网; 2. reticular tissue 网状组织; **endoplasmic r.,** an ultramicroscopic organelle of all eukaryotic cells, consisting of an interconnecting network of tubules, flat saccules, and vesicles, extending from the nuclear envelope to the cell surface. There are three compartments: *rough,* bearing ribosomes on the outer surface of its membrane and specialized for protein synthesis; *smooth,* which lacks ribosomes and is associated with many metabolic processes; and *transitional,* from which vesicles bud during the transport of proteins to the Golgi complex 内质网; **sarcoplasmic r.,** a form of agranular reticulum in the sarcoplasm of striated muscle, comprising a system of smooth-surfaced tubules surrounding each myofibril 肌浆网; **stellate r.,** the soft center part of the enamel organ of a developing tooth 星网状层，牙釉质器官柔软的中心部分

re·ti·form (re'tĭ-form) (ret'ĭ-form) plexiform 网状的

ret·i·na (ret'ĭ-nə) [L.] the innermost tunic of the eyeball, containing the neural elements for reception and transmission of visual stimuli 视网膜

ret·i·nac·u·lum (ret″ĭ-nak'u-ləm) pl. *retina'cula* [L.] a structure that retains an organ or tissue in place 支持带，系带; **extensor r. of hand,** the distal part of the antebrachial fascia, overlying the extensor tendons 手部伸肌支持带; **flexor r. of foot,** a strong band of fascia that extends from the medial malleolus down onto the calcaneus, holding in place the tendons of the posterior tibial and flexor muscles as they pass to the sole of the foot and protecting the posterior tibial vessels and tibial nerve 足部屈肌支持带; **flexor r. of hand,** a fibrous band forming the carpal canal through which pass the tendons of the flexor muscles of the hand and fingers 手部屈肌支持带; **inferior extensor r. of foot,** a Y-shaped band of fascia passing from the lateral side of the upper surface of the calcaneus across the foot to attach by one arm to the medial malleolus and by the other to the medial side of the plantar aponeurosis 足部伸肌下支持带; **inferior fibular r., inferior peroneal r.,** a fibrous band that arches over the tendons of the fibular muscles and holds them in position on the lateral side of the calcaneus 腓骨下支持带; **superior extensor r. of foot,** the thickened lower portion of the fascia on the front of the leg, attached to the tibia on one side and the fibula on the other, and holding in place the extensor tendons that pass beneath it 足部伸肌上支持带; **superior fibular r., superior peroneal r.,** a fibrous band that arches over the tendons of the fibular muscles and helps to hold them in place below and behind the lateral malleolus 腓骨上支持带

ret·i·nal (ret'ĭ-nəl) 1. pertaining to the retina 视网膜的; 2. the aldehyde of retinol, derived from absorbed dietary carotenoids or esters of retinol and having vitamin A activity. In the retina, retinal combines with opsins to form visual pigments. The two isomers 11-*cis* retinal and all-*trans* retinal are interconverted in the visual cycle 视黄醛

ret·i·ni·tis (ret″ĭ-ni'tis) inflammation of the retina 视网膜炎; **r. circina'ta, circinate r.,** circinate retinopathy 环状视网膜炎; **exudative r.,** 渗出性视网膜炎，参见 *retinopathy* 下词条; **r. pigmento'sa,** a group of diseases, often hereditary, marked by progressive loss of retinal response, retinal atrophy, attenuation of retinal vessels, clumping of pigment, and contraction of the visual field 色素性视网膜炎; **r. prolif'erans, proliferating r.,** a condition sometimes due to intraocular hemorrhage, with neovascularization and the formation of fibrous tissue extending into the vitreous from the retinal surface; retinal detachment may be a sequel 增生性视网膜炎; **suppurative r.,** that due to pyemic infection 化脓性视网膜炎

R

ret·i·no·blas·to·ma (ret″ĭ-no-blas-to′mə) a malignant congenital blastoma, hereditary or sporadic, composed of tumor cells arising from the retinoblasts 视网膜母细胞瘤；**endophytic r., r. endo′phytum,** a retinoblastoma that begins in the inner layers of the retina and spreads toward the center of the globe 内生型视网膜母细胞瘤；**exophytic r., r. exo′phytum,** a retinoblastoma that begins in the outer layers of the retina and spreads away from the center of the globe 外生型视网膜母细胞瘤

ret·i·no·cer·e·bral (ret″i-no-sə-re′brəl) (-ser′ə-brəl) affecting both the retina and cerebrum 视网膜脑的

ret·i·no·cho·roi·di·tis (ret″ĭ-no-kor-oi-di′tis) inflammation of the retina and choroid 视网膜脉络膜炎；**r. juxtapapilla′ris,** a small area of inflammation on the fundus near the papilla; seen in young healthy individuals 近视乳头性脉络膜视网膜炎

ret·i·no·ic ac·id (ret″ĭ-no′ik) an oxidized derivative of retinol, believed to be the form of vitamin A that plays a role in the development and growth of bone and in the maintenance of normal epithelial structures. In pharmacology, it often denotes the all-*trans* isomer (tretinoin); the 13-*cis* isomer is usually called *isotretinoin* 视黄酸，维甲酸，维生素 A 酸

ret·i·noid (ret′ĭ-noid) 1. resembling the retina 视网膜样的；2. retinal, retinol, or any structurally similar natural derivative or synthetic compound, with or without vitamin A activity 类维生素 A

ret·i·nol (ret′ĭ-nol) vitamin A$_1$; a 20-carbon primary alcohol in several isomers that is the form of vitamin A found in mammals and that 视黄醇，维生素 A$_1$

ret·i·no·ma·la·cia (ret″i-no-mə-la′shə) softening of the retina 视网膜软化

ret·i·no·pap·il·li·tis (ret″i-no-pap″ĭ-li′tis) inflammation of the retina and optic papilla 视网膜乳头炎

ret·i·nop·a·thy (ret″ĭ-nop′ə-the) any noninflammatory disease of the retina 视网膜病变；**circinate r.,** a condition in which a circle of white spots encloses the macula, leading to complete foveal blindness 环状视网膜病变；**diabetic r.,** retinopathy associated with diabetes mellitus, which may be of the nonproliferative type, progressively characterized by microaneurysms, intraretinal punctate hemorrhages, yellow, waxy exudates, cotton-wool patches, and macular edema, or of the proliferative type, characterized by neovascularization of the retina and optic disk, which may project into the vitreous, proliferation of fibrous tissue, vitreous hemorrhage, and retinal detachment 糖尿病视网膜病变；**exudative r.,** that marked by masses of white or yellowish exudate in the posterior part of

the fundus oculi, with deposit of cholesterin and blood debris from retinal hemorrhage, and leading to destruction of the macula and blindness 渗出性视网膜变；**hypertensive r.,** that associated with essential or malignant hypertension; changes may include irregular narrowing of the retinal arterioles, hemorrhages in the nerve fiber layers and the outer plexiform layer, exudates and cotton-wool patches, arteriosclerotic changes, and, in malignant hypertension, papilledema 高血压性视网膜病变；**r. of prematurity,** a bilateral retinopathy typically occurring in premature infants treated with high concentrations of oxygen, characterized by vascular dilatation, proliferation, tortuosity, edema, retinal detachment, and fibrous tissue behind the lens 早产儿视网膜病变；**proliferative r.,** retinopathy with neovascularization of the retina and optic disk, proliferation of fibrous tissue, vitreous hemorrhage, and later retinal detachment with blindness; seen in inflammatory conditions and diabetes mellitus 增生性视网膜病变；**renal r.,** a retinopathy associated with renal and hypertensive disorders and presenting the same symptoms as hypertensive retinopathy 肾性视网膜病变；**stellate r.,** a retinopathy not associated with hypertensive, renal, or arteriosclerotic disorders, but presenting the same symptoms as hypertensive retinopathy 星状视网膜病变

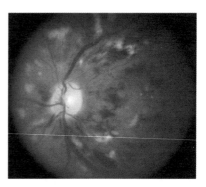

▲ 糖尿病患者的严重增生性视网膜病变，可见弥漫性视网膜出血和新生血管形成

ret·i·no·pexy (ret′ĭ-no-pek″se) restoring of the retina to its proper anatomic location 视网膜固定术；**pneumatic r.,** treatment of retinal detachment by injection of gas into the posterior vitreous cavity such that the gas bubble presses against the area of torn retina, forcing it back into place 充气性视网膜固定术

ret·i·nos·chi·sis (ret″i-nos′kĭ-sis) splitting of the

retina, occurring in the nerve fiber layer *(juvenile form)* or in the external plexiform layer *(adult form)* 视网膜裂

ret·i·no·scope (ret″ĭ-no-skōp″) an instrument for performing retinoscopy 检影镜，视网膜镜

ret·i·nos·co·py (ret″ĭ-nos′kə-pe) observation of the pupil under a beam of light projected into the eye, as a means of determining refractive errors 检影（法），视网膜镜检影法

ret·i·no·sis (ret″ĭ-no′sis) any degenerative, noninflammatory condition of the retina 视网膜变性

ret·i·no·top·ic (ret″ĭ-no-top′ik) relating to the organization of the visual pathways and visual area of the brain 视局部的

re·to·the·li·um (re″to-the′le-əm) reticuloendothelium 网状上皮组织

re·trac·tile (re-trak′təl) able to be drawn back 可收缩的，可退缩的

re·trac·tion (re-trak′shən) the act of drawing back, or condition of being drawn back 退缩，收缩；**clot r.,** the drawing away of a blood clot from the wall of a vessel, a stage of wound healing caused by contraction of platelets 血块收缩

re·trac·tor (re-trak′tər) 1. an instrument for holding open the lips of a wound 牵开器；2. a muscle that retracts 缩肌

re·triev·al (re-tre′vəl) in psychology, the process of obtaining memory information from wherever it has been stored（记忆内容的）随意再现

ret·ro·ac·tion (ret″ro-ak′shən) action in a reversed direction 反作用

ret·ro·bul·bar (ret″ro-bul′bər) 1. behind the medulla oblongata 延髓后的；2. behind the eyeball 眼球后的

ret·ro·cer·vi·cal (ret″ro-sur′vĭ-kəl) behind the cervix uteri 子宫颈后部的

ret·ro·ces·sion (ret″ro-sesh′ən) a going backward; backward displacement 后退，后移

ret·ro·coch·le·ar (ret″ro-kok′le-ər) 1. behind the cochlea 耳蜗后的；2. denoting the eighth cranial nerve and cerebellopontine angle as opposed to the cochlea 与耳蜗相对的第Ⅷ对脑神经和小脑脑桥角

ret·ro·col·lic (ret″ro-kol′ik) nuchal 颈的，颈后的

ret·ro·col·lis (ret″ro-kol′is) hyperextension of the neck and head associated with increased tonicity of the posterior cervical muscles in cervical dystonia 颈后倾

ret·ro·cur·sive (ret″ro-kur′siv) marked by stepping backward 退走的，退奔的

ret·ro·de·vi·a·tion (ret″ro-de″ve-a′shən) retrodisplacement; any displacement backwards, such as

retroversion or retroflexion 后偏

ret·ro·dis·place·ment (ret″ro-dis-plās′mənt) retrodeviation 后移位

ret·ro·flex·ion (ret″ro-flek′shən) the bending of an organ or part so that its top is thrust backward, particularly, the bending posteriorly of the body of the uterus toward the cervix 后屈（尤指子宫后屈）

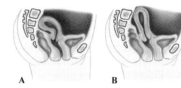

▲ 子宫的后屈（A）和后倾（B）

ret·ro·gas·se·ri·an (ret″ro-gə-sēr′e-ən) pertaining to the sensory (posterior) root of the trigeminal (gasserian) ganglion 半月神经节（三叉神经节）后根的

ret·ro·gnath·ism (ret″ro-nath′iz-əm) retrusion of the mandible 缩颌，颌退缩；**retrognath′ic** *adj.*

ret·ro·grade (ret′ro-grād) going backward; retracing a former course; catabolic 退行性的，逆行的；衰退的，退化的

ret·ro·gres·sion (ret″ro-gresh′ən) degeneration; deterioration; regression; return to an earlier, less complex condition 退化，变性；退行（指退行至发育早期不太复杂的状态）

ret·ro·lab·y·rin·thine (ret″ro-lab″ə-rin′thēn) posterior to the labyrinth 迷路后的

ret·ro·len·tal (ret″ro-len′təl) behind the lens of the eye 晶状体后的

ret·ro·mo·lar (ret″ro-mo′lər) behind a molar 磨牙后的

ret·ro·peri·to·ne·al (ret″ro-per″ĭ-to-ne′əl) posterior to the peritoneum 腹膜后的

ret·ro·peri·to·ne·um (ret″ro-per″ĭ-to-ne′əm) retroperitoneal space 腹膜后腔

ret·ro·peri·to·ni·tis (ret″ro-per″ĭ-to-ni′tis) inflammation of the retroperitoneal space 腹膜后间隙炎

ret·ro·pha·ryn·ge·al (ret″ro-fə-rin′je-əl) 1. pertaining to the posterior part of the pharynx 咽后部的；2. posterior to the pharynx 咽后的

ret·ro·phar·yn·gi·tis (ret″ro-far″in-ji′tis) inflammation of the posterior part of the pharynx 咽后炎

ret·ro·pla·sia (ret″ro-pla′zhə) retrograde metaplasia; degeneration of a tissue or cell into a more primitive type 退行性化生，指组织或细胞变性为更原始的类型

ret·ro·posed (ret′ro-pōzd″) displaced backward

后移的

ret·ro·po·si·tion (ret″ro-pə-zish′ən) retrodeviation 后移，后位

ret·ro·pu·bic (ret″ro-pu′bik) posterior to the pubic arch 耻骨后的

ret·ro·pul·sion (ret″ro-pul′shən) 1. a driving back, as of the fetal head in labor 推回，向后压（如分娩时的胎头）；2. tendency to walk backward, as in some cases of tabes dorsalis 后退倾向；3. an abnormal gait in which the body is bent backward 后退步态

ret·ro·sig·moid·al (ret″ro-sig-moi′dəl) posterior to the sigmoid sinus 乙状窦后的

ret·ro·spec·tive (ret″ro-spek′tiv) looking backward, or directed toward the past 回顾的，回想的，追溯的

ret·ro·uter·ine (ret″ro-u′tər-in) behind the uterus 子宫后的

ret·ro·ver·sion (ret″ro-vur′zhən) the tipping backward of an entire organ or part 后倾，整个或部分器官向后倾斜

ret·ro·ves·i·cal (ret″ro-ves′ĭ-kəl) posterior to the urinary bladder 膀胱后的

Ret·ro·vir·i·dae (ret″ro-vir′ĭ-de) the retroviruses, a large family of RNA viruses that carry reverse transcriptase. Genera that infect humans include *Deltaretrovirus* and *Lentivirus* 逆转录病毒科

ret·ro·vi·rus (ret″ro-vi″rəs) any virus of the family Retroviridae 逆转录病毒；**BLV-HTLV r's,** former name for the genus *Deltaretrovirus* BLV-HTLV 逆转录病毒

re·tru·sion (re-troo′zhən) the state of being located posterior to the normal position, such as the mandible or a tooth displaced in the line of occlusion 后移（如牙齿在咬合线后的位置不良）；下颌后移；**retru′sive** *adj.*

re·up·take (re-up′tāk) reabsorption of a previously secreted substance 重摄取

re·vas·cu·lar·iza·tion (re-vas″ku-lər-ĭ- za′shən) 1. the restoration of blood supply, as after a wound 血管重建，如创伤后血管重建；2. the restoration of an adequate blood supply to a part by means of a blood vessel graft, as in aortocoronary bypass 血管重建术，通过移植血管恢复对器官的充足血液供应的手术，如主动脉冠动脉旁路术

re·ver·ber·a·tion (re-vur″bə-ra′shən) duration of neuronal activity well beyond an initial stimulus due to transmission of impulses along branches of nerves arranged in a circle, permitting positive feedback 反射

re·verse tran·scrip·tase (re-vurs′tran-skrip′tās) an enzyme that catalyzes the template-directed, step-by-step addition of deoxyribonucleotides to the end

of a DNA or RNA primer or growing DNA chain, using a single-stranded RNA template; it occurs in retroviruses, and the DNA formed is an intermediate in the formation of progeny RNA 逆转录酶

re·ver·sion (re-vur′zhən) 1. 同 regression (1)；2. in genetics, the mutation of a mutant phenotype so that the original function is restored, as by mutation of the DNA back to the parental base sequence (reverse mutation) or by suppression 回复突变

RF rheumatoid factor 类风湿因子

RFA right frontoanterior (position of the fetus) 右额前位（胎位）

RFLP restriction fragment length polymorphism 限制性片断长度多态性

RFP right frontoposterior (position of the fetus) 右额后位（胎位）

RFT right frontotransverse (position of the fetus) 右额横位（胎位）

Rh rhodium 元素铑的符号

Rh$_{null}$ symbol for a rare blood type in which all Rh factors are lacking Rh 因子缺乏，无 Rh 因子血型，一种用于标记稀有血液类型的符号，血液中缺乏所有的 Rh 因子

Rhab·di·tis (rab-di′tis) a genus of minute nematodes found mostly in damp earth and as an accidental parasite in humans 小杆线虫属

rhab·doid (rab′doid) resembling a rod; rodshaped 杆状的

rhab·do·myo·blast (rab″do-mi′o-blast″) a pathologic racket-shaped or spindle-shaped myoblast occurring in rhabdomyosarcoma 成横纹肌细胞；**rhabdomyoblas′tic** *adj.*

rhab·do·myo·blas·to·ma (rab″do-mi″o-blasto′mə) 同 rhabdomyosarcoma

rhab·do·my·ol·y·sis (rab″do-mi-ol′ĭ-sis) disintegration of striated muscle fibers with excretion of myoglobin in the urine 横纹肌溶解

rhab·do·my·o·ma (rab″do-mi-o′mə) a benign tumor derived from striated muscle; the cardiac form is considered to be a hamartoma and is often associated with tuberous sclerosis 横纹肌瘤

rhab·do·myo·sar·co·ma (rab″do-mi″o-sahrko′mə) a highly malignant tumor of striated muscle derived from primitive mesenchymal cells 横纹肌肉瘤；**alveolar r.,** a type having dense proliferations of small round cells among fibrous septa that form alveoli, seen mainly in adolescents and young adults 腺泡状横纹肌肉瘤；**embryonal r.,** a type having alternating loosely cellular areas with myxoid stroma and densely cellular areas with spindle cells, seen mainly in infants and small children 胚胎性横纹肌肉瘤；**pleo-morphic r.**, a type having large cells with bizarre hyperchromatic nuclei, seen in the skeletal muscles, usually in the limbs of adults 多形性横纹肌肉瘤

rhab·do·sphinc·ter (rab″do-sfingk′tər) a sphincter consisting of striated muscle fibers 横纹肌纤维括约肌

Rhab·do·vi·ri·dae (rab″do-vir′ĭ-de) the rhabdoviruses, a family of RNA viruses that includes the genera *Lyssavirus* and *Vesiculovirus* 弹状病毒科

rhab·do·vi·rus (rab′do-vi″rəs) any virus of the family Rhabdoviridae 弹状病毒，棒状病毒

Rhad·in·o·vi·rus (rad′ĭ-no-vi″rus) a genus of viruses of the family Herpesviridae; it includes the species human herpesvirus 8 猴病毒属，参见 *herpesvirus* 下表

rhag·a·des (rag′ə-dēz) fissures, cracks, or fine linear scars in the skin, such as those around the mouth or in other regions where the skin moves frequently （皮肤）皲裂

Rham·nus (ram′nəs) [L.] a genus of trees and shrubs often having a cathartic bark and fruit. *R. purshia′na* D.C. is the source of cascara sagrada（植物学）鼠李属

rha·phe (ra′fe) 同 raphe

rheg·ma (reg′mə) a rupture, rent, or fracture 破裂，裂损

rheg·ma·tog·e·nous (reg″mə-toj′ə-nəs) arising from or caused by a rhegma or tear 裂孔源性的

rhe·ni·um (Re) (re′ne-əm) a heavy, silvery white, noble metallic element; at. no. 75, at. wt. 186.207 铼（化学元素）；**r. 186,** a radioisotope of rhenium having a half-life of 3.78 days and emitting beta particles (1.077, 0.933 MeV) and gamma rays (0.137, 0.632, 0.768 MeV); used in the palliative treatment of disseminated bone metastases and injected into joints for radiation synovectomy ^{186}Re；**r. 188,** a radioisotope of rhenium having a half-life of 16.9 hours and emitting beta particles (2.12, 1.96 MeV) and gamma rays (0.155 MeV); used in the palliative treatment of disseminated bone metastases, in liver cancer, and for inhibition of arterial restenosis following balloon angioplasty ^{188}Re

rhe·ol·o·gy (re-ol′ə-je) the science of the deformation and flow of matter, such as the flow of blood through the heart and blood vessels 流变学（如研究血液在心脏和血管的流动）

rhe·os·to·sis (re″os-to′sis) a condition of hyperostosis marked by the presence of streaks in the bones 条纹状骨肥厚，另参见 *melorheostosis*

rheo·tax·is (re″o-tak′sis) the orientation of an organism in a stream of liquid, with its long axis parallel with the direction of flow, designated *negative* (moving in the same direction) or *positive* (moving in the opposite direction) 向流性，生物体在流动中的液体中的方向，其长轴与液体的流动方向平行，分为负向流性（沿相同方向移动）或正向流性（沿相反方向移动）

rheum (room) a watery discharge 稀黏液

rheu·ma·tal·gia (roo″mə-tal′jə) chronic rheumatic pain 风湿痛

rheu·ma·tism (roo′mə-tiz-əm) any of a variety of disorders marked by inflammation, degeneration, or metabolic derangement of the connective tissue structures, especially the joints and related structures, and attended by pain, stiffness, or limitation of motion 风湿病；**rheumat′ic, rheumatis′mal** *adj.*；**muscular r.**, fibrositis 肌风湿病；**palindromic r.**, repeated attacks of arthritis and periarthritis without fever and without causing irreversible joint changes 复发性风湿病

rheu·ma·toid (roo′mə-toid) 1. resembling rheumatism 类风湿的；2. associated with rheumatoid arthritis 风湿性关节炎的

rheu·ma·tol·o·gist (roo″mə-tol′ə-jist) a specialist in rheumatology 风湿病学家

rheu·ma·tol·o·gy (roo″mə-tol′ə-je) the branch of medicine dealing with rheumatic disorders, their causes, pathology, diagnosis, treatment, etc. 风湿病学

rhex·is (rek′sis) the rupture of a blood vessel or of an organ（血管或器官的）破裂

rhi·go·sis (rĭ-go′sis) [Gr.] the ability to feel cold 寒觉

rhi·nal·gia (ri-nal′jə) rhinodynia; pain in the nose 鼻痛

rhin·en·ceph·a·lon (ri″nən-sef′ə-lon) 1. the part of the brain once thought to be concerned entirely with olfactory mechanisms, including olfactory nerves, bulbs, tracts, and subsequent connections (all olfactory in function) and the limbic system (not primarily olfactory in function); homologous with olfactory portions of the brain in certain other animals 嗅脑；2. formerly, the area of the brain comprising the anterior perforated substance, band of Broca, subcallosal area, and paraterminal gyrus 以前指大脑区域包括前穿质、Broca 区、胼胝体下区和终板旁回的脑部区域；3. one of the portions of the embryonic cerebrum 菱脑

rhin·i·on (rin′e-on) [Gr.] the lower end of the suture between the nasal bones 鼻尖点

rhi·ni·tis (ri-ni′tis) inflammation of the nasal mucous membrane 鼻炎；**allergic r.**, any allergic reaction of the nasal mucosa, occurring perennially *(nonseasonal allergic r.)* or seasonally *(hay fever)*

R

变应性鼻炎；**atrophic r.,** chronic rhinitis with wasting of the mucous membrane and glands 萎缩性鼻炎；**r. caseo′sa,** that with a caseous, gelatinous, and fetid discharge 干酪性鼻炎；**fibrinous r.,** membranous r. 纤维蛋白性鼻炎；**hypertrophic r.,** that with thickening and swelling of the mucous membrane 肥大性鼻炎；**membranous r.,** fibrinous r.; chronic rhinitis with the formation of a false membrane, as in nasal diphtheria 膜性鼻炎；**nonseasonal allergic r., perennial r.,** allergic rhinitis occurring continuously or intermittently all year round, due to exposure to a more or less ever-present allergen, marked by sudden attacks of sneezing, swelling of the nasal mucosa with profuse watery discharge, itching of the eyes, and lacrimation 非季节性变应性鼻炎，常年性鼻炎；**seasonal allergic r.,** hay fever 季节性变应性鼻炎；**vasomotor r.,** 1. nonallergic rhinitis in which symptoms like those of allergic rhinitis are brought on by such stimuli as chilling, fatigue, anger, or anxiety 血管运动性鼻炎；2. any condition of allergic or nonallergic rhinitis, as opposed to infectious rhinitis 与感染性鼻炎相对的过敏性或非过敏性鼻炎

rhi·no·an·tri·tis (ri″no-ən-tri′tis) inflammation of the nasal cavity and maxillary sinus 鼻上颌窦炎

rhi·no·cele (ri′no-sēl) 同 rhinocoele

rhi·no·ceph·a·ly (ri″no-sef′ə-le) a developmental anomaly characterized by the presence of a proboscis-like nose above eyes partially or completely fused into one 喙状鼻

rhi·no·chei·lo·plas·ty (ri″no-ki′lo-plas″te) plastic surgery of the lip and nose 鼻唇成形术

rhi·no·coele (ri′no-sēl) the ventricle of the olfactory lobe of the brain 嗅叶腔

rhi·no·dyn·ia (ri″no-din′e-ə) 同 rhinalgia

rhi·no·en·to·moph·tho·ro·my·co·sis (ri″noen″to-mof″thə-ro-mi-ko′sis) conidiobolomycosis 鼻藻菌病

rhi·nog·e·nous (ri-noj′ə-nəs) arising in the nose 鼻源的，鼻性的

rhi·no·ky·pho·sis (ri″no-ki-fo′sis) an abnormal hump on the ridge of the nose 鼻后凸

rhi·no·la·lia (ri″no-la′le-ə) rhinophonia; a nasal quality of the voice from some disease or defect of the nasal passages, such as undue patency *(r. aper′ta)* or undue closure *(r. clau′sa)* of the posterior nares 鼻音，来自某些疾病或鼻腔缺陷的声音，如后鼻孔的开放性鼻音（r.perta）和闭合性鼻音（r.clau′sa）

rhi·no·lar·yn·gi·tis (ri″no-lar″in-ji′tis) inflammation of the mucosa of the nose and larynx 鼻喉炎

rhi·no·lith (ri′no-lith) a nasal stone or concretion 鼻石

rhi·no·li·thi·a·sis (ri″no-lī-thi′ə-sis) a condition associated with formation of rhinoliths 鼻石病

rhi·nol·o·gist (ri-nol′ə-jist) a specialist in rhinology 鼻科专家，鼻科医生

rhi·nol·o·gy (ri-nol′ə-je) the medical specialty that deals with the nose and its diseases 鼻科学

rhi·no·ma·nom·e·try (ri″no-mə-nom′ə-tre) measurement of the airflow and pressure within the nose during respiration; nasal resistance or obstruction can be calculated from the figures obtained 鼻腔测压（法）

rhi·nom·mec·to·my (ri″no-mek′tə-me) excision of the inner canthus of the eye 内眦切除术

rhi·no·ne·cro·sis (ri″no-nə-kro′sis) necrosis of the nasal bones 鼻（骨）坏死

rhi·nop·a·thy (ri-nop′ə-the) any disease of the nose 鼻病

rhi·no·phar·yn·gi·tis (ri″no-far″in-ji′tis) nasopharyngitis 鼻咽炎

rhi·no·pho·nia (ri″no-fo′ne-ə) 同 rhinolalia

rhi·no·phy·ma (ri″no-fi′mə) a form of rosacea marked by redness, sebaceous hyperplasia, and nodular swelling and congestion of the skin of the nose 鼻赘，肥大性酒渣鼻

rhi·no·plas·ty (ri′no-plas″te) plastic surgery of the nose 鼻成形术

rhi·nor·rha·gia (ri″no-ra′jə) epistaxis 鼻出血，鼻衄

rhi·nor·rhea (ri″no-re′ə) the free discharge of a thin nasal mucus 鼻漏，鼻液溢；**cerebrospinal fluid r.,** discharge of cerebrospinal fluid through the nose 脑脊液鼻漏

rhi·no·sal·pin·gi·tis (ri″no-sal-pin-ji′tis) inflammation of the mucosa of the nose and eustachian tube 鼻咽鼓管炎

rhi·no·scle·ro·ma (ri″no-sklə-ro′mə) a granulomatous disease, ascribed to *Klebsiella rhinoscleromatis,* involving the nose and nasopharynx; the growth forms hard patches or nodules, which tend to enlarge and are painful to the touch 鼻硬结病

rhi·no·scope (ri′no-skōp) a speculum for use in nasal examination 鼻镜，鼻腔镜

rhi·nos·co·py (ri-nos′kə-pe) examination of the nose with a speculum, either through the anterior nares *(anterior r.)* or the nasopharynx *(posterior r.)* 鼻镜检查

rhi·no·si·nus·itis (ri″no-si″nəs-itis) inflammation of the paranasal sinuses 鼻窦炎

rhi·no·spo·rid·i·o·sis (ri″no-spor-id″e-o′sis) a fungal disease caused by *Rhinosporidium seeberi,* marked by large polyps on the mucosa of the nose, eyes, ears, and sometimes the penis and vagina 鼻孢

R

子菌病

rhi·not·o·my (ri-not′ə-me) incision into the nose 鼻切开术

Rhi·no·vi·rus (ri′no-vi″rəs) the rhinoviruses, a genus of the family Picornaviridae that infect the upper respiratory tract and cause the common cold. Over 100 antigenically distinct varieties infect humans 鼻病毒属

rhi·no·vi·rus (ri′no-vi″rəs) any virus belonging to the genus *Rhinovirus* 鼻病毒

Rhi·pi·ceph·a·lus (ri″pĭ-sef′ə-ləs) a genus of cattle ticks, many species of which transmit disease-producing organisms, such as *Babesia ovis*, *B. canis, Rickettsia rickettsii,* and *R. conorii* 扇头蜱属

Rhi·zo·bi·a·ceae (ri-zo″be-a′se-e) a phenotypically diverse family of bacteria of the order Rhizobiales 根瘤菌科

Rhi·zo·bi·a·les (ri-zo″be-a′lēz) a heterogeneous order of gram-negative bacteria of the class Alphaproteobacteria 根瘤菌目

Rhi·zo·bi·um (ri-zo′be-əm) a genus of gramnegative, aerobic, rod-shaped bacteria of the family Rhizobiaceae; organisms are symbionts that produce nodules on the roots of leguminous plants and fix free nitrogen. *R. radiobac′ter* is an occasional opportunistic human pathogen 根瘤菌属

rhi·zoid (ri′zoid) 1. resembling a root 根样的；2. a filamentous structure of fungi and some algae that extends into the substrate 假根

rhi·zol·y·sis (ri-zol′ə-sis) percutaneous radiofrequency rhizotomy; percutaneous rhizotomy performed using radio waves 射频神经切断术

rhi·zo·mel·ic (ri-zo-mel′ik) pertaining to or involving the proximal part of a limb 肢根的

Rhi·zop·o·da (ri-zop′ə-də) a superclass of protozoa of the subphylum Sarcodina, comprising the amebae 根足（虫）亚纲；肉足（虫）纲

Rhi·zo·pus (ri′zo-pəs) a genus of fungi (order Mucorales); some species, including *R. arrhi′zus* and *R. rhizopodofor′mis,* cause mucormycosis 根霉菌属

rhi·zot·o·my (ri-zot′ə-me) interruption of a cranial or spinal nerve root, such as by chemicals or radio waves 脊神经根切断术；**percutaneous r.,** that performed without brain surgery, such as by means of glycerol or radio waves 经皮神经根切断术

rho·da·mine (ro′də-mēn) any of a group of red fluorescent dyes used to label proteins in various immunofluorescence techniques 罗丹明，在各种免疫荧光技术中用于标记蛋白质的一种红色荧光

染料

rho·di·um (Rh) (ro′de-əm) a very rare, silvery white, hard, noble metallic element; at. no. 45, at. wt. 102.906 铑（化学元素）

Rhod·ni·us (rod′ne-əs) a genus of winged hemipterous insects of South America. *R. prolix′us* transmits *Trypanosoma cruzi,* the cause of Chagas disease 红猎蝽属

Rho·do·coc·cus (ro″do-kok′əs) a widespread genus of gram-positive, aerobic bacteria of the family Nocardiaceae; *R. e′qui* causes bronchopneumonia in foals and can infect immunocompromised humans 红球菌属

rho·do·gen·e·sis (ro″do-jen′ə-sis) regeneration of rhodopsin after its bleaching by light 视紫红质生成

rho·do·phy·lax·is (ro″do-fə-lak′sis) the ability of the retinal epithelium to regenerate rhodopsin 视紫红质保护性；**rhodophylac′tic** *adj.*

rho·dop·sin (ro-dop′sin) visual purple; a photosensitive purple-red chromoprotein in the retinal rods that is bleached to visual yellow (all*trans* retinal) by light, thereby stimulating retinal sensory endings 视紫红质

Rho·do·spi·ril·la·les (ro″do-spi″rĭ-la′lēz) a morphologically, metabolically, and ecologically diverse order of bacteria of the class Alphaproteobacteria 红螺菌目

rhomb·en·ceph·a·lon (rom″ben-sef′ə-lon) hindbrain. 1. the part of the brain developed from the posterior of the three primary brain vesicles of the embryonic neural tube; it comprises the cerebellum, pons, and medulla oblongata 后脑；2. the most caudal of the three primary brain vesicles in the embryo, later dividing into the pons, cerebellum, and medulla oblongata 菱脑

rhom·bo·coele (rom′bo-sēl) the terminal expansion of the canal of the spinal cord 脊髓终室

rhom·boid (rom′boid) having a shape similar to a rectangle that has been skewed to one side so that the angles are oblique 菱形的

rhon·chus (rong′kəs) pl. *rhon′chi* [L.] a continuous snorelike sound in the throat or bronchial tubes, due to a partial obstruction 鼾音，干啰音；**rhon′chal, rhon′chial** *adj.*

r-HuEPO epoetin (recombinant human erythropoietin)（重组人肾）红细胞生成素

Rhus (rus) a genus of trees and shrubs; contact with certain species produces a severe dermatitis in sensitive persons. The most important toxic species are: *R. diversilo′ba* and *R. toxicoden′dron,* or poison oak; *R. ra′dicans,* or poison ivy; and *R. ver′nix,* or poison sumac 漆树属

rhythm (rith′əm) a measured movement; the recurrence of an action or function at regular intervals 节奏；节律；**rhyth′mic, rhyth′mical** adj.; **alpha r.**, electroencephalographic waves having a uniform rhythm and average frequency of 10 per second, typical of a normal person awake in a quiet resting state α 节律，平均每秒 10 次的均匀脑电波节律，可见于处于安静状态下清醒的正常人；**atrial escape r.**, a cardiac dysrhythmia occurring when sustained suppression of sinus impulse formation causes other atrial foci to act as cardiac pacemakers 心房逸律；**atrioventricular (AV) junctional r.**, the heart rhythm that results when the atrioventricular junction acts as pacemaker 房室节律；**atrioventricular (AV) junctional escape r.**, a cardiac rhythm of four or more AV junctional escape beats at a rate below 60 beats per minute 房室交界区逸搏节律；**beta r.**, electroencephalographic waves having a frequency of 18 to 30 per second, typical during periods of intense activity of the nervous system β 节律，频率为每秒 18 至 30 次的脑电波节律，可见于神经系统剧烈活动期间；**circadian r.**, the regular recurrence in cycles of approximately 24 hours from one stated point to another, e.g., certain biologic activities that occur at that interval regardless of constant darkness or other conditions of illumination 昼夜节律；**coupled r.**, heartbeats occurring in pairs, the second beat usually being a ventricular premature beat; see also *bigeminal pulse* 二联律；**delta r.**, rhythm on the electroencephalogram consisting of delta waves δ 节律，由 δ 组成的脑电波节律；**ectopic r.**, a heart rhythm initiated by a focus outside the sinoatrial node 异位心律；**escape r.**, a heart rhythm initiated by lower centers when the sinoatrial node fails to initiate impulses, when its rhythmicity is depressed, or when its impulses are completely blocked 逸搏心律；**gallop r.**, an auscultatory finding of three *(triple r.)* or four *(quadruple r.)* heart sounds; the extra sounds occur in diastole and are related either to atrial contraction *(S$_4$ gallop)*, to early rapid filling of a ventricle *(S$_3$ gallop)*, or to concurrence of both events *(summation gallop)* （心脏）奔马律；**idioventricular r.**, a sustained series of impulses propagated by an independent pacemaker within the ventricles, with a rate of 20 to 50 beats per minute 心室自主心律；**infradian r.**, the regular recurrence in cycles of more than 24 hours, e.g., certain biologic activities that occur at such intervals, regardless of conditions of illumination 超昼夜节律；**nodal r.**, atrioventricular junctional r. （房室）结性心律；**pendulum r.**, alternation in the rhythm of the heart

sounds in which the diastolic and systolic sounds are nearly identical and the heartbeat resembles the tick of a watch 钟摆状节律；**quadruple r.**, the gallop rhythm cadence produced when all four heart sounds recur in successive cardiac cycles 四联律；**reciprocal r.**, a cardiac dysrhythmia established by a sustained reentrant mechanism in which impulses traveling back toward the atria also travel forward to reexcite the ventricles, so that each cycle contains a reciprocal beat, with two ventricular contractions 折反心律；**reciprocating r.**, a cardiac dysrhythmia in which an impulse initiated in the atrioventricular node travels toward both the atria and ventricles, followed by cycles of bidirectional propagation of the impulse alternately initiating from those impulses traveling up and those traveling down 交互节律；**reentrant r.**, an abnormal cardiac rhythm resulting from reentry 折返心律；**sinoatrial r., sinus r.**, the normal heart rhythm originating in the sinoatrial node 窦性心律；**supraventricular r.**, any cardiac rhythm originating above the ventricles 心室上节律；**theta r.**, rhythm on the electroencephalogram consisting of theta waves θ 节律，由 θ 波组成的脑电波节律；**triple r.**, the cadence produced when three heart sounds recur in successive cardiac cycles 三联律；另参见 *gallop r.*；**ultradian r.**, the regular recurrence in cycles of less than 24 hours, e.g., certain biologic activities that occur at such intervals, regardless of conditions of illumination 短昼夜律；**ventricular r.**, 1. 同 idioventricular r.；2. any cardiac rhythm controlled by a focus within the ventricles 室性节律

rhyth·mic·i·ty (rith-mis′ĭ-te) 1. the state of having rhythm 节律性；2. automaticity (2) 自律性

rhy·tid (ri′tid) pl. *rhy′tides*. A wrinkle in the skin 皱纹

rhyt·i·dec·to·my (rit″ĭ-dek′tə-me) excision of skin for elimination of wrinkles 除皱术

rhyt·i·do·plas·ty (rit″ĭ-do-plas″te) 同 rhytidectomy

rhyt·i·do·sis (rit″ĭ-do′sis) a wrinkling, as of the cornea 角膜皱缩

rib (rib) any one of the paired bones, 12 on either side, extending from the thoracic vertebrae toward the median line on the ventral aspect of the trunk, forming the major part of the thoracic skeleton. The upper seven are *true r′s;* the lower five are *false r′s,* with the lowest two of the latter also called *floating r′s* 肋（骨），见图1；**abdominal r′s, asternal r′s,** false r′s 腹皮肋，弓肋；**cervical r.**, a supernumerary rib arising from a cervical vertebra 颈肋；**false r′s**, the five lower ribs on either side, not attached directly to the sternum 假肋；**floating r′s**, the two lower false ribs on either side, usually without anterior attachment 浮肋; **slipping r.,** one whose attaching cartilage is repeatedly dislocated 肋骨滑脱; **true r's,** the seven upper ribs on either side, connected to the sternum by their costal cartilages 真肋

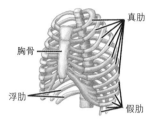

真肋

胸骨

浮肋

假肋

▲ 肋

ri·ba·vi·rin (ri″bə-vi′rin) a broad-spectrum antiviral used in the treatment of severe viral pneumonia caused by respiratory syncytial virus, particularly in high-risk infants; also used in conjunction with interferon alfa-2b in the treatment of chronic hepatitis C 利巴韦林，用于治疗由呼吸道合胞病毒引起的严重病毒性肺炎的广谱抗病毒药，尤其可用于高危婴儿，也可联合干扰素 α-2b 用于治疗慢性丙型肝炎

ri·bo·fla·vin (ri′bo-fla″vin) vitamin B₂; a heat-stable, water-soluble flavin of the vitamin B complex, found in milk, organ meats, eggs, leafy green vegetables, whole grains and enriched cereals and breads, and various algae; it is an essential nutrient for humans and is a component of two coenzymes, FAD and FMN, of flavoproteins, which function as electron carriers in oxidation-reduction reactions. Deficiency of the vitamin is known as ariboflavinosis 核黄素，维生素 B₂

ri·bo·nu·cle·ase (ri″bo-noo′kle-ās) an enzyme that catalyzes the depolymerization of ribonucleic acid 核糖核酸酶

ri·bo·nu·cle·ic ac·id (RNA) (ri″bo-noo-kle′ik) the nucleic acid in which the sugar is ribose, constituting the genetic material in the RNA viruses and playing a role in the flow of genetic information in all cells; it is a linear polymer which on hydrolysis yields adenine, guanine, cytosine, uracil, ribose, and phosphoric acid and which may contain an extensive secondary structure. For specific types of RNA, see under *RNA* 核糖核酸

ri·bo·nu·cleo·pro·tein (RNP) (ri″bo-noo″kleo-pro′tēn) a complex of protein and ribonucleic acid 核糖核蛋白; **small nuclear r. (snRNP),** any of a group of ribonucleoproteins, each composed of a small nuclear RNA (snRNA) associated with

approximately 10 to 20 polypeptides; involved in posttranscriptional RNA processing 核内小分子核糖核蛋白

ri·bo·nu·cleo·side (ri″bo-noo′kle-o-sīd) a nucleoside in which the purine or pyrimidine base is combined with ribose 核糖核苷

ri·bo·nu·cleo·tide (ri″bo-noo′kle-o-tīd) a nucleotide in which the purine or pyrimidine base is combined with ribose 核糖核苷酸

ri·bose (ri′bōs) an aldopentose present in ribonucleic acid (RNA) 核糖

ri·bo·some (ri′bo-sōm) any of the intracellular ribonucleoprotein particles concerned with protein synthesis; they consist of reversibly dissociable units and are found either bound to cell membranes or free in the cytoplasm. They may occur singly or occur in clusters (polyribosomes) 核糖体; **riboso′mal** *adj.*

ri·bo·syl (ri′bo-səl) a glycosyl radical formed from ribose 核糖基

ri·bo·zyme (ri′bo-zīm″) an RNA molecule with catalytic activity; the reactions catalyzed may be intramolecular, e.g., self-splicing, or intermolecular 核酶

ri·cin (ri′sin) a phytotoxin in the seeds of the castor oil plant *(Ricinus communis),* used in the synthesis of immunotoxins 蓖麻毒素

Ric·i·nus (ris′ĭ-nəs) a genus of plants, including *R. commu′nis,* or castor oil plant, whose seeds contain castor oil and ricin 蓖麻属

rick·ets (rik′əts) a condition due to vitamin D deficiency, especially in infancy and childhood, with disturbance of normal ossification, marked by bending and distortion of the bones, nodular enlargements on the ends and sides of the bones, delayed closure of the fontanelles, muscle pain, and sweating of the head 佝偻病; **adult r.,** osteomalacia 成年性佝偻病; **familial hypophosphatemic r.,** any of several inherited disorders of proximal renal tubule function causing phosphate loss, hypophosphatemia, and skeletal deformities, including rickets and osteomalacia 家族性低磷酸盐血症佝偻病; **fetal r.,** achondroplasia 胎性佝偻病; **hereditary hypophosphatemic r. with hypercalciuria,** a form of familial hypophosphatemic rickets; hypophosphatemia is accompanied by elevated serum 1,25-dihydroxyvitamin D, increased intestinal absorption of calcium and phosphate, and hypercalciuria 遗传性低血磷性佝偻病伴高钙尿症; **hypophosphatemic r.,** any of a group of disorders characterized by rickets associated with hypophosphatemia, resulting from dietary phosphorus deficiency or due to defects in renal tubular function; skeletal deformities are present, but hypocalcemia, myopathy, and tetany are absent and serum parathyroid hormone is normal 低血磷性佝偻病；**oncogenous r.,** oncogenous osteomalacia occurring in children 瘤原性佝偻病；**pseudovitamin D-deficiency r.,** vitamin D-dependent r., sometimes specifically the type Ⅰ form 假性维生素 D 缺乏性佝偻病；**refractory r.,** vitamin D-resistant r. 难治性佝偻病；**vitamin D-dependent r.,** either of two (types Ⅰ and Ⅱ) inherited disorders characterized by myopathy, hypocalcemia, moderate hypophosphatemia, secondary hyperparathyroidism, and subnormal serum concentrations of 1,25-dihydroxyvitamin D; type Ⅰ can be overcome by high doses of vitamin D, but type Ⅱ cannot 维生素 D 依赖性佝偻病；**vitamin D-resistant r.,** 1. X-linked hypophosphatemia 伴 X 遗传低磷酸血症；2. any of a group of disorders characterized by rickets but not responding to high doses of vitamin D; most are forms of familial hypophosphatemic rickets 抗维生素 D 佝偻病

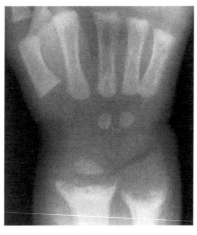

▲ 佝偻病。图示桡骨和尺骨的干骺端的特征性圆窝和磨损

Rick·ett·sia (rĭ-ket′se-ə) a genus of bacteria of the family Rickettsiaceae, transmitted by lice, fleas, ticks, and mites to humans and other animals, causing various diseases 立克次体属；*R. afri'cae,* a species occurring in southern Africa, spread by the ticks of the genus *Amblyomma;* it causes African tick-bite fever 非洲立克次体；*R. a'kari,* the etiologic agent of rickettsialpox, transmitted by the mite *Allodermanyssus sanguineus* from the reservoir of infection in house mice 小蛛立克次体；*R. austra'-lis,* the etiologic agent of Queensland tick typhus, transmitted by *Ixodes* ticks 澳大利亚立克次体；

R. cono'rii, the etiologic agent of boutonneuse fever and possibly other tickborne illnesses; transmitted by *Rhipicephalus* and *Haemaphysalis* ticks 康氏立克次体；*R. japo'nica,* the etiologic agent of Japanese spotted fever, transmitted by *Ixodes* ticks 日本立克次体；*R. prowaze'kii,* the etiologic agent of epidemic typhus and Brill-Zinsser disease, transmitted by *Pediculus humanus* 普氏立克次体；*R. rickett'sii,* the etiologic agent of Rocky Mountain spotted fever, transmitted by *Dermacentor, Rhipicephalus, Haemaphysalis, Amblyomma,* and *Ixodes* ticks 立氏立克次体

rick·ett·sia (rĭ-ket′se-ə) pl. *rickett'siae.* An individual organism of the Rickettsiaceae 立克次体；**rickett'sial** *adj.*

Rick·ett·si·a·ceae (rĭ-ket″se-a′se-e) a family of bacteria of the order Rickettsiales 立克次体科

rick·ett·si·al (rĭ-ket′se-əl) pertaining to or caused by rickettsiae 立克次体的

Rick·ett·si·a·les (rĭ-ket″se-a′lēz) an order of gram-negative bacteria of the class Alphaproteobacteria. Organisms are parasites of vertebrates and invertebrates and multiply only inside cells of the host; some are pathogenic 立克次体目

rick·ett·si·al·pox (rĭ-ket′se-əl-poks″) a febrile disease with a vesiculopapular eruption, resembling chickenpox clinically, caused by *Rickettsia akari* 立克次体痘

rick·ett·si·ci·dal (rĭ-ket″sĭ-si′dəl) lethal to rickettsiae 杀立克次体的

rick·ett·si·o·sis (rĭ-ket″se-o′sis) infection with rickettsiae 立克次体病

ridge (rij) a linear projection or projecting structure; a crest 隆起，嵴；**dental r.,** any linear elevation on the crown of a tooth 牙嵴；**dermal r's,** cristae cutis 皮嵴；**genital r., gonadal r.,** a bulge on the medial side of the embryonic mesonephros; the primordial germ cells become embedded in it, forming the primordium of the testis or ovary 生殖嵴；**healing r.,** an indurated ridge that normally forms deep to the skin along the length of a healing wound 愈合嵴；**interureteric r.,** a fold of mucous membrane extending across the bladder between the ureteric orifices 输尿管间嵴；**mammary r.,** a ridge of thickened epithelium from axilla to inguinal region on each side in the mammalian embryo, along which nipples and mammary glands develop, all but one pair usually disappearing in the human 乳嵴；**mesonephric r.,** the more lateral portion of the urogenital ridge, giving rise to the mesonephros 中肾嵴；**rete r's,** inward projections of the epidermis into the dermis, as seen histologically in vertical sections 网嵴；**synaptic r.,** a wedge-shaped projection of a cone pedicle or of a rod spherule, on either side of which lie the horizontal cells whose dendrites are inserted into the ridge 突触嵴; **urogenital r.,** a longitudinal ridge in the embryo, lateral to the mesentery, which later divides into the mesonephric and gonadal ridges 尿生殖嵴

rif·a·bu·tin (rif′ə-bu′tin) an antibacterial used for the prevention of disseminated *Mycobacterium avium* complex (MAC) disease in patients with advanced HIV infection 利福布汀，用于预防晚期 HIV 感染患者播散性鸟分枝杆菌复合体（MAC）疾病的抗菌药物

rif·am·pi·cin (rif′am-pī-sin) 同 rifampin

rif·am·pin (rif-am′pin) a semisynthetic derivative of rifamycin, with the antibacterial actions and uses of the rifamycin group 利福平，利福霉素的半合成衍生物，具有利福霉素类的抗菌作用和用途

rif·a·my·cin (rif″ə-mi′sin) any of a family of antibiotics biosynthesized by a strain of *Streptomyces mediterranei,* effective against a broad spectrum of bacteria, including gram-positive cocci, some gram-negative bacilli, and *Mycobacterium tuberculosis* and certain other mycobacteria; used for the treatment of tuberculosis and the prophylaxis of meningococcal infections 利福霉素，由地中海链霉菌（*Streptomyces mediterranei*）菌株生物合成的抗生素，对广谱细菌有效，包括革兰阳性球菌、部分革兰阴性杆菌、结核分枝杆菌和某些其他分枝杆菌；用于治疗结核病和预防脑膜炎球菌感染

rif·a·pen·tine (rif″ə-pen′tēn) a synthetic rifamycin antibiotic used in the treatment of pulmonary tuberculosis 利福喷丁，一种合成的利福霉素抗生素，用于治疗肺结核

rif·ax·i·min (rif-ak′sī-min) a semisynthetic derivative of rifamycin, used for the treatment of traveler's diarrhea caused by noninvasive strains of *Escherichia coli* 利福昔明，利福霉素的半合成衍生物，用于治疗由非侵入性大肠杆菌（*Escherichia coli*）菌株引起的旅行者腹泻

ri·gid·i·ty (rĭ-jid′ĭ-te) inflexibility or stiffness 僵硬；强直；**clasp-knife r.,** increased tension in the extensors of a joint when it is passively flexed, giving way suddenly on exertion of further pressure 折刀样强直；**cogwheel r.,** tension in a muscle that gives way in little jerks when the muscle is passively stretched 齿轮样强直；**decerebrate r.,** rigid extension of an animal's legs as a result of decerebration; occurring in humans as a result of lesions in the upper brainstem 去大脑强直

rig·or (rig′or) (ri′gor) [L.] chill; rigidity 寒战；强直；**r. mor′tis,** the stiffening of a dead body accompanying depletion of adenosine triphosphate in the muscle fibers 尸僵，死后强直，伴随着肌纤维中

三磷酸腺苷消耗而产生的尸体僵硬

ril·pi·vir·ine (ril′pi-vir″in) nonnucleoside reverse transcriptase inhibitor used as an antiretroviral agent in combination therapies to treat human immunodeficiency virus infection; administered orally in tablet formulation for treatment-naïve patients 一种非核苷酸逆转录酶抑制药，用于治疗人类免疫缺陷病毒感染的联合疗法中的抗逆转录病毒药物；口服给予片剂，可用于治疗首治患者

ril·u·zole (ril′u-zōl) a compound used to prolong survival time in the treatment of amyotrophic lateral sclerosis 一种用于延长肌萎缩侧索硬化症治疗存活时间的药物

rim (rim) a border or edge 边，缘；**bite r., occlusion r., record r.,** a border constructed on temporary or permanent denture bases in order to record the maxillomandibular relation and for positioning of the teeth 𬌗堤，𬌗缘，在临时或永久性义齿基托上构建的边界，以记录上颌下颌关系和牙齿定位

ri·ma (ri′mə) pl. *ri′mae* [L.] a cleft or crack 裂；**r. glot′tidis,** the elongated opening between the true vocal cords and between the arytenoid cartilages 声门裂；**r. o′ris,** the opening of the mouth 口裂；**r. palpebra′rum,** palpebral fissure 睑裂

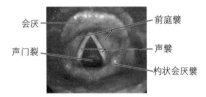

会厌　前庭襞
声门裂　声襞
杓状会厌襞

▲　声门裂的喉镜观

rima·bot·u·li·num·tox·in B (rim″ə-boch″uli′nəm-tok″sin) a preparation of botulinum toxin type B, used to treat cervical dystonia 肉毒杆菌素 B，B 型肉毒杆菌毒素的制剂，用于治疗颈肌张力障碍

ri·man·ta·dine (ri-man′tə-dēn) an antiviral agent used in the prophylaxis and treatment of influenza A 金刚乙胺，一种用于预防和治疗甲型流感的抗病毒药物

ri·mex·o·lone (rĭ-mek′sə-lōn″) a corticosteroid used as a topical antiinflammatory in the treatment of inflammation following eye surgery and of uveitis affecting the anterior structures of the eye 双甲丙酰龙，一种皮质类固醇，可用作局部抗炎药，用于治疗眼部手术后的炎症和影响眼前部结构的葡萄膜炎

rim·u·la (rim′u-lə) pl. *ri′mulae* [L.] a minute fissure, especially of the spinal cord or brain 小裂

ring (ring) 1. any annular or circular organ or area 环，环状物；2. in chemistry, a collection of atoms united in a continuous or closed chain（化学）环；**Albl r.**, a ring-shaped shadow in radiographs of the skull, caused by aneurysm of a cerebral artery Albl 环，脑动脉瘤在 X 线片上的环状阴影；**Bandl r.**, pathologic retraction r. Bandl 环，一种病理性收缩环，参见 *retraction r.*；**benzene r.**, the closed hexagon of carbon atoms in benzene, from which different benzene compounds are derived by replacement of hydrogen atoms 苯环；**Cannon r.**, a focal contraction seen radiographically at the mid-third of the transverse colon, marking an area of overlap between the superior and inferior nerve plexuses Cannon 环；**common tendinous r.**, the annular ligament of origin common to the recti muscles of the eye, attached to the edge of the optic canal and the inner part of the superior orbital fissure 总腱环；**conjunctival r.**, a ring at the junction of the conjunctiva and cornea 结膜环；**constriction r.**, a contracted area of the uterus, where the resistance of the uterine contents is slight, as over a depression in the contour of the fetus or below the presenting part 痉挛性狭窄环；**femoral r.**, the abdominal opening of the femoral canal, normally closed by the crural septum and peritoneum 股环；**fibrous r's, of heart**, 心脏纤维环，参见 *anulus fibrosus* (1)；**greater r. of iris**, the less coarsely striated outer concentric circle on the anterior surface of the iris 虹膜大环；**inguinal r., deep**, an aperture in the transverse fascia for the spermatic cord or the round ligament 腹股沟深环；**inguinal r., superficial**, an opening in the aponeurosis of the external abdominal oblique muscle for the spermatic cord or the round ligament 腹股沟浅环；**Kayser-Fleischer r.**, a gray-green to red-gold pigmented ring at the outer margin of the cornea, resulting from copper deposition in Wilson disease and other liver disorders 凯-弗环，角膜色素环；**Landolt r's**, broken rings used in testing visual acuity 蓝道环，用于测试视力的环；**lesser r. of iris**, the more coarsely striated inner concentric circle on the anterior surface of the iris 虹膜小环；**mitral r.**, 二尖瓣环，参见 *anulus fibrosus*；**retraction r.**, a ringlike thickening and indentation occurring in normal labor at the junction of the isthmus and corpus uteri, delineating the upper contracting portion and the lower dilating portion *(physiologic retraction r.)* or a persistent retraction ring in abnormal or prolonged labor that obstructs expulsion of the fetus *(pathologic retraction r.)* 子宫收缩环，在子宫峡部和子宫交界处的正常分娩中发生的环状增厚和压痕，描绘上部收缩部分和下部扩张部分（生理性收缩环）或者在异常和长时间分娩中阻止胎儿娩出的持续收缩环（病理性收缩环）；**Schwalbe r.**, a circular ridge composed of collagenous fibers surrounding the outer margin of the Descemet membrane Schwalbe 环，由围绕德塞梅膜外缘的胶原纤维组成的圆形脊；**scleral r.**, a white ring seen adjacent to the optic disk in ophthalmoscopy when the retinal pigment epithelium and choroid do not extend to the disk 巩膜环；**tracheal r's**, tracheal cartilages: the 16 to 20 incomplete rings which, held together and enclosed by a strong, elastic, fibrous membrane, constitute the wall of the trachea 气管环；**tricuspid r.**, 三尖瓣环，参见 *anulus fibrosus*；**tympanic r.**, the bony ring forming part of the temporal bone at birth and developing into the tympanic plate 鼓环；**umbilical r.**, the aperture in the fetal abdominal wall through which the umbilical cord communicates with the fetus 脐环；**vascular r.**, a developmental anomaly of the aortic arch wherein the trachea and esophagus are encircled by vascular structures, many variations being possible 血管环

ring·worm (ring′worm) popular name for dermatophyte infections 癣，参见 *tinea* 和 *onychomycosis*；**black dot r.**, tinea capitis with endothrix invasion of the hair shaft, usually caused by *Trichophyton tonsurans;* multiple areas of alopecia are studded with black dots representing infected hairs broken off at or below the scalp surface 黑（点）癣；**gray patch r.**, tinea capitis with ectothrix invasion of the hair shaft, caused by species of *Microsporum;* characterized by multiple gray scaly lesions and stubs of dry, lusterless, broken hairs 灰斑癣

ris·ed·ro·nate (ris-ed′rə-nāt″) an inhibitor of bone resorption used as the sodium salt in the treatment of osteitis deformans and for the prevention and treatment of osteoporosis 一种骨吸收抑制药，其钠盐用于治疗变形性骨炎以及预防和治疗骨质疏松症

ris·per·i·done (ris-per′ĭ-dōn) an antipsychotic agent, which may act by a combination of dopamine and serotonin antagonism 利培酮，一种抗精神病药，可以通过多巴胺和 5- 羟色胺拮抗作用起效

RIST radioimmunosorbent test 放射免疫吸附试验

ri·sus (ri′səs) [L.] laughter 笑，大笑；**r. sardo′nicus**, a grinning expression produced by spasm of facial muscles 苦笑面容

rit·o·drine (rit′o-drēn) a beta$_2$-adrenergic agonist used as the hydrochloride salt as a smooth muscle (uterine muscle) relaxant to delay uncomplicated premature labor 利托君，一种 β$_2$- 肾上腺素能药，其盐酸盐可作为平滑肌（子宫肌）松弛药，以延缓不复杂的早产

ri·to·na·vir (ri-to′nə-vir) an HIV protease inhibitor used in treatment of HIV infection and AIDS 利

托那韦，一种用于治疗艾滋病病毒感染和艾滋病的 HIV 蛋白酶抑制药

ri·tux·i·mab (rī-tuk′sĭ-mab) a monoclonal antibody that binds the antigen CD20; used as an antineoplastic in the treatment of CD20-positive, B-cell non-Hodgkin lymphoma 利妥昔单抗，一种结合抗原 CD20 的单克隆抗体；用作抗肿瘤药物治疗 CD20 阳性的 B 细胞非霍奇金淋巴瘤

ri·val·ry (ri′vəl-re) a state of competition or antagonism 竞争，敌对；抗拮；**sibling r.**, competition between siblings for the love, affection, and attention of one or both parents or for other recognition or gain 同胞竞争，兄弟姐妹之间为了争取双亲或双亲之一的抚爱、感情和注意，或为了得到其他承认或利益而进行的竞争

riv·a·rox·a·ban (riv″ə-rok′sə-bən) a selective inhibitor of coagulation factor Xa, used to prevent stroke and embolism in nonvalvular atrial fibrillation and deep venous thrombosis following knee or hip replacement surgery 一种凝血因子Ⅹa 的选择性抑制药，可用于预防膝关节或髋关节置换术后非瓣膜性心房颤动和深静脉血栓形成的中风和栓塞

riv·a·stig·mine (riv″ə-stig′mēn) a cholinesterase inhibitor used as the tartrate salt as an adjunct in the treatment of dementia of the Alzheimer type 利凡斯的明，一种胆碱酯酶抑制药，其酒石酸盐作为治疗阿尔茨海默型痴呆的辅助手段

ri·za·trip·tan (ri″zə-trip′tan) a selective serotonin receptor agonist used as the benzoate salt in the acute treatment of migraine 一种选择性 5- 羟色胺受体激动药，其苯甲酸盐可用于偏头痛的急性治疗

riz·i·form (riz′ĭ-form) resembling grains of rice 米粒形的

RLF retinopathy of prematurity (retrolental fibroplasia) 早产儿视网膜病变（晶体后纤维增生症）

RLL right lower lobe (of lungs) 右肺下叶

RMA right mentoanterior (position of the fetus) 颏右前（胎位）

RML right middle lobe (of lungs) 右肺中叶

RMP right mentoposterior (position of the fetus) 颏右后（胎位）

RMT right mentotransverse (position of the fetus) 颏右横（胎位）

RN registered nurse 注册护士

Rn radon. 氡

RNA ribonucleic acid 核糖核酸；**complementary RNA (cRNA)**, viral RNA that is transcribed from negative-sense RNA and serves as a template for protein synthesis 互补 RNA；**heterogeneous nuclear RNA (hnRNA)**, a diverse group of long primary transcripts formed in the eukaryotic nucleus, many of which will be processed to mRNA molecules by splicing 核内不均一 RNA，核内异质 RNA，不均一核 RNA；**messenger RNA (mRNA)**, RNA molecules, usually 400 to 10,000 bases long, that serve as templates for protein synthesis (translation) 信使 RNA；**negative-sense RNA**, viral RNA with a base sequence complementary to that of mRNA; during replication it serves as a template for the transcription of viral complementary RNA 反义 RNA；**positive-sense RNA**, viral RNA with the same base sequence as mRNA; during replication it functions as mRNA, serving as a template for protein synthesis 正义 RNA；**ribosomal RNA (rRNA)**, that which together with proteins forms the ribosomes, playing a structural role and also a role in ribosomal binding of mRNA and tRNAs 核糖体 RNA；**small nuclear RNA (snRNA)**, any of a class of small RNA molecules found in the nucleus, usually as small nuclear ribonucleoproteins (snRNP's) and involved in posttranscriptional RNA processing 核内小 RNA；**transfer RNA (tRNA)**, 20 or more varieties of small RNA molecules functioning in translation; each variety carries a specific amino acid to a site specified by an RNA codon, binding to amino acid, to ribosome, and to the codon via an anticodon region 转运 RNA

RNase ribonuclease 核糖核酸酶

RNP ribonucleoprotein 核糖核蛋白

RNT radionuclide therapy 放射性核素治疗

ROA right occipitoanterior (position of the fetus) 右枕前（胎位）

Ro·cha·li·maea (ro″kə-li-me′ə) a former genus of bacteria, now merged with *Bartonella* 罗克利马体属

ro·cu·ro·ni·um (ro″ku-ro′ne-əm) a nondepolarizing neuromuscular blocking agent, used as the bromide salt as an adjunct in general anesthesia to facilitate endotracheal intubation and as a skeletal muscle relaxant during surgery or mechanical ventilation 罗库溴铵，一种非去极化神经肌肉阻滞药，其溴盐作为全身麻醉中的辅助剂，以促进气管插管，在手术或机械通气期间作为骨骼肌松弛药

rod (rod) 1. a straight, slim mass of substance 杆，棒；2. 同 retinal r.；**Corti's r's**, pillar cells 柯蒂杆，柱细胞；**enamel r's**, the approximately parallel rods or prisms forming the enamel of the teeth 釉柱；**olfactory r.**, the slender apical portion of an olfactory bipolar neuron, a modified dendrite extending to the surface of the epithelium 嗅杆；**retinal r.**, a specialized cylindrical segment of the visual cells containing rhodopsin; the rods serve night vision and detection of motion, and together with the ret-

R

inal cones form the light-sensitive elements of the retina 视杆细胞

ro·dent (ro'dənt) 1. an order of mammals characterized by large chisel-shaped incisors, including the rats, mice, and squirrels, many of which are reservoirs for infectious diseases 啮齿动物; 2. gnawing; corroding 咬的，啮的；侵蚀性的

ro·den·ti·cide (ro-den'tĭ-sīd) 1. destructive to rodents 杀啮齿类的；2. an agent destructive to rodents 杀鼠剂

roent·gen (R) (rent'gən) the international unit of x-or γ-radiation; it is the quantity of x- or γ- radiation such that the associated corpuscular emission per 0.001293 g of dry air produces in air ions carrying 1 electrostatic unit of electrical charge of either sign 伦琴（X 线或 γ 辐射的国际单位）

roent·gen·og·ra·phy (rent″gən-og′rə-fe) radiography 放射摄影术；X 线检查；射线照相术；**roentgenograph′ic** adj.

roent·gen·ol·o·gist (rent″gən-ol′ə-jist) 同 radiologist

roent·gen·ol·o·gy (rent″gən-ol′ə-je) radiology 放射学

roent·gen·o·scope (rent-gen′o-skōp) fluoroscope X 线透视仪

roent·gen·os·co·py (rent″gən-os′kə-pe) fluoroscopy X 线透视检查

ro·fe·cox·ib (ro″fə-cok′sib) a nonsteroidal antiinflammatory drug used in the treatment of osteoarthritis, acute pain, and dysmenorrhea 一种非甾体类抗炎药，用于治疗骨关节炎、急性疼痛和痛经

ro·flu·mi·last (ro-floo″mĭ-last) a selective phosphodiesterase inhibitor used in the treatment of severe chronic obstructive pulmonary disease associated with chronic bronchitis 一种选择性磷酸二酯酶抑制药，用于治疗与慢性支气管炎相关的严重慢性阻塞性肺疾病

role (rōl) the behavior pattern that an individual presents to others 角色；**gender r.**, the public expression of gender; the image projected by a person that identifies their maleness or femaleness, which need not correspond to their gender identity 性别角色

Rol·fing (rawl′fing) service mark for a bodywork technique consisting of systematic manipulation of the connective tissue in order to improve posture and relieve chronic musculoskeletal pain and stress 罗尔芬，一家健身服务公司，其健身法包括通过对结缔组织系统操纵的手法，以改善姿势和缓解慢性肌肉骨骼疼痛和压力

rom·berg·ism (rom′bərg-iz-əm) Romberg sign 闭目难立征

ron·geur (raw-zhur′) [Fr.] a forceps-like instrument for cutting tough tissue, particularly bone 咬骨钳，修骨钳

room (room) a place in a building, enclosed and set apart for occupancy or for performance of certain procedures 房间，室；**operating r.**, one especially equipped for the performance of surgical operations 手术室；**recovery r.**, postanesthesia care unit 复苏室，麻醉后恢复室

room·ing-in (room′ing-in) the practice of keeping a newborn infant in a crib near the mother's bed instead of in a nursery during the hospital stay 母婴同室

root (root) that portion of an organ, such as a tooth, hair, or nail, that is buried in the tissues, or by which it arises from another structure 根；**anterior r. of spinal nerve**, the anterior, or motor, division of each spinal nerve, attached centrally to the spinal cord and joining peripherally with the posterior root to form the nerve before it emerges from the intervertebral foramen 脊神经前根；**motor r. of spinal nerve**, anterior r. of spinal nerve 脊神经运动根；**nerve r's**, the series of paired bundles of nerve fibers that emerge at each side of the spinal cord, termed posterior (or dorsal) or anterior (or ventral) according to their position. There are 31 pairs (8 cervical, 12 thoracic, 5 lumbar, 5 sacral, and 1 coccygeal), each corresponding posterior and anterior root joining to form a spinal nerve. Certain cranial nerves, e.g., the trigeminal, also have nerve roots 神经根；**posterior r. of spinal nerve**, the posterior, or sensory, division of each spinal nerve, attached centrally to the spinal cord and joining peripherally with the anterior root to form the nerve before it emerges from the intervertebral foramen 脊神经后根；**sensory r. of spinal nerve**, posterior r. of spinal nerve 脊神经感觉根；**r. of tongue**, the posterior part of the tongue, attached inferiorly to the hyoid bone 舌根

ROP right occipitoposterior (position of the fetus) 右枕后（胎位）

ro·pin·i·role (ro-pin′ĭ-rōl″) a dopamine agonist used as the hydrochloride salt as an antidyskinetic in the treatment of Parkinson disease 罗匹尼罗，一种多巴胺激动剂，其盐酸盐可作为抗运动障碍药物治疗帕金森病

ro·pi·va·caine (ro-piv′ə-kān) a local anesthetic of the amide type, used as the hydrochloride salt for percutaneous infiltration anesthesia, peripheral nerve block, and epidural block 罗哌卡因，一种酰胺类局部麻醉药，其盐酸盐用作经皮浸润麻醉、周围神经阻滞和硬膜外阻滞

ro·sa·cea (ro-za′she-ə) a chronic condition of the skin of the face, marked by flushing, followed by red coloration due to dilatation of the capillaries, often with papules and acnelike pustules. Lesions are caused by an abnormal peptide formed when there is an excess of cathelicidin and stratum corneum tryptic enzyme 酒渣鼻

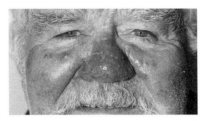

▲ 酒渣鼻

ro·san·i·line (ro-zan′ĭ-lin) a triphenylmethane derivative, the basis of various dyes and a component of basic fuchsin 玫瑰苯胺，一种三苯甲烷衍生物，是各种染料的基础和碱性品红的组成成分

ro·sa·ry (ro′zə-re) a structure resembling a string of beads 串珠样结构; **rachitic r.,** 串珠肋，参见 *bead* 下词条

ro·se·o·la (ro-ze′o-lə) (ro″ze-o′lə) [L.] 1. any rose-colored rash 玫瑰疹; 2. exanthema subitum 幼儿急疹; **r. infan′tum,** exanthema subitum 婴儿玫瑰疹幼儿急疹

Ro·se·o·lo·vi·rus (ro″ze-o′lo-vi″rəs) a genus of viruses of the family Herpesviridae, containing the species human herpesviruses 6 and 7. See table at *herpesvirus* 玫瑰疹病毒属

Ro·seo·mo·nas (ro″ze-o-mo′nəs) a genus of gram-negative, aerobic bacteria of the family Acetobacteraceae that produce a pale pink pigment; members of this genus are occasional pathogens, chiefly in immunocompromised or debilitated patients 玫瑰单胞菌

ro·sette (ro-zet′) [Fr.] any structure or formation resembling a rose, such as the clusters of polymorphonuclear leukocytes around a globule of lipid nuclear material, as observed in the test for disseminated lupus erythematosus 玫瑰花结，玫瑰花形（任何类似玫瑰花的结构或形成物，如播散性红斑狼疮试验时所见的溶化核质小球周围有多形核白细胞簇; **Flexner-Wintersteiner r.,** a spoke-and-wheel–shaped cell formation seen in retinoblastoma and certain other ophthalmic tumors 弗 - 温菊形环，一种可在视网膜母细胞瘤和某些其他眼科肿瘤中看到的轮辐和轮状细胞形成; **Homer Wright r.,** a circular or spherical grouping of dark tumor cells around a pale, eosinophilic, central area that contains neurofibrils but lacks a lumen; seen in some medulloblastomas, neuroblastomas, and retinoblastomas or other ophthalmic tumors 霍 - 赖玫瑰花结，在苍白的、嗜酸性的中心区域周围的黑色肿瘤细胞的圆形或球形组，包含神经纤维但缺乏管腔; 可见于一些髓母细胞瘤、神经母细胞瘤、视网膜母细胞瘤及其他眼科肿瘤

ro·sig·lit·a·zone (ro-sig-lit′ə-zōn) an antidiabetic agent that increases insulin sensitivity, used as the maleate salt in the treatment of type 2 diabetes mellitus 罗格列酮，一种增加胰岛素敏感性的抗糖尿病药，其马来酸盐用于治疗 2 型糖尿病

ro·sin (roz′in) a solid resin obtained from species of *Pinus*; it is used in preparation of ointments and plasters and in many products such as chewing gum, polishes, and varnishes, but is a common cause of contact allergy 松香

ros·tel·lum (ros-tel′əm) pl. *rostel′lae* [L.] a small protuberance of beak, especially the fleshy protuberance of the scolex of a tapeworm, which may or may not bear hooks 顶突

ros·trad (ros′trad) 1. toward a rostrum; nearer the rostrum in relation to a specific point of reference 向嘴侧; 2. cephalad 向头侧

ros·tral (ros′trəl) 1. pertaining to or resembling a rostrum; having a rostrum or beak 似喙的，有喙的; 2. in human anatomy, toward or nearer the oronasal region, which may mean superior (for areas of the spinal cord) or anterior or ventral (for brain areas)（解剖学）嘴侧的

ros·tra·lis (ros-tra′lis) [L.] 同 rostral (2)

ros·trate (ros′trāt) having a beaklike process 有嘴的，有喙的

ros·trum (ros′trəm) pl. *ros′tra, rostrums* [L.] a beak-shaped process 嘴，喙

rot (rot) decay 腐烂，腐败; **liver r.,** a disease of sheep, and sometimes of humans, due to *Fasciola hepatica* 肝双盘吸虫病，由肝片吸虫（*Fasciola hepatica*）引起，见于绵羊或人类

ro·tab·la·tion (ro″tab-la′shən) an atherectomy technique in which a rotating burr is inserted through a catheter into an artery; the burr rotates and debulks atherosclerotic plaque 旋转切除术，一种粥样斑块切除术，将旋转毛刺通过导管插入动脉，旋转毛刺以去除动脉粥样硬化斑块

ro·ta·tion (ro-ta′shən) the process of turning around an axis. In obstetrics, the turning of the fetal head (or presenting part) for proper orientation to the pelvic axis 旋转转动; **ro′tary, ro′tatory** *adj.*; **optical r.,** the quality of certain optically active substances whereby the plane of polarized light is changed, so that it is rotated in an arc the length of which is characteristic of the substance 旋光性旋光度; **van Ness r.,** fusion of the knee joint and rotation of the ankle to function as the knee; done to

R

correct a congenitally missing femur 凡·耐斯转动，融合膝关节并旋转脚踝以起到膝盖的功能，用于纠正先天性股骨缺失

ro·ta·tion·plas·ty (ro-ta'shən-plas″te) replacement of a knee joint using the ipsilateral distal segment of the leg and foot, rotating the lower portion 180 degrees and positioning the ankle at the level of the opposite knee 旋转成形术

Ro·ta·vi·rus (ro'tə-vi″rəs) rotaviruses; a genus of viruses of the family Reoviridae, having a wheel-like appearance, that cause acute infantile gastro-enteritis and cause diarrhea in young children and many animal species 轮状病毒属

ro·ta·vi·rus (ro'tə-vi″rəs) any member of the genus *Rotavirus* 轮状病毒；**ro'taviral** *adj.*

ro·te·none (ro'tə-nōn) a poisonous compound from derris root and other roots; used as an insecticide 鱼藤酮，一种来自鱼藤根和其他植物根的有毒化合物，可用作杀虫药

Roth·ia (roth'e-ə) a genus of aerobic, grampositive, non–spore-forming bacteria of the family Micrococcaceae. *R. dentocario'sa* and *R. mucilagino'sa* are inhabitants of the oral cavity and can cause infective endocarditis 罗思氏菌属

rough·age (ruf'əj) indigestible material such as fibers or cellulose in the diet 粗糙食物，饮食中难消化的食物，如纤维、纤维素等

rou·leau (roo-lo') pl. *rouleaux'* [Fr.] an abnormal group of red blood cells adhering together like a roll of coins 红细胞钱串

round·worm (round'wərm) any worm of the class Nematoda; a nematode 线虫（动物）

RPF renal plasma flow 肾血浆流量

rPFS radiographic progression-free survival 放射学无进展生存率

R Ph Registered Pharmacist 注册药师

rpm revolutions per minute 每分钟转数

RQ respiratory quotient 呼吸商

RRA Registered Record Administrator 注册病案管理员

RRB restricted repetitive behaviors, interests, and activities 受限制的重复行为、兴趣和活动

rRNA ribosomal RNA 核糖体 RNA

RSA right sacroanterior (position of the fetus) 右骶前位（胎位）

RScA right scapuloanterior (position of the fetus) 右肩前（胎位）

RScP right scapuloposterior (position of the fetus) 右肩后（胎位）

RSNA Radiological Society of North America 北美放射学会

RSP right sacroposterior (position of the fetus) 右骶后（胎位）

RST right sacrotransverse (position of the fetus) 右骶横（胎位）

RSV respiratory syncytial virus 呼吸道合胞病毒；Rous sarcoma virus 劳斯肉瘤病毒

RTF resistance transfer factor 耐药传递因子

Ru ruthenium 元素钌的符号

RU-486 mifepristone 米非司酮

rub (rub) 1. to move something over a surface with friction 摩擦；2. the action of such movement 摩擦；3. 同 friction r.；**friction r.**, an auscultatory sound caused by the rubbing together of two serous surfaces, as in pericardial rub 摩擦音；**pericardial r., pericardial friction r.**, a scraping or grating friction rub heard with the heartbeat, usually a to-and-fro sound, associated with pericarditis or other pathologic condition of the pericardium 心包摩擦音；**pleural r., pleuritic r.**, a friction rub caused by friction between the visceral and costal pleurae 胸膜摩擦音

ru·be·fa·cient (roo″bə-fa'shənt) 1. causing reddening of the skin by producing hyperemia 使皮肤发红的；2. an agent that so acts 发红药

ru·bel·la (roo-bel'ə) German measles: a mild viral infection marked by a pink macular rash, fever, and lymph node enlargement most often affecting children and nonimmune young adults; transplacental infection of the fetus in the first trimester may produce death of the conceptus or severe developmental anomalies 风疹，另参见 *syndrome* 下 *congenital rubella syndrome*

ru·be·o·la (roo-be'o-lə) (roo-be·o'lə) a synonym for measles in English and for German measles in French and Spanish 麻疹

ru·be·o·sis (roo″be-o'sis) redness 发红，红变；**r. i'ridis**, a condition characterized by a new formation of vessels and connective tissue on the surface of the iris, frequently seen in diabetics 虹膜发红

ru·ber (roo'bər) [L.] red 红色，红色的

ru·bes·cent (roo-bes'ənt) growing red; reddish 发红的，变红的

ru·bid·i·um (Rb) (roo-bid'e-əm) a rare, soft, silvery white, alkali metal element; at. no. 37, at. wt. 85.468 铷（化学元素）；**r. 82**, a radioactive isotope of rubidium having a half-life of 1.273 minutes and decaying by positron emission; used as a tracer in positron emission tomography ^{82}Rb

Ru·bi·vi·rus (roo″bĭ-vi″rəs) rubella virus; a genus of viruses of the family Togaviridae that contains the cause of rubella 风疹病毒；风疹病毒属

ru·bor (roo'bor) [L.] redness, one of the cardinal signs of inflammation 红，发红，炎症主要表现之一

ru·bra (roo'brə) [L.] 同 red

ru·bri·blast (roo′brĭ-blast) proerythroblast 原红细胞

ru·bric (roo′brik) red; specifically, pertaining to the red nucleus 红色的；红核的

ru·bri·cyte (roo′brĭ-sīt) polychromatophilic erythroblast 中幼红细胞

ru·bro·spi·nal (roo″bro-spi′nəl) pertaining to the red nucleus and the spinal cord 红核脊髓的

ru·bro·tha·lam·ic (roo″bro-thə-lam′ik) pertaining to the red nucleus and the thalamus 红核丘脑的

Ru·bu·la·vi·rus (roo′bu-lə-vi″rəs) a genus of viruses of the subfamily Paramyxovirinae (family Paramyxoviridae); it includes several human parainfluenza viruses and mumps virus 腮腺炎病毒属

ru·di·ment (roo′dĭ-mənt) 1. a structure that has remained undeveloped, or one with little or no function at present but which was functionally developed earlier 萌芽；雏形；2. primordium 原基

ru·di·men·ta·ry (roo″dĭ-men′tə-re) 1. imperfectly developed 未充分发展的，原始的；2. vestigial 残留的，退化的

ru·di·men·tum (roo″dĭ-men′təm) pl. rudimen′ta [L.] 同 rudiment

ru·fin·a·mide (roo-fin′ə-mīd) an anticonvulsant used as an adjunct in the treatment of seizures associated with Lennox-Gastaut syndrome 一种抗惊厥药，用作治疗与 Lennox-Gastaut 综合征有关的癫痫发作的辅助药物

ru·ga (roo′gə) pl. ru′gae [L.] a ridge or fold 皱襞；ru′gose adj.

ru·gos·i·ty (roo-gos′ĭ-te) 1. a condition of being rugose 皱褶状态；2. a fold, wrinkle, or ruga 皱褶

RUL right upper lobe (of lung) (肺的) 右上叶

rule (rool) a statement of conditions commonly observed in a given situation, or of a prescribed procedure, to obtain a given result 规定，规则，条例；Durham r., a definition of criminal responsibility from a federal appeals court case, *Durham vs. United States,* holding that "an accused is not criminally responsible if his unlawful act was the product of mental disease or mental defect." In 1972 the same court reversed itself and adopted the American Law Institute Formulation Durham 规律；M'Naghten r., a definition of criminal responsibility formulated in 1843 by English judges questioned by the House of Lords as a result of the acquittal of Daniel M'Naghten on grounds of insanity. It holds that "to establish a defense on the ground of insanity, it must be clearly proved that at the time of committing the act the party accused was laboring under such a defect of reason from disease of the mind as not to know the nature and quality of the act he was doing, or, if he did know it, that he did not know that what he was doing was wrong." M'Naghten 规则；Nägele r.,

(for predicting day of labor) subtract 3 months from the first day of the last menstruation and add 7 days Nägele 法则，用于预测分娩日期；r. of nines, a method of estimating the extent of body surface that has been burned in an adult, dividing the body into sections of 9% or multiples of 9% 九分法，一种烧伤面积和深度估计方法；van't Hoff r., the velocity of chemical reactions is increased twofold or more for each rise of 10℃ in temperature; generally true only when temperatures approximate those normal for the reaction 范托夫定律，即每升高10℃，化学反应的速度增加两倍或更多；通常仅当温度接近反应的正常温度时成立

ru·mi·nant (roo′mĭ-nənt) 1. chewing the cud 反刍的；2. one of the order of animals, including cattle, sheep, goats, deer, and antelopes, which have a stomach with four complete cavities (rumen, reticulum, omasum, abomasum) through which the food passes in digestion 反刍动物

ru·mi·na·tion (roo″mĭ-na′shən) 1. the casting up of the food to be chewed thoroughly a second time, as in cattle 反刍；2. in humans, the regurgitation of food after almost every meal, part of it being vomited and the rest swallowed: a condition sometimes seen in infants *(rumination disorder)* or in mentally retarded individuals 反刍症；3. repeated, excessive thinking about an event or situation 沉思，深思熟虑

rump (rump) the buttock or gluteal region 臀部，臀

ru·pia (roo′pe-ə) thick, dark, raised, lamellated, adherent crusts on the skin, somewhat resembling oyster shells, as in late recurrent secondary syphilis. 蛎壳疮；ru′pial adj.

rup·ture (rup′chər) 1. tearing or disruption of tissue 破裂；2. to forcibly disrupt tissue (使) 破裂，(使) 裂开；3. hernia 疝

rush (rush) peristaltic rush; a powerful wave of contractile activity that travels very long distances down the small intestine, caused by intense irritation or unusual distention 冲感

ru·the·ni·um (Ru) (roo-the′ne-əm) a rare, very hard, silvery white, noble metallic element; at. no. 44, at. wt. 101.07 钌 (化学元素)；r. 106, a radioisotope of ruthenium having a half-life of 373.59 days and emitting beta particles (3.54 MeV); used in brachytherapy of ocular tumors, particularly uveal melanomas [106]Ru

ruth·er·ford (ruth′ər-fərd) a unit of radioactive disintegration, representing one million disintegrations per second 卢 (瑟福) (放射性物质的蜕变单位，每秒蜕变一百万次)

rux·o·li·ti·nib (rux″o-li′tih-nib) selective

smallmolecule inhibitor of JAK1 and JAK2 that reduces interleukins and other inflammatory markers; used to treat polycythemia vera and multiple types of myelofibrosis 一 种 JAK1 和 JAK2 的选择性小分子抑制药，可减少白细胞介素和其他炎症标志物，可用于治疗真性红细胞增多症和多种类型的骨髓纤维化

RV residual volume 残气量；*Rotavirus* (or rotavirus) 轮状病毒属（或轮状病毒）；rotavirus vaccine 轮状病毒疫苗

RVAD right ventricular assist device 右心室辅助装置，参见 device 下 ventricular assist device

S

S [符号] heart sound (S_1 to S_4) 心音（S_1 至 S_4）；sacral vertebrae (S_1 to S_5) 骶椎（S_1 至 S_5）；serine 丝氨酸；siemens 西门子；spherical lens 球面镜片；substrate 酶作用物；sulfur 硫；Svedberg unit 斯维德伯格单位

S. [L.] sig′na (mark) 标记

S entropy 熵的符号

S- a stereodescriptor used to specify the absolute configuration of compounds having asymmetric carbon atoms; opposed to *R-* 左的

s second 秒的符号

s. [L.] se′mis (half) 半，一半；sinis′ter (left) 左的

s̄ [L.] si′ne (without) 无

SA sinoatrial 窦房的

sab·u·lous (sab′u-ləs) gritty or sandy 沙样的，有沙的

sa·bur·ra (sə-bur′ə) foulness of the mouth or stomach 口垢；**sabur′ral** *adj.*

sac (sak) a pouch or bag 囊；袋，**air s′s**, alveolar s′s 气囊；**allantoic s.**, the dilated portion of the allantois, becoming a part of the placenta in many mammals; it becomes the urachus in humans 尿囊；**alveolar s′s**, the spaces into which the alveolar ducts open distally, and with which the alveoli communicate 肺泡囊；**amniotic s.**, that formed by the amnion, containing the amniotic fluid 羊膜囊；**chorionic s.**, that formed by the vertebrate chorion, surrounding the embryo, amniotic cavity, and amniotic sac and contributing to the fetal part of the placenta 绒毛膜囊；**conjunctival s.**, the potential space, lined by conjunctiva, between the eyelids and eyeball 结膜囊；**dental s.**, the dense fibrous layer of mesenchyme surrounding the enamel organ and dental papilla 牙囊；**dural s.**, 1. the portion of the spinal dura mater extending caudally from the upper lumbar level to the attachment at the filum terminale externum; sometimes used more broadly for the entire length of the spinal dura mater from the foramen magnum to its caudal attachment 硬膜囊；2. more broadly, the entire length of the spinal dura mater from the foramen magnum to the attachment at the filum terminale externum; located in the vertebral canal and containing the spinal cord, spinal roots, and contents of the lumbar cistern 硬膜腔；**endolymphatic s.**, the blind, flattened cerebral end of the endolymphatic duct 内淋巴囊；**gestational s.**, that comprising the extraembryonic membranes that envelop the embryo or fetus; in humans, that formed by the fused amnion and chorion 妊娠囊；**heart s.**, pericardium 心包；**hernial s.**, the peritoneal pouch enclosing a hernia 疝囊；**Hilton s.**, laryngeal saccule 喉室；**lacrimal s.**, the dilated upper end of the nasolacrimal duct 泪囊；**yolk s.**, the extraembryonic membrane that connects with the midgut; formed during the development of higher vertebrates. In human embryos it contains no yolk and does not serve a primary nutritive function. It is the first hematopoietic organ of the embryo and produces a complete vitelline circulation, its endoderm is incorporated into the embryo as the primordial gut, and it is the site of origin of the primordial germ cells 卵黄囊

sac·cade (sə-kād′) [Fr.] the series of involuntary, abrupt, rapid, small movements or jerks of both eyes simultaneously in changing the point of fixation 眼球跳动，眼急动；**saccad′ic** *adj.*

sac·cate (sak′āt) 1. saccular 囊状的；2. contained in a sac 有囊的

sac·cha·ride (sak′ə-rīd) one of a series of carbohydrates, including the sugars 糖类

sac·cha·rin (sak′ə-rin) a white, crystalline compound several hundred times sweeter than sucrose; used as the base or the calcium or sodium salt as a flavor and nonnutritive sweetener 糖精

sac·cha·ro·lyt·ic (sak″ə-ro-lit′ik) capable of breaking the glycosidic bonds in saccharides 可分解糖的

sac·cha·ro·me·tab·o·lism (sak″ə-ro-mə-tab′oliz-əm) metabolism of sugar 糖代谢；**saccharometabol′ic** *adj.*

Sac·cha·ro·mo·no·spo·ra (sak″ə-ro-mon″ospor′ə) a genus of gram-positive, spore-forming actinomycetes of the family Pseudonocardiaceae; *S. vi′ridis* causes hypersensitivity pneumonitis 糖单孢菌属

Sac·cha·ro·my·ces (sak″ə-ro-mi′sēz) a genus of yeasts, including *S. cerevi′siae* (brewers' or bakers' yeast) 酵母属

sac·cha·ro·pine (sak′ə-ro-pēn″) an intermediate in the metabolism of lysine, accumulating abnormally in some disorders of lysine degradation 酵母氨酸

sac·cha·ro·pin·emia (sak″ə-ro-pī-ne′me-ə) an excess of saccharopine in the blood 酵母氨酸血症

sac·cha·ro·pin·uria (sak″ə-ro-pĭ-nu′re-ə) 1. excretion of saccharopine in the urine 酵母氨酸尿症; 2. a variant form of hyperlysinemia, clinically similar but having higher urinary saccharopine and lower lysine levels 赖氨酸血症的一个变种，临床上与赖氨酸血症类似，但尿中酵母氨酸水平更高，赖氨酸水平更低

Sac·cha·ro·poly·spo·ra (sak″ə-ro-pol″espor′ə) a genus of gram-positive, aerobic actinomycetes of the family Pseudonocardiaceae; *S. rectivir′gula* is the principal cause of farmer's lung 糖多孢菌属

sac·ci·form (sak′sī-form) 同 saccular

sac·cu·lar (sak′u-lər) pertaining to or resembling a sac 囊状的

sac·cu·lat·ed (sak′u-lāt″əd) containing saccules 囊状的，成囊的，有小囊的

sac·cu·la·tion (sak″u-la′shən) 1. a saccule or pouch 小囊，袋; 2. the quality of being sacculated 成囊

sac·cule (sak′ūl) 1. a little bag or sac 小囊，球囊; 2. 同 vestibular s.; **alveolar s's,** 肺泡囊，参见 sac 下词条; **laryngeal s.,** a diverticulum extending upward from the front of the laryngeal ventricle 喉囊; **vestibular s.,** the smaller of the two divisions of the membranous labyrinth of the ear 前庭球囊

sac·cu·lo·coch·le·ar (sak″u-lo-kok′le-ər) pertaining to the saccule and cochlea 球囊耳蜗的

sac·cu·lus (sak′u-ləs) pl. *sac′culi* [L.] 同 saccule

sac·cus (sak′əs) pl. *sac′ci* [L.] 同 sac

sa·crad (sa′krad) toward the sacrum 向骶骨，向骶侧

sa·cral (sa′krəl) pertaining to the sacrum 骶骨的

sacral anterior root stimulation stimulation applied via an externally controlled implanted device, used to assist with defecation and urination 骶前根刺激

sa·cral·gia (sa-kral′jə) pain in the sacrum 骶骨痛

sa·cral·iza·tion (sa″krəl-ĭ-za′shən) anomalous fusion of the fifth lumbar vertebra with the first segment of the sacrum 骶骨化，第五腰椎与骶骨第一节的异常融合

sa·crec·to·my (sa-krek′tə-me) excision or resection of the sacrum 骶骨切除术

sa·cro·coc·cy·ge·al (sa″kro-kok-sij′e-əl) pertaining to the sacrum and coccyx 骶尾的

sa·cro·col·po·pexy (sa″kro-kol′po-pek″se) correction of prolapse of the vaginal fornix by securing the fornix to the anterior surface of the sacrum 阴道-骶骨固定术

sa·cro·dyn·ia (sa″kro-din′e-ə) 同 sacralgia

sa·cro·il·i·ac (sa″kro-il′e-ak) pertaining to the sacrum and ilium, or to their articulation 骶髂的

sa·cro·lum·bar (sa″kro-lum′bər) (-bahr) pertaining to the sacrum and loins 骶腰的

sa·cro·sci·at·ic (sa″kro-si-at′ik) pertaining to the sacrum and ischium 骶骨坐骨的

sac·ro·sid·ase (sak-ro′sĭ-dās) an enzyme used as a substitute to replace the sucrase activity lacking in sucrase-isomaltase deficiency 蔗糖酶的替代品用于蔗糖酶-异麦芽糖酶缺乏症

sa·cro·spi·nal (sa″kro-spi′nəl) pertaining to the sacrum and the vertebral column 骶棘的；骶脊的

sa·cro·ver·te·bral (sa″kro-vur′tə-brəl) pertaining to the sacrum and vertebrae 骶骨椎骨的

sa·crum (sa′krəm) [L.] the wedge-shaped bone just below the lumbar vertebrae, formed usually by five fused vertebrae that are lodged dorsally between the two coxal bones 骶骨，参见 图 1; **scimitar s.,** a congenitally deformed sacrum resembling a scimitar, usually accompanied by other defects such as anorectal or neural anomalies 先天骶骨变形，一种先天性变形的骶骨，形似弯刀，通常伴有其他缺陷，如肛门直肠畸形或神经异常

SAD seasonal affective disorder 季节性情感障碍

sa·dism (sa′diz-əm) (sad′iz-əm) the act or instance of gaining pleasure from inflicting physical or psychological pain on another; the term is usually used to denote *sexual s.* 施虐癖，施虐待症; **sa·dis′tic** *adj.* ; **sexual s.,** a paraphilia in which sexual gratification is derived from inflicting physical or psychological pain on another 性虐待

sa·do·ma·so·chism (sa″do-mas′ə-kiz-əm) a state characterized by both sadistic and masochistic tendencies 施虐受虐症; **sadomasochis′tic** *adj.*

sage (sāj) *Salvia officinalis,* an herb whose leaves contain a volatile oil and are sudorific, carminative, and astringent; they are used as an antisecretory agent in hyperhidrosis, sialorrhea, pharyngitis, and bronchitis 洋苏草

sag·it·tal (saj′ĭ-təl) 1. shaped like an arrow 矢状的; 2. of, relating to, or situated in the plane of the sagittal suture or parallel to it 矢状位的

sag·it·ta·lis (saj″ĭ-ta′lis) [L.] 同 sagittal

St. John's wort (sānt jonz wort) any of various species of the genus *Hypericum; H. perforatum* is used as a mild antidepressant, sedative, and anxiolytic and is also used topically for inflammation of the skin, contusions, myalgia, and first-degree burns 金丝桃属

Sak·se·naea (sak″sə-ne′ə) a genus of fungi of the order Mucorales, characterized by flaskshaped sporangia; *S. vasifor'mis* can cause severe opportunistic mucormycosis in debilitated or immunocompromised patients 毛霉属

sal·a·bra·sion (săl″uh-bray″zhen) use of salt or a salt solution to abrade the skin; used in tattoo and permanent makeup removal 盐摩擦术，使用盐或盐溶液来磨损皮肤；用于文身和永久卸妆

sal·bu·ta·mol (sal-bu′tə-mol) albuterol 沙丁胺醇

sal·i·cin (sal′ĭ-sin) a precursor of salicylic acid, contained in the bark of the willow and poplar, that is responsible for the antiinflammatory and antipyretic effects of willow bark 水杨甙，水杨醇葡萄糖甙

sal·i·cyl·am·ide (sal″ĭ-səl-am′ĭd) an amide of salicylic acid used as an analgesic and antipyretic 水杨酰胺

sal·i·cyl·ate (sal″ĭ-sil′āt) (sə-lis′ə-lāt) 1. asalt, anion, or ester of salicylic acid 水杨酸盐，水杨酸阴离子，水杨酸酯；2. any of a group of related compounds derived from salicylic acid, which inhibit prostaglandin synthesis and have analgesic, antipyretic, and antiinflammatory activity; included are *acetylsalicylic acid, choline s., magnesium s.,* and *sodium s.* 水杨酸衍生物；**methyl** s.，水杨酸甲酯，参见 *methyl* 下词条

sal·i·cyl·ic ac·id (sal′ĭ-sil′ĭk) a topical keratolytic and caustic 水杨酸，另参见 *salicylate*

sal·i·cyl·ism (sal′ĭ-sil′iz-əm) toxic effects of overdosage with salicylic acid or its salts, usually marked by tinnitus, nausea, and vomiting 水扬酸中毒

sal·i·cyl·ur·ic ac·id (sal′ĭ-səl-ūr′ĭk) the glycine conjugate of salicylic acid, a form in which salicylates are excreted in the urine 水杨尿酸，水杨酸甘氨酸

sal·i·fi·a·ble (sal′ĭ-fi″ə-bəl) capable of combining with an acid to form a salt（能变）成盐的

sa·line (sa′lēn) (sa′līn) salty; of the nature of a salt; containing a salt or salts 咸的，盐的，含盐的
normal s., physiologic s., physiologic saline soliution 生理盐水

sa·li·va (sə-li′və) the enzyme-containing secretion of the salivary glands 唾液；**sal′ivary** *adj.*

sal·i·va·tion (sal″ĭ-va′shən) 1. the secretion of saliva 流涎；2. ptyalism. 多涎

sal·met·er·ol (sal-met′er-ol) a β₂-adrenergic receptor agonist, used as *s. xinafoate* as a bronchodilator 沙美特罗

Sal·mo·nel·la (sal″mo-nel′ə) a genus of gramnegative, facultatively anaerobic, non–sporeforming, usually motile bacteria of the family Enterobacteriaceae. This genus is very complex; it comprises two species, *S. bon'gori* and *S. ente'rica,* the latter containing six subspecies, and is separable into over 2400 serovars. Pathogenic members are widely distributed in the animal kingdom and cause enteric fevers (typhoid and paratyphoid), septicemia, and gastroenteritis. In reporting *Salmonella* infections, the full taxonomic designation may be abbreviated, so that *S. enterica* subsp. *enterica* serovar Typhi can become *Salmonella* serovar Typhi or *Salmonella* Typhi 沙门菌属；*S. bon'gori,* a species isolated mainly from cold-blooded animals and the environment 邦戈沙门菌；*S. ente'rica,* a species containing most of the serovars of *Salmonella,* divided into six subspecies; most infections of warm-blooded animals are caused by the subspecies *S. enterica* subsp. *enterica.* Pathogenic serovars of this subspecies include *S.* Choleraesuis (paratyphoid fever, gastroenteritis, and septicemia), *S.* Enteritidis (enteritis), *S.* Paratyphi (paratyphoid fever), *S.* Sendai (septicemia and typhoid fever), *S.* Typhi (typhoid fever), and *S.* Typhimurium (food poisoning and paratyphoid fever) 肠道沙门菌

sal·mo·nel·la (sal″mo-nel′ə) pl. *salmonel'lae.* Any organism of the genus *Salmonella* 沙门菌；**salmonel′lal** *adj.*

sal·mo·nel·lo·sis (sal″mo-nəl-o′sis) infection with *Salmonella* 沙门菌病

sal·pin·gec·to·my (sal″pin-jek′tə-me) tubectomy; excision of a uterine tube 输卵管切除术

sal·pin·gem·phrax·is (sal″pin-jəm-frak′sis) obstruction of an auditory tube 咽鼓管阻塞

sal·pin·gi·an (sal-pin′je-ən) tubal 输卵管的；咽鼓管的

sal·pin·gi·tis (sal″pin-ji′tis) inflammation of an auditory or a uterine tube 咽鼓管炎；输卵管炎；**salpingit′ic** *adj.*

sal·pin·go·cele (sal-ping′go-sēl) hernial protrusion of a uterine tube 输卵管疝

sal·pin·gog·ra·phy (sal″ping-gog′rə-fe) radiography of the uterine tubes after injection of a radiopaque medium 输卵管造影术

sal·pin·gol·y·sis (sal″ping-gol′ĭ-sis) surgical separation of adhesions involving the uterine tubes 输卵管粘连分离术

sal·pin·go-ooph·o·rec·to·my (sal-ping″goo-of″ə-rek′tə-me) excision of a uterine tube and ovary 输卵管卵巢切除术

sal·pin·go-ooph·o·ri·tis (sal-ping″go-o-of″ə-ri′tis) inflammation of a uterine tube and ovary 输卵管卵巢炎

sal·pin·go-ooph·oro·cele (sal-ping″go-oof′ə-ro-sēl) hernia of a uterine tube and ovary 输卵管卵巢疝

sal·pin·go·pexy (sal-ping′go-pek″se) fixation of a uterine tube 输卵管固定术

sal·pin·go·pha·ryn·ge·al (sal-ping″go-fə- rin′-je-əl) pertaining to the auditory tube and the pharynx 咽鼓管咽的

sal·pin·go·plas·ty (sal-ping′go-plas″te) plastic repair of a uterine tube 输卵管成形术

sal·pin·gos·co·py (sal″ping-gos′kə-pe) endoscopic visualization of the uterine tubes via the fimbrial ends of the tubes 输卵管镜检查

sal·pin·gos·to·my (sal″ping-gos′tə-me) 1. formation of an opening or fistula into a uterine tube 输卵管造口术；2. surgical restoration of the patency of a uterine tube 输卵管复通术

sal·pin·got·o·my (sal″ping-got′ə-me) surgical incision of a uterine tube 输卵管切开术

sal·pinx (sal′pinks) [Gr.] a tube, particularly an auditory tube or a uterine tube 管，尤指咽鼓管或输卵管

sal·sa·late (sal′sə-lāt) a salicylate with analgesic, antipyretic, and antiinflammatory actions; used in the treatment of osteoarthritis and rheumatoid arthritis 双水杨酯，水杨酰水杨酸，双水杨酸，水杨酸水杨酸酯（用于治疗骨关节炎和类风湿关节炎）

salt (sawlt) 1. sodium chloride, or common salt 氯化钠，食盐；2. any compound of a base and an acid; any compound of an acid some of whose replaceable atoms have been substituted 盐；3. (in the pl.) a saline cathartic（用于复数）泻盐，bile s's, conjugates of glycine or taurine with bile acids, formed in the liver and secreted in the bile. They are powerful detergents that break down fat globules, making them to be digested 胆盐；Epsom s., magnesium sulfate 硫酸镁；Glauber s., sodium sulfate 硫酸钠；oral rehydration s's (ORS), a dry mixture of sodium chloride, potassium chloride, dextrose, and either sodium citrate or sodium bicarbonate; dissolved in water for use in treatment of dehydration 口服补液盐；smelling s's, aromatized ammonium carbonate; stimulant and restorative 嗅盐

sal·ta·tion (sal-ta′shən) 1. the action of leaping 跳跃；2. the jerky dancing or leaping that sometimes occurs in chorea 出现于舞蹈症的跳动；3. saltatory conduction 跳跃式传导；4. in genetics, a dramatic and abrupt inherited change in the phenotype of an organism due to a mutation（遗传学）由于突变导致的生物表型的显著和突然的遗传变化；5. sudden increases or changes in the course of an illness 病情的突然进展或变化；**sal′tatory** adj.

salt·ing out (sawl′ting out) the precipitation of proteins by raising the salt concentration 盐析

sa·lu·bri·ous (sə-loo′bre-əs) conducive to health; wholesome 有益健康的，适于卫生的

sal·ure·sis (sal″u-re′sis) urinary excretion of sodi-um and chloride ions 尿氯盐排泄（尿中钠和氯根离子的排泄）

sal·uret·ic (sal″u-ret′ik) 1. pertaining to, characterized by, or promoting saluresis（促）尿氯盐排泄的；2. an agent that so acts 促尿氯盐排泄药

salve (sav) ointment 药膏，软膏，油膏

sa·mar·i·um (Sm) (sə-mar′e-əm) a heavy, lustrous, silvery, rare earth element; at. no. 62, at. wt. 150.36 钐（化学元素）；s. 153, a radioisotope of samarium having a half-life of 46.70 hours and emitting beta particles (0.81, 0.71, 0.64 MeV) and gamma rays (0.103, 0.070 MeV); used in radiation synovectomy. As the complex s. Sm 153 lexidronam, it is used in the palliative treatment of bone pain associated with osteoblastic metastatic bone lesions [153]S

SAMHSA Substance Abuse and Mental Health Services Administration 药物滥用和心理健康服务管理局

sam·pling (sam′pling) the selection or making of a sample 采样，取样；chorionic villus s. (CVS), any of several procedures for obtaining fetal tissue to use in prenatal diagnosis, performed at 9 to 12 weeks' gestation, usually by means of a catheter passed through the cervix or by a needle inserted through the abdominal and uterine walls 绒毛活检术；percutaneous umbilical blood s. (PUBS), cordocentesis 经皮脐血管穿刺

san·a·tive (san′ə-tiv) curative; healing 治愈的

san·a·to·ry (san′ə-tor″e) 同 salubrious

sanc·tu·ary (sangk′choo-ar″e) an area in the body where a drug tends to collect and to escape metabolic breakdown 庇护区，体内药物倾向于聚集并避免被代谢分解的区域

sand (sand) material occurring in small, gritty particles 砂，细小的颗粒；brain s., corpora arenacea 脑砂

sand·fly (sand′fli) any of various two-winged flies, especially of the genus *Phlebotomus* 白蛉

sane (sān) sound in mind 神志正常的，精神健全的

san·guin·e·ous (sang-gwin′e-əs) pertaining to or containing blood; bloody 含血的，血的

san·guin·o·lent (sang-gwin′ə-lənt) of a bloody tinge 含血的，血色的

san·gui·no·pu·ru·lent (sang″gwī-no-pu′roolənt) containing both blood and pus 脓血的

san·guis (sang′gwis) [L.] blood 血，血液

sa·ni·es (sa′ne-ēz) a fetid ichorous discharge containing serum, pus, and blood 腐液，腐脓液；**sa′nious** adj.

san·i·tar·i·an (san″ī-tar′e-ən) one skilled in sanitation and public health science 公共卫生学家

san·i·tar·i·um (san″ĭ-tar′e-əm) an institution for the promotion of health 疗养院

san·i·tary (san′ĭ-tar″e) promoting or pertaining to health 卫生的，保健的

san·i·ta·tion (san″ĭ-ta′shən) the establishment of conditions favorable to health 卫生，卫生设施体系

san·i·ti·za·tion (san″ĭ-tĭ-za′shən) the process of making or the quality of being made sanitary 卫生处理

san·i·ty (san′ĭ-te) soundness, especially of mind 精神健全，神志正常

SAP sphingolipid activator protein 鞘脂激活蛋白

sa·phe·na (sə-fe′nə) [L.] the small saphenous or the great saphenous vein 隐静脉

sa·phe·nous (sə-fe′nəs) pertaining to or associated with a saphena; applied to certain arteries, nerves, veins, etc. 隐静脉的，隐的

sa·po·na·ceous (sap″o-na′shəs) soapy; of soaplike feel or quality 肥皂性的，肥皂般的

sa·pon·i·fi·ca·tion (sə-pon″ĭ-fĭ-ka′shən) conversion of an oil or fat into a soap by combination with an alkali. In chemistry, the term now denotes hydrolysis of an ester by an alkali, producing a free alcohol and an alkali salt of the ester acid 皂化（作用）

sap·o·nin (sap′o-nin) any of a group of glycosides widely distributed in plants, which form a durable foam when their watery solutions are shaken and which even in high dilutions dissolve erythrocytes 皂苷

Sapo·vi·rus (sap′o-vi″rəs) a genus of viruses of the family Caliciviridae that cause self-limited acute gastroenteritis 札幌病毒

sap·robe (sap′rōb) an organism, usually referring to a fungus, that feeds on dead or decaying organic matter 腐生生物 ; **sapro′bic** *adj.*

Sap·ro·chae·te (sap″ro-ke′te) a genus of yeast-like anamorphic fungi, environmental saprobes and also part of the normal microbial flora of the skin and the gastrointestinal and respiratory tracts. *S. capita′ta* is an emerging opportunistic pathogen causing severe systemic infection in immunocompromised individuals, particularly those with hematologic malignancies 腐生螺旋体属

sap·ro·phyte (sap′ro-fīt) any organism living upon dead or decaying organic matter. For fungi, the preferred term is *saprobe* 腐生物 ; **saprophyt′ic** *adj.*

sap·ro·zo·ic (sap″ro-zo′ik) living on decayed organic matter; said of animals, especially protozoa 腐物寄生生物，尤指寄生于腐物的原虫

sa·quin·a·vir (sah-kwin′ah-vir) an HIV protease inhibitor that causes formation of immature, noninfectious viral particles; used as the base or the mesylate salt in treatment of HIV infection and AIDS 沙奎那韦，一种 HIV 蛋白酶抑制药，可导致病毒形成未成熟的非传染性病毒颗粒；其碱或甲磺酸盐用于治疗 HIV 感染和艾滋病

SAR Society of Abdominal Radiology 腹部放射学会

sar·al·a·sin (sə-ral′ə-sin) an angiotensin Ⅱ antagonist, used in the form of the acetate ester as an antihypertensive in the treatment of severe hypertension and in the diagnosis of renindependent hypertension 沙拉新，一种血管紧张素 Ⅱ 拮抗药，其醋酸酯的形式用于治疗严重高血压和诊断肾上腺素依赖性高血压

sar·co·blast (sahr′ko-blast) myoblast 成肌细胞

sar·co·cyst (sahr′ko-sist) 1. a protozoan of the genus *Sarcocystis* 肉孢子虫，肉孢子虫属的一种原虫 ; 2. a cylindrical cyst containing parasitic spores, found in muscles of those infected with *Sarcocystis* 肉孢子虫囊

Sar·co·cys·tis (sahr″ko-sis′tis) a genus of parasitic protozoa that occur as sporocysts in the muscle tissue of mammals, birds, and reptiles 肉孢子虫属

sar·co·cys·to·sis (sahr″ko-sis-to′sis) infection with protozoa of the genus *Sarcocystis*, which in humans is usually asymptomatic or manifested by muscle cysts associated with myositis or myocarditis or by intestinal infection. It is usually transmitted by eating undercooked beef or pork containing sporocysts or by ingestion of sporocysts from the feces of an infected animal 肉孢子虫病

Sar·co·di·na (sahr″ko-di′nə) a subphylum of protozoa consisting of organisms that alter their body shape and that move about and acquire food either by means of pseudopodia or by protoplasmic flow without producing discrete pseudopodia 肉足纲

sar·coid (sahr′koid) 1. 同 sarcoidosis ; 2. a sarcoma-like tumor 肉瘤样肿瘤 ; 3. fleshlike. 肉样的，似肉的

sar·coi·do·sis (sahr″koi-do′sis) a chronic, progressive, generalized granulomatous reticulosis involving almost any organ or tissue, characterized by hard tubercles 结节病

sar·co·lem·ma (sahr″ko-lem′ə) the membrane covering a striated muscle fiber 肌膜 ; **sarcolem′mic**, **sarcolem′mous** *adj.*

sar·co·ma (sahr-ko′mə) pl. *sarcomas, sarco′mata.* Any of a group of tumors usually arising from connective tissue, although the term now includes some of epithelial origin; most are malignant 肉瘤，通常指由结缔组织引起的一组肿瘤，现在该术语包括一些上皮来源的肿瘤；大多数是恶性的；

S

alveolar soft part s., a well-circumscribed, painless, highly metastatic neoplasm with a distinctive alveolar pattern, usually in the limbs, head, and neck of young adults 腺泡状软组织肉瘤; **ameloblastic s.,** 成釉细胞肉瘤，造肉细胞内瘤，参见 *fibrosarcoma* 下词条; **botryoid s., s. botryoi′des,** an embryonal rhabdomyosarcoma arising in submucosal tissue, usually in the upper vagina, cervix uteri, or neck of urinary bladder in young children and infants, presenting grossly as a polypoid grapelike structure 葡萄状肉瘤; **clear cell s. of kidney,** a malignant kidney tumor similar to a Wilms tumor but having a poorer prognosis; it often metastasizes to bone 肾透明细胞肉瘤; **endometrial stromal s.,** a pale, polypoid, fleshy, malignant tumor of the endometrial stroma 子宫内膜间质肉瘤; **Ewing s.,** a primary malignant tumor of the bone, closely related to a primitive neuroectodermal tumor, arising in medullary tissue, usually of cylindrical bones. Prominent symptoms are pain, fever, and leukocytosis 尤因肉瘤; **giant cell s.,** 1. a form of giant cell tumor of bone arising malignant de novo rather than transforming to malignancy 骨巨细胞肉瘤; 2. sarcoma characterized by large anaplastic (giant) cells 巨细胞肉瘤; **immunoblastic s. of B cells,** large cell immunoblastic lymphoma composed predominantly of B cells B 细胞免疫母细胞肉瘤; **immunoblastic s. of T cells,** large cell immunoblastic lymphoma composed predominantly of T cells T 细胞免疫母细胞肉瘤; **Kaposi s.,** a multicentric, malignant neoplastic vascular proliferation, characterized by blue to red nodules on the skin, sometimes with widespread visceral involvement; a particularly virulent, disseminated form occurs in immunocompromised patients; it is caused by human herpesvirus 8 卡波西肉瘤; **Kupffer cell s.,** hepatic angiosarcoma 库普弗细胞肉瘤; **osteogenic s.,** osteosarcoma 骨肉瘤; **pseudo–Kaposi s.,** unilateral subacute to chronic dermatitis occurring in association with an underlying arteriovenous fistula and closely resembling Kaposi sarcoma clinically and histologically 假性卡波西肉瘤; **reticulum cell s.,** histiocytic lymphoma 网状细胞肉瘤; **Rous s.,** a virus-induced sarcomalike growth of fowls 劳斯肉瘤; **soft tissue s.,** a general term for a malignant tumor derived from extraskeletal connective tissue, including fibrous, fat, smooth muscle, nerve, vascular, histiocytic, and synovial tissue; almost all lesions arise from primitive mesoderm 软组织肉瘤; **spindle cell s.,** 1. any sarcoma composed of spindle cells 梭形细胞肉瘤; 2. a type of soft tissue sarcoma whose cells are spindle-shaped; it is usually resistant to radiation therapy 软组织肉瘤

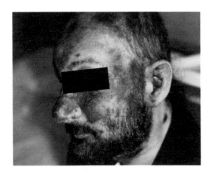

▲　卡波西肉瘤

sar·co·ma·toid (sahr-ko′mə-toid) resembling a sarcoma 肉瘤样的

sar·co·ma·to·sis (sahr″ko-mə-to′sis) a condition characterized by development of many sarcomas at various sites 肉瘤病

sar·co·ma·tous (sahr-ko′mə-təs) pertaining to or of the nature of a sarcoma 肉瘤的

sar·co·mere (sahr′ko-mēr) the contractile unit of a myofibril; sarcomeres are repeating units, delimited by the Z bands, along the length of the myofibril 肌（小）节

sar·co·pe·nia (sahr″ko-pe′ne-ə) age-related reduction in skeletal muscle mass in the elderly 肌肉减少症

sar·co·plasm (sahr′ko-plaz″əm) the interfibrillary matter of striated muscle 肌质; **sarcoplas′mic** *adj.*

sar·co·plast (sahr′ko-plast) an interstitial cell of muscle, itself capable of being transformed into muscle 肌间质细胞

sar·co·poi·et·ic (sahr″ko-poi-et′ik) producing flesh or muscle 生肌的

Sar·cop·tes (sahr-kop′tēz) a genus of mites, including *S. scabie′i,* the cause of scabies in humans 疥螨属

sar·co·si·ne·mia (sahr″ko-sī-ne′me-ə) accumulation of plasma sarcosine and elevated urinary excretion, caused by deficiency of activity of sarcosine dehydrogenase; the deficiency can be caused by mutation in the gene encoding the apoenzyme, a defect in electron transfer flavoprotein, or severe folate deficiency 肌氨酸血症

sar·co·sis (sahr-ko′sis) abnormal increase of flesh 肉瘤病；肉过多

sar·co·spo·rid·i·an (sahr″ko-spor-id′e-ən) similar to or caused by protozoa of the genus *Sarcocystis* 肉孢子虫

sar·co·spo·rid·i·o·sis (sahr″ko-spor-id″e-o′sis) 同 sarcocystosis 肉孢子虫病

S

sar·cos·to·sis (sahr″kos-to′sis) ossification of fleshy tissue 肌骨化

sar·co·tu·bules (sahr″ko-too′būlz) the membrane-limited structures of the sarcoplasm, forming a canalicular network around each myofibril 肌浆小管

sar·cous (sahr′kəs) pertaining to flesh or muscle tissue 肉的，肌（肉组织）的

sar·gram·os·tim (sahr-gram′o-stim) granulocyte-macrophage colony-stimulating factor developed by recombinant technology; used to enhance neutrophil function, stimulating hematopoiesis and decreasing neutropenia 一种重组的粒细胞－巨噬细胞集落刺激因子，用于增强中性粒细胞功能、刺激造血功能和缓解中性粒细胞减少

SARS severe acute respiratory syndrome 严重急性呼吸综合征

sar·sa·pa·ril·la (sahr″sə-pə-ril′ə) (sas″pə- ril′ə) [Sp. zarzaparrilla, fr. zarza briar + parrilla vine] 1. any of various plants of the genus *Smilax* 菝葜；2. the dried root of any of various species of *Smilax;* used as a flavoring in beverages, in the treatment of psoriasis and other skin conditions, and in homeopathy 菝葜根

sat·el·lite (sat′ə-līt) 1. a vein that closely accompanies an artery, such as the brachial 伴行静脉；2. a minor, or attendant, lesion situated near a larger one 卫星病灶；3. a globoid mass of chromatin attached at the secondary constriction to the ends of the short arms of acrocentric autosomes 随体，指在次级收缩处连接到中心常染色体短臂末端的球状染色质团块；4. exhibiting satellitism 卫星现象，卫星状共栖

sat·el·li·tism (sat′ə-li-tiz-əm) the phenomenon in which certain bacterial species grow more vigorously in the immediate vicinity of colonies of other unrelated species, owing to the production of an essential metabolite by the latter species 卫星现象，某些细菌物种在其他无关菌种的菌落附近由于后者产生必需代谢物而生长得更加剧烈的现象

sat·el·li·to·sis (sat″ə-li-to′sis) accumulation of neuroglial cells about neurons; seen whenever neurons are damaged（神经细胞的）卫星现象，在神经元受损时发生的神经胶质细胞在神经元周围积聚的现象

satt·va (sahth′və) [Sanskrit] according to ayurveda, the purest aspect of the three gunas, characterized by equilibrium; responsible for health and contentment of mind and body and associated with the mind, consciousness, or intelligence that maintains health 悦性，根据阿育吠陀的说法，为人的三个属性中最纯净的方面，以平衡为特征；负责身心的健康和满足，并与维持健康的思想、意识或智慧有关

sat·u·rat·ed (sach′ə-rāt-əd) 1. denoting a chemical compound that has only single bonds and no double or triple bonds between atoms（化学）饱和的；2. unable to hold in solution any more of a given substance（溶液）饱和的

sat·u·ra·tion (sach″ə-ra′shən) 1. the state of being saturated, or the act of saturating 饱和，饱和度；2. in radiotherapy, the delivery of a maximum tolerable tissue dose within a short period; then maintenance of the dose by additional smaller fractional doses over a prolonged period 饱和剂量，放射治疗时，先短时间内给予组织能耐受的最大剂量，然后在一段时间内分次给予较小剂量以维持生物效应；**oxy·gen s.**, the amount of oxygen bound to hemoglobin in the blood expressed as a percentage of the maximal binding capacity 氧饱和

sat·y·ri·a·sis (sat″ĭ-ri′ə-sis) abnormal, excessive, insatiable sexual desire in the male 男子色情狂，求雌狂

sau·cer·iza·tion (saw″sər-ī-za′shən) 1. the excavation of tissue to form a shallow shelving depression, usually performed to facilitate drainage from infected areas of bone 碟形手术，治疗创伤时，将组织挖出后，局部形成一较浅的倾斜形碟形凹陷，通常用于促进骨感染区域的引流；2. the shallow saucerlike depression on the upper surface of a vertebra that has suffered a compression fracture 碟形凹陷，当脊椎受压骨折时，其椎骨上面形成的碟状凹陷

saw (saw) a cutting instrument with a serrated edge 带有锯齿状边缘的切割工具；**Gigli wire s.**, a flexible wire with saw teeth 季格利线锯，带锯齿的柔性线

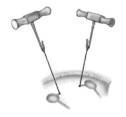

▲ 季格利线锯用于截断一段颅骨

saw pal·met·to (saw pal-met′o) a small creeping palm of the southeastern United States, *Serenoa repens,* or its fruit, which is used for urination problems associated with benign prostatic hyperplasia 锯叶棕，一种生长在美国东南部的棕榈科小灌木，锯叶棕或其果实可用于治疗与良性前列腺增生相关的

排尿问题

sax·a·glip·tin (sak″sə-glip′tin) an agent that in response to elevated blood sugar slows the inactivation of incretins, thereby increasing insulin release and decreasing circulating glucagon levels; used as the hydrochloride in the treatment of type 2 diabetes mellitus 一种响应血糖升高的药物，可通过减缓肠促胰岛素失活，从而增加胰岛素的释放及降低胰高血糖素的循环水平；其盐酸盐用于治疗Ⅱ型糖尿病

saxi·tox·in (sak′sĭ-tok″sin) a powerful neurotoxin synthesized and secreted by certain dinoflagellates, which accumulates in the tissues of shellfish feeding on the dinoflagellates and may cause a severe toxic reaction in persons consuming contaminated shellfish 石房蛤毒素，一种由某些甲藻类植物合成和分泌的强大神经毒素，该毒素在以甲藻为食的贝类组织中积累，可能对食用受污染贝类的人造成严重的毒性反应

Sb antimony ([L.] *sti′bium*) 元素锑符号

SBMA spinobulbar muscular atrophy 椎间盘肌肉萎缩

Sc scandium 元素钪符号

scab (skab) 1. the crust of a superficial sore 痂；2. to become covered with a crust or scab 结痂

sca·bi·cide (ska′bĭ-sīd) 1. lethal to *Sarcoptes scabiei* 杀疥螨的；2. an agent lethal to *Sarcoptes scabiei* 杀疥螨药

sca·bies (ska′bēz) a contagious skin disease due to the itch mite, *Sarcoptes scabiei;* the female bores into the stratum corneum, forming burrows (cuniculi), attended by intense itching and eczema caused by scratching 疥疮，一种由疥癣虫、疥螨引起的传染性皮肤病；雌性疥螨钻入角质层形成的隆起的洞穴，伴随着强烈的瘙痒和因抓伤引起的湿疹；**scabiet′ic** *adj.;* **Norwegian s.,** a rare, severe form associated with an immense number of mites, with marked scales and crusts, usually accompanied by lymphadenopathy and eosinophilia 结痂性疥疮，一种罕见的严重的疥疮，伴有大量螨虫，有明显的鳞屑和硬痂，通常伴有淋巴结病和嗜酸性粒细胞增多

sca·la (ska′lə) pl. *sca′lae* [L.] a stairlike structure 阶梯状结构，尤指耳蜗的各种通道；**s. me′dia,** cochlear duct 耳蜗导管，中阶；**s. tym′pani,** the part of the cochlea below the lamina spiralis 鼓室阶，螺旋板下耳蜗的一部分；**s. vesti′buli,** the part of the cochlea above the lamina spiralis 前庭阶，螺旋板上耳蜗的一部分

sca·lar (ska′lər) 1. a quantity that has magnitude only (as opposed to also having direction), such as mass or temperature 纯量（的），标量的，无向量的。Cf. *vector*; 2. pertaining to such a quantity 与数量

相关的

scald (skawld) to burn with hot liquid or steam 烫；a burn so produced 烫伤

scale (skāl) 1. a thin flake or compacted platelike structure, as of cornified epithelial cells on the body surface 鳞屑，指皮肤上一种薄而致密的片状组织，如体表的角化上皮细胞；2. a thin fragment of tartar or other concretion on the surface of a tooth 齿垢，牙齿表面的薄牙垢或其他结石；3. to remove such material from the tooth surface 除去……的积垢；4. a scheme or device by which some property may be measured (as hardness, weight, linear dimension) 标，标度，刻度；**absolute temperature s.,** a temperature scale with its zero at absolute zero (-273.15 ℃, -459.67°F) 绝对温标；**Brazelton behavioral s.,** a method for assessing infant behavior by responses to environmental stimuli 布拉兹尔顿行为表，一种通过环境刺激的反应评估婴儿行为的方法；**Celsius s. (C),** a temperature scale on which 0° is officially 273.15 kelvins and 100° is 373.15 kelvins. Formerly (and still, unofficially), the degree Celsius was called the degree centigrade, with 0° at the freezing point of fresh water and 100° at the boiling point under normal atmospheric pressure 摄氏温标；参见 *temperature* 下附表；**centigrade s.,** a scale in which the interval between two fixed points is divided into 100 equal units, such as the Celsius scale 百分温标；**Fahrenheit s. (F),** a temperature scale with the ice point at 32 degrees and the normal boiling point of water at 212 degrees (212°F) 华氏温度；参见 *temperature* 下附表；**French s.,** a scale used for denoting the size of catheters, sounds, etc., each unit (symbol F) being roughly equivalent to 0.33 mm in diameter 法兰西标度，用于表示导管、声音等尺寸的刻度，每个单位（符号 F）的直径大致相当于 0.33mm；**Glasgow Coma S.,** a standardized system for assessing response to stimuli in a neurologically impaired patient; reactions are given a numerical value in three categories (eye opening, verbal responsiveness, and motor responsiveness), and the three scores are then added together. The lowest values are the worst clinical scores 格拉斯哥昏迷量表；**gray s.,** a representation of intensities in shades of gray, as in gray scale ultrasonography 灰阶，灰阶中灰度强度的表示，如灰阶超声；**Kelvin s.,** an absolute temperature scale whose unit of measurement, the kelvin, is equivalent to the degree Celsius, the ice point therefore being at 273.15 kelvins 开尔文温标；**temperature s.,** one for expressing degree of heat, based on absolute zero as a reference point, or with a certain value arbitrarily assigned to such temperatures as the ice point and boiling point of water 温标；参见 *temperature* 下附表

sca·lene (ska′lēn) 1. uneven; unequally threesided 不等边的（指三角形），偏三角的；2. pertaining to one of the scalene muscles 斜角肌的；参见 *muscle* 下词条

sca·le·nec·to·my (ska″lə-nek′tə-me) resection of the scalenus muscle 斜角肌切除术

sca·le·not·o·my (ska″lə-not′ə-me) division of the scalenus muscle 斜角肌切开术

scal·er (ska′lər) a dental instrument for removal of calculus from teeth 刮器，用于去除牙结石的牙科器械

scalp (skalp) the skin covering the cranium 头皮

scal·pel (skal′pəl) a small surgical knife usually having a convex edge 解剖刀，手术刀

sca·ly (ska′le) pertaining to or characterized by scales 有鳞屑的；鳞状的

scan (skan) 1. to examine or map the body, or one or more organs or regions of it, by gathering information with a sensing device 扫 描；2. the data or image so obtained 扫描图；通过上述方式获得的数据或图像；3. *scintiscan* 的缩写；**A-s.**, display on a cathode ray tube of ultrasonic echoes, in which one axis represents the time required for return of the echo and the other corresponds to the strength of the echo A 型扫描；**B-s.**, display on a cathode ray tube of ultrasonic echoes, depicting time elapsed and echo strength and producing two-dimensional cross-sectional displays by movement of the transducer B 型扫描；**CAT s., CT s.**, computed tomography, or the image obtained from it 电子计算机断层扫描；**M-mode s.**, the image obtained using M-mode echocardiography, showing the motion (M) over time of a monodimensional ("icepick") section of the heart 运动式扫描；**PET s.**, positron emission tomography, or the image obtained from it 正电子发射断层摄影术；**ventilation-perfusion s., V/Q s.**, a scintigraphic technique for demonstrating perfusion defects in normally ventilated areas of the lung in the diagnosis of pulmonary embolism 换气－灌注扫描

scan·di·um (Sc) (skan′de-əm) a silvery white, ductile, rare earth element; at. no. 21, at. wt. 44.956 元素钪的符号

scan·ning (skan′ing) 1. the act of examining by passing over an area or organ with a sensing device 扫描（术）；2. scanning speech 断续语言；**MUGA s., multiple gated acquisition s.**, equilibrium radionuclide angiocardiography 多门电路探测扫描，平衡放射性核素心血管造影

sca·pha (ska′fə) [L.] the curved depression separating the helix of the ear from the anthelix 耳舟，

舟状窝

scapho·ceph·a·ly (skaf″o-sef′ə-le) anteroposterior elongation of the skull, with bitemporal narrowing, usually resulting from premature closure of the sagittal suture 舟状头，头骨的前后延伸，双颞部变窄，通常由矢状缝过早闭合引起；**scaphocephal′ic, scaphoceph′alous** adj.

scaph·oid (skaf′oid) 1. boat-shaped. 舟状的；2. scaphoid bone 舟状骨

scaph·oid·itis (skaf″oi-di′tis) inflammation of the scaphoid bone. 舟骨炎

scap·u·la (skap′u-lə) pl. *scap′ulae* [L.] shoulder blade; the flat, triangular bone in the back of the shoulder, articulating with the ipsilateral clavicle and humerus 肩胛骨，参见图 1；**scap′ular** adj.

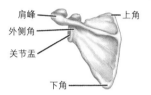

▲ 肩胛骨，显示外侧角、上角和下角

scap·u·lal·gia (skap″u-lal′jə) pain in the scapular region 肩胛痛

scap·u·lec·to·my (skap″u-lek′tə-me) excision or resection of the scapula 肩胛骨切除术

scap·u·lo·cla·vic·u·lar (skap″u-lo-klə-vik′ulər) pertaining to the scapula and clavicle 肩胛骨锁骨的

scap·u·lo·hu·mer·al (skap″u-lo-hu′mər-əl) pertaining to the scapula and humerus 肩胛骨肱骨的

scap·u·lo·pexy (skap′u-lo-pek″se) surgical fixation of the scapula 肩胛固定术

sca·pus (ska′pəs) pl. *sca′pi* [L.] shaft 干、体、柄

scar (skahr) cicatrix; a mark remaining after the healing of a wound or other morbid process. By extension, any visible manifestation of an earlier event 瘢痕；

scar·i·fi·ca·tion (skar″ĭ-fĭ-ka′shən) production in the skin of many small superficial scratches or punctures, as for introduction of vaccine 划破，划痕

scar·i·fi·ca·tor (skar′ĭ-fĭ-ka″tər) 同 scarifier

scar·i·fi·er (skar′ĭ-fi″ər) an instrument with many sharp points, used in scarification 划痕器

scar·la·ti·na (skahr″lə-te′nə) scarlet fever 猩红热；**scarlat′inal** adj.

scar·la·tin·i·form (skahr″lə-tin′ĭ-form) re - sembling scarlet fever 猩红热样的

SCAT sheep cell agglutination test 绵羊细胞凝集试验

sca·tol·o·gy (skah-tol′ə-je) 1. study and analysis

of feces, as for diagnosis 粪便学；2. a preoccupation with feces, filth, and obscenities 对粪便、污秽和淫秽的迷恋；**scatolog′ic, scatolog′ical** *adj.*

sca·tos·co·py (skə-tos′kə-pe) examination of the feces 粪便检视法

ScD [L.] Scien′tiae Doc′tor (Doctor of Science) 理学博士

scDNA   single-copy DNA 单拷贝 DNA

Sce·do·spo·ri·um (se-do-spor′e-əm) a genus of anamorphic fungi. *S. angisper′mum* is usually described as its teleomorph, *Pseudallescheria boydii. S. proli′ficans* causes infections ranging from localized, often osteoarticular, to disseminated 足放线病菌属

SCFA   short-chain fatty acids 短链脂肪酸

schin·dy·le·sis (skin″də-le′sis) an articulation in which one bone is received into a cleft in another 夹合连接，将一块骨板插入另一骨裂缝中的一种接合方式

schis·to·cor·mus (shis″-) (skis″to-kor′məs) a fetus with a cleft lower trunk 躯裂畸胎

schis·to·cyte (shis′-) (skis′to-sīt) helmet cell; a fragment of an erythrocyte, commonly observed in the blood in hemolytic anemia 裂红细胞

schis·to·cy·to·sis (shis″-) (skis″to-si-to′sis)an accumulation of schistocytes in the blood 裂细胞症

Schis·to·so·ma (shis″-) (skis″to-so′mə) the blood flukes, a genus of parasitic trematodes.Species that cause schistosomiasis in humans include *S. haemato′bium* and *S. intercala′tum* in Africa, *S. japon′icum* in East Asia and nearby islands, and *S. manso′ni* in Africa, South America, and the West Indies. The invertebrate hosts are snails. Infection follows penetration of the skin in those coming in contact with infected waters 裂体吸虫属，血吸虫属；**schistoso′mal** *adj.*

schis·to·some (shis′-) (skis′to-sōm) an individual fluke of the genus *Schistosoma* 血吸虫

schis·to·so·mi·a·sis (shis″-) (skis″to-so-mi′ə- sis) infection with *Schistosoma* 血吸虫病；**s. haemato′bia,** urinary s. 同 urinary s.，尿路血吸虫病 **intestinal s.,** the chronic form of schistosomiasis mansoni and japonica in which the intestinal tract is involved; usually asymptomatic 肠血吸虫病；**s. japo′nica,** infection with *Schistosoma japonicum.* The acute form is marked by fever, allergic symptoms, and diarrhea; chronic effects, which may be severe, are due to fibrosis around eggs deposited in the liver, lungs, and central nervous system 日本血吸虫病；**s. manso′ni,** infection with *Schistosoma mansoni,* which live chiefly in the mesenteric veins but migrate to deposit eggs in venules, primarily of the large intestine; eggs that lodge in the liver may lead to peripheral fibrosis, hepatosplenomegaly,

and ascites 曼氏血吸虫病；**urinary s., vesical s.,** infection with *Schistosoma haematobium* involving the urinary tract and causing cystitis and hematuria 尿路血吸虫病，膀胱血吸虫病

schis·to·so·mi·cide (shis″-) (skis″to-so′mĭ- sīd) an antischistosomal agent that kills the parasites 杀血吸虫药

schiz·am·ni·on (skiz-am′ne-ən) an amnion formed by cavitation over or in the embryoblast, as in human development 裂隙羊膜

schizo·af·fec·tive (skit″so-ə-fek′tiv) pertaining to or exhibiting features of both schizophrenic and mood disorders 情感性分裂的

schizo·gen·e·sis (skiz″o-jen′ə-sis) fission (2). 裂殖；**schizog′enous** *adj.*

schi·zog·o·ny (skī-zog′ə-ne) the asexual reproduction of a sporozoan parasite (sporozoite) by multiple fission of the nucleus of the parasite followed by segmentation of the cytoplasm, giving rise to merozoites 裂殖生殖；**schizogon′ic** *adj.*

schizo·gy·ria (skiz″o-ji′re-ə) a condition in which there are wedge-shaped cracks in the cerebral convolutions 脑回裂畸形

schiz·oid (skit′soid) 1. denoting the traits that characterize the schizoid personality 精神分裂样的； 2. denoting any of a variety of schizophrenia-related characteristics, including traits said to indicate a predisposition to schizophrenia as well as disorders other than schizophrenia either occurring in a relative of a schizophrenic or occurring more commonly than average in families of schizophrenics 类精神分裂症的

schiz·ont (skiz′ont) the multinucleate stage in the development of some members of the Sarcodina and some sporozoans during schizogony 裂殖体

schizo·nych·ia (skiz″o-nik′e-ə) splitting of the nails（指或趾）甲裂

schizo·pha·sia (skit″so-fa′zhə) word salad 分裂性言语，言语杂乱，参见 *W.* 下词条

schizo·phre·nia (skit″so-fre′ne-ə) a mental disorder characterized by various combinations of disturbances in the form and content of thought (e.g., delusions, hallucinations), in mood (e.g., inappropriate affect), in sense of self and relationship to the external world (e.g., loss of ego boundaries, withdrawal), and in behavior (e.g., bizarre or apparently purposeless behavior), which cause marked decrease in functioning 精神分裂症；**schizophren′ic** *adj.* **catatonic s.,** a form characterized by psychomotor disturbance, which may be manifested by a marked decrease in reactivity to the environment and in spontaneous activity, by excited, uncontrollable, and apparently purposeless motor activity, by resis-

S

tance to instructions or attempts to be moved, or by maintenance of a rigid posture or of fixed bizarre postures 紧张型精神分裂症 ; **childhood s.**, former name for schizophrenia-like symptoms with onset before puberty, marked by autistic, withdrawn behavior, failure to develop an identity separate from the mother's, and gross developmental immaturity, now classified as pervasive developmental disorders 儿童期精神分裂症，曾称精神分裂症样症状，现归类为普遍性发育障碍 ; **disorganized s.**, a form marked by disorganized and incoherent thought and speech, shallow, inappropriate, and silly affect, and regressive behavior without systematized delusions 错乱型精神分裂症 ; **paranoid s.**, a form characterized by delusions, often with auditory hallucinations, with relative preservation of affect and cognitive functioning 偏执型精神分裂症 ; **residual s.**, a condition manifested by individuals with symptoms of schizophrenia who, after a psychotic schizophrenic episode, are no longer psychotic 残余型精神分裂症 ; **undifferentiated s.**, a type characterized by the presence of prominent psychotic symptoms but not classifiable as catatonic, disorganized, or paranoid 混合型精神分裂症

schizo·phren·i·form (skit″so-fren′ĭ-form) resembling schizophrenia 精神分裂症样的

schizo·trich·ia (skiz″o-trik′e-ə) splitting of the hairs at the ends 毛发端分裂

schizo·ty·pal (skit″so-ti′pəl) exhibiting abnormalities in behavior and communication similar to those of schizophrenia, but less severe 精神分裂型的, 参见 *personality* 下词条

schizo·zo·ite (skiz″o-zo′ĭt) merozoite 裂殖子

schwan·no·ma (shwah-no′mə) a neoplasm originating from Schwann cells (of the myelin sheath) of neurons; schwannomas include neurofibromas and neurilemomas 神经鞘瘤 ; **granular cell s.**, 颗粒细胞神经鞘瘤, 参见 *tumor* 下词条

sci·at·ic (si-at′ik) 1. near or related to the sciatic nerve or vein 关于或靠近坐骨神经或静脉的；2. ischial 坐骨的

sci·at·i·ca (si-at′ĭ-kə) neuralgia along the course of the sciatic nerve, most often with pain radiating into the buttock and lower limb, most commonly due to herniation of a lumbar disk 坐骨神经痛

SCID severe combined immunodeficiency (disease); 严重联合免疫缺陷病；参见 *immunodeficiency* 下词条

sci·ence (si′əns) 1. the systematic observation of natural phenomena for the purpose of discovering laws governing those phenomena 科学 ; 2. the body of knowledge accumulated by such means 学科 ; **scientif′ic** *adj.*

sci·er·opia (si-ər-o′pe-ə) defect of vision in which objects appear in a shadow 雾视，一种所见物体出现在阴影中的视觉缺陷

scin·ti·gram (sin′tĭ-gram) the graphic record obtained by scintigraphy 闪烁图，通过闪烁扫描获得的图形记录

scin·tig·ra·phy (sin-tig′rə-fe) the production of two-dimensional images of the distribution of radioactivity in tissues after the internal administration of a radiopharmaceutical imaging agent, the images being obtained by a scintillation camera 闪烁成像，闪烁显像，受检者内服放射性药物显像剂后，通过闪烁照相机拍摄的组织内放射性分布的二维影像 ; **scintigraph′ic** *adj.*; **exercise thallium s.**, myocardial perfusion using thallium 201 as a tracer and performed in conjunction with an exercise stress test 运动铊闪烁造影法 ; **gated blood pool s.**, equilibrium radionuclide angiocardiography 门电路血池闪烁照相术，平衡放射性核素心血管造影术 ; **infarct avid s.**, that performed following myocardial infarction to confirm infarction as well as detect, localize, and quantify areas of myocardial necrosis by means of a radiotracer that concentrates in necrotic regions 心肌梗死闪烁法，在心肌梗死后，通过集中在坏死区域的放射性示踪剂来确认梗死以及检测、定位和量化心肌坏死区域 ; **myocardial perfusion s.**, that performed using a radiotracer that traverses the myocardial capillary system; immediate and delayed images are obtained to assess regional blood flow and cell viability 心肌灌注闪烁扫描，使用放射性示踪剂穿过心肌毛细血管系统进行的检查；获得即时和延迟图像，以评估局部血流和细胞活力

scin·til·la·tion (sin″tĭ-la′shən) 1. an emission of sparks 发出火花 ; 2. a subjective visual sensation, as of seeing sparks 光闪视 ; 3. a particle emitted in disintegration of a radioactive element 闪烁粒，放射性元素蜕变时放射的微粒 ; 另参见 *counter* 下词条

scin·ti·scan (sin′tĭ-skan) a two-dimensional representation of the radiation emitted by a radioisotope, revealing its concentration in specific organs or tissues 闪烁扫描，放射性同位素放射出的射线产生的二维图像，显示其在特定器官或组织中的浓度

scir·rhoid (skir′oid) resembling scirrhous carcinoma 硬癌样的

scir·rhous (skir′əs) hard or indurated 硬癌的；参见 *carcinoma* 下词条

scle·ra (sklēr′ə) pl. **scle·rae** [L.] the tough white outer coat of the eyeball, covering approximately the posterior five-sixths of its surface, continuous anteriorly with the cornea and posteriorly with the external sheath of the optic nerve 巩膜，眼球的白色坚韧被膜，覆盖眼球表面后方约 5/6 部分，向前延续于角膜，向后延伸于视神经外鞘; **scler′al** *adj.*

scle·rad·e·ni·tis (sklēr″ad-ə-ni′tis) inflammation and hardening of a gland 巩膜炎

scle·rec·ta·sia (sklēr″ək-ta′zhə) a bulging state of the sclera 巩膜膨胀

scle·rec·to·iri·dec·to·my (sklə-rek″to-ir″ĭ- dek′tə-me) excision of part of the sclera and of the iris 巩膜虹膜切除术

scle·rec·to·iri·do·di·al·y·sis (sklə-rek″toir″ĭ-do-di-al′ĭ-sis) sclerectomy and iridodialysis 巩膜切除虹膜分离术

scle·rec·to·my (sklə-rek′tə-me) excision of part of the sclera 巩膜切除术

scle·re·de·ma (sklēr″ə-de′mə) diffuse, symmetric, woodlike, nonpitting induration of the skin of unknown etiology, typically beginning on the head, face, or neck and spreading to involve the shoulders, arms, and thorax and sometimes extracutaneous sites 硬化病，一种见于皮肤的弥散，对称、木质样、无凹陷的硬结，病因不明，典型病变始于面部、头或颈部，逐渐不断蔓延到肩部、手臂、胸部，有时亦扩散到皮肤以外部位

scle·re·ma (sklə-re′mə) a severe, sometimes fatal disorder of adipose tissue seen in preterm, sick, debilitated infants, with induration of involved tissue and skin that is cold, yellowish white, mottled, boardlike, and inflexible 硬化病，一种严重的，有时是致命的脂肪组织病，主要见于早产、患病的或衰弱的婴儿，表现为受侵及组织和皮肤硬化、变冷、呈黄白色、花斑状、板样僵硬、不能屈曲

scle·ri·rit·o·my (sklēr″ĭ-rit′ə-me) incision of the sclera and iris in anterior staphyloma 巩膜虹膜切开术，一种治疗前葡萄肿巩膜虹膜切口的手术

scle·ri·tis (sklə-ri′tis) inflammation of the sclera; it may involve the part adjoining the limbus of the cornea *(anterior s.)* or the underlying retina and choroid *(posterior s.);* the former may take diffuse, nodular, or necrotizing forms, or a related necrotizing form without inflammation (scleromalacia perforans) 巩膜炎，可能累及角膜边缘附近的部分（前巩膜炎）或视网膜下层和脉络膜（后巩膜炎）；前者可呈弥漫性、结节状或坏死状，或无炎症坏死状（巩膜穿孔）

scle·ro·blas·te·ma (sklēr″o-blas-te′mə) the embryonic tissue from which bone is formed 生骨胚组织，成骨胚组织; **scleroblaste′mic** *adj.*

scle·ro·cho·roi·di·tis (sklēr″o-ko″roi-di′tis) inflammation of the sclera and choroid 巩膜脉络膜炎

scle·ro·cor·nea (sklēr″o-kor′ne-ə) the sclera and choroid regarded as forming a single layer 硬化性角膜

scle·ro·cor·ne·al (sklēr″o-kor′ne-əl) pertaining to the sclera and the cornea 巩（膜）角膜的

scle·ro·dac·ty·ly (sklēr″o-dak′tə-le) localized scleroderma of the digits 指（趾）硬皮病

scle·ro·der·ma (sklēr″o-dur′mə) hardening and thickening of the skin, a finding in various different diseases, occurring in localized and general forms 硬皮病; **circumscribed s.**, morphea 局限性硬皮病; **systemic s.**, a systemic disorder of connective tissue with skin hardening and thickening, blood vessel abnormalities, and fibrotic degenerative changes in various body organs 全身性硬皮病，一种侵犯身体各部位结缔组织的全身性疾病，其特征为皮肤出现硬结和增厚，血管异常和各种身体器官的纤维变性

scle·rog·e·nous (sklə-roj′ə-nəs) producing sclerosis or sclerous tissue 致硬化的

scle·ro·iri·tis (sklēr″o-i-ri′tis) inflammation of the sclera and iris 巩膜虹膜炎

scle·ro·ker·a·ti·tis (sklēr″o-ker″ə-ti′tis) in - flammation of the sclera and cornea 巩膜角膜炎

scle·ro·ma (sklə-ro′mə) a hardened patch or induration, especially of the nasal or laryngeal tissues 硬结，（尤指鼻或喉组织）

scle·ro·ma·la·cia (sklēr″o-mə-la′shə) degeneration and thinning (softening) of the sclera 巩膜软化; **s. per′forans**, a nodular form of anterior scleritis in which necrosis and atrophy, usually painless, occur without inflammation; marked thinning of the sclera exposes the underlying uvea, and perforation of the globe readily occurs 穿孔性巩膜软化，一种结节状的前巩膜炎，坏死和萎缩，通常无痛，无炎症; 巩膜明显变薄，暴露葡萄膜下层，球体容易穿孔

scle·ro·mere (sklēr′o-mēr) 1. any segment or metamere of the skeletal system 骨节; 2. the caudal half of a sclerotome (3) 生骨板

scle·ro·myx·ede·ma (sklēr″o-mik″sə- de′mə) 1. lichen myxedematosus 黏液水肿性苔藓; 2. a term sometimes used to refer to lichen myxedematosus associated with scleroderma 有时用来指与硬皮病有关的黏液水肿性苔藓

scle·ro·nyx·is (sklēr″o-nik′sis) surgical puncture of the sclera 巩膜穿刺术

scle·ro·ooph·o·ri·tis (sklēr″o-o-of′ə-ri′tis) sclerosing inflammation of the ovary 硬化性卵巢炎

scle·roph·thal·mia (sklēr″of-thal′me-ə) a condition, resulting from imperfect differentiation of the sclera and cornea, in which only the central part of the cornea remains clear 巩膜化角膜，巩膜眼症，因角膜和巩膜分化不完全，致角膜周围不透明，仅中央部清晰

角膜

S

scle·ro·pro·tein (sklēr″o-pro′tēn) a simple protein characterized by its insolubility and fibrous structure and usually serving a supportive or protective function in the body 硬蛋白，一种单纯蛋白，其特性为不溶性及纤维结构，通常对身体起支特及保护作用

scle·ro·sant (sklə-ro′sənt) sclerosing agent 组织硬化剂

scle·rose (sklə-rōs′) to become, or cause to become, hardened or sclerotic 变硬、硬化

scle·ros·ing (sklə-rōs′ing) causing or undergoing sclerosis 致硬化的

scle·ro·sis (sklə-ro′sis) an induration or hardening, especially from inflammation and in diseases of the interstitial substance; applied chiefly to such hardening of the nervous system or to hardening of the blood vessels 硬化，尤指间质组织疾病与炎症引起的部分硬化，主要用于神经系统硬化或血管硬化；**amyotrophic lateral s.,** Lou Gehrig disease: progressive degeneration of the neurons that give rise to the corticospinal tract and of the motor cells of the brainstem and spinal cord, resulting in a deficit of upper and lower motor neurons; it usually has a fatal outcome within 2 to 3 years 肌萎缩侧索硬化；**arterial s.,** arteriosclerosis 动脉硬化；**arteriolar s.,** arteriolosclerosis 小动脉硬化；**diffuse cerebral s.,** the infantile form of metachromatic leukodystrophy 弥漫性脑硬化；**glomerular s.,** glomerulosclerosis 肾小球硬化；**hippocampal s.,** loss of neurons in the region of the hippocampus, with gliosis; sometimes seen in epilepsy 海马硬化；**lateral s.,** degeneration of the lateral columns of the spinal cord, leading to spastic paraplegia. See *amyotrophic lateral s.* and *primary lateral s.* 侧索硬化，参见 *amyotrophic lateral s.* 和 *primary lateral s.*；**Mönckeberg s.,** Mönckeberg 硬化症，参见 *arteriosclerosis* 下词条；**multiple s. (MS),** demyelination occurring in patches throughout the white matter of the central nervous system, sometimes extending into the gray matter; symptoms of lesions of the white matter are weakness, incoordination, paresthesias, speech disturbances, and visual complaints 多发性硬化（症）；**primary lateral s.,** a form of motor neuron disease in which the degenerative process is limited to the corticospinal pathways 原发性侧索硬化；**tuberous s.,** 结节性硬化（症），参见 *complex* 下词条

scle·ro·ste·no·sis (sklēr″o-stə-no′sis) induration or hardening combined with contraction 硬化性狭窄，硬缩

scle·ros·to·my (sklə-ros′tə-me) surgical creation of an opening in the sclera; usually performed in treatment of glaucoma 巩膜造口术

scle·ro·ther·a·py (sklēr″o-ther′ə-pe) injection of a chemical irritant into a vein to produce inflammation and eventual fibrosis and obliteration of the lumen, as for treatment of hemorrhoids 硬化疗法

scle·rot·ic (sklə-rot′ik) 1. hard or hardening; affected with sclerosis 硬的、硬化的；2. scleral 巩膜

scle·ro·ti·tis (sklēr″o-ti′tis) 同 scleritis

scle·ro·ti·um (sklə-ro′she-əm) a structure formed by fungi and certain protozoa in response to adverse environmental conditions, which will germinate under favorable conditions; in fungi, it is a hard mass of intertwined mycelia, usually with pigmented walls, and in protozoa it is a multinucleated hard cyst into which the plasmodium divides 菌核，真菌和某些原生动物在恶劣的环境条件下形成的结构，在适宜的条件下会发芽；在真菌中，它是一个硬的交织的菌丝团，通常带有色素壁；在原生动物中，它是一个多核的硬囊，分裂形成多核硬囊

scle·ro·tome (sklēr′o-tōm) 1. an instrument used in the incision of the sclera 巩膜刀；2. the area of a bone innervated from a single spinal segment 由单一脊髓节支配的骨区域；3. one of the paired masses of mesenchymal tissue, separated from the ventromedial part of a somite, which develop into vertebrae and ribs 生骨节

scle·rot·o·my (sklə-rot′ə-me) incision of the sclera 巩膜切开术

scle·rous (sklēr′əs) hard; indurated 硬的；硬化的

sco·lex (sko′leks) pl. *sco′leces, sco′lices* [Gr.] the attachment organ of a tapeworm, generally considered the anterior, or cephalic, end 头节，指绦虫的吸附器官，通常指绦虫的前端，即头端

sco·lio·ky·pho·sis (sko″le-o-ki-fo′sis) combined lateral (scoliosis) and posterior (kyphosis) curvature of the spine 脊柱后侧凸

sco·li·o·si·om·e·try (sko″le-o-se-om′ə-tre) measurement of spinal curvature 脊柱凸度测量法

sco·li·o·sis (sko″le-o′sis) lateral curvature of the vertebral column 脊柱侧凸；**scoliot′ic** *adj.*

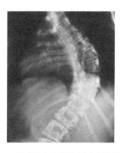

▲ 严重胸部脊柱侧凸（后前凸）

scom·broid (skom′broid) 1. of or pertaining to the suborder Scombroidea 鲭亚目的；2. a fish of the suborder Scombroidea 鲭，另参见 *poisoning* 下词条

Scom·broi·dea (skom-broi′de-ə) a suborder of larger, bony marine fish having oily flesh, including tunas, bonitos, mackerels, albacores, and skipjacks; their flesh may contain a toxic histamine-like substance and, if ingested, can cause scombroid poisoning 鲭亚目

sco·pol·amine (sko-pol′ə-mēn) an anticholinergic alkaloid obtained from various solanaceous plants; used as the base or the hydrobromide salt as an antiemetic and as the hydrobromide salt as a preanesthetic antisialagogue, adjunct to general anesthesia, and topical mydriatic and cycloplegic 东莨菪碱（抗胆碱能药）

sco·po·phil·ia (sko-po-fil′e-ə) usually, voyeurism, but it is sometimes divided into active and passive forms, *active s.* being *voyeurism* and *passive s.* being *exhibitionism* 窥淫癖，露阴癖

sco·po·pho·bia (sko″po-fo′be-ə) irrational fear of being seen 被窥视恐怖

scor·bu·tic (skor-bu′tik) pertaining to or affected with scurvy 坏血病的

scor·bu·ti·gen·ic (skor-bu″tī-jen′ik) causing scurvy 致坏血病的

score (skor) a rating, usually expressed numerically, based on specific achievement or the degree to which certain qualities or conditions are present 得分；评分，分数；**APACHE s.**, a widely used method for assessing severity of illness in acutely ill patients in intensive care units, taking into account a variety of routine physiologic parameters APACHE 评分，一种广泛应用的评估重症监护病房急病患者病情严重程度的方法，考虑各种常规生理参数；**Apgar s.**, a numerical expression of an infant's condition, usually determined at 60 seconds after birth, based on heart rate, respiratory effort, muscle tone, reflex irritability, and color 阿普加评分，一种用数字来表示新生儿产后 60 秒时的身体状况，通常是评定新生儿的心率、呼吸力、肌张力、反射应激性和肤色所得的总分；**Bishop s.**, a score for estimating the prospects of induction of labor, arrived at by evaluating the extent of cervical dilation and effacement, station of the fetal head, consistency of the cervix, and cervical position in relation to the vaginal axis 毕晓普评分，通过评价子宫颈的扩张程度、宫颈消失、胎头的姿势、子宫颈的坚松度及宫颈位置与阴道轴的关系等以预测引产术前的情况

sco·to·chro·mo·gen (sko″to-kro′mo-jən) a microorganism whose pigmentation develops in the dark as well as in the light 黑暗产色菌类，一种既能在光中又能在暗中形成色素沉着的微生物；**scoto-chromogen′ic** *adj.*

sco·to·din·ia (sko″to-din′e-ə) dizziness with blurring of vision and headache 暗点性眩晕，伴有视物模糊及头痛

sco·to·ma (sko-to′mə) pl. *scoto′mata*. 1. an area of depressed vision in the visual field, surrounded by an area of less depressed or of normal vision 暗点，盲点，视野中视觉消失或受到抑制的区域，周围抑制程度较差甚或视力正常；2. 同 mental s.; **scotom′atous** *adj.*; **annular s.**, circular area of depressed vision surrounding the point of fixation 环状暗点，视野中固定点周围形成的环状视觉抑制区；**central s.**, an area of depressed vision corresponding with the point of fixation and interfering with central vision 中心暗点，与固定点相当的视觉抑制区，可干扰中心视觉或完全使之丧失；**centrocecal s.**, a horizontal oval defect in the field of vision situated between and embracing both the point of fixation and the blind spot 哑铃形暗点，视野中位于固定点与盲点之间并将两者完全包绕的一水平卵圆形视觉缺损区；**color s.**, an isolated area of depressed or defective vision for color 色盲暗点，视野中色视觉抑制或缺损的孤立性区域；**hemianopic s.**, depressed or lost vision affecting half of the central visual field 偏盲暗点，影响中心视野一半的视觉抑制区或缺损区；**mental s.**, a figurative blind spot in a person's psychological awareness, the person being unable to gain insight into and to understand their mental problems; lack of insight 精神盲点，精神病学上指人心理意识的盲点，患者不能自知、认识自己精神上的问题，即缺乏自省力；**negative s.**, one that appears as a blank spot or hiatus in the visual field, the patient being unaware of it 负性暗点：视野中出现空白斑点的暗点，但患者本人不能察觉；**peripheral s.**, an area of depressed vision toward the periphery of the visual field, distant from the point of fixation 外周暗点，远离固定点并接近视野外周的视觉抑制；**physiologic s.**, the area of the visual field corresponding with the optic disk, in which the photosensitive receptors are absent 生理暗点，视野中相当于视神经乳头的区域，该区无光敏感接受器；**positive s.**, one that appears as a dark spot in the visual field, the patient being aware of it 正性暗点，患者能主观察觉的视野中的一个黑点；**relative s.**, an area of the visual field in which perception of light is only diminished, or loss is restricted to light of certain wavelengths 相对暗点，视野中一个光感只是减弱或只是对某些波长的光感消失的区域；**ring s.**, 同 annular s.; **scintillating s.**, teichopsia 闪光暗点

sco·to·ma·graph (sko-to′mə-graf) an instrument

for recording a scotoma 暗点描记器

sco·tom·e·try (sko-tom′ə-tre) the measurement of scotomas 暗点测量法

sco·to·pho·bia (sko″to-fo′be-ə) irrational fear of darkness 恐暗症，黑暗恐怖

sco·to·pia (sko-to′pe-ə) 1. night vision 暗视；2. dark adaptation 暗适应；**scotop′ic** *adj.*

sco·top·sin (sko-top′sin) the opsin of the retinal rods that combines with 11-cis retinal to form rhodopsin 视暗蛋白：视网膜杆体中的蛋白质部分，与视黄醛（11-顺式视黄醛）结合为视紫质；参见 *retinal* (2)

scra·pie (skra′pe) a prion disease occurring in sheep and goats, characterized by severe pruritus, debility, and muscular incoordination, ending in death 羊瘙痒病，一种见于绵羊及山羊的一种朊病毒病，表现为严重瘙痒、衰弱及肌肉运动失调，最终结局为死亡

scratch (skrach) 1. to scrape or rub a surface lightly, such as to relieve itching 轻轻地刮或擦表面，如减轻瘙痒；2. to make shallow cuts on a surface 在表面上做浅的划痕；3. a slight wound 轻微的伤口；4. to make a thin grating sound 发出细的摩擦声

screen (skrēn) 1. a structure resembling a curtain or partition, used as a protection or shield, e.g., against excessive radiation exposure 一种类似于窗帘或隔板的结构，用作防护或屏蔽，例如防止过度辐射暴露；2. a large flat surface upon which light rays are projected 荧光屏；3. protective (2) 保护剂；4. to examine by fluoroscopy (Great Britain) 荧光屏检查（英国用语）；5. to separate well individuals in a population from those with an undiagnosed pathologic condition by means of tests, examinations, or other procedures 筛选检查，通过试验、检查或其他方法，将人群中为未诊断的疾病的高危者与正常人分离开；**skin s.,** a substance applied to the skin to protect it from the sun's rays or other noxious agents 皮肤保护剂；**solar s., sun s.,** sunscreen 遮光剂

screen·ing (skrēn′ing) 1. examination of a group to separate well persons from those who have an undiagnosed pathologic condition or who are at high risk 筛选检查，通过检查或试验，从人群中将罹患某种疾病、缺陷或属于某种疾病高危组的人与正常人分开；2. fluoroscopy (Great Britain) 荧光屏检查（英国用语）；**antibody s.,** a method of determining the presence and amount of anti-HLA antibodies in the serum of a potential allograft recipient: aliquots of the recipient's serum are mixed with a panel of leukocytes from well-characterized cell donors, complement is added, and the percentage of cells that lyse (referred to as the *panel-reactive antibody*) indicates the degree of sensitization of the recipient 抗体筛查

screw·worm (skroo′wərm) the larva of *Cochliomyia hominivorax* 螺旋虫

scro·bic·u·late (skro-bik′u-lāt) marked with pits 有小凹的

scrof·u·la (skrof′u-lə) tuberculous cervical lymphadenitis 淋巴腺结核

scrof·u·lo·der·ma (skrof″u-lo-dur′mə) a type of cutaneous tuberculosis representing either direct extension of tuberculosis into the skin from underlying structures (e.g., cervical lymph nodes, bone, lung) or contact exposure to tuberculosis; manifested by painless subcutaneous swellings that evolve into cold abscesses, ulcers, and draining sinus tracts 瘰疬性皮肤结核，一种皮肤结核，表现为结核分枝杆菌从皮下组织（如颈部淋巴结、骨、肺）直接扩散至皮肤所致，或接触结核病人也可发病。其表现为形成无痛性皮下肿胀，并进而发展为寒性脓疡、多发性溃疡及引流窦道

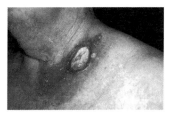

▲ 瘰疬性皮肤结核：病变来自皮下淋巴结扩散

scro·tal (skro′təl) pertaining to the scrotum 阴囊的

scro·tec·to·my (skro-tek′tə-me) partial or complete excision of the scrotum 阴囊切除术

scro·to·plasty (skro′to-plas″te) plastic reconstruction of the scrotum 阴囊成形术

scro·tum (skro′təm) the pouch containing the testes and their accessory organs 阴囊

scu-PA single-chain urokinase–type plasminogen activator 单链尿激酶型纤溶酶原激活剂；参见 *prourokinase*

scur·vy (skur′ve) a disease due to deficiency of ascorbic acid (vitamin C), marked by anemia, spongy gums, a tendency to mucocutaneous hemorrhages, and brawny induration of calf and leg muscles 坏血病

scute (skūt) any squama or scalelike structure, especially the bony plate separating the upper tympanic cavity and mastoid cells *(tympanic s.)* 鳞；鼓室盾板

scu·ti·form (sku′tĭ-form) shaped like a shield 盾状的

scu·tu·lum (sku′tu-ləm) pl. *scu′tula* [L.] one of the

disklike or saucerlike crusts characteristic of favus 黄癣痂，具黄癣特征的一种盘形或碟状痂皮

scu·tum (sku′təm) 1. 同 scute; 2. a hard chitinous plate on the anterior dorsal surface of hardbodied ticks 盾片（指蜱科或硬体蜱）

scy·ba·lum (sib′ə-ləm) pl. *scy′bala* [Gr.] a hard mass of fecal matter in the intestines 硬粪块; **scy′balous** *adj.*

SD skin dose 皮肤量; standard deviation 标准差

SDMS Society of Diagnostic Medical Sonographers 诊断医学超声医师学会

SDS sodium dodecyl sulfate 十二烷基硫酸钠

SE standard error 标准误

Se selenium 元素硒的符号

sealed source (seeld sŏrs) a radiation source sealed in a small implant holder; used in brachytherapy 密封（放射）源

seam (sēm)a line of union 接缝; **osteoid s.**, on the surface of a bone, the narrow region of newly formed organic matrix not yet mineralized 骨接缝

sea·sick·ness (se′sik-nis) motion sickness malaise caused by the motion of a ship 晕船

sea·son·al (se′zən-əl) of, depending on, or occurring in a particular season of the year 季节性的

seat·worm (sēt′wərm) oxyurid 蛲虫

se·ba·ceous (sə-ba′shəs) pertaining to or secreting sebum 皮脂的，脂肪的; 分泌皮脂的

seb·or·rhea (seb″o-re′ə) 1. excessive secretion of sebum 皮脂溢出; 2. seborrheic dermatitis 脂溢性皮炎; **seborrhe′al, seborrhe′ic** *adj.*; **s. sic′ca,** dry, scaly seborrheic dermatitis 干性皮脂溢

sebo·tro·pic (seb″o-tro′pik) having an affinity for sebaceous glands 亲皮脂的

se·bum (se′bəm) the oily secretion of the sebaceous glands, composed of fat and epithelial debris 皮脂

seco·bar·bi·tal (sek″o-bahr′bĭ-təl) a short-acting barbiturate used as the sodium salt as a hypnotic and sedative and as an anticonvulsant in tetanus 司可巴比妥（短效巴比妥酸盐）

sec·ond·ary (sek′ən-dar″e) 1. second or inferior in order of time, place, or importance 次等的; 第二的; 2. derived from or consequent to a primary event or thing 继发的

se·cret·a·gogue (se-krēt′ə-gog) stimulating secretion, or an agent that so acts 促分泌的; 促分泌素

se·crete (se-krēt′) to elaborate and release a secretion 分泌

se·cre·tin (se-kre′tin) a hormone secreted by the duodenal and jejunal mucosa when acid chyme enters the intestine; it stimulates secretion of pancreatic juice and, to a lesser extent, bile and intestinal secretion 促胰液素

se·cre·tion (se-kre′shən) 1. the cellular process of elaborating and releasing a specific product; this activity may range from separating a specific substance of the blood to the elaboration of a new chemical substance 分泌（作用）; 2. material that is secreted 分泌物

se·cret·o·gran·in (suh″crēt′ō-grăn-ən) a family of acidic secretory proteins found in the secretory granules of many endocrine cells and neurons 分泌粒蛋白

se·cre·to·in·hib·i·to·ry (se-kre″to-in-hib′ĭ- tor″e) antisecretory 抑制分泌的

se·cre·to·mo·tor (se-kre″to-mo′tər) stimulating secretion; said of nerves 刺激分泌的（指神经）

se·cre·tor (se-kre′tər) 1. an individual expressing the autosomal dominant phenotype of secreting the ABH antigens of the ABO blood group in the saliva and other body fluids 分泌者，在遗传学中指在唾液和其他体液中含有 ABO 血型的 ABH 抗原的人; 2. the gene determining this phenotype 分泌（者）基因，决定分泌者遗传特性的基因

se·cre·to·ry (se-kre′tə-re) (se′krə-tor″e) pertaining to secretion or affecting the secretions 分泌作用的，分泌性的

sec·tio (sek′she-o) pl. *sectio′nes* [L.] section 切开术; 切断面; 切片; 节

sec·tion (sek′shən) 1. an act of cutting 切开术; 2. a cut surface 切断面，截面; 切片; 3. a segment or subdivision of an organ 节，（器官的）部分; 4. a supplemental taxonomic category subordinate to a subgenus but superior to a species or series 科; **abdominal s.,** laparotomy 剖腹术; **cesarean s.,** delivery of a fetus by incision through the abdominal wall and uterus 剖宫产; **frozen s.,** a specimen cut by microtome from tissue that has been frozen 冰冻切片; **perineal s.,** external urethrotomy 尿道外切开术; **serial s.,** histologic sections made in consecutive order and so arranged for the purpose of microscopic examination 连续切片

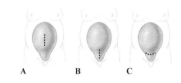

▲ 剖宫产切口（**A**）经典式;（**B**）子宫下段纵向式;（**C**）子宫下段横向式

se·cun·di·grav·i·da (sə-kun″dĭ-grav′ĭ-də) a woman pregnant the second time; gravida Ⅱ 第二次孕妇

se·cun·dines (sek′ən-dēnz) (se-kun′dēnz) afterbirth 产后物

se·cun·dip·a·ra (se″kən-dip′ə-rə) a woman who

has had two pregnancies that resulted in viable off-spring; para Ⅱ 二产妇

SED skin erythema dose 皮肤红斑剂量；参见 *dose.* 下 *erythema dose*

se·da·tion (sə-da′shən) 1. the allaying of irritability or excitement, especially by administration of a sedative 镇静药；2. the state so induced 镇静状态；**conscious s.,** a state of anesthesia in which the patient is conscious but is rendered free of fear and anxiety 清醒镇静

sed·a·tive (sed′ə-tiv) 1. allaying irritability and excitement 镇静的；2. a drug that so acts 镇静药

sed·en·tary (sed′ən-tar″e) 1. sitting habitually; of inactive habits 静坐的，惯于久坐的；2. pertaining to a sitting posture 坐式的

sed·i·ment (sed′ĭ-mənt) a precipitate, especially that formed spontaneously 沉淀，沉积物

sed·i·men·ta·tion (sed″ĭ-mən-ta′shən) the settling out of sediment 沉积，沉降

seed (sēd) 1. the mature ovule of a flowering plant 种子，籽；2. a small cylindrical shell of gold or other suitable material, used in application of radiation therapy 种子形小管（用于放射治疗）；3. to inoculate a culture medium with microorganisms 接种，将微生物接种在培养基上；**grape s.,** a preparation of the seeds of grapes, having antioxidant, antimutagenic, and antiinflammatory properties; used for the prevention of atherosclerosis and cancer and in folk medicine for the treatment of circulatory disorders 葡萄籽；**plantago s., psyllium s.,** cleaned, dried ripe seed of species of *Plantago;* used as a bulk-forming laxative 车前子

SEGA subependymal giant cell astrocytoma 室管膜下巨细胞性星形细胞瘤

seg·ment (seg′mənt) a demarcated portion of a whole 段；**anterior s. of eye, anterior s. of eyeball,** the sclera, conjunctiva, cornea, anterior chamber, iris, and lens 眼前半段；**bronchopulmonary s's,** some of the smaller subdivisions of the lobes of the lungs, separated by connective tissue septa and supplied by branches of the respective lobar bronchi 支气管肺段，肺叶的一些较小的分支，由结缔组织隔开，由各自的肺叶支气管分支供应，见图 26; **posterior s. of eye, posterior s. of eyeball,** the vitreous, retina, and optic nerve 眼后半段；**renal s's,** subdivisions of the kidney that have an independent blood supply from branches of the renal artery, including the *superior, anterior superior, inferior, anterior inferior,* and *posterior* segments 肾段，由肾动脉分支提供独立血液供应的肾的分支，包括上段、上前段、下段、下前段和后段；**spinal s's, s's of spinal cord,** the regions of the spinal cord to each of which is attached anterior and posterior

roots of the 31 pairs of spinal nerves: 8 *cervical,* 12 *thoracic,* 5 *lumbar,* 5 *sacral,* and 3 *coccygeal* 脊髓节段；**ST s.,** the interval from the end of ventricular depolarization to the onset of the T wave ST 节段（心电图），从心室去极化结束到 T 波开始的时间间隔；**uterine s.,** either of the portions into which the uterus differentites in early labor; the upper contractile portion (corpus uteri) becomes thicker as labor advances, and the lower noncontractile portion (the isthmus) is expanded and thin-walled 子宫节段

seg·men·tal (seg-men′təl) 1. pertaining to or forming a segment or a product of division, especially into serially arranged or nearly equal parts 与节段有关或形成节段、产生分节的，尤指形成连续排列或几乎相等的部分；2. undergoing segmentation 分割的

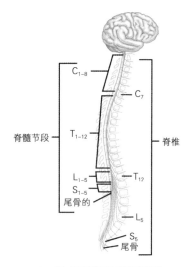

▲ 相对于脊椎显示的脊髓节段

seg·men·ta·tion (seg″mən-ta′shən) 1. division into similar parts 分节；2. cleavage 分裂

seg·men·tum (seg-men′təm) pl. *segmen′ta* [L.] 同 segment

seg·re·ga·tion (seg″rə-ga′shən) 1. the separation of allelic genes during meiosis as homologous chromosomes begin to migrate toward opposite poles of the cell, so that the members of each pair of allelic genes go to separate gametes 分离，遗传学上，在细胞减数分裂过程中，当同源染色体开始向细胞极迁移时，出现等位基因分离现象，从而使每对等位基因分向不同的配子中；2. the progressive restriction of potencies in the zygote to the various regions of the forming embryo 分离，分异，将合

子中的效能逐渐限制于胚胎形成中的不同区域

sei·zure (se′zhər) 1. the sudden attack or recurrence of a disease（疾病的）发作；2. a single episode of epilepsy, often named for the type it represents 癫痫发作；**absence s.**, the seizure of absence epilepsy, marked by a momentary break in consciousness of thought or activity and accompanied by a symmetric 3-cps spike and wave activity on the electroencephalogram 失神发作；**adversive s.**, a type of focal motor seizure in which there is forceful, sustained turning to one side by the eyes, head, or body 扭转性癫痫发作 **atonic s.**, an absence seizure characterized by sudden loss of muscle tone 失张性癫痫发作；**automatic s.**, a type of complex partial seizure characterized by automatisms, often ambulatory and involving quasipurposeful acts 自发性癫痫发作；**clonic s.**, one in which there are generalized clonic contractions without a preceding tonic phase 阵挛性发作；**complex partial s.**, a type of partial seizure associated with disease of the temporal lobe and characterized by varying degrees of impairment of consciousness and automatisms, for which the patient is later amnestic 复杂部分发作；**febrile s's,** 高热惊厥，参见 *convulsion* 下词条；**generalized tonic-clonic s.**, the seizure of grand mal epilepsy, consisting of a loss of consciousness and generalized tonic convulsions followed by clonic convulsions 全身性强直–阵挛性发作；**myoclonic s.**, one characterized by a brief episode of myoclonus 肌阵挛性发作；**partial s.**, any seizure due to a lesion in a specific, known area of the cerebral cortex 部分性发作；**reflex s.**, an episode of reflex epilepsy 反射性（癫痫）发作；**sensory s.**, 1. a simple partial seizure manifested by paresthesias or other hallucinations, including several types of aura 一种简单的部分性发作，表现为感觉异常或其他幻觉，包括几种类型的先兆；2. a reflex seizure in response to a sensory stimulus 感觉性癫痫发作，对感觉刺激作出反应的反射性癫痫；**simple partial s.**, a localized type of partial seizure, without loss of consciousness; if it progresses to another type of seizure it is called an *aura* 单纯部分性（癫痫）发作；**tonic s.**, one characterized by tonic but not clonic contractions 强直发作

se·lec·tion (sə-lek′shən) the play of forces that determines the relative reproductive performance of the various genotypes in a population 选择，决定种群中各种基因型的相对繁殖性能；**natural s.**, the survival in nature of those individuals and their progeny best equipped to adapt to environmental conditions 自然选择；**sexual s.**, natural selection in which certain characteristics attract male or female members of a species, thus ensuring survival of those characteristics 性选择

se·lec·tive (sə-lek′tiv) 1. having a high degree of selectivity 有选择力的；2. discriminating; making a choice from multiple alternatives; singling out in preference 选择的，挑选的

se·lec·tiv·i·ty (sə-lek-tiv′ĭ-te) in pharmacology, the degree to which a dose of a drug produces the desired effect in relation to adverse effects 选择性，在药理学上，指药物产生所需效应与不良效应的剂量关系

se·le·gil·ine (sə-lej′ə-lēn) an inhibitor of monoamine oxidase type B; adminstered transdermally in the treatment of major depressive disorder; also used orally as the hydrochloride salt in conjunction with levodopa and carbidopa as an antiparkinsonian agent 司来吉兰，一种 B 型单胺氧化酶抑制药；经皮给药治疗严重的抑郁症；其盐酸盐口服与左旋多巴和卡比多巴联合治疗帕金森病

se·le·ni·ous ac·id (sə-le′ne-əs) monohydrated selenium dioxide, a source of elemental selenium 亚硒酸

se·le·ni·um (Se) (sə-le′ne-əm) a nonmetallic element occurring in various allotropes; at. no. 34, at. wt. 78.96.; it is an essential mineral, forming the active center of several antioxidant enzymes 硒（化学元素）；**s. sulfide**, a topical antiseborrheic and antifungal, used in the treatment of seborrheic dermatitis and dandruff of the scalp and of tinea versicolor 硫化硒

self-an·ti·gen (self-an′tĭ-jən) autoantigen 自身抗原

self-lim·it·ed (self″lim′it-əd) limited by its own peculiarities and not by outside influence; said of a disease that runs a definite limited course 自身限制（性）的，（病程）自限的

self-tol·er·ance (self″tol′ər-əns) immunologic tolerance to self-antigens 自身耐受

sel·la (sel′ə) pl. *sel′lae* [L.] 1. a saddle-shaped depression 鞍形凹窝；2. s. turcica 蝶鞍；**sel′lar** *adj.*; **s. tur′cica**, a depression on the upper surface of the sphenoid bone, lodging the pituitary gland 蝶鞍，蝶骨体上面通过中线的横向凹窝，其内含有脑垂体

sem·a·phor·in (sem-ə-for′ĭn) a class of secreted, transmembrane, and GPI-linked proteins, defined by cysteine-rich semaphorin protein domains 信号素，一类分泌的、跨膜的和 GPI 连接的蛋白质，由富含半胱氨酸的信号蛋白结构域定义

se·men (se′mən) [L.] fluid discharged at ejaculation in the male, consisting of secretions of glands associated with the urogenital tract and containing spermatozoa 精液；**sem′inal** *adj.*

semi·ca·nal (sem″e-kə-nal′) a channel open at one

S

side 半管

semi·co·ma (sem″e-ko′mə) a stupor from which the patient may be aroused 轻昏迷、半昏迷; **semico′matose** adj.

semi·dom·i·nance (sem′e-dom′ĭ-nəns) in - complete dominance 半显性

semi·flex·ion (sem″e-flek′shən) position of a limb midway between flexion and extension; the act of bringing to such a position 半屈位

semi·lu·nar (sem″e-loo′nər) resembling a crescent or half-moon 半月形的

sem·i·nif·er·ous (sem″ĭ-nif′ər-əs) producing or conveying semen 生精子的、输精子的

sem·i·no·ma (sem″ĭ-no′mə) a radiosensitive, malignant neoplasm of the testis, thought to be derived from primordial germ cells of the sexually undifferentiated embryonic gonad 精原细胞瘤。Cf. *germinoma*; **classical s.**, the most common type, composed of well-differentiated sheets or cords of polygonal or round cells (seminoma cells) 典型精原细胞瘤; **ovarian s.**, dysgerminoma 卵巢精原细胞瘤; **spermatocytic s.**, a less malignant form characterized by cells resembling maturing spermatogonia with filamentous chromatin 精母细胞性精原细胞瘤

se·mi·nu·ria (se′mĭ-nu′re-ə) the presence of semen in the urine 精液尿

se·mi·ot·ic (se″me-ot′ik) 1. pertaining to signs or symptoms 症状的; 2. pathognomonic 特殊病征的

se·mi·ot·ics (se″me-ot′iks) symptomatology 症状学

semi·per·me·a·ble (sem″e-pur′me-ə-bəl) permitting passage only of certain molecules 半（渗）透性的

semi·quan·ti·ta·tive (sem″e-kwahn′tĭ-ta″tiv) yielding an approximation of the quantity or amount of a substance; between a qualitative and a quantitative result 半定量的

se·mis (ss.) (se′mis) [L.] half 半，一半

semi·sul·cus (sem″e-sul′kəs) a depression that, with an adjoining one, forms a sulcus 半沟，半月板的一种凹陷，与相邻的凹陷形成沟

semi·su·pi·na·tion (sem″e-soo″pĭ-na′shən) a position of partial supination 半仰卧位; 半旋后

semi·syn·thet·ic (sem″e-sin-thet′ik) produced by chemical manipulation of naturally occurring substances 半合成的

se·nes·cence (sə-nes′əns) the process of growing old, especially the condition resulting from the transitions and accumulations of the deleterious aging processes 衰老，老化

se·nile (se′nīl) pertaining to old age; manifesting senility 衰老的

se·nil·ism (se′nil-iz-əm) premature old age 早衰

se·nil·i·ty (sə-nil′ĭ-te) the physical and mental deterioration associated with old age 衰老

sen·na (sen′ə) the dried leaflets of *Cassia acutifolia* or *C. angustifolia;* used chiefly as a cathartic 番泻叶

sen·no·side (sen′o-sīd) either of two anthraquinone glucosides, sennoside A and B, found in senna as the calcium salts; a mixture of the two is used as a cathartic 番泻苷

sen·sa·tion (sen-sa′shən) an impression produced by impulses conveyed by an afferent nerve to the sensorium 感知，知觉; **girdle s.**, zonesthesia 束带感; **referred s., reflex s.**, one felt elsewhere than at the site of application of a stimulus 牵涉性感觉，反射性感觉; **subjective s.**, one perceptible only to the subject, and not connected with any object external to the body 主观感觉

sense (sens) 1. any of the physical processes by which stimuli are received, transduced, and conducted as impulses to be interpreted to the brain 一种物理过程，通过这种物理过程，刺激被接收、转导和传导为脉冲，并向大脑解释; 2. to perceive by one of these processes 感知上述过程; 3. in molecular genetics, referring to the strand of a nucleic acid that directly specifies the product 在分子遗传学中，指的是直接指定产物的核酸链; **body s.**, somatognosis 躯体觉; **color s.**, the faculty by which colors are perceived and distinguished 色觉; **s. of equilibrium,** the sense that maintains awareness of being or not being in an upright position, controlled by receptors in the vestibule of the ear 平衡觉; **joint s.,** arthresthesia 关节感觉; **kinesthetic s.,** 1. kinesthesia 运动觉; 2. 同 muscle s.; **light s.,** the sense by which degrees of brilliancy are distinguished 光觉; **motion s., movement s.,** the awareness of motion by the head or body 运动觉; **muscle s., muscular s.,** 1. sensory impressions, such as movement and stretch, that come from the muscles 肌肉感觉; 2. 同 movement s.; **pain s.,** the ability to feel pain, caused by stimulation of a nociceptor 痛觉; **position s., posture s.,** the awareness of the position of the body or its parts in space, a combination of the sense of equilibrium and kinesthesia 位置（感）觉; **pressure s.,** the sense by which pressure upon the surface of the body is perceived 压觉; **sixth s.,** somatognosis 第六感觉; **somatic s's,** senses other than the special senses, including touch, pressure, pain, and temperature, kinesthesia, muscle sense, visceral sense, and sometimes sense of equilibrium 躯体感觉; **space s.,** the sense by which relative positions and relations of objects in space are perceived 空间觉; **special s's,** those of seeing, hearing, taste, smell, and sometimes sense of equilibrium 特殊感觉; **stereognostic s.,** the sense by which form and solidity are perceived 实体觉；**temperature s.,** the sense by which differences of temperature are distinguished by the thermoreceptors 温度觉；**vestibular s.,** s. of equilibrium 前庭感；**vibration s.,** pallesthesia 震动觉；**visceral s.,** the awareness of sensations that arise from the viscera and stimulate the interoceptors; sensations include pain, pressure or fullness, and organ movement 内脏感觉

sen·si·bil·i·ty (sen″sĭ-bil′ĭ-te) susceptibility of feeling; ability to feel or perceive 敏感性；感觉，感觉能力；**deep s.,** sensibility to stimuli such as pain, pressure, and movement that activate receptors below the body surface but not in the viscera 深部感觉；**epicritic s.,** the sensibility of the skin to gentle stimulations permitting fine discriminations of touch and temperature 精细感觉（区别皮肤触觉和温度的能力）；**proprioceptive s.,** proprioception 本体感觉；**protopathic s.,** sensibility to pain and temperature that is low in degree and poorly localized 粗觉；**splanchnesthetic s.,** visceral sense 内脏感觉

sen·si·ble (sen′sĭ-bəl) 1. capable of sensation 感觉的能力；2. perceptible to the senses 能被感知的

sen·si·tive (sen′sĭ-tiv) 1. able to receive or respond to stimuli 能接受刺激或对刺激发生反应的；2. unusually responsive to stimulation, such as too quickly or acutely 敏感：常指对刺激反应异常，如过快的或迅猛的

sen·si·tiv·i·ty (sen″sĭ-tiv′ĭ-te) 1. the state or quality of being sensitive 感受性、敏感性；2. the smallest concentration of a substance that can be reliably measured by a given analytical method 分析敏感性，用特定分析方法可靠地测得最低的物质浓度；3. the probability that a person having a disease will be correctly identified by a clinical test 诊断敏感性，通过临床试验，正确鉴定某人患某病的条件概率

sen·si·ti·za·tion (sen″sĭ-tĭ-za′shən) 致敏（作用）；1. admin - istration of an antigen to an induce a primary immune response 给予抗原以诱导初级免疫反应；2. exposure to an allergen that results in the development of hypersensitivity 接触过敏原导致过敏 **autoerythrocyte s.,** 自体红细胞致敏，参见 *syndrome* 下 *painful bruising syndrome*

sen·si·tized (sen′sĭ-tīzd) rendered sensitiveu 致敏的

sen·so·mo·tor (sen″so-mo′tər) 同 sensorimotor

sen·so·ri·al (sen-sor′e-əl) pertaining to the sensorium 感觉中枢的

sen·so·ri·mo·tor (sen″sə-re-mo′tər) both sensory and motor 感觉运动的

sen·so·ri·neu·ral (sen″sə-re-noor′əl) of or pertaining to a sensory nerve or mechanism 感觉神经的

sen·so·ri·um (sən-sor′e-əm) 1. a sensory nerve center 感觉中枢；2. the state of an individual as regards consciousness or mental awareness 神志，感觉，知觉

sen·so·ry (sen′sə-re) pertaining to sensation 感觉的

sen·ti·ent (sen′she-ənt) able to feel; sensitive 能感觉的；敏感的

sen·ti·nel (sen′tĭ-nəl) an individual or object that gives a warning or indicates danger 发出警告或表示危险的个人或物体

Seph·a·dex (sef′ə-deks) trademark for crosslinked dextran beads. Various forms are used in chromatography 交联葡聚糖（商品名，作为分子筛色谱法的介质）

sep·sis (sep′sis) 1. presence in the blood or other tissues of pathogenic microorganisms or their toxins 脓毒症；2. 同 septicemia.; **catheter s.,** sepsis occurring as a complication of intravenous catheterization 导管脓毒症；**puerperal s.,** 产后脓毒症，参见 *fever* 下词条

sep·ta (sep′tə) [L.] 隔膜 *septum* 的复数

sep·tal (sep′təl) pertaining to a septum 中隔的，间隔的

sep·tate (sep′tāt) divided by a septum 有隔的，分隔的

sep·tec·to·my (sep-tek′tə-me) excision of part of the nasal septum 鼻中隔切除术

sep·tic (sep′tik) pertaining to sepsis 脓毒性的

sep·ti·ce·mia (sep″tĭ-se′me-ə) blood poisoning; systemic disease associated with the presence and persistence of pathogenic microorganisms or their toxins in the blood 败血症；**septice′mic adj.**; **cryptogenic s.,** septicemia in which the focus of infection is not evident during life 隐原性败血病；**puerperal s.,** 产后败血症，参见 *fever* 下词条

sep·ti·co·py·emia (sep″tĭ-ko-pi-e′me-ə) septicemia and pyemia combined 脓毒败血病；**septicopye′mic** *adj.*

sep·to·mar·gi·nal (sep″to-mahr′jĭ-nəl) pertaining to the margin of a septum 隔缘的

sep·to·na·sal (sep″to-na′zəl) pertaining to the nasal septum 鼻中隔的

sep·to·plas·ty (sep″to-plas″te) surgical reconstruction of the nasal septum 鼻中隔成形术

sep·tos·to·my (sep-tos′tə-me) surgical creation of an opening in a septum 隔膜造口术

sep·tot·o·my (sep-tot′ə-me) incision of the nasal septum 鼻中隔切开术

sep·tu·lum (sep′tu-ləm) pl. *sep′tula* [L.] a small separating wall or partition 小隔

sep·tum (sep′təm) pl. *sep′ta* [L.] a dividing wall or partition 中隔，间隔，隔膜；**alveolar s.,** interalveolar s. 参见 interalveolar s. **atrioventricular s.**

of heart, the part of the membranous portion of the interventricular septum between the left ventricle and the right atrium 房室隔 ; **Cloquet s., crural s., femoral s.,** the thin fibrous membrane that helps close the femoral ring 克洛凯氏隔，股环隔，帮助闭合股骨环的薄纤维膜 **gingival s.,** the part of the gingiva interposed between adjoining teeth 龈中隔 ; **interalveolar s.,** 1. one of the thin plates of bone separating the alveoli of the different teeth in the mandible and maxilla 牙槽中隔 ; 2. one of the thin septa separating adjacent pulmonary alveoli 肺泡隔 ; **interatrial s. of heart,** the partition separating the right and left atria of the heart 房间隔 ; **interdental s.,** interalveolar s. 参 见 interalveolar s. **interradicular s.,** 同 interalveolar s. (1); **interventricular s. of heart,** the partition separating the right and left ventricles of the heart 室 间 隔 ; **lingual s.,** the median vertical fibrous part of the tongue 舌中隔 ; **nasal s.,** the partition between the two nasal cavities 鼻中隔 ; **s. pectinifor′me,** 同 s. penis; **pellucid s., s. pellu′cidum,** the double membrane separating the anterior horns of the lateral ventricles of the brain 透明隔 ; **s. pe′nis,** the fibrous sheet between the corpora cavernosa of the penis 梳状隔 ; **s. pri′mum,** the first septum in the embryonic heart, dividing the primordial atrium into right and left chambers 第一房间隔 ; **rectovaginal s.,** the membranous partition between the rectum and vagina 直肠阴道隔 ; **rectovesical s.,** a membranous partition separating the rectum from the prostate and urinary bladder 直肠膀胱隔 ; **scrotal s.,** the partition between the two chambers of the scrotum 阴囊隔 ; **s. secun′dum,** the second septum in the embryonic heart, to the right of the septum primum; after birth it fuses with the septum primum to close the foramen ovale and form the interatrial septum 第二房间隔

sep·tup·let (sep-tup′lət) one of seven offspring produced at one birth 一胎七儿

se·que·la (sə-kwel′ə) pl. *seque′lae* [L.] a morbid condition following or occurring as a consequence of another condition or event 后遗症，后发病，遗患；又称 *sequel*

se·quence (se′kwəns) 1. a connected series of events or things 一系列相互联系的事件或事物；2. in dysmorphology, a pattern of multiple anomalies derived from a single prior anomaly or mechanical factor 系列畸形，畸形学上，指已知的或设想的一个异常或机械因素衍生的多发异常；3. the order of arrangement of residues or constituents in a biologic polymer, such as the order of nucleotides in DNA or RNA, or of amino acids in a protein 生物聚合物中残基或组分的排列顺序，如 DNA 或 RNA 中核苷酸的排列顺序，或蛋白质中氨基酸

的排列顺序；4. a specific fragment or segment of a biologic polymer, with a known arrangement of its residues 生物聚合物的特定片段，具有其残基的已知排列；5. to ascertain the order of the residues of a biologic polymer 确定生物聚合物残留的顺序；**amniotic band s.,** early rupture of the amnion with formation of strands of amnion that may adhere to or compress parts of the fetus, resulting in a wide variety of deformities 羊膜索系列畸形，羊膜早期破裂，形成羊膜束，可能粘附或压缩胎儿的部分，导致各种畸形；**insertion s. (IS),** a small bacterial transposable element encoding transposition functions and terminating in inverted repeated sequences; it can act alone, or a pair can form the ends of a more complex transposon 插入序列，一种编码换位功能并以反向重复序列终止的小的细菌转座元件；它可以单独作用，也可以形成一对更复杂的转座子；**oligohydramnios s.,** a group of anomalies, usually fatal shortly after birth, caused by compression of the fetus secondary to oligohydramnios, which may result from renal agenesis or other urinary tract defects or from leakage of amniotic fluid; infants have characteristic flattened facies *(Potter facies),* skeletal abnormalities, and often hypoplasia of the lungs 羊水过少序列征，一组由羊水过少导致胎儿压迫的异常现象，通常在出生后不久死亡，可能由肾发育不全或其他尿路缺陷或羊水渗漏引起；婴儿具有特征性的扁平面容（波特相），骨骼异常，常有肺发育不全；**Pierre Robin s.,** Pierre Robin syndrome; a congenital triad of micrognathia, cleft palate, and glossoptosis, occurring alone or in combination with another syndrome 罗班序列征，皮埃尔·罗班综合征，先天性三联症，腭裂和神经胶质细胞凋亡，单独发生或与另一种综合征联合发生

se·ques·ter (sə-kwes′tər) 1. to detach or separate abnormally a small portion from the whole 使隔离；*sequestration* 和 *sequestrum*; 2. to isolate a constituent of a chemical system by chelation or other means 螯合

se·ques·trant (sə-kwes′trənt) a sequestering agent, as, for example, cholestyramine resin, which binds bile acids in the intestine, thus preventing their absorption 多价螯合剂，如胆甾醇胺树脂，它能使胆汁酸在肠内结合，从而阻止它们的吸收

se·ques·tra·tion (se″kwəs-tra′shən) 1. the formation of a sequestrum 死骨形成；2. the isolation of a patient 隔离（病人）；3. a net increase in the quantity of blood within a limited vascular area, occurring physiologically, with forward flow persisting or not, or produced artificially by the application of tourniquets 血管内血量净增，局部血管内血量净增或为生理情况，或为用止血带造成的；**pulmo-**

nary s., loss of connection of lung tissue with the bronchial tree and the pulmonary veins 肺隔离，肺组织与支气管树和肺静脉连接丢失

se·ques·trec·to·my (se″kwəs-trek′tə-me) excision of a sequestrum 死骨摘除术

se·ques·trum (sə-kwes′trəm) pl. *seques'tra* [L.] 1. any sequestered tissue 任何隔离组织；2. a piece of dead bone separated from the sound bone in the process of necrosis 骨坏死过程中，自健康骨骨分离的死骨片

se·quoi·o·sis (se″kwoi-o′sis) hypersensitivity pneumonitis due to inhalation of and tissue reaction to dust from moldy redwood bark 过敏性肺泡炎，由于吸入和组织对发霉的红木树皮灰尘的反应引起的红斑狼疮过敏性肺炎

Ser serine 丝氨酸

se·ra (se′rə) [L.] *serum* 的复数

se·ries (sēr′ēz) a group or succession of events, objects, or substances arranged in regular order or forming a kind of chain; in electricity, parts of a circuit connected successively end to end to form a single path for the current 连续、系列；系、列、组、族、型；串联；**se'rial** *adj.*; **erythrocytic s.**, the succession of morphologically distinguishable cells that are stages in erythrocyte development: proerythroblast, basophilic erythroblast, polychromatophilic erythroblast, orthochromatic erythroblast, reticulocyte, and erythrocyte 红细胞系；**granulocytic s.**, the succession of morphologically distinguishable cells that are stages in granulocyte development; there are distinct basophil, eosinophil, and neutrophil series, but the morphologic stages are the same 粒细胞系；**lymphocytic s.**, a series of morphologically distinguishable cells once thought to represent stages in lymphocyte development; now known to represent various forms of mature lymphocytes 淋巴细胞系；**monocytic s.**, the succession of developing cells that ultimately culminates in the monocyte 单核细胞系；**thrombocytic s.**, the succession of developing cells that ultimately culminates in the blood platelets (thrombocytes) 血小板系；

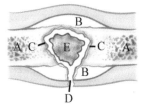

▲ 死骨的形成：**A**，健骨；**B**，新骨；**C**，包被上的肉芽；**D**，窦道；**E**，死骨

ser·ine (Ser) (S) (sēr′ēn) a naturally occurring nonessential amino acid present in many proteins 丝氨酸

ser·mo·rel·in (sur″mo-rel′in) a synthetic peptide corresponding to a portion of growth hormone–releasing hormone; used as the acetate salt in the treatment of growth hormone deficiency 一种与生长激素释放激素的一部分相对应的合成肽，其醋酸盐用于治疗生长激素缺乏

se·ro·con·ver·sion (sēr″o-kən-vur′zhən) the change of serologic test results from negative to positive, indicating development of antibodies in response to immunization or infection 血清转化，血清学检查结果由阴性变为阳性，表明免疫或感染后抗体产生

se·ro·di·ag·no·sis (sēr″o-di″əg-no′sis) diagnosis of disease based on serologic tests 血清学诊断，基于血清学试验的疾病诊断；**serodiagnos'tic** *adj.*

se·ro·en·ter·i·tis (sēr″o-en″tə-ri′tis) inflammation of the serous coat of the intestine 肠浆膜炎

se·ro·fib·rin·ous (sēr″o-fi′brin-əs) composed of serum and fibrin, as is a serofibrinous exudate 浆液纤维蛋白性的

se·ro·group (sēr′o-groop) 血清群 1. an unofficial designation denoting a group of bacteria containing a common antigen, possibly including more than one serovar, species, or genus 含有共同抗原的一群细菌，可能包括一种或一属以上的血清型，血清型是一种暂定非正式名称；2. a group of viral species that are closely related antigenically 在抗原上密切相关的一群病毒种

se·rol·o·gy (sēr-ol′ə-je) the study of antigenantibody reactions in vitro 血清学，在体外研究抗体抗原反应的科学；**serolog'ic, serolog'ical** *adj.*

se·ro·ma (sēr-o′mə) a tumorlike collection of serum in the tissues 血清肿，组织内有肿瘤样的血清血液性积液

se·ro·mem·bra·nous (sēr″o-mem′brə-nəs) pertaining to or composed of serous membrane 浆液膜性的，浆膜的

se·ro·mu·cous (sēr″o-mu′kəs) both serous and mucous 浆液黏液性的

se·ro·mus·cu·lar (sēr″o-mus′ku-lər) pertaining to the serous and muscular coats of the intestine (肠道) 浆膜肌膜的

se·ro·neg·a·tive (sēr″o-neg′ə-tiv) showing negative results on serologic examination; showing a lack of antibody 血清阴性的

se·ro·pos·i·tive (sēr″o-poz′ĭ-tiv) showing positive results on serologic examination; showing a high level of antibody 血清阳性的

se·ro·pu·ru·lent (sēr″o-pu′roo-lənt) both serous and purulent 浆液脓性的

S

se·ro·re·ac·tion (sēr″o-re-ak′shən) a reaction occurring in serum or as a result of the action of a serum 血清反应

se·ro·re·ver·sion (sēr″o-re-ver′zhən) spontaneous or induced conversion from a seropositive to a sero-negative state 血清还原，自发或诱导的从血清阳性状态到血清阴性状态的转变

se·ro·sa (sē-ro′sə) (sēr-o′zə) tunica serosa; the membrane lining the external walls of the body cavities and reflected over the surfaces of protruding organs; it secretes a watery exudate 浆膜；**sero′sal** adj.

se·ro·san·guin·e·ous (sēr″o-sang-gwin′e-əs) composed of serum and blood 血清血液的

se·ro·se·rous (sēr″o-sēr′əs) pertaining to two or more serous membranes 浆膜与浆膜的

se·ro·si·tis (sēr″o-si′tis) pl. serosi′tides. Inflammation of a serous membrane 浆膜炎

se·ro·sur·vey (sēr″o-sur′va) a screening test of the serum of persons at risk to determine susceptibility to a particular disease 血清学调查

se·ro·ther·a·py (sēr″o-ther′ə-pe) treatment of infectious disease by injection of immune serum or antitoxin 血清疗法

sero·to·nin (ser″o-to′nin) a hormone and neuro-transmitter, 5-hydroxytryptamine (5-HT), found in many tissues, including blood platelets, intestinal mucosa, the pineal body, and the central nervous system; it has many physiologic properties, including inhibition of gastric secretions, stimulation of smooth muscles, and production of vasoconstriction 5-羟色胺，血清素

sero·to·nin·er·gic (ser″o-to″nin-ur′jik) 1. containing or activated by serotonin 含血清素的；血清素激活的；2. pertaining to neurons that secrete serotonin 分泌血清素的神经元的

se·ro·type (sēr′o-tīp″) 1. the type of a microorganism determined by its constituent antigens; a taxonomic subdivision based thereon 血清分型；2. 同 serovar

se·rous (sēr′əs) 1. pertaining to or resembling serum 血清的；2. producing or containing serum 浆液的

se·ro·vac·ci·na·tion (sēr″o-vak″sĭ-na′shən) injection of serum combined with bacterial vaccination to produce passive immunity by the former and active immunity by the latter 血清疫苗接种

se·ro·var (sēr′o-var) a taxonomic subdivision of bacteria based on the kinds and combinations of constituent antigens present in the cell 血清型，又称 serotype

ser·pig·i·nous (sər-pij′ĭ-nəs) creeping; having a wavy or much indented border 匐行的，匐行性的

ser·pin (sur′pin) any of a superfamily of serine protease inhibitors, found in plasma and tissues; they are homologous single-chain glycoproteins targeting specific serine proteases involved in coagulation, complement activation, fibrinolysis, inflammation, and tissue remodeling 丝氨酸抑制蛋白，血浆和组织中发现的任何丝氨酸蛋白酶抑制药超家族；它们是同源的单链糖蛋白，靶向参与凝血、补体激活、纤维蛋白溶解、炎症和组织重塑的特定丝氨酸蛋白酶

ser·rat·ed (ser′āt-ed) having a sawlike edge 锯齿状

Ser·ra·tia (sə-ra′she-ə) a genus of bacteria made up of motile gram-negative rods that produce a white, pink, or red pigment. For the most part, they are free-living saprophytes, but they cause a variety of infections in immunocompromised patients 沙雷菌属，由活动的革兰阴性杆菌组成的一个细菌属，产生白色、粉色或红色色素。在大多数情况下，它们是自由生活的腐生细胞，但它们会引起免疫综合征患者的各种感染

ser·ra·tion (sə-ra′shən) 1. the state of being serrated 锯齿状；2. a serrated structure or formation 锯齿构造

ser·tra·line (sur′trə-lēn) a selective serotonin reuptake inhibitor used as the hydrochloride salt in the treatment of depression, obsessive-compulsive disorder, and panic disorder 舍曲林，一种 5-羟色胺再摄取的选择性抑制药，其盐酸盐用于治疗抑郁症、强迫症和惊恐障碍

se·rum (sēr′əm) pl. serums, se′ra [L.] 1. the clear portion of any liquid separated from its more solid elements 浆液，指任何体液中与有形成份分离的透明部分；2. 同 blood s.; 3. antiserum 抗血清，**antilymphocyte s. (ALS),** antiserum derived from animals immunized against human lymphocytes; a powerful nonspecific immunosuppressive agent that causes destruction of circulating lymphocytes 抗淋巴细胞血清；**antirabies s.,** antiserum obtained from the blood serum or plasma of animals immunized with rabies vaccine; used for postexposure prophylaxis against rabies if rabies immune globulin is unavailable 抗狂犬病血清；**blood s.,** the clear liquid that separates from blood when it is allowed to clot completely, and is therefore blood plasma from which fibrogen has been removed during clotting 血清；**foreign s.,** 同 heterologous s.; **heterologous s.,** 异种血清 1. that obtained from an animal belonging to a species different from that of the recipient 从与受体不同种属动物制取的血清；2. that prepared from an animal immunized by an organism differing from that against which it is to be used 从经某种有机体免疫动物制取的血清，该有机体与此血清用来对抗的有机体不同；**homol-**

ogous s., 同种血清 1. that obtained from an animal belonging to the same species as the recipient 从与受体同一种属的动物制取的血清；2. that prepared from an animal immunized by the same organism against which it is to be used 从经某种细菌免疫动物制备的血清，该菌与血清所对抗的致病菌相同；**immune s.**, antiserum 免疫血清；**polyvalent s.**, antiserum containing antibody to more than one kind of antigen 多价血清；**pooled s.**, the mixed serum from a number of individuals 混合血清

se·ru·mal (sēr-oo′məl) pertaining to or formed from serum 血清的

se·rum-fast (sēr′əm-fast″) resistant to the effects of serum 抗血清的

ses·a·moid (ses′ə-moid) 1. denoting a small nodular bone embedded in a tendon or joint capsule 籽样的，种子样的，指腱或关节囊内的骨性小结节的；2. a sesamoid bone 籽骨

ses·sile (ses′il) attached by a broad base, as opposed to being pedunculated or stalked 无柄的，无蒂的；固定的

se·ta·ceous (se-ta′shəs) bristlelike 刚毛状的

Se·ta·ria (se-tar′e-ə) a genus of filarial nematodes 鬃丝虫属

set-point (set′point) the target value of a controlled variable that is maintained physiologically by bodily control mechanisms for homeostasis 调定点，自控系统维持的控制变量的目标值

se·vel·a·mer (sə-vel′ə-mər) a phosphate-binding substance used as the hydrochloride salt to reduce serum phosphorus concentrations in hyperphosphatemia associated with end-stage renal disease 一种磷酸盐结合剂，用于降低终末期肾病相关的高磷酸盐血症中的血清磷浓度

sex (seks) 1. a distinctive character of most animals and plants, based on the type of gametes produced by the gonads, ova (macrogametes) being typical of the female and spermatozoa (microgametes) of the male, or the category in which the individual is placed on such a basis 性别，性；2. 性别认同，参见 *identity* 下 *gender identity*；3. sexual intercourse 性交；4. to determine whether an organism is male or female 区别（生物体的性别）；**chromosomal s.**, **genetic s.**, sex as determined by the presence of the XX (female) or the XY (male) genotype, without regard to phenotypic manifestations 染色体性别，遗传性别；**gonadal s.**, that part of the phenotypic sex that is determined by the gonadal tissue present (ovarian or testicular) 性腺性别；**morphologic s.**, that part of the phenotypic sex that is determined by the morphology of the external genitals 形态性别；**phenotypic s.**, the phenotypic manifestations of sex determined by endocrine in-

fluences 表型性别

sex·duc·tion (seks-duk′shən) the process whereby part of the bacterial chromosome is attached to the autonomous F (sex) factor and thus is transferred from donor (male) bacterium to recipient (female) 性导，在细菌遗传中，指一种性遗传过程，部分细菌染色体附着于常染色体 F 因子（性因子），从而以高频率从授体（雄性）细菌转移到受体（雌性）细菌

sex-in·flu·enced (seks-in′floo-ənst) pertaining to a trait carried on an autosome but expressed differently, in either frequency or degree, in males and females, e.g., androgenetic alopecia 从性的

sex-lim·it·ed (seks-lim′it-əd) pertaining to a trait caried on an autosome but expressed in one sex only, e.g., lactation 限性的，限于一性的

sex-linked (seks′linkt) carried on one of the sex chromosomes, as a gene; by extension, sexually determined, as an inherited trait determined by such a gene 性联锁的

sex·ol·o·gy (sek-sol′ə-je) the scientific study of sex and sexual relations 性学

sex·tup·let (seks-tup′lət) any one of six offspring produced at the same birth 六胎儿

sex·u·al (sek′shoo-əl) 1. pertaining to, characterized by, involving, or endowed with sex, sexuality, the sexes, or the sex organs and their functions 性的；2. characterized by the property of maleness or femaleness 两性的；3. pertaining to reproduction involving both male and female gametes 生殖的；4. implying or symbolizing erotic desires or activity 性欲的

sex·u·al·i·ty (sek″shoo-al′ĭ-te) 1. the characteristic of the male and female reproductive elements 性别；2. the constitution of an individual in relation to sexual attitudes and behavior 性欲；**infantile s.**, in freudian theory, the erotic life of infants and children, encompassing the oral, anal, and phallic stages of psychosexual development 幼稚性欲，据弗洛伊德学说，婴儿和儿童的性活动，包括心理发育的口欲期、肛欲期和阳具期

SGOT serum glutamic-oxaloacetic transaminase 血清谷氨酸草酰乙酸转氨酶，参见 *aspartate transaminase*

SGPT serum glutamic-pyruvic transaminase 血清谷氨酸丙酮酸转氨酶，参见 *alanine transaminase*

shad·ow-cast·ing (shad′o-kast′ing) application of a coating of gold, chromium, or other metal to ultramicroscopic structures to increase their visibility under the microscope 阴影定型，定影法，将金、铬或其他金属涂层涂覆到超显微结构上以增加其在显微镜下的可见度

shaft (shaft) a long slender part, such as the diaph-

S

ysis of a long bone 干，柄，体，轴

shag·gy (shag′e) 1. covered with, having, or resembling rough long hair or wool 长有或类似粗糙的长毛或羊毛的 ; 2. having a rough texture or surface or hairlike processes 有粗糙的纹理、表面或毛发状突起的

sham (sham) 1. a hoax; a fraudulent imitation 假冒，骗子 ; 2. not genuine; fraudulent; marked by falseness 假的，虚伪的

sha·man·ism (shah′-) (sha′mə-niz″əm) a traditional system, occurring in tribal societies, in which certain individuals (shamans) are believed to be gifted with access to an invisible spiritual world and are able to mediate between it and the physical world to heal, divine, and affect events in the latter 萨满教

shank (shangk) 1. leg (1) 小腿 ; 2. crus (2) 脚

shap·ing (shāp′ing) a technique in behavior therapy in which new behavior is produced by providing reinforcement for progressively closer approximations of the final desired behavior 塑造法，用于行为疗法的一种操作性条件反射技术，通过循序渐进以接近最后要求的方法产生新行为

shave (shāv) 1. to cut at or parallel to the surface of the skin 擦 过 ; 2. to remove the beard or other body hair by such a process 剃，刮 ; 3. to cut thin slices from or to cut into thin slices 削去……的薄薄一层

SHBG sex hormone–binding globulin 性激素结合球蛋白

sheath (shēth) a tubular case or envelope 护套；鞘；**arachnoid s.,** the continuation of the arachnoidea mater around the optic nerve, forming part of its internal sheath 蛛网膜鞘；**carotid s.,** a portion of the cervical fascia enclosing the carotid artery, the internal jugular vein, and the vagus nerve 颈动脉鞘；**crural s.,** 同 femoral s.；**dentinal s.,** the layer of tissue forming the wall of a dentinal tubule 牙质小管鞘；**dural s.,** the external investment of the optic nerve 硬脑膜鞘；**femoral s.,** the investing fascia of the proximal portion of the femoral vessels 股鞘；**Henle s.,** endoneurium Henle 鞘；**Hertwig s.,** root s. (1) 赫特维希上皮根鞘；**s. of Key and Retzius,** endoneurium Key-Retzius 结缔组织鞘；**lamellar s.,** the perineurium 神经束膜；**Mauthner s.,** axolemma Mauthner 鞘；**medullary s., myelin s.,** the sheath surrounding the axon of myelinated nerve cells, consisting of concentric layers of myelin formed in the peripheral nervous system by the plasma membrane of Schwann cells, and in the central nervous system by oligodendrocytes. It is interrupted at intervals along the length of the axon by gaps known as *nodes of Ranvier*. Myelin is an electrical insulator that serves to speed the conduction of nerve impulses 髓 鞘；**periarterial lymphatic s., periarteriolar lymphoid s. (PALS),** any of the sheaths of lymphatic tissue surrounding the splenic arteries, mainly composed of T lymphocytes and at intervals expanding to form the malpighian corpuscles; together they compose the white pulp of the spleen 动脉周围淋巴鞘；**pial s.,** the continuation of the pia mater around the optic nerve, forming part of its internal sheath 软膜鞘；**root s.,** 1. an investment of epithelial cells around the unerupted tooth and inside the dental follicle 根鞘，位于未出牙的周围及由齿釉质组织分化的牙囊内侧的一种上皮细胞膜 ; 2. the epithelial layer of a hair follicle, divided into an *inner* and an *outer root sheath* 毛囊的上皮部分，可分为内根鞘和产生皮脂腺的外根鞘；**s. of Schwann,** neurilemma Schwann 鞘，神经鞘；**synovial s.,** a double-layered, fibrous sheath with synovial fluid present between the layers, such as surrounds a tendon 滑膜鞘；**tendon s.,** the fibrous sheath covering a tendon 肌腱鞘

sheet (shēt) 1. an oblong piece of cotton, linen, etc., for a bed covering 单 ; 2. any structure resembling such a covering 类似于这种覆盖物的任何结构；**draw s.,** one folded and placed under a patient's body so it may be removed with minimal disturbance of the patient 抽单，折叠放在病人身体下面，以便在病人不受干扰的情况下取出

shen (shen) one of the basic substances that according to traditional Chinese medicine pervade the body, usually translated "spirit," encompassing both the mind of the individual and healthy mental and physical function 神，根据中医说法，它包含了个体的精神和健康的身心功能

shi·at·su (she-ot′soo) [Japanese] a Japanese form of acupressure, in which pressure is applied using the thumb, elbow, or knee, perpendicularly to the skin at acupoints, combined with passive stretching and rotation of the joints 日本的一种穴位按压法，用拇指、肘部或膝盖在穴位垂直于皮肤施加压力，结合被动伸展和关节旋转

shield (shēld) any protecting structure 盾，罩，屏；防护物；**Buller s.,** a watch glass fitted over the eye to guard it from infection Buller 眼罩，为保护眼睛，防止感染用的刚好遮住眼睛的一种玻璃罩；**nipple s.,** a device to protect the nipple of a nursing woman 乳头罩，用于保护哺乳妇女的乳头

shift (shift) a change or deviation 替换；转移；移 位 ; **chloride s.,** the exchange of chloride (Cl^-) and bicarbonate (HCO_3^-) between plasma and the erythrocytes occurring whenever HCO_3^- is generated

or decomposed within the erythrocytes 氯离子转移；
Doppler s., the magnitude of frequency change due to the Doppler effect 多普勒频移；**s. to the left**, an increase in the percentage of neutrophils having only one or a few lobes 核左移；**s. to the right**, an increase in the percentage of multilobed neutrophils 核右移

Shi·gel·la (shĭ-gel′ə) a genus of gram-negative, facultatively anaerobic bacteria of the family Enterobacteriaceae; its members cause dysentery. It contains the species *S. boy′dii*, *S. dysente′riae*, *S. flexne′ri*, and *S. son′nei* 志贺菌属

shi·gel·la (shĭ-gel′ə) pl. *shigel′lae*. An individual organism of the genus *Shigella* 志贺菌

shi·gel·lo·sis (shĭ′gə-lo′sis) intestinal infection with *Shigella*, such as bacillary dysentery 志贺菌病

shin (shin) the prominent anterior edge of the tibia or the leg 胫，胫部；**saber s.**, marked anterior convexity of the tibia, seen in congenital syphilis and in yaws 军刀状胫，胫骨前凸，见于先天性梅毒和雅司病

shin·gles (shing′gəlz) herpes zoster 带状疱疹

shiv·er·ing (shiv′ər-ing) 1. involuntary shaking of the body, as with cold 战栗，肌肉收缩引起的不随意颤抖，如在寒冷天气；2. a disease of horses, with trembling or quivering of various muscles 肌肉异常抽搐，一种马病

shock (shok) 1. a sudden disturbance of mental equilibrium 冲击，心理平衡的突然紊乱；2. a profound hemodynamic and metabolic disturbance due to failure of the circulatory system to maintain adequate perfusion of vital organs 休克，以血液循环系统不能维持生命器官的充分灌注为特征的严重血液动力性及代谢性障碍；**anaphylactic s.**, shock occurring as a consequence of anaphylaxis 过敏性休克；**cardiogenic s.**, shock resulting from inadequate cardiac function, as from myocardial infarction or mechanical obstruction; characteristics include hypovolemia, hypotension, cold skin, weak pulse, and confusion 心源性休克，心脏功能不全引起的休克，如心肌梗死或机械性梗阻，特征包括低血容量、低血压、皮肤寒冷、脉搏无力和精神混乱；**endotoxic s., endotoxin s.**, septic shock due to release of endotoxins by gram-negative bacteria 内毒素性休克，由革兰阴性菌释放的内毒素引起的败血症性休克；**hypovolemic s.**, shock due to insufficient blood volume, either from hemorrhage or other loss of fluid or from widespread vasodilation so that normal blood volume cannot maintain tissue perfusion; symptoms are like those of cardiogenic shock 低血容量性休克，由于血容量不足引起的休克，可能是由于出血或其他液体损失，也可能是由于广泛的血管扩张导致正常血

容量不能维持组织灌注；症状与心源性休克相似；**insulin s.**, a hypoglycemic reaction to overdosage of insulin, a skipped meal, or strenuous exercise in an insulin-dependent diabetic, with tremor, dizziness, cool moist skin, hunger, and tachycardia, sometimes progressing to coma and convulsions 胰岛素休克，胰岛素依赖性患者胰岛素过量、误餐或剧烈运动的一种低血糖反应；早期症状是震颤、兴奋、头晕、皮肤湿冷、饥饿及心动过速，如不治疗，可发展为昏迷及惊厥；**septic s.**, shock associated with overwhelming infection, most commonly infection with gram-negative bacteria, thought to result from the actions of endotoxins and other products of the infectious agent that cause sequestration of blood in the capillaries and veins 败血性休克，与重度感染有关的休克，最常见的是革兰阴性细菌的感染，有人认为是内毒素或传染原的其他产物作用于血管系统，使大量血液淤积在毛细血管和静脉中；**serum s.**, anaphylactic shock resulting from administration of foreign serum to a sensitized individual 血清性休克，对致敏个体血清所致的过敏性休克

shot·ty (shot′e) like shot; resembling the pellets used in shotgun cartridges; as to describe the feel of lymph nodes during palpation 像弹丸的，用来描述触诊时淋巴结的感觉

shoul·der (shōl′dər) the area where the arm joins the trunk and the clavicle meets the scapula 肩；**frozen s.**, adhesive capsulitis 冻肩

shoul·der-blade (shōl′dər-blād) 同 scapula

show (sho) 1. a tiny amount or appearance of something 显露；外观；2. 同 bloody s.；**bloody s.**, vaginal discharge of blood-tinged mucus, usually meaning that the cervix has begun to dilate and the onset of labor is imminent 见红，分娩的前兆出血；

shunt (shunt) 1. to turn to one side; to bypass 移（或）转向一边；绕过；2. a passage or anastomosis between two natural channels, especially between blood vessels, formed physiologically or anomalously 分流，两自然管道尤其是血管间的通路；这类结构可能是生理上或结构异常形成的；3. a surgically created anastomosis; also, the operation of forming a shunt 吻合，一种通过外科手术建立的吻合，或一种作成旁路的手术；**arteriovenous s.**, 1. arteriovenous anastomosis (1) 动静脉短路；2. a U-shaped plastic tube inserted between an artery and a vein; usually to allow repeated access to the arterial system for hemodialysis 插入动脉和静脉之间的 U 形塑料管，通常允许反复进入动脉系统进行血液透析；**Blalock-Taussig s.**, 布莱洛克 - 陶西格分流术，参见 *operation* 下词条；**cardiovascular s.**, diversion of the blood flow through an anomalous opening from the left side of the heart to the right side or from the systemic to the pulmonary circulation *(left-to-right s.),* or from the right side to the left side or from the pulmonary to the systemic circulation *(right-to-left s.)* 心肺分流，从心脏左侧到右侧，或从体循环到肺循环（左向右分流），或从右侧到左侧，或从肺到体循环（右向左分流）；**left-to-right s.**, 左向右分流，参见 *cardiovascular s.*; **LeVeen s.**, 同 peritoneovenous s.; **peritoneovenous s.**, a surgically implanted subcutaneous plastic tube for continuous shunting of ascites fluid from the peritoneal cavity to the jugular vein; a pressureactivated valve buried in the abdominal wall ensures one-way flow 腹腔静脉分流术；**portacaval s.**, surgical anastomosis of the portal vein and the vena cava 门腔静脉分流术；**right-to-left s.**, 右向左分流，参见 *cardiovascular s.*; **splenorenal s.**, removal of the spleen with anastomosis of the splenic vein to the left renal vein 脾肾分流术；**ventriculoatrial s.**, the surgical creation of a communication between a cerebral ventricle and a cardiac atrium by means of a plastic tube, to permit drainage of cerebrospinal fluid for relief of hydrocephalus 脑室心房分流术；**ventriculoperitoneal s.**, a communication between a cerebral ventricle and the peritoneum by means of plastic tubing; done for the relief of hydrocephalus 脑室腹膜分流术

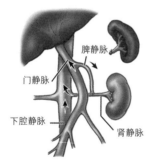

▲ 脾肾分流术

SI Système International d'Unités, or International System of Units 国际单位制，参见 *unit* 下 *SI unit*

Si silicon 元素硅的符号

SIADH syndrome of inappropriate antidiuretic hormone 抗利尿激素分泌失调综合征

si·al·ad·e·ni·tis (si″əl-ad′ə-ni′tis) inflammation of a salivary gland 涎腺炎

si·al·ad·e·no·ma (si″əl-ad″ə-no′mə) a benign tumor of the salivary glands 涎腺瘤

si·al·ad·e·nop·a·thy (si″əl-ad″ən-op′ə- the) 同 sialadenosis

si·al·ad·e·no·sis (si″əl-ad″ə-no′sis) sialadenopa-

thy; a disease of a salivary gland 唾液腺肿大症

si·al·a·gogue (si-al′ə-gog) an agent that stimulates the flow of saliva 催涎剂；**sialagog′ic** *adj.*

si·al·ec·ta·sia (si″əl-ek-ta′zhə) dilatation of a salivary duct 涎管扩张

si·al·ic ac·id (si-al′ik) any of a group of acetylated derivatives of neuraminic acid; they occur in many polysaccharides, glycoproteins, and glycolipids in animals and bacteria 唾液酸

si·al·i·dase (si-al′ĭ-dās) neuraminidase 唾液酸酶

si·al·i·do·sis (si-al″ĭ-do′sis) an autosomal recessive lysosomal storage disorder caused by mutation in the gene encoding neuraminidase. There is a less severe type I form, with later onset, myoclonus, ocular cherry red spot with progressive loss of visual acuity, and storage of sialyloligosaccharides. The more severe type II form additionally shows somatic abnormalities, coarse facies, and dysostosis multiplex; it occurs as several variants, infantile and congenital, of increased severity with earlier age of onset 涎酸贮积症，一种由编码神经氨酸酶的基因突变引起的常染色体隐性溶酶体储存障碍。I 型较轻，起病晚，肌阵挛，眼樱桃红斑，视力逐渐丧失，唾液低寡糖储存。更严重的 II 型表现为躯体畸形、粗糙面容和骨发育不全，多发性；多发性变种，婴儿和先天性变种，发病年龄越早，其严重程度越高

si·a·li·tis (si″ə-li′tis) inflammation of a salivary gland or duct 涎腺（或涎管）炎

si·a·lo·ad·e·nec·to·my (si″ə-lo-ad″ə-nek′tə- me) excision of a salivary gland 涎腺切除术

si·a·lo·ad·e·ni·tis (si″ə-lo-ad″ə-ni′tis) 同 sialadenitis

si·a·lo·ad·e·not·o·my (si″ə-lo-ad″ə-not′o- me) incision and drainage of a salivary gland 涎腺切开引流术

si·a·lo·aer·oph·a·gy (si″ə-lo-ār-of′ə-je) the swallowing of saliva and air 咽气涎癖

si·a·lo·an·gi·ec·ta·sis (si″ə-lo-an″je-ek′tə- sis) sialectasia 涎管扩张

si·a·lo·an·gi·itis (si″ə-lo-an″je-i′tis) sialoductitis; inflammation of a salivary duct 涎管炎

si·a·lo·an·gi·og·ra·phy (si″ə-lo-an″je-og′rə- fe) radiography of the ducts of the salivary glands after injection of a radiopaque medium 涎管放射造影术

si·a·lo·cele (si′ə-lo-sēl″) a salivary cyst 涎腺囊肿

si·a·lo·do·chi·tis (si″ə-lo-do-ki′tis) 同 sialoangiitis

si·a·lo·do·cho·plas·ty (si″ə-lo-do′ko-plas″te) plastic repair of a salivary duct 涎管成形术

si·a·lo·duc·ti·tis (si″ə-lo-dək-ti′tis) 同 sialoangiitis

si·a·log·e·nous (si″ə-loj′ə-nəs) producing saliva 生涎的

si·a·log·ra·phy (si″ə-log′rə-fe) 同 sialoangiography

si·a·lo·lith (si-al′o-lith) a calcareous concretion or calculus in the salivary ducts or glands, usually the submaxillary gland and its duct 涎石，涎腺体或涎管内的一种结石，最常见于颌下腺体及腺管

si·a·lo·li·thi·a·sis (si″ə-lo-lĭ-thi′ə-sis) the formation of salivary calculi 涎石病

si·a·lo·li·thot·o·my (si″ə-lo-lĭ-thot′ə-me) excision of a salivary calculus 涎石摘除术

si·a·lo·meta·pla·sia (si″ə-lo-met″ə-pla′zhə) metaplasia of the salivary glands 涎腺化生；**necrotizing s.**, a benign inflammatory condition of the salivary glands, simulating mucoepidermoid and squamous cell carcinoma 坏死性涎腺化生，一种小腺体的良性炎症病变，类似黏液表皮样及磷状细胞癌

si·a·lo·mu·cin (si″ə-lo-mu′sin) a mucin whose carbohydrate groups contain sialic acid 唾液酸黏蛋白

si·a·lor·rhea (si″ə-lo-re′ə) ptyalism 流涎

si·a·los·che·sis (si″ə-los′kə-sis) suppression of secretion of saliva 涎液分泌抑制

si·a·lo·ste·no·sis (si″ə-lo-stə-no′sis) stenosis of a salivary duct 涎管狭窄

si·a·lo·sy·rinx (si″ə-lo-sir′inks) 1. salivary fistula 涎腺瘘；2. a syringe for washing out the salivary ducts, or a drainage tube for the salivary ducts 涎管注射器，涎管引流管

sib (sib) 1. a blood relative; one of a group of persons all descended from a common ancestor 亲族；2. 同 sibling

sib·i·lant (sib′ĭ-lənt) whistling or hissing 咝音的

sib·ling (sib′ling) any of two or more offspring of the same parents; a brother or sister 同胞（兄弟姊妹）

sib·ship (sib′ship) 1. relationship by blood 血缘关系；2. a group of persons all descended from a common ancestor 同胞关系；3. a group of siblings 一群同胞（兄弟姊妹）

sic·cus (sik′əs) [L.] dry 干燥的

sick (sik) 1. not in good health; afflicted by disease; ill 不舒服的，患病的；2. nauseated 恶心的

sick·le·mia (sik-le′me-ə) sickle cell anemia 镰状细胞性贫血

sick·ling (sik′ling) the development of sickle cells in the blood 镰状化，血内镰状细胞形成

sick·ness (sik′nis) disease 疾病；**African sleeping s.**, African trypanosomiasis 非洲昏睡病，非洲锥虫病；**air s.**, airsickness 晕机；**altitude s.**, a condition due to difficulty adjusting to lowered oxygen pressure at high altitudes; it may take the form of mountain sickness, high-altitude pulmonary edema, or cerebral edema 高原病，一种由于难以适应高海拔地区氧压降低而引起的疾病，可能表现为高山病、高海拔肺水肿或脑水肿；**cars., carsickness** 晕车病 **decompression s.**, one or more symptoms of joint pain, respiratory manifestations, skin lesions, and neurologic signs in association with overly rapid reduction of ambient pressure, which causes gases dissolved in the blood and body fluids under high pressure to be released as bubbles 减压病，一种或多种关节疼痛、呼吸症状、皮肤损伤和神经症状的症状，与环境压力的过快下降有关，导致高压下血液和体液中溶解的气体以气泡形式释放；**green tobacco s.**, transient, recurring nicotine poisoning in tobacco harvesters 烟草萎黄病，烟草收割者患的短暂反复的尼古丁中毒；**high-altitude s.**, 同 altitude s.；**milk s.**, an acute, often fatal disease in humans after they ingest milk, milk products, or flesh of cattle or sheep who have eaten certain toxic plants; human disease is marked by weakness, anorexia, vomiting, and sometimes muscular tremors 乳毒病，一种急性的，通常是致命的疾病，在人摄入牛奶、奶制品或吃过某些有毒植物的牛或羊的肉之后发病，以虚弱、厌食、呕吐和肌肉震颤为特征；**morning s.**, nausea of early pregnancy 孕妇晨吐；**motion s.**, nausea and malaise due to the motions of travel, as by airplane, automobile, ship, or train 晕动病，因乘交通工具引起的眩晕病，如晕船、晕车（火车、汽车）及晕机；**mountain s.**, a type of high-altitude sickness with oliguria, dyspnea, blood pressure and pulse rate changes, and neurologic disorders 高山病，一种伴有少尿、呼吸困难、血压和脉搏变化以及神经系统疾病的高海拔病；**radiation s.**, a condition resulting from exposure to a whole-body dose of over 1 gray of ionizing radiation and characterized by the symptoms of the acute radiation syndrome 放射病；**sea s.**, seasickness 晕船病；**serum s.**, a hypersensitivity reaction after administration of foreign serum or serum proteins, marked by urticaria, arthralgia, edema, and lymphadenopathy 血清病；**sleeping s.**, 1. African trypanosomiasis 昏睡病，非洲锥虫病；2. increasing lethargy and drowsiness due to a disease process such as African trypanosomiasis or types of encephalomyelitis 昏睡病，由于疾病过程（如非洲锥虫病或脑脊髓炎）导致的嗜睡和嗜睡增加

s.i.d. [L.] sem′el in di′e (once a day) 每日一次

sid·ero·blast (sid′ər-o-blast″) a nucleated erythrocyte containing iron granules in its cytoplasm 铁粒幼红细胞；**sideroblas′tic** adj.；**ringed s.**, an abnormal sideroblast with many iron granules in its mitochondria, found in a ring around the nucleus;

S

seen in sideroblastic anemia 环形铁粒幼红细胞

sid·ero·cyte (sid″ər-o-sīt″) an erythrocyte containing nonhemoglobin iron 高铁红细胞

sid·ero·der·ma (sid″ər-o-dur′mə) bronzed coloration of the skin due to disordered iron metabolism 铁色皮症

sid·ero·fi·bro·sis (sid″ər-o-fi-bro′sis) fibrosis of the spleen with deposits of iron 铁末沉着性纤维变性，以含铁沉积物为特征的脾纤维变性；**siderofibrot′ic** *adj.*

sid·ero·my·cin (sid″ər-o-mi′sin) any of a class of antibiotics, synthesized by certain actinomycetes, that inhibit bacterial growth by interfering with iron uptake 高铁霉素，含铁抗生素，由某些放线菌合成，通过干扰铁的吸收来抑制细菌的生长

sid·ero·pe·nia (sid″ər-o-pe′ne-ə) iron deficiency 铁质缺乏；**siderope′nic** *adj.*

sid·ero·phil (sid′ər-o-fil″) 1. 同 siderophilous；2. a siderophilous cell or tissue 嗜铁组织，嗜铁体

sid·er·oph·i·lous (sid″ər-of′ī-ləs) tending to absorb iron 嗜铁的

sid·ero·phore (sid′ər-o-for″) a macrophage containing hemosiderin 含铁血黄素巨噬细胞

sid·er·o·sil·i·co·sis (sid″ər-o-sil″ī-ko′sis) pneumoconiosis from inhalation of dust-containing particles of iron ore and silica 铁硅末沉着病

sid·er·o·sis (sid″ər-o′sis) 1. pneumoconiosis due to inhalation of iron particles 肺铁末沉着病；2. hyperferremia 高铁血症；3. hemosiderosis 含铁血黄素沉着症；**hepatic s.,** the deposit of an abnormal quantity of iron in the liver 肝铁质沉着；**urinary s.,** hemosiderinuria 尿铁质沉着

SIDS sudden infant death syndrome 婴儿猝死综合征

sie·mens (S) (se′mənz) the SI unit of conductance; the conductance of 1 ampere per volt in a body with 1 ohm resistance 西门子，电导的国际单位

sig. [L.] sig′na (mark) 标记

sight (sīt) vision (1, 2) 视觉，视；**far s.,** hyperopia 远视；**near s.,** myopia 近视；**night s.,** hemeralopia 夜视症

sig·ma·tism (sig′mə-tiz-əm) faulty enunciation or too frequent use of the *s* sound s 发音困难，滥用 s 音

sig·moid (sig′moid) 1. shaped like the letter C or S 形的；C 形的；2. sigmoid colon 乙状结肠

sig·moid·ec·to·my (sig″moi-dek′tə-me) excision of part or all of the sigmoid colon 乙状结肠切除术

sig·moid·itis (sig″moi-di′tis) inflammation of the sigmoid colon 乙状结肠炎

sig·moido·pexy (sig-moi′do-pek″se) fixation of the sigmoid colon, as for rectal prolapse 乙状结肠固定术

sig·moido·proc·tos·to·my (sig-moi″do-prok-tos′tə-me) surgical anastomosis of the sigmoid colon to the rectum 乙状结肠直肠吻口术

sig·moid·os·co·py (sig″moi-dos′kə-pe) direct examination of the interior of the sigmoid colon 乙状结肠镜

sig·moido·sig·moi·dos·to·my (sig-moi″dosig-moi-dos′tə-me) surgical anastomosis of two portions of the sigmoid colon; the opening so created 乙状结肠吻合术

sig·moid·os·to·my (sig″moi-dos′tə-me) creation of an artificial opening from the sigmoid colon to the body surface; the opening so created 乙状结肠造口术

sig·moid·ot·o·my (sig″moi-dot′ə-me) incision of the sigmoid colon 乙状结肠切开术

sig·moido·ves·i·cal (sig-moi″do-ves′ĭ-kəl) pertaining to or communicating with the sigmoid colon and the urinary bladder 乙状结肠膀胱的

sign (sīn) an indication of the existence of something; any objective evidence of a disease, i.e., such evidence as is perceptible to the examining physician, as opposed to the subjective sensations (symptoms) of the patient 征兆，迹象；征，体征；**Abadie s.,** insensibility of the Achilles tendon to pressure in the tabes dorsalis 阿巴迪氏征，肌腱在脊髓背侧的压力不敏感；**Babinski s.,** 巴宾斯基征 1. loss or lessening of the triceps surae reflex in organic sciatica 坐骨神经痛时，跟腱反射减弱或消失；2. 参见 *reflex* 下词条；3. in organic hemiplegia, failure of the platysma muscle to contract on the affected side in opening the mouth, whistling, etc. 偏瘫时，令患者开口、吹气、吹哨等，可见到健侧颈阔肌比患侧有力；4. in organic hemiplegia, flexion of the thigh and lifting of the heel from the ground when the patient tries to sit up from a supine position with arms crossed upon the chest 患者仰卧，双臂交叉于胸前，然后令其坐起，此时偏瘫侧大腿向骨盆屈曲，脚跟离地面，而健侧肢体不动；5. in organic paralysis, when the affected forearm is placed in supination, it turns over to pronation 将偏瘫侧前臂置于旋后位时，该臂又回到旋前位；**Battle s.,** ecchymosis in the mastoid region, in the line of the posterior auricular artery, appearing first near the tip of the mastoid process; seen in fracture of the base of the skull 巴特尔征，耳后淤血斑，乳突区域中的瘀斑，在耳后动脉的线上，出现在乳突突起的尖端附近；见于头骨基部骨折；**Beevor s.,** 比弗征 1. in functional paralysis, inability to inhibit the antagonistic muscles 功能性麻痹时，病人不能抑制对抗肌；2. in paralysis of the lower abdominal muscles due to a spinal cord lesion in the region of the lower thoracic vertebrae, there is upward excursion of the umbilicus on attempting to lift the head 由于下胸椎区域的脊髓损伤导致下腹部肌肉瘫痪，试图抬起头部时脐向上偏移；**Bergman s.,** in urologic radiography, *(a)* the ureter is dilated immediately below a neoplasm, rather than collapsed as below an obstructing stone, and *(b)* the ureteral catheter tends to coil in this dilated portion of the ureter Bergman 征，尿路放射线照相所见，(a) 紧邻肿瘤下部的输尿管膨胀，而结石梗阻的下部为塌陷；(b) 导尿管在输尿管膨胀部往往呈卷曲状；**Biernacki s.,** analgesia of the ulnar nerve in general paresis and tabes dorsalis Biernacki 征，麻痹性痴呆及脊髓痨患者尺神经痛觉缺失；**Blumberg s.,** pain on abrupt release of steady pressure (rebound tenderness) over the site of a suspected abdominal lesion, indicative of peritonitis Blumberg 征，以一定压力压迫腹部可疑病变处突然放松，如有剧痛（反跳痛），则表示存在腹膜炎；**Branham s.,** bradycardia produced by digital closure of an artery proximal to an arteriovenous fistula 布拉纳姆征，用手指压迫动静脉瘘近侧的动脉可引起心动徐缓；**Braxton Hicks s.,** Braxton Hicks 征，参见 *contraction* 下词条；**Broadbent s.,** retraction on the left side of the back, near the eleventh and twelfth ribs, related to pericardial adhesion 布罗德本特征，与心包粘连有关的背部左侧第十一、十二肋附近凹陷；**Brudzinski s.,** 布鲁津斯基征 1. in meningitis, flexion of the neck usually causes flexion of the hip and knee 脑膜炎患者屈颈时常可导致髋膝屈曲；2. in meningitis, on passive flexion of one lower limb, the contralateral limb shows a similar movement 使脑膜炎患者一侧下肢屈曲时，对侧肢也发生同样的运动；**Chaddock s.,** 查多克征，参见 *reflex* 下词条；**Chadwick s.,** a dark blue to purplish red congested appearance of the vaginal mucosa, an indication of pregnancy 查德韦克征，阴道黏膜呈深蓝色至紫红色充血，提示妊娠；**Chvostek s., Chvostek-Weiss s.,** spasm of the facial muscles elicited by tapping the facial nerve in the region of the parotid gland; seen in tetany 低钙击面征，轻叩腮腺部面神经可引起面肌痉挛；**cogwheel s.,** muscle rigidity that releases in a series of small jerks rather than in a smooth range of motion when passively stretched. Seen in Parkinson disease. Called also *cogwheel rigidity* and *cogwheel phenomenon* 齿轮征，肌肉刚度，当被动拉伸时，会以一系列小的急促动作释放，而不是以平稳的运动范围释放，见于帕金森病。又称齿轮样强直和齿轮现象；**Cullen s.,** bluish discoloration around the umbilicus sometimes associated with intraperitoneal hemorrhage, especially after rupture of the uterine tube in ectopic pregnancy; similar discoloration occurs in acute hemorrhagic pancreatitis 卡伦征，脐周皮肤颜色变蓝，有时与腹膜内出血，尤与宫外孕输卵管破裂后出血有关；另亦见于急性出血性胰腺炎；**Dalrymple s.,** abnormal wideness of the palpebral opening in Graves disease 达尔林普耳征，在格雷夫斯病中，眼裂异常扩大；**Delbet s.,** in aneurysm of a limb's main artery, if nutrition of the part distal to the aneurysm is maintained despite absence of the pulse, collateral circulation is sufficient Delbet 征，一条肢体的主要动脉发生动脉瘤时，若动脉瘤远端仍能维持营养，尽管脉搏已消失，仍表示侧支循环充足；**de Musset s.,** 同 Musset s.；**Ewart s.,** bronchial breathing and dullness on percussion at the lower angle of the left scapula, a sign of pericardial effusion 心包积液征，左肩胛下角叩诊时呈浊音，可听到支气管呼吸音，提示心包积液；**fabere s.,** 屈展旋伸征，参见 *Patrick test*；**Friedreich s.,** diastolic collapse of the cervical veins due to adhesion of the pericardium Friedreich 征，由粘连性心包炎引起的心舒张期颈静脉塌陷；**Goodell s.,** softening of the cervix; a sign of pregnancy 古德耳征，子宫颈变软，提示妊娠；**Gorlin s.,** the ability to touch the tip of the nose with the tongue, often a sign of Ehlers-Danlos syndrome Gorlin 征，用舌头触摸鼻尖的能力，通常是 Ehlers-Danlos 综合征的症状；**Graefe s.,** tardy or jerky downward movement of the upper eyelids when the gaze is directed downward; noted in thyrotoxicosis 格雷费征，当向下注视时上眼睑的缓慢或急促向下运动；见于甲状腺毒症；**halo s.,** a halo effect produced in the radiograph of the fetal head between the subcutaneous fat and the cranium; said to indicate intrauterine death of the fetus 晕轮征，胎儿头颅 X 线照片上，皮下脂肪与颅骨间呈现晕轮现象，提示宫内死胎；**harlequin s.,** reddening of the lower half of the laterally recumbent body and blanching of the upper half, due to temporary vasomotor disturbance in newborn infants 丑角征，新生儿因暂时性血管运动障碍，身体侧卧时下半身变红，上半身变白；**Hegar s.,** softening of the lower uterine segment; indicative of pregnancy 黑加征，子宫下段变软，提示妊娠；**Hoffmann s.,** 霍夫曼征 1. increased mechanical irritability of the sensory nerves in tetany; the ulnar nerve is usually tested 手足搐搦时，感觉神经对机械性刺激的敏感性增强；通常测试尺神经；2. a sudden nipping of the nail of the index, middle, or ring finger produces flexion of the terminal phalanx of the thumb and of the second and third phalanges of some other finger 快速弹拨示指、中指或无名指指甲时，拇指末节及其他指的第二、第三指节屈曲；**Homans s.,** discomfort behind the knee on forced dor-

S

siflexion of the foot, due to thrombosis in the calf veins 霍曼斯征，由于小腿静脉血栓形成，导致脚被迫背屈时膝后不适；**Hoover s.**, 胡佛征 1. in the normal state or in true paralysis, when the supine patient presses one leg against the surface on which he or she is lying, their other leg will lift 见于正常人或真性偏瘫患者，令病人仰卧用一条腿下压时，可见另一腿有向上的活动，而癔病及诈病者则不出现此现象；2. movement of the costal arches toward the midline in inhalation, bilaterally in pulmonary emphysema and unilaterally in conditions causing flattening of the respiratory diaphragm 吸气时肋骨缘向中线移动，肺气肿时双侧均有此征，而由胸腔积液和气胸使膈变平伏则仅限于单侧；**Kernig s.**, in meningitis, inability to completely extend the leg when sitting or lying with the thigh flexed upon the abdomen; when in the dorsal decubitus position, the leg can be easily and completely extended 克尼格征，仰卧时病人易将腿完全伸直，而坐位或大腿屈向腹部仰卧时，则不能完全伸直，为脑膜炎的体征；**Klippel-Weil s.**, in pyramidal tract disease, flexion and adduction of the thumb when the flexed fingers are quickly extended by the examiner 克－威二氏征，迅速将患者屈曲的手指扳直时，如拇指屈曲内收，提示锥体束病；**Lasègue s.**, in sciatica, flexion of the hip is painful when the knee is extended, but painless when the knee is flexed 拉塞格征，坐骨神经痛时伸膝屈髋可引起疼痛，但屈膝时则无痛；**Léri s.**, absence of normal flexion of the elbow on passive flexion of the hand at the wrist of the affected side in hemiplegia Léri 征，被动屈曲偏瘫者患侧的手与腕时，不能显示正常的肘部弯曲；**Lhermitte s.**, electric-like shocks spreading down the body on flexing the head forward; seen mainly in multiple sclerosis but also in compression and other cervical cord disorders 莱尔米特征，病人低头时，引起短暂迅速的电击样感觉，由上向下传播，主要见于多发性硬化症，但也可见于颈髓受压及其他疾病；**Macewen s.**, a more resonant note than normal on percussion of the skull behind the junction of the frontal, temporal, and parietal bones in internal hydrocephalus and cerebral abscess 麦克尤恩征，脑积水和脑脓肿时，叩诊额、顶及颞骨接缝后的颅骨时，叩诊音较正常叩诊音响；**McMurray s.**, occurrence of a cartilage click on manipulation of the knee; indicative of meniscal injury 麦氏征，用手活动膝部时听到软骨的咔嗒声，提示半月板损伤；**Möbius s.**, in Graves disease, inability to keep the eyes converged due to insufficiency of the internal rectus muscles. Möbius 征，在格雷夫斯病中，由于内直肌功能不全，不能使眼睛集中；**Musset s.**, rhythmic jerking of the head in aortic aneurysm

and aortic insufficiency 谬塞征，节律性地点头，见于主动脉瘤和主动脉瓣关闭不全患者；**Nikolsky s.**, ready separation of the outer layer of the epidermis from the basal layer with sloughing of the skin produced by minor trauma such as a sliding or rubbing pressure on the skin; it can occur in certain skin disorders, infection, and thermal burns 尼科利斯基征，轻微外伤（如皮肤上的滑动或摩擦压力）即将表皮外层从基底层擦离而脱失，见于某些皮肤疾病、感染和热烧伤；**Oliver s.**, tracheal tugging 奥利弗征，气管牵拉感，参见 tugging；**Oppenheim s.**, 奥本海姆征，参见 reflex 下词条；**Queckenstedt s.**, when the veins in the neck are compressed on one or both sides in healthy persons, there is a rapid rise in the pressure of the cerebrospinal fluid, which then returns quickly to normal when compression ceases. In obstruction of the vertebral canal, the pressure of the cerebrospinal fluid is little or not at all affected 奎肯施泰特征，当健康人的颈部静脉一侧或两侧受到压迫时，脑脊液压力迅速升，当压迫停止时，脑脊液压力迅速恢复正常。在椎管阻塞时，脑脊液的压力很少或根本不受影响；**Romberg s.**, swaying of the body or falling when the eyes are closed while standing withthe feet close together; observed in tabes dorsalis 龙贝格征，闭目难立征，闭目并足站立时身体不稳、为共济失调表现，见于脊髓痨；**Rossolimo s.**, 罗索利莫征，参见 reflex 下词条；**setting sun s.**, downward deviation of the eyes so that each iris appears to "set" beneath the lower lid, with white sclera exposed between it and the upper lid; indicative of increased intracranial pressure or irritation of the brainstem 落日征，眼睛向下偏斜，使每个虹膜似乎都位于下眼睑下方，白色巩膜暴露在虹膜和上眼睑之间；提示颅内压增高或脑干刺激；**Stellwag s.**, infrequent or incomplete blinking, a sign of Graves disease 施特尔瓦格征，突眼性甲状腺肿时、眼裂增大、瞬目运动稀少，是 Graves 病的征兆；**string of beads s.**, a series of rounded shapes resembling a string of beads on a radiograph of the small intestine, indicating bubbles of trapped gas within the fluid of an obstructed and distended bowel 串珠征，小肠 X 线片上的一串圆形串珠状物，提示肠阻塞或膨胀时，液体中有气泡；**Tinel s.**, a tingling sensation in the distal end of a limb when percussion is made over the site of a divided nerve. It indicates a partial lesion or the beginning regeneration of the nerve 蒂内尔征，当敲击神经分裂部位时，肢体远端产生的刺痛感。它表明神经的部分损伤或开始再生；**Trousseau s.**, tache cérébrale 低钙束臂征；**vital s's**, the pulse, respiration, and temperature 生命体征，脉搏、呼吸和体温

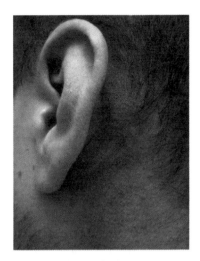

▲ 巴特尔征

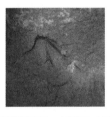

▲ 尼科利斯基征阳性：中毒性表皮坏死松解时，因机械压力对红斑皮肤区域造成的表皮脱离

sig·na (sig′nə) [L.] write or make a mark; abbreviated S. or sig. in prescriptions 书写或标记，在处方中缩写为 S. 或 sig.

sig·na·ture (sig′nə-chər) the part of a prescription that gives directions as to the taking of the medicine 用法签，标记，处方中指导患者服药方法的部分

sig·nif·i·cant (sig-nif′ĭ-kənt) in statistics, probably resulting from something other than chance 有意义的，统计学上指可能不是由某种偶然事物引起的

sign·ing (sīn′ing) dactylology; use of a system of hand movements for communication 手语

Si·las·tic (sī-las′tik) trademark for polymeric silicone substances that have the properties of rubber but are biologically inert; used in surgical prostheses 硅化橡胶（商品名，用于外科修复）

sil·den·a·fil (sil-den′ə-fil″) a phosphodiesterase inhibitor that relaxes the smooth muscle of the penis, facilitating blood flow to the corpus cavernosum; used as the citrate salt to treat erectile dysfunction 西地那非

si·len·cing (si′lən-sing) the process of making or keeping something silent 沉默；**gene s.,** negative regulation of gene expression, including processes that inhibit transcription of genes, such as DNA methylation, and posttranscriptional processes 基因沉默，基因表达的负调控，包括抑制基因转录的过程，如 DNA 甲基化和转录后过程

si·lent (si′lənt) 1. noiseless 无症状的；2. producing no detectable signs or symptoms 无声的

sil·i·ca (sil′ĭ-kə) silicon dioxide, SiO$_2$, occurring in various allotropic forms, some of which are used in dental materials 硅石，二氧化硅，另参见 *silicosis*

sil·i·ca·to·sis (sil″ĭ-kə-to′sis) pneumoconiosis caused by inhalation of the dust of silicates such as those in asbestos, kaolin, mica, or talc 硅酸盐尘肺

sil·i·co·an·thra·co·sis (sil″ĭ-ko-an″thrə-ko′sis) anthracosilicosis 石末沉着病，硅肺

sil·i·con (Si) (sil′ĭ-kon) an abundant, gray, crystalline, metalloid element usually occurring in nature as forms of silicon dioxide (silica) or silicates; at. no. 14, at. wt. 28.085 硅（化学元素）；**s. carbide,** a compound of silicon and carbon used in dentistry as an abrasive agent 金刚砂；**s. dioxide,** silica 二氧化硅

sil·i·cone (sil′ĭ-kōn) any of a large group of organic compounds comprising alternating silicon and oxygen atoms linked to organic radicals, particularly methyl groups; uses have included wetting agents and surfactants, sealants, coolants, contact lenses, and surgical membranes and implants 聚硅酮

sil·i·co·sid·er·o·sis (sil″ĭ-ko-sid″ər-o′sis) 同 siderosilicosis

sil·i·co·sis (sil″ĭ-ko′sis) pneumoconiosis due to inhalation of the dust of stone, sand, or flint containing silica, with generalized nodular fibrotic changes in the lungs 硅沉着病，硅肺病；**silicot′ic** *adj.*

sil·i·quose (sil′ĭ-kwōs) pertaining to or resembling a pod or husk 长角状的，长壳状的

silk (silk) the protein filament produced by the larvae of various insects; braided, degummed silk obtained from the cocoons of the silkworm *Bombyx mori* is used as a nonabsorbable suture material 丝，丝线

si·lox·ane (si-lok′sān) any of various compounds based on a substituted backbone of alternating silica and oxygen molecules; in polymeric form they are polysiloxanes, and when the side chain substituents are organic radicals, they are silicones 硅氧烷

sil·ver (Ag) (sil′vər) a soft, white, malleable and ductile, lustrous metallic element; at. no. 47, at. wt. 107.868 银；**s. nitrate,** used as a local antiinfective, as in the prophylaxis of ophthalmia neonatorum 硝酸盐，用作局部抗感染药，如预防新生儿眼炎；

s. protein, silver made colloidal by the presence of, or combination with, protein; it may be *mild*, used as a topical antiinfective, or *strong*, used as an active germicide with a local irritant and astringent effect 蛋白银，银通过蛋白质的存在或与蛋白质的结合而制成的胶状物；它可以是温和的，用作局部抗感染剂，也可以是强性的，用作具有局部刺激和收敛作用的活性杀菌剂；**s. sulfadiazine,** the silver derivative of sulfadiazine, having bactericidal activity against many gram-positive and gram-negative organisms, as well as being effective against yeasts; used as a topical antiinfective for the prevention and treatment of wound sepsis in patients with second- and third-degree burns 磺胺嘧啶银，磺胺的银衍生物，对酵母菌和很多革兰阳性、革兰阴性菌有杀菌作用，用作局部抗感染药物，用于预防和治疗二度和三度烧伤创面化脓；**toughened s. nitrate,** a compound of silver nitrate, hydrochloric acid, sodium chloride, or potassium nitrate; used as a caustic, applied topically after being dipped in water 增韧硝酸银，由硝酸银、盐酸、氯化钠或硝酸钾组成的化合物；用作腐蚀剂，浸在水中后局部使用

si·meth·i·cone (sĭ-meth′ĭ-kōn) an antifoaming and antiflatulent agent consisting of a mixture of dimethicones and silicon dioxide 二甲硅油，消泡净，聚二甲硅氧烷，胃镜检查时用作消泡沫药

SIMFE severe infantile multifocal epilepsy 严重婴儿多灶性癫痫

sim·i·an (sim′e-ən) of, pertaining to, or resembling an ape or a monkey 猴的，似猿的

si·mi·lia si·mi·li·bus cu·ran·tur (sĭ-mĭl′e-ə sĭ-mĭl′lĭ-bəs ku-ran′tər) [L. "likes are cured by likes"] the doctrine, which lies at the foundation of homeopathy, that a disease is cured by those remedies that produce effects resembling the disease itself 类病类治，顺势疗法的一种理论，即认为药物作用如与某病表现相似，即可以该药治疗

si·mil·li·mum (sĭ-mil′ĭ-məm) [L.] the homeopathic remedy that most exactly reproduces the symptoms of any disease 顺势疗法药物

sim·ple (sim′pəl) neither compound nor complex; single 简单的；单的，单一的

Sim·plex·vi·rus (sim′pleks-vi″rəs) a genus of ubiquitous viruses of the family Herpesviridae; it includes the species human herpesviruses 1 and 2 单纯疱疹病毒属，参见 *herpesvirus* 表

sim·ul (sim′əl) [L.] at the same time as 同时

sim·u·la·tion (sim″u-la′shən) 1. an imitation or pretense 模仿，假装；2. the act of counterfeiting a disease; malingering 诈病，装病；3. the mimicking of one disease by another 模仿，模拟，一种疾病模拟另一种疾病；4. a health care education meth-od involving scenarios designed to replicate real health encounters, using lifelike manikins, physical models, standardized patients, or computers 一种医疗保健教育方法，设计用于复制真实健康遭遇的场景，使用逼真的人体模型，物理模型，标准化患者或计算机

sim·u·la·tor (sim″u-la′tər) something that simulates, such as an apparatus that simulates conditions that will be encountered in real life 模拟装置

Si·mu·li·um (si-mu′le-əm) a genus of biting gnats; some species are intermediate hosts of *Onchocerca volvulus* 蚋属

si·mul·tan·ag·no·sia (si″məl-tān″əg-no′zhah) partial visual agnosia, consisting of the inability to comprehend more than one element of a visual scene at the same time or to integrate the parts as a whole 画片中动作失认

sim·va·stat·in (sim′və-stat″in) an antihyperlipidemic agent that acts by inhibiting cholesterol synthesis, used in the treatment of hypercholesterolemia and other forms of dyslipidemia and to lower the risks associated with atherosclerosis and coronary heart disease 西伐他汀，一种通过抑制胆固醇合成而起作用的降血脂药物，用于治疗高胆固醇血症和其他形式的血脂异常，并降低与动脉粥样硬化和冠状动脉粥样硬化性心脏病相关的风险

sin·ci·put (sin′sĭ-pət) forehead 前头，前顶；**sincip′ital** *adj.*

sin·ew (sin′u) a tendon of a muscle 腱；**weeping s.,** an encysted ganglion, chiefly on the back of the hand, containing synovial fluid 腱鞘囊肿，内含滑液外有包膜的腱鞘囊肿，主要发生于手背

sin·gle blind (sing′gəl blīnd) pertaining to an experiment in which subjects do not know which treatment they are receiving 单盲法的

sin·gul·tus (sing-gul′təs) [L.] hiccup 呃逆

si·nis·ter (sĭ-nis′tər) [L.] left; on the left side 左，左侧的

si·nis·trad (sĭ-nis′trad) to or toward the left 左旋，向左

sin·is·tral (sin′is-trəl) pertaining to the left side 左侧的；左利的

sin·is·tral·i·ty (sin″is-tral′ĭ-te) lateral dominance on the left side 左利（善用左侧器官）

sin·is·tro·cer·e·bral (sin″is-tro-ser′ə-brəl) pertaining to or situated in the left cerebral hemisphere 左大脑（半球）的

sin·is·troc·u·lar (sin″is-trok′u-lər) having the left eye dominant 左利眼的

sin·is·tro·man·u·al (sin″is-tro-man′u-əl) left-handed 左利手的

sin·is·trop·e·dal (sin″is-trop′ə-dəl) using the left foot in preference to the right 左利足的

sin·is·tro·tor·sion (sin″is-tro-tor′shən) levoclination 左旋（主要指眼）

si·no·atri·al (si″no-a′tre-əl) pertaining to the sinus venosus and the atrium of the heart 窦房的

si·no·bron·chi·tis (si″no-brong-ki′tis) chronic paranasal sinusitis with recurrent bronchitis 鼻窦支气管炎

si·no·pul·mo·nary (si″no-pool′mə-nar″e) involving the paranasal sinuses and the lungs 窦肺的

sinu·at·ri·al (sin″u-a′tre-əl) 同 sinoatrial

sin·u·ous (sin′u-əs) bending in and out; winding 弯曲的，纤曲的

si·nus (si′nəs) pl. *si′nus*, *sinuses* [L.] 1. a recess, cavity, or channel, as *(a)* one in bone or *(b)* a dilated channel for venous blood 窦，一种凹处、腔或通道，如（a）骨中的凹处或（b）静脉血的扩张通道；2. an abnormal channel or fistula permitting escape of pus 窦道，脓液流出的异常管道或瘘管；**si′nusal** *adj.*; **air s.**, an air-containing space within a bone 含气窦，骨本质内的含气腔；**anal s's**, furrows, with pouchlike openings at the distal end, separating the rectal columns 肛窦，直肠窦，与直肠柱分开，下端带有袋状隐窝的沟；**aortic s.**, a dilatation between the aortic wall and each of the semilunar leaflets of the aortic valve; from two of these sinuses the coronary arteries originate 主动脉窦，主动脉壁和主动脉瓣半月叶之间的扩张，冠状动脉起源于其中两个窦；**branchial s.**, an abnormal cavity or space opening externally on the inferior third of the neck; usually a result of persistence of the second pharyngeal groove and cervical sinus 鳃窦，颈部下三分之一的异常开口，通常是第二咽沟和颈窦持续存在的结果；**carotid s.**, a dilatation of the proximal portion of the internal carotid or distal portion of the common carotid artery, containing in its wall pressoreceptors that are stimulated by changes in blood pressure 颈动脉窦，颈内动脉近端或颈总动脉远端部分的扩张，其壁内含有受血压变化刺激的压力感受器；**cavernous s.**, either of two irregularly shaped sinuses of the dura mater, located at either side of the body of the sphenoid bone and communicating across the midline; it contains the internal carotid artery and abducens nerve and, in its lateral wall, the oculomotor, trochlear, ophthalmic, and maxillary nerves 海绵窦，两个不规则形状的硬脑膜鼻窦，位于蝶骨体的两侧，与中线连通；包含颈内动脉和外展神经，在其侧壁包含动眼神经、滑车神经、眼神经和上颌神经；**cervical s.**, a temporary depression caudal to the second pharyngeal arch, containing the succeeding pharyngeal arches; it is overgrown by the second pharyngeal arch and closes off as the cervical vesicle 颈窦，位于第二咽弓尾部的暂时性凹陷，包括随后的咽弓，

它在第二咽弓处过度生长，并在颈部囊泡处关闭；**circular s.**, the venous channel encircling the hypophysis, formed by the two cavernous sinuses and the anterior and posterior intercavernous sinuses 环状窦，由两个海绵窦及前、后海绵窦围绕垂体形成的静脉环；**coccygeal s.**, a sinus or fistula just over or close to the tip of the coccyx 骶尾瘘，尾骨尖端或上方的窦或瘘；**coronary s.**, the terminal portion of the great cardiac vein, lying in the coronary sulcus between the left atrium and ventricle, and emptying into the right atrium 冠状窦，心脏大静脉的终末部，位于左心房和心室间的冠状沟，流入右心房；**cortical s's**, lymph sinuses in the cortex of a lymph node, which arise from the marginal sinuses and continue into the medullary sinuses 皮质窦，淋巴结皮质内的淋巴窦，起于缘窦，延续进入髓窦；**dermal s.**, a congenital sinus tract extending from the surface of the body, between the bodies of two adjacent lumbar vertebrae, to the spinal canal 皮窦，皮洞，位于相邻两腰椎体之间，由体表向椎管延伸的先天性窦道；**dural s's**, large venous channels forming an anastomosing system between the layers of the cranial dura mater, draining the cerebral veins and some diploic and meningeal veins into the veins of the neck 硬脑膜窦，大静脉通道在颅硬脑膜层之间形成吻合系统，将脑静脉和一些脑干和脑膜静脉引流至颈静脉；**s. of epididymis**, a long, slitlike serous pocket between the upper part of the testis and the overlying epididymis 附睾窦，位于睾丸上部和附睾冠部之间的裂缝状长浆液囊；**ethmoid s's, ethmoidal s's**, 筛窦，参见 *cell* 下词条；**frontal s.**, one of the paired paranasal vsinuses in the frontal bone, each communicating with the middle meatus of the ipsilateral nasal cavity 额窦，额窦中成对的鼻旁窦之一，每个都与同侧鼻腔的中鼻沟相连；**intercavernous s's**, two sinuses of the dura mater connecting the two cavernous sinuses, one passing anterior and the other posterior to the infundibulum of the hypophysis 海绵间窦；**lacteal s's, lactiferous s's**, enlargements of the lactiferous ducts just before they open on the mammary papilla 输乳窦，输乳管汇入乳头前的膨大部；**lymphatic s's**, irregular, tortuous spaces within lymphoid tissue (nodes) through which lymph passes, to enter efferent lymphatic vessels 淋巴窦，淋巴结内不规则的纤曲腔隙，淋巴液经此不断流入输出淋巴管；**marginal s's**, 1. see under *lake* 缘窦，参见 lake; 2. bowl-shaped lymph sinuses separating the capsule from the cortical parenchyma, and from which lymph flows into the cortical sinuses 分隔淋巴结皮质和囊的弓形淋巴窦，淋巴液由此流入皮质窦 **maxillary s.**, one of the paired paranasal sinuses in the body of the maxilla on either side, and opening into the middle meatus of the ipsilateral nasal cavity 上颌窦，两侧上颌骨体内成对的鼻旁窦之一，并通向同侧鼻腔的中鼻道；**medullary s's,** lymph sinuses in the medulla of a lymph node, which divide the lymphoid tissue into a number of medullary cords 髓质淋巴窦，髓窦，位于淋巴结髓质部的淋巴窦，将淋巴组织分隔成许多髓索；**occipital s.,** one of the sinuses of the dura mater, passing upward along the midline of the cerebellum 枕窦，硬脑膜的一个窦，沿小脑中线向上延伸；**oral s.,** stomodeum 口道；**paranasal s's,** mucosa-lined air cavities in bones of the skull, communicating with the nasal cavity and including ethmoidal, frontal, maxillary, and sphenoidal sinuses 鼻旁窦，颅骨内与鼻腔相通且衬附黏膜的含气腔，包括筛窦、额窦、上颌窦及蝶窦；**petrosal s.,** either of two sinuses of the dura mater, arising from the cavernous sinus and draining into the internal jugular vein *(inferior petrosal s.)* or into the transverse sinus *(superior petrosal s.)* 岩窦，硬脑膜的两个窦中的一个，由海绵窦形成，引流至颈内静脉（岩下窦）或横窦（岩上窦）；**pilonidal s.,** a suppurating sinus containing hair, occurring chiefly in the coccygeal region 藏毛窦，一种含毛发的化脓窦，主要发生于尾骨区；**prostatic s.,** the posterolateral recess between the seminal colliculus and the wall of the urethra 前列腺窦，精阜与尿道壁之间的后外侧隐窝；**s. of pulmonary trunk,** a slight dilatation between the wall of the pulmonary trunk and each of the semilunar leaflets of the pulmonary trunk valve 肺动脉窦，肺动脉干壁和肺动脉干的每个半月瓣之间轻微扩张；**renal s.,** a recess in the substance of the kidney, occupied by the renal pelvis, calices, vessels, nerves, and fat 肾窦，肾实质内的一个腔隙，内有肾盂、肾盏、血管、神经及脂肪等；**sagittal s., inferior,** a small venous sinus of the dura mater, opening into the straight sinus 下矢状窦，硬脑膜的小静脉窦，通向直窦；**sagittal s., superior,** a venous sinus of the dura mater that ends in the confluence of sinuses, usually in the right transverse sinus 上矢状窦，硬脑膜的静脉窦，终止于鼻窦的汇合处，通常在右侧横窦；**sigmoid s.,** a venous sinus of the dura mater on either side, continuous with the transverse sinus and draining into the internal jugular vein of the same side 乙状窦，硬脑膜内与横窦相连的两个静脉窦，各从小脑幕弯曲向下而与颈内静脉上球相连；**sphenoid s., sphenoidal s.,** one of the paired paranasal sinuses in the body of the sphenoid bone and opening into the highest meatus of the ipsilateral nasal cavity 蝶窦，蝶骨体中成对的鼻旁窦之一，通向同侧鼻腔最高的鼻窦；**sphenoparietal s.,** either of two sinuses of the dura mater, draining into

the anterior part of the cavernous sinus 碟顶窦，硬脑膜的两个窦中的任一个，流入海绵窦的前部；**splenic s.,** a dilated venous sinus in the substance of the spleen 脾窦，脾脏内扩张的静脉窦；**straight s.,** one of the sinuses of the dura mater formed by the junction of the great cerebral vein and inferior sagittal sinus, ending in a transverse sinus, usually the left, at the confluence of the sinuses 直窦，由大脑静脉和下矢状窦交界处形成的硬脑膜的一个鼻窦，终止于鼻窦汇合处的横窦，通常是左窦；**tarsal s.,** a space between the calcaneus and talus 跗骨窦，跟骨与距骨间的腔隙，内含骨间韧带；**tentorial s.,** 同 straight s.；**terminal s.,** a vein that encircles the vascular area in the blastoderm 终窦，胚叶内环绕血管区的一条静脉；**transverse s.,** 横窦 1. either of two large sinuses of the dura mater. At their origin in the confluence of sinuses, one, usually the right, is continuous with the superior sagittal sinus and the other, usually the left, with the straight sinus 硬脑膜横窦，硬脑膜两大静脉窦之一，在两窦汇合的起点处，一个通常是右窦，与上矢状窦相连，另一个，通常是左窦，与直窦相连；2. a passage behind the aorta and pulmonary trunk and in front of the atria 心包横窦，位于主动脉和肺动脉干后及心房前的一条通道；**tympanic s.,** a deep recess in the posterior part of the tympanic cavity 鼓窦，鼓室后部的一个深凹陷；**urogenital s.,** an elongated sac formed by division of the cloaca in the early embryo, forming most of the bladder, the female vestibule, urethra, and vagina, and most of the male urethra 尿生殖窦，由早期胚胎泄殖腔分化而成的长形囊，与中肾管及膀胱相通，以后该部女性形成前庭、尿道和阴道，男性则形成尿道的一部分；**uterine s's,** venous channels in the wall of the uterus in pregnancy 子宫静脉窦，妊娠时子宫壁内的静脉管道；**s. of venae cavae,** the portion of the right atrium into which the inferior and the superior venae cavae open 腔静脉窦，右心房的一部分，上下腔静脉均流入其中；**s. veno'-sus,** 1. the common venous receptacle in the embryonic midheart, attached to the mastoid wall of the primordial atrium 为胚胎中心总静脉接受器，连接原始心房后壁；2. 同 venous s. (1)；3. 同 s. of venae cavae；**venous s.,** 1. a large vein or channel for the circulation of venous blood 静脉窦，静脉血循环的一个大静脉道；2. 同 s. venosus (1)；**venous s's of dura mater,** large channels for venous blood forming an anastomosing system between the layers of the dura mater of the brain, receiving blood from the brain and draining into the veins of the scalp or deep veins at the base of the skull 硬脑膜静脉窦，是在硬脑膜各层之间形成一个吻合系统的大静脉通道，从大脑接收血液并流入头皮静脉

或颅底深静脉；**venous s. of sclera,** a branching, circumferential vessel in the internal scleral sulcus, a major component of the drainage pathway for aqueous humor 巩膜静脉窦，巩膜深部的环行小管，是房水回流通道

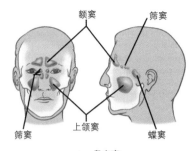

额窦　　　筛窦

筛窦　　上颌窦　　蝶窦

▲ **鼻旁窦**

si·nus·itis (si″nəs-i′tis) inflammation of a sinus 鼻窦炎

si·nus·oid (si′nə-soid) 1. resembling a sinus 窦状的；2. a form of terminal blood channel consisting of a large, irregular anastomosing vessel having a lining of reticuloendothelium and found in the liver, heart, spleen, pancreas, and adrenal, parathyroid, and carotid glands 窦状隙，一种终末血液通道，由一个大的、不规则的吻合血管组成，具有内衬网状内皮，存在于肝脏、心脏、脾脏、胰腺和肾上腺、甲状旁腺和颈动脉腺中

si·nus·oi·dal (si″nə-soi′dəl) 1. located in a sinusoid or affecting the circulation in the region of a sinusoid 窦状隙的；2. shaped like or pertaining to a sine wave 正弦（曲线）样的

si·nus·ot·o·my (si″nə-sot′ə-me) incision of a sinus 窦切开术

si·phon (si′fən) a bent tube with two arms of unequal length, used to transfer liquids from a higher to a lower level by the force of atmospheric pressure 虹吸管，一种弯管，两端不等长，通过大气压作用可将高水位的液体输送到低位处

si·phon·age (si′fon-əj) the use of the siphon, as in gastric lavage or in draining the bladder 虹吸法；虹吸作用

si·reno·me·lia (si″rən-o-me′le-ə) apodal symmelia 并肢畸形

si·ren·om·e·lus (si″rən-om′ə-ləs) a fetus with sirenomelia 并腿畸胎

si·ro·li·mus (sī-ro′lī-məs) a macrolide antibiotic having immunosuppressant properties; used to prevent rejection of kidney transplants 西罗莫司，一种具有免疫抑制特性的大环内酯类抗生素；用于防止肾移植排斥反应

Sir·tu·ro (sir-toor′ō) trademark for a preparation

of bedaquiline 贝达奎林制剂的商品名

SISI short increment sensitivity index 短增量敏感指数

sis·ter (sis′tər) the nurse in charge of a hospital ward (Great Britain) 病房护士长（英国用语）

Sis·tru·rus (sis-troo′rəs) a genus of small rattlesnakes of the family Crotalidae; they occur throughout the United States and have symmetric plates covering their heads. *S. catena′tus* is the massasauga and *S. milia′rius* is the *pygmy rattlesnake* 小响尾蛇属

si·ta·glip·tin (si″tə-glip′tin) an agent that in response to elevated blood sugar slows the inactivation of incretins, thereby increasing insulin release and decreasing circulating glucagon levels; used as the phosphate salt in the treatment of type 2 diabetes mellitus 西他列汀，一种对血糖升高作出反应，减缓肠促胰岛素失活，从而增加胰岛素释放和降低循环胰高血糖素水平的药物；其磷酸盐用于治疗Ⅱ型糖尿病

site (sīt) a place, a position, or locus 地点，位置，部位；**active s.,** the three-dimensional region of an enzyme or other catalyst at which the reaction occurs, binding the substrate and facilitating its conversion to a reaction product 活性部位；**allosteric s.,** a site on a multisubunit enzyme that is not the substrate binding site but that when reversibly bound by an effector induces a conformational change in the enzyme, altering its catalytic properties 别构部位；**antigen-binding s., antigen-combining s.,** the region of the antibody molecule that binds to antigens 抗原结合部位；**binding s.,** in an enzyme or other protein, the threedimensional configuration of specific groups on specific amino acids that binds specific compounds, such as substrates or effectors, with high affinity and specificity 结合部位；**catalytic s.,** in an enzyme, the portion of the active site that converts the substrate to a reaction product or otherwise interacts with it 催化部位；**restriction s.,** a base sequence in a DNA segment recognized by a particular restriction endonuclease 限制（酶切）位点

si·tos·ter·ol (si-tos′tər-ol) any of a group of closely related plant sterols, having anticholesterolemic activity 谷甾醇，一种具有抗胆固醇活性的植物甾醇

si·tos·ter·ol·emia (si-tos″tər-ol-e′me-ə) the presence of excessive sitosterols in the blood, especially β -sitosterol, from dietary vegetables. Written also β -*sitosterolemia* 谷甾醇血症

si·tot·ro·pism (si-tot′ro-piz-əm) response of living cells to the presence of nutritive elements 向食性，趋食性，活细胞对营养成分的一种反应

S

si·tus (si′təs) pl. *si′tus* [L.] site or position 位置，部位；**s. inver′sus, s. inver′sus vis′cerum,** lateral transposition of the viscera of the thorax and abdomen; a familial pattern and consanguineous parents have been reported. Complete transposition of the viscera in the absence of other defects is structurally sound, but see *dextrocardia, levocardia,* and *Kartagener syndrome* 内脏逆位，内脏反位；**s. transver′sus,** 同 s. inversus

SIV simian immunodeficiency virus 猴免疫缺陷病毒

skat·ole (skat′ōl) a strong-smelling crystalline amine from human feces, produced by protein decomposition in the intestine and directly from tryptophan by decarboxylation 3– 甲基吲哚，类臭素，一种具有强烈气味的结晶胺，由人体粪便中的蛋白质在肠道中分解而成，直接由色氨酸脱羧而成

skel·e·tal (skel′ə-təl) pertaining to the skeleton 骨骼的

skel·e·ti·za·tion (skel″ə-tī-za′shən) 1. extreme emaciation 极度消瘦；2. removal of soft parts from the skeleton 骨骼剥制法，去除附着于骨骼的软组织的方法

skel·e·tog·e·nous (skel″ə-toj′ə-nəs) producing skeletal or bony structures 成骨骼的

skel·e·ton (skel′ə-tən) [Gr.] the hard framework of the animal body, especially that of higher vertebrates; the bones of the body collectively 骨骼，参见图 1；**appendicular s.,** the bones of the limbs and supporting thoracic (pectoral) and pelvic girdles 四肢骨骼；**axial s.,** the bones of the body axis, including the skull, vertebral column, ribs, and sternum 中轴骨骼，指颅骨、脊椎骨、肋骨以及胸骨；**cardiac s.,** the fibrous or fibrocartilaginous framework that supports and gives attachment to the cardiac muscle fibers and valves, and the roots of the aorta and pulmonary trunk 心骨骼，支持和附着于心肌纤维和瓣膜，以及主动脉和肺干根部的纤维或纤维软骨框架

ske·ni·tis (ske-ni′tis) inflammation of the paraurethral (Skene) glands（女）尿道旁腺炎

skin (skin) the outer protective covering of the body, consisting of the dermis and epidermis 皮肤，由真皮和表皮组成的身体外部保护层；**farmers' s.,** actinic elastosis 慢性光化性皮炎

skin·fold (skin′fōld) the layer of skin and subcutaneous fat raised by pinching the skin and letting the underlying muscle fall back to the bone; used to estimate the percentage of body fat 皮褶

SKSD streptokinase-streptodornase 双链酶

skull (skul) the skeleton of the head, including the cranium and the mandible 颅，见图 1；**cloverleaf s.,**

kleeblattschädel 分页状颅

slant (slant) 1. a sloping surface of agar in a test tube 斜面，指试管内的琼脂斜面；2. slant culture 斜面培养

SLE systemic lupus erythematosus 系统性红斑狼疮

sleep (slēp) a period of rest for the body and mind, during which volition and consciousness are in abeyance and bodily functions are partially suspended; also described as a behavioral state, with characteristic immobile posture and diminished but readily reversible sensitivity to external stimuli 睡眠，躯体和精神休息期，其间意志和意识部分或完全消失，人体部分功能暂停；也认为睡眠是一种行为状态，特征为特有的不动姿势，对外界刺激的感觉降低但易恢复；**NREM s.,** non–rapid eye movement sleep; the deep, dreamless period of sleep during which the brain waves are slow and of high voltage, and autonomic activities, such as heart rate and blood pressure, are low and regular 非快速眼动睡眠、无梦期，在此期间，脑电波缓慢而高电压，自主活动（如心率和血压）低而有规律；**REM s.,** the period of sleep during which the brain waves are fast and of low voltage, and autonomic activities, such as heart rate and respiration, are irregular. This type of sleep is associated with dreaming, mild involuntary muscle jerks, and rapid eye movements (REM). It usually occurs three to four times each night at intervals of 80 to 120 minutes, each occurrence lasting from 5 minutes to more than an hour 快速眼动睡眠，指脑电波快速、低电压的睡眠期，心率、呼吸等自主活动不规则。这种睡眠与做梦、轻微的不自主肌肉痉挛和快速眼动（REM）有关。通常每晚发生 3～4 次，间隔 80～120 分钟，每次持续 5 分钟到 1 小时以上

sleep·walk·ing (slēp′wawk-ing) somnambulism 梦游，睡行（症）

slide (slīd) a glass plate on which objects are placed for microscopic examination（显微镜用）载玻片

sling (sling) a bandage or suspensory for supporting a part 悬带；**mandibular s.,** a structure suspending the mandible, formed by the medial pterygoid and masseter muscles and aiding in mandibulomaxillary articulation 下颌带；**pubovaginal s.,** a supporting strip placed underneath the bladder in the treatment of stress incontinence; it may be constructed of autologous or allogeneic tissue or of synthetic material 阴道吊带；**suburethral s.,** a support constructed surgically from muscle, ligament, or synthetic material that elevates the bladder from underneath in the treatment of stress incontinence

S

尿道下悬带

slough (sluf) 1. necrotic tissue in the process of separating from viable portions of the body 腐肉，腐痂；2. to shed or cast off 脱落

sludg·ing (sluj'ing) settling out of solid particles from solution 淤沉，沉积；**s. of blood**, intravascular agglutination（血管内）血液沉积

Sm samarium 元素钐的符号

small·pox (smawl'poks) variola; an acute, highly contagious, often fatal infectious disease, now eradicated worldwide by vaccination programs, caused by an orthopoxvirus and marked by fever and distinctive progressive skin eruptions 天花

smear (smēr) a specimen for microscopic study prepared by spreading the material across the slide 涂片；**Pap s., Papanicolaou s.,** 巴氏涂片，参见 *test* 下词条

SMEB severe myoclonic epilepsy borderline 严重肌阵挛性癫痫

smeg·ma (smeg'mə) a type of secretion of sebaceous glands, found chiefly beneath the prepuce; it consists principally of desquamated epithelial cells and sometimes has a cheesy consistency 包皮垢，皮脂腺分泌物，尤指呈干酪状者，主要含脱屑上皮细胞，多见于包皮内；**smegmat'ic** *adj.*

smell (smel) olfaction 嗅觉

Sn tin ([L.] *stan'num*) 元素锡的符号

SNA State Nurses Association 国家护士协会

SNAC scaphoid nonunion advanced collapse; a complication that can occur with a scaphoid fracture 舟状骨不连晚期塌陷

snake (snāk) 1. a limbless reptile of the suborder Ophidia, some of which are poisonous 蛇；2. any of various worms that resemble members of Ophidia 任何一种类似蛇的蠕虫；3. to insert a long, flexible object 插入一个长而灵活的物体；**black s.,** blacksnake 乌梢蛇；**brown s.,** a venomous elapid snake of Australia and New Guinea belonging to the genus *Demansia* 褐蛇；**coral s.,** any of various venomous snakes of the genera *Micrurus* and *Micruroides* 珊瑚蛇；**crotalid s.,** crotalid (1) 响尾蛇；**elapid s.,** elapid (1)眼镜蛇；**harlequin s.,** coral s. 花斑眼镜蛇；**poisonous s's,** 1. real venomous s's; 2. snakes that contain poison, either in venom glands or in other organs or tissues 毒液腺或其他器官或组织中含有毒素的蛇；**sea s.,** a snake of the family Hydrophiidae 海蛇；**tiger s.,** *Notechis scutatus* 虎蛇；**venomous s's,** snakes that secrete venoms capable of producing a deleterious effect on either the blood (hemotoxin) or the nervous system (neurotoxin), with the venom injected into the body of the victim by the snake's bite 毒蛇；**viperine s.,** true viper 蝰蛇

snap (snap) a short, sharp sound 短而尖锐的声音；**opening s.,** a short, sharp sound in early diastole caused by abrupt halting at its maximal opening of an abnormal atrioventricular valve 二尖瓣开瓣音

snare (snār) a wire loop for removing polyps and tumors by encircling them at the base and closing the loop 勒除器，将息肉和肿瘤环绕在底部并闭合环，从而去除息肉和肿瘤的金属环

sneeze (snēz) 1. to expel air forcibly and spasmodically through the nose and mouth 打喷嚏；2. an involuntary, sudden, violent, and audible expulsion of air through the mouth and nose 喷嚏

SNMTS Society of Nuclear Medicine—Technologists Section 核医学技师学会分会

snow (sno) a freezing or frozen mixture consisting of discrete particles or crystals 雪；**carbon dioxide s.,** solid carbon dioxide, formed by rapid evaporation of liquid carbon dioxide; it gives a temperature of about −79°C (−110°F). It is used in cryotherapy to freeze and anesthetize the skin and, in the form of a slush (carbon dioxide slush), as an escharotic to destroy skin lesions and as a peeling agent for chemabrasion 干冰，固体二氧化碳，由液态二氧化碳快速蒸发形成；温度约为 −79°C（−110°F）。在冷冻疗法中用于冷冻和麻醉皮肤，以泥浆（二氧化碳泥浆）的形式作为破坏皮肤损伤的无症状药物和用于化学清洗的剥离剂

snow·blind·ness (sno'blīnd-nis) 雪盲症，参见 *blindness* 下词条

SNP (snip) single-nucleotide polymorphism 单核苷酸多态性

SNRI serotonin-norepinephrine reuptake inhibitor 血清素去甲肾上腺素再摄取抑制药，另参见 *selective norepinephrine reuptake inhibitor*

snRNA small nuclear RNA 核内小 RNA

snRNP (snurp) small nuclear ribonucleoprotein 核小核糖核蛋白颗粒

SNS sympathetic nervous system 交感神经系统

snuf·fles (snuf'əlz) catarrhal discharge from the nasal mucous membrane in infants, generally in congenital syphilis 婴儿鼻塞，婴儿的鼻黏膜卡他性溢液；常见于先天梅毒

SOAP (sōp) a device for conceptualizing the process of recording the progress notes in the *problem-oriented record* (see under *record*): S indicates subjective data obtained from the patient and others close to him; O designates objective data obtained by observation, physical examination, diagnostic studies, etc.; A refers to assessment of the patient's status through analysis of the problem, possible interaction of the problems, and changes in the status of the problems; P designates the plan for patient care SOAP 护理计划，在面向问题记录中使病程记录程概念化的方案：S 表示从病人及其亲近者获得的主观数据；O 表示由观察、体格检查、诊断学方法等获得的客观数据；A 指分析问题、问题之间相互影响和问题状况的变化所获得的对病人情况的评价；P 为对病人的护理计划

soap (sōp) any compound of one or more fatty acids, or their equivalents, with an alkali; it is detergent and is used as a cleanser 肥皂

SOB shortness of breath 气短

so·cial·iza·tion (so″shəl-ī-za′shən) the process by which society integrates the individual and the individual learns to behave in socially acceptable ways 社会化

so·cio·bi·ol·o·gy (so″se-o-bi-ol′ə-je) the branch of theoretical biology that proposes that animal (including human) behavior has a biologic basis controlled by the genes 社会生物学；**sociobiolog′ic, sociobiolog′ical** adj.

so·ci·om·e·try (so″se-om′ə-tre) the branch of sociology concerned with the measurement of human social behavior 社会测验学

so·cio·ther·a·py (so″se-o-ther′ə-pe) any treatment emphasizing modification of the environment and improvement in interpersonal relationships rather than intrapsychic factors 社会疗法

sock·et (sok′ət) a hollow into which a corresponding part fits 槽，臼，窝；**dry s.,** a condition sometimes occurring after tooth extraction, with exposure of bone, inflammation of an alveolar crypt, and severe pain 干槽症，拔牙后有时发生的一种疾病，有骨外露、牙槽隐窝发炎和严重疼痛；**eye s., orbit** 眼眶；**tooth s.,** dental alveolus 牙槽

so·da (so′də) a term loosely applied to sodium bicarbonate, sodium hydroxide, or sodium carbonate 苏打，泛指碳酸氢钠、氢氧化钠或碳酸钠；**baking s., bicarbonate of s.,** sodium bicarbonate 小苏打碳酸氢钠，重碳酸钠；**s. lime,** calcium hydroxide with sodium or potassium hydroxide, or both; used as adsorbent of carbon dioxide in equipment for metabolism tests, inhalant anesthesia, or oxygen therapy 碱石灰

so·di·um (Na) (so′de-əm) an abundant, soft, silvery white, alkali metal element; at. no. 11, at. wt. 22.990; the chief cation of extracellular body fluids. For sodium salts not listed here, see under the acid or the active ingredient 钠；**s. acetate,** a source of sodium ions for hemodialysis and peritoneal dialysis, also a systemic and urinary alkalizer 醋酸钠，是血液透析和腹膜透析的钠离子来源，也是一种全身性与泌尿系统的尿碱化剂；**s. ascorbate,** an antiscorbutic vitamin and nutritional supplement;

also used as an aid to deferoxamine therapy in the treatment of chronic iron toxicity 抗坏血酸钠，一种抗坏血酸维生素和营养补充剂；也可作为慢性铁中毒的辅助治疗手段；**s. benzoate,** an antifungal agent also used in a test of liver function 苯甲酸钠，一种抗真菌药，也用于肝功能测试；**s. bicarbonate,** the monosodium salt of carbonic acid, used as a gastric and systemic anatacid and to alkalize urine; also used, in solution, for washing the nose, mouth, and vagina, as a cleansing enema, and as a dressing for minor burns 碳酸氢钠，用于碱化尿液；在溶液中用于清洗鼻腔、口腔和阴道，作为清洁灌肠剂，也用作轻微烧伤的敷料；**s. biphosphate,** 同 monobasic s. phosphate；**s. borate,** the sodium salt of boric acid, used as an alkalizing agent in pharmaceuticals 硼酸钠（碱化剂）**s. carbonate,** the disodium salt of carbonic acid, used as an alkalizing agent in pharmaceuticals 碳酸钠（碱化剂）**s. chloride,** common table salt, a necessary constituent of the body and therefore of the diet, involved in maintaining osmotic tension of blood and tissues; uses include replenishment of electrolytes in the body, irrigation of wounds and body cavities, enema, inhaled mucolytic, topical osmotic ophthalmic agent, and preparation of pharmaceuticals 氯化钠，普通食盐，是人体必需的组成部分，因此也是饮食的组成部分，用于维持血液和组织的渗透性张力；用途包括补充体内电解质、冲洗伤口和体腔、灌肠、吸入溶解黏液、局部渗透性眼用制剂以及药物的制备；**s. chromate Cr 51,** the disodium salt of chromic acid prepared using the radioactive isotope chromium 51; used to tag erythrocytes or platelets for studies of red cell disease, gastrointestinal bleeding, and platelet survival 铬（⁵¹Cr）酸钠；**s. citrate,** the trisodium salt of citric acid, used as an anticoagulant for blood or plasma for transfusion; also used as a urinary alkalizer 枸橼酸钠，作为血液或血浆的抗凝剂时用于输血，也用作碱化剂；**dibasic s. phosphate,** an electrolyte replenisher, laxative, urinary acidifier, and antiurolithic, often used in combination with other phosphate compounds. Labeled with radiophosphorus (s. phosphate P 32), it is used as an antineoplastic in the treatment of polycythemia vera, chronic lymphocytic or myelogenous leukemia, and metastatic bone lesions 二元磷酸钠，电解质补充剂、泻药、尿酸化剂和抗尿路结石药，经常与其他磷酸盐化合物结合使用。用放射性磷标记，用于治疗真性红细胞增多症、慢性淋巴细胞性或髓性白血病以及转移性骨损伤；**s. dodecyl sulfate (SDS),** the more usual name for sodium lauryl sulfate when used as an anionic detergent to solubilize proteins 十二烷基硫酸钠，作为一种阴离子洗涤剂用于溶解蛋白质时更常用的名称；**s.**

fluoride, a dental caries prophylactic, NaF; used in the fluoridation of water and applied topically to the teeth 氟化钠, 用于水的氟化, 局部用于牙齿, 预防龋齿 ; **s. glutamate,** monosodium glutamate 谷氨酸钠 ; **s. hydroxide,** NaOH, a strongly alkaline and caustic compound; used as an alkalizing agent in pharmaceuticals 氢氧化钠, 一种强碱性和腐蚀性的化合物; 在药品中用作碱性剂 ; **s. hypochlorite,** the sodium salt of hypochlorous acid, NaClO, having germicidal and disinfectant properties 次氯酸钠, 具有杀菌和消毒剂的特性 ; **s. hyposulfite,** 同 s. thiosulfate; **s. iodide,** a binary haloid, used as a source of iodine. Labeled with radioactive iodine, it is used in thyroid function tests and thyroid imaging and to treat hyperthyroidism and thyroid carcinoma 碘化钠, 一种二元类卤代物, 用作碘的来源。用放射性碘标记, 用于甲状腺功能测试和甲状腺成像, 治疗甲状腺功能亢进和甲状腺癌 ; **s. lactate,** the sodium salt of racemic or inactive lactic acid, used as a fluid and electrolyte replenisher to combat acidosis 乳酸钠, 作为液体和电解质补充物以对抗酸中毒 ; **monobasic s. phosphate,** the monohydrate, dihydrate, or anhydrous monosodium salt of phosphoric acid; used in buffer solutions. Used alone or in combination with other phosphate compounds, given intravenously as an electrolyte replenisher, orally or rectally as a laxative, and orally as a urinary acidifier and as an antiurolithic 磷酸二氢钠, 磷酸的一水合物、二水合物或无水单钠盐; 用于缓冲溶液中。单独使用或与其他磷酸盐化合物结合使用, 作为电解质补充剂时静脉给药, 作为泻药时口服或直肠给药, 作为尿酸化剂和抗尿石剂时口服给药 ; **s. monofluorophosphate,** a dental caries prophylactic applied topically to the teeth 氟磷酸二钠, 预防龋齿局部应用于牙齿 ; **s. nitrite,** an antidote for cyanide poisoning; also used as a preservative in cured meats and other foods 亚硝酸钠, 氰化物中毒的解毒剂; 也可用于腌制肉类和其他食品的防腐剂 ; **s. nitroprusside,** an antihypertensive used in the treatment of acute congestive heart failure and of hypertensive crisis and to produce controlled hypotension during surgery; also used as a reagent 硝普钠, 一种降压药, 用于治疗急性充血性心力衰竭和高血压危象, 并在手术中产生控制性低血压; 也用作试剂 ; **s. phenylbutyrate,** an agent used as adjunctive treatment to control the hyperammonemia of urea cycle enzyme disorders 苯丁酸钠, 一种用于控制尿素循环酶紊乱的高氨血症的辅助治疗剂 ; **s. phosphate,** any of various compounds of sodium and phosphoric acid; usually specifically *dibasic s. phosphate* 磷酸钠, 通常是二元磷酸钠 ; **s. polystyrene sulfonate,** a cation exchange resin used as an antihyperkalemic 聚丙乙烯磺酸钠, 一种用作抗高血钾的阳离子交换树脂 ; **s. propionate,** the sodium salt of propionic acid, having antifungal properties; used as a topical antifungal; also used as a preservative 丙酸钠, 具有抗真菌特性; 用作局部抗真菌药; 也用作防腐剂 ; **s. salicylate,** 水杨酸钠, 参见 *salicylate*; **s. sulfate,** an osmotic laxative 硫酸钠, 渗透性泻药; **s. tetradecyl sulfate,** an anionic surfactant with sclerosing properties; used as a wetting agent and in the treatment of varicose veins 十四羟基硫酸钠, 一种具有硬化特性的阴离子表面活性剂, 用作湿润剂和治疗静脉曲张 ; **s. thiosulfate,** a compound used as an antidote (with s. nitrite) to cyanide poisoning, in the prophylaxis of ringworm (added to foot baths), topically in tinea versicolor, and in some tests of renal function 硫代硫酸钠, 用作氰化物中毒的解毒剂（与亚硝酸钠一起）, 用于预防环虫（添加到脚浴中）, 局部用于花斑癣和一些肾功能测试

so·do·ku (so′do-koo) Japanese name for the spirillary form of rat-bite fever 螺菌型鼠咬热的日本名称

sod·o·my (sod′ə-me) 1. anal intercourse 肛交 ; 2. any of various nonreproductive sexual acts, particularly anal intercourse 任何一种非生殖性的性行为, 特别是肛交

so·fos·bu·vir (soe-fos′-bue-vir) a nucleotide analogue inhibitor of the RNA polymerase nonstructural protein 5B, used in combination therapy to treat hepatitis C virus; available in formulations alone or in a fixed dose with ledipasvir 一种 RNA 聚合酶非结构蛋白 5B 的核苷酸类似物抑制药, 用于治疗丙型肝炎病毒的联合治疗; 可单独或以固定剂量 ledipasvir 配伍

sof·ten·ing (sof′en-ing) malacia 使软化

sol (sol) a colloid system in which the dispersion medium is liquid or gas; the latter is usually called an *aerosol* 溶胶

so·lar (so′lər) denoting the great sympathetic plexus and its principal ganglia (especially the celiac); so called because of their radiating nerves 太阳神经丛的, 指大的交感神经丛及其主要的神经节（尤其是腹腔神经丛）, 因其神经由中心呈辐射状发出而得名

sol·a·tion (sol-a′shən) the conversion of a gel into a sol 溶胶化

sole (sōl) the bottom of the foot 足底, 跖

sol·i·tary (sol′ĭ-tar″e) 1. alone; separated from others 单独的 ; 2. living alone or in pairs only 独居的; 仅成对居住的

sol·u·bil·i·ty (sol″u-bil′ĭ-te) quality of being soluble; susceptibility of being dissolved 可溶性, 溶解度

sol·u·ble (sol′u-bəl) susceptible of being dissolved

可溶的

so·lute (sol′ūt) the substance dissolved in solvent to form a solution 溶质

so·lu·tion (sə-loo′shən) 1. a homogeneous mixture of one or more substances (solutes) dispersed molecularly in a sufficient quantity of dissolving medium (solvent) 溶液，一种由一种或多种物质（溶质）组成的均匀混合物，分子分散在足量的溶解介质（溶剂）中；2. in pharmacology, a liquid preparation of one or more soluble chemical substances usually dissolved in water 在药理学上指一种液体制剂，内含一种或几种通常是溶于水的可溶性化学物质；3. the process of dissolving 溶解，物质溶解的过程；**acetic acid otic s.**, a solution of glacial acetic acid in a nonaqueous solvent, used to treat otitis externa caused by various fungi 醋酸洗耳液；**aluminum acetate topical s.**, a preparation of aluminum subacetate solution, glacial acetic acid, and water; an astringent applied topically to the skin as a wet dressing and used as a gargle or mouthwash 醋酸铝外用溶液作为湿敷料外用在皮肤上的收敛剂，用作漱口液；**aluminum subacetate topical s.**, a solution of aluminum sulfate, acetic acid, precipitated calcium carbonate, and water; applied topically as an astringent, and also as an antiseptic and a wet dressing 碱式醋酸铝溶液，次醋酸铝外用液，局部用作收敛剂，也用作防腐剂和湿敷料；**anisotonic s.**, one having tonicity differing from that of the standard of reference 不等渗溶液；**anticoagulant citrate dextrose s.**, a solution of citric acid, sodium citrate, and dextrose in water for injection, used for preservation of whole blood 枸橼酸盐葡萄糖抗凝溶液，用于保存全血；**anticoagulant citrate phosphate dextrose s.**, a solution containing citric acid, sodium citrate, monobasic sodium phosphate, and dextrose in water for injection; used for preservation of whole blood 抗凝枸橼磷酸盐葡萄糖溶液用于保存全血；**anticoagulant citrate phosphate dextrose adenine s.**, a solution consisting of anticoagulant citrate phosphate dextrose solution and adenine; used for the preservation of whole blood 抗凝枸橼酸盐磷酸盐葡萄糖腺嘌呤溶液，用于保存全血；**anticoagulant heparin s.**, a sterile solution of heparin sodium in sodium chloride, used as an anticoagulant in the preservation of whole blood 肝素抗凝液，用作抗凝血剂以保存全血；**anticoagulant sodium citrate s.**, a solution of sodium citrate in water for injection, used for the storage of whole blood, preparation of blood for fractionation, and preparation of citrated human plasma 抗凝枸橼酸钠溶液，用于保存全血、分馏血液制备、枸橼酸化人血浆制备；**APF s.**, sodium fluoride and acidulated phosphate topical s. APF 溶液；**aqueous**

s., one in which water is the solvent 水溶液；**Benedict s.**, a sodium citrate, sodium carbonate, and cupric sulfate aqueous solution; used to determine the presence of glucose in urine 一种枸橼酸钠、碳酸钠和硫酸铜水溶液；用于测定尿液中葡萄糖的存在；**buffer s.**, one that resists appreciable change in its hydrogen ion concentration upon addition of acid or alkali 缓冲溶液；**cardioplegic s.**, a cold solution injected into the aortic root or the coronary ostia to induce cardiac arrest and protect the heart during open heart surgery, usually potassium in an electrolyte solution or in blood 心脏停搏液；**colloid s.**, **colloidal s.**, imprecise term for a *colloidal system* 胶体溶液，胶体系统的不精确术语，参见 *colloid* (2)；**Dakin s.**, a diluted sodium hypochlorite solution, which has been used as a topical antiinfective for skin and wounds 次氯酸钠消毒液，用作皮肤和伤口的局部抗感染剂 **formaldehyde s.**, an aqueous solution containing not less than 37 percent formaldehyde; used as a disinfectant and as a preservative and fixative for pathologic specimens 甲醛溶液，一种含有不少于37%甲醛的水溶液，用作消毒剂和病理标本的防腐剂和固定剂；**hyperbaric s.**, one having a greater specific gravity than a standard of reference 高比重溶液；**hypobaric s.**, one having a specific gravity less than that of a standard of reference 轻比重溶液；**iodine topical s.**, a solution prepared with purified water, each 100 ml containing 1.8 to 2.2 g of iodine and 2.1 to 2.6 g of sodium iodide; a local antiinfective 外用碘溶液；**isobaric s.**, a solution having the same specific gravity as a standard of reference 等比重溶液；**lactated Ringer s.**, 乳酸林格液，参见 *injection*；**Lugol s.**, 同 strong iodine s.；**molar s.**, a solution each liter of which contains 1 mole of the dissolved substance; designated 1 M. The concentration of other solutions may be expressed in relation to that of molar solutions as tenth-molar (0.1 M), etc. 摩尔溶液，容积克分子溶液；**Monsel s.**, a reddish-brown aqueous solution of basic ferric sulfate; astringent and hemostatic 蒙塞尔溶液；**normal s.**, a solution each liter of which contains 1 equivalent weight of the dissolved substance; designated 1 N 当量溶液，每升含 1 克当量溶解物质的溶液，以 1N 表示；**normal saline s.**, **normal salt s.**, 同 physiologic salt s.；**ophthalmic s.**, a sterile solution, free from foreign particles, for instillation into the eye 洗眼液；**physiologic saline s.**, **physiologic salt s.**, **physiologic sodium chloride s.**, a 0.9 percent aqueous solution of sodium chloride, which is isotonic with blood serum 生理盐水溶液，生理盐水，生理氯化钠溶液，一种 0.9% 的氯化钠水溶液，与血清等渗；**Ringer s.**, 林格（溶）液，参见 *injection* 和 *irrigation* 下词条；

saline s., salt s., a solution of sodium chloride in purified water 盐溶液 ; **saturated s.,** one containing all of the solute that can be held in solution by the solvent 饱 和 溶 液 ; **sclerosing s.,** a solution of a sclerosing agent, for use in sclerotherapy 硬 化 溶 液，用于硬化疗法 ; **Shohl s.,** an aqueous solution of citric acid and sodium citrate; used to correct electrolyte imbalance in renal tubular acidosis Shohl 溶液，用于纠正肾小管酸中毒的电解质失衡 ; **sodium fluoride and acidulated phosphate topical s.,** a solution of sodium fluoride, acidulated with phosphoric acid, pH of 3.0 to 3.5; applied topically to the teeth as a dental caries prophylactic 氟 化 钠 和酸化磷酸盐局部溶液，一种氟化钠溶液，用 磷酸酸化，pH 值为 3.0 到 3.5；局部应用于牙 齿以预防龋齿 ; **sodium hypochlorite s.,** a solution containing 4 to 6 percent by weight of sodium hypochlorite; used to disinfect utensils. In dilution, usually containing approximately 0.5 percent free chlorine, it is used for skin disinfection and wound irrigation 次氯酸钠溶液 ; **standard s.,** a solution that contains in each liter a definitely stated amount of reagent; usually expressed in terms of normality (equivalent weights of solute per liter of solution) or molarity (moles of solute per liter of solution) 标 准溶液 ; **strong iodine s.,** a solution containing, in each 100 ml, 5 g of iodine and 10 g of potassium iodide; a source of iodine 浓碘溶液 ; **supersaturated s.,** an unstable solution containing more of the solute than it can permanently hold 过饱和溶 液 ; **TAC s.,** a solution of tetracaine, epinephrine (or adrenaline), and cocaine, used as a local anesthetic in the emergency treatment of uncomplicated lacerations TAC 溶液，一种丁卡因、肾上腺素和可 卡因组成的溶液，在简单裂伤的紧急治疗中用 作局部麻醉剂 ; **volumetric s.,** one that contains a specific quantity of solvent per stated unit of volume 滴定液

sol·vent (sol′vənt) 1. dissolving; effecting a solution 溶解 ; 2. a substance, usually a liquid, that dissolves or is capable of dissolving; the component of a solution present in greater amount 溶剂，溶媒

so·ma (so′mə) 1. the body as distinguished from the mind 体，躯体，有别于精神 ; 2. the body tissue as distinguished from the germ cells 体组织，有别于生殖细胞 ; 3. the cell body of a neuron（神 经元）胞体

so·ma·tal·gia (so″mə-tal′jə) generalized bodily pain 躯体痛

so·mat·es·the·sia (so″mat-es-the′zhə) 同 somatognosis

so·mat·ic (so-mat′ik) 1. pertaining to or character-

istic of the soma or body 躯体的 ; 2. pertaining to the body wall in contrast to the viscera 体壁的

so·ma·ti·za·tion (so″mə-tĭ-za′shən) the conversion of mental experiences or states into bodily symptoms 躯体化，指在精神病学中，精神症状 转化为躯体症状

so·mato·chrome (so-mat′o-krōm) any neuron that has cytoplasm completely surrounding the nucleus and easily stainable Nissl bodies 体染色细 胞（的）

so·mato·form (so-mat′o-form) denoting physical symptoms that cannot be attributed to organic disease and appear to be psychogenic 躯体型症状，指不能归因于器质性疾病并表现为精神性的身体 症状

so·ma·to·gen·ic (so″mə-to-jen′ik) originating in the cells of the body, as opposed to *psychogenic* 躯 体原的，与精神原的相反

so·ma·tog·no·sis (so″mə-tog-no′sis) the general feeling of the existence of one's body and of the functioning of the organs 躯体感觉

so·ma·tol·o·gy (so″mə-tol′ə-je) the sum of what is known about the body; the study of anatomy and physiology 躯体学，身体学，躯体解剖学与生理 学的研究

so·ma·to·me·din (so″mə-to-me′din) any of a group of peptides found in plasma, complexed with binding proteins; they stimulate cellular growth and replication as second messengers in the somatotropic actions of growth hormone and also have insulin-like activities. Two such peptides have been isolated, insulin-like growth factors Ⅰ and Ⅱ 生长调 节肽，生长调节素，生长素介质

so·ma·tom·e·try (so″mə-tom′ə-tre) measurement of the body 活体测量（法）

so·ma·to·mo·tor (so″mə-to-mo′tər) pertaining to movements of the body 躯体运动的

so·mato·pleure (so-mat′o-ploor) the embryonic body wall, formed by ectoderm and somatic mesoderm 胚体壁，由外胚层和体壁中胚层形成 ; **somatopleur′al** *adj.*

so·ma·to·psy·chic (so″mə-to-si′kik) pertaining to both mind and body; relating to the effects of the body on the mind 躯体精神的 ; 身心的

so·ma·tos·co·py (so″mə-tos′kə-pe) examination of the body 体格检查

so·ma·to·sen·so·ry (so″mə-to-sen′sə-re) pertaining to sensations received in the skin and deep tissues 躯体感觉的

so·ma·to·sex·u·al (so″mə-to-sek′shoo-əl) pertaining to both physical and sex characteristics, or to physical manifestations of sexual development 体征 与性征的，性发育与身体现象的

S

so·ma·to·stat·in (so″mə-tō-stat′in) a polypeptide elaborated primarily by the median eminence of the hypothalamus and by the delta cells of the islets of Langerhans; it inhibits release of thyrotropin, somatotropin, and corticotropin by the anterior lobe of the pituitary, of insulin and glucagon by the pancreas, of gastrin by the gastric mucosa, of secretin by the intestinal mucosa, and of renin by the kidney 促生长素，抑制素，生长抑素

so·ma·to·stat·in·oma (som″ə-to-stat″ĭ-no′- mə) an islet cell tumor that secretes somatostatin 生长抑（制）素瘤

so·ma·to·ther·a·py (so″mə-to-ther′ə-pe) biologic treatment of mental disorders, as with electric shock or drug therapy 躯体疗法

so·ma·to·top·ic (so″mə-to-top′ik) related to particular areas of the body; describing organization of the motor area of the brain, control of the movement of different parts of the body being centered in specific regions of the cortex 躯体定位的，与身体特定区域有关的；描述大脑运动区的组织及身体不同部位运动的控制在大脑皮质特定区中的定位

so·ma·to·trope (so-mat′o-trōp) 同 somatotroph

so·ma·to·troph (so-mat′o-trōf) a type of acidophil of the anterior lobe of the pituitary that secretes growth hormone 生长激素细胞，垂体前叶分泌生长激素的一种嗜酸细胞

so·ma·to·tro·phic (so″mə-to-tro′fik) somatotropic 促生长的

so·ma·to·tro·phin (so′mə-to-tro″fin) growth hormone 生长激素

so·ma·to·tro·pic (so″mə-to-tro′pik) 1. having an affinity for or attacking the body cells 亲躯体的，亲躯体细胞的；2. having a stimulating effect on nutrition and growth 促生长的；3. having the properties of somatotrophin 有生长激素特性的

so·ma·to·tro·pin (so′mə-to-tro″pin) growth hormone 生长激素

so·ma·to·type (so-mat′o-tīp) a particular type of body build 体型

so·ma·trem (so′mə-trem) biosynthetic human growth hormone, prepared by recombinant technology and differing from the natural human hormone in containing an additional methionine residue at the terminus; used to treat growth failure and AIDS-associated cachexia or weight loss 基因重组人生长激素

so·mat·ro·pin (so-mat′ro-pin) biosynthetic human growth hormone, prepared by recombinant means and having the same amino acid sequence as the natural hormone; used to treat growth failure and AIDS-associated cachexia or weight loss 生长激素

so·mes·the·sia (so″mes-the′zhə) 同 somatognosis

so·mite (so′mīt) one of the paired, blocklike masses of mesoderm, arranged segmentally alongside the neural tube of the embryo, forming the vertebral column and segmental musculature 体节

som·nam·bu·lism (som-nam′bu-liz-əm) sleepwalking; rising out of bed and walking about or performing other complex motor behavior during an apparent state of sleep 睡行（症），梦游（症）

som·ni·fa·cient (som″nĭ-fa′shənt) hypnotic (1, 2) 眠的，催眠药

som·nif·er·ous (som-nif′ər-əs) hypnotic (1) 催眠的

som·nil·o·quism (som-nil′o-kwiz-əm) talking in one's sleep 梦语

som·no·lence (som′nə-ləns) drowsiness or sleepiness, particularly in excess 嗜睡

som·no·len·tia (som″nə-len′shə) [L.] 1. drowsiness, or somnolence 嗜睡，瞌睡；2. sleep drunkenness 醉梦状态

son·i·ca·tion (son″ĭ-ka′shən) exposure to sound waves; disruption of bacteria exposure to high-frequency sound waves 声波处理，超声波降解

so·nog·ra·phy (sə-nog′rə-fe) ultrasonography 超声检查；**sonograph′ic** *adj.*

sono·lu·cent (son″o-loo′sənt) anechoic; in ultrasonography, permitting the passage of ultrasound waves without reflecting them back to their source (without giving off echoes) 超声透过，透声的

SOPHE Society for Public Health Education 公共卫生教育学会

so·por (so′por) [L.] unnaturally deep or profound sleep 昏迷，昏睡

sop·o·rif·ic (sop″o-rif′ik) (so′po-rif′ik) 1. producing deep sleep 催眠的；2. hypnotic (2) 催眠药

so·por·ous (so′por-əs) associated with coma or profound sleep 迷睡的

sorb (sorb) to attract and retain substances by absorption or adsorption 吸收，吸附

sor·be·fa·cient (sor″bə-fa′shənt) absorbefacient 促吸收的；吸收剂

sor·bent (sor′bənt) an agent that sorbs 吸着剂，参见 *absorbent* 和 *adsorbent*

sor·bic ac·id (sor′bik) a fungistat used as an antimicrobial inhibitor in pharmaceuticals 山梨酸

sor·bi·tan (sor′bĭ-tən) any of the anhydrides of sorbitol, the fatty acids of which are surfactants used as emulsifiers in pharmaceutical preparations 山梨聚糖，另参见 *polysorbate 80*

sor·bi·tol (sor′bĭ-tol) a 6-carbon sugar alcohol from a variety of fruits, found in lens deposits in diabetes mellitus. A pharmaceutical preparation is used as a sweetening agent and osmotic laxative, and in drugs as a tablet excipient, humectant, and stabilizer 山梨糖醇

sor·des (sor'dēz) debris, especially the encrustations of food, epithelial matter, and bacteria that collect on the lips and teeth during a prolonged fever 口垢

sore (sor) 1. popularly, almost any lesion of the skin or mucous membranes 溃疡；2. painful 疼痛的；**bed s.,** decubitus ulcer 压疮；**canker s.,** recurrent aphthous stomatitis 口腔溃疡；**cold s.,** herpes febrilis 唇疱疹

sorp·tion (sorp'shən) the process or state of being sorbed; absorption or adsorption 吸收作用，吸附作用

SOS sinusoidal obstruction syndrome 肝窦阻塞综合征

S.O.S. [L.] si o'pus sit (if it is necessary) 必要时

so·ta·lol (so'tə-lol) a noncardioselective betaadrenergic blocking agent used as the hydrochloride salt in the treatment of life-threatening cardiac arrhythmias 心得怡，甲磺胺心定

souf·fle (soo'fəl) a soft, blowing auscultatory sound 杂音，吹气音；**cardiac s.,** any cardiac or vascular murmur of a blowing quality 心脏杂音；**funic s., funicu-lar s.,** hissing souffle synchronous with fetal heart sounds, probably from the umbilical cord 脐带杂音；**mammary s.,** a functional cardiac murmur with a blowing sound, heard over the breasts in late pregnancy and during lactation 乳房杂音；**placental s.,** the sound supposed to be produced by the blood current in the placenta 胎盘杂音；**uterine s.,** a sound made by the blood within the arteries of the gravid uterus 子宫杂音

sound (sound) 1. a pressure wave propagating through an elastic medium; waves with a frequency of 20 to 20 000 Hz cause the sensation of hearing 声（音）；2. the effect produced on the organ of hearing by vibrations of the air or other medium 声音；3. a noise, normal or abnormal, heard within the body 听诊；4. an instrument to be introduced into a cavity to detect a foreign body or to dilate a stricture 探子；**adventitious s's,** abnormal auscultatory sounds heard over the lung, such as rales, rhonchi, or abnormal resonance 附加音；**aortic second s. (A₂),** the audible vibrations related to the closure of the aortic valve 主动脉瓣第二心音；**auscultatory s's,** those vheard on auscultation, such as breath sounds, heart sounds, and adventitious sounds 听诊音；**breath s's,** respiratory s's; sounds heard on auscultation over the respiratory tract; bronchial and ventricular ones are heard normally at certain places, whereas a cavernous one indicates a lung cavity 呼吸音；**continuous s's,** adventitious sounds lasting longer than 0.2 second, such as wheezes and rhonchi 连续附加音；**discontinuous s's,** adventitious sounds lasting less than 0.2 second and coming in a series; the most common are rales 非连续附加音，乱序附加音；**ejection s's,** high-pitched clicking sounds heard just after the first heart sound, at maximal opening of the semilunar valves; seen in patients with valvular abnormalities or dilatations of aortic or pulmonary arteries 喷射音；**friction s.,** 摩擦音，参见 *rub* 下词条；**heart s's,** sounds heard over the cardiac region, produced by the functioning of the heart. The *first,* at the beginning of ventricular systole, is dull, firm, and prolonged, and heard as a "lubb" sound; the *second,* produced mainly by closure of the semilunar valves, is shorter and sharper than the first and is heard as a "dupp" sound; the *third* is usually audible only in youth; and the *fourth* is normally inaudible 心音；**hippocratic s's,** succussion s's 希波克拉底振荡音；**Korotkoff s's,** sounds heard during auscultatory determination of blood pressure 科罗特科夫音，科氏音；**percussion s.,** any sound obtained by percussion 叩诊音；**pulmonic second s. (P₂),** the audible vibrations related to the closure of the pulmonary valve 肺动脉瓣第二心音；**respiratory s's,** 同 breath s's；**speech s.,** one of the minimal elements of a spoken language, such as a consonant or vowel 语音；**succussion s's,** splashing sounds heard on succussion over a distended stomach or in hydropneumothorax 振荡音；**to-and-fro s.,** 风箱音，参见 *murmur* 下词条；**urethral s.,** a long, slender instrument for exploring and dilating the urethra 尿道探子；**valvular ejection s.,** an ejection sound resulting from abnormality of one or both semilunar valves 瓣膜喷射音；**vascular ejection s.,** an ejection sound resulting from abnormality of the pulmonary artery or aorta without abnormality of either semilunar valve 脉管喷射音；**voice s's,** auscultatory sounds heard over the lungs or airways when the patient speaks; increased resonance indicates consolidation or effusion 患者讲话时在肺或气道的语音共鸣音；**white s.,** a mixture of all frequencies of mechanical vibration perceptible as sound 白声，所有频率的机械振动混合而成的可被察觉的声音

soy (soi) 同 soybean

soy·bean (soi'bēn) the bean of the leguminous plant *Glycine max,* which contains little starch but is rich in protein and phytoestrogens 大豆；又称 *soy*

space (spās) 1. a delimited area 空间；2. an actual or potential cavity of the body 隙，间隙，腔；**spa'tial** *adj.*；**apical s.,** the region between the wall of the alveolus and the apex of the root of a tooth 根尖隙；**Bowman s.,** capsular s. 肾小囊腔，参

见 capsular s. **capsular s.,** a narrow chalice-shaped cavity between the glomerular and capsular epithelium of the glomerular capsule of the kidney 肾 小 囊腔；**cartilage s's,** the spaces in hyaline cartilage containing the cartilage cells 软骨间隙；**corneal s's,** the spaces between the lamellae of the substantia propria of the cornea containing corneal cells and interstitial fluid 角膜间隙；**cupular s.,** the part of the attic above the malleus 顶隙，鼓室上隐窝顶部；**danger s.,** a subdivision of the retropharyngeal space, extending from the base of the skull to the level of the respiratory diaphragm; it provides a route for the spread of infection from the pharynx to the mediastinum 危险间隙，咽后空间的一部分，从颅骨基底延伸到呼吸膈；为从咽到纵隔感染的播散提供路径；**dead s.,** 1. the space remaining after incomplete closure of surgical or other wounds, permitting accumulation of blood or serum and resultant delay in healing 手术切口或其他伤口不完全的关闭遗留的空间，允许血液或血清积聚而导致延迟愈合；2. in the respiratory tract: (1) *anatomical dead s.,* those portions, from the nose and mouth to the terminal bronchioles, not participating in oxygen–carbon dioxide exchange, and (2) *physiologic dead s.,* which reflects nonuniformity of ventilation and perfusion in the lung, is the anatomical dead space plus the space in the alveoli occupied by air that does not participate in oxygen–carbon dioxide exchange 无效腔，（1）解剖无效腔，指从口鼻到终末支气管，不参与氧气－二氧化碳交换的部分；（2）生理无效腔，反映肺通气与灌注的不一致性，指解剖无效腔和肺泡无效腔无法参加氧气－二氧化碳交换的肺泡空间；**epidural s.,** 硬膜外腔 1. the space between the dura mater and the lining of the vertebral canal 硬脑膜与椎管内壁之间的间隙；2. an artifactual space created between the dura and the inner table of the skull as a result of trauma or a pathologic process 由于创伤或病理过程导致的硬膜与颅骨内板之间形成的人造成空间；**episcleral s.,** the space between the bulbar fascia and the eyeball 巩膜外隙；**iliocostal s.,** the area between the twelfth rib and the crest of the ilium 髂肋间隙；**intercostal s.,** the space between two adjacent ribs 肋 间 隙；**interglobular s's,** small irregular spaces on the outer surface of the dentin in the tooth root 球间隙；**interproximal s.,** the space between the proximal surfaces of adjoining teeth 邻面间隙，相邻牙齿的临近表面之间的间隙；**intervillous s.,** the space of the placenta into which the chorionic villi project and through which the maternal blood circulates 绒毛间隙；**Kiernan s's,** the triangular spaces bounded by the invaginated Glisson capsule between the liver

lobules, containing the larger interlobular branches of the portal vein, hepatic artery, and hepatic duct Kiernan 间隙，肝小叶间淋巴间隙，包含门静脉，肝动脉和肝管较大的小叶间分支；**lymph s.,** any space in tissue occupied by lymph 淋巴隙；**Meckel s.,** a recess in the dura mater that lodges the gasserian ganglion Meckel 隙，固定半月神经节的硬膜凹陷；**medullary s.,** the central cavity and the intervals between the trabeculae of bone that contain the marrow 髓腔；**palmar s.,** a large fascial space in the hand, divided by a fibrous septum into a mid-palmar and a thenar space 掌间隙；**parasinoidal s's,** lateral lacunae 窦旁间隙（外侧陷窝）**periaxial s.,** a fluid-filled cavity surrounding the nuclear bag and myotubule regions of a muscle spindle 轴周围间隙；**perilymphatic s.,** the fluid-filled space separating the membranous from the osseous labyrinth 外 淋巴隙，骨迷路和膜迷路之间的间隙；**perineal s's,** spaces on either side of the inferior fascia of the urogenital diaphragm, the *deep* between it and the superior fascia, the *superficial* between it and the superficial perineal fascia 会阴间隙；**perinuclear s.,** a space, approximately 30 nm wide and continuous with the lumen of the endoplasmic reticulum, separating the inner and outer membranes of the nuclear envelope 核周隙；**periplasmic s.,** a zone between the plasma membrane and the outer membrane of the cell wall of gram-negative bacteria 周质间隙；**perivascular s's,** spaces, often only potential, that surround blood vessels for a short distance as they enter the brain（脑）血管周隙，脑血管周围间隙；**perivitelline s.,** a space between the oocyte and the zona pellucida 卵周隙；**pneumatic s.,** a portion of bone occupied by air-containing cells, especially the spaces constituting the paranasal sinuses 含气腔；**Poiseuille s.,** that part of the lumen of a tube, at its periphery, where no flow of liquid occurs Poiseuille 间隙，血管腔的边缘部，此处红细胞不流动；**Reinke s.,** a potential space between the vocal ligament and the overlying mucosa Reink 间隙，声带与其上黏膜之间潜在的腔；**retroperitoneal s.,** the space between the peritoneum and the posterior abdominal wall 腹膜后隙；**retropharyngeal s.,** the space behind the pharynx, containing areolar tissue 咽后间隙；**retropubic s.,** the areolar space bounded by the reflection of peritoneum, symphysis pubis, and bladder 耻 骨 后 隙；**Retzius s.,** 1. retropubic s. 雷丘斯间隙；2. 同 perilymphatic s.；**subarachnoid s.,** the space between the arachnoid and the pia mater 蛛网膜下腔，蛛网膜下隙；**subdural s.,** an artifactual space between the dura mater and the arachnoid; normally the arachnoid is attached to the dura and space exists only as the result of trauma or a pathologic process 硬膜下隙；**subgingival s.,** gingival crevice 龈下隙；**subphrenic s.,** the space between the respiratory diaphragm and subjacent organs 膈下隙；**subumbilical s.,** a somewhat triangular space in the body cavity beneath the umbilicus 脐下隙；**Tenon s.,** episcleral s. 眼球筋膜隙；**thenar s.,** the palmar space lying between the middle metacarpal bone and the tendon of the flexor pollicis longus 鱼际间隙；**zonular s's,** the lymph-filled spaces between the fibers of the ciliary zonule 小带间隙

spar·flox·a·cin (spahr-flok′sə-sin) a synthetic, broad-spectrum antimicrobial agent 施怕沙星，一种合成广谱抗菌药

spar·ga·no·sis (spahr″gə-no′sis) infection with the larvae (spargana) of any of several species of tapeworms, which invade the superficial fascia, causing inflammation and fibrosis 裂头蚴病

spar·ga·num (spahr′gə-nəm) pl. *spar′gana* [Gr.] the larval stage of certain tapeworms, especially of the genera *Diphyllobothrium* and *Spirometra;* see also *sparganosis.* Also, a genus name applied to such larvae, usually when the adult stage is unknown 裂头蚴属

spasm (spaz′əm) 1. a sudden, violent, involuntary muscular contraction 突然的，暴力的，非自愿的肌肉收缩；2. a sudden transitory constriction of a passage, canal, or orifice 管道，腔道或孔的突然短暂的收缩 **bronchial s.,** bronchospasm 支气管痉挛；**carpopedal s.,** spasm of the hand or foot, or of the thumbs or great toes, seen in tetany 腕足痉挛；**clonic s.,** a spasm consisting of clonic contractions 阵挛性痉挛；**facial s.,** tonic spasm of the muscles supplied by the facial nerve, involving the entire side of the face or confined to a limited area about the eye 面痉挛；**habit s.,** 习惯性痉挛，参见 *tic* 下词条；**infantile s's,** a syndrome of severe myoclonus appearing in infancy and associated with general cerebral deterioration 婴儿痉挛（症）；**intention s.,** muscular spasm on attempting voluntary movement 意向性痉挛；**myopathic s.,** spasm accompanying disease of the muscles 肌病性痉挛；**nodding s.,** a nodding motion of the head accompanied by nystagmus, seen in infants and young children 点头状痉挛；**saltatory s.,** clonic spasm of the muscles of the legs, producing a peculiar jumping or springing motion when standing 痉跳病；**tetanic s., tonic s.,** tetanus (2) 强直性痉挛，破伤风痉挛；**toxic s.,** spasm caused by a toxin 中毒性痉挛

spas·mod·ic (spaz-mod′ik) of the nature of a spasm; occurring in spasms 痉挛性的；痉挛的

spas·mol·y·sis (spaz-mol′ĭ-sis) the arrest of spasm 解痉（作用）；**spasmolyt′ic** *adj.*

spas·mus (spaz′məs) [L.] spasm 痉挛；**s. nu′tans,** nodding spasm 点头状痉挛

spas·tic (spas′tik) 1. of the nature of or characterized by spasms 痉挛的；2. hypertonic, so that the muscles are stiff and movements awkward 僵硬的，强直的

spas·tic·i·ty (spas-tis′ĭ-te) the state of being spastic 痉挛状态，参见 *spastic* (2)

spa·tial (spa′shəl) pertaining to space 空间的；隙的，间隙的，腔的

spa·ti·um (spa′she-əm) pl. *spa′tia* [L.] space 隙，间隙，腔

spat·u·la (spach′ə-lə) [L.] 1. a wide, flat, blunt, usually flexible instrument of little thickness, used for spreading material on a smooth surface 抹刀，刮铲，（调软膏用的）药刀，软膏刀；压舌板；2. a spatulate structure 竹片状结构

spat·u·late (spach′ə-lāt) 1. having a flat blunt end 药刀状的，铲形的；2. to mix or manipulate with a spatula 调拌，用抹刀混合或操作；3. to make an enlarged opening in a tubular structure by means of a longitudinal incision that is then spread open 通过纵向切口在管状结构中做一个扩大的开口，然后展开

SPCA serum prothrombin conversion accelerator (coagulation factor Ⅶ) 血清凝血酶原转变加速因子（凝血因子Ⅶ）

spe·cial·ist (spesh′əl-ist) a physician whose practice is limited to a particular branch of medicine or surgery, especially one who, by virtue of advanced training, is certified by a specialty board as being qualified to so limit it 专家，专科医师；**clinical nurse s., nurse s.,** 护理专家，临床护理专业人员，参见 *nurse* 下词条

spe·cial·ty (spesh′əl-te) the field of practice of a specialist 专业，特长

spe·ci·a·tion (spe″se-a′shən) the evolutionary formation of new species 物种形成

spe·cies (spe′shēz) (spe′sēz) a taxonomic category subordinate to a genus (or subgenus) and superior to a subspecies or variety 物种，种；**type s.,** the original species from which the description of the genus is formulated 模式种

spe·cies-spe·cif·ic (spe″sēz-spə-sif′ik) 1. characteristic of a particular species 特定特种的特征；2. having a characteristic effect on, or interaction with, cells or tissues of members of a particular species; said of an antigen, drug, or infective agent 对特定物种成员的细胞或组织有特征有特征性影响或相互作用；指抗原、药物或传染物

spe·cif·ic (spə-sif′ik) 1. pertaining to a species 种的；2. produced by a single kind of microorganism 由一种病菌引起的；3. restricted in application, effect, etc., to a particular structure, function, etc. 特异的，在应用、效果等方面限于特定的结构、功能等；4. a remedy specially indicated for a particular disease 特效药；5. in immunology, pertaining to the special affinity of antigen for the corresponding antibody 特异性的，专一性的，在免疫学上用于修饰或说明抗原对相应抗体的特殊亲和力

spec·i·fic·i·ty (spes″ĭ-fis′ĭ-te) 1. the quality or state of being specific 特异性，特殊性；2. the probability that a person who does not have a disease will be correctly identified by a clinical test 特性，特征

spec·i·men (spes′ĭ-mən) a small sample or part taken to show the nature of the whole, as a small quantity of urine for analysis, or a small fragment of tissue for microscopic study 标本；样品，（检验用）抽样

SPECT single-photon emission computed tomography 单光子发射计算机体层摄影

spec·ta·cles (spek′tə-kəlz) glasses 眼镜

spec·ti·no·my·cin (spek″tĭ-no-mi′sin) an antibiotic derived from *Streptomyces spectabilis*, used as the hydrochloride salt in the treatment of gonorrhea 壮观霉素，大观霉素

spec·tral (spek′trəl) pertaining to a spectrum; performed by means of a spectrum 光谱的

spec·trin (spek′trin) 血影蛋白 1. a contractile protein attached to glycophorin at the cytoplasmic surface of the cell membrane of erythrocytes, important in maintaining cell shape 红细胞细胞膜细胞质表面附着在糖激素上的收缩蛋白，对维持细胞形状很重要；2. a contractile protein that with actin, glycophorin, and other cytoskeleton proteins forms a fibrous network beneath the plasma membrane of erythrocytes that maintains cell shape and flexibility 与活性素、糖激素和其他细胞骨架蛋白一起形成红细胞血浆膜下的纤维网络，维持细胞形状和灵活性的收缩蛋白

spec·trom·e·try (spek-trom′ə-tre) determination of the wavelengths or frequencies of the lines in a spectrum 度（光）谱术

spec·tro·pho·tom·e·ter (spek″tro-fo-tom′ə-tər) 1. an apparatus for measuring light sense by means of a spectrum 光谱光度计；2. an apparatus for determining the quantity of coloring matter in solution by measurement of transmitted light 分光光度计

spec·tro·scope (spek′trə-skōp) an instrument for developing and analyzing spectra 分光镜；**spec·troscop′ic** *adj.*

spec·trum (spek′trəm) pl. *spec′tra* [L.] 1. a charted band of wavelengths of electromagnetic radiation obtained by refraction or diffraction 光谱，通过折射或衍射获得的电磁辐射波长的图表带；2. by extension, a measurable range of activity, as the range of bacteria affected by an antibiotic *(antibacterial s.)* or the complete range of manifestations of a disease 谱，一个可测量的活动范围，作为受抗生素影响的细菌范围（抗菌谱）或疾病的临床表现；**absorption s.,** that afforded by light which has passed through various gaseous media, each gas absorbing those rays of which its own spectrum is composed 吸收光谱；**broad-s.,** effective against a wide range of microorganisms; said of an antibiotic 广谱；**electromagnetic s.,** the range of electromagnetic energy from cosmic rays to electric waves, including gamma, x- and ultraviolet rays, visible light, infrared waves, and radio waves 电磁波谱；**fortification s.,** a form of migraine aura characterized by scintillating or zigzag bands of colored light forming the edge of an area of teichopsia 闪光暗点；**visible s.,** the portion of the range of wavelengths of electromagnetic vibrations (from 770 to 390 nm) that is capable of stimulating specialized sense organs and is perceptible as light 可见光谱

spec·u·lum (spek′u-ləm) pl. *spec′ula* [L.] an instrument for opening or distending a body orifice or cavity to permit visual inspection 窥器

speech (spēch) the expression of thoughts and ideas by vocal sounds 言语，谈话，发言；**esophageal s.,** that produced by vibration of the column of air in the esophagus against the contracting cricopharyngeal sphincter; used after laryngectomy 食管言语；**explosive s.,** speech uttered with more force than necessary 爆炸式语言；**mirror s.,** a speech abnormality in which the order of syllables in a sentence is reversed 倒语；**pressured s.,** logorrhea 强制言语，多言症；**scanning s.,** that in which syllables of words are separated by noticeable pauses 断续言语；**staccato s.,** that in which each syllable is uttered separately 断音言语；**telegraphic s.,** that consisting of only certain prominent words and lacking articles, modifiers, and other ancillary words, a form of agrammaticism in other than young children 电报式言语

sperm (spurm) 1. 同 spermatozoon；2. 同 semen

sper·mat·ic (spər-mat′ik) 1. seminal 精液的；2. pertaining to spermatozoa 精子的

sper·ma·tid (spur′mə-tid) a cell derived from a secondary spermatocyte by fission, and developing into a spermatozoon 精子细胞

sper·ma·to·blast (spur′mə-to-blast″) 同 spermatid

sper·ma·to·cele (spur′mə-to-sēl″) cystic distention of the epididymis or rete testis, containing spermatozoa 精液囊肿

sper·ma·to·ce·lec·to·my (spər-mat″o-sə- lek′tə-me) excision of a spermatocele 精液囊肿切除术

sper·ma·to·ci·dal (spur″mə-to-si′dəl) spermicidal. 杀精子的，参见 *spermicide*

sper·ma·to·cide (spər-mat′o-sīd″) 同 spermicide

sper·ma·to·cyst (spur′mə-to-sist″) 同 spermatocele

sper·ma·to·cyte (spər-mat′o-sīt) a cell developed from a spermatogonium in spermatogenesis 精母细胞；**spermatocy′tal, spermatocyt′ic** *adj.*; **primary s,** a diploid cell that has been derived from a spermatogonium and can subsequently begin meiosis and divide into two haploid secondary spermatocytes 初级精母细胞，**secondary s,** one of the two haploid cells into which a primary spermatocyte divides, and which in turn gives origin to spermatids 次级精母细胞

sper·ma·to·cy·to·gen·e·sis (spur″mə-tosi″to-jen′ə-sis) the first stage of formation of spermatozoa, in which the spermatogonia develop into spermatocytes and then into spermatids 精母细胞发生

sper·ma·to·gen·e·sis (spur″mə-to-jen′ə-sis) the process of formation of spermatozoa, including both spermatocytogenesis and spermiogenesis 精子发生

sper·ma·to·ge·net·ic (spur″mə-to-jə-net″- ik) 1. pertaining to spermatogenesis 精子发生的；2. 同 spermatogenic

sper·ma·to·gen·ic (spur″mə-to-jen′ik) producing semen or spermatozoa 生成精子的

sper·ma·to·go·ni·um (spur″mə-to-go′ne- əm) pl. *spermatogo′nia.* An undifferentiated male germ cell, originating in a seminiferous tubule and dividing into two primary spermatocytes 精原细胞

sper·ma·tol·y·sis (spur″mə-tol′ĭ-sis) destruction or dissolution of spermatozoa 精子破坏，精子溶解；**spermatolyt′ic** *adj.*

sper·ma·to·tox·ic (spur″mə-to-tok″sik) 1. spermicidal 杀精子的，参见 *spermicide*; 2. having a destructive or toxic effect on spermatozoa 对精子有破坏性或者毒性作用

sper·ma·to·zo·on (spur″mə-to-zo′on) pl. *spermatozo′a.* A mature male germ cell, which fertilizes the oocyte in sexual reproduction and contains the genetic information for the zygote from the male. Spermatozoa, formed in the seminiferous tubules, are derived from spermatogonia, which first develop into spermatocytes; these in turn produce spermatids by meiosis, which then differentiate into spermatozoa 精子；**spermatozo′al** *adj.*

sper·ma·tu·ria (spur″mə-tu′re-ə) 同 seminuria

sper·mi·a·tion (spur″me-a′shən) the release of mature spermatozoa from the Sertoli cells 精子释放

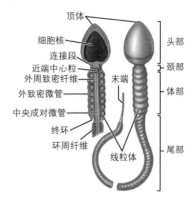

顶体
细胞核
连接段
近端中心粒
外周致密纤维
外致密微管
中央成对微管
终环
环周纤维
末端
线粒体
头部
颈部
体部
尾部

▲ 人类精子

sper·mi·cide (spur′mĭ-sīd) an agent destructive to spermatozoa 杀精子剂；**spermici′dal** *adj.*

sper·mi·duct (spur′mĭ-dukt″) the ejaculatory duct and ductus deferens together 输精管

sper·mio·gen·e·sis (spur″me-o-jen′ə-sis) the second stage in the formation of spermatozoa, when spermatids transform into spermatozoa 精子形成

sp gr specific gravity 比重

sphe·no·eth·moi·dal (sfe″no-eth-moi′d- əl) pertaining to the sphenoid and ethmoid bones 蝶筛骨的

sphe·noid (sfe′noid) 1. wedge-shaped 楔形的，楔状的，参见 *bone* 下 sphenoid bone; 2. 同 sphenoidal

sphe·noi·dal (sfe-noi′dəl) pertaining to the sphenoid bone; sphenoid 蝶骨的

sphe·noi·di·tis (sfe″noi-di′tis) inflammation of a sphenoidal sinus 蝶窦炎

sphe·noi·dot·o·my (sfe″noi-dot′ə-me) incision of a sphenoidal sinus 蝶窦切除术

sphe·no·max·il·lary (sfe″no-mak″sĭ-lar″e) pertaining to the sphenoid bone and the maxilla 蝶上颌骨的

sphe·no·oc·cip·i·tal (sfe″no-ok-sip′ĭ-təl) pertaining to the sphenoid and occipital bones 蝶枕骨的

sphe·no·pal·a·tine (sfe″no-pal′ə-tīn) pertaining to the sphenoid and palatine bones 蝶腭骨的

sphe·no·pa·ri·e·tal (sfe″no-pə-ri′ə-təl) pertaining to the sphenoid and parietal bones 蝶顶骨的

sphere (sfēr) ball or globe; a three-dimensional round body 球；圆体；**spher′ical** *adj.*

sphe·ro·cyte (sfēr′o-sīt) a small, globular, completely hemoglobinated erythrocyte without the usual central pallor characteristically found in hereditary spherocytosis but also in acquired hemolytic anemia 球形细胞；**spherocyt′ic** *adj.*

sphe·ro·cy·to·sis (sfēr″o-si-to′sis) the presence of spherocytes in the blood 球形细胞增多症 **hereditary s.**, a group of clinically and genetically heterogeneous hereditary disorders characterized by the presence of spherocytes, hemolytic anemia, abnormal fragility of erythrocytes, jaundice, and splenomegaly 遗传性球形细胞增多症

sphe·roid (sfēr′oid) a spherelike body 球状体

sphe·roi·dal (sfēr-oi′dəl) resembling a sphere 球形的，球状的

sphe·ro·plast (sfēr′o-plast) a membranebound, spherical cell that results after partial or complete removal of the cell wall from a bacterial, yeast, or fungal cell; it is dependent for its integrity on an isotonic or hypertonic medium 原生质球

sphinc·ter (sfingk′tər) [L.] a ringlike muscle that closes a natural orifice or passage 括 约 肌；**sphinc′teral, sphincter′ic** *adj.*; **anal s., external,** external sphincter muscle of anus: a muscle surrounding the anal canal, originating at the tip of the coccyx and the anococcygeal ligament and inserting into the perineal body; it closes the anus 肛门外括约肌；**anal s., internal,** internal sphincter muscle of anus: a thickening of the circular lamina of the tunica muscularis at the caudal end of the rectum 肛门内括约肌；**s. a′ni,** 肛门括约肌，参见 *external anal s.* 和 *internal anal s.*; **s. of bile duct, s. of Boyden,** an annular sheath of muscle that invests the bile duct within the wall of the duodenum 胆管括约肌；**cardiac s.,** lower esophageal s. 贲门括约肌；**cricopharyngeal s.,** upper esophageal s. 环咽括约肌；**esophageal s., lower (LES),** the terminal few centimeters of the esophagus, which prevents reflux of gastric contents into the esophagus 食管下括约肌；**esophageal s., upper (UES),** the upper 3 to 5 cm of the esophagus, including the cricopharyngeus muscle, which prevents the aspiration of air from the pharynx into the esophagus 食管上括约肌；**gastroesophageal s.,** lower esophageal s. 胃食管括约肌；**hepatic s.,** a thickened portion of the muscular coat of the hepatic veins near their entrance into the inferior vena cava 肝静脉括约肌；**O′Beirne s.,** a band of muscle at the junction of the sigmoid colon and rectum. O′Beirne 括约肌；**s. of Oddi,** muscle fibers investing the hepatopancreatic ampulla in the wall of the duodenum Oddi 括约肌；**palatopharyngeal s.,** a transverse band of muscle fibers in the mastoid wall of the pharynx, derived from the superior pharyngeal constrictor muscle or palatopharyngeus muscle, which contracts during swallowing to seal shut the isthmus between the nasopharynx and oropharynx 腭咽部括约肌；**pan-**creatic s.,** a muscle that surrounds the pancreatic duct just above the hepatopancreatic ampulla 胰管括约肌；**pharyngoesophageal s.,** a region of higher muscular tone at the junction of the pharynx and esophagus, which is involved in movements of swallowing 食管咽括约肌；**precapillary s.,** a smooth muscle fiber encircling a true capillary where it originates from the arterial capillary, which can open and close the capillary entrance 前毛细血管前括约肌；**preprostatic s.,** 同 internal urethral s.; **s. pupil′lae,** sphincter muscle of pupil: circular fibers of the iris, innervated by the ciliary nerves (parasympathetic), and acting to contract the pupil 瞳孔括约肌；**pyloric s.,** pyloric sphincter muscle: a thickening of the circular muscle of the stomach around its opening into the duodenum 幽门括约肌；**rectal s.,** an incomplete band or thickening of the muscle fibers in the rectum a few inches above the anus in the upper part of the rectal ampulla 直肠括约肌；**rectosigmoid s.,** O′Beirne s. 直肠乙状结肠括约肌；**tubal s.,** an encircling band of muscle fibers at the junction of the uterine tube and the uterus 输卵管括约肌；**urethral s., external,** the external sphincter muscle of the urethra, originating at the ramus of the pubis and inserting at the median raphe behind and in front of the urethra, innervated by the perineal nerve; it compresses the central part of the urethra in females and the membranous part in males 尿道外括约肌；**urethral s., internal,** the internal sphincter muscle of the urethra, occurring only in males; it is a circular layer of smooth muscle fibers surrounding the internal urethral orifice, innervated by the vesical nerve, and acting to close the orifice 尿道内括约肌；**vesical s.,** 同 internal urethral s.

sphinc·ter·ec·to·my (sfingk″tər-ek′tə-me) excision of a sphincter 括约肌切除术

sphinc·ter·is·mus (sfingk″tər-iz′məs) spasm of a sphincter 括约肌痉挛

sphinc·ter·itis (sfingk″tər-i′tis) inflammation of a sphincter 括约肌炎

sphinc·ter·ol·y·sis (sfingk″tər-ol′ĭ-sis) surgical separation of the iris from the cornea in anterior synechia 虹膜前粘连分离术

sphinc·tero·plas·ty (sfingk′tər-o-plas″te) plastic reconstruction of a sphincter 括约肌成形术

sphinc·ter·ot·o·my (sfingk″tər-ot′ə-me) incision of a sphincter 括约肌切开术

sphin·ga·nine (sfing′gə-nēn) a dihydroxy derivative of sphingosine, commonly occurring in sphingolipids 二氢神经鞘氨醇

sphin·go·lip·id (sfing′go-lip′id) a lipid in which the backbone is sphingosine or a related base, the basic unit being a ceramide attached to a polar head group; it includes sphingomyelins, cerebrosides, and gangliosides 鞘脂，神经鞘脂质

sphin·go·lip·i·do·sis (sfing″go-lip″ĭ-do′sis) any of various lysosomal storage diseases characterized by abnormal storage of sphingolipids 神经鞘脂类沉积症

Sphin·go·mo·na·da·ceae (sfing″go-mo″nə-da′se-e) a family of gram-negative bacteria of the order Sphingomonadales 鞘脂单胞菌科

Sphin·go·mo·na·da·les (sfing″go-mo″nə- da′lēz) an order of gram-negative, mainly aerobic, non–spore-forming bacteria of the class Alphaproteobacteria 鞘脂单胞菌目

Sphin·go·mo·nas (sfing″go-mo′nəs) a genus of free-living, gram-negative, aerobic, non–sporeforming bacteria of the family Sphingomonadaceae; *S. paucimo'bilis* is widely distributed in soil and water and causes opportunistic infections 鞘脂单胞菌属

sphin·go·my·elin (sfing″go-mi′ə-lin) any of the sphingolipids in which the head group is phosphorylated choline; they occur in membranes, primarily in nervous tissue, and accumulate abnormally in Niemann-Pick disease 鞘磷脂

sphin·go·sine (sfing′go-sēn) a long-chain, monounsaturated, aliphatic amino alcohol found in sphingolipids 鞘氨醇 **s. 1-phosphate, (S1P),** a bioactive lipid mediator that regulates a variety of cell processes, acting as both a second messenger and a receptor ligand active in cell signaling via a set of at least five G protein–coupled receptors 1- 磷酸 - 鞘氨醇，一种生物活性脂质介质，调节各种细胞过程，通过至少 5 个 G 蛋白耦合受体在细胞信号中充当第二信使和活跃于细胞信号的受体配体

sphyg·mic (sfig′mik) pertaining to the pulse 脉搏的

sphyg·mo·dy·na·mom·e·ter (sfig″mo-di″nə-mom′ə-tər) an instrument for measuring the force of the pulse 脉力计

sphyg·mo·gram (sfig′mo-gram) a record or tracing made by a sphygmograph 脉搏图

sphyg·mo·graph (sfig′mo-graf) apparatus for registering the movements, form, and force of the arterial pulse 脉搏描记器; **sphygmograph'ic** *adj.*

sphyg·moid (sfig′moid) resembling the pulse 脉搏样的

sphyg·mo·ma·nom·e·ter (sfig″mo-mə-nom′-ə-tər) an instrument for measuring arterial blood pressure 血压计

sphyg·mom·e·ter (sfig-mom′ə-tər) an instru - ment for measuring the pulse 脉搏计

sphyg·mo·scope (sfig′mo-skōp) a device for rendering the pulse beat visible 脉搏检视器

sphyg·mo·to·nom·e·ter (sfig″mo-to-nom′ə- tər) an instrument for measuring elasticity of arterial walls 动脉管弹性计，脉张力计

spi·ca (spi′kə) [L.] a figure-of-8 bandage, with turns crossing each other 人字形绷带

spic·ule (spik′ūl) a sharp, needle-like body 针，刺; 针状体; 交合刺

spic·u·lum (spik′u-ləm) pl. *spic'ula* [L.] spicule 针，刺; 交合刺

spi·der (spi′dər) 1. an arthropod of the class Arachnida 蜘蛛; 2. spider angioma 蜘蛛痣; **black widow s.,** a spider, *Latrodectus mactans,* whose bite causes severe poisoning 黑寡妇蜘蛛，致命红斑蜘蛛; **vascular s.,** spider angioma 蜘蛛痣

spike (spīk) a sharp upward deflection in a curve or tracing, as on the encephalogra（曲线的）峰

spi·na (spi′nə) pl. *spi'nae* [L.] 同 spine; **s. bi'fida,** a neural tube defect marked by defective closure of the vertebral arch, through which the meninges may *(s. bi'fida cys'tica)* or may not *(s. bi'fida occul'ta)* protrude 脊柱裂; **s. vento'sa,** dactylitis, usually in infants and young children, with enlargement of digits, caseation, sequestration, and sinus formation 真性指 / 趾炎

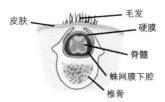

皮肤　毛发　硬膜　脊髓　蛛网膜下腔　椎骨

▲　隐性脊柱裂（脊柱横断面）

spi·nal (spi′nəl) 1. pertaining to a spine or to the vertebral column 脊柱的; 2. pertaining to the spinal cord's functioning independently from the brain 与独立于大脑功能的脊髓功能有关

spi·nate (spi′nāt) having thorns; thorn-shaped 有棘的，棘状的

spin·dle (spin′dəl) 1. a pin tapered at both ends 梭; 2. the fusiform figure occurring during metaphase of cell division, composed of microtubules radiating from the centrioles and connecting to the chromosomes at their centromeres 纺锤体; 3. a type of brain wave occurring on the electroencephalogram in groups at a frequency of about 14 per second, usually while the patient is falling asleep 梭形波，脑电图上以大约每秒 14 次的频率发生脑电波，通常是在病人入睡时发生的; 4. 同 muscle s.; **Krukenberg s.,** a spindle-shaped, brownish-red opacity of the cornea 克鲁肯贝格梭，角膜的主轴形、棕红色不透明的浊嵌; **mitotic s.,** spindle (2) 有丝分裂纺锤体; **muscle s.,** a fusiform end organ arranged in parallel between the fibers of skeletal muscle and acting as a mechanoreceptor, being the receptor of impulses responsible for the stretch reflex 肌梭；**nuclear s.,** spindle (2) 核纺锤体；**tendon s.,** Golgi tendon organ 腱梭

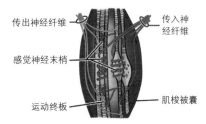

传出神经纤维
传入神经纤维
感觉神经末梢
运动终板
肌梭被囊

▲ 肌梭的横截面，显示梭内肌纤维以及传入和传出神经末梢

spine (spīn) 1. a slender, thornlike process or projection 棘，刺；2. vertebral column 脊柱；**alar s., angular s.,** s. of sphenoid bone 角棘，蝶骨棘；**bamboo s.,** the rigid spine produced by ankylosing spondylitis, so called from its radiographic appearance 竹节样脊柱，强直性脊柱炎导致的脊柱僵硬而出现的竹节样变；**cervical s.,** that portion of the spine comprising the cervical vertebrae 颈椎；**cleft s.,** spina bifida 脊柱裂；**s. of helix,** a small, forward-projecting cartilaginous process on the anterior portion of the helix at about the junction of the helix and its crus, just above the tragus 耳轮棘；**ischial s.,** a bony process projecting backward and medialward from the posterior border of the ischium 坐骨棘突 **lumbar s.,** that portion of the spine comprising the lumbar vertebrae 腰椎；**mental s., inferior,** the lower part of a small bony projection on the internal surface of the mandible, near the lower end of the midline, serving for attachment of the geniohyoid muscle 颏下棘；**mental s., superior,** the upper part of a small bony projection on the internal surface of the mandible, near the lower end of the midline, serving for attachment of the genioglossus muscle 颏上棘；**nasal s., anterior,** the sharp anterosuperior projection at the anterior extremity of the nasal crest of the maxilla 鼻前棘；**nasal s., posterior,** a sharp, backward-projecting bony spine forming the medial posterior angle of the horizontal part of the palatine bone 鼻后棘；**neural s.,** the spinous process of a vertebra 椎骨棘突；**palatine s's,** laterally placed ridges on the lower surface of the maxillary part of the hard palate, separating the palatine sulci 腭棘；**poker s., rigid s.,** the ankylosed spine produced by rheumatoid spondylitis 脊柱强直，类风湿性脊

柱炎导致的脊柱强直；**s. of scapula,** a triangular bony plate attached by one end to the back of the scapula 肩胛冈；**sciatic s.,** 同 ischial s.; **s. of sphenoid bone,** the posterior and downward projection from the lower aspect of the greater wing of the sphenoid bone 蝶骨棘；**thoracic s.,** that part of the spine comprising the thoracic vertebrae 胸椎；**s. of tibia,** a longitudinally elongated, raised and roughened area on the anterior crest of the tibia 胫骨粗隆；**trochlear s.,** a bony spicule on the anteromedial part of the orbital surface of the frontal bone for attachment of the trochlea of the superior oblique muscle 滑车棘

spi·nip·e·tal (spi-nip′ə-təl) conducting or moving toward the spinal cord 向脊髓的

spinn·bar·keit (spin′bahr-kīt) [Ger.] the formation of an elastic thread by mucus of the uterine cervix when it is drawn out; the time of maximum elasticity usually precedes or coincides with ovulation 宫颈黏液成丝现象

spi·no·bul·bar (spi″no-bul′bər) pertaining to the spinal cord and medulla oblongata 脊髓延髓的

spi·no·cer·e·bel·lar (spi″no-ser″ə-bel′ər) pertaining to the spinal cord and cerebellum 脊髓小脑的

spi·no·cer·e·bel·lum (spi″no-ser″ə-bel′əm) the portion of the cerebellum serving as the primary site of termination of the major spinocerebellar afferents; sometimes equated with paleocerebellum (q.v.) 脊髓小脑

spin·o·sad (spin′o-sad) a pediculicide applied topically to treat head lice 多杀霉素，多杀菌素

spi·no·tha·lam·ic (spi″no-thə-lam′ik) pertaining to or extending between the spinal cord and the thalamus 脊髓丘脑的

spinous (spi′nəs) pertaining to or like a spine 棘状的；棘的，刺的；棘突的

spir·ad·e·no·ma (spīr″ad-ə-no′mə) a benign adnexal tumor of the sweat glands, particularly of the coil portion 螺旋腺瘤

spi·ral (spi′rəl) 1. helical; winding like the thread of a screw 螺旋形的；2. helix; a winding structure 螺旋；**Curschmann s's,** coiled mucinous fibrils sometimes found in the sputum in bronchial asthma Curschmann 螺旋物，在支气管哮喘患者的痰中有时可见卷曲的黏液纤维

spi·ril·la (spi-ril′ə) [L.] *spirillum* 的复数

Spi·ril·la·ceae (spi″ril-a′se-e) a family of gramnegative, spiral bacteria of the order Nitrosomonadales occurring in stagnant fresh water 螺菌科

spi·ril·lo·sis (spi″rĭ-lo′sis) a disease caused by presence of spirilla 螺菌病

Spi·ril·lum (spi-ril′əm) a genus of gram-negative bacteria of the family Spirillaceae. *S. mi′nus* is pathogenic for guinea pigs, rats, mice, and monkeys and causes the spirillary form of ratbite fever (sodoku) in humans 螺菌属

spi·ril·lum　(spi-ril′əm) pl. *spiril′la* [L.] an organism of the genus *Spirillum* 螺菌

spir·it　(spir′it) 1. any volatile or distilled liquid 任何挥发性或可蒸馏液体 ; 2. an alcoholic or hydroalcoholic solution of a volatile material 醇剂 ; 3. in traditional Chinese medicine, shen (q.v.) 神 ; **aromatic ammonia s.,** an ammonia-containing preparation used as a respiratory stimulant in syncope, weakness, or threatened faint 芳香氨醑 ; **camphor s.,** a solution of camphor and alcohol, used topically as a local counterirritant 樟脑醑

spir·it·u·al　care (spir′ich-ūəl cair) 1. the use of spiritual practices, such as prayer, for the purpose of effecting a cure of or an improvement in an illness 使用祈祷等修持方法，以达到治愈或改善疾病的目的 ; 2. health care provision focusing on holistic treatment of mind, body, and spirit to effect improved outcomes in health and quality of life 提供保健服务，重点是对心理、身体和精神进行整体治疗，以改善健康和生活质量的结果

Spi·ro·chae·ta·ce·ae　(spi″ro-ke-ta′se-e) a family of slender, coiled, undulating, motile bacteria of the order Spirochaetales; it includes the pathogenic genera *Borrelia* and *Treponema* 螺旋体科

Spi·ro·chae·ta·les　(spi″ro-ke-ta′lēz) the spirochetes, an order of free-living, commensal, or parasitic bacteria of the class Spirochaetes 螺旋体目

Spi·ro·chae·tes　(spi″ro-ke′tēz) 1. a phylum of gram-negative, motile, highly flexible, helical bacteria. Members are free-living or associated with animal hosts, and some are pathogenic 螺旋体属 ; 2. the sole class of the order Spirochaetes 螺旋体目中的独立分类

spi·ro·chete　(spi′ro-kēt) any microorganism of the order Spirochaetales 螺旋体 ; **spiroche′tal** *adj.*

spi·ro·che·to·sis　(spi″ro-ke-to′sis) infection with spirochetes 螺旋体病

spi·ro·gram　(spi′ro-gram) a tracing or graph of respiratory movements 呼吸描记图

spi·ro·graph　(spi′ro-graf) an instrument for registering respiratory movements 呼吸描记器

spi·rog·ra·phy　(spi-rog′rə-fe) pneumography; the graphic measurement of breathing, including breathing movements and breathing capacity 呼吸描记法

spi·roid　(spi′roid) resembling a spiral 类螺旋的

spi·ro·lac·tone　(spi″ro-lak′tōn) any of a group of compounds capable of opposing the action of sodium-retaining steroids on renal transport of sodium and potassium 螺旋内酯固醇，螺甾内酯

spi·rom·e·ter　(spi-rom′ə-tər) an instrument for measuring the air taken into and exhaled by the lungs 肺量计

Spi·ro·me·tra　(spi″ro-me′trə) a genus of tapeworms parasitic in fish-eating cats, dogs, and birds; larval infection (sparganosis) in humans is caused by ingestion of inadequately cooked fish 迭宫绦虫属

spi·rom·e·try　(spi-rom′ə-tre) the measurement of the breathing capacity of the lungs, such as in pulmonary function tests 肺量计法，另参见 *spirography*; **spiromet′ric** *adj.*

spir·o·no·lac·tone　(spi″rə-no-lak′tōn) one of the spirolactones, an aldosterone inhibitor that blocks the aldosterone-dependent exchange of sodium and potassium in the distal tubule, thus increasing excretion of sodium and water and decreasing excretion of potassium; used in the treatment of edema, hypokalemia, primary aldosteronism, and hypertension 螺内酯（醛固酮拮抗药）

spis·sat·ed　(spis′āt-ed) inspissated 浓缩的；蒸浓的；凝结的

splanch·nic　(splank′nik) pertaining to the viscera 内脏的

splanch·ni·cec·to·my　(splank″nĭ-sek′tə- me) resection of one or more of the splanchnic nerves for the treatment of hypertension or intractable pain 内脏神经切除术

splanch·ni·cot·o·my　(splank″nĭ-kot′ə-me) splanchnicectomy 内脏神经切断术

splanch·no·coele　(splank′no-sēl) that portion of the coelom from which the visceral cavities are formed 体腔，胸腹腔

splanch·nol·o·gy　(splank-nol′ə-je) the scientific study of the viscera of the body; applied also to the body of knowledge relating thereto 内脏学

splanch·no·pleure　(splank′no-ploor) the layer formed by union of the splanchnic mesoderm with endoderm; from it are developed the muscles and the connective tissue of the digestive tube 胚脏壁 ; **splanchnopleu′ral** *adj.*

splay·foot　(spla′foot) flatfoot 平跖外翻足

spleen　(spl ē n) a large, glandlike organ situated in the upper left part of the abdominal cavity, lateral to the cardiac end of the stomach. Among its functions are the disintegration of erythrocytes and the setting free of hemoglobin, which the liver converts into bilirubin; the genesis of new erythrocytes during fetal life and in the newborn; serving as a blood reservoir; and production of lymphocytes and plasma cells 脾 ; **accessory s.,** a connected or detached outlying portion, or exclave, of the spleen 副脾 ; **floating s., movable s.,** one displaced and abnormally movable 游走脾 ; **lardaceous s.,** one with amyloid degeneration in which deposits diffusely infiltrate the red pulp adjacent to sinus walls and around small vessels 蜡样脾; **sago s.,** one with amyloid degeneration in which deposits surround cells in the white pulp, giving the cut surface the appearance of pearls of sago or tapioca 西米脾; **wandering s.,** 同 floating s.

splen (splen) [Gr.] 同 spleen

sple·nal·gia (sple-nal'jə) pain in the spleen 脾痛

sple·nec·to·my (sple-nek'tə-me) excision of the spleen 脾切除术

splen·ic (splen'ik) pertaining to the spleen 脾的

sple·ni·tis (sple-ni'tis) inflammation of the spleen 脾炎

sple·ni·um (sple'ne-um) [L.] 1. a bandlike structure 带状结构; 2. a bandage or compress 绷带，压布; 3. 同 s. corporis callosi; **s. cor'poriscallo'si,** the posterior, rounded end of the corpus callosum 胼胝体压部

sple·no·cele (sple'no-sēl) hernia of the spleen 脾疝

sple·no·col·ic (sple"no-kol'ik) pertaining to the spleen and colon 脾结肠的

sple·no·cyte (sple'no-sīt) the monocyte characteristic of splenic tissue 脾细胞

sple·nog·ra·phy (sple-nog'rə-fe) radiography of the spleen 脾 X 线照相术

sple·no·hep·a·to·meg·a·ly (sple"no-hep"ə- tomeg'ə-le) hepatosplenomegaly 脾肝肿大

sple·noid (sple'noid) resembling the spleen 脾样的

sple·nol·y·sis (sple-nol'ĭ-sis) destruction of splenic tissue 脾溶解，脾组织破坏

sple·no·ma (sple-no'mə) pl. *splenomas, spleno'mata.* A splenic tumor 脾瘤

sple·no·med·ul·lary (sple"no-med'u-lar"e) of or pertaining to the spleen and bone marrow 脾骨髓的

sple·no·meg·a·ly (sple"no-meg'ə-le) enlargement of the spleen 脾（肿）大; **congestive s.,** Banti disease: splenomegaly secondary to portal hypertension 充血性脾大; **hemolytic s.,** that associated with any disorder causing increased erythrocyte degradation 溶血性脾大

sple·no·my·elog·e·nous (sple"no-mi"ə-loj'ə- nəs) formed in the spleen and bone marrow 脾骨髓性的

sple·no·pan·cre·at·ic (sple"no-pan"kreat'ik) pertaining to the spleen and pancreas 脾胰的

sple·nop·a·thy (sple-nop'ə-the) any disease of the spleen 脾病

sple·no·pexy (sple'no-pek"se) surgical fixation of the spleen 脾固定术

sple·nop·to·sis (sple"nop-to'sis) downward displacement of the spleen 脾下垂

sple·no·re·nal (sple"no-re'nəl) pertaining to the spleen and kidney, or to splenic and renal veins 脾肾的，脾肾静脉的

sple·nor·rha·phy (sple-nor'ə-fe) surgical repair of the spleen 脾缝术

sple·no·sis (sple-no'sis) the occurrence of multiple ectopic splenic implants, usually secondary to trauma that ruptures the splenic capsule 脾组织植入

sple·no·tox·in (sple'no-tok"sin) a toxin that acts on the spleen 脾毒素

splic·ing (spli'sing) the joining together of two nucleic acid segments so as to form a new genetic combination, as DNA to DNA in immunoglobulin gene rearrangement or in recombinant DNA technology, or RNA to RNA in processing of primary transcripts to form mature RNA 剪接; **alternative s.,** the splicing of RNA at variable positions on the primary transcript under different conditions, removing varying introns to yield distinct mRNAs 可变剪接，选择性剪接

splint (splint) 1. a rigid or flexible appliance for fixation of displaced or movable parts 夹板; 2. the act of fastening or confining with such an appliance 用夹板夹; **airplane s.,** one that holds the splinted limb suspended in the air 飞机式夹; **anchor s.,** one for fracture of the jaw, with metal loops fitting over the teeth and held together by a rod 锚状夹，用于下颌骨折; **Angle s.,** one for fracture of the mandible Angle 夹，用于下颌骨折; **coaptation s's,** small splints adjusted around a fractured limb for the purpose of approximating the fragments 接合夹; **Denis Browne s.,** a splint consisting of a pair of metal foot splints joined by a cross bar; used in talipes equinovarus Denis Browne 夹 用 于 马蹄内翻足; **dynamic s., functional s.,** 动力性夹板，功能性夹板，参见 *orthosis* 下词条; **shin s's,** an overuse injury seen in athletes, with strain of the flexor digitorum longus muscle and pain along the shin bone 外胫夹，运动员在趾长屈肌劳损后，沿胫骨出现疼痛; **Thomas s.,** a leg splint consisting of two rigid rods attached to an ovoid ring that fits around the thigh; it can be combined with other apparatuses to provide traction 托马斯夹板

splin·ter (splin'tər) 1. a small slender fragment 裂片，碎片; 2. to break into small fragments 使成碎片，使分裂

splint·ing (splin'ting) 1. application of a splint, or treatment by use of a splint 夹板疗法，夹板用法; 2. in dentistry, the application of a fixed restoration to join two or more teeth into a single rigid unit 齿固定法，应用固定修复将两颗或多颗牙齿连接到单个刚性单元中; 3. rigidity of muscles occurring as a means of avoiding pain caused by movement of the part 肌僵直，作为避免运动引起的疼痛的手段时而导致肌肉的僵硬

split·ting (split'ing) 1. the division of a single object into two or more objects or parts 分裂，分解，将单个对象划分为两个或多个对象或部分；2. in psychoanalytic theory, a primitive defense mechanism, in which "objects" (persons) are perceived as "all good" or "all bad" rather than as an intermediate or mixture 在精神分析理论中，一种原始的防御机制，其中人被视为非好即坏，而非中间或混合型；**s. of heart sounds,** the presence of two components in the first or second heart sound complexes; particularly denoting separation of the elements of the second sound into two, representing aortic valve closure and pulmonic valve closure 心音分裂

spon·dy·lal·gia (spon″də-lal'jə) 同 spondylodynia

spon·dyl·ar·thri·tis (spon″dəl-ahr-thri'tis) arthritis of the spine 脊椎关节炎

spon·dy·lit·ic (spon″də-lit'ik) pertaining to or marked by spondylitis 脊椎炎的

spon·dy·li·tis (spon″də-li'tis) inflammation of vertebrae 脊椎炎；**ankylosing s.,** a chronic multisystem inflammatory disorder associated with the presence of the HLA-B27 antigen; it usually initially affects the sacroiliac joints and often later other axial skeletal joints and peripheral joints, causing pain and progressive stiffness and restricted range of motion. Extraskeletal manifestations include ocular, pulmonary, cardiovascular, renal, and neurologic complications 强直性脊柱炎

spon·dy·li·ze·ma (spon″də-li-ze'mə) downward displacement of a vertebra because of destruction or softening of the one below it 脊椎下移

spon·dy·loc·a·ce (spon″də-lok'ə-se) tuberculosis of the vertebrae 脊柱结核

spon·dy·lo·dyn·ia (spon″də-lo-din'e-ə) pain in a vertebra 脊椎痛

spon·dy·lo·lis·the·sis (spon″də-lo-lis-the'sis) forward displacement of a vertebra over a lower segment, usually of the fourth or fifth lumbar vertebra due to a developmental defect in the pars interarticularis 脊椎前移；**spondylolisthet'ic** adj.

spon·dy·lol·y·sis (spon″də-lol'ĭ-sis) the breaking down of a vertebra 椎骨滑脱

spon·dy·lop·a·thy (spon″də-lop'ə-the) any disease of the vertebrae 脊椎病，脊柱病

spon·dy·lo·py·o·sis (spon″də-lo-pi-o'sis) suppuration of a vertebra 脊椎化脓

spon·dy·los·chi·sis (spon″dĭ-los'kĭ-sis) rachischisis 椎弓裂

spon·dy·lo·sis (spon″də-lo'sis) 1. ankylosis of a vertebral joint 脊椎关节僵硬；2. degenerative spinal changes due to osteoarthritis 骨关节炎性退行变

spon·dy·lo·syn·de·sis (spon″də-lo-sin-de'sis) spinal fusion 脊柱融合术

spon·dy·lot·ic (spon″də-lot'ik) pertaining to or due to spondylosis 椎关节强硬的

sponge (spunj) 1. a porous, absorbent mass, as a pad of gauze or cotton surrounded by gauze 纱布；2. the elastic fibrous skeleton of certain species of marine animals 海绵（动物）**absorbable gelatin s.,** a sterile, absorbable, water-insoluble, gelatin-base material, used as a local hemostatic 可吸收性明胶海绵

spon·gi·form (spun'jĭ-form) resembling a sponge 海绵状的

spon·gio·blast (spun'je-o-blast) 1. any of the embryonic epithelial cells that develop near the neural tube and later become transformed, some into neuroglial and some into ependymal cells 成胶质细胞；2. amacrine cell 无轴索细胞

spon·gio·blas·to·ma (spun″je-o-blas-to'mə) a tumor containing spongioblasts; considered to be one of the neuroepithelial tumors 成胶质细胞瘤

spon·gio·cyte (spun'je-o-sīt) 1. neuroglial cell 神经胶质细胞；2. one of the cells with spongy vacuolated protoplasm in the adrenal cortex 肾上腺皮质海绵状细胞

spon·gi·oid (spun'je-oid) resembling a sponge 海绵样的

spon·gio·sa (spun'je-o'sə) 1. 同 spongy 海绵样的；2. cancellous bone 松质骨

spon·gio·sa·plas·ty (spun″je-o'sə-plas″te) autoplasty of cancellous bone to encourage formation of new bone or to cover bone defects 骨松质成形术

spon·gi·o·sis (spun″je-o'sis) intercellular edema within the epidermis 皮肤海绵层细胞间水肿

spon·gy (spun'je) of a spongelike appearance or texture 海绵状的

spon·ta·ne·ous (spon-ta'ne-əs) 1. voluntary; instinctive 自发的，本能的；2. occurring without external influence 特发的，自生的

spo·rad·ic (spə-rad'ik) occurring singly; widely scattered; not epidemic or endemic 散在的，散发的

spo·ran·gi·um (spə-ran'je-əm) pl. *sporan'gia*. Any encystment containing spores or sporelike bodies, as in certain fungi 孢子囊

spore (spor) 1. a refractile, oval body formed within bacteria, especially *Bacillus* and *Clostridium*, which is regarded as a resting stage during the life history of the cell and is characterized by its resistance to environmental changes 芽孢，细菌内部形成的折射的椭圆形体体，尤指杆菌和梭菌，在细胞生命史中被视为休息阶段，其特征是其对环境变化的抵抗力；2. the reproductive element, produced sexually or asexually, of one of the lower organisms, such as protozoa, fungi, algae, etc. 孢子，低等生物的一种有性或无性的生殖元素，比如原生动物、真菌、藻类等

spo·ri·cide (spor'ĭ-sīd) an agent that destroys spores 杀孢子剂；**sporici'dal** adj.

spo·ro·blast (spor'o-blast) one of the bodies formed in the oocyst of the malarial parasite in the mosquito and from which the sporozoite later develops; also, similar stages in certain other sporozoa 孢子母细胞

spo·ro·cyst (spor'o-sist) 1. any cyst or sac containing spores or reproductive cells 孢子囊；2. a germinal saclike stage in the life cycle of digenetic trematodes, produced by metamorphosis of a miracidium and giving rise to rediae 孢蚴；3. a stage in the life cycle of certain coccidian protozoa, contained within the oocyst, produced by a sporoblast, and giving rise to sporozoites 子孢子发育

spo·ro·gen·ic (spor″o-jen'ik) producing spores 能产孢子的，孢子能形成的

spo·rog·o·ny (spə-rog'ə-ne) sporulation involving multiple fission of a sporont, resulting in the formation of sporocysts and sporozoites 孢子生殖，孢子发生；**sporogon'ic** adj.

spo·ront (spor'ont) a zygote of coccidian protozoa enclosed in an oocyst, which undergoes sporogony to produce sporoblasts 产孢体

spo·ro·plasm (spor'o-plaz″əm) 1. the protoplasm of spores 孢子质；2. in certain protozoa, the central mass of cytoplasm that leaves the spores as an amebula to infect the host 孢原质

Spo·ro·thrix (spor'o-thriks) a genus of fungi, including *S. schen'ckii* (see *sporotrichosis*) and *S. car'nis,* which causes formation of white mold on meat in cold storage 孢子丝菌属

spo·ro·tri·cho·sis (spor″o-trī-ko'sis) a chronic fungal disease caused by *Sporothrix schenckii,* most commonly characterized by nodular lesions of the cutaneous and subcutaneous tissues and adjacent lymphatics that suppurate, ulcerate, and drain; it may remain localized or be disseminated by the bloodstream 孢子丝菌病

spo·ro·zo·an (spor″o-zo'ən) 1. any protozoan of the phyla Apicomplexa, Ascetospora, Microspora, and Myxozoa 孢子虫；2. pertaining or relating to protozoa of these phyla 孢子虫的

spo·ro·zo·ite (spor″o-zo'ĭt) the motile, infective stage of certain protozoa that results from sporogony 子孢子

spo·ro·zo·on (spor″o-zo'on) pl. *sporozo'a.* Sporozoan (1) 孢子虫

spor·u·la·tion (spor″u-la'shən) formation of

spores 孢子形成

spor·ule (spor'ūl) a small spore 小孢子

spot (spot) a circumscribed, usually discolored area 点，斑点；**Bitot s's,** foamy, gray, triangular spots of keratinized epithelium on the conjunctivae, seen with vitamin A deficiency 比托斑，结膜角化上皮上的泡沫状灰色三角形斑点，见于维生素 A 缺乏；**blind s.,** 1. optic disk 盲点（视网膜）；2. mental scotoma 精神性盲点；**café au lait s's,** macules of a distinctive light brown color, such as occur in neurofibromatosis and Albright syndrome 咖啡（牛奶）斑，主要见于神经纤维瘤病和奥尔布赖特综合征；**cayenne pepper s's,** red angiomatous puncta within or on the border of the lesions of the chronic pigmented purpuras 辣椒斑，慢性色素性紫癜的病损中或病损边缘的红色血管瘤；**cherry-red s.,** the choroid appearing as a red circular area surrounded by gray-white retina, as viewed through the fovea centralis in Tay-Sachs disease and other disorders causing accumulation of sphingolipids 樱桃红斑，脉络膜呈现出红色圆形区域并被灰白色视网膜包绕，见于泰-萨克斯病及其他引起鞘脂类积聚的疾病；**cold s.,** 冷点，参见 **cotton-wool s's,** white or gray softedged opacities in the retina, seen in hypertensive retinopathy, lupus erythematosus, and other conditions 棉絮状渗出点，视网膜上白色或灰色的边缘模糊的浊斑，在高血压视网膜病变、红斑狼疮和其他疾病中可见；**focal s.,** a small area of an x-ray target that receives the main electron stream 焦点，X 线检查时接受主要电流的小区域；**germinal s.,** the nucleolus of an oocyte 胚斑 **hot s.,** 热点 1. 参见 *temperature s's;* 2. the sensitive area of a neuroma 神经瘤点，神经瘤的敏感区域；3. an area of increased density on an x-ray or thermographic film 阳性区，X 线片或热象图胶片上的密度增高区；4. a region of a genome that has a particularly high tendency for recombination or mutation 基因组中具有特别高的重组或突变倾向的区域；**Koplik s's,** irregular, bright red spots on the buccal and lingual mucosa, with tiny bluish white specks in the center of each; seen in the prodromal stage of measles 科氏斑，麻疹黏膜斑；**liver s.,** solar lentigo 雀斑；**milky s's,** aggregations of macrophages in the subserous connective tissue of the pleura and peritoneum 乳色斑，胸膜和腹膜的浆膜下结缔组织中巨噬细胞的积聚点；**mongolian s.,** a smooth, brown to grayish blue nevus, consisting of an excess of melanocytes, typically found at birth in the sacral region in Asians and dark-skinned races; it usually disappears during childhood 蒙古斑，胎斑，骶斑，臀斑；**pain s's,** spots on the skin where alone the sense of pain can be produced by a stimulus 痛点；**rose s's,** an eruption of rose-colored spots on the abdomen and thighs during the first 7 days of typhoid fever 玫瑰疹，伤寒热发病的前 7 天中在腹部和大腿暴发性出现的玫瑰色斑点；**Roth s's,** round or oval white spots sometimes seen in the retina early in the course of subacute bacterial endocarditis 罗特斑，亚急性细菌性心内膜炎早期在视网膜上出现的圆形或卵圆形白点；**Tardieu s's,** spots of ecchymosis under the pleura after death by suffocation Tardieu 斑，窒息而死后在胸膜上出现的淤斑；**temperature s's,** spots on the skin normally anesthetic to pain and pressure but sensitive, respectively, to heat and cold 温度点，皮肤上对痛觉和压力觉缺失但对冷热刺激敏感的点

SPR Society for Pediatric Radiology 儿科放射学会

sprain (sprān) a joint injury in which some of the fibers of a supporting ligament are ruptured but the continuity of the ligament remains intact 扭伤

SPRM selective progesterone receptor modulator 选择性孕酮受体调节剂

sprue (sproo) 1. a chronic form of malabsorption syndrome, occurring in both tropical and nontropical forms 口炎性腹泻，热带和非热带慢性吸收不良综合征；2. in dentistry, the hole through which metal or other material is poured or forced into a mold 铸道，在牙科学上指金属或其他材料被浇铸或压入铸模时所经的孔道；**celiac s.,** 乳糜泻，参见 *disease* 下词条；**collagenous s.,** an often fatal condition resembling celiac sprue but unresponsive to withdrawal of dietary gluten, characterized by extensive deposition of collagen in the lamina propria of the colon 胶原性口炎性腹泻；**nontropical s.,** celiac disease 非热带性口炎性腹泻；**tropical s.,** a malabsorption syndrome occurring in the tropics and subtropics, marked by stomatitis, diarrhea, and anemia 热带口炎性腹泻

Spu·ma·vi·rus (spu'mə-vi"rəs) foamy viruses; a genus of nonpathogenic viruses of the subfamily Spumavirinae (family Retroviridae) that induce persistent infection in humans and many other mammals 泡沫病毒属

spur (spur) 1. a projecting body, as from a bone 骨刺；2. in dentistry, a piece of metal projecting from a plate, band, or other appliance（口腔器械上的）金属突出片；**calcaneal s.,** an abnormal bony projection on the calcaneus, most often the posterior or plantar surface, which frequently causes pain on walking 跟骨刺；**olecranon s.,** an abnormal bony process at the insertion of the triceps muscle 鹰嘴刺；**scleral s.,** the posterior lip of the venous sinus of the sclera to which most of the fibers of the trabecular reticulum of the iridocorneal angle and the meridional fibers of the ciliary muscle are attached 巩膜距

spu·tum (spu'təm) [L.] expectoration; matter ejected from the trachea, bronchi, and lungs through the mouth 痰；**nummular s.,** sputum in rounded coinlike disks 钱币状痰；**rusty s.,** sputum stained with blood or blood pigments 铁锈色痰

SQ subcutaneous 皮下的

squa·ma (skwa'mə) pl. *squa'mae* [L.] 1. a flat platelike structure, as of bone 扁平的盘状结构；2. 同 scale (1)

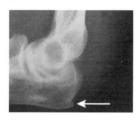

▲ 鹰嘴骨刺（箭）

squa·mate (skwa'māt) 1. scaly 有鳞的；2. 同 squamous (2)

squame (skwām) 1. 同 squama (1); 2. 同 scale (1)

squa·mo·oc·cip·i·tal (skwa"mo-ok-sip'ĭ-təl) pertaining to the squamous portion of the occipital bone 枕鳞的

squa·mo·pa·ri·e·tal (skwa"mo-pə-ri'ə-təl) pertaining to the squamous portion of the temporal bone and the parietal bone 鳞部顶骨的

squa·mo·so·pa·ri·e·tal (skwa-mo"so-pə-ri'ə-təl) 同 squamoparietal

squa·mous (skwa'məs) 1. scaly 有鳞的；2. resembling a squama; flattened or platelike 鳞状的

squat·ting (skwaht'ing) a position with hips and knees flexed, the buttocks resting on the heels; sometimes adopted by the parturient at delivery or by children with certain types of cardiac defects 蹲坐；蹲位

squill (skwil) any of various plants of the genus *Urginea*, particularly *U. maritima* or *U. indica,* or the fleshy inner scales of their bulbs 海葱；**red s.,** a variety of *Urginea maritima* with red bulbs, or the fleshy inner scales of its bulb, a source of the cardiac glycoside scilliroside; it can cause convulsions or cardiac arrest and is used as a rodenticide 红海葱；**white s.,** a variety of *Urginea maritima* with white bulbs, or the fleshy inner scales of its bulb, a source of several cardiac glycosides; used as a cardiotonic; also used in folk medicine 白海葱

squint (skwint) 同 strabismus

Sr strontium 元素锶的符号

SRH somatotropin-releasing hormone 生长激素释放激素，参见 *hormone* 下 *growth hormone–*

releasing hormone

SROM spontaneous rupture of membrane 自发性胞膜破裂

sro·ta (sro′tə) [Sanskrit] in ayurveda, channels in the body through which nutrients and waste flow for body function, ranging from the gross to the imperceptible and classified by their origin and by the substances that they carry 在阿育吠陀中，体内的通道中流动着维持体能的营养物质与废物，这些通道大小不等，并按照他们的起源和他们所携带的物质进行分类

SRS-A slow-reacting substance of anaphylaxis 过敏反应迟缓反应物质，参见 *substance* 下词条

SS somatostatin 生长抑素

ss. [L.] se′mis (half) 半，一半

SSH Society for Simulation in Healthcare 医学仿生学会

SSRI selective serotonin reuptake inhibitor 选择性 5- 羟色胺再摄取抑制药

ST sinus tachycardia 窦性心动过速

stab¹ (stab) 1. to pierce or wound with a pointed instrument 刺，刺伤；2. to thrust a pointed instrument into something 穿刺；3. stab culture 穿刺培养

stab² (stab) shaped like or resembling a staff or rod 杆

sta·bile (sta′bəl) (sta′bīl) stable; stationary; resistant to change; opposed to *labile* 稳定的；不动的；不变的；安定的；与 labile 相对

sta·ble (sta′bəl) 1. not moving, fixed, firm 稳定的，坚固的；2. constant (1) 不变的

stac·ca·to (stə-kah′to) delivered in quick, jerky bursts 断续的（地），不连贯的（地）

staff (staf) 1. a wooden rod or rodlike structure 杆，棒；2. a grooved director used as a guide for the knife in surgery 探杆，引导探子；3. the professional personnel of a hospital 医务人员；**s. of Aesculapius,** the rod or staff with entwining snake, symbolic of the god of healing, official insignia of the American Medical Association 医杖，另参见 *caduceus;* **attending s.,** the corps of attending physicians and surgeons of a hospital 内外科主治医师；**consulting s.,** specialists associated with a hospital and acting in an advisory capacity to the attending staff 会诊医师；**house s.,** the resident physicians and surgeons of a hospital 住院医师

stage (stāj) 1. a definite period or distinct phase, as of development of a disease or of an organism 阶段，时期；2. the platform of a microscope on which the slide containing the object to be studied is placed 镜台，载物台；**anal s.,** in psychoanalytic theory, the second stage of psychosexual development, occurring between the ages of 1 and 3 years, during which the infant's activities, interests, and concerns are on the anal zone 肛门期；**cold s.,** the period of chill or rigor in a malarial paroxysm 发冷期；**first s. of labor,** 第一产程，参见 *labor.;* **fourth s. of labor,** 第四产程，参见 *labor;* **genital s.,** in psychoanalytic theory, the final stage in psychosexual development, occurring during puberty, during which the person can receive sexual gratification from genital-to-genital contact and is capable of a mature relationship with a member of the opposite sex 生殖期；**hot s.,** period of pyrexia in a malarial paroxysm 发热期；**latency s.,** 1. in psychoanalytic theory, the period of relative quiescence in psychosexual development, lasting from age 5 to 6 years to adolescence, during which interest in persons of the opposite sex ceases and association is mainly with other children of the same sex 相对静止期，精神分析理论中人的性心理发展的第 4 期；2. latent period 潜伏期；**oral s.,** in psychoanalytic theory, the earliest stage of psychosexual development, from birth to about 18 months, during which the infant's needs, expression, and pleasurable experiences center on the oral zone 口欲期；**phallic s.,** in psychoanalytic theory, the third stage of psychosexual development, lasting from age 2 or 3 years to 5 or 6 years, during which sexual interest, curiosity, and pleasurable experiences center on the penis in boys and the clitoris in girls 生殖器期；**second s. of labor,** 第二产程，参见 *labor.;* **third s. of labor,** 第三产程，参见 *labor*

stag·gers (stag′ərz) a form of vertigo occurring in decompression sickness 减压眩晕，减压病中的一种眩晕表现

stag·ing (stāj′ing) 1. the determination of distinct phases or periods in the course of a disease, the life history of an organism, or any biologic process 疾病分期；2. the classification of neoplasms according to the extent of the tumor 肿瘤分类；**TNM s.,** staging of tumors according to three basic components: primary tumor (T), regional nodes (N), and metastasis (M). Adscripts are used to denote size and degree of involvement; for example, 0 indicates undetectable, and 1, 2, 3, and 4 a progressive increase in size or involvement. Thus, a tumor may be described as T1, N2, M0 TNM 分期系统

stag·nant (stag′nənt) 1. motionless; not flowing or moving 不流动的；2. inactive; not developing or progressing 停滞的

stain (stān) 1. a substance used to impart color to tissues or cells, to facilitate microscopic study and identification 染剂，一种用于给组织或细胞染色的物质，以利于微观研究和鉴定；2. an area of discoloration of the skin 色素斑；**acid-fast s.,** a staining procedure for demonstrating acid-fast microorganisms, e.g., *auramine-rhodamine s., Kinyoun carbolfuchsin s.,* and *Ziehl-Neelsen carbolfuchsin s.* 抗酸染色剂；**auramine-rhodamine s.,** an acid-fast stain using the fluorescent dyes auramine O and rhodamine B, with a potassium permanganate counterstain; under ultraviolet light, acid-fast organisms glow with a yellow-orange color 金胺－若丹明染剂；**differential s.,** one that facilitates differentiation of various elements in a specimen 鉴别染色液，帮助鉴别样本中不同元素的染剂；**Giemsa s.,** a solution containing azure Ⅱ-eosin, azure Ⅱ, glycerin, and methanol; used for staining protozoan parasites, such as *Plasmodium* and *Trypanosoma,* for *Chlamydiaceae,* for differential staining of blood smears, and for viral inclusion bodies 吉姆萨液，由天青Ⅱ伊红、天青Ⅱ、甘油和甲醇配成的复合染色剂；用于原生动物寄生虫、血液涂片，以及病毒包含体的染色；**Gram s.,** a staining procedure in which microorganisms are stained with crystal violet, treated with strong iodine solution, decolorized with ethanol or ethanol-acetone, and counterstained with a contrasting dye; those retaining the stain are *gram-positive,* and those losing the stain but staining with the counterstain are *gram-negative* 革兰染剂；**hematoxylin-eosin s.,** a mixture of hematoxylin in distilled water and aqueous eosin solution, employed universally for routine tissue examination 苏木精-伊红染色剂；**Kinyoun carbolfuchsin s.,** an acid-fast stain using carbolfuchsin but not requiring heat; generally counterstained with methylene red. Acid-fast organisms appear red against a blue background Kinyoun 石炭酸品红染色剂；**metachromatic s.,** one that produces in certain elements colors different from that of the stain itself 异染性染剂；**port-wine s.,** 焰色痣，参见 *nevus flammeus;* **supravital s.,** a stain introduced in living tissue that has been removed from the body, but before cessation of the chemical life of the cells 活体外染剂；**tumor s.,** an area of increased density in a radiograph, due to collection of contrast material in distorted and abnormal vessels, prominent in the capillary and venous phase of arteriography, and presumed to indicate neoplasm 肿瘤显染；**vital s.,** a stain introduced into the living organism and taken up selectively by various tissues or cellular elements 活体染料；**Wright s.,** a mixture of eosin and methylene blue, used for demonstrating blood cells and malarial parasites 瑞特染液，由伊红和亚甲蓝配成的复合染色剂，用于红细胞和疟原虫染色；**Ziehl-Neelsen s.,** an acidfast stain using carbolfuchsin and heat; generally counterstained with methylene blue. Acid-fast organisms appear red against a blue background 齐-内染剂，使用石炭酸品红液且需加热的抗酸染色剂

stain·ing (stān′ing) 1. artificial coloration of a substance to facilitate examination of tissues, microorganisms, or other cells under the microscope. For various techniques, see under *stain* 染色法，物质的人工着色，如引入或应用染料使组织、微生物或其他细胞在显微镜下易于检查，有关技术参见 stain; 2. in dentistry, the modification of the color of a tooth or denture base 染色，改变牙或托牙基板的颜色，使之更像活体的外观

stal·ag·mom·e·ter (stal″əg-mom′ə-tər) an instrument for measuring surface tension by determining the exact number of drops in a given quantity of a liquid（表面张力）滴重计

stalk (stawk) an elongated anatomic structure resembling the stem of a plant 茎，柄，蒂；**allantoic s.,** the slender tube interposed between the urogenital sinus and allantoic sac; it is the precursor of the urachus 尿囊茎；**body s., connecting s.,** a bridge of mesoderm connecting the caudal end of the young embryo with the trophoblastic tissues; the precursor of part of the umbilical cord 体蒂，中胚层中连接幼胚的尾末端与滋养层组织的桥梁；脐带的前体；**pineal s.,** habenula (2) 松果体柄；**yolk s.,** a narrow duct connecting the yolk sac (umbilical vesicle) with the midgut of the early embryo 卵黄蒂

stam·mer·ing (stam′ər-ing) a disorder of speech behavior marked by involuntary pauses in speech; sometimes used synonymously with stuttering, especially in Great Britain 口吃

stan·dard (stan′dərd) something established as a measure or model to which other similar things should conform 标准，水准，规格，规范

stand·ard·ized pa·tient (stan′dər-dīzd pa′sh- ənt) a person trained to portray patient scenarios for the instruction, practice, and assessment of the professional and interpersonal skills of medical students, nurses, and other health care professionals 标准化病人

stand·still (stand′stil) cessation of activity, as of the heart *(cardiac s.)* or chest *(respiratory s.)* 停顿，停止

stan·nous (stan′əs) containing tin as a bivalent element 亚锡的，二价锡的；**s. fluoride,** a dental caries prophylactic, SnF_2, applied topically to the teeth 氟化亚锡

stan·o·lone (stan′o-lōn) a semisynthetic form of dihydrotestosterone, which has been used as an androgenic and anabolic steroid 二氢睾酮

stan·o·zo·lol (stan′o-zo-lol″) an androgenic anabolic steroid, used to prevent attacks of hereditary angioedema 康力龙，一种雄激素性合成类固醇，特别用于某些再生障碍性贫血病人以提高血红蛋

白的水平

sta·pe·dec·to·my (sta″pə-dek′tə-me) excision of the stapes 镫骨足板切除术

sta·pe·di·al (stə-pe′de-əl) pertaining to the stapes 蹬骨

sta·pe·dio·te·not·o·my (stə-pe″de-o-tə-not′ə-me) cutting of the tendon of the stapedius muscle 镫骨肌腱切断术

sta·pe·dio·ves·tib·u·lar (stə-pe″de-o-vəs-tib′ulər) pertaining to the stapes and vestibule 镫骨前庭的

sta·pe·dot·o·my (sta″pə-dot′ə-me) the surgical creation of a small opening in the footplate of the stapes 镫骨足板造孔术

sta·pes (sta′pēz) [L.] the innermost of the auditory ossicles, shaped somewhat like the stirrup used in horse riding; it articulates with the incus, and its base is inserted into the vestibular window 镫骨, 见 图 29

staph·y·line (staf′ə-līn) 1. uvular 悬雍垂的; 2. botryoid 葡萄状的

Sta·phy·lo·coc·ca·ceae (staf″ə-lo-kŏ-ka′se-e) a family of gram-positive, facultatively anaerobic bacteria of the order Bacillales 葡萄球菌科

staph·y·lo·coc·ce·mia (staf″ə-lo-kok-se′me-ə) staphylococci in the blood 葡萄球菌菌血症

Sta·phy·lo·coc·cus (staf″ə-lo-kok′əs) a genus of gram-positive, mainly facultatively anaerobic, non-motile, coccoid bacteria of the family Staphylococcaceae. Staphylococci are important inhabitants of the skin, cutaneous glands, and mucous membranes, and several species are important pathogens 葡萄球菌属; *S.au′reus*, a yellow-pigmented species that causes serious suppurative infections and systemic disease and whose toxins cause food poisoning and toxic shock 金黄色葡萄球菌; *S. epider′midis*, a species commonly found on normal skin; it includes many pathogenic strains and causes mainly nosocomial infections 表皮葡萄球菌; *S. lugdunen′sis*, a transient inhabitant of the skin that is a potential pathogen, associated with skin and soft tissue infections, bacteremia, and endocarditis 一种皮肤上的潜在病原体, 与皮肤和软组织感染、菌血症和心内膜炎有关; *S. saprophy′ticus*, an inhabitant of the genitourinary skin that is usually nonpathogenic but that can cause urinary tract infections 腐生葡萄球菌

staph·y·lo·coc·cus (staf″ə-lo-kok′əs) pl. *staphylococ′ci*. Any organism of the genus *Staphylococcus* 葡萄球菌; **staphylococ′cal, staphylococ′cic** *adj.*

staph·y·lo·der·ma (staf″ə-lo-dur′mə) pyogenic skin infection caused by staphylococci 葡萄球菌性

皮肤化脓

staph·y·lol·y·sin (staf″ə-lol′ə-sin) a hemolysin produced by staphylococci 葡萄球菌溶血素

staph·y·lo·ma (staf″ə-lo′mə) protrusion of the cornea or the sclera and the underlying uveal tissue 葡萄肿; **staphylom′atous** *adj.*

staph·y·lor·rha·phy (staf″ə-lor′ə-fe) palatorrhaphy 悬雍垂缝术

starch (stahrch) 淀粉 1. any of a group of polysaccharides of the general formula ($C_6H_{10}O_5$); it is the chief storage form of carbohydrates in plants 淀粉, 植物中碳水化合物的主要储存形式; 2. granules separated from mature corn, wheat, or potatoes; used as a dusting powder and pharmaceutical aid 从成熟的玉米、小麦或土豆中提取的淀粉物质, 用作除尘粉和药物辅助剂

star·tle (stahr′təl) 1. to make a quick involuntary movement as in alarm, surprise, or fright 惊起, 惊跳起来; 2. to become alarmed, surprised, or frightened 使大吃一惊

star·va·tion (stahr-va′shən) long-continued and extreme deprivation of food and resulting morbid effects 饥饿, 绝食

sta·sis (sta′sis) 1. a stoppage or diminution of flow, as of blood or other body fluid 停滞, 淤滞, 血液或其他体液的停止或减少流动; 2. a state of equilibrium among opposing forces 对抗力量之间的平衡状态; **stat′ic** *adj.*; **intestinal s.**, impairment of the normal passage of intestinal contents, due to mechanical obstruction or to impaired intestinal motility 便秘, 肠停滞; **urinary s.**, stoppage of the flow or discharge of urine, at any level of the urinary tract 尿淤滞; **venous s.**, impairment or cessation of venous flow 静脉淤滞

stat. [L.] sta′tim (at once, immediately) 立即

state (stāt) condition or situation 状态, 情况; **alpha s.**, the state of relaxation and peaceful wakefulness, associated with prominent alpha brain wave activity α 脑波状态, 松弛和宁静的觉醒状态, 脑电波以 α 型为主; **minimally conscious s.**, a level of consciousness higher than the vegetative state, characterized by limited but discernible evidence of awareness of self or the environment 微意识状态; **persistent vegetative s.**, the presence of a vegetative state 1 month after acute brain damage 持续性植物状态; **refractory s.**, a condition of subnormal excitability of muscle and nerve following excitation 不应状态, 激发后肌肉和神经的亚正常兴奋状态; **resting s.**, the physiologic condition achieved by complete bed rest for at least 1 hour 静息状态; **steady s.**, dynamic equilibrium 动力平衡, 稳态; **vegetative s.**, a condition of profound nonresponsiveness in a state of apparent wakefulness, characterized by complete lack of awareness of the self or of the environment and no evidence of purposeful behavior, although sleep/wake cycles occur and hypothalamic and brainstem autonomic functions are at least partially preserved 植物状态

sta·tim (sta′tim) [L.] at once 立即

sta·tion (sta′shən) 1. a position or location 站 立 姿 势；站，所；2. the location of the presenting part of the fetus in the birth canal, designated as −5 to −1 according to the number of centimeters the part is above an imaginary plane passing through the ischial spines, 0 when at the plane, and +1 to +5 according to the number of centimeters the part is below the plane 产位

sta·tis·tics (stə-tis′tiks) 1. a collection of numerical data 统 计；2. a discipline devoted to the collection, analysis, and interpretation of numerical data using the theory of probability 统计学；**vital s.**, data detailing the rates of birth, death, disease, marriage, and divorce in a population 生命统计，详细说明人口出生率、死亡率、疾病、婚姻率和离婚率

stato·acous·tic (stat″o-ə-koos′tik) pertaining to balance and hearing 平衡听觉的

stato·co·nia (stat″o-ko′ne-ə) sing. **statoco′nium.** Minute calciferous granules within the gelatinous membrane surrounding the acoustic maculae 耳石，位觉砂

stato·lith (stat′o-lith) a granule of the statoconia 位觉砂，耳石；平衡石（动物耳囊内）

sta·tom·e·ter (stə-tom′ə-tər) an apparatus for measuring the degree of exophthalmos 眼球突出计

sta·ture (stach′oor) the natural height of an individual in the upright position. *Short* and *tall statures* are generally defined as being greater than 2 standard deviations from the mean 身高；**stat′ural** *adj.*

sta·tus (sta′təs) [L.] state; particularly used in reference to a morbid condition 状态，情况（特指疾病状况）；体质；**s. asthma′ticus,** a particularly severe asthmatic attack that does not respond adequately to usual therapy and may require hospitalization 哮喘持续状态；**complex partial s.,** status epilepticus consisting of a series of complex partial seizures without return to full consciousness in between 复杂部分发作；**s. epilep′ticus,** a prolonged series of seizures without return to consciousness between them; subdivided into convulsive and nonconvulsive types 癫痫持续状态；**s. lympha′ticus, s. thymicolympha′ticus,** hyperplasia of lymphoid tissue and the thymus 淋巴体质；**s. verruco′sus,** a

wartlike appearance of the cerebral cortex, produced by disorderly arrangement of the neuroblasts so that the formation of fissures and sulci is irregular and unpredictable 疣状脑

stav·u·dine (stav′u-dēn) a nucleoside analogue of thymidine that inhibits human immunodeficiency virus (HIV) replication, used in the treatment of HIV infection 司他夫定，胸腺嘧啶的核苷类似物，抑制人体免疫缺陷病毒 (HIV) 复制，用于治疗 HIV 感染

stax·is (stak′sis) [Gr.] hemorrhage 滴流，渗血

steal (stē l) diversion, as of blood flow, of something from its normal course, as in occlusive arterial disease 盗血，血流从正常的流程迂回分流，见于闭塞性动脉疾病；**subclavian s.,** in occlusive disease of the subclavian artery, a reversal of blood flow in the ipsilateral vertebral artery from the basilar artery to the subclavian artery beyond the point of occlusion 锁骨下动脉盗血，锁骨下动脉闭塞性疾病时，同侧椎动脉血流逆转（可使脑血流缺失），即在闭塞点上方，从基底动脉转向锁骨下动脉

ste·a·rate (ste′ə-rāt) any salt (soap), ester, or anionic form of stearic acid 硬脂酸盐，硬脂酸酯，硬脂酸阴离子

ste·a·ric ac·id (ste-ar′ik) a saturated 18-carbon fatty acid occurring in most fats and oils, particularly of tropical plants and land animals; used pharmaceutically as a tablet and capsule lubricant and as an emulsifying and solubilizing agent 硬脂酸，十八烷酸

ste·a·ti·tis (ste″ə-ti′tis) inflammation of adipose tissue 脂肪织炎

ste·a·to·cys·to·ma (ste″ə-to-sis-to′mə) an epidermal cyst having an intricately infolded thin epidermal lining, without a granular layer, containing an oily liquid and often abortive hair follicles, lanugo hair, and sebaceous apocrine, or eccrine, glands 皮脂囊肿；**s. mul′tiplex,** development of numerous steatocystomas; often an autosomal dominant disorder chiefly affecting males at birth or presenting about the time of puberty 多发性皮脂囊肿，皮脂囊肿病

ste·a·tog·e·nous (ste″ə-toj′ə-nəs) lipogenic 产 生脂肪的

ste·a·to·ma·to·sis (ste″ə-to-mə-to′sis) 1. lipomatosis 脂肪瘤病；2. 同 steatocystoma multiplex

ste·a·to·ne·cro·sis (ste″ə-to-nə-kro′sis) fat necrosis 脂肪坏死

ste·a·to·pyg·ia (ste″ə-to-pij′e-ə) excessive fatness of the buttocks 臀脂过多；**steatop′ygous** *adj.*

ste·a·tor·rhea (ste″ə-to-re′ə) excess fat in feces 脂肪泻，从粪便中排出过量的脂肪，见于吸收不

良综合征

ste·a·to·sis (ste″ə-to′sis) fatty change 脂肪变性

steg·no·sis (steg-no′sis) constriction; stenosis 缩窄；狭窄；**stegnot′ic** *adj.*

stel·late (stel′āt) star-shaped; arranged in rosettes 星状的，排列呈玫瑰花形的

stel·lec·to·my (stə-lek′tə-me) excision of a portion of the stellate ganglion 星状神经节切除术

STEM science, technology, engineering, and mathematics 科学，技术，工程和数学

stem (stem) a supporting structure comparable to the stalk of a plant 茎，干，类似于植物茎的支持结构；**brain s.,** brainstem 脑干，参见 *B.* 下词条

STEMI ST-elevation myocardial infarction ST 段抬高型心肌梗死

steno·cho·ria (sten″o-kor′e-ə) 同 stenosis

steno·pe·ic (sten″o-pe′ik) having a narrow opening or slit 狭隙的，裂隙的，小孔的

ste·nosed (stə-nōzd′) narrowed; constricted 狭窄的，缩窄的

ste·no·sis (stə-no′sis) pl. *steno′ses* [Gr.] stricture; an abnormal narrowing or contraction of a duct or canal 狭窄；**aortic s. (AS),** a narrowing of the aortic orifice of the heart or of the aorta near the valve 主动脉瓣狭窄；**hypertrophic pyloric s.,** narrowing of the pyloric canal due to muscular hypertrophy and mucosal edema, usually in infants 肥大性幽门狭窄；**hypertrophic subaortic s., idiopathic hypertrophic subaortic s. (IHSS),** a form of hypertrophic cardiomyopathy in which the left ventricle is hypertrophied and the cavity is small; it is marked by obstruction to left ventricular outflow 肥厚型主动脉瓣瓣下狭窄，特发性肥厚性主动脉瓣瓣下狭窄；**infantile hypertrophic gastric s.,** congenital hypertrophy and hyperplasia of the musculature of the pyloric sphincter, leading to partial obstruction of the gastric outlet 婴儿肥大性胃狭窄；**mitral s.,** a narrowing of the left atrioventricular orifice 二尖瓣狭窄；**pulmonary s. (PS),** narrowing of the opening between the pulmonary artery and the right ventricle, usually at the level of the valve leaflets 肺动脉瓣狭窄；**pyloric s.,** obstruction of the pyloric orifice of the stomach; it may be congenital or acquired 幽门狭窄；**renal artery s.,** narrowing of one or both renal arteries, so that renal function is impaired, resulting in renal hypertension and, if stenosis is bilateral, chronic renal failure 肾动脉狭窄；**subaortic s.,** aortic stenosis due to an obstructive lesion in the left ventricle below the aortic valve, causing a pressure gradient across the obstruction within the ventricle 主动脉瓣下狭窄；**tricuspid s. (TS),** narrowing or stricture of the tricuspid orifice of the heart 三尖瓣狭窄

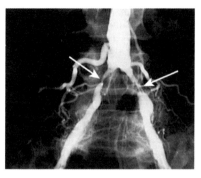

▲ 血管造影图中可见双侧髂总动脉严重狭窄（箭）

steno·ther·mal (sten″o-thur′məl) 同 stenothermic

steno·ther·mic (sten″o-thur′mik) developing only within a narrow range of temperature; said of bacteria 耐狭温的，指仅能耐小范围温度的细菌

steno·tho·rax (sten″o-thor′aks) abnormal narrowness of the chest 胸狭窄

ste·not·ic (stə-not′ik) marked by stenosis; abnormally narrowed 狭窄的，异常狭窄的

Steno·tro·pho·mo·nas (sten″o-tro″fo-mo′nəs) a genus of gram-negative, aerobic, rod-shaped bacteria of the family Xanthomonadaceae. *S. maltophi′lia* is a widespread, antibiotic-resistant species that is an opportunistic pathogen 寡养单胞菌属

stent (stent) 1. a device or mold of a suitable material, used to hold a skin graft in place 移植片固定膜，适当材料的装置或模具，用于将皮肤移植物固定在原位；2. a slender rodlike or threadlike device used to provide support for tubular structures that are being anastomosed, or to induce or maintain their patency 细长的棒状或线状装置，用于为被吻合的管状结构提供支持，或诱导或保持其开放；3. to apply or insert a stent. 应用或插入支架 **Palmaz s.,** an intravascular stent made of rigid wire mesh; it is introduced by a guidewire and expanded into place by a balloon 帕尔马滋支架，有坚硬的金属网制成的血管内支架，由导丝引入并且由球囊扩张到位；**pigtail s.,** one with a curl near the end like that of a pig's tail to maintain it in place 猪尾状支架

ste·pha·ni·on (stə-fa′ne-ən) [Gr.] intersection of the superior temporal line and the coronal suture 冠状点，上颞线与冠状缝的交点；**stepha′nial** *adj.*

ster·co·bi·lin (stur″ko-bi′lin) a bile pigment derivative formed by air oxidation of stercobilinogen; it is a brown-orange-red pigmentation contributing to the color of feces and urine 粪胆素

ster·co·bi·lin·o·gen (stur″ko-bi-lin′o-jən) a bilirubin metabolite and precursor of stercobilin, formed by reduction of urobilinogen 粪胆素原

ster·co·lith (stur′ko-lith) fecalith 粪石

ster·co·ra·ceous (stur″kə-ra′shəs) fecal 粪的，含粪的

ster·co·ral (stur″kə-rəl) fecal 粪的，含粪的

ster·co·ro·ma (stur″kə-ro′mə) a tumor-like mass of fecal matter in the rectum 粪结，粪瘤（肠内积粪）

ster·co·rous (stur′kə-rəs) fecal 粪的，含粪的

ster·eo·ar·throl·y·sis (ster″e-o-ahr-throl′ĭ-sis) operative formation of a movable new joint in cases of bony ankylosis 关节松解术

ster·eo·aus·cul·ta·tion (ster″e-o-aws″kəltə′shən) auscultation with two stethoscopes, on different parts of the chest 实体听诊法

ster·eo·chem·is·try (ster″e-o-kem′is-tre) the branch of chemistry concerned with the space relations of atoms in molecules 立体化学；**stereochem′ical** adj.

ster·eo·cine·flu·o·rog·ra·phy (ster″e-osin″ə-floo-rog′rə-fe) recording by a motion picture camera of images observed by stereoscopic fluoroscopy 立体荧光电影摄像术

ster·e·og·no·sis (ster″e-og-no′sis) 1. the faculty of perceiving and understanding the form and nature of objects by the sense of touch 实体觉，立体辨别，通过触觉感知和理解物体的形状和性质的能力；2. perception by the senses of the solidity of objects 感知物体固体特性的能力；**stereognos′tic** adj.

ster·eo·iso·mer (ster″e-o-i′so-mər) one of a group of compounds showing stereoisomerism 立体异构体

ster·eo·isom·er·ism (ster″e-o-i-som′ər-iz-əm) isomerism in which the isomers have the same structure (same linkages between atoms) but different spatial arrangements of the atoms 立体异构；**stereoisomer′ic** adj.

Ster·eo-or·thop·ter (ster″e-o-or-thop′tər) trademark for a mirror-reflecting instrument for correcting strabismus 视轴矫正实体镜（商品名）

ster·eo·scope (ster′e-o-skōp″) an instrument for producing the appearance of solidity and relief by combining the images of two similar pictures of an object 立体镜

ster·eo·scop·ic (ster′e-o-skop′ik) having the effect of a stereoscope; giving objects a solid or three-dimensional appearance 立体镜的

ster·eo·spe·cif·ic (ster′e-o-spə-sif′ik) exhibiting marked specificity for one of several stereoisomers of a substrate or reactant; said of enzymes or of synthetic organic reactions 立体特异性的

ster·eo·tac·tic (ster′e-o-tak′tik) 1. characterized by precise positioning in space; said especially of discrete areas of the brain that control specific func-

tions 立体定位的，尤指控制特定功能的大脑分立各区的定位；2. pertaining to stereotactic surgery 立体定向手术的；3. pertaining to thigmotaxis (thigmotactic) 趋触性的

ster·eo·tax·ic (ster″e-o-tak′sik) 1. stereotactic 立体定位的；2. pertaining to or exhibiting thigmotaxis (thigmotactic) 趋实体的

ster·eo·tax·is (ster″e-o-tak′sis) 1. stereotactic surgery 脑立体定位；2. thigmotaxis 趋触性

ster·e·ot·ro·pism (ster″e-ot′rə-piz-əm) tropism in response to contact with a solid or rigid surface 向实体性，亲实体性；**stereotrop′ic** adj.

ster·eo·typ·ic (ster″e-o-tip′ik) having a fixed, unvarying form 定型的

ster·eo·ty·py (ster′e-o-ti″pe) persistent repetition or sameness of acts, ideas, or words 刻板症

ster·ic (ste′rik) pertaining to the arrangement of atoms in space; pertaining to stereochemistry 空间原子排列的；立体化学的

ster·ile (ster′il) 1. unable to produce offspring 不生育的；2. aseptic 无菌的，消毒的

ster·il·i·ty (stə-ril′ĭ-te) 1. inability to produce offspring, i.e., either to conceive (female s.) or to induce conception (male s.) 不孕，不育；2. asepsis 无菌

ster·i·li·za·tion (ster″ĭ-lĭ-za′shən) 1. the complete elimination or destruction of all living microorganisms 灭菌，消毒；2. any procedure by which an individual is made incapable of reproduction 绝育

ster·i·lize (ster′ĭ-līz) 1. to render sterile; to free from microorganisms 灭菌，把……消毒；2. to render incapable of reproduction 使绝育

ster·i·liz·er (ster′ĭ-līz″ər) an apparatus for the destruction of microorganisms 灭菌器

ster·nal (ster′nəl) of or relating to the sternum 胸骨的

ster·nal·gia (stər-nal′jə) pain in the sternum 胸骨痛

ster·ne·bra (stur′nə-brə) pl. *ster′nebrae*. Any of the segments of the sternum in early life, which later fuse to form the body of the sternum 胸骨节，指幼年期的胸骨节，以后才融合为胸骨体

ster·no·cla·vic·u·lar (stur″no-klə-vik′u-lər) pertaining to the sternum and clavicle 胸骨锁的

ster·no·clei·do·mas·toid (stur″no-kli″domas′toid) pertaining to the sternum, clavicle, and mastoid process 胸锁乳突的

ster·no·cos·tal (stur″no-kos′təl) pertaining to the sternum and ribs 胸肋的

ster·no·hy·oid (stur″no-hi′oid) pertaining to the sternum and hyoid bone 胸骨舌骨的

ster·noid (stur′noid) resembling the sternum 胸骨样的

ster·no·mas·toid (stur″no-mas′toid) pertaining to

the sternum and mastoid process 胸骨乳突的

ster·no·peri·car·di·al (stur″no-per′ĭ-kahr′de-əl) pertaining to the sternum and pericardium 胸骨心包的

ster·nos·chi·sis (stər-nos′kĭ-sis) congenital fissure of the sternum 胸骨裂

ster·no·thy·roid (stur″no-thi′roid) pertaining to the sternum and thyroid cartilage or gland 胸骨甲状软骨的；胸骨甲状腺的

ster·not·o·my (stər-not′ə-me) the operation of cutting through the sternum 胸骨切开术

ster·num (stur′nəm) [L.] a longitudinal unpaired plate of bone forming the middle of the anterior wall of the thorax; it articulates above with the clavicles and along its sides with the cartilages of the first seven ribs. Its three parts are the manubrium, body, and xiphoid process 胸骨，见图 1

ster·nu·ta·to·ry (stər-nu′tə-tor″e) 1. causing sneezing 催嚏的；2. an agent that causes sneezing 催嚏剂

ster·oid (ster′oid) any of a group of lipids with a specific 7-carbon–atom ring system as a nucleus, such as progesterone, adrenocortical and gonadal hormones, bile acids, sterols, toad poisons, and some carcinogenic hydrocarbons 类固醇；**steroi′dal** adj.; **anabolic s.,** any of a group of synthetic derivatives of testosterone having pronounced anabolic properties and relatively weak androgenic properties; they are used clinically mainly to promote growth and repair of body tissues in diseases or states promoting catabolism or tissue wasting 促蛋白合成类固醇

ste·roi·do·gen·e·sis (stə-roi″do-jen′ə-sis) production of steroids, as by the suprarenal glands 类固醇生成；**steroidogen′ic** adj.

ster·ol (ster′ol) any of a group of steroids with a long (8 to 10 carbons) aliphatic side-chain at position 17 and at least one alcoholic group; they have lipidlike solubility 甾醇，固醇

steth·om·e·ter (steth-om′ə-tər) an instrument for measuring the circular dimension or expansion of the chest 胸围计

stetho·scope (steth′o-skōp) an instrument for performing mediate auscultation 听诊器；**stethoscop′ic** adj.

steth·os·co·py (steth-os′kə-pe) examination with the stethoscope 听诊器检查

sthe·nia (sthe′ne-ə) a condition of strength and activity 强壮，壮健，有力

sthen·ic (sthen′ik) active; strong 强壮的，有力的

STI systolic time intervals 收缩时间间期

stig·ma (stig′mə) pl. **stigmas, stig′mata** [Gr.] 1. any mental or physical mark or peculiarity that aids in identification or diagnosis of a condition 特征，有助于识别或诊断疾病的任何心理或身体标记或特点；2. a mark, spot, or pore on the surface of an organ or organism 小斑，器官或有机体表面的标记、斑点或小孔；3. 同 follicular s.; 4. a distinguishing personal trait that is perceived as or actually is physically, socially, or psychologically disadvantageous 个性，被认为或实际上在身体、社会或心理上处于不利地位的显著个人特质；5. (in the pl.) purpuric or hemorrhagic lesions of the hands and/or feet, resembling crucifixion wounds （复数形式）出血病灶，手和／或脚的紫癜或出血性病变，类似于十字架伤口；**stig′mal, stigmat′ic** adj.; **follicular s.,** a spot on the surface of an ovary where the vesicular follicle will rupture vand permit passage of the secondary oocyte during ovulation 卵泡斑，卵巢表面囊状滤泡即将破裂处的斑点，排卵时经此排出卵子；**malpighian s's,** the points where the smaller veins enter into the larger veins of the spleen Malpighi 小孔，脾静脉上小静脉进入大静脉处

stig·ma·ti·za·tion (stig″mə-tĭ-za′shən) 1. the developing of or being identified as possessing one or more stigmata 痕迹形成，被确定为拥有一种或多个红斑，或者红斑的发生过程；2. the act or process of negatively labeling or characterizing another 使他人蒙受耻辱的过程或行为；3. the condition due to or marked by stigmata 羞辱，受辱（的状态）

sti·let (sti-let′) stylet 管心针，通管丝

still·birth (stil′burth″) delivery of a dead child 死产

still·born (stil′born″) born dead 死产的

stim·u·lant (stim′u-lənt) 1. producing stimulation 引起兴奋的，产生刺激；2. an agent that stimulates 刺激剂，兴奋剂；**central s.,** a stimulant of the central nervous system 中枢兴奋剂；**diffusible s.,** a stimulant that acts quickly and strongly but transiently 弥散性兴奋剂；**general s.,** a stimulant that acts upon the whole body 全身兴奋剂；**local s.,** a stimulant that affects only, or mainly, the part to which it is applied 局部兴奋剂

stim·u·late (stim′u-lāt) to excite functional activity 激发功能活动

stim·u·la·tion (stim″u-la′shən) the act or process of stimulating; the condition of being stimulated 兴奋，刺激作用；**deep brain s. (DBS),** patient-controlled, continuous, high-frequency electrical stimulation of a specific area of the thalamus, globus pallidus, or subthalamic nucleus by means of an electrode implanted in the brain 脑深部电刺激；**functional electrical s. (FES),** the application of an electric current by means of a prosthesis to stimulate and restore partial function to a muscle disabled by neurologic lesions 功能性电刺激疗法；**transcutaneous electrical nerve s. (TENS),** transcutaneous nerve s. (TNS), electrical stimulation of nerves for relief of pain by delivering a current through the skin 经皮神经电刺激疗法

stim·u·la·tor (stim′u-la″tər) 1. any agent that excites functional activity 刺激质；2. in electrodiagnosis, an instrument that applies pulses of current to stimulate a nerve, muscle, or area of the central nervous system 刺激器，在电诊断手段中，使用电流脉冲刺激神经、肌肉或中枢神经系统区域的仪器；**long-acting thyroid s. (LATS),** thyroid-stimulating antibody associated with Graves disease; it is an autoantibody reactive against thyroid cell receptors for thyroid-stimulating hormone and thus mimics the effects of the hormone 长时程作用甲状腺刺激物

stim·u·la·to·ry (stim′u-lə-tor″e) capable of stimulating or causing stimulation 刺激性

stim·u·lus (stim′u-ləs) pl. *stim′uli* [L.] any agent, act, or influence that produces a functional or trophic reaction in a receptor or an irritable tissue 刺激物，刺激；**adequate s.,** a stimulus of the specific form of energy to which a given receptor is sensitive 适宜刺激物；**aversive s.,** one that, when applied following the occurrence of a response, decreases the strength of that response on later occurrences 后抑刺激；**conditioned s.,** a stimulus that acquires the capacity to evoke a particular response on repeated pairing with another stimulus naturally capable of eliciting the response 条件刺激；**discriminative s.,** a stimulus, associated with reinforcement, that exerts control over a particular form of behavior; the subject discriminates between closely related stimuli and responds positively only in the presence of that stimulus 辨别刺激；**eliciting s.,** any stimulus, conditioned or unconditioned, that elicits a response 诱发刺激；**heterologous s.,** one that produces an effect or sensation when applied to any part of a nerve tract 异种刺激物；**homologous s.,** 同 adequate s.; **threshold s.,** a stimulus that is just strong enough to elicit a response 阈刺激物；**unconditioned s.,** any stimulus naturally capable of eliciting a specific response 非条件刺激

sting (sting) 1. injury due to a biotoxin introduced into an individual or with which they come in contact, together with the mechanical trauma incident to its introduction 蜇伤；2. the organ used to inflict such injury（动植物的）蜇针

stip·pled (stip′əld) marked by small spots or flecks 斑点状的

stip·pling (stip′ling) a spotted condition or appearance, as an appearance of the retina as if dotted with light and dark points, or the appearance of red blood cells in basophilia 点彩

stir·rup (stur′əp) 1. a structure or device resembling the stirrup of a saddle, or the portion of an apparatus on which to rest the feet 镫；2. stapes 镫骨

stitch (stich) 1. a sudden, transient cutting pain 刺痛；2. a suture（缝的）一针

Sti·var·ga (stī-var′gə) trademark for a preparation of regorafenib 瑞格非尼制剂的商品名

sto·chas·tic (sto-kas′tik) pertaining to a random process, particularly a time series of random variables 随机的

stoi·chi·ol·o·gy (stoi″ke-ol′ə-je) the science of elements, especially the physiology of the cellular elements of tissues 细胞生理学；**stoichiolog′ic** *adj.*

stoi·chi·om·e·try (stoi″ke-om′ə-tre) the determination of the relative proportions of the compounds involved in a chemical reaction 化学计量学，化学计算学；**stoichiomet′ric** *adj.*

sto·ma (sto′mə) pl. *sto′mas, sto′mata* [Gr.] a mouthlike opening, particularly an incised opening that is kept open for drainage or other purposes 口，小孔；人造口；**sto′mal** *adj.*

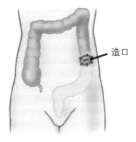

造口

▲　降结肠造瘘术的造口

stom·ach (stum′ək) the musculomembranous expansion of the alimentary canal between the esophagus and duodenum, consisting of a cardiac part, a fundus, a body, and a pyloric part. Its (gastric) glands secrete the gastric juice that, when mixed with food, forms chyme, a semifluid substance suitable for further digestion by the intestine 胃，见图 27；**stom′achal** *adj.*; **cascade s.,** an atypical form of hourglass stomach, characterized radiographically by a drawing up of the mastoid wall; an opaque medium first fills the upper sac and then cascades into the lower sac 瀑布形胃；**hourglass s.,** one more or less completely divided into two parts, resembling an hourglass in shape, due to scarring that complicates chronic gastric ulcer 葫芦胃；**leather bottle s.,** linitis plastica 革袋胃，皮革样胃

sto·mach·ic (sto-mak′ik) 1. gastric 胃 的；2. a medicine that promotes the functional activity of the stomach 健胃药

S

sto·ma·tal·gia (sto″mə-tal′jə) pain in the mouth 口腔痛

sto·ma·ti·tis (sto″mə-ti′tis) pl. *stomati′tides*. Generalized inflammation of the oral mucosa 口炎；**angular s.**, perlèche 口角炎；**aphthous s.**, 同 recurrent aphthous s.; **gangrenous s.**, 坏疽性口炎，参见 *noma*; **herpetic s.**, herpes simplex involving the oral mucosa and lips, with yellowish vesicles that rupture and produce ragged painful ulcers covered by a gray membrane and surrounded by an erythematous halo 疱疹性口炎，口溃疡；**mycotic s.**, thrush 鹅口疮，真菌性口炎；**recurrent aphthous s.**, a recurrent stomatitis of unknown etiology characterized by the appearance of small ulcers on the oral mucosa, covered by a grayish exudate and surrounded by a bright red halo; they heal without scarring in 7 to 14 days 复发性阿弗他口疮；**ulcerative s.**, stomatitis with shallow ulcers on the cheeks, tongue, and lips 溃疡性口炎；**Vincent s.**, necrotizing ulcerative gingivitis 急性坏死溃疡性龈炎

sto·ma·to·dyn·ia (sto″mə-to-din′e-ə) 同 stomatalgia

sto·ma·tog·nath·ic (sto″mə-tog-nath′ik) denoting the mouth and jaws collectively 口颌的

sto·ma·tol·o·gy (sto″mə-tol′ə-je) the branch of medicine that deals with the mouth and its diseases 口腔学；**stomatological** *adj.*

sto·ma·to·ma·la·cia (sto″mə-to-mə-la′she-ə) softening of the structures of the mouth 口腔软化

sto·ma·to·me·nia (sto″mə-to-me′ne-ə) bleeding from the mouth at the time of menstruation 月经期口出血

sto·ma·top·a·thy (sto″mə-top′ə-the) any disorder of the mouth 口腔病

sto·ma·to·plas·ty (sto′mə-to-plas″te) plastic reconstruction of the mouth 口腔成形术

sto·ma·tor·rha·gia (sto″mə-to-ra′jə) hemorrhage from the mouth 口腔出血

sto·mo·de·um (sto″mo-de′əm) an invagination of the surface ectoderm of the embryo, at the point where later the mouth is formed 口道，口凹，胚胎外胚层内陷处以后即形成口；**stomode′al** *adj.*

stone (stōn) 1. calculus. 石，结石 2. a unit of weight in Great Britain, the equivalent of 14 pounds (avoirdupois), or about 6.34 kg 英石，英制重量单位，用来表示体重时，相当于 14 磅或约 6.34kg

stool (stool) feces 粪便；**rice-water s's**, the watery diarrhea of cholera 米泔水样便，出现在霍乱的水样腹泻；**silver s.**, feces with a silver color from a mixture of melena and white fatty material, seen in tropical sprue, in children with diarrhea who are given sulfonamides, and with carcinoma of the ampulla of Vater 银色粪，见于热带性口炎性腹泻

stor·i·form (stor′ĭ-form) having an irregularly whorled pattern somewhat like that of a straw mat; said of the microscopic appearance of dermatofibrosarcomas 席纹状的

storm (storm) a sudden and temporary increase in symptoms 暴发，发作，症状骤增；**thyroid s.**, **thyrotoxic s.**, 甲状腺危象，参见 *crisis* 下词条

STR short tandem repeat 短串联重复序列

stra·bis·mom·e·ter (stra″biz-mom′ə-tər) an apparatus for measuring strabismus 斜视计

stra·bis·mus (strə-biz′məs) a condition in which the visual axes cannot be directed at the same point of fixation 斜视；**strabis′mal, strabis′mic** *adj.*; **concomitant s.**, that due to faulty insertion of the eye muscles, resulting in the same amount of deviation regardless of the direction of the gaze 共同性斜视；**convergent s.**, esotropia 会聚性斜视，内斜视；**divergent s.**, exotropia 散开性斜视，外斜视；**nonconcomitant s.**, that in which the amount of deviation of the squinting eye varies according to the direction of gaze 非共同性斜视；**vertical s.**, that in which the visual axis of the squinting eye deviates in the vertical plane (hypertropia or hypotropia) 垂直斜视

stra·bot·o·my (strə-bot′ə-me) section of an ocular tendon in treatment of strabismus 斜视手术

strad·dle (strad′əl) 1. to extend over or across, to be on both sides 延伸或交叉到两边；2. to have one leg on each opposite side of something 叉开腿坐于，跨立

strain (strān) 1. to overexercise 过度训练；2. excessive effort or exercise 过劳，劳损；3. an overstretching or overexertion of some part of the musculature 拉紧；4. to filter 被过滤；5. change in the size or shape of a body as the result of an externally applied force 应变；6. a group of organisms within a species or variety, characterized by some particular quality 菌系，品系；**wild-type s.**, that used as a standard for a given species or variety of organism, usually assumed to be the one found in nature 野生型菌株

strait (strāt) a narrow passage 窄道，狭口；**s's of pelvis**, the pelvic inlet (*superior pelvic s.*) and pelvic outlet (*inferior pelvic s.*) 骨盆，骨盆入口（上骨盆）和骨盆出口（下骨盆）

strait·jack·et (strāt′jak″ət) a device for restraining the limbs, especially the arms, of a violently disturbed person; it consists of a canvas jacket with long sleeves that can be fastened behind the back of the patient 约束衣尤指用以约束疯人的臂而言

stra·mo·ni·um (strə-mo′ne-əm) the flowering plant *Datura stramonium* or a preparation of its dried leaf and flowering or fruiting tops; it is a source of hyoscyamine and scopolamine and has anticholinergic and parasympatholytic effects. It is used in folk medicine, Chinese medicine, and homeopathy 曼陀罗

stran·gle (strang'gəl) choke (1) 使窒息

stran·gu·lat·ed (strang'gu-lāt″əd) congested by reason of constriction or hernial stricture 绞窄的

stran·gu·la·tion (strang″gu-la'shən) 1. choke (2) 勒颈、勒颈窒息; 2. arrest of circulation in a part due to compression 绞窄, 参见 *hemostasis* (2)

stran·gu·ry (strang'gu-re) slow and painful discharge of the urine, due to spasm of the urethra and bladder 痛性尿淋沥

strap (strap) 1. a band or slip, as of adhesive plaster, used in attaching parts to each other 带, 条, 胶布; 2. to bind down tightly 绑扎; **Montgomery s's,** straps of adhesive tape used to secure dressings that must be changed frequently Montgomery 带, 用于固定经常更换的敷料的胶带

strat·i·fied (strat'ĭ-fīd) formed or arranged in layers 分层的

strat·i·form (strat'ĭ-form) having a layered structure 层状的

stra·tum (strat'əm) (stra'təm) pl. *stra'ta* [L.] 1. a layer or lamina 层; 2. in anatomy, a sheetlike mass of substance 解剖学里的片状物质; **s. basa'le,** basal layer: the deepest layer, as of the endometrium or epidermis 基底层; **s. cor'neum,** horny layer: the outermost layer of the epidermis, consisting of dead and desquamating cells 角质层; **s. functiona'le,** functional layer of endometrium: the layer of endometrium facing the uterine lumen, overlying the stratum basale. Its cells are cast off at menstruation and parturition. It is called the *decidua* during pregnancy 子宫内膜功能层; **s. germinati'vum,** 1. germinative layer: the stratum basale and stratum spinosum of the epidermis considered as a single layer 表皮生发层; 2. stratum basale 表皮基层; **s. granulo'sum,** granular layer 颗粒层 1. the layer of epidermis between the stratum lucidum and stratum spinosum, containing keratohyalin granules 表皮颗粒层, 位于皮肤表皮棘层上方一层, 胞质内含有角质透明颗粒; 2. the layer of follicle cells lining the theca of the vesicular ovarian follicles 颗粒层, 卵泡腔周围密集排列的卵泡细胞; **s. lu'cidum,** clear layer: in the epidermis, the clear translucent layer just beneath the stratum corneum 透明层; **s. spino'sum,** spinous or prickle cell layer: in the epidermis, the layer between the stratum granulosum and stratum basale, characterized by the presence of prickle cells 棘细胞层

streak (strēk) a line, stria, or stripe. 线条, 条纹,

划痕 **angioid s's,** red to black irregular bands in the ocular fundus running outward from the optic disk 血管样条纹纹, 从视盘向外延伸的眼底红色至黑色不规则带; **fatty s.,** a small, flat, yellow-gray area, composed mainly of cholesterol, in an artery; possibly an early stage of atherosclerosis 脂纹, 动脉中小的、扁平的黄灰色的区域, 主要由胆固醇组成; 可能是动脉粥样硬化早期损伤的表现; **meningitic s.,** tache cérébrale 脑膜性划痕, 脑病性划痕; **Moore lightning s's,** vertical flashes of light sometimes seen on the peripheral side of the field of vision when the eyes are moved, a benign condition Moore 亮线, 当眼睛移动时, 有时会在视野的外围侧看到垂直闪烁的光线, 这是一种良性状态; **primitive s.,** a faint white trace at the caudal end of the embryonic disc, formed by movement of cells at the onset of mesoderm formation and providing the first evidence of the embryonic axis 原条, 指在胚盘的尾端有一条微弱的白色痕迹, 由中胚层形成开始时细胞的运动形成, 是胚轴的初始迹象

stream (strēm) a current or flow of water or other fluid 流, 水流或其他流体的流动; **blood s.,** bloodstream 血流

strepho·sym·bo·lia (stref″o-sim-bo'le-ə) 1. a perceptual disorder in which objects seem reversed as in a mirror 视象倒反, 一种感知障碍, 物体和在镜子中的象看起来像是一样的; 2. a type of dyslexia in which letters are perceived as if in a mirror; it begins with confusion between similar but oppositely oriented letters (b-d, q-p) and there may be a tendency to read backward 读字倒反, 一种阅读障碍, 就像字母被映在镜子中

Strep·to·ba·cil·lus (strep″to-bə-sil'əs) a genus of gram-negative, facultatively anaerobic, nonmotile, non–spore-forming bacteria of the family Fusobacteriaceae; organisms are highly variable in form. *S. monilifor'mis* is a cause of ratbite fever 链杆菌属

strep·to·ba·cil·lus (strep″to-bə-sil'əs) pl. *streptobacil'li.* An organism of the genus *Streptobacillus* 链杆菌

strep·to·cer·ci·a·sis (strep″to-sər-ki'ə-sis) infection with *Mansonella streptocerca,* whose microfilariae produce a pruritic rash resembling that in onchocerciasis; transmitted by midges of the genus *Culicoides,* it occurs in Central Africa 链尾丝虫病

Strep·to·coc·ca·ceae (strep″to-kok-a'se-e) a family of gram-positive, facultatively anaerobic cocci of the order Lactobacillales 链球菌科

strep·to·coc·cal (strep″to-kok'əl) pertaining to or caused by a streptococcus 链球菌的

strep·to·coc·ce·mia (strep″to-kok-se'me-ə) occurrence of streptococci in the blood 链球菌血症

Strep·to·coc·cus (strep″to-kok'əs) a genus of

gram-positive, facultatively anaerobic cocci of the family Streptococcaceae, occurring in pairs or chains. Streptococci are most often classified according to patterns of hemolysis on blood agar (see *hemolytic streptococci,* under *streptococcus*), or by antigenic composition (see *Lancefield classification,* under *classification*) 链球菌属；*S. bo'vis,* a species that is found in the bovine alimentary tract and is associated with human infective endocarditis and urinary tract infections 牛链球菌；*S. mu'tans,* a species that has been implicated in the formation of dental caries 突变链球菌；*S. pneumo'niae,* the *pneumococci,* a species that is the usual cause of lobar pneumonia; it also causes other serious, acute, pyogenic disorders 肺炎链球菌；*S. pyo'genes,* a toxigenic and pyogenic species that causes a number of diseases, including pharyngitis, scarlet fever, rheumatic fever, puerperal sepsis, poststreptococcal acute glomerulonephritis, and necrotizing fasciitis 酿脓链球菌；*S. san'guinis,* a species found in dental plaque and the blood, it is a cause of subacute bacterial endocarditis 血链球菌，在牙菌斑和血液中发现的一种细菌，它是亚急性细菌性心内膜炎的病因

strep·to·coc·cus (strep″to-kok′əs) pl. *streptococ'-ci.* An organism of the genus *Streptococcus* 链球菌；**streptococ′cal, streptococ′cic** *adj.;* **hemolytic s.,** any streptococcus capable of hemolyzing erythrocytes, classified as either α -hemolytic (producing a small greenish zone around the colony on blood agar) or β *-hemolytic* (producing a clear zone of hemolysis around the colony on blood agar). The most virulent streptococci are β -hemolytic. On immunologic grounds, the β -hemolytic streptococci may be divided into groups A through T; most human pathogens belong to groups A through G 溶血性链球菌；**nonhemolytic s.,** any streptococcus that does not cause a change in the medium when cultured on blood agar 非溶血性链球菌；**viridanss treptococci,** in one classification, a group of streptococci other than *S. pneumoniae,* usually α -hemolytic but sometimes nonhemolytic; some are found normally in the respiratory tract and others cause dental caries, bacterial endocarditis, or opportunistic infections 草绿色链球菌

strep·to·dor·nase (strep″to-dor′nās) a deoxyribonuclease produced by hemolytic streptococci 链球菌 DNA 酶

strep·to·ki·nase (strep″to-ki′nās) a protein produced by β -hemolytic streptococci, which produces fibrinolysis by binding to plasminogen and causing its conversion to plasmin; used as a thrombolytic agent 链激酶；**s.-streptodornase (SKSD),** a mix-

ture of enzymes elaborated by hemolytic streptococci; used as a proteolytic and fibrinolytic agent 双链酶，链激酶 – 链道酶，用作蛋白分解剂和纤维蛋白溶解剂

strep·tol·y·sin (strep-tol′ĭ-sin) the hemolysin of hemolytic streptococci 链球菌溶血素

Strep·to·my·ces (strep″to-mi′sēz) a large genus of aerobic, gram-positive bacteria of the family Streptomycetaceae. Most species are soil forms, but some are parasitic on plants and animals; many are sources of various antibiotics. *S. somalien'sis* is a cause of mycetoma 链霉菌属

Strep·to·my·ce·ta·ceae (strep″to-mi″sə- ta′se-e) a family of aerobic, gram-positive bacteria of the order Actinomycetales 链霉菌科

strep·to·my·cin (strep″to-mi′sin) an aminoglycoside antibiotic produced by *Streptomyces griseus* and effective against a wide variety of aerobic gram-negative bacilli and some grampositive bacteria, including mycobacteria, but to which many of the former have developed resistance; used as the sulfate salt in the treatment of tuberculosis, tularemia, plague, and brucellosis 链霉素

Strep·to·spo·ran·gi·neae (strep″to-spor″an-jin′e-e) a suborder of gram-positive, aerobic bacteria of the order Actinomycetales that produce an aerial mycelium 链孢素菌亚目

strep·to·zo·cin (strep″to-zo′sin) an antineoplastic antibiotic derived from *Streptomyces achromogenes;* used principally in the treatment of islet cell and other tumors of the pancreas 链脲菌素

stress (stres) 1. forcibly exerted influence; pressure 压力；2. force per unit area 应力；3. in dentistry, the pressure of the upper teeth against the lower in mastication 口腔科中，咀嚼时产生的上牙对下牙的压力；4. a state of physiologic or psychological strain caused by adverse stimuli, physical, mental, or emotional, internal or external, that tend to disturb the functioning of an organism and that the organism naturally desires to avoid 应激，参见 *reaction* 下词条；5. the stimuli that elicit such a state or stress reactions 引起这种状态或应激反应的刺激

stretch·er (strech′ər) a contrivance for carrying the sick or wounded 担架

stria (stri′ə) pl. *stri'ae* [L.] 1. a band, line, streak, or stripe 带，条纹；2. in anatomy, a longitudinal collection of nerve fibers in the brain 在解剖学中，大脑中的神经纤维的纵向聚集；**stri'aeatro'phi-cae, stri'aedisten'sae,** atrophic, pink to purple, scarlike lesions on the breasts, thighs, abdomen, or buttocks, due to weakening of elastic tissues, associated with pregnancy *(striae gravidarum),* overweight, rapid growth during puberty and adolescence, Cushing syndrome, and topical or prolonged treatment with corticosteroids 萎缩纹，白纹；**stri′aegrav·ida′rum**, 妊娠纹，参见 *striae atrophicae*

stri·ate (stri′āt) 1. 同 striated; 2. to mark with stripes or striae 在……上加条纹（或线条）

stri·at·ed (stri′āt-əd) having stripes or striae 纹状的

stri·a·tion (stri-a′shən) 1. the quality of being marked by stripes or striae 纹，条纹；2. a streak or scratch, or a series of streaks 划痕

stri·a·to·ni·gral (stri″ə-to-ni′grəl) projecting from the corpus striatum to the substantia nigra 纹黑突，纹黑突的

stri·a·tum (stri-a′təm) corpus striatum 纹状体；**stria′tal** *adj.*

stric·ture (strik′chər) stenosis 狭窄

stric·ture·plas·ty (strik′chər-plas″te) surgical enlargement of the caliber of a constricted bowel segment by means of longitudinal incision and transverse suturing of the stricture 狭窄缝术，通过狭窄的纵向切口和横向缝合手术扩大狭窄肠段的直径

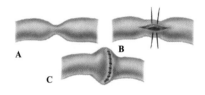

▲ 狭窄缝术 **A.** 狭窄。**B.** 纵切口。**C.** 横向闭合

stric·tur·iza·tion (strik″chər-ī-za′shən) the process of decreasing in caliber or of becoming constricted 狭窄化

stri·dor (stri′dər) [L.] a harsh, high-pitched breath sound 喘鸣；**stri′dent, strid′ulous** *adj.*; **laryngeal s.**, that due to laryngeal obstruction. A *congenital* form with dyspnea is due to infolding of a congenitally flabby epiglottis and aryepiglottic folds during inhalation; it is usually outgrown by 2 years of age 喉喘鸣

strio·cer·e·bel·lar (stri″o-ser″ə-bel′ər) pertaining to the corpus striatum and cerebellum 纹状体小脑的

strip (strip) 1. to press the contents from a canal, such as the urethra or a blood vessel, by running the finger along it 挤出，如用手指沿血管压挤其内容物；2. to excise lengths of large veins and incompetent tributaries after subcutaneous dissection 剥

离，剥脱，在皮下解剖后切除大静脉和无用的静脉分支；3. to remove tooth structure or restorative material from the mesial or distal surfaces of teeth utilizing abrasive strips; usually done to alleviate crowding 磨光，缩小牙齿近中远中的宽度

stro·bi·la (stro-bi′lə) pl. *strobi′lae* [L.] the chain of proglottids constituting the bulk of the body of adult tapeworms 链体，构成绦虫成虫虫体大部分的节片链

stroke (strōk) 1. a sudden and severe attack 打，击；2. stroke syndrome 中风；3. a pulsation 搏动；**completed s.**, stroke syndrome reflecting the infarction of the vascular territory that is put at risk by a stenosis or occlusion of a feeding vessel 完成性发作，反映血管区域梗塞的中风，这些营养血管的狭窄或闭塞状态使人处于危险之中；**embolic s.**, stroke syndrome due to cerebral embolism 栓塞发作，脑栓塞引起的中风症状；**s. in evolution,** a preliminary, unstable stage in stroke syndrome in which the blockage is present but the syndrome has not progressed to the stage of completed stroke 渐进性发作，卒中症状的初期；**heat s.**, a condition due to excessive exposure to heat, with dry skin, vertigo, headache, thirst, nausea, and muscular cramps; the body temperature may be dangerously elevated 热射病，中暑；**ischemic s.**, stroke syndrome caused by ischemia of an area of the brain 缺血性发作；**thrombotic s.**, stroke syndrome due to cerebral thrombosis, most often superimposed on a plaque of atherosclerosis 血栓性发作

stro·ma (stro′mə) pl. *stro′mata* [Gr.] the matrix or supporting tissue of an organ 基质；**stro′mal, stro·mat′ic** *adj.*

stro·muhr (shtro′moor) [Ger.] an instrument for measuring the velocity of blood flow.Ludwi 血流速度计

Stron·gy·loi·des (stron″jə-loi′dēz) a genus of widely distributed nematodes parasitic in the intestine of humans and other mammals. *S. stercora′lis* is found in the tropics and subtropics and causes strongyloidiasis 类圆线虫属

stron·gy·loi·di·a·sis (stron″jə-loi-di′ə-sis) infection with *Strongyloides stercoralis*. In the small intestine it causes mucosal ulceration and diarrhea. In the lungs it causes hemorrhaging 类圆线虫病

stron·gy·loi·do·sis (stron″jə-loi-do′sis) strongyloidiasis 类圆线虫病

stron·gy·lo·sis (stron″jə-lo′sis) infection with *Strongylus* 圆线虫病

Stron·gy·lus (stron′jə-ləs) a genus of nematode parasites 圆线虫属

stron·ti·um (Sr) (stron′she-əm) a soft, silvery white or yellowish, highly reactive, alkaline earth metal element; at. no. 38, at. wt. 87.62 锶（化学元素）; **s. 89,** a radioisotope of strontium having a half-life of 50.55 days and decaying by beta emission; used in the form of the chloride as a radiation source in palliation of bone pain caused by metastatic lesions ^{89}Sr **s. 90,** a radioisotope of strontium having a half-life of 28.5 years and decaying by emission of beta particles; used in radiotherapy and the treatment of a variety of benign ophthalmologic conditions ^{90}Sr

stroph·u·lus (strofʹu-ləs) papular urticaria 小儿丘疹性荨麻疹

stru·ma (strooʹmə) [L.] goiter 甲状腺肿 ; **struʹmous** *adj.*; **Hashimoto s., s. lymphomatoʹsa,** Hashimoto disease 桥本甲状腺肿，淋巴瘤性甲状腺肿 ; **s. maligʹna,** carcinoma of the thyroid gland 恶性甲状腺肿 ; **s. ovaʹrii,** a teratoid ovarian tumor composed of thyroid tissue 卵巢甲状腺肿 ; **Riedel s.,** Riedel thyroiditis 木样甲状腺炎，慢性纤维性甲状腺炎

stru·mec·to·my (stroo-mekʹtə-me) excision of a goiter 甲状腺肿切除术

stru·mi·tis (stroo-miʹtis) thyroiditis 甲状腺炎

strych·nine (strikʹnīn) a very poisonous alkaloid, obtained chiefly from *Strychnos nux-vomica* and other species of *Strychnos,* which causes excitation of all portions of the central nervous system by blocking postsynaptic inhibition of neural impulses 士的宁，番木鳖碱

STTI Sigma Theta Tau International 国际荣誉护理学会

stump (stump) the distal end of a limb left after amputation 残肢

stun (stun) to knock senseless; to render unconscious by a blow or other force 打昏，震晕

stun·ning (stunʹing) loss of function, analogous to unconsciousness 失去功能 ; **myocardial s.,** temporarily impaired myocardial function, resulting from a brief episode of ischemia and persisting for some period afterward 心肌顿抑

stupe (stoop) a hot, wet cloth or sponge, charged with a medication for external application 热敷布

stu·pe·fa·cient (stooʺpə-faʹshənt) 1. inducing stupor 致木僵的，麻醉的 ; 2. an agent that induces stupor 麻醉药

stu·por (stooʹpər) [L.] 1. a lowered level of consciousness 昏迷 ; 2. in psychiatry, a disorder marked by reduced responsiveness 木僵，在精神病学中，指应答性降低 ; **stuʹporous** *adj.*

stut·ter·ing (stutʹər-ing) a speech problem characterized chiefly by spasmodic repetition of sounds, especially of initial consonants, by prolongation of sounds and hesitation, and by anxiety and tension on the part of the speaker about perceived speech difficulties. Cf. *stammering.* Called also *childhoodonset fluency disorder* 口吃

stye (sti) hordeolum 睑腺炎，麦粒肿

sty·let (stiʹlət) 1. a wire run through a catheter or cannula to render it stiff or to remove debris from its lumen 通管丝，管心针 ; 2. a slender probe 细探针

sty·lo·hy·oid (stiʺlo-hiʹoid) pertaining to the styloid process and hyoid bone 茎突舌骨的

sty·loid (stiʹloid) resembling a pillar; long and pointed; relating to the styloid process 柱样的，长而尖的，茎状的

sty·loid·itis (stiʺloi-diʹtis) inflammation of tissues around the styloid process of the temporal bone 茎突炎

sty·lo·mas·toid (stiʺlo-masʹtoid) pertaining to the styloid and mastoid processes of the temporal bone 茎突乳突的

sty·lo·max·il·lary (stiʺlo-makʹsĭ-larʺe) pertaining to the styloid process of the temporal bone and the maxilla 茎突上颌的

sty·lus (stiʹləs) 1. 同 stylet; 2. a pencil-shaped medicinal preparation, as of caustic 药笔剂，一种铅笔状的药用制剂

styp·sis (stipʹsis) [Gr.] the action or application of a styptic 收敛疗法，收敛作用

styp·tic (stipʹtik) 1. contracting the tissues or blood vessels; used particularly to denote that arresting hemorrhage or resulting in hemostasis 收敛的，止血的 ; 2. an agent that so acts 收敛止血药

sub·ab·dom·i·nal (subʺab-dŏmʹĭ-nəl) below the abdomen 腹下的

sub·acro·mi·al (subʺə-kroʹme-əl) below the acromion 肩峰下的

sub·acute (subʺə-kūtʹ) somewhat acute; between acute and chronic 亚急性的

sub·al·i·men·ta·tion (subʺal-ĭ-mən-taʹshən) hypoalimentation 营养不良

sub·aor·tic (subʺa-orʹtik) below the aorta or the aortic valve 主动脉下

sub·apo·neu·rot·ic (subʺap-o-noo-rotʹik) below an aponeurosis 腱膜下的

sub·arach·noid (subʺə-rakʹnoid) between the arachnoid and the pia mater 蛛网膜下的

sub·ar·cu·ate (səb-ahrʹku-āt) somewhat arched or bent 微弯的，稍呈弓状的

sub·are·o·lar (subʺə-reʹə-lər) beneath the areola 乳晕下的

sub·as·trag·a·lar (subʺəs-tragʹə-lər) below the astragalus 距骨下的

sub·atom·ic (subʺə-tomʹik) of or pertaining to the constituent parts of an atom 亚原子的

sub·au·ral (səb-awʹrəl) below the ear 耳下的

sub·au·ra·le (sub″aw-ra′le) the lowest point on the inferior border of the ear lobule when the person is looking straight ahead 耳廓下点

sub·cal·lo·sal (sub″kə-lo′səl) inferior to the corpus callosum 胼胝体下的

sub·cap·su·lar (səb-kap′su-lər) below a capsule, especially the capsule of the cerebrum 囊下的，被膜下的

sub·car·ti·lag·i·nous (sub″kahr-tĭ-laj′ĭ-nəs) 1. beneath a cartilage 软骨下的；2. partly cartilaginous 部分软骨的

sub·chon·dral (səb-kon′drəl) 同 subcartilaginous (1)

sub·cho·ri·al (səb-kor′e-əl) beneath the chorion or some part of the chorion 绒毛膜下的

sub·class (sub′klas″) a taxonomic category subordinate to a class and superior to an order 亚纲（生物分类）

sub·cla·vi·an (səb-kla′ve-ən) below the clavicle 锁骨下的

sub·cla·vic·u·lar (sub″klə-vik′u-lər) 同 subclavian

sub·clin·i·cal (səb-klin′ĭ-kəl) without clinical manifestations 亚临床的，临床症状不明显的

sub·clone (sub′klōn) 1. the progeny of a mutant cell arising in a clone 亚克隆，在克隆中产生的突变型细胞的后代；2. each new DNA population produced by cleaving DNA from a clonal population into fragments and cloning them 通过将克隆群体中的 DNA 分裂成片段并进行克隆而产生的每个新的 DNA 群体

sub·con·junc·ti·val (sub″kən-junk′tĭ-vəl) beneath the conjunctiva 结膜下的

sub·con·scious (səb-kon′shəs) 1. imperfectly or partially conscious 下意识的；2. a lay term used to include the preconscious and unconscious 一种外行术语，包括前意识和无意识

sub·con·scious·ness (səb-kon′shəs-nis) the state of being partially conscious 潜意识，下意识

sub·cor·a·coid (səb-kor′ə-koid) situated under the coracoid process 喙突下的

sub·cor·ne·al (səb-kor′ne-əl) 1. beneath the cornea 角膜下的；2. beneath the stratum corneum of the skin 皮肤角质层下的

sub·cor·tex (səb-kor′təks) the brain substance underlying the cortex 皮质下

sub·cor·ti·cal (səb-kor′tĭ-kəl) beneath a cortex, such as the cerebral cortex 皮质下的

sub·cos·tal (səb-kos′təl) below a rib or ribs 肋骨下的

sub·cra·ni·al (səb-kra′ne-əl) below the cranium 颅下的

sub·crep·i·tant (səb-krep′ĭ-tənt) pertaining to a rale that is slightly more coarse than a crepitant rale 亚捻发音的，比捻发音略粗糙的一种啰音

sub·cul·ture (sub′kul″chər) a culture of bacteria derived from another culture 次代培养物，次代培养

sub·cu·ta·ne·ous (sub″ku-ta′ne-əs) hypodermic; beneath the skin 皮下注射的；皮下的

sub·cu·tic·u·lar (sub″ku-tik′u-lər) 同 subepidermal

sub·de·lir·i·um (sub″də-lēr′e-əm) mild delirium 轻度谵妄

sub·del·toid (səb-del′toid) beneath the deltoid muscle 三角肌下的

sub·di·a·phrag·mat·ic (sub″di-ə-frag-mat′ik) subphrenic 膈下的

sub·duct (səb-dukt′) to draw down 下转

sub·du·ral (səb-doo′rəl) between the dura mater and the arachnoid 硬膜下的

sub·en·do·car·di·al (sub″en-do-kahr′de-əl) beneath the endocardium 心内膜下的

sub·en·do·car·di·um (sub″en-do-kahr′de-əm) subendocardial layer 心内膜下层

sub·en·do·the·li·al (sub″en-do-the′le-əl) beneath the endothelium 内皮下的

sub·epi·car·di·al (sub″ep-ĭ-kahr′de-əl) situated below the epicardium 心外膜下的

sub·epi·car·di·um (sub″ep-ĭ-kahr′de-əm) subepicardial layer 心外膜下层

sub·epi·der·mal (sub″ep-ĭ-dur′məl) beneath the epidermis 表皮下的

sub·epi·the·li·al (sub″ep-ĭ-the′le-əl) beneath the epithelium 上皮下的

sub·fam·i·ly (sub′fam″ĭ-le) a taxonomic division between a family and a tribe 亚科（生物分类）

sub·fas·cial (səb-fash′əl) beneath a fascia 筋膜下的

sub·fer·til·i·ty (sub″fər-til′ĭ-te) hypofertility; diminished reproductive capacity 低生育力；**sub·fer′tile** adj.

sub·fron·tal (səb-frun′təl) situated or extending underneath the frontal lobe 额叶下的

sub·ge·nus (sub′je″nəs) a taxonomic category between a genus and a species 亚属（生物分类）

sub·gin·gi·val (səb-jin′jĭ-vəl) beneath the gingiva 龈下的

sub·gle·noid (səb-gle′noid) beneath the glenoid fossa 关节盂下的

sub·glos·sal (səb-glos′əl) 同 sublingual

sub·glot·tic (səb-glot′ik) inferior to the glottis 声门下的

sub·gron·da·tion (sub″gron-da′shən) [Fr.] a type of depressed skull fracture, with depression of one fragment of bone beneath another 骨嵌凹，一种颅

骨凹陷骨折，一块碎骨片下陷于另一骨片下

sub·he·pat·ic (sub″hə-pat′ik) below the liver 肝下的

sub·hy·oid (səb-hi′oid) below the hyoid bone 舌骨下的

su·bic·u·lum (sə-bik′u-ləm) an underlying or supporting structure 下托

sub·il·i·ac (səb-il′e-ak) below the ilium 髂骨下的

sub·il·i·um (səb-il′e-əm) the lowest portion of the ilium 髂骨下部

sub·in·vo·lu·tion (sub″in-vo-loo′shən) incomplete involution 复旧不全

sub·ja·cent (səb-ja′sənt) located beneath 在下的，下邻的

sub·ject[1] (səb-jekt′) to cause to undergo or submit to; to render subservient 忍受或使服从；使屈从

sub·ject[2] (sub′jəkt) 1. a person or animal subjected to treatment, observation, or experiment 受试者；2. a body for dissection 用于解剖的尸体

sub·jec·tive (səb-jek′tiv) pertaining to or perceived only by the affected individual; not perceptible to the senses of another person 主观的，自觉的，主觉性的

sub·ju·gal (səb-joo′gəl) below the zygomatic bone 颧骨下的

sub·le·thal (səb-le′thəl) insufficient to cause death 亚致死的，不致引起死亡的

sub·li·mate (sub′lĭ-māt) 1. a substance obtained by sublimation 升华物；2. to accomplish sublimation（使）升华

sub·li·ma·tion (sub″lĭ-ma′shən) 1. the conversion of a solid directly into the gaseous state 升华（作用），把固态直接转变成气态的过程；2. an unconscious defense mechanism by which consciously unacceptable instinctual drives are expressed in personally and socially acceptable channels（心理学）升华，将意识上不能接受的本能冲动转为可被个人和社会所接受的无意识的防御机制

sub·lime (səb-līm′) to volatilize a solid body by heat and then to collect it in a purified form as a solid or powder（使）升华；（使）纯化

sub·lim·i·nal (səb-lim′ĭ-nəl) below the threshold of sensation or conscious awareness（感觉）阈下的

sub·lin·gual (səb-ling′gwəl) hypoglossal; beneath the tongue 舌下的

sub·lin·gui·tis (sub″ling-gwi′tis) inflammation of the sublingual gland 舌下腺炎

sub·lob·u·lar (səb-lob′u-lər) beneath a lobule 小叶下的

sub·lux·a·tion (sub″lək-sa′shən) 1. incomplete or partial dislocation 半脱位；2. in chiropractic, any mechanical impediment to nerve function; originally, a vertebral displacement believed to impair nerve function 在脊椎按摩治疗中，对神经功能的任何机械损害；最初脊椎移位被认为会损害神经功能

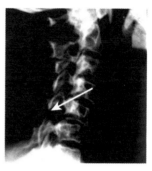

▲ C₅、C₆ 的严重半脱位，图中可见 "坐落征"（箭）

sub·mam·ma·ry (səb-mam′ə-re) below the mammary gland 乳腺下的

sub·man·dib·u·lar (sub″man-dib′u-lər) below the mandible 下颌下的

sub·max·il·lar·itis (səb-mak″sĭ-lər-i′tis) inflammation of the submaxillary gland 颌下腺炎

sub·max·il·lary (səb-mak′sĭ-lar″e) below the maxilla 颌下的

sub·men·tal (səb-men′təl) beneath the chin 颏下的

sub·meta·cen·tric (sub″met-ə-sen′trik) having the centromere near, but not at, the center of the chromosome, so that one arm is shorter than the other 亚中间着丝粒的，具近中间着丝粒的

sub·mi·cro·scop·ic (sub″mi-kro-skop′ik) too small to be visible with the light microscope 亚微观的，亚显微的

sub·mor·phous (səb-mor′fəs) neither amorphous nor perfectly crystalline 亚晶形的

sub·mu·co·sa (sub″mu-ko′sə) the layer of loose connective tissue between the mucosa and the tunica muscularis in most parts of the digestive, respiratory, urinary, and genital tracts. 黏膜下层

sub·mu·co·sal (sub″mu-ko′səl) 1. pertaining to the submucosa 黏膜下层；2. beneath a mucous membrane 黏膜下的

sub·mu·cous (səb-mu′kəs) beneath a mucous membrane 黏膜下的

sub·nar·cot·ic (sub″nahr-kot′ik) moderately narcotic 中度麻醉的

sub·na·sal (səb-na′zəl) inferior to the nose 鼻下的

sub·na·sa·le (sub″na-sa′le) the point at which the nasal septum merges, in the midsagittal plane, with the upper lip 鼻中隔下点，鼻中隔以中矢状平面方向与上唇会合处所成之点

sub·neu·ral (sŭb-noor′əl) beneath a nerve 神经下的

sub·nor·mal (sŭb-nor′məl) below normal 低于正常的，正常下的

sub·nu·cle·us (sŭb-noo′kle-əs) a partial or secondary nucleus 亚核

sub·oc·cip·i·tal (sŭb″ok-sip′ĭ-təl) below the occiput 枕骨下的

sub·or·bi·tal (sŭb-or′bĭ-təl) infraorbital 眶下的

sub·or·der (sŭb′or″dər) a taxonomic category between an order and a family 亚目（生物分类）

Sub·ox·one (sŭb-oks′ōn) trademark for a combination preparation of buprenorphine hydrochloride and naloxone hydrochloride 盐酸丁丙诺啡和盐酸纳洛酮联合制剂的商品名

sub·pa·tel·lar (sŭb″pə-tel′ər) infrapatellar 髌下的

sub·peri·car·di·al (sŭb″per-ĭ-kahr′de-əl) beneath the pericardium 心包下的

sub·peri·os·te·al (sŭb″per-e-os′te-əl) beneath the periosteum 骨膜下的

sub·peri·to·ne·al (sŭb″per-ĭ-to-ne′əl) beneath or deep to the peritoneum 腹膜下的，腹腔腹膜下的

sub·pha·ryn·ge·al (sŭb″fə-rin′je-əl) beneath the pharynx 咽下的

sub·phren·ic (sŭb-fren′ik) beneath the respiratory diaphragm 膈下的

sub·phy·lum (sŭb-fi′ləm) pl. *subphy′la*. A taxonomic category between a phylum and a class 亚门（生物分类）

sub·pla·cen·ta (sŭb″plə-sen′tə) decidua basalis 基蜕膜

sub·pleu·ral (sŭb-ploor′əl) beneath the pleura 胸膜下的

sub·pre·pu·tial (sŭb″pre-pu′shəl) beneath the prepuce 包皮下的

sub·pu·bic (sŭb-pu′bik) beneath the pubic bone 耻骨下的

sub·pul·mo·nary (sŭb-pool′mo-nar″e) beneath the lung 肺下的

sub·ret·i·nal (sŭb-ret′ĭ-nəl) beneath the retina 视网膜下的

sub·scap·u·lar (sŭb-skap′u-lər) below the scapula 肩胛骨下的

sub·scrip·tion (sŭb-skrip′shən) that part of a prescription giving directions for compounding the ingredients 调配法，处方中说明如何调配成分的部分

sub·se·ro·sa (sŭb″sēr-o′sə) a layer of loose areolar tissue underlying the serosa of various organs 浆膜下层

sub·se·ro·sal (sŭb″sēr-o′səl) 1. pertaining to the subserosa 浆膜下层的；2. 同 subserous

sub·se·rous (sŭb-sēr′əs) beneath a serous membrane 浆膜下的

sub·spe·cies (sŭb′spe″sēz) a taxonomic category subordinate to a species, differing morphologically from others of the species but capable of interbreeding with them; a variety or race 亚种（生物分类）

sub·spi·na·le (sŭb″spi-na′le) point A; the deepest midline point on the maxilla on the concavity between the anterior nasal spine and the prosthion 上颌牙槽座点

sub·spi·nous (sŭb-spi′nəs) inferior to a spinous process 棘突下的

sub·stance (sŭb′stəns) 1. matter with a particular set of characteristics 物，物质；2. material constituting an organ or body 实质，本质；3. 同 psychoactive s.; **black s.**, substantia nigra 黑质；**controlled s.**, any drug regulated under the Controlled Substances Act 管制药，受控药；**gelatinous s.**, substantia gelatinosa 胶状质；**gray s.**, substantia grisea 灰质；**ground s.**, the gel-like material in which connective tissue cells and fibers are embedded 基质；**H s.**, H antigen (2) H 物质；**medullary s.**, 1. substantia alba 白质；2. the soft marrowlike substance of the interior of an organ 髓质；**s. P**, an 11–amino acid peptide, present in nerve cells throughout the body and in special endocrine cells of the intestine. It increases contraction of gastrointestinal smooth muscle, causes vasodilatation, and is a sensory neurotransmitter P 物质，一种 11- 氨基酸多肽，存在于全身的神经细胞和肠道的特殊内分泌细胞中，增加胃肠道平滑肌的收缩，引起血管舒张，是一种感觉神经递质；**perforated s.**, 1. *anterior perforated s.*, an area anterolateral to each optic tract, pierced by branches of the anterior and middle cerebral arteries 前穿质；2. *posterior perforated s.*, an area between the cerebral peduncles, pierced by branches of the posterior cerebral arteries 后穿质；**psychoactive s., psychotropic s.**, any chemical compound that affects the mind or mental processes; used particularly for drugs used therapeutically in psychiatry, the major classes being the antipsychotic, antidepressant, anxiolytic-sedative, and mood-stabilizing drugs 精神活性物质；**reticular s.**, 1. 网状结构，参见 *formation* 下词条；2. the netlike mass seen in red blood cells after vital staining 网状物质；**Rolando gelatinous s.**, substantia gelatinosa 胶状质；**slow-reacting s. of anaphylaxis (SRS-A)**, an inflammatory agent released by mast cells in the anaphylactic reaction, inducing a slow, prolonged contraction of certain smooth muscles and acting as an important mediator of allergic bronchial asthma 过敏反应迟缓反应物质，炎症细胞在过敏反应中释放的一种炎症介质，可引起平滑肌长时间缓慢收缩，是过敏性支气管哮喘的重要介质；**white s.**, substantia alba 白质

sub·stan·tia (səb-stan′she-ə) pl. *substan′tiae* [L.] 同 substance; **s. al′ba,** the white nervous tissue, constituting the conducting portion of the brain and spinal cord, composed mostly of myelinated nerve fibers 白质; **s. gelatino′sa,** the gelatinousappearing cap forming the posterior part of the posterior horn of the spinal cord and lining its central canal 胶状质; **s. gri′sea,** gray substance; the gray nervous tissue composed of nerve cell bodies, unmyelinated nerve fibers, and supportive tissue 灰质; **s. ni′gra,** the layer of neurons separating the tegmentum of the midbrain from the crus cerebri, composed of a posterior compact part packed with melanin-containing dopaminergic cells and an anterior reticular part whose cells have little pigment 黑质; **s. pro′pria,** 1. the tough, fibrous, transparent main part of the cornea, between the Bowman and Descemet membranes 角膜固有质; 2. the main part of the sclera, between the episcleral lamina and the lamina fusca 巩膜固有质

sub·ster·nal (səb-stur′nəl) below the sternum 胸骨下的

sub·stit·u·ent (səb-stich′u-ənt) 1. of or pertaining to substitution 取代的; 2. 同 substitute (2); 3. the component substituted in a substitution reaction 取代基

sub·sti·tute (sub′stĭ-toot) 1. to put one thing in place of another 用……代替; 取代 2. a material used in place of another 代替物

sub·sti·tu·tion (sub″stĭ-too′shən) 1. the act of putting one thing in place of another 取代, 置换; 2. an unconscious defense mechanism in which an unattainable or unacceptable goal, emotion, or object is replaced by one that is attainable or acceptable （心理学）替代

sub·strate (sub′strāt) 1. a substance upon which an enzyme acts 底物; 2. a neutral substance containing a nutrient solution 基质; 3. a surface upon which a different material is deposited or adhered, usually in a coating or layer 储存着不同物质或被不同物质黏附(通常在包衣和层中)的表面

sub·struc·ture (sub′struk″chər) the underlying or supporting portion of an organ or appliance; that portion of an implant denture embedded in the tissues of the jaw 下部结构, 器官或组织的基础部分或支持部分; 植入性下部结构, 如骨膜下植入义齿

sub·syl·vi·an (səb-sil′ve-ən) situated deep in the lateral sulcus (sylvian fissure) 大脑侧裂下的

sub·tar·sal (səb-tahr′səl) below the tarsus 跗骨下的

sub·ten·to·ri·al (sub″ten-tor′e-əl) beneath the tentorium of the cerebellum（小脑）幕下的

sub·tha·lam·ic (sub″thə-lam′ik) 1. inferior to the thalamus 丘脑下的; 2. pertaining to the subthalamus 底丘脑的

sub·thal·a·mus (sub-thal′ə-məs) the ventral thalamus or subthalamic tegmental region: a transitional region of the diencephalon interposed between the (dorsal) thalamus, the hypothalamus, and the tegmentum of the midbrain; it includes the subthalamic nucleus, Forel fields, and zona incerta 底丘脑; **subthalam′ic** *adj.*

sub·to·tal (səb-to′təl) less than, but often almost, complete 次全的, 几乎全部的

sub·tribe (sub′trīb″) a taxonomic category between a tribe and a genus 亚族（生物）分类

sub·tro·chan·ter·ic (sub″tro-kan-ter′ik) below the trochanter 转子下的

sub·um·bil·i·cal (sub″əm-bil′ĭ-kəl) inferior to the umbilicus 脐下的

sub·un·gual (səb-ung′gwəl) beneath a nail 指(趾)甲下的

sub·ure·thral (sub″u-re′thrəl) inferior to the urethra 尿道下的

sub·vag·i·nal (səb-vaj′ĭ-nəl) under a sheath, or below the vagina 鞘下的, 阴道下的

sub·ver·te·bral (səb-vur′tə-brəl) on the ventral side of the vertebrae 脊柱前的

sub·vo·lu·tion (sub″vo-loo′shən) the operation of turning over a flap to prevent adhesions 翻转术（一种皮瓣反转术）

suc·cen·tu·ri·ate (suk″sən-tu′re-āt) accessory; serving as a substitute 副的, 替代的

suc·ces·sion·al (sək-sesh′ən-əl) pertaining to that which follows in order or sequence 连续的

suc·ci·mer (DMSA) (suk′sĭ-mər) a heavy metal–chelating agent that is an analogue of dimercaprol, used in the treatment of lead poisoning; also complexed with technetium ^{99m}Tc and used in renal function testing 琥巯酸, 一种螯合剂, 二巯丙醇的类似物, 用于治疗铅中毒, 一种与 ^{99m}Tc 的合剂用作肾功能试验的诊断用药

suc·ci·nate (suk′sĭ-nāt) any salt or ester of succinic acid 丁二酸盐, 琥珀酸盐; **s. semialdehyde,** γ-hydroxybutyric acid 半缩醛琥珀酸盐

suc·ci·nate-semi·alde·hyde·hy·dro·gen·ase (suk′sĭ-nāt sem″e-al′də-hīd de-hi′- dro-jən-ās) an oxidoreductase catalyzing the final step in γ-aminobutyric acid (GABA) inactivation; deficiency (succinic semialdehyde dehydrogenase deficiency) causes increased levels of GABA and γ-hydroxybutyric acid in urine, plasma, and cerebrospinal fluid, intellectual disability, hypotonia, and ataxia 琥珀酸–半醛脱氢酶

suc·cin·ic　ac·id (sək-sin′ik) an intermediate in the tricarboxylic acid cycle 丁二酸，琥珀酸

suc·ci·ni·mide　(sək-sin′ĭ-mīd) 1. an organic compound comprising a pyrrole ring with two carbonyl substitutions 琥珀酰亚胺；2. any of a class of anti-convulsants with such a basic structure 任何有这种基础结构的抗惊厥药

suc·ci·nyl·cho·line　(suk″sī-nəl-ko′lēn) a depolarizing neuromuscular blocking agent used as the chloride salt as an anesthesia adjunct and in convulsive therapy 氯化琥珀胆碱，神经肌肉阻断剂

suc·ci·nyl　CoA (suk′sī-nəl ko-a′) a high-energy intermediate formed in the tricarboxylic acid cycle from α -ketoglutaric acid; it is also a precursor in the synthesis of porphyrins 琥珀酰辅酶 A，琥珀酰 CoA

suc·cor·rhea　(suk″o-re′ə) excessive flow of a natural secretion 分泌液溢，分泌过多

suc·cus·sion　(sə-kush′ən) 1. the shaking of the body during an examination, a splashing sound indicating the presence of fluid and air in a body cavity 振荡法，查体时摇晃身体的方法，振水音为体腔内存在液体和空气的表现；2. the vigorous shaking of a diluted homeopathic preparation in order to activate the medicinal substance 剧烈摇动稀释的顺势疗法制剂来激活药物

su·cral·fate　(soo-kral′fāt) a complex of aluminum and a sulfated polysaccharide, used as a gastrointestinal antiulcerative 硫糖铝

su·crase　(soo′krās) a hydrolase that catalyzes the cleavage of the disaccharides sucrose and maltose to their component monosaccharides; it occurs complexed with α -dextrinase in the brush border of the intestinal mucosa, and deficiency of the complex causes the disaccharide intolerance sucrase-isomaltase deficiency 蔗糖酶

suc·rase-iso·mal·tase　de·fi·cien·cy (soo′krās i″so-mawl′tās) a hereditary disaccharidase deficiency in which deficiency of the sucrase-isomaltase enzyme complex causes malabsorption of sucrose and starch dextrins, with watery, osmotic-fermentative diarrhea, sometimes leading to dehydration and malnutrition, manifest in infancy (congenital sucrose intolerance) 蔗糖酶-异麦芽糖酶缺乏症

su·crose　(soo′krōs) a disaccharide of glucose and fructose from sugar cane, sugar beet, or other sources; used as a food and sweetening agent and pharmaceutical aid 蔗糖

su·cros·uria　(soo″kro-su′re-ə) excessive sucrose in the urine 蔗糖尿（症）

suc·tion　(suk′shən) aspiration of gas or fluid by mechanical means 抽吸，吸入；posttussive s., a sucking sound heard over a lung cavity just after a cough 咳后回吸声

suc·to·ri·al　(sək-tor′e-əl) adapted for sucking 适于吸吮的

su·da·men　(soo-da′mən) pl. suda′mina [L.] 1. a whitish vesicle caused by the retention of sweat in the sweat ducts or the layers of the epidermis 粟疹，痱子，汗疹；2. (in the pl.) miliaria crystallina 白痱

Su·dan　(soo-dan′) a group of azo compounds used as biologic stains for fats 苏丹，用作脂肪染色的一组偶氮化合物；S. black B, a black, fat-soluble diazo dye, used as a stain for fats 苏丹黑 B，一种黑色、脂溶性的重氮染料，用作脂肪染色剂

su·dano·phil·ia　(soo-dan″o-fil′e-ə) affinity for Sudan stain 染苏丹性，嗜苏丹性；sudanophil′ic adj.

su·do·mo·tor　(soo″do-mo′tər) stimulating the sweat glands 促汗的，催汗的

su·do·rif·er·ous　(soo″də-rif′ər-əs) 1. conveying sweat. 分泌汗的；2. 同 sudoriparous

su·do·rif·ic　(soo″də-rif′ik) diaphoretic 生汗的；发汗药

su·do·rip·a·rous　(soo″də-rip′ə-rəs) secreting or producing sweat 生汗的，出汗的

su·et　(soo′ət) the fat from the abdominal cavity of ruminants, especially the sheep, used in preparing cerates and ointments and as an emollient 兽脂，牛羊脂，获自反刍动物腹腔脂肪，特别是绵羊腹内脂肪，用于制备蜡膏与软膏，也用作润肤剂

su·fen·ta·nil　(soo-fen′tə-nil) an opioid analgesic derived from fentanyl, used as the citrate salt as an anesthetic or anesthesia adjunct; also used for the treatment of obstetric pain 舒芬太尼，噻哌苯胺(镇痛药)

suf·fo·ca·tion　(suf″ə-ka′shən) asphyxiation 窒息；suf′focative adj.

suf·fu·sion　(sə-fu′zhən) 1. the process of overspreading, or diffusion 充满，弥漫；2. the condition of being moistened or of being permeated through, as by blood 溢血

sug·ar　(shoog′ər) any of a class of sweet water-soluble carbohydrates, the monosaccharides and smaller oligosaccharides; often specifically sucrose 糖；blood s., glucose occurring in the blood, or the amount of glucose in the blood 血糖；invert s., a mixture of equal amounts of dextrose and fructose, obtained by hydrolyzing sucrose; used in solution as a parenteral nutrient 转化糖

sug·ges·tion　(səg-jes′chən) 1. the act of offering an idea for action or for consideration of action 建议，提出想法以供行动或参考的行为；2. an idea so offered 建议，意见，提出的以供行动或者参考的想法；3. in psychiatry, the process of causing uncritical acceptance of an idea 暗示，在精神病学

S

中，不加批判地接受一个想法】; **hypnotic s.**, one imparted to a person in the hypnotic state, by which the person is induced to alter perceptions or memory or to perform actions 催眠暗示; **posthypnotic s.**, implantation in the mind of a person during hypnosis of a suggestion to be acted upon after recovery from the hypnotic state 催眠后暗示

sug·gil·la·tion (sug″jĭ-la′shən) 1. ecchymosis 紫斑，瘀斑; 2. contusion 尸斑

su·i·cide (soo′ĭ-sīd) the taking of one's own life 自杀; **assisted s.**, suicide with the help of another person, such as when an incurably ill patient intentionally ingests a toxic substance or an overdose of a medication that was prescribed; the choice to die must always be made by the patient 爱助自杀，另参见 *euthanasia*

su·i·ci·dol·o·gy (soo″ĭ-sīd-ol′ə-je) the study of the causes and prevention of suicide 自杀学，研究自杀的原因及预防

sul·bac·tam (səl-bak′təm) a β-lactamase inhibitor used as the sodium salt to increase the antibacterial activity of penicillins and cephalosporins against β-lactamase–producing organisms 舒巴坦（β– 内酰胺酶抑制药）

sul·cate (sul′kāt) furrowed; marked with sulci 有沟的

sul·con·a·zole (səl-kon′ə-zōl) a broad-spectrum imidazole antifungal, used as the nitrate salt in the treatment of various forms of tinea and cutaneous candidiasis 氯苄硫咪唑，硫康唑

sul·cus (sul′kəs) pl. *sul′ci* [L.] a long groove or furrow, especially one of the cerebral sulci 沟，尤指脑沟; **arterial sulci**, grooves on the internal surfaces of the cranial bones for the meningeal arteries 动脉沟; **calcarine s.**, a sulcus of the medial surface of the occipital lobe, separating the cuneus from the lingual gyrus 距状沟; **central s. of cerebrum**, one between the frontal and parietal lobes of the cerebral hemisphere 大脑中央沟; **cerebral sulci**, the furrows between the cerebral gyri 大脑沟; **cingulate s.**, a long, irregularly shaped sulcus on the medial surface of a hemisphere, separating the cingulate gyrus below from the medial surface of the superior frontal gyrus and the paracentral lobule above 扣带沟，大脑半球内侧面长而形状不规则的沟，该沟在下方将扣带回与额中回隔开，在上方把旁中央小叶隔开; **collateral s.**, one on the inferior surface of the cerebral hemisphere between the fusiform and parahippocampal gyri 侧副沟，大脑半球下表面梭状回和海马回之间的纵沟; **coronary s.**, the transverse groove separating the atria of the heart from the ventricles 冠状沟，房室沟; **sul′ci cu′tis**, the fine depressions on the surface of the skin between

the dermal ridges 皮沟; **gingival s.**, the groove between the surface of the tooth and the epithelium lining the free gingiva 龈沟; **hippocampal s.**, one extending from the splenium of the corpus callosum almost to the tip of the temporal lobe 海马沟; **interlobar sulci**, the sulci that separate the lobes of the brain from each other 叶间沟; **intraparietal s.**, a sulcus separating the inferior and superior parietal lobules 顶内沟; **lateral s. of cerebrum**, 大脑外侧沟，参见 *fissure* 下词条; **parietooccipital s.**, one marking the boundary between the cuneus and precuneus, and also between the parietal and occipital lobes of the cerebral hemisphere 顶枕沟; **posterior median s.**, 1. a shallow vertical groove in the closed part of the medulla oblongata, continuous with the posterior median sulcus of the spinal cord 延髓后正中沟; 2. a shallow vertical groove dividing the spinal cord throughout its whole length in the midline posteriorly 脊髓后正中沟; **precentral s.**, one separating the precentral gyrus from the remainder of the frontal lobe 中央前沟; **scleral s.**, a slight groove at the junction of the sclera and cornea 巩膜沟

sul·fa·cet·a·mide (sul″fə-set′ə-mīd) a sulfonamide used topically as the sodium salt to treat ophthalmic infections and acne vulgaris 磺胺醋酰

sul·fa·di·a·zine (sul″fə-di′ə-zēn) a sulfonamide antibacterial, used as the base or the sodium salt in the treatment of infections, including nocardiosis, toxoplasmosis, otitis media, and chloroquine-resistant falciparum malaria 磺胺嘧啶，参见 *silver* 下词条

sul·fa·dox·ine (sul″fə-dok′sēn) a long-acting sulfonamide used in combination with pyrimethamine in the prophylaxis and treatment of chloroquine-resistant falciparum malaria 周效磺胺，磺胺邻二甲氧嘧啶，一种长效磺胺类药，用于预防和治疗对氯喹有耐药性的疟原虫所致的恶性疟疾

sul·fa·meth·i·zole (sul″fə-meth′ĭ-zōl) a sulfonamide used in urinary tract infections 磺胺甲噻二唑

sul·fa·meth·ox·a·zole (sul″fə-mə-thok′sə-zōl) a sulfonamide antibacterial and antiprotozoal, particularly used in acute urinary tract infections 磺胺甲噁唑

sul·fa·pyr·i·dine (sul″fə-pir′ĭ-dēn) a sulfonamide used as an oral suppressant for dermatitis herpetiformis 磺胺吡啶

sul·fa·sal·a·zine (sul″fə-sal′ə-zēn) a sulfonamide used in the treatment and prophylaxis of inflammatory bowel disease and the treatment of rheumatoid arthritis 柳氮磺胺吡啶

sul·fa·tase (sul′fə-tās) an enzyme that catalyzes the hydrolytic cleavage of inorganic sulfate from sulfate esters 硫酸酯酶

sul·fate (sul′fāt) a salt of sulfuric acid 硫酸盐

sul·fa·tide (sul′fə-tīd) any of a class of cerebroside sulfuric esters; they are found largely in the medullated nerve fibers and may accumulate in metachromatic leukodystrophy 硫（脑）苷脂

sulf·he·mo·glo·bin (sulf″he′mo-glo″bin) sulfmethemoglobin 硫血红蛋白

sulf·he·mo·glo·bin·emia (sulf″he″-mo-glo″bine′me-ə) sulfmethemoglobin in the blood 硫血红蛋白血症

sulf·hy·dryl (səlf-hi′drəl) the univalent radical, − SH 硫氢基，巯基

sul·fide (sul′fīd) any binary compound of sulfur; a compound of sulfur with another element or radical or base 硫化物

sul·fin·py·ra·zone (sul″fin-pi′rə-zōn) a uricosuric agent used in the treatment of gout 磺吡酮，苯磺唑酮，用于治疗痛风的促尿酸排泄药

sul·fi·sox·a·zole (sul″fə-sok′sə-zōl) a shortacting sulfonamide antibacterial, used particularly as the base or *s. acetyl* for infections of the urinary tract and as *s. diolamine* as a topical ophthalmic antibacterial 磺胺异噁唑，一种短效磺胺类抗菌药，乙酰基磺胺异噁唑用于泌尿道感染，二胺基磺胺异噁唑作为外用眼科抗菌药

sul·fite (sul′fīt) any salt of sulfurous acid 亚硫酸盐

sul·fite ox·i·dase (sul′fīt ok′sĭ-dās) an oxidoreductase that catalyzes the oxidation of sulfite to sulfate as well as the detoxification of sulfite and sulfur dioxide from exogenous sources. It is a mitochondrial hemoprotein containing molybdenum; deficiency results in progressive neurologic abnormalities, lens dislocation, and intellectual disability 亚硫酸氧化酶（此酶先天缺乏，可致进行性神经系统异常、晶状体脱位和智力迟钝）

sulf·met·he·mo·glo·bin (sulf″mət-he′moglo″bin) a greenish substance formed by treating the blood with hydrogen sulfide or by absorption of this gas from the intestinal tract 硫血红蛋白

sul·fon·amide (səl-fon′ə-mīd) a compound containing the −SO₂NH₂ group. The sulfonamides, or sulfa drugs, are derivatives of sulfanilamide, competitively inhibit folic acid synthesis in microorganisms, and formerly were bacteriostatic against a wide variety of bacteria and some protozoa. Because many microbes are now resistant, sulfonamides have largely been supplanted by more effective and less toxic antibiotics 磺胺，氨苯磺胺，（磺胺类药，已大部被更有效而毒性低的抗菌素所取代）

sul·fone (sul′fōn) 1. the radical SO₂ SO₂ 基团，也称磺（基）; 2. a compound containing two hydrocarbon radicals attached to the −SO₂− group, especially dapsone and its derivatives, which are potent antibacterials effective against many gram-positive and gram-negative organisms and are widely used as leprostatics 砜，含有两个连接在 −SO₂− 基团上的烃基化合物，尤其是氨苯砜及其衍生物，是对许多革兰阳性和革兰阴性菌有效的强效抗菌药，被广泛用作抑菌剂

sul·fo·nyl·urea (sul″fə-nəl-u-re′ə) any of a class of compounds that exert hypoglycemic activity by stimulating the islet tissue to secrete insulin; used to control hyperglycemia in patients with type 2 diabetes mellitus who cannot be treated solely by diet and exercise 磺酰脲，用于对不能单靠饮食与运动治疗的非胰岛素依赖性糖尿病患者控制高血糖

sul·fur (S) (sul′fər) [L.] a nonmetallic element existing in many allotropic forms, notably a bright yellow crystalline solid characteristic of elemental sulfur; at. no. 16, at. wt. 32.06. It occurs in several amino acids and as part of both organic and inorganic cofactors, and is used in diseases of the skin 硫（化学元素）; **s. dioxide**, a colorless, nonflammable gas used as a pharmaceutical antioxidant; also an important air pollutant, irritating the eyes and respiratory tract 二氧化硫; **precipitated s.**, a topical scabicide, antiparasitic, antibacterial, antifungal, and keratolytic 沉淀硫，一种局部杀疥剂，抗寄生虫，抗菌，抗真菌和角化剂; **sublimed s.**, a topical scabicide and antiparasitic 升华硫，一种局部杀疥剂和抗寄生虫药

sul·fu·rat·ed (sul′fu-rāt″ed) combined with or charged with sulfur 含硫的，硫化的

sul·fur·ic ac·id (səl-fūr′ik) an oily, highly caustic, poisonous acid, H₂SO₄, widely used in chemistry, industry, and the arts 硫酸

sul·fur·ous ac·id (səl-fūr′əs) 1. a solution of sulfur dioxide in water, H₂SO₃; used as a reagent 亚硫酸，二氧化硫的水溶液，化学式为 H₂SO₃; 作为试剂; 2. sulfur dioxide 二氧化硫

sul·in·dac (səl-in′dak) 舒林酸 1. a nonsteroidal antiinflammatory drug, analgesic, and antipyretic, used in treatment of rheumatic disorders 一种非甾体抗炎药、止痛药和解热药，用于治疗风湿性疾病; 2. a nonsteroidal antiinflammatory drug used in the treatment of various rheumatic and nonrheumatic inflammatory disorders 用于多种风湿性和非风湿性炎症性疾病的治疗

su·mac (soo′mak) name of various trees and shrubs of the genus *Rhus* 漆树; **poison s.**, a species, *Rhus vernix*, which causes an itching rash on contact with the skin 美国毒漆（Rhus vernix），与皮肤接触会引起瘙痒皮疹

su·ma·trip·tan (soo″mə-trip′tan) a selective serotonin receptor agonist used as the succinate salt in the acute treatment of migraine and cluster headaches 舒马普坦，一种选择性 5- 羟色胺受体激动剂，其琥珀酸盐，用于治疗偏头痛和丛集性头痛

sum·ma·tion (sə-ma'shən) the cumulative effect of a number of stimuli applied to a muscle, nerve, or reflex arc 总和，总合，多数刺激作用于肌肉、神经或反射弧的累积效应

sun·block (sun'blok″) a topical protective agent that prevents sunlight from reaching the skin; the term is often used interchangeably with *sunscreen* 防晒霜，防止阳光照射皮肤的局部保护剂

sun·burn (sun'burn″) injury to the skin, with erythema, tenderness, and sometimes blistering, after excessive exposure to sunlight, produced by unfiltered ultraviolet rays 晒伤，晒斑，过度暴露在阳光下，由未经过滤的紫外线产生的皮肤伤害，有红斑、触痛、有时产生水疱

sun·down·ing (sun'doun-ing) confusion, agitation, and other severely disruptive behavior coupled with inability to remain asleep, occurring solely or markedly worsening at night; sometimes seen in older patients with dementia or other mental disorders 日落现象，混乱、激动和其他严重破坏性的行为加上无法保持睡眠，在夜间发生单独或明显恶化，有时见于老年痴呆症或其他精神障碍患者

su·ni·ti·nib (soo-nī'tĭ-nib) a tyrosine kinase inhibitor used as the malate salt in the treatment of advanced renal cell carcinoma, gastrointestinal stromal tumors, and pancreatic neuroendocrine tumors 一种酪氨酸激酶抑制药，其苹果酸盐用于治疗晚期肾细胞癌，胃肠道间质瘤和胰腺神经内分泌肿瘤

sun·screen (sun'skrēn″) a topical agent that protects the skin from the effects of the sun's rays, either by absorbing ultraviolet radiation or by reflecting the incident light, or both. The term is often used interchangeably with *sunblock* 遮光剂

sun·stroke (sun'strōk″) a condition caused by excessive exposure to the sun, marked by high skin temperature, convulsions, and coma 中暑，日射病，由过度暴露在阳光下引起的病症，以高温、抽搐和昏迷为特征

su·per·al·i·men·ta·tion (soo″pər-al″ĭ-mənta'shən) treatment of wasting diseases by feeding beyond appetite requirements 管饲法

su·per·al·ka·lin·i·ty (soo″pər-al″kə-lin'ĭ-te) excessive alkalinity 碱性过度

su·per·an·ti·gen (soo″pər-an'tĭ-jən) any of a group of powerful antigens occurring in various bacteria and viruses that binds outside of the normal T-cell receptor site, reacting with multiple T-cell receptor molecules and activating T cells nonspecifically 超抗原，在各种细菌和病毒中发生的强大的抗原，它们与正常的 T 细胞受体位点结合，

与多种 T 细胞受体分子反应，并且非特异性地激活 T 细胞

su·per·cen·te·nar·ian (soo″pər-sen-te-nər′-ē-ən) a person who lives to be at least 110 years of age 寿命超过 110 岁的人

su·per·cil·ia (soo″pər-sil'e-ə) 1. eyebrow (2) 眉毛 ; 2. plural of *supercilium* [eyebrow (1)], i.e., the elevations upon which the hairs grow 眉（supercilium 的复数）

su·per·cil·i·um (soo″pər-sil'e-əm) pl. *superci'lia* [L.] eyebrow (1) 眉

su·per·class (soo′pər-klas″) a taxonomic category between a phylum and a class 总纲（生物分类）

su·per·ego (soo″pər-e'go) in psychoanalysis, the aspect of the personality that acts as a monitor and evaluator of ego functioning, comparing it with an ideal standard 超我

su·per·fam·i·ly (soo′pər-fam″ĭ-le) 1. a taxonomic category between an order and a family 总科，介于目和科之间的生物分类阶元 ; 2. any of a group of proteins having similarities such as areas of structural homology and believed to descend from the same ancestral gene 超家族，一组具有共同特征并被认为从统一一祖先基因而来的蛋白质中的任何一种

su·per·fe·cun·da·tion (soo″pər-fe″kəndə′ shən) fertilization of two or more oocytes during the same ovulatory cycle by separate coital acts 同期复孕，通过单独的性交行为在同一排卵周期中有两个或更多个卵细胞受精

su·per·fi·cial (soo″pər-fish'əl) 1. pertaining to or situated near or nearer the surface 浅的，表面的；2. external to the outermost layer of deep fascia 在深筋膜的最外层外部

su·per·fi·ci·a·lis (soo″pər-fish″e-a'lis) [L.] superficial 浅的，表面的

su·per·fi·ci·es (soo″pər-fish'e-ēz) [L.] an outer surface 表面

su·per·in·duce (soo″pər-in-doos′) to bring on in addition to an already existing condition 重复诱导

su·per·in·fec·tion (soo″pər-in-fek'shən) a new infection occurring in a patient having a preexisting infection, such as bacterial superinfection in viral respiratory disease or infection of a chronic hepatitis B carrier with hepatitis D virus 重叠感染

su·per·in·vo·lu·tion (soo″pər-in″vo-loo′ shən) prolonged involution of the uterus, after delivery, to a size much smaller than the normal, occurring in nursing mothers 复旧过度，指分娩后，子宫长时间退化使得其复旧延长，使其比哺乳期母亲的子宫小得多

su·pe·ri·or (soo-pēr′e-ər) situated above, or directed upward; in anatomy, used in reference to the upper surface of a structure, or to a structure closer to the vertex 上的，在上的；在解剖学中，用于结构的上表面，或用于更靠近顶点的结构

su·per·ja·cent (soo″pər-ja′sənt) located just above 压在上面的，盖在上面的

su·per·lac·ta·tion (soo″pər-lak-ta′shən) hyperlactation 泌乳过多

su·per·mo·til·i·ty (soo″pər-mo-til′ĭ-te) excess of motility 运动过度

su·per·na·tant (soo″pər-na′tənt) the liquid lying above a layer of precipitated insoluble material 上清液（离心沉淀后的上层液）

su·per·nu·mer·ary (soo″pər-noo′mər-ar″e) in excess of the regular or normal number 额外的，超数的

su·per·nu·tri·tion (soo″pər-noo-trĭ′shən) excessive nutrition 营养过度

su·pero·lat·er·al (soo″pər-o-lat′ər-əl) above and to the side 上外侧的

su·per·ov·u·la·tion (soo″pər-ov″u-la′shən) extraordinary acceleration of ovulation, producing a greater than normal number of oocytes 超排卵

su·per·ox·ide (soo″pər-ok′sīd) any compound containing the highly reactive and extremely toxic oxygen radical O_2^-, a common intermediate in numerous biologic oxidations 过氧化物

su·per·sat·u·rate (soo″pər-sach′ər-āt) to add more of an ingredient than can be held in solution permanently 使过饱和

su·per·scrip·tion (soo″pər-skrip′shən) the heading of a prescription, i.e., the symbol ℞ or the word Recipe, meaning "take." 取，处方标记，处方上的符号℞

su·per·struc·ture (soo″pər-struk″chər) the overlying or visible portion of a structure 嵌于上部的结构，结构上方

su·per·vas·cu·lar·iza·tion (soo″pər-vas″kulər-ĭ-za′shən) in radiotherapy, the relative increase in vascularity that occurs when tumor cells are destroyed so that the remaining tumor cells are better supplied by the (uninjured) capillary stroma 血管形成过度，在放射治疗中，指肿瘤细胞被破坏时血管供应相对增加，致使残留的肿瘤细胞得以经由未损伤的毛细血管基质提供较好的血流供应

su·per·vol·tage (soo″pər-vōl″təj) in radiotherapy, voltage between 500 kilovolts and 1 megavolt, in contrast to orthovoltage and megavoltage 超电压，高电压

su·pi·nate (soo′pĭ-nāt) to assume or place in a supine position 仰卧；旋后

su·pi·na·tion (soo″pĭ-na′shən) the act of assuming the supine position, or the state of being supine. Applied to the hand, the act of turning the palm forward (anteriorly) or upward, performed by lateral rotation of the forearm. Applied to the foot, it generally impliesmovements resulting in raising of the medial margin of the foot, hence of the longitudinal arch 仰卧，采取仰卧姿势或仰卧状态的行为；旋后应用于手部，将手掌向前或向上翻转的动作，由前臂外侧旋转完成；应用于足部，一段是指运动导致足内侧缘抬高，从而引起纵弓抬高

su·pine (soo′pīn) (soo-pīn′) lying with the face upward, or on the dorsal surface 仰卧的，旋后的

sup·port (sə-port′) 1. to prevent weakening or failing 供养；维持；2. a structure that bears the weight of something else 支柱，支持器；3. a mechanism or arrangement that helps keep something else functioning 支持；**suppor′tive** *adj.*; **extracorporeal life s. (ECLS),** a technique for providing respiratory support for newborns and for adult respiratory distress syndrome, in which the blood is circulated through an artificial lung consisting of two compartments separated by a gas-permeable membrane, with the blood on one side and the ventilating gas on the other. Called also *extracorporeal membrane oxygenation* 一种为新生儿和成人呼吸窘迫综合征提供呼吸支持的技术，其中血液通过人工肺循环，人工肺由两个透气膜隔开的隔室组成，一侧为血液，另一侧为通气气体。又称体外膜氧合

sup·pos·i·to·ry (sə-poz′ĭ-tor-e) an easily fusible medicated mass to be introduced into a body orifice, as the rectum, urethra, or vagina 栓剂

sup·pres·sant (sə-pres′ənt) 1. inducing suppression 诱导抑制；2. an agent that stops secretion, excretion, or normal discharge 抑制药

sup·pres·sion (sə-presh′ən) 1. the act of holding back or checking 抑制，制止；2. sudden stoppage of a secretion, excretion, or normal discharge 突然停止分泌、排泄或正常排出；3. in psychiatry, conscious inhibition of an unacceptable impulse or idea as contrasted with repression, which is unconscious 压抑，在精神病学中，有意识地抑制一种不可接受的冲动或想法，与无意识的压抑有鲜明对比；4. in genetics, masking of the phenotypic expression of a mutation by the occurrence of a second (suppressor) mutation at a different site from the first; the organism appears to be reverted but is in fact doubly mutated 阻抑，在遗传学中，通过在与第一个位点不同的位点发生第二个(抑制子)突变来掩盖突变的表型表达；有机体似乎已经恢复，但事实上是双重变异；5. cortical inhibition of perception of objects in all or part of the visual field of one eye during binocular vision 在双眼视觉期间，皮质抑制一只眼睛的全部或部分视野中的物体感知；**bone marrow s.,** suppression of bone marrow activity, resulting in reduction in the number of platelets, red cells, and white cells 骨髓抑制；**over-**

drive s., transient suppression of automaticity in a cardiac pacemaker following a period of stimulation by a more rapidly discharging pacemaker 超速驱动阻抑，超驱动压抑

sup·pu·rant (sup'u-rənt) 1. suppurative 化脓的；2. an agent that causes suppuration 催脓剂

sup·pu·ra·tion (sup"u-ra'shən) pyogenesis 化脓；**sup'purative** adj.

su·pra·acro·mi·al (soo"prə-ə-kro'me-əl) above the acromion 肩峰上的

su·pra·au·ric·u·lar (soo"prə-aw-rik'u-lər) above the auricle of the ear 耳上的

su·pra·bulge (soo'prə-bulj") the surface of the crown of a tooth sloping toward the occlusal surface from the height of contour 上膨出

su·pra·cer·e·bel·lar (soo"prə-ser-ə-bel'ər) superior to the cerebellum 小脑上的

su·pra·chi·as·mat·ic (soo"prə-ki-az-mat'ik) above the optic chiasm 视交叉上的

su·pra·cho·roid (soo"prə-kor'oid) above or upon the choroid 脉络膜上的

su·pra·cla·vic·u·lar (soo"prə-klə-vik'u-lər) above the clavicle 锁骨上的

su·pra·clu·sion (soo"prə-kloo'zhən) projection of a tooth beyond the normal occlusal plane 越𬌗，超咬合

su·pra·con·dy·lar (soo"prə-kon'də-lər) above a condyle 髁上的

su·pra·cos·tal (soo"prə-kos'təl) above or upon the ribs 肋上的，肋外的

su·pra·cot·y·loid (soo"prə-kot'ə-loid) above the acetabulum 髋臼上的

su·pra·di·a·phrag·mat·ic (soo"prə-di"ə-frag-mat'ik) above the respiratory diaphragm 隔上的

su·pra·duc·tion (soo"prə-duk'shən) upward rotation of an eye around its horizontal axis 上转，眼上转

su·pra·epi·con·dy·lar (soo"prə-ep"ĭ-kon'də-lər) above an epicondyle 上髁上的

su·pra·gin·gi·val (soo"prə-jin'jĭ-vəl) superior to the gingiva or to the gingival margin 龈缘上的

su·pra·gle·noid (soo"prə-gle'noid) superior to the glenoid fossa 关节盂上的

su·pra·glot·tis (soo"prə-glot'is) the area of the pharynx above the glottis as far as the epiglottis 声门上的

su·pra·glot·ti·tis (soo"prə-glŏ-ti'tis) inflammation of the supraglottis, which can lead to lifethreatening upper airway obstruction 声门上炎，可导致生命危急上呼吸道阻塞

su·pra·hy·oid (soo"prə-hi'oid) above the hyoid bone 舌骨上的

su·pra·lim·i·nal (soo"prə-lim'ĭ-nəl) above the threshold of sensation（感觉）阈上的

su·pra·lum·bar (soo"prə-lum'bər) (-bahr) above the loin 腰上的

su·pra·mal·le·o·lar (soo"prə-mə-le'o-lər) above a malleolus 踝上的

su·pra·mar·gi·nal (soo"prə-mahr'jĭ-nəl) superior to a margin or border 缘上的

su·pra·mas·toid (soo"prə-mas'toid) superior to the mastoid process（颞骨）乳突上的

su·pra·max·il·lary (soo"prə-mak'sĭ-lar"e) above the maxilla 上颌的；上颌骨上的

su·pra·me·a·tal (soo"prə-me-a'təl) above a meatus 道上的，口上的

su·pra·men·ta·le (soo"prə-mən-ta'le) point B 下颌牙槽座点，又称 B 点

su·pra·oc·clu·sion (soo"prə-ŏ-kloo'zhən) supraclusion 超咬合，超𬌗

su·pra·op·tic (soo"prə-op'tik) superior to the optic chiasm 视上的

su·pra·or·bi·tal (soo"prə-or'bĭ-təl) above the orbit 眶上的

su·pra·pel·vic (soo"prə-pel'vik) above the pelvis 骨盆上的

su·pra·phar·ma·co·log·ic (soo"prə-fahr"mə-ko-loj'ik) much greater than the usual therapeutic dose or pharmacologic concentration of a drug 超药理学的，超出一般治疗剂量或药物的药理浓度

su·pra·pon·tine (soo"prə-pon'tīn) above or in the upper part of the pons 脑桥上（部）的

su·pra·pu·bic (soo"prə-pu'bik) superior to the pubic arch 耻骨弓上的

su·pra·re·nal (soo"prə-re'nəl) 1. above a kidney 肾上的；2. adrenal 肾上腺的

su·pra·scap·u·lar (soo"prə-skap'u-lər) above the scapula 肩胛上的

su·pra·scle·ral (soo"prə-sklēr'əl) on the outer surface of the sclera 巩膜外的

su·pra·sel·lar (soo"prə-sel'ər) above the sella turcica 蝶鞍上的

su·pra·spi·nal (soo"prə-spi'nəl) above the spine 脊柱上的；棘上的

su·pra·spi·nous (soo"prə-spi'nəs) 1. supraspinal 棘上的；2. superior to a spinous process 棘突上的

su·pra·ster·nal (soo"prə-stur'nəl) above the sternum 胸骨上的

su·pra·troch·le·ar (soo"prə-trok'le-ər) situated above a trochlea 滑车上的

su·pra·vag·i·nal (soo"prə-vaj'ĭ-nəl) outside or above a sheath; specifically, above the vagina 鞘上的，鞘外的；阴道上的

su·pra·val·var (soo"prə-val'vər) situated above a valve, particularly the aortic or pulmonary valve 瓣膜上的，尤其是主动脉瓣或肺动脉瓣

su·pra·ven·tric·u·lar (soo″prə-vən-trik′u-lər) situated or occurring above the ventricles, especially in an atrium or atrioventricular node 室上的，尤指在心房或房室结

su·pra·ver·gence (soo″prə-vur′jəns) disjunctive reciprocal movement of the eyes in which one eye rotates upward while the other one stays still 上转，眼上转

su·pra·ver·sion (soo″prə-vur′zhən) 1. abnormal elongation of a tooth from its socket 超𬌗错位；2. 同 sursumversion

su·pra·vi·tal (soo″prə-vi′təl) beyond living, as in supravital staining 体外活体的，超活体的，例如体外活体染色

su·pra·zy·go·mat·ic (soo″prə-zi″go-mat′ik) situated above the zygomatic bone 颧骨上的

su·preme (soo-prēm′) ultimate, greatest; highest; used in anatomy for the one in a group having the most superior location 极度的，最重要的；最高的

su·pro·fen (soo-pro′fən) a nonsteroidal antiinflammatory drug applied topically to the conjunctiva to inhibit miosis during ophthalmic surgery 舒洛芬，一种非甾体类抗炎药，局部应用于结膜，在眼科手术中抑制瞳孔缩小

su·ra (soo′rə) [L.] calf 腓肠（小腿肚）；**su′ral** *adj.*

sur·fac·tant (sər-fak′tənt) 1. surface-active agent 表面活性剂，表面活化剂；2. in pulmonary physiology, a mixture of phospholipids that reduces the surface tension of pulmonary fluids and thus contributes to the elastic properties of pulmonary tissue 表面活性物质，在肺生理学中，一种磷脂混合物，可降低肺液的表面张力，从而增加肺组织弹性

sur·geon (sur′jən) 1. a physician who specializes in surgery 外科医师；2. the senior medical officer of a military unit 军事单位的高级医官

sur·gery (sur′jər-e) 1. the branch of medicine that treats diseases, injuries, and deformities by manual or operative methods 外科学；2. the place in a hospital, or doctor's or dentist's office, where surgery is performed 外科；3. in Great Britain, a room or office where a doctor sees and treats patients（英国）医生诊疗室；4. the work performed by a surgeon 外科手术；**antiseptic s.**, surgery using antiseptic methods 抗菌外科；**aseptic s.**, that performed in an environment so free from microorganisms that significant infection or suppuration does not supervene 无菌外科；**bench s.**, surgery performed on an organ that has been removed from the body, after which it is reimplanted 离体外科；**conservative s.**, surgery designed to preserve, or to remove with minimal risk, diseased or injured organs, tissues, or limbs 保守性手术；**cytoreductive s.**, debulking 减瘤术；

dental s., oral and maxillofacial s. 牙外科；**general s.**, that which deals with surgical problems of all kinds, rather than those in a restricted area, as in a surgical specialty such as neurosurgery 普通外科学；**major s.**, surgery involving the more important, difficult, and hazardous operations 大外科；**minimally invasive s.**, surgery done with only a small incision or no incision at all, such as that done through a cannula with a laparoscope or endoscope 微创手术；**minor s.**, surgery restricted to management of minor problems and injuries 小外科；**Mohs s.**, microscopically controlled excision of highrisk, nonmelanoma skin cancers in which serial excisions of fresh tissue are done with examination of each sample Mohs（莫氏）显微手术，是用显微镜控制来切除高风险的非黑色素瘤皮肤癌，通过检查每个样本进行新鲜组织的连续切除；**oral and maxillofacial s.**, the branch of dentistry that deals with the diagnosis and surgical and adjunct treatment of diseases and defects of the mouth and dental structures 口腔及颌面外科；**plastic s.**, surgery concerned with restoration, reconstruction, correction, or improvement in shape and appearance of body structures that are defective, damaged, or misshapen by injury, disease, or growth and development 成形外科，整形外科；**radical s.**, surgery designed to extirpate all areas of locally extensive disease and adjacent zones of lymphatic drainage 根治外科手术；**stereotactic s., stereotaxic s.**, any of several techniques for the production of sharply circumscribed lesions in specific tiny areas of pathologic tissue in deep-seated brain structures after locating the discrete structure by means of three-dimensional coordinates 立体定向手术

sur·gi·cal (sur′jĭ-kəl) of, pertaining to, or correctable by surgery 外科（术）的，外科（手术）用的

Sur·gi·cel (sur′jĭ-sel) trademark for an absorbable knitted fabric prepared by controlled oxidation of cellulose, used to control intraoperative hemorrhage when other conventional methods are impractical or ineffective 氧化纤维素，为纤维素在控制氧化作用下制成的可吸收性编织物的商品名，用作止血剂，以控制当其他常规方法不能实施或无效时的术中出血

sur·ro·gate (sur′o-gət) a substitute; a thing or person that takes the place of something or someone else, as a drug used in place of another, or a person who takes the place of another in someone's affective existence 替代品，替代物

sur·sum·duc·tion (sur″səm-duk′shən) 同 supraduction 上转，眼上转

sur·sum·ver·gence (sur″səm-vur′jəns) 同 supravergence

sur·sum·ver·sion (sur″səm-vur′zhən) the simultaneous and equal upward turning of the eyes 上转，眼上转

sus·vi·val (sər-vi′vəl) the act or process of remaining alive; the continuation of life 幸存，生存，存活

sus·cep·ti·bil·i·ty (sə-sep″tĭ-bil′ĭ-te) the state of being susceptible 易感性，敏感性，感受性；**antibiotic s., antimicrobial s.,** the vulnerability of a strain of a microorganism to being inhibited or killed by a given antibiotic or antimicrobial 抗菌药物敏感性

sus·cep·ti·ble (sə-sep′tĭ-bəl) 1. readily affected or acted upon 易感的，易受影响的；2. lacking immunity or resistance and thus at risk of infection 易感者

sus·pen·sion (səs-pen′shən) 1. a condition of temporary cessation, as of animation, of pain, or of any vital process 暂停，如兴奋、疼痛或任何生命过程的暂停状态；2. attachment of an organ or other body part to a supporting structure, as of the uterus or bladder in the correction of a hernia or prolapse 悬吊（术）在矫正疝气或脱垂时将器官或其他身体部位附着在支撑结构上，如子宫或膀胱；3. a liquid preparation consisting of solid particles dispersed throughout a liquid phase in which they are not soluble 悬浮液，某些很细药物在使用前将其悬浮在适合的液体媒介物中；**bladder neck s.,** any of various methods of surgical fixation of the urethrovesical junction area and bladder neck to restore the neck to a high retropubic position for relief of stress incontinence 膀胱颈悬吊术；**colloid s.,** a colloid system; see *colloid* (2). Sometimes used specifically for a sol in which the dispersed phase is solid and the particles are large enough to settle out of solution 胶体悬浮液

sus·pen·soid (səs-pen′soid) lyophobic colloid 悬浮液，悬胶体

sus·pen·so·ry (səs-pen′sə-re) 1. serving to hold up a part 悬的，提举的；2. a ligament, bone, muscle, sling, or bandage that serves to hold up a part 悬吊物，悬带

sus·ten·tac·u·lum (sus″tən-tak′u-ləm) pl. *sustentac′ula* [L.] a support 支柱；支撑物；**sustentac′u-lar** *adj.*

su·tu·ra (soo-tu′rə) pl. *sutu′rae* [L.] suture; in anatomy, a type of joint in which the apposed bony surfaces are united by fibrous tissue, permitting no movement; found only between bones of the skull 缝，骨缝；**s. denta′ta,** s. serrata 齿状缝；**s. pla′na,** a type in which there is simple apposition of the contiguous surfaces, with no interlocking of the edges of the participating bones 直缝；**s. serra′ta,** a type in which the participating bones are

united by interlocking processes resembling the teeth of a saw 锯缝；**s. squamo′sa,** a type formed by overlapping of the broad beveled edges of the participating bones 鳞缝；**s. ve′ra,** sutura. 真缝，真骨缝

su·ture (soo′chər) 1. 同 sutura. 2. a stitch or series of stitches made to secure apposition of the edges of a surgical or traumatic wound 一针，线迹；3. to apply such stitches 缝合；4. material used in closing a wound with stitches 缝线；**su′tural** *adj.*；**absorbable s.,** a strand of suture material that is dissolved by tissue fluids after the wound heals 可吸收，缝线；**apposition s.,** a superficial type for exact approximation of cutaneous edges of a wound 对位缝合；**approximation s.,** a deep suture for securing apposition of the deep tissue of a wound 接近缝合术；**buried s.,** one placed deep in the tissues and concealed by the skin 埋藏缝合术；**catgut s.,** 肠线，参见 *gut* 下 *surgical gut*；**coaptation s.,** 同 apposition s；**cobbler's s.,** one in which suture material is threaded through a needle at each end 鞋匠缝术；**continuous s.,** one using a continuous, uninterrupted length of material 连续缝合（法）；**coronal s.,** the line of junction of the frontal bone with the two parietal bones 冠状缝；**cranial s's,** the lines of junction between the bones of the skull 颅缝；**Czerny s.,** Czerny 缝术. 1. an intestinal suture in which the thread is passed through the mucous membrane only 肠管缝术，缝线只穿过黏膜；2. union of a ruptured tendon by splitting one of the ends and suturing the other end into the slit 筋膜末端修补缝术，将断裂的肌腱一端切开并将另一端缝合到狭缝中而愈合；**alse s.,** a line of junction between apposed surfaces without fibrous union of the bones 假缝；**figure-of eight s.,** one in which the threads follow the contours of the figure 8 8字形缝合；**Gély s.,** a continuous stitch for wounds of the intestine, made with a thread having a needle at each end Gely 缝术；**Halsted s.,** a modification of the Lembert suture 褥式浆肌层缝合；**interrupted s.,** one in which each stitch is made with a separate piece of material 间断缝合；**Lembert s.,** an inverting suture used in gastrointestinal surgery 间断浆肌层缝合；**locked s., lock-stitch s.,** a continuous suture in which the suture loop falls over the point where the needle emerges from the skin to form a self-locking stitch when the strand is pulled taut 连锁缝术；**loop s.,** 同 interrupted s；**mattress s.,** a method in which the stitches are parallel with *(horizontal mattress s.)* or at right angles to *(vertical mattress s.)* the wound edges 褥式缝合（法）**non-absorbable s.,** suture material that is not absorbed in the body 不吸收缝线；**purse-string s.,** a continuous, circular inverting suture, such as is used to bury the stump of the appendix 荷包缝合；**relaxation s.,** any suture that can be loosened to relieve tension if necessary 减张缝合；**subcuticular s.,** a method of skin closure involving placement of stitches in the subcuticular tissues parallel with the line of the wound 皮内缝合（法）；**uninterrupted s.,** 同 continuous s.

SV sinus venosus 静脉窦；stroke volume 心搏排血量

svas·tha (swus′thyə) [Sanskrit] the term for health used in ayurveda 阿育吠陀所用的健康术语

sved·berg (sfed′bərg) Svedberg unit 斯韦德贝里单位（沉降系数单位）

SVT superficial venous thrombosis; supraventricular tachycardia 室上性心动过速

SVU Society for Vascular Ultrasound 血管超声学会

swab (swahb) a wad of cotton or other absorbent material attached to the end of a wire or stick, used for applying medication, removing material, collecting bacteriologic material, etc. 拭子，药签

swage (swāj) 1. to shape metal by hammering or by adapting it to a die 压膜，通过锤击或使之与模具相适应而使金属成形；2. to fuse, as suture material to the end of a suture needle 把缝合材料熔到缝合针的末端

swal·low·ing (swahl′o-ing) the taking in of a substance through the mouth and pharynx, past the cricopharyngeal sphincter, through the esophagus, and into the stomach 吞咽

sway·back (swa′bak) lordosis (2) 脊柱前凸

sweat (swet) perspiration; the clear liquid secreted by the sweat glands 出汗；**night s's,** sweating during sleep, a symptom frequently occurring in tuberculosis and acquired immune deficiency syndrome 盗汗，睡眠时出汗，为肺结核和获得性免疫缺陷综合征的常见症状

sweat·ing (swet′ing) perspiration; the functional secretion of sweat 出汗，排汗

swell·ing (swel′ing) 1. transient abnormal enlargement of a body part or area not due to cell proliferation 肿胀，膨胀，非细胞增生引起的身体部位或区域的短暂异常增大；2. an eminence or elevation 隆凸；**cloudy s.,** an early stage of toxic degenerative changes, especially in protein constituents of organs in infectious diseases, in which the tissues appear swollen, parboiled, and opaque but revert to normal when the cause is removed 浊肿，细胞肿胀

SWI susceptibility-weighted imaging 敏感加权成像

sy·co·si·form (si-ko′sĭ-form) resembling sycosis 须疮样的

sy·co·sis (si-ko′sis) papulopustular inflammation of hair follicles, especially of the beard 须疮；**s. bar′bae,** inflammation of hair follicles, usually seen on the neck of a male with tightly curled beard hair 寻常须疮；**lupoid s.,** a chronic, scarring form of deep sycosis barbae 狼疮样须疮；**s. vulga′ris,** 同 s. barbae

syl·vat·ic (sil-vat′ik) sylvan; pertaining to, located in, or living in the woods 森林的

sym·bal·lo·phone (sim-bal′o-fōn) a stethoscope with two chest pieces, making possible the comparison and localization of sounds 定向听诊器

sym·bi·ont (sim′bi-ont) (sim′be-ont) an organism living in a state of symbiosis 共生生物

sym·bi·o·sis (sim″bi-o′sis) pl. *symbio′ses* [Gr.] 1. in parasitology, the close association of two dissimilar organisms, classified as mutualism, commensalism, parasitism, amensalism, or synnecrosis, depending on the advantage or disadvantage derived from the relationship 共生关系，在寄生学中，两种不同生物之间的密切联系；2. in psychiatry, a mutually reinforcing relationship between persons who are dependent on each other; a normal characteristic of the relationship between mother and infant 依赖关系，在精神病学中，相互依赖的人之间相互加强的关系；母婴关系的正常特征

sym·bi·ote (sim′bi-ōt) symbiont 共生体

sym·bi·ot·ic (sim″bi-ot′ik) associated in symbiosis; living together 共生的；共同生活的

sym·bleph·a·ron (sim-blef′ə-ron) adhesion of the eyelid to the eyeball 睑球粘连

▲ 睑球粘连

sym·bleph·a·rop·ter·yg·i·um (sim-blef″ə-rotər-ij′e-əm) symblepharon in which the adhesion is a cicatricial band resembling a pterygium 翼状睑球粘连

sym·bol (sim′bəl) 1. something, particularly an object, that represents something else 标记，符号，

象征；2. in psychoanalytic theory, a representation or perception that replaces unconscious mental content 在精神病学中，代替无意识心理内容的一种象征或知觉；**phallic s.**, in psychoanalytic theory, any pointed or upright object that may represent the phallus or penis 阳具象征，在精神分析中，任何尖形或直立的物体都可象征阴茎

sym·bo·lia (sim-bo′le-ə) ability to recognize the nature of objects by the sense of touch 形体感觉，通过触觉识别物体本质的能力

sym·bol·ism (sim′bəl-iz-əm) 1. the act or process of representing something by a symbol 用符号表示某物的行为或过程；2. in psychoanalytic theory, a mechanism of unconscious thinking characterized by substitution of a symbol for a repressed or threatening impulse or object so as to avoid censorship by the superego 象征表示，在精神分析上，潜意识思维的一种机制，其特征是用一个符号代替被压抑或威胁的冲动或物体，以避免超我的审查

sym·bol·iza·tion (sim″bəl-ĭ-za′shən) a type of defense mechanism in which one idea or object comes to represent another because of similarity or association between them 象征化，象征作用

sym·brachy·dac·ty·ly (sim-brak″e-dak′tə-le) a condition in which the fingers or toes are short and webbed 短指粘连畸形

sym·me·lia (sĭ-me′le-ə) a developmental anomaly characterized by an apparent fusion of the lower limbs, having three feet *(tripodial s.)*, two feet *(dipodial s.)*, one foot *(monopodial s.)*, or no feet *(apodal s.* or *sirenomelia)* 并腿畸形，以下肢明显融合为特征的发育异常，可以是三足并腿畸形，两足并腿畸形，单足并腿畸形，或无足并腿畸形

sym·me·lus (sim′ə-ləs) a fetus exhibiting symmelia 并腿畸胎

sym·me·try (sim′ə-tre) correspondence in size, form, and arrangement of parts on opposite sides of a plane or around an axis 对称（性），均称；**symmet′ric, symmet′rical** *adj.*；**bilateral s.**, the configuration of an irregularly shaped body (as the human body or that of higher animals) that can be divided by a longitudinal plane into halves that are mirror images of each other 两侧对称；**helical s.**, an arrangement of capsomers seen in viruses with a rodlike or filamentous capsid, in which subunits form a coiled structure, with each subunit forming bonds with the subunit in each of the adjoining turns to provide stability 螺旋对称，衣壳病毒中的一种衣壳排列，具有棒状或丝状衣壳，其中亚单位形成一个螺旋结构，每个亚单位与相邻的每个转弯处的亚单位形成键以提供稳定性；**inverse s.**, correspondence as between a part and its mirror

image, wherein the right (or left) side of one part corresponds with the left (or right) side of the other 反面对称；**radial s.**, that in which the body parts are arranged regularly around a central axis 辐射对称

sym·pa·thec·to·my (sim″pə-thek′tə-me) transection, resection, or other interruption of some portion of the sympathetic nervous pathway 交感神经切除术；**chemical s.**, that accomplished by means of a chemical agent 化学性交感神经阻断术

sym·pa·thet·ic (sim″pə-thet′ik) 1. pertaining to, exhibiting, or caused by sympathy 同情的，同感的；2. pertaining to the sympathetic nervous system or one of its nerves 交感神经的

sym·path·i·co·blast (sim-path′ĭ-ko-blast″) 同 sympathoblast

sym·path·i·co·blas·to·ma (sim-path″ĭ-ko-blasto′mə) a neuroblastoma arising in one of the ganglia of the sympathetic nervous system 成交感神经细胞瘤

sym·path·i·co·trip·sy (sim-path″ĭ-ko-trip′se) the surgical crushing of a nerve, ganglion, or plexus of the sympathetic nervous system 交感神经压轧术

sym·path·i·co·tro·pic (sim-path″ĭ-ko-tro′pik) 1. having an affinity for the sympathetic nervous system 向交感神经的，趋交感神经的；2. an agent having an affinity for or exerting its principal effect on the sympathetic nervous system 向交感神经药，趋交感神经药

sym·pa·tho·ad·re·nal (sim″pə-tho-ə-dre′nəl) 1. pertaining to the sympathetic nervous system and the adrenal medulla 交感肾上腺的；2. involving the sympathetic nervous system and the suprarenal glands, especially increased sympathetic activity that causes increased secretion of epinephrine and norepinephrine 交感肾上腺性，涉及交感神经系统和肾上腺，尤指交感神经活动增强，引起肾上腺素和去甲肾上腺素分泌增加

sym·patho·blast (sim-path′o-blast″) a pluripotential cell in the embryo that will develop into a sympathetic nerve cell or a chromaffin cell 成交感神经细胞

sym·pa·tho·go·nia (sim″pə-tho-go′ne-ə) sing. *sympathogo′nium.* [Gr.] undifferentiated embryonic cells that develop into sympathetic neurons 交感神经原细胞

sym·pa·tho·lyt·ic (sim″pə-tho-lit′ik) 1. antiadrenergic; opposing the effects of impulses conveyed by adrenergic postganglionic fibers of the sympathetic nervous system 抗交感神经的；交感神经阻滞的；2. an agent that so acts 抗交感神经药；交感神经阻滞药

sym·pa·tho·mi·met·ic (sim″pə-tho-mi-met′ik) 1. mimicking the effects of impulses conveyed by adrenergic postganglionic fibers of the sympathetic nervous system 拟交感神经的，类交感神经的；2. an agent that produces such an effect 拟交感神经药

sym·pa·thy (sim′pə-the) 1. compassion for another person's thoughts, feelings, and experiences 同情；2. an influence produced in any organ by disease, disorder, or other change in another part 感 应；3. a relation that exists between people or things such that change in the state of one is reflected in the other 同感（作用）

sym·pha·lan·gia (sim″fə-lan′jə) congenital end-to-end fusion of contiguous phalanges of a digit 指（趾）关节粘连

sym·phys·e·al (sim-fiz′e-əl) pertaining to a symphysis. Spelled also *symphysial* 联合的

sym·phys·i·or·rha·phy (sim-fiz″e-or′ə-fe) suture of a divided symphysis 耻骨联合缝合术

sym·phys·i·ot·o·my (sim-fiz″e-ot′ə-me) division of the symphysis pubis to facilitate delivery 耻骨联合切开术

sym·phy·sis (sim′fĭ-sis) pl. *sym′physes* [Gr.] a type of joint in which the apposed bony surfaces are firmly united by a plate of fibrocartilage 联合，为软骨关节的一种类型，其骨对合面由纤维软骨板紧密连接；**pubic s.,** the line of union of the bodies of the pubic bones in the median plane 耻骨联合

sym·po·dia (sim-po′de-ə) symmelia 无足并腿畸形

sym·port (sim′port) a mechanism of transporting two compounds simultaneously across a cell membrane in the same direction, one compound being transported down a concentration gradient, the other against a gradient 同向转运，通过细胞膜往相同方向同时转运两种物质的过程，被转运的化合物之一是顺浓度梯度转运而另一种化合物则是逆浓度梯度转运

symp·tom (simp′təm) any subjective evidence of disease or of a patient's condition, i.e., such evidence as perceived by the patient; a change in a patient's condition indicative of some bodily or mental state 症 状；**objective s.,** one that is evident to the observer 客观症状，参见 *sign*；**presenting s.,** the symptom or group of symptoms about which the patient complains or from which they seek relief 主要症状，主诉；**subjective s.,** one perceptible only to the patient. 自觉症状，主观症状；**withdrawal s's,** substance withdrawal 戒断症状，脱瘾症状

symp·to·mat·ic (simp″tə-mat′ik) 1. pertaining to or of the nature of a symptom 症状的；2. indicative (of a particular disease or disorder) 提示的，表明的；

exhibiting the symptoms of a particular disease but having a different cause 征候的，征兆的，显示不同原因引起的疾病；4. directed at the allaying of symptoms, as symptomatic treatment 针对症状的，旨在缓解症状的

symp·to·ma·tol·o·gy (simp″tə-mə-tol′ə-je) 1. the branch of medicine dealing with symptoms 症状学；2. the combined symptoms of a disease 疾病的复合症状

symp·to·ma·to·lyt·ic (simp″tə-mat″o-lit′ik) causing the disappearance of symptoms 消除症状的

sym·pus (sim′pəs) symmelus 无足并腿畸胎

syn·apse (sin′aps) the site of functional apposition between neurons, where an impulse is transmitted from one to another, usually by a chemical neurotransmitter released by the axon terminal of the presynaptic neuron. The neurotransmitter diffuses across the gap to bind with receptors on the postsynaptic cell membrane and cause electrical changes in that neuron (depolarization/excitation or hyperpolarization/inhibition) 突触

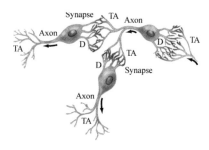

▲ 三个突触。神经冲动用箭表示，表明神经冲动通路从末梢分枝（**TA**），或从一个神经元的轴突神经末梢传递到另一个神经元的树突（**D**）
Axon. 轴突；Synapse. 突触

syn·ap·sis (sĭ-nap′sis) the intimate association of homologous chromosomes that occurs during the zygotene stage of meiosis Ⅰ 联会，减数分裂合子期发生的同源染色体的密切联系

syn·ap·tic (sĭ-nap′tik) 1. pertaining to or affecting a synapse 突触的；2. pertaining to synapsis 联会的

syn·ap·to·some (sĭ-nap′to-sōm″) any of the membrane-bound sacs that break away from axon terminals at a synapse after brain tissue has been homogenized in sugar solution; it contains synaptic vessels and mitochondria 突触体

syn·ar·thro·dia (sin″ahr-thro′de-ə) a fibrous joint 不动关节；**synarthro′dial** *adj.*

syn·ar·thro·phy·sis (sin-ahr″thro-fi′sis) any ankylosing process 关节粘连

syn·ar·thro·sis (sin″ahr-thro′sis) pl. *synarthro′ses.* A bony junction that is immovable and is connected by solid connective tissue, comprising the fibrous joints and the cartilaginous joints 不动关节

syn·can·thus (sin-kan′thəs) adhesion of the eyeball to the orbital structures 眶球粘连

syn·ceph·a·lus (sin-sef′ə-ləs) conjoined twins with one head and a single face with four ears, two on the back of the head 并头联胎，单头双畸胎，有一张脸，四只耳，其中二只耳在头的背面

syn·chi·ria (sin-ki′re-ə) dyschiria in which a stimulus applied to one side of the body is felt on both sides 两侧错觉，施刺激于身体一侧，引起的感觉却遍涉及两侧的一种状态

syn·chon·dro·sis (sin″kon-dro′sis) pl. *synchondro′ses* [Gr.] a type of cartilaginous joint in which the cartilage is usually converted into bone before adult life 软骨结合

syn·chon·drot·o·my (sin″kon-drot′ə-me) division of a synchondrosis 软骨结合切开术

syn·chro·nism (sing′krə-niz-əm) 同 synchrony

syn·chro·ny (sing′krə-ne) the occurrence of two events simultaneously or with a fixed time interval between them 同时性，同步现象；**synchron′ic, syn′chronous** *adj.*; **atrioventricular (AV) s.,** in the heart, the physiologic condition of atrial electrical activity followed by ventricular electrical activity 房室同步；**bilateral s.,** the occurrence of a secondary synchronous discharge at a location in the brain exactly contralateral to a discharge caused by a lesion 同侧同步

syn·chy·sis (sin′ki-sis) [Gr.] a softening or fluid condition of the vitreous body of the eye 玻璃体液化；**s. scintillans,** floating cholesterol crystals in the vitreous, developing as a secondary degenerative change 闪光性玻璃体液化，玻璃状体液内发生胆固醇结晶，是炎症或其他眼病后的蜕变

syn·clit·ism (sin′klit-izm) 1. parallelism between the planes of the fetal head and those of the maternal pelvis 胎头均倾，头盆倾势匀匀；2. normal synchronous maturation of the nucleus and cytoplasm of blood cells 同时成熟，指血细胞和胞浆 **syn·clit′ic** *adj.*

syn·clo·nus (sin′klo-nəs) muscular tremor or successive clonic contraction of various muscles together 共同阵挛，肌肉震颤或不同肌肉共同连续的阵挛性收缩

syn·co·pe (sing′kə-pe) a faint, temporary loss of consciousness due to generalized cerebral ischemia 晕厥；**syn′copal, syncop′ic** *adj.*; **cardiac s.,** sudden loss of consciousness, with momentary premonitory symptoms or without warning, due to cerebral anemia caused by obstructions to cardiac output or arrhythmias such as ventricular asystole, extreme bradycardia, or ventricular fibrillation 心脏性晕厥；**carotid sinus s.,** 颈动脉窦性晕厥，参见 *syndrome* 下 词条；**convulsive s.,** syncope with convulsive movements that are milder than those seen in epilepsy 抽搐性晕厥；**laryngeal s.,** tussive s. 喉性晕厥；**stretching s.,** syncope associated with stretching the arms upward with the spine extended 伸展性晕厥；**swallow s.,** syncope associated with swallowing, a disorder of atrioventricular conduction mediated by the vagus nerve 吞咽性晕厥；**tussive s.,** brief loss of consciousness associated with paroxysms of coughing 咳嗽晕厥；**vasovagal s.,** a transient vascular and neurogenic reaction marked by pallor, nausea, sweating, bradycardia, and rapid fall in arterial blood pressure, which may result in syncope 血管迷走性晕厥

syn·cy·tial (sin-sish′əl) of or pertaining to a syncytium 合胞体的

syn·cyt·i·o·ma (sin-sit″e-o′mə) syncytial endometritis 合胞体瘤

syn·cyt·io·tro·pho·blast (sin-sit″e-o-tro′foblast) the outer syncytial layer of the trophoblast 合胞体滋养层；**syncytiotrophoblas′tic** *adj.*

syn·cy·ti·um (sin-sish′e-əm) a multinucleate mass of protoplasm produced by the merging of cells 合胞体

syn·dac·ty·ly (sin-dak′tə-le) persistence of webbing between distal phalanges of adjacent digits of the hand or foot, so that they are more or less completely fused together 并指（趾）；**syndac′tylous** *adj.*

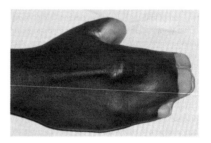

▲　并指（趾）

syn·dec·to·my (sin-dek′tə-me) peritectomy 球结膜环切术

syn·de·sis (sin′də-sis) (sin-de′sis) 1. arthrodesis 关节固定术；2. synapsis（染色体）联会

syn·des·mec·to·my (sin″dəz-mek′tə-me) surgical removal of part or all of a ligament 韧带切除术

syn·des·mec·to·pia (sin″dəz-mək-to′pe-ə) unusual situation of a ligament 韧带异位

syn·des·mi·tis (sin″dez-mi′tis) 1. inflammation of a ligament 韧带炎；2. conjunctivitis 结膜炎

syn·des·mog·ra·phy (sin″dez-mog′rə-fe) a description of the ligaments 韧带论

syn·des·mol·o·gy (sin″dəz-mol′ə-je) arthrology 韧带学

syn·des·mo·plas·ty (sin-dez′mo-plas″te) plastic repair of a ligament 韧带成形术

syn·des·mo·sis (sin″dəz-mo′sis) pl. *syndesmo′ses* [Gr.] a type of fibrous joint in which the intervening connective tissue forms an interosseous membrane or ligament 韧带联合，一种纤维关节，介于其间的纤维性结缔组织形成一层骨间膜或韧带

syn·des·mot·o·my (sin″dəz-mot′ə-me) incision of a ligament 韧带切开术

syn·drome (sin′drōm) a set of symptoms occurring together; the sum of signs of any morbid state; a symptom complex 综合征，另参见 *disease* 下词条；**22q11 deletion s.,** hemizygous deletion of a 1.5 to 3.0 Mb region of chromosome 22q11.2 as a result of defective recombination in meiosis. Its manifestations are so variable they are often grouped into different named syndromes, including DiGeorge syndrome and velocardiofacial syndrome (qq.v.) 22q11 微缺失综合征，染色体 22q11.2 1.5-3.0 Mb 区域的半合子缺失，是减数分裂中重组缺陷的结果；**Aarskog s., Aarskog-Scott s.,** an X-linked condition due to mutation of a protein involved in signaling during embryonic development and characterized by ocular hypertelorism, anteverted nostrils, broad upper lip, scrotal "shawl" above the penis or other genital anomalies, and small hands 阿 - 斯综合征，有 X - 连锁遗传特性的征群，以眼距增宽、鼻孔前、上唇宽、特有的阴囊 "围巾" 包在阴茎上方及手小等为特征；**abdominal compartment s.,** increased intraabdominal pressure resulting in impaired organ function, most often affecting the cardiovascular, pulmonary, and renal systems 腹腔间隔综合征，腹内压升高导致器官功能受损，最常影响心血管、肺和肾系统；**abstinence s.,** a mental disorder that follows cessation of use of a substance that had been regularly used to induce a state of intoxication 脱瘾综合征；**acquired immune deficiency s., acquired immunodeficiency s.,** the most severe manifestation of clinical disease due to infection with human immunodeficiency virus (HIV). The CDC criteria include (1) presence of certain opportunistic infections indicating an underlying defect in cell-mediated immunity in the absence of known causes of underlying immunodeficiency or other host defense defects; or (2) CD4$^+$ cell count of less than 200/ml; or (3) CD4$^+$ cell percentage of less than 14 percent 获得性免疫缺陷综合征（艾滋病），参见 *infection.* 下 *human immunodeficiency virus infection*；**acute coronary s.,** a classification encompassing clinical presentations ranging from unstable angina through non–Q wave infarction, sometimes also including Q wave infarction 急性冠脉综合征；**acute radiation s.,** a syndrome caused by exposure to a whole-body dose of over 1 gray of ionizing radiation; symptoms, whose severity and time of onset depend on the size of the dose, include erythema, nausea and vomiting, fatigue, diarrhea, petechiae, bleeding from the mucous membranes, hematologic changes, gastrointestinal hemorrhage, epilation, hypotension, tachycardia, and dehydration; death may occur within hours or weeks of exposure 急性放射性综合征，全身照射的电离辐射剂量超过 1Gy 所引起的症候群。各种症状的严重程度和发生时间与剂量的大小有关，这些症状包括红斑、恶心呕吐、疲劳、腹泻、发热、瘀点、黏膜出血、淋巴细胞和粒细胞以及血小板减少、胃肠道出血、脱毛（发）、低血压、心搏过速及脱水；死亡可发生于照射后数小时或数周内；**Acute respiratory distress s. (ARDS),** fulminant pulmonary interstitial and alveolar edema, which usually develops within a few days after the initiating trauma, thought to result from alveolar injury that has led to increased capillary permeability 急性呼吸窘迫综合征；**Adams-Stokes s.,** episodic cardiac arrest and syncope due to failure of normal and escape pacemakers, with or without ventricular fibrillation; the principal manifestation of severe heart attack 阿 - 斯综合征（心源性脑缺血综合征），由于正常起搏器和逃逸起搏器故障引起的阵发性心脏骤停和晕厥，伴有或不伴有心室颤动；严重心脏病发作的主要表现；**addisonian s.,** the complex of symptoms resulting from adrenocortical insufficiency 艾迪生综合征，由肾上腺功能不全引起的综合症状，参见 *disease* 下 *Addison disease*；**Adie s.,** Holmes-Adie s.; tonic pupil associated with absence or diminution of certain tendon reflexes 阿迪综合征（瞳孔紧张症），与某些肌腱反射消失或减弱有关的强直性瞳孔；**adrenogenital s.,** a group of syndromes in which inappropriate virilism or feminization results from disorders of adrenal function that also affect gonadal steroidogenesis 肾上腺性征综合征；**adult respiratory distress s. (ARDS),** 同 acute respiratory distress s.；**AEC s.,** 同 Hay-Wells s.；**afferent loop s.,** chronic partial obstruction of the proximal loop (duodenum and jejunum) after gastrojejunostomy, resulting in duodenal distention, pain, and nausea following ingestion of food 输入襻综合征，部分胃切除和胃空肠吻合术后，十二指肠和空肠近端肠襻发生慢性部分性梗阻，导致进食后十二指肠膨胀、疼痛及恶心；

Ahumada-del Castillo s., galactorrhea-amenorrhea syndrome with low gonadotropin secretion 乳溢闭经综合征，一种非产后三联症，包括乳溢、经闭及促性腺激素分泌减少；**akinetic-rigid s.,** muscular rigidity with varying degrees of slowness of movement; seen in parkinsonism and disorders of the basal ganglia 运动不能 - 强直综合征；**Alagille s.,** an autosomal dominant disorder characterized by a paucity of intrahepatic bile ducts in association with cholestasis, cardiac disease, skeletal and ocular abnormalities, and an unusual facies; sometimes with renal or vascular manifestations 先天性肝内胆管发育不良征，阿拉日明综合征，一种常染色体显性疾病，以肝内胆管缺乏为特征，伴有胆汁淤积、心脏病、骨骼和眼部异常以及异常面容；有时伴有肾或血管表现；**Albright s.,** McCune-Albright s. 奥尔布赖特综合征；**Aldrich s.,** Wiskott-Aldrich s. 奥尔德里奇综合征；**Allgrove s.,** triple A s.; autosomal recessive adrenal insufficiency with achalasia and alacrima; sometimes with neurologic abnormalities Allgrove 综合征；**Alport s.,** a hereditary disorder of the basement membrane, characterized by progressive sensorineural hearing loss, progressive pyelonephritis et glomerulonephritis, and variable ocular defects 奥尔波特综合征（遗传性肾炎），一种遗传性征群，以进行性感神经性听觉丧失及进行性肾盂肾炎或肾小球肾炎为特征，偶有眼异常；**Alström s.,** an autosomal recessive disorder of retinitis pigmentosa with nystagmus and early loss of central vision, deafness, early childhood obesity, and type 2 diabetes mellitus 先天性黑矇，遗传性先天性视网膜病，一种常见色素性视网膜炎隐性遗传病，伴有眼球震颤和早期视力丧失、耳聋、儿童早期肥胖和 2 型糖尿病；**amnestic s.,** a mental disorder characterized by impairment of memory occurring in a normal state of consciousness; the most common cause is thiamine deficiency associated with alcohol abuse 遗忘综合征，以正常意识状态下发生的记忆障碍为特征的精神障碍；最常见的原因是与酗酒有关的硫胺素缺乏；**amniotic band s.,** 羊膜带综合征，参见 *sequence* 下词条；**Andersen-Tawil s.,** an autosomal dominant disorder due to mutation of an inwardly rectifying potassium channel, characterized by periodic paralysis, cardiac arrhythmias, and skeletal dysmorphism Andersen-Tawil 综合征，一种由内向整流钾通道突变引起的常染色体显性疾病，以周期性麻痹、心律失常和骨骼畸形为特征；**androgen insensitivity s.,** resistance of target organs to the action of androgens; the result in XY males is any of a spectrum ranging from normal-appearing male (*mild* to *partial* forms) to female external genitalia and habitus (*complete* form). In most cases,

testes are present, often abdominal. It is an X-linked disorder due to mutation in the androgen receptor gene 雄激素不敏感综合征；**Angelman s.,** an autosomal recessive syndrome inherited via a maternal mutation or deletion; characterized by jerky puppetlike movements, frequent laughter, mental and motor retardation, peculiar openmouthed facies, and seizures 快乐木偶综合征，一种通过母体突变或缺失遗传的常染色体隐性综合征，特征是木偶样动作急促、频繁大笑、精神和运动迟缓、特有的张口相和癫痫发作；**angular gyrus s.,** a syndrome resulting from an infarction or other lesion of the angular gyrus on the dominant side, often characterized by alexia or agraphia 角回综合征；**ankyloblepharon–ectodermal dysplasia–clefting s.,** 同 Hay-Wells s.；**anorexia-cachexia s.,** a systemic response to cancer and certain other conditions, occurring as a result of a poorly understood relationship between anorexia and cachexia, manifested by malnutrition, weight loss, muscular weakness, acidosis, and toxemia 厌食 - 恶病质综合征，机体对肿瘤的一种全身性反应，系因食欲缺乏与恶病质之间的某种关系而产生，但对这种关系尚所知甚少；其表现为营养不良、体重减轻、肌肉软弱无力、酸中毒及毒血症；**anterior cord s.,** anterior spinal artery s. 脊髓前索综合征；**anterior interosseous s.,** a complex of symptoms caused by a lesion of the anterior interosseous nerve, usually resulting from a fracture or laceration 前骨间综合征，由前骨间神经损伤引起的综合征，通常由骨折或裂伤引起；**anterior spinal artery s.,** localized injury to the anterior portion of the spinal cord, characterized by complete paralysis and hypalgesia and hypesthesia to the level of the lesion, but with relative preservation of posterior column sensations of touch, position, and vibration 脊髓前动脉综合征，脊髓前部的局部损伤，其特征是完全瘫痪、痛觉减退和对病变水平的感觉减退，但对后柱感觉的触摸、位置和振动有相对保留；**Apert s.,** an autosomal dominant disorder due to mutation of a fibroblast growth factor receptor, characterized by oxycephaly and syndactyly, often with other skeletal deformities and intellectual disability 阿佩尔综合征，尖头并指（趾），由于成纤维细胞生长因子受体突变引起的一种常染色体显性疾病，以头畸形和间指畸形为特征，常伴有其他骨骼畸形和智力障碍；**Asherman s.,** persistent amenorrhea and secondary sterility due to intrauterine adhesions and synechiae, usually as a result of uterine curettage 子宫腔粘连综合征，由于子宫内粘连和闭锁引起的持续闭经与继发性不孕，通常为子宫刮术的不良后果；**Asperger s.,** a pervasive developmental disorder resembling autistic disorder, being characterized by severe impairment of social interactions and by restricted interests and behaviors; however, patients are not delayed in development of language, cognitive function, and self-help skills 阿斯佩格综合征，一种类似孤独症的普遍性发展障碍，其特征为严重的社会交往障碍，兴趣和行为受到限制；然而，患者在语言、认知功能和自助技能的发展上没有延迟；**Bannayan-Riley-Ruvalcaba s.**, a clinically heterogeneous autosomal dominant disorder, characterized predominantly by hamartomatous intestinal polyps, hemangiomas, lipomas, macrocephaly, café-au-lait spots on the penis, and thyroid problems BRR 综合征，一种临床上不均一的常染色体显性遗传疾病，主要表现为错构瘤性肠息肉、血管瘤、脂肪瘤、大头畸形、阴茎上的咖啡色斑点和甲状腺问题；**Bannayan-Zonana s.**, 同 Bannayan-Riley-Ruvalcaba s；**Bardet-Biedl s.**, a genetically and clinically heterogeneous autosomal recessive disorder of ciliary function, with pigmentary retinopathy, truncal obesity, cognitive impairment, polydactyly, male hypogonadism or female genitourinary malformations, and renal abnormalities 巴尔得 - 别德尔综合征，一种遗传和临床上不均一的常染色体隐性纤毛功能紊乱，伴有色素性视网膜病变、躯干肥胖、认知障碍、多指畸形、男性性腺功能减退或女性生殖泌尿系统畸形以及肾异常；**Barrett s.**, peptic ulcer of the lower esophagus, often with stricture, due to the presence of columnar-lined epithelium, which may contain functional mucous cells, parietal cells, or chief cells in the esophagus instead of normal squamous cell epithelium 巴雷特综合征，为食管下段消化性溃疡，常伴有狭窄，系由于食管内存在柱状上皮细胞，其中可能含有功能性黏液细胞、壁细胞或主细胞，取代了正常的鳞状上皮细胞所致；**Bart s.**, a clinical variant of dominant epidermolysis bullosa dystrophica, characterized by congenital localized absence of the skin, blister formation after mechanical trauma, and nail dystrophy 巴氏综合征，一种显性大疱性营养不良性表皮松解的临床变异，其特征是先天性局部皮肤缺失、机械创伤后形成水疱和指甲营养不良；**Bartter s.**, a group of autosomal recessive disorders of impaired salt reabsorption in the thick ascending loop of Henle, characterized by pronounced salt wasting, hypokalemic metabolic alkalosis, growth retardation, and hypercalciuria. It is often subdivided into more severe, earlyonset, antenatal forms; less severe "classic" forms; and Gitelman syndrome 巴特综合征（先天性醛固酮增多症），一组常染色体隐性疾病；**basal cell nevus s.**, an autosomal dominant syndrome characterized by the development in early life of numerous basal cell carcinomas, in association with abnormalities of the

skin, bone, nervous system, eyes, and reproductive tract 基底细胞痣综合征，为常染色体显性遗传性症候群，特征为生命早期发生多发性基底细胞癌，伴发有皮肤异常（尤其是手和足的一种特殊的红斑性凹陷水肿），及骨、神经系统、眼和生殖道的异常；**Bassen-Kornzweig s.**, abetalipoproteinemia 棘状红细胞 - β - 脂蛋白缺乏症；**battered child s.**, multiple traumatic lesions of the bones and soft tissues of children, often accompanied by subdural hematomas, willfully inflicted by an adult 受虐儿童综合征，儿童出现的无法解释或不适当解释的身体创伤及其他严重表现，为累遭（通常系父母）虐待所致；**Beckwith-Wiedemann s.**, a congenital hereditary disorder of overgrowth with predisposition to tumor formation, usually characterized by exomphalos, macroglossia, and gigantism, often associated with organomegaly, adrenocortical cytomegaly, and renal medullary dysplasia 贝 - 维综合征，表现度不等的先天性常染色体显性遗传综合征，特征有脐疝、巨舌、巨大发育，常伴有内脏肥大，肾上腺皮质细胞肥大，及肾髓质发育不良；**Behçet s.**, severe uveitis and retinal vasculitis, optic atrophy, and aphtha-like lesions of the mouth and genitalia, often with other signs and symptoms suggesting a diffuse vasculitis; it most often affects young males 白塞综合征，贝赫切特综合征，严重的葡萄膜炎和视网膜血管炎、视神经萎缩、口腔和生殖器的口疮样病变，常伴有其他症状和体征，提示弥漫性血管炎；最常见于年轻男性；**Bernard-Soulier s.**, a hereditary coagulation disorder marked by mild thrombocytopenia, giant and morphologically abnormal platelets that lack the receptor necessary for binding von Willebrand factor, hemorrhagic tendency, prolonged bleeding time, and purpura 巨血小板综合征，一种遗传性凝血障碍，以轻度血小板减少、巨血小板和形态异常血小板为特征；**Bing-Neel s.**, the central nervous system manifestations of Waldenström macroglobulinemia, possibly including encephalopathy, hemorrhage, stroke, convulsions, delirium, and coma 宾 - 尼综合征（神经精神病巨球蛋白症综合征）；**Birt-Hogg-Dube s.**, an autosomal dominant disorder of proliferation of ectodermal and mesodermal components, due to mutation of a tumor suppressor protein and occurring as multiple fibrofolliculomas on the head, chest, back, and arms; kidney tumors; spontaneous pneumothorax; and intestinal polyposis Birt-Hogg-Dube 综合征，一种常染色体显性遗传的外胚层和中胚层成分增殖障碍，由于肿瘤抑制蛋白的突变，在头部、胸部、背部和手臂、肾肿瘤、自发性气胸和肠息肉上发生多发性纤维滤泡瘤；**Björnstad s.**, an autosomal recessive disorder due to mutation of a mitochondrial respiratory chain protein, characterized by congenital sensorineural deafness and pili torti Björnstad 综合征，一种由线粒体呼吸链蛋白突变引起的常染色体隐性疾病，以先天性感音神经性耳聋和毛滴虫为特征；**Blackfan-Diamond s.,** Diamond-Blackfan anemia 布 - 戴综合征（纯红细胞再生障碍性贫血）；**blind loop s.,** stasis s. 盲襻综合征；**Bloom s.,** an autosomal recessive disorder with chromosome instability due to mutation of a DNA helicase; there are erythema and telangiectasia in a butterfly distribution on the face, photosensitivity, well-proportioned dwarfism, abnormal immunoglobulins, and a high incidence of malignancy 布卢姆综合征（面部红斑侏儒综合征），为常染色体隐性遗传病，在婴儿期逐步显现，包括面部蝶形分布的毛细血管扩张性红斑，对光敏感，及出生前发生的侏儒症。染色体结构及免疫球蛋白有异常，而且恶性肿瘤发生率高；**blue toe s.,** skin necrosis and ischemic gangrene manifest as a blue color of the toes, resulting from arterial occlusion, usually caused by emboli, thrombi, or injury 蓝趾综合征，皮肤坏死和缺血性坏疽表现为脚趾呈蓝色，由动脉阻塞引起，通常由栓塞、血栓或损伤引起；**Boerhaave s.,** spontaneous rupture of the esophagus 布尔哈弗综合征；（特发性食管破裂综合征）；**BOR s.,** 同 branchio-oto-renal s.；**Börjeson s., Börjeson-Forssman-Lehmann s.,** an X-linked recessive disorder characterized by severe intellectual disability, epilepsy, hypogonadism, hypometabolism, marked obesity, swelling of the subcutaneous tissues of the face, and large ears 布 - 弗 - 勒综合征，一种以严重智力残疾、癫痫、性腺功能减退、新陈代谢不足、明显肥胖、面部皮下组织肿胀和大耳朵为特征的 X 连锁隐性疾病；**bowel bypass s.,** a syndrome of dermatosis and arthritis occurring some time after jejunoileal bypass, probably caused by immune reponse to bacterial overgrowth in the bypassed bowel 肠旁路综合征，空肠旁路术后一段时间发生的皮肤病和关节炎综合征，可能是由旁路肠细菌过度生长的免疫反应引起的；**Bradbury-Eggleston s.,** a progressive syndrome of postural hypotension without tachycardia but with visual disturbances, impotence, hypohidrosis, lowered metabolic rate, dizziness, syncope, and slow pulse; due to impaired peripheral vasoconstriction Bradbury-Eggleston 综合征，无心动过速的体位性低血压进行性综合征，但伴有视觉障碍、阳痿、多汗、代谢率降低、头晕、晕厥和脉搏缓慢；由周围血管收缩受损引起；**bradycardia-tachycardia s., bradytachy s.,** a clinical manifestation of the sick sinus syndrome characterized by alternating periods of bradycardia and tachycardia 心动过缓 - 心动过速综合征；**branchio-oto-renal s.,** BOR s.; an autosomal dominant disorder due to mutation in any of several genes involved in embryonic development; characterized by branchial arch anomalies, hearing loss, and structural and functional renal abnormalities 鳃 - 耳 - 肾综合征，一种常染色体显性遗传疾病，由胚胎发育中的几个基因突变引起，以鳃弓异常、听力丧失、肾结构和功能性异常为特征；**Brown-Séquard s.,** ipsilateral paralysis and loss of discriminatory and joint sensation, and contralateral loss of pain and temperature sensation; due to damage to one-half of the spinal cord 布朗 - 塞卡综合征，脊髓半切综合征；**Brown-Vialetto-van Laere s.,** an autosomal recessive disorder of progressive bulbar palsy with any of several cranial nerve disorders 布 - 维 - 范综合征，一种进行性延髓麻痹的常染色体隐性遗传病，伴有多种颅神经疾病；**Brugada s.,** an autosomal dominant, genetically heterogeneous ion channelopathy characterized by sudden, idiopathic ventricular fibrillation in an apparently healthy person, often resulting in death 布鲁加达综合征，一种常染色体显性遗传异质性离子通道病，特征是明显健康的人发生突发性特发性室颤，常导致死亡；**Budd-Chiari s.,** symptomatic obstruction or occlusion of the hepatic veins, causing hepatomegaly, abdominal pain and tenderness, intractable ascites, mild jaundice, and eventually portal hypertension and liver failure 巴德 - 基亚里综合征，布 - 加综合征，症状性肝静脉阻塞或闭塞，引起肝肿大、腹痛和压痛、顽固性腹水、轻度黄疸，最终导致门静脉高压和肝衰竭；**burning mouth s.,** any of various conditions of burning sensations in the mouth, such as in perimenopausal women or in persons using antibiotics for long periods. Canada-Cronkhite s., 同 Cronkhite-Canada s.；**capillary leak s.,** extravasation of plasma fluid and proteins into the extravascular space, resulting in sometimes fatal hypotension and reduced organ perfusion; an adverse effect of interleukin-2 therapy 毛细血管渗漏综合征，血浆和蛋白质外渗到血管外，有时导致致命的低血压和器官灌注减少；白细胞介素 -2 治疗的副作用；**carcinoid s.,** a symptom complex associated with carcinoid tumors, marked by attacks of cyanotic flushing of the skin and by watery diarrhea, bronchoconstrictive attacks, lesions of the heart valves, edema, and ascites. Symptoms are caused by tumor secretion of serotonin, prostaglandins, and other biologically active substances 类癌综合征，一种与类癌肿瘤相关的综合症状，以皮肤发绀、腹泻、支气管收缩、心脏瓣膜病变、水肿和腹水为特征。症状是由肿瘤分泌的血清素、前列腺素和其他生物活性物质引起的；**carotid sinus s.,** syncope sometimes associated with convulsions due to overactivity of the carotid sinus reflex when pressure is applied to one or both carotid sinuses 颈动脉窦综合征当对一个或两个颈动脉窦施加压力时，有时由于颈动脉窦反射过度活动而导致抽搐；**carpal tunnel s.,** pain and burning or tingling paresthesias in the fingers and hand, sometimes extending to the elbow, due to compression of the median nerve in the carpal tunnel 腕管综合征，由于腕管正中神经的压迫，手指和手的疼痛和灼痛或刺痛感觉一直延伸到肘部；**Carpenter s.,** acrocephalopolysyndactyly, type Ⅱ; an autosomal recessive disorder due to mutation of a negative regulator involved in developmental signaling; characterized by acrocephaly, polysyndactyly, brachydactyly, mild obesity, intellectual disability, hypogonadism, and other anomalies 尖头多趾并趾（畸形）；**cat-eye s. (CES),** partial trisomy or tetrasomy of chromosome 22, which may be mosaic; characterized by coloboma and down-slanting palpebral fissures ("cat eye"), with variable additional manifestations, including analatresia, preauricular skin tags or fistulas, hypertelorism, congenital heart disease, skeletal abnormalities, and renal malformations 猫眼综合征，22号染色体的部分三体或四体，可能呈镶嵌状；特征为缺损和下斜的眼睑裂口（"猫眼"），具有可变的附加表现，包括肛门闭锁、耳前皮肤标签或瘘管、高色素血症、先天性心脏病、骨骼畸形和肾畸形；**central cord s.,** a syndrome resulting from injury to the cervical or upper thoracic spinal cord that damages the central cord while sparing the more external fibers, characterized by disproportionately more weakness or paralysis in the upper extremity than in the lower 脊髓中央损伤综合征，颈或胸上脊髓损伤引起的综合征，在保留更多外部纤维的同时损伤中心脊髓，其特征是上肢比下肢更虚弱或瘫痪；**cerebrocostomandibular s.,** a rare congenital anomaly of severe micrognathia and costovertebral abnormalities, with palatal defects, prenatal and postnatal growth deficiencies, and intellectual disability secondary to neonatal respiratory distress 脑、肋骨、下颌骨综合征，一种罕见的先天性畸形，表现为严重的小颌骨和肋椎畸形，伴有腭部缺陷、产前和产后生长缺陷以及继于新生儿呼吸窘迫的智力障碍；**cerebrohepatorenal s.,** 同 Zellweger s.; **cervical rib s.,** inferior thoracic aperture syndrome caused by a cervical rib 颈肋综合征；**Cestan-Chenais s.,** an association of contralateral hemiplegia, contralateral hemianesthesia, ipsilateral lateropulsion and hemiasynergia, Horner syndrome, and ipsilateral laryngoplegia, due to scattered lesions of the pyramid, sensory tract, inferior cerebellar peduncle, nucleus ambiguus, and oculopupillary center Cestan-Chenais 综合征，因

锥体、感觉束、小脑下脚、疑核和眼瞳孔中枢的散在病变，而产生对侧偏瘫、对侧半身感觉异常、同侧横行与偏身协同不能、Horner 征及同侧喉麻痹；**Charcot s.,** 1. amyotrophic lateral sclerosis 肌萎缩侧索硬化综合征；2. intermittent claudication 间歇性跛行；**CHARGE s.,** a syndrome of associated defects, including coloboma of the eye, heart anomaly, choanal atresia, retardation, and genital and ear anomalies, and often including facial palsy, cleft palate, and dysphagia CHARGE 综合征，一种相关缺陷综合征，包括眼缺损、心脏异常、后鼻孔闭锁、发育迟缓和生殖器和耳异常，通常包括面瘫、腭裂及吞咽困难；**Chédiak-Higashi s.,** a usually lethal autosomal recessive disorder due to mutation in a regulator of lysosomal trafficking; characterized by oculocutaneous albinism, massive leukocyte inclusions (giant lysosomes), histiocytic infiltration of multiple body organs, pancytopenia, hepatosplenomegaly, recurrent or persistent bacterial infections, and predisposition to malignant lymphoma Chédiak-Higashi 综合征，一种致死性常染色体隐性遗传病，由溶酶体运输调节因子的突变引起以眼皮肤白化病，大量白细胞内含物（巨型溶酶体）、多种器官的组织浸润，全血细胞减少、肝脾胀、反复或持续性细胞感染和恶性淋巴瘤易感性为特征；**Chinese restaurant s.,** transient arterial dilatation due to ingestion of monosodium glutamate, which is sometimes used liberally in seasoning Chinese food, marked by throbbing head, light-headedness, tightness of the jaw, neck, and shoulders, and backache 味精综合征，一种与动脉扩张有关的暂时性症候群，系因食入食物中大量应用的味精谷氨酸钠所致；其特征为头震颤，头昏眼花，颌、颈与肩部紧缩感及背痛；**Chotzen s.,** 同 Saethre-Chotzen s.; **Christ-Siemens-Touraine s.,** anhidrotic ectodermal dysplasia 基 - 西 - 都氏综合征；**chronic fatigue s.,** persistent debilitating fatigue of recent onset, with greatly reduced physical activity and some combination of muscle weakness, sore throat, mild fever, tender lymph nodes, headaches, and depression, not attributable to any other known causes; it is of controversial etiology 慢性疲劳综合征，近期发作的持续性虚弱性疲劳，体力活动大大减少，并伴有肌肉无力、咽喉痛、轻度发热、淋巴结肿痛、头痛和抑郁等症状，并非由任何其他已知原因引起；其病因有争议；**Churg-Strauss s.,** allergic granulomatous angiitis; a systemic form of necrotizing vasculitis in which there is prominent lung involvementytf 许尔许斯特劳斯综合征，变应性肉芽肿病脉管炎，一种系统性的坏死性血管炎，其中有明显的肺部受累；**chylomicronemia s.,** familial hyperchylomicronemia 乳糜微粒血症综合征；**Coffin-Lowry s.,** an X-linked

S

dominant syndrome of severe intellectual disability, growth retardation, and muscle, ligament, and skeletal abnormalities 科 - 洛综合征，严重智力残疾、生长迟缓、肌肉、韧带和骨骼异常的 X 连锁显性综合征；**Coffin-Siris s.**, hypoplasia or absence of the nails of the fifth fingers and toes associated with growth and mental deficiencies, coarse facies, mild microcephaly, hypotonia, lax joints, and mild hirsutism 科 - 西综合征第五指（趾）的指（趾）甲发育不全或缺失，与生长和精神缺陷、面容粗糙、轻度小头畸形、张力减退、关节松弛和轻度多毛有关；**compartmental s.**, a condition in which increased tissue pressure in a confined anatomic space causes decreased blood flow leading to ischemia and dysfunction of contained myoneural elements, marked by pain, muscle weakness, sensory loss, and palpable tenseness in the involved compartment; ischemia can lead to necrosis resulting in permanent impairment of function 腔隙综合征，在有限的解剖空间内组织内压力增加，使所包含的肌神经成分因血流减少导致缺血及功能障碍而产生的症状，特点为疼痛，肌肉软弱无力，感觉丧失及触痛。缺血可导致坏死而发生功能永久性损害；**complex regional pain s. (CRPS)**, a chronic pain syndrome, usually affecting an extremity, and characterized by intense burning pain, changes in skin color and texture, increased skin temperature and sensitivity, sweating, edema, and, in some cases, osteoporosis. It is categorized as type 1 (without demonstrable nerve injury; called also *reflex sympathetic dystrophy*), and type 2 (with nerve injury; called also *causalgia*) 复合性区域疼痛综合征，一种慢性疼痛综合征，通常影响肢体，以剧烈的灼痛、皮肤颜色和质地的变化、皮肤温度和敏感性升高、出汗、水肿和骨质疏松为特征。分为 1 型（无明显神经损伤）也称为反射性交感神经营养不良）和 2 型（有神经损伤；也称为致痛）；**compulsive hoarding s.**, a compulsive urge to acquire possessions and an inability to voluntarily discard them, even when they have no practical value, resulting in a long-term accumulation of clutter that makes living and work spaces unavailable 强迫囤积综合征；**congenital rubella s.**, transplacental infection of the fetus with rubella, usually in the first trimester of pregnancy, as a consequence of maternal infection, resulting in various developmental anomalies in the newborn infant 先天性风疹综合征，胎儿经胎盘感染风疹，通常在妊娠早期，由于母体感染，导致新生儿出现各种发育异常；**Conn s.**, primary aldosteronism Conn 综合征；**Cornelia de Lange s. (CdLS)**, de Lange s.; a congenital genetic syndrome, usually arising as a de novo mutation; characterized by severe intellectual

disability; developmental and growth retardation; characteristic facies, including depressed nasal bridge and anteverted nares, synophrys, long, curly eyelashes, and low anterior hairline; and often upper limb anomalies 阿姆斯特丹型侏儒征，德朗热综合征，一种先天性遗传综合征，以严重智力障碍发育和生长迟缓为特征，表现为特征性面容，包括鼻梁凹陷和前倾鼻孔、连眉、长而卷曲的睫毛和低前倾的发际线，常有上肢畸形；**cri du chat s.**, a congenital syndrome characterized by hypertelorism, microcephaly, severe mental deficiency, and a plaintive catlike cry, due to deletion of a variably sized portion of the short arm of hromosome 5 猫叫综合征，一种遗传性先天性症候群，特征为器官距离过远，小头，严重智能缺陷及痛苦的猫叫样哭泣，由于 5 号染色体短臂缺失引起；**Crigler-Najjar s.**, an autosomal recessive nonhemolytic jaundice due to absence of the hepatic enzyme glucuronosyltransferase, marked by excessive unconjugated bilirubin in the blood, kernicterus, and severe central nervous system disorders 克里格勒 - 纳贾尔综合征，先天性非梗阻性非溶血性黄疸；**s. of crocodile tears**, spontaneous lacrimation occurring parallel with the normal salivation of eating, and associated with facial paralysis; it seems to be due to straying of regenerating nerve fibers, some of those destined for the salivary glands going to the lacrimal glands 鳄泪综合征；**Cronkhite-Canada s.**, multiple polyps of the gastrointestinal tract associated with ectodermal defects such as alopecia and onychodystrophy 卡纳达 - 克朗凯特综合征；**Crouzon s.**, a hereditary disorder characterized by acrocephaly, exophthalmos, hypertelorism, strabismus, parrot-beaked nose, and hypoplastic maxilla Crouzon 综合征，一种遗传性疾病，特征是头端畸形、眼球突出、高眼压、斜视、鹦鹉喙鼻和上颌骨发育不全；**Crow-Fukase s.**, 同 POEMS s.；**crush s.**, the edema, oliguria, and other symptoms of renal failure that follow crushing of a part, especially a large muscle mass 挤压综合征；**Cruveilhier-Baumgarten s.**, cirrhosis with portal hypertension associated with congenital patency of the umbilical and paraumbilical veins 克 - 鲍综合征，肝硬化合并门静脉高压与脐静脉及脐旁静脉先天性未闭有关；**Currarino s.**, a complex of congenital anomalies in the anococcygeal region, consisting of partial sacral agenesis, presacral mass, and rectal malformations, often accompanied by gynecologic and renal malformations Currarino 综合征，一种肛门区的先天性异常，由部分骶骨发育不全、骶前肿块和直肠畸形组成，常伴有妇科和肾脏畸形；**Cushing s.**, a condition more often seen in females, due to hyperadrenocorticism resulting from neoplasms of the adrenal cortex or anterior pituitary; or to prolonged excessive intake of glucocorticoids for therapeutic purposes (*iatrogenic Cushing s. or Cushing s. medicamentosus*). Symptoms may include adiposity of the face, neck, and trunk, kyphosis from softening of the spine, amenorrhea, hypertrichosis (in females), impotence (in males), dusky complexion with purple markings, hypertension, polycythemia, abdominal and back pain, and muscular weakness 库欣综合征，皮质醇增多症；**Da Costa s.**, neurocirculatory asthenia 达科斯塔综合征；**Dandy-Walker s.**, 丹迪 - 沃克综合征，参见 *malformation* 下词条；**Dejerine-Sottas s.**, 代 - 索尔综合征，参见 *disease* 下词条；**de Lange s.**, 同 Cornelia de Lange s.；**Denys-Drash s. (DDS)**, an autosomal dominant disorder due to mutation of a zinc finger DNA-binding protein required for normal formation of the genitourinary system and mesothelial tissues; characterized by nephropathy leading to renal failure, Wilms tumor, and disorders of sex development 德尼 - 德拉什综合征，一种常染色体显性遗传疾病，由生殖泌尿系统和间皮组织正常形成所需的锌指 DNA 结合蛋白突变引起；以肾病导致肾衰竭、Wilms 肿瘤和性发育障碍为特征；**dialysis disequilibrium s.**, symptoms such as headache, nausea, muscle cramps, nervous irritability, drowsiness, and convulsions during or after overly rapid hemodialysis or peritoneal dialysis, resulting from an osmotic shift of water into the brain 透析失衡综合征，由于水渗透进入大脑而引起的过度快速血液透析或腹膜透析期间或之后出现头痛、恶心、肌肉痉挛、神经过敏、嗜睡和抽搐等症状；**DiGeorge s.**, a congenital disorder in which defective development of the third and fourth pharyngeal pouches results in hypoplasia or aplasia of the thymus and parathyroid glands, often with congenital heart defects, anomalies of the great vessels, esophageal atresia, and abnormalities of facial structures. There may be hypocalcemic tetany or seizures due to lack of parathyroid hormone and deficiency of cell-mediated immunity. It is usually a phenotype of 22q11 deletion syndrome 迪格奥尔格综合征，第三、四咽囊综合征，一种先天性疾病，系第三和第四咽囊发育缺陷，导致胸腺与甲状旁腺发育不全或缺如，常伴有先天性心脏缺陷、大血管异常、食管闭锁畸形及面部结构异常。依甲状旁腺与胸腺发育不全的程度，可因甲状旁腺激素缺乏而产生低血钙手足搐搦或癫痫发作；通常是 22q11 缺失综合征的一种表现形式；**disconnection s.**, any neurologic disorder caused by an interruption in impulse transmission along cerebral fiber pathways 分离综合征，任何因脑纤维传导脉冲中断而引起的神经系统疾病；**Donohue s.**, a rare, lethal, autosomal recessive condition caused by defects in the insulin receptor and characterized by slow physical and mental development, elfin facies, and endocrine abnormalities such as hyperinsulinemia and precocious puberty 矮妖精貌综合征，一种罕见的致死性的常染色体隐性疾病，其特征是体格和智力均发育迟缓、精灵面容和内分泌异常如高胰岛素血症和性早熟；又称 *leprechaunism*；**Down s.**, small, anteroposteriorly flattened skull, short, flat-bridge nose, epicanthal fold, short phalanges, widened spaces between the first and second digits of hands and feet, and moderate to severe intellectual disability, with Alzheimer disease developing in the fourth or fifth decade; due to trisomy of chromosome 21 唐氏综合征，21 三体综合征；**Duane s. (DS), Duane retraction s. (DRS) (DURS)**, a clinically heterogeneous, congenital eye movement disorder, usually unilateral, due to a defect in the development of cranial nerve VI and characterized by some combination of limitation or absence of abduction and restriction of adduction, with retraction of the globe and narrowing of the palpebral fissure on attempted adduction 杜安后缩综合征，眼球后缩综合征，为遗传性先天性综合征，一种临床上不均一的先天性眼球运动障碍，通常是单侧的，由于脑神经Ⅵ发育缺陷，其特征是有局限性或无外展和内收受限的组合，并伴有视网膜病变，尝试内收时眼球牵引及睑裂变窄；**Dubin-Johnson s.**, an autosomal recessive form of conjugated hyperbilirubinemia characterized by jaundice, deposition of melanin-like pigment in hepatocytes, and in some cases hepatosplenomegaly, with otherwise normal liver function 杜宾 - 约翰逊综合征，一种常染色体隐性遗传的结合性高胆红素血症，以黄疸、肝细胞内黑色素样色素沉积为特征，在某些情况下还伴有肝功能正常的肝脾肿大；**dumping s.**, nausea, weakness, sweating, palpitation, syncope, often a sensation of warmth, and sometimes diarrhea, occurring after ingestion of food in patients who have undergone partial gastrectomy 倾倒综合征，部分胃切除或行胃空肠吻合术后的患者，在进食之后表现恶心、乏力、出汗、心悸、不同程度的晕厥，常有热感，有时有腹泻等；**dyscontrol s.**, a pattern of episodic abnormal and often violent and uncontrollable social behavior with little or no provocation; it may have an organic cause or be associated with abuse of a psychoactive substance 控制障碍综合征，一种偶发性异常的、经常是暴力的、不可控制的社会行为，很少或没有挑衅；它可能有器质性原因或与滥用精神活性物质有关；**dysmaturity s.**, 同 postmaturity s.；**Eaton-Lambert s.**, 同 Lambert-Eaton myasthenic s.；**ectrodactyly–ectodermal dysplasia–clefting s., EEC s.**, an autosomal dominant disorder of ectodermal tissue development, characterized by ectrodactyly, ectodermal dysplasia with hypopigmentation of skin and hair, and other hair, nail, tooth, lip, and palate abnormalities; hearing loss and genitourinary anomalies are also frequent 缺指（趾）- 外胚层发育异常 - 唇腭裂综合征，一种外胚层组织发育的常染色体显性疾病，特征为多发性外胚层发育不良，皮肤和头发色素沉着不足，以及其他头发、指甲、牙齿、嘴唇和腭部异常；听力丧失和生殖泌尿系统异常也很常见；**Ehlers-Danlos s.**, a group of inherited disorders of connective tissue, varying clinically and biochemically, in mode of inheritance, and in severity. Manifestations include hyperextensible skin and joints, easy bruisability, friability of tissues, bleeding, and poor wound healing; some types also show cardiovascular, orthopedic, intestinal, or ocular defects 埃勒斯 - 当洛斯综合征，皮肤弹性过度综合征，一组遗传性结缔组织疾病，在临床和生物化学上有不同的遗传方式，主要表现为皮肤和关节过度伸展、组织脆性增加、容易损伤出血、伤口难以愈合，有些类型还表现为心血管、骨科、肠道或眼部缺损；**Eisenmenger s.**, ventricular septal defect with pulmonary hypertension and cyanosis due to right-to-left (reversed) shunting of blood. Sometimes defined as pulmonary hypertension (pulmonary vascular disease) and cyanosis with the shunt being at the atrial, ventricular, or great vessel area 艾森门格综合征，为室间隔缺损合并肺动脉高压及因血液自右至左分流（反向流动）引起的紫绀；有时为肺动脉高压（肺血管性疾病）及主动脉、心室或大血管区存在分流而引起；**EMG s.**, 同 BeckwithWiedemann s.Escobar s., 同 multiple pterygium s.; **excited skin s.**, nonspecific cutaneous hyperirritability of the back, sometimes occurring when multiple positive reactions are elicited in patch test screening of a battery of substances 激发性皮肤综合征，背部非特异性皮肤过敏，有时在对一组物质进行贴片试验筛选时引发多重阳性反应；**exomphalos-macroglossia-gigantism s.**, 同 Beckwith-Wiedemann s.；**extrapyramidal s.**, any of a group of clinical disorders considered to be due to malfunction in the extrapyramidal system and marked by abnormal involuntary movements; included are parkinsonism, athetosis, and chorea 锥体外综合征，任何一组被认为是由于锥体外系功能紊乱引起的临床疾病，以异常的非自愿运动为特征；包括帕金森病、动脉粥样硬化和舞蹈病；**Faber s.**, hypochromic anemia Faber 综合征，胃液缺乏性贫血；**Fanconi s.**, any of a broad group of disorders marked by generalized dysfunction of proximal renal tubule transport, with impaired reabsorption of sodium, bicarbonate, calcium, magne-

sium, potassium, chloride, phosphate, glucose, amino acids, uric acid, low-molecular-weight proteins and peptides, and organic acids; it may be either complete or partial, and both primary (genetic or sporadic) and secondary (genetic or secondary to exogenous agents) forms exist 范科尼综合征，以近端肾小管转运功能障碍为特征的一大类失调症，包括钠、碳酸氢盐、钙、镁、钾、氯化物、磷酸盐、葡萄糖、氨基酸、尿酸、低分子量蛋白质和肽以及有机酸的重吸收受损；它可以是完全的或部分的，既有原发性（遗传性或散发性）也有继发性（遗传性或继发性）形式；**Felty s.**, a syndrome of splenomegaly with chronic rheumatoid arthritis and leukopenia; there are usually pigmented spots on the skin of the lower extremities, and sometimes there is other evidence of hypersplenism, such as anemia or thrombocytopenia 费尔蒂综合征，类风湿关节炎伴脾大白细胞减少，血蛋白过少性贫血，慢性类风湿关节炎和白血球减少症脾肿大的综合征；下肢皮肤上通常有色素斑点，有时还有其他脾功能亢进的症状，如贫血或血小板减少症；**fetal alcohol s.**, a syndrome of altered prenatal growth and morphogenesis, occurring in infants born of women who were chronically alcoholic during pregnancy; it includes maxillary hypoplasia, prominence of the forehead and mandible, short palpebral fissures, microophthalmia, epicanthal folds, severe growth retardation, intellectual disability, and microcephaly 胎儿酒精综合征，一种产前生长和形态发生改变的综合征，见于怀孕期间长期酗酒的妇女所生的婴儿，包括上颌发育不全、前额和下颌骨突出、眼睑短裂、微眼、花被皱褶、严重生长缓、智力障碍和小头畸形；**fetal hydantoin s.**, poor growth and development with craniofacial and skeletal abnormalities, caused by prenatal exposure to hydantoin analogues, including phenytoin 胎儿乙内酰脲综合征，由于产前暴露于海因类似物（包括苯妥英钠）而导致的颅面和骨骼异常的生长发育不良；**floppy infant s.**, abnormal posture in an infant suspended prone, the limbs and head hanging down; due to any of numerous conditions, particularly perinatal injury to the brain or spinal cord, spinal muscular atrophy, and various genetic disorders 婴儿松弛综合征，婴儿的姿势异常，呈悬垂的俯卧姿势，四肢和头部下垂；由多种情况导致，特别是围产期脑或脊髓损伤、脊髓肌肉萎缩和各种遗传性疾病；**Foix-Alajouanine s.**, a fatal necrotizing myelopathy characterized by necrosis of the gray matter of the spinal cord, thickening of the walls of the spinal vessels, and abnormal spinal fluid 亚急性坏死性脊髓炎，一种致命的坏死性脊髓病，以脊髓灰质坏死、脊髓血管壁增厚和脊髓液异常为特征；**fragile X s.**, an X-linked syndrome char-

S

acterized by intellectual disability, enlarged testes, high forehead, and enlarged jaw and ears in most males and mild intellectual disability in many heterozygous females. It is a triplet repeat disorder, associated with expansion of CGG sequences in the promoter region of a gene expressed in brain cells and believed to be involved in translation 脆性 X 染色体综合征，一种 X 连锁综合征，以大多数男性的智力障碍、睾丸增大、前额高、下颌和耳朵增大，以及许多杂合子女性的轻度智力残疾为特征。这是一种三重态重复障碍，与 CGG 序列的扩增有关；**Franceschetti s.,** the complete form of mandibulofacial dysostosis 下颌颜面部发育不全综合征；**galactorrhea-amenorrhea s.,** amenorrhea and galactorrhea, sometimes associated with increased levels of prolactin 乳溢 - 闭经综合征，有时与催乳素水平升高有关；**Ganser s.,** the giving of approximate answers to questions, commonly associated with amnesia, disorientation, perceptual disturbances, fugue, and conversion symptoms 甘瑟综合征，对问题给出近似的答案，通常与健忘、定向障碍、知觉障碍、神游和转换症状有关；**Garcin s.,** unilateral paralysis of most or all of the cranial nerves due to a tumor at the base of the skull or in the nasopharynx 加桑综合征，由于颅底或鼻咽肿瘤导致的大部分或全部脑神经的单侧瘫痪；**Gardner s.,** a phenotypic variant of familial adenomatous polyposis characterized additionally by extracolonic lesions, including osteomas and skin and soft tissue tumors 加德纳综合征，遗传性肠肠肉综合征，主要表现为结肠息肉、软组织肿瘤和骨瘤三联征的综合征；**general adaptation s.,** the total of all nonspecific reactions of the body to prolonged systemic stress, comprising alarm, resistance, and exhaustion 一般适应综合征，全身对长期全身应激的所有非特异性反应的总和；**Gerstmann-Sträussler s., Gerstmann-Sträussler- Scheinker s.,** a rare autosomal dominant prion disease caused by any of numerous mutations in the gene encoding prion protein, having the common characteristics of multicentric amyloid plaques in the brain, with cognitive and motor disturbances 格 - 施综合征，一种罕见的常染色体显性遗传的朊病毒病，由编码朊病毒蛋白的基因突变引起，具有脑内多中心淀粉样斑块的共同特征，伴有以死亡为终点的认知和运动障碍；**Gianotti-Crosti s.,** monomorphous, usually nonpruritic, tan to red, flat-topped, firm papules forming a symmetric eruption on the face, buttocks, and limbs, including palms and soles, with malaise and low-grade fever; seen in young children and associated with viral infection 儿童丘疹性肢端皮炎，单态的，通常为非临床，棕褐色至红色，顶部平坦，在面部、臀部和四肢

（包括手掌和足底）形成不对称的丘疹，伴有不适和低热；见于幼儿，与病毒感染有关；**Gilbert s.,** an autosomal recessive disorder of bilirubin metabolism caused by mutation of the hepatic enzyme glucuronosyltransferase, characterized by a benign elevation of unconjugated bilirubin without liver damage or hematologic abnormalities 吉尔伯特综合征，一种由肝酶葡萄糖醛酸转移酶突变引起的常染色体隐性胆红素代谢紊乱遗传病，以未结合胆红素的良性升高为特征，无肝损伤或血液学异常；**Gilles de la Tourette s.,** a childhood-onset syndrome comprising both multiple motor and one or more vocal tics, often associated with obsessions, compulsions, hyperactivity, distractibility, and impulsivity; it may diminish or even remit in adolescence or adulthood 日勒德拉图雷特综合征，抽动秽语综合征，一种儿童期发病的综合征，包括多运动性抽搐和一次或多次发声性抽搐，常与强迫症、强迫、多动症、分心和冲动有关；可能在青春期或成年时减弱或减轻；**Gitelman s.,** a later-onset, milder variant form of Bartter syndrome, specifically characterized by hypocalciuria and hypomagnesemia Gitelman 综合征，一种后来发病的轻度巴特综合征变种，以低钙尿和低镁血症为特征；**Goodpasture s.,** glomerulonephritis with pulmonary hemorrhage and circulating antibodies against basement membranes, usually seen in young men and with a course of rapidly progressing renal failure, with hemoptysis, pulmonary infiltrates, and dyspnea 古德帕斯丘综合征，肺出血肾炎综合征，肾小球肾炎伴肺出血和基底膜循环抗体，通常见于年轻男性，并伴有进展迅速的肾衰竭、咯血、肺单胞浸润和呼吸困难；**Gradenigo s.,** sixth nerve palsy and unilateral headache in suppurative disease of the middle ear, due to involvement of the abducens and trigeminal nerves by direct spread of the infection 格拉代尼戈综合征，岩骨尖综合征，急性化脓性中耳炎累及外展神经和三叉神经；**gray s.,** a potentially fatal condition seen in neonates, particularly premature infants, due to a reaction to chloramphenicol, characterized by an ashen gray cyanosis, listlessness, weakness, and hypotension 灰婴综合征，一种可能致命的疾病，见于新生儿，特别是早产儿，由于对氯霉素的反应，表现为灰白发绀、无精打采、虚弱和低血压；**Guillain-Barré s.,** an acute, rapidly progressive, ascending motor neuron paralysis, beginning in the feet and ascending to the other muscles, often occurring after an enteric or respiratory infection 吉兰 - 巴雷综合征，一种急性的、快速进行的、上升的运动神经元麻痹，从脚开始上升到其他肌肉，通常发生在肠胃或呼吸道感染后；**Gunn s.,** unilateral ptosis of the eyelid, with movements of the affected eyelid associated with those of the jaw 联氏颌目瞬目综合征; **Hamman-Rich s.**, the acute form of idiopathic pulmonary fibrosis 阿曼 - 里奇综合征，急性间质性肺炎; **hantavirus pulmonary s.**, a sometimes fatal febrile illness caused by a hantavirus, characterized by variable respiratory symptoms followed by acute respiratory distress, sometimes progressing to respiratory failure 汉坦病毒肺综合征，一种由汉坦病毒引起的有时致命的发热性疾病，其特征是呼吸系统症状多变，随后伴有急性呼吸窘迫，有时发展为呼吸衰竭; **Harada s.**, 同 Vogt-Koyanagi-Harada s.; **Hay-Wells s.**, an autosomal dominant syndrome of ectodermal dysplasia, cleft lip and palate, and adhesions of the margins of the eyelids, accompanied by tooth, skin, and hair abnormalities 海 - 威综合征（睑缘粘连 - 外胚层发育不全 - 唇腭裂综合征）; **HELLP s.**, *h*emolysis, *e*levated *l*iver enzymes, and *l*ow *p*latelet count occurring in association with preeclampsia. HELLP 综合征，与子痫前期相关的溶血、肝酶升高和血小板计数降低; **Helweg-Larsen s.**, an inherited syndrome of anhidrosis present from birth and labyrinthitis occurring late in life 先天性无汗，迷走神经炎综合征; **hemolytic uremic s.**, a form of thrombotic microangiopathy with renal failure, hemolytic anemia, and severe thrombocytopenia and purpura 溶血尿毒症综合征，一种伴有肾衰竭、溶血性贫血和严重血小板减少和紫癜的血栓性微血管病; **Herrmann s.**, an inherited syndrome initially characterized by photomyogenic seizures and progressive deafness, with later development of diabetes mellitus, nephropathy, and mental deterioration Herrmann 综合征，一种遗传综合征，最初表现为光肌源性和进行性耳聋，随后发展为糖尿病、肾病和精神恶化; **HHH s.**, 同 hyperornithinemia-hyperammonemia-homocitrullinuria s.; **Hinman s.**, a psychogenic disorder seen in children, imitating a neurogenic bladder, consisting of detrusorsphincter dyssynergia without evidence of neural lesion 欣曼综合征，一种见于儿童的精神性疾病，类似于神经性膀胱，由逼尿肌、括约肌协同障碍组成，无神经损伤迹象; **Holmes-Adie s.**, 同 Adie s.; **Horner s., Horner-Bernard s.**, sinking in of the eyeball, ptosis of the upper lid, slight elevation of the lower lid, miosis, narrowing of the palpebral fissure, and anhidrosis and flushing of the affected side of the face; due to a brainstem lesion on the ipsilateral side that interrupts descending sympathetic nerves 霍纳综合征表现为病变侧眼球内陷、上睑下垂、下睑轻度抬高、瞳孔缩小眼裂变小伴同侧面部少汗和潮红; 见于颈上交感神经通路损伤及脑干网状结构的交感神经纤维损害; **Hughes-Stovin s.**, thrombosis of the pulmonary arteries and peripheral veins, characterized by headache, fever, cough, papilledema, and hemoptysis 休 - 斯综合征，肺动脉栓塞综合征，肺动脉和外周静脉血栓形成，以头痛、发热、咳嗽、乳头水肿和咯血为特征; **hungry bone s.**, a condition seen after parathyroidectomy in patients who had had hyperparathyroidism; rapid deposition of calcium in bones leads to hypocalcemia 骨饥饿综合征，甲状旁腺切除术后出现甲状旁腺功能亢进; 由于骨骼中钙的快速沉积导致低钙血症; **Hunter s.**, an X-linked recessive mucopolysaccharidosis due to deficiency of iduronate-2-sulfatase, characterized by excretion of dermatan sulfate and heparan sulfate in the urine; it resembles Hurler syndrome clinically but is less severe and does not involve corneal clouding 黏多糖贮积症 II 型综合征，一种由艾杜糖醛酸 -2- 硫酸酯酶缺乏引起的 X 连锁隐性黏多糖症，以尿液中硫酸皮肤素和硫酸乙酰肝素的排泄为特征; 临床上与黏多糖贮积症 IH 型相似，但病情较轻，不涉及角膜混浊; **Hurler s.**, an autosomal recessive mucopolysaccharidosis due to deficiency of the enzyme α-l-iduronidase, characterized by gargoyle-like facies, dwarfism, severe somatic and skeletal changes, severe intellectual disability, cloudy corneas, deafness, cardiovascular defects, hepatosplenomegaly, joint contractures, and death in childhood 黏多糖贮积症 IH 型，一种由于 α-L- 艾杜糖苷酸酶缺乏而引起的常染色体隐性黏多糖症，特征为畸形面容、侏儒症、严重的躯体和骨骼变化、严重的智力障碍、角膜混浊、耳聋、心血管缺陷、肝脾肿大、关节挛缩和儿童期死亡; **Hurler-Scheie s.**, a form of mucopolysaccharidosis I, allelic with the Hurler and Scheie syndromes and clinically intermediate between them; characterized by short stature, corneal clouding, stiff joints, and hepatosplenomegaly, without intellectual dysfunction 胡 - 沙综合征，α-L- 艾杜糖苷酶缺乏综合征，黏多糖贮积症 I 型的一种，与黏多糖贮积症 IH 型和黏多糖贮积症 IS 型等位，临床上介于两者之间; 特征是身材矮小、角膜混浊、关节僵硬、肝脾肿大、智力障碍; **Hutchinson-Gilford s., progeria** 哈 - 吉二氏综合征，早老症; **hypereosinophilic s.**, any of several diseases characterized by a massive increase in the number of eosinophils in the blood and bone marrow, with infiltration of other organs. Symptoms vary from mild to the often fatal outcome of eosinophilic leukemia 嗜酸细胞增多综合征，一种以血液和骨髓中嗜酸性粒细胞大量增多为特征的疾病，并伴有其他器官的浸润; 嗜酸粒细胞性白血病的症状从轻微到致命不等; **hyperornithinemia-hyperammonemia-homocitrullinuria s.**, an autosomal recessive disorder in which a defect in the mitochondrial ornithine transporter disturbs the cycle of ureagenesis; characterized by elevated plasma ornithine, postprandial hyperammonemia and homocitrullinuria, and aversion to protein ingestion; variable symptoms often include growth and developmental delays, learning disabilities, and periodic confusion and ataxia 高鸟氨酸血症 - 高氨血症 - 高瓜氨酸尿综合征，一种常染色体隐性遗传病，其中，线粒体鸟氨酸转运体的缺陷干扰了尿毒症的周期；其特征是血浆鸟氨酸升高、餐后高氨血症和高瓜氨酸尿，以及对蛋白质摄入的厌恶；可变症状通常包括生长和发育迟缓、学习障碍、周期性混乱和共济失调；**hyperventilation s.,** a complex of symptoms that accompany hypocapnia caused by hyperventilation, including palpitations, shortness of breath, light-headedness, heavy sweating, tingling sensations, and eventually vasomotor collapse and loss of consciousness 通气过度综合征，一种伴随由通气过度引起的低碳酸血症的复杂症状，包括心悸、呼吸短促、头昏、大汗、刺痛感，最终血管舒缩崩溃和意识丧失；**hypoplastic left heart s.,** congenital hypoplasia or atresia of the left ventricle, aortic or left atrioventricular valve, and ascending aorta, with respiratory distress, cardiac failure, and death in infancy 左心发育不全综合征，先天性左心室、主动脉或左房室瓣、升主动脉发育不全或闭锁，伴有呼吸窘迫、心力衰竭和婴儿期死亡；**impingement s.,** an overuse injury in the shoulder region resulting from the impingement of the acromion, coracoacromial ligament, coracoid process, or acromioclavicular joint on the rotator cuff 撞击综合征，肩峰、喙肩韧带、喙突或肩锁关节撞击肩袖造成肩关节过度使用性损 伤；**s. of inappropriate antidiuretic hormone (SIADH),** persistent hyponatremia, inappropriately elevated urine osmolality, caused by release of vasopressin (antidiuretic hormone) without a discernible stimulus 抗利尿激素分泌失调综合征，持续性低钠血症，尿渗透压不适当升高，由在无明显刺激的情况下释放血管升压素（抗利尿激素）引起；**inferior thoracic aperture s.,** any of several neurovascular syndromes due to compression of the subclavian artery, the brachial plexus nerve trunks, or the axillary vein or subclavian vein, by inferior thoracic aperture abnormalities such as a drooping pectoral girdle, a cervical rib or fibrous band, an abnormal first rib, or compression of the edge of the scalenus anterior muscle; characterized by muscle wasting, weakness, pain, and vascular abnormalities in the hand and arm 胸廓下口综合征，由于锁骨下动脉、臂丛神经干、腋静脉或锁骨下静脉的压迫而引起的几种神经血管综合征，由胸下开口异常引起，如胸带下垂、颈肋或纤维带、第一根肋

骨异常或斜角肌前肌边缘的压迫；以手和手臂的肌肉萎缩、无力、疼痛和血管异常为特征；**irritable bowel s.,** a chronic noninflammatory disease with a psychophysiologic basis, characterized by abdominal pain, diarrhea or constipation or both, and no detectable pathologic change 肠易激综合征，一种具有心理生理基础的慢性非炎症性疾病，以腹痛、腹泻或便秘或两者兼有为特征，无明显病理变化；**Isaacs s., Isaacs-Mertens s.,** an autoimmune disorder characterized by progressive muscle stiffness and spasms, with continuous muscle fiber activity similar to that seen with neuromyotonia 艾 - 梅综合征，一种自身免疫性疾病，以进行性肌肉僵硬和痉挛为特征，具有与神经性肌强直相似的持续性肌纤维活动；**Jacod s.,** chronic arthritis after rheumatic fever, with fibrous changes in the joint capsules leading to deformities that may resemble rheumatoid arthritis but lack bone erosion 雅可综合征，岩蝶间隙综合征，风湿热后的慢性关节炎，关节囊中的纤维改变可导致类似风湿性关节炎的畸形，但无骨侵蚀；**Jarcho-Levin s.,** an autosomal recessive disorder of multiple vertebral defects, short thorax, rib abnormalities, camptodactyly, syndactyly, and sometimes urogenital abnormalities, usually fatal in infancy 贾 - 勒综合征，一种常染色体隐性遗传病，表现为多发性脊椎缺损、胸短、肋骨畸形、先天性指屈曲、并指（趾）、有时伴有泌尿生殖系统畸形，通常在婴儿期致命；**Jervell and Lange-Nielsen s.,** a rare, autosomal recessive form of long QT syndrome, characterized by neural hearing loss and syncope, sometimes with ventricular fibrillation and sudden death; due to mutations that disrupt potassium voltage-gated channels 耶韦尔和朗格 - 尼尔森综合征，一种罕见的常染色体隐性长 QT 综合征，以神经性听力丧失和晕厥为特征，同时伴有室颤和猝死；由于突变而中断钾电压门控通道；**Joubert s.,** a genetically and clinically heterogeneous autosomal recessive syndrome, usually fatal in infancy, of partial to complete agenesis of the cerebellar vermis, with hypotonia, episodic hyperpnea, and intellectual disability. Renal anomalies and abnormal eye movements are sometimes present 先天性小脑蚓部发育不全，一种遗传和临床上不同的常染色体隐性遗传病，通常在婴儿期致命，小脑蚓部部分或完全发育不全，伴有张力减退、阵发性高通气和智力障碍；有时伴有肾脏异常和眼球运动异常；**Kallmann s.,** hypogonadotropic hypogonadism resulting from failure of gonadotropin-releasing hormone (GnRH) neurons to migrate from the olfactory bulb into the hypothalamus during fetal development, usually associated with anosmia or hyposmia secondary to defective development of the olfactory bulb 卡尔曼综

合征，由于促性腺激素释放激素（GnRH）神经元在胎儿发育过程中未能从嗅球迁移到下丘脑而引起的促性腺激素功能减退，通常与嗅球发育不良而继发的嗅觉缺失或嗅觉减退有关；**Kartagener s.**, situs inversus occurring in association with primary ciliary dyskinesia; absence of the normal ciliary movement necessary to create normal visceral asymmetry during embryogenesis results in left–right positioning of the viscera depending on chance 卡塔格内综合征；**Kimmelstiel-Wilson s.**, intercapillary glomerulosclerosis in which the lesions are nodular 基 - 威综合征，毛细血管间肾小球硬化症，病变呈结节状；**kinky hair s.**, Menkes disease 卷发综合征；**Klinefelter s.**, smallness of testes with fibrosis and hyalinization of seminiferous tubules, variable degrees of masculinization, azoospermia, and infertility, and increased urinary gonadotropins. It is associated typically with an XXY chromosome complement, although variants include XXYY, XXXY, XXXXY, and various mosaic patterns 克兰费尔特综合征，细精管发育障碍症，伴有纤维化和生精小管透明化的睾丸变小，不同程度的男性化、无精子症和不孕，以及尿促性腺激素增加；通常与 XXY 染色体补体有关，尽管变体包括 XXYY、XXXY、XXXY 和各种嵌合体；**Klippel-Feil s.**, shortness of the neck due to reduction in the number of cervical vertebrae or the fusion of multiple hemivertebrae into one osseous mass, usually with limitation of neck motion and low posterior hairline 克利佩尔 - 费尔综合征，先天性短颈综合征，由于颈椎数量减少或多节半椎骨融合而导致的短颈，通常伴有颈部运动受限和后发际低下；**Korsakoff s.**, a syndrome of anterograde and retrograde amnesia with confabulation associated with alcoholic or nonalcoholic polyneuritis, currently used synonymously with the term amnestic syndrome or, more narrowly, to refer to the amnestic component of the Wernicke-Korsakoff syndrome 科萨科夫综合征，一种与酒精性或非酒精性多神经炎相关的顺行性和逆行性健忘综合征，目前健忘综合征同义，或更狭义地指韦尼克 - 科尔萨科夫综合征的健忘症状；**Kostmann s.**, an inherited disorder of hematopoiesis, characterized by recurrent, severe pyogenic infections of the skin and lung with onset in infancy, absence of neutrophils in the blood, and early death Kostmann 综合征，一种遗传性造血障碍，特征为皮肤和肺部反复出现严重的化脓性感染，婴儿期发病，血液中无中性粒细胞，早期死亡；**Kugelberg-Welander s.**, the least severe type of spinal muscular atrophy, with onset after age 18 months, with atrophy and weakness of the proximal muscles of the lower limbs and pelvic girdle, followed by involvement of the distal muscles and muscular twitching Kugelberg-Welander 综合征，最轻的脊髓性肌肉萎缩类型，18 个月后发病，伴有下肢和骨盆带近端肌肉萎缩和无力，其次累及远端肌肉受累和肌肉抽搐；**Lambert-Eaton myasthenic s.**, a myasthenia-like syndrome in which the weakness usually affects the limbs and ocular and bulbar muscles are spared; often associated with oat-cell carcinoma of the lung 兰伯特 - 伊顿肌无力综合征，一种类似肌无力的综合征，累及四肢、眼和延髓肌肉；常与小胞肺癌有关；**Landau-Kleffner s.**, an epileptic syndrome of childhood with partial or generalized seizures, psychomotor abnormalities, and aphasia progressing to mutism 兰道 - 克勒夫纳综合征，获得性癫痫性失语，表现为部分或全身性癫痫发作、精神运动异常和失语发展为缄默症；**Laron s.**, an autosomal recessive disorder of skeletal growth retardation due to impaired ability to synthesize insulin-like growth factor I despite normal to elevated levels of growth hormone, usually as a result of mutation in the gene encoding growth hormone receptorLaron 综合征，一种常染色体隐性遗传病，尽管生长激素水平正常或升高，但由于合成类似胰岛素样生长因子 I 的能力受损而导致的骨骼生长迟缓，通常是由于编码生长激素受体的基因突变所致；**Laurence-Moon s.**, an autosomal recessive disorder sharing many of the characteristics of Bardet-Biedl syndrome; considered by many to be the same disorder 劳 - 穆综合征，一种常染色体隐性遗传病，具有巴尔得 - 别德尔综合征的特征，被认为是同一种疾病；**lazy leukocyte s.**, a syndrome in children, marked by recurrent lowgrade infections with a defect in neutrophil chemotaxis and deficient random mobility of neutrophils 懒惰白细胞综合征，以反复出现的低度感染为特征的儿童综合征，伴有中性粒细胞趋化性缺陷和中性粒细胞迁移率不足；**left atrioventricular valve prolapse s.**, prolapse of the left atrioventricular valve, often with regurgitation; a common, usually benign, often asymptomatic condition characterized by midsystolic clicks and late systolic murmurs on auscultation 左房室瓣膜脱垂综合征，左房室瓣脱垂，常伴有反流；一种常见的，通常是良性的、无症状的病症，其特征是听诊时出现单次收缩期咔哒声和晚期收缩期杂音；**Lennox-Gastaut s.**, an atypical form of absence epilepsy characterized by onset in early childhood with frequent seizures of multiple types, often with developmental delays and behavioral disorders 伦诺克斯 - 加斯托特综合征，一种非典型的失神癫痫，以儿童早期发病为特征，发作形式多样，常伴有发育迟缓和行为障碍；**LEOPARD s.**, an autosomal dominant, genetically heterogeneous syndrome of multiple *l*entigines, asymptomatic *electrocardiographic* abnormalities, and often *oc*-ular hypertelorism, *p*ulmonary stenosis, *a*bnormal genitalia, growth *r*etardation, and sensorineural *d*eafness 豹斑综合征，一种常染色体显性遗传的遗传异质性综合征，表现为多发性痣，无症状心电图异常，常有眼距过宽、肺动脉狭窄、生殖器异常、生长迟缓和感音神经性耳聋；**Leriche s.**，lower limb fatigue on exercising, lack of femoral pulse, impotence, and often pale, cold lower limbs, usually seen in males due to obstruction of the terminal aorta 勒里施综合征，运动时下肢乏力、股动脉搏动乏力、阳痿、下肢常苍白冰冷，多见于男性因主动脉末端梗阻所致；**Lesch-Nyhan s.**, an X-linked disorder of purine metabolism, characterized by physical growth retardation and intellectual disability, compulsive self-mutilation of fingers and lips by biting, choreoathetosis, spastic cerebral palsy, and impaired renal function, and by excessive purine synthesis and consequent hyperuricemia and uricaciduria 莱施 - 奈恩综合征，一种 X 染色体连锁的嘌呤代谢紊乱，其特征是身体发育迟缓和智力残疾，因咬伤、舞蹈病、痉挛性脑瘫和肾功能受损而导致手指和嘴唇的强迫自残，嘌呤合成过多并导致高尿酸血症和尿毒症；**levator ani s.**, chronic or recurrent episodes of vague, dull aching or pressure high in the rectum, occurring chiefly in women under 45 years of age; symptoms last 20 minutes or more and are often worse when the person is sitting. Cf. *proctalgia fugax* 肛提肌综合征，直肠隐痛、钝痛或高压的慢性或反复发作，主要发生在 45 岁以下的女性；症状持续 20 分钟或更长时间，当患者坐位时症状更严重；**Li-Fraumenis.**, a clinically and genetically heterogeneous, autosomal dominant cancer syndrome with early onset of tumors, particularly soft tissue sarcomas, osteosarcomas, and breast cancer; multiple tumors in individuals; and multiple affected family members; it is most often due to mutation in the p53 tumor suppressor gene 利 - 弗劳梅尼综合征，临床和遗传异质性常染色体显性癌症综合征，伴有肿瘤的早期发病，特别是软组织肉瘤、骨肉瘤和乳腺癌；具有家族聚集性；最常见的原因是 p53 肿瘤抑制基因的突变；**locked-in s.**, quadriplegia and mutism with intact consciousness and preservation of some eye movements; usually due to a vascular lesion of the anterior pons 闭锁综合征，表现为四肢瘫痪和缄默症，意识完整，保留一些眼球运动；通常因前脑桥血管病变引起；**long QT s.**, prolongation of the Q-T interval combined with torsades de pointes and manifest in several forms, either acquired or congenital, the latter with or without deafness; it may lead to serious arrhythmia and sudden death 长 QT 间期综合征，Q-T 间期延长与尖端

扭转型室性心动过速并呈现多种形式，既可以是后天性的，也可以是先天性的，后者伴或不伴耳聋；均可导致严重的心律失常和猝死；**Lowe s.**，同 oculocerebrorenal s.；**Lown-Ganong-Levine s.**, a preexcitation syndrome of electrocardiographic abnormality characterized by a short P–R interval with a normal QRS complex, accompanied by atrial tachycardia Lown-Ganong-Levine 综合征，一种心电图异常的预激综合征，特征是 P-R 间期短，QRS 波群正常，伴有房性心动过速；**Lutembacher s.**, atrial septal defect with mitral stenosis (usually rheumatic) 卢滕巴赫综合征，房间隔缺损伴二尖瓣狭窄（通常为风湿性）；**lymphadenopathy s.**, unexplained lymphadenopathy for 3 or more months at extrainguinal sites, revealing on biopsy nonspecific lymphoid hyperplasia, possibly a prodrome of acquired immunodeficiency syndrome 淋巴结病综合征，腹股沟外 3 个月或 3 个月以上不明原因的淋巴结肿大，活检显示非特异性淋巴组织增生，可能是获得性免疫缺陷的前驱症状；**Maffucci s.**, enchondromatosis with multiple cutaneous or visceral hemangiomas 马富奇综合征，内生软骨瘤伴多发性皮肤或内脏血管瘤；**malabsorption s.**, a group of disorders marked by subnormal absorption of dietary constituents, and thus excessive loss of nutrients in the stool, which may be due to a digestive defect, mucosal abnormality, or lymphatic obstruction 吸收不良综合征，一组以饮食成分的吸收低于正常水平，从而导致粪便中营养物质过度流失为特征的疾病，这可能是由消化缺陷、黏膜异常或淋巴阻塞引起；**male Turner s.**, Noonan s. 男性特纳综合征；**Marfan s.**, an autosomal dominant connective tissue disorder due to mutation of fibrillin, with skeletal, cardiovascular, and ocular manifestations, particularly abnormally long limbs, pectus excavatum or carinatum, subluxation of the lens, mitral valve prolapse, and dilatation of the ascending aorta 马方综合征，由于原纤维蛋白突变引起的常染色体显性遗传性结缔组织疾病，伴有骨骼、心血管和眼部表现，特别是异常长肢，漏斗胸或角膜，晶状体半脱位，二尖瓣脱垂和升主动脉扩张；**Maroteaux-Lamy s.**, mucopolysaccharidosis Ⅵ; an autosomal recessive disorder characterized by dermatan sulfate in the urine, coarse metachromatic granules in the leukocytes, and clinical signs ranging from a severe form, resembling Hurler syndrome but with normal intelligence, to a mild form, resembling Scheie syndrome 黏多糖贮积症Ⅵ型一种常染色体隐性遗传病，以尿液中的硫酸皮肤素，白细胞中的粗异染色颗粒为特征，临床症状从类似 Hurler 综合征，但智力正常的严重型到类似于 Scheie 综合征的轻型均可发生；**maternal deprivation s.**, failure to

S

thrive with severe growth retardation, unresponsiveness to the environment, depression, retarded mental and emotional development, and behavioral problems resulting from loss, absence, or neglect of the mother or other primary caregiver 失母爱综合征，由于严重的生长迟缓、对环境无反应、抑郁、智力和情绪发育迟缓以及因母亲或其他主要照顾者的失去、缺席或疏忽而导致的行为问题而未能茁壮成长；**McCune-Albright s.**, polyostotic fibrous dysplasia, large irregular café au lait spots, and endocrine dysfunction; due to an embryonic somatic activating mutation that results in a mosaic state of a gene involved in signal transduction (*GNAS*) 纤维性骨营养不良综合征，多发性纤维异常增生，大型不规则咖啡斑，内分泌功能障碍；由于胚胎体细胞激活突变导致参与信号转导（GNAS）的基因的嵌合状态；**Meckel s.**, an autosomal recessive syndrome, with sloping forehead, posterior meningoencephalocele, polydactyly, polycystic kidneys, and death in the perinatal period 麦克尔综合征，一种常染色体隐性遗传病，伴前额倾斜、后脑膜脑膨出、多发性肾、多囊肾、围产期死亡；**meconium aspiration s.**, the respiratory complications resulting from the passage and aspiration of meconium prior to or during delivery 胎粪吸入综合征，分娩前或分娩中胎粪通过和吸入引起的呼吸并发症；**megacystis-megaureter s.**, chronic ureteral dilatation (megaureter) associated with hypotonia and dilatation of the bladder (megacystis) and gaping of ureteral orifices, permitting vesicoureteral reflux of urine, and resulting in chronic pyclonephritis 巨膀胱 - 巨输尿管综合征，慢性输尿管扩张伴有张力减退和膀胱扩张和输尿管口间隙增宽，允许膀胱输尿管反流，导致慢性肾盂肾炎；**megacystis-microcolon–intestinal hypoperistalsis s. (MMIHS)**, enlarged bladder (megacystis), small colon with decreased or absent peristalsis (microcolon and intestinal hypoperistalsis), and the same abdominal muscle defect as occurs in prune-belly syndrome 巨膀胱 - 小结肠 - 肠蠕动迟缓综合征，膀胱肿大，蠕动减少或不存在的小结肠，以及与干梅状腹部综合征相同的腹部肌肉缺损；**Meige s.**, dystonia of facial and oromandibular muscles with blepharospasm, grimacing mouth movements, and protrusion of the tongue 梅热杰综合征，面部和口下颌肌肉肌张力障碍伴眼睑痉挛、噘嘴缩唇、吐舌；**MELAS s.**, a maternally inherited multisystem disorder of *m*itochondrial myopathy, *e*ncephalopathy, *l*actic *a*cidosis, and *s*troke-like episodes, with variable additional features; due to mutation in any of several mitochondrial genes encoding transfer RNA MELAS 综合征，母系遗传多系统疾病的线粒体病，即脑病、乳酸性酸中毒和中风样发作，具有可变的附加特征；由于编码转移 RNA 的几个线粒体基因中的任何一个发生突变引起；**MERRF s.**, a maternally inherited syndrome of *my*oclonic *e*pilepsy with *r*agged *r*ed *f*ibers, caused by mutation in a mitochondrial gene 伴有癫痫和粗糙红纤维的肌痉挛综合征，由线粒体基因突变引起的具有不规则红纤维的肌阵挛性癫痫的母系遗传综合征；**metabolic s.**, a combination including at least three of the following: abdominal obesity, hypertriglyceridemia, low level of high-density lipoproteins, hypertension, and high fasting glucose level 代谢综合征，至少包括以下三种疾病的综合征：中心性肥胖、高甘油三酯血症、低密度脂蛋白水平、高血压和高空腹血糖水平；**methionine malabsorption s.**, an inborn aminoacidopathy marked by white hair, intellectual disability, convulsions, attacks of hyperpnea, and urine with an odor like an oasthouse (for drying hops) due to α-hydroxybutyric acid formed by bacterial action on the unabsorbed methionine 甲硫氨酸吸收不良综合征，一种先天性氨基酸病，由于细菌作用于未被吸收的甲硫氨酸而形成 α- 羟基丁酸，以白发、智力障碍、惊厥、呼吸过度发作为特征，尿液中有臭味物质（用于干燥啤酒花）；**middle lobe s.**, lobar atelectasis in the right middle lobe of the lung, with chronic pneumonitis 中叶综合征，右肺中叶肺不张伴慢性肺炎；**Mikulicz s.**, chronic bilateral hypertrophy of the lacrimal, parotid, and salivary glands, associated with chronic lymphocytic infiltration; it may be associated with other diseases 米库利兹综合征，泪腺、腮腺和唾液腺的慢性双侧肥大，与慢性淋巴细胞浸润有关；也可能与其他疾病有关；**milkalkali s.**, hypercalcemia without hypercalciuria or hypophosphatemia and with only mild alkalosis and other symptoms attributed to ingestion of milk and absorbable alkali for long periodsmilkalkali 综合征，高钙血症、无高钙尿症或低磷血症，仅有轻微的碱中毒和其他症状，可归因于长期摄入牛奶和可吸收碱；**Milkman s.**, a generalized bone disease marked by multiple transparent stripes of absorption in the long and flat bones Milkman 综合征，一种全身性骨疾病，特征是长而扁平的骨头上有多条透明的吸收条纹；**Miller s.**, an inherited syndrome of extensive facial and limb defects, sometimes accompanied by heart defects and hearing loss 米勒综合征，广泛性面部和肢体缺陷的遗传综合征，有时伴有心脏缺陷和听力损失；**Miller-Dieker s.**, an autosomal dominant, contiguous gene deletion syndrome (locus 17p13.3) characterized by lissencephaly, microcephaly, mental retardation, dysmorphic facial appearance, polydactyly, cryptorchidism, and variable malformations of other organs Miller-Dieker 综合征，

S

常染色体显性遗传性相邻基因缺失综合征（17p13.3 位点），其特征为脑裂、小头畸形、智力低下、面部畸形、多指畸形、隐睾症和其他器官的可变畸形；**MMIH s.,** 同 megacystis-microcolon–intestinal hypoperistalsis s.；**Möbius s.,** agenesis or aplasia of cranial nerve motor nuclei in congenital bilateral facial palsy, with unilateral or bilateral paralysis of abductors of the eye and sometimes cranial nerve involvement and limb anomalies MÖbius 综合征，先天性面肌双瘫，先天性双侧面瘫脑神经运动核发育不全或再生障碍，伴眼外展肌单侧或双侧麻痹，脑神经有时受累及肢体异常；**Mohr s.,** an autosomal recessive disorder characterized by brachydactyly, clinodactyly, polydactyly, syndactyly, and bilateral hallucal polysyndactyly; by cranial, facial, lingual, palatal, and mandibular anomalies; and by episodic neuromuscular disturbances 莫尔综合征，一种常染色体隐性遗传病，特征为指（趾）过短、指（趾）弯曲、多指（趾）畸形，并指（趾）畸形和双侧拇多指畸形；颅、面部、舌、腭和下颌畸形；以及阵发性神经肌肉紊乱；**Morquio s.,** two biochemically distinct but clinically nearly indistinguishable forms of mucopolysaccharidosis, marked by genu valgum, pigeon breast, progressive flattening of the vertebral bodies, short neck and trunk, progressive deafness, mild corneal clouding, and excretion of keratan sulfate in the urine 莫基奥综合征，黏多糖贮积症Ⅳ型，两种生物化学上不同但临床上几乎无法区分的黏多糖症，表现为膝外翻、鸡胸、椎体逐渐变平、颈干短缩、进行性耳聋、轻度角膜混浊和尿液中硫酸角化钙的排泄；**mucocutaneous lymph node s.,** Kawasaki disease 黏膜皮肤淋巴结综合征，川崎病；**multiple endocrine deficiency s.,multiple glandular deficiency s.,** failure of any combination of endocrine glands, often accompanied by nonendocrine autoimmune abnormalities 多发性内分泌缺陷综合征，多腺体缺乏综合征；**multiple pterygium s.,** an inherited syndrome characterized by pterygia of the neck, axillae, and various body fold areas, with facial, skeletal, and genital abnormalities 多发性翼状胬肉综合征，一种遗传综合征，特征是颈部、腋下和身体各折叠部位的翼状胬肉，面部、骨骼和生殖器异常；**Munchausen s.,** a subtype of factitious disorder; habitual seeking of hospital treatment for apparent acute illness, the patient giving a plausible and dramatic history, all of which is false 蒙肖森综合征，人为障碍的一种亚型；习惯性地寻求医院治疗以治疗明显的急性疾病，病人给出了一个可信的和戏剧性的病史，而所有这些都是错误的；**Munchausen s. by proxy,** 代理性蒙肖森综合征，参见 disorder 下 *factitious disorder by proxy*；**MVP s.,** 同 left atrioventricular valve (formerly mitral valve) prolapse s；**myelodysplastic s.,** any of a group of related bone marrow disorders of varying duration preceding the development of overt acute myelogenous leukemia; characterized by abnormal hematopoietic stem cells, anemia, neutropenia, and thrombocytopenia 骨髓增生异常综合征，在明显急性髓性白血病发展之前不同持续时间的一组相关骨髓疾病中的任何一种；特征在于异常的造血干细胞，贫血，中性粒细胞减少和血小板减少症；**Negri-Jacod s.,** 同 Jacod s.；**Nelson s.,** the development of an ACTH-producing pituitary tumor after bilateral adrenalectomy in Cushing syndrome; it is characterized by aggressive growth of the tumor and hyperpigmentation of the skin 纳尔逊综合征，库欣综合征双侧肾上腺切除术后产生促肾上腺皮质激素的垂体肿瘤的发展征；其特征是肿瘤生长旺盛，皮肤色素沉着过多；**neonatal respiratory distress s.,** a condition seen in infants born prematurely, by cesarean section, or to diabetic mothers, marked by dyspnea and cyanosis; a common, usually fatal subtype is hyaline membrane disease 新生儿呼吸窘迫综合征，见于早产儿剖宫产儿或新生儿的母亲患有呼吸困难和发绀；常见的、通常致命的亚型为肺透明膜疾病；**nephrogenic s. of inappropriate antidiuresis (NSIAD),** an inherited syndrome, clinically resembling the syndrome of inappropriate diuretic hormone, caused by inability of the renal collecting tubules to absorb water in response to antidiuretic hormone 抗利尿不适肾病综合征，一种遗传综合征，临床上类似于不适当的利尿激素综合征，是由于肾小管对抗利尿激素反应而无法吸收水分引起的；**nephrotic s.,** any of a group of diseases involving defective kidney glomeruli, with massive proteinuria, lipiduria with edema, hypoalbuminemia, and hyperlipidemia 肾病综合征，任何涉及肾小球缺陷的疾病，伴有大量蛋白尿，伴有水肿的血尿，低蛋白血症和高脂血症；**nerve compression s.,** entrapment neuropathy 神经压迫综合征；**Noonan s.,** webbed neck, ptosis, hypogonadism, and short stature, i.e., the phenotype of Turner syndrome without the gonadal dysgenesis 努南综合征，假特纳综合征，表典型特征为蹼、上睑下垂、性腺功能减退和身材矮小，如无性腺发育不全的特纳综合征表型；**obesity-hypoventilation s.,** pickwickian syndrome; a syndrome of obesity, somnolence, hypoventilation, and erythrocytosis 肥胖通气低下综合征，伴有肥胖、嗜睡、通气不足和红细胞增多的综合征；**occipital horn s.,** a variant of Menkes disease, characterized by hyperelastic and bruisable skin, hernias, bladder diverticula and dysfunction, hyperextensible joints, varicosities, multiple skeletal abnormalities, and exostoses at the sites of muscular attachment to

S

the occipital skull 枕骨角综合征, 门克斯病的一种变体, 其特征是过度弹性和可擦伤的皮肤, 疝气, 膀胱憩室和功能障碍, 过度伸展的关节, 静脉曲张, 多发骨骼异常, 以及在枕骨肌肉附着部位的外生骨疣; **oculocerebrorenal s.,** an X-linked disorder due to mutation of an enzyme involved in actin polymerization and membrane trafficking; marked by vitamin D–refractory rickets, hydrophthalmia, congenital glaucoma and cataracts, intellectual disability, and renal tubule dysfunction with hypophosphatemia, acidosis, and aminoaciduria 脑 - 肾综合征, 由于肌动蛋白聚合和膜运输相关酶的突变而导致的 X 连锁疾病; 以维生素 D 难治性佝偻病、嗜盐血症、先天性青光眼和白内障、智力障碍和肾小管功能障碍为特征, 伴有低磷血症,酸中毒和氨基酸尿症; **oculodentodigital s.,** 眼 - 齿 - 指（趾）综合征, 参见 *dysplasia.* 下词条; **oculoglandular s.,** 同 Parinaud oculoglandular s.; **OFD s.,** 同 oral-facial-digital s.; **Opitz s., Opitz G/BBB s.,** a hereditary disorder occurring in X-linked and autosomal dominant forms, involving midline anomalies and consisting of hypertelorism and hernias, and in males also hypospadias, cryptorchidism, and bifid scrotum. Cardiac, laryngotracheal, pulmonary, anal, and renal abnormalities may also be present 奥皮茨综合征, 以 X 连锁和常染色体显性遗传为特征的遗传疾病, 包括中线中线畸形、器官距离过远和疝组成, 男性也有尿道下裂、隐睾和阴囊裂, 也可能存在心脏、喉气管、肺、肛门和肾脏异常; **oral-facial-digital s.,** OFD s.; any of a group of congenital syndromes characterized by oral, facial, and digital anomalies. *Type I,* a male-lethal X-linked dominant disorder, is characterized by camptodactyly, polydactyly, and syndactyly; by cranial, facial, lingual, and dental anomalies; and by intellectual disability, familial trembling, alopecia, and seborrhea of the face and milia; *type II is Mohr s.; type III,* an autosomal recessive disorder, is characterized by postaxial hexadactyly; ocular, lingual, and dental anomalies; and profound intellectual disability 口 - 面 - 指综合征, 以口腔、面部和手指异常为特征的一组先天性综合征。I 型是一种男性致死性 X 连锁显性疾病, 特点为先天性指屈曲、多指（趾）、并指, 颅骨、面部、语言和牙齿异常, 智力残疾、家族性颤抖、脱发、面部脂溢、粟粒疹为特征; II 型为 Mohr 综合征; III 型为一种常见隐性遗传病, 以轴后六指畸形、眼、舌、牙畸形, 以及严重的智力残疾为特征; **organic anxiety s.,** in a former system of classification, an organic mental syndrome with prominent, recurrent panic attacks or generalized anxiety caused by a specific organic factor and not associated with delirium 器质性焦虑综合征, 在以前的分类系统中, 一种由特定的器质因素引起的显著的、反复发作的惊恐发作或全身性焦虑而与谵妄无关的器质性精神综合征; **organic brain s.,** organic mental s. 器质性脑病综合征; **organic delusional s.,** in a former system of classification, an organic mental syndrome marked by delusions caused by a specific organic factor and not associated with delirium 器质性在以前的分类系统中, 一种有机的精神综合征, 以特定的有机因素引起的错觉为特征, 与谵妄无关; **organic mental s.,** former term for a constellation of psychological or behavioral signs and symptoms associated with brain dysfunction of unknown or unspecified etiology and grouped according to symptoms rather than etiology 器质性精神综合征, 指与未知或不明病因的脑功能障碍有关的一系列心理或行为体征和症状, 并按症状而不是病因学分组, 参见 *disorder* 下词条; **organic mood s.,** in a former system of classification, an organic mental syndrome marked by manic or depressive mood disturbance caused by a specific organic factor and not associated with delirium 器质性心境综合征, 在以前的分类系统中, 一种有机心理的综合征, 其特征是由特定的有机因素引起的躁狂或抑郁性心境障碍, 与谵妄无关; **organic personality s.,** in a former system of classification, an organic mental syndrome characterized by a marked change in behavior or personality, caused by a specific organic factor and not associated with delirium or dementia 器质性人格综合征, 在以前的分类系统中, 一种有机的精神综合征, 其特征是行为或个性的显著变化, 由特定的有机因素引起, 与精神错乱或痴呆无关; **orofaciodigital s.,;** 同 oral-facial-digital s.**Ortner s.,** laryngeal paralysis associated with heart disease, due to compression of the recurrent laryngeal nerve between the aorta and a dilated pulmonary artery 心脏 - 声带综合征, 因主动脉和扩张的肺动脉之间的喉返神经压迫导致的与心脏疾病相关的喉麻痹; **ovarian hyperstimulation s.,** mild to severe ovarian enlargement with exudation of fluid and protein, leading to ascites, pleural or pericardial effusion, azotemia, oliguria, and thromboembolism in women undergoing ovulation induction 卵巢过度刺激综合征, 轻度至重度卵巢增大伴液体和蛋白质渗出, 导致接受排卵诱导的妇女出现腹水、胸膜或心包积液、氮质血症、少尿和血栓栓塞; **ovarian vein s.,** obstruction of the ureter due to compression by an enlarged or varicose ovarian vein; typically the vein becomes enlarged during pregnancy 卵巢静脉综合征, 由于卵巢静脉扩大或静脉曲张压迫输尿管阻塞, 通常在怀孕期间静脉扩大; **overlap s.,** any of a group of connective tissue disorders that either combine scleroderma with polymyositis or systemic lupus erythematosus or combine systemic lupus erythematosus with rheumatoid arthritis or polymyositis 重叠综合征，一组结缔组织疾病，或合并硬皮病和多发性红斑狼疮或合并系统性红斑狼疮和类风湿性关节炎或多发性肌炎；**overwear s.,** extreme photophobia, pain, and lacrimation associated with contact lenses, particularly non–gas-permeable hard lenses, usually caused by wearing them excessively 过度疲劳综合征，与隐形眼镜有关的极度畏光、疼痛和流泪，尤其是不透气的硬镜片，通常是由于过度佩戴而引起的；**pacemaker s.,** vertigo, syncope, and hypotension, often accompanied by dyspnea, cough, nausea, peripheral edema, and palpitations, all exacerbated or caused by pacemakers that stimulate the ventricle and therefore do not maintain normal atrioventricular synchrony 起搏器综合征，表现为眩晕、晕厥和低血压，常伴有呼吸困难、咳嗽、恶心、周围水肿和心悸，均由刺激心室的起搏器加剧引起，因此不能维持正常的房室同步；**pacemaker twiddler s.,** twiddler's syndrome in a patient with an artificial cardiac pacemaker 起搏器旋弄综合征；**painful bruising s.,** occurrence of one or more spontaneous, chronic, recurring painful ecchymoses without antecedent trauma or after insufficient trauma; sometimes precipitated by emotional stress. Because certain patients exhibit autoerythrocyte sensitization in which intradermal injection of their own erythrocytes produces a painful ecchymosis, some consider the condition to be an autosensitivity to a component of the erythrocyte membrane; others consider it to be of psychosomatic or factitious origin 痛性瘀紫综合征，一个或多个自发性、慢性、复发性疼痛性瘀斑的发生，无先兆创伤或创伤不足，有时因情绪紧张而发生；由于某些患者表现出自身红细胞致敏，皮内注射自己的红细胞会产生疼痛性瘀斑，有人认为这种情况是对红细胞膜某种成分的自敏也有人认为这是心身或人为的；**Pancoast s.,** 潘科斯特综合征 1. neuritic pain and muscle atrophy in the upper limb, and Horner syndrome, seen with a tumor near the apex of the lung when it involves the brachial plexus 上肢神经炎性疼痛和肌肉萎缩，以及霍纳综合征，当累及臂丛时，在肺尖部附近见到肿瘤；2. osteolysis in the posterior part of a rib or ribs, sometimes spreading to adjacent vertebrae 骨质溶解发生于一肋或多肋的后部，有时也累及邻近的脊椎；**paraneoplastic s.,** a symptom complex arising in a cancer-bearing patient that cannot be explained by local or distant spread of the tumor 副肿瘤综合征，肿瘤伴随综合征，癌症患者出现的复杂症状，不能用肿瘤的局部或远处扩散来解释；**Parinaud s.,** paralysis of conjugate upward movement of the eyes without paralysis of convergence; associated with tumors of the midbrain 帕里诺综合征，眼球向上运动的共轭性麻痹，无会聚性麻痹；与中脑肿瘤有关；**Parinaud oculoglandular s.,** conjunctivitis followed by tenderness and enlargement of the pre-auricular lymph nodes; it is often associated with other infections 帕里诺眼淋巴结综合征，结膜炎伴耳前淋巴结压痛和肿大；常与其他感染有关；**parkinsonian s.,** any disorder manifesting the symptoms of Parkinson disease 震颤麻痹综合征；**Patau s.,** 同 trisomy 13 s.；**persistent müllerian duct s.,** a hereditary syndrome in males of persistence of müllerian structures in addition to male genital ducts. There may be cryptorchidism on just one side with a contralateral inguinal hernia that contains a testis, uterus, and uterine tube *(hernia uteri inguinalis)* 米勒管永存综合征，男性除男性生殖道以外还有米勒结构持续存在的遗传性综合征。可能只有一侧隐睾，伴对侧腹股沟疝，包括睾丸、子宫和输卵管（子宫腹股沟疝）；**Peters-plus s.,** an autosomal recessive congenital disorder caused by mutation of a specific glycosyltransferase and consisting of Peters anomaly in association with characteristic facial features, cleft lip and palate, short stature, limb shortening, brachydactyly, and developmental delay Peters-plus 综合征，一种常染色体隐性遗传病，由特异性糖基转移酶突变引起的先天性疾病，包括与特征性面容、唇腭裂、身材矮小、肢体缩短、短指和发育迟缓相关的 Peters 异常；**Peutz-Jeghers s.,** familial adenomatous polyposis, especially in the small intestine, associated with mucocutaneous pigmentation 波伊茨 - 耶格综合征，家族性腺瘤性息肉病，尤其是小肠，与黏膜皮肤色素沉着有关；**Pfeiffer s.,** acrocephalosyndactyly, type V; an autosomal dominant disorder with variable expressivity, characterized by acrocephaly with midface hypoplasia and hypertelorism and mild syndactyly associated with broad short thumbs and great toes Pfeiffer 综合征，尖头并指（趾）V 型，一种常染色体显性遗传病，常表现为肢端发育不全，伴面中部发育不良和畸形，伴拇指宽大、趾长大的轻度并指（趾）畸形；**pickwickian s.,** obesity-hypoventilation s. 皮克威克综合征；**Pierre Robin s.,** 皮埃尔 - 罗班综合征，参见 *sequence* 下词条；**plica s.,** pain, tenderness, swelling, and crepitus of the knee joint, sometimes with weakness or locking of the joint, caused by fibrosis and calcification of the synovial fold (plica) 襞综合征，膝关节疼痛、压痛、肿胀弹响，有时伴有关节无力或闭锁，由滑膜皱襞纤维化和钙化引起；**Plummer-Vinson s.,** dysphagia with glossitis, hypochromic anemia, splenomegaly, and atrophy in the mouth, pharynx, and upper end of the esophagus 普 - 文二氏综合征，吞咽困难伴舌炎，低色

S

素性贫血，脾肿大，口腔、咽和食道上端萎缩；**POEMS s.,** *p*olyneuropathy, *o*rganomegaly, *e*ndocrinopathy, *M* component, and *s*kin changes, sometimes linked to a dysproteinemia such as the presence of unusual monoclonal proteins and light chains POEMS综合征，多发性神经病、器官肿大、内分泌疾病、M组分和皮肤变化与异常蛋白血症有关，如异常单克隆蛋白和轻链的存在；**polyangiitis overlap s.,** a form of systemic necrotizing vasculitis resembling polyarteritis nodosa and Churg-Strauss syndrome but also showing features of hypersensitivity vasculitis 多脉管炎重叠综合征，系统性坏死性血管炎的一种形式，类似于结节性多动脉炎和许尔许斯特劳斯综合征，但也显示过敏性血管炎的特征；**polycystic ovary s. (PCOS),** a symptom complex associated with polycystic ovaries, characterized by oligomenorrhea or amenorrhea, anovulation (hence infertility), and hirsutism; both hyperestrogenism and hyperandrogenism are present 多囊卵巢综合征，一种与多囊卵巢相关的症状复合体，以月经过少或闭经、无排卵（因此不孕）和多毛为特征；同时存在高雌激素和高雄激素血症；**polysplenia s.,** a congenital syndrome of multiple splenic masses, abnormal position and development of visceral organs, complex cardiovascular defects, and abnormal, usually bilobate, lungs 多脾综合征，多发脾肿物、内脏器官位置和发育异常、复杂的心血管缺陷和通常为双叶的肺异常的先天综合征；**popliteal pterygium s.,** an autosomal dominant disorder with webbing behind the knees, cleft palate, lower lip pits, hypodontia, and epidermal and genital anomalies; due to mutation in interferon regulatory factor 6, a cooperative transcriptional activator 腘翼状赘蹼综合征，一种常染色体显性病由于干扰素调节因子6（一种协同转录激活物）的突变，导致膝盖后有蹼、腭裂、下唇凹陷、缺牙、表皮和生殖器异常；**post-cardiac injury s.,** fever, chest pain, pleuritis, and pericarditis weeks after injury to the heart, including that due to surgery *(postpericardiotomy s.)* and that due to myocardial infarction *(post–myocardial infarction s.).* 心脏损伤后综合征，心脏损伤后、发热、胸痛、胸膜炎和心包炎，包括手术（心包切开术后）和心肌梗塞（心肌梗塞后）引起的 **postcardiotomy s., postcommissurotomy s.,** 同 postpericardiotomy s.；**postconcussional s.,** physical and personality changes that may occur after concussion of the brain, including amnesia, headache, dizziness, tinnitus, irritability, fatigability, sweating, heart palpitations, insomnia, and difficulty concentrating 脑震荡后综合征，脑震荡后可能发生的身体和人格变化，包括遗忘症、头痛、头晕、耳鸣、易怒、疲劳、出汗、心悸、失眠和注意力

不集中；**postgastrectomy s.,** dumping s. 胃切除术后综合征；**post-lumbar puncture s.,** the lumbar puncture headache and other symptoms, which may include pain at the back of the neck, vomiting, sweating, and malaise, occurring when the person is upright and relieved upon lying down, due to lowering of intracranial pressure by leakage of cerebrospinal fluid through the needle tract 腰椎穿刺后综合征，表现为腰椎穿刺后头痛和其他症状，可能包括颈部疼痛、呕吐、出汗和不适，发生于患者直立时，由于脑脊液经针道漏出而降低颅内压，卧床后缓解；**postmaturity s.,** a syndrome due to placental insufficiency that causes chronic stress and hypoxia, seen in fetuses and neonates in postterm pregnancies, characterized by decreased subcutaneous fat, skin desquamation, and long fingernails, often with yellow meconium staining of the nails, skin, and vernix 过度成熟综合征，胎盘功能不全引起慢性应激和缺氧的综合征，见于足月后妊娠的胎儿和新生儿，表现为皮下脂肪减少、皮肤脱皮和指甲长，常伴有指甲、皮肤和胎脂的黄色胎粪染色；**post-myocardial infarction s.,** post–cardiac injury s. after myocardial infarction 心肌梗死后综合征；**postpericardiotomy s.,** post–cardiac injury s. after surgery with opening of the pericardium 心包切开术后综合征；**postphlebitic s.,** *postthrombotic s.* 静脉炎后综合征；**postpolio s., postpoliomyelitis s.,** symptoms of unknown etiology seen in patients several to many years after they have recovered from the major illness of poliomyelitis 脊髓灰质炎后综合征，从脊髓灰质炎的主要疾病中恢复几年至五年后，患者出现不明病因的症状；**postthrombotic s.,** long-term complications of deep venous thrombosis, including destruction of the valves and lack of recanalization of the veins, resulting in chronic venous insufficiency, marked by edema, stasis dermatitis, and ulceration 血栓后综合征，深静脉血栓形成的长期并发症，包括瓣膜破坏和静脉再通不足，导致慢性静脉功能不全，以水肿、瘀血性皮炎和溃疡为特征；**Potter s.,** oligohydramnios sequence 波特综合征，羊水过少序列征；**Prader-Willi s.,** congenital obesity, short stature, lack of muscle tone, hypogonadism, and central nervous system dysfunction 普拉德-威利综合征，表现为先天性肥胖、身材矮小、肌肉张力不足、性腺功能减退和中枢神经系统功能障碍；**preexcitation s.,** any syndrome with electrocardiographic signs of preexcitation, such as Wolff-Parkinson-White syndrome; sometimes used synonymously with it 预激综合征，任何具有预激的心电图体征的综合征，如Wolff-Parkinson-White综合征；有时与之同义；**premenstrual s.,** some or all of the symptoms of depressed, anxious, angry, or irritable mood, emotional lability, bloating, edema, headache, increased fatigue or lethargy, altered appetite or food cravings, breast swelling and tenderness, constipation, and decreased ability to concentrate during the time between ovulation and onset of menstruation 经前期综合征; **prune-belly s.,** a congenital syndrome of deficient or absent anterior abdominal wall musculature, urinary tract anomalies, and undescended testicles. The abdomen is protruding and thin-walled, with wrinkled skin 腹肌发育异常损综合征，前腹壁肌肉组织缺乏或缺失、尿路异常和睾丸未发育的先天综合征；腹部突出、壁薄、皮肤起皱；**Putnam-Dana s.,** subacute combined degeneration of the spinal cord 普 - 达综合征，亚急性脊髓联合变性；**Raeder s., Raeder paratrigeminal s.,** unilateral paroxysmal neuralgic pain in the face associated with Horner syndrome 雷德综合征，三叉神经旁综合征，单侧阵发性面部神经痛伴 Horner 综合征；**Ramsay Hunt s.,** 1. geniculate neuralgia; herpes zoster involving the facial and vestibulocochlear nerves, often with transitory ipsilateral facial paralysis and herpetic vesicles of the external ear or tympanic membrane 带状疱疹病毒累及面神经和前庭耳蜗神经，常伴有短暂的同侧面瘫和外耳或鼓膜疱疹性水疱；2. juvenile paralysis agitans 幼年型震颤麻痹；3. dyssynergia cerebellaris progressiva 拉姆齐 - 亨特综合征，肌阵挛性小脑协调障碍；**Reiter s.,** the triad of aseptic arthritis, nongonococcal urethritis, and conjunctivitis, frequently with mucocutaneous lesions; often now considered to be part of reactive arthritis and not named separately 莱特尔综合征，结膜 - 尿道 - 滑膜综合征，常伴有皮肤黏膜损伤；现在常被认为是反应性关节炎的一部分，不单独命名；**respiratory distress s. of newborn,** 同 neonatal respiratory distress s；**Reye s.,** a rare, often fatal encephalopathy of childhood, marked by acute brain swelling with hypoglycemia, fatty infiltration of the liver, hepatomegaly, and disturbed consciousness and seizures, usually seen as a sequela of varicella or an upper airway viral infection 瑞氏综合征，脑病合并内脏脂肪变性综合征，一种罕见的、通常是致命的儿童脑病，以急性脑肿胀伴低血糖、肝脏脂肪浸润、肝肿大、意识紊乱和癫痫为特征，通常被视为水痘或上呼吸道病毒感染的后遗症；**Rh-null s.,** chronic hemolytic anemia affecting individuals who lack all Rh factors (Rhnull); it is marked by spherocytosis, stomatocytosis, and increased osmotic fragility Rh 因子缺乏综合征，慢性溶血性贫血，影响缺乏所有 Rh 因子的个体（rhnull）；其特征是球形细胞增多、气孔增多和渗透脆弱性增加；**Riley-Day s.,** familial dysautonomia 赖利 - 戴综合征，家族性自主神经功能

障碍；**Riley-Smith s.,** 同 Bannayan-Riley-Ruvalcaba s.；**Robinow s.,** dwarfism associated with increased interorbital distance, malaligned teeth, bulging forehead, depressed nasal bridge, genital abnormalities, and short limbs; autosomal dominant and recessive forms exist 胎儿面容综合征，与眶间距离增加、牙齿不齐、前额隆起、鼻梁凹陷、生殖器异常和四肢短小相关的侏儒症；常染色体显性和隐性形式存在；**Rosenberg-Bergstrom s.,** an inherited syndrome of hyperuricemia, renal insufficiency, ataxia, and deafness Rosenberg-Bergstrom 综合征，表现为高尿酸血症、肾功能不全、共济失调和耳聋的遗传综合征；**Rundles-Falls s.,** hereditary sideroblastic anemia 拉 - 法综合征，遗传性铁幼粒细胞贫血；**Ruvalcaba s.,** abnormal shortness of the metacarpal or metatarsal bones, hypoplastic genitalia, and mental and physical retardation of unknown etiology, present from birth in males R 综合征，男性出生时出现的掌骨或跖骨异常短促、生殖器发育不全和不明病因的精神和身体发育迟缓；**Ruvalcaba-Myhre-Smith s.,** 同 Bannayan-RileyRuvalcaba s.；**Saethre-Chotzen s.,** acrocephalosyndactyly, type Ⅲ; an autosomal dominant disorder characterized by craniosynostosis and brachycephaly, cutaneous syndactyly, hypertelorism, ptosis, and sometimes intellectual disability 塞 - 乔综合征，尖头并指（趾）Ⅲ型，一种常染色体显性遗传病，以颅缝早闭、短头畸形、并指（趾）畸形、眼距过宽、上睑下垂为特征，有时伴有智力障碍；**salt depletion s., salt-losing s.,** vomiting, dehydration, hypotension, and sudden death due to very large sodium losses from the body. It may be seen in abnormal losses of sodium into the urine (as in congenital adrenal hyperplasia, adrenocortical insufficiency, or one of the forms of salt-losing nephritis) or in large extrarenal sodium losses, usually from the gastrointestinal tract 失盐综合征；**Sanfilippo s.,** four biochemically distinct but clinically indistinguishable forms of mucopolysaccharidosis, characterized by urinary excretion of heparan sulfate, rapid mental deterioration, and mild Hurler-like symptoms, with death usually occurring before 20 years of age 黏多糖贮积症Ⅲ型；**scalenus s., scalenus anticus s.,** a type of inferior thoracic aperture syndrome due to compression of the nerves and vessels between a cervical rib and the scalenus anticus muscle, with pain over the shoulder, often extending down the arm or radiating up the back 斜角肌综合征，一种由颈肋和斜角肌之间的神经和血管压迫引起的胸廓下开口综合征，肩上疼痛，常向下延伸至手臂或向上放射至背部；**Schaumann s.,** sarcoidosis 绍曼综合征（全身播散性结节病）；**Scheie s.,** a mild allelic variant of Hurler syndrome,

S

marked by corneal clouding, clawhand, aortic valve involvement, wide-mouthed facies, genu valgus, and pes cavus; stature, intelligence, and life span are normal 黏多糖贮积症 IS 型，黏多糖贮积症 IH 型的一种轻度等位基因变体，以角膜混浊、爪手、主动脉瓣受累、宽口面容、膝外翻和腔静脉畸形为特征；身高、智力和寿命正常；**Schwartz-Jampel s.,** an autosomal recessive skeletal dysplasia characterized by varying levels of myotonia and chondrodysplasia, with muscle abnormalities, dwarfism, blepharophimosis, joint contractures, and flat facies; due to mutation of a proteoglycan of the basement membrane 施瓦茨 - 杨佩尔综合征，软骨营养不良性肌强直，常染色体隐性遗传性骨骼发育不良，以不同程度的肌强直和软骨发育不良为特征，伴有肌肉异常、侏儒症、上睑下垂、关节挛缩和扁平面容；由于基底膜蛋白多糖的突变；**second impact s.,** acute, usually fatal, brain swelling and increased cranial pressure, caused by repeated head trauma in a short space of time, so that a second concussion occurs before recovery from a previous concussion is complete 二次脑损伤综合征，急性的，通常是致命的脑肿胀和颅压升高，由短时间内反复的头部创伤引起，在先前的脑震荡完全恢复之前发生第二次脑震荡；**Sertoli-cell–only s.,** congenital absence of the germinal epithelium of the testes, the seminiferous tubules containing only Sertoli cells, marked by testes slightly smaller than normal, azoospermia, and elevated titers of folliclestimulating hormone and sometimes of luteinizing hormone 单纯塞托利细胞综合征，睾丸生殖细胞先天性缺失，曲细精管仅含支持细胞，以睾丸略小于正常、无精子为标志、卵泡刺激素滴度升高，有时伴有黄体生成素滴度升高；**severe acute respiratory s. (SARS),** an infectious respiratory illness caused by a coronavirus and characterized by fever, dry cough, and breathing difficulties, often accompanied by headache and body aches 严重急性呼吸综合征，一种由冠状病毒引起的传染性呼吸道疾病，以发热、干咳和呼吸困难为特征，常伴有头痛和身体疼痛；**Sézary s.,** a form of cutaneous T-cell lymphoma manifested by exfoliative erythroderma, intense pruritus, peripheral lymphadenopathy, and Sézary cells in the skin, lymph nodes, and peripheral blood 塞扎里综合征，一种皮肤 T 细胞淋巴瘤，表现为剥脱性红皮病、严重瘙痒、周围淋巴结病和皮肤、淋巴结和外周血中的塞扎里细胞；**Sheehan s.,** postpartum pituitary necrosis 希恩综合征，产后大出血导致腺垂体坏死；**short bowel s., short gut s.,** any of the malabsorption conditions resulting from massive resection of the small intestine, the degree and kind of malabsorption depending on the site and extent of the resection; it is characterized by diarrhea, steatorrhea, and malnutrition 短肠综合征，小肠大量切除引起的任何一种吸收不良的情况，其程度和种类取决于切除的部位和程度；以腹泻、脂肪热和营养不良为特征；**shoulder-hand s.,** complex regional pain syndrome type 1 limited to the upper limb 肩 - 手综合征，局限于上肢的复杂局部疼痛综合征 1 型；**Shprintzen s.,** 同 velocardiofacial s.；**Shwachman s., Shwachman-Diamond s.,** primary pancreatic insufficiency and bone marrow failure, characterized by normal sweat chloride values, pancreatic insufficiency, and neutropenia; it may be associated with dwarfism and metaphyseal dysostosis of the hips Shwachman 综合征，Shwachman-Diamond 综合征，原发性胰腺功能不全和骨髓功能衰竭，以正常的氯化汗值、胰腺功能不全和中性粒细胞减少为特征；可能与侏儒症和髋部干骺端发育不全有关；**sick sinus s.,** intermittent bradycardia, sometimes with episodes of atrial tachyarrhythmias or periods of sinus arrest, due to malfunction originating in the supraventricular portion of the cardiac conducting system 病态窦房结综合征，间歇性心动过缓，有时伴有房性心动过速发作或窦性停搏，由于心脏传导系统室上部分的功能障碍引起；**Silver-Russell s.,** a syndrome of low birth weight despite normal gestation duration, and short stature, lateral asymmetry, and some increase in gonadotropin secretionSilver-Russell 综合征，一种低出生体重综合征，尽管妊娠期正常，出生后以身材矮小、躯体偏身不对称、促性腺激素分泌增加为特征；**Sjögren s.,** a symptom complex usually in middle-aged or older women, marked by keratoconjunctivitis sicca, xerostomia, and enlargement of the parotid glands; it is often associated with rheumatoid arthritis and sometimes with systemic lupus erythematosus, scleroderma, or polymyositis 干燥综合征，一种通常在中年或老年妇女中出现的症状综合征，以干眼症、干燥症和腮腺肿大为特征；常与类风湿关节炎有关，有时与系统性红斑狼疮、硬皮病或多发性肌炎有关；**sleep apnea s.,** sleep apnea 睡眠呼吸暂停综合征；**Smith-Lemli-Opitz s.,** an autosomal recessive syndrome of microcephaly, intellectual disability, hypotonia, incomplete development of male genitalia, short nose with anteverted nostrils, and syndactyly of second and third toes Smith-Lemli-Opitz 综合征，小头 - 小颌 - 并趾综合征，一种常染色体隐性遗传综合征，包括小头畸形、智力障碍、张力减退、男性生殖器发育不全、鼻孔前倾的短鼻、第二趾和第三趾的并趾畸形；**social breakdown s.,** deterioration of social and interpersonal skills, work habits, and behavior seen in chronically institutionalized persons who have little productive activity, such as long-term psychiatric patients or prisoners 社交能力衰退综合征，社会和人际交往技能、工作习惯和行为的恶化，见于长期缺乏生产活动的精神病患者或囚犯等；**stagnant loops.,** 同 stasis；**staphylococcal scalded skin s.,** an infectious disease, usually affecting infants and young children, following infection with certain strains of *Staphylococcus aureus,* characterized by localized to widespread bullous eruption and exfoliation of the skin, leaving raw, denuded areas that make the skin look scalded 葡萄球菌烫伤样皮肤综合征，一种感染性疾病，通常影响婴幼儿，感染某些金黄色葡萄球菌菌株后，其特征是局部出现广泛的大疱和皮肤脱落，留下粗糙、脱皮的区域，使皮肤看起来像烫伤；**stasis s.,** overgrowth of bacteria in the small intestine secondary to various disorders causing stasis; it is characterized by malabsorption of vitamin B_{12}, steatorrhea, and anemia 停滞综合征，小肠中细菌的过度生长，继发于各种引起停滞的疾病；其特征为维生素 B_{12} 吸收不良、脂肪热和贫血；**Steele-Richardson-Olszewski s.,** a progressive neurologic disorder with onset during the sixth decade, characterized by supranuclear ophthalmoplegia, especially paralysis of the downward gaze, pseudobulbar palsy, dysarthria, dystonic rigidity of the neck and trunk, and dementia Steele-Richardson-Olszewski 综合征，于 60 岁发病的进行性神经病，主要表现为核上性眼肌麻痹，尤其是向下凝视的麻痹、假球性麻痹、构音障碍、颈和躯干的张力障碍性僵硬和痴呆；**Stein-Leventhal s.,** 同 polycystic ovary s.；**Stevens-Johnson s.,** a sometimes fatal form of erythema multiforme presenting with a flulike prodrome and characterized by severe mucocutaneous lesions; pulmonary, gastrointestinal, cardiac, and renal involvement may occur 重症多形性红斑，一种有时致命的多形性红斑，表现为流感样前驱症状，以严重的黏膜皮肤损伤为特征；可能发生肺部、胃肠道、心脏和肾脏受累；**Stewart-Treves s.,** lymphangiosarcoma occurring as a late complication of severe lymphedema of the arm after excision of the lymph nodes, usually in radical mastectomy 乳腺癌切除术后淋巴管肉瘤，切除淋巴结后手臂严重淋巴水肿的晚期并发症，通常在根治性乳房切除术中发生；**stiff-man s.,** a condition of unknown etiology marked by progressive fluctuating rigidity of axial and limb muscles in the absence of signs of cerebral and spinal cord disease but with continuous electromyographic activity 僵人综合征，一种病因不明的疾病，其特征是在没有脑脊髓病迹象的情况下，躯干和肢体肌肉的硬度逐渐波动，但肌电图活动持续；**stroke s.,** stroke; a condition with sudden onset due to acute vascular lesions of the brain (hemorrhage, embolism, thrombosis, rupturing aneurysm), which may be marked by hemiplegia or hemiparesis, vertigo, numbness, aphasia, and dysarthria, and often followed by permanent neurologic damage 中风综合征，由于大脑的急性血管损伤（出血、栓塞、血栓形成、动脉瘤破裂）而突然发作的一种疾病，可能以偏瘫或轻偏瘫、眩晕、麻木、失语症和构音障碍为特征，常伴有永久性神经损伤；**Sturge-Weber s.,** a congenital syndrome consisting of a port-wine stain type of nevus flammeus distributed over the trigeminal nerve accompanied by a similar vascular disorder of the underlying meninges and cerebral cortex 斯特奇 - 韦伯综合征，脸面血管瘤病，脑三叉神经血管瘤综合征，一种先天性综合征，由分布在三叉神经上的红痣型葡萄酒色斑构成，伴随着下半月板和大脑皮质的类似血管疾病；**subclavian steal s.,** cerebral or brainstem ischemia due to vertebrobasilar insufficiency in cases of subclavian steal 锁骨下动脉盗血综合征，椎基底动脉供血不足致脑或脑干缺血；**sudden infant death s.,** sudden and unexpected death of an infant who had previously been apparently well, and which is unexplained by careful postmortem examination 婴儿猝死综合征，健康的婴儿突然死亡，尸检无法解释；**supine hypotension s.,** partial occlusion of the inferior vena cava and the descending aorta by the uterus, especially when a woman is pregnant, resulting in hypotension when in a supine position 仰卧位低血压综合征，子宫对下腔静脉和降主动脉的部分阻塞，尤其是孕妇，在仰卧位时引起低血压；**Swyer-James s.,** acquired unilateral hyperlucent lung, with severe airway obstruction during exhalation, oligemia, and a small hilum Swyer-James 综合征，获得性单侧高透光肺，呼气时有严重的气道阻塞；**tarsal tunnel s.,** a syndrome of overuse injury with a complex of symptoms resulting from compression of the posterior tibial nerve or of the plantar nerves in the tarsal tunnel, with pain, numbness, and tingling paresthesia of the sole of the foot 跗管综合征，踝管卡压症，伴随着胫后神经或跗管内足底神经压迫引起的复杂症状，伴有足底疼痛、麻木和刺痛性感觉异常；**Taussig-Bing s.,** transposition of the great vessels of the heart and a ventricular septal defect straddled by a large pulmonary artery 陶 - 宾综合征，心脏大血管转位和由大肺动脉跨接的室间隔缺损；**temporomandibular joint s.,** temporomandibular disorder 颞下颌关节紊乱；**Tolosa-Hunt s.,** unilateral ophthalmoplegia associated with pain behind the orbit and in the area supplied by the first division of the trigeminal nerve; it is thought to be due to nonspecific inflammation and granulation tissue in the superior orbital fissure or cavernous sinus 托洛萨 - 亨特综合征，痛性眼肌麻痹，单侧眼肌麻痹，伴有眶后及三叉神经第一节区疼痛；据认为是由于眶上裂或海绵窦内非特异性炎症和肉芽组织所致；**TORCH s.**, any of a group of infections seen in neonates as a result of the infectious agent having crossed the placental barrier TORCH 综合征，由于感染性生物质穿过胎盘屏障而在新生儿中发现的一组传染病；**Tourette s.**, 同 Gilles de la Tourette s；**Townes s.**, an inherited disorder of auricular anomalies, anal defects, limb and digit anomalies, and renal deficiencies, occasionally including cardiac disease, deafness, or cystic ovary Townes 综合征，遗传性耳廓异常、肛门缺陷、四肢和手指异常以及肾功能不全的遗传性疾病，有时包括心脏疾病、耳聋或卵巢囊性病变；**toxic shock s.**, sudden high fever, vomiting, diarrhea, and myalgia, followed by hypotension and, in severe cases, shock; a sunburnlike rash with skin peeling, especially on palms and soles, occurs during the acute phase. Formerly observed mainly in menstruating women using tampons, caused by *Staphylococcus aureus* infection, it has now been observed in other women and in males, caused by infection with *Streptococcus* 中毒性休克综合征；**transurethral resection s.**, hyponatremia caused by absorption of fluids used to irrigate the bladder during transurethral resection of the prostate 经尿道电切除综合征术中吸收用于冲洗膀胱的液体引起的低钠血症；**Treacher Collins s.**, the incomplete form of mandibulofacial dysostosis 特雷彻·柯林斯综合征，下颌颜面发育不全；**triple A s.**, Allgrove s. 三联 A 综合征，贲门弛缓不能—无泪—肾上腺功能低下综合征；**trisomy 8 s.**, a syndrome due to an extra chromosome 8, usually mosaic (trisomy 8/ normal), with mild to severe intellectual disability, prominent forehead, deep-set eyes, thick lips, prominent ears, and camptodactyly 8 三体综合征，由额外的 8 号染色体引起的综合征，通常为嵌合体（8 号三体 / 正常），有轻度到重度智力障碍、前额突出、眼睛深陷、嘴唇厚、耳朵突出、先天性指屈曲；**trisomy 13 s.**, holoprosencephaly due to an extra chromosome 13, in which central nervous system defects are associated with intellectual disability, along with cleft lip and palate, polydactyly, and dermal pattern anomalies, and abnormalities of the heart, viscera, and genitalia 13 三体综合征，由 13 号染色体引起的无前脑畸形，其中中枢神经系统缺陷与智力障碍有关，伴有唇腭裂、多指畸形和皮肤形态异常，以及心脏、内脏和生殖器异常；**trisomy 18 s.**, neonatal hepatitis, mental retardation, scaphocephaly or other skull abnormality, micrognathia, blepharoptosis, low-set ears, corneal opacities, deafness, webbed

neck, short digits, ventricular septal defects, Meckel diverticulum, and other deformities. It is due to an extra chromosome 18 18 三体综合征，新生儿肝炎、精神发育迟滞、舟头畸形或其他颅骨异常、小颌骨、上睑下垂、低置耳、角膜混浊、耳聋、蹼颈、短指、室间隔缺损、梅克尔憩室等畸形由额外的 18 号染色体引起；**trisomy 21 s.**, 同 Down s.；**Trousseau s.**, spontaneous venous thrombosis of upper and lower limbs associated with visceral carcinoma Trousseau 综合征，内脏癌并发上下肢自发性静脉血栓形成；**tumor lysis s.**, severe hyperphosphatemia, hyperkalemia, hyperuricemia, and hypocalcemia after effective induction chemotherapy of rapidly growing malignant neoplasms 肿瘤溶解综合征，对快速生长的恶性肿瘤进行有效诱导化疗后出现严重的高磷血症、高钾血症、高尿酸血症和低钙血症；**TUR s.**, transurethral resection syndrome 经尿道电切综合征；**Turcot s.**, familial polyposis of the colon associated with gliomas of the central nervous sytem 特科特综合征，与中枢神经系统胶质瘤相关的家族性结肠息肉病；**Turner s.**, gonadal dysgenesis with short stature, undifferentiated (streak) gonads, and variable abnormalities such as webbing of the neck, low posterior hairline, increased carrying angle of elbow, cubitus valgus, and cardiac defects. The genotype is XO (45, X) or X/XX or X/XXX mosaic. The phenotype is female 特纳综合征，性腺发育障碍症，患者性腺发育不全伴身材矮小、性腺未分化（条状）、蹼状颈、后发际低、肘部抬角增大、肘外翻和心脏缺陷等；基因型为 XO（45，X）或 X/XX 或 X/XXX 嵌合；表型为女性；**twiddler's s.**, dislodgement, breakdown, or other malfunction of an implanted diagnostic device as a result of unconscious or habitual manipulation by the patient 起搏器旋弄综合征，由于患者无意识或习惯性操作导致植入诊断设备移位、故障或其他故障；**twin transfusion s.**, **twin–twin transfusion s.**, one caused by twin-to-twin transfusion (q.v.); the donor twin is small, pale, and anemic, whereas the recipient is large and polycythemic, with an overloaded cardiovascular system 双胎间输血综合征，双胎对双胎输血引起的；供体双胎小、苍白、贫血，而受体大、红细胞增多，心血管系统负荷过重；**urethral s.**, symptoms associated with a urethral problem other than infection, including suprapubic aching and cramping, urinary frequency, and bladder complaints such as dysuria, tenesmus, and low back pain 尿道综合征，与感染以外的尿道问题相关的症状，包括耻骨上疼痛和痉挛、尿频和膀胱不适，如排尿困难、尿急和膀痛；**Usher s.**, an inherited syndrome of congenital deafness with retinitis pigmentosa, often ending in blindness; intellectual dis-

S

ability and gait disturbances may also occur 乌谢尔综合征，先天性聋视网膜色素变性综合征，先天性耳聋合并色素性视网膜炎的遗传综合征，常以失明告终；也可发生智力障碍和步态障碍；**Van der Woude s. (VWS)**, an autosomal dominant syndrome consisting of cleft lip with or without cleft palate, with cysts of the lower lip Van der Woude 综合征，一种常染色体显性综合征，包括唇裂伴或不伴腭裂；下唇囊肿；**velocardiofacial s.**, Shprintzen s.; an inherited syndrome of cardiac defects and craniofacial anomalies; learning disabilities often occur, and less often other abnormalities. It is a phenotype of 22q11 deletion syndrome 腭心面综合征，施普因岑综合征，常表现为学习困难，为 22q11 缺失综合征的一种表现形式；**Verner-Morrison s.**, profuse watery diarrhea, hypokalemia, and achlorhydria, usually with excess levels of vasoactive intestinal polypeptide from a VIPoma in the pancreas 弗纳 - 莫里森综合征，胰性霍乱综合征，表现为大量水样腹泻、低钾血症和低胃酸，通常伴有胰腺内血管活性肠多肽水平过高；**Vernet s.**, paralysis of the glossopharyngeal, vagus, and spinal accessory nerves due to a lesion in the region of the jugular foramen 颈动脉孔综合征，颈静脉孔区损伤导致的舌咽神经、迷走神经和脊髓副神经麻痹；**Villaret s.**, unilateral paralysis of the glossopharyngeal, vagus, spinal accessory, and hypoglossal nerves and sometimes the facial nerve, due to a lesion behind the parotid glands 间隙综合征，由于腮腺后的病变而造成的舌咽、迷走神经、脊柱附件和舌下神经及面部神经的单侧麻痹；**Vogt-Koyanagi-Harada s.**, bilateral uveitis with iridocyclitis, exudative choroiditis, meningism, and retinal detachment, accompanied by alopecia, vitiligo, poliosis, loss of visual acuity, headache, vomiting, and deafness; possibly an inflammatory autoimmune disorder 福格特 - 小柳 - 原田综合征，双侧葡萄膜炎伴虹膜睫状体炎、渗出性脉络膜炎、脑膜炎和视网膜脱离，伴有脱发、白癜风、脊髓灰质炎、视力丧失、头痛、呕吐和耳聋；可能为炎症性自身免疫性疾病；**Vohwinkel s.**, an autosomal dominant, progressive, dystrophic form of palmoplantar keratoderma beginning in childhood, sometimes with scarring alopecia and deafness 残毁性皮肤角化病综合征，一种常染色体显性、进行性、营养不良型掌跖角化病，从儿童期开始，伴有瘢痕性脱发和耳聋；**Waardenburg s.**, any of several inherited conditions characterized principally by pigmentary abnormalities of the eyes, skin, and hair, including iris heterochromia and white forelock, and hearing loss. In some forms, there is lateral displacement of the inner canthi of the eyes with a widened bridge of the nose Waardenburg 综合征，一种主要表现为眼睛、皮肤和头发的色素异常的遗传病，包括虹膜异色和白色前锁和听力损失；在某些情况下，眼角内侧有横向位移、鼻梁加宽；**WAGR s.**, a syndrome of Wilms tumor, aniridia, genitourinary abnormalities or gonadoblastoma, and retardation, due to a deletion in chromosome 11 11p 缺失综合征，临床表现为肾母细胞瘤、无虹膜、泌尿生殖系统异常或性腺母细胞瘤和发育迟缓；**Walker-Warburg s.**, a genetically and clinically heterogeneous, autosomal recessive syndrome, usually fatal in infancy, of hydrocephalus, agyria with cerebellar malformations, retinal dysplasia and other ocular anomalies, muscular dystrophy, and sometimes encephalocele 沃 - 华综合征，一种遗传和临床上的异质性、常染色体隐性遗传病，通常在婴儿期致命，包括脑积水、小脑畸形的无脑畸形、视网膜发育不良和其他眼部异常、肌肉营养不良，有时伴有脑膨出；**Waterhouse-Friderichsen s.**, a fulminating complication of meningococcemia, with bilateral adrenal hemorrhages, cyanosis, petechiae on the skin and mucous membranes, shock, collapse, and coma 华 - 弗综合征，暴发型脑膜炎球菌败血症，脑膜炎球菌血症的严重并发症，伴有双侧肾上腺出血、发绀、皮肤和黏膜瘀点、休克、虚脱和昏迷；**Weber s.**, paralysis of the oculomotor nerve on the same side as the lesion, causing ptosis, strabismus, and loss of light reflex and accommodation; also spastic hemiplegia on the side opposite the lesion with increased reflexes and loss of superficial reflexes 韦伯综合征，大脑脚综合征，临床表现为病变同侧动眼神经麻痹，对侧上下肢瘫痪；**Weil s.**, a severe form of leptospirosis, marked by jaundice usually accompanied by azotemia, hemorrhage, anemia, disturbances of consciousness, and continued fever 魏尔综合征，一种严重的钩端螺旋体病，以黄疸为特征，通常伴有氮质血症、出血、贫血、意识障碍和持续发热；**Werner s.**, premature aging of an adult, with early graying and some hair loss, cataracts, hyperkeratinization, muscular atrophy, scleroderma-like changes in the skin of the limbs, and a high incidence of neoplasm 沃纳综合征，成人早老综合征，成人早衰，早期灰白，部分脱发，白内障，角化过度，肌肉萎缩，四肢皮肤硬皮病样改变，肿瘤发生率高；**Wernicke-Korsakoff s.**, a neuropsychiatric disorder caused by thiamine deficiency, most often due to alcohol abuse, combining the features of Wernicke encephalopathy and Korsakoff syndrome 韦尼克 - 科尔萨夫综合征一种由硫胺素缺乏引起的神经精神疾病，通常由酗酒引起，结合了韦尼克脑病和科尔萨夫综合征的特征 **whiplash shake s.**, subdural hematomas, retinal hemorrhage, and sometimes cerebral contusions caused by the stretching and tearing of cerebral vessels and brain substance, sometimes seen when a very young child is shaken vigorously by the limbs or trunk with the head unsupported; paralysis, visual disturbances, blindness, convulsions, and death may result 头部摇摆综合征，硬膜下血肿 - 视网膜出血，有时因脑血管和脑实质的拉伸和撕裂而导致脑挫伤，有时在剧烈摇晃无头部支撑的幼儿四肢或躯干时发生；可能导致瘫痪、视觉障碍、失明、抽搐和死亡；**white clot s.**, heparin-induced thrombocytopenia 白色血凝块综合征，肝素诱导的血小板减少；**Williams s.**, supravalvular aortic stenosis, intellectual disability, elfin facies, and idiopathic hypercalcemia in infants Williams 综合征，婴儿主动脉瓣上狭窄，智力障碍、小精灵面容和特发性高钙血症；**Wilson-Mikity s.**, a rare form of pulmonary insufficiency in low birth-weight infants, with hyperpnea and cyanosis during the first month of life, sometimes ending in death; there are also radiologic abnormalities 威 - 米综合征，低出生体重儿肺功能不全的一种罕见形式，在出生后的第一个月内出现高通气和发绀，有时以死亡告终；也有放射学异常；**Wiskott-Aldrich s.**, chronic eczema with chronic suppurative otitis media, anemia, and thrombocytopenic purpura, an immunodeficiency syndrome transmitted as an X-linked recessive trait, with poor antibody response to polysaccharide antigens and dysfunction of cell-mediated immunity 威斯科特 - 奥尔德里奇综合征，湿疹 - 血小板减少 - 免疫缺陷综合征，一种 X 连锁隐性性状传播的免疫缺陷综合征，对多糖抗原抗体反应差，细胞免疫功能紊乱；**Wolf-Hirschhorn s.**, a syndrome due to partial deletion of the short arm of chromosome 4, with microcephaly, ocular hypertelorism, epicanthus, cleft palate, micrognathia, low-set ears simplified in form, cryptorchidism, and hypospadias 沃尔夫 - 赫希霍恩综合征，4p 部分单体综合征，第 4 染色体短臂缺失导致的综合征，伴有小头畸形，眼距宽宽、内眦赘皮、腭裂、小颌畸形、形态简化的低耳畸形、隐睾和尿道下裂；**Wolff-Parkinson-White (WPW) s.**, the association of paroxysmal tachycardia (or atrial fibrillation) and preexcitation, in which the electrocardiogram displays a short P–R interval and a wide QRS complex that characteristically shows an early QRS vector (delta wave) 沃 - 帕 - 怀综合征，预激综合征，阵发性心动过速（或心房颤动）与预激的关联，其中心电图显示短 P-R 间期和宽 QRS 波群，其特征性显示早期 QRS 向量（δ 波）；**Wyburn-Mason s.**, arteriovenous aneurysms on one or both sides of the brain, with ocular anomalies, facial nevi, and sometimes intellectual disability Wyburn-Mason 综合征，大脑一侧或两侧的动静脉瘤，

伴有眼部异常，面部痣，有时伴有智力障碍；**s. X**, angina pectoris or anginalike chest pain associated with a normal arteriographic appearance of the coronary arteries X 综合征，心绞痛或心绞痛样胸痛与冠状动脉的正常动脉造影相关；**Zellweger s.**, an autosomal recessive disorder characterized by craniofacial abnormalities, hypotonia, hepatomegaly, polycystic kidneys, jaundice, and usually death in early infancy; due to mutations affecting peroxisome biosynthesis 泽尔韦格综合征，脑肝肾综合征，一种常染色体隐性遗传病，以颅面畸形、张力减退、肝肿大、多囊肾、黄疸为特征，通常在婴儿期早期死亡；**Zollinger-Ellison s.**, the association of atypical, intractable, sometimes fulminating peptic ulcers with extreme gastric hyperacidity and benign or malignant gastrinomas in the pancreas 佐林格 - 埃利森综合征，以难治性、反复发作的消化性溃疡和高胃酸分泌为临床特征；由一种少见的神经内分泌肿瘤（胃泌瘤）或胃泌素细胞增生所致

syn·drom·ic (sin-drom′ik) occurring as a syndrome or as part of a syndrome 综合征的

syn·drom·ol·o·gy (sin″drə-mol′ə-je) the field concerned with the taxonomy, etiology, and patterns of congenital malformations 综合征学，与先天畸形的分类、病因和类型有关的领域

syn·ech·ia (sĭ-nek′e-ə) pl. **syne′chiae** [Gr.] adhesion, as of the iris to the cornea or lens 粘连，尤指虹膜与角膜或虹膜与晶状体的粘连；**s. vulvae**, a congenital condition in which the labia minora are sealed in the midline, with only a small opening below the clitoris through which urination and menstruation may occur 外阴粘连，一种先天性疾病，其中小阴唇密封在中线，阴蒂下方只有一个小开口，通过它可以发生排尿和月经

syn·echot·o·my (sin″ə-kot′ə-me) incision of a synechia 虹膜粘连切开术

syn·er·e·sis (sĭ-ner′ə-sis) a drawing together of the particles of the dispersed phase of a gel, with separation of some of the dispersed medium and shrinkage of the gel 离浆作用，脱水收缩，将凝胶分散相的颗粒拉近，分离一些分散介质和凝胶收缩

syn·er·gic (sin-ur′jik) acting together or in harmony 协作的，协同的，又称 *synergetic*

syn·er·gism (sin′ər-jizm) synergy 协同，增效

syn·er·gist (sin′ər-jist) a muscle or agent that acts with another 增效剂，协作剂

syn·er·gis·tic (sin″ər-jis′tik) 1. acting together 协作的；2. enhancing the effect of another force or agent 协同作用的

syn·er·gy (sin′ər-je) 1. correlated action or cooperation on the part of two or more structures or drugs 协同作用（指药物）；2. in neurology, the faculty by which movements are properly grouped for the performance of acts requiring special adjustments 协同作用，在神经学中，各种运动适当组合以执行需要调节的动作

syn·es·the·sia (sin″es-the′zhə) 联　觉 1. a secondary sensation accompanying an actual perception 伴随着实际感知的第二感觉；2. a dysesthesia in which a stimulus of one sense is perceived as sensation of a different sense, as when a sound produces a sensation of color 一种感觉障碍，一种感觉刺激被感知为不同感觉的感觉，如声音产生颜色的感觉；3. a dysesthesia in which a stimulus to one part of the body is experienced as being at a different location 一种感觉障碍，其中对身体某一部分的刺激被体验为处于不同的位置

syn·es·the·si·al·gia (sin″es-the″ze-al′jə) a painful synesthesia 痛联觉，痛性牵连感觉

syn·ga·my (sing′gə-me) 1. sexual reproduction 有性生殖；2. the union of two gametes to form a zygote in fertilization 配子配合，受精时两个配子结合形成合子；**syn′gamous** adj.

syn·ge·ne·ic (sin″jə-ne′ik) denoting individuals or tissues that have identical genotypes and thus could participate in a syngraft 同基因的，同源的，同系的，同质的，指具有相同基因型的个体或组织，因此可以参与同种移植

syn·gen·e·sis (sin-jen′ə-sis) 1. the origin of an individual from a germ cell derived from both parents and not from either one alone 有性生殖，个体起源于双亲的生殖细胞而非单独一方；2. the state of having descended from a common ancestor 共生，同生，来自同一共同祖先

syn·graft (sin′graft) isograft; a graft between genetically identical individuals, typically between identical twins or between animals of a single highly inbred strain 同种同基因移植

syn·i·ze·sis (sin″ĭ-ze′sis) 1. occlusion. 闭合；2. a mitotic stage in which the nuclear chromatin is massed 终变期，浓缩期

syn·ki·ne·sis (sin″kĭ-ne′sis) an involuntary movement accompanying a volitional movement 联带运动，伴随意向运动的无意运动；**synkinet′ic** adj.

syn·ne·cro·sis (sin″ə-kro′sis) symbiosis in which the relationship between populations (or individuals) is mutually detrimental 双损共生，群体（或个体）间导致相互抑制或死亡的关系

syn·oph·thal·mia (sin″of-thal′me-ə) the usual form of cyclopia, in which the two eyes are more or less completely fused into one 并眼（畸形），独眼（畸形）

syn·os·che·os (sin-os′ke-os) adhesion between the penis and scrotum 阴囊阴茎粘连

syn·os·te·ot·o·my (sin″os-te-ot′ə-me) dissection of the joints 关节切开术

syn·os·to·sis (sin″os-to′sis) pl. *synosto′ses*. 1. a union between adjacent bones or parts of a single bone formed by osseous material 骨连接；2. the osseous union of bones that are normally distinct 骨性（融）合；**synostot′ic** adj.; **sagittal s.,** premature fusion of the sagittal suture, usually sporadic but sometimes of autosomal dominant inheritance; it results in anteroposterior elongation and reduction in width of the skull (scaphocephaly), often with bossing and a ridge along the suture 矢状缝间骨性结合

sy·no·tia (sĭ-no′she-ə) persistence of the ears in their initial fetal position (horizontal, beneath the mandible) 并耳（畸形）

syn·o·vec·to·my (sin″o-vek′tə-me) excision of a synovial membrane. The analogous destruction of the membrane performed using chemicals *(chemical s.)* or radiation *(radiation s.)* may be called synoviorthesis, particularly the latter 滑膜切除术

sy·no·via (sĭ-no′ve-ə) synovial fluid 滑液

sy·no·vi·al (sĭ-no′ve-əl) 1. pertaining to a synovial membrane 滑膜的；2. pertaining to or secreting synovia 滑液的

sy·no·vi·a·lis (sĭ-no″ve-a′lis) [L.] synovial 滑液的

sy·no·vi·o·ma (sĭ-no″ve-o′mə) a tumor of synovial membrane origin 滑膜瘤

sy·no·vi·or·the·sis (sĭ-no″ve-or-the′sis) 放射性滑膜切除术，参见 *synovectomy*

syno·vi·tis (sin″o-vi′tis) inflammation of a synovial membrane, usually painful, particularly on motion, and characterized by fluctuating swelling, due to effusion in a synovial sac 滑膜炎 **dry s., s. sic′ca,** that with little effusion 干性滑膜炎；**simple s.,** that with clear or but slightly turbid effusion 单纯性滑膜炎；**tendinous s.,** tenosynovitis 腱鞘炎；**villonodular s.,** proliferation of synovial tissue, especially of the knee joint, composed of synovial villi and fibrous nodules infiltrated by giant cells and macrophages 绒毛结节性滑膜炎

sy·no·vi·um (sĭ-no′ve-əm) synovial membrane 滑膜

syn·poly·dac·ty·ly (sin-pol″e-dak′tə-le) association of polydactyly and syndactyly of varying degrees of the hand and foot 并指多指，并趾多趾

Syn·ri·bo (sĭn-rye′bow) trademark for a preparation of omacetaxine mepesuccinate 高三尖杉酯碱制剂的商品名

syn·tax·in (sin-tak′sin) a transmembrane protein anchored in the target area of the presynaptic membrane of the nerve terminal and playing a role in synaptic vesicle fusion and neurotransmitter release 突触融合蛋白，跨膜蛋白锚定在神经末梢突触前膜的目标区域，在突触小泡融合和神经递质释放中发挥作用

syn·te·ny (sin′tə-ne) 1. the presence together on the

same chromosome of two or more gene loci whether or not in such proximity that they may be subject to linkage 同线性；2. conservation of gene order between the chromosomes of different species 同源模块；**synten′ic** *adj*

syn·thase (sin′thās) a term used in the names of some enzymes, particularly lyases, when the synthetic aspect of the reaction is dominant or emphasized 合酶

syn·the·sis (sin′thə-sis) 1. the creation of an integrated whole by the combining of simpler parts or entities 合成；2. the formation of a chemical compound by the union of its elements or from other suitable components（化学）合成；3. in psychiatry, the integration of the various elements of the personality 综合，在精神病学中，人格各要素的整合；**synthet′ic** *adj.*

syn·the·tase (sin′thə-tās) a term used in the names of some of the ligases, no longer favored because of its similarity to the term synthase and its emphasis on reaction products 合成酶

syn·tro·pho·blast (sin-trof′o-blast) syncytiotrophoblast 合胞体滋养层

syn·tro·pic (sin-tro′pik) 1. turning or pointing in the same direction 同向的，转向或指向同一方向；2. denoting correlation of several factors, as the relation of one disease to the development or incidence of another 同调的，指若干因素的相关性，如一种疾病与另一种疾病的发展或发病率的关系

syn·tro·py (sin′trə-pe) the state of being syntropic 同向；同调

sy·nuc·le·in (sĭ-noo′kle-in) a family of structurally related brain proteins, comprising three types designated α, β, and γ. Abnormal aggregations of α-synuclein are characteristic of certain neurodegenerative diseases 突触核蛋白，一个与结构相关的脑蛋白家族，包括三种类型，即α、β和γ。α-突触核蛋白异常聚集是某些神经退行性疾病的特征

syph·i·lid (sif′ĭ-lid) any of the skin lesions of secondary syphilis 梅毒疹

syph·i·lis (sif′ĭ-lis) a subacute to chronic infectious disease caused by *Treponema pallidum*, leading to many structural and cutaneous lesions, usually transmitted by direct sexual contact or acquired in utero 梅毒，参见 *primary s., secondary s.,tertiary s.*；**syphilit′ic** *adj.*；**cardiovascular s.**, tertiary syphilis in which obliterative endarteritis of the aorta causes damage to the intima and media of the great vessels 心血管梅毒，为三期梅毒的一种类型，表现为主动脉瓣关闭不全发生闭塞性动脉内膜炎，使大血管的内膜及中层受损；**congenital s.**, syphilis acquired in utero, manifested by any of several characteristic malformations of teeth or bones, by mucocutaneous

lesions at birth or shortly thereafter, and by ocular or neurologic changes 胎性梅毒，先天性梅毒，在子宫内获得的梅毒，有不同的表现，可以是某种牙或骨的典型畸形，也可以是出生时或出生后不久发生的活动性黏膜皮肤梅毒，眼的改变如间质性角膜炎，或神经方面的改变如耳聋等；**endemic s., nonvenereal s.**, a chronic inflammatory infection caused by a subspecies of *Treponema pallidum,* transmitted nonsexually; it has an early stage with mucous patches and moist papules in axillae and skin folds; a latent stage; and then late complications such as gummata 地方性梅毒，非性病梅毒，一种慢性炎症性传染病，非性传播的螺旋体感染，早期在腋窝和皮肤皱褶处有黏液斑和湿丘疹，经过一段潜伏期出现晚期并发症，如梅毒瘤；**late benign s.**, tertiary syphilis characterized mainly by gummata and responding rapidly to treatment 晚期良性梅毒，三期梅毒的一种类型，治疗收效迅速，典型损害为梅毒瘤；**primary s.**, syphilis in its first stage, with a chancre that is infectious and painless, and adjacent hard, swollen lymph nodes 一期梅毒，下疳具有传染性和无痛性，并邻近硬而肿胀的淋巴结；**secondary s.**, syphilis in the second of three stages, with fever, multiform skin eruptions (syphilids), iritis, alopecia, mucous patches, and severe pain in the head, joints, and periosteum 二期梅毒，伴有发热、多种形式的皮疹（梅毒疹）、虹膜炎、脱发、黏液斑和头部、关节和骨膜剧烈疼痛；**tertiary s.**, the third and last stage of syphilis; marked by destructive lesions involving many tissues and organs and occurring in three principal forms: *cardiovascular s., late benign s.,* and *neurosyphilis* 三期梅毒，以破坏性损伤为特征，累及多种组织和器官，以三种主要形式出现，心血管梅毒、晚期良性梅毒和神经梅毒

sy·ringe (sĭ-rinj′) (sir′inj) an instrument for injecting liquids into or withdrawing them from any vessel or cavity 注射器；**air s., chip s.**, a small, finenozzled syringe, used to direct an air current into a tooth cavity being excavated, to remove small fragments, or to dry the cavity 吹干器，气枪；**bulb s.**, one with a bulb on one end, which is compressed to create a vacuum for gentle suction of small amounts of bodily drainage; also used for intraoperative irrigation 球注射器；**dental s.**, a small syringe used in operative dentistry, containing an anesthetic solution 牙科注射器，一种用于牙科手术的小注射器，含有麻醉溶液；**hypodermic s.**, one for introduction of liquids through a hollow needle into superficial fascia 皮下注射器

syr·in·gec·to·my (sir″in-jek′tə-me) excision of the walls of a fistula 瘘管切除术

syr·in·gi·tis (sir″in-ji′tis) inflammation of the auditory tube 咽鼓管炎

sy·rin·go·bul·bia (sĭ-ring′go-bul′be-ə) the presence of cavities in the medulla oblongata 延髓空洞症

sy·rin·go·cele (sĭ-ring′go-sēl) 1. a cystlike swelling in a tubular structure of the body 空洞性脊髓突出；2. myelocele 脊髓膨出

sy·rin·go·coele (sĭ-ring′go-sēl) the central canal of the spinal cord 脊髓中央管

sy·rin·go·cys·tad·e·no·ma (sĭ-ring″go-sistad″ə-no′mə) a benign adnexal tumor of the sweat glands 汗腺腺瘤

sy·rin·go·ma (sir″ing-go′mə) a benign tumor believed to originate from the ductal portion of the eccrine sweat glands, characterized by dilated cystic sweat ducts in a fibrous stroma 汗腺腺瘤，一种良性肿瘤，被认为是起源于小汗腺的导管部分，特征是纤维间质中的囊性汗管扩张

sy·rin·go·my·elia (sĭ-ring″go-mi-e′le-ə) a slowly progressive syndrome of varying etiology, in which cavitation occurs in the central segments of the spinal cord, generally in the cervical region, with resulting neurologic defects; thoracic scoliosis is often present 脊髓空洞症

sy·rin·got·o·my (sir″in-got′ə-me) fistulotomy 瘘管切开术

syr·inx (sir′inks) [Gr.] 1. a tube or pipe 管；2. fistula 瘘，瘘管

syr·up (sir′əp) a concentrated solution of a sugar, such as sucrose, in water or other aqueous liquid, sometimes with a medicinal agent added; usually used as a flavored vehicle for drugs. The meaning is commonly expanded to include any liquid dosage form (e.g., oral suspension) in a sweet and viscid vehicle 糖浆剂

sys·tal·tic (sis-tawl′tik) alternately contracting and dilating; pulsating 舒缩交替的

sys·tem (sis′təm) 1. a set or series of interconnected or interdependent parts or entities (objects, organs, or organisms) that act together for a common purpose or produce results impossible by action of one alone 系统，系；2. a school or method of practice based on a specific set of principles 学派；**alimentary s.,** 同 digestive s.；**auditory s.,** the series of structures by which sounds are received from the environment and conveyed as signals to the central nervous system; it consists of the outer, middle, and inner ear and the tracts in the auditory pathways 听觉系统；**autonomic nervous s.,** the portion of the nervous system concerned with regulation of activity of cardiac muscle, smooth muscle, and glandular epithelium, usually restricted to the sympathetic and parasympathetic nervous systems 自主神经系统；**Bethesda S.,** a classification of cervical and vaginal cytology used in cytopathologic diagnosis Bethesda 分类系统，在细胞病理学诊断中使用的宫颈和阴道细胞学分类体系；**cardiovascular s.,** the heart and blood vessels, by which blood is pumped and circulated through the body 心血管系统，见图 15 至图 24；**CD s.,** a system for classifying cell surface markers expressed by lymphocytes based on a computer analysis grouping similar monoclonal antibodies raised against human leukocyte antigens 群簇命名体系，一种基于计算机分析对人类白细胞抗原产生的类似单克隆抗体分组的淋巴细胞表达的细胞表面标志物分类系统；**centimeter-gram-second s. (CGS) (cgs),** a system of measurements in which the units are based on the centimeter as the unit of length, the gram as the unit of mass, and the second as the unit of time 厘米 - 克 - 秒制，以厘米为长度单位，克为质量单位，秒为时间单位的测量系统；**central nervous s. (CNS),** the brain and spinal cord 中枢神经系统；**centrencephalic s.,** the neurons in the central core of the brainstem from the thalamus to the medulla oblongata, connecting the two hemispheres 中央脑系，位于上脑干中心的神经元系统，从丘脑向下至延髓及大脑两半球的连接部分；**chromaffin s.,** the chromaffin cells of the body considered collectively 嗜铬系统；**circulatory s.,** the cardiovascular and lymphatic systems considered together; occasionally, used to denote one of the systems only, particularly the former 循环系统；**colloid s., colloidal s.,** 胶体系统，参见 *colloid* (2) **conduction s. of heart,** a system of specialized muscle fibers that generate and transmit cardiac impulses and coordinate cardiac contractions, comprising the sinoatrial and atrioventricular nodes, bundle of His and its bundle branches, and subendocardial branches of Purkinje fibers 心传导系，一种产生和传送心脏脉冲并协调收缩的专门肌肉纤维系统，包括窦房结和房室结、希氏束及其束支和浦肯野纤维的心内膜下支；**digestive s.,** the organs concerned with ingestion, digestion, and absorption of food or nutritional elements 消化系统 **endocrine s.,** the glands and other structures that elaborate and secrete hormones that are released directly into the circulatory system, influencing metabolism and other body processes; included are the pituitary, thyroid, parathyroid, and suprarenal glands, pineal body, gonads, pancreas, and paraganglia 内分泌系统；**enteric nervous s.,** the enteric plexus, sometimes considered separately from the autonomic nervous system because it has independent local reflex activity 肠神经系统；**extrapyramidal s.,** a functional, rather than anatomic, unit comprising the nuclei and fibers (excluding those of the pyramidal tract) involved in motor activities; they control and coordinate especially the postural, static, supporting, and locomotor mechanisms. It includes the corpus striatum, subthalamic nu-

S

cleus, substantia nigra, and red nucleus, along with their interconnections with the reticular formation, cerebellum, and cerebrum 锥体外系统; **genitourinary s.,** 同 urogenital s.; **haversian s.,** a haversian canal and its concentrically arranged lamellae, constituting the basic unit of structure in compact bone (osteon) 骨单位, 哈弗斯系统, 为 Havers 管及其以同心圆排列的板层, 是构成密质骨结构的基本单位; **hematopoietic s.,** the tissues concerned in production of the blood, including the bone marrow, liver, lymph nodes, spleen, and thymus 造血系统; **heterogeneous s.,** a system or structure made up of mechanically separable parts, as an emulsion or a suspension 非均匀系, 多相系, 组成部分可用机械方法分开的结构或系统, 如乳剂; **His-Purkinje s.,** a portion of the conducting system of the heart, usually referring specifically to the segment beginning with the bundle of His and ending at the terminus of the Purkinje fiber network within the ventricles 希 - 浦系统; **homogeneous s.,** a system or structure made up of parts that cannot be mechanically separated, as a solution 均相系统, 组成部分不能以机械方法分开的结构或系统, 如溶液; **hypophysioportal s., hypothalamo-hypophysial portal s.,** the venules connecting the capillaries (gomitoli) in the median eminence of the hypothalamus with the sinusoidal capillaries of the anterior lobe of the pituitary 垂体门脉系统; **immune s.,** a complex system of cellular and molecular components having the primary functions of distinguishing self from not self and of defense against foreign organisms or substances 免疫系统; **integumentary s.,** integument (2) 体被系统; **International S. of Units,** 国际单位制, 参见 *unit* 下 *SI unit*; **limbic s.,** a group of brain structures (including the hippocampus, gyrus fornicatus, and amygdala) common to all mammals; it is associated with olfaction, autonomic functions, and certain aspects of emotion and behavior 边缘系统, 指一切哺乳动物共有的一组脑结构(包括海马、穹窿回和杏仁核); 它与嗅觉、自主神经功能以及情感和行为的某些方面有关; **locomotor s.,** the structures in a living organism responsible for locomotion, in humans consisting of the muscles, joints, and ligaments of the lower limbs as well as the arteries and nerves that supply them 运动系统; **lymphatic s., lymphoid s.,** the lymphatic vessels and lymphoid tissue considered collectively 淋巴系统; **lymphoreticular s.,** the tissues of the lymphoid and reticuloendothelial systems considered together as one system 淋巴网状系统; **masticatory s.,** the bony and soft structures of the face and mouth involved in mastication, and the vessels and nerves supplying them 咀嚼系统; **metric s.,** a decimal system of weights and measures based on the meter 米制, 见 *weight* 下附表;

mononuclear phagocyte s. (MPS), the set of cells consisting of macrophages and their precursors (blood monocytes and their precursor cells in bone marrow). The term has been proposed to replace reticuloendothelial system, which does not include all macrophages and does include other unrelated cell types 单核吞噬细胞系统; **muscular s.,** the muscles of the body considered collectively; generally restricted to the voluntary, skeletal muscles 肌肉系统; **nervous s.,** the organ system that, along with the endocrine system, correlates the adjustments and reactions of the organism to its internal and external environment, comprising the central and peripheral nervous systems 神经系统, 见图 8 至图 14; **neuroendocrine s.,** the APUD cells considered as a system, having endocrine effects on the structures of the central and peripheral nervous systems 神经内分泌系统; **parasympathetic nervous s.,** the craniosacral portion of the autonomic nervous system, its preganglionic fibers traveling with cranial nerves Ⅲ, Ⅶ, Ⅸ, and Ⅹ and with the second to fourth sacral ventral roots; it innervates the heart, smooth muscle and glands of the head and neck, and thoracic, abdominal, and pelvic viscera 副交感神经系统; **peripheral nervous s. (PNS),** all elements of the nervous system (nerves and ganglia) outside the brain and spinal cord 周围神经系统; **portal s.,** an arrangement by which blood collected from one set of capillaries passes through a large vessel or vessels and another set of capillaries before returning to the systemic circulation, as in the pituitary gland and liver 门静脉系统; **Purkinje s.,** a portion of the conducting system of the heart, usually referring specifically to the Purkinje network 浦肯野系统; **respiratory s.,** respiratory tract; the tubular and cavernous organs that allow atmospheric air to reach the membranes across which gases are exchanged with the blood 呼吸系统, 见图 25 和图 26; **reticular activating s. (RAS),** the system of cells of the reticular formation of the medulla oblongata that receive collaterals from the ascending sensory pathways and project to higher centers; they control the overall degree of central nervous system activity, including wakefulness, attentiveness, and sleep 网状激动系统, 延髓网状结构的细胞系统, 接收上行的感觉通路侧支并向更高级中枢投射, 它全面控制中枢神经系统的活动性, 包括醒觉、专心及睡眠; **reticuloendothelial s. (RES),** a group of cells having the ability to take up and sequester inert particles and vital dyes, including macrophages and macrophage precursors; specialized endothelial cells lining the sinusoids of the liver, spleen, and bone marrow; and reticular cells of lymphatic tissue (macrophages) and bone marrow (fibroblasts) 网状内皮系统, 另参见 *mononuclear phagocytes*; **SI s.,** 国际单

位制，参见 unit 下词条；**stomatognathic s.**, structures of the mouth and jaws, considered collectively, as they subserve the functions of mastication, deglutition, respiration, and speech 口颌系统；**stress s.**, the parts of the neuroendocrine system that mediate the physiologic changes that occur in response to stress 应激系统；**sympathetic nervous s. (SNS)**, the thoracolumbar part of the autonomic nervous system, the preganglionic fibers of which arise from cell bodies in the thoracic and first three lumbar segments of the spinal cord; postganglionic fibers are distributed to the heart, smooth muscle, and glands of the entire body 交感神经系统；**urinary s.**, the organs and passageways concerned with the production and excretion of urine, including the kidneys, ureters, urinary bladder, and urethra 泌尿系统；**urogenital s.**, the urinary system considered together with the organs of reproduction 泌尿生殖系统，见图28；**vascular s.**, the blood and lymphatic vessels of the body and all their ramifications, considered collectively; sometimes used specifically for either those of the blood or of the lymph, particularly the former 脉管系统；**visual s.**, the series of structures by which visual sensations are received from the environment and conveyed as signals to the central nervous system; it consists of the photoreceptors in the retina and the afferent fibers in the optic nerve, chiasm, and tract 视觉系统；

sys·te·ma (sis-te′mə) [Gr.] system 系，系统

sys·tem·ic (sis-tem′ik) pertaining to or affecting the body as a whole 属于或影响全身的

sys·to·le (sis′to-le) the contraction, or period of contraction, of the heart, especially of the ventricles 心脏收缩期；**systol′ic** adj.；**aborted s.**, a weak systole, usually premature, not associated with pulsation of a peripheral artery 顿挫性收缩，不伴有外周动脉搏动的收缩，通常为过早收缩；**atrial s.**, the contraction of the atria by which blood is propelled from them into the ventricles 心房收缩期；**extra s.**, extrasystole 期前收缩；**ventricular s.**, the contraction of the cardiac ventricles by which blood is forced into the aorta and pulmonary artery 心室收缩期

sys·trem·ma (sis-trem′ə) a cramp in the muscles of the calf of the leg 腓肠痉挛

syz·y·gy (siz′ĭ-je) the conjunction and fusion of organs without the loss of identity（器官）融合；**syzyg′ial** adj.

T

T [符号] intraocular tension 眼压（参见 pressure 下词条）；tera- 垓；tesla 特斯拉；tetanus toxoid 破伤风类毒素；thoracic vertebrae (T1 to T12) 胸椎；threonine 苏氨酸；thymine or thymidine 胸腺嘧啶或胸苷

T [符号] absolute temperature 绝对温度

T₁/₂ [符号] half-life 半衰期

T2DM type 2 diabetes mellitus 2 型糖尿病

T₃ [符号] triiodothyronine 三碘甲腺原氨酸

T₄ [符号] thyroxine 甲状腺素

Tₘ [符号] transport maximum. In kidney function tests, it is expressed as T_m with inferior letters representing the substance used in the test, e.g., T_{mPAH} for p-aminohippuric acid 肾小管最大转运率，用于报告肾功能检查结果，用下标字母代表实验用物质，如 $T_{m_{PAH}}$ 表示肾小管排泄对氨基马尿酸的最大量

2,4,5-T a toxic chlorphenoxy herbicide (2,4,5- trichlorophenoxyacetic acid), a component of Agent Orange 2，4，5- 三氯苯氧乙酸，245 涕（除莠剂）

t [符号] translocation 易位

t [符号] temperature 温度；time 时间

t₁/₂ [符号] half-life 半衰期

TA Terminologia Anatomica 解剖学术语；toxin-antitoxin 毒素 - 抗毒素

Ta tantalum 元素钽的符号

TAA tumor-associated antigen 肿瘤相关抗原

tab·a·nid (tab′ə-nid) any gadfly of the family Tabanidae, including the horseflies and deerflies 虻

Ta·ba·nus (tə-ba′nəs) a genus of biting, bloodsucking horse flies that transmit trypanosomes and anthrax to various animals 虻属

ta·bes (ta′bēz) 1. wasting of the body or a part of it 消耗，消瘦；2. 同 t. dorsalis；**t. dorsa′lis**, parenchymatous neurosyphilis marked by degeneration of the posterior columns and posterior roots and ganglion of the spinal cord, with muscular incoordination, paroxysms of intense pain, visceral crises, disturbances of sensation, and various trophic disturbances, especially of bones and joints 脊髓痨，实质性神经梅毒，表现为脊髓后柱、后根和神经节退化、肌肉不协调、剧烈疼痛发作、内脏危象、感觉障碍，以及各种营养障碍，尤其是骨骼和关节

ta·bes·cent (tə-bes′ənt) wasting away 消瘦的，干瘪的

ta·bet·ic (tə-bet′ik) pertaining to or affected with tabes 脊髓痨的

ta·bet·i·form (tə-bet′ĭ-form) resembling tabes 脊髓痨样的

tab·la·ture (tab′lə-chər) separation of the chief cranial bones into inner and outer tables, separated by a diploë 颅骨分层

ta·ble (ta′bəl) a flat layer or surface 平面，平的表面 **inner t. of calvaria,** the inner compact layer of the bones covering the brain 颅骨内板；**outer t. of calvaria.,** the outer compact layer of the bones covering the brain. 颅骨外板

tab·let (tab′lət) a solid dosage form containing a medicinal substance with or without a suitable diluent 药片，片剂；**buccal t.,** one that dissolves when held between the cheek and gum, permitting direct absorption of the active ingredient through the oral mucosa 口腔片；**enteric-coated t.,** a tablet coated with material that delays release of the medication until after it leaves the stomach 肠溶片；**sublingualt.,** one that dissolves when held beneath the tongue, permitting direct absorption of the active ingredient by the oral mucosa 舌下片

tache (tahsh) [Fr.] spot 斑点；**t. cérébrale,** a congested streak produced by drawing the nail across the skin; a concomitant of various nervous or cerebral diseases 脑病性划痕，以指甲划过皮肤时出现的充血性条痕，见于各种神经病和脑病；**t. noire,** an ulcer covered with a black crust, a characteristic local reaction at the presumed site of the infective bite in certain tickborne rickettsioses 黑斑，一种被黑色结皮覆盖的溃疡，在某些蜱传播立克次体中，在假定的感染性咬伤部位有特征性的局部反应

tach·og·ra·phy (tə-kog′rə-fe) the recording of the movement and speed of the blood current 血流速度描记法

tachy·ar·rhyth·mia (tak″e-ə-rith′me-ə) any disturbance of the heart rhythm in which the heart rate is abnormally increased 快速心律失常

tachy·car·dia (tak″ĭ-kahr′de-ə) abnormally rapid heart rate 心动过速；**tachycar′diac** *adj.*；**atrial t.,** tachycardia, usually 160 to 190 beats per minute, originating from an atrial locus 房性心动过速；**atrioventricular nodal reentrant t.,** that resulting from reentry in or around the atrioventricular node; it may be *antidromic,* in which conduction is anterograde over the accessory pathway and retrograde over the normal conduction pathway, or *orthodromic,* in which conduction is anterograde over the normal conduction pa-thway and retrograde over the accessory pathway 房室结内折返性心动过速；**atrioventricular reciprocating t. (AVRT),** a reentrant tachycardia in which the reentrant circuit contains both the normal conduction pathway and an accessory pathway as integral parts 房室折返性心动过速；**chaotic atrial t.,** a type having atrial rates of 100 to 130 beats per minute, markedly variable P-wave morphology, and irregular P–P intervals, often leading to atrial fibrillation 混乱性房性心动过

速；**circus movement t.,** 同 reentrant t.；**ectopic t.,** tachycardia in response to impulses arising outside the sinoatrial node 异位性心动过速；**junctional t.,** that arising in response to impulses originating in the atrioventricular junction, i.e., in the atrioventricular node, with a heart rate greater than 75 beats per minute 交接区性心动过速；**multifocal atrial t. (MAT),** chaotic atrial t. 多源性房性心动过速；**nodal t.,** junctional t. 结性心动过速；**nonparoxysmal junctional t.,** a junctional tachycardia of slow onset, with a heart rate of 70 to 130 beats per minute; due to enhanced automaticity of the atrioventricular junctional tissue, often secondary to disease or trauma 非阵发性交接区性心动过速；**paroxysmal t.,** tachycardia that starts and stops abruptly 阵发性心动过速；**paroxysmal supraventricular t. (PSVT),** supraventricular tachycardia occurring in attacks of rapid onset and cessation, usually owing to a reentrant circuit 阵发性室上性心动过速；**reciprocating t.,** a tachycardia due to a reentrant mechanism and characterized by a reciprocating rhythm 反复性心动过速，由折返机制引起的一种心动过速，以反复心律为特征 **reentrant t.,** any tachycardia characterized by a reentrant circuit 折返性心动过速；**sinus t. (ST),** tachycardia originating in the sinus node; normal during exercise or anxiety but also associated with shock, hypotension, hypoxia, congestive heart failure, fever, and various high-output states 窦性心动过速；**supraventricular t. (SVT),** any regular tachycardia in which the point of stimulation is above the bundle branches; it may also include those arising from large reentrant circuits that encompass both atrial and ventricular sites 室上性心动过速；**ventricular t.,** an abnormally rapid ventricular rhythm with aberrant ventricular excitation, usually above 150 beats per minute, generated within the ventricle, and most often associated with atrioventricular dissociation 室性心动过速

tachy·dys·rhyth·mia (tak″e-dis-rith′me-ə) an abnormal heart rhythm with a rate greater than 100 beats per minute in an adult; the term *tachyarrhythmia* is usually used instead 快速性心律紊乱，成人心律每分钟大于100次的异常心律；常用 tachyarrhythmia 代替

tachy·gas·tria (tak″ĭ-gas′tre-ə) a sequence of electric potentials at abnormally high frequencies in the gastric antrum 胃窦电活动亢进

tachy·ki·nin (tak″e-ki′nin) any of a family of peptides structurally and functionally similar to substance P; all are potent, rapidly acting secretagogues and cause smooth muscle contraction and vasodilation 速激肽可引起平滑肌收缩和血管扩张

tachy·pha·gia (tak″ĭ-fa′je-ə) rapid eating 速食癖

tachy·phy·lax·is (tak″e-fə-lak′sis) 1. rapid immunization against the effect of toxic doses of an extract or serum by previous injection of small doses of it 快速免疫，先前注射小剂量的提取物或血清以抵抗毒性剂量的影响；2. rapidly decreasing response to a drug or physiologically active agent after administration of a few doses 快速减敏，服用某些药物后，机体迅速减低对某种药物或生理学活性物质的反应；**tachyphylac′tic** adj.

tach·yp·nea (tak″ip-ne′ə) very rapid respiration 呼吸急促

tachy·rhyth·mia (tak″ĭ-rith′me-ə) 同 tachycardia

tach·ys·te·rol (tak-is′tə-rol) an isomer of ergosterol produced by irradiation 速固醇

tac·rine (tak′rēn) a cholinesterase inhibitor used to improve cognitive performance in dementia of the Alzheimer type; used as the hydrochloride salt 他克林，一种胆碱酯酶抑制药，用于改善阿尔茨海默性痴呆症的认知功能；用其盐酸盐；

tac·ro·li·mus (tak″ro-li′məs) a macrolide immunosuppressant having actions similar to those of cyclosporine; used to prevent rejection of organ transplants; also used topically to treat moderate to severe atopic dermatitis 他克莫司，一种大环内酯类免疫抑制药，与环孢菌素有相似的药物活性，用来防止器官移植排异，也用于中度至重度特应性皮炎的局部治疗

tac·tile (tak′til) pertaining to touch 触觉的

Tae′nia (te′ne-ə) a genus of tapeworms 绦虫属，带绦虫属；*T. echinococ′cus, Echinococcus granulosus* 细粒棘球绦虫 *T. sagina′ta,* a species 4 to 8 meters long, found in the adult form in the human intestine and in the larval state in muscles and other tissues of cattle and other ruminants; human infection usually results from eating inadequately cooked beef 牛肉绦虫，无钩绦虫，人类最常见的一种绦虫，长 4～8m。成虫寄生于人体肠道内，囊尾蚴（幼虫期）则在牛和其他反刍动物肌肉及其他组织中发育；人类感染通常是由于食用煮熟不充分的牛肉造成的；*T. so′lium,* a species 1 to 2 meters long, found in the adult intestine; the larval form most often is found in muscle and other tissues of the pig; human infection results from eating inadequately cooked pork 猪肉绦虫，此种绦虫长 1～2m，发现于成人的肠道中；其囊尾蚴（幼虫期）最常见于猪的肌肉和其他组织中；人类因食用未经充分烹调的猪肉而感染；

tae·nia (te′ne-ə) pl. *tae′niae* [L.] 1. a flat band or strip of soft tissue 带；2. a tapeworm of the genus *Taenia* 绦虫；**tae′niae co′li,** three thickened bands formed by the longitudinal fibers in the muscular tunic of the large intestine and extending from the vermiform appendix to the rectum 结肠带

tae·ni·a·cide (te′ne-ə-sīd″) 1. destruction of tapeworms 杀绦虫的；2. an agent lethal to tapeworms 杀绦虫药

tae·ni·a·fuge (te′ne-ə-fūj″) an agent that expels tapeworms 驱绦虫药；**taeniafu′gal** adj.

tae·ni·a·sis (te-ni′ə-sis) infection with tapeworms of the genus *Taenia* 绦虫病

ta·flu·prost (ta′floo-prost) a prostaglandin analogue that selectively stimulates the prostanoid FP receptor to reduce intraocular pressure and treat progressive open-angle glaucoma and ocular hypertension 他氟前列素，一种前列腺素类似物，选择性地刺激前列腺素 FP 受体，以降低眼压，治疗进行性开角型青光眼和高眼压

tag (tag) 1. a small appendage, flap, or polyp 附属物；2. label 签条，标签；**skin t.,** acrochordon 皮赘，软疣

tai chi (ti′ che′) [Chinese] a system of postures linked by elegant and graceful movements, originating in China, whose purpose is to balance yin and yang, creating inner and outer harmony. It improves cardiovascular, musculoskeletal, and respiratory function and increases central nervous system function, and can be used for treating various conditions 太极

tail (tāl) any slender appendage 尾；尾状物；**t. of spermatozoon,** the flagellum of a spermatozoon, which contains the axonema; it has four regions: the neck, middle piece, principal piece, and end piece 精子尾

talc (talk) a native hydrous magnesium silicate, sometimes with a small amount of aluminum silicate; in purified form, used as a dusting powder and pharmaceutical aid 滑石

tal·co·sis (tal-ko′sis) talc pneumoconiosis 滑石病

tal·i·glu·cer·ase (tal-i-gloo′ser-ase) a recombinant alfa analogue of β-glucocerebrosidase; used as enzyme replacement therapy to treat type 1 Gaucher disease β- 葡萄糖脑苷脂酶的重组 α 类似物，用于 I 型戈谢病的酶替代治疗

tal·i·pes (tal′ĭ-pēz) a congenital deformity in which the foot is twisted out of shape or position; it may be in dorsiflexion *(t. calca′neus)*, in plantarflexion *(t. equi′nus)*, abducted and everted *(t. val′gus or flatfoot)*, abducted and inverted *(t. va′rus)*, or various combinations *(t. calcaneoval′gus, t. calcaneova′rus, t. equinoval′gus,* or *t. equinova′rus)* 畸形足，足的先天性畸形，足形和足位向外扭转，可能是背屈（仰趾足），跖屈（马蹄足），外展和外翻（外翻足或扁平足），外展和倒转（内翻足）或各种组合（仰趾外翻足，仰趾内翻足，马蹄外翻足或马蹄内翻足）

tal·i·pom·a·nus (tal″ĭ-pom′ə-nəs) clubhand 畸形手

ta·lo·cal·ca·ne·al (ta″lo-kal-ka′ne-əl) pertaining to the talus and calcaneus 距骨跟骨的

ta·lo·cru·ral (ta″lo-kroo′rəl) pertaining to the talus and the leg bones 距骨小腿骨的

ta·lo·fib·u·lar (ta″lo-fib′u-lər) pertaining to the talus and fibula 距骨腓骨的

ta·lo·na·vic·u·lar (ta″lo-nə-vik′u-lər) pertaining to the talus and navicular bone 距骨舟骨的

ta·lus (ta′ləs) pl. *ta′li* [L.] the highest of the tarsal bones, articulating with the tibia and fibula to form the ankle joint 距骨, 见图 1

ta·mas (tah-mus′) [Sanskrit] according to ayurveda, one of the three gunas, characterized by inertia and responsible for stability, lethargy, and retentiveness in the mind and body 惰性, 根据阿育吠陀 (ayuveda), 三种属性 (gunas) 中的一个, 以惰性为特征 (其余两个为悦性 sattva 及变性 rajas), 司稳定、嗜睡眠和维持身心健康

tam·bour (tam-boor′) a drum-shaped appliance used in transmitting movements in a recording instrument 气鼓, 鼓形装置用于传送运动的记录仪器

ta·mox·i·fen (tə-mok′sī-fən) a nonsteroidal anti-estrogen used as the citrate salt in the prophylaxis and treatment of breast cancer 三苯氧胺, 他莫昔芬, 一种非甾体类抗雌激素, 其枸橼酸盐用于乳腺癌的预防和治疗

tam·pon (tam′pon) [Fr.] a pack, pad, or plug made of cotton, sponge, or other material, variously used in surgery to plug the nose, vagina, etc., for the control of hemorrhage or the absorption of secretions 塞子, 以棉花、海绵或其他材料制成的包、块或塞, 用于各种手术中的鼻腔及阴道等处的填塞, 以控制出血或吸收分泌物

tam·pon·ade (tam″pon-ād′) 1. surgical use of a tampon 填塞, 压紧, 手术中填塞物 (塞子) 的应用; 2. pathologic compression of a part 病变的病理性压迫; **balloon t.,** esophagogastric tamponade by means of a device with a triple-lumen tube and two inflatable balloons, the third lumen providing for aspiration of blood clots 气囊填塞, 用三腔二囊管对胃和食管进行的填塞; **cardiac t.,** compression of the heart caused by increased intrapericardial pressure due to collection of blood or fluid in the pericardium 心脏压塞, 心包填塞, 因心包内积血或积液引起心包内压力增高而致的心脏压迫; **esophagogastric t.,** the exertion of direct pressure against bleeding esophageal varices by insertion of a tube with a balloon in the esophagus and another in the stomach and inflating them 胃食管压塞, 将分别带有两个气囊的管插入食道和胃中, 对其充气以直接施加压力, 控制食管静脉曲张出血

tam·su·lo·sin (tam-soo′lo-sin) an α₁-adrenergic blocking agent specific for the receptors in the pros-tate; used as the hydrochloride salt in the treatment of benign prostatic hyperplasiaα₁- 肾上腺素能阻断药, 特异作用于前列腺的受体; 其盐酸盐用于治疗良性前列腺增生症

tan·gen·ti·al·i·ty (tan-jen″she-al′ĭ-te) a pattern of speech characterized by oblique, digressive, or irrelevant replies to questions; the responses never approach the point of the questions 接触性离题, 一种说话方式, 其特点为转弯抹角、远离正题或答非所问; 其回应决不触及问题的实质

tan·gle (tang′gəl) a knot or snarl 结或缠结; **neu-rofibrillary t's,** intracellular knots or clumps of neurofibrils seen in the cerebral cortex in Alzheimer disease 神经原纤维缠结, 阿尔茨海默病时, 在大脑皮质中所见细胞内结或神经纤维错乱缠结

tan·nate (tan′āt) any of the salts of tannic acid, all of which are astringent 鞣酸盐

tan·nic ac·id (tan′ik) a substance obtained from nutgalls, used as an ingredient of dermatologic preparations and formerly used as an astringent 鞣酸, 从五倍子中提取的一种物质, 用作皮肤科制剂的原料, 以前也用作收敛剂

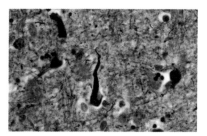

▲ 神经元细胞质内的神经纤维缠结 (银染色)

tan·nin (tan′in) 同 tannic acid

tan·ta·lum (Ta) (tan′tə-ləm) a blue-gray, heavy, very hard, nonreactive, noncorrosive, transition metal element; at. no. 73, at. wt. 180.948; it has been used in medical equipment and prostheses 钽 (化学元素)

tan·y·cyte (tan′ĭ-sīt) a modified cell of the ependyma of the infundibulum of the hypothalamus; its function is unknown, but it may transport hormones from the cerebrospinal fluid into the hypophyseal circulation or from the hypothalamic neurons to the cerebrospinal fluid 伸长细胞, 下丘脑漏斗部一种产生了变化的室管膜细胞; 其功能尚不详, 可能是把激素由脑脊液输送到门脉循环中, 或由下丘脑神经元输送到脑脊液中

tap (tap) 1. a quick, light blow 轻叩; 2. to drain off fluid by paracentesis 穿刺放液; **spinal t.,** lumbar puncture 腰椎穿刺;

tape (tāp) a long, narrow strip of fabric or other flexible material 带；胶带；**adhesive t.**, a strip of fabric or other material evenly coated on one side with a pressure-sensitive adhesive material 胶带，将压敏胶剂涂布于带状载体得到的制品

tap·ei·no·ceph·a·ly (tap″ī-no-sef′ə-le) flatness of the skull, with a vertical index below 72 矮型头，低型头，颅骨低平，颅长高指数低于 72；**tapeinocephal′ic** adj.

ta·pe·to·ret·i·nal (tə-pe″to-ret′ī-nəl) pertain - ing to the pigmented layer of the retina 视网膜色层的，视网膜的

ta·pe·tum (tə-pe′təm) pl. *tape′ta* [L.] 1. a covering structure or layer of cells 毯，覆盖结构或细胞层；2. a stratum of fibers of the corpus callosum on the superolateral aspect of the occipital horn of the lateral ventricle 胼胝体毯，侧脑室枕骨角上外侧的一层侧胼胝体纤维

tape·worm (tāp′wərm) cestode; a parasitic intestinal worm with a flattened, bandlike form 绦虫；**armed t.**, 同 *Taenia solium* beef t., 同 *Taenia saginata*；**broad t.**, *Diphyllobothrium latum* 阔节裂头绦虫；latum dog t., *Dipylidium caninum* 犬绦虫；**fish t.**, *Diphyllobothrium latum* 鱼绦虫；**hydatid t.**, *Echinococcus granulosus* 细粒棘球绦虫；**pork t.**, 同 *Taenia solium* unarmed t., 同 *Taenia saginata*

ta·pote·ment (tah-pōt-maw′) [Fr.] a tapping or percussing movement in massage 叩抚法

tar (tahr) a dark-brown or black, viscid liquid obtained from various species of pine or from bituminous coal *(coal t.)*. It is used for topical treatment of skin conditions, including eczema, psoriasis, and dandruff, but is toxic and carcinogenic by inhalation or ingestion 焦油，一种暗棕色或黑色枯稠液体，从各种松木或烟煤中提取，其用于皮肤病的局部治疗，包括湿疹、银屑病和头皮屑，但吸入或摄入具有毒性和致癌性

ta·ran·tu·la (tə-ran′tu-lə) a venomous spider whose bite causes local inflammation and pain, usually not to a severe extent, including *Eurypelma hentzii* (American t.), *Sericopelma communis* (black t.) of Panama, and *Lycosa tarentula* (European wolf spider) 狼蛛，一种毒蛛，咬伤后引起局部发炎和疼痛，一般并不严重，包括 Eurypelma hentzii（美洲狼蛛），Sericopelma communis（黑狼蛛），和 Lycosa tarentula（欧洲狼蛛）

tar·dive (tahr′div) [Fr.] tardy; late 迟发的，延迟的

tar·get (tahr′gət) 1. an object or area toward which something is directed, such as the area of the anode of an x-ray tube where the electron beam collides, causing the emission of x-rays 某物所指向的目标或区域，如 X 线管的金属板，电子撞击此板并由此发出 X 线；2. a cell or organ that is affected by a particular agent, e.g., a hormone or drug 靶，屏极 选择性接受某种特定物质（如激素或药物）作用的细胞或器官

tar·ich·a·tox·in (tar′ik-ə-tok″sin) name given to the lethal neurotoxin tetrodotoxin when it comes from the newt *Taricha torosa* 蝾螈毒素

tar·ry (tahr′e) 1. filled with or covered by tar 用焦油填充或覆盖；2. thick, dark; resembling tar 稠厚的，暗黑色的，像焦油状的

tar·sad·e·ni·tis (tahr″sad-ə-ni′tis) inflammation of the meibomian glands and tarsus 睑板腺炎

tar·sal (tahr′səl) pertaining to a tarsus 睑板的，跗骨的

tar·sal·gia (tahr-sal′jə) pain in a tarsus 跗骨痛

tar·sa·lia (tahr-sa′le-ə) the bones of the tarsus 跗骨

tar·sa·lis (tahr-sa′lis) [L.] tarsal 睑板的；跗骨的

tar·sec·to·my (tahr-sek′tə-me) 1. excision of a bone or bones of the tarsus of the foot 跗骨切除术；2. excision of the tarsus of an eyelid 睑板切除术

tar·si·tis (tahr-si′tis) blepharitis 睑缘炎，睑板炎

tar·soc·la·sis (tahr-sok′lə-sis) surgical fracturing of the tarsus of the foot 跗骨折骨术

tar·so·con·junc·ti·val (tahr″so-kən-junk′tī-vəl) pertaining to the tarsus of an eyelid and the conjunctiva 睑板结膜的

tar·so·ma·la·cia (tahr″so-mə-la′shə) softening of the tarsus of an eyelid 睑板软化

tar·so·meta·tar·sal (tahr″so-met″ə-tahr′səl) pertaining to the tarsus and metatarsus 跗骨跖骨的

tar·so·plas·ty (tahr′so-plas″te) blepharoplasty 睑成形术

tar·sor·rha·phy (tahr-sor′ə-fe) suture of a portion of or the entire upper and lower eyelids together; done to shorten or entirely close the palpebral fissure 睑缝合术

tar·sot·o·my (tahr-sot′ə-me) blepharotomy 睑板切开术

tar·sus (tahr′səs) 1. ankle; the region of the foot adjacent to the articulation between the foot and the leg, composed of seven tarsal bones 跗骨；2. a plate of connective tissue forming the framework of an eyelid, one on the upper and and one on the lower eyelid 睑板

tar·tar (tahr′tər) dental calculus 牙石，牙垢

tar·tar·ic ac·id (tahr-tar′ik) any of several isomers of the dicarboxylic acid $HOOC(CHOH)_2COOH$, occurring especially in grapes 酒石酸

tar·trate (tahr′trāt) a salt of tartaric acid 酒石酸盐

tas·tant (tās′tənt) any substance, e.g., salt, capable of eliciting gustatory excitation, i.e., stimulating the sense of taste 促味剂，任何能诱发味觉刺激即刺激味觉的物质，如盐

taste (tāst) 1. the sense effected by the gustatory

receptors in the tongue. Four qualities are distinguished: sweet, sour, salty, and bitter 味觉; 2. the act of perceiving by this sense 尝

tast·er (tās'tər) an individual capable of tasting a particular test substance (e.g., phenylthiourea, used in genetic studies) 尝味者，在遗传学研究中指对一种特别的试验物质如苯硫脲能辨别出苦味的人

tat·too·ing (tă-too'ing) the introduction, by punctures, of permanent colors in the skin 文身术; **t, of the cone,** permanent coloring of the cornea, chiefly to conceal leukomatous spots 角膜墨针术，角膜染色术，使角膜长久着色，主要为了遮盖角膜白斑

tau·rine (taw'rēn) an oxidized sulfur-containing amine occurring conjugated in the bile, usually as cholyltaurine or chenodeoxycholyltaurine; it may also be a central nervous system neurotransmitter or neuromodulator 牛磺酸，氨基乙磺酸

tau·to·mer (taw'to-mər) a chemical compound exhibiting, or capable of exhibiting, tautomerism 互变异构体

tau·tom·er·al (taw-tom'ər-əl) pertaining to the same part; said especially of neurons and neuroblasts sending processes to aid in formation of the white matter in the same side of the spinal cord 同侧的，尤指发出胞突以助脊髓同侧白质形成的细胞，如某些神经元和神经母细胞

tau·tom·er·ase (taw-tom'ər-ās) any enzyme catalyzing the interconversion of tautomers 互变异构酶，催化互变异构体间相互转化的酶

tau·tom·er·ism (taw-tom'ər-iz-əm) the relationship that exists between two constitutional isomers (those having the same atoms linked in different structures) that are in chemical equilibrium and freely change from one to the other 互变异构; **tautomer'ic** adj.

TAVR transcatheter aortic valve replacement 经导管主动脉瓣置换术

tax·is (tak'sis) [Gr.] 1. an orientation movement of a motile organism in response to a stimulus, either toward (positive) or away from (negative) the source of the stimulus 趋性，一种能动生物对某一外部刺激做出反应时的定向运动。这样的反应可为阳性（趋向刺激物）或阴性（离开刺激物）; 2. exertion of force in manual replacement of a displaced organ or part 整复法，以手法施力使脱位器官或组织结构复位

tax·on (tak'son) pl. *tax'a.* 分类单位，分类单元，分类群 1. a particular taxonomic grouping, e.g., a species, genus, family, order, class, phylum, or kingdom 相关生物被划分的特定类别，如：种、属、科、目、纲、门和界; 2. the name applied to a taxonomic grouping 应用于分类分组的名称

tax·on·o·my (tak-son'ə-me) the orderly classification of organisms into appropriate categories (taxa),

with application of suitable and correct names 分类学; **taxonom'ic** adj.; **numerical t.,** a method of classifying organisms solely on the basis of the number of shared phenotypic characters, each character usually being given equal weight; used primarily in bacteriology 数值分类法，一种仅根据共有表型特征的数量对生物体进行分类的方法，每个特征通常具有同等权重；主要用于细菌学

ta·zar·o·tene (tə-zar'o-tēn) a retinoid prodrug used topically in the treatment of acne vulgaris and psoriasis 他扎罗汀，一种局部使用以治疗寻常痤疮和银屑病的维生素 A 类前体药物

taz·o·bac·tam (taz″o-bak'tam) a β-lactamase inhibitor having antibacterial actions and uses similar to those of sulbactam; used as the sodium salt 他唑巴坦，一种具有抗菌作用的β-内酰胺酶抑制药，使用类于舒巴坦；常用其钠盐

Tb terbium 元素铽的符号

TBM tracheobronchomalacia 气管支气管软化症

Tc technetium 元素锝的符号

TCM traditional Chinese medicine 中医学，中医，传统中药

TD₅₀ median toxic dose 半数中毒量

Td tetanus and diphtheria toxoids 成人型破伤风及白喉类毒素

Tdap tetanus toxoid, reduced diphtheria toxoid, and acellular pertussis vaccine 破伤风类毒素、减量白喉类毒素、非细胞性百日咳疫苗

tDCS transcranial direct current stimulation 经颅直流电刺激

Te tellurium 元素碲的符号

tea (te) 1. *Camellia sinensis* or its dried leaves, which contain caffeine, theophylline, tannic acid, and a volatile oil. Tea is either *green* or *black,* depending on the curing method 茶; 2. a decoction of these leaves, used as a stimulating beverage or soothing drink for various abdominal discomforts. Green tea has been used for prevention of dental caries and is also used in traditional Chinese medicine, ayurveda, and homeopathy 茶剂; 3. any decoction or infusion 煎剂，浸剂

tears (tērz) the watery, slightly alkaline and saline secretion of the lacrimal glands, which moistens the conjunctiva 眼泪

tease (tēz) to pull apart gently with fine needles to permit microscopic examination（用针）拨开，挑开（组织）

teat (tēt) nipple (1)（乳房）乳头

tea tree (te' tre″) a tree, *Melaleuca alternifolia,* native to eastern Australia, from whose leaves and branches tea tree oil is obtained 茶树

teb·u·tate (teb'u-tāt) USAN contraction for tertiary butyl acetate 醋酸特丁酯 tertiarybutyl acetate 的

USAN 缩 约 词；**tech·ne·ti·um (Tc)** (tek-ne′she-əm) a radioactive, silvery white, transition metal element; at. no. 43, at. wt. 98; virtually always synthetic 锝（化学元素）；**t. 99m,** the most frequently used radioisotope in nuclear medicine, a gamma emitter (0.141 MeV) having a half-life of 6.01 hours 锝 99m，是核医学中最常用的放射性同位素，作为一种伽马射线发射器（0.141 MeV），其半衰期为 6.01h

tech·ni·cian (tek-nish′ən) a person skilled in the performance of the technical or procedural aspects of a health care profession, usually with at least an associate's degree, working under the supervision of a physician, therapist, technologist, or other health care professional 技术员，技师，指在医疗保健行业，对技术或程序方面工作能力熟练的人员，其在医师、治疗师、技术专家或其他卫生保健专家的监督下工作，并通常至少具备大专文凭

tech·nique (tek-nēk′) a maneuver, method, or procedure 术，技术，操作法；**fluorescent antibody t.,** an immunofluorescence technique in which antigen in tissue sections is located by homologous antibody labeled with fluorochrome or by treating the antigen with unlabeled antibody followed by a second layer of labeled antiglobulin that is reactive with the unlabeled antibody 荧光抗体技术，一种免疫荧光技术，即以荧光色素标记的同种抗体来为组织切片中的抗原定位（单层法），或先以未标记的抗体处理抗原，再以标记的抗球蛋白作二层处理，该抗球蛋白与未经标记的抗体共起反应（双层法）；**isolation-perfusion t.,** a technique for administering high doses of a chemotherapy agent to a region while protecting the patient from toxicity; the region is isolated and perfused with the drug by means of a pump-oxygenator 分离 - 灌注法，一种在保护病人免受毒性的同时向某一区域注射大剂量化疗药物的技术，该区域通过泵氧器隔离并灌注药物；**Jerne plaque t.,** a hemolytic technique for detecting antibody-producing cells: a suspension of presensitized lymphocytes is mixed in an agar gel with erythrocytes; after a period of incubation, complement is added and a clear area of lysis of red cells can be seen around each of the antibody-producing cells 热内尔斑块技术，溶血法检测抗体生成细胞，即将预先致敏的淋巴细胞悬液在琼脂凝胶中与红细胞混合，经过一段孵育期后加入补体，即可在每一抗体生成细胞周围见到清晰的红细胞溶解区；**Mohs' t.,** 莫斯手术，参见 *surgery* 下词条 **Pomeroy t.,** sterilization by ligation of a loop of fallopian tube and resection of the tied loop Pomeroy 手术，输卵管套圈结扎切除绝育术

tech·nol·o·gist (tek-nol′ə-jist) a person skilled in the theory and practice of a technical profession, usually with at least a baccalaureate degree; in several allied health fields, technologist is the highest professional rank 技术人员，精通理论和实践技术专业，通常至少具备学士学位；在数个相关的健康领域，技术人员的专业级别最高

tech·nol·o·gy (tek-nol′ə-je) scientific knowledge; the sum of the study of a technique 技术学；**assisted reproductive t. (ART),** any procedure involving the manipulation of eggs or sperm to establish pregnancy in the treatment of infertility 辅助生殖技术，辅助生育技术；**recombinant DNA t.,** a body of techniques that isolate specific DNA sequences, create and amplify recombinant DNA molecules, and employ them in a variety of analytic, therapeutic, and industrial applications 重组 DNA 技术

tec·ton·ic (tek-ton′ik) pertaining to construction 整复的，成型的

tec·to·ri·al (tek-tor′e-əl) of the nature of a roof or covering 覆膜的，顶盖的

tec·to·ri·um (tek-tor′e-əm) pl. *tecto′ria* [L.] Corti membrane 覆膜，耳蜗覆膜

tec·to·spi·nal (tek″to-spi′nəl) extending from the tectum of the midbrain to the spinal cord 顶盖脊髓的

tec·tum (tek′təm) [L.] a rooflike structure 顶盖；**t. of mesencephalon, t. of midbrain,** the dorsal portion of the midbrain 中脑顶盖，中脑的背侧部分

TEE transesophageal echocardiography 经食管超声心动图

teeth·ing (tēth′ing) the entire process resulting in eruption of the teeth 出牙，生牙

Tef·lon (tef′lon) trademark for preparations of polytef (polytetrafluoroethylene) 特氟隆，聚四氟乙烯制剂的商品名

teg·men (teg′mən) pl. *teg′mina* [L.] a covering structure or roof 盖；**t. tym′pani,** the thin layer of bone that forms the roof of the tympanic cavity, separating it from the cranial cavity 鼓室盖

teg·men·tal (təg-men′təl) pertaining to or of the nature of a tegmen or tegmentum 盖的

teg·men·tum (təg-men′təm) pl. *tegmen′ta* [L.] 1. a covering 盖，被盖；2. tegmentum of mesencephalon 中脑盖；3. the dorsal part of each cerebral peduncle 大脑脚盖；**t. of midbrain,** the dorsal part of the midbrain, formed by continuation of the dorsal parts of the cerebral peduncles across the median plane, and extending on each side from the substantia nigra to the level of the mesencephalic aqueduct 中脑被盖，中脑的背侧部分，由大脑脚的背侧部分沿正中平面延伸而形成，自黑质向两侧延伸至中脑导水管

teg·u·ment (teg′u-ment) 1. integument 体被组织；2. a complex, heterogeneous, protein-containing

T

structure lying between the capsid and envelope of herpesviruses 疱疹病毒壳体与外壳间的一种复杂的、异质的、含蛋白质的结构

tei·cho·ic ac·id (ti-ko′ik) any of a diverse group of antigenic polymers of glycerol or ribitol phosphates found attached to the cell walls or in intracellular association with membranes of gram-positive bacteria; they determine group specificity of some species, e.g., the staphylococci 磷壁酸，从革兰阳性细菌的细胞壁上或细胞膜内与细胞膜结合时，发现的甘油或核糖醇磷酸盐的各种抗原聚合物；他们决定一些物种的群体特异性，如葡萄球菌

tei·chop·sia (ti-kop′se-ə) the sensation of a luminous appearance before the eyes, with a zigzag, wall-like outline. It may be a migraine aura 闪光暗点，眼前出现的发亮感觉，带有 z 字形的墙样轮廓；可能为偏头痛先兆

tei·co·pla·nin (ti-ko-pla′nin) a glycopeptide antibiotic used as a less toxic alternative to vancomycin in the treatment of infections caused by gram-positive bacteria 替考拉宁，一种糖肽类抗生素，在治疗革兰阳性细菌引起的感染时，作为万古霉素的一种毒性较低的替代药

te·la (te′lə) pl. *te′lae* [L.] any weblike tissue 组织；**t. elas′tica,** elastic tissue 弹性组织；**t. subcuta′nea,** superficial fascia 皮下组织

tel·al·gia (tə-lal′jə) referred pain 牵涉痛

tel·an·gi·ec·ta·sia (tə-lan″je-ək-ta′zhə) permanent dilation of preexisting small blood vessels to form focal, discolored lesions 毛细血管扩张；**hereditary hemorrhagic t.,** a hereditary condition marked by multiple small telangiectases of the skin, mucous membranes, and other organs, associated with recurrent episodes of bleeding from affected sites and gross or occult melena 遗传性出血性毛细血管扩张，一种遗传性疾病，特征为皮肤、黏膜其他器官出现多发性小血管扩张，与病变部位屡有出血并有显性或潜血黑粪有关；**spider t.,** *angioma* 下词条

tel·an·gi·ec·ta·sis (tə-lan″je-ek′tə-sis) pl. *telangiec′tases.* 1. the lesion produced by telangiectasia, which may present as a coarse or fine red line or as a punctum with radiating limbs (spider) 毛细血管扩张症；2. 同 telangiectasia

tel·an·gi·o·sis (tə-lan″je-o′sis) any disease of the capillaries 毛细血管病

tel·a·van·cin (tel″uh-van′sǐn) an antibiotic active against gram-positive bacteria, including methicillin-resistant *Staphylococcus aureus;* administered by intravenous injection 一种具有革兰阳性抗菌活性药物，覆盖耐甲氧西林金黄色葡萄球菌，通过静脉注射给药

tele·can·thus (tel″ə-kan′thəs) abnormally increased

distance between the medial canthi of the eyelids 内眦距过宽

tele·car·di·og·ra·phy (tel″ə-kahr″de-og′rə-fe) the recording of an electrocardiogram by transmission of impulses to a site at a distance from the patient 远距心电描记法，心电遥测法

tele·car·dio·phone (tel″ə-kahr′de-o-fōn) an apparatus for making heart sounds audible at a distance from the patient 远距心音听诊器

tele·cep·tor (tel′ə-sep″tər) a sensory nerve terminal, such as those in the eyes, ears, and nose, that is sensitive to distant stimuli 距离感受器，对产生于远处的刺激具有敏感性的感觉神经末梢，见于眼、耳及鼻等处

tele·di·ag·no·sis (tel″ə-di″əg-no′sis) determination of the nature of a disease at a site remote from the patient on the basis of transmitted telemonitoring data or closed-circuit television consultation 远距诊断，依据被传送的遥测监护资料或闭路电视会诊，在远离患者处确定疾病性质

tele·flu·o·ros·co·py (tel″ə-floo-ros′kə-pe) television transmission of fluoroscopic images for study at a distant location 远距荧光屏检查，利用电视传送荧光屏影像在远距离进行研究

tele·ki·ne·sis (tel″ə-ki-ne′sis) 1. movement of an object produced without contact 感应运动；2. the ability to produce such movement 感应运动性；**telekinet′ic** *adj.*

tele·med·i·cine (tel″ə-med′ĭ-sin) the provision of consultant services by off-site physicians to health care professionals on the scene, as by means of closed-circuit television 远距医学，远距会诊，借助闭路电视的方式请异地医师为现场医疗专业人员提供会诊服务

te·lem·e·try (tə-lem′ə-tre) the making of measurements at a distance from the subject, the measurable evidence of phenomena under investigation being transmitted by radio signals, wires, or other means 远距离测定法，遥测术，远距患者进行的检测，可测定的调研中现象的数据由无线电信号、电报或其他媒介传送

tel·en·ceph·a·lon (tel″en-sef′ə-lon) endbrain 端脑 1. one of the two divisions of the forebrain, composing the cerebrum (q.v.) 前脑的两个部分之一，为大脑的组成部分；2. the anterior of the two vesicles formed by specialization of the forebrain in embryonic development; from it the cerebral hemispheres are derived 胚胎发育时期由前脑泡向两侧膨出而成的结构，后演化为左右大脑半球；**telencephal′ic** *adj.*

tele·neu·rite (tel″ə-noor′ĭt) an end expansion of an axon 终轴突

tele·neu·ron (tel″ə-noor′on) a nerve ending 神经

末端

te·le·ol·o·gy (te″le-ol′ə-je) the doctrine of final causes or of adaptation to a definite purpose 目的论，认为任何事物有其最终目标或适应于一定的目标

te·leo·morph (te′le-o-morf″) the state of a fungus in which reproduction is sexual; as opposed to anamorph 有性型，真菌的有性状态；与无性型相对

tele·op·sia (tel″e-op′se-ə) a visual disturbance in which objects appear to be farther away than they actually are 视物显远症

te·ler·gan·ic (te″ler-gan′ik) necessary to life 生命必需的

Tele·paque (tel′ə-pāk) trademark for a preparation of iopanoic acid 碘番酸制剂的商品名

tele·pa·thol·o·gy (tel″ə-pə-thol′ə-je) the practice of pathology at a remote location by means of video cameras, monitors, and a remotecontrolled microscope 远距病理学

tele·ra·di·og·ra·phy (tel″ə-ra″de-og′rə-fe) 1. interpretation of images transmitted over telephone lines or by satellite 远距离照相术；2. radiography with the radiation source 6.5 to 7 feet from the subject to maximize the parallelism of the rays and minimize distortion 远距X线照相术，以辐射源在距患者6.5至7英尺处拍照X线片，该方法更能确保射线的平行及使失真减小至最低限度

tele·ther·a·py (tel″ə-ther′ə-pe) treatment in which the source of the therapeutic agent, e.g., radiation, is at a distance from the body 远程放射治疗，治疗物（如放射线）在远离患者躯体处发出的疗法

tel·lu·ric (tə-lu′rik) 1. pertaining to tellurium 碲化的；2. pertaining to or originating from the earth 地球的

tel·lu·ri·um (Te) (tə-lu′re-əm) a very rare, brittle, silvery white, lustrous, metalloid element; at. no. 52, at. wt. 127.60 碲（化学元素）

tel·mi·sar·tan (tel″mī-sahr′tan) an angiotensin II antagonist used as an antihypertensive 替米沙坦，一种为血管紧张素II拮抗药的降压药

telo·cen·tric (tel″o-sen′trik) having the centromere at the extreme end of the chromosome, which thus has only one arm 端着丝点，着丝点位于染色体的末端，故该染色体为单臂

telo·den·dron (tel″o-den′dron) any of the fine terminal branches of an axon 终树突，轴突终末分出的纤细分支

tel·o·gen (tel′o-jən) the quiescent or resting phase of the hair cycle, following catagen; the hair has become a club hair and does not grow further 毛发生长终期，毛发生长周期中的静止期，此时毛发已发育成杵状毛，不再生长

tel·og·no·sis (tel″og-no′sis) diagnosis based on interpretation of radiographs transmitted by telera*diography* 远距诊断，电讯诊断，依据远程放射学传输的X线片判读而进行的诊断

telo·lec·i·thal (tel″o-les′ĭ-thəl) having a medium to large amount of yolk, with the yolk concentrated toward one pole (the vegetal pole); as in the eggs of fish, amphibians, birds, and reptiles 端黄卵的，具有中至大量的卵黄，其卵黄向卵的一极（植物极）集中；如鱼、两栖动物、鸟类和爬行动物的卵

telo·mer·ase (tə-lo′mər-ās) a DNA polymerase involved in the formation of telomeres and the maintenance of telomere sequences during replication 端粒酶

telo·mere (tel′o-mēr) either of the ends of a eukaryotic chromosome, consisting of many repeats of a short DNA sequence in specific orientation; it protects the chromosomal end and facilitates its replication 端粒，指真核生物染色体的末端，许多重复的短DNA序列组成的特殊定位；保护染色体末端并促进其复制

telo·phase (tel′o-fāz) the final stage of mitosis and meiosis, following metaphase and immediately preceding cytokinesis; the daughter chromatids separate from the kinetochore microtubules and the nuclear membrane reforms 末期，有丝分裂和减数分裂的最后阶段，中期后胞质迅速分裂；子染色粒从着丝点微管和核膜中更新分离出来

te·maz·e·pam (tə-maz′ə-pam) a benzodiazepine used as a sedative and hypnotic in the treatment of insomnia 羟基安定，在治疗失眠症中用以镇静和催眠的一种苯二氮草类药物

tem·o·zo·lo·mide (tem″ə-zo′lə-mīd) a cytotoxic alkylating agent used as an antineoplastic in the treatment of refractory anaplastic astrocytoma 一种细胞毒性烷化剂，用作抗肿瘤药物，治疗难治性星形细胞瘤

tem·per·ate (tem′pər-ət) restrained; characterized by moderation; as a temperate bacteriophage, which infects but does not lyse its host 有节制的，适度的，温和的表示物体冷热程度的物理量，是物体分子热运动的剧烈程度，作为一种温和的噬菌体，感染宿主但不分解宿主

tem·per·a·ture (tem′pər-ə-chər) 1. an expression of heat or coldness in terms of a specific scale; a measure of the average kinetic energy due to thermal agitation of the particles in a system. Symbol t. See accompanying tables 温度，符号t见附表；2. the level of heat natural to a living being 体温；3. colloquial term for *fever* 发热的俗称 **absolute t.** (*T*), that reckoned from absolute zero (−273.15°C or −459.67°F), expressed on an absolute scale 绝对温度；**basal body t. (BBT),** the temperature of the body under conditions of absolute rest 基础体温，处于绝对静息状态下的体温；**core t.,** the temperature of structures deep within the body, as opposed to a peripheral temperature such as that of the skin 体核温度，人体深部结构的温度；**critical t.**, that below which a gas may be converted to a liquid by increased pressure 临界温度，在该温度以下，气体可通过加压而被液化；**normal t.**, that of the human body in health, about 98.6 ℉ or 37℃ when measured orally 正常体温

tem·plate (tem′plət) 1. a pattern or mold 模板，样板；2. in genetics, the strand of DNA or RNA that specifies the base sequence of the strand of DNA or RNA to be synthesized, the newly synthesized strand being complementary to it 遗传学中指 DNA 或 RNA 的一条链，因其新合成的 DNA 或 RNA 特定碱基序列要与之互补的模板链；3. in dentistry, a curved or flat plate used as an aid in setting teeth in a denture 牙科安装义齿时，作为辅助而使用的弯板或平板

tem·ple (tem′pəl) the lateral region on either side of the head, above the zygomatic arch 颞颥，颞部

tem·po·ra (tem′pə-rə) [L.] the temples 颞颥，颞部（复数）

tem·po·ral (tem′pə-rəl) 1. pertaining to the temple 颞的；2. pertaining to time; limited as to time; temporary 暂时的，时间时

tem·po·ro·man·dib·u·lar (tem″pə-ro-mandib′u-lər) pertaining to the temporal bone and mandible 颞下颌的

tem·po·ro·max·il·lary (tem″pə-ro-mak′sĭ- lar″e) pertaining to the temporal bone and maxilla 颞上颌的

tem·po·ro·oc·cip·i·tal (tem″pə-ro-ok-sip′ĭ-təl) per-

taining to the temporal and occipital bones 颞枕的

tem·po·ro·sphe·noid (tem″pə-ro-sfe′noid) pertaining to the temporal and sphenoid bones 颞蝶的

te·nac·u·lum (tə-nak′u-ləm) a hooklike surgical instrument for grasping and holding parts 持钩（外科手术用）

te·nal·gia (te-nal′jə) pain in a tendon 腱痛

te·nas·cin (ten-as′in) a glycoprotein of the extracellular matrix, isolated from a variety of embryo and adult tissues, including epithelial sites, smooth muscles, and some tumors 生腱蛋白，一种细胞外基质的糖蛋白，可从多种胚胎和成熟组织中分离出来，包括上皮部位、平滑肌和一些肿瘤组织

ten·der·ness (ten′dər-nis) a state of unusual sensitivity to touch or pressure 触痛，压痛；**rebound t.**, a state in which pain is felt on the release of pressure over a part 反跳痛

ten·di·ni·tis (ten″dĭ-ni′tis) inflammation of tendons and of tendon-muscle attachments 腱炎；**calcific t.**, inflammation and calcification of the subacromial or subdeltoid bursa, resulting in pain, tenderness, and limitation of motion in the shoulder 钙化性肌腱炎，肩峰下囊或三角肌下囊的炎症和钙化，导致肩关节疼痛、压痛及活动受限

ten·di·no·plas·ty (ten′dĭ-no-plas″te) 同 tenoplasty

ten·di·no·su·ture (ten″dĭ-no-soo′chər) 同 tenorrhaphy

ten·di·nous (ten′dĭ-nəs) pertaining to, resembling, or of the nature of a tendon 腱的，腱状的，腱性的

ten·do (ten′do) pl. *ten′dines* [L.] 同 tendon

ten·don (ten′dən) a fibrous cord of connective tissue

温度值换算：摄氏温度换算为华氏温度

Temperature Equivalents: Celsius to Fahrenheit

℃	℉	℃	℉	℃	℉	℃	℉
−40	−40.0	−3	26.6	34	93.2	71	159.8
−39	−38.2	−2	28.4	35	95.0	72	161.6
−38	−36.4	−1	30.2	36	96.8	73	163.4
−37	−34.6	0	32.0	37	98.6	74	165.2
−36	−32.8	+1	33.8	38	100.4	75	167.0
−35	−31.0	2	35.6	39	102.2	76	168.8
−34	−29.2	3	37.4	40	104.0	77	170.6

℃	℉	℃	℉	℃	℉	℃	℉
−33	−27.4	4	39.2	41	105.8	78	172.4
−32	−25.6	5	41.0	42	107.6	79	174.2
−31	−23.8	6	42.8	43	109.4	80	176.0
−30	−22.0	7	44.6	44	111.2	81	177.8
−29	−20.2	8	46.4	45	113.0	82	179.6
−28	−18.4	9	48.2	46	114.8	83	181.4
−27	−16.6	10	50.0	47	116.6	84	183.2
−26	−14.8	11	51.8	48	118.4	85	185.0
−25	−13.0	12	53.6	49	120.2	86	186.8
−24	−11.2	13	55.4	50	122.0	87	188.6
−23	−9.4	14	57.2	51	123.8	88	190.4
−22	−7.6	15	59.0	52	125.6	89	192.2
−21	−5.8	16	60.8	53	127.4	90	194.0
−20	−4.0	17	62.6	54	129.2	91	195.8
−19	−2.2	18	64.4	55	131.0	92	197.6
−18	−0.4	19	66.2	56	132.8	93	199.4
−17	+1.4	20	68.0	57	134.6	94	201.2
−16	3.2	21	69.8	58	136.4	95	203.0
−15	5.0	22	71.6	59	138.2	96	204.8
−14	6.8	23	73.4	60	140.0	97	206.6
−13	8.6	24	75.2	61	141.8	98	208.4
−12	10.4	25	77.0	62	143.6	99	210.2
−11	12.2	26	78.8	63	145.4	100	212.0
−10	14.0	27	80.6	64	147.2	101	213.8
−9	15.8	28	82.4	65	149.0	102	215.6

T

℃	℉	℃	℉	℃	℉	℃	℉
−8	17.6	29	84.2	66	150.8	103	217.4
−7	19.4	30	86.0	67	152.6	104	219.2
−6	21.2	31	87.8	68	154.4	105	221.0
−5	23.0	32	89.6	69	156.2	106	222.8
−4	24.8	33	91.4	70	158.0		

温度值换算：华氏温度换算为摄氏温度

Temperature Equivalents: Fahrenheit to Celsius

℉	℃	℉	℃	℉	℃	℉	℃
−40	−40.0	11	−11.7	62	16.7	112	44.4
−39	−39.4	12	−11.1	63	17.2	113	45.0
−38	−38.9	13	−10.6	64	17.8	114	45.5
−37	−38.3	14	−10.0	65	18.3	115	46.1
−36	−37.8	15	−9.4	66	18.9	116	46.6
−35	−37.2	16	−8.9	67	19.4	117	47.2
−34	−36.7	17	−8.3	68	20.0	118	47.7
−33	−36.1	18	−7.8	69	20.6	119	48.3
−32	−35.6	19	−7.2	70	21.1	120	48.8
−31	−35.0	20	−6.6	71	21.7	121	49.4
−30	−34.4	21	−6.1	72	22.2	122	50.0
−29	−33.9	22	−5.6	73	22.8	123	50.5
−28	−33.3	23	−5.0	74	23.3	124	51.1
−27	−32.8	24	−4.4	75	23.8	125	51.6
−26	−32.2	25	−3.8	76	24.4	126	52.2
−25	−31.7	26	−3.3	77	25.0	127	52.7
−24	−31.1	27	−2.8	78	25.6	128	53.3

T

℉	℃	℉	℃	℉	℃	℉	℃
−23	−30.6	28	−2.2	79	26.1	129	53.8
−22	−30.0	29	−1.7	80	26.6	130	54.4
−21	−29.4	30	−1.1	81	27.2	131	55.0
−20	−28.9	31	−0.5	82	27.8	132	55.5
−19	−28.3	32	0	83	28.3	133	56.1
−18	−27.8	33	+0.5	84	28.9	134	56.6
−17	−27.2	34	1.1	85	29.4	135	57.2
−16	−26.7	35	1.6	86	30.0	136	57.7
−15	−26.1	36	2.2	87	30.5	137	58.3
−14	−25.6	37	2.7	88	31.0	138	58.8
−13	−25.0	38	3.3	89	31.6	139	59.4
−12	−24.4	39	3.8	90	32.2	140	60.0
−11	−23.9	40	4.4	91	32.7	141	60.5
−10	−23.3	41	5.0	92	33.3	142	61.1
−9	−22.8	42	5.5	93	33.8	143	61.6
−8	−22.2	43	6.1	94	34.4	144	62.2
−7	−21.7	44	6.6	95	35.0	145	62.7
−6	−21.1	45	7.2	96	35.5	146	63.3
−5	−20.6	46	7.7	97	36.1	147	63.8
−4	−20.0	47	8.3	98	36.6	148	64.4
−3	−19.4	48	8.8	98.6	37.0	149	65.0
−2	−18.9	49	9.4	99	37.2	150	65.5
−1	−18.3	50	10.0	100	37.7	155	68.3
0	−17.8	51	10.6	101	38.3	160	71.1
+1	−17.2	52	11.1	102	38.8	165	73.8
2	−16.7	53	11.7	103	39.4	170	76.6

T

℉	℃	℉	℃	℉	℃	℉	℃
3	−16.1	54	12.2	104	40.0	175	79.4
4	−15.6	55	12.7	105	40.5	180	82.2
5	−15.0	56	13.3	106	41.1	185	85.0
6	−14.4	57	13.9	107	41.6	190	87.7
7	−13.9	58	14.4	108	42.2	195	90.5
8	−13.3	59	15.0	109	42.7	200	93.3
9	−12.8	60	15.5	110	43.3	205	96.1
10	−12.2	61	16.1	111	43.8	212	100.0

continuous with the fibers of a muscle and attaching the muscle to bone or cartilage 腱；**Achilles t.**, **calcaneal t.**, the powerful tendon at the back of the heel, attaching the triceps surae muscle to the calcaneus 跟腱，足跟后部强有力的肌腱，将腓肠三头肌与跟骨连接在一起；**t. of conus, t. of infundibulum**, a collagenous band connecting the posterior surface of the pulmonary valve and the muscular infundibulum with the root of the aorta 动脉圆锥腱，连接肺动脉瓣后表面和主动脉根部动脉圆锥肌部之间的胶原带

ten·do·ni·tis (ten″də-ni′tis) 同 tendinitis

ten·do·vag·i·nal (ten″do-vaj′ĭ-nəl) pertaining to a tendon and its sheath 腱鞘的

te·nec·te·plase (tə-nek′tə-plās) a modified form of human tissue plasminogen activator produced by recombinant DNA technology; used as a thrombolytic agent in the treatment of myocardial infarction 通过 DNA 重组技术生产的改良人组织纤溶酶原激活物所产生的；其用作治疗心肌梗死的溶栓剂

te·nec·to·my (tə-nek′tə-me) excision of a lesion of a tendon or of a tendon sheath 肌腱病变切除术，腱鞘切除术

te·nes·mus (tə-nez′məs) straining, especially ineffectual and painful straining at stool or urination 里急后重；**tenes′mic** adj.

te·nia (te′ne-ə) pl. te′niae. Taenia 绦虫

te·ni·a·cide (te′ne-ə-sīd″) 同 taeniacide

ten·i·a·fuge (te′ne-ə-fūj″) 同 taeniafuge

te·ni·a·sis (te-ni′ə-sis) 同 taeniasis

ten·i·po·side (ten-ĭ-po′sīd) a semisynthetic antineoplastic used in the treatment of neuroblastoma, non-Hodgkin lymphoma, and acute lymphoblastic leukemia 替尼泊甙，一种半合成抗肿瘤药物，其用于治疗神经细胞瘤、非霍奇金淋巴瘤和急性淋巴细胞性白血病

te·nod·e·sis (tə-nod′ə-sis) suture of the end of a tendon to a bone 腱固定术

ten·odyn·ia (ten″o-din′e-ə) 同 tenalgia

te·no·fo·vir (tə-no′fo-vir″) an antiretroviral agent that inhibits reverse transcriptase; used as **t. disoproxil fumarate** in the treatment of HIV-1 (human immunodeficiency virus-1) infection 替诺福韦，一种抗逆转录病毒药物，可以抑制逆转录酶；替诺福韦富马酸酯，用于治疗 HIV-1 感染

te·nol·y·sis (tə-nol′ĭ-sis) the operation of freeing a tendon from adhesions 肌腱粘连松解术

teno·myo·plas·ty (ten″o-mi′o-plas″te) plastic repair of a tendon and muscle 腱肌成形术

teno·my·ot·o·my (ten″o-mi-ot′o-me) excision of a portion of a tendon and muscle 腱肌切除术

teno·nec·to·my (ten″o-nek′tə-me) excision of part of a tendon to shorten it 腱切除术

teno·ni·tis (ten″o-ni′tis) 1. tendinitis 腱 炎；2. inflammation of the Tenon capsule 眼球囊炎

ten·on·tol·o·gy (ten″on-tol′ə-je) the sum of what is known about the tendons 腱学

teno·phyte (ten′o-fīt) a growth or concretion in a tendon 腱赘，腱中赘生物

teno·plas·ty (ten′o-plas″te) plastic repair of a tendon 腱成形术；**tenoplas′tic** adj.

teno·re·cep·tor (ten′o-re-sep″tər) a proprioreceptor in a tendon 腱感受器

te·nor·rha·phy (tə-nor′ə-fe) suture of a tendon 腱缝术

ten·os·to·sis (ten″os-to′sis) conversion of a tendon

into bone 腱骨化

teno·su·ture (ten″o-soo′chər) 同 tenorrhaphy

teno·syn·o·vec·to·my (ten″o-sin″o-vek′tə-me) surgical removal of a tendon sheath 腱鞘切除术

teno·syn·o·vi·tis (ten″o-sin″o-vi′tis) inflammation of a tendon sheath 腱鞘炎; **villonodular t.,** a condition marked by exaggerated proliferation of synovial membrane cells, producing a solid tumor-like mass, commonly occurring in periarticular soft tissues and less frequently in joints 绒毛结节性腱鞘炎, 其特征为滑膜细胞过度增生, 形成实体肿瘤样团块, 常见于关节周围软组织, 在关节中较少见

te·not·o·my (tə-not′ə-me) transection of a tendon 腱切断术

teno·vag·i·ni·tis (ten″o-vaj″ĭ-ni′tis) 同 tenosynovitis

TENS transcutaneous electrical nerve stimulation 经皮电神经刺激

ten·sion (ten′shən) 1. the act of stretching 拉伸; 2. the condition of being stretched or strained 张力; 3. the partial pressure of a component of a gas mixture 分压; 4. mental, emotional, or nervous strain 紧张; 5. hostility between two or more individuals or groups 紧张关系; **arterial t.,** blood pressure (2) 动脉压; **intraocular t. (T),** 眼压, 参见 *pressure* 下词条; **intravenous t.,** venous pressure 静脉压; **surface t.,** tension or resistance that acts to preserve the integrity of a surface 表面张力; **tissue t.,** a state of equilibrium between tissues and cells that prevents overaction of any part 组织张力

ten·sor (ten′sor) any muscle that stretches or makes tense 张肌

tent (tent) 1. a fabric covering for enclosing an open space 帷幕; 帐篷; 2. a conical, expansible plug of soft material for dilating an orifice, or keeping a wound open to prevent its healing except at the bottom 塞条, 以软料制成的锥形可膨胀塞条, 以扩张孔以或保持伤口开放, 利于伤口底部自下而上的愈合; **oxygen t.,** one above a patient's bed for administering oxygen by inhalation 氧帐

ten·to·ri·um (ten-tor′e-əm) pl. *tento′ria* [L.] an anatomic part resembling a tent or covering 幕; **tento′rial** *adj.*; **t. cerebel′li, t. of cerebellum,** the process of the dura mater supporting the occipital lobes and covering the cerebellum 小脑幕

ter·a·tism (ter′ə-tiz-əm) an anomaly of formation or development 畸胎畸形; **terat′ic** *adj.*

ter·a·to·blas·to·ma (ter″ə-to-blas-to′mə) 同 teratoma

ter·a·to·car·ci·no·ma (ter″ə-to-kahr″sĭ-no′mə) a malignant neoplasm consisting of elements of teratoma with those of embryonal carcinoma or choriocarcinoma, or both; occurring most often in the testis 畸胎癌

ter·a·to·gen (ter′ə-to-jən) any agent or factor that induces or increases the incidence of abnormal prenatal development 致畸剂, 致畸原, 致畸因子; 生率的药物或因素 **teratogen′ic** *adj.*

ter·a·to·gen·e·sis (ter″ə-to-jen′ə-sis) the production of birth defects in embryos and fetuses 畸形; **teratogenet′ic** *adj.*

ter·a·tog·e·nous (ter″ə-toj′ə-nəs) developed from fetal remains 畸形性的

ter·a·toid (ter′ə-toid) teratomatous 畸胎样的

ter·a·tol·o·gy (ter″ə-tol′ə-je) that division of embryology and pathology dealing with abnormal development and the production of congenital anomalies 畸形学, 畸胎学; **teratolog′ic, teratolog′ical** *adj.*

ter·a·to·ma (ter″ə-to′mə) pl. *terato′mata, teratomas.* A true neoplasm made up of different types of tissue, none of which is native to the area in which it occurs; usually found in the ovary or testis 畸胎瘤; **teratom′atous** *adj.*; **malignant t.,** 1. a solid, malignant ovarian tumor resembling a dermoid cyst but composed of immature embryonal and/or extraembryonal elements derived from all three germ layers 卵巢的恶性畸胎瘤, 卵巢的一种实性恶性肿瘤, 与皮样囊肿相似, 但由源于三个胚层的非成熟型胚性和(或)胚外成分构成; 2. 同 teratocarcinoma

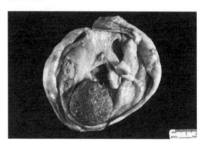

▲ 切开的卵巢成熟性畸胎瘤, 内含有混合性组织, 可见毛发(底部)

ter·a·to·sis (ter″ə-to′sis) 同 teratism

ter·a·zo·sin (tər-a′zo-sin) an alpha₁-adrenergic blocking agent used as the hydrochloride salt in the treatment of hypertension and of benign prostatic hyperplasia 特拉唑嗪, 一种 α₁ 受体阻断药, 其盐酸盐用于治疗高血压和良性前列腺增生

ter·bin·a·fine (tur′bĭ-nə-fēn″) a synthetic antifungal used as the hydrochloride salt in the treatment of tinea and onychomycosis 阿莫罗芬, 一种合成抗真菌药, 其盐酸盐用于治疗癣、甲癣

ter·bi·um (Tb) (tur′be-əm) a heavy, soft, silvery white, malleable and ductile, rare earth element; at. no. 65, at. wt. 158.925 铽(化学元素)

T

ter·bu·ta·line (tər-bu′tə-lēn) a β₂-adrenergic receptor agonist; used as the sulfate salt as a bronchodilator and as a tocolytic in the prevention of premature labor 特布他林，一种 β₂ 肾上腺素受体激动药，其硫酸盐作为支气管扩张药和预防早产的宫缩抑制药

ter·co·na·zole (tər-kon′ə-zōl) an imidazole antifungal used in the treatment of vulvovaginal candidiasis 酮康唑，咪唑类抗真菌药，置于阴道内以治疗外阴阴道念珠病

ter·e·bra·tion (ter″ə-bra′shən) a boring pain 锥痛

te·res (te′rēz) [L.] long and round 长而圆的；圆肌

term (turm) a definite period, especially the period of gestation, or pregnancy 期，尤指妊娠期或怀孕期

ter·mi·nal (tur′mĭ-nəl) 1. forming or pertaining to an end; placed at the end 终末的；末端的；2. a termination, end, or extremity 终点，末端

ter·mi·na·tio (tur″mĭ-na′she-o) pl. *terminatio′nes* [L.] an ending; the site of discontinuation of a structure, as the free nerve endings *(terminatio′nes nervo′rum li′berae),* in which the peripheral fiber divides into fine branches that terminate freely in connective tissue or epithelium 终止；末端

Ter·mi·no·lo·gia Ana·to·mi·ca (TA) (tur″mĭ-no-lo′je-ə an″ə-tom′ĭ-kə) [L.] *International Anatomical Terminology:* the internationally approved official body of anatomical nomenclature, superseding the *Nomina Anatomica* (NA) 人体解剖学术语

ter·mi·nol·o·gy (tur″mĭ-nol′o-je) 1. the vocabulary of an art or science 术语，人文学科或理工（自然）学科所用词汇；2. the science that deals with the investigation, arrangement, and construction of terms 术语学，涉及（专有）名词的研究、分类及编排的科学；**International Anatomical T.,** *Terminologia Anatomica* 国际人体解剖学术语

ter·mi·nus (tur′mĭ-nəs) pl. *ter′mini* [L.] an ending 末端

ter·na·ry (tur′nə-re) 1. third in order 第三的；2. made up of three distinct chemical elements 三元的，由 3 种不同的化学元素构成的

ter·pene (tur′pēn) any hydrocarbon of the formula $C_{10}H_{16}$ 萜

ter·ri·to·ry (ter′ĭ-tor″e) an area or region 范围；地区；**chromosome t′s,** discrete, compact regions within the cell nucleus that are occupied by individual chromosomes during interphase and separated by the interchromosomal domain 染色体域，细胞核内被单个的间期染色体占据的离散的、紧密的区域，由染色体间域分隔开

terror (ter′ər) intense fright 恐怖，惊吓，惊悸；**night t′s,** pavor nocturnus 夜惊

ter·tian (tur′shən) recurring every third day (counting the day of occurrence as the first day) 第三日复

发的，间日的，参见 *malaria* 下词条

ter·ti·ary (tur′she-ar-e) third in order 第三的；第三期的

ter·ti·grav·i·da (tər-tĭ-grav′ĭ-də) a woman pregnant for the third time; gravida Ⅲ 第三胎孕妇

ter·tip·a·ra (tər-tip′ə-rə) a woman who has had three pregnancies that resulted in viable offspring; para Ⅲ 三产妇

tesa·mo·rel·in (tes″ə-mo-rel′in) a synthetic analogue of human growth hormone–releasing hormone, used as the acetate salt to reduce excess abdominal fat associated with HIV infection 替莫瑞林，一种合成的人生长激素释放激素类似物，其醋酸盐用于减少与艾滋病病毒感染有关的腹部脂肪过多

tes·la (T) (tes′lə) the SI unit of magnetic flux density, a vector quantity that measures the magnitude of a magnetic field. It is equal to 1 weber per square meter 特斯拉，磁通量密度的 SI 单位

tes·sel·lat·ed (tes′ə-lāt″əd) divided into squares, like a checker board 棋盘格状的，分成方格的

test (test) 1. an examination or trial 试验，测验；2. a significant chemical reaction 化验，化验结果；3. a reagent 试剂；**abortus Bang ring t., ABR t.,** an agglutination test for brucellosis in cattle, performed by mixing a drop of stained brucellae with 1 ml of milk and incubating for 1 hour at 37 ℃；agglutinated bacteria rise to the surface to form a colored ring 牛流产布鲁菌环试验，即牛布鲁菌病凝集试验，将一滴染色的布鲁氏杆菌滴入 1ml 牛奶中，37℃孵育 1h；被凝集的布鲁氏杆菌升至表层，形成一个彩环；**acid elution t.,** air-dried blood smears are fixed in 80% methanol and immersed in a pH 3.3 buffer; all hemoglobins are eluted except fetal hemoglobin, which is seen in red cells after staining 酸洗脱试验，风干后的血液涂片用 80% 的甲醇固定，浸泡在 pH3.3 的缓冲剂里；所有血红蛋白均被洗脱，只有胎儿血红蛋白仍固定于红细胞中，染色后即可检出；**acidified serum t.,** incubation of red cells in acidified serum; after centrifugation, the supernatant is examined by colorimetry for hemolysis, which indicates paroxysmal nocturnal hemoglobinuria 酸化血清试验，将红细胞在酸化血清中培养；离心后取上清液用比色法检查溶血，如有则提示阵发性夜间血红蛋白尿；**acoustic reflex t.,** measurement of the acoustic reflex threshold; used to differentiate between conductive and sensorineural deafness and to diagnose acoustic neuroma 听反射试验，听反射阈值的测量；用于区分传导性耳聋和感觉神经性耳聋，以及听神经瘤的诊断；**Adson t.,** one for inferior thoracic aperture syndrome; with the patient in a sitting position, hands on thighs, the examiner palpates both radial pulses as the patient rapidly fills the lungs by deep inhalation and, holding the breath, hyperextends the neck, turning the head toward the affected side. If the radial pulse on that side is markedly or completely obliterated, the result is positive 爱德生试验，斜角肌压迫试验，一种诊断胸廓出口综合征的试验，当病人坐位，双手放在大腿上时，检查者触诊双侧桡动脉，嘱患者深吸气使肺部快速充满，同时屏息，过度伸颈，将头转向患侧，如果一侧桡动脉搏动明显或完全被阻塞，试验结果为阳性 **agglutination t.,** cells containing antigens to a given antibody are mixed into the solution being tested for a particular antibody, with agglutination indicative of antibody presence 凝集试验，含有特定抗体抗原的细胞被混合到测试特定抗体的溶液中，如有凝集反应则表明抗体存在; **alkali denaturation t.,** a spectrophotometric method for determining the concentration of fetal (F) hemoglobin 碱变性试验，用分光光度法测定胎儿血红蛋白浓度; **Ames t.,** a strain of *Salmonella typhimurium* that lacks the enzyme necessary for histidine synthesis is cultured in the absence of histidine and in the presence of the suspected mutagen and certain enzymes known to activate procarcinogens. If the substance causes DNA damage resulting in mutations, some of the bacteria will regain the ability to synthesize histidine and will proliferate to form colonies; almost all of the mutagenic substances are also carcinogenic 埃姆斯试验，一株缺乏组氨酸合成酶的鼠伤寒沙门菌，在无组氨酸有某种可疑的诱变剂和已知的前致癌物活化酶的情况下进行培养。如果这种物质引起因 DNA 损伤导致的突变，这些细菌将重新获得合成组氨酸的能力，并增殖形成菌落；几乎所有的诱变物质都是致癌的; **antibiotic sensitivity t., antibiotic susceptibility t.,** 同 antimicrobial susceptibility t.; **anti-DNA t., anti–double-stranded DNA t.,** an immunoassay that uses native doublestranded DNA as an antigen to detect and monitor increased serum levels of anti-DNA antibodies; used in the detection and management of systemic lupus erythematosus 抗脱氧核糖核酸试验，一种酶免疫测定法，即以天然双链 DNA 作为抗原来检查并监测抗 DNA 抗体在血清中的增加程度；用于监测和管理系统性红斑狼疮; **antiglobulin t. (AGT),** a test for nonagglutinating antibodies against red cells, using antihuman globulin antibody to agglutinate red cells coated with the nonagglutinating antibody. The *direct antiglobulin test* detects antibodies bound to circulating red cells in vivo. It is used in the evaluation of autoimmune and drug-induced hemolytic anemia and hemolytic disease of the newborn. The *indirect antiglobulin test* detects serum antibodies that bind to red cells in an in vitro incubation step. It is used in typing of erythrocyte antigens and in compatibility testing (crossmatch) 抗球蛋白试验，摩姆斯试验，以抗人球蛋白抗体凝集有非凝集性抗体包被的红细胞，以检测抗红细胞的非凝集性抗体之有无。直接球蛋白试验系检测体内与循环中红细胞结合的抗体，用于新生儿自体免疫及药物诱发的溶血性贫血和溶血病的评估；间接球蛋白试验系检测与体外孵育的红细胞结合的血清抗体，用于红细胞抗原的分型及相容性检验（交叉配试）; **antimicrobial susceptibility t.,** any of numerous tests of how susceptible bacteria are to antimicrobial agents; the bacteria are classified as either *sensitive* or *susceptible, indeterminate* or *intermediate,* or *resistant* 抗菌药物敏感性试验，关于细菌对抗菌剂有敏度的测试；将这些细菌可分为：敏感或可疑敏感的，不确定的或中间的，或者耐药的类型; **aptitude t's,** tests designed to determine ability to undertake study or training in a particular field 能力倾向测验，测定从事某一特定领域的研究或训练的资质或能力的一些测验项目; **association t.,** one based on associative reaction, usually by mentioning words to a patient and noting what other words the patient thinks of and gives in reply 联想测验，根据联想反应建立的一种测验法，即通常向被测者提出一些词，注意在他心中唤起和回复的是其他什么词; **automated reagin t. (ART),** a modification of the rapid plasma reagin test for syphilis, used with automated analyzers in clinical chemistry 自动化反应素试验，以用于临床化学的自动分析仪对血浆快速反应素试验所做的改进; **basophil degranulation t.,** an in vitro procedure testing allergic sensitivity to a specific allergen at the cellular level by measuring staining of basophils after exposure to the allergen; a reduced number of granular cells is a positive result 嗜碱性粒细胞脱粒试验，检测在细胞水平下对某一特异变应原的过敏程度的一种体外过程，即测定嗜碱细胞在接触变应原后的染色；细胞数量的减少代表阳性结果 **Benedict t.,** a qualitative or quantitative test for the determination of glucose content of urine Benedict 试验，定性或定量检测尿液中葡萄糖含量的试验; **Binet t., Binet-Simon t.,** a method of ascertaining a child's or youth's mental age by asking a series of questions adapted to, and standardized on, the capacity of normal children at various ages 比奈测验，一种测试儿童及青少年智能的方法，即提出一系列适合于不同年龄组正常儿童的能力的问题，依照回答来确定受试者的心理年龄; **Bing t.,** a vibrating tuning fork is held to the mastoid process and the auditory meatus is alternately occluded and left open; an increase and decrease in loudness is perceived by the normal ear and in sensorineural hearing loss, whereas the hearing of no difference occurs in conductive hearing loss 宾氏试验，振动的音叉置于乳突，交替堵塞和开放外耳道：听力正常和感觉神经性耳聋者可听到音量的增强和减弱（阳性宾氏试验），但传导性耳聋者则听不到音量的差异；**caloric t.,** irrigation of the normal ear with warm water produces a rotatory nystagmus toward that side; irrigation with cold water produces a rotatory nystagmus away from that side 冷热试验，以热水灌注正常耳产生朝被灌注耳一侧的旋转性眼球震颤，以冷水灌注则产生远离灌注耳一侧的旋转性眼球震颤；**chi-square t.,** any statistical hypothesis test employing the chi-square ($\chi 2$) distribution, measuring the difference between theoretical and observed frequencies and hypothesized to approach the $\chi 2$-distribution as the sample size increases 卡方(χ^2)检验，以卡方分布进行的任何一种假设检验，用于测量理论和观测频率之间的区别，并被假设认为随着样本容量的增加更趋近于χ^2分布；**cis-trans t.,** one used to determine whether two mutations are in the same gene (alleles) or different genes (pseudoalleles) by examining the phenotypes of heterozygotes carrying the mutations in cis (same chromosome) and in *trans* (different chromosomes) configurations 顺反测定，该试验测定杂合子表型携带的顺式（同一染色体）和反式（不同染色体）的突变，确定两个突变是否存在于相同的基因（等位基因）或不同的基因（拟等位基因）；**clomiphene citrate challenge t.,** measurement of fertility potential in a woman by examination of the response of the folliclestimulating hormone level to administration of clomiphene citrate early in the menstrual cycle 枸橼酸氯芪酚试验，在月经周期早期给予枸橼酸氯芪酚，通过检测促卵泡激素水平对其的反应来测量妇女的生育潜力；**complement fixation t.,** 补体结合试验，参见 *fixation* 下词条；**contraction stress t. (CST),** the monitoring of the response of the fetal heart rate to spontaneous or induced uterine contractions by cardiotocography, with deceleration indicating possible fetal hypoxia 宫缩应激试验，通过胎心分娩力描记法监测胎儿心率对子宫收缩的反应，如有胎心减速，可提示胎儿缺氧；**Coombs t.,** 同 antiglobulin t.；**Denver Developmental Screening t.,** a test for identification of infants and preschool children with developmental delay 丹佛儿童发展筛选测验，婴幼儿发育迟缓；鉴定试验；**DFA-TP t.,** 同 direct florescent antibody-*Treponemal pallidum t.*；**direct fluorescent antibody-*Treponema pallidum t.,*** DFA-TP t.; a serologic test for syphilis using direct immunofluorescence 直接荧光抗体 - 苍白密螺旋体试验；**disk diffusion t.,** a test for antibiotic sensitivity in bacteria; agar plates are inoculated with a standard-ized suspension of a microorganism. Antibiotic-containing disks are applied to the agar surface. Following overnight incubation, the diameters of the zones of inhibition are interpreted as sensitive (susceptible), indeterminate (intermediate), or resistant 平板扩散药敏试验，检细菌中抗生素的敏感性，琼脂平板接种标准微生物悬液；含抗生素的小盘置于琼脂面上，孵育一夜后，按其抑制区的直径大小分为敏感、中间及耐药三种情况；**drawer t's,** tests for the integrity of the cruciate ligaments of the knee; with the knee flexed 90 degrees, if the tibia can be drawn too far forward there is rupture of the anterior ligaments *(anterior drawer t.),* if too far back then the rupture is of the posterior ligaments *(posterior drawer t.)* 抽屉试验，用以检查膝交叉韧带的完整性，仰卧屈膝90°，若胫骨向前拉的过远，则存在前韧带撕裂（前抽屉试验），而向后拉的过远，则存在后韧带撕裂（后抽屉试验）；**early pregnancy t.,** a do-it-yourself immunologic test for pregnancy based on an increase in urinary levels of human chorionic gonadotropin after fertilization and performed as early as 1 day after menstruation was expected 早孕试验，可在家自测的一种妊娠免疫学试验，其依据是受精后尿中人绒毛膜促性腺激素水平增高，早在预期月经后1日即可检出；**EP t., erythrocyte protoporphyrin t.,** determination of erythrocyte protoporphyrin levels as a screening test for lead toxicity; levels are increased in lead poisoning and iron deficiency 红细胞原卟啉试验，铅中毒筛选试验，在铅中毒和铁缺乏时水平增高；**exercise t's, exercise stress t's,** any of various stress tests in which exercise is used in the electrocardiographic assessment of cardiovascular health and function, particularly in the diagnosis of myocardial ischemia. The most widely used forms are the treadmill and bicycle ergometer exercise tests; they are usually graded, consisting of a series of incrementally increasing workloads sustained for defined intervals 运动试验，运动负荷试验；**FAB t.,** 同 fluorescent antibody t.；**finger-nose t.,** one for coordinated limb movements; with the upper limb extended to one side the patient is asked to try to touch the end of the nose with the tip of the index finger 指鼻试验，检测四肢的协调运动，患者上肢伸展于一侧，嘱其以食指尖缓慢碰触鼻尖；**Finn chamber t.,** a type of patch test in which the materials being tested are held in shallow aluminum cups (Finn chambers) that are taped against the skin, usually for a few days 芬恩斑试验，一种斑片试验，将待检物置于浅铝杯（芬恩杯）中，通常铝杯贴于皮肤数日；**Fishberg concentration t.,** determination of the ability of the kidneys to maintain excretion of solids under conditions of reduced water intake and a high protein diet, in which urine samples are collected and tested for specific gravity 菲什伯格浓缩试验，测定肾脏在减少水分摄入和高蛋白饮食条件下维持固体排泄的能力，在这种情况下，收集尿液样本并测试尿比重；**flocculation t.,** any serologic test in which a flocculent agglomerate is formed; usually applied to a variant form of the precipitin reaction 絮状沉淀试验，絮凝试验；**fluorescent antibody t., FAB t.,** a test for the distribution of cells expressing a specific protein by binding antibody specific for the protein and detecting complexes by fluorescent labeling of the antibody 荧光抗体试验，通过结合对蛋白特异性抗体和荧光标记抗体检测复合物来检测表达特定蛋白的细胞的分布；**fluorescent treponemal antibody absorption t., FTA-ABS t.,** the standard treponemal antigen serologic test for syphilis, using fluorescein-labeled antihuman globulin to demonstrate specific treponemal antibodies in patient serum 荧光密螺旋体抗体吸收试验，特异性梅毒螺旋体抗原血清试验，通过间接免疫荧光技术检测血清中抗梅毒螺旋体 IgG 抗体；**gel diffusion t.,** 凝胶扩散试验，参见 *immunodiffusion* **glaucoma hemifield t.,** used to evaluate single static threshold visual field test results in glaucoma 青光眼半视野试验，用于评价青光眼单静态阈视野的检查；**glucose tolerance t.,** a test of the body's ability to utilize carbohydrates by measuring the plasma glucose level at stated intervals after ingestion or intravenous injection of a large quantity of glucose 葡萄糖耐量试验，检测机体利用糖的能力，其通过在摄入或静脉注射大量葡萄糖后，在规定的时间间隔测定血糖水平；**glycosylated hemoglobin t.,** measurement of the percentage of hemoglobin A molecules that have formed a stable keto–amine linkage between the terminal amino acid position of the β -chains and a glucose group; in normal persons this is about 7% of the total and in diabetics about 14.5% 糖基血红蛋白试验，测定 β 链末端氨基酸位与葡萄糖基因间形成稳定酮胺链的血红蛋白 A 分子百分比；在正常人中约为总量的 7%，糖尿病患者则为 14.5% 左右；**guaiac t.,** one for occult blood; glacial acetic acid and a solution of gum guaiac are mixed with the specimen; on addition of hydrogen peroxide, the presence of blood is indicated by a blue tint 愈创木脂试验，冰醋酸和愈创木脂溶液与标本混合；加过氧化氢后，若显蓝色即提示潜血；**Ham t.,** acidified serum t. 哈姆试验；**heterophil antibody t., heterophile antibody t.,** any of several tests for heterophile antibodies associated with infectious mononucleosis 嗜异性抗体试验，检测与传染性单核细胞增多症有关的嗜异性抗体的试验；**histamine t.,** 组胺试验 1. subcutaneous injection of 0.1% solution of histamine to stimulate gastric secretion 皮下注射 0.1% 组胺溶液 1ml 以刺激胃液分泌；2. after rapid intravenous injection of histamine phosphate, normal persons experience a brief fall in blood pressure, but in those with pheochromocytoma, after the fall, there is a marked rise in blood pressure 快速静脉注射磷酸组胺后，正常人即出现血压短暂降低，但嗜铬细胞瘤患者在血压一度降低后又明显增高；**Huhner t.,** 同 postcoital t.；**hydrogen breath t.,** a test for deficiency of lactase or other hydrolases or for colonic overgrowth of bacteria, in which the exhalations are trapped and measured after administration of carbohydrate, with excess carbohydrate fermentation in the colon resulting in high levels of exhaled hydrogen 氢呼吸试验，检测乳糖酶或其他水解酶的缺乏，或结肠细菌生长过度；服用已知量的碳水化合物后，呼出的气体被收集并测定，过量的碳水化合物滞留在患者结肠中，导致呼出的氢增多；**hypo-osmotic swelling t.,** determination of sperm viability by placing a sample in a hypo-osmotic solution, which causes swelling and curling of the tails of spermatozoa with normal plasma membranes 低渗肿胀试验，通过将样本置于低渗溶液中以测定精子活力，因低渗溶液会导致精子尾部肿胀和卷曲，但质膜正常；**immobilization t.,** detection of antibody based on its ability to inhibit the motility of a bacterial cell or protozoan 制动试验，依照抗体抑制细菌细胞或原生动物能动性的能力检测抗体；**inkblot t.,** Rorschach t. 墨迹测验；**intelligence t.,** a set of problems or tasks posed to assess an individual's innate ability to judge, comprehend, and reason 智力测验；**intracutaneous t., intradermal t.,** skin test in which the antigen is injected intradermally 皮内试验，皮内注射抗原的一种皮肤试验；**Kveim t.,** an intradermal test for the diagnosis of sarcoidosis 克韦姆试验，用于诊断结节病的皮内试验；**latex agglutination t., latex fixation t.,** a type of agglutination test in which antigen to a given antibody is adsorbed to latex particles and mixed with a test solution to observe for agglutination of the latex 乳胶凝集试验，乳胶结合试验，一种凝集试验，即针对某一特定抗体的抗原被吸附到乳胶颗粒中，同某一种溶液混合以观察乳胶凝集情况；**limulus t.,** an extract of blood cells from the horseshoe crab *(Limulus polyphemus)* is exposed to a blood sample from a patient; if gram-negative endotoxin is present in the sample, it will produce gelation of the extract of blood cells 鲎蛛试验，鲎血细胞提取液接触患者血液标本，若后者含革兰阴性杆菌内毒素则发生血细胞提取液的胶凝作用；**Lundh t.,** a test for pancreatic function in which trypsin concentrations in the duode-

T

num after a test meal are measured, with owered levels of trypsin indicating low pancreatic secretion 伦德试验，检查胰腺功能的试验，即测定餐后数小时期间十二指肠中的胰蛋白酶浓度，若胰蛋白浓度减低则提示胰腺分泌减低；**lupus band t.,** an immunofluorescence test to determine the presence and extent of immunoglobulin and complement deposits at the dermal-epidermal junction of skin specimens from patients with systemic lupus erythematosus 狼疮带试验，一种免疫荧光试验，测定系统性红斑狼疮患者皮肤标本的真皮与表皮接合处有无免疫球蛋白和补体沉积及其程度；**Mantoux t.,** an intracutaneous tuberculin test 芒图试验，即结核菌素皮内试验; **Master "two-step" exercise t.,** an early exercise test for coronary insufficiency in which electrocardiograms were recorded while and after the subject repeatedly ascended and descended two steps 马斯特二级梯运动试验，早期检测冠状动脉供血不足的运动试验，受试者反复上、下两个阶梯，运动停止后立即记录心电图；**McMurray t.,** as the patient lies supine with one knee fully flexed, the examiner rotates the patient's foot fully outward and the knee is slowly extended; a painful "click" indicates a tear of the medial meniscus of the knee joint; if the click occurs when the foot is rotated inward, the tear is in the lateral meniscus 半月板回旋挤压试验，患者仰卧，充分屈膝，检查者将患者的一足向外充分转动，并使其膝部慢慢伸展，如患者感到疼痛且有咔嗒声，则说明膝关节内侧半月板撕裂，如在足内旋时听到咔嗒声，则为外侧半月板撕裂；**Moloney t.,** one for detection of delayed hypersensitivity to diphtheria toxoid 莫洛尼试验，检测白喉类毒素的迟发型过敏反应；**monospot t.,** a type of heterophile antibody test based on the Paul-Bunnell-Davidsohn test but using erythrocytes from horses instead of sheep, so that the test is much faster 单斑试验（检测与传染性单核细胞增多症有关的抗体），基于 Paul-Bunnell-Davidaohn 试验的嗜异抗体试验，但用马红细胞代替绵羊红细胞，所以检测速度要快得多；**multiple-puncture t.,** a skin test in which the material used (e.g., tuberculin) is introduced into the skin by pressure of several needles or pointed tines or prongs 多刺试验，皮内试验的一种，即以刺针或叉针数次刺压，将物品（如结核菌素）接种于皮内；**neostigmine t.,** on injection of neostigmine methylsulfate mixed with atropine sulfate, lessening of myasthenic symptoms indicates myasthenia gravis 新斯的明试验，注射硫酸阿托品的甲硫酸新斯的明的混合物后，如肌无力症状减轻，则说明患有重症肌无力；**neutralization t.,** a test for the power of an antiserum, antibiotic, antitoxin, antiviral, or other substance to antagonize the pathogenic

properties of a microorganism, virus, bacteriophage, or toxic substance 中和试验，检测抗血清、抗菌素、抗毒素、抗病毒或其他物质，拮抗微生物、毒素、病毒、噬菌体或毒性物质的试验；**nocturnal penile tumescence (NPT) t.,** monitoring of erections occurring during sleep; used in the differential diagnosis of psychogenic and organic impotence 夜间阴茎勃起试验，监测睡眠中阴茎勃起的情况；用于鉴别心因性阳痿和器质性阳痿；**nonstress t. (NST),**the monitoring of the response of the fetal heart rate to fetal movements by cardiotocography 无激惹试验，通过心脏分娩力描记法持续胎心监护；监听胎儿的心率对胎动的反应；**nontreponemal antigen t.,** any of various tests detecting serum antibodies to reagin (cardiolipin and lecithin) derived from host tissues in the diagnosis of the *Treponema pallidum* infection of syphilis 非密螺旋体抗原试验，在梅毒螺旋体感染诊断中，检测血清中源于宿主组织的反应素抗体（心磷脂和卵磷脂）；**NPT t.,** 同 nocturnal penile tumescence t.；**osmotic fragility t.,** heparinized or defibrinated blood is placed in sodium chloride solutions of varying concentrations; increased fragility, measured as hemolysis, indicates spherocytosis 渗透脆性试验，肝素化或去纤维化的血液放置在不同浓度的氯化钠溶液中，如脆性增加（可以溶血来衡量），则表明存在球形红细胞症；**oxytocin challenge t. (OCT),** a contraction stress test in which the uterine contractions are stimulated by intravenous infusion of oxytocin 催产素激惹试验，一种收缩应力试验，即以静脉内注射催产素来刺激子宫收缩；**Pap t., Papanicolaou t.,** an exfoliative cytologic staining procedure for detection and diagnosis of various conditions, particularly malignant and premalignant conditions of the female genital tract; also used in evaluating endocrine function and in the diagnosis of malignancies of other organs 帕普试验，宫颈刮片检查，用于检测和诊断脱落细胞学染色方法，尤其是女性生殖道的恶性和癌前状态；也用于内分泌功能评估及诊断其他器官的恶性肿瘤；**pareidolia t.,** a test that evokes and measures pareidolias (an imagined perception of a representational pattern or meaning that does not actually exist); used as a tool in diagnosing Lewy body dementia 空想性错觉测试，唤起并衡量幻想性错觉（对实际上并不存在的表征模式或意义的想象感知）的测试；用于诊断路易体痴呆；**patch t's,** tests for hypersensitivity, performed by observing the reaction to application to the skin of filter paper or gauze saturated with the substance in question 斑贴试验，主要用于诊断过敏反应的皮肤试验；**Patrick t.,** thigh and knee of the supine patient are flexed, the external malleolus rests on the patella on the oppo-

T

site leg, and the knee is depressed; production of pain indicates arthritis of the hip. Also known as *fabere sign,* from the first letters of movements that elicit it (*f*lexion, *ab*duction, *e*xternal *r*otation, *ex*tension) 骶髋关节分离试验，患者仰卧，健侧下肢伸直，患侧下肢屈膝屈髋，并将外踝置于健侧膝上，下压膝部，如感疼痛即提示髋关节炎。也称此为 "屈展旋伸征"，由完成以上检查动作的起始字母屈（flexion）、展（abduction）、旋（external rotation）、伸（extension）组成；**Paul-Bunnell-Davidsohn t.,** a type of heterophile antibody test that differentiates among three types of heterophile sheep agglutinins: those associated with infectious mononucleosis and serum sickness and natural antibodies against Forssman antigen Paul-Bunnell-Davidsohn 试验，可鉴别三种异种抗体的异种抗体检测方法，检测与传染性单核分裂症和血清病相关的异种抗体，以及针对嗜异性抗原的天然抗体；**postcoital t.,** determination of the number and condition of spermatozoa in mucus aspirated from the cervical canal soon after intercourse 性交后试验，性交后不久测定从宫颈管抽出的黏液中的精子数量和状况 **precipitin t.,** any serologic test based on a precipitin reaction 沉淀素试验，任何基于沉淀素反应的血清学试验；**projective t.,** any of various tests in which an individual interprets ambiguous stimulus situations according to their own unconscious dispositions, yielding information about their personality and possible psychopathology 投射测验，让受试者对性质含糊的刺激信号作出臆想解释的试验，从而获知其个性和可能的精神病理学的信息；**psychological t.,** any test to measure a subject's development, achievement, personality, intelligence, thought processes, etc. 心理测验，检测受实验者的发育、成就、性格、能力、思维过程等的试验；**psychomotor t.,** a test that assesses the subject's ability to perceive instructions and perform motor responses 精神运动测验；**Queckenstedt t.,** 奎肯施泰特试验，参见 *sign* 下词条；**Quick t.,** 1. a test for liver function based on excretion of hippuric acid after administration of sodium benzoate 快速测验用于检测肝功能，即测试应用苯甲酸钠后马尿酸的排出量；2. prothrombin time 凝血酶原时间；**Radioallergosorbent t. (RAST),** a radioimmunoassay test for the measurement of specific IgE antibody in serum, using allergen extract antigens fixed in a solid-phase matrix and radiolabeled anti-human IgE 放射性变应原吸附试验借助放射免疫方法测定被固相载体上变应原吸附的特异性 IgE 抗体的技术；**radioimmunosorbent t. (RIST),** a radioimmunoassay technique for measuring serum IgE concentration, using radiolabeled IgE and anti-

human IgE bound to an insoluble matrix 放射免疫吸附试验，测定血清中总 IgE 浓度的试验；**rapid plasma reagin t., RPR test;** a screening flocculation test for syphilis, using a modified VDRL antigen 快速血浆反应素试验，RPR 试验，筛查梅毒的絮凝试验，VDRL 抗原；**Rinne t.,** a test of hearing made with tuning forks of 256, 512, and 1024 Hz, comparing the duration of perception by bone and by air conduction 林纳试验，鉴别感觉性神经性耳聋和传导性耳聋，以 256Hz、512Hz 和 1024Hz 音叉测试听力，比较骨和空气传导感知的持续时间；**rollover t.,** comparison of the blood pressure of a pregnant woman lying on her back versus on her side; an excessive increase when she rolls to the supine position indicates increased risk of preeclampsia 滚动试验，比较妊娠妇女左侧卧和仰卧时的血压，当滚动到仰卧位时，血压过度升高，提示痫前期发病风险增加；**Rorschach t.,** an association technique for personality testing based on the patient's response to a series of inkblot designs 罗夏测验，让受实验者讲述其对一系列墨迹图的反应，进行性格测试的联想测验；**RPR t.,** 同 rapid plasma reagin test；**Rubin t.,** one for patency of the uterine tubes, performed by transuterine inflation with carbon dioxide gas 输卵管通气术，经子宫二氧化碳充气测定输卵管的通畅；**Schick t.,** an intradermal test for determination of susceptibility to diphtheria 锡克试验，测定白喉是否有免疫性的皮内试验；**Schiller t.,** one for early squamous cell carcinoma of the cervix, performed by painting the uterine cervix with a solution of iodine and potassium iodide, diseased areas being revealed by a failure to take the stain 宫颈黏膜碘试验，用于早期宫颈鳞状细胞癌，在宫颈上涂抹碘和碘化钾溶液，未着色的则为病变区域；**Schilling t.,** a test for vitamin B_{12} absorption employing cyanocobalamin tagged with Co-57; used in the diagnosis of pernicious anemia and other disorders of vitamin B_{12} metabolism 希林试验，使用带有 ^{57}Co 标记的维生素 B_{12}（氰钴胺）检测胃肠道对维生素 B_1 的吸收；其结果用于诊断恶性贫血和其他维生素 B_{12} 代谢疾病；**Schirmer t.,** a test of tear production in keratoconjunctivitis sicca, performed by measuring the area of moisture on a piece of filter paper inserted over the conjunctival sac of the lower lid, with the end of the paper hanging down on the outside 希尔默试验，测试角结膜炎泪液生成情况，于下眼睑结膜囊上方置一小片滤纸，未端垂悬于外，测量湿润区的面积；**Schober t.,** a test to determine the range of motion of the lumbar spine Schober 试验，测定腰椎运动范围的试验；**Schwabach t.,** a hearing test made, with the opposite ear masked, placing the stems of vibrating tuning forks on the mastoid process first of the patient and then of the examiner. If heard longer by the patient it indicates conductive hearing loss and if heard longer by the examiner it indicates sensorineural hearing loss in the patient 施瓦赫试验，患者对侧耳掩盖，将振动中的音叉柄交替置于患者和检查者本人（听力应正常）的颞骨乳突上，如患者听音时间长，则提示传导性耳聋，如检查者听音时间长，则提示感觉神经性耳聋; **scratch t.,** a skin test in which the antigen is applied to a superficial scratch 划痕试验，把抗原用于浅层划痕上的一种皮肤试验; **serologic t.,** a laboratory test involving seroreactions, especially one measuring serum antibody titer 血清学试验，涉及到血清学反应的检验项目，尤指其中测定血清抗体效价的试验; **sheep cell agglutination t. (SCAT),** any agglutination test using sheep erythrocytes 绵羊红细胞凝集试验，任何使用绵羊红细胞的凝集试验; **sickling t.,** one for demonstration of abnormal hemoglobin and the sickling phenomenon in erythrocytes 镰变试验，揭示红细胞中血红蛋白异常和镰变现象; **skin t.,** any test in which an antigen is applied to the skin in order to observe the patient's reaction; used to determine exposure or immunity to infectious diseases, to identify allergens producing allergic reactions, and to assess ability to mount a cellular immune response 皮肤试验，把抗原用于皮肤以观察病人反应的试验，皮肤试验被用于测定对传染病的暴露和免疫力，鉴别产生过敏反应的过敏原以及评定发动细胞免疫反应的能力; **sperm agglutination t.,** any of various tests for the presence of antisperm antibodies as a cause of infertility, based on the ability of large multivalent isotypes such as IgM or secretory IgA to cross-link and agglutinate spermatozoa with such antibodies 精子凝集试验，不孕症病因中检测是否存在抗精子抗体，基于测定大分子多价同种抗体（如 IgM 或分泌型 IgA）与此类抗体交联并凝集精子的能力; **stress t's,** any of various tests that assess cardiovascular health and function after application of a stress, usually exercise, to the heart 应激试验，一种评估压力（通常是运动）作用于心脏后心血管健康和功能的测试; **swinging flashlight t.,** with the eyes fixed at a distance and a strong light shining before the intact eye, a crisp bilateral contraction of the pupil is noted; on moving the light to the affected eye, both pupils dilate for a short period, and on moving it back to the intact eye, both pupils contract promptly and remain contracted; indicative of minimal damage to the optic nerve or retina 摆动闪光试验，在与患者有一固定距离处用强光照射其患侧眼，可见其两侧瞳孔收缩活跃，当用强光照射健侧眼时，两个瞳孔均在短时间内扩大，之后

再使强光照射健侧眼，两个瞳孔都迅速收缩，并保持收缩的状态，以上情况表明视神经或视网膜有微小损伤; **Thematic apperception t. (TAT),** a projective test in which the subject tells a story based on each of a series of standard ambiguous pictures, so that the responses reflect a projection of some aspect of the subject's personality and current psychological preoccupations and conflicts 主题统觉试验，一种投射试验，受试者根据一套标准而内容含糊的图片讲述一个故事，自受试者的回应可窥悉其性格的某些方面以及当前的心理关注和冲突; **thyroid suppression t.,** after administration of liothyronine for several days, radioactive iodine uptake is decreased in normal persons but not in those with hyperthyroidism 甲状腺抑制试验，检测甲状腺功能亢进; **tine t.,** a tuberculin test in which four small tines coated with dip-dried tuberculin are pressed into the forearm skin; the test is positive if after 48 to 72 hours there is induration of at least 2 mm in diameter around one or more of the puncture wounds 结核菌素叉刺试验，带 4 个尖的尖叉浸蘸浸干结核菌素后，压入前臂掌侧皮内; 48～72h 后检查，如在划刺处周围有 1 个或更多的直径为 2mm 或更大的硬结，即为阳性; **treponemal antigen t.,** any of various tests detecting specific antitreponemal antibodies in serum in the diagnosis of the *Treponema pallidum* infection of syphilis 螺旋体抗原试验; **tuberculin t.,** any of a number of skin tests for tuberculosis using a variety of different types of tuberculin and methods of application 结核菌素试验; **unheated serum reagin t., USR t.,** a modification of the VDRL test using unheated serum; used primarily for screening 不加热血清反应素试验，改良的 VDRL 试验，使用未加热血清，主要用于筛查 **VDRL t.,** a flocculation test for syphilis using VDRL antigen, which contains cardiolipin, cholesterol, and lecithin, to test heat-inactivated serum VDRL 试验，性病研究实验室试验，检验梅毒的试验，以含心磷脂、胆固醇和卵磷脂的 VDRI 抗原进行的玻片絮凝试验，测定热灭活血清; **Weber t.,** the stem of a vibrating tuning fork is placed on the vertex or midline of the forehead. If the sound is heard better in the affected ear, it suggests conductive hearing loss; if heard better in the normal ear, it suggests sensorineural hearing loss 韦伯试验，鉴别传导性和感觉神经性耳聋，置振动中的音叉柄于头顶或前额中线处，如患耳更易听到，则可能为传导性听力丧失，如健耳更易听到，则可能为感觉神经性耳聋; **Widal t.,** a test for agglutinins to O and H antigens of *Salmonella typhi* and *Salmonella paratyphi* in the serum of patients with suspected *Salmonella* infection 肥达试验，肥达凝集试验，对疑似沙门菌感染患者

血清中伤寒沙门菌和副伤寒沙门菌的 O 抗原及 H 抗原凝集素的检测

tes·tal·gia (tes-tal′jə) orchialgia 睾丸痛

test card (test kahrd) a card printed with various letters or symbols, used in testing vision 视力卡

tes·tes (tes′tēz) [L.] *testis* 的复数

tes·ti·cle (tes′tĭ-kəl) 同 testis

tes·tic·u·lar (tes-tik′u-lər) pertaining to a testis 睾丸的

tes·tis (tes′tis) pl. *tes′tes* [L.] the male gonad; either of the paired egg-shaped glands normally situated in the scrotum, in which the spermatozoa develop. Specialized interstitial cells (Leydig cells) secrete testosterone 睾丸; **abdominal t.**, an undescended testis in the abdominal cavity 腹腔睾丸，腹腔内未下降的睾丸; **ectopic t.**, one outside the normal pathway of descent 异位睾丸; **obstructed t.**, one whose normal descent is blocked, so that it goes into an inguinal pouch 睾丸受阻; **retained t.**, 同 undescended t.; **retractile t.**, one that can descend fully into the scrotum but then moves freely up into the inguinal canal 可回缩的睾丸; **undescended t.**, one that has failed to descend into the scrotum, as in cryptorchidism 睾丸未降，隐睾

tes·ti·tis (tes-ti′tis) orchitis 睾丸炎

tes·tos·te·rone (tes-tos′tə-rōn) the principal androgenic hormone, produced by the interstitial (Leydig) cells of the testes in response to stimulation by the luteinizing hormone of the anterior pituitary gland; it is thought to be responsible for regulation of gonadotropic secretion, spermatogenesis, and wolffian duct differentiation. It is also responsible for other male characteristics after its conversion to dihydrotestosterone. In addition, testosterone possesses protein anabolic properties. It is used as replacement therapy for androgen deficiency in males, in the treatment of delayed male puberty or hypogonadism, and in the palliation of certain breast cancers in females; used as the base or various esters (e.g., cypionate, enanthate, propionate) 睾酮

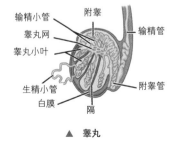

▲ 睾丸

test type (test tīp) printed letters of varying size, used in the testing of visual acuity 视力试标型视力

表，视力标型

TET treadmill exercise test 踏板运动试验; tubal embryo transfer 胚胎输卵管内移植

te·tan·ic (tə-tan′ik) pertaining to tetanus 破伤风的，强直性的

te·tan·i·form (tə-tan′ĭ-form) 同 tetanoid

tet·a·nize (tet′ə-nīz) to induce tetanic convulsions or symptoms 使强直，致强直

tet·a·node (tet′ə-nōd) the unexcited stage occurring between the tetanic contractions in tetanus 手足搐搦静止期

tet·a·noid (tet′ə-noid) resembling tetanus 破伤风样的，强直样的

tet·a·nol·y·sin (tet″ə-nol′ĭ-sin) the hemolytic exotoxin produced by *Clostridium tetani;* its importance in the pathogenesis of tetanus is uncertain 破伤风菌素溶血素。Cf. *tetanospasmin*

tet·a·no·spas·min (tet″ə-no-spaz′min) *tetanus toxin;* the exotoxin produced by *Clostridium tetani,* which blocks the synaptic terminals of the central nervous system, causing the typical muscle spasms of tetanus 破伤风菌痉挛毒素

tet·a·nus (tet′ə-nəs) 1. an acute, often fatal, infectious disease caused by the bacillus *Clostridium tetani,* usually entering the body through a contaminated puncture wound or laceration 破伤风; 2. a state of muscular contraction without periods of relaxation 强直收缩; **tetan′ic** *adj.;* **cephalic t.**, a rare, sometimes fatal form of tetanus sometimes seen after injury to the head or face or otitis media; it is characterized by dysfunction of the cranial nerves, especially the seventh cranial nerve, and may remain localized or progress to generalized tetanus 脑破伤风，一种罕见类型的破伤风，有时是致命的，可发生于头面部外伤或中耳炎后；以脑神经功能失常为特征，特别是第七脑神经，可以保持局限型，亦可发展为全身型破伤风; **generalized t.**, the most common type of *Clostridium tetani* infection, characterized by tetanic muscular contractions and hyperreflexia, resulting in trismus, laryngospasm, generalized muscle spasm, opisthotonos, respiratory spasm, seizures, and paralysis that can be fatal 全身型破伤风，是最常见的破伤风梭菌感染类型，以强直性肌挛缩和反射亢进为特征，引起牙关紧闭、声门痉挛、全身肌痉挛、角弓反张、呼吸痉挛、惊厥发作和麻痹，这些都可能是致命的; **localized t.**, *Clostridium tetani* infection characterized by localized muscular twitching and spasms near the site of injury; it may progress to generalized tetanus 局限性强直，破伤风梭菌感染以局限的肌肉抽动和损伤部位附近的肌群痉挛为特征；亦可发展为全身型; **neonatal t.**, **t. neonato′rum**, tetanus of neonates, usually due to umbilical infection 新生儿破伤风，通常因脐部残

端感染所致；**physiologic t.,** 同 tetanus (2)

tet·a·ny (tet′ə-ne) a syndrome of sharp flexion of the wrist and ankle joints (carpopedal spasm), muscle twitching, cramps, and convulsions, sometimes with attacks of stridor; due to hyperexcitability of nerves and muscles caused by decreased extracellular ionized calcium in parathyroid hypofunction, vitamin D deficiency, or alkalosis, or following ingestion of alkaline salts 手足搐搦；**duration t.,** a continuous tetanic contraction in response to a strong continuous current, seen especially in degenerated muscles 持续性搐搦；**gastric t.,** a severe form due to disease of the stomach, with difficult respiration and painful tonic spasms of limbs 胃病性手足搐搦；**hyperventilation t.,** tetany produced by forced inhalation and exhalation over a period of time 通气过度性手足搐搦；**latent t.,** tetany elicited by the application of electrical and mechanical stimulation 潜在性手足搐搦；**neonatal t. of newborn,** hypocalcemic tetany in the first few days of life, often marked by irritability, muscle twitchings, jitteriness, tremors, and convulsions, and less often by laryngospasm and carpopedal spasm 新生儿手足搐搦，生后数日发生的低血钙性手足搐搦，常以激惹、肌抽搐、躁动、震颤、惊厥等症象为主，其次如喉痉挛、手足痉挛等；**parathyroid t., parathyroprival t.,** tetany due to removal or hypofunction of the parathyroids 甲状旁腺缺乏性手足搐搦

tet·ar·ta·no·pia (tet″ər-tə-no′pe-ə) 1. quadrantanopia 象限盲，四分之一盲；2. a rare type of dichromatic vision of doubtful existence, characterized by perception of red and green only, with blue and yellow perceived as an achromatic (gray) band 黄蓝色盲，第四型色盲，一种罕见的疑难型色觉缺陷，其特点为患者保留对红、绿两色的感受机制，而缺乏蓝、黄色觉，在光谱上代之以一种无色（灰）带

tet·ra·caine (tet′rə-kān) a local, topical, and spinal anesthetic, used as the base or the hydrochloride salt 丁卡因，一种可用于局部、表面和脊髓的麻醉剂，用其碱或盐酸盐

tet·ra·chlo·ro·eth·y·lene (tet″rə-klor″o-eth′- ə-lēn) a moderately toxic chlorinated hydrocarbon used as a dry-cleaning solvent and for other industrial uses 四氯乙烯

tet·ra·crot·ic (tet″rə-krot′ik) having four sphygmographic elevations to 1 beat of the pulse 四波脉的

tet·ra·cyc·lic (tet″rə-sik′lik) (-si′klik) containing four fused rings or closed chains in the molecular structure 四环的

tet·ra·cy·cline (tet″rə-si′klēn) a semisynthetic antibiotic produced from chlortetracycline; used as the base or the hydrochloride salt. The term is also used to denote any of the group of related antibiotics, isolated from species of *Streptomyces* or produced semisynthetically 四环素

tet·rad (tet′rad) a group of four similar or related entities, as (1) any element or radical having a valence, or combining power, of four; (2) a group of four chromosomal elements formed in the pachytene stage of the first meiotic prophase; (3) a square of cells produced by division into two planes of certain cocci (*Sarcina*) 四价元素；四分体（染色体）；四裂体（细菌）；**Fallot t.,** tetralogy of Fallot 法洛四联症

tet·ra·dac·ty·ly (tet″rə-dak′tə-le) the presence of four digits on the hand or foot 四指（趾）

tet·ra·go·num (tet″rə-go′nəm) [L.] a quadrilateral 方形，四边形；四边形间隙；**t. lumba′le,** the area bounded by the four lumbar muscles 腰四边形间隙

tet·ra·hy·dro·bi·op·ter·in (BH₄, BH₄) (tet″rə-hi″dro-bi-op′tər-in) a coenzyme in the reactions hydroxylating phenylalanine, tryptophan, and tyrosine; defects in its biosynthesis or regeneration affect all three hydroxylation reactions, interfere with production of the corresponding neurotrans mitter precursors, and result in hyperphenylalaninemia 四氢生物蝶呤，在苯丙氨酸、色氨酸和酪氨酸羟基化反应中作为辅酶；生物合成的缺乏或辅酶的再生影响这三种羟基化作用，妨碍对应的神经递质前体的产生，并导致高苯丙氨酸血症

tet·ra·hy·dro·can·nab·i·nol (THC) (tet″rə- hi″dro-kə-nab′ĭ-nol) the active principle of cannabis, occurring in two isomeric forms, both considered psychomimetically active 四氢大麻酚，大麻的活性成分，有两种异构体，都被认为是拟精神活性药物

tet·ra·hy·dro·fo·lic ac·id (THF) (tet″rə-hi″drofo′- lik) a form of folic acid in which the pteridine ring is fully reduced; it is the parent compound of a variety of coenzymes that serve as carriers of 1-carbon groups in metabolic reactions; in dissociated form, called *tetrahydrofolate* 四氢叶酸，一种叶酸，蝶呤环在其中充分还原；它是各种辅酶的母体化合物，在新陈代谢作用中充当单碳族的载体；其解离形式被称为四氢叶酸

tet·ra·hy·droz·o·line (tet″rə-hi-droz′ə-lēn) an adrenergic applied topically as the hydrochloride salt to the nasal mucosa and to the conjunctiva to produce vasoconstriction 四氢唑啉，肾上腺素能药，其盐酸盐可局部用于鼻黏膜及结膜以促使血管收缩

te·tral·o·gy (tĕ-tral′ə-je) a group or series of four 四联症；**t. of Fallot,** a complex of congenital heart defects consisting of pulmonary stenosis, interventricular septal defect, hypertrophy of the right ventricle, and dextroposition of the aorta 法洛四联症，一种复杂的先天性心脏病，包括肺动脉狭窄、室间隔缺损、右心室肥大和主动脉骑跨

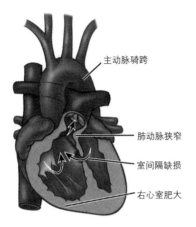

主动脉骑跨

肺动脉狭窄

室间隔缺损

右心室肥大

▲ 法洛四联症

tet·ra·mer·ic (tet″rə-mer′ik) having four parts 四部分的，四聚体的

tet·ra·nop·sia (tet″rə-nop′se-ə) quadrantanopia 象限盲

tet·ra·pa·re·sis (tet″rə-pə-re′sis) muscular weakness of all four limbs 四肢轻瘫

tet·ra·pep·tide (tet″rə-pep′tīd) a peptide that on hydrolysis yields four amino acids 四肽

tet·ra·ple·gia (tet″rə-ple′jə) quadriplegia 四肢麻痹，四肢瘫

tet·ra·ploid (tet′rə-ploid″) 1. pertaining to or characterized by tetraploidy 四倍的；2. an individual or cell having four sets of chromosomes 四倍体，有四套染色体的个体或细胞

tet·ra·ploi·dy (tet′rə-ploi″de) the state of having four sets of chromosomes (4*n*) 四倍性

tet·ra·pus (tet′rə-pəs) a human fetus having four feet 四足畸胎

tet·ra·pyr·role (tet″rə-pə-rōl′) a compound containing four pyrrole rings, e.g., heme or chlorophyll 四吡咯

te·tras·ce·lus (tĕ-tras′ə-ləs) a human fetus with four lower limbs 四腿畸胎

tet·ra·so·my (tet′rə-so″me) the presence of two extra chromosomes of one type in an otherwise diploid cell 四体性；**tetraso′mic** *adj.*

tet·ra·va·lent (tet″rə-va′lənt) having a valence of four 四价的

tet·ro·do·tox·in (tet′ro-do-tok″sin) a highly lethal neurotoxin present in numerous species of puffer fish and in certain newts (in which it is called *tarichatoxin*); ingestion rapidly causes malaise, dizziness, and tingling about the mouth, which may be followed by ataxia, convulsions, respiratory paralysis, and death 河鲀毒素，高度致死性神经毒性物质，鲀鱼亚目中很多种属的河豚鱼以及蝾螈属中的某些蝾螈都有此毒素，后者称蝾螈毒素；食后数分钟内即感不适、头晕、口周刺痛，随后可出现共济失调、惊厥、呼吸麻痹和死亡

tex·ti·form (teks′tĭ-form) formed like a network 网状的；组织状的

TGF transforming growth factor 转化生长因子

Th thorium 元素钍的符号

THA total hip arthroplasty 全髋关节置换术

tha·lam·ic (thə-lam′ik) pertaining to the thalamus 丘脑的

thal·a·mo·cor·ti·cal (thal″ə-mo-kor′tĭ-kəl) pertaining to the thalamus and cerebral cortex 丘脑和大脑皮质的

thal·a·mo·len·tic·u·lar (thal″ə-mo-lən-tik′ulər) pertaining to the thalamus and lenticular nucleus 丘脑豆状核的

thal·a·mot·o·my (thal″ə-mot′ə-me) a stereotaxic surgical technique for the discrete destruction of specific groups of cells within the thalamus, as for the relief of pain, for relief of tremor and rigidity in paralysis agitans, or in the treatment of certain psychiatric disorders 丘脑切开术

thal·a·mus (thal′ə-məs) pl. *thal′ami* [L.] either of two large ovoid masses, consisting chiefly of gray matter, situated one on either side of and forming part of the lateral wall of the third ventricle. Each is divided into dorsal and ventral parts; the term *thalamus* without a modifier usually refers to the dorsal thalamus, which functions as a relay center for sensory impulses to the cerebral cortex 丘脑，背侧丘脑；**optic t.**, lateral geniculate body 视丘脑

thal·as·se·mia (thal″ə-se′me-ə) a heterogeneous group of hereditary hemolytic anemias marked by a decreased rate of synthesis of one or more hemoglobin polypeptide chains, classified according to the chain involved (α, β, δ); the two major categories are α- and β-thalassemia 地中海贫血，一组异质性的遗传性溶血性贫血，其共同特点为都有一种以上血红蛋白多肽链的合成速率减低，按其受累多肽链（α, β, δ）分类；α型和β型是地中海贫血的两大类；**α-t.**, that caused by diminished synthesis of alpha chains of hemoglobin. The *homozygous* form is incompatible with life, the stillborn infant displaying severe hydrops fetalis. The *heterozygous* form may be asymptomatic or marked by mild anemia α-珠蛋白生成障碍性贫

血，α- 地中海贫血，由血红蛋白 α 链合成减慢所致，纯合子难以生存，死婴表现为严重的胎儿水肿，杂合子可能表现为无症状或轻度贫血；β-t., that caused by diminished synthesis of beta chains of hemoglobin. The homozygous form is called *t. major* and the heterozygous form is called *t. minor* β-珠蛋白生成障碍性贫血，β- 地中海贫血，为血红蛋白 β 链合成减慢所致。纯合子称为重型地中海贫血，杂合子称为轻型地中海贫血；**t. ma'jor**, the homozygous form of β -thalassemia, in which hemoglobin A is completely absent; it appears in the newborn period and is marked by hemolytic, hypochromic, microcytic anemia, hepatosplenomegaly, skeletal deformation, mongoloid facies, and cardiac enlargement 重型地中海贫血，为β- 地中海贫血的纯合子，患者血红蛋白 A 完全缺乏，新生儿期即发病者病情严重，表现为溶血性、低色素和小细胞性贫血，肝脾肿大，骨畸形，先天愚型样面容，心脏肥大；**t. mi'nor**, the heterozygous form of β-thalassemia, usually asymptomatic, although there is sometimes mild anemia 轻型地中海贫血，为β- 地中海贫血的杂合子，通常无症状，但有时有轻度贫血；**sickle cell-t.**, a hereditary anemia involving simultaneous heterozygosity for hemoglobin S and thalassemia 镰形细胞 - 地中海贫血，一种同时包括血红蛋白 S 和地中海贫血的杂合体型

tha·lid·o·mide (thə-lid'o-mīd) a sedative and hypnotic, commonly used in Europe in the early 1960s, and discovered to cause serious congenital anomalies in the fetus, notably amelia and phocomelia, when taken during early pregnancy; now used in the treatment of erythema nodosum leprosum 沙 利 度胺，镇静安眠药，六十年代初欧洲常用，后来发现，妇女妊娠早期应用本药可使胎儿发生严重先天性畸形，主要表现为无肢及海豹肢畸形；现用于治疗结节红斑性麻风病

thal·li·um (Tl) (thal'e-əm) a heavy, soft, bluish white, malleable metallic element; at. no. 81, at. wt. 204.38. It is highly toxic, absorbed from the gut and through intact skin, causing a variety of neurologic and psychic symptoms and liver and kidney damage 铊（化学元素）；**t. 201**, a radioactive isotope of thallium having a half-life of 3.05 days and decaying by electron capture with emission of gamma rays (0.135, 0.167 MeV); it is used as a diagnostic aid in the form of thallous chloride Tl 201 ^{201}Tl

thal·lous (thal'əs) of, pertaining to, or containing thallium 亚 铊 的；**t. chloride Tl 201**, the form in which thallium 201 in solution is injected intravenously for imaging of myocardial disease, parathyroid disorder, or neoplastic disease 氯化亚铊（^{201}Tl）静脉注射以用于心肌疾病、甲状旁腺疾病或肿瘤的成像

than·a·to·gno·mon·ic (than"ə-to-no-mon'ik) indicating the approach of death 死征的，濒死的

than·a·to·pho·bia (than"ə-to-fo'be-ə) irrational fear of death 死亡恐惧，对死亡的不合情理的恐惧

than·a·to·pho·ric (than"ə-to-for'ik) deadly; lethal 致死的

THC tetrahydrocannabinol 四氢大麻酚

thea·ism (the'ə-iz-əm) caffeinism resulting from ingestion of excessive quantities of tea 茶中毒

the·baine (the-ba'in) a crystalline, poisonous, and anodyne alkaloid from opium, having properties similar to those of strychnine 蒂巴因，二甲基吗啡，鸦片的一种，具有止痛作用的毒性、晶体性生物碱，性质与士的宁相似

the·ca (the'kə) pl. *the'cae* [L.] a case or sheath 膜，鞘 **the'cal** *adj.*; **t. folli'culi**, an envelope of condensed connective tissue surrounding a vesicular ovarian follicle, comprising an internal vascular layer (*t. interna*) and an external fibrous layer (*t. externa*) 卵泡膜，囊状卵泡周围由致密结缔组织构成的包膜，由内膜和外膜组成

the·co·ma (the-ko'mə) theca cell tumor 卵 泡 膜 细胞瘤

the·co·steg·no·sis (the"ko-stəg-no'sis) contraction of a tendon sheath 腱鞘窄狭

the·lal·gia (the-lal'jə) pain in the nipples 乳头痛

the·lar·che (the-lahr'ke) the beginning of development of the breasts at puberty 乳房初发育

The·la·zia (the-la'zhə) a genus of nematode worms parasitic in the eyes of mammals, including, rarely, humans 吸吮线虫属，一种在哺乳动物眼内寄生的线虫属，罕见寄生于人类

the·le·plas·ty (the'le-plas"te) a plastic operation on the nipple 乳头成形术

the·ler·e·thism (thə-ler'ə-thiz"əm) erection of the nipple 乳头膨起

the·li·tis (the-li'tis) inflammation of a nipple 乳头炎

the·lor·rha·gia (the"lo-ra'jə) hemorrhage from the nipple 乳头出血

the·nar (the'nər) 1. the fleshy part of the hand at the base of the thumb 鱼际，拇指基部的掌侧隆起；2. pertaining to the palm 掌的

the·oph·yl·line (the-of'ə-lin) a xanthine derivative found in tea leaves and prepared synthetically; its salts and derivatives act as smooth muscle relaxants, central nervous system and cardiac muscle stimulants, and bronchodilators; used as a bronchodilator in asthma and in bronchitis, emphysema, or other chronic obstructive pulmonary disease. Its choline salt is oxtriphylline 茶碱

the·o·ry (the'ə-re) (thēr'e) 1. the doctrine or the principles underlying an art as distinguished from

T

the practice of that particular art 理论，学说；2. a formulated hypothesis or, loosely speaking, any hypothesis or opinion not based upon actual knowledge 假想，臆想；**cell t.,** all organic matter consists of cells, and cell activity is the essential process of life 细胞学说，认为一切生物都是细胞构成的，细胞活动就是生命的本质；**clonal deletion t.,** a theory of immunologic self-tolerance according to which "forbidden clones" of immunocytes, those reactive with self antigens, are eliminated on contact with antigen during fetal life 克隆缺失理论，对自体抗原具有免疫耐受的理论，认为与自体抗原反应的免疫细胞因"禁忌克隆"，在胚胎期间与抗原接触而被清除；**clonal selection t.,** there are several million clones of antibody-producing cells in each adult, each programmed to make an antibody of a single specificity and carrying cell-surface receptors for specific antigens; exposure to antigen induces cells with receptors for that antigen to proliferate and produce large quantities of specific antibody 克隆选择学说，认为每个成年者体内都有数百万产生抗体细胞的克隆，每个克隆都被安排产生一种品系（特异性）的抗体；细胞表面则带有能与特定抗原反应的受体；暴露于抗原后，带有该抗原受体的细胞即增殖以产生大量特定抗体；**information t.,** a system for analyzing, chiefly by statistical methods, the characteristics of communicated messages and the systems that encode, transmit, distort, receive, and decode them 信息论，主要通过统计学方法，对交流的信息进行分析的系统，以及对此进行编码、传输、变异、接收和破译的系统；**overflow t.,** one similar to the underfilling theory but that proposes that the primary event in ascites formation is sodium and water retention, with portal hypertension resulting; plasma volume expansion to the point of overflow from the hepatic sinusoids then causes ascites formation 溢流学说，与未充满学说相似的学说，但此说认为，腹水形成时所发生的主要事件是钠和水的滞留，并伴有门静脉高血压产生；血浆量增加至溢出肝窦状隙，然后造成腹水形成；**quantum t.,** radiation and absorption of energy occur in quantities (quanta) that vary in size with the frequency of the radiation 量子理论，能量的辐射和吸收是以明确的数量（量子）发生的，量子在辐射频率上大小不一；**recapitulation t.,** ontogeny recapitulates phylogeny, i.e., an organism in the course of its development goes through the same successive stages (in abbreviated form) as did the species in its evolutionary development 重演论，个体发育是种系发生的重演，即个体在其发育过程中，要经历早年种系经历过的同样连续过程（以简短的形式）；**underfilling t.,** a theory that ascites associated with portal hypertension causes

hypovolemia and so both a lowering of portal pressure and retention of sodium and water. The higher sodium concentration causes increases in the plasma volume and portal pressure, and the subsequent formation of ascites renews the cycle 未充满学说，认为与门静脉高血压有密切联系的腹水会造成（循环）血容量减少，这样既会降低门静脉压，又会导致钠水潴留。较高浓度的钠会增加血浆量和门静脉压，随后形成的腹水就会使这一循环得到恢复；**Young-Helmholtz t.,** color vision depends on three sets of retinal receptors, corresponding to the colors red, green, and violet 扬 - 亥理论，认为色觉是由三套视网膜受体产生的，分别对应红、绿、蓝三色

ther·a·peu·tic (ther″ə-pu′tik) 1. pertaining to therapy 治疗学的；2. tending to overcome disease and promote recovery 治疗的

ther·a·pist (ther′ə-pist) a person skilled in the treatment of disease or other disorder 治疗学家；**physical t.,** a person skilled in the techniques of physical therapy and qualified to administer treatment prescribed by a physician 物理治疗师；**speech t.,** a person specially trained and qualified to assist patients in overcoming speech and language disorders 言语治疗师

ther·a·py (ther′ə-pe) the treatment of disease 治疗，疗法，另见 *treatment* **ablation t.,** the destruction of small areas of myocardial tissue, usually by application of electrical or chemical energy, in the treatment of some tachyarrhythmias 烧蚀疗法，在治疗一些快速心律失常疾病时，常应用电能或化学能对小面积心肌组织进行破坏；**adjuvant t.,** the use of chemotherapy or radiotherapy in addition to surgical resection in the treatment of cancer 辅助疗法，佐药疗法，除手术切除外，在癌症治疗中使用化疗或放疗的方法；**antiplatelet t.,** the use of platelet-modifying agents to inhibit platelet adhesion or aggregation and so prevent thrombosis, alter the course of atherosclerosis, or prolong vascular graft patency 抗血小板治疗，用改变血小板的药物抑制血小板的黏附或凝集，可预防血栓形成，改变动脉粥样硬化的进程或延长脉管移植物开放的时间；**art t.,** the use of art, the creative process, and patient response to the products created for the treatment of psychiatric and psychological conditions and for rehabilitation 艺术疗法，运用艺术、创作过程及患者对作品的反应，创造治疗精神疾病和心理疾病的条件，有利于患者的康复；**aversion t., aversive t.,** that using aversive conditioning to reduce or eliminate undesirable behavior or symptoms; sometimes used synonymously with *aversive conditioning* 厌恶疗法，用劣性刺激减少或消除不良习性或综合征的治疗方法；有时也表述为"厌

恶条件反射" aversive conditioning **behavior t.,** a therapeutic approach that focuses on modifying the patient's observable behavior, rather than on the conflicts and unconscious processes presumed to underlie the behavior 行为疗法，即着重注意病人可观察到的行为；而不是那些被认为是造成不良行为的内心冲突及不自觉的心理过程；**bile acid t.,** administration of bile acids for treatment of hyperlipidemia 胆汁酸疗法，给予胆汁酸以治疗高脂血症；**biologic t.,** treatment of disease by injection of substances that produce a biologic reaction in the organism 生物治疗，通过注射能在体内引起生物学反应的物质进行治疗；**chelation t.,** the use of a chelating agent to remove toxic metals from the body, used in the treatment of heavy metal poisoning. In complementary medicine, also used for the treatment of atherosclerosis and other disorders 络合剂治疗，运用螯合剂清除体内有毒金属，以治疗重金属中毒；在补充疗法中，也用于治疗动脉粥样硬化等疾病；**cognitive t., cognitive-behavioral t.,** that based on the theory that emotional problems result from distorted attitudes and ways of thinking that can be corrected, the therapist guiding the patient to do so 认知疗法，认知行为疗法，是基于歪曲的态度和思维方式导致的感情问题可以被纠正的理论，治疗学家应用行为治疗的方法积极地引导病人；**convulsive t.,** treatment of mental disorders, primarily depression, by induction of convulsions; now it is virtually always by electric shock (*electroconvulsive t.*) 惊厥疗法，以诱发惊厥的方法治疗精神病，现在常用电休克疗法；**couples t.,** 1. 同 marital t.；2. a form of therapy that parallels marital therapy but also includes the treatment of two unmarried adults in a committed relationship 类似于婚姻疗法，但也包括对承诺关系的两个未婚成人的治疗；**dance t.,** the therapeutic use of movement to further the emotional, social, cognitive, and physical integration of the individual in the treatment of a variety of social, emotional, cognitive, and physical disorders 舞蹈疗法，利用运动将个体的情感、社会、认知和身体整合起来的疗法，用于多种社会、情感、认知和身体障碍的治疗中；**electroconvulsive t. (ECT),** a treatment for mental disorders, primarily depression, in which convulsions and loss of consciousness are induced by application of brief pulses of low-voltage alternating current to the brain via scalp electrodes 电休克疗法，一种治疗精神障碍的方法，主要是抑郁症，即通过头皮电极向脑引入低压交流电诱导惊厥和意识丧失；**electroshock t. (EST),** 同 electroconvulsive t.；**endocrine t.,** treatment of disease by the use of hormones 内分泌疗法，通过使用激素达到治疗的目的；**enzyme t.,** in complementary medicine, the oral administration of proteolytic enzymes to improve immune system function; used for a wide variety of disorders and as adjunctive therapy in cancer treatment 酶疗法，在补充医学中，口服蛋白水解酶以改善免疫系统功能；用于多种疾病和癌症的辅助治疗；**estrogen replacement t.,** administration of an estrogen to treat estrogen deficiency, as that following menopause; in women with a uterus, a progestational agent is usually included to prevent endometrial hyperplasia 雌激素替代治疗，补充雌激素以治疗雌激素缺乏，如绝经后(低雌激素)；对于有子宫的妇女，其方案通常也包含孕激素，以防止子宫内膜增生；**family t.,** group therapy of the members of a family, exploring and improving family relationships and processes and thus the mental health of the collective unit and of individual members 家庭疗法，对家庭成员进行团体治疗，探索和改善家庭关系，从而改善集体和个人的心理健康；**fibrinolytic t.,** the use of fibrinolytic agents (e.g., prourokinase) to lyse thrombi in patients with acute peripheral arterial occlusion, deep venous thrombosis, pulmonary embolism, or acute myocardial infarction 溶解纤维蛋白疗法，应用纤维蛋白溶解药物（如尿激酶原）来溶解血栓，用于治疗急性周围动脉闭塞、深部静脉血栓形成、肺栓塞或急性心肌梗死；**gene t.,** manipulation of the genome of an individual to prevent, mask, or lessen the effects of a genetic disorder 基因治疗，通过改造个体的基因组，以预防、掩盖或减轻遗传疾病的影响；**group t.,** psychotherapy carried out regularly with a group of patients under the guidance of a group leader, usually a therapist 团体测验，精神治疗的一种，即在一位组长，通常是治疗师的指导下，集合一组患者进行的治疗；**highly active antiretroviral t. (HAART),** the aggressive use of extremely potent antiretroviral agents in the treatment of human immunodeficiency virus infection 高效抗反转录病毒治疗，积极应用高效的抗逆转录病毒药物治疗人类免疫缺陷病毒感染；**hormonal t., hormone t., endocrine t.** 激素；**hormone replacement t.,** the administration of hormones to correct a deficiency, such as postmenopausal estrogen replacement therapy 激素替代治疗，补充激素以纠正激素缺乏，如绝经后雌激素替代治疗；**immunosuppressive t.,** treatment with agents, such as x-rays, corticosteroids, or cytotoxic chemicals, that suppress the immune response to antigen(s); used in conditions such as organ transplantation, autoimmune disease, allergy, multiple myeloma, and chronic nephritis 免疫抑制治疗，以 X 线、皮质激素和细胞毒性化学药物抑制机体对抗原的免疫反应，用于器官移植、自体免疫病、变态反应、多发性骨髓瘤、慢性肾炎等情况；

inhalation t., respiratory care (2) 吸入疗法; **light t.**, 1. phototherapy (1); 2. 同 photodynamic t.; **marital t., marriage t.**, a type of family therapy aimed at understanding and treating one or both members of a couple in the context of a distressed relationship; it may be used more generally to include unmarried couples in a committed relationship, i.e., *couples t.* 婚姻疗法, 一种家庭疗法, 旨在理解并治疗处于苦恼关系中的夫妻, 并可更广泛用于关系稳定的未婚夫妇中; **massage t.**, the manipulation of the soft tissues of the body for the purpose of normalizing them, thereby enhancing health and healing 按摩疗法; **milieu t.**, treatment, usually in a psychiatric hospital, that emphasizes the provision of an environment and activities appropriate to the patient's emotional and interpersonal needs 环境疗法, 通常在精神病院进行的治疗, 强调为病人提供适合其精神和人际关系的环境及活动以利于恢复; **music t.**, the use of music to effect positive changes in the psychological, physical, cognitive, or social functioning of individuals with health or educational problems 音乐疗法; **occupational t.**, the therapeutic use of self-care, work, and play activities to increase function, enhance development, and prevent disabilities 作业疗法; **oral rehydration t. (ORT)**, oral administration of a solution of electrolytes and carbohydrates in the treatment of dehydration 口服补液疗法; **orthomolecular t.**, treatment of disease based on the theory that restoration of optimal concentrations of substances normally present in the body, such as vitamins, trace elements, and amino acids, will effect a cure 分子矫治疗法, 指治疗疾病恢复的理论依据为, 只要使体内正常存在的物质, 如维生素、微量元素及氨基酸, 恢复最适浓度即可求得治愈; **photodynamic t.**, intravenous administration of a hematoporphyrin derivative, which concentrates selectively in metabolically active tumor tissue, followed by exposure to the tumor tissue to red laser light to produce cytotoxic free radicals that destroy hematoporphyrin-containing tissue 光动力疗法, 静脉注射血卟啉衍生物后, 即选择性集中于代谢活跃的瘤组织, 再使瘤组织接受红激光照射, 以促使细胞毒性游离基团的生成, 破坏含血卟啉组织; **physical t.**, 1. treatment by physical means 以物理方法进行治疗; 2. the health profession concerned with the promotion of health, the prevention of disability, and the evaluation and rehabilitation of patients disabled by pain, disease, or injury, and with treatment by physical therapeutic measures as opposed to medical, surgical, or radiologic measures 物理疗法, 一种卫生专业, 内容为促进健康, 防止病残, 对因疼痛或病伤所致功能丧失情况进行评估并使其康复, 并以

物理疗法而不是药物、手术或放射等方式进行治疗; **poetry t.**, a form of bibliotherapy in which a poem, sometimes one composed by the patient, is used to evoke feelings and responses for discussion in a therapeutic setting 诗歌疗法; **PUVA t.**, a form of photochemotherapy for skin disorders such as psoriasis and vitiligo; oral psoralen administration is followed 2 hours later by exposure to ultraviolet light 补骨脂素加长波紫外线疗法补骨脂素光化学疗法, 口服补骨脂素 2h 后, 紫外线 A 照射皮肤治疗银屑病、白癜风等皮肤病变; **radiation t.**, radiotherapy 放射治疗; **relaxation t.**, any of a number of techniques for inducing the relaxation response, used for the reduction of stress; useful in the management of a wide variety of chronic illnesses caused or exacerbated by stress 放松疗法, 一种诱导松弛反应的技术, 用以减轻压力; 其适于治疗各种由压力引起或加重的慢性疾病; **replacement t.**, 1. treatment to replace deficiencies in body products by administration of natural or synthetic substitutes 补偿疗法, 以天然产物或合成代用品补偿体内某种产物的缺失; 2. treatment that replaces or compensates for a nonfunctioning organ, e.g., hemodialysis 替代疗法, 取代或补偿一个失去功能的器官, 如血液透析; **respiratory t.**, 呼吸疗法, 参见 *care* 下词条; **substitution t.**, the administration of a hormone to compensate for glandular deficiency 替代疗法, 以某一激素代偿该内分泌腺的分泌缺乏; **thrombolytic t.**, fibrinolytic t. 溶栓疗法, 血栓溶解疗法; **thyroid replacement t.**, treatment with a preparation of a thyroid hormone 甲状腺激素替补治疗

therm (thurm) a unit of heat. The word has been used as equivalent to *(a)* large calorie; *(b)* small calorie; *(c)* 1000 large calories; *(d)* 100,000 British thermal units 克卡（热单位旧称）, 曾作为以下表述的等价概念(a)大卡; (b)小卡; (c)1000大卡; (d)10万英国热量单位 (BTU)

ther·mal (thur′məl) pertaining to or characterized by heat 热的, 热量的

ther·mal·ge·sia (thur″məl-je′ze-ə) a dysesthesia in which application of heat causes pain 热性痛觉

ther·mal·gia (thər-mal′jə) causalgia 灼痛

therm·an·al·ge·sia (thurm″an-əl-je′ze-ə) 同 thermoanesthesia

therm·an·es·the·sia (thurm″an-es-the′zhə) 同 thermoanesthesia

therm·es·the·sia (thurm″es-the′zhə) temperature sense 温度觉

therm·es·the·si·om·e·ter (thurm″əs-the″zeo-m′ə-tər) an instrument for measuring sensibility to heat 温度觉测量器

therm·hy·per·es·the·sia (thurm″hi-pər-esthe′zhə)

同 thermohyperesthesia

therm·hy·pes·the·sia (thurm″hi-pes-the′zhə) 同 thermohypesthesia

ther·mic (thur′mik) pertaining to heat 热的

ther·mo·an·es·the·sia (thur″mo-an″es-the′- zhə) inability to recognize sensations of heat and cold; loss or lack of temperature sense 温度觉缺失

ther·mo·cau·tery (thur″mo-kaw′tər-e) cauterization by a heated wire or point 热烙术

ther·mo·chem·is·try (thur″mo-kem′is-tre) the aspect of physical chemistry dealing with heat changes that accompany chemical reactions 热化学

ther·mo·co·ag·u·la·tion (thur″mo-ko-ag″ula′shən) tissue coagulation with high-frequency currents 热凝固术

ther·mo·dif·fu·sion (thur″mo-dĭ-fu′zhən) diffusion due to a temperature gradient 热扩散

ther·mo·dy·nam·ics (thur″mo-di-nam′iks) the branch of science dealing with heat, work, and energy, their interconversion, and problems related thereto 热力学

ther·mo·ex·ci·to·ry (thur″mo-ek-si′tə-re) stimulating production of bodily heat 刺激生热的

ther·mo·gen·e·sis (thur″mo-jen′ə-sis) the production of heat, especially within the animal body 产热; **thermogenet′ic, thermogen′ic** adj.

ther·mo·gram (thur′mo-gram) 1. a graphic record of temperature variations 温度记录图; 2. the visual record obtained by thermography 热象图

ther·mo·graph (thur′mo-graf) 1. an instrument for recording temperature variations 温度记录器; 2. 同 thermogram (2); 3. the apparatus used in thermography 温度描记器

ther·mog·ra·phy (thər-mog′rə-fe) a technique wherein an infrared camera photographically portrays the body's surface temperature, based on self-emanating infrared radiation; sometimes used as a means of diagnosing underlying pathologic conditions, such as breast tumors 热成像术

ther·mo·hy·per·al·ge·sia (thur″mo-hi″pəralje′ze-ə) extreme thermalgesia 热性痛觉过敏

ther·mo·hy·per·es·the·sia (thur″mo-hi″pəresthe′zhə) a dysesthesia with increased sensibility to heat and cold 温度觉过敏

ther·mo·hy·pes·the·sia (thur″mo-hi″pesthe′zhə) a dysesthesia with decreased sensibility to heat and cold 温度觉迟钝

ther·mo·in·hib·i·to·ry (thur″mo-in-hib′ĭ-tor-e) retarding generation of bodily heat 抑制生热的

ther·mo·la·bile (thur″mo-la′bəl) (-la′bīl) easily affected by heat 不耐热的

ther·mol·y·sis (thər-mol′ĭ-sis) 1. chemical dissociation by means of heat 热分解; 2. dissipation of

bodily heat by radiation, evaporation, etc. 散热; **thermolyt′ic** adj.

ther·mo·mas·sage (thur″mo-mə-sahzh′) massage with heat 热按摩法

ther·mom·e·ter (thər-mom′ə-tər) an instrument for determining temperatures, in principle making use of a substance with a physical property that varies with temperature and is susceptible of measurement on some defined scale (see tables accompanying *temperature*) 温度计; **clinical t.**, one used to determine the temperature of the human body 玻璃体温计; **infrared tympanic t.**, a clinical thermometer inserted into the external acoustic meatus to determine the body temperature by measuring the infrared radiation emanating from the tympanic membrane 红外耳式体温计; **oral t.**, a clinical thermometer that is placed under the tongue 口腔温度计; **recording t.**, a temperature-sensitive instrument by which the temperature to which it is exposed is continuously recorded 记录温度计; **rectal t.**, a clinical thermometer that is inserted into the rectum 直肠温度计; **tympanic t.**, 同 infrared

Ther·mo·no·spo·ra·ceae (thur″mo-monos″pə-ra′se-e) a family of aerobic, gram-positive bacteria (suborder Streptosporangineae), that produce a branched substrate mycelium bearing aerial hyphae 高温单孢菌科

ther·mo·phile (thur′mo-fīl) an organism that grows best at elevated temperatures 嗜热生物; **thermo-phil′ic** adj.

ther·mo·phore (thur′mo-for) a device or ap-paratus for retaining heat, used in therapeutic local application 保热器; 温度觉检测器, 一种用于局部治疗的保温装置或设备

ther·mo·plac·en·tog·ra·phy (thur″mo-plas″ əntog′rə-fe) use of thermography for determination of the site of placental attachment 胎盘温度记录法, 以温度记录法测定胎盘附着部位

ther·mo·re·cep·tor (thur″mo-re-sep′tər) a nerve ending sensitive to stimulation by heat 温度感受器

ther·mo·reg·u·la·tion (thur″mo-reg″u-la′- shən) the regulation of heat, as of the body heat of a warm-blooded animal 体温调节; **thermoreg′ula-tory** adj.

ther·mo·sta·bile (thur″mo-sta′bəl) (-sta′bīl) not affected by heat 耐热的

ther·mo·sys·tal·tic (thur″mo-sis-tawl′tik) contracting under the stimulus of heat 温度性收缩的

ther·mo·tax·is (thur″mo-tak′sis) 1. normal adjustment of bodily temperature 体温调节; 2. movement of an organism in response to an increase in temperature 趋温性; **thermotac′tic, thermotax′ic**

ther·mo·ther·a·py (thur″mo-ther′ə-pe) treatment of disease by the application of heat 热 疗 法; **transurethral microwave t. (TUMT),** delivery of microwave energy to the prostate through the urethra, to destroy hyperplastic tissue in the treatment of benign prostatic hyperplasia 经尿道微波热疗, 通过尿道将微波能量输送到前列腺，破坏增生组织，治疗良性前列腺增生

ther·mo·to·nom·e·ter (thur″mo-to-nom′ə- tər) an instrument for measuring the amount of muscular contraction produced by heat 热性肌张力计

ther·mot·ro·pism (thər-mot′ro-piz-əm) tropism in response to an increase in temperature 向 温 性; **thermotrop′ic** adj.

THF tetrahydrofolic acid 四氢叶酸

thi·a·ben·da·zole (thi″ə-ben′də-zōl) a broadspectrum anthelmintic used in the treatment of strongyloidiasis, trichinosis, and cutaneous or visceral larva migrans 噻苯达唑，广谱驱肠虫药，用于蛲虫、线虫、鞭虫、圆虫和钩虫感染以及皮肤幼虫游走病

thi·a·mine (thi′ə-min) vitamin B_1; a watersoluble component of the B-vitamin complex, found particularly in pork, organ meats, legumes, nuts, and whole-grain or enriched breads and cereals. The active form is *thiamine pyrophosphate (TPP),* which serves as a coenzyme in various reactions. Deficiency can result in beriberi and is a factor in alcoholic neuritis and WernickeKorsakoff syndrome. Written also *thiamin* 硫胺素，维 生 素 B_1; **t. pyrophosphate (TPP),** the active form of thiamine, serving as a coenzyme in a variety of reactions, particularly in carbohydrate metabolism 硫胺素焦磷酸

thi·a·zide (thi′ə-zīd) any of a group of diuretics that act by inhibiting the reabsorption of sodium in the proximal renal tubule and stimulating chloride excretion, with resultant increase in excretion of water 噻嗪化物，噻嗪类（利尿药）

thick·ness (thik′nis) a measurement across the smallest dimension of an object 厚，厚度; **triceps skinfold (TSF) t.,** a measurement of subcutaneous fat taken by measuring a fold of skin running parallel to the length of the arm over the triceps muscle midway between the acromion and olecranon 三 头 肌皮褶度

thi·emia (thi-e′me-ə) sulfur in the blood 硫血症

thi·eth·yl·per·a·zine (thi-eth″əl-par′ə-zēn) an antiemetic, used as the malate or maleate salt in the treatment and prophylaxis of nausea and vomiting 硫乙哌丙嗪，止吐药，其苹果酸或马来酸盐用于治疗和预防恶心和呕吐

thigh (thi) the portion of the lower extremity ex-tending from the hip above to the knee below; 股，大腿，另参见 *femur*

thig·mes·the·sia (thig″mes-the′zhə) 同 touch (1)

thig·mo·tax·is (thig″mo-tak′sis) taxis of an organism in response to contact or touch 趋触性，对触摸刺激作出的反应; **thigmotac′tic** adj.

thig·mot·ro·pism (thig-mot′ro-piz-əm) tropism of an organism elicited by touch or by contact with a solid or rigid surface 向触性，机体对坚硬表面触摸或接触的趋向反应; **thigmotrop′ic** adj.

thi·mero·sal (thi-mer′o-səl) an organomercurial antiseptic that is antifungal and bacteriostatic for many nonsporulating bacteria, used as a topical antiinfective and as a pharmaceutical preservative 硫柳汞，硫汞柳酸钠，邻乙汞硫基苯酸钠，有机汞防腐剂，有效抗霉菌，对很多无芽胞细菌亦有抑制作用，局部抗感染，并可用作制剂的保存药

think·ing (thingk′ing) ideational mental activity (as opposed to emotional activity) 思 维; **autistic t.,** preoccupation with inner thoughts, daydreams, fantasies, private logic; egocentric, subjective thinking lacking objectivity and connection with external reality 我向思维，不顾外部现实世界因素，由内心愿望或欲求所控制的思维活动; **dereistic t.,** thinking not in accordance with the facts of reality and experience and following illogical, idiosyncratic reasoning 空 想; **magical t.,** that characterized by the belief that thinking or wishing something can cause it to occur 奇幻思维，特征为相信思考或希望某事就会使其发生

thio·bar·bi·tu·ric ac·id (thi″o-bahr″bĭ-tu′rik) a condensation of malonic acid and thiourea, closely related to barbituric acid. It is the parent compound of a class of drugs, the thiobarbiturates, which are analogous in their effects to barbiturates 硫 巴 比 妥酸

thio·cy·a·nate (thi″o-si′ə-nāt) a salt analogous in composition to a cyanate, but containing sulfur instead of oxygen 硫氰酸根，硫氰酸盐; 硫氰酸酯

thio·es·ter (thi″o-es′tər) a carboxylic acid and a thiol group in ester linkage, e.g., acetyl coenzyme A 硫醚

thio·gua·nine (thi″o-gwah′nēn) an antineoplastic derived from mercaptopurine; used in the treatment of acute myelogenous leukemia 硫鸟嘌呤，由巯基嘌呤衍生的抗肿瘤药，用于急性髓性白血病的治疗

thio·ki·nase (thi″o-ki′nās) any of the ligases that catalyze the formation of a thioester in a reaction coupled to cleavage of a high-energy phosphate bond 硫激酶

thi·ol (thi′ol) 1. sulfhydryl. 巯基，硫氢基; 2. any organic compound containing the −SH group 巯 基

化合物

thi·o·nine (thi′o-nēn) a dark-green powder, purple in solution, used as a metachromatic stain in microscopy 硫堇，暗绿色粉末，溶液呈紫色，用作镜检异色染色剂

thio·pen·tal (thi″o-pen′təl) an ultrashort-acting barbiturate; the sodium salt is used intravenously to induce general anesthesia, as an adjunct to general or local anesthesia, and as an anticonvulsant 硫喷妥，超短效巴比妥盐；其钠盐静脉注射可诱导全身麻醉，作为全麻或局麻的辅助用药，以及作为抗惊厥药

thi·o·rid·a·zine (thi″o-rid′ə-zēn) a tranquilizer with antipsychotic and sedative effects, used as the base or hydrochloride salt 硫利达嗪，甲硫哒嗪，有抗精神病和镇静作用，用其碱或盐酸盐

thio·sul·fate (thi″o-sul′fāt) the $S_2O_3^{2-}$ anion, or a salt containing this ion; produced in cysteine metabolism 硫代硫酸离子，硫代硫酸盐，半胱氨酸代谢产物

thio·tepa (thi″o-tep′ə) a cytotoxic alkylating agent, used as an antineoplastic in the treatment of breast, ovarian, or bladder cancer, Hodgkin disease, and malignant pleural or pericardial effusion 噻替哌，一种细胞毒性烷化药，抗肿瘤药，现用于乳腺癌、卵巢癌、膀胱癌、霍奇金病、恶性胸腔积液或心包积液的治疗

thio·thix·ene (thi″o-thik′sēn) a thioxanthene derivative, used as the base or the hydrochloride salt for the treatment of psychotic disorders 氨砜噻吨，甲哌硫丙硫蒽，噻吨衍生物，其碱或盐酸盐用于治疗精神疾病

Thio·tri·cha·les (thi″o-trī-ka′lēz) a diverse order of bacteria of the class Gammaproteobacteria; some members are obligate parasites of animals 硫发菌目

thio·xan·thene (thi″o-zan′thēn) 噻吨，硫蒽；1. a threering compound structurally related to phenothiazine 一种结构上与吩噻嗪有关的三环化合物；2. any of a class of structurally related antipsychotic agents, e.g., thiothixene 任何一类结构上有关的抗精神病药，如氨砜噻吨

thirst (thurst) a sensation, often referred to the mouth and throat, associated with a craving for drink; ordinarily interpreted as a desire for water 渴感

this·tle (this′əl) any of a number of weedy plants of the family Compositae, having spiny leaves and flower heads surrounded by spiny bracts 蓟；蓟属植物；**blessed t.**, the thistlelike herb *Cnicus benedictus*, or its dried flowers, leaves, and upper stems; used for dyspepsia and loss of appetite; used also in folk medicine for fever and colds and as a diuretic 圣蓟，蓟状草本植物藏掖花，或指其干燥的花、

叶和上茎；用于消化不良及食欲不振的治疗；在民间医药中用于治疗发热和感冒，并作为利尿药；**milk t.**, the thistle, *Silybum marianum*, or its dried ripe fruit; used for loss of appetite and for supportive treatment in gallbladder and liver disorders 奶蓟，蓟、水飞蓟或其干燥或热的果实；用于食欲不振及肝胆疾病的支持治疗

thix·ot·ro·pism (thik-sot′ro-piz-əm) 同 thixotropy

thix·ot·ro·py (thik-sot′rə-pe) the property of certain gels of becoming fluid when shaken and then becoming semisolid again 触变性，摇溶性，某些凝胶在震荡时变成液，后又变成半固体的特性；**thixotrop′ic** *adj.*

tho·ra·cal·gia (thor″ə-kal′jə) thoracodynia; pain in the chest 胸痛

tho·ra·cec·to·my (thor″ə-sek′tə-me) thoracotomy with resection of part of a rib 胸廓部分切除术

tho·ra·cen·te·sis (thor″ə-sen-te′sis) pleurocentesis; surgical puncture of the chest wall into the parietal cavity for aspiration of fluids 胸腔穿刺术

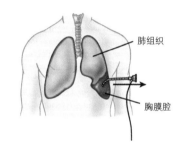

肺组织

胸膜腔

▲ 胸腔穿刺

tho·ra·ces (tho′rə-sēz) [Gr.] thorax 的复数

tho·rac·ic (thə-ras′ik) pectoral; pertaining to the thorax (chest) 胸的，胸廓的

tho·ra·co·acro·mi·al (thor″ə-ko-ə-kro′me-əl) pertaining to the chest and acromion 胸肩峰的

tho·ra·co·cyr·to·sis (thor″ə-ko-sir-to′sis) abnormal curvature of the thorax or unusual prominence of the chest 胸变曲，胸部异常弯曲或隆起

tho·ra·co·dyn·ia (thor″ə-ko-din′e-ə) 同 thoracalgia

tho·ra·co·gas·tros·chi·sis (thor″ə-ko-gastros′kī-sis) congenital fissure of the thorax and abdomen 胸腹裂畸形

tho·ra·co·lum·bar (thor″ə-ko-lum′bər) pertaining to thoracic and lumbar vertebrae 胸腰的，脊柱胸腰段的

tho·ra·col·y·sis (thor″ə-kol′ĭ-sis) the freeing of adhesions of the chest wall 胸壁粘连松解术

tho·ra·com·e·ter (tho″rə-kom′ə-tər) stethometer 胸围计，胸廓张度计

tho·ra·cop·a·gus (thor″ə-kop′ə-gəs) conjoined twins united in or near the sternal region 胸部联胎，两个接近完整的个体在胸骨区或其附近相连的双联畸胎

tho·ra·cop·a·thy (thor″ə-kop′ə-the) any disease of the thoracic organs or tissues 胸部疾病

tho·ra·cos·chi·sis (thor″ə-kos′kī-sis) congenital fissure of the thorax 胸裂畸形

tho·raco·scope (thə-rak′o-skōp) an endoscope for examining the pleural cavity through an intercostal space 胸腔镜

tho·ra·co·ste·no·sis (thor″ə-ko-stə-no′sis) abnormal contraction of the thorax 胸廓狭窄

tho·ra·cos·to·my (thor″ə-kos′tə-me) 1. incision of the chest wall, with maintenance of the opening for drainage 胸膜腔造口术；2. the incision so created 胸膜腔造口

tho·ra·cot·o·my (thor″ə-kot′ə-me) pleurotomy; incision of the chest wall 开胸术

tho·rax (thor′aks) pl. *tho′races* [Gr.] chest; the part of the body between the neck and respiratory diaphragm, encased by the ribs 胸，胸廓；**Peyrot t.,** an obliquely oval thorax associated with massive pleural effusions 佩罗胸，胸呈斜卵圆形，见于大量胸膜渗出时

tho·ri·um (Th) (thor′e-əm) a heavy, gray, naturally radioactive, rare earth element; at. no. 90, at. wt. 232.038. Its most stable isotope, 232Th, has a half-life of 1.4×10^{10} years and is the parent element of a radioactive disintegration series 钍（化学元素）

thought broad·cast·ing (thawt brawd′kasting) the feeling that one's thoughts are being broadcast to the environment 思维散播，认为自己的思想正被广播于众

thought in·ser·tion (thawt in-sur′shən) the delusion that thoughts that are not one's own are being inserted into one's mind 思维插入，认为思想不是自己的，而是被强行插入个人意念中的一种妄想

thought with·draw·al (thawt with-draw′əl) the delusion that someone or something is removing thoughts from one's mind 思维被夺，认为某人或某物正从自己脑中把思想抽走的一种妄想

Thr threonine 苏氨酸

thread·worm (thred′wərm) any long slender nematode, especially *Enterobius vermicularis* 线虫，尤指蛲虫

thready (thred′e) weak, thin; shallow 纤细的；微弱的

thre·o·nine (Thr, T) (thre′o-nēn) a naturally occurring amino acid essential for human metabolism 苏氨酸

thresh·old (thresh′ōld) the level that must be reached for an effect to be produced, as the degree of intensity of a stimulus that just produces a sensation, or the concentration that must be present in the blood before certain substances are excreted by the kidney (*renal t.*) 阈

thrill (thril) a vibration felt by the examiner on palpation 震颤；**diastolic t.,** one felt over the precordium during ventricular diastole in advanced aortic insufficiency 舒张期震颤；**hydatid t.,** one sometimes felt on percussing over a hydatid cyst 包虫囊震颤，棘球蚴囊肿震颤；**apresystolic t.,** one felt just before the systole over the apex of the heart 收缩期前震颤；**systolic t.,** one felt over the precordium during systole in aortic stenosis, pulmonary stenosis, and ventricular septal defect 收缩期震颤

throat (thrōt) 1. pharynx 咽；2. fauces 喉头，咽喉；3. anterior aspect of the neck 颈前部；**sore t.,** 1. faucitis 咽门炎，咽峡炎；2. pharyngitis 咽炎；**streptococcal sore t.,** septic sore throat; severe sore throat occurring in epidemics, usually caused by *Streptococcus pyogenes,* with local hyperemia and sometimes a gray exudate and enlargement of cervical lymph nodes 链球菌性扁桃体炎，化脓性咽喉炎

throm·bas·the·nia (throm″bəs-the′ne-ə) a platelet abnormality characterized by defective clot retraction and impaired ADP-induced platelet aggregation; clinically manifested by epistaxis, inappropriate bruising, and excessive posttraumatic bleeding 血小板功能不全；**Glanzmann t.,** thrombasthenia 格兰兹曼（氏）血小板功能不全，参见 thrombasthenia

throm·bec·to·my (throm-bek′tə-me) surgical removal of a clot from a blood vessel 血栓切除术

throm·bi (throm′bi) *thrombus* 的复数

throm·bin (throm′bin) 1. the activated form of coagulation factor II (prothrombin); it catalyzes the conversion of fibrinogen to fibrin 凝血酶，凝血因子 II（凝血酶原）的活化形式；2. a preparation derived from prothrombin of bovine origin together with thromboplastin and calcium; used therapeutically as a local hemostatic 外用凝血酶，由牛凝血酶原制取，加凝血激酶及钙离子制备的药剂，用于局部止血

throm·bo·an·gi·itis (throm″bo-an″je-i′tis) inflammation of a blood vessel, with thrombosis 血栓性脉管炎；**t. obli′terans,** Buerger disease; an inflammatory and obliterative disease of the blood vessels of the limbs, primarily the legs, leading to ischemia and gangrene 血栓闭塞性脉管炎

throm·bo·ar·ter·i·tis (throm″bo-ahr″tər-i′tis) thrombosis associated with arteritis 血栓性动脉炎

throm·boc·la·sis (throm-bok′lə-sis) the dissolution of a thrombus 血栓碎裂，血栓溶解；**thrombo-clas′tic** adj.

throm·bo·cyst (throm′bo-sist) a chronic sac formed around a thrombus in a hematoma 血栓囊

throm·bo·cys·tis (throm″bo-sis′tis) 同 thrombocyst

throm·bo·cy·ta·phe·re·sis (throm″bo-si″tə- fə-re′-sis) the selective separation and removal of platelets from withdrawn blood, the remainder of the blood then being retransfused into the donor 血小板提取法

throm·bo·cyte (throm′bo-sīt) platelet 血小板

throm·bo·cy·the·mia (throm″bo-si-the′me-ə) 同 thrombocytosis；**essential t., hemorrhagic t.,** a syndrome of repeated spontaneous hemorrhages, either external or into the tissues, and greatly increased numbers of circulating platelets.a syndrome of repeated spontaneous hemorrhages, either external or into the tissues, and greatly increased numbers of circulating platelets 原发性血小板增多症

throm·bo·cyt·ic (throm″bo-sit′ik) 1. pertaining to, characterized by, or of the nature of a platelet (thrombocyte) 血小板的；2. pertaining to the thrombocytic series 血小板系的

throm·bo·cy·tol·y·sis (throm″bo-si-tol′ĭ-sis) destruction of platelets 血小板溶解

throm·bo·cy·top·a·thy (throm″bo-si-top′ə- the) any qualitative disorder of platelets 血小板病

throm·bo·cy·to·pe·nia (throm″bo-si″to-pe′- ne-ə) decrease in number of platelets in circulating blood 血小板减少；**thrombocytope′nic** *adj.*；**heparin-induced t.,** a complication of heparin therapy in certain persons, characterized by intravascular clots composed of platelet aggregates 肝素诱发的血小板减少症，某些患者在接受肝素治疗时发生的一种并发症，其特征是血小板聚集形成血管内血块；**immune t.,** that associated with the presence of antiplatelet antibodies (IgG) 免疫性血小板减少症，与存在抗血小板抗体（IgG）有关

throm·bo·cy·to·poi·e·sis (throm″bo-si″topoi-e′sis) the production of platelets 血小板生成；**thrombo-cytopoiet′ic** *adj.*

throm·bo·cy·to·sis (throm″bo-si-to′sis) thrombocythemia; an increase in the number of circulating platelets 血小板增多

throm·bo·em·bo·lism (throm″bo-em′bo-liz- əm) obstruction of a blood vessel with thrombotic material carried by the blood from the site of origin to plug another vessel 血栓栓塞

throm·bo·end·ar·ter·ec·to·my (throm″boend″ahr-tər-ek′tə-me) excision of an obstructing thrombus together with a portion of the inner lining of the obstructed artery 血栓动脉内膜切除术

throm·bo·end·ar·ter·i·tis (throm″bo-endahr′tər-i′-tis) inflammation of the innermost coat of an artery, with thrombus formation 血栓性动脉内膜炎，血

栓性动脉炎

throm·bo·en·do·car·di·tis (throm″bo-en″do-kahr-di′tis) a term formerly used for nonbacterial thrombotic endocarditis or sometimes incorrectly for nonbacterial verrucous endocarditis 血栓性心内膜炎，该定义先前用于描述非细菌性血栓性心内膜炎，或有时错误地用于非细菌性疣状心内膜炎

throm·bo·gen·e·sis (throm″bo-jen′ə-sis) clot formation 血栓形成；**thrombogen′ic** *adj.*

β-throm·bo·glob·u·lin (throm″bo-glob′u-lin) a platelet-specific protein released with platelet factor 4 on platelet activation; it mediates several reactions of the inflammatory response, binds and inactivates heparin, and blocks endothelial cell release of prostacyclin β-血小板球蛋白，在血小板活化中伴随血小板因子Ⅵ而释放的一种血小板特异蛋白；在炎症反应中它调节其中的几个反应步骤，及灭活肝素并阻止内皮细胞释放前列环素

throm·boid (throm′boid) resembling a thrombus 血栓样的

throm·bo·ki·nase (throm″bo-ki′nās) activated factor X 促凝血酶原激酶，参见 *factor* 下 *coagulation factors*

throm·bo·ki·net·ics (throm″bo-kĭ-net′iks) the dynamics of blood coagulation 血凝动力学

throm·bol·y·sis (throm-bol′ĭ-sis) dissolution of a thrombus 血栓溶解

throm·bo·lyt·ic (throm″bo-lit′ik) dissolving or splitting up a thrombus, or an agent that so acts 血栓溶解的；血栓溶解剂

throm·bo·phil·ia (throm″bo-fil′e-ə) a tendency to the occurrence of thrombosis 血栓形成倾向

throm·bo·phle·bi·tis (throm″bo-flə-bi′tis) inflammation of a vein (phlebitis) associated with thrombus formation (thrombosis) 血栓性静脉炎；**t. mi′grans,** a recurring thrombophlebitis involving different vessels simultaneously or at intervals 游走性血栓性静脉炎 一种复发性静脉炎，可同时在多处发生，亦可间断先后发生；**postpartum iliofemoral t.,** thrombophlebitis of the iliofemoral vein following childbirth 产后髂股血栓性静脉炎

throm·bo·plas·tic (throm″bo-plas′tik) causing or accelerating clot formation in the blood 血栓形成的，促血凝的

throm·bo·plas·tin (throm″bo-plas′tin) coagulation factor Ⅲ 促凝血酶原激酶；**tissue t.,** coagulation factor Ⅲ 组织凝血激酶

throm·bo·poi·e·sis (throm″bo-poi-e′sis) 1. 同 thrombogenesis；2. 同 thrombocytopoiesis；**thrombopoiet′ic** *adj.* 血栓形成的

throm·bo·re·sis·tance (throm″bo-re-zis′təns) resistance by a blood vessel to thrombus formation 抗血栓，抗血栓性

throm·bosed (throm′bōzd) affected with thrombosis 形成血栓的

throm·bo·sis (throm-bo′sis) the formation or presence of a thrombus 血栓形成; **thrombot′ic** adj.; **cerebral t.**, thrombosis of a cerebral vessel, which may result in cerebral infarction 脑血栓形成, 脑血管内血栓形成, 可致脑梗死; **coronary t.**, thrombosis of a coronary artery, usually associated with atherosclerosis and often causing sudden death or myocardial infarction 冠状动脉血栓形成, 冠状动脉中形成的阻塞性血栓, 常致猝死或心肌梗死; **deep vein t.**, **deep venous t.**, thrombosis of one or more deep veins, usually of the lower limb, with swelling, warmth, and erythema, frequently a precursor of pulmonary embolism 深静脉血栓形成, 一条或多条深静脉血栓形成, 通常位于下肢, 伴肿胀、发热和红斑, 通常是肺栓塞的先兆

throm·bo·spon·din (throm″bo-spon′din) a glycoprotein that interacts with a wide variety of molecules, including heparin, fibrin, fibrinogen, platelet cell membrane receptors, collagen, and fibronectin, and plays a role in platelet aggregation, tumor metastasis, adhesion of *Plasmodium falciparum,* vascular smooth muscle growth, and tissue repair in skeletal muscle following crush injury 血小板应答蛋白, 一种与各种各样的分子相互作用的糖蛋白, 包括肝素、纤维蛋白、纤维蛋白原、血小板细胞膜受体、胶原蛋白及纤连蛋白, 在血小板聚集、肿瘤转移、恶性疟原虫附着、血管平滑肌生长和挤压伤后骨骼肌组织修复中起作用

throm·bos·ta·sis (throm-bos′tə-sis) stasis of blood in a part with formation of a thrombus 血栓性瘀血

throm·bot·ic (throm-bot′ik) pertaining to or affected with thrombosis 血栓形成的

throm·box·ane (throm-bok′sān) either of two compounds, one designated A_2 and the other B_2. Thromboxane A_2 is synthesized by platelets and is an inducer of platelet aggregation and platelet release functions and is a vasoconstrictor; it is very unstable and is hydrolyzed to thromboxane B_2 血栓烷, 包括血栓烷 A_2 和血栓烷 B_2, 前者由血小板合成, 是血小板凝聚和促使血小板释出的诱导剂, 并有血管收缩作用; 其性质极不稳定, 水解为 B_2 而灭活

throm·bus (throm′bəs) pl. *throm′bi*. A stationary blood clot along the wall of a blood vessel, frequently causing vascular obstruction. Some authorities differentiate thrombus formation from simple coagulation or clot formation 血栓; **mural t.**, one attached to the wall of the endocardium in a diseased area or to the aortic wall overlying an intimal lesion 附壁血栓; **occluding t.**, **occlusive t.**, one that occupies the entire lumen of a vessel and obstructs

blood flow 闭塞性血栓; **parietal t.**, one attached to a vessel or heart wall 附壁血栓

thrush (thrush) candidiasis of the oral mucous membranes, usually seen in sick, weak infants or in persons who are debilitated or immunocompromised, characterized by creamy white plaques resembling milk curds, which if stripped away leave raw bleeding surfaces 鹅口疮

thryp·sis (thrip′sis) comminuted fracture 粉碎性骨折

thu·ja (thu′jə) the fresh tops of *Thuja occidentalis* (arbor vitae); used in some topical dermatologic preparations and also in homeopathy 金钟柏, 侧柏

thu·li·um (Tm) (thoo′le-əm) a lustrous, silvery gray, rare earth element; at. no. 69, at. wt. 168.934 铥 (化学元素)

thumb (thum) the radial or first digit of the hand 拇指; **tennis t.**, tendinitis of the tendon of the long flexor muscle of the thumb, with calcification 网球员拇病, 因打网球时反复磨损所致拇长屈肌的肌腱发炎并钙化

thumb·print·ing (thum′print″ing) a radiographic sign appearing as smooth indentations on the barium-filled colon, as though made by depression with the thumb 指压征, 结肠充钡时出现的匀称的压迹, 像是拇指压成

thump·ver·sion (thump-vur′zhən) delivery of one or two blows to the chest in initiating cardiopulmonary resuscitation, in order to initiate a pulse or to convert ventricular fibrillation to a normal rhythm 拳击复律, 开始心脏复苏术时, 给胸部一至二次叩击, 以此激发心脏搏动或将心室纤颤转变为正常心律

THV transcatheter heart valve 经导管心瓣膜

thyme (t ī m) 1. any plant of the genus *Thymus* 百里香、麝香草; 2. a preparation of the leaves and flowers of garden thyme (*T. vulgaris*), used as an antitussive and expectorant 百里香制剂, 用作镇咳和祛痰剂

thy·mec·to·my (thi-mek′tə-me) excision of the thymus 胸腺切除术

thy·mic (thi′mik) pertaining to the thymus 胸腺的

thy·mi·co·lym·phat·ic (thi″mĭ-ko-lim-fat′ik) pertaining to the thymus and lymphatic nodes 胸腺淋巴结的

thy·mi·dine (T) (thi′mĭ-dēn) thymine linked to ribose, a rarely occurring base in rRNA and tRNA; frequently used incorrectly to denote deoxythymidine 胸苷, 胸腺嘧啶与核糖结合, 偶尔作为碱基出现于核糖体 RNA (rRNA) 和转移 RNA (tRNA) 中; 常被错误地表达为脱氧胸苷

thy·mine (T) (thi′mēn) a pyrimidine base, in animal cells usually occurring condensed with deoxyribose

T

to form deoxythymidine, a component of DNA. The corresponding compound with ribose, thymidine, is a rare constituent of RNA 胸腺嘧啶，一种嘧啶碱基，在动物细胞中通常与脱氧核糖发生聚合形成脱氧胸苷，后者为 DNA 的成分。与核糖相对应的化合物——胸苷，是一种稀有的 RNA 成分

thy·mi·tis (thi-mi′tis) inflammation of the thymus 胸腺炎

thy·mo·cyte (thi′mo-sīt) a lymphocyte arising in the thymus 胸腺细胞

thy·mo·lep·tic (thi″mo-lep′tik) any drug that favorably modifies mood in serious affective disorders such as depression or mania; categories include tricyclic antidepressants, monoamine oxidase inhibitors, and lithium compounds 抗抑郁药

thy·mo·ma (thi-mo′mə) a tumor derived from the epithelial or lymphoid elements of the thymus 胸腺瘤

thy·mop·a·thy (thi-mop′ə-the) any disease of the thymus 胸腺病；**thymopath′ic** adj.

thy·mo·poi·e·tin (thi″mo-poi′ĕ-tin) a polypeptide hormone secreted by thymic epithelial cells that induces differentiation of precursor lymphocytes into thymocytes 胸腺生成素，由胸腺上皮细胞分泌，可诱导淋巴细胞前体分化为胸腺细胞的多肽激素

thy·mop·ri·vous (thi-mop′rĭ-vəs) pertaining to or resulting from removal or atrophy of the thymus 胸腺缺乏的

thy·mo·sin (thi′mo-sin) a humoral factor secreted by the thymus, which promotes the maturation of T lymphocytes 胸腺素，胸腺分泌的一种体液因子，能促使 T 淋巴细胞成熟

thy·mus (thi′məs) a bilaterally symmetric lymphoid organ consisting of two pyramidal lobules situated in the anterior superior mediastinum, each lobule consisting of an outer cortex, rich in lymphocytes (thymocytes), and an inner medulla, rich in epithelial cells. The thymus is the site of production of T lymphocytes: precursor cells migrate to the outer cortex, where they proliferate. They then move through the inner cortex, where T-cell surface markers are acquired, and they finally move into the medulla, where they become mature T cells. Maturation is controlled by hormones produced by the thymus, including thymopoietin and thymosin. The thymus reaches maximal development at about puberty and then undergoes gradual involution 胸腺

thy·ro·ad·e·ni·tis (thi″ro-ad″ə-ni′tis) 同 thyroiditis

thy·ro·apla·sia (thi″ro-ə-pla′zhə) defective development of the thyroid gland with hypothyroidism 甲状腺发育不全

thy·ro·ar·y·te·noid (thi″ro-ar″ĭ-te′noid) pertaining to the thyroid and arytenoid cartilages 甲杓软骨的

thy·ro·car·di·ac (thi″ro-kahr′de-ak) pertaining to the thyroid gland and heart 甲状腺与心脏的

thy·ro·chon·drot·o·my (thi″ro-kon-drot′ə-me) median laryngotomy 甲状软骨切开术

thy·ro·cri·cot·o·my (thi″ro-kri-kot′ə-me) incision of the cricothyroid membrane 环甲膜切开术

thy·ro·epi·glot·tic (thi″ro-ep″ĭ-glot′ik) pertaining to the thyroid gland and epiglottis 甲状会厌的

thy·ro·gen·ic (thi″ro-jen′ik) 同 thyrogenous

thy·rog·e·nous (thi-roj′ə-nəs) originating in the thyroid gland 甲状腺源的，甲状腺性的

thy·ro·glob·u·lin (thi-ro-glob′u-lin) an iodine-containing glycoprotein of high molecular weight, occurring in the colloid of the follicles of the thyroid gland; the iodinated tyrosine moieties of thyroglobulin form the active hormones thyroxine and triiodothyronine 甲状腺球蛋白

thy·ro·glos·sal (thi″ro-glos′əl) pertaining to the thyroid gland and tongue 甲状舌管的

thy·ro·hy·al (thi″ro-hi′əl) pertaining to the thyroid cartilage and the hyoid bone 甲状舌骨的，甲状软骨和舌骨的

thy·ro·hy·oid (thi″ro-hi′oid) pertaining to the thyroid gland or cartilage and the hyoid bone 甲状舌骨的，甲状腺或甲状软骨和舌骨的

thy·roid (thi′roid) 1. the thyroid gland 甲状腺，参见 gland 下词条；2. pertaining to the thyroid gland 甲状腺的；3. scutiform 甲状的；4. a preparation of thyroid gland from domesticated food animals, containing levothyroxine and liothyronine and used as replacement therapy in the diagnosis and treatment of hypothyroidism and the prophylaxis and treatment of goiter and thyroid carcinoma 甲状腺制剂，甲状腺粉，从家养食用动物中提取的一种甲状腺制剂，含有左甲状腺素和三碘甲状原氨酸，用于甲状腺功能减退的诊断性和治疗性替代治疗及甲状腺肿和甲状腺癌的预防和治疗

thy·roid·ec·to·mize (thi″roid-ek′tə-mīz) to excise the thyroid gland 切除甲状腺

thy·roid·ec·to·my (thi″roid-ek′tə-me) excision of the thyroid gland, or suppression of its function 甲状腺切除术

thy·roid·itis (thi″roid-i′tis) inflammation of the thyroid gland 甲状腺炎；**atrophic t.**, a type of autoimmune thyroiditis with atrophy of the follicles and without goiter 萎缩性甲状腺炎，自身免疫性甲状腺炎的一种，伴滤泡萎缩且无甲状腺肿；**autoimmune t.**, any of various types characterized by autoantibodies against the thyroid, resulting in hypothyroidism; the two major types are Hashimoto disease and atrophic thyroiditis; Riedel thyroiditis is a less common type 自身免疫性甲状腺炎，机体

免疫功能异常，导致甲状腺功能减退；主要的两种类型为桥本甲状腺炎和萎缩性甲状腺炎，木样甲状腺炎较为罕见；**Hashimoto t.,** 桥本甲状腺炎，参见 *disease* 下词条；**Riedel t.,** a chronic type of autoimmune thyroiditis with a proliferating, fibrosing, inflammatory process involving usually one but sometimes both lobes of the thyroid gland, as well as the trachea and other adjacent structures 木样甲状腺炎，一种慢性增生性纤维化炎症性疾病，通常累及甲状腺其中一叶，有时为两叶，且波及邻近的气管及其腺体结构

thy·roid·ot·o·my (thi″roid-ot′ə-me) median laryngotomy 甲状软骨切开术，喉正中切开术

thy·ro·lin·gual (thi″ro-ling′gwəl) 同 thyroglossal

thy·ro·meg·a·ly (thi″ro-meg′ə-le) goiter 甲状腺肿大

thy·ro·mi·met·ic (thi″ro-mi-met′ik) producing effects similar to those of thyroid hormones or the thyroid gland 拟甲状腺素的，拟甲状腺的

thy·ro·para·thy·roid·ec·to·my (thi″ro-par″ə-thi″roi-dek′tə-me) excision of the thyroid and parathyroids 甲状腺甲状旁腺切除术

thy·rop·to·sis (thi″rop-to′sis) downward displacement of the thyroid gland into the thorax 甲状腺下移，低位甲状腺

thy·ro·ther·a·py (thi″ro-ther′ə-pe) thyroid replacement therapy 甲状腺制剂疗法

thy·rot·o·my (thi-rot′o-me) 1. median laryngotomy 甲状软骨切开术；2. the operation of cutting the thyroid gland 甲状腺切开术；3. biopsy of the thyroid gland 甲状腺活体组织检查

thy·ro·tox·ic (thi″ro-tok″sik) 1. pertaining to the effects of thyroid hormone excess 甲状腺毒性的，与甲状腺激素过多作用有关的；2. describing a patient suffering from thyrotoxicosis 描述甲状腺毒症患者的

thy·ro·tox·i·co·sis (thi″ro-tok″sĭ-ko′sis) a morbid condition due to overactivity of the thyroid gland, such as Graves disease 甲状腺毒症

thy·ro·trope (thi′ro-trōp) 同 thyrotroph

thy·ro·troph (thi′ro-trōf) a type of basophil found in the anterior lobe of the pituitary that secretes thyrotropin 促甲状腺细胞

thy·ro·tro·phic (thi″ro-tro′fik) 同 thyrotropic

thy·ro·troph·in (thi-rot′rə-fin) 同 thyrotropin

thy·ro·tro·pic (thi″ro-tro′pik) 1. pertaining to or marked by thyrotropism 关于或明显以甲状腺功能亢进为特征的；2. having an influence on the thyroid gland 促甲状腺的，对甲状腺有影响的

thy·rot·ro·pin (thi-rot′rə-pin) thyroid-stimulating hormone; a hormone of the anterior pituitary gland having an affinity for and specifically stimulating the thyroid gland 促甲状腺激素；**t. alfa,** a recombinant form of thyrotropin used as a diagnostic adjunct in serum thyroglobulin testing in followup of patients with thyroid cancer 促甲状腺素 α，一种重组促甲状腺素，用作甲状腺癌随访时检测患者血清甲状腺球蛋白的诊断辅助用药

thy·rox·ine (T₄) (thi-rok′sin) an iodine-containing hormone secreted by the thyroid gland, occurring naturally as l-thyroxine; its chief function is to increase the rate of cell metabolism. It is deiodinated in peripheral tissues to form triiodothyronine, which has greater biologic activity. A preparation of thyroxine, levothyroxine, is used pharmaceutically 甲状腺素

Ti titanium 元素钛的符号

TIA transient ischemic attack 短暂性脑缺血发作

ti·ag·a·bine (ti-ag′ə-bēn) an anticonvulsant agent used as the hydrochloride salt as an adjunct in the treatment of partial seizures 噻加宾，一种抗惊厥药，其盐酸盐用于辅助治疗部分性癫痫发作

tib·ia (tib′e-ə) [L.] shin bone: the more medial and larger bone of the leg below the knee; it articulates with the femur and head of the fibula above and with the talus below 胫骨，见图 1；**t. val′ga,** bowing of the leg in which the angulation is away from the midline 胫骨外翻，小腿弯曲角度背离躯体中线；**t. va′ra,** medial angulation of the tibia in the metaphyseal region, due to a growth disturbance of the medial aspect of the proximal tibial epiphysis 胫骨内翻，胫骨近端骺部内侧生长紊乱而于干骺区内侧形成的角度畸形

tib·i·al (tib′e-əl) pertaining to the tibia or to the medial aspect of the leg 胫骨的

tib·i·a·lis (tib″e-a′lis) [L.] 同 tibial

tib·io·fem·or·al (tib″e-o-fem′ə-rəl) pertaining to the tibia and femur 胫骨股骨的

tib·io·fib·u·lar (tib″e-o-fib′u-lər) pertaining to the tibia and fibula 胫骨腓骨的

tib·io·tar·sal (tib″e-o-tahr′səl) pertaining to the tibia and tarsus 胫骨跗骨的

TIC tubal intraepithelial carcinoma 输卵管上皮内癌

tic (tik) (Fr. tēk) an involuntary, compulsive, rapid, repetitive, stereotyped movement or vocalization, experienced as irresistible although it can be suppressed for some length of time 抽搐；**t. doulou-reux,** (doo-loo-roo′) trigeminal neuralgia 三叉神经痛；**facial t.,** 面肌抽搐，参见 *spasm* 下词条；**habit t.,** any tic that is psychogenic in origin 习惯性抽搐

ti·car·cil·lin (ti″kahr-sil′in) a semisynthetic broad-spectrum penicillin effective against both gram-negative and gram-positive organisms; used as the disodium salt 羧噻吩青霉素，铁卡青霉素，一

种半合成广谱青霉素，对革兰阴性菌和革兰阳性菌均有效；常用其二钠盐

tick (tik) a blood-sucking acarid parasite of the superfamily Ixodoidea, divided into *soft-bodied ticks* and *hard-bodied ticks.* Some ticks are vectors and reservoirs of disease-causing agents 蜱，壁虱

ti·clo·pi·dine (ti-klo′pĭ-dēn) a platelet inhibitor used as the hydrochloride salt in the prophylaxis of stroke syndrome 噻氯匹定，血小板抑制药，其盐酸盐用于预防中风综合征

t.i.d. [L.] ter in di′e (three times a day) 每天三次

ti·dal (ti′dəl) ebbing and flowing like the waters of the oceans 潮汐的，变异的

tide (tīd) a physiologic variation or increase of a certain constituent in body fluids 潮，变异，体液中某种成分的生理变异或增加；**acid t.,** temporary increase in the acidity of the urine, which sometimes follows fasting 酸潮尿，禁食后，尿液酸度的暂时性增高；**alkaline t.,** temporary increase in the alkalinity of the urine during gastric digestion 碱潮尿，胃消化过程中尿碱度的暂时性增高

ti·ge·cy·cline (ti″gə-si′klēn) an antibiotic effective against a variety of gram-positive and gramnegative bacteria, used in the treatment of skin and intra-abdominal infections 替加环素，一种有效对抗各种革兰阳性菌和革兰阴性菌的抗生素，用于治疗皮肤和腹腔内感染

ti·lu·dro·nate (ti-loo′drə-nāt) an inhibitor of bone resorption, used as the disodium salt in the treatment of osteitis deformans 替鲁膦酸盐，骨吸收抑制药，其二钠盐用于治疗变形性骨炎

tim·bre (tam′bər) [Fr.] musical quality of a tone or sound 音色，音品

time (t) (t ī m) a measure of duration 时间，时期；**activated partial thromboplastin t. (APTT) (aPTT) (PTT),** the period required for clot formation in recalcified blood plasma after contact activation and the addition of platelet substitutes; used to address the intrinsic and common pathways of coagulation 活化部位凝血活酶时间，血浆在加入钙后，经过接触激活和加入血小板替代物后，形成血液块所需的时间；**bleeding t.,** the duration of bleeding after controlled, standardized puncture of the earlobe or forearm; a relatively inconsistent measure of capillary and platelet function 出血时间，耳垂或前臂标准化穿刺后出血的持续时间，但以此测试毛细血管和血小板功能并不可信；**circulation t.,** the time required for blood to flow between two given points 循环时间，血液流经两个给定标记点所需时间；**clotting t., coagulation t.,** the time required for blood to clot in a glass tube 凝血时间，血液在试管中凝固所需的时间；**inertia t.,** the time required to overcome the inertia of

a muscle after reception of a stimulus from a nerve 惰性时间，肌肉从神经接受一次刺激后克服其本身的惰性所需的时间；**one-stage prothrombin t.,** 同 prothrombin t.；**prothrombin t. (PT),** the rate at which prothrombin is converted to thrombin in citrated blood with added calcium; used to assess the extrinsic coagulation system of the blood 凝血酶原时间，在加钙的枸橼酸血中，凝血酶原转化为凝血酶的速率；用于评估血液的外源性凝血系统；**reaction t.,** the time elapsing between the application of a stimulus and the resulting reaction 反应时，给予刺激到反应出现所需的时间；**stimulus-response t.,** 同 reaction t.；**thrombin t. (TT),** the time required for plasma fibrinogen to form thrombin, measured as the time for clot formation after exogenous thrombin is added to citrated plasma 凝血酶时间，血浆纤维蛋白原形成凝血酶所需的时间，通过测量外源性凝血酶加入枸橼酸盐血浆后形成血块的时间

ti·mo·lol (ti′mo-lol) a nonselective beta-adrenergic blocking agent used as the maleate salt in the treatment of hypertension, the treatment and prophylaxis of recurrent myocardial infarction, and the prophylaxis of migraine; also used as the hemihydrate or the maleate salt to relieve intraocular pressure in treatment of glaucoma 噻吗洛尔，噻吗心安，一种非选择性 β 肾上腺素能阻滞药，其马来酸盐用于治疗高血压，治疗和预防复发性心肌梗死，以及预防偏头痛；其半水合物或马来酸盐，也用于减轻眼压治疗青光眼

tin (Sn) (tin) a heavy metal element occurring in several forms; it is silvery white, metallic, and malleable at room temperature; at. no. 50, at. wt. 118.710 锡（化学元素）

tinct. [L.] tinctura (tincture) 酊，酊剂

tinc·to·ri·al (tink-tor′e-əl) pertaining to dyeing or staining 染色的

tinc·ture (tink′chər) an alcoholic or hydroalcoholic solution prepared from vegetable materials or chemical substances 酊，酊剂；**iodine t.,** a preparation of iodine and sodium iodide in diluted alcohol, used as a topical antiinfective 碘酊，局部抗感染药

tine (tīn) a prong or pointed projection on an implement, as on a fork 叉，尖齿

tin·ea (tin′e-ə) ringworm; any of various dermatophytoses, types being designated according to appearance, etiology, or site 癣；**t. bar′bae,** tinea of the beard area, caused by species of *Trichophyton* and associated with contact with farm animals; it is most often a severe inflammatory pustular folliculitis, with a less common, milder form characterized by circular, erythematous, scaly lesions 须癣，由发癣菌属引起的胡须癣，与农场动物接触有关；通

常为一种严重的炎性脓疱性毛囊炎，以圆形、红斑及鳞状病变为特征的轻型较少见；t. ca′pitis, tinea of the scalp, due to species of *Trichophyton* or *Microsporum*, beginning as one or more patches of scale or alopecia that may progress to inflammation, ulceration, scarring, and permanent alopecia 头癣，由发癣菌属或小孢子菌属感染引起，最初表现为一块或多块斑片或脱发，可发展为炎症、溃疡、瘢痕和永久性脱发；t. circina′ta, tinea corporis, sometimes specifically that occurring in the classic, typical presentation 圆癣，体癣；t. cor′poris, tinea involving the skin of the trunk and extremities, excluding the nails, palms, soles, and groin; usually due to *Microsporum canis, Trichophyton rubrum,* or *T. mentagrophytes.*The typical lesion is a well-demarcated, circular, erythematous, scaly macule with a raised border; progressive central healing leaves an annular outline 体癣，常累及躯干和四肢皮肤，不包括指甲、手掌、脚底和腹股沟；最常见的病原菌为大小孢子菌、红色毛癣菌或须毛癣菌；典型者表现为边界明显的鳞屑性红斑性损害，边缘凸起，中心痊愈后呈环形轮廓；t. cru′ris, tinea of the inguinal region and adjacent areas, more common in males and often associated with tinea pedis; usually caused by *Epidermophyton floccosum, Trichophyton rubrum,* or *T. mentagrophytes* 股癣，多见于男性，累及腹股沟、会阴等处，常伴有足癣；通常由絮状麦皮癣菌、红色毛癣菌、或须毛癣菌引起；t. fa′ciei, tinea of nonhairy areas of the face, usually similar in presentation and etiology to tinea corporis 面癣，面部除须区以外的癣，在表现和病因上与体癣相似；t. imbrica′ta, a chronic type of tinea corporis seen in the tropics, due to *Trichophyton concentricum;* the early lesion is annular with a circle of scales at the periphery 叠瓦癣，同心性发癣菌所致的慢性热带皮癣，早期病变为环状，周围有一圈鳞屑；t. ma′nuum, tinea of the hands, often specifically interdigital or palmar infection; usually unilateral and accompanied by tinea pedis of the soles having the same etiologic agent; it typically presents as hyperkeratosis with dry scaling 鹅掌风，累及指间和手掌，通常单侧并伴有病原相同的足底癣，典型表现为干性鳞屑伴角化过度；t. ni′gra, a minor fungal infection caused by *Hortaea werneckii,* having dark spatterlike lesions on the skin of the hands or occasionally other areas 掌黑癣，小毛菌感染，病原为威尼克外霉，在手部皮肤或偶尔其他部位有深色的散斑样病变；t. pe′dis, athlete's foot; usually interdigital or plantar and most often due to *Trichophyton rubrum, T. mentagrophytes,* or *Epidermophyton floccosum;* intensely pruritic lesions vary from mild, chronic, and scaling to acute, exfoliative, pustular, and bullous 足癣，

常累及指间或足底，最常见的病原是红色毛癣菌、须癣菌或絮状麦皮癣菌，临床表现自轻微的慢性脱屑到急性剥脱性脓疱及大疱性损害不等，伴剧痒，参见 *dermatophytosis*；t. profun′da, a variant form of tinea corporis resulting from an excessive inflammatory response and having deep, kerion-like lesions 深癣，一种体癣的变体，由过度的炎症反应和深的类脓疱病变引起；t. un′guium, onychomycosis caused by dermatophytes; because this describes most cases of onychomycosis, the two terms are often used interchangeably 甲癣，由皮肤真菌引起的甲真菌病；因该词描述了大多数甲真菌病的情况，故可与 onychomycosis 互换使用；t. versi′color, a chronic, usually asymptomatic disorder with multiple macular patches, seen in tropical regions and caused by *Malassezia,* particularly *M. furfur* 花斑癣，一种常见的慢性非炎症性疾病，常无症状而只表现为多发性斑疹损害，见于热带地区，由马拉色菌引起，尤其是糠秕马拉色菌

tin·ni·tus (tin′ĭ-təs) (tĭ-ni′təs) [L.] a noise in the ears, such as ringing, buzzing, roaring, or clicking 耳鸣

tin·zap·a·rin (tin-zap′ə-rin) a low-molecular-weight heparin of porcine origin, having antithrombotic activity and used with warfarin in the treatment of deep vein thrombosis with or without pulmonary embolism 亭扎肝素，替扎帕灵，猪来源的低分子量肝素，有抗血栓活性和与华法林合用治疗深静脉血栓或肺栓塞

ti·o·con·a·zole (tiʺo-kon′ə-zōl) an imidazole antifungal used in the treatment of vulvovaginal candidiasis 噻康唑，咪唑类衍生物，作为抗真菌药治疗外阴阴道念珠病

ti·o·pro·nin (ti-o′pro-nin) a thiol compound used in the treatment of cystinuria and the prophylaxis of cystine renal calculi 硫普罗宁，一种硫醇类化合物，用于治疗胱氨酸尿症和预防胱氨酸肾结石

ti·ro·fi·ban (tiʺro-fi′ban) a platelet inhibitor, used as the hydrochloride salt in prophylaxis of thrombosis in unstable angina or in myocardial infarction that is not characterized by abnormal Q waves 替罗非班，一种血小板抑制药，其盐酸盐用于预防无异常 Q 波不稳定心绞痛或心肌梗死患者的血栓形成

tis·sue (tish′oo) an aggregation of similarly specialized cells that together perform certain special functions 组织；**adipose t.,** connective tissue made of fat cells in meshwork of areolar tissue 脂肪组织，蜂窝组织网状结构中脂肪细胞构成的结缔组织；**areolar t.,** connective tissue made up largely of interlacing fibers 蜂窝组织，主要由交叉纤维构成的结缔组织；**bony t.,** bone 骨组织；**brown adipose t.,** a thermogenic type of adipose tissue containing a dark pigment. It arises during embryonic life in certain specific areas in many mammals, including humans; it is prominent in the newborn 棕色脂肪组织，含深色色素的产热的脂肪组织，出现于包括人类在内的某些哺乳动物胚胎期身体的特定区域；新生儿期显著；**cancellous t.**, the spongy tissue of bone 海绵骨组织 **cartilaginous t.**, the substance of cartilage 软骨组织；**chromaffin t.**, a tissue composed largely of chromaffin cells, well supplied with nerves and vessels; it occurs in the adrenal medulla and also forms the paraganglia of the body 嗜铬组织，主要由嗜铬细胞构成的组织，神经和血管供应丰厚，见于肾上腺髓质，另亦构成副神经节（嗜铬体）；**cicatricial t.**, the dense fibrous tissue forming a cicatrix, derived directly from granulation tissue 瘢痕组织，由致密纤维组织构成的瘢痕，直接由肉芽组织衍变而来；**connective t.**, the stromatous or nonparenchymatous tissues of the body; that which binds together and is the ground substance of the various parts and organs of the body 结缔组织，间质或非实质的身体组织；其结合在一起，是身体的各个部分和器官的基质；**elastic t., elastic t., yellow,** connective tissue made up of yellow elastic fibers, frequently massed into sheets 弹性组织，由黄色弹力纤维构成的结缔组织，常集合成片；**endothelial t.**, endothelium 内皮组织；**epithelial t.**, epithelium 上皮组织；**erectile t.**, spongy tissue that expands and becomes hard when filled with blood 勃起组织，可以充血扩张变硬的海绵组织；**extracellular t.**, the total of tissues and body fluids outside the cells 细胞外组织，一切位于细胞外的组织和体液；**fatty t.**, 同 adipose t.；**fibrous t.**, the common connective tissue of the body, composed of yellow or white parallel fibers 纤维组织，体内的普遍结缔组织，主要由黄色或白色的平行纤维构成；**gelatinous t.**, 同 mucous t.；**glandular t.**, an aggregation of epithelial cells that elaborate secretions 腺组织，有分泌功能的上皮细胞会集成的组织；**granulation t.**, the newly formed vascular tissue normally produced in the healing of wounds of soft tissue, ultimately forming the cicatrix 肉芽组织，新形成的血管组织，通常在软组织创口愈合时形成、最终形成瘢痕；**gut-associated lymphoid t. (GALT)**, lymphoid tissue associated with the gut (primordial digestive tube), including the tonsils, Peyer patches, lamina propria of the gastrointestinal tract, and appendix 肠相关淋巴组织，与肠管伴随的淋巴组织，包括集合淋巴样组织、肠道集合淋巴结，胃肠道黏膜固有层和阑尾等；**indifferent t.**, undifferentiated embryonic tissue 未分化组织；**interstitial t.**, stroma 间质组织，间质 **lymphoid t.**, a latticework of reticular tissue, whose interspaces

contain lymphocytes 淋巴组织，网状组织的网络间隙中，含有淋巴细胞 **mesenchymal t.**, mesenchyme 间叶组织；**mucosa-associated lymphoid t. (MALT)**, a type of specialized lymphoid tissue found in association with certain types of epithelia; it usually has prominent B-cell follicles and sometimes has zones of T cells 黏膜相关淋巴组织，在特定上皮中的一类特殊的淋巴样组织；通常有明显的 B 细胞滤泡，有时有 T 细胞区；**mucous t.**, a jellylike connective tissue, as occurs in the umbilical cord 黏液组织，胶冻状结缔组织，分布于脐带等处；**muscle t., muscular t.**, the substance of muscle, consisting of muscle fibers, muscle cells, connective tissue, and extracellular material 肌肉组织，即肌肉，由肌纤维、肌细胞、结缔组织和细胞外组织组成；**myeloid t.**, red bone marrow 骨髓组织，指红骨髓；**nerve t., nervous t.**, the specialized tissue making up the central and peripheral nervous systems, consisting of neurons with their processes, other specialized or supporting cells, and extracellular material 神经组织，由中枢神经系统和周围神经系统组成，它是由神经元和其突触构成的，另一特点是由骨架细胞如神经胶质和细胞外物质构成；**osseous t.**, the specialized tissue forming the bones 骨组织；**reticular t., reticulated t.**, connective tissue consisting of reticular cells and fibers 网状组织，由网状细胞和纤维构成的结缔组织；**scar t.**, 同 cicatricial t.；**skeletal t.**, the bony, ligamentous, fibrous, and cartilaginous tissue forming the skeleton and its attachments 骨骼组织，由骨、韧带、纤维和软骨等组织形成的骨骼及其附着组织；**subcutaneous t.**, the layer of loose connective tissue directly under the skin 皮下组织，位于皮下的疏松结缔组织层；**white adipose t., yellow adipose t.**, the adipose tissue comprising the bulk of the body fat 白脂肪组织，黄脂肪组织，组成体内脂肪的主体

ti·ta·ni·um (Ti) (ti-ta′ne-əm) a lustrous, white, strong, ductile, corrosion-resistant, biocompatible, metallic element; at. no. 22, at. wt. 47.867; its uses include implants, prostheses, and surgical implements 钛（化学元素）；**t. dioxide**, an oxide of titanium used as a topical skin protectant and in sunscreens, and as a white pigment for artificial teeth. Industrial exposure via inhalation may lead to a mild pneumoconiosis 二氧化钛，钛白粉，用作局部皮肤保护剂和防晒霜，也用作义齿的白色色素；工业吸入可能导致轻度尘肺

ti·ter (ti′tər) the quantity of a substance required to react with or to correspond to a given amount of another substance 效价，滴度，值；**agglutination t.**, the highest dilution of a serum that causes agglutination (clumping) of microorganisms or other particulate antigens 凝集反应效价，可使微生物或其他颗粒抗原发生凝集的血清最高稀释度

ti·tra·tion (ti-tra′shən) determination of a given component in solution by addition of a liquid reagent of known strength until the end point is reached when the component has been consumed by reaction with the reagent 滴定法

tit·u·ba·tion (tit″u-ba′shən) 1. the act of staggering or reeling 步态蹒跚；2. a tremor of the head and sometimes trunk, commonly seen in cerebellar disease 头与躯体颤动，常见于小脑病变时

TIV trivalent inactivated influenza vaccine 流行性感冒灭活疫苗，参见 *vaccine* 下 *influenza virus vaccine* (1)

ti·zan·i·dine (ti-zan′ĭ-dēn″) an antispastic used as the hydrochloride salt in the treatment of spasticity related to multiple sclerosis or spinal cord injury 替扎尼定，其盐酸盐用于治疗多发性硬化症或脊髓损伤的痉挛状态

TJC The Joint Commission 联合委员会

Tl thallium 元素铊的符号

TLC thin-layer chromatography 薄层色谱法；total lung capacity 肺总量

Tm thulium 元素铥的符号

TMD temporomandibular disorder 颞下颌关节紊乱

TMJ temporomandibular joint 颞下颌关节

TMJD temporomandibular joint disorder 颞下颌关节紊乱症

TNM tumor-nodes-metastasisTNM 分类，参见 *staging* 下词条

TNT trinitrotoluene 三硝基甲苯

to·bac·co (tə-bak′o) 1. any of various plants of the genus *Nicotiana*, especially *N. tabacum* 烟草，任何烟草属植物，尤指茄科植物烟草；2. the dried prepared leaves of *N. tabacum*, the source of various alkaloids, principally nicotine; it is sedative and narcotic, emetic and diuretic, antispasmodic, and a cardiac depressant 烟叶，烟草的干燥制备的叶子，是多种生物碱的来源，主要是烟碱；可作为镇静药、麻醉药、催吐剂、利尿药、镇痉药和心抑制药；**mountain t.**, arnica 山金车花

to·bra·my·cin (to″brə-mi′sin) an aminoglycoside antibiotic derived from a complex produced by *Streptomyces tenebrarius*, bactericidal against many gram-negative and some gram-positive organisms; also used as the sulfate salt 妥布霉素，由黑暗链霉菌产生的氨基糖苷类抗生素复合体中提取的一种成分，对很多革兰阴性菌和部分革兰阳性菌有杀菌作用；用其硫酸盐

to·cai·nide (to-ka′nīd) an antiarrhythmic agent, used as the hydrochloride salt in the treatment of ventric-

ular arrhythmias 妥卡胺，抗心律失常药；其盐酸盐用于治疗室性心律失常

to·ci·liz·u·mab (taw-sih-liz′-ū-mab) an antiinflammatory that targets and blocks the interleukin-6 receptor to treat inflammatory autoimmune conditions, including rheumatoid arthritis, types of juvenile arthritis, and giant cell arteritis 抗炎靶向药，可阻断白介素-6受体以治疗炎症性自身免疫性疾病，包括类风湿关节炎，多种少年（慢性类风湿性）关节炎及巨细胞动脉炎

to·col (to′kol) the basic unit of the tocopherols and tocotrienols, hydroquinone with a saturated side chain; it is an antioxidant 母生育酚，生育酚和生育三烯酚的基本单位，是具有饱和侧链的氢醌；是一种抗氧化剂

to·col·y·sis (to-kol′ĭ-sis) inhibition of uterine contractions 子宫收缩抑制药

to·co·lyt·ic (to″ko-lit′ik) 1. pertaining to or causing tocolysis 抗分娩的；2. an agent having such an action 抗分娩药

to·com·e·ter (to-kom′ə-tər) 同 tokodynamometer

to·coph·er·ol (to-kof′ər-ol) any of a series of structurally similar compounds, some of which have biologic vitamin E activity 生育酚，一系列维生素E类似物的总称，具有多种亚型，具有抗氧化特性；**α-t., alpha t.**, the most prevalent form of vitamin E in the body and that administered as a supplement; often used synonymously with vitamin E. Also used as the acetate and acid succinate esters α-生育酚，维生素E在体内最普遍的形式，也称醋酸酯和琥珀酸酯

to·co·pho·bia (to″ko-fo′be-ə) irrational fear of childbirth 分娩恐怖

toe (to) a digit of the foot 足趾；**claw t.**, a toe deformity in which the metatarsophalangeal joint is held in extension while the proximal interphalangeal joint is fixed in flexion and the distal joint is held in the neutral or slightly flexed position 爪状趾，跖趾关节伸直，近端趾间关节固定屈曲，远端趾间关节保持中性或轻微弯曲的脚趾畸形；**hammer t.**, deformity of a toe, most often the second, in which the proximal phalanx is extended and the second and distal phalanges are flexed, giving a clawlike appearance 锤状趾，一种最常见于第二趾的脚趾畸形，近节趾骨伸展，第二节和远节趾骨弯曲，呈爪状外观；**Morton t.**, Morton 趾，参见 *neuralgia*；**pigeon t.**, permanent toeing-in position of the feet 鸽趾，足部永久趾尖位置；**tennis t.**, a painful toe or toes from subungual hematoma, such as from trauma in vigorous tennis playing 网球趾，足趾甲下血肿引起的脚趾痛，如在激烈的网球比赛中所受的创伤；**webbed t's**, syndactyly of the toes 蹼状趾

toe·nail (to′nāl) the nail on a toe 趾甲；**ingrown t.**, 嵌甲，参见 *nail* 下词条

To·ga·vi·ri·dae (to″gə-vir′ĭ-de) the togaviruses, a family of RNA viruses that includes the genera *Alphavirus* and *Rubivirus* 披膜病毒科，是一种 RNA 病毒，包括 α 病毒属和风疹病毒属

to·ga·vi·rus (to′gə-vi′rəs) any virus of the family Togaviridae 披膜病毒

toi·let (toi′lət) the cleansing and dressing of a wound 清洗创口

to·ko·dy·na·graph (to″ko-di′nə-graf) a tracing obtained by the tokodynamometer 分娩力描记图

to·ko·dy·na·mom·e·ter (to″ko-di″nə-mom′ə- tər) an instrument for measuring and recording the expulsive force of uterine contractions 分娩力计

tol·az·a·mide (tol-az′ə-mīd) a sulfonylurea used as a hypoglycemic in the treatment of type 2 diabetes mellitus 妥拉磺脲，一种用于治疗 2 型糖尿病的磺脲类药物

tol·az·o·line (tol-az′o-lēn) an adrenergic blocking agent and peripheral vasodilator; used as the hydrochloride salt in the treatment of peripheral vascular disorders due to vasospasm and as a vasodilator in pharmacoangiography 妥拉唑啉，一种肾上腺素能阻断药和外周血管扩张药，其盐酸盐用于治疗因血管痉挛引起的周围血管疾病和药物血管造影术中的血管扩张药

tol·bu·ta·mide (tol-bu′tə-mīd) a sulfonylurea used as a hypoglycemic in the treatment of type 2 diabetes mellitus; the monosodium salt is used to test for insulinoma and diabetes mellitus 甲磺丁脲，一种磺脲类药物，用于治疗 2 型糖尿病，单钠盐用于检测胰岛素瘤和糖尿病

tol·ca·pone (tōl′kə-pōn″) an antidyskinetic used as an adjunct to levodopa and carbidopa in the treatment of Parkinson disease 托卡朋，一种抗运动障碍药物，在治疗帕金森病时作为左旋多巴和卡比多帕的辅助药物

tol·er·ance (tol′ər-əns) 1. diminution of response to a stimulus after prolonged exposure 耐受性；2. the ability to endure unusually large doses of a poison or toxin 耐药性；3. 同 drug t.；4. 同 immunologic t.；**tol′erant** *adj.*；**drug t.**, decrease in susceptibility to the effects of a drug due to its continued administration 药物耐受性，由于持续给药，机体对药物作用的敏感性降低；**immunologic t.**, the development of specific nonreactivity of lymphoid tissues to a particular antigen capable under other conditions of inducing immunity, resulting from previous contact with the antigen and having no effect on the response to non–cross-reacting antigens 免疫耐受性，淋巴组织对特定抗原产生特异性反应缺乏现象，而在其他情况下可诱导免疫，原因是过去接触过该抗原，非交叉反应性抗原的效应则不受影响；**impaired glucose t. (IGT)**, a term denoting values of fasting plasma glucose or results of an oral glucose tolerance test that are abnormal but not high enough to be diagnostic of diabetes mellitus 糖耐量减低，代表空腹血糖值或口服葡萄糖耐量试验结果异常，但并没有高到足以诊断为糖尿病

tol·ero·gen (tol′ər-o-jən) an antigen that induces a state of specific immunologic unresponsiveness to subsequent challenging doses of the antigen 耐受原，可诱导特定的免疫状态，但对随后具有挑战性的抗原剂量反应迟缓

tol·le cau·sam (tol′ə kaw′zam) [L. "remove the cause"] a principle of naturopathic medicine, stating that the goal of treatment is to identify and remove the cause of the disease, often involving the removal of multiple causes in the proper order 自然疗法中的一种原则，说明治疗的目的是确定和消除疾病的病因，通常包括要按适当的顺序消除多种病因

tol·met·in (tol′met-in) a nonsteroidal antiinflammatory drug used as the sodium salt in the treatment of various rheumatic inflammatory disorders 托美汀，一种非甾体抗炎药，其钠盐用于治疗各种风湿性炎症性疾病

tol·naf·tate (tol-naf′tāt) a synthetic topical antifungal, used in the treatment of tinea 托萘酯，发癣退，一种合成的局部抗真菌药物，用于治疗癣

tol·ter·o·dine (tol-ter′ə-dēn) an antispasmodic used as *t. tartrate* in the treatment of bladder hyperactivity 托特罗定，一种酒石酸托特罗定解痉药，通常用于治疗膀胱亢进

tol·u·ene (tol′u-ēn) the hydrocarbon C7H8; it is an organic solvent that can cause poisoning by ingestion or by inhalation of its vapors 甲苯

to·mac·u·lous (to-mak′u-ləs) resembling a sausage, usually because of swelling 香肠状的

to·mo·gram (to′mo-gram) an image of a tissue section produced by tomography X 线断层照片

to·mo·graph (to′mo-graf) an apparatus for moving an x-ray source in one direction as the film is moved in the opposite direction, thus showing in detail a predetermined plane of tissue while blurring or eliminating detail in other planes X 线断层照相机

to·mog·ra·phy (to-mog′rə-fe) the recording of internal body images at a predetermined plane by means of the tomograph 层析 X 线照相术 **computed t. (CT), computerized axial t. (CAT)**, an imaging method in which a cross-sectional image of the structures in a body plane is reconstructed by a computer program from the x-ray absorption of beams projected through the body in the image plane 计算机体层成像，计算机断层扫描；**optical coherence t.**, the creation of high-resolution cross-sectional images of body structures by recording the reflection of infrared waves from the tissues 光学相干层析术；**positron emission t. (PET)**, a nuclear medicine imaging method similar to computed tomography, except that the image shows the tissue concentration of a positron-emitting radioisotope 正电子发射体层成像；**singlephoton emission computed t. (SPECT)**, a type in which gamma photon–emitting radionuclides are administered and then detected by one or more gamma cameras rotated around the patient, using the series of two-dimensional images to recreate a three-dimensional view 单光子发射计算机断层成像；**ultrasonic t.**, the ultrasonographic visualization of a cross-section of a predetermined plane of the body 超声显像术

tone (tōn) 1. normal degree of vigor and tension; in muscle, the resistance to passive elongation or stretch 紧张性；2. a healthy state of a part; tonus 身体（各器官的）健康状况；3. a particular quality of sound or of voice 音，音调

tongue (tung) the movable muscular organ on the floor of the mouth; it is the chief organ of taste and aids in mastication, swallowing, and speech 舌；**bifid t.**, one with an anterior lengthwise cleft 舌裂，舌前部因纵裂而分裂；**black t., black hairy t.**, hairy tongue in which the papillae are brown or black 黑毛舌，舌乳头呈棕色或黑色；**cleft t.**, bifid t. 舌裂，参见 bifid t.；**coated t.**, one covered with a whitish or yellowish layer consisting of desquamated epithelium, debris, bacteria, fungi, etc. 舌苔，舌面上披覆着的一层由脱落的上皮细胞、碎片、细菌、真菌等组成的白色或黄色的被膜；**fissuredt., furrowed t.**, a tongue with numerous furrows or grooves on the dorsal surface, often radiating from a groove on the midline; it is sometimes a familial condition 裂缝舌，舌背表面有许多沟或槽，通常从舌中线上的凹槽放射出来，有时具有家庭遗传倾向；**geographict.**, benign migratory glossitis 地图样舌；**hairy t.**, one with the papillae elongated and hairlike 毛舌，具有细长的、毛发状的乳头；**raspberry t.**, a red, uncoated tongue, with elevated papillae, as seen a few days after the onset of the rash in scarlet fever 草莓舌，一种红色的、无舌苔的舌头，有乳突状突起，见于猩红热皮疹发作后几天 red strawberry t., 同 raspberry）；**scrotal t.**, 同 fissured t.；**white strawberry t.**, the whitecoated tongue with prominent red papillae characteristic of the early stage of scarlet fever 草莓舌，舌乳头显著发红，且有白膜覆盖，是猩红热早期的典型表现

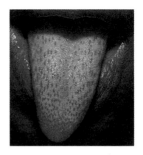

▲ 早期猩红热的草莓舌

tongue-tie (tung'ti″) abnormal shortness of the frenum of the tongue, interfering with its motion; ankyloglossia 结舌，舌系带短缩

ton·ic (ton'ik) 1. producing and restoring normal tone 恢复正常音调的；2. characterized by continuous tension 紧张的；强直的

to·nic·i·ty (to-nis'ĭ-te) 1. the state of tissue tone or tension 紧张性，张力；2. in body fluid physiology, the effective osmotic pressure equivalent 渗透性在体液生理学中，指有效渗透压当量

ton·i·co·clon·ic (ton″ĭ-ko-klon'ik) both tonic and clonic; said of a spasm or seizure consisting of a convulsive twitching of muscles 强直阵挛性的

tono·clon·ic (ton″o-klon'ik) 同 tonicoclonic

tono·fi·bril (ton'o-fi″bril) a bundle of tonofilaments occurring in epithelial cells, the individual strands of which traverse the cytoplasm in all directions and extend into the cell processes to converge and insert on the desmosomes 张力原纤维，上皮细胞中存在的一束张力丝，这些张力丝的单链从各个方向穿过细胞质，伸入胞突，汇合并插入到桥粒上

tono·fil·a·ment (ton″o-fil'ə-mənt) an intermediate filament composed of keratin, occurring in epithelial cells, particularly those of the epidermis, and participating in the formation of desmosomes 张力丝，一种由角蛋白组成的中间丝，存在于上皮细胞中，尤指表皮细胞，并参与桥粒的形成

to·nog·ra·phy (to-nog'rə-fe) recording of changes in intraocular pressure due to sustained pressure on the eyeball 眼压描记检查法；**carotid compression t.**, a test for occlusion of the carotid artery by measuring intraocular pressure and pulse before, during, and after the proximal portion of the carotid artery is compressed by the fingers 颈动脉加压张力描记法，用手指在颈动脉近端加压，记录加压前、中、后的眼压和脉搏，以此测试颈动脉有无阻塞的一种试验方法

to·nom·e·ter (to-nom'ə-tər) an instrument for measuring tension or pressure, particularly intraocular pressure 眼 压 计; **air-puff t.,** an instrument for measuring intraocular pressure by sensing deflections of the cornea in reaction to a puff of pressurized air 气压眼压计; **applanation t.,** an instrument that measures intraocular pressure by determination of the force necessary to flatten a corneal surface of constant size 压平式眼压计; **impression t., indentation t.,** an instrument that measures intraocular pressure by direct pressure on the eyeball 压 陷 眼 压 计

to·nom·e·try (to-nom′ə-tre) measurement of tension or pressure, particularly intraocular pressure 眼压测量法; **digital t.,** estimation of the degree of intraocular pressure by pressure exerted on the eyeball by the examiner's finger 指触眼压测量法

ton·sil (ton′sil) a small, rounded mass of tissue, especially of lymphoid tissue; generally used alone to designate the palatine tonsil 扁桃体; **t. of cerebellum,** a rounded mass of tissue forming part of each hemisphere in the posterior lobe of the cerebellum 小脑扁桃体; **faucial t.,** 同 palatine t.; **lingual t.,** an aggregation of lymph follicles at the root of the tongue 舌扁桃体; **palatine t.,** a small mass of lymphoid tissue between the pillars of the fauces on either side of the pharynx 腭 扁 桃 体; **pharyngeal t.,** the diffuse lymphoid tissue and follicles in the roof and mastoid wall of the nasopharynx 咽部桃体

ton·sil·la, (ton-sil′ə) pl. *tonsil'lae* [L.] 同 tonsil

ton·sil·lar (ton′sĭ-lər) of or pertaining to a tonsil 扁桃体的

ton·sil·lec·to·my (ton″sĭ-lek′tə-me) excision of a tonsil 扁桃体切除术

ton·sil·li·tis (ton″sĭ-li′tis) inflammation of the tonsils, especially the palatine tonsils 扁桃体炎, 尤指腭扁桃体的化脓性炎症; **follicular t.,** tonsillitis especially affecting the crypts 滤泡扁桃体炎, 尤其累及隐窝的扁桃体炎

ton·sil·lo·lith (ton-sil′o-lith) a calculus in a tonsil 扁桃体石

ton·sil·lot·o·my (ton″sĭ-lot′ə-me) incision of a tonsil 扁桃体切开术

to·nus (to′nəs) tone or tonicity; the slight, continuous contraction of a muscle, which in skeletal muscles aids in the maintenance of posture and in the return of blood to the heart 紧张, 张力, 一种有助于维持姿势和血液回流到心脏的轻微的肌肉收缩

tooth (tooth) pl. *teeth*. One of the hard, calcified structures set in the alveolar processes of the jaws for the biting and mastication of food 牙齿; **accessional teeth,** those having no deciduous predecessors: the permanent molars 恒 磨 牙; **artificial t.,**

one made of porcelain or other synthetic compound in imitation of a natural tooth 人 工 牙; **auditory teeth of Huschke,** toothlike projections in the cochlea 听 牙, 耳蜗中的齿状突起; **bicuspid teeth,** 同 premolar t.; **canine t. (C), cuspid t.,** the third tooth on either side from the midline in each jaw 尖牙, 位于上下颌中线两侧的第三颗牙齿; **deciduous teeth,** primary teeth; the 20 teeth of the first dentition, which are shed and replaced by the permanent teeth 乳牙, 人萌出的第一副牙, 一共20颗, 脱落后被恒牙所取代; **eye t.,** a canine tooth of the upper jaw 眼牙上颌的尖牙; **Hutchinson teeth,** notched, narrow-edged permanent incisors, sometimes but not always a sign of congenital syphilis 哈钦森牙, 有缺口、边缘狭窄的恒切牙, 有时为先天性梅毒的症状; **impacted t.,** one prevented from erupting by a physical barrier 阻生牙, 由于物理因素障碍而不能萌生的牙; **incisor t. (I),** one of the four front teeth, two on each side of the midline, in each jaw 切牙, 上下颌中线两侧的牙, 共四颗; **milk teeth,** 同 deciduous teeth; **molar teeth (M),** any of the posterior teeth on either side in each jaw, numbering three in the permanent dentition and two in the deciduous 磨牙, 臼齿, 上、下颌两侧的任何一颗后牙, 其中恒牙有三颗, 乳牙有两颗, 见图31; **peg t., pegshaped t.,** a tooth whose sides converge or taper together incisally 钉状牙, 牙两侧向中会聚或逐渐变细的牙齿; **permanent teeth,** the 32 teeth of the second dentition 恒牙, 人萌出的第二副牙, 一共32颗; **premolar teeth (P),** bicuspid tooth; either of two permanent teeth found between the canine and molar teeth 前磨牙, 双尖牙, 见 bicuspid tooth **primary teeth,** 同 deciduous teeth; **stomach t.,** a canine tooth of the lower jaw 胃牙; **successional teeth,** the permanent teeth that have deciduous predecessors 继承牙, 恒牙, 指第一副牙脱落后再长出的牙; **temporary teeth,** 同 deciduous; **wisdom t.,** the last molar tooth on either side in each jaw 智齿, 第三磨牙

tooth·ache (tooth′āk″) pain in a tooth 牙痛

to·pal·gia (to-pal′jə) pain localized or fixed in one spot; often a symptom of conversion disorder 局部痛

to·pec·to·my (to-pek′tə-me) ablation of a small and specific area of the frontal cortex in the treatment of certain forms of epilepsy and psychiatric disorders 额叶皮质局部切除术, 切除额叶皮质的特定区域, 以治疗癫痫和精神病

top·es·the·sia (top″es-the′zhə) ability to recognize the location of a tactile stimulus 位置觉

to·pha·ceous (to-fa′shəs) gritty or sandy; pertaining to tophi 砂砾性的

to·phus (to′fəs) pl. *to'phi* [L.] a deposit of sodium

urate in the tissues about the joints or in the outer ear in gout, producing a chronic, foreign-body inflammatory response 痛风石

top·i·cal (top'ĭ-kəl) pertaining to a particular area, as a topical antiinfective applied to a certain area of the skin and affecting only the area to which it is applied 表面的，局部的，指特定的表面，如应用于皮肤某区的局部抗感染药，其作用仅限于用药区

to·pi·ra·mate (to-pi'rə-māt) a substituted monosaccharide used as an anticonvulsant in the treatment of partial seizures 托吡酯，在治疗部分性癫痫发作中用作抗惊厥药的一种代替性单糖

to·pog·ra·phy (to-pog'rə-fe) the description of an anatomic region or a special part 局部解剖，局部记载，对解剖区或特定部位的描述；**topograph'ic, topograph'ical** adj.

topo·scop·ic (to″po-skop'ik) pertaining to endoscopic delivery to a specific site 内镜局部定位的

to·po·te·can (to″po-te'kan) an antineoplastic that inhibits DNA topoisomerase; used as the hydrochloride salt in the treatment of metastatic ovarian carcinoma and small cell lung carcinoma 一种抑制 DNA 拓扑酶的抗肿瘤药物，其盐酸盐用于治疗转移性卵巢癌及小细胞肺癌

to·re·mi·fene (tor'ə-mĭ-fēn″) an analogue of tamoxifen that acts as an estrogen antagonist; used as the citrate salt in the palliative treatment of metastatic breast carcinoma 托瑞米芬，一种类似他莫昔芬的雌激素拮抗药，其枸橼酸盐用于转移性乳腺癌的缓解性治疗

tor·por (tor'pər) [L.] sluggishness 迟钝，不活泼；**tor'pid** adj.；**t. re'tinae,** sluggish response of the retina to the stimulus of light 视网膜迟钝

torque (tork) 1. a rotary force causing part of a structure to twist about an axis. Symbol τ 旋力，符号 τ；2. in dentistry, the rotation of a tooth on its long axis, especially the movement of the apical portions of the teeth by use of orthodontic appliances 扭转力，在牙科中，尤指用正畸矫治器使牙齿沿长轴旋转

tor·se·mide (tor'sə-mīd) a diuretic related to sulfonylurea, used in the treatment of edema and hypertension 一种与磺脲药物有关的利尿药，用于治疗水肿和高血压

tor·sion (tor'shən) 1. the act or process of being twisted or rotated about an axis 旋转，扭转；2. a type of mechanical stress, whereby the external forces twist an object about its axis 机械性应力，扭力，通过外力使物体绕轴旋转；3. in ophthalmology, any rotation of the vertical corneal meridians 在眼科学中，任何垂直角膜径线的旋转；**tor'sional** adj.

tor·si·ver·sion (tor″sĭ-vur'zhən) turning of a tooth on its long axis out of normal position 扭转位牙，牙沿其长轴扭转而脱离其正常位置

tor·so (tor'so) 同 trunk (1)

tor·ti·col·lis (tor″tĭ-kol'is) 斜颈 1. abnormal twisted position of the neck 颈部异常扭曲，斜颈；2. cervical dystonia 颈肌张力障碍；**spasmodic t.,** cervical dystonia 痉挛性斜颈

tor·ti·pel·vis (tor″tĭ-pel'vis) dystonia musculorum deformans 骨盆扭转，变形性肌张力障碍

tor·u·lus (tor'u-ləs) pl. **tor'uli** [L.] a small elevation; a papilla 隆凸，小圆凸；**to'ruli tac'tiles,** small tactile elevations in the skin of the palms and soles 触觉隆凸，触觉小珠，掌、跖皮肤上的小突起，富含感觉神经末梢

to·rus (tor'əs) pl. **to'ri** [L.] a swelling or bulging projection 隆突，圆枕

to·sy·late (to'sə-lāt) USAN contraction for p-toluenesulfonate 甲苯磺酸盐，p-toluenesulfonate 为 USAN 的缩约词

to·ti·po·ten·cy (to″tĭ-po'tən-se) the ability to differentiate along any line or into any type of cell 全能性，细胞具有能重复个体的全部发育阶段和产生所有细胞类型的能力；**totip'otent, totipoten'tial** adj.

to·ti·po·ten·ti·al·i·ty (to″tĭ-po-ten″she-al'ĭ-te) 同 totipotency

touch (tuch) 1. the sense by which contact with objects gives evidence as to certain of their qualities 触觉；2. palpation with the finger 触诊，指诊；**therapeutic t. (TT),** a healing method based on the premise that the body possesses an energy field that can be affected by the focused intention of the healer. The practitioner uses the hands to assess the patient's energy field, to release areas where the free flow of energy is blocked, and to balance the patient's energy, by transferring energy from a universal life energy force to the patient 治疗性接触

Tou·je·o (too'jay-o) trademark for a preparation of insulin glargine 甘精胰岛素制剂的商品名

tour·ni·quet (toor'nĭ-kət) a band to be drawn tightly around a limb for the temporary arrest of circulation in the distal area 止血带，在肢体周围拉紧的带子，用于在身体远端区域暂时阻断血液循环

tox·emia (tok-se'me-ə) any condition resulting from spread of bacterial products (toxins) by the bloodstream 毒血症；**toxe'mic** adj. 毒血症的

tox·ic (tok'sik) 1. poisonous 有毒的；2. sometimes extended to mean injurious by other means 有时引申为通过其他方式受到伤害

tox·i·cant (tok'sĭ-kənt) 1. poisonous 有毒的；2. poison 毒物

tox·ic·i·ty (tok-sis′ĭ-te) the quality of being poisonous, especially the degree of virulence of a toxic microbe or of a poison 毒力，毒性；**developmental t.**, the extent to which a toxin crosses the placental barrier and produces adverse effects on a developing embryo or fetus 发育毒性，毒素穿过胎盘屏障对发育中的胚胎或胎儿产生不利影响的程度；**O2 t., oxygen t.**, serious, sometimes irreversible, damage to the pulmonary capillary endothelium associated with breathing high partial pressures of oxygen for prolonged periods 氧毒性，严重的肺毛细血管内皮损害，有时不可逆，与长时间吸入高分压氧有关

tox·i·co·gen·ic (tok″sĭ-ko-jen′ik) 同 toxigenic

tox·i·col·o·gy (tok″sĭ-kol′ə-je) the science or study of poisons 毒理学，毒物学；**toxicolog′ic** adj.

tox·i·cop·a·thy (tok″sĭ-kop′ə-the) 同 toxicosis；**toxicopath′ic** adj.

tox·i·co·pex·is (tok″sĭ-ko-pek′sis) the fixation or neutralization of a poison in the body 毒物中和；**toxicopec′tic, toxicopex′ic** adj.

tox·i·co·pho·bia (tok″sĭ-ko-fo′be-ə) irrational fear of being poisoned 毒物恐怖

tox·i·co·sis (tok″sĭ-ko′sis) any diseased condition due to poisoning 中毒

tox·i·drome (tok′sĭ-drōm) a specific group of symptoms associated with exposure to a given poison 中毒综合征

tox·if·er·ous (tok-sif′ər-əs) conveying or producing a poison 有毒的，产毒的

tox·i·gen·ic (tok″sĭ-jen′ik) 1. producing or elaborating toxins 产毒素的；2. derived from or containing toxins 源于或含有毒素的

tox·i·ge·nic·i·ty (tok″sĭ-jə-nis′ĭ-te) the property of producing toxins 产毒性

tox·in (tok′sin) a poison, especially a protein or conjugated protein produced by some higher plants, certain animals, and pathogenic bacteria, that is highly poisonous for other living organisms 毒素，通常是指某些高等植物、某些动物和致病菌产生的蛋白质或结合蛋白，对其他生物体有很强的毒性；**bacterial t's**, toxins produced by bacteria, including exotoxins, endotoxins, and toxic enzymes 细菌毒素，细菌产生的毒素，包括外毒素、内毒素和有毒酶；**botulinum t.**, an exotoxin produced by *Clostridium botulinum* that produces paralysis by blocking the release of acetylcholine in the central nervous system; there are seven immunologically distinct types (A to G), several of which have therapeutic uses 肉毒毒素，一种由肉毒梭菌产生的外毒素，通过抑制乙酰胆碱在中枢神经系统的释放而导致瘫痪，有 7 种不同的免疫型类型（A 到 G），其中一些具有治疗作用；**cholera t.**, choleragen;

the enterotoxin that causes cholera 霍乱毒素；**clostridial t.**, one produced by species of *Clostridium*, including those causing botulinus, gas gangrene, and tetanus 梭菌毒素，一种由梭状芽胞杆菌产生的毒素，包括引起肉毒杆菌、气性坏疽和破伤风的梭状芽胞杆菌；**diphtheria t.**, a protein exotoxin produced by *Corynebacterium diphtheriae* that is primarily responsible for the pathogenesis of diphtheritic infection; it is an enzyme that inhibits protein synthesis 白喉毒素，白喉棒状杆菌产生的一种蛋白外毒素，引起白喉感染，是一种抑制蛋白质合成的酶；**extracellular t.**, exotoxin 细胞外毒素；**gas gangrene t.**, an exotoxin produced by *Clostridium perfringens* that causes gas gangrene; at least 10 types have been identified 气性坏疽毒素，产气荚膜梭菌产生的一种外毒素，可引起气性坏疽，目前至少有 10 种确定的类型；**intracellular t.**, endotoxin 细胞内毒素；**tetanus t.**, tetanospasmin 破伤风毒素

tox·in·an·ti·tox·in (TA) (tok″sin-an′tĭ-tok″sin) a nearly neutral mixture of diphtheria toxin with its antitoxin; used for diphtheria immunization 毒素抗毒素合剂，一种近乎中性的白喉毒素和其抗毒素的混合物，用于白喉免疫处理

tox·in·ol·o·gy (tok″sin-ol′ə-je) the science dealing with the toxins produced by certain higher plants and animals and by pathogenic bacteria 毒素学

Tox·o·ca·ra (tok″so-kar′ə) a genus of nematode parasites of the dog (*T. ca′nis*) and cat (*T. ca′ti*); they can infect humans, usually causing ocular or visceral larva migrans 弓蛔虫属

tox·o·car·i·a·sis (tok″so-kə-ri′ə-sis) infection by worms of the genus *Toxocara* 弓蛔虫病

tox·oid (tok′soid) a modified or inactivated exotoxin that has lost toxicity but retains the ability to combine with, or stimulate the production of, antitoxin 类毒素，经过处理或灭活的细菌外毒素，已失去其毒性，但仍能与抗毒素结合或促使抗毒素生成；**diphtheria t.**, the formaldehyde-inactivated toxin of *Corynebacterium diphtheriae*, used as an active immunizing agent against diphtheria, usually in mixtures with tetanus toxoid and acellular pertussis vaccine (DTaPor Tdap) or with tetanus toxoid alone (DT or Td) when pertussis vaccine is contraindicated 白喉类毒素，经甲醛灭活的白喉棒状杆菌毒素，通常与破伤风类毒素和无细胞百日咳疫苗联合使用，或单独与破伤风毒素联合使用，用作对抗白喉的主动免疫处理；**diphtheria and tetanus t's adsorbed (DT)**, a combination of full-strength doses of diphtheria toxoid and tetanus toxoid; used for immunization of pediatric patients under 7 years of age when pertussis vaccine is contraindicated 吸附白喉破伤风类毒素，用于 7 岁以

下儿童白喉和破伤风的免疫处理 tetanus t. (T), the formaldehyde-inactivated toxins of *Clostridium tetani;* each is used as an active immunizing agent, usually in mixtures with diphtheria toxoid and acellular pertussis vaccine 破伤风类毒素，经甲醛灭活的破伤风梭菌毒素，每一种都被用作一种有效的免疫剂，通常与白喉类毒素和无细胞百日咳疫苗混合使用；**tetanus and diphtheria t's (Td)**, a combination of tetanus toxoid and (reduced) diphtheria toxoid used for immunization of patients at least 7 years of age when pertussis vaccine is contraindicated 破伤风白喉类毒素，破伤风类毒素和白喉类毒素（剂量减少）的组合物，用于 7 岁以上患者的免疫接种

toxo·phil·ic (tok″so-fil′ik) easily susceptible to poison; having affinity for toxins 亲毒的，易感毒素的

toxo·phore (tok′so-for) the group of atoms in a toxin molecule that produces the toxic effect 毒簇，毒性基团，毒素分子中起毒素作用的原子基团；**toxoph′orous** *adj.*

Toxo·plas·ma (tok″so-plaz′mə) a genus of sporozoa that are intracellular parasites of many organs and tissues of birds and mammals, including humans. *T. gon′dii* is the etiologic agent of toxoplasmosis 弓形体属

toxo·plas·mic (tok″so-plaz′mik) pertaining to *Toxoplasma* or to toxoplasmosis 弓形体的

tox·o·plas·mo·sis (tok″so-plaz-mo′sis) an acute or chronic widespread disease of animals and humans caused by *Toxoplasma gondii* and transmitted by oocysts in the feces of cats. Most human infections are asymptomatic; when symptoms occur, they range from a mild, self-limited disease resembling mononucleosis to a disseminated, fulminating disease that may damage the brain, eyes, muscles, liver, and lungs. Severe manifestations are seen principally in immunocompromised patients and in fetuses infected transplacentally as a result of maternal infection. Chorioretinitis may be associated with all forms, but it is usually a late sequela of congenital disease 弓形体病，由弓形虫引起的在人类和动物中广泛传播急慢性疾病，虫卵随猫便排出。大多数人类感染时是无症状的；当症状出现时，范围从类似单核细胞增多症的轻度自限性疾病到可能损害大脑、眼睛、肌肉、肝脏和肺的播散性暴发性疾病。严重的表现主要见于免疫功能缺陷者和因母体感染而经胎盘感染的胎儿。各种弓形体病都可伴有脉络膜视网膜炎，但通常为先天性弓形体病的晚期后遗症

TPA t-PA tissue plasminogen activator 组织型纤溶酶原激活物

t-plas·min·o·gen ac·ti·va·tor (plaz-min′o-jən″ ak′tǐ-va-tər) 组织纤维蛋白溶酶原激活剂 *activator* 下词条

TPM tropomyosin 原肌球蛋白

TPN total parenteral nutrition 全胃肠外营养

TPP thiamine pyrophosphate 硫胺素焦磷酸

tra·be·cu·la (trə-bek′u-lə) pl. *trabec′culae* [L.] a little beam; in anatomy, a general term for a supporting or anchoring strand of connective tissue, e.g., a strand extending from a capsule into the substance of the enclosed organ 小梁，柱；**trabec′ular** *adj.*; **trabeculae of bone,** anastomosing bony spicules in cancellous bone that form a meshwork of intercommunicating spaces that are filled with bone marrow 骨小梁，骨松质中互相吻合的骨板，形成网状结构，腔隙互通，内充骨髓；**trabe′culae car′neae,** irregular bundles and bands of muscle projecting from a great part of the interior walls of the ventricles of the heart 肉柱，从大部分心室壁内部突出的肌束或肌带；**septomarginal t.,** a bundle of muscle at the apical end of the right cardiac ventricle, connecting the base of the superoposterior papillary muscle to the interventricular septum 隔缘肉柱，右心室顶端的一束肌肉，连接着前乳头肌和室间隔

tra·bec·u·late (trə-bek′u-lāt) marked with transverse or radiating bars or trabeculae 有小梁的

tra·bec·u·lo·plas·ty (trə-bek′u-lo-plas″te) plastic surgery of a trabecula 小梁成形术；**laser t.,** the placing of surface burns in the trabecular network of the eye to lower intraocular pressure in openangle glaucoma 激光小梁成形术，在开角型青光眼中，通过灼伤小梁网的表面以降低眼压

trac·er (trās′ər) 1. a means or agent by which certain substances or structures can be identified or followed 示踪物，鉴定或追查某些物质或结构的方法或药物；2. a mechanical device for graphically recording the outline of an object or the direction and extent of movement of a part 示踪器，描记器，一种机械装置，用于以图形方式记录物体的轮廓或部件的运动方向和程度；3. a dissecting instrument for isolating vessels and nerves 分离器，用于隔离血管和神经的解剖器械；**radioactive t.,** a radioactive isotope replacing a stable chemical element in a compound and so able to be followed or tracked through one or more reactions or systems; generally one that is introduced into and followed through the body 放射性示踪物

tra·chea (tra′ke-ə) pl. *tra′cheae* [L.] windpipe; the cartilaginous and membranous tube descending from the larynx and branching into the left and right main bronchi 气管，见图 25 和图 26；**tra′cheal** *adj.*

tra·che·al·gia (tra″ke-al′jə) pain in the trachea 气管痛

tra·che·itis (tra″ke-i′tis) inflammation of the trachea 气管炎；**bacterial t.,** membranous or pseudomembranous croup; an acute crouplike bacterial infection of the upper airway in children, with coughing and high fever 细菌性气管炎

tra·che·lec·to·my (tra″kə-lek′tə-me) cervicectomy 宫颈切除术

tra·che·lism (tra′kə-liz-əm) spasm of the neck muscles; spasmodic retraction of the head in epilepsy 颈肌痉挛

tra·che·lis·mus (tra″kə-liz′məs) 同 trachelism

tra·che·li·tis (tra″kə-li′tis) cervicitis 子宫颈炎

tra·che·lo·pexy (tra′kə-lo-pek″se) fixation of the uterine cervix 子宫颈固定术

tra·che·lo·plas·ty (tra′kə-lo-plas″te) plastic repair of the uterine cervix 宫颈成形术

tra·che·lor·rha·phy (tra″kə-lor′ə-fe) suture of the uterine cervix 宫颈修补术

tra·che·lot·o·my (tra″kə-lot′ə-me) incision of the uterine cervix 宫颈切开术

tra·cheo·bron·chi·al (tra″ke-o-brong′ke-əl) pertaining to the trachea and bronchi 气管支气管的

tra·cheo·bron·chi·tis (tra″ke-o-brong-ki′tis) inflammation of the trachea and bronchi 气管支气管炎

tra·cheo·bron·chos·co·py (tra″ke-o-brongkos′kə-pe) inspection of the interior of the trachea and bronchi 气管支气管镜检查

tra·cheo·cele (tra′ke-o-sēl″) hernial protrusion of tracheal mucous membrane 气管黏膜疝样突出

tra·cheo·esoph·a·ge·al (tra″ke-o-ə-sof″ə-je′əl) pertaining to the trachea and esophagus 气管食管的

tra·cheo·la·ryn·ge·al (tra″ke-o-lə-rin′je-əl) pertaining to the trachea and larynx 气管喉的

tra·cheo·ma·la·cia (tra″ke-o-mə-la′shə) softening of the tracheal cartilages 气管软化

tra·che·op·a·thy (tra″ke-op′ə-the) disease of the trachea 气管病

tra·cheo·pha·ryn·ge·al (tra″ke-o-fə-rin′je-əl) pertaining to the trachea and pharynx 气管咽的

tra·che·oph·o·ny (tra″ke-of′o-ne) a voice sound heard over the trachea 气管音

tra·cheo·plas·ty (tra′ke-o-plas″te) plastic repair of the trachea 气管成形术

tra·che·or·rha·gia (tra″ke-o-ra′jə) hemorrhage from the trachea 气管出血

tra·che·os·chi·sis (tra″ke-os′kĭ-sis) fissure of the trachea 气管裂

tra·che·os·co·py (tra″ke-os′kə-pe) inspection of interior of the trachea 气管镜检查；**tracheoscop′ic** *adj.*

tra·cheo·ste·no·sis (tra″ke-o-stə-no′sis) constriction of the trachea 气管狭窄

tra·che·os·to·my (tra″ke-os′tə-me) creation of an opening into the trachea through the neck, with the tracheal mucosa being brought into continuity with the skin; also, the opening so created 气管造口术

tra·che·ot·o·my (tra″ke-ot′ə-me) incision of the trachea through the skin and muscles of the neck 气管切开术；**inferior t.,** that performed below the isthmus of the thyroid 气管下部切开术；**superior t.,** that performed above the isthmus of the thyroid 气管上部切开术

tra·cho·ma (trə-ko′mə) pl. *tracho′mata* [Gr.] a contagious disease of the conjunctiva and cornea, producing photophobia, pain, and lacrimation, caused by a strain of *Chlamydia trachomatis*. It progresses from a mild infection with tiny follicles on the eyelid conjunctiva to invasion of the cornea, with scarring and contraction that may end in blindness 沙眼；**tracho′matous** *adj.*

tra·chy·onych·ia (tra″ke-o-nik′e-ə) roughness of nails, with brittleness and splitting 指甲粗糙脆裂

tract (trakt) 1. a region, principally one of some length 束，一个区域，特指一定长度的区域；2. a bundle of nerve fibers having a common origin, function, and termination 神经束，具有共同起源、功能和终止的神经纤维束；3. a number of organs, arranged in series and serving a common function. 道，担负某一共同功能的若干脏器的有序组合；**alimentary t.,** 消化道，参见 canal 下词条；**atriohisian t's,** myocardial fibers that bypass the physiologic delay of the atrioventricular node and connect the atrium directly to the bundle of His, allowing preexcitation of the ventricle 心房希氏束，心肌纤维绕过房室结的生理延迟，并将心房直接连接到希氏束，预先激发心室；**biliary t.,** the organs, ducts, etc., participating in secretion (the liver), storage (the gallbladder), and delivery (hepatic and bile ducts) of bile into the duodenum 胆道；**digestive t.,** alimentary canal 消化管；**dorsolateral t.,** a group of nerve fibers in the lateral funiculus of the spinal cord dorsal to the posterior column 脊柱背侧神经束，背外侧束；**extracorticospinal t.,** **extrapyramidal t.,** extrapyramidal system 锥体外束；**Flechsig t.,** posterior spinocerebellar t. 脊髓小脑后束；**flow t's of the heart,** the paths of the blood within the chambers of the heart. In the *left flow tract,* oxygenated blood from the pulmonary circulation enters the left atrium through the pulmonary veins, flows through the left atrioventricular valve into the left ventricle, and passes out through the aortic valve into the aorta and systemic circulation. In the *right flow tract,* deoxygenated blood from the systemic circulation enters the right atrium through the venae cavae, flows through the right atrioventricular valve into the right ventricle, and passes through the pulmonary valve and on into the pulmonary artery and the pulmonary circulation 心脏血流途径; **gastrointestinal t.,** the stomach and intestine in continuity 消 化 道; **genitourinary t.,** urogenital system 生殖泌尿道; **Gowers t.,** anterior spinocerebellar t. 脊 髓 小 脑 前 束; **iliotibial t.,** a thickened longitudinal band of fascia lata extending from the tensor muscle downward to the lateral condyle of the tibia 髂胫束，阔筋膜增厚的纵筋膜带，从张力肌向下延伸到胫骨外侧髁; **intestinal t.,** the small and large intestines in continuity 肠道; **nigrostriatal t.,** a bundle of nerve fibers extending from the substantia nigra to the globus pallidus and putamen in the corpus striatum; injury to it may be a cause of parkinsonism 黑质纹状体束，起至黑质，延伸到纹状体苍白球和壳核的神经传导束，其损伤可能是导致帕金森病的原因之一; **optic t.,** the nerve tract proceeding backward from the optic chiasm, around the cerebral peduncle, and dividing into lateral and medial roots, which end in the superior colliculus and lateral geniculate body, respectively 视束，神经束从视交叉向后延伸，分内侧根和外侧根，绕大脑脚后终止于上丘和外侧膝状体; **pyramidal t.,** several groups of fibers arising chiefly in the sensorimotor regions of the cerebral cortex and descending in the internal capsule, cerebral peduncle, and pons to the medulla oblongata and downward to synapse with internuncial and motor neurons in the spinal cord. It provides for direct cortical control and initiation of skilled movements, especially those related to speech and involving the hand and fingers 椎体束，起源于大脑皮质的感觉运动区，下行经内囊、大脑脚和脑桥通向延髓，向下与脊髓中间神经元和运动神经元形成突触。其参与皮质随意动作的控制，特别是有关言语与手的运动; **respiratory t.,** 呼吸道，参见 *system* 下词条; **reticulospinal t.,** a group of fibers arising mostly from the reticular formation of the pons and medulla oblongata; chiefly homolateral, the fibers descend in the ventral and lateral funiculi to most levels of the spinal cord 网状脊髓束，起自脑桥和延髓网状结构的下行传导束，位于脊髓水平的腹侧和腹外侧; **spinocerebellar t., anterior,** a group of nerve fibers in the lateral funiculus of the spinal cord, arising mostly in the gray matter of the opposite side and ascending to the cerebellum through the superior cerebellar peduncle 脊髓小脑前束，脊髓外侧索中的一组神经纤维，主要起源于对侧的灰质，通过上小脑脚上升至小脑; **spinocerebellar t., posterior,** a group of nerve fibers in the later-

al funiculus of the spinal cord, arising mostly from the thoracic column and ascending to the cerebellum through the inferior cerebellar peduncle 脊髓小脑后束，位于脊髓外侧索的后外缘，起源于胸柱，经小脑下脚上升至小脑; **spinothalamic t.,** either of two groups of nerve fibers, anterior or lateral; the anterior are found in the anterior funiculus of the spinal cord and the lateral in the lateral funiculus, each arising in the contralateral gray matter and ascending to the thalamus. The anterior carry sensory impulses activated by light touch, and the lateral carry those activated by pain and temperature 脊髓丘脑束，起源于脊髓对侧脊髓灰质，前侧束位于脊髓前索，外侧束位于脊髓侧索，均上行至丘脑。前侧束传导轻触激活的感觉冲动，而外侧束传导由疼痛和温度激活的感觉冲动; **urinary t.,** 1. 泌尿道，参见 *system* 下词条; 2. sometimes more specifically the conduits leading from the pelvis of the kidneys to the urinary meatus 有时更确切地说，是从肾盂到尿道的管道; **urogenital t.,** 泌尿生殖道，参见 *system* 下词条; **uveal t.,** the vascular tunic of the eye, comprising the choroid, ciliary body, and iris 葡萄膜，眼睛的血管束膜，包括脉络膜、睫状体和虹膜

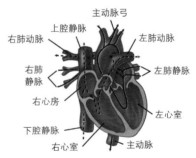

▲ 心脏血液流动轨迹，左（实线）和右（虚线）

trac·tion (trak'shən) the act of drawing or pulling 牵 引; **elastic t.,** traction by an elastic force or by means of an elastic appliance 弹力牵引; **skeletal t.,** traction applied directly upon long bones by means of pins, wires, etc. 骨 牵 引; **skin t.,** traction on a body part maintained by an apparatus affixed by dressings to the body surface 皮肤牵引

trac·tot·o·my (trak-tot'ə-me) surgical severing or incising of a nerve tract 神经束切断术

trac·tus, (trak'təs) pl. *trac'tus* [L.] 同 tract

tra·gus, (tra'gəs) pl. *tra'gi* [L.] 1. the cartilaginous projection anterior to the external opening of the ear 耳屏; 2. *(in the pl.)* hairs growing on the pinna of the external ear, especially on the cartilaginous projection anterior to the external opening 耳毛；**tra′gal** *adj.*

train·ing (trān′ing) a system of instruction or teaching; preparation by instruction and practice 训练，锻炼，培养；**assertiveness t.,** a form of behavior therapy in which individuals are taught appropriate interpersonal responses, involving direct expression of their feelings, both negative and positive 决断力训练，自信训练，一种行为疗法，引导患者恰当的人际反应，比如直接表达他们的感情，这些感情中有消极和积极的成分；**bladder t.,** the training of a child or an incontinent adult in habits of urinary continence 膀胱训练；**bowel t.,** the training of a child or incontinent adult in the habits of fecal continence 排便训练

trait (trāt) 1. any genetically determined characteristic 由基因决定的特征，性状；2. sometimes, more specifically, the condition prevailing in the heterozygous state of a recessive disorder, as sickle cell trait 有时指隐性遗传病的杂合状态下普遍存在的病症，如镰形细胞性状；3. a distinctive behavior pattern 独特的行为模式；**sex-linked t.,** an inherited trait determined by a gene on a sex (X or Y) chromosome and therefore having a different pattern of expression in males and females 伴性性状，由性（X 或 Y）染色体上的基因决定的遗传特征，因此在男性和女性中有不同的表达模式；**sickle cell t.,** the condition, usually asymptomatic, due to heterozygosity for hemoglobin S 镰形细胞性状，由血红蛋白 S 的杂合性所致，通常无明显症状

tra·ma·dol (tram′ə-dol″) an opioid analgesic used as the hydrochloride salt for the treatment of pain following surgical procedures and oral surgery 曲马多，阿片类镇痛药，其盐酸盐用于外科手术和口腔外科手术后镇痛

trance (trans) a sleeplike state of altered consciousness marked by heightened focal awareness and reduced peripheral awareness 迷睡，恍惚，迷睡性木僵，意识改变的一种睡眠状态，以局灶性警觉增高和外周性警觉降低为特征

tran·do·la·pril (tran-do′lə-pril″) an angiotensinconverting enzyme inhibitor used in the treatment of hypertension and post–myocardial infarction congestive heart failure or left ventricular dysfunction 一种血管紧张素转换酶抑制药，用于治疗高血压和心肌梗死后充血性心力衰竭或左心室功能障碍

tran·ex·am·ic ac·id (tran″ək-sam′ik) an antifibrinolytic that competitively inhibits activation of plasminogen; used as a hemostatic in the prophylaxis and treatment of severe hemorrhage associated with excessive fibrinolysis 氨甲环酸，一种竞争性抑制

纤溶酶原活化的抗纤溶酶，用于预防和治疗因过度纤溶而引起的严重出血

tran·qui·liz·er (trang″kwĭ-līz′ər) a drug with a calming, soothing effect; usually a *minor tranquilizer* 镇静药，安定药，通常是一种弱安定药；**major t.,** former name for antipsychotic agent 强安定药，参见 *antipsychotic*；**minor t.,** antianxiety agent 弱安定药，参见 *antianxiety*

trans (tranz) 1. in organic chemistry, having certain atoms or radicals on opposite sides of a nonrotatable parent structure 在有机化学中指对侧的某些原子或基团；2. in genetics, denoting two or more loci occurring on opposite chromosomes of a homologous pair 遗传学中指同源染色体上拟等位基因的两个突变基因中的一个。Cf. *cis*

trans·ab·dom·i·nal (trans″ab-dom′ĭ-nəl) across the abdominal wall or through the abdominal cavity 经腹壁的

trans·ac·e·tyl·a·tion (trans″ə-set′ə-la′shən) a chemical reaction involving the transfer of the acetyl radical 转乙酰基作用

trans·ac·y·lase (trans-a′sə-lās) an enzyme that catalyzes transacylation 转酰基酶

trans·ac·y·la·tion (trans-a″sə-la′shən) a chemical reaction involving the transfer of an acyl radical 转酰基作用

trans·am·i·nase (trans-am′ĭ-nās) aminotransferase 氨基转移酶

trans·am·i·na·tion (trans″am-ĭ-na′shən) the reversible exchange of amino groups between different amino acids 转氨基作用

trans·am·i·ni·tis (trans″ami-nite′əs) elevated levels of transaminases 转氨酶水平升高，又称 *transaminasemia*

trans·an·tral (trans-an′trəl) performed across or through an antrum 经窦的

trans·aor·tic (trans″a-or′tik) performed through the aorta 经主动脉的，尤指经主动脉进行的手术操作

trans·au·di·ent (trans-aw′de-ənt) penetrable by sound waves 透声的

trans·ax·i·al (trans-ak′se-əl) directed at right angles to the long axis of the body or a part 经轴的，与人体或某一局部的长轴垂直的

trans·ba·sal (trans-ba′səl) through the base, as a surgical approach through the base of the skull 经基底的，如经颅底的手术

trans·cal·lo·sal (trans-kə-lo′səl) performed across or through the corpus callosum 经胼胝体的

trans·cal·var·i·al (trans″kal-var′e-əl) through or across the calvaria 经颅盖的

trans·cath·e·ter (trans-kath′ə-tər) performed through the lumen of a catheter 经导管的

trans·co·bal·a·min (TC) (trans″ko-bal′ə-min) any of three plasma proteins (transcobalamins Ⅰ, Ⅱ, and Ⅲ) that bind and transport cobalamin (vitamin B₁₂) 钴胺传递蛋白，三种血浆蛋白（转钴胺素Ⅰ、转钴胺素Ⅱ和转钴胺素Ⅲ）中的任何一种，它们结合并运载钴胺（维生素 B₁₂）

trans·cor·ti·cal (trans-kor′tĭ-kəl) connecting two parts of the cerebral cortex 经皮质的

trans·cor·tin (trans-kor′tin) an α-globulin that binds and transports biologically active, unconjugated cortisol in plasma 皮质激素传递蛋白，一种 α-球蛋白，结合并运输血浆中具有生物活性、游离的皮质醇

trans·cra·ni·al (trans-kra′ne-əl) performed through the cranium 经颅的

trans·cript (trans′kript) a strand of nucleic acid that has been synthesized using another nucleic acid strand as a template 转录本，以另一条核酸链作为模板合成的核酸链

trans·crip·tase (trans-krip′tās) a DNA-directed RNA polymerase; an enzyme that catalyzes the synthesis (polymerization) of RNA from ribonucleoside triphosphates, with DNA serving as a template 转录酶，一种 DNA 指导的 RNA 聚合酶；一种催化以 DNA 作为模板，核糖核苷三磷酸腺苷为原料合成 RNA 的酶；**reverse t.**，逆转录酶，RNA 指导的 DNA 聚合酶，参见 R.

trans·crip·tion (trans-krip′shən) the synthesis of RNA using a DNA template, catalyzed by an RNA polymerase; the base sequences of the RNA and DNA are complementary 转录，利用聚合酶催化 DNA 模板合成 RNA 的过程；其中生成的 RNA 和模板 DNA 的碱基序列是互补的；**reverse t.**, the synthesis of a DNA molecule complementary to an RNA molecule, the RNA acting as a template; catalyzed by reverse transcriptase 反转录，逆转录，以 RNA 为模板，由转录酶催化合成与 RNA 分子互补的 DNA 分子

trans·crip·tome (trans-krip′tōm) the complete population of mRNA transcripts produced by a genome 转录物组，由基因组转录产生的全部 mRNA 分子

trans·cu·ta·ne·ous (trans″ku-ta′ne-əs) 同 transdermal

trans·der·mal (trans-dur′məl) entering through the dermis, or skin, as in administration of a drug via ointment or patch 经皮的

trans·dif·fer·en·ti·a·tion (trans-dif″ər-en″shea′shən) the irreversible conversion of differentiated cells of one type to normal cells of another type 转分化，横向分化，一种类型的细胞分化为另一种类型的细胞，通常不可逆

trans·du·cer (trans-doo′sər) a device that translates

one form of energy to another, e.g., the pressure, temperature, or pulse to an electrical signal 换能器，将一种形式的能量转换为另一种形式能量的装置，如将压力、温度或脉冲电流转化为电信号；**neuroendocrine t.**, a neuron, such as a neurohypophyseal neuron, that on stimulation secretes a hormone, thereby translating neural information into hormonal information 神经内分泌换能器，兼具神经和腺体特性的神经元，例如神经垂体神经元，受刺激时产生分泌激素，从而将神经信息转化为激素信息

trans·du·cin (trans-doo′sin) a G protein of the disk membrane of the retinal rods that interacts with activated rhodopsin and participates in the triggering of a nerve impulse in vision 转导蛋白，视网膜杆盘膜上的种 G 蛋白，其与活化的视紫红质相互作用并参与触发视觉冲动

trans·duc·tion (trans-duk′shən) 1. the transfer of genetic information from one bacterium to another via a bacteriophage vector 转导，遗传信息通过噬菌体载体从一种细菌转移到另一种细菌；2. the transforming of one form of energy into another, as by the sensory mechanisms of the body 能量转换，如通过机体的感觉机制，将一种能量形式转化为另一种形式；**sensory t.**, the process by which a sensory receptor converts a stimulus from the environment to an action potential for transmission to the brain 感觉转导，感觉感受器将环境中的刺激转化为动作电位传递给大脑的过程

trans·du·ral (trans-doo′rəl) through or across the dura mater 经硬膜的

tran·sec·tion (tran-sek′shən) a cross-section; division by cutting transversely 横断

trans·esoph·a·ge·al (trans″ə-sof″ə-je′əl) through or across the esophagus 经食道的

trans·eth·moi·dal (trans-eth-moi′dəl) performed across or through the ethmoid bone 经筛骨的

trans·fec·tion (trans-fek′shən) originally, the artificial infection of bacterial cells by uptake of viral nucleic acid, resulting in the production of mature virus particles. Now it includes any means of artificial introduction of foreign DNA into cultured eukaryotic cells; stable integration of the DNA into the recipient genome may be denoted *stable t.* 转染，既往是指人工感染细菌细胞通过摄取病毒核酸，产生成熟的病毒颗粒；现指任何将外来 DNA 人工导入培养的真核细胞的方法。DNA 与受体基因组的稳定整合称为稳定转染

trans·fem·o·ral (trans-fem′ə-rəl) 1. across or through the femur 经股的；2. through the femoral artery 经股动脉

trans·fer (trans′fər) the taking or moving of something from one place to another 转 移；**gamete intrafallopian t. (GIFT)**, retrieval of oocytes from the ovary, followed by laparoscopic placement of the oocytes and sperm in the fallopian tubes; used in the treatment of infertility 输卵管内配子移植术，从卵巢取出卵母细胞，然后用腹腔镜将卵母细胞和精子植入输卵管，用来治疗不孕；**passive t.**, the conferring of immunity to a nonimmune host by injection of antibody or lymphocytes from an immune or sensitized donor 被动转移，通过注射抗体或淋巴细胞赋予非免疫宿主免疫力；**tubal embryo t. (TET)**, 胚胎输卵管内移植 1. retrieval of oocytes from the ovary, fertilization and culture in vitro, and then laparoscopic placement of resulting embryos in the fallopian tubes more than 24 hours after oocyte retrieval; used in the treatment of infertility 从卵巢中取出卵母细胞，并在体外受精和培养，在卵母细胞取出超过24h后用腹腔镜将胚胎置于输卵管中；2. laparoscopic transfer of cryopreserved embryos to the fallopian tubes 将冷冻保存的胚胎经腹腔镜转移至输卵管；**zygote intrafallopian t. (ZIFT)**, retrieval of oocytes from the ovary, fertilization and culture in vitro, and then laparoscopic placement of the resulting zygotes in the fallopian tubes 24 hours after oocyte retrieval; used in the treatment of infertility 输卵管内合子移植术，从卵巢中取出卵母细胞，并在体外受精和培养，在卵母细胞取出超过24h后用腹腔镜将所得胚胎置于输卵管中，用于治疗不孕

trans·fer·ase (trans′fər-ās) a class of enzymes that transfer a chemical group from one compound to another 转移酶

trans·fer·ence (trans-fer′əns) in psychotherapy, the unconscious tendency to assign to others in one's present environment feelings and attitudes associated with significance in one's early life, especially the patient's transfer to the therapist of feelings and attitudes associated with a parent 移情，在心理治疗中，存在一种无意识的倾向，即患者将自己早年生活中与重要意义相关的情感和态度分配给所处环境中的其他人，特别是患者将与父母相关的情感和态度转移给治疗师；**counter t.**, 反向移情，参见 *countertransference*

trans·fer·rin (trans-fer′in) a glycoprotein mainly produced in the liver, binding and transporting iron, closely related to the *apoferritin* of the intestinal mucosa 转铁球蛋白，运铁蛋白，一种主要在肝脏中产生，结合并运输铁，与肠黏膜上的去铁蛋白密切相关的糖蛋白

trans·fix·ion (trans-fik′shən) a cutting through from within outward, as in amputation 切断术，从内而外地切断，如截肢

trans·for·ma·tion (trans″for-ma′shən) 1. change of form or structure; conversion from one form to another 变形，转化，转形变异，形式或结构的变化，即从一种形式转换为另一种形式；2. in oncology, the change that a normal cell undergoes as it becomes malignant 在肿瘤学中，正常细胞向癌细胞的演变；3. in eukaryotes, the conversion of normal cells to malignant cells in cell culture 在真核生物中，细胞培养中正常细胞向恶性细胞的转化；4. 同 bacterial t.；**bacterial t.**, the exchange of genetic material between strains of bacteria by the transfer of a fragment of naked DNA from a donor cell to a recipient cell, followed by recombination in the recipient chromosome 细菌转化，通过将裸DNA 片段从供体细胞转移到受体细胞，随后在受体染色体中重组，以此在细菌菌株之间交换遗传物质

trans·fron·tal (trans-frun′təl) through the frontal bone 经额的

trans·fu·sion (trans-fu′zhən) the introduction of whole blood or blood components directly into the bloodstream 输血；**direct t.**, 同 immediate t.；**exchange t.**, repetitive withdrawal of small amounts of blood and replacement with donor blood, until a large proportion of the original volume has been replaced 交换输血，换血输血，重复抽取少量血液并用供体血液替代，直至更新原始血液的大部分；**immediate t.**, transfer of blood directly from a vessel of the donor to a vessel of the recipient 直接输血，将血液直接从供者的血管转移到受血者的血管；**indirect t., mediate t.**, introduction of blood that has been stored in a suitable container after withdrawal from the donor 间接输血，引入从供体中取出后储存在合适容器中的血液；**placental t.**, return to an infant after birth, through the intact umbilical cord, of the blood contained in the placenta 胎盘输血，分娩后将残留胎盘中的血液通过脐带回输到新生儿体内；**replacement t., substitution t.**, 同 exchange t.；**twin-to-twin t.**, an abnormality of fetal circulation occurring between two monozygotic twins, in which blood is shunted directly from one twin to the other 孪生输血，一卵双生胎中的胎循环异常，血液直接由一个胎儿分流至另一个胎儿

trans·gene (trans′jēn) a segment of recombinant DNA that has been transferred from one genome to another; sometimes specifically one that has been integrated into the germline of the recipient and is transmissible 转基因，来自一个基因组的DNA 片段剪接到不同基因组DNA 片段上，有时专指已经被整合到接受者的种系中并且具有遗传特性的DNA；**transgen′ic** *adj.*

trans·glu·tam·in·ase (trans″gloo-tam′in-ās) an

enzyme, formed by cleavage and activation of pro-transglutaminase, which forms stabilizing covalent bonds within fibrin strands. It is the activated form of coagulation factor Ⅹ Ⅲ 转谷氨酰胺酶

trans·il·i·ac (trans-il′e-ak) across the two ilia 经髂骨的

trans·il·lu·mi·na·tion (trans″ĭ-loo″mĭ-na′shən) the passage of strong light through a body structure, to permit inspection by an observer on the opposite side 透照法

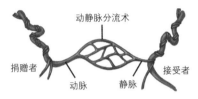

动静脉分流术

捐赠者　　动脉　　静脉　　接受者

▲ 单绒毛膜双胞胎在共用胎盘中通过动静脉分流进行双胎血液输送

tran·si·tion (tran-zĭ′shən) 1. a passage or change from one state or condition to another 过渡；2. in molecular genetics, a point mutation in which a purine base replaces a pyrimidine base or vice versa 转换在分子遗传学中，嘌呤碱基取代嘧啶碱基或嘧啶碱基取代嘌呤碱基的点突变；**transi′tional** *adj.*

trans·la·tion (trans-la′shən) 1. conversion or transformation 转化，转移；2. in genetics, the process by which the series of codons in a messenger RNA (mRNA) is converted to the ordered sequence of amino acids that constitutes a specific polypeptide chain 翻译，转译，在遗传学中，mRNA 中的一系列密码子被转化为具有特定多肽链的有序氨基酸序列的过程，**nick t.**, a process by which radiolabeled nucleotides are incorporated into duplex DNA at single-strand nicks or cleavage points created enzymatically along its two strands 切口平移，切口移位，放射性标记的核苷酸掺入双链 DNA 中的过程，常从双链切口或沿酶促链产生的切割点掺入

trans·lo·case (trans-lo′kās) transport protein 移位酶

trans·lo·ca·tion (trans″lo-ka′shən) 1. movement of a substance from one place to another 移位，物质从一个地方到另一个地方的运动；2. movement of the ribosome from one codon to the next along the messenger RNA (mRNA) in protein synthesis 核糖体沿着合成蛋白质的 mRNA 从一个密码子到另一个密码子的运动；3. the transfer of a fragment of one chromosome to a nonhomologous chromosome. Abbreviated t 易位，将一条染色体的片段转到非同源染色体上，缩写为 t；**reciprocal t.(rcp)**,

the complete mutual exchange of fragments between two broken nonhomologous chromosomes 相互易位，两个断裂的非同源染色体之间染色体片段的完全相互交换；**robertsonian t.**, translocation involving two acrocentric chromosomes, which fuse at the centromere region and lose their short arms 罗伯逊易位，端点着丝粒易位，主要指两个近端着丝粒染色体的融合，它们在着丝粒区域融合并失去短臂

trans·lo·con (tranz-lo′kon) a complex of proteins in the membrane of the endoplasmic reticulum, through which nascent polypeptides pass during protein synthesis 易位子，转运体，易位蛋白质

trans·lu·mi·nal (trans-loo′mĭ-nəl) through or across a lumen, particularly of a blood vessel 经腔的，特别指经过血管腔

trans·man·dib·u·lar (trans″man-dib′u-lər) through or across the mandible 经下颌的

trans·mem·brane (trans-mem′brān) crossing a membrane 透膜的

trans·meth·y·la·tion (trans″məth-ə-la′shən) the transfer of a methyl group (CH_3) from one compound to another 甲基转移作用

trans·mis·si·ble (trans-mis′ĭ-bəl) capable of being transmitted 可传播的

trans·mis·sion (trans-mish′ən) 1. the transfer, as of a disease, from one person to another 传播；2. the communication of genetic traits from parent to offspring 传递，从父母到后代的基因特征的传递；**horizontal t.**, the spread of infection from one individual to another, usually through contact with bodily excretions or fluids containing the pathogen 水平传播，传染病从一个人传播到另一个人，通常是通过接触身体排泄物或含有病原体的液体而传播；**vertical t.**, transmission from one generation to another. The term is restricted by some to genetic transmission and extended by others to include transmission of infection from one generation to the next, as by maternal milk or through the placenta 垂直传播，有学者将其局限于遗传传播，也将其扩展到包括感染的代代相传，如通过母乳或胎盘的传播

trans·mu·co·sal (trans″mu-ko′səl) entering through, or across, a mucous membrane 转化黏液质的

trans·mu·ral (trans-mu′rəl) through the wall of an organ; extending through or affecting the entire thickness of the wall of an organ or cavity 透壁的

trans·mu·ta·tion (trans″mu-ta′shən) 1. evolutionary change of one species into another 衍变，进化过程中物种的演变；2. the change of one chemical element into another 蜕变，一种元素成为另一种

元素的变化

trans·neu·ro·nal (trans-noor′ə-nəl) between or across neurons 经神经元的

trans·par·ent (trans-par′ənt) permitting the passage of rays of light, so that objects may be seen through the substance 透明的

trans·phos·phor·y·la·tion (trans-fos″for-ə- la′shən) the exchange of phosphate groups between organic phosphates, without their going through the stage of inorganic phosphates 磷酸转移作用

tran·spi·ra·tion (tran″spī-ra′shən) discharge of air, vapor, or sweat through the skin 不显性出汗

trans·pla·cen·tal (trans″plə-sen′təl) through the placenta 经胎盘的

trans·plant[1] (trans′plant) 1. graft: an organ or tissue taken from the body for grafting into another area of the same body or into another individual 移植物，移植片；2. 同 transplantation

trans·plant[2] (trans-plant′) to transfer tissue from one part to another 移植

trans·plan·ta·tion (trans″plan-ta′shən) the grafting of tissues taken from the patient's own body or from another 移植术；**allogeneic t.**, allotransplantation; transplantation of an allograft; it may be from a cadaveric, living related, or living unrelated donor 同种异体移植术；**bone marrow t. (BMT)**, intravenous infusion of autologous, syngeneic, or allogeneic bone marrow or stem cells 骨髓移植；**heterotopic t.**, transplantation of tissue typical of one area to a different recipient site 异位移植术；**homotopic t., orthotopic t.**, transplantation of tissue from a donor into its normal anatomic position in the recipient 同位移植术，原位移植术；**stem cell t.**, infusion of new hematopoietic stem cells after therapeutic high-dose irradiation or chemotherapy has destroyed the patient's original ones 干细胞移植；**syngeneic t.**, transplantation of a syngraft 同质移植术；**xenogeneic t.**, transplantation of a xenograft 异种移植术

trans·port (trans′port) movement of materials in biologic systems, particularly into and out of cells and across epithelial layers 转运，生物系统中的物质的运动，尤指进出细胞和跨越上皮质的运动；**active t.**, the movement of substances across the cell membrane, usually up a concentration gradient, produced by the expenditure of metabolic energy 主动转运，主动运输，物质的跨膜运动，通常是逆浓度梯度的，需要消耗代谢能量；**passive t.**, the movement of substances, usually across cell membranes, by processes not requiring expenditure of metabolic energy 被动转运，通常指通过不需要消耗代谢能量的方式穿过细胞膜

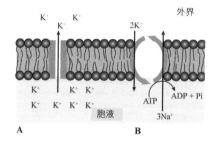

▲ 被动转运和主动转运示例（A）被动转运：钾离子通过特定的离子通道沿着浓度梯度扩散穿过质膜（B）主动转运：细胞钠泵利用三磷酸腺苷（ATP）水解在质膜上产生浓度梯度使得钠离子和钾离子穿过质膜

trans·pos·a·ble (trans-poz′ə-bəl) capable of being interchanged or put in a different place or order 转座的，可互换或放在不同的位置或顺序的

trans·po·si·tion (trans″po-zi′shən) 1. any of various congenital anomalies in which organs are displaced to the opposite side from normal 错位，反位，先天性异常中的任何一种，其中器官移位到正常位置的相反侧；2. the operation of carrying a tissue flap from one situation to another without severing its connection entirely until it is united at its new location 转位，将组织瓣移位至另一处；3. the exchange of position of two atoms within a molecule 换位，移位，分子内两个原子的位置交换；4. movement of genetic information from one locus to another, as via a transposable element 转座，通过转座因子将遗传信息从一个基因座移动到另一个基因座；**t. of great arteries, t. of great vessels**, a congenital cardiovascular malformation in which the position of the chief blood vessels of the heart is reversed. Life then depends on a crossflow of blood between the right and left sides of the heart, as through a ventricular septal defect 大动脉错位，大血管错位，是一种先天性心血管畸形，患者的生命活动依赖于心脏左右两侧的血液相互流动，例如通过室间隔缺损进行

trans·po·son (tranz-po′zon) a transposable element that carries additional genes besides merely those for transposition, particularly a complex one occurring in prokaryotes. Sometimes used interchangeably with *transposable element* 转座子，一种除了携带用于转位的基因外，还可携带其他基因的转位因子，尤指发生在原核生物中的复杂基因；有时与转座因子互换使用

trans·pu·bic (trans-pu′bik) performed through the pubic bone after removal of a segment of the bone 经耻骨的

trans·sa·cral (tran-sa′krəl) through or across the sacrum 经骶骨的

trans·seg·men·tal (tran″səg-men′təl) extending across segments 经肢节的

trans·sep·tal (tran-sep′təl) extending or performed through or across a septum 经中隔的

trans·sex·u·al·ism (tran-sek′shoo-əl-iz-əm) 1. the most severe manifestation of gender identity disorder in adults, being a prolonged, persistent desire to relinquish their primary and secondary sex characteristics and acquire those of the opposite sex 易性癖；2. the state of being a transsexual 易性癖的状态

trans·tha·lam·ic (trans″thə-lam′ik) across the thalamus 经丘脑的，横过丘脑的

trans·tho·rac·ic (trans″thə-ras′ik) through the thoracic cavity or across the chest wall 经胸腔的

trans·thy·re·tin (trans″thi-ret′in) an α-globulin secreted by the liver that transports retinol-binding protein and thyroxine in the blood. Numerous mutations have been associated with the ATTR form of familial amyloidosis 甲状腺素视黄质运载蛋白，一种由肝脏分泌的 α-球蛋白，在血液中转运视黄醇结合蛋白和甲状腺素；其许多突变与家族性淀粉样变性的 ATTR 形式有关

trans·tib·i·al (trans-tib′e-əl) across or through the tibia 经胫骨的

trans·tym·pan·ic (trans″tim-pan′ik) across the tympanic membrane or cavity 经鼓室的

tran·su·date (trans′u-dāt) a fluid substance that has passed through a membrane or has been extruded from a tissue; in contrast to an exudate, it is of high fluidity and has a low content of protein, cells, or solid materials derived from cells 漏出液，一种通过膜或从组织中排出的流体物质，与渗出液相比，它具有高流动性、蛋白质、细胞或来自细胞的固体物质等含量少

trans·ure·thral (trans″u-re′thrəl) performed through the urethra 经尿道的

trans·vag·i·nal (trans-vaj′ĭ-nəl) through the vagina 经阴道的

trans·ve·nous (trans-ve′nəs) performed or inserted through a vein 经静脉的

trans·ver·sa·lis (trans″vər-sa′lis) [L.] 同 transverse 横的；横肌

trans·verse (trans-vurs′) placed crosswise; at right angles to the long axis 横向的

trans·ver·sec·to·my (trans″vər-sek′tə-me) excision of a transverse process of a vertebra 椎骨横突切除术

trans·ver·sion (trans-vur′zhən) 1. displacement of a tooth from its proper numerical position in the jaw 易位牙；2. in molecular genetics, a point mutation in which a purine base replaces a pyrimidine base or vice versa 颠换，分子遗传学中的点突变，即一嘌呤碱基取代一嘧啶碱基或反之

trans·ver·sus (trans-vur′səs) [L.] 同 transverse 横的；横肌

trans·ves·i·cal (trans-ves′ĭ-kəl) through the bladder 经膀胱的

trans·ves·tism (trans-ves′tiz-əm) 1. the practice of wearing articles of clothing and assuming the appearance, manner, or roles of the opposite sex 异装癖；2. transvestic fetishism 易物癖

tran·yl·cy·pro·mine (tran″əl-si′pro-mēn) a monoamine oxidase inhibitor; the sulfate salt is used as an antidepressant and in the prophylaxis of migraine 反苯环丙胺，一种单胺氧化酶抑制药，其硫酸盐用作抗抑郁药并用于预防偏头痛

tra·pe·zi·al (trə-pe′ze-əl) pertaining to a trapezium 斜方形的

tra·pe·zi·um (trə-pe′ze-əm) [L.] 1. an irregular, four-sided figure 斜方形；2. the most lateral bone of the distal row of carpal bones 大多角骨

trap·e·zoid (trap′ə-zoid) 1. having the shape of a four-sided plane, with two sides parallel and two diverging 斜方形的；2. trapezoid bone 小多角骨

tras·tuz·u·mab (tras-tuz′u-mab) a monoclonal antibody that binds to a protein overexpressed in some breast cancers; used as an antineoplastic in the treatment of metastatic breast cancer with such overexpression 群伏珠单抗，一种可与某些乳腺癌中过表达的蛋白结合单克隆抗体，用于治疗转移性乳腺癌

trau·ma (traw′mə) (trou′mə) pl. *traumas, trau′mata* [Gr.] 1. injury 创伤，外伤；2. psychological or emotional damage 精神创伤；**traumat′ic** *adj.*；**birth t.,** 1. an injury to the infant during the process of being born 产伤；2. the psychic shock produced in an infant by the experience of being born 出生创伤；**psychic t.,** a psychologically upsetting experience that produces a mental disorder or otherwise has lasting negative effects on a person's thoughts, feelings, or behavior 精神创伤

trau·ma·tism (traw′mə-tiz-əm) 1. the physical or psychic state resulting from an injury or wound 创伤病，外伤病；2. a wound or injury 伤口，损伤

trau·ma·tol·o·gy (traw″mə-tol′ə-je) the branch of surgery dealing with wounds and disability from injuries 创伤学

trav·o·prost (trav′o-prost) a synthetic prostaglandin analogue used in the treatment of elevated intraocular pressure in open-angle glaucoma or ocular hypertension 曲伏前列素，一种合成的前列腺素类似物，用于治疗开角型青光眼患者的高眼压

tray (tra) a flat-surfaced utensil for the conveyance

of various objects or material 托盘；**impression t.**, a contoured container to hold the material for making an impression of the teeth and associated structures 印模托盘，一种用于容纳对牙齿和相关结构进行印模的材料的成形容器

tra·zo·done (tra′zo-dōn) an antidepressant, used as the hydrochloride salt to treat major depressive episodes with or without prominent anxiety 曲唑酮，一种抗抑郁药，盐酸曲唑酮用来治疗伴或不伴明显焦虑的重度抑郁发作

treat·ment (trēt′mənt) management and care of a patient or the combating of disease or disorder 治疗，疗法；**active t.**, that directed immediately to the cure of the disease or injury 直接疗法，积极疗法；**causal t.**, treatment directed against the cause of a disease 病因疗法；**conservative t.**, that designed to avoid radical medical therapeutic measures or operative procedures 保守疗法；**empirical t.**, treatment by means that experience has proved to be beneficial 经验疗法；**expectant t.**, treatment directed toward relief of untoward symptoms, leaving cure of the disease to natural forces 期待疗法；**palliative t.**, treatment designed to relieve pain and distress with no attempt to cure 姑息疗法；**preventive t., prophylactic t.**, that in which the aim is to prevent the occurrence of the disease; prophylaxis 预防疗法；**specific t.**, treatment particularly adapted to the disease being treated 特效治疗；**supportive t.**, treatment that is mainly directed to sustaining the strength of the patient 支持疗法；**symptomatic t.** 同 expectant t.

tree (tre) an anatomic structure with branches resembling a tree 树；**bronchial t.**, the bronchi and their branching structures 支气管树；**dendritic t.**, the branching arrangement of a dendrite 树突的树；**tracheobronchial t.** the trachea, bronchi, and their branching structures 气管支气管树

Trem·a·to·da (trem″ə-to′də) the flukes, a class of Platyhelminthes; they are parasitic in humans and other animals, infection usually resulting from ingestion of inadequately cooked fish, crustaceans, or vegetation containing their larvae 吸虫纲

trem·a·tode (trem′ə-tōd) an individual of the class Trematoda 吸虫

trem·or (trem′ər) an involuntary trembling or quivering 震颤；**action t.**, rhythmic, oscillatory, involuntary movements of the outstretched upper limb; it may also affect the voice and other parts 动作性震颤，伸展的肢体有节奏地、不自主地震颤，也可能影响声音和身体其他部分；**coarse t.**, one in which the vibrations are slow 粗大震颤；**essential t.**, a hereditary tremor with onset usually at about 50 years of age, beginning with a fine rapid tremor of the hands, followed by tremor of the head, tongue, limbs, and trunk 特发性震颤，通常在50岁左右发病，发作时从手的快速震颤开始，后累及头部、舌头、四肢和躯干；**fine t.**, one in which the vibrations are rapid 频细震颤；**flapping t.**, asterixis 扑翼样震颤；**intention t.**, action t. 意向震颤；**parkinsonian t.**, the resting tremor seen with parkinsonism, consisting of slow regular movements of the hands and sometimes the legs, neck, face, or jaw; it typically stops upon voluntary movement of the part and is intensified by stimuli such as cold, fatigue, and strong emotions 震颤性麻痹，帕金森病中所见的静止性震颤，包括缓慢规则的手震颤，有时也包括腿、颈、睑和下颌的震颤，以上部位有自主性运动时震颤停止，当受寒冷、饥饿和强烈的精神刺激时震颤加剧；**physiologic t.**, a rapid tremor of extremely low amplitude found in the legs and sometimes the neck or face of normal individuals; it may become accentuated and visible under certain conditions 生理性震颤，低振幅的快速震颤，见于正常人的腿部，有时见于颈部或面部；**pill-rolling t.**, a parkinsonian tremor of the hand consisting of a flexion and extension of the fingers in connection with adduction and abduction of the thumb 捻丸样震颤，手部的麻痹性震颤，包括手指的屈曲和伸展动作，与拇指的内收和外展动作相关；**resting t.**, tremor occurring in a relaxed and supported limb or other bodily part; it is sometimes abnormal, as in parkinsonism 静止性震颤，肢体休息时发生的震颤，有时是非正常的，常见于帕金森病；**senile t.** that due to the infirmities of old age 老年震颤；**volitional t.**, action t. 意向性震颤

trem·u·lous (trem′u-ləs) pertaining to or characterized by tremors 震颤的

treph·i·na·tion (tref″ĭ-na′shən) the operation of trephining 环钻术

tre·phine (trə-fīn′) (trə-fēn′) 1. a crown saw for removing a disk of bone, chiefly from the skull 环钻，一种用来锯去骨头的冠锯，主要用于锯颅骨；2. an instrument for removing a circular area of cornea 角膜移植术时在角膜上钻取圆形所用的器具；3. to remove with a trephine 以环钻施行手术

trep·i·dant (trep′ĭ-dənt) tremulous 震颤性的

trep·i·da·tion (trep″ĭ-da′shən) 1. tremor 震颤，抖颤；2. nervous anxiety and fear 悸惧；**trep′idant adj.**

Trep·o·ne·ma (trep″o-ne′mə) a genus of gramnegative, microaerophilic, motile, spiral bacteria of the family Spirochaetaceae, often pathogenic and parasitic; it includes the etiologic agents of pinta (*T. cara′teum*), syphilis (*T. pal′lidum* subspecies *pal′l-idum*), and yaws (*T. pal′lidum* subspecies *perte′nue*) 密螺旋体属，螺旋体目密螺旋科所属细菌，为

革兰阴性螺旋形微需氧微生物，具有致病性和寄生性，包括品他病（品他密螺旋体），梅毒（苍白密螺旋体苍白亚种）和雅司病（苍白密螺旋体细弱密螺旋体亚种）的病原菌

trep·o·ne·ma (trep″o-ne′mə) an organism of the genus *Treponema* 密螺旋体；**trepone′mal** *adj*.

trep·o·ne·ma·to·sis (trep″o-ne-mə-to′sis) infection with *Treponema* 密螺旋体病

tre·pop·nea (tre″pop-ne′ə) dyspnea that is relieved when the patient is in the lateral recumbent position 转卧呼吸，取卧位时最舒适的呼吸状态

trep·pe (trep′ə) [Ger.] the gradual increase in muscular contraction following rapidly repeated stimulation 阶梯现象，肌肉经快速反复刺激后收缩幅度逐渐增加的现象

tret·i·noin (tret′ĭ-noin″) the all-*trans* stereoisomer of retinoic acid, used as a topical keratolytic in the treatment of acne vulgaris and disorders of keratinization and administered orally in the treatment of acute promyelocytic leukemia 全反维生素 A 酸，维甲酸，用于治疗寻常痤疮、角质化紊乱和急性早幼粒细胞白血病

TRH thyrotropin-releasing hormone 促甲状腺激素释放激素

tri·ac·e·tin (tri-as′ə-tin) an antifungal agent used topically in the treatment of superficial fungal infections of the skin 三乙酰甘油，乙酸甘油酯，一种抗真菌药，局部用药治疗皮肤浅表真菌感染

tri·ad (tri′ad) 1. any trivalent element 三价元素；2. a group of three associated entities or objects 三征，三联三联征；**Beck t.,** rising venous pressure, falling arterial pressure, and small quiet heart; characteristic of cardiac tamponade 贝克三体征，静脉压升高、动脉压下降、心音遥远，属于心脏压塞的特征；**Currarino t.,** 参见 *syndrome* 下词条；**Cushing t.,** decreased pulse, increased blood pressure, and a widening pulse pressure associated with increased intracranial pressure; it is a late clinical sign and may indicate brainstem herniation 库欣三联征，与颅内压增高相关的脉搏减慢、血压升高、脉压增大，为晚期临床症状，可提示脑干疝形成；**Hutchinson t.,** diffuse interstitial keratitis, labyrinthine disease, and Hutchinson teeth, seen in congenital syphilis 哈钦森三联征，弥漫性间质性角膜炎、迷路疾病和哈钦森齿，见于先天性梅毒；**Saint t.,** hiatal hernia, colonic diverticula, and cholelithiasis 圣氏三联征，食管裂孔疝、结肠憩室和胆石症同时发生

tri·age (tre-ahzh′) (tre′ahzh) [Fr.] 1. the sorting out of casualties of war or other disaster to determine priority of need and proper place of treatment 伤员鉴别分类，对战伤或其他灾难造成的伤员进行甄别分类，从而决定哪些优先处理和送往何处治疗为宜；2. by extension, the sorting and prioritizing of nonemergency patients for treatment 分诊

tri·al (tri′əl) (trīl) a test or experiment 试用，试验；**clinical t.,** an experiment performed on human beings in order to evaluate the comparative efficacy of two or more therapies 临床试验

tri·am·cin·o·lone (tri″am-sin′ə-lōn) a synthetic glucocorticoid used in replacement therapy for adrenocortical insufficiency and as an antiinflammatory and immunosuppressant in a wide variety of disorders 氟羟强的松龙，一种合成糖皮质激素，用于肾上腺皮质功能不全的替代治疗，并作为抗炎和免疫抑制药治疗多种疾病

tri·am·ter·ene (tri-am′tər-ēn) a potassium-sparing diuretic that blocks the reabsorption of sodium in the distal convoluted tubules; used in the treatment of edema and hypertension 氨苯蝶啶，一种可阻止钠在远曲小管中的重吸收的保钾利尿药，用于治疗水肿和高血压

tri·an·gle (tri′ang-gəl) trigone; a three-cornered figure or area, such as one on the surface of the body 三角；**triang′ular** *adj.*；**anal t.,** the portion of the perineal region surrounding the anus 肛三角；**carotid t.,** the triangular region bounded by the posterior belly of the digastric muscle and the stylohyoid, the sternocleidomastoid muscle, and the superior belly of the omohyoid 颈动脉三角，由二腹肌的后腹部和甲状腺、胸锁乳突肌和舌骨肌的上腹部界定的三角区域；**cephalic t.,** one on the anteroposterior plane of the skull, between lines from the occiput to the forehead and to the chin, and from the chin to the forehead 头三角，在颅骨正后面上的三角，居枕骨及枕颏连线之间，第三边是从颏至前额的连线；**Codman t.,** a triangular area visible radiographically where the periosteum, elevated by a bone tumor, rejoins the cortex of normal bone Codman 三角，骨膜三角区，在放射学上可见的被骨肿瘤顶起的骨膜与正常骨皮质间的三角区；**digastric t.,** 同 submandibular t.；**t. of elbow,** in front, the supinator longus on the outside and pronator teres inside, the base toward the humerus 肘三角，外侧为肱桡肌，内侧为旋前圆肌，底为肱骨；**facial t.,** a triangle whose points are the basion and alveolar and nasal points 面三角，由颅府点、上齿槽前点和颅骨鼻根点所组成的三角；**Farabeuf t.,** a triangle in the upper part of the neck bounded by the internal jugular vein, the facial vein, and the hypoglossal nerve 法拉伯夫三角，颈上部三角，由颈内静脉、面静脉和作为底边的舌下神经组成的三角区域；**femoral t.,** the area formed superiorly by the inguinal ligament, laterally by the sartorius muscle, and medially by the adductor longus muscle 股三角，上部为腹股沟韧带，外侧为缝匠肌，

内侧为长内收肌构成的三角区域；**frontal t.,** a triangular area bounded by the maximum frontal diameter and the lines to the glabella 额三角，以最大额径和该直径两端与眉间的连线组成的三角区域；**Grynfeltt-Lesshaft t.,** 同 superior lumbar t.；**Hesselbach t.,** inguinal t. (1) 海氏三角；**iliofemoral t.,** a triangle formed by the Nélaton line, a second line through the superior iliac spine, and a third from this to the greater trochanter 布莱恩特三角，髂骨三角，由通过髂前上棘的 Nélaton 线和曲髂前上棘延伸至股骨大转子的线围成的三角区域；**infraclavicular t.,** one formed by the clavicle above, upper border of the pectoralis major on the inside, and anterior border of the deltoid on the outside 锁骨下三角，上侧为锁骨，内侧为胸大肌的上边界，外侧为三角肌的前边界组成的三角区域；**inguinal t.,** 1. the area on the inferoanterior abdominal wall bounded by the rectus abdominis muscle, inguinal ligament, and inferior epigastric vessels 腹股沟三角，下腹壁上由腹直肌、腹股沟韧带和腹壁下血管组成的三角区域；2. 同 femoral t.(1)；**t. of Koch,** a roughly triangular area on the septal wall of the right atrium, bounded by the right atrioventricular valve, coronary sinus orifice, and tendon of Todaro, that marks the site of the atrioventricular node 科赫三角，位于右心房隔膜壁，由三尖瓣的中隔瓣基部，冠状窦开口的前正中缘和托达罗腱组成的三角区域，标志着房室结的部位；**Langenbeck t.,** a triangular area whose apex is the anterior superior iliac spine, its base the anatomic neck of the femur, and its external side the external base of the greater trochanter Langenbeck 三角，股骨颈三角，顶端是髂前上棘，底部是股骨解剖颈，其外侧是大转子外侧的三角区域；**Lesser t.,** a triangle formed by the hypoglossal nerve above and the two bellies of the digastricus on the two sides 莱塞三角，由上方的舌下神经和两侧二腹肌两腹组成的三角区域；**lumbar t., inferior,** one between the inferolateral margin of the latissimus dorsi muscle and the external abdominal oblique muscles, just superior to the ilium 腰下三角，由髂骨上、背阔肌下缘与腹外斜肌的三角区域；**lumbar t., superior,** one bounded by the twelfth rib and the serratus posterior inferior, erector spinae, and internal abdominal oblique muscles 腰上三角，由第十二肋和下后锯肌、竖脊肌和腹内斜肌组成的三角区域；**lumbocostoabdominal t.,** one between the obliquus externus, the serratus posterior inferior, the erector spinae, and the obliquus internus 腰肋腹三角，腹外斜肌、下后锯肌、竖脊肌和内斜肌之间的间隙；**Macewen t.,** mastoid fossa 麦克尤恩三角，外耳道上三角；**occipital t.,** one having the sternomastoid in front, the trapezius behind, and the omohyoid below 枕三角，前界为胸锁乳突肌，后界为斜方肌，下界为肩胛舌骨肌下腹；**occipital t., inferior,** one having a line between the two mastoid processes as its base and the inion its apex 枕下三角，以两乳突的连线为底，枕骨隆突作为顶点形成的三角区域；**omoclavicular t.,** 同 subclavian t.；**Petit t.,** 同 inferior lumbar t.；**Scarpa t.,** 同 femoral t.；**subclavian t.,** a deep region of the neck: the triangular area bounded by the clavicle, sternocleidomastoid, and omohyoid 肩锁三角，颈深区，以锁骨、胸锁乳突肌和舌骨肌为界形成的三角形区域；**submandibular t., submaxillary t.,** the triangular region of the neck bounded by the mandible, the stylohyoid muscle and posterior belly of the digastric muscle, and the anterior belly of the digastric muscle 下颌三角，二腹肌三角；颈部的三角形区域，由下颌骨、舌骨肌和二腹肌的后腹部以及二腹肌的前腹部组成的三角区域；**suboccipital t.,** one between the rectus capitis posterior major and superior and inferior oblique muscles 枕下三角；**supraclavicular t.,** subclavian t. 锁骨上三角；**suprameatal t.,** mastoid fossa 道上三角
tri·an·gu·la·ris (tri-ang″gu-lar′is) [L.] triangular 三角的

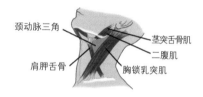

颈动脉三角
茎突舌骨肌
二腹肌
肩胛舌骨
胸锁乳突肌

▲　**颈动脉三角示意图**

Tri·at·o·ma (tri-at′o-mə) a genus of bugs (order Hemiptera), the cone-nosed bugs, important in medicine as vectors of *Trypanosoma cruzi* 锥蝽属
tri·atom·ic (tri″ə-tom′ik) containing three atoms 三原子的
tri·a·zo·lam (tri-a′zə-lam) a benzodiazepine used as a sedative and hypnotic in the treatment of insomnia 三唑苯二氮䓬，用于治疗失眠症的镇静催眠药
tri·a·zole (tri-a′zōl) (tri-a′zōl) 1. a five-membered heterocyclic ring containing two carbon and three nitrogen atoms 三唑；2. any of a class of antifungal compounds containing this structure 任何一种含有这种结构的抗真菌化合物
tribe (trīb) a taxonomic category subordinate to a family (or subfamily) and superior to a genus (or subtribe) 族（生物分类）
tri·bra·chi·us (tri-bra′ke-əs) 1. a fetus having three upper limbs 三臂畸胎；2. conjoined twins having only three upper limbs 三臂联胎

tri·ceph·a·lus (tri-sef'ə-ləs) a fetus with three heads. (tri-sef'ə-ləs) a fetus with three heads 三头畸胎

tri·ceps (tri'seps) three-headed, as a triceps muscle 三头的；三头肌的；参见 *muscle* 下词条

tri·chi·a·sis (trĭ-ki'ə-sis) 1. a condition of ingrowing hairs about an orifice, or ingrowing eyelashes 倒毛，倒睫；2. appearance of hairlike filaments in the urine 毛尿症

trich·i·lem·mal (trik″ĭ-lem'əl) pertaining to the outer root sheath 毛膜的

trich·i·lem·mo·ma (trik″ĭ-ləm-o'mə) a benign adnexal tumor of the lower outer root sheath of the hair 毛根鞘瘤

tri·chi·na (trĭ-ki'nə) pl. *trichi'nae*. an individual organism of the genus *Trichinella* 毛线虫

Trich·i·nel·la (trik″ĭ-nel'ə) a genus of nematode parasites, including *T. spira'lis,* the etiologic agent of trichinosis, found in the muscles of rats, pigs, and humans 毛线虫属

trich·i·no·sis (trik″ĭ-no'sis) a disease due to eating inadequately cooked meat infected with *Trichinella spiralis,* attended by diarrhea, nausea, colic, and fever, and later by stiffness, pain, muscle swelling, fever, sweating, eosinophilia, circumorbital edema, and splinter hemorrhages 旋毛虫病，毛线球病

trich·i·nous (trik'ĭ-nəs) affected with or containing trichinae 含旋毛虫的

tri·chlor·me·thi·a·zide (tri-klor″mə-thi'ə- zīd) a thiazide diuretic used in the treatment of hypertension and edema 三氯甲噻嗪，一种噻嗪类利尿药，用于治疗高血压和水肿

tri·chlo·ro·ace·tic ac·id (tri-klor″o-ə-se'tik) an extremely caustic acid, used in clinical chemistry to precipitate proteins and applied topically in chemabrasion and to remove warts 三氯乙酸，一种极碱酸，临床化学中用作蛋白质沉淀剂，也用作腐蚀剂去除皮疣

tri·chlo·ro·eth·y·lene (tri-klor″o-eth'ə-lēn) a clear, mobile liquid used as an industrial solvent; formerly used as an inhalant anesthetic 三氯乙烯，一种用作工业溶剂的透明流动液体，曾用作吸入性麻醉剂

tricho·ad·e·no·ma (trik″o-ad″ə-no'mə) a benign adnexal tumor on the face or trunk, with large cystic spaces lined by squamous epithelium and squamous cells 毛发腺瘤

tricho·be·zoar (trik″o-be'zor) a concretion within the stomach or intestines formed of hairs 毛石

tricho·blas·to·ma (trik″o-blas-to'mə) any of a large group of benign adnexal tumors that differentiate toward hair germ epithelium 透明性毛基细胞瘤

Tricho·der·ma (trik″o-dur'mə) [*tricho-* + Gr. *derma* skin] a genus of anamorphic fungi found in soil, wood, and decaying vegetation, with corresponding teleomorphs in *Hypocrea*. *T. longibrachia'tum* and other species are opportunistic pathogens 木霉属

tricho·dis·co·ma (trik″o-dis-ko'mə) a benign adnexal tumor arising from the mesodermal portion of the hair disk, probably a variety of fibrofolliculoma 毛盘状瘤

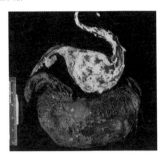

▲ 毛石，由胃腔内的毛发、食物和黏液组成的毛团

tricho·epi·the·li·o·ma (trik″o-ep″ĭ-the-leo'mə) a benign adnexal tumor originating in the hair follicles, usually on the face; it may occur as an inherited condition with multiple tumors *(multiple t.)* or as a noninherited solitary lesion *(solitary t.)* 毛发上皮瘤

tricho·es·the·sia (trik″o-es-the'zhə) the perception that one of the hairs of the skin has been touched, caused by stimulation of a hair follicle receptor 毛发感觉

tricho·fol·lic·u·lo·ma (trik″o-fə-lik″u-lo'mə) a benign, usually solitary, dome-shaped adnexal tumor with a central pore that frequently contains a hairlike tuft; it is derived from a hair follicle and is usually on the head or neck 毛囊瘤

tricho·glos·sia (trik″o-glos'e-ə) hairy tongue 毛舌

tri·chome (tri'kōm) a filamentous or hairlike structure 毛状体丝状

tricho·meg·a·ly (trik″o-meg'ə-le) elongation of the eyelashes 多毛病，长睫毛

tricho·mo·nad (trik″o-mo'nad) (trik″omon'ad) a parasite of the genus *Trichomonas* 毛滴虫

Tricho·mo·nas (trik″o-mo'nəs) a genus of flagellate protozoa. It includes *T. ho'minis,* a nonpathogenic human intestinal parasite, *T. te'nax,* a nonpathogenic species found in the human mouth, and *T. vagina'lis,* the cause of trichomoniasis 毛滴虫属；**trichomo'nal** *adj.*

tricho·mo·ni·a·sis (trik″o-mo-ni'ə-sis) infection by species of *Trichomonas,* usually in the vagina or male genital tract by *T. vagi'nalis,* with pruritus and a refractory discharge 毛滴虫病，滴虫病；

tricho·my·co·sis (trik″o-mi-ko′sis) any disease of the hair caused by fungi 毛发真菌病；**t. axilla′ris,** infection of axillary and sometimes pubic hair by *Corynebacterium tenuis,* a microorganism of uncertain affiliation, with colored clumps of bacteria on the hairs 腋毛真菌病

tricho·no·do·sis (trik″o-no-do′sis) a condition characterized by apparent or actual knotting of the hair 结节性脆发病

trich·op·a·thy (trī-kop′ə-the) 同 trichosis

tricho·phyt·ic (trik″o-fit′ik) pertaining to trichophytosis 发癣菌病的

tri·choph·y·tin (trī-kof′ĭ-tin) a filtrate from cultures of *Trichophyton;* used in testing for trichophytosis 发癣菌素

tricho·phy·to·be·zoar (trik″o-fi″to-be′zor) a bezoar composed of animal hair and vegetable fiber 毛植物石

Tri·choph·y·ton (tri-kof′ĭ-ton) a genus of filamentous, dermatophytic, anamorphic fungi that colonize keratinized tissues and may cause diseases of the skin, hair, and nails. It includes anthropophilic *(T. concern′tricum, T. ru′brum, T. schoenlei′nii, T. tonsu′rans, T. viola′ceum),* zoophilic *(T. si′mii, T. verruco′sum),* and geophilic species; the species *T. mentagrophy′tes* has both zoophilic and anthropophilic subgroups. Teleomorphs are classified in the genus *Arthroderma* 发癣菌属

tricho·phy·to·sis (trik″o-fi-to′sis) infection with fungi of the genus *Trichophyton* 发癣菌病，毛癣菌病

trich·op·ti·lo·sis (trik″o-tī-lo′sis) splitting of hairs at the end 毛发纵裂病

trich·or·rhex·is (trik″o-rek′sis) the condition in which the hairs break 脆发症；**t.nodo′sa,** a condition in which hairs fracture and split into strands with the appearance of nodes that can be easily broken 结节性脆发病

trich·os·chi·sis (trik-os′kĭ-sis) 同 trichoptilosis

tri·cho·sis (trī-ko′sis) any disease of the hair 毛发病，又称 *richopathy*

Tri·chos·po·ron (tri-kos′pə-ron) a genus of fungi that are normal flora of the respiratory and digestive tracts of humans and other animals and may infect the hair 毛孢子菌属

tricho·spo·ro·sis (trik″o-spə-ro′sis) infection with *Trichosporon* 毛孢子菌病，参见 *piedra*

tri·chos·ta·sis spin·u·lo·sa (trī-kos′tə-sis spin″-u-lo′sə) a condition in which the hair follicles contain a dark, horny plug that contains a bundle of vellus hair 小棘毛壅病

tricho·stron·gy·li·a·sis (trik″o-stron″jə-li′ə- sis) infection with *Trichostrongylus* 毛圆线虫病

Tricho·stron·gy·lus (trik″o-stron′jə-ləs) a genus of nematodes parasitic in animals and humans 毛圆线虫属

tricho·thio·dys·tro·phy (trik″o-thi″o-dis″trə- fe) any of several autosomal recessive disorders in which hair is sparse and brittle, has an unusually low sulfur content, and has a banded appearance under polarized light; ichthyotic skin and physical and intellectual disability are also present. The disorders are categorized on the basis of whether photosensitivity is also present 毛发硫营养不良

tricho·til·lo·ma·nia (trik″o-til″o-ma′ne-ə) compulsive pulling out of one's hair 拔毛狂，拔毛症

tri·chot·o·mous (tri-kot′ə-məs) divided into three parts 分三部的，三分法的

tri·chro·ism (tri′kro-iz-əm) the exhibition of three different colors in three different aspects 三色现象；**trichro′ic** *adj.*

tri·chro·ma·cy (tri-kro′mə-se) trichromatic vision 三色视

tri·chro·mat·ic (tri″kro-mat′ik) 1. pertaining to or exhibiting three colors 三色的，又称 *trichromic;* 2. able to distinguish three colors 三色视的，能够区分三原色（红、蓝、绿）的，有正常色觉的

trich·u·ri·a·sis (trik″u-ri′ə-sis) infection with *Trichuris,* often asymptomatic in adults but with gastrointestinal symptoms in children 鞭虫病

Tri·chu·ris (trī-ku′ris) the whipworms, a genus of intestinal nematode parasites. *T. trichiu′ra* causes trichuriasis in humans 鞭虫属

tri·cip·i·tal (tri-sip′ĭ-təl) 1. three-headed 三头的；2. relating to the triceps muscle 三头肌的

tri·cit·rates (tri-sit′rāts) a solution of sodium citrate, potassium citrate, and citric acid; used as a systemic or urinary alkalizer, antiurolithic, and neutralizing buffer 柠檬酸钠、柠檬酸钾和柠檬酸的混合溶液，可用作全身性尿碱化剂、抗尿路结石药和中和缓冲液

tri·cor·nute (tri-kor′nūt) having three horns, cornua, or processes 有三个角的，三突的

tri·cro·tism (tri′kro-tiz-əm) quality of having three sphygmographic waves or elevations to one beat of the pulse 三脉波；**tricrot′ic** *adj.*

tri·cus·pid (tri-kus′pid) having three points or cusps, as a valve of the heart 三尖的；三尖瓣的

tri·cyc·lic (tri-sik′lik) (-si′klik) containing three fused rings or closed chains in the molecular structure 三环的，在分子结构中含有三个融合环或闭合链的，另参见 *antidepressant* 下词条

tri·dac·ty·lism (tri-dak′tə-liz-əm) presence of only three digits on the hand or foot 三指（趾）畸形

tri·den·tate (tri-den′tāt) having three prongs 三叉的，三尖的

tri·der·mic (tri-dur′mik) derived from all three germ layers (ectoderm, endoderm, and mesoderm) 三胚层的（来自外胚层、内胚层和中胚层的）

tri·en·tene (tri′en-tēn) a chelating agent used as the hydrochloride salt for chelation of copper in the treatment of Wilson disease 一种螯合剂，其盐酸盐用于治疗威尔逊病

tri·fa·cial (tri-fa′shəl) designating the trigeminal (fifth cranial) nerve 三叉神经的

tri·fas·cic·u·lar (tri″fə-sik′u-lər) pertaining to three bundles, or fasciculi 三束的

tri·fid (tri′fid) split into three parts 三裂的

tri·flu·o·per·a·zine (tri-floo″o-per′ə-zēn) a phenothiazine derivative used as the hydrochloride salt as an antipsychotic 三氯拉嗪，一种吩噻嗪类化合物，其盐酸盐用作抗精神病药

tri·flur·i·dine (tri-floor′ĭ-dēn) an antiviral compound that interferes with viral DNA synthesis, used topically in the treatment of keratitis and keratoconjunctivitis caused by human herpesviruses 1 and 2 三氟胸苷，一种干扰病毒 DNA 合成的抗病毒化合物，局部用药用于治疗由人类疱疹病毒 1 型和 2 型引起的角膜炎和结膜炎

tri·fo·cal (tri-fo′-) (tri′fo-kəl) 1. having three foci 三焦点的；2. containing one part for near vision, one for intermediate vision, and a third for distant vision, as does a trifocal lens 包含一部分适用于近视眼，一部分用于中视力，第三部分用于远视的镜片，如三焦透镜

tri·fo·cals (tri′fo-kəlz) trifocal glasses 三焦眼镜

tri·fur·ca·tion (tri″fər-ka′shən) division, or the site of separation, into three branches 三叉分支

tri·gem·i·nal (tri-jem′ĭ-nəl) 1. triple 三倍；2. pertaining to the trigeminal (fifth cranial) nerve 三叉神经的；3. pertaining to trigeminy 三联的

tri·gem·i·ny (tri-jem′ĭ-ne) 1. occurrence in threes 三发性；2. the occurrence of a trigeminal pulse 三联脉；**ventricular t.,** an arrhythmia consisting of the repetitive sequence of one ventricular premature complex followed by two normal beats 室性三联脉

tri·glyc·er·ide (tri-glis′ər-īd) a compound consisting of three molecules of fatty acid esterified to glycerol; a neutral fat that is the usual storage form of lipids in animals 甘油三酯，三酰甘油

tri·go·nal (tri′go-nəl) 1. 同 triangular；2. pertaining to a trigone 三角区的

tri·gone (tri′gōn) 1. 同 triangle 三角，三角区；2. the first three cusps of an upper molar tooth 三尖，上磨牙的前三尖；**t. of bladder,** 同 vesical t.；**olfactory t.,** the triangular area of gray matter between the roots of the olfactory tract 嗅三角；**vesical t.,** the smooth triangular portion of the mucosa at the base of the bladder, bounded behind by the interureteric fold, ending in front in the uvula of the bladder 膀胱三角

trig·o·ni·tis (trig″o-ni′tis) inflammation or localized hyperemia of the vesical trigone 膀胱三角炎

trig·o·no·ceph·a·lus (trig″o-no-sef′ə-ləs) an individual exhibiting trigonocephaly 三角头畸胎

trig·o·no·ceph·a·ly (trig″o-no-sef′ə-le) triangular shape of the head due to sharp forward angulation at the midline of the frontal bone 三角头畸形；**trigonocephal′ic** adj.

tri·go·num (tri-go′nəm) pl. trigo′na [L.] triangle 三角，三角区

tri·hex·y·phen·i·dyl (tri-hek″sĭ-fen′ĭ-dəl) an antidyskinetic used as the hydrochloride salt in the treatment of parkinsonism and for the control of drug-induced extrapyramidal reactions 安坦，苯海索，一种治疗帕金森病和控制药物诱导的锥体外系反应的抗运动障碍药

tri·io·do·thy·ro·nine (T₃) (tri-i″o-do-thi′ronēn) one of the thyroid hormones, an organic iodine-containing compound liberated from thyroglobulin by hydrolysis. It has several times the biologic activity of thyroxine 三碘甲腺原氨酸

tri·kates (tri′kāts) a combination of potassium acetate, potassium bicarbonate, and potassium citrate used in the treatment and prophylaxis of hypokalemia 一种由醋酸钾、碳酸氢钾和枸橼酸钾组成的化合物，用于治疗和预防低钾血症

tri·lam·i·nar (tri-lam′ĭ-nər) three-layered 三层的

tri·lo·bate (tri-lo′bāt) having three lobes 三叶的

tri·loc·u·lar (tri-lok′u-lər) having three compartments or cells 三室的，三细胞的

tri·l·o·gy (tril′ə-je) a group or series of three 三联，三联症；**t.of Fallot,** a term sometimes applied to concurrent pulmonic stenosis, atrial septal defect, and right ventricular hypertrophy 法洛三联症

tri·mep·ra·zine (tri-mep′rə-zēn) a phenothiazine derivative antihistamine; used as the tartrate salt as an antipruritic 异丁嗪，吩噻嗪类衍生物，一种抗组胺药，酒石酸异丁嗪可用作止痒药

tri·mes·ter (tri-mes′tər) a period of 3 months 三个月，三月期

tri·meth·a·di·one (tri″meth-ə-di′ōn) an anticonvulsant with analgesic properties, used for the control of petit mal seizures 三甲双酮，一种抗惊厥药，用于控制癫痫小发作

tri·meth·a·phan (tri-meth′ə-fan) a short-acting ganglionic blocking agent, used as the camsylate ester to produce controlled hypotension during surgery and for the emergency treatment of hypertensive crises and pulmonary edema due to hypertension 咪噻芬，一种短效神经节阻滞药，用于在手术过程中产生控制性低血压，特别用于高血压危象和高

T

血压引起的肺水肿的紧急治疗

tri·meth·o·ben·za·mide (tri-meth″o-ben′zə- mīd) an antiemetic, used as the hydrochloride salt 曲美苄胺，三甲氧苯酰胺，其盐酸盐用作止吐药

tri·meth·o·prim (tri-meth′o-prim) an antibacterial closely related to pyrimethamine; almost always used in combination with a sulfonamide, primarily for the treatment of urinary tract infections. The sulfate salt is used in combination with polymyxin B sulfate in the topical treatment of ocular infections 甲氧苄啶，甲氧苄氨嘧啶，常与磺胺联用，主要用于治疗尿路感染，与多黏霉素 B 联用治疗眼部感染

tri·me·trex·ate (tri″mə-trek′sāt) a folic acid antagonist structurally related to methotrexate, used as the glucuronate salt, in combination with leukovorin, to treat pneumocystis pneumonia in AIDS 曲美沙特，三甲蝶呤，一种与氨甲蝶呤结构相关的叶酸拮抗药，与白细胞介素联合用于治疗艾滋病患者的肺囊虫肺炎

tri·mip·ra·mine (tri-mip′rə-mēn) a tricyclic antidepressant of the dibenzazepine class; used as the maleate salt in the treatment of depression as well as peptic ulcer and severe chronic pain 三甲丙咪嗪，曲米帕明，三环类抑郁药，用作治疗抑郁症以及消化性溃疡和严重慢性疼痛

tri·mor·phous (tri-mor′fəs) existing in three different forms 三形的

tri·ni·tro·phe·nol (tri″ni-tro-fe′nol) a yellow substance used as a dye and a tissue fixative; it can be detonated on percussion or by heating above 300℃ 三硝基酚，苦味酸

tri·ni·tro·tol·u·ene (TNT) (tri″ni-tro-tol′u-ēn) a high explosive derived from toluene; it sometimes causes poisoning in those who work with it, marked by dermatitis, gastritis, abdominal pain, vomiting, constipation, and flatulence 三硝基甲苯

tri·or·chi·dism (tri-or′ki-diz-əm) the condition of having three testes 三睾畸形；**trior′chid** adj.

tri·ose (tri′ōs) a monosaccharide containing three carbon atoms in the molecule 丙糖

tri·ox·sa·len (tri-ok′sə-lən) a psoralen used in conjunction with ultraviolet exposure in the treatment of vitiligo 三甲沙林，三甲呋豆素，三甲呋苯吡喃酮，三甲补骨脂内酯，合成补骨脂素，口服本品联合紫外线照射可治疗白癜风

tri·pe·len·na·mine (tri″pə-len′ə-min) an antihistamine with anticholinergic and sedative effects, used as the citrate and hydrochloride salts 曲吡那敏，苄吡二胺，吡苄明，一种具有抗胆碱能作用和镇静作用的抗组胺药

tri·pep·tide (tri-pep′tid) a peptide that on hydrolysis yields three amino acids 三肽

tri·phal·an·gism (tri-fal′ən-jiz-əm) three phalanges in a digit normally having only two 拇指三指节畸形

tri·pha·sic (tri-fa′zik) having three phases 三相的

tri·phen·yl·meth·ane (tri-fen″əl-meth′ān) a substance from coal tar, the basis of various dyes and stains, including rosaniline, basic fuchsin, and gentian violet 三苯甲烷

tri·phos·phate (tri-fos′fāt) a salt containing three phosphate radicals 三磷酸盐

trip·le blind (trip′əl blīnd) pertaining to an experiment in which neither the subject nor the person administering the treatment nor the person evaluating the response to treatment knows which treatment any particular subject is receiving 三盲法，临床或其他实验时受试者、治疗者、评估治疗反应者都不知道任何一位受试者接受的是何种治疗

trip·le·gia (tri-ple′jə) paralysis of three limbs 三肢麻痹，三瘫

trip·let (trip′lət) 1. one of three offspring produced at one birth 三胞胎中的一个；2. a combination of three objects or entities acting together, as three lenses 三联组，同时发生或起作用的三个物体或实体的组合，如构成显微镜目镜或物镜的三合透镜；3. codon 密码子，三联密码；4. a triple discharge 三联放电

trip·lex (tri′pleks) (trip′leks) triple or threefold 三倍的，三联的

trip·loid (trip′loid) having triple the haploid number of chromosomes (3n) 三倍的，三倍体

trip·lo·pia (trip-lo′pe-ə) the perception of three images of a single object 三重复视，一物在眼中成三个物象

tri·pro·li·dine (tri-pro′lĭ-dēn) an antihistamine with anticholinergic and sedative effects, used as the hydrochloride salt 盐酸苯丙烯啶，一种具有抗胆碱能作用和镇静作用的抗组胺药

trip·to·rel·in (trip″to-rel′in) a synthetic gonadorelin analogue that on prolonged administration suppresses gonadotropin release; used as *t. pamoate* as an antineoplastic in the treatment of prostatic carcinoma 曲普瑞林，一种促性腺激素合成类似物，长期服用可抑制促性腺激素的释放；用作治疗前列腺癌的抗肿瘤药

tri·pus (tri′pəs) conjoined twins with tripodial symmelia 三足畸胎

TRIS tromethamine 氨基丁三醇，缓血酸胺，三羟甲基氨基甲烷

Tris (tris) 1. 同 tromethamine；2. 同 tris (2,3-dibromopropyl) phosphate

tri·sal·i·cyl·ate (tri″sal-ĭ-sil′āt) (tri″sə-lis′ə-lāt) a compound containing three salicylate ions 三水杨酸酯，一种含有三个水杨酸根离子的化合物；

T

choline magnesium t., a combination of choline and magnesium salicylates, used as an analgesic, antipyretic, antiinflammatory, and antirheumatic 三柳胆镁，一种胆碱和水杨酸镁的混合物，用作止痛药、解热药、消炎药和抗风湿药

tris. (2,3-di·bro·mo·pro·pyl) phos·phate (tris″-di-bro″mo-pro′pəl fos′fāt) a yellow liquid flame retardant, formerly used in children's clothing but now restricted in use because it is carcinogenic 三（2,3-二溴丙基）磷酸盐，一种黄色液态阻燃剂，曾用于制作儿童服装，由于具有致癌性，现已禁止使用

tris·mus (triz′məs) motor disturbance of the trigeminal nerve, especially spasm of the masticatory muscles, with difficulty in opening the mouth (lockjaw); a characteristic early symptom of tetanus 牙关紧闭，三叉神经的运动障碍，尤指咀嚼肌痉挛、张口困难；为破伤风早期的特征性症状

tri·so·my (tri′so-me) the presence of an additional (third) chromosome of one type in an otherwise diploid cell (2n + 1) 三体性，二倍体中某一对同源染色体增加了一条染色体的现象，染色体数目为 2n+1 *syndrome* 下词条；**triso′mic** *adj.*

tri·splanch·nic (tri-splangk′nik) pertaining to the three great visceral cavities 三大体腔的

tri·sul·cate (tri-sul′kāt) having three furrows 有三沟的

tri·sul·fide (tri-sul′fīd) a sulfur compound containing three atoms of sulfur to one of the base 三硫化物

tri·ta·nom·a·ly (tri″tə-nom′ə-le) a rare type of anomalous trichromatic vision in which the third, blue-sensitive, cones have decreased sensitivity 蓝色弱，黄蓝色弱，一种罕见的异常三色视觉，病人的蓝色感即第三锥体细胞的敏感性降低

tri·ta·nope (tri′tə-nōp″) a person exhibiting tritanopia 蓝色盲者

tri·ta·no·pia (tri″tə-no′pe-ə) a rare type of dichromatic vision marked by retention of the sensory mechanism for two hues only (red and green), with blue and yellow being absent 蓝色盲，一种罕见的二色视觉，以仅保留两种色调（红色和绿色）的感觉机制，以蓝色和黄色的感觉机制的缺失为特征；**tritanop′ic** *adj.*

tri·ti·ceous (tri-tish′əs) resembling a grain of wheat 麦粒样的

trit·i·um (trit′e-əm) 氚，参见 *hydrogen*

trit·ur·a·tion (trich″ər-a′shən) 1. reduction to powder by friction or grinding 研制，研磨，以持续研磨的方法将固体物质变成粉末；2. a drug so created, especially one rubbed up with lactose 研制剂，尤指以乳糖研制而成的药物；3. the creation of a homogeneous whole by mixing, as the combining of particles of an alloy with mercury to form dental amalgam 齐化，通过混合形成的均匀的整体，如将合金颗粒与汞结合形成牙科用汞合金

tri·va·lent (tri-va′lənt) 1. having a valence of 3 三价的；2. effective against three different entities, as diseases or strains of a pathogen 疫苗三联的，有效对抗三种不同的实体，如病原体的疾病种类或菌株

tRNA transfer RNA 转移 RNA

tro·car (tro′kahr) a sharp-pointed instrument equipped with a cannula, used to puncture the wall of a body cavity and withdraw fluid 套针

tro·chan·ter (tro-kan′tər) a broad, flat process on the femur, at the upper end of its lateral surface *(greater t.),* or a short conical process on the posterior border of the base of its neck *(lesser t.)* 转子，股骨外侧面上端的宽而平的突起（大转子），和股骨颈基部后缘下部向内的短圆锥形突起（小转子）；**trochanter′ian, trochanter′ic** *adj.*

tro·che (tro′ke) lozenge (1) 锭剂，糖锭

troch·lea (trok′le-ə) pl. *troch′leae* [L.] a pulley-shaped part or structure; used in anatomic nomenclature to designate a bony or fibrous structure through which a tendon passes or with which other structures articulate 滑车，滑轮形部件或结构；解剖学上用于表示肌腱穿过或与其他结构进行关节运动的骨或纤维结构；**troch′lear** *adj.*

tro·cho·ceph·a·ly (tro″ko-sef′ə-le) a rounded appearance of the head due to synostosis of the frontal and parietal bones 轮状头畸形，圆头畸形，由额骨和顶骨的骨性结合导致的圆头畸形

tro·choid (tro′koid) pivot-like, or pulley-shaped 车轴状的，滑车状的

tro·choi·des (tro-koi′dēz) a pivot joint 车轴关节

Trog·lo·tre·ma (trog″lo-tre′mə) a genus of flukes, including *T. salmin′cola* (salmon fluke), a parasite of various fish, especially salmon and trout, which is a vector of *Neorickettsia helminthoeca* 隐孔吸虫属，包括鲑隐孔吸虫，是各种鱼类的寄生虫，尤其是鲑鱼和鳟鱼，是蠕虫样新立克次体的传播媒介

tro·le·an·do·my·cin (tro″le-an-do-mi′sin) a macrolide antibiotic used in the treatment of pneumococcal pneumonia and Group A β -hemolytic streptococcal infections 三乙酰竹桃霉素，一种大环内酯类抗生素，用于治疗肺炎球菌肺炎和 A 组 β -溶血性链球菌感染

Trom·bic·u·la (trom-bik′u-lə) a genus of acarine mites (family Trombiculidae), including *T. akamu′shi, T. delien′sis, T. fletch′eri, T. interme′dia, T. pal′lida,* and *T. scutella′ris,* whose larvae (chiggers) are vectors of *Orientia tsutsugamushi,* the cause of scrub typhus 恙螨属，包括红恙螨、地里恙螨、弗恙螨、居中恙螨、苍白恙螨和小板恙螨，

T

其幼虫是恙虫热立克次体的传播媒介，可引起恙虫病

trom·bic·u·li·a·sis (trom-bik″u-li′ə-sis) infestation with mites of the genus *Trombicula* 恙螨病

Trom·bic·u·li·dae (trom-bik′u-lī″de) a family of mites cosmopolitan in distribution, whose parasitic larvae (chiggers) infest vertebrates 恙螨科

tro·meth·amine (tro-meth′ə-mēn) a proton acceptor used as an alkalizer in the treatment of metabolic acidosis; also used to make buffer solutions 氨基丁三醇，缓血酸胺，三羟甲基氨基甲烷，一种质子受体，用作碱化剂治疗代谢性酸中毒，也用于制作缓冲溶液

troph·ede·ma (trof″ə-de′mə) a chronic disease with permanent edema of the feet or legs 营养性水肿，以足或小腿持续性浮肿为特征的疾病

Tro·phe·ry·ma (tro-fer′ĭ-mə) a genus of grampositive, aerobic, soil-dwelling bacteria of the family Cellulomonadaceae. *T. whippe′lii* is the cause of Whipple disease 属于纤维单胞菌科的一种革兰阳性好氧土壤细菌，惠普尔养障体感染引起惠普尔病

tro·phic (tro′fik) pertaining to nutrition 营养的

tro·pho·blast (tro′fo-blast) the peripheral cells of the blastocyst, which attach the blastocyst to the uterine wall and become the placenta and the membranes that nourish and protect the developing organism 滋养层; **trophoblas′tic** *adj.*

tro·pho·neu·ro·sis (tro″fo-noo-ro′sis) any functional disease due to failure of nutrition in a part because its nerve supply is defective 营养神经功能病，由于神经作用的缺陷致使营养缺乏而发生的各种神经疾患; **trophoneurot′ic** *adj.*

tro·phont (tro′font) the active, motile, feeding stage in the life cycle of certain ciliate protozoa 营养体，某些纤毛虫原虫生命周期中的活跃、能动和摄食的阶段

tro·pho·tax·is (tro″fo-tak′sis) taxis in response to nutritive materials 趋营养性

tro·pho·zo·ite (tro″fo-zo′īt) the active, motile feeding stage of a sporozoan parasite 滋养体，原生动物的活跃、能动和摄食的阶段

tro·pia (tro′pe-ə) strabismus 斜视，斜眼

tro·pism (tro′piz-əm) the turning, bending, movement, or growth of an organism or part of an organism elicited by an external stimulus, either toward (*positive t.*) or away from (*negative t.*) the stimulus; used as a word element combined with a stem indicating the nature of the stimulus (e.g., phototropism) or material or entity for which an organism (or substance) shows a special affinity (e.g., neurotropism). Usually applied to nonmotile organisms 向性，趋向性，机体或其某部对外界刺激所作出的转向、

屈曲、运动或生长反应，这种反应或为正（趋向刺激）或为负（背离刺激）；也扩展用作构词成分，与词干相连，表示刺激的性质（如，向光性）或以有机体或物质对之有特殊亲和力的物质或实体（如，嗜中性），通常指无活动性的有机体

tro·po·col·la·gen (tro″po-kol′ə-jən) the basic structural unit of all forms of collagen; it is a helical structure of three polypeptides wound around each other 原胶原，各种形式胶原蛋白的基本结构单元，为 3 条多肽链彼此缠绕形成的螺旋结构

tro·po·my·o·sin (tro″po-mi′o-sin) a muscle protein of the I band that inhibits contraction by blocking the interaction of actin and myosin, except when influenced by troponin 原肌球蛋白

tro·po·nin (tro′po-nin) a complex of muscle proteins that, when combined with Ca²⁺, influences tropomyosin to initiate contraction 肌钙蛋白

tro·spi·um (tro′spe-əm″) an antispasmodic used as *t. chloride* in the treatment of bladder hyperactivity 一种解痉药，用于治疗膀胱亢进

trough (trof) a shallow longtudinal depression 沟，槽; **synaptic t.**, an invagination of the membrane of a striated muscle fiber, surrounding a motor end plate at a neuromuscular junction 突触裂隙，神经肌肉接头处包绕运动终板的横纹肌纤维膜的内陷

tro·va·flox·a·cin (tro″və-flok′sə-sin) an antibacterial effective against a broad spectrum of gram-positive and gram-negative organisms; used as the mesylate salt 对革兰阳性菌和革兰阴性菌均有抗菌作用的体外广谱抗菌药

Trp tryptophan 色氨酸

Tru·li·ci·ty (troo″lih′sitee) trademark for a preparation of dulaglutide 一种降糖药物的商品名

trun·cal (trung′kəl) pertaining to the trunk 躯干的，干的

trun·cate (trung′kāt) 1. to amputate; to deprive of limbs 截肢; 2. ha ving the end cut squarely off 截断的

trun·cus (trung′kəs) pl. *trun′ci* [L.] 同 trunk; **t. arterio′sus**, an arterial trunk, especially the artery connected with the embryonic heart, which gives off the arteries of the pharyngeal arches and develops into the aortic and pulmonary arteries 动脉干，尤指与胚胎心脏相连的动脉，由此发出咽弓动脉并发育成主动脉和肺动脉

trunk (trungk) 1. torso; the main part of the body, to which head and limbs are attached 躯干; 2. a major, undivided, and often short part of a nerve, vessel, or duct 干，神经、血管或导管的一个主要的、不可分割的部分，通常较短; **brachiocephalic t.**, a vessel arising from the arch of the aorta; giving rise to the right common carotid and right subclavian arteries; and supplying the right side of the head and neck and the right arm 头臂干; **celiac t.**, the arterial trunk arising from the abdominal aorta; giving origin to the left gastric, common hepatic, and splenic arteries; and supplying the esophagus, stomach, duodenum, spleen, pancreas, liver, and gallbladder 腹腔干; **costocervical t.**, a vessel arising from the subclavian artery; giving rise to the deep cervical and highest intercostal arteries; and supplying the first two intercostal spaces, vertebral column, back muscles, and deep neck muscles 肋颈干; **lumbosacral t.**, a trunk formed by union of the lower part of the anterior branch of the fourth lumbar nerve with the anterior branch of the fifth lumbar nerve 腰骶干; **lymphatic t's**, the lymphatic vessels that drain lymph from the various regions of the body into the right lymphatic or the thoracic duct 淋巴干; **pulmonary t.**, a vessel arising from the conus arteriosus of the right ventricle and bifurcating into the right and left pulmonary arteries, conveying unaerated blood toward the lungs 肺动脉干; **sympathetic t.**, two long ganglionated nerve strands, one on each side of the vertebral column, extending from the base of the skull to the coccyx 交感干; **thyrocervical t.**, a vessel arising from the subclavian artery; giving rise to the inferior thyroid, transverse cervical, and suprascapular arteries; and supplying the thyroid, neck, and scapular regions 甲状颈干

TRUS transrectal ultrasonography 经直肠超声检查

truss (trus) an elastic, canvas, or metallic device for retaining a reduced hernia within the abdominal cavity 疝带, 疝还纳腹腔后, 为防其脱出而应用的弹性、粗帆布或金属的保持器具

try·pano·cide (tri-pan′o-sīd) an agent lethal to trypanosomes 杀锥虫药; **trypanoci′dal** adj.

try·pan·ol·y·sis (tri″pan-ol′ĭ-sis) the destruction of trypanosomes by lysis 溶锥虫作用; **trypanolyt′ic** adj.

Try·pano·so·ma (tri-pan″o-so′mə) a genus of protozoa parasitic in the blood and lymph of invertebrates and vertebrates, including humans. *T. bru'cei gambien'se* and *T. bru'cei rhodesien'se* cause types of African trypanosomiasis, and *T. cru'zi* causes Chagas disease 锥虫属, 包括寄生于无脊椎动物和脊椎动物（包括人类）的血液和淋巴中; 感染布氏冈比亚锥虫和布氏罗德西亚锥虫后引起非洲锥体虫病, 而感染克氏锥虫则引起美洲锥体虫病

try·pano·so·mal (tri-pan″o-so′məl) pertaining to or caused by trypanosomes 锥虫的

try·pano·so·ma·tid (tri-pan″o-so′mə-tid) 1. any protozoan of the suborder Trypanosomatina 锥虫亚目原虫的; 2. 同 trypanosomal

Try·pano·so·ma·ti·na (tri-pan″o-so″mə-ti′nə) a suborder of parasitic protozoa (order Kinetoplastida, class Zoomastigophorea), comprising hemoflagellates that are found in the hosts' blood, lymph, and tissues. They have a leaflike or rounded body with one nucleus, one flagellum that is free or attached to the body by an undulating membrane, and a relatively small, compact kinetoplast, and pass through at least two morphologically distinct stages in their life cycles 锥虫亚目

try·pano·some (tri-pan′o-sōm) an individual of the genus *Trypanosoma* or of the suborder Trypanosomatina 锥虫

try·pano·so·mi·a·sis (tri-pan″o-si-mi′ə-sis) infection with trypanosomes 锥虫病; **African t.**, human trypanosomiasis endemic in areas of tropical Africa, due to infection with *Trypanosoma gambiense* (West African t.) or *T. rhodesiense* (East African t.); it is transmitted by the bite of species of *Glossina* (tsetse flies) and in advanced stages attacks the central nervous system, resulting in meningoencephalitis that leads to lethargy, tremors, convulsions, and eventually coma and death 非洲锥虫病, 因感染冈比亚锥虫（西非锥虫病）或罗得西亚锥虫（东非锥虫病）而在非洲热带地区流行的人类锥虫病; 该病主要通过舌蝇咬伤传播, 侵犯中枢神经系统, 导致脑膜脑炎, 出现嗜睡、颤抖、抽搐, 最终昏迷和死亡; **American t., South American t.**, Chagas disease 美洲锥虫病, 南美洲锥虫病

try·pano·so·mi·cide (tri-pan″o-si-mĭ-sīd) 同 trypanocide

try·pano·so·mid (tri-pan′o-so-mid) 1. a skin eruption occurring in trypanosomiasis 锥虫病疹; 2. 同 trypanosomal

try·po·mas·ti·gote (tri″po-mas′tĭ-gōt) a morphologic stage in the life cycle of certain trypanosomatid protozoa, characterized by a kinetoplast and basal body at the posterior end and a flagellum running anteriorly along an undulating membrane to become a free-flowing structure 锥鞭毛体

tryp·sin (trip′sin) an enzyme of the hydrolase class, secreted as trypsinogen by the pancreas and converted to the active form in the small intestine, that catalyzes the cleavage of peptide linkages involving the carboxyl group of either lysine or arginine; a purified preparation derived from ox pancreas is used for its proteolytic effect in débridement and in the treatment of empyema 胰蛋白酶; **tryp′tic** adj.

tryp·sin·o·gen (trip-sin′o-jən) the inactive precursor of trypsin, secreted by the pancreas and activated in the duodenum by cleavage by enteropeptidase 胰蛋白酶原

tryp·ta·mine (trip′tə-mēn) a product of the decarboxylation of tryptophan, occurring in plants and

T

certain foods such as cheese; it raises blood pressure via vasoconstriction by causing the release of norepinephrine at postganglionic nerve endings 色胺

tryp·to·phan (Trp, W) (trip′to-fan) a naturally occurring amino acid, existing in proteins and essential for human metabolism. It is a precursor of serotonin. Adequate levels may mitigate pellagra by compensating for deficiencies of niacin 色氨酸

tryp·to·phan·uria (trip″to-fə-nu′re-ə) excessive urinary excretion of tryptophan 色氨酸尿

TS tricuspid stenosis 三尖瓣狭窄

TSA tumor-specific antigen 肿瘤特异性抗原

TSC tuberous sclerosis complex 结节性硬化症

TSD Tay-Sachs disease 泰萨克斯病，家族黑蒙性痴呆

tset·se (tset′se) an African fly of the genus *Glossina*, which transmits trypanosomiasis 采采蝇，舌蝇属的一种非洲舌蝇，可传播锥虫病

TSH thyroid-stimulating hormone 促甲状腺激素，参见 *thyrotropin*

T-spine thoracic spine 胸椎

TT therapeutic touch; thrombin time 治疗性触摸；thrombin time 凝血酶时间

tu·ba (too′bə) pl. *tu′bae* [L.] 同 tube 管

tu·bal (too′bəl) pertaining to or occurring in a tube 管的，尤指输卵管的

tube (toob) a hollow cylindrical organ or instrument 管，解剖学上指细长、中空的柱状器官或结构；**auditory t.**, eustachian tube; the narrow channel connecting the middle ear and the nasopharynx 咽鼓管；**drainage t.**, a tube used in surgery to facilitate escape of fluids 引流管；**Durham t.**, a jointed tracheotomy tube 德拉姆管，有接头的气管切开插管；**endobronchial t.**, a double-lumen tube inserted into the bronchus of one lung to deflate the other lung for anesthesia or thoracic surgery 支气管导管；**endotracheal t.**, an airway catheter inserted in the trachea in endotracheal intubation 气管导管；**esophageal t.**, stomach t. 食管导管，参见 stomach t **eustachian t.**, 同 auditory t.；**fallopian t.**, 同 uterine t.；**feeding t.**, one for introducing high-caloric fluids into the stomach 饲管；**Miller-Abbott t.**, a double-channel intestinal tube with an inflatable balloon at its distal end, for use in treatment of obstruction of the small intestine and occasionally as a diagnostic aid 米 - 艾管，双腔肠管，远端带有可充气的气囊，用于治疗小肠阻塞，偶尔用作诊断辅助装置；**nasogastric t.**, a stomach tube inserted through a nostril and into the stomach, for instilling liquids or other substances or for withdrawing gastric contents 鼻胃管；**nasotracheal t.**, an endotracheal tube that passes through the nose 鼻气管插管；**neural t.**, the epithelial tube developed from

the neural plate and forming the central nervous system of the embryo 神经管，从神经板发育而形成胚胎的中枢神经系统；**orotracheal t.**, an endotracheal tube that passes through the mouth 经口气管导管；**Sengstaken-Blakemore t.**, a multilumen tube used for tamponade of bleeding esophageal varices 森斯塔肯 - 布莱克莫尔管，三腔二气囊管；**stomach t.**, a tube for feeding or for stomach irrigation; the most common kind is the nasogastric tube 胃管；**test t.**, a tube of thin glass, closed at one end; used in chemical tests and other laboratory procedures 试管；**tracheal t.**, 同 endotracheal t.；**tracheostomy.**, a curved endotracheal tube that is inserted into the trachea through a tracheostomy 气管切开插管；**uterine t.**, fallopian tube; a slender tube extending from the uterus toward the ovary on the same side, for passage of oocytes to the cavity of the uterus and the usual site of fertilization 输卵管；**Wangensteen t.**, a small nasogastric tube connected with a special suction apparatus to maintain gastric and duodenal decompression 旺根斯藤管，连接有一个特殊的抽吸设备的鼻胃管，以维持胃和十二指肠减压 **x-ray t.**, a vacuum tube used for the production of x-rays; when a suitable current is applied, highspeed electrons travel from the cathode to the anode, where they are suddenly arrested, giving rise to x-rays X 射线管

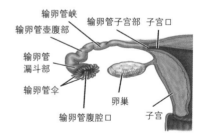

▲ 子宫输卵管，可分为漏斗部、伞部、壶腹部、峡部

tu·bec·to·my (too-bek′tə-me) salpingectomy 输卵管部分切除术

tu·ber (too′bər) pl. *tu′bera, tubers* [L.] 1. a swelling or protuberance 肿起，隆突；2. the essential lesion of tuberous sclerosis, occurring as a pale, firm, nodular, phakomalike glial hamartomatous brain lesion 结节，结节性硬化症的主要病变，表现为苍白、坚实、结节状、晶体瘤样胶质错构瘤样脑病变；**t. cine′reum**, a layer of gray matter forming part of the floor of the third ventricle, to which the infundibulum of the hypothalamus is attached 灰结节，下丘脑的灰质层，形成第三脑室底的一部分，下

丘脑漏斗部附着于其上；**t. ver′mis, t. of vermis,** the part of the vermis of the cerebellum between the folium vermis and the pyramid of vermis 蚓结节，小脑蚓叶和锥体之间的蚓部

tu·ber·cle (too′bər-kəl) 1. a nodule or small eminence, especially one on a bone for attachment of a tendon 结节或小隆起，如骨骼上肌腱附着处的结节；2. the characteristic lesion of tuberculosis, a small round gray translucent granulomatous lesion, usually with central caseation 结核结节，结核病的特征性病变，小圆形灰色半透明肉芽肿样病变，常伴中央干酪样坏死；**anatomic t.,** tuberculosis verrucosa cutis 剖尸疣，尸毒性疣；**auricular t., auricular t. of Darwin, darwinian t.,** a small projection sometimes found on the edge of the helix; conjectured by some to be a relic of simioid ancestry 耳廓结节，达尔文结节；**Farre t′s,** masses beneath the capsule of the liver in some cases of hepatocellular carcinoma 法尔氏结节，在某些肝细胞癌病例中，在肝被膜下方存在的肿块；**genial t., inferior,** inferior mental spine 下颏棘；**genial t., superior,** superior mental spine 上颏棘；**genital t.,** an eminence ventral to the cloaca in the early embryo; the primordium of the penis or clitoris 生殖结节；**Ghon t.,** 冈氏结节，参见 *focus* 下词条；**gracile t.,** an enlargement of the fasciculus gracilis in the medulla oblongata, produced by the underlying nucleus gracilis 薄束结节；**hard t.,** a noncaseating tubercle, characteristic of sarcoidosis; composed of aggregations of large, pale-staining, epithelioid cells intermingled with histiocytes, lymphocytes, and Langhans giant cells, sometimes surrounded by a band of lymphocytes 硬结节；**intervenous t.,** a ridge across the inner surface of the right atrium between the openings of the venae cavae 静脉间结节；**Lisfranc t.,** an eminence on the first rib, for attachment of the anterior scalene muscle 前斜角肌结节；**Lower t.,** 同 intervenous t.；**mental t.,** a prominence on the inner border of either side of the mental protuberance of the mandible 颏结节；**miliary t.,** one of the many minute tubercles formed in many organs in acute miliary tuberculosis 粟粒性结核结节；**pubic t.,** a prominent tubercle at the lateral end of the pubic crest 耻骨结节；**scalene t.,** 同 Lisfranc t.；**supraglenoid t.,** one on the scapula for attachment of the long head of the biceps 盂上结节

tu·ber·cu·lar (too-bur′ku-lər) 1. pertaining to or resembling tubercles 结节的，结节状的；2. 同 tuberculous

tu·ber·cu·lid (too-bur′ku-lid) recurrent eruptions of the skin, usually with spontaneous involution, considered by some authorities to be hyperergic

reactions to mycobacteria or their antigens 结核疹；**papulonecrotic t.,** a grouped, symmetric eruption of symptomless papules, appearing in successive crops and healing spontaneously with superficially depressed scars 丘疹坏死性结核疹，对称发生的无症状丘疹簇，连续分批发生，伴有浅表凹陷性瘢痕，自行愈合

tu·ber·cu·lin (too-bur′ku-lin) a sterile solution containing the growth products of, or specific substances extracted from, *Mycobacterium tuberculosis* or *M. bovis;* used in the diagnosis of tuberculosis; see also under test. It is provided as a culture filtrate *(Old t.)* or as a further purified protein fraction *(purified protein derivative* or *PPD t.)* 结核菌素，含有从结核分枝杆菌或牛分枝杆菌中提取的生长产物的无菌溶液，用于结核病的诊断，另见 test 下词条；用作为培养滤液（旧结核菌素）或纯化蛋白（纯蛋白衍化物结核菌素）

tu·ber·cu·li·tis (too-bur″ku-li′tis) inflammation of or near a tubercle 结核结节炎

tu·ber·cu·loid (too-bur′ku-loid) resembling a tubercle or tuberculosis 结核结节样的，结核病样的

tu·ber·cu·lo·ma (too-bur″ku-lo′mə) a tumorlike mass resulting from enlargement of a caseous tubercle 结核瘤

tu·ber·cu·lo·sis (too-bur″ku-lo′sis) any of the infectious diseases of humans and other animals due to species of *Mycobacterium* and marked by formation of tubercles and caseous necrosis in tissues of any organ; in humans the lung is the major seat of infection and the usual portal through which infection reaches other organs 结核病；**tuber′cular, tuber′culous** adj.；**avian t.,** a form affecting birds, due to *Mycobacterium avium,* transmissible to humans and other animals 鸟结核，禽结核；**bovine t.,** an infection of cattle due to *Mycobacterium bovis,* transmissible to humans and other animals 牛结核；**cutaneous t., t. cu′tis,** tuberculosis of the skin, which may be from an external cause or from spread of an existing infection, manifesting with any of numerous different clinical expressions 皮肤结核；**disseminated t.,** an acute form of miliary t. 播散性结核；**genital t.,** tuberculosis of the genital tract, e.g., tuberculous endometritis 生殖系统结核；**t. of lungs,** 同 pulmonary t.；**miliary t.,** a form varying in severity, with minute tubercles in different organs due to dissemination of bacilli through the body by the bloodstream 粟粒性结核；**open t.,** 1. a type with lesions that discharge tubercle bacilli from the body 开放性结核；2. pulmonary tuberculosis with cavitation 有空洞形成的肺结核；**pulmonary t.,** infection of the lungs by *Mycobacterium tuberculosis,* with tuberculous pneumonia, formation of tuberculous granulation tissue, caseous necrosis, calcification, and cavity formation. Symptoms include weight loss, fatigue, night sweats, purulent sputum, hemoptysis, and chest pain 肺结核；**renal t.**, renal disease due to *Mycobacterium tuberculosis* 肾结核；**spinal t.**, osteitis or caries of vertebrae, usually as a complication of pulmonary tuberculosis 脊柱结核；**t. verruco′sa cu′tis, warty t.**, cutaneous tuberculosis from external inoculation of tubercle bacilli into the skin, with wartlike patches having a red, inflamed border 疣状皮肤结核

tu·ber·cu·lo·stat·ic (too-bur″ku-lo-stat′ik) 1. inhibiting growth of *Mycobacterium tuberculosis* 抑制结核菌的；2. an agent that so acts 结核菌抑制药

tu·ber·cu·lous (too-bur′ku-ləs) pertaining to or affected with tuberculosis; caused by *Mycobacterium tuberculosis* 患结核病的；结核性的

tu·ber·cu·lum (too-bur′ku-ləm) pl. *tuber′cula* [L.] tubercle (2) 结节；**t.arthri′ticum**, a gouty concretion in a joint 痛风结节

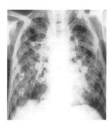

▲ 导致呼吸衰竭的广泛性肺结核

tu·ber·o·sis (too″bər-o′sis) a condition characterized by the presence of nodules 结节形成

tu·be·ros·i·tas (too″bə-ros′ĭ-təs) pl. *tuberosita′tes* [L.] tuber 粗隆

tu·be·ros·i·ty (too″bə-ros′ĭ-te) an elevation or protuberance, especially one on a bone where a muscle is attached 顶结节，粗隆

tu·ber·ous (too′bər-əs) covered with tubers; knobby 有结节的，结节状的，隆凸的；有块茎的，块茎状的

tubo- word element [L.], *tube[* 构词成分] 管

tu·bo·ab·dom·i·nal (too″bo-ab-dom′ĭ-nəl) pertaining to the uterine tube and the abdomen 输卵管腹腔的

tu·bo·cu·ra·rine (too″bo-ku-rah′rēn) an alkaloid from the bark and stems of *Chondrodendron tomentosum;* it is the active principle of curare and is a nondepolarizing neuromuscular blocking agent; used as the chloride salt as a skeletal muscle relaxant and as an aid in the diagnosis of myasthenia gravis 筒箭毒碱，一种从马钱子属植物的树皮和茎中提取的生物碱；是一种非去极化的神经肌肉阻断药；也作为骨骼肌松弛药，是诊断重症肌无力的辅助药物

tu·bo·lig·a·men·tous (too″bo-lig″ə-men′təs) pertaining to the uterine tube and broad ligament 输卵管阔韧带的

tu·bo·ovar·i·an (too″bo-o-var′e-ən) of or pertaining to a uterine tube and ovary 输卵管卵巢的

tu·bo·peri·to·ne·al (too″bo-per″ĭ-to-ne′əl) pertaining to the uterine tube and the peritoneum 输卵管腹膜的

tu·bo·plas·ty (too′bo-plas″te) plastic repair of a tube, such as the uterine tube or auditory tube 管成形术，对管道的成形修复，如输卵管成形术，咽鼓管成形术

tu·bo·tym·pa·num (too″bo-tim′pə-nəm) the auditory tube and tympanic cavity considered together 咽鼓管鼓室

tu·bo·uter·ine (too″bo-u′tər-in) pertaining to a uterine tube and the uterus 输卵管子宫的

tu·bu·lar (too′bu-lər) 1. shaped like a tube 管状的；2. of or pertaining to a tubule 小管的

tu·bule (too′būl) a small tube 小管，细管；**collecting t.**, one of the terminal channels of the nephrons that open on the summits of the renal pyramids in the renal papillae 集合小管；**connecting t.**, 同 junctional t.；**dental t's, dentinal t's**, dental canaliculi 牙本质小管；**distal convoluted t.**, a distal, convoluted part of the ascending limb of the renal tubule, extending from the distal straight tubule to the junctional tubule 远曲小管；**distal straight t.**, part of the renal tubule primarily on the ascending limb, extending from the thin tubule to the distal convoluted tubule 远直小管；**junctional t.**, a short, curved part of the distal end of the renal tubule, extending from the distal convoluted tubule to a collecting duct 接合小管；**mesonephric t's**, those constituting the mesonephros of the embryo of an amniote 中肾小管；**metanephric t's**, those constituting the metanephros of an amniote 后肾小管；**pronephric t's**, the rudimentary tubules constituting the pronephros of an amniote 前肾小管；**proximal convoluted t.**, the most proximal part of the renal tubule, extending from the glomerular capsule to the proximal straight tubule 近曲小管；**proximal straight t.**, part of the descending limb of the renal tubule, extending from the proximal convoluted tubule to the thin tubule 近直小管；**renal t.**, the minute reabsorptive canals made up of basement membrane and lined with epithelium, composing the substance of the kidney and secreting, collecting, and conducting the urine 肾小管，另参见 *nephron*；**seminiferous t's**, channels in the testis in which the spermatozoa develop and through which they leave the gland, each comprising a convoluted portion and a straight terminal portion 生精小管; **T t's,** the transverse intracellular tubules invaginating from the cell membrane and surrounding the myofibrils of the T system of skeletal and cardiac muscle, serving as a pathway for the spread of electrical excitation within a muscle cell 横小管, 由细胞膜反折而成的胞内横行小管, 位于横纹肌骨骼肌和心肌 T 系统的肌原纤维周围, 是肌细胞内电兴奋扩散的通路; **thin t.,** part of the renal tubule where the walls are especially thin, extending from the proximal straight tubule to the distal straight tubule 肾小管细段; **uriniferous t.,** 同 renal t's

tu·bu·lin (too′bu-lin) the constituent protein of microtubules 微管蛋白

tu·bu·lo·in·ter·sti·tial (too″bu-lo-in″tər-stī′- shəl) pertaining to the renal tubules and interstitial tubules 小管间质的, 包括肾小管和间质组织

tu·bu·lor·rhex·is (too″bu-lo-rek′sis) rupture of the renal tubules 肾小管破裂

tu·bu·lo·ve·sic·u·lar (too″bu-lo-və-sik′u-lər) composed of small tubes and sacs; used particularly of the cytoplasmic membranes of the resting parietal cell 管状囊泡的, 由小管和囊组成; 尤其用于描述静止状态壁细胞的细胞质膜

tu·bu·lus (too′bu-ləs) pl. *tu′buli* [L.] tubule; a minute canal 小管, 细管

tuft (tuft) a small clump or cluster; a coil 丛, 簇; 螺旋

tuft·sin (tuft′sin) a tetrapeptide cleaved from IgG that stimulates phagocytosis by neutrophils 吞噬肽素, IgG 中裂解生成的四肽（苏氨酸 - 赖氨酸 - 脯氨酸 - 精氨酸）, 可激发嗜中性粒细胞的吞噬作用

tug·ging (tug′ing) a pulling sensation, as a pulling sensation in the trachea *(tracheal t.),* due to aneurysm of the arch of the aorta 牵引感, 如因主动脉弓动脉瘤引起的气管牵拉感

tui na (too′e nah′) [Chinese] a Chinese system of massage, acupoint stimulation, and manipulation using forceful maneuvers, including pushing, rolling, kneading, rubbing, and grasping, sometimes in conjunction with acupuncture 推拿; **tu·la·re·mia** (too″lə-re′me-ə) a plaguelike disease of squirrels, rabbits, and other small mammals, caused by *Francisella tularensis* and transmissible to humans by the bites of deer flies, fleas, and ticks 土拉菌病, 兔热病, 松鼠、兔子和其他小型哺乳动物患的一种瘟疫性疾病, 由土拉热弗朗西斯菌引起, 并通过斑虻、蚤和蜱的叮咬传染给人类; **oculoglandular t.,** a type whose primary site of infection is the conjunctival sac, with conjunctivitis, corneal lesions,

and enlargement of preauricular lymph nodes 眼腺型土拉菌病, 病原主要经结膜囊侵入的一型土拉菌病, 其症状有结膜炎、角膜病变和耳前淋巴结肿大; **pulmonary t.,** that with involvement of the lungs by spread of primary infection or inhalation of the pathogen, with cough, fever, chest pain, and bloody sputum 肺土拉菌病, 通过原发感染或吸入病原体引起肺部受累的土拉菌病, 伴有咳嗽、发热、胸骨下疼痛和咳血痰; **typhoidal t.,** the most serious type, caused by swallowing the pathogen; symptoms are similar to those of typhoid fever 伤寒性土拉菌病, 为各型土拉菌病中最严重的一型, 由吞咽病原菌引起, 表现为腹痛、高热等类似于伤寒的症状; **ulceroglandular t.,** the most common type in humans, beginning with a painful red papule at the point of inoculation, later forming a shallow ulcer; lymphadenopathy, hepatosplenomegaly, and pneumonia may also occur 溃疡淋巴腺型土拉菌病, 人体最常见的土拉菌病类型, 开始为感染处的疼痛性红色丘疹, 后形成浅溃疡, 也可能发生淋巴结肿大、肝脾肿大和肺炎

tul·si (tool′se) a type of basil, *Ocimum sanctum,* considered sacred in India and having immunostimulant, antibacterial, antifungal, and antiviral properties, used in ayurvedic medicine 一种罗勒属植物, 其在印度被认为是神圣的, 具有免疫刺激、抗菌、抗真菌和抗病毒的特性, 用于阿育吠陀医学

tu·me·fa·cient (too″mə-fa′shənt) producing swelling 致肿胀的

tu·me·fac·tion (too″mə-fak′shən) swelling 肿胀, 肿大

tu·mes·cence (too-mes′əns) swelling 肿胀, 肿大

tu·mid (too′mid) swollen; edematous 肿胀的, 水肿的

tu·mor (too′mər) 1. swelling, one of the cardinal signs of inflammation; morbid enlargement 肿胀, 肿块; 2. neoplasm; a new growth of tissue in which cell multiplication is uncontrolled and progressive 肿瘤, 瘤; **adenomatoid odontogenic t.,** a benign odontogenic tumor with ductlike or glandlike arrangements of columnar epithelial cells, usually occurring in the anterior jaw region 牙源性腺瘤样瘤, 通常发生在前颌骨区域的一种良性的牙源性肿瘤, 有管状或腺状排列的柱状上皮细胞; **adnexal t's,** neoplasms of the skin adnexa, a large group including benign hamartomas and adenomas as well as malignant adnexal carcinomas 皮肤附件肿瘤, 包括良性错构瘤和腺瘤以及恶性附件癌; **Askin t,** a malignant small-cell tumor of soft tissue in the thoracopulmonary region in children; one of the peripheral neuroectodermal tumors Askin 瘤, 儿童胸肺区软组织恶性小细胞瘤, 是一种周围神经外胚层肿瘤; **benign t.,** one lacking the properties of invasion and metastasis and showing a lesser degree of anaplasia than do malignant tumors; it is usu ally surrounded by a fibrous capsule 良性瘤，无侵袭和转移特性，且癌细胞退行发育程度低于恶性肿瘤，周围通常被纤维囊包裹；**Brenner t.**, a rare, usually benign, tumor of the ovary characterized by groups of epithelial cells lying in a fibrous connective tissue stroma 布伦纳瘤，一种罕见的，良性的卵巢肿瘤，以位于纤维结缔组织基质中的上皮细胞群为特征；**brown t.**, a giant-cell granuloma produced in and replacing bone, occurring in osteitis fibrosa cystica and due to hyperparathyroidism 棕色瘤，甲状腺功能亢进所致囊状纤维性骨炎时在骨内发生并取代骨质的一种巨细胞肉芽肿；**Buschke-Löwenstein t.**, a large, destructive, penetrating, cauliflower-like mass on the prepuce, especially in uncircumcised males, and also in the perianal region 巨大尖锐湿疣，包皮上的一个大的，具有破坏性、穿透性、花椰菜样的肿块，尤其容易出现在未进行包皮环切术的男性，也可出现于肛周区域；**carcinoid t.**, a small, slow-growing neuroendocrine tumor arising from enterochromaffin cells and occurring most often in the gastrointestinal tract and lung. Escape of humoral mediators produced by the tumor into the bloodstream causes the carcinoid syndrome 类癌瘤，由肠嗜铬细胞产生的小的、生长缓慢的神经内分泌肿瘤，最常发生在胃肠道和肺部，肿瘤产生的体液介质逃逸到血液导致类癌综合征；**carcinoma ex mixed t.**, carcinoma ex pleomorphic adenoma 混合性肿瘤，多形性腺瘤；**carotid body t.**, a chemodectoma of the carotid body, a firm, round mass at the bifurcation of the common carotid artery 颈动脉体化学感受器瘤，颈总动脉分叉处的一个坚实的圆形肿块；**connective tissue t.**, any tumor arising from a connective tissue structure, e.g., fibroma, sarcoma 结缔组织肿瘤，如纤维瘤、肉瘤；**dermal duct t.**, a small, intradermal, papular, eccrine lesion occurring on the head and neck in older adults 真皮管肿瘤，皮内丘疹样由外分泌物引起的病变，易发生于中老年人的头颈部；**desmoid t.**, an unencapsulated locally invasive fibromatous tumor arising in the musculoaponeurotic tissue, usually the abdominal wall, and often resembling fibrosarcoma 硬纤维瘤，一种无包膜的局部侵袭性纤维瘤，发生于肌肉筋膜组织，通常位于腹壁，类似于纤维肉瘤；**endodermal sinus t.**, yolk sac t. 内胚窦瘤；**Ewing t.**, 尤因肉瘤，参见 *sarcoma* **false t.**, structural enlargement due to extravasation, exudation, echinococcus, or retained sebaceous matter 假性瘤，由于血液外渗，液体渗出，棘球蚴或皮脂物潴留等原因形成的肿胀；**feminizing t.**, a functional tumor that produces feminization in boys and men or pre-cocious puberty in girls, e.g., germinoma 女性化瘤，一种功能性肿瘤，可使男性（青少年及成人）女性化，或使女孩性早熟，如生殖细胞瘤；**fibrohistiocytic t.**, one containing cells resembling histiocytes and others resembling fibroblasts, such as a benign or malignant fibrous histiocytoma.one containing cells resembling histiocytes and others resembling fibroblasts, such as a benign or malignant fibrous histiocytoma 纤维组织细胞肿瘤，一种以不同比例含有似结缔组织细胞和似间质细胞的肿瘤，通常表现是良性或恶性的纤维组织细胞瘤；**fibroid t.**, 1. fibroma 纤维瘤；2. leiomyoma uteri 子宫肌瘤；**functional t.**, **functioning t.**, a hormone-secreting tumor in an endocrine gland 功能性肿瘤，通常发生在内分泌腺内，是激素分泌性肿瘤；**germ cell t.**, any of a group of tumors arising from primitive germ cells, usually of the testis or ovary 生殖细胞肿瘤，起源于原始生殖细胞的一类肿瘤，通常发生于睾丸或卵巢；**giant cell t.**, 1. a bone tumor, ranging from benign to frankly malignant, composed of cellular spindle cell stroma containing multinucleated giant cells resembling osteoclasts 骨巨细胞瘤，一种骨肿瘤，从良性到严重恶性不等，由含有类似破骨细胞的多核巨细胞和梭形细胞组成；2. a benign, small, yellow, tumor-like nodule of tendon sheath origin, most often of the wrist and fingers or ankle and toes, laden with lipophages and containing multinucleated giant cells 腱鞘巨细胞瘤，腱鞘起源的良性结节样肿瘤，最常见于腕部和手指或脚踝和脚趾，富含嗜脂细胞，并含有多核巨细胞；**glomus t.**, 1. a benign, blue-red, painful tumor involving a glomus body 血管球瘤，血管神经肌瘤，一种良性、蓝红色的痛性肿瘤，常累及血管球体；2. chemodectoma 非嗜铬性副神经节瘤，化学感受器瘤；**glomus jugulare t.**, a chemodectoma involving the jugular body (glomus jugulare) 颈静脉球瘤，一种涉及颈静脉体的非嗜铬性副神经节瘤；**granular cell t.**, a usually benign, circumscribed, tumorlike lesion of soft tissue, particularly of the tongue, composed of large cells with prominent granular cytoplasm; the histiogenesis is uncertain, but Schwann cell derivation is favored 颗粒细胞瘤，通常为良性、局限性、软组织肿瘤样病变，易发生在舌部，由具有突出颗粒状细胞质的大细胞组成，发生机制不明确，可能与施万细胞有关；**granulosa t.**, **granulosa cell t.**, an ovarian tumor originating in the cells of the membrana granulosa 颗粒细胞癌，起源于颗粒细胞的卵巢肿瘤；**granulosa-theca cell t.**, an ovarian tumor composed of granulosa (follicular) cells and theca cells; either form may predominate 颗粒-卵泡膜细胞瘤，由颗粒（卵泡）细胞和卵泡膜细胞组成的卵巢肿瘤，两种细胞所占比例不定，任何

细胞的含量都可居多；**heterologous t.,** a tumor made up of tissue different from the tissue it is growing in 异源性瘤，癌组织与其生长处相比组织不同的肿瘤；**hilar cell t.,** a rare benign neoplasm of the hilum of the ovary, histologically resembling a Leydig cell tumor of the testis 门细胞瘤，卵巢门上一种罕见的良性肿瘤，组织学表现类似睾丸间质细胞瘤；**homologous t.,** a tumor that resembles the surrounding parts in its structure 同型瘤，同种瘤，一种在结构上与周围部分组织相似的肿瘤；**Hürthle cell t.,** new growth of the thyroid gland composed predominantly of Hürthle cells; it is usually benign (Hürthle cell adenoma) but may be locally invasive or metastasize (Hürthle cell carcinoma or malignant Hürthle cell tumor) 许特莱细胞瘤，由大量颗粒性酸性胞浆的大细胞构成的甲状腺肿瘤；通常为良性（许特莱细胞腺瘤），但可能有局部浸润或转移（许特莱细胞癌或恶性许特莱细胞瘤）**islet cell t.,** a tumor of the pancreatic islets; many secrete excessive amounts of hormones. Types include gastrinoma, glucagonoma, insulinoma, somatostatinoma, and VIPoma 胰岛细胞瘤；**Krukenberg t.,** carcinoma of the ovary, usually metastatic from gastrointestinal cancer, marked by areas of mucoid degeneration and by the presence of signet-ring–like cells 库肯勃瘤，通常由胃肠道癌转移而来的卵巢肿瘤，以出现黏液样变性和印戒样细胞为特征；**Leydig cell t.,**1. a usually benign, nongerminal tumor of the Leydig cells of the testis 睾丸间质细胞瘤；2. 同 hilar cell t.；**lipoid cell t. of ovary,** a usually benign ovarian tumor composed of eosinophilic cells or cells with lipoid vacuoles; it causes masculinization 卵巢类脂质细胞瘤，一种良性肿瘤，通常由嗜酸性细胞或含有脂类空泡的细胞组成，可导致男性化；**malignant t.,** one having the properties of invasion and metastasis and showing a high degree of anaplasia 恶性瘤；**mast cell t.,** mastocytosis 肥大细胞瘤；**melanotic neuroectodermal t.,** a benign, rapidly growing, dark tumor of the jaw and occasionally of other sites; seen almost exclusively in infants 黑色素神经外胚瘤，生长迅速，着色深浓的颌骨良性肿瘤，偶见其他部位，但几乎发生于婴儿 **mixed t.,** a tumor composed of more than one type of neoplastic tissue 混合瘤，由多种新生组织形成的肿瘤；**müllerian mixed t.,** a malignant mixed tumor of the uterus containing both endometrioid adenocarcinoma and sarcomatous cells that may be either of uterine or extrauterine origin 米勒管混合瘤，一种子宫恶性混合肿瘤，包括子宫内皮腺瘤和肉瘤细胞，可能起源于宫内或宫外；**neuroendocrine t., neuroendocrine cell t.,** any of a diverse group of tumors containing neurosecretory cells that cause endocrine

dysfunction; most are carcinoids or carcinomas 神经内分泌肿瘤含有内分泌细胞并引起内分泌功能紊乱的肿瘤，大多数是类癌或癌；**nonfunctional t., nonfunctioning t.,** a tumor located in an endocrine gland but not secreting hormones 无功能性肿瘤，一种位于内分泌腺但不分泌激素的肿瘤；**odontogenic t.,** a lesion derived from mesenchymal or epithelial elements, or both, that are associated with the development of the teeth; it occurs in the mandible or maxilla, or occasionally the gingiva 牙源性肿瘤，一种由牙间质或上皮成分或两者兼有的肿瘤，与牙齿的发育程度有关；它发生在下颌或上颌，有时发生在牙龈；**papillary t.,** papilloma 乳头状瘤；**pearly t.,** cholesteatoma 珠光瘤；**peripheral neuroectodermal t.,** a primitive neuroectodermal tumor occurring outside of the central nervous system, e.g., on the pelvis, a limb, or the chest wall 周围神经外胚层瘤，发生在肢体、骨盆或胸壁等在中枢神经系统外的原始神经外胚层肿瘤；**phyllodes t.,** a large, locally aggressive, sometimes metastatic fibroadenoma in the breast, with an unusually cellular, sarcomalike stroma 分叶状瘤，乳腺中一种巨大纤维腺瘤，由异常细胞的肉瘤样间质组成，具有局灶侵袭性和转移性；**primitive neuroectodermal t. (PNET),** a heterogeneous group of neoplasms thought to derive from undifferentiated cells of the neural crest 原始神经外胚叶肿瘤，起源于神经嵴的未分化细胞的异质性肿瘤；**proliferating trichilemmal t.,** a large, solitary, multilobulated lesion of the hair follicle, occurring on the scalp, usually in middle-aged or older women; often confused with squamous cell carcinoma 增殖性毛囊肿瘤，一种发生在头皮毛囊的大而单发的分叶病变，通常发生在中老年妇女身上，常与鳞状细胞癌混淆；**squamous odontogenic t.,** a benign odontogenic epithelial neoplasm occurring in the mandible or maxilla and believed to derive from transformation of the rests of Malassez 牙源性鳞状细胞瘤，一种发生于下颌骨或上颌上的良性牙源性上皮性肿瘤，被认为是由马拉瑟残体转变而来；**stromal t's,** a diverse group of tumors derived from the ovarian stroma, many of which secrete sex hormones 间质肿瘤；**testicular t.,** any tumor of the testes; in adults these are almost always malignant germinomas, whereas in children many are yolk sac tumors or benign varieties such as teratomas or androblastomas 睾丸肿瘤，在成年人中，几乎总是恶性生殖细胞瘤，而在儿童中，则许多是卵黄囊瘤或良性肿瘤如畸胎瘤或胚细胞瘤；**theca cell t.,** a fibroid-like ovarian tumor containing yellow areas of lipoid material derived from theca cells 泡膜细胞瘤，卵巢的纤维样癌，含有来自卵泡膜细胞中类脂性黄色区域；**turban t.,**

T

multiple cylindromas of the scalp 头巾样瘤，头皮的多圆柱瘤；**virilizing t.,** a functional tumor that produces virilization in girls and women or precocious puberty in boys 男性化瘤，一种功能性肿瘤，可使女孩和妇女身上出现男性化特征，或使男性出现性早熟现象；**Warthin t.,** adenolymphoma 沃辛瘤，淋巴瘤性乳头状囊腺瘤；**Wilms t.,** a rapidly developing malignant mixed tumor of the kidneys, made up of embryonal elements, usually affecting children before the fifth year 肾母细胞瘤，一种由胚胎成分组成的的恶性肾脏肿瘤，进展迅速，常见于五岁前儿童；**yolk sac t.,** a germ cell tumor that represents a proliferation of both yolk sac endoderm and extraembryonic mesenchyme; it produces α-fetoprotein and is usually in the testes 卵黄囊瘤，由卵黄囊内胚层和胚胎外间质增殖而成的肿瘤，产生 α-甲胎蛋白，通常位于睾丸中

tu·mor·i·ci·dal (too″mər-ĭ-si′dal) oncolytic 破坏癌细胞的

tu·mor·i·gen·e·sis (too″mər-ĭ-jen′ə-sis) the production of tumors 肿瘤发生

tu·mor·let (too′mər-lət) a type of tiny, often microscopic, benign neoplasm occurring singly or multiply in bronchial and bronchiolar mucosa of middle-aged to elderly people, often in areas of scarring 微小肿瘤，通常为微小的良性肿瘤，在中老年人的支气管和支气管黏膜中呈单发或多发，常发生在瘢痕区域

TUMT transurethral microwave thermotherapy 经尿道微波热疗法

TUNA transurethral needle ablation 经尿道针刺消融术

Tun·ga (tung′gə) a genus of fleas, including T. *pe′netrans*, the chigoe (q.v.) 潜蚤属

tung·sten (W) (tung′stən) a steel-gray, corrosion-resistant, metallic element, ductile when pure; at. no. 74, at. wt. 183.84 钨（化学元素）

tu·ni·ca (too′nĭ-kə) pl. *tu′nicae* [L.] coat, layer; a membrane or other structure covering or lining a body part or organ 膜，被膜；**t. adventi′tia,** the outer coat of various tubular structures, made up of connective tissue and elastic fibers 血管外膜；**adventi′tia vaso′rum,** 同 t. externa vasorum；**t. albugi′nea,** a dense, white, fibrous sheath enclosing a part or organ 白膜；**t. dar′tos,** the thin layer of superficial fascia underlying the skin of the scrotum, consisting mainly of the dartos muscle. The term may be used to denote the dartos muscle specifically 肉膜，特指肌肉膜；**t. exter′na vaso′rum,** the outer, fibroelastic coat of the blood vessels 血管外膜；**t. fibro′sa,** fibrous coat; an enveloping fibrous membrane or capsule 纤维膜；**t. in′tima vaso′rum,** the innermost coat of blood vessels 血

管内膜；**t. me′dia vaso′rum,** the middle coat of blood vessels 血管中膜；**t. muco′sa,** mucosa 黏膜；**t. muscula′ris,** the muscular coat or layer surrounding the submucosa in most portions of the digestive, respiratory, urinary, and genital tracts 肌层；**t. sero′sa,** serosa 浆膜；**t. vagina′lis tes′tis,** the serous membrane covering the front and sides of the testis and epididymis 睾丸鞘膜；**t. vasculo′sa,** a vascular coat, or a layer well supplied with blood vessels 血管膜

tun·nel (tun′əl) a passageway of varying length through a solid body, completely enclosed except for the open ends, permitting entrance and exit 隧道；**carpal t.,** the osseofibrous passage for the median nerve and the flexor tendons, formed by the flexor retinaculum and the carpal bones 腕管；**Corti t.,** inner t. 科蒂隧道；**flexor t.,** carpal t. 屈肌管；**inner t.,** a canal extending the length of the cochlea, formed by the pillar cells of the organ of Corti 内隧道；**tarsal t.,** the osseofibrous passage for the posterior tibial vessels, tibial nerve, and flexor tendons, formed by the flexor retinaculum and the tarsal bones 跗管

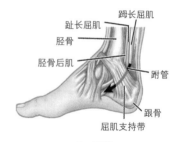

趾长屈肌
拇长屈肌
胫骨
胫骨后肌
跗管
跟骨
屈肌支持带

▲ 跗管

tur·bi·dim·e·ter (tur″bĭ-dim′ə-tər) an apparatus for measuring turbidity of a solution 浊度仪

tur·bid·i·ty (tər-bid′ĭ-te) cloudiness; disturbance of solids (sediment) in a solution, so that it is not clear 浊度；**tur′bid** *adj*

tur·bi·nal (tur′bĭ-nəl) 同 turbinate

tur·bi·nate (tur′bĭ-nāt) 1. shaped like a top 甲介形的；2. any of the nasal conchae 鼻甲； Called also turbinal

tur·bi·nec·to·my (tur″bĭ-nek′tə-me) excision of a turbinate bone (nasal concha) 鼻甲切除术

tur·bi·not·o·my (tur″bĭ-not′ə-me) incision of a turbinate bone 鼻甲切开术

tur·ges·cence (tər-jes′əns) swelling 肿胀，肿大

tur·gid (tur′jid) swollen and congested 肿胀的，浮肿的；充满的，胀满的

tur·gor (tur′gər) condition of being turgid; normal

or other fullness 充盈，充满，胀满

tu·ris·ta (too-rēs′tah) Mexican name for *traveler's diarrhea* 墨西哥对旅游者腹泻的称呼

tur·mer·ic (too′mər-ik) (tur′mər-ik) *Curcuma longa* or its rhizome, which is used to treat dyspepsia and anorexia and has a wide variety of uses in traditional Chinese medicine, ayurveda, and folk medicine 姜黄

turm·schä·del (toorm′sha-dəl) [Ger.] a developmental anomaly in which the head is high and rounded, due to early synostosis of the three major sutures of the skull 颅骨高圆畸形，由于颅骨三条主要骨缝过早闭合而呈现的头部高而圆的发育异常

turn·over (turn′o-vər) the movement of something into, through, and out of a place; the rate at which a thing is depleted and replaced 更新，周转，转换；**erythrocyte iron t. (EIT)**, the rate at which iron moves from the bone marrow into circulating red cells 红细胞铁周转率；**plasma iron t. (PIT)**, the rate at which iron moves from the blood plasma to the bone marrow or other tissues 血浆铁周转率

TURP transurethral resection of the prostate 经尿道前列腺切除术

tur·ri·ceph·a·ly (tur″ĭ-sef′ə-le) an abnormally tall skull with a short anteroposterior length, giving it a domed shape 尖头畸形

tus·si·gen·ic (tus″ĭ-jen′ik) causing cough 致咳的

tus·sis (tus′is) [L.] cough 咳嗽；**tus′sal, tus′sive** *adj.*

tu·ta·men (tu-ta′mən) pl. *tu′tamina* [L.] a protective covering or structure 保护器，防御物

TWBC terminal warm blood cardioplegia 末期温血心肌灌注

twig (twig) a final ramification, as of branches of a nerve or blood vessel 小支，细支，解剖上指神经或血管的分支

twin (twin) one of two offspring produced in the same pregnancy 双胞胎之一的；双胎，双生；**allantoidoangiopagous t's**, twins united by the umbilical vessels only 脐血管联胎；**conjoined t's**, monozygotic twins whose bodies are joined to a varying extent 联胎；**diamniotic t's**, twins developing within separate amniotic cavities; they may be monochorionic or dichorionic 双羊膜双胎，在不同的羊膜腔内发育的双胎，可以是单绒毛膜或双绒毛膜的；**dichorionic t's**, twins having distinct chorions, including monozygotic twins separated within 72 hours of fertilization and all dizygotic twins 双卵性双胎；**dizygotic t's, fraternal t's, heterologous t's**, twins developed from two separate oocytes fertilized at the same time 二卵双生，异卵双生，双卵双胎；**identical t's**, 同 monozygotic t's；**impacted t's**, twins so situated during delivery that the

pressure of one against the other prevents simultaneous engagement of both 阻生双胎；**monoamniotic t's**, twins developing within a single amniotic cavity; they are always monozygotic and monochorionic 单羊膜双胎；**monochorionic t's**, twins developing with a single chorion; they are always monozygotic and may be monoamniotic or diamniotic 单绒毛膜双胎；**monozygotic t's**, two individuals developed from a single zygote; they have identical genomes 单卵双生，同卵双生；**omphaloangiopagous t's**, 脐血管联胎，参见 allantoidoangiopagous t's.Siamese t's, 同 conjoined t's；**similar t's**, 同 monozygotic t's

twin·ning (twin′ing) 1. the production of symmetric structures or parts by division 对裂，成对；2. the simultaneous intrauterine production of two or more embryos 双生，孪生

twitch (twich) a brief, contractile response of a skeletal muscle elicited by a single maximal volley of impulses in the neurons supplying it 抽搐，颤搐，肌肉因所属运动神经元的一系列最大冲动而发生的短时收缩反应

ty·lec·to·my (ti-lek′tə-me) lumpectomy 肿块切除术

tyl·i·on (til′e-on) a point on the anterior edge of the optic groove in the median line 交叉沟中点，视交叉沟前缘的正中点

ty·lo·sis (ti-lo′sis) callus formation 胼胝形成；**tylot′ic** *adj.*

ty·lox·a·pol (ti-lok′sə-pol) a nonionic liquid polymer used as a surfactant to aid liquefaction and removal of mucopurulent bronchopulmonary secretions, administered by inhalation 泰洛沙泊，一种非离子液体聚合体，用作表面活性剂促使支气管和肺中黏液脓性分泌物的液化和清除

tym·pa·nal (tim′pə-nəl) 同 tympanic

tym·pa·nec·to·my (tim″pə-nek′tə-me) myringectomy; excision of the tympanic membrane 鼓膜切除术

tym·pan·ic (tim-pan′ik) 1. tympanal; of or pertaining to the tympanum 鼓室的；鼓膜的；2. bell-like; resonant 鼓响的

tym·pa·nism (tim′pə-niz-əm) 同 tympanites

tym·pa·ni·tes (tim″pə-ni′tēz) abnormal distention from gas or air in the intestine or peritoneal cavity 气鼓，鼓胀

tym·pa·nit·ic (tim″pə-nit′ik) 1. pertaining to or affected with tympanites 气鼓的；2. bell-like; tympanic 鼓响的

tym·pa·no·cen·te·sis (tim″pə-no-sen-te′sis) surgical puncture of the tympanic membrane or tympanum 鼓膜穿刺术

tym·pa·no·gen·ic (tim″pə-no-jen′ik) arising from the tympanum or middle ear 鼓室源的

tym·pa·no·gram (tim-pan′o-gram″) a graphic representation of the relative compliance and impedance of the tympanic membrane and ossicles of the middle ear obtained by tympanometry 鼓室导抗图

tym·pa·no·mas·toid·itis (tim″pə-no-mas″toidi′tis) otitis media accompanied by inflammation of the mastoid air cells 鼓室乳突炎

tym·pa·nom·e·try (tim″pə-nom′ə-tre) indirect measurement of the compliance (mobility) and impedance of the tympanic membrane and ossicles of the middle ear 鼓室测压法 tym·pa·no·plas·ty (tim′pə-no-plas″te) surgical reconstruction of the tympanic membrane and establishment of ossicular continuity from the tympanic membrane to the vestibular window 鼓室成形术; **tympanoplas′tic** adj.

tym·pa·no·scle·ro·sis (tim″pə-no-sklə-ro′sis) a condition characterized by the presence of masses of hard, dense connective tissue around the auditory ossicles in the tympanic cavity 鼓室硬化; **tympanosclerot′ic** adj.

tym·pa·not·o·my (tim″pə-not′ə-me) myringotomy 鼓室探查术

tym·pa·nous (tim′pə-nəs) distended with gas 气鼓的, 鼓胀的

tym·pa·num (tim′pə-nəm) 1. tympanic membrane 鼓膜; 2. tympanic cavity 鼓室

tym·pa·ny (tim′pə-ne) 1. 同 tympanites; 2. a tympanic, or bell-like, percussion note 鼓响, 鼓音

type (tīp) the general or prevailing character of any particular case of disease, person, substance, etc. 型, 类型, 式; **blood t.**, 血型, 参见 blood group; **mating t.**, in ciliate protozoa, certain bacteria, and certain fungi, the equivalent of a sex 交配型; **phage t.**, an intraspecies type of bacterium demonstrated by phage typing 噬菌体类型; **wild t.**, the typical form occurring in a natural population or in the standard laboratory stock, as a strain, phenotype, or gene, and therefore designated as representative of the group 野生型, 遗传学中指任何自然群体或试验体的标准表型, 亦指决定标准表型性状的基因

ty·phoid (ti′foid) 1. resembling typhus 似斑疹伤寒的; 2. typhoid fever 伤寒; 3. 同 typhoidal

ty·phoid·al (ti-foid′əl) resembling typhoid fever 伤寒的, 伤寒样的

ty·phus (ti′fəs) a group of closely related, acute, arthropod-borne rickettsial diseases that differ in the intensity of certain signs and symptoms, severity, and fatality rate; all are characterized by headache, chills, fever, stupor, and a macular, maculopapular, petechial, or papulovesicular eruption. Often used alone in English-speaking countries to refer to epidemic typhus, and in several European languages to refer to typhoid fever 斑疹伤寒; **ty′phous** adj.; **endemic t.**, murine t. 地方性斑疹伤寒; **epidemic t.**, the classic form, due to Rickettsia prowazekii and transmitted between humans by body lice 流行性斑疹伤寒; **flying squirrel t.**, an acute infectious disease seen in the southeastern United States, similar to epidemic typhus, caused by Rickettsia prowazekii, and transmitted by fleas and lice of the flying squirrel 鼠型斑疹伤寒; **murine t.**, an infectious disease similar to epidemic typhus but milder, due to Rickettsia typhi, transmitted from rat to human by the rat flea 鼠型斑疹伤寒; **Queensland tick t.**, an acute spotted fever caused by Rickettsia australis; it has a characteristic primary lesion (tache noire) and is transmitted by Australian ticks of the genus Ixodes 昆士兰蜱传斑疹伤寒; **recrudescent t.**, Brill-Zinsser disease 变发性斑疹伤寒; **scrub t.**, an acute, typhus-like infectious disease caused by Orientia tsutsugamushi and transmitted by chiggers, characterized by a primary skin lesion at the site of inoculation and development of a rash, regional lymphadenopathy, and fever 恙虫病

ty·pol·o·gy (ti-pol′ə-je) the study of types; the science of classifying, as bacteria according to type 类型学, 血型学

Tyr tyrosine 酪氨酸

ty·ro·ma·to·sis (ti″ro-mə-to′sis) a condition characterized by caseous degeneration 干酪变性, 干酪化

ty·ro·pa·no·ate (ti″ro-pə-no′āt) a radiopaque medium used as the sodium salt in oral cholecystography 丁酰碘番酸钠, 胆囊造影剂

ty·ro·sine (Tyr) (ti′ro-sēn) a naturally occurring, nonessential amino acid present in most proteins; it is a product of phenylalanine metabolism and a precursor of thyroid hormones, catecholamines, and melanin 酪氨酸

ty·ro·sin·e·mia (ti″ro-sĭ-ne′me-ə) any of several disorders of tyrosine metabolism, most genetic, with elevated blood levels of tyrosine and urinary excretion of related metabolites. Type I shows inhibition of some liver enzymes and renal tubular function. Type II is marked by crystallization of the accumulated tyrosine in the epidermis and cornea and is frequently accompanied by intellectual disability. Neonatal t. is nongenetic, transitory, and usually asymptomatic 铬氨酸血症, 另参见 hawkinsinuria

ty·ro·syl·uria (ti″ro-səl-u′re-ə) increased urinary secretion of compounds derived from tyrosine 酪氨酰基尿

ty·vel·ose (ti′vəl-ōs) an unusual sugar that is a polysaccharide somatic antigen of certain Salmonella serovars 泰威糖

tzet·ze (tset′se) 同 tsetse 采采蝇

U

U[符号] international unit of enzyme activity 酶活性国际单位；unit (on The Joint Commission "Do Not Use" List) 单位；uracil 尿嘧啶；uranium 元素铀；uridine 尿苷

u[符号] atomic mass unit 原子质量单位

ubi·qui·nol (u″bĭ-kwĭ-nol′) the reduced form of ubiquinone 泛醌醇，泛醌的还原型

ubi·qui·none (Q, Q₁₀) (u″bĭ-kwĭ-nōn′) a quinone derivative with an unsaturated branched hydrocarbon side chain occurring in the lipid core of inner mitochondrial membranes and functioning in the electron transport chain. In naturopathic practice it is used for a wide variety of indications; also used as a dietary supplement for its antioxidant properties 泛醌，辅酶 Q

ubiq·ui·tin (u-bik′wĭ-tin) a polypeptide that is attached to proteins during intracellular proteolysis, marking them for degradation by protea - somes 泛素

UCBT umbilical cord blood transplantation 脐带血移植

UDP uridine diphosphate 尿苷二磷酸

UK urokinase 尿激酶

ul·cer (ul′sər) a local defect, or excavation of the surface, of an organ or tissue, produced by sloughing of necrotic inflammatory tissue 溃疡；aphthous u., the ulcerative lesion of recurrent aphthous stomatitis 口疮性溃疡；corneal u., ulcerative keratitis 角膜溃疡；decubital u., decubitus u., bedsore; an ulceration due to an arterial occlusion or prolonged pressure, as when a patient is confined to a bed or a wheelchair 压疮；duodenal u., a peptic ulcer in the duodenum 十二指肠溃疡；gastric u., a peptic ulcer of the gastric mucosa 胃溃疡；Hunner u., one involving all layers of the bladder wall, occurring in chronic interstitial cystitis 洪纳溃疡；hypertensive ischemic u., a manifestation of infarction of the skin due to arteriolar occlusion as part of a long-standing vascular disease, seen as a red painful plaque on the lower limb 高血压缺血性溃疡；jejunal u., a rare type of peptic ulcer in the jejunum 空肠溃疡；marginal u., 同 stomal u.；peptic u., one in the mucous membrane of the gastrointestinal tract, usually the stomach or duodenum but sometimes the lower esophagus, due to action of acidic gastric juice 消化性溃疡；perforating u., one involving the entire thickness of an organ or of the wall of an organ, creating an opening on both surfaces 穿孔性溃疡，穿通性溃疡；phagedenic u., 1.a necrotic lesion associated with tissue destruction, due to bacterial invasion of an existing cutaneous lesion or of intact skin in a person with impaired resistance because of systemic disease 崩蚀性溃疡；2. 同 tropical phagedenic u.；plantar u., a deep neurotrophic ulcer of the sole of the foot, resulting from repeated injury because of lack of sensation in the part; seen with diseases such as diabetes mellitus and leprosy 足底溃疡；pressure u., 同 decubitus u.；rodent u., ulcerating basal cell carcinoma of the skin 侵蚀性溃疡；stasis u., venous u 瘀积性溃疡；stercoraceous u., one caused by pressure of impacted feces; also, a fistulous ulcer through which fecal matter escapes 粪性溃疡；stomal u., a jejunal ulcer near the margin of a gastroenterostomy stoma 吻合口溃疡；stress u., a peptic ulcer resulting from stress 应激性溃疡；trophic u., one due to imperfect nutrition of the part 营养不良性溃疡；tropical u., 1. a lesion of cutaneous leishmaniasis 热带性溃疡；2. 同 tropical phagedenic u.；tropical phagedenic u., a chronic, painful, phagedenic ulcer of unknown cause, usually on the lower limbs of malnourished children in the tropics 热带性腐离性溃疡；varicose u., an ulcer on the leg due to varicose veins 静脉曲张性溃疡；venereal u., one around the external genitalia, resembling chancre or chancroid 生殖器溃疡；venous u., ulceration on the skin of the ankle due to venous insufficiency and venous stasis 静脉性溃疡

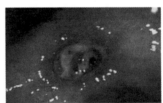

▲　角切迹处的胃溃疡

ul·cer·ate (ul′sər-āt) to undergo ulceration （使）形成溃疡

ul·cer·a·tion (ul″sər-a′shən) 1. the formation or development of an ulcer 溃疡形成；2. an ulcer 溃疡

ul·cer·a·tive (ul′sə-ra″tiv) (ul′sər-ə-tiv) pertaining to or characterized by ulceration 溃疡的，溃疡性的

ul·cero·gen·ic (ul″sər-o-jen′ik) causing ulceration; leading to the production of ulcers 产生溃疡的，致溃疡的

ul·cero·mem·bra·nous (ul″sər-o-mem′brə- nəs) characterized by ulceration and a membranous exudation 溃疡膜性的，以溃疡和膜性渗出为特征

ul·cer·ous (ul′sər-əs) 同 ulcerative

ul·cus (ul′kəs) pl. *ul′cera* [L.] 同 ulcer

ulec·to·my (u-lek′tə-me) 1. excision of scar tissue 瘢痕切除术；2. gingivectomy 龈切除术

uler·y·the·ma (u-ler″ə-the′mə) an erythematous skin disease with scarring and atrophy 瘢痕性红斑，一种以瘢痕形成和萎缩为特征的红斑性皮肤病；**u. ophryo′genes,** a hereditary form in which keratosis pilaris involves the hair follicles of the eyebrows 眉部瘢痕性红斑，一种累及眉毛毛囊的毛囊角化病，是一种遗传病

uli·pris·tal (u″lī-pris′təl) a selective progesterone receptor modulator, used as *u. acetate* for emergency postcoital contraception 一种选择性黄体酮受体调节药，用于紧急避孕

ul·na (ul′nə) pl. *ul′nae* [L.] the inner and larger bone of the forearm, on the side opposite that of the thumb; it articulates with the humerus and radius at its proximal end and with the radius and bones of the carpus at the distal end 尺骨

ul·nad (ul′nad) toward the ulna 向尺侧

ul·nar (ul′nər) pertaining to the ulna or to the medial aspect of the forearm as compared with the lateral (radial) aspect 尺骨的，尺侧的

ul·na·ris (əl-na′ris) [L.] 同 ulnar

ul·no·car·pal (ul″no-kahr′pəl) pertaining to the ulna and carpus 尺腕的

ul·no·ra·di·al (ul″no-ra′de-əl) pertaining to the ulna and radius 尺桡的

ulot·o·my (u-lot′ə-me) 1. incision of scar tissue 瘢痕切开术；2. incision of the gums 龈切开术

ul·tra·cen·trif·u·ga·tion (ul″trə-sən-trif″u-ga′-shən) subjection of material to an exceedingly high centrifugal force, which will separate and sediment the molecules of a substance 超速离心法

ul·tra·di·an (ul″trə-de′ən) pertaining to a period of less than 24 hours; applied to the rhythmic repetition of certain phenomena in living organisms occurring in cycles of less than a day *(ultradian rhythm)* 超日，是生物体内某些以高于昼夜频率的周期重复出现的现象，即每日不止出现一次

ul·tra·fil·tra·tion (ul″trə-fil-tra′shən) filtration through a filter capable of removing very minute (ultramicroscopic) particles 超滤法

ul·tra·mi·cro·scope (ul″trə-mi′kro-skōp) a special darkfield microscope for the examination of particles of colloidal size 超显微镜；**ultramicroscop′ic** *adj.*

ul·tra·son·ic (ul″trə-son′ik) beyond the upper limit of perception by the human ear; relating to sound waves having a frequency of more than 20,000 Hz 超声波的

ul·tra·son·ics (ul″trə-son′iks) the science dealing with ultrasonic sound waves 超声学

ul·tra·so·nog·ra·phy (ul″trə-sə-nog′rə-fe) the imaging of deep structures of the body by recording the echoes of pulses of ultrasonic waves directed into the tissues and reflected by tissue planes where there is a change in density. Diagnostic ultrasonography uses 1–10 megahertz waves 超声检查，超声成像；**ultrasonograph′ic** *adj.*; **Doppler u.,** that in which the shifts in frequency between emitted ultrasonic waves and their echoes are used to measure the velocities of moving objects, based on the principle of the Doppler effect. The waves may be continuous or pulsed; the technique is frequently used to examine cardiovascular blood flow (Doppler echocardiography) 多普勒超声检查；**duplex u.,** the combination of real-time and Doppler ultrasonography 双功能超声检查；**gray-scale u.,** a B-scan technique in which the strength of echoes is indicated by a proportional brightness of the displayed dots 灰阶超声检查；**real-time u.,** a series of ultrasound images produced in rapid succession so that the video display shows motion of an organ or part 实时成像超声波检查法；**transrectal u. (TRUS),** that using an endorectal probe to visualize structures adjacent to the rectum, such as the prostate 经直肠超声检查

ul·tra·sound (ul′trə-sound) 1. sound waves of a frequency greater than 20,000 Hz. 超声，频率大于20000 Hz 的声波；2. ultrasonography 超声波检查

ul·tra·struc·ture (ul′trə-struk″chər) the structure beyond the resolution power of the light microscope, i.e., visible only under the ultramicroscope and electron microscope 超微结构，指超出光学显微镜分辨能力的结构，即仅显微镜下可见

ul·tra·vi·o·let (UV) (ul″trə-vi′ə-lət) denoting electromagnetic radiation between violet light and x-rays, having wavelengths of 200 to 400 nm 紫外线；**u. A (UVA),** ultraviolet radiation with wavelengths between 320 and 400 nm, comprising over 99 percent of that reaching the surface of the earth. It enhances the harmful effects of UVB, is responsible for some photosensitivity reactions, and is used therapeutically in the treatment of various skin disorders 紫外线 A 段，近紫外线，长波紫外线，**u. B(UVB),** ultraviolet radiation with wavelengths between 290 and 320 nm, comprising 1 per cent of that reaching the surface of the earth. It causes sunburn and a number of damaging photochemical changes within cells, including damage to DNA leading to premature aging of the skin, premalignant and malignant changes, and various photosensitivity reactions; it is also used therapeutically in the treatment of skin disorders 紫外线 B（段），远紫外线，中波紫外线；**u. C(UVC),** ultraviolet radiation with wavelengths between 200 and 290 nm, all of which is filtered out by the ozone layer and does not reach the surface of the earth; it is germicidal and is also used in ultraviolet phototherapy 紫外线 C（段），超短紫外线，短波紫外线

um·bil·i·cal (əm-bil′ĭ-kəl) pertaining to the umbilicus 脐的

um·bil·i·ca·tion (əm-bil″ĭ-ka′shən) a depression resembling the umbilicus 脐样凹陷

um·bil·i·cus (əm-bil′ĭ-kəs) [L.] the navel; the scar marking the site of attachment of the umbilical cord in the fetus 脐

um·bo (um′bo) pl. *umbo′nes* [L.] 1. a rounded elevation 圆头；2. the slight projection at the center of the outer surface of the tympanic membrane 鼓膜突

UMP uridine monophosphate 尿苷（一磷）酸

uña de ga·to (oo′nyah da gah′to) [Sp.] cat's claw 猫爪

un·cal (ung′kəl) of or pertaining to the uncus 钩的

un·ci·form (un′sĭ-form) 同 uncinate (1)

un·ci·na·ri·al (un″sĭ-nar′e-əl) of, pertaining to, or caused by a hookworm 钩虫的

un·ci·nate (un′sĭ-nāt) 1. shaped like a hook 钩形的，钩状的；2. relating to or affecting the uncinate gyrus 钩回的

un·ci·pres·sure (un′sĭ-presh″ər) pressure with a hook to stop hemorrhage 钩压止血法

un·con·di·tioned (un″kən-dish′ənd) not a result of conditioning; unlearned; occurring naturally or spontaneously 无条件的，绝对的

un·con·scious (ən-kon′shəs) 1. insensible; incapable of responding to sensory stimuli and of having subjective experiences 不省人事的，意识丧失的；2. the part of the mind not readily accessible to conscious awareness but whose existence may be manifested in symptom formation, in dreams, or under the influence of drugs 无意识的，潜意识的；**collective u.,** the elements of the unconscious that are theoretically common to mankind 集体无意识，集体潜意识

un·co·ver·te·bral (ung″ko-vur′tə-brəl) pertaining to the uncinate processes of a vertebra 椎骨钩突的

un·cus (ung′kəs) 1. hook 钩状；2. the medially curved anterior end of the parahippocampal gyrus 海马回钩；**un′cal** *adj.*

un·dec·yl·en·ic ac·id (un″des-əl-en′ik) an unsaturated fatty acid used as a topical antifungal agent 十一烯酸

un·der·bite (un′dər-bīt) retrognathism 缩颌，颌退缩，咬颌不足

un·der·drive (un′dər-drīv″) pertaining to a rate less than normal 亚速；参见 *pacing*

un·der·sens·ing (un′dər-sens″ing) missed sensing

of cardiac electrical signals by an artificial pacemaker, resulting in too frequent or irregular delivery of stimuli 失敏，人工心脏起搏器无法感应到心脏电信号，导致刺激太频繁或不规则地传递

un·dif·fer·en·ti·at·ed (ən-dif″ər-en′she-āt-əd) anaplastic 未分化的

un·du·lant (un′jə-) (un′dyə-lənt) characterized by wavelike fluctuations 波动的，波状的

un·du·late (un′jə-) (un′dyə-lāt) 1. to move in waves or in a wavelike motion （使）波动，（使）起伏；2. to have a wavelike appearance, outline, or form （使）成波浪形；**un′dulate, un′dulatory** *adj.*

un·du·la·tion (un′jə-) (un″dyə-la′shən) 1. a wavelike motion 波动，参见 *pulsation*；2. a wavelike appearance, outline, or form 波浪形

ung. [L.] unguen′tum (ointment) 软膏，油膏

un·gual (ung′gwəl) pertaining to the nails 指（趾）甲的

un·guent (ung′gwənt) ointment 软膏，油膏

un·guic·u·late (əng-gwik′u-lāt) having claws or nails; clawlike 有爪的，爪样的

un·guis (ung′gwis) pl. *un′gues* [L.] nail (1) 指（趾）甲

uni·ax·i·al (u″ne-ak′se-əl) 1. having only one axis 单轴的；2. developing in an axial direction only 单轴向的

uni·cam·er·al (u″nĭ-kam′ər-əl) having only one cavity or compartment 单腔的

uni·cel·lu·lar (u″nĭ-sel′u-lər) made up of a single cell, as the bacteria 单细胞的

uni·cor·nu·ate (u″nĭ-kor′nu-āt) having only one horn or cornu 单角的，独角的

uni·fas·cic·u·lar (u″nĭ-fə-sik′u-lər) pertaining to a single bundle, or fasciculus 单束支传导

uni·glan·du·lar (u″nĭ-glan′du-lər) affecting only one gland 单腺的

uni·lat·er·al (u″nĭ-lat′ər-əl) affecting only one side 一侧的，单侧的

uni·loc·u·lar (u″nĭ-lok′u-lər) having but one cavity or compartment 单房的

un·in·hib·it·ed (un″in-hib′ĭ-təd) free from usual constraints; not subject to normal inhibitory mechanisms 无拘束的；不受禁止的

uni·nu·cle·at·ed (u″nĭ-noo′kle-āt″əd) mononuclear (1) 单核的

uni·oc·u·lar (u″ne-ok′u-lər) monocular 单眼的

un·ion (ūn′yən) the renewal of continuity in a broken bone or between the edges of a wound 愈合；连接；联合

uni·ov·u·lar (u″ne-ov′u-lər) 1. monozygotic 单合子的；2. monovular 单卵的

uni·pa·ren·tal (u″nĭ-pə-ren′təl) pertaining to one of the parents only 单亲的

unip·a·rous (u-nip′ə-rəs) 1. producing only one offspring or egg at one time 产一卵的，产一子的；2. primiparous 初产的；参见 *primipara*

uni·po·lar (u″nĭ-po′lər) 1. having a single pole or process, as a nerve cell 单极的，仅有单极的或单突的，如神经细胞；2. pertaining to mood disorders in which only depressive episodes occur（指精神错乱）仅有抑郁发作的

uni·po·ten·cy (u″nĭ-po′tən-se) the ability of a part to develop in one manner only, or of a cell to develop into only one type of cell 单能性，只能以一种方式发育的能力，或者某细胞只发育成一型细胞的能力 unip′otent, unipoten′tial *adj.*

unit (U) (u′nit) 1. a single thing 单元；2. a quantity assumed as a standard of measurement 单位；Angström u., angstrom 埃 单位；atomic mass u. (u) (amu), the unit mass equal to one-twelfth the mass of the nuclide of carbon-12 原子质量单位，又称 *dalton*；Bethesda u., a measure of the level of inhibitor to coagulation factor Ⅷ; equal to the amount of inhibitor in patient plasma that will inactivate 50 percent of factor Ⅷ in an equal volume of normal plasma following a 2-hour incubation period 贝 特斯达单位；Bodansky u., the quantity of alkaline phosphatase that liberates 1 mg of phosphate ion from glycerol 2-phosphate in 1 hour under standard conditions Bodansky 单位；British thermal u. (BTU), the amount of heat necessary to raise the temperature of 1 pound of water 1 degree Fahrenheit, usually from 39 ℉ to 40 ℉英热单位；CGS u., any unit in the centimeter-gramsecond system 厘米 - 克 - 秒制单位；CH50 u., the amount of complement that will lyse 50 percent of a standard preparation of sheep red blood cells coated with antisheep erythrocyte antibody CH50 单位，可溶解 50% 覆有抗绵羊红细胞抗体的绵羊红细胞标准液的补体量；coronary care u., a specially designed and equipped hospital area containing a small number of private rooms, with all facilities necessary for constant observation and possible emergency treatment of patients with severe heart disease 冠心病监护治疗病房；intensive care u. (ICU), a hospital unit in which are concentrated special equipment and skilled personnel for the care of seriously ill patients requiring immediate and continuous attention 加强监护病房，重症监护室，重症监护治疗病房；International u. (IU), a unit of biologic material, such as enzymes, hormones, vitamins, etc., established by the International Conference for the Unification of Formulas 国际单位；motor u., the unit of motor activity formed by a motor nerve cell and its many innervated muscle fibers 运动单位；pilosebaceous u., the complex consisting of a hair follicle,

its sebaceous gland, and the arrector pili muscle 毛囊皮脂腺单位；postanesthesia care u. (PACU), a specialized unit adjoining an operating room, equipped and staffed for giving postoperative care to patients recovering from anesthesia and intravenous sedation 麻醉后恢复室，又称 *recovery room*；SI u., any of the units of the Système International d'Unités (International System of Units) adopted in 1960 at the Eleventh General Conference of Weights and Measures 国际单位制；见附表；Somogyi u., that amount of amylase which will liberate reducing equivalents equal to 1 mg of glucose per 30 minutes under defined conditions Somogyi 单 位；Svedberg u. (S), a unit equal to 10⁻13 second used for expressing sedimentation coefficients of macromolecules 斯韦德贝里单位；terminal respiratory u., the anatomic and functional unit of the lung, including a respiratory bronchiole, alveolar ducts and sacs, and alveoli 终末呼吸单位，见图 25；toxic u., toxin u., the smallest dose of a toxin that will kill a guinea pig weighing about 250 g in 3 to 4 days 毒素单位，能使大约 250g 重的豚鼠在 3~4 天内死亡的最小的毒素量；USP u., one used in the *United States Pharmacopeia* in expressing potency of drugs and other preparations 美国药典单位

Unit·ed States Phar·ma·co·peia (USP) a legally recognized compendium of standards for drugs, published by The United States Pharmacopeial Convention, Inc., and revised periodically. It includes also assays and tests for the determination of strength, quality, and purity 美国药典

uni·va·lent (u″nĭ-va′lənt) having a valence of 1 单价的，一价的

un·my·eli·nat·ed (ən-mi′ə-lĭ-nāt″əd) not having a myelin sheath; said of a nerve fiber 无髓鞘的

uno·pros·tone (u″no-pros′tōn) an antiglaucoma agent that decreases elevated intraocular pressure; used as u. isopropyl in the treatment of open-angle glaucoma and ocular hypertension 乌诺前列酮，用于治疗原发性开角型青光眼及高眼压症

un·phys·i·o·log·ic (un″fiz-e-o-loj′ik) not physiologic in character 非生理性的

un·sat·u·rat·ed (ən-sach′ə-rāt″əd) 1. not holding all of a solute that can be held in solution by the solvent （溶液）不饱和的；2. denoting compounds in which two or more atoms are united by double or triple bonds 不饱和化合物的

un·stri·at·ed (ən-stri′āt-əd) having no striations, as smooth muscle 无横纹的，平滑的

UP urticaria pigmentosa 色素性荨麻疹

upa·dha·tu (oo″pə-thū′too) according to ayurveda, secondary, temporary tissue that arises from the metabolism and waste of primary tissues (dhatus) 次生

组织，根据阿育吠陀的说法继发的，临时性的组织产生于初级组织的代谢和废物中

u·plas·min·o·gen ac·ti·va·tor (plaz-min′ə-jən″ ak′tĭ-va″tər) formal name for *urokinase* 尿纤维溶酶原激活剂；尿激酶的正式名

UPPP uvulopalatopharyngoplasty 悬雍垂咽成形术

up·reg·u·la·tion (up″reg-u-la′shən) increase in expression of a gene; most narrowly, that due to increased transcription of a specific mRNA, but also used more broadly for increase in mRNA levels for the gene by any means 基因表达的上调，最狭义的解释是由于特定 mRNA 的转录增加，但也可以更广泛地用于以任何方式提高该基因的 mRNA 水平

up·stream (up′strēm) in molecular biology, a term used to denote a region of nucleic acid to the 5′ side of a gene or region of interest 上游区，在分子生物学中，用于表示位于基因的 5′ 位的核酸区或感兴趣区

up·take (up′tāk) absorption and incorporation of a substance by living tissue 摄入，摄取

ura·chus (u′rə-kəs) a fetal canal connecting the bladder with the allantois, persisting throughout life as a cord (median umbilical ligament) 脐尿管；**u′rachal** *adj.*

ura·cil (U) (ūr′ə-sil) a pyrimidine base, in animal cells usually occurring condensed with ribose to form the ribonucleoside uridine; the corresponding deoxyribonucleoside is deoxyuridine 尿嘧啶

ura·ni·um (U) (u-ra′ne-əm) a hard, silvery white, lustrous, heavy, radioactive metallic element; at. no. 92, at. wt. 238.029; it has both natural (^{234}U, ^{235}U, and ^{238}U) and synthetic isotopes. Both ^{235}U and ^{238}U are parent compounds of natural decay series 铀（化

SI Units 国际单位制

Quantity 量	Unit 单位	Symbol 符号	Derivation 推出单位
Base Units 基本单位			
Length 长度	meter 米	m	
Mass 质量	kilogram 千克	kg	
Time 时间	second 秒	s	
Electric current 电流	ampere 安培	A	
Temperature 热力学温度	kelvin 开尔文	K	
Luminous intensity 发光强度	candela 坎德拉	cd	
Amount of substance 物质的量	mole 摩尔	mol	
Supplementary Units 辅助单位			
Plane angle 平面角	radian 弧度	rad	
Solid angle 立体角	steradian 立体弧度	sr	
Derived Units 导出单位			
Force 力	newton 牛顿	N	$kg \cdot m/s^2$
Pressure 压力、压强	pascal 帕斯卡	Pa	N/m^2
Energy, work 能，功	joule 焦耳	J	$N \cdot m$
Power 功率	watt 瓦特	W	J/s

U

Quantity 量	Unit 单位	Symbol 符号	Derivation 推出单位
Electric charge 电荷	coulomb 库仑	C	A•s
Electric potential 电位	volt 伏特	V	J/C
Electric capacitance 电容	farad 法拉	F	C/V
Electric resistance 电阻	ohm 欧姆	Ω	V/A
Electric conductance 电导	siemens 西门子	S	Ω^{-1}
Magnetic flux 磁通量	weber 韦伯	Wb	V•s
Magnetic flux density 磁通密度，磁感应强度	tesla 特斯拉	T	Wb/m^2
Inductance 电感	henry 亨利	H	Wb/A
Frequency 频率	hertz 赫兹	Hz	s^{-1}
Luminous flux 光通量	lumen 流明	lm	cd•sr
Illumination 光照度	lux 勒克斯	lx	lm/m^2
Temperature 摄氏温度	degree celsius 摄氏度	℃	K-273.15
Radioactivity 放射性活度	becquerel 贝可勒尔	Bq	S^{-1}
Absorbed dose 吸收剂量	gray 戈瑞	Gy	J/kg
Absorbed dose equivalent 剂量当量	sievert 希沃特	Sv	J/kg

学元素）

urar·thri·tis (u″rahr-thri′tis) gouty arthritis 痛风性关节炎

urate (ūr′āt) any salt or anion of uric acid (q.v.) 尿酸盐

ura·to·ma (u″rə-to′mə) a concretion made up of urates; tophus 痛风石，尿酸盐结石

ura·tu·ria (u″rə-tu′re-ə) hyperuricosuria 尿酸（盐）

ur·ce·i·form (ər-se′ĭ-form) pitcher-shaped 壶形的

urea (u-re′ə) 1. the chief nitrogenous end product of protein metabolism, formed in the liver from amino acids and from ammonia compounds; found in urine, blood, and lymph 脲，尿素；2. a pharmaceutical preparation of urea used to lower intracranial or intraocular pressure, to induce abortion, and as a topical skin moisturizer 尿素制剂；**ure′al** adj.；

u. nitrogen, the urea concentration of serum or plasma, conventionally specified in terms of nitrogen content and called *blood urea nitrogen (BUN);* an important indicator of renal function 尿素氮

urea·gen·e·sis (u-re″ə-jen′ə-sis) formation of urea 脲生成，尿素生成；**ureagenet′ic** adj.

Urea·plas·ma (u-re″ə-plaz′mə) a genus of gramnegative, microaerophilic, nonmotile bacteria of the family Mycoplastaceae, including *U. urealyt′i-cum,* a normal inhabitant of the genitourinary tract that is an opportunistic pathogen, causing genitourinary and respiratory infections 脲原体属

urea·poi·e·sis (u-re″ə-poi-e′sis) 同 ureagenesis；**ureapoiet′ic** adj.

ure·ase (u′re-ās) an enzyme that catalyzes the hydrolysis of urea to ammonia and carbon dioxide; it is a nickel protein of microorganisms and plants that is used in clinical assays of plasma urea concentrations

脲酶，尿素酶

ure·mia (u-re′me-ə) 1. azotemia; an excess of the nitrogenous end products of protein and amino acid metabolism in the blood 氮质血症; 2. the entire constellation of signs and symptoms of chronic renal failure 尿毒症. **ure′mic** *adj*.

ure·mi·gen·ic (u-re″mĭ-jen′ik) 1. caused by uremia 尿毒症性的; 2. causing uremia 致尿毒症的

ureo·tel·ic (u″re-o-tel′ik) having urea as the chief excretory product of nitrogen metabolism 排尿素（氮代谢）的

ure·ter (u-re′tər) (u′rə-tər) the fibromuscular tube through which urine passes from kidney to bladder 输尿管; **ure′teral, ureter′ic** *adj*.

ure·ter·al·gia (u-re″tər-al′jə) pain in the ureter 输尿管痛

ure·ter·ec·ta·sis (u-re″tər-ek′tə-sis) distention of the ureter 输尿管扩张

ure·ter·ec·to·my (u-re″tər-ek′tə-me) excision of a ureter 输尿管切除术

ure·ter·itis (u-re″tər-i′tis) inflammation of a ureter 输尿管炎

ure·tero·cele (u-re′tər-o-sēl″) sacculation of the terminal portion of the ureter into the bladder, as a result of stenosis of the ureteral meatus 输尿管疝，因输尿管口狭窄而导致的输尿管末端囊泡进入膀胱

ure·tero·ce·lec·to·my (u-re″tər-o-se-lek′tə- me) excision of a ureterocele 输尿管疝切除术

ure·tero·co·los·to·my (u-re″tər-o-kə-los′tə- me) anastomosis of a ureter to the colon 输尿管结肠吻合术

ure·tero·cys·tos·to·my (u-re″tər-o-sis-tos′tə- me) ureteroneocystostomy. 输尿管膀胱吻合术

ure·ter·en·ter·os·to·my (u-re″tər-o-en″təros′tə- me) anastomosis of one or both ureters to the wall of the intestine 输尿管肠吻合术

ure·ter·og·ra·phy (u-re″tər-og′rə-fe) radiography of the ureter after injection of a contrast medium 输尿管造影术

ure·tero·il·e·os·to·my (u-re″tər-o-il″e-os′tə- me) anastomosis of the ureters to an isolated loop of the ileum drained through a stoma on the abdominal wall 输尿管回肠吻合术

ure·tero·lith (u-re′tər-o-lith) a calculus in the ureter 输尿管石

ure·tero·li·thi·a·sis (u-re″tər-o-li-thi′ə-sis) formation or presence of calculi in the ureter 输尿管石病

ure·tero·li·thot·o·my (u-re″tər-o-li-thot′ə- me) incision of a ureter for removal of calculus 输尿管石切除术

ure·ter·ol·y·sis (u-re″tər-ol′ĭ-sis) 1. the op - eration of freeing the ureter from adhesions 输尿管松解术; 2. rupture of the ureter 输尿管破裂

ure·tero·neo·cys·tos·to·my (u-re″tər-o-ne″osis-tos′tə-me) surgical transplantation of a ureter to a different site in the bladder 输尿管膀胱吻合术

ure·tero·ne·phrec·to·my (u-re″tər-o-nə-frek′- tə-me) nephroureterectomy 输尿管肾切除术

ure·ter·op·a·thy (u-re″tər-op′ə-the) any disease of the ureter 输尿管病

ure·tero·pel·vic (u-re″tər-o-pel′vik) pertaining to or affecting the ureter and the renal pelvis 输尿管肾盂的

ure·tero·plas·ty (u-re′tər-o-plas″te) plastic surgery of a ureter 输尿管成形术

ure·tero·py·elog·ra·phy (u-re″tər-o-pi-ə- log′rə-fe) radiography of the ureter and renal pelvis 输尿管肾盂造影术

ure·tero·py·elo·plas·ty (u-re″tər-o-pi′ə-loplas″te) ureteropyelostomy 输尿管肾盂成形术

ure·tero·py·elos·to·my (u-re″tər-o-pi′ə- los′tə-me) surgical creation of a new communication between a ureter and the renal pelvis 输尿管肾盂吻合术

ure·tero·py·o·sis (u-re″tər-o-pi-o′sis) pyoureter 输尿管化脓

ure·tero·re·nos·co·py (u-re″tər-o-re-nos′kə- pe) visual inspection of the interior of the ureter and kidney by means of a fiberoptic endoscope (ureter-orenoscope), as for biopsy or removal or crushing of stones 输尿管肾镜检查

ure·ter·or·rha·gia (u-re″tər-o-ra′jə) discharge of blood from a ureter 输尿管出血

ure·ter·or·rha·phy (u-re″tər-or′ə-fe) suture of a ureter 输尿管缝合术

ure·ter·os·copy (u-re″tər-os′kə-pe) examination of the ureter by means of a fiberoptic endoscope (ureteroscope) 输尿管镜

ure·tero·sig·moi·dos·to·my (u-re″tər-o-sig″-moi-dos′tə-me) anastomosis of a ureter to the sigmoid colon 输尿管乙状结肠吻合术

ure·ter·os·to·my (u-re″tər-os′tə-me) creation of a new outlet for a ureter 输尿管造口术

ure·ter·ot·o·my (u-re″tər-ot′ə-me) incision of a ure-ter 输尿管切开术

ure·tero·ure·ter·os·to·my (u-re″tər-o-u-re″-tər-os′tə-me) end-to-end anastomosis of the two portions of a transected ureter 输尿管输尿管吻合术

ure·tero·vag·i·nal (u-re″tər-o-vaj′ĭ-nəl) pertaining to or communicating with a ureter and the vagina 输尿管阴道的

ure·tero·ves·i·cal (u-re″tər-o-ves′ĭ-kəl) pertaining to a ureter and the bladder 输尿管膀胱的

ure·thra (u-re′thrə) the membranous canal through which urine is discharged from the bladder to the exterior of the body 尿道; **ure′thral** *adj*.; **membranous u.**, a short portion of the urethra between the prostatic urethra and spongy urethra 尿道膜部;

U

Multiples and Submultiples of the Metric System
度量系统的倍数和约数

Multiples and Submultiples 倍数和约数	Power 幂	Prefix 词头	Symbol 符号
1,000,000,000,000	(10^{12})	tera- 太（拉）	T
1,000,000,000	(10^{9})	giga- 吉（咖）	G
1,000,000	(10^{6})	mega- 兆	M
1,000	(10^{3})	kilo- 千	k
100	(10^{2})	hecto- 百	h
10	(10)	deca- 十	da
0.1	(10^{-1})	deci- 分	d
0.01	(10^{-2})	centi- 厘	c
0.001	(10^{-3})	milli- 毫	m
0.000 001	(10^{-6})	micro- 微	μ
0.000 000 001	(10^{-9})	nano- 纳（诺）	n
0.000 000 000 001	(10^{-12})	pico- 皮（可）	p
0.000 000 000 000 001	(10^{-15})	femto- 飞（母托）	f
0.000 000 000 000 000 001	(10^{-18})	atto- 阿（托）	a

prostatic u., that part of the urethra passing through the prostate 尿道前列腺部；**Spongy u.,** the portion of the urethra within the corpus spongiosum penis 尿道海绵体部

ure·thral·gia (u″re-thral′jə) pain in the urethra 尿道痛

ure·thra·tre·sia (u-re″thrə-tre′zhə) urethral atresia 尿道闭锁

ure·threc·to·my (u″rə-threk′tə-me) surgical removal of all or part of the urethra 尿道（部分）切除术

ure·thri·tis (u″rə-thri′tis) inflammation of the urethra 尿 道 炎；**nongonococcal u., nonspecific u.,** urethritis without evidence of gonococcal infection 非淋菌性尿道炎，非特异性尿道炎

ure·thro·bul·bar (u-re″thro-bul′bər) bulbourethral 尿道球的

ure·thro·cele (u-re′thro-sēl) 1. prolapse of the urethral mucosa（女性）尿道突出；2. a diverticulum of the urethral walls encroaching upon the vaginal

canal（女性）尿道憩室

ure·thro·cys·ti·tis (u-re″thro-sis-ti′tis) in - flammation of the urethra and bladder 尿道膀胱炎

ure·thro·dyn·ia (u-re″thro-din′e-ə) 同 urethralgia

ure·throg·ra·phy (u″rə-throg′rə-fe) radiography of the urethra 尿道造影（术）

ure·throm·e·try (u″rə-throm′ə-tre) 1. determination of the resistance of various segments of the urethra to retrograde flow of fluid 尿道阻力测定法；2. measurement of the urethra 尿道测量法

ure·thro·pe·nile (u-re″thro-pe′nīl) pertaining to the urethra and penis 尿道阴茎的

ure·thro·peri·ne·al (u-re″thro-per″ĭ-ne′əl) pertaining to the urethra and perineum 尿道会阴的

ure·thro·peri·neo·scro·tal (u-re″thro-per″ĭ- ne″o-skro′təl) pertaining to the urethra, perineum, and scrotum 尿道会阴阴囊的

ure·thro·pexy (u-re′thro-pek″se) bladder neck suspension 尿道固定术

ure·thro·plas·ty (u-re′thro-plas″te) plastic surgery of the urethra 尿道成形术

ure·thro·pros·tat·ic (u-re″thro-pros-tat′ik) pertaining to the urethra and prostate 尿道前列腺的

ure·thro·rec·tal (u-re′thro-rek′təl) rectourethral 尿道直肠的

ure·thror·rha·gia (u-re″thro-ra′jə) flow of blood from the urethra 尿道出血

ure·thror·rha·phy (u″rə-thror′ə-fe) suture of the urethra 尿道缝合术

ure·thror·rhea (u-re″thro-re′ə) abnormal discharge from the urethra 尿道液溢

ure·thro·scope (u-re′thro-skōp) an endoscope for viewing the interior of the urethra 尿道镜

ure·thro·scop·ic (u-re″thro-skop′ik) 1. pertaining to a urethroscope 尿道镜的；2. pertaining to urethroscopy 尿道镜检查的

ure·thros·co·py (u″rə-thros′kə-pe) inspection of the interior of the urethra with a urethroscope 尿道镜检查

ure·thro·stax·is (u-re″thro-stak′sis) oozing of blood from the urethra 尿道渗血

ure·thro·ste·no·sis (u-re″thro-stə-no′sis) stricture or stenosis of the urethra 尿道狭窄

ure·thros·to·my (u″rə-thros′tə-me) surgical formation of a permanent opening of the urethra at the perineal surface 尿道造口术

ure·thro·tome (u-re′thro-tōm) an instrument for cutting a urethral stricture 尿道刀

ure·throt·o·my (u″rə-throt′ə-me) incision of the urethra, either through the perineum (external u.) or from within (internal u.) 尿道切开术

ure·thro·tri·go·ni·tis (u-re″thro-tri″go-ni′tis) inflammation of the urethra and trigone of the bladder 尿道膀胱三角炎

ure·thro·vag·i·nal (u-re″thro-vaj′ĭ-nəl) pertaining to the urethra and vagina 尿道阴道的

ure·thro·ves·i·cal (u-re″thro-ves′ĭ-kəl) vesicourethral 尿道膀胱的

ur·gen·cy (ur′jən-se) a sudden compelling need to do something 尿急，紧急；bowel u., the sudden need to defecate 肠急症；urinary u., the sudden need to urinate 尿急

urhi·dro·sis (u″rĭ-dro′sis) the presence in the sweat of urinous materials, chiefly uric acid and urea 尿汗症

uric ac·id (u′rik) the end product of purine catabolism in primates; elevated levels are associated with gout and nephrolithiasis. Its salts, urates, are insoluble in water and can form crystals, stones, or calculi 尿酸

uric·ac·i·de·mia (u″rik-as″ĭ-de′me-ə) hyperurice-

mia 尿酸血症

uric·ac·i·du·ria (u″rik-as″ĭ-du′re-ə) hyperuricosuria 尿酸尿

uri·ce·mia (u″rĭ-se′me-ə) hyperuricemia 尿酸血症

uri·co·su·ria (u″rĭ-ko-su′re-ə) excretion of uric acid in the urine 尿酸尿

uri·co·su·ric (u″rĭ-ko-su′rik) 1. pertaining to, characterized by, or promoting uricosuria 促尿酸尿的；2. an agent that so acts 促尿酸尿药

uri·dine (U) (ūr′ĭ-dēn) a pyrimidine nucleoside containing uracil and ribose; it is a component of nucleic acid, and its nucleosides are involved in the biosynthesis of polysaccharides 尿苷，尿嘧啶核苷；u. diphosphate (UDP), a pyrophosphate-containing nucleotide that serves as a carrier for hexoses, hexosamines, and hexuronic acids in the synthesis of glycogen, glycoproteins, and glycosaminoglycans 尿苷二磷酸；u. monophosphate (UMP), uridylic acid; a nucleotide, uridine 5′-phosphate 尿苷一磷酸；u. triphosphate (UTP), a nucleotide involved in RNA synthesis 尿苷三磷酸

uri·dyl·ic ac·id (u″rĭ-dil′ik) phosphorylated uridine; uridine monophosphate unless otherwise specified 尿苷酸

uri·nal (u′rĭ-nəl) a receptacle for urine 尿壶，贮尿器

uri·nal·y·sis (u″rĭ-nal′ĭ-sis) analysis of the urine 尿分析（法）

uri·nary (u′rĭ-nar″e) pertaining to, containing, or secreting urine 尿的，含尿的；泌尿的

uri·nate (u′rĭ-nāt) to discharge urine 排尿

uri·na·tion (u″rĭ-na′shən) the discharge of urine 排尿

urine (u′rin) the fluid excreted by the kidneys, stored in the bladder, and discharged through the urethra 尿；residual u., urine remaining in the bladder after urination 剩余尿，残余尿

uri·nif·er·ous (u″rĭ-nif′ər-əs) transporting or conveying urine 输尿的

uri·nog·e·nous (u″rĭ-noj′ə-nəs) of urinary origin 生尿的，尿原的

uri·no·ma (u″rĭ-no′mə) 尿性囊肿 1. a cyst containing urine 含有尿液的囊肿；2. a collection of urine surrounded by fibrous tissue, from leakage through a tear in the ureter, renal pelvis, or renal calix due to obstruction, or from trauma 由于输尿管、肾盂或肾盏因梗阻或外伤撕裂而漏出的由纤维组织包围的尿液的集合

uri·nom·e·ter (u″rĭ-nom′ə-tər) an instrument for determining the specific gravity of urine 尿比重计

uri·nom·e·try (u″rĭ-nom′ə-tre) determination of the specific gravity of urine 尿比重测量法

uro·bi·lin (u″ro-bi′lin) a brown pigment formed by

U

oxidation of urobilinogen, found in feces 尿胆素

uro·bil·in·emia (u″ro-bil″ĭ-ne′me-ə) urobilin in the blood 尿胆素血症

uro·bi·lino·gen (u″ro-bĭ-lin′o-jən) a colorless compound formed in the intestines by reduction of bilirubin 尿胆素原

uro·can·ic ac·id (u″ro-kan′ik) an intermediate metabolite of histamine, convertible normally to glutamic acid 尿酸，组氨酸的一种中间代谢产物，一般可转换成谷氨酸

uro·che·zia (u″ro-ke′zhə) the discharge of urine in the feces 肛门排尿

uro·chrome (u′ro-krōm) the end product of hemoglobin breakdown, found in the urine and responsible for its yellow color 尿色素，尿色肽

uro·cys·ti·tis (u″ro-sis-ti′tis) cystitis 膀胱炎

uro·dy·nam·ics (u″ro-di-nam′iks) the dynamics of the propulsion and flow of urine in the urinary tract 尿动力学；**urodynam′ic** *adj.*

uro·dyn·ia (u″ro-din′e-ə) pain accompanying urination 排尿痛

uro·ede·ma (u″ro-ə-de′mə) edema due to infiltration of urine 尿液性水肿

uro·flow·me·ter (u″ro-flo′me-tər) a device for the continuous recording of urine flow in milliliters per second 尿流（量）计

uro·fol·li·tro·pin (u″ro-fol′ĭ-tro″pin) a preparation of gonadotropins from the urine of postmenopausal women, containing follicle-stimulating hormone and used in conjunction with human chorionic gonadotropin to induce ovulation 尿促卵泡，一种由绝经后妇女的尿液制得的促性腺激素，用于诱导排卵

uro·gas·trone (u″ro-gas′trōn) a urinary peptide derived from epidermal growth factor, with which it shares substantial homology and similar effects on the stomach 尿抑胃素

uro·gen·i·tal (u″ro-jen′ĭ-təl) genitourinary 泌尿生殖的

urog·e·nous (u-roj′ə-nəs) 1. producing urine 生尿的；2. produced from or in the urine 尿源的

uro·gram (u′ro-gram) a film obtained by urography 尿路造影照片

urog·ra·phy (u-rog′rə-fe) radiography of any part of the urinary tract 尿路造影（术）；**ascending u., cystoscopic u.**, retrograde u 逆行性尿路造影术；**descending u., excretion u., excretory u., intravenous u.**, urography after intravenous injection of an opaque medium that is rapidly excreted in the urine 排泄性尿路造影术静脉尿路造影；**retrograde u.**, urography after injection of a contrast medium into the bladder through the urethra 逆行肾盂造影（术）

uro·gy·ne·col·o·gy (u″ro-gi″nə-kol′ə-je) a subspecialty of gynecology that deals with pelvic diaphragm disorders, such as fecal or urinary incontinence or prolapse of the bladder or uterus 女性泌尿妇科学

uro·ki·nase (UK) (u″ro-ki′nās) u-plasminogen activator; an enzyme in the urine of humans and other mammals, elaborated by the parenchymal cells of the human kidney and acting as a plasminogen activator. It is used as a therapeutic thrombolytic agent 尿激酶

uro·lith (u′ro-lith) urinary calculus 尿路结石，尿石症；**urolith′ic** *adj.*

uro·li·thi·a·sis (u″ro-lĭ-thi′ə-sis) the formation of urinary calculi, or the condition associated with urinary calculi 尿石形成，尿石病

urol·o·gy (u-rol′ə-je) the medical specialty concerned with the urinary system in the male and female and genital organs in the male 泌尿外科学；**urolog′ic, urolog′ical** *adj.*

urop·a·thy (u-rop′ə-the) any disease or other pathologic change in the urinary tract 尿路病

uro·poi·e·sis (u″ro-poi-e′sis) the formation of urine 尿生成；**uropoiet′ic** *adj.*

uro·por·phyr·ia (u″ro-por-fir′e-ə) porphyria with excessive excretion of uroporphyrin 尿卟啉症

uro·por·phy·rin (u″ro-por′fə-rin) any of several porphyrins produced by oxidation of uroporphyrinogen; one or more are excreted in excess in the urine in several of the porphyrias 尿卟啉

uro·por·phy·rin·o·gen (u″ro-por″fə-rin′ə-jən) a porphyrinogen formed from porphobilinogen; it is a precursor of uroporphyrin and coproporphyrinogen 尿卟啉原

uro·pro·tec·tion (u″ro-pro-tek′shən) protection of the urinary tract, especially against urotoxic chemicals 一种泌尿道保护药，尤指对有毒化学物质的防护；**uroprotec′tive** *adj.*

uro·psam·mus (u″ro-sam′əs) sediment or gravel in the urine 尿沙

uro·ra·di·ol·o·gy (u″ro-ra″de-ol′ə-je) radiology of the urinary tract 尿路放射学

uros·co·py (u-ros′kə-pe) diagnostic examination of the urine 尿检查；**uroscop′ic** *adj.*

uro·sep·sis (u″ro-sep′sis) a term used imprecisely to denote infection ranging from urinary tract infection to generalized sepsis that may result from such infection 尿脓毒症；**urosep′tic** *adj.*

uro·tox·ic (u′ro-tok″sik) harmful to the bladder 尿毒素的

ur·so·di·ol (ur″so-di′ol) the secondary bile acid ursodeoxycholic acid used as an anticholelithic to dissolve radiolucent, noncalcified gallstones 抗胆石药

Ur·ti·ca (ər-ti′kə) [L.] 荨麻属，参见 *nettle*

ur·ti·cant (ur′tĭ-kənt) producing urticaria 刺痒的，引起风团的

ur·ti·ca·ria (ur″tĭ-kar′e-ə) hives; a vascular reaction of the upper dermis with transient, slightly elevated patches (wheals) that are redder or paler than the surrounding skin; there is often severe itching. Common causes are foods, drugs, infections, and emotional stress 荨麻疹；**urticar′ial, urticar′ious** *adj.*；**acute u.,** urticaria taking place within hours to a few days of the stimulus; some cases evolve into chronic urticaria 急性荨麻疹；**cholinergic u.,** a type of physical urticaria, usually evoked by exertion, stress, cold, or heat; thought to be a non-immunologic hypersensitivity reaction 胆碱能性荨麻疹；**chronic u.,** urticaria that either is continuous or develops over a period of 6 weeks or more; most cases are idiopathic 慢性荨麻疹；**cold u.,** physical urticaria caused by cold air, water, or objects, occurring in a hereditary and an acquired form 寒冷性荨麻疹；**contact u.,** immune-mediated urticaria as a form of allergic reaction 接触性荨麻疹；**drug-induced u.,** immune-mediated urticaria in reaction to a medication 药物性荨麻疹；**heat u.,** cholinergic urticaria produced by something hot on the skin or a high environmental temperature 热性荨麻疹；**immune-mediated u.,** acute urticaria that is an immune response to antigenic stimulation 免疫介导性荨麻疹；**u. medicamentosa,** 同 drug-induced u.；**papular u.,** a hypersensitivity reaction to insect bites, with small papules and wheals 丘疹性荨麻疹；**physical u.,** acute urticaria caused by a physical stimulus such as heat, cold, sunlight, or rubbing or light scratching of the skin 物理性荨麻疹；**u. pigmentosa,** the most common form of mastocytosis, characterized by small, reddish brown macules or papules that occur mainly on the trunk and tend to urtication upon mild mechanical trauma or chemical irritation 色素性荨麻疹；**solar u.,** a type of rapidly developing physical urticaria occurring in reaction to ultraviolet radiation 日光性荨麻疹；**stress u.,** cholinergic urticaria caused by emotional stress 压力性荨麻疹

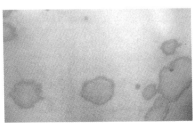

▲ 荨麻疹

ur·ti·ca·tion (ur″tĭ-ka′shən) 1. the development or formation of urticaria 荨麻疹形成；2. a burning sensation as of stinging with nettles 刺痒

uru·shi·ol (u-roo′she-ol) the toxic irritant principle of poison ivy and various related plants 漆酚

US ultrasound 采用超声

USAN (u′san) United States Adopted Name 美国采用药名

USP *United States Pharmacopeia* 美国药典

USPHS United States Public Health Service 美国公共卫生署

uter·al·gia (u″tər-al′jə) hysteralgia 子宫痛

uter·ine (u′tər-in) pertaining to the uterus 子宫的

utero·ab·dom·i·nal (u″tər-o-ab-dom′ĭ-nəl) pertaining to the uterus and abdomen 子宫腹部的

utero·cer·vi·cal (u″tər-o-ser′vĭ-kəl) pertaining to the uterus and cervix uteri 子宫宫颈的

utero·lith (u′tər-o-lith″) uterine calculus 子宫石

uter·om·e·ter (u″tər-om′ə-tər) an instrument for measuring the uterus 子宫测量器

utero-ovar·i·an (u″tər-o-o-var′e-ən) pertaining to the uterus and ovary 子宫卵巢的

utero·pel·vic (u″tər-o-pel′vik) pertaining to or connecting the uterus and the pelvis 子宫骨盆的

utero·pla·cen·tal (u″tər-o-plə-sen′təl) pertaining to the placenta and uterus 子宫胎盘的

utero·rec·tal (u″tər-o-rek′təl) rectouterine 子宫直肠的

utero·sa·cral (u″tər-o-sa′krəl) pertaining to the uterus and sacrum 子宫骶骨的

utero·ton·ic (u″tər-o-ton′ik) 1. increasing the tone of uterine muscle 子宫收缩的；2. an agent that so acts 子宫收缩药

utero·tu·bal (u″tər-o-too′bəl) tubouterine 子宫输卵管的

utero·vag·i·nal (u″tər-o-vaj′ĭ-nəl) pertaining to the uterus and vagina 子宫阴道的

uter·o·ves·i·cal (u″tər-o-ves′ĭ-kəl) vesicouterine 子宫膀胱的

uter·us (u′tər-əs) pl. *u′teri* [L.] the hollow muscular organ in female mammals in which the blastocyst normally becomes embedded and in which the developing embryo and fetus is nourished. Its cavity opens into the vagina below and into a uterine tube on either side 子宫；**bicornuate u.,** one with two horns, or cornua 双角子宫；**u. didelphys,** the existence of two distinct uteri in the same individual 双子宫；**gravid u.,** one containing a developing fetus 妊娠子宫；**septate u.,** a uterus whose cavity is divided into two parts by a septum 纵隔子宫；**unicornuate u.,** one with a single horn, or cornu 单角子宫

UTI urinary tract infection 尿路感染

U

UTP uridine triphosphate 尿苷三磷酸

utri·cle (u'trĭ-kəl) 1. any small sac 小囊；2. the larger of the two sacs of the vestibule of the internal ear 椭圆囊；prostatic u., urethral u., a small blind pouch in the substance of the prostate 前列腺小囊

utric·u·lar (u-trik'u-lər) 1. pertaining to the utricle 囊状的；2. bladderlike 膀胱样的

utric·u·li·tis (u-trik"u-li'tis) inflammation of the prostatic utricle or the utricle of the ear 前列腺囊炎，椭圆囊炎

utric·u·lo·sac·cu·lar (u-trik"u-lo-sak'u-lər) pertaining to the utricle and saccule of the labyrinth 椭圆囊球囊的

utric·u·lus (u-trik'u-ləs) pl. utri'culi [L.] 同 utricle；u. masculinus, u. prostaticus, 同 prostatic utricle

UV ultraviolet 紫外线

UVA ultraviolet 紫外线 A，参见 ultraviolet

uva ur·si (u'vah ur'se) Arctostaphylos uva-ursi or its leaves, which are used medicinally and homeopathically for urinary tract inflammation 熊果

UVB ultraviolet B 紫外线 B，参见 ultraviolet

UVC ultraviolet C 紫外线 C，参见 ultraviolet

uvea (u've-ə) the tunica vasculosa of the eyeball, consisting of the iris, ciliary body, and choroid 眼色素层，葡萄膜；u'veal adj.

uve·itis (u"ve-i'tis) inflammation of all or part of the uvea 葡萄膜炎；uveit'ic adj.；heterochromic u., 异色性葡萄膜炎，参见 iridocyclitis sympathetic

u., 交感性葡萄膜炎，参见 ophthalmia

uveo·scle·ri·tis (u"ve-o-sklə-ri'tis) scleritis due to extension of uveitis 色素层巩膜炎，葡萄膜巩膜炎

uvi·form (u'vĭ-form) shaped like a grape 葡萄形的

uvu·la (u'vu-lə) pl. u'vulae [L.] 1. a pendant, fleshy mass 下垂的肉块；2. 同 palatine u；u'vular adj.；u. of bladder, a rounded elevation at the bladder neck, formed by convergence of muscle fibers terminating in the urethra 膀胱悬雍垂；u. of cerebellum, 同 u. vermis；palatine u., the small, fleshy mass hanging from the soft palate above the root of the tongue 悬雍垂；u. vermis, the lobule of the vermis of the cerebellum between the pyramid and nodule 小脑悬雍垂，蚓

uvu·lec·to·my (u"vu-lek'tə-me) excision of the uvula 悬雍垂切除术

uvu·li·tis (u"vu-li'tis) inflammation of the uvula 悬雍垂炎

uvu·lo·pal·a·to·phar·yn·go·plas·ty (UPPP) (u"vu-lo-pal"ə-to"fə-ring'go-plas"te) an operation performed on the soft tissues of the soft palate and pharyngeal area in the treatment of sleep apnea 悬雍垂咽成形术

uvu·lop·to·sis (u"vu-lop-to'sis) a relaxed, pendulous state of the uvula 悬雍垂下垂

uvu·lot·o·my (u"vu-lot'ə-me) the cutting off of the uvula or a part of it 悬雍垂（部分）切除术，悬雍垂切开术

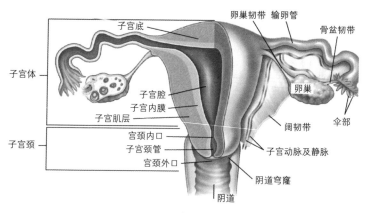

▲ 子宫

V[符号] valine 缬氨酸；vanadium 钒；visual acuity 视敏度；volt 伏特；volume 容积

V[符号] volume 容量，容积，体积

v. [L.] ve'na (vein) 静脉

VA Veterans Administration (now the Department of Veterans Affairs [DVA]) 退伍军人管理局（现称退

伍军人事务部）；visual acuity 视敏度

VABP ventilator-associated bacterial pneumonia 呼吸机相关性细菌性肺炎

VAC a regimen of vincristine, dactinomycin, and cyclophosphamide, used in cancer therapy 长春新碱 - 放线菌素 D- 环磷酰胺（联合化疗治癌方案）

vac·ci·nal (vak′sĭ-nəl) 1. pertaining to vaccine or to vaccination 疫苗的；接种的；2. having protective qualities when used by way of inoculation 有预防力的

vac·ci·na·tion (vak″sĭ-na′shən) the introduction of vaccine into the body to produce immunity 预防接种，疫苗接种，种痘

vac·cine (vak-sēn′) a suspension of attenuated or killed microorganisms (viruses, bacteria, or rickettsiae), or of antigenic proteins derived from them, administered for prevention, amelioration, or treatment of infectious diseases 菌苗，疫苗；**acellular v.**, a cell-free vaccine prepared from purified antigenic components of cell-free microorganisms, carrying less risk than whole-cell preparations 无细胞菌苗；**acellular pertussis v.**, a preparation of purified antigenic components of *Bordetella pertussis;* used in combination preparations with diphtheria and tetanus toxoids. See *diphtheria and tetanus toxoids and acellular pertussis v.* and *tetanus toxoid, reduced diphtheria toxoid, and acellular pertussis v.* 无细胞百日咳疫苗；**anthrax v.**, a cell-free filtrate of cultures of an avirulent nonencapsulated strain of *Bacillus anthracis,* adsorbed on aluminum hydroxide; used for immunization against anthrax 炭疽疫苗；**attenuated v.**, a vaccine prepared from live microorganisms or viruses cultured under adverse conditions leading to loss of their virulence but retention of their ability to induce protective immunity 减毒疫苗；**autogenous v.**, a vaccine prepared from a culture of microorganisms taken from the person to be treated with it 自身疫苗；**BCG v.**, a preparation used as an active immunizing agent against tuberculosis and in treatment of bladder cancer, consisting of a dried, living, avirulent culture of the Calmette-Guérin strain of *Mycobacterium bovis* 卡介苗；**diphtheria and tetanus toxoids and acellular pertussis v.**, DTaP vaccine; a combination of diphtheria toxoid, tetanus toxoid, and acellular pertussis vaccine; adsorbed on an aluminum-adsorbing agent. It is administered intramuscularly to children younger than 7 years of age, for simultaneous triple immunization 白喉、破伤风类毒素、无细胞百日咳疫苗；**diphtheria and tetanus toxoids and pertussis v.**, DTP vaccine; a combination of diphtheria and tetanus toxoids and whole-cell pertussis vaccine, which has been used for simultaneous triple immunization 白喉、破伤风类毒素、百日咳菌苗混合制剂，百白破三联制剂；**DTaP v.**, 同 diphtheria and tetanus toxoids and acellular pertussis v.; **DTP v.**, 同 diphtheria and tetanus toxoids and pertussis v.; *Haemophilus* **b conjugate v. (HbCV)**, a preparation of *Haemophilus influenzae* type b capsular polysaccharide covalently bound to a specific diphtheria or meningococcal protein or tetanus toxoid; used as an immunizing agent in infants and young children 流感嗜血杆菌 b 结合疫苗；**hepatitis A v. inactivated**, an inactivated whole-virus vaccine derived from an attenuated strain of hepatitis A virus grown in cell culture 甲型肝炎灭活疫苗；**hepatitis B v. (recombinant)**, an inactivated virus vaccine derived by recombination from hepatitis B surface antigen and cloned in yeast cells 乙型肝炎疫苗（重组）；**heterologous v.**, a vaccine that confers protective immunity against a pathogen that shares cross-reacting antigens with the microorganisms in the vaccine 异种疫苗；**human diploid cell v. (HDCV)**, 人二倍体细胞疫苗，参见 *rabies v.*; **human papillomavirus quadrivalent v.**, recombinant, a vaccine prepared from the viruslike particles of the major capsid protein of human papillomavirus (HPV) types 6, 11, 16, and 18, which are responsible for most cases of condyloma acuminatum and cervical cancer; used to immunize girls and young women 重组人乳头瘤病毒四价疫苗；**influenza virus v.**, a trivalent virus vaccine against influenza, containing two influenza A virus strains and one influenza B virus strain. The composition of the vaccine is changed each year in response to antigenic shifts and changes in prevalence of influenza virus strains. It is available in killed (trivalent inactivated influenza vaccine or TIV) and live attenuated forms (live, attenuated influenza vaccine or LAIV) 流感病毒疫苗；**Japanese encephalitis virus v.**, a formaldehyde-inactivated vaccine prepared from infected mouse brains, used for immunization against Japanese encephalitis 乙型脑炎病毒疫苗；**live v.**, one prepared from live microorganisms that have been attenuated but that retain their immunogenic properties 活疫苗；**live, attenuated influenza v. (LAIV)**, a live, attenuated influenza virus vaccine containing temperature-sensitive type A and B strains that can replicate in the nasal passages but not in the lower respiratory tract; for intranasal administration 减毒活流感疫苗；**measles, mumps, rubella, and varicella virus v. live (MMRV)**, a combination of live attenuated measles, mumps, rubella, and human herpesvirus 3 (varicella-zoster virus), administered subcutaneously for simultaneous immunization against measles, mumps, rubella, and varicella in children between

V

the ages of 12 months and 12 years 麻疹、腮腺炎、风疹和水痘病毒活疫苗；**measles, mumps, and rubella virus v. live (MMR)**, a combination of live attenuated measles, mumps, and rubella viruses, used for simultaneous immunization against measles, mumps, and rubella in persons 12 months of age or older 麻疹、腮腺炎和风疹病毒活疫苗；**measles virus v. live**, a live attenuated virus vaccine used for immunization against measles; usually administered as the combination measles, mumps, and rubella virus vaccine 麻疹病毒活疫苗；**meningococcal conjugate v. (MCV) (MCV4)**, a preparation of capsular polysaccharide antigens of *Neisseria meningitidis* serovars A, C, Y, and W-135, covalently bound to diphtheria toxoid; used for the prevention of meningococcal disease 脑膜炎球菌结合疫苗；**meningococcal polysaccharide v. (MPSV)**, a preparation of capsular polysaccharide antigens of *Neisseria meningitidis* serovars A, C, Y, and W-135; used for the prevention of meningococcal disease 脑膜炎球菌多糖菌苗；**mixed v.**, polyvalent v. 混合疫苗；**mumps virus v. live**, a live attenuated virus vaccine used for immunization against mumps; usually administered as the combination measles, mumps, and rubella virus vaccine 腮腺炎病毒活疫苗；**pertussis v.**, a preparation of killed *Bordetella pertussis* bacilli (whole-cell vaccine) or of purified antigenic components thereof (acellular pertussis v.); only the latter is currently available in the United States 百日咳菌苗；**pneumococcal conjugate v., pneumococcal 7-valent conjugate v. (PCV7)**, a preparation of capsular polysaccharides from the seven serovars of *Streptococcus pneumoniae* most commonly isolated from young children, coupled to a nontoxic variant of diphtheria toxin; used as an active immunizing agent for infants and toddlers 肺炎球菌结合疫苗，7 价肺炎球菌结合疫苗；**pneumococcal v. polyvalent (PPSV)**, a preparation of purified capsular polysaccharides from the 23 serovars of *Streptococcus pneumoniae* causing the majority of pneumococcal diseases; used as an active immunizing agent 多价肺炎球菌疫苗；**poliovirus v. inactivated (IPV)**, Salk v.; a suspension of formalin-inactivated polioviruses used for immunization against poliomyelitis 灭活脊髓灰质炎病毒疫苗，索尔克疫苗；**poliovirus v. live oral (OPV)**, Sabin v.; a preparation of live, attenuated polioviruses for oral administration as an active immunizing agent against poliomyelitis; no longer used in the United States 口服脊髓灰质炎病毒疫苗，萨宾疫苗；**polyvalent v.**, one prepared from cultures or antigens of more than one strain or species 多价疫苗；**purified chick embryo cell v. (PCECV)**, 纯化鸡胚

细胞疫苗，参见 *rabies v.*；**rabies v.**, an inactivated viral vaccine used for pre- and postexposure immunization against rabies; it may be prepared from rabies virus grown in human diploid cell culture *(human diploid cell v.)* or that grown in cultures of chicken fibroblasts *(purified chick embryo cell v.)* 狂犬病疫苗；**replicative v.**, any vaccine containing organisms that are able to reproduce, including live and attenuated viruses and bacteria 增殖性疫苗；**rotavirus v. (RV)**, a live attenuated virus vaccine produced from one or more rotavirus strains; administered orally to immunize infants against rotaviral gastroenteritis 轮状病毒疫苗；**rubella virus v. live**, a live attenuated virus vaccine used for immunization against rubella, usually administered as the combination measles, mumps, and rubella virus vaccine 风疹病毒活疫苗 **Sabin v.**, 同 poliovirus v. live oral；**Salk v.**, 同 poliovirus v. inactivated；**smallpox v.**, a live viral vaccine prepared from vaccinia virus; used for immunization against smallpox. Now only used in laboratory workers with potential exposure to smallpox virus and military forces of certain countries 天花疫苗；**subunit v.**, a vaccine produced from specific protein subunits of a virus and thus having less risk of adverse reactions than whole-virus vaccines 亚单位疫苗；**Tdap v.**, 同 tetanus toxoid, reduced diphtheria toxoid, and acellular pertussis v；**tetanus toxoid, reduced diphtheria toxoid, and acellular pertussis v.**, Tdap vaccine; a combination of tetanus toxoid, a reduced dose of diphtheria toxoid, and acellular pertussis vaccine; adsorbed on an aluminum-adsorbing agent. It is administered intramuscularly to adolescents and adults, for simultaneous triple immunization 破伤风类毒素、白喉减毒素、无细胞百日咳疫苗；**trivalent inactivated influenza v. (TIV)**, an inactivated influenza virus vaccine for intramuscular administration 三价灭活流感病毒疫苗；**typhoid v.**, any of several preparations of *Salmonella enterica* subsp. *enterica* serovar Typhi used for immunization against typhoid fever, including an oral live vaccine prepared from an attenuated strain *(typhoid v. live oral)* and a parenteral vaccine prepared from typhoid Vi capsular polysaccharide *(typhoid Vi polysaccharide v.)* 伤寒疫苗；**varicella virus v. live**, a live attenuated viral vaccine prepared from human herpesvirus 3 (varicella-zoster virus); used for immunization against varicella 水痘病毒活疫苗；**yellow fever v.**, a live viral vaccine prepared from an attenuated strain of yellow fever virus; used to immunize against yellow fever 黄热病疫苗；**zoster v. live**, a live attenuated virus vaccine prepared from human herpesvirus 3 (varicella-zoster virus); administered subcutaneously in older adults to prevent herpes zoster 带状疱疹活疫苗

vac·cin·ia (vak-sin′e-ə) the cutaneous and sometimes systemic reactions associated with vaccination with smallpox vaccine 牛痘；**generalized v.,** a condition of widespread vaccinal lesions resulting from a sensitivity response to smallpox vaccination and delayed production of neutralizing antibodies 泛化痘，全身性牛痘；**progressive v.,** generalized vaccinia with failure to develop antibodies against the virus (due to agammaglobulinemia), with spreading necrosis at the site and metastasis of lesions throughout the body; the condition is often fatal 进行性痘

vac·u·o·lar (vak″u-o′lər) pertaining to or of the nature of vacuoles 空泡的

vac·u·o·lat·ed (vak′u-o-lāt″əd) containing vacuoles 有空泡的

vac·u·o·la·tion (vak″u-o-la′shən) the process of forming vacuoles; the condition of being vacuolated 空泡形成

vac·u·ole (vak′u-ōl) any membrane-bound space or cavity within a cell 空泡，液泡

vac·u·um (vak′ūm) [L.] a space devoid of air or of other gas; a space from which the air has been exhausted 真空

VAD ventricular assist device 心室辅助装置

va·gal (va′gəl) pertaining to the vagus nerve 迷走神经的

va·gi·na (və-ji′nə) pl. *vagi′nae* [L.] 1. a sheath or sheathlike structure 鞘，鞘样结构；2. the canal in the female, from the vulva to the cervix uteri, that receives the penis in copulation 阴道；**vag′inal** *adj.*

vag·i·nate (vaj′ĭ-nāt) enclosed in a sheath 有鞘的

vag·i·nec·to·my (vaj″ĭ-nek′tə-me) excision of the vagina 睾丸鞘膜切除术；阴道切除术

vag·i·nis·mus (vaj″ĭ-niz′məs) painful spasm of the vagina due to involuntary muscular contraction, usually severe enough to prevent intercourse; the cause may be organic or psychogenic 阴道痉挛

vag·i·ni·tis (vaj″ĭ-ni′tis) 1. inflammation of the vagina 阴道炎；2. inflammation of a sheath 鞘炎；**adhesive v.,** atrophic vaginitis marked by formation of superficial erosions, which often adhere to opposing surfaces, obliterating the vaginal canal 粘连性阴道炎；**atrophic v.,** vaginitis with tissue atrophy occurring in postmenopausal women and associated with estrogen deficiency 萎缩性阴道炎；**candidal v.,** vulvovaginal candidiasis 念珠菌（性）阴道炎；**desquamative inflammatory v.,** a form resembling atrophic vaginitis but affecting women with normal estrogen levels 脱屑性阴道炎；**emphysematous v.,** inflammation of the vagina and adjacent cervix,

characterized by numerous, asymptomatic, gas-filled cystlike lesions 气肿性阴道炎；**senile v.,** adhesive v. 老年性阴道炎

vag·i·no·ab·dom·i·nal (vaj″ĭ-no-ab-dom′ĭ- nəl) pertaining to the vagina and abdomen 阴道腹的

vag·in·odyn·ia (vaj″ĭ-no-din′e-ə) pain in the vagina 阴道痛

vag·i·no·fix·a·tion (vaj″ĭ-no-fik-sa′shən) suture of the vagina to the abdominal wall 阴道固定术

vag·i·no·la·bi·al (vaj″ĭ-no-la′be-əl) pertaining to the vagina and labia 阴道阴唇的

vag·i·nop·a·thy (vaj″ĭ-nop′ə-the) any disease of the vagina 阴道病

vag·i·no·per·i·ne·al (vaj″ĭ-no-per″ĭ-ne′əl) pertaining to the vagina and perineum 阴道会阴的

vag·i·no·peri·ne·or·rha·phy (vaj″ĭ-no-per″ĭ- ne-or′ə-fe) suture repair of the vagina and perineum 阴道会阴缝合术

vag·i·no·peri·ne·ot·o·my (vaj″ĭ-no-per″ĭ-neot′ə-me) paravaginal incision 阴道会阴切开术

vag·i·no·peri·to·ne·al (vaj″ĭ-no-per″ĭ-to-ne′əl) pertaining to the vagina and peritoneum 阴道腹膜的

vag·i·no·pexy (vaj″ĭ-no-pek″se) □vaginofixation

vag·i·no·plas·ty (vaj″ĭ-no-plas″te) plastic surgery of the vagina 阴道成形术

vag·i·no·scope (vaj″ĭ-no-skōp) colposcope 阴道镜

vag·i·not·o·my (vaj″ĭ-not′ə-me) colpotomy 阴道切开术

vag·i·no·ves·i·cal (vaj″ĭ-no-ves′ĭ-kəl) vesicovaginal 阴道膀胱的

va·gi·tus (və-ji′təs) [L.] the cry of an infant 婴儿哭声；**v. uterinus,** the cry of an infant in the uterus 子宫内儿哭

va·gol·y·sis (va-gol′ĭ-sis) surgical destruction of the vagus nerve 迷走神经撕脱术

va·go·lyt·ic (va″go-lit′ik) 1. pertaining to or caused by vagolysis 迷走神经松弛的；2. having an effect resembling that produced by interruption of impulses transmitted by the vagus nerve 消除迷走神经作用的

va·go·mi·met·ic (va″go-mĭ-met′ik) having an effect resembling that produced by stimulation of the vagus nerve 类迷走神经的，拟迷走神经的

va·got·o·my (va-got′ə-me) interruption of the impulses carried by the vagus nerve or nerves 迷走神经切断术；**highly selective v.,** division of only those vagal fibers supplying the acid-secreting glands of the stomach, with preservation of those supplying the antrum as well as the hepatic and celiac branches 高选择性迷走神经切断术；**medical v.,** that accomplished by administration of suitable drugs 迷走神经药物切断术；**parietal cell v.,** selective severing of the vagus nerve fibers sup-

V

plying the proximal two-thirds (parietal area) of the stomach; done for duodenal ulcer 胃壁细胞迷走神经切断术; **selective v.**, division of the vagal fibers to the stomach with preservation of the hepatic and celiac branches 选择性迷走神经切断术; **truncal v.**, surgical division of the two main trunks of the abdominal vagus nerve 迷走神经干切断术

va·go·tro·pic (va″go-tro′pik) having an effect on the vagus nerve 向迷走神经的

va·go·va·gal (va″go-va′gəl) arising as a result of afferent and efferent impulses mediated through the vagus nerve 经迷走神经反射的

va·gus (va′gəs) pl. *va′gi* [L.] the vagus nerve 迷走神经

vai·dya (vi′dyah) [Sanskrit] in ayurveda, a physician（在阿育吠陀中指）医生

Val valine 缬氨酸

val·a·cy·clo·vir (val″a-si′klo-vir) an ester of acyclovir, to which it is metabolized; used as the hydrochloride salt as an antiviral agent in the treatment of genital herpes and herpes zoster in immunocompetent adults 伐昔洛韦

val·de·cox·ib (val″də-kok′sib) a nonsteroidal anti-inflammatory drug of the COX-2 inhibitors group, used for the treatment of osteoarthritis, rheumatoid arthritis, and primary dysmenorrhea COX-2 抑制药组的非甾体类抗炎药，用于治疗骨关节炎、类风湿关节炎、原发性痛经

va·lence (va′lens) 1. a positive number that represents the number of bonds that each atom of an element makes in a chemical compound; now replaced by the concept "oxidation number" but still used to denote *(a)* the number of covalent bonds formed by an atom in a covalent compound or *(b)* the charge on a monatomic or polyatomic molecule 原子价，化合价；2. in immunology, *(a)* the number of antigen-binding sites possessed by an antibody molecule or *(b)* the number of antigenic determinants possessed by an antigen 效价

va·le·ri·an (və-lēr′e-ən) 1. a plant of the genus *Valeriana* 缬草属植物；2. the dried roots, rhizome, and stolons of *V. officinalis,* which are antispasmodic and sedative and are used for nervousness and insomnia 缬草的干根、根茎和匍匐茎，具有抗痉挛和镇静作用，用于治疗紧张和失眠

val·gan·ci·clo·vir (val″gan-si′klo-vir) a prodrug of ganciclovir, used as the hydrochloride salt in the treatment of cytomegalovirus retinitis in patients with AIDS 缬更昔洛韦

val·gus (val′gəs) [L.] bent out, twisted; denoting a deformity in which the angulation is away from the midline of the body, as in talipes valgus. The meanings of valgus and varus are often reversed 外翻的（足），外偏的（手）

val·ine (Val, V) (va′lēn) (val′ēn) a naturally occurring amino acid, essential for human metabolism 缬氨酸

Val·i·um (val′e-əm) trademark for preparations of diazepam 安定，地西泮制剂的商品名

val·late (val′āt) having a wall or rim; cupshaped 轮廓形的，杯状的

val·lec·u·la (və-lek′u-lə) pl. *valle′culae* [L.] a depression or furrow 谷；**vallec′ular** *adj.*；v. **cerebel′li**, the longitudinal fissure on the inferior cerebellum, in which the medulla oblongata rests 小脑谷

val·pro·ate (val-pro′āt) a salt of valproic acid; the sodium salt has the same uses as the acid 丙戊酸盐

val·pro·ic ac·id (val-pro′ik) an anticonvulsant used particularly for the control of absence seizures 丙戊酸（抗惊厥药）

val·ru·bi·cin (val-roo′bĭ-sin″) an antineoplastic that interferes with nucleic acid metabolism and other related biologic functions; used intravesically for treatment of bladder carcinoma 戊柔比星，一种干扰核酸代谢的抗增生药，用于治疗膀胱癌

val·sar·tan (val-sahr′tan) an angiotensin Ⅱ antagonist used as an antihypertensive 缬沙坦，一种血管紧张素Ⅱ拮抗药，用于抗高血压

val·ue (val′u) a measure of worth or efficiency or of the activity, concentration, etc., of something 价值，值；**normal v's**, the range in concentration of specific substances found in normal healthy tissues, secretions, etc. 正常值；*P* **v.**, *p* **v.**, the probability of obtaining by chance a result at least as extreme as that observed, even when the null hypothesis is true and no real difference exists; if it is ≤ 0.05, the sample results are usually deemed statistically significant and the null hypothesis is rejected P 值；**reference v's**, a set of values of a quantity measured in the clinical laboratory that characterize a specified population in a defined state of health 参考值

val·va (val′və) pl. *val′vae* [L.] a valve 瓣，瓣膜

valve (valv) a membranous fold in a canal or passage that prevents backward flow of material passing through it 瓣，瓣膜；**anal v's**, archlike folds of mucous membrane connecting the caudal ends of the anal columns 肛瓣；**aortic v.**, valve guarding the entrance to the aorta from the left ventricle 主动脉瓣；**artificial cardiac v.**, **artificial heart v.**, 同 prosthetic heart v.；**atrioventricular v's**, cardiac valves connecting an atrium and a ventricle 房室瓣，参见 *tricuspid v.* 和 *mitral v.*；**Béraud v.**, a fold of mucous membrane sometimes occurring at the beginning of the nasolacrimal duct 贝罗德瓣，泪囊瓣；**Bicuspid v.,** 同 mitral v.；**bileaflet v.,** a prosthetic heart valve consisting of a sewing ring to which are attached two semicircular occluding disks that swing open and closed 双叶瓣; **bioprosthetic v.,** a prosthetic heart valve composed of biologic tissue, usually porcine 生物瓣; **caged-ball v.,** a prosthetic heart valve comprising a sewing ring attached to a cage composed of curved struts that contains a free-floating ball 笼罩球瓣; **cardiac v's,** those controlling the flow of blood through and from the heart 心瓣膜; **coronary v.,** that at the entrance of the coronary sinus into the right atrium 冠状窦瓣; **flail mitral v.,** a cardiac valve having a leaflet that has lost its normal support (as in ruptured chordae tendineae) and flutters in the bloodstream 连枷状心房瓣; **Houston v's,** permanent transverse folds, usually numbering three, in the rectum 直肠瓣; **ileocecal v.,** the valvelike structure in the cadaver corresponding to the ileal papilla of a living person 回盲瓣; **left atrioventricular v.,** mitral v. 左房室瓣; **mitral v.,** that between the left atrium and left ventricle, usually having two leaflets (anterior and posterior) 二尖瓣; **prosthetic heart v.,** a substitute, mechanical or composed of tissue, for a cardiac valve 人工心脏瓣膜; **pulmonary v.,** that at the entrance of the pulmonary trunk from the right ventricle 肺动脉瓣; **pyloric v.,** a prominent fold of mucous membrane at the pyloric orifice of the stomach 幽门瓣; **right atrioventricular v.,** tricuspic v. 右房室瓣; **semilunar v.,** 1. one having semilunar leaflets (i.e., the aortic and pulmonary valves) 半月形小叶（即主动脉瓣和脉动脉瓣）; 2. one of the semilunar leaflets composing such a valve 半月瓣; **thebesian v.,** 同 coronary v. **tilting-disk v.,** a prosthetic heart valve consisting of a sewing ring and valve housing containing a suspended disk that swings between open and closed positions 倾斜盘形瓣; **tricuspid v.,** that between the right atrium and right ventricle 三尖瓣; **ureteral v.,** a congenital transverse fold across the lumen of the ureter, composed of redundant mucosa made prominent by circular muscle fibers; it usually disappears in time but may rarely cause urinary obstruction 输尿管襞

val·vot·o·my (val-vot′ə-me) incision of a valve 瓣膜切开术

val·vu·la (val′vu-lə) pl. *val′vulae* [L.] valvule; a small valve; formerly used in official nomenclature for any valve but now restricted to certain small valves and leaflets of heart valves 瓣，瓣膜

val·vu·lar (val′vu-lər) pertaining to, affecting, or of the nature of a valve 瓣的，瓣膜的

val·vule (val′vūl) 参见 *valvula*

val·vu·li·tis (val″vu-li′tis) inflammation of a valve, especially of a heart valve 心瓣膜炎

val·vu·lo·plas·ty (val′vu-lo-plas″te) plastic repair of a valve, especially a heart valve 瓣膜成形术; **balloon v.,** dilation of a stenotic cardiac valve by means of a balloon-tipped catheter that is introduced into the valve and inflated 球囊瓣膜成形术

val·vu·lo·tome (val′vu-lo-tōm″) an instrument for cutting a valve 瓣膜刀

va·na·di·um (V) (və-na′de-əm) a soft, silvery gray, transition metal element; at. no. 23, at. wt. 50.942. Although considered a dietary trace element, it is toxic at higher doses; absorption, particularly by inhalation, can cause respiratory tract irritation, pneumonitis, conjunctivitis, and anemia 钒（化学元素）

van·co·my·cin (van″ko-mi′sin) an antibiotic produced by the soil bacillus *Amycolatopsis orientalis,* highly effective against gram-positive bacteria, especially against staphylococci; used as the hydrochloride salt 万古霉素

van·det·a·nib (van-det′ə-nib) a kinase inhibitor used as an antineoplastic in the treatment of advanced medullary thyroid carcinoma 一种激酶抑制药，用作治疗晚期甲状腺髓样癌的抗肿瘤药物

va·nil·lism (və-nil′iz-əm) acarodermatitis and rhinitis in persons working with raw vanilla, due to a mite found on the plant 香草中毒，香子兰中毒

va·nil·lyl·man·del·ic ac·id (VMA) (və-nil′əlmən-del′ik) an excretory product of the catecholamines; urinary levels are used in screening patients for pheochromocytoma 香草基扁桃酸，尿内 VMA 浓度可用于筛选嗜铬细胞瘤病人

va·por (va′pər) [L.] an atmospheric dispersion of a substance that in its normal state is liquid or solid 汽，蒸气

va·por·iza·tion (va″pər-ĭ-za′shən) 1. the conversion of a solid or liquid into a vapor without chemical change 汽化，参见 *nebulization*; 2. distillation 蒸馏

var·i·a·ble (var′e-ə-bəl) 1. changing from time to time 可变的; 2. in mathematics, a symbol that represents an arbitrary number or an arbitrary element of a set 变量

var·i·ance (var′e-əns) a measure of the variation shown by a set of observations: the average of the squared deviations from the mean; it is the square of the standard deviation 方差

var·i·ant (var′e-ənt) 1. something that differs in some characteristic from the class to which it belongs 变异体，变型; 2. exhibiting such variation 变异的

var·i·a·tion (var″e-a′shən) 1. the act or process of changing 变化; 2. the state or fact of differing 改变; 3. in genetics, deviation in phenotype of an indi-

V

vidual from that typical of the group to which it belongs; also, deviation in phenotype of the offspring from that of its parents（遗传学）变异；**antigenic v.**, a mechanism by which parasites can escape the immune surveillance of a host by modifying or completely altering their surface antigens 抗原性变异；**microbial v.**, the range of characteristics with a species used in identification and differentiation 微生物变异

var·i·ca·tion (var″ĭ-ka′shən) 1. formation of a varix 静脉曲张形成；2. 同 varicosity (1)

var·i·ce·al (var′ĭ-se′əl) varicose 静脉曲张的

var·i·cel·la (var′ĭ-sel′ə) [L.] chickenpox 水痘

var·i·cel·li·form (var′ĭ-sel′ĭ-form) resembling varicella 水痘样的

Var·i·cel·lo·vi·rus (var′ĭ-sel′o-vi″rəs) a genus of viruses of the family Herpesviridae; it includes the species human herpesvirus 3. See table at herpesvirus 水痘病毒属；见 herpesvirus 下附表；**varicellovi′ral** adj. 水

var·i·ces (var′ĭ-sēz) [L.] varix 的复数

var·i·co·bleph·a·ron (var″ĭ-ko-blef′ə-ron) a varicose swelling of the eyelid 睑静脉曲张

var·i·co·cele (var′ĭ-ko-sēl″) 1. varicosity of the pampiniform plexus of the spermatic cord, forming a scrotal swelling that feels like a "bag of worms." 精索静脉曲张；2. a similar condition in females, with varicosity of the veins of the broad ligament of the uterus 子宫阔韧带静脉曲张

var·i·co·ce·lec·to·my (var″ĭ-ko-sə-lek′tə-me) ligation and excision of a varicocele 曲张精索静脉切除术

var·i·cog·ra·phy (var″ĭ-kog′rə-fe) x-ray visualization of varicose veins 曲张静脉造影术，曲张静脉照相术

var·i·com·pha·lus (var″ĭ-kom′fə-ləs) a varicose tumor of the umbilicus 脐静脉曲张

var·i·co·phle·bi·tis (var″ĭ-ko-flə-bi′tis) varicose veins with inflammation 曲张静脉炎

var·i·cose (var′ĭ-kōs) variceal or variciform; of the nature of or pertaining to a varix; unnaturally and permanently distended 曲张的，静脉曲张的；不自然的；持续扩张的

var·i·cos·i·ty (var′ĭ-kos′ĭ-te) 1. the quality or fact of being varicose 静脉曲张；2. 同 varix；3. varicose vein 曲张静脉

var·i·cot·o·my (var″ĭ-kot′ə-me) excision of a varix or of a varicose vein 曲张静脉切除术

va·ric·u·la (və-rik′u-lə) a varix of the conjunctiva 结膜静脉曲张

var·i·e·gate (var′e-ĭ-gāt″) 1. marked by variety; diversified 使多样化；2. having patchy spots or streaks of different colors 使玫驳，使成杂色

va·ri·e·ty (və-ri′ə-te) in taxonomy, a subcategory of a species 变种

va·ri·o·la (və-ri′o-lə) smallpox 天花；**vari′olar**, **vari′olous** adj

va·ri·o·late (var′e-o-lāt) having the nature or appearance of smallpox 天花样的

va·ri·ol·i·form (var″e-ol′ĭ-form) 同 varioloid

va·ri·o·loid (və-ri′o-loid″) varioliform; resembling smallpox 天花样的

va·rix (var′iks) pl. *va′rices* [L.] an enlarged tortuous vein, artery, or lymphatic vessel 脉管曲张；**aneurysmal v.**, a markedly dilated tortuous vessel 动静脉瘤性静脉曲张；**arterial v.**, a racemose aneurysm or varicose artery 曲张状动脉瘤，动脉曲张；**esophageal varices**, varicosities of branches of the azygos vein that anastomose with tributaries of the portal vein in the lower esophagus, due to portal hypertension in cirrhosis 食管静脉曲张

va·ro·li·an (və-ro′le-ən) pertaining to the pons 脑桥的

va·rus (var′əs) [L.] bent inward; denoting a deformity in which the angulation of the part is toward the midline of the body, as in talipes varus. The meanings of *varus* and *valgus* are often reversed 内翻的

vas (vas) pl. *va′sa* [L.] 同 vessel；**va′sal** adj.；**v.aber′rans**, 1. a blind tubule sometimes connected with the epididymis; a vestigial mesonephric tubule 上迷管（附睾）；2. any anomalous or unusual vessel 任何异常的管；**va′sa bre′via**, short gastric arteries 短管；**v. de′ferens**, the excretory duct of the testis, which joins the excretory duct of the seminal vesicle to form the ejaculatory duct 输精管，又称 *ductus deferens*；**va′sa prae′via**, presentation, in front of the fetal head during labor, of the blood vessels of the umbilical cord where they enter the placenta 前置血管；**va′sa rec′ta re′nis**, straight arterioles of kidney（肾）直小管；**va′sa vaso′rum**, the small nutrient arteries and veins in the walls of the larger blood vessels 营养血管

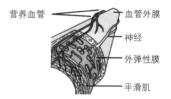

▲ 营养血管进入一条动脉

vas·cu·lar (vas′ku-lər) 1. pertaining to vessels, particularly blood vessels 脉管的，（尤指）血管的；2. indicative of a copious blood supply 供血丰富的

vas·cu·lar·iza·tion (vas″ku-lər-ĭ-za′shən) 1. the process of becoming vascular 血管形成；2. angiogenesis 血管化；3. the surgically induced development of vessels in a tissue 血管增生手术诱导组织中血管的发育 vas·cu·la-ture (vas′ku-lə-chər) the vascular system of the body, or any specific part of it 脉管系统，血管系统

vas·cu·li·tis (vas″ku-li′tis) pl. *vasculi'tides*. Inflammation of a blood or lymph vessel 脉管炎，血管炎；**vasculit'ic** *adj*.; **hypersensitivity v.,** a subgroup of systemic necrotizing vasculitis including several types of hypersensitivity reactions, such as to drugs, infectious agents, or exogenous or endogenous proteins; all disorders in this group involve the small vessels 过敏性脉管炎；**nodular v.,** vasculitis of superficial fascia of the lower legs, a condition almost identical to erythema induratum but without evidence of tuberculosis 结节性血管炎；**systemic necrotizing v.,** any of a group of disorders characterized by inflammation and necrosis of blood vessel walls 系统性坏死性血管炎

vas·cu·lo·gen·e·sis (vas″ku-lo-jen′ə-sis) angiogenesis 血管发生

vas·cu·lo·gen·ic (vas″ku-lo-jen′ik) angiogenic (1) 形成血管的，血管化的

vas·cu·lop·a·thy (vas″ku-lop′ə-the) any disorder of blood vessels 血管病

va·sec·to·my (və-sek′tə-me) surgical removal of all or part of the ductus deferens 输精管切除术

vas·i·form (vas′ĭ-form) resembling a vessel 脉管状的

va·si·tis (və-si′tis) deferentitis 输精管炎

vaso·ac·tive (va″zo-) (vas″o-ak′tiv) exerting an effect upon the caliber of blood vessels（化学物质）作用于血管的

vaso·con·stric·tion (va″zo-) (vas″o-kənstrik′shən) decrease in the caliber of blood vessels 血管收缩；**vasoconstric'tive** *adj*.

vaso·con·stric·tor (va″zo-) (vas″o-kən-strik′- tər) 1. causing constriction of blood vessels 血管收缩的；2. a nerve or agent that does this 血管收缩药

vaso·de·pres·sion (va″zo-) (vas″o-de-presh′ən) decrease in vascular resistance with hypotension 血管减压

vaso·de·pres·sor (va″zo-) (vas″o-de-pres′ər) 1. having the effect of lowering the blood pressure through reduction in peripheral resistance 血管减压的；2. an agent that causes vasodepression 血管减压药

vaso·di·la·ta·tion (va″zo-) (vas″o-dī-lə-ta′shən) vasodilation 血管舒张

vaso·di·la·tion (va″zo-) (vas″o-di-la′shən) 1. increase in caliber of blood vessels 血管舒张；2. a state of increased caliber of blood vessels 血管舒张状态；**vasodi'lative** *adj*.

vaso·di·la·tor (va″zo-) (vas″o-di′la-tər) 1. causing dilatation of blood vessels 血管舒张的；2. a nerve or agent that does this 血管扩张药；血管舒张神经

vaso·epi·did·y·mog·ra·phy (va″zo-) (vas″oep″ĭ-did″ĭ-mog′rə-fe) radiography of the ductus deferens and epididymis after injection of a contrast medium 输精管附睾造影术

vaso·epi·did·y·mos·to·my (va″zo-) (vas″oep″ĭ-did-ĭ-mos′tə-me) anastomosis of the ductus deferens and the epididymis 输精管附睾吻合术

vaso·for·ma·tive (va″zo-) (vas″o-for′mə-tiv) angiogenic (1) 血管形成的

vaso·gan·gli·on (va″zo-) (vas″o-gang′gle-on) a vascular ganglion or rete 血管网

vaso·gen·ic (va″zo-jen′ik) originating in the blood vessels 血管源的

vaso·hy·per·ton·ic (va″zo-) (vas″o-hi″pər-ton′ik) vasoconstrictor (1) 血管增压的

vaso·hy·po·ton·ic (va″zo-) (vas″o-hi″po-ton′ik) vasodilator (1) 血管减压的

vaso·in·hib·i·tor (va″zo-) (vas″o-in-hib′ĭ- tər) an agent that inhibits the action of the vasomotor nerves 血管抑制药；**vasoinhib'itory** *adj*.

vaso·li·ga·tion (va″zo-) (vas″o-li-ga′shən) ligation of the ductus deferens 输精管结扎术

vaso·mo·tor (va″zo-) (vas″o-mo′tər) 1. affecting the caliber of blood vessels 血管舒缩的；2. a vasomotor agent or nerve 血管舒缩药；血管舒缩神经

vaso·neu·ro·sis (va″zo-) (vas″o-noo-ro′sis) angioneuropathy 血管神经病

vaso·oc·clu·sion (va″zo-) (vas″o-ə-kloo′zhən) occlusion of a blood vessel or vessels 血管闭塞；**vasoocclu'sive** *adj*.

vaso·pa·re·sis (va″zo-) (vas″o-pə-re′sis) partial paralysis of vasomotor nerves 血管轻瘫

vaso·per·me·a·bil·i·ty (va″zo-) (vas″o-pur″me-ə-bil′ĭ-te) the extent to which a blood vessel is permeable 血管通透性

vaso·pres·sin (va″zo-) (vas″o-pres′in) a hormone secreted by cells of the hypothalamic nuclei and stored in the posterior pituitary for release as necessary; it constricts blood vessels, raising the blood pressure, and increases peristalsis, exerts some influence on the uterus, and influences resorption of water by the kidney tubules, resulting in concentration of urine. In most mammals, including humans, it exists as the arginine form, a synthetic preparation of which is used as an antidiuretic and in tests of hypothalamo-neurohypophysial-renal function in the diagnosis of central diabetes insipidus. A lysine form occurs in pigs; the synthetic pharmaceutical preparation is lypressin 血管升压素

vaso·pres·sor (va"zo-) (vas"o-pres'ər) 1. stimulating contraction of the muscular tissue of the capillaries and arteries 血管加压的；2. an agent that so acts 血管加压药

vaso·re·flex (va"zo-) (vas"o-re'fleks) a reflex involving a blood vessel 血管反射

vaso·re·lax·a·tion (va"zo-) (vas"o-re-lak-sa'- shən) decrease of vascular pressure 血管舒张

vaso·sec·tion (va"zo-) (vas"o-sek'shən) severing of a vessel or vessels 输精管切断术

vaso·sen·so·ry (va"zo-) (vas"o-sen'sər-e) supplying sensory filaments to the vessels 血管感觉的

vaso·spasm (va'zo-) (vas'o-spaz"əm) angiospasm; spasm of blood vessels, causing vasoconstriction 血管痉挛；**vasospas'tic** adj.

vaso·stim·u·lant (va"zo-) (vas"o-stim'u-lənt) stimulating vasomotor action 促血管舒缩的，刺激血管的

va·sos·to·my (vas-os'tə-me) 1. surgical formation of an opening into the ductus deferens 输精管造口术；2. fined vasotomy

va·sot·o·my (va-zot'ə-me) incision of the ductus deferens 输精管切断术

vaso·to·nia (va"zo-) (vas"o-to'ne-ə) tone or tension of the vessels 血管紧张；**vasoton'ic** adj.

vaso·tro·phic (va"zo-) (vas"o-tro'fik) pertaining to the nutrition of blood vessels 血管营养的

vaso·tro·pic (va"zo-) (vas"o-tro'pik) tending to act on blood vessels 促血管的，向血管的

vaso·va·gal (va"zo-) (vas"o-va'gəl) vascular and vagal 血管迷走神经的，另参见 attack 下词条

vaso·va·sos·to·my (va"zo-) (vas"o-va-zos'tə- me) reanastomosis of the ends of the severed ductus deferens 输精管吻合术

vaso·ve·sic·u·lec·to·my (va"zo-) (vas"o-ve- sik"u- lek'tə-me) excision of the ductus deferens and seminal vesicles 输精管精囊切除术

vas·tu (vahs'too) [Sanskrit] a traditional Hindu system of space design whose purpose is to promote well-being by constructing buildings in harmony with natural forces 印度传统的空间设计体系，其目的是通过与自然力量和谐地建造建筑来增进幸福感

vas·tus (vas'təs) [L.] great 巨大的；describes muscles（指肌肉）股肌

va·ta (vah'tah) [Sanskrit] in ayurveda, one of the three doshas, condensed from the elements air and space. It is the principle of kinetic energy in the body, is concerned with the nervous system and with circulation, movement, and pathology, and is eliminated from the body through defecation 在 阿育吠陀中，doshas 中的一种，由空气和空间元素

浓缩而成。它是人体动能的原理，与神经系统、循环、运动和病理有关，通过排便排出体外

VC vital capacity 肺活量

VCG vectorcardiogram 心电向量图

VD venereal disease 性病

VDH valvular disease of the heart 心瓣膜病

VDRL Venereal Disease Research Laboratory 性病研究所

vec·tor (vek'tər) 1. a carrier, especially the animal (usually an arthropod) that transfers an infective agent from one host to another 媒 介 物，尤 指 动物（常为节肢动物）传病媒介；2. cloning v.; a DNA molecule that can carry a fragment of foreign DNA into a host cell and create many copies of itself and the foreign DNA 载体；3. a quantity possessing magnitude, direction, and sense (positivity or negativity) 向量，矢量；**vecto'rial** adj.；biologic v., an animal vector in whose body the infecting organism develops or multiplies before becoming infective to the recipient individual 生物性媒介物；**mechanical v.**, an animal vector not essential to the life cycle of the parasite 机械性媒介物

vec·tor·car·dio·gram (VCG) (vek"tər-kahr'deo- gram") the record, usually a photograph, of the loop formed on the oscilloscope in vectorcardiography 心电向量图

vec·tor·car·di·og·ra·phy (vek"tər-kahr"deog'rə- fe) the registration, usually by formation of a loop display on an oscilloscope, of the direction and magnitude (vector) of the moment-tomoment electromotive forces of the heart during one complete cycle 心电向量描记法；**vectorcardiograph'ic** adj.

ve·cu·ro·ni·um (vek"u-ro'ne-um) a nondepolarizing neuromuscular blocking agent used as the bromide salt as an adjunct to anesthesia 维库溴铵，一种非去极化神经肌肉阻断药，用作麻醉辅助剂

VEE Venezuelan equine encephalomyelitis 委内瑞拉马脑脊髓炎

ve·gan (ve'gən) (vej'ən) 1. a diet that excludes all food of animal origin 绝对素食；2. a person who does not eat food of animal origin and who seeks to avoid exploitation of animals 绝对素食者

veg·e·tal (vej'ə-təl) 同 vegetative (1, 2, 3)

veg·e·tar·i·an (vej"ə-tar'e-ən) 1. one who practices vegetarianism 素食者；2. pertaining to vegetarianism 素食主义的，素食者的，素食的

veg·e·tar·i·an·ism (vej"ə-tar'e-ən-iz"əm) restriction of the diet to disallow some or all foods of animal origin, consuming mainly or wholly foods of plant origin 素食主义

veg·e·ta·tion (vej"ə-ta'shən) any plantlike fungoid neoplasm or growth; a luxuriant fungus-like growth of pathologic tissue 增殖体，赘生物，赘疣；生

长，增殖；**marantic v's,** small, sterile, verrucous, fibrinous excrescences occurring in the left-side heart valves in nonbacterial thrombotic (marantic) endocarditis 衰弱性赘生物

veg·e·ta·tive (vej'ə-ta″tiv) 1. of, pertaining to, or characteristic of plants 植物的，植物性的；2. concerned with growth and nutrition, as opposed to reproduction 生长的，营养的；3. of or pertaining to asexual reproduction, as by budding or fission 无性生殖的；4. functioning involuntarily or unconsciously 本能的，无意识的

VEGF vascular endothelial growth factor 血管内皮生长因子

ve·hi·cle (ve′ĭ-kəl) excipient 赋形剂

veil (vāl) 1. a covering structure 帆，帘，幕，盖；2. a caul or piece of amniotic sac occasionally covering the face of a newborn child 胎膜；羊膜

Veil·lon·el·la (va″on-el′ə) a genus of gramnegative bacteria of the family Acidaminococcaceae; they are normal inhabitants of the mouth, gastrointestinal tract, and vagina and are opportunistic pathogens 韦荣球菌属

vein (vān) a vessel through which blood passes from various organs or parts back to the heart; all veins except the pulmonary veins carry blood low in oxygen 静脉；**accompanying v.,** vena comitans 伴行静脉；**accompanying v. of hypoglossal nerve,** a vessel, formed by union of the deep lingual vein and the sublingual vein, that accompanies the hypoglossal nerve; it empties into the facial, lingual, or internal jugular vein 舌下神经伴行静脉，又称 *vena comitans nervi hypoglossi;* **afferent v's,** veins that carry blood to an organ 传入静脉；**allantoic v's,** paired vessels that accompany the allantois; they enter the body stalk of the early embryo with the allantois and later form the umbilical veins 尿囊静脉；**anastomotic v., inferior,** a vein that interconnects the superficial middle cerebral vein and the transverse sinus 下吻合静脉（大脑中浅静脉所属），又称 *vena anastomotica inferior;* **anastomotic v., superior,** a vein that interconnects the superficial middle cerebral vein and the superior sagittal sinus 上吻合静脉（大脑中浅静脉所属），又称 *vena anastomotica superior;* **angular v.,** a short vein between the eye and the root of the nose; it is formed by union of the supratrochlear and supraorbital veins and continues inferiorly as the facial vein 内　　静脉，又称 *vena angularis;* **antebrachial v., median,** a vein that arises from a palmar venous plexus and passes up the forearm between the cephalic and the basilic veins to the elbow, where it either joins one of these, bifurcates to join both, or joins the median cubital vein 前臂正中静脉，又称 *vena mediana antebrachii;* **anterior v's of right ventricle,** small veins that drain blood from the anterior aspect of the right ventricle, ascend in subepicardial tissue to cross the right part of the atrioventricular sulcus, and empty into the right atrium 右室前静脉，又称 *venae ventriculi dextri anteriores;* **anterior v. of septum pellucidum,** a vein that drains the anterior septum pellucidum into the superior thalamostriate vein 透明隔前静脉，又称 *vena anterior septi pellucidi;* **apical v.,** a vein draining the apical segment of the superior lobe of the right lung and emptying into the right superior pulmonary vein 心尖静脉，又称 *vena apicalis;* **apicoposterior v.,** a vein draining the apicoposterior segment of the superior lobe of the left lung and emptying into the left superior pulmonary vein 尖后静脉，又称 *vena apicoposterior;* **appendicular v.,** the accompanying vein of the appendicular artery; it drains into the ileocolic vein 阑尾静脉，又称 *vena appendicularis;* **arcuate v's of kidney,** a series of complete arches across the bases of the renal pyramids; they are formed by union of the interlobular veins and the straight venules and drain into the interlobar veins 肾弓状静脉，又称 *venae arcuatae renis;* **articular v's,** small vessels that drain the plexus around the temporomandibular joint into the retromandibular vein. 颞下颌关节静脉，又称 *venae articulares;* **atrial v's of heart, left,** inconstant smallest cardiac veins emptying into the left atrium of the heart 左心房静脉，又称 *venae atriales sinistrae;* **atrial v's of heart, right,** the smallest cardiac veins emptying into the right atrium of the heart 右心房静脉，又称 *venae atriales dextrae;* **auditory v's, internal,** 同 labyrin thine v's; **auricular v's, anterior,** branches from the anterior part of the pinna that enter the superficial temporal vein 耳前静脉，又称 *venae auriculares anteriores;* **auricular v., posterior,** a vein that begins in a plexus on the side of the head, passes down behind the pinna, and joins with the retromandibular vein to form the external jugular vein 耳后静脉，又称 *vena auricularis posterior;* **axillary v.,** the venous trunk of the upper limb; it begins at the lower border of the teres major muscle by junction of the basilic and brachial veins, and at the lateral border of the first rib is continuous with the subclavian vein 腋静脉，又称 *vena axillaris;* **azygos v.,** an intercepting trunk for the right intercostal veins as well as a connecting branch between the superior and inferior venae cavae: it arises from the ascending lumbar vein, passes up in the posterior mediastinum, arches over the root of the right lung, and empties into the superior vena cava 奇静脉，又称 *vena azygos;* **basal v.,** a vein that arises at the anterior perforated sub-

V

stance, passes backward and around the cerebral peduncle, and empties into the internal cerebral vein 基底静脉，又称 *vena basalis*; **basal v., anterior,** either of two veins, each draining the anterior basal segment of the inferior lobe of a lung and emptying into the corresponding superior basal vein 前基底静脉，又称 *vena basalis anterior*; **basal v., common,** either of two veins, each draining the inferior lobe of a lung, via the superior and inferior basal veins, and emptying into the corresponding inferior pulmonary vein 总基底静脉，又称 *vena basalis communis*; **basal v., inferior,** either of two veins, each draining the medial and posterior basal segments of the inferior lobe of a lung and emptying into the corresponding common basal vein 下基底静脉，又称 *vena basalis inferior*; **basal v., superior,** either of two veins, each draining the lateral and anterior basal segments of the inferior lobe of a lung and emptying into the corresponding common basal vein 上基底静脉，又称 *vena basalis superior*; **basilic v.,** the superficial vein that arises from the ulnar side of the dorsal rete of the hand, passes up the forearm, and joins with the brachial veins to form the axillary vein 贵要静脉，又称 *vena basilica*; **basilic v., median,** a vein sometimes present as the medial branch, ending in the basilic vein, of a bifurcation of the median antebrachial vein 贵要正中静脉，又称 *vena basilica antebrachii*; **basivertebral v's,** venous sinuses in the cancellous tissue of the bodies of the vertebrae, which communicate with the plexus of veins on the anterior surface of the vertebrae and with the anterior internal and anterior external vertebral plexuses 椎体静脉，又称 *venae basivertebrales*; **brachial v's,** the accompanying veins of the brachial artery, which join with the basilic vein to form the axillary vein 肱静脉，又称 *venae brachiales*; **brachiocephalic v.,** either of the two veins (right and left) that drain blood from the head, neck, and upper limbs, and unite to form the superior vena cava. Each is formed at the root of the neck by union of the ipsilateral internal jugular and subclavian veins. The right vein passes almost vertically downward in front of the brachiocephalic artery, and the left vein passes from left to right behind the upper part of the sternum. Each vein receives the vertebral, deep cervical, deep thyroid, and internal thoracic veins. The left vein also receives numerous branches as well as the thoracic duct, and the right vein receives the right lymphatic duct 头臂静脉，又称 *vena brachiocephalica*; **bronchial v's,** vessels that drain blood from the larger subdivisions of the bronchi; on the left they drain into the azygos vein and on the right they drain into the hemiazygos vein or

superior intercostal vein 支气管静脉，又称 *venae bronchiales*; **v. of bulb of penis,** a vein draining blood from the bulb of the penis into the internal pudendal vein 尿道球静脉，又称 *vena bulbi penis*; **v. of bulb of vestibule,** a vein draining blood from the bulb of the vestibule of the vagina into the internal pudendal vein 前庭球静脉，又称 *vena bulbi vestibuli*; **cardiac v's, anterior,** anterior v's of right ventricle 心前静脉；**cardiac v., great,** a vein that collects blood from the anterior surface of the ventricles, follows the anterior longitudinal sulcus, and empties into the coronary sinus 左大静脉，又称 *vena cardiaca magna*; **cardiac v., middle,** a vein that collects blood from the diaphragmatic surface of the ventricles, follows the posterior longitudinal sulcus, and empties into the coronary sinus 心中静脉，又称 *vena cardiaca media*; **cardiac v., small,** a vein that collects blood from both parts of the right heart, follows the coronary sulcus to the left, and opens into the coronary sinus 心小静脉，又称 *vena cardiaca parva*; **cardiac v's, smallest,** numerous small veins arising in the muscular walls and draining independently into the cavities of the heart, particularly the right atrium and ventricle 心最小静脉 *venae cardiacae minimae*; **cardinal v's,** embryonic vessels that include the precardinal, postcardinal, and common cardinal veins 主静脉；**cardinal v's, common,** two short venous trunks in the embryo that open into the primordial atrium of the heart; the right one combines with the anterior cardinal vein to become the superior vena cava 总主静脉；**v's of caudate nucleus,** veins within the corpus striatum that drain into the superior thalamostriate vein 尾状核静脉，又称 *venae nuclei caudati*; **cavernous v's of penis,** veins that return the blood from the corpora cavernosa to the deep veins and the dorsal vein of the penis 阴茎海绵体静脉，又称 *venae cavernosae penis*; **central v's of liver,** veins in the middle of the hepatic lobules, draining into the hepatic vein 肝中央静脉，又称 *venae centrales hepatis*; **central v. of retina,** the vein that is formed by union of the retinal veins; it passes out of the eyeball in the optic nerve to empty into the superior ophthalmic vein 视网膜中央静脉，又称 *vena centralis retinae*; **central v. of suprarenal gland,** the large single vein into which the various veins within the substance of the gland empty, and which continues at the hilum as the suprarenal vein 肾上腺中央静脉，又称 *vena centralis glandulae suprarenalis*; **cephalic v.,** the superficial vein that arises from the radial side of the dorsal rete of the hand, and winds anteriorly to pass along the anterior border of the brachioradialis muscle; above the elbow it ascends along the lateral border of the biceps muscle and the pectoral border of the deltoid muscle and opens into the axillary vein 头静脉，又称 *vena cephalica*; **cephalic v., accessory,** 副头静脉; **cephalic v., median,** a vein arising from the dorsal rete of the hand, passing up the forearm to join the cephalic vein just above the elbow 头正中静脉，又称 *vena cephalica accessoria*; **cerebellar v's, inferior,** a vein sometimes present as the diagonal branch, ending in the cephalic vein, of a bifurcation of the median antebrachial vein 小脑下静脉，又称 *vena cephalica antebrachii*; **cerebellar v., precentral,** veins that drain the inferior surface of the cerebellum and empty into the straight or sigmoid sinus, or into the inferior petrosal and occipital sinuses 小脑中央前静脉，又称 *venae inferiores cerebelli*; **cerebellar v's, superior,** a vein arising in the precentral cerebellar fissure and passing anterior and superior to the culmen, terminating in the great cerebral vein 小脑上静脉，又称 *vena precentralis cerebelli*; **cerebral v's, anterior,** veins that accompany the anterior cerebral artery and join the basal vein 大脑前静脉，又称 *venae anteriores cerebri*; **cerebral v., deep middle,** the vein that accompanies the middle cerebral artery in the floor of the lateral sulcus, and joins the basal vein 大脑中深静脉，又称 *vena media profunda cerebri*; **cerebral v., great,** a short median trunk formed by union of the two internal cerebral veins, which curves around the splenium of the corpus callosum and empties into, or is continued as, the straight sinus 大脑大静脉，又称 *vena magna cerebri*; **cerebral v's, inferior,** superficial cerebral veins that ramify on the base and the inferolateral surface of the brain: those on the inferior surface of the frontal lobe drain into the inferior sagittal sinus and the cavernous sinus; those on the temporal lobe, into the superior petrosal sinus and the transverse sinus; those on the occipital lobe, into the straight sinus 大脑下静脉，又称 *venae inferiores cerebri*; **cerebral v's, internal,** two veins that arise at the interventricular foramen by the union of the thalamostriate and the choroid veins; they pass backward through the tela choroidea, collecting blood from the basal nuclei, and unite at the splenium of the corpus callosum to form the great cerebral vein 大脑内静脉，又称 *venae internae cerebri*; **cerebral v's, superficial middle,** either of the two veins, one in each hemisphere, that drain the lateral surface of the cerebrum, follow the lateral cerebral fissure, and empty into the cavernous sinus; they are fed by the inferior and superior anastomotic veins 大脑浅中静脉，又称 *vena media superficialis cerebri*; **cerebral v's, superior,** the 8 to 12 superficial cerebral veins (prefrontal, frontal, parietal, and occipital) that drain the superior, lateral, and medial surfaces of the cerebrum toward the longitudinal cerebral fissure, where they open into the superior sagittal sinus 大脑上静脉，又称 venae superiores cerebri; **cervical v., deep,** a vein that arises from a plexus in the suboccipital triangle, follows the deep cervical artery down the neck, and empties into the vertebral or the brachiocephalic vein 颈深静脉，又称 *vena cervicalis profunda*; **cervical v's, transverse,** veins that follow the transverse cervical artery and open into the subclavian vein 颈横静脉，又称 *venae transversae cervicis*; **choroid v., inferior,** a vein that drains the inferior choroid plexus into the basal vein 脉络膜下静脉，又称 *vena choroidea inferior*; **choroid v., superior,** the vein that runs along the whole length of the choroid plexus, draining it and the hippocampus, fornix, and corpus callosum; it unites with the superior thalamostriate vein to form the internal cerebral vein 脉络膜上静脉，又称 *vena choroidea superior*; **ciliary v's,** veins that arise inside the eyeball by branches from the ciliary muscle and drain into the superior ophthalmic vein. The *anterior ciliary v's* follow the anterior ciliary arteries, and receive branches from the sinus venosus, sclerae, episcleral veins, and conjunctiva of the eyeball. The *posterior ciliary v's* follow the posterior ciliary arteries and empty also into the inferior ophthalmic vein 睫状静脉，又称 *venae ciliares*; **circumflex femoral v's, lateral,** accompanying veins of the lateral circumflex femoral artery, emptying into the femoral or the deep femoral vein 旋股外侧静脉，又称 *venae circumflexae femoris laterales*; **circumflex femoral v's, medial,** accompanying veins of the medial circumflex femoral artery, emptying into the femoral or the deep femoral vein 旋股内侧静脉，又称 *venae circumflexae femoris mediales*; **circumflex iliac v., deep,** a common trunk formed from the accompanying veins of the homonymous artery and emptying into the external iliac vein 旋髂深静脉，又称 *vena circumflexa ilium profunda*; **circumflex iliac v., superficial,** a vein that follows the homonymous artery and empties into the great saphenous vein 旋髂浅静脉，又称 *vena circumflexa ilium superficialis*; **v. of cochlear aqueduct, v. of cochlear canaliculus,** a vein along the aqueduct of the cochlea that empties into the superior bulb of the internal jugular vein 蜗水管静脉，蜗小管静脉，又称 *vena aqueductus cochleae*; **colic v., left,** a vein that follows the left colic artery and opens into the inferior mesenteric vein 左结肠静脉，又称 *vena colica sinistra*; **colic v., middle,** a vein that follows the distribution of the middle colic artery and empties into the superior mesenteric vein

中结肠静脉，又称 *vena colica media*; **colic v., right,** a vein that follows the distribution of the right colic artery and empties into the superior mesenteric vein 右结肠静脉，又称 *vena colica dextra*; **communicating v's,** 同 perforating v's; **conjunctival v's,** small veins that drain blood from the conjunctiva to the superior ophthalmic vein 结膜静脉，又称 *venae conjunctivales*; **coronary v., left,** the portion of the great cardiac vein lying in the coronary sulcus; it receives blood from the anterior interventricular vein and empties into the coronary sinus 心大静脉，左冠状静脉; **coronary v., right,** the portion of the middle cardiac vein that receives blood from the posterior interventricular vein and empties into the coronary sinus 右冠状静脉; **cortical radiate v's of kidney,** 同 interlobular v's of kidney; **cutaneous v.,** one of the small veins that begin in the papillae of the skin, form subpapillary plexuses, and open into the subcutaneous veins 皮静脉，又称 *vena cutanea*; **cystic v.,** a small vein that returns the blood from the gallbladder to the right branch of the portal vein, within the substance of the liver 胆囊静脉，又称 *vena cystica*; **deep v's of clitoris,** small veins of the clitoris that drain into the vesical venous plexus 阴蒂深静脉，又称 *venae profundae clitoridis*; **deep v's of lower limb,** veins that drain the lower limb, found accompanying homonymous arteries, and anastomosing freely with the superficial veins; the principal ones are the femoral and popliteal veins 下肢深静脉; **deep v's of penis,** veins that follow the distribution of the homonymous artery and empty into the dorsal vein of the penis 阴茎深静脉，又称 *venae profundae penis*; **deep v's of upper limb,** veins that drain the upper limb, found accompanying homonymous arteries, and anastomosing freely with the superficial veins; they include the brachial, ulnar, and radial veins, and their tributaries, all of which ultimately drain into the axillary vein 上肢深静脉; **digital v's, palmar,** the accompanying veins of the proper and common palmar digital arteries, which join the superficial palmar venous arch 指掌侧静脉，又称 *venae digitales palmares*; **digital v's, plantar,** veins from the plantar surfaces of the toes that unite at the clefts to form the plantar metatarsal veins of the foot 趾足底静脉，又称 *venae digitales plantares*; **digital v's of foot, dorsal,** the veins on the dorsal surfaces of the toes that unite in pairs around each cleft to form the dorsal metatarsal veins 趾背静脉，又称 *venae digitales dorsales pedis*; **diploic v's,** veins of the skull, including the frontal, occipital, anterior temporal, and posterior temporal diploic veins, which form sinuses in the cancellous tissue between the laminae of the cranial bones and communicate with meningeal veins, dural sinuses, pericranial veins, and each other 板障静脉; **diploic v., anterior temporal,** a vein that drains the lateral portion of the frontal and the anterior part of the parietal bone, opening internally into the sphenoparietal sinus and externally into a deep temporal vein 颞前板障静脉，又称 *vena diploica temporalis anterior*; **diploic v., frontal,** a vein that drains the frontal bone, emptying externally into the supraorbital vein and internally into the superior sagittal sinus 额板障静脉，又称 *vena diploica frontalis*; **diploic v., occipital,** the largest of the diploic veins, which drains blood from the occipital bone and empties into the occipital vein or the transverse sinus 枕板障静脉，又称 *vena diploica occipitalis*; **diploic v., posterior temporal,** a vein that drains the parietal bone and empties into the transverse sinus 颞后板障静脉，又称 *vena diploica temporalis posterior*; **dorsal v. of clitoris, deep,** a vein that follows the course of the dorsal artery of clitoris and opens into the vesical plexus 阴蒂背深静脉，又称 *vena dorsalis profunda clitoridis*; **dorsal v's of clitoris, superficial,** veins that collect blood subcutaneously from the clitoris and drain into the external pudendal vein 阴蒂背浅静脉，又称 *venae dorsales superficiales clitoridis*; **dorsal v. of corpus callosum,** a vein that drains the superior surface of the corpus callosum into the great cerebral vein 胼胝体背侧静脉，又称 *vena dorsalis corporis callosi*; **dorsal v. of penis, deep,** a vein lying subfascially in the midline of the penis between the dorsal arteries; it begins in small veins around the corona of the glans, is joined by the deep veins of the penis as it passes proximally, and passes between the arcuate pubic and transverse perineal ligaments, where it divides into left and right veins to join the prostatic plexus 阴茎背深静脉，又称 *vena dorsalis profunda penis*; **dorsal v's of penis, superficial,** veins that collect blood subcutaneously from the penis and drain into the external pudendal vein 阴茎背浅静脉，又称 *venae dorsales superficiales penis*; **dorsal scapular v.,** an occasional branch that contributes to the subclavian vein 肩胛背静脉，又称 *vena scapularis dorsalis*; **dorsal v's of tongue,** 同 lingual v's, dorsal; **emissary v.,** one of the small, valveless veins that pass through foramina of the skull, connecting the dural venous sinuses with scalp veins or with deep veins below the base of the skull 导静脉，又称 *vena emissaria*; **emissary v., condylar,** a small vein running through the condylar canal of the skull, connecting the sigmoid sinus with the vertebral or the internal jugular vein 髁导静脉，又称 *vena emissaria condylaris*; **emissary v., mastoid,** a small vein passing through the mastoid foramen of the skull and connecting the sigmoid sinus with the occipital or the posterior auricular vein 乳突导静脉, 又称 *vena emissaria mastoidea*; **emissary v., occipital,** an occasional small vein running through a minute foramen in the occipital protuberance of the skull and connecting the confluence of the sinuses with the occipital vein 枕骨导静脉, 又称 *vena emissaria occipitalis*; **emissary v., parietal,** a small vein passing through the parietal foramen of the skull and connecting the superior sagittal sinus with the superficial temporal veins 顶导静脉, 又称 *vena emissaria parietalis*; **v's of encephalic trunk,** the veins that drain the brainstem and empty into the basal or great cerebral vein; see *anterior pontomesencephalic v., v. of lateral recess of fourth ventricle, v's of medulla oblongata,* and *pontine v's* 脑干静脉, 又称 *venae trunci encephalici*; **epigastric v., inferior,** a vein that accompanies the inferior epigastric artery and opens into the external iliac vein 腹壁下静脉, 又称 *vena epigastrica inferior*; **epigastric v., superficial,** a vein that follows its homonymous artery and opens into the great saphenous or the femoral vein 腹壁浅静脉, 又称 *vena epigastrica superficialis*; **epigastric v's, superior,** the accompanying veins of the superior epigastric artery, which open into the internal thoracic vein 腹壁上静脉, 又称 *venae epigastricae superiores*; **episcleral v's,** the veins that ring the cornea and drain into the vorticose and ciliary veins 巩膜外静脉, 又称 *venae episclerales*; **esophageal v's,** small veins that drain blood from the esophagus into the hemiazygos and azygos veins, or into the left brachiocephalic vein 食管静脉, 又称 *venae oesophageales*; **ethmoidal v's,** veins that follow the anterior and posterior ethmoidal arteries, emerge from the ethmoidal foramina, and empty into the superior ophthalmic vein 筛静脉, 又称 *venae ethmoidales*; **facial v.,** the vein that begins at the medial angle of the eye as the angular vein, descends behind the facial artery, and usually ends in the internal jugular vein; it sometimes joins the retromandibular vein to form a common trunk 面静脉, 又称 *vena facialis*; **facial v., deep,** a vein draining from the pterygoid plexus to the facial vein 面深静脉, 又称 *vena profunda faciei*; **facial v., posterior,** retromandibular v. 面后静脉; **facial v., transverse,** a vein that passes backward with the transverse facial artery just below the zygomatic arch to join the retromandibular vein 面横静脉, 又称 *vena transversa faciei*; **femoral v.,** a vein that lies in the proximal twothirds of the thigh; it is a direct continuation of the popliteal vein, follows the course of the femoral artery, and at the in-guinal ligament becomes the external iliac vein. note: The portion of the femoral vein proximal to the branching of the deep femoral vein is sometimes referred to as the *common femoral v.* and its continuation distal to the branching as the *superficial femoral v.* 股静脉, 又称 *vena femoralis*; **femoral v., deep,** a vein that follows the distribution of the deep femoral artery and opens into the femoral vein 股深静脉, 又称 *vena profunda femoris*; **fibular v's,** the accompanying veins of the fibular artery, emptying into the posterior tibial vein 腓静脉, 又称 *venae fibulares*; **frontal v's,** a group of superior cerebral veins, superficial cerebral veins that drain the cortex of the frontal lobe 额叶静脉, 又称 *venae frontales*; **gastric v., left,** the accompanying vein of the left gastric artery, emptying into the portal vein 胃左静脉, 又称 *vena gastrica sinistra*; **gastric v., right,** the accompanying vein of the right gastric artery, emptying into the portal vein 胃右静脉, 又称 *vena gastrica dextra*; **gastric v's, short,** small vessels draining the left portion of the greater curvature of the stomach and emptying into the splenic vein 胃短静脉, 又称 *venae gastricae breves*; **gastroepiploic v.,** gastro-omental v. (left or right) 胃网膜静脉; **gastro-omental v., left,** a vein that follows the distribution of its homonymous artery and empties into the splenic vein 胃网膜左静脉, 又称 *vena gastroomentalis sinistra*; **gastro-omental v., right,** a vein that follows the distribution of its homonymous artery and empties into the superior mesenteric vein 胃网膜右静脉, 又称 *vena gastroomentalis dextra*; **genicular v's,** veins accompanying the genicular arteries and draining into the popliteal vein 膝静脉, 又称 *venae geniculares*; **gluteal v's, inferior,** accompanying veins of the inferior gluteal artery; they drain the superficial fascia of the back of the thigh and the muscles of the buttock, unite into a single vein after passing through the greater sciatic foramen, and empty into the internal iliac vein 臀下静脉, 又称 *venae gluteae inferiores*; **gluteal v's, superior,** accompanying veins of the superior gluteal artery; they drain the muscles of the buttock, pass through the greater sciatic foramen, and empty into the internal iliac vein 臀上静脉, 又称 *venae gluteae superiores*; **gonadal v's,** the ovarian veins and testicular veins 性腺静脉; **hemiazygos v.,** an intercepting trunk for the lower left posterior intercostal veins; it arises from the ascending lumbar vein, passes up on the left side of the vertebrae to the eighth thoracic vertebra, where it may receive the accessory branch, and crosses over the vertebral column to open into the azygos vein 半奇静脉, 又称 *vena hemiazygos*; **hemiazygos v., accessory,** the de-

V

scending intercepting trunk for the upper, often the fourth through the eighth, left posterior intercostal veins. It lies on the left side and at the eighth thoracic vertebra joins the hemiazygos vein or crosses to the right side to join the azygos vein directly; above, it may communicate with the left superior intercostal vein 副半奇静脉, 又称 *vena hemiazygos accessoria*; **hemorrhoidal v's,** rectal v's 直肠静脉; **hepatic v's,** veins that receive blood from the central veins of the liver. The upper group usually consists of three large veins *(left, middle, and right hepatic veins)*, and the lower group consists of six to twenty small veins, which come from the right and caudate lobes; all are contiguous with the hepatic tissue and valveless, and open into the inferior vena cava on the posterior aspect of the liver 肝静脉, 又称 *venae hepaticae*; **hepatic v., left,** the large hepatic vein that drains the central veins in the left side of the liver and empties into the inferior vena cava 肝左静脉, 又称 *vena hepatica sinistra*; **hepatic v., middle,** the large hepatic vein that drains the central veins in the transverse part of the liver and empties into the inferior vena cava 肝中间静脉, 又称 *vena hepatica intermedia*; **hepatic v., right,** the large hepatic vein that drains the central veins in the right side of the liver and empties into the inferior vena cava 肝右静脉, 又称 *vena hepatica dextra*; **hepatic portal v.,** 同 portal v.; **hypophysioportal v's,** a system of venules connecting capillaries in the hypothalamus with sinusoidal capillaries in the anterior lobe of the hypophysis 垂体门静脉, 又称 *venae portales hypophysiales*; **ileal v's,** veins draining blood from the ileum into the superior mesenteric vein 回肠静脉, 又称 *venae ileales*; **ileocolic v.,** a vein that follows the distribution of its homonymous artery and empties into the superior mesenteric vein 回结肠静脉, 又称 *vena ileocolica*; **iliac v., common,** a vein that arises at the sacroiliac joint by union of the external iliac and the internal iliac veins, and passes upward to the right side of the fifth lumbar vertebra where it unites with its fellow of the opposite side to form the inferior vena cava 髂总静脉, 又称 *vena iliaca communis*; **iliac v., external,** the continuation of the femoral vein from the inguinal ligament to the sacroiliac joint, where it joins with the internal iliac vein to form the common iliac vein 髂外静脉, 又称 *vena iliaca externa*; **iliac v., internal,** a short trunk formed by union of parietal branches; it extends from the greater sciatic notch to the brim of the pelvis, where it joins the external iliac vein to form the common iliac vein 髂内静脉, 又称 *vena iliaca interna*; **iliolumbar v.,** a vein that follows the distribution of the iliolumbar artery and

opens into the internal iliac or the common iliac vein, or it may divide to end in both 髂腰静脉, 又称 *vena iliolumbalis*; **inferior v. of vermis,** a vein that drains the inferior surface of the cerebellum; it runs backward on the inferior vermis to empty into the straight sinus or one of the sigmoid sinuses 蚓下静脉, 又称 *vena inferior vermis*; **innominate v.,** brachiocephalic v. 无名静脉; **insular v's,** veins that drain the insula and join the deep middle cerebral vein 岛静脉, 又称 *venae insulares*; **intercapitular v's of foot,** veins at the clefts of the toes that pass between the heads of the metatarsal bones and establish communication between the dorsal and plantar venous systems of the foot 足小头间静脉, 又称 *venae intercapitulares pedis*; **intercapitular v's of hand,** veins at the clefts of the fingers that pass between the heads of the metacarpal bones and establish communication between the dorsal and palmar venous systems of the hand 手小头间静脉, 又称 *venae intercapitulares manus*; **intercostal v's, anterior,** the twelve paired accompanying veins of the anterior thoracic arteries, which drain into the internal thoracic veins 肋间前静脉, 又称 *venae intercostales anteriores*; **intercostal v., highest,** the first posterior intercostal vein of either side, which passes over the apex of the lung and ends in the brachiocephalic, vertebral, or superior intercostal vein 肋间最上静脉, 又称 *vena intercostalis suprema*; **intercostal v., left superior,** the common trunk formed by union of the second, third, and sometimes fourth posterior intercostal veins, which crosses the arch of the aorta and joins the left brachiocephalic vein 左肋间上静脉, 又称 *vena intercostalis superior sinistra*; **intercostal v's, posterior,** the veins that accompany the corresponding intercostal arteries and drain the intercostal spaces posteriorly; the first ends in the brachiocephalic or the vertebral vein, the second and third join the superior intercostal vein, and the fourth to eleventh join the azygos vein on the right and the hemiazygos or accessory hemiazygos vein on the left 肋间后静脉, 又称 *venae intercostales posteriores*; **intercostal v., right superior,** a common trunk formed by union of the second, third, and sometimes fourth posterior intercostal veins, which drains into the azygos vein 右肋间上静脉, 又称 *vena intercostalis superior dextra*; **interlobar v's of kidney,** veins that drain the arcuate veins, pass down between the renal pyramids, and unite to form the renal vein 肾叶间静脉, 又称 *venae interlobares renis*; **interlobular v's of kidney,** veins that collect blood from the capillary network of the renal cortex and empty into the arcuate veins 肾小叶间静脉, 又称 *venae corticales radia-*

tae renis; **interlobular v's of liver,** veins that arise as tributaries of the hepatic veins between the hepatic lobules 肝小叶间静脉，又称 *venae interlobulares hepatis*; **interosseous v's, anterior,** the veins accompanying the anterior interosseous artery, which join the ulnar veins near the elbow 骨间前静脉，又称 *venae interosseae anteriores*; **interosseous v's, posterior,** the veins accompanying the posterior interosseous artery, which join the ulnar veins near the elbow 骨间后静脉，又称 *venae interosseae posteriores*; **interventricular v., anterior,** the portion of the great cardiac vein ascending in the anterior interventricular sulcus and emptying into the left coronary vein 前室间静脉，又称 *vena interventricularis anterior*; **interventricular v., posterior,** middle cardiac v. 后室间静脉; **intervertebral v.,** any one of the veins that drain the vertebral plexuses, passing out through the intervertebral foramina and emptying into the regional veins: in the neck, into the vertebral; in the thorax, the intercostal; in the abdomen, the lumbar; and in the pelvis, the lateral sacral veins 椎间静脉，又称 *vena intervertebralis*; **intrarenal v's,** the veins within the kidney, including the interlobar, arcuate, interlobular, and stellate veins, and the straight venules 肾内静脉，又称 *venae intrarenales*; **jejunal v's,** veins draining blood from the jejunum into the superior mesenteric vein 空肠静脉，又称 *venae jejunales*; **jugular v., anterior,** a vein that arises under the chin, passes down the neck, and opens into the external jugular or the subclavian vein or into the jugular venous arch 颈前静脉，又称 *vena jugularis anterior*; **jugular v., external,** a vein that begins in the parotid gland behind the angle of the jaw by union of the retromandibular and the posterior auricular veins, passes down the neck, and opens into the subclavian, internal jugular, or brachiocephalic vein 颈外静脉，又称 *vena jugularis externa*; **jugular v., internal,** the vein that begins as the superior bulb in the jugular fossa, draining much of the head and neck; it descends with first the internal carotid artery and then the common carotid artery in the neck, and joins with the subclavian vein to form the brachiocephalic vein 颈内静脉，又称 *vena jugularis interna*; **labial v's, anterior,** veins that collect blood from the anterior aspect of the labia and drain into the external pudendal vein; they are homologues of the anterior scrotal veins in the male 阴唇前静脉，又称 *venae labiales anteriores*; **labial v's, inferior,** veins that drain the region of the lower lip into the facial vein 阴唇下静脉，又称 *venae labiales inferiores*; **labial v's, posterior,** small branches from the labia that open into the vesical venous plexus;

they are homologues of the posterior scrotal veins in the male 阴唇后静脉，又称 *venae labiales posteriores*; **labial v., superior,** a vein that drains blood from the region of the upper lip into the facial vein 阴唇上静脉，又称 *vena labialis superior*; **labyrinthine v's,** several small veins that pass through the internal acoustic meatus from the cochlea into the inferior petrosal or transverse sinus 迷路静脉，又称 *venae labyrinthi*; **lacrimal v.,** the vein that drains blood from the lacrimal gland into the superior ophthalmic vein 泪腺静脉，又称 *vena lacrimalis*; **laryngeal v., inferior,** a vein draining blood from the larynx into the inferior thyroid vein 喉下静脉，又称 *vena laryngea inferior*; **laryngeal v., superior,** a vein that drains blood from the larynx into the superior thyroid vein 喉上静脉，又称 *vena laryngea superior*; **lateral direct v's,** veins of the lateral ventricle, draining into the great cerebral vein 外直静脉，又称 *venae directae laterales*; **v. of lateral recess of fourth ventricle,** a small vein arising in the tonsil of the cerebellum, passing the lateral recess of the fourth ventricle, and terminating in the petrosal vein 第四脑室外侧隐窝静脉，又称 *vena recessus lateralis ventriculi quarti*; **v. of lateral ventricle, lateral,** a vein passing through the lateral wall of the lateral ventricle to drain the temporal and parietal lobes into the superior thalamostriate vein 侧脑室外侧静脉，又称 *vena lateralis ventriculi lateralis*; **v. of lateral ventricle, medial,** a vein passing through the labyrinthine wall of the lateral ventricle to drain the parietal and occipital lobes into the internal cerebral or great cerebral vein 侧脑室内侧静脉，又称 *vena medialis ventriculi lateralis*; **lingual v.,** the deep vein that follows the distribution of the lingual artery and empties into the internal jugular vein 舌静脉，又称 *vena lingualis*; **lingual v., deep,** a vein that drains blood from the deep aspect of the tongue and joins the sublingual vein to form the accompanying vein of the hypoglossal nerve 舌深静脉，又称 *vena profunda linguae*; **lingual v's, dorsal,** veins that unite with a small accompanying vein of the lingual artery and join the main lingual trunk 舌背静脉，又称 *venae dorsales linguae*; **lingular v.,** a vein draining the lingular segments of the superior lobe of the left lung, emptying into the left superior pulmonary vein and formed by the union of superior and inferior parts 舌静脉，又称 *vena lingularis*; **lumbar v's,** the veins, four or five on each side, that accompany the corresponding lumbar arteries and drain the mastoid wall of the abdomen, vertebral canal, spinal cord, and meninges; the first four usually end in the inferior vena cava, although the first may end in the ascending lumbar vein; the fifth is a tributary of the iliolumbar or of the common iliac vein; and all are generally united by the ascending iliac vein 腰静脉，又称 *venae lumbales*; **lumbar v., ascending,** an ascending intercepting vein for the lumbar veins of either side; it begins in the lateral sacral veins and passes up the spine to the first lumbar vertebra, where by union with the subcostal vein it becomes on the right side the azygos vein, and on the left side, the hemiazygos vein 腰升静脉，又称 *vena lumbalis ascendens*; **marginal v., lateral,** a vein running along the lateral side of the dorsum of the foot, returning blood from the dorsal venous arch, dorsal venous network, and superficial veins of the sole and draining into the small saphenous vein 外侧缘静脉，又称 *vena marginalis lateralis.* **marginal v., left,** a vein ascending along the left margin of the heart, draining the left ventricle and emptying into the great cardiac vein 左缘静脉; **marginal v., medial,** a vein running along the medial side of the dorsum of the foot, returning blood from the dorsal venous arch, dorsal venous network, and superficial veins of the sole and draining into the great saphenous vein 内侧缘静脉，又称 *vena marginalis medialis*; **marginal v., right,** a vein ascending along the right margin of the heart, draining adjacent parts of the right ventricle and opening into the right atrium or anterior cardiac veins 右缘静脉，又称 *vena marginalis dextra*; **masseteric v's,** veins from the masseter muscle that empty into the facial vein 咬肌静脉; **maxillary v's,** veins from the pterygoid plexus, usually forming a single short trunk, passing back and uniting with the superficial temporal vein in the parotid gland to form the retromandibular vein 上颌静脉，又称 *venae maxillares*; **median cubital v.,** the large connecting branch that arises from the cephalic vein below the elbow and passes obliquely upward over the cubital fossa to join the basilic vein 肘正中静脉，又称 *vena mediana cubiti*; **mediastinal v's,** numerous small branches that drain blood from the anterior mediastinum into the brachiocephalic vein, azygos vein, or superior vena cava 纵隔静脉，又称 *venae mediastinales*; **v's of medulla oblongata,** the veins that drain the medulla oblongata, which empty into the veins of the spinal cord, the adjacent dural venous sinuses, the inferior petrosal sinus, or the superior bulb of the jugular vein 延髓静脉，又称 *venae medullae oblongatae*; **meningeal v's,** the accompanying veins of the meningeal arteries, which drain the dura mater, communicate with the lateral lacunae, and empty into the regional sinuses and veins 脑膜静脉，又称 *venae meningeae*; **meningeal v's, middle,** the accompanying veins of the middle meningeal artery,

which end in the pterygoid venous plexus 脑膜中静脉，又称 *venae meningeae mediae*; **mesenteric v., inferior,** a vein that follows the distribution of its homonymous artery and empties into the splenic vein 肠系膜下静脉，又称 *vena mesenterica inferior*; **mesenteric v., superior,** a vein that follows the distribution of its homonymous artery and joins with the splenic vein to form the hepatic portal vein 肠系膜上静脉，又称 *vena mesenterica superior*; **metacarpal v's, dorsal,** veins that arise from the union of dorsal veins of adjacent fingers and pass proximally to join in forming the dorsal venous rete of the hand 掌背静脉，又称 *venae metacarpales dorsales*; **metacarpal v's, palmar,** the accompanying veins of the palmar metacarpal arteries, which open into the deep palmar venous arch 掌心静脉，又称 *venae metacarpales palmares*; **metatarsal v's, dorsal,** veins that are formed by the dorsal digital veins of the toes at the clefts of the toes, joining the dorsal venous arch 跖背静脉，又称 *venae metatarsales dorsales*; **metatarsal v's, plantar,** deep veins of the foot that arise from the plantar digital veins at the clefts of the toes and pass back to open into the plantar venous arch 跖底静脉，又称 *venae metatarsales plantares*; **middle lobe v.,** a vein draining the middle lobe of the right lung, emptying into the right superior pulmonary vein and formed by the union of lateral and medial parts 中部叶静脉，又称 *vena lobi medii*; **musculophrenic v's,** the accompanying veins of the musculophrenic artery, draining blood from parts of the respiratory diaphragm and from the wall of the thorax and abdomen and emptying into the internal thoracic veins 肌膈静脉，又称 *venae musculophrenicae*; **nasal v's, external,** small ascending branches from the nose that open into the angular and facial veins 鼻外静脉，又称 *venae nasales externae*; **nasofrontal v.,** a vein that begins at the supraorbital vein, enters the orbit, and joins the superior ophthalmic vein 鼻额静脉，又称 *vena nasofrontalis*; **oblique v. of left atrium,** a small vein from the left atrium that opens into the coronary sinus 左房斜静脉，又称 *vena obliqua atrii sinistri*; **obturator v's,** veins that drain the hip joint and the regional muscles, enter the pelvis through the obturator canal, and empty into the internal iliac vein or inferior epigastric vein, or both 闭孔静脉，又称 *venae obturatoriae*; **occipital v.,** 枕静脉 1. a vein in the scalp that follows the distribution of the occipital artery and opens under the trapezius muscle into the suboccipital venous plexus; it may continue with the occipital artery and end in the internal jugular vein. 2. any of the group of superficial superior cerebral veins that drain the cortex of the occipital lobe. 又称 *vena occipitalis*; **v. of olfactory gyrus**, a vein that drains the olfactory gyrus into the basal vein 嗅回静脉, 又称 *vena gyri olfactorii*; **ophthalmic v., inferior**, a vein formed by confluence of muscular and ciliary branches, and running backward either to join the superior ophthalmic vein or to open directly into the cavernous sinus; it sends a communicating branch through the inferior orbital fissure to join the pterygoid venous plexus 眼下静脉, 又称 *vena ophthalmica inferior*; **ophthalmic v., superior**, a vein that begins at the medial angle of the eye, where it communicates with the frontal, supraorbital, and angular veins; it follows the distribution of the ophthalmic artery, and may be joined by the inferior ophthalmic vein at the superior orbital fissure before opening into the cavernous sinus 眼上静脉, 又称 *vena ophthalmica superior*; **v's of orbit**, the veins that drain the orbit and its structures, including the superior ophthalmic vein and its tributaries and the inferior ophthalmic vein 眶静脉; **ovarian v., left**, a vein that drains the left pampiniform plexus of the broad ligament and empties into the left renal vein 左卵巢静脉, 又称 *vena ovarica sinistra*; **ovarian v., right**, a vein that drains the right pampiniform plexus of the broad ligament and empties into the inferior vena cava 右卵巢静脉, 又称 *vena ovarica dextra*; **palatine v., external**, a vein that drains blood from the tonsils and the soft palate into the facial vein 腭外静脉, 又称 *vena palatina externa*; **palpebral v's**, small branches from the eyelids that open into the superior ophthalmic vein 眼睑静脉, 又称 *venae palpebrales*; **palpebral v's, inferior**, branches that drain the blood from the lower eyelid into the facial vein 下睑静脉, 又称 *venae palpebrales inferiores*; **palpebral v's, superior**, branches that drain the blood from the upper eyelid to the angular vein 上睑静脉, 又称 *venae palpebrales superiores*; **pancreatic v's**, numerous branches from the pancreas that open into the splenic and superior mesenteric veins 胰静脉, 又称 *venae pancreaticae*; **pancreaticoduodenal v's**, four veins that drain blood from the pancreas and duodenum, closely following the homonymous arteries. A superior and an inferior vein originate from both an anterior and a posterior venous arcade. The anterior superior vein joins the right gastro-omental vein; the posterior superior vein joins the portal vein. The anterior and posterior inferior veins join, sometimes as one trunk and other times singly, the uppermost jejunal vein or the superior mesenteric vein 胰十二指肠静脉, 又称 *venae pancreaticoduodenales*; **paraumbilical v's**, veins that communicate with the portal vein and anastomose with the superior and inferior epigastric and the superior vesical veins in the region of the umbilicus. They form a part of the collateral circulation of the portal vein in the event of hepatic obstruction 附脐静脉, 又称 *venae paraumbilicales*; **parietal v's**, a group of superior cerebral veins, superficial cerebral veins that drain the cortex of the parietal lobe 顶叶静脉, 又称 *venae parietales*; **parotid v's**, small veins from the parotid gland that open into the facial vein or the retromandibular vein 腮腺静脉, 又称 *venae parotideae*; **pectoral v's**, a collective term for branches of the subclavian vein that drain the pectoral region 胸肌静脉, 又称 *venae pectorales*; **peduncular v's**, veins that drain the cerebral peduncle into the basal vein 大脑脚静脉, 又称 *venae pedunculares*; **perforating v's**, valved veins that drain blood from the superficial to the deep veins in the leg and foot 穿静脉, 又称 *venae perforantes*; **pericardiacophrenic v's**, small veins that drain blood from the pericardium and respiratory diaphragm into the left brachiocephalic vein 心包膈静脉, 又称 *venae pericardiacophrenicae*; **pericardial v's**, numerous small branches that drain blood from the pericardium into the brachiocephalic, inferior thyroid, and azygos veins, and the superior vena cava 心包静脉, 又称 *venae pericardiacae*; **peroneal v's**, 同 fibular v's; **petrosal v.**, a short trunk arising from the union of four or five cerebellar and pontine veins opposite the middle cerebellar peduncle and terminating in the superior petrosal sinus 岩静脉, 又称 *vena petrosa*; **pharyngeal v's**, veins that drain the pharyngeal plexus and empty into the internal jugular vein 咽静脉, 又称 *venae pharyngeae*; **phrenic v's, inferior**, veins that follow the homonymous arteries, the one on the right entering the inferior vena cava and the one on the left entering the left suprarenal or renal vein or the inferior vena cava 膈下静脉, 又称 *venae phrenicae inferiores*; **phrenic v's, superior**, small veins on the superior surface of the respiratory diaphragm that drain into the azygos and hemiazygos veins 膈上静脉, 又称 *venae phrenicae superiores*; **pontine v's**, the veins that drain the pons, which empty into the basal vein, cerebellar veins, petrosal or venous sinuses, or venous plexus of the foramen ovale 脑桥静脉, 又称 *venae pontis*; **pontomesencephalic v., anterior**, a vein lying on the superior and anterior aspects of the pons in the midline of the interpeduncular fossa, communicating superiorly with the basal vein and inferiorly with the petrosal vein 脑桥中脑前静脉, 又称 *vena pontomesencephalica anterior*; **popliteal v.**, a vein following the popliteal artery and formed by union of the accompanying veins of the anterior and posterior tibial arteries; at the adductor hiatus it becomes continuous with the femoral vein 腘静脉，又称 *vena poplitea*; **portal v.**, a short thick trunk formed by union of the superior mesenteric and the splenic veins behind the neck of the pancreas; it passes upward to the right end of the porta hepatis, where it divides into successively smaller branches, following the branches of the hepatic artery, until it forms a capillarylike system of sinusoids that permeates the entire substance of the liver 门静脉，又称 *vena portae hepatis*; **Postcardinal v's**, paired vessels in the early embryo caudal to the heart 后主静脉; **posterior v. of corpus callosum**, a vein that drains the posterior surface of the corpus callosum into the great cerebral vein 胼胝体后静脉，又称 *vena posterior corporis callosi*; **posterior v. of left ventricle**, the vein that drains blood from the posterior surface of the left ventricle into the coronary sinus 左室后静脉，又称 *vena ventriculi sinistri posterior*; **posterior v. of septum pellucidum**, a vein that drains the posterior septum pellucidum into the superior thalamostriate vein 透明隔后静脉，又称 *vena posterior septi pellucidi*; **precardinal v's**, paired venous trunks in the embryo cranial to the heart 前主静脉; **prefrontal v's**, a group of superior cerebral veins, superficial cerebral veins that drain the prefrontal area of the cerebral cortex 额叶前静脉，又称 *venae prefrontales*; **prepyloric v.**, a vein that accompanies the prepyloric artery, passing upward over the anterior surface of the junction between the pylorus and the duodenum and emptying into the right gastric vein 幽门前静脉，又称 *vena prepylorica*; **v. of pterygoid canal**, one of the veins that pass through the pterygoid canal and empty into the pterygoid plexus 翼管静脉，又称 *vena canalis pterygoidei*; **pudendal v's, external**, veins that follow the distribution of the external pudendal arteries, drain anterior parts of the labia or scrotum, and open into the great saphenous vein and femoral vein 阴部外静脉，又称 *venae pudendae externae*; **pudendal v., internal**, a vein that follows the course of the internal pudendal artery and drains into the internal iliac vein 阴部内静脉，又称 *vena pudenda interna*; **pulmonary v's**, the four veins, right and left superior and right and left inferior, that return aerated blood from the lungs to the left atrium of the heart 肺静脉，又称 *venae pulmonales*; **pulmonary v., left inferior**, the vein that returns blood from the lower lobe of the left lung (from the superior segmental and common basal veins) to the left atrium of the heart 左下肺静脉，又称 *vena pulmonalis sinistra inferior*; **pulmonary v., left superior**, the vein that returns blood from the upper lobe of the

left lung (from the apicoposterior, anterior segmental, and lingular veins) to the left atrium of the heart 左肺上静脉，又称 *vena pulmonalis sinistra superior*; **pulmonary v., right inferior**, the vein that returns blood from the lower lobe of the right lung (from the superior segmental and common basal veins) to the left atrium of the heart 右下肺静脉，又称 *vena pulmonalis dextra inferior*; **pulmonary v., right superior**, the vein that returns blood from the upper and middle lobes of the right lung (from the middle lobe, apical, anterior segmental, and posterior segmental veins) to the left atrium of the heart 右上肺静脉，又称 *vena pulmonalis dextra superior*; **pulp v's**, vessels draining the splenic sinuses 髓静脉; **pyloric v.**, 同 right gastric v.; **radial v's**, the accompanying veins of the radial artery, which open into the brachial veins 桡静脉，又称 *venae radiales*; **ranine v.**, 同 sublingual v.; **rectal v's, inferior**, veins that drain the rectal plexus into the internal pudendal vein 直肠下静脉，又称 *venae rectales inferiores*; **rectal v's, middle**, veins that drain the rectal plexus and empty into the internal iliac and superior rectal veins 直肠中静脉，又称 *venae rectales mediae*; **rectal v., superior**, the vein that drains the upper part of the rectal plexus into the inferior mesenteric vein and thus establishes connection between the portal system and the systemic circulation 直肠上静脉，又称 *vena rectalis superior*; **renal v's**, 1. two veins, one from each kidney, that receive blood from the interlobar veins, with the left also receiving blood from the left testicular (or ovarian), left suprarenal, and (sometimes) inferior phrenic veins; they empty into the inferior vena cava at the level of the second lumbar vertebra 肾静脉，又称 *venae renales*. 2. 同 intrarenal v's; **retromandibular v.**, the vein that is formed in the upper part of the parotid gland behind the neck of the mandible by union of the maxillary and superficial temporal veins; it passes downward through the gland, communicates with the facial vein, and, emerging from the gland, joins with the posterior auricular vein to form the external jugular vein 下颌后静脉，又称 *vena retromandibularis*; **sacral v's, lateral**, veins that follow the homonymous arteries, help to form the lateral sacral plexus, and empty into the internal iliac vein or the superior gluteal veins 骶外侧静脉，又称 *venae sacrales laterales*; **sacral v., median**, a vein that follows the median sacral artery and opens into the common iliac vein 骶正中静脉，又称 *vena sacralis mediana*; **saphenous v., accessory**, a vein that, when present, drains the medial and posterior superficial parts of the thigh and opens into the great saphenous vein 副隐静脉，又称 *vena saphena ac-*

cessoria; saphenous v., great, the longest vein in the body, extending from the dorsum of the foot to just below the inguinal ligament, where it opens into the femoral vein. It drains the foot and leg through many tributaries 大隐静脉，又称 vena saphena magna; saphenous v., small, the vein that continues the lateral marginal vein from behind the malleolus and passes up the back of the leg to the knee joint, where it opens into the popliteal vein 小隐静脉，又称 vena saphena parva; scleral v's, tributaries of the anterior ciliary veins that drain the sclera 巩膜静脉，又称 venae sclerales; scrotal v's, anterior, veins that collect blood from the anterior aspect of the scrotum and drain into the external pudendal vein 阴囊前静脉，又称 venae scrotales anteriores; scrotal v's, posterior, small branches from the posterior aspect of the scrotum that open into the vesical venous plexus 阴囊后静脉，又称 venae scrotales posteriores; segmental v., anterior, either of two veins, each draining the anterior segment of the superior lobe of a lung and emptying into the corresponding superior pulmonary vein 肺上叶前静脉，又称 vena anterior lobi superioris pulmonis; segmental v., apical, 同 apical v.; segmental v., apicoposterior, apicoposterior v; segmental v., posterior, a vein draining the posterior segment of the superior lobe of the right lung and emptying into the right superior pulmonary vein 肺上叶后静脉，又称 vena posterior lobi superioris pulmonis dextri; segmental v., superior, either of two veins, each draining the superior segment of the inferior lobe of a lung and emptying into the corresponding inferior pulmonary vein 肺上叶静脉，又称 vena superior lobi inferioris pulmonis; sigmoid v's, veins from the sigmoid colon that empty into the inferior mesenteric vein 乙状结肠静脉，又称 venae sigmoideae; spinal v's, anterior, a group of longitudinal veins (one median and two anterolateral) forming a plexus on the anterior surface of the spinal cord; they drain the anterior spinal cord 脊髓前静脉，又称 venae spinales anteriores; spinal v's, posterior, a group of longitudinal, usually discontinuous, veins (one median and two posterolateral) forming a plexus on the posterior surface of the spinal cord; they drain the posterior spinal cord 脊髓后静脉，又称 venae spinales posteriores; splenic v., the vein formed by union of several branches at the hilum of the spleen, passing from left to right to the neck of the pancreas, where it joins the superior mesenteric vein to form the portal vein 脾静脉，又称 vena splenica; stellate v's of kidney, veins on the surface of the kidney that collect blood from the superficial parts of the renal cortex and empty into the interlobular veins 肾

星状静脉，又称 venae stellatae renis; sternocleidomastoid v., a vein that follows the course of the homonymous artery and opens into the internal jugular vein 锁乳突肌静脉，又称 vena sternocleidomastoidea; stylomastoid v., a vein following the stylomastoid artery and emptying into the retromandibular vein 茎乳静脉，又称 vena stylomastoidea; subcardinal v's, paired vessels in the embryo, replacing the postcardinal veins and persisting to some degree as definitive vessels 下主静脉; subclavian v., the vein that continues the axillary as the main venous stem of the upper member, follows the subclavian artery, and joins with the internal jugular vein to form the brachiocephalic vein 锁骨下静脉，又称 vena subclavia; subcostal v., the accompanying vein of the subcostal artery on the left or right side; it joins the ascending lumbar vein to form the azygos vein on the right or the hemiazygos vein on the left 肋下静脉，又称 vena subcostalis; subcutaneous v's of abdomen, the superficial veins of the abdominal wall 腹皮下静脉，又称 venae subcutaneae abdominis; sublingual v., a vein that follows the sublingual artery and opens into the lingual vein 舌下静脉，又称 vena sublingualis; sublobular v's, tributaries of the hepatic veins that receive the central veins of liver 小叶下静脉; submental v., a vein that follows the submental artery and opens into the facial vein 颏下静脉，又称 vena submentalis; superficial v's of lower limb, veins that drain the lower limb, found immediately beneath the skin, and anastomosing freely with the deep veins; the principal ones are the great and small saphenous veins 下肢浅静脉; superficial v's of upper limb, veins that drain the upper limb, found immediately beneath the skin, and anastomosing freely with the deep veins; they include the cephalic, basilic, and median cubital and antebrachial veins and their tributaries, all of which ultimately drain into the axillary vein 上肢浅静脉; superior v. of vermis, a vein that drains the superior surface of the cerebellum; it runs forward and medially across the superior vermis to empty into the straight sinus or the great cerebral vein 上蚓静脉，又称 vena superior vermis; supracardinal v's, paired vessels in the embryo, developing later than the subcardinal veins and persisting chiefly as the inferior segment of the inferior vena cava 上主静脉; supraorbital v., the vein that passes down the forehead lateral to the supratrochlear vein, joining it at the root of the nose to form the angular vein 眶上静脉，又称 vena supraorbitalis; suprarenal v., left, the vein that returns blood from the left suprarenal gland to the left renal vein 左肾上腺静脉，又称 vena suprarenalis sinistra; supra-

V

renal v., right, a vein that drains the right suprarenal gland into the inferior vena cava 右肾上腺静脉，又称 *vena suprarenalis dextra*; **suprascapular v.**, the vein that accompanies the homonymous artery (sometimes as two veins that unite), opening usually into the external jugular vein or occasionally into the subclavian vein 肩胛上静脉，又称 *vena suprascapularis*; **supratrochlear v's**, two veins, each beginning in a venous plexus high up on the forehead and descending to the root of the nose, where each joins with the supraorbital vein to form the angular vein 滑车上静脉，又称 *venae supratrochleares*; **sural v's**, veins that ascend with the sural arteries and drain blood from the calf into the popliteal vein 腓肠静脉，又称 *venae surales*; **temporal v's, deep**, veins that drain the deep portions of the temporalis muscle and empty into the pterygoid plexus 颞深静脉，又称 *venae temporales profundae*; **temporal v., middle**, a vein that arises in the substance of the temporalis muscle and passes down under the fascia to the zygoma, where it breaks through to join the superficial temporal vein 颞中静脉，又称 *vena temporalis media*; **temporal v's, superficial**, veins that drain the lateral part of the scalp in the frontal and parietal regions, the tributaries forming a single superficial temporal vein in front of the ear, just above the zygoma. This descending vein receives the middle temporal and transverse facial veins and, entering the parotid gland, unites with the maxillary vein deep to the neck of the mandible to form the retromandibular vein 颞浅静脉，又称 *venae temporales superficiales*; **testicular v., left**, a vein that drains the left pampiniform plexus and empties into the left renal vein 左睾丸静脉，又称 *vena testicularis sinistra*; **testicular v., right**, a vein that drains the right pampiniform plexus and empties into the inferior vena cava 右睾丸静脉，又称 *vena testicularis dextra*; **thalamostriate v's, inferior**, veins that pass through the anterior perforated substance and join the deep middle cerebral and anterior cerebral veins to form the basal vein 丘纹下静脉，又称 *venae thalamostriatae inferiores*; **Thalamostriate v., superior**, a vein that collects blood from the corpus striatum and thalamus and joins with the choroid vein to form the internal cerebral vein 丘纹上静脉，又称 *vena thalamostriata superior*; **Thebesian v's**, 同 smallest cardiac v's; **thoracic v's, internal**, two veins formed by junction of the accompanying veins of the internal thoracic artery of either side; each continues along the artery to open into the brachiocephalic vein 胸廓内静脉，又称 *venae thoracicae internae*; **thoracic v., lateral**, a large vein accompanying the lateral thoracic artery and draining into the axillary vein 胸外侧静脉，又称 *vena thoracica lateralis*; **thoracoacromial v.**, the vein that follows the homonymous artery and opens into the subclavian vein 胸肩峰静脉，又称 *vena thoracoacromialis*; **thoracoepigastric v's**, long longitudinal, superficial veins in the anterolateral superficial fascia of the trunk, which empty superiorly into the lateral thoracic and inferiorly into the femoral vein 胸腹壁静脉，又称 *venae thoracoepigastricae*; **thymic v's**, small branches from the thymus gland that open into the left brachiocephalic vein 胸腺静脉，又称 *venae thymicae*; **thyroid v., inferior**, either of two veins, left and right, that drain the thyroid plexus into the left and right brachiocephalic veins; occasionally they may unite into a common trunk to empty, usually, into the left brachiocephalic vein 甲状腺下静脉，又称 *vena thyroidei inferioris*; **thyroid v's, middle**, veins that drain blood from the thyroid gland into the internal jugular vein 甲状腺中静脉，又称 *venae thyroideae mediae*; **thyroid v., superior**, a vein arising from the upper part of the thyroid gland on either side, opening into the internal jugular vein, occasionally in common with the facial vein 甲状腺上静脉，又称 *vena thyroidea superior*; **tibial v's, anterior**, accompanying veins of the anterior tibial artery, which unite with the posterior tibial veins to form the popliteal vein 胫前静脉，又称 *venae tibiales anteriores*; **tibial v's, posterior**, accompanying veins of the posterior tibial artery, which unite with the anterior tibial veins to form the popliteal vein 胫后静脉，又称 *venae tibiales posteriores*; **trabecular v's**, vessels coursing in splenic trabeculae, formed by tributary pulp veins 小梁静脉; **tracheal v's**, small branches that drain blood from the trachea into the brachiocephalic vein 气管静脉，又称 *venae tracheales*; **tympanic v's**, small veins from the tympanic cavity that pass through the petrotympanic fissure, open into the plexus around the temporomandibular joint, and finally drain into the retromandibular vein 鼓室静脉，又称 *venae tympanicae*; **ulnar v's**, the accompanying veins of the ulnar artery, which unite with the radial veins at the elbow to form the brachial veins 尺静脉，又称 *venae ulnares*; **umbilical v's**, the two veins *(left umbilical v. and right umbilical v.)* that carry blood from the placenta to the sinus venosus of the heart in the early embryo; the right later degenerates, leaving the left as a single umbilical vein that carries the blood from the placenta to the ductus venosus 脐静脉; **v. of uncus**, a vein that drains the uncus into the ipsilateral inferior cerebral vein 钩回静脉，又称 *vena uncalis*; **uterine v's**, veins that drain the uterine plexus into the internal iliac veins 子宫静脉，又称 *venae uterinae*; **varicose v.**, a dilated, tortuous vein, usually in the superficial fascia of the leg; incompetency of the venous valve is associated 曲张静脉; **ventricular v., inferior**, a vein that drains the temporal lobe into the basal vein 侧脑室下静脉，又称 *vena ventricularis inferior*; **vertebral v.**, a vein that arises from the suboccipital venous plexus, passes with the vertebral artery through the foramina of the transverse processes of the upper six cervical vertebrae, and opens into the brachiocephalic vein 椎静脉，又称 *vena vertebralis*; **vertebral v., accessory**, a vein that sometimes arises from a plexus formed around the vertebral artery by the vertebral vein, descends with the vertebral vein, and emerges through the transverse foramen of the seventh cervical vertebra to empty into the brachiocephalic vein 副椎静脉，又称 *vena vertebralis accessoria*; **vertebral v., anterior**, a small vein accompanying the ascending cervical artery; it arises in a venous plexus adjacent to the more cranial cervical transverse processes, and descends to end in the vertebral vein 椎前静脉，又称 *vena vertebralis anterior*; **v's of vertebral column**, a plexiform venous network extending the entire length of the vertebral column, outside or inside the vertebral canal; the anterior and posterior external and anterior and posterior internal groups freely anastomose and end in the intervertebral veins 脊柱静脉，又称 *venae columnae vertebralis*; **vesalian v.**, Vesalian 静脉; **vesical v's**, veins passing from the vesical plexus to the internal iliac vein 膀胱静脉，又称 *venae vesicales*; **vestibular v's**, branches draining blood from the vestibule into the labyrinthine veins 前庭静脉，又称 *venae vestibulares*; **v. of vestibular aqueduct**, a small vein from the internal ear that passes through the aqueduct of the vestibule and empties into the superior petrosal sinus 前庭水管静脉，又称 *vena aqueductus vestibuli*; **vitelline v's**, veins that return the blood from the yolk sac to the primordial heart of the early embryo 卵黄静脉; **vorticose v's**, four veins that pierce the sclera and carry blood from the choroid to the superior ophthalmic vein 涡静脉，又称 *venae vorticosae*

ve·la·men (ve-la′mən) pl. *vela′mina* [L.] a membrane, meninx, or velum 膜，帆，脑（脊）膜（体被）

vel·a·men·tous (vel″ə-men′təs) membranous and pendant; like a veil 膜状的，帆状的

vel·lus (vel′əs) [L.] 1. the fine hair that succeeds the lanugo over most of the body 毫毛; 2. a structure resembling this fine hair 细毛结构

ve·lo·cim·e·try (ve″lo-sim′ə-tre) measurement of speed, such as speed of flow 速度测量法

ve·lo·pha·ryn·ge·al (ve″lo-fə-rin′je-əl) pertaining to the soft palate and pharynx 腭咽的，腭帆与咽的

ve·lum (ve′ləm) pl. *ve′la* [L.] a covering structure or veil 帆; **ve′lar** *adj.* **v. interpositum cerebri**, membranous roof of the third ventricle 第三脑室脉络组织，大脑中帆; **medullary v.**, one of the two portions (*superiormedullary v.* and *inferior medullary v.*) of the white substance that form the roof of the fourth ventricle 髓帆; **v. palatinum**, soft palate 腭帆

ve·na (ve′nə) pl. *ve′nae* [L.] 同 vein; **v. comitans**, accompanying vein: a vein that closely follows its homonymous artery 并行静脉，伴行静脉; **inferior v. cava**, the venous trunk for the lower extremities and for the pelvic and abdominal viscera; it begins at the level of the fifth lumbar vertebra by union of the common iliac veins, passes upward on the right of the aorta, and empties into the right atrium of the heart 下腔静脉; **superior v. cava**, the venous trunk draining blood from the head, neck, upper extremities, and chest; it begins by union of the two brachiocephalic veins, passes directly downward, and empties into the right atrium of the heart 上腔静脉; **venae vasorum**, small veins that return blood from the tissues making up the walls of the blood vessels themselves 脉管静脉

ve·na·ca·vo·gram (ve″nə-ka′vo-gram) a film obtained by venacavography 腔静脉照相

ve·na·ca·vog·ra·phy (ve″nə-ka-vog′rə-fe) radiography of a vena cava, usually the inferior vena cava 腔静脉造影（术）

ve·nec·ta·sia (ve″nək-ta′zhə) a varicosity of a vein 静脉扩张

ve·nec·to·my (ve-nek′tə-me) phlebectomy 静脉切除术

ve·ne·re·al (və-nēr′e-əl) due to or propagated by sexual intercourse 性病的，性交的

ve·ne·re·ol·o·gist (və-nēr″e-ol′ə-jist) a specialist in venereology 性病学家

ve·ne·re·ol·o·gy (və-nēr″e-ol′ə-je) the study and treatment of venereal diseases 性病学

vene·sec·tion (ven″ə-sek′shən) phlebotomy 静脉切开术

veni·punc·ture (ven″ĭ-punk″chər) surgical puncture of a vein 静脉穿刺

veni·su·ture (ven″ĭ-soo′chər) phleborrhaphy 静脉缝术

ven·la·fax·ine (ven″lə-fak′sēn) a serotonin-norepinephrine reuptake inhibitor; used as the hydrochloride salt as an antidepressant and antianxiety agent 5-羟色胺 - 去甲肾上腺素再摄取抑制药; 其盐酸盐作为抗抑郁药和抗焦虑药

V

ve·nog·ra·phy (ve-nog′rə-fe) phlebography 静脉造影术

ven·om (ven′əm) a poison, especially one normally secreted by a serpent, insect, or other animal 毒（物），毒液，动物毒素；**ven′omous** *adj.*

ve·no·mo·tor (ve″no-mo′tər) controlling dilation or constriction of the veins 静脉舒缩的

ve·no·oc·clu·sive (ve″no-ə-kloo′siv) characterized by obstruction of the veins 静脉闭塞的

ve·no·peri·to·ne·os·to·my (ve″no-per″ĭ-to″neos′to-me) anastomosis of the saphenous vein with the peritoneum for drainage of ascites 隐静脉腹膜造口引流术

ve·no·pres·sor (ve″no-pres′ər) 1. pertaining to venous blood pressure 静脉血压的；2. an agent that causes venous constriction 静脉收缩药

ve·nor·rha·phy (ve-nor′ə-fe) suture of a vein 静脉缝合术

ve·no·scle·ro·sis (ve″no-sklə-ro′sis) phlebosclerosis 静脉硬化

ve·nos·i·ty (ve-nos′ĭ-te) 1. the condition of being venous 静脉血性充血；2. excess of venous blood in a part 静脉血过多；3. a plentiful supply of veins 血管或静脉血供应充裕

ve·no·sta·sis (ve″no-sta′sis) venous stasis 静脉瘀滞

ve·not·o·my (ve-not′ə-me) phlebotomy 静脉切开放血术

ve·nous (ve′nəs) pertaining to the veins 静脉的

ve·no·ve·nos·to·my (ve″no-ve-nos′tə-me) phlebophlebostomy 静脉静脉吻合术

vent (vent) an opening or outlet, such as an opening that discharges pus, or the anus 孔，口（如排脓口、肛门）

ven·ter (ven′tər) pl. *ven′tres* [L.] 1. a fleshy contractile part of a muscle 肌，腹；2. abdomen 腹；3. a hollowed part or cavity 凹，窝

ven·ti·la·tion (ven″tĭ-la′shən) 1. breathing; the exchange of air between the lungs and the environment, including inhalation and exhalation 通气，换气；2. circulation, replacement, or purification of the air or other gas in a space 通风；3. the equipment with which this is done 通风设备；4. verbalization of one's problems, emotions, or feelings 公开讨论；**alveolar v.,** the amount of air that reaches the alveoli and is available for gas exchange with the blood per unit time 肺泡通气量；**high-frequency v.,** mechanical ventilation in which small tidal volumes are delivered at a high respiration rate 高频通气；**maximum voluntary v.,** maximal breathing capacity; the greatest volume of gas that can be breathed per minute by voluntary effort 最大随意通气量；**mechanical v.,** that accomplished by extrinsic means; usually either *negative pressure v.*

or *positive pressure v.* 机械通气；**minute v.,** total v.; the total volume of gas in liters exhaled from the lungs per minute 每分通气量，总通气量；**negative pressure v.,** mechanical ventilation in which negative pressure is generated on the outside of the patient's chest and transmitted to the interior to expand the lungs and allow air to flow in; used with weak or paralyzed patients 负压通气；**positive pressure v.,** mechanical ventilation in which air is delivered into the airways and lungs under positive pressure, usually via an endotracheal tube, producing positive airway pressure during inspiration 正压通气；**pulmonary v.,** a measure of the rate of ventilation, referring to the total exchange of air between the lungs and the ambient air 肺通气量；**total v.,** 同 minute v.

ven·ti·la·tor (ven′tĭ-la″tər) 1. an apparatus for qualifying the air breathed through it 通风机；2. a device for giving artificial respiration or aiding in pulmonary ventilation 呼吸机，**cuirass v.,** one applied only to the chest, either completely surrounding the trunk or only on the front of the chest and abdomen 胸甲式负压呼吸机

ven·ti·la·to·ry (ven′tĭ-lə-tor″e) pertaining to ventilation 通风的，换气的

ven·trad (ven′trad) toward a belly, venter, or ventral aspect 向腹侧，向前

ven·tral (ven′trəl) 1. pertaining to the abdomen or to any venter 腹的；2. denoting a position more toward the belly surface than some other object of reference; opposite of dorsal 腹侧的，前侧的

ven·tra·lis (vən-tra′lis) [L.] 同 ventral

ven·tri·cle (ven′trĭ-kəl) a small cavity or chamber, as in the brain or heart 室（如脑室、心室）；**ventric′ular** *adj.*；**v. of Arantius,** the rhomboid fossa, especially its lower end 菱形窝；**double-inlet v.,** a congenital anomaly in which both atrioventricular valves, or a single common atrioventricular valve, open into a single ventricle, which usually resembles the left ventricle morphologically *(double-inlet left v.)* but may resemble the right *(double-inlet right v.)* or neither or both ventricles 心室双入口；**double-outlet left v.,** a rare anomaly in which both great arteries arise from the left ventricle, often associated with a hypoplastic right ventricle, ventricular septal defect, and other cardiac malformations 左心室双出口；**double-outlet right v.,** incomplete transposition of the great ventricles in which both the aorta and the pulmonary artery arise from the right ventricle, associated with a ventricular septal defect 右心室双出口；**fifth v.,** the median cleft between the two laminae of the septum pellucidum 第五脑室；**fourth v.,** a median cavity in the hindbrain, containing cerebrospinal fluid 第 四 脑 室; **laryngeal v.,** the space between the true and false vocal cords 喉室; **lateral v.,** the cavity in each cerebral hemisphere, derived from the cavity of the embryonic neural tube and containing cerebrospinal fluid 侧脑室; **left v. of heart,** the lower chamber of the left side of the heart, which pumps oxygenated blood out through the aorta into the systemic arteries 左心室; **Morgagni v.,** 同 laryngeal v.; **pineal v.,** an extension of the third ventricle into the stalk of the pineal body 松果体室; **right v. of heart,** the lower chamber of the right side of the heart, which pumps venous blood through the pulmonary trunk and arteries to the capillaries of the lungs 右心室; **third v.,** a narrow cleft in the diencephalon, below the corpus callosum and between the two thalami 第三脑室; **Verga v.,** an occasional space between the corpus callosum and fornix Verga 室, 穹窿与胼胝体间的裂隙

ven·tric·u·li·tis (ven-trik″u-li′tis) inflammation of a ventricle, especially a cerebral ventricle 室炎，尤指脑室炎

ven·tric·u·lo·atri·al (ven-trik″u-lo-a′tre- əl) connecting a cerebral ventricle with a cardiac atrium, as a shunt in the treatment of hydrocephalus 房室的

ven·tric·u·lo·atri·os·to·my (ven-trik″u-loa″tre-os′tə-me) ventriculoatrial shunt 脑室心房造口（引流）术

ven·tric·u·lo·en·ceph·a·li·tis (ven-trik″u-loen-sef″ə-li′tis) ventriculitis accompanied by encephalitis 脑室脑炎

ven·tric·u·log·ra·phy (ven-trik″u-log′rə-fe) 1. radiography of the cerebral ventricles after introduction of air or other contrast medium 脑室造影术; 2. radiography of a ventricle of the heart after injection of a contrast medium 心室造影术; **first-pass v.,** 首通心室造影术，参见 *angiocardiography* 下词条 **gated blood pool v.,** equilibrium radionuclide angiocardiography 门控血池心室造影术; **radio-nuclide v.,** 放射性核素心室造影术，参见 *angiocardiography* 下词条

ven·tric·u·lom·e·try (ven-trik″u-lom′ə-tre) measurement of intracranial pressure 脑室压测量法

ven·tric·u·lo·peri·to·ne·al (ven-trik″u-lo-per″ĭ- to-ne′əl) connecting a cerebral ventricle with the peritoneum, as a shunt in the treatment of hydrocephalus 脑室腹膜分流术

ven·tric·u·lo·punc·ture (ven-trik′u-lo-pungk″-chər) ventricular puncture 脑室穿刺术

ven·tric·u·los·co·py (ven-trik″u-los′kə-pe) endoscopic or cystoscopic examination of cerebral ventricles 脑室镜检查

ven·tric·u·los·to·my (ven-trik″u-los′tə-me) surgical creation of a free communication or shunt between the third ventricle and the interpeduncular cistern for relief of hydrocephalus 脑室造口（引流）术

ven·tric·u·lo·sub·arach·noid (ven-trik″ulo-sub″ə-rak′noid) pertaining to the cerebral ventricles and subarachnoid space 脑室与蛛网膜下腔的

ven·tric·u·lot·o·my (ven-trik″u-lot′ə-me) incision of a ventricle of the brain or heart 脑室切开术; 心室切开术

ven·tric·u·lus (ven-trik′u-ləs) pl. *ventri′culi* [L.] 1. 同 ventricle; 2. stomach 胃

ven·tri·duct (ven′trĭ-dukt) to bring or carry ventrad 引向腹侧

ven·tro·fix·a·tion (ven″tro-fik-sa′shən) fixation of a viscus, e.g., the uterus, to the abdominal wall 子宫悬吊术

ven·tro·hys·tero·pexy (ven″tro-his′tər-opek″se) ventrofixation 腹壁子宫固定术

ven·tro·lat·er·al (ven″tro-lat′ər-əl) both ventral and lateral 腹外侧的

ven·tro·me·di·an (ven″tro-me′de-ən) both ventral and median 腹侧正中的

ven·tro·pos·te·ri·or (ven″tro-pos-tēr′e-ər) both ventral and posterior (caudal) 腹侧后部的

ven·trose (ven′trōs) having a bellylike expansion 腹状膨凸的

ven·tro·sus·pen·sion (ven″tro-səs-pen′shən) ventrofixation 子宫悬吊术

ven·u·la (ven′u-lə) pl. *ve′nulae* [L.] 同 venule

ven·ule (ven′ūl) any of the small vessels that collect blood from the capillary plexuses and join to form veins 微 静 脉; **ven′ular** *adj.*; **postcapillary v.,** venous capillary 毛细血管后微静脉; **stellate v's of kidney,** 肾星状小静脉，参见 *vein* 下词条; **straight v's of kidney,** venules that drain the papillary part of the kidney and empty into the arcuate veins 肾直小静脉

ven·u·li·tis (ven″u-li′tis) inflammation of the venules 小静脉炎

ve·rap·a·mil (və-rap′ə-mil) a calcium channel blocker that dilates coronary arteries and decreases myocardial oxygen demand, used as the hydrochloride salt in the treatment of angina pectoris and of hypertension and the treatment and prophylaxis of supraventricular tachyarrhythmias 维拉帕米，一种钙通道阻滞药，扩张冠脉并减少心肌的耗氧量，其盐酸盐用于治疗和预防心绞痛、高血压病、室上性快速性心律失常

ver·big·er·a·tion (vər-bij″ər-a′shən) stereotyped and meaningless repetition of words and phrases 重复言语

verge (vurj) a circumference or ring 环, 圆周; **anal v.,** the opening of the anus on the surface of the

V

body 痔环

ver·gence (vur′jəns) 1. the amount of convergence or divergence of a bundle of light rays entering or leaving a lens or mirror, expressed as the reciprocal of the distance from the lens or mirror to the focus of the rays 聚散度，一束光线的会聚或发散量进入或离开镜头或镜子，表示作为镜头距离的倒数或镜像到光线的焦点。2. a disjunctive reciprocal rotation of both eyes so that the axes of fixation are not parallel; the kind of vergence is indicated by a prefix, e.g., convergence, divergence 眼转向，双眼的分离相互旋转使得固定轴不平行；聚散的类型由前缀表示。

ver·mi·cide (vur′mĭ-sīd) anthelmintic (2) 杀蠕虫药

ver·mic·u·lar (vər-mik′u-lər) wormlike in shape or appearance 蠕虫样的

ver·mic·u·la·tion (vər-mik″u-la′shən) 1. wormlike movement 蠕动；2. peristalsis 肠蠕动

ver·mic·u·lous (vər-mik′u-ləs) 1. 同 vermicular；2. verminous 患蠕虫病的

ver·mi·form (vur′mĭ-form) 同 vermicular

ver·mi·fuge (vur′mĭ-fūj) anthelmintic (2) 驱蠕虫药，**vermifu′gal** adj.

ver·mil·ion·ec·to·my (vər-mil″yon-ek′to-me) excision of the vermilion border of the lip 唇红缘切除术

ver·min (vur′min) 1. any small animal, insect, or worm that is a nuisance to humans; sometimes limited to parasitic animals 任何对人类有害的小动物、昆虫或蠕虫；或仅指寄生生物；2. nuisance animals or ectoparasites collectively 虫，体外寄生虫；**ver′minous** adj.

ver·mis (vur′mis) [L.] a wormlike structure, particularly the vermis cerebelli 蚓部；cerebellar v., v. cerebel′li, the median part of the cerebellum, between the two lateral hemispheres 小脑蚓部

ver·nal (vur′nəl) pertaining to or occurring in the spring 春天的，春天发生的

ver·nix (vur′niks) [L.] varnish 清漆，护漆；v. caseo′sa, an unctuous substance composed of sebum and desquamated epithelial cells, which covers the skin of the fetus 胎脂，由皮脂和脱落的上皮细胞组成的油性物质

ver·ru·ca (və-roo′kə) pl. verru′cae [L.] wart 疣；**ver′rucose, verru′cous** adj; v. pla′na, flat wart 扁平疣；v. vulga′ris, common wart 寻常疣

ver·ru·ci·form (və-roo′sĭ-form) wartlike 疣状的

ver·ru·cous (və-roo′kəs) rough; warty 有疣的，疣的

ver·ru·ga (və-roo′gə) [Sp.] wart 疣，猴；v. peru·a′na, the second or chronic stage of bartonellosis 秘鲁疣

ver·si·co·lor (vur″si-kul′ər) variegated; having a variety of colors, or changing in color 杂色的，多色的，花斑的

ver·sion (vur′zhən) 1. the act or process of turning or changing direction 转动，行为或方向改变的过程；2. the situation of an organ or part in relation to an established normal position（器官）转位；3. in gynecology, misalignment or tilting of the uterus 子宫倾侧；4. in obstetrics, the manual turning of the fetus（胎位）倒转术，转胎位术；5. in ophthalmology, rotation of the eyes in the same direction（双眼）共轭旋转；**bimanual v.**, version by combined external and internal manipulation 内外倒转术；**bipolar v.**, turning effected by acting upon both poles of the fetus, either by external or combined version 两极倒转术；**cephalic v.**, turning of the fetus so that the head presents 胎头倒转术；**combined v.**, 同 bimanual v.；**external v.**, turning effected by outside manipulation 外倒转术；**internal v.**, turning effected by the hand or fingers inserted through the dilated cervix 内倒转术；**pelvic v.**, version by manipulation of the breech 臀部倒转术；**podalic v.**, conversion of a more unfavorable presentation into a footling presentation 胎足倒转术；**spontaneous v.**, one that occurs without aid from any extraneous force 自动倒转

ver·te·bra (vur′tə-brə) pl. ver′tebrae [L.] any of the 33 bones of the vertebral (spinal) column, comprising 7 cervical, 12 thoracic, 5 lumbar, 5 sacral, and 4 coccygeal vertebrae. 椎骨，见 1；**ver′tebral** adj.；**basilar v.**, the lowest lumbar vertebra 末腰椎，基椎；**cervical vertebrae (C1 to C7)**, the seven vertebrae closest to the skull, constituting the skeleton of the neck 颈椎；**coccygeal vertebrae**, the lowest segments of the vertebral column, comprising three to five rudimentary vertebrae that form the coccyx 尾椎；**dorsal vertebrae**, thoracic vertebrae 胸椎；**false vertebrae**, those vertebrae which normally fuse with adjoining segments; the sacral and coccygeal vertebrae 假椎；**lumbar vertebrae (L1 to L5)**, the five segments of the vertebral column between the twelfth thoracic vertebra and the sacrum 腰椎；**odontoid v.**, the second cervical vertebra (axis) 枢椎，第二颈椎；**v. pla′na**, a condition of spondylitis in which the body of the vertebra is reduced to a sclerotic disk 扁平椎，椎体扁平症；**sacral vertebrae(S1 to S5)**, the segments (usually five) below the lumbar vertebrae, which are normally fused, forming the sacrum 骶椎；**sternal v.**, sternebra 胸骨节，胸杠；**thoracic vertebrae (T1 to T12)**, the 12 segments of the vertebral column between the cervical and the lumbar vertebrae, giving attachment to the ribs and forming part of the mastoid wall of the thorax 胸椎；**true vertebrae**, those segments of the vertebral column that normally remain unfused throughout life: the cervical, thoracic, and lumbar vertebrae 真椎

Ver·te·bra·ta (vur″tə-bra′tə) a subphylum of the Chordata, comprising all animals having a vertebral column, including mammals, birds, reptiles, amphibians, and fishes 脊椎动物亚门

ver·te·brate (vur′tə-brāt) 1. having a vertebral column 有脊椎的；2. any member of the subphylum Vertebrata 脊椎动物

ver·te·brec·to·my (vur″tə-brek′tə-me) excision of a vertebra 椎骨切除术

ver·te·bro·bas·i·lar (vur″tə-bro-bas′ĭ-lər) pertaining to or affecting the vertebral and basilar arteries 脊椎基底动脉的

ver·te·bro·chon·dral (vur″tə-bro-kon′drəl) pertaining to a vertebra and a costal cartilage 椎骨肋软骨的

ver·te·bro·cos·tal (vur″tə-bro-kos′təl) pertaining to a vertebra and a rib 椎肋的

ver·te·bro·gen·ic (vur″tə-bro-jen′ik) arising in a vertebra or in the vertebral column 脊椎所致的

ver·te·bro·ster·nal (vur″tə-bro-stur′nəl) pertaining to a vertebra and the sternum 椎骨胸骨的

ver·te·por·fin (vur″tə-por′fin) a photosensitizing agent that accumulates preferentially in blood vessels formed by neovascularization, including those in the choroid; used, together with appropriate laser irradiation of the lesion, in the treatment of neovascularization due to age-related macular degeneration, to presumed ocular histoplasmosis, or to pathologic myopia 一种优先聚集在新生血管中的光敏剂，药物配合使用，并用适当的激光照射病灶，治疗与年龄相关的黄斑变性，假定的眼组织胞浆菌病，或病理性的近视中新生血管形成

ver·tex (vur′teks) pl. *ver′tices* [L.] the summit or top, especially the top of the head 顶，头顶

ver·ti·cal (vur′tĭ-kəl) 1. perpendicular to the plane of the horizon 垂直的；2. relating to the vertex 顶的；3. relating to or occupying different levels in a hierarchy, as the spread from one generation to another in vertical transmission 垂直传输的

ver·ti·ca·lis (vur″tĭ-ka′lis) [L.] 同 vertical (1)

ver·tic·il·late (vər-tis′ĭ-lāt) arranged in whorls 轮生的，环生的

ver·ti·go (vur′tĭ-go) [L.] a sensation of rotation or movement of one's self (*subjective v.*) or of one's surroundings (*objective v.*) in any plane; sometimes used erroneously to mean any form of dizziness 眩晕；**vertig′inous** *adj.*；**alternobaric v.**, a transient, true, whirling vertigo sometimes affecting those subjected to large, rapid variations in barometric pressure 变压性眩晕；**benign paroxysmal**

postural v., recurrent brief periods of vertigo and nystagmus occurring when the head is placed in certain positions, due to otolithiasis that causes exaggerated movement of the endolymph 良性阵发性体位性眩晕；**cerebral v.**, a type resulting from a brain lesion 大脑性眩晕；**cervical v.**, vertigo after injury to the neck such as whiplash 颈椎性眩晕；**disabling positional v.**, constant positional vertigo or dysequilibrium and nausea with the head in the upright position, without hearing disturbance or loss of vestibular function 体位性失能眩晕；**labyrinthine v.**, Meniere disease 迷路性眩晕；**objective v.**, 物体旋转性眩晕，参见 *vertigo*；**ocular v.**, a form due to eye disease 眼病性眩晕；**organic v.**, cerebral v. 器质性眩晕；**positional v., postural v.**, that associated with a specific position of the head in space or with changes in position of the head in space 体位性眩晕；**subjective v.**, 主观眩晕，自体性眩晕，参见 *vertigo*；**vestibular v.**, vertigo due to disturbances of the vestibular system 前庭性眩晕

ve·ru·mon·ta·num (ver″u-mon-ta′nəm) seminal colliculus 精阜

ve·sa·li·a·num (və-sa″le-a′nəm) a sesamoid bone in the tendon of origin of the gastrocnemius muscle, or in the angle between the cuboid and fifth metatarsal 韦萨留斯骨，几种籽骨的名称，一块在骰骨与第五跖骨之间的足外缘，一块在腓肠肌的腱起处

ve·si·ca (və-si′kə) pl. *vesi′cae* [L.] bladder 囊，泡；膀胱；**v. bilia′ris, v. fel′lea**, gallbladder 胆囊；**v. urina′ria**, urinary bladder 膀胱

ves·i·cal (ves′ĭ-kəl) pertaining to the urinary bladder 膀胱的。Cf. *cystic*

ves·i·cant (ves′ĭ-kənt) 1. producing blisters 起疱的，发疱的；2. an agent that so acts 起疱剂

ves·i·ca·tion (ves″ĭ-ka′shən) vesiculation 起疱，发疱；疱

ves·i·cle (ves′ĭ-kəl) 1. a small bladder or sac containing liquid 囊，泡；2. a small circumscribed elevation of the epidermis containing a serous fluid; a small blister 小 疱；3. a small membrane-bound sac, derived mainly from the plasma membrane, Golgi complex, or endoplasmic reticulum, occurring in eukaryotic cells 囊泡，小泡；**acrosomal v.**, a membrane-bounded vacuolelike structure that spreads over the upper two-thirds of the head of a spermatozoon to form the head cap 顶体泡；**auditory v.**, 同 otic v.；**brain v's, cephalic v's, cerebral v's**, the five divisions of the closed neural tube in the head of the developing embryo, including the cerebrum, diencephalon, midbrain, pons and cerebellum, and medulla oblongata 脑 泡；**chorionic v.**, 绒毛膜，参见 *sac* 下词条；**encephalic v's**, 同 brain v's；**germinal v.**, the fluid-filled nucleus of an oocyte toward the end of prophase of its first meiotic division 发生泡; **lens v.**, a vesicle formed from the lens pit of the embryo, developing into the crystalline lens 晶状体泡; **matrix v's**, small membranelimited structures at sites of calcification of the cartilage matrix 基质小泡; **olfactory v.**, 1. the vesicle in the embryo that later develops into the olfactory bulb and tract 嗅泡, 胚胎中发育成嗅球、嗅束的囊泡; 2. a bulbous expansion at the distal end of an olfactory cell, from which the olfactory hairs project 嗅细胞小泡, 嗅细胞远端扩大成小球, 由此伸出嗅毛; **optic v.**, an evagination on either side of the forebrain of the early embryo, from which the percipient parts of the eye develop 视泡; **otic v.**, a detached ovoid sac formed by closure of the otic pit in embryonic development of the external ear 听泡; **primary brain v's**, the three earliest subdivisions of the embryonic neural tube, including the forebrain, midbrain, and hindbrain 初级脑泡; **secondary brain v's**, the five brain vesicles formed by specialization of the forebrain (cerebrum and diencephalon), midbrain, and hindbrain (pons, cerebellum, and medulla oblongata) in later embryonic development 次级脑泡; **seminal v.**, either of the paired sacculated pouches attached to the posterior urinary bladder; the duct of each joins the ipsilateral ductus deferens to form the ejaculatory duct 精囊; **synaptic v's**, small membrane-bound structures behind a presynaptic membrane, containing neurotransmitters; when depolarization occurs they fuse with the presynaptic membrane and release the neurotransmitter into the synaptic cleft. transport v., a vesicle that carries substances between intracellular compartments 突触囊泡, 突触小泡; **umbilical v.**, yolk sac 脐囊, 胚胎发育至第四周末, 卵黄囊梨形膨大进入绒膜腔, 以卵黄蒂与胚胎中肠连接

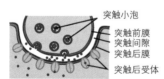

突触小泡
突触前膜
突触间隙
突触后膜
突触后受体

▲ **突触内的突触小泡**

ves·i·co·cer·vi·cal (ves″ĭ-ko-sur′vĭ-kəl) pertaining to the bladder and cervix uteri, or communicating with the bladder and cervical canal 膀胱宫颈的

ves·i·co·en·ter·ic (ves″ĭ-ko-en-ter′ik) enterovesical 膀胱肠的

ves·i·co·in·tes·ti·nal (ves″ĭ-ko-in-tes′tĭ-nəl) enterovesical 膀胱肠的

ves·i·co·pros·tat·ic (ves″ĭ-ko-pros-tat′ik) pertaining to the urinary bladder and the prostate 膀胱前列腺的

ves·i·co·pu·bic (ves″ĭ-ko-pu′bik) pubovesical; pertaining to the urinary bladder and the hypogastric region 膀胱耻骨的

ves·i·co·sig·moid·os·to·my (ves″ĭ-ko-sig″-moi-dos′tə-me) surgical creation of an opening between the urinary bladder and the sigmoid colon 膀胱乙状结肠吻合术

ves·i·co·spi·nal (ves″ĭ-ko-spi′nəl) pertaining to the urinary bladder and the spinal cord 膀胱脊椎的

ves·i·cos·to·my (ves″ĭ-kos′tə-me) cystostomy 膀胱造口术; **cutaneous v.**, surgical anastomosis of the bladder mucosa to an opening in the skin below the umbilicus, creating a stoma for bladder drainage 膀胱皮肤造口术

ves·i·cot·o·my (ves″ĭ-kot′ə-me) cystotomy 膀胱切开术

ves·i·co·um·bil·i·cal (ves″ĭ-ko-əm-bil′ĭ-kəl) pertaining to the urinary bladder and the umbilicus 膀胱脐的

ves·i·co·ure·ter·al (ves″ĭ-ko-u-re′tər-əl) ureterovesical 膀胱输尿管的

ves·i·co·ure·ter·ic (ves″ĭ-ko-u″rə-ter′ik) ureterovesical 膀胱输尿管的

ves·i·co·ure·thral (ves″ĭ-ko-u-re′thrəl) pertaining to the urinary bladder and urethra 膀胱尿道的

ves·i·co·uter·ine (ves″ĭ-ko-u′tər-in) pertaining to or connecting the bladder and uterus 膀胱子宫的

ves·i·co·vag·i·nal (ves″ĭ-ko-vaj′ĭ-nəl) pertaining to or connecting the bladder and vagina 膀胱阴道的

ve·sic·u·la (və-sik′u-lə) pl. *vesi′culae* [L.] 同 vesicle

ve·sic·u·lar (və-sik′u-lər) 1. pertaining to or made up of vesicles on the skin 囊状的, 泡状的; 2. having a low pitch, such as the normal breath sound over the lung during ventilation 水疱的

ve·sic·u·la·tion (və-sik″u-la′shən) 1. the process of blistering 水疱形成; 2. a blistered spot or surface 起疱

ve·sic·u·lec·to·my (və-sik″u-lek′tə-me) excision of a vesicle, especially the seminal vesicles 囊切除术, 尤指精囊切除术

ve·sic·u·li·tis (və-sik″u-li′tis) inflammation of a vesicle, especially a seminal vesicle *(seminal v.)* 囊炎, 尤指精囊炎

ve·sic·u·lo·cav·er·nous (və-sik″u-lo-kav′ərnəs) both vesicular and cavernous 肺泡空洞性的

ve·sic·u·log·ra·phy (və-sik″u-log′rə-fe) radiography of the seminal vesicles 精囊造影术

ve·sic·u·lo·pus·tu·lar (və-sik″u-lo-pus′tu-lər) both vesicular and pustular 水疱脓疱的

ve·sic·u·lot·o·my (və-sik″u-lot′ə-me) incision into a

vesicle, especially the seminal vesicles 囊切开术，尤指精囊切开术

Ves·ic·u·lo·vi·rus (və-sik′u-lo-vi″rəs) vesicular stomatitis-like viruses; a genus of viruses of the family Rhabdoviridae that includes viruses that cause vesicular stomatitis in swine, cattle, and horses and related viruses that infect humans and other animals 水疱性病毒属

ves·sel (ves′əl) any channel for carrying a fluid, such as blood or lymph 管，脉管；**blood v.**, one of the vessels conveying the blood, comprising arteries, capillaries, and veins 血 管；**chyliferous v.** lacteal (2) 乳糜管；**collateral v,** 1. a vessel that parallels another vessel, nerve, or other structure 并行管，与其他血管，神经或其他结构平行的管道；2. a vessel important in establishing and maintaining a collateral circulation 侧副管，建立和维持侧支循环的重要血管；**great v's,** the large vessels entering the heart, including the aorta, the pulmonary arteries and veins, and the venae cavae 大血管；**lacteal v.,** lacteal (2) 乳糜管；**lymphatic v.,** one of the vessels that collect lymph from the tissues and carry it to the bloodstream 淋巴管；**nutrient v's,** vessels supplying nutritive elements to special tissues, such as arteries entering the substance of bone or the walls of large blood vessels 营养血管，血管滋养管

ves·ti·bule (ves′tĭ-būl) a space or cavity at the entrance to a canal 前庭；**vestib′ular adj.; v. of aorta,** a small space at the root of the aorta 主动脉前庭；**v. of ear,** an oval cavity in the middle of the bony labyrinth 耳前庭；**v. of mouth,** the portion of the oral cavity bounded on the one side by teeth and gingivae, or residual alveolar ridges, and on the other by the lips *(labial v.)* and cheeks *(buccal v.)* 口腔前庭；**nasal v., v. of nose,** the anterior part of the nasal cavity 鼻前庭；**v. of vagina, v. of vulva,** the space between the labia minora into which the urethra and vagina open 阴道前庭

ves·tib·u·li·tis (ves-tib″u-li′tis) inflammation of the vulvar vestibule and the periglandular and subepithelial stroma, resulting in a burning sensation and dyspareunia 前庭炎

ves·tib·u·lo·gen·ic (vəs-tib″u-lo-jen′ik) arising in a vestibule, as that of the ear 前庭形成的，源于前庭的

ves·tib·u·lo·oc·u·lar (vəs-tib″u-lo-ok′u-lər) 1. pertaining to the vestibular and oculomotor nerves 前庭眼的，前庭与动眼神经的；2. pertaining to the maintenance of visual stability during head movements 头部运动时维持视力稳定性的

ves·tib·u·lo·plas·ty (vəs-tib″u-lo-plas″te) surgical modification of gingival–mucous membrane relationships in the vestibule of the mouth 口腔前庭成形术

ves·tib·u·lot·o·my (vəs-tib″u-lot′ə-me) surgical opening of the vestibule of the ear（耳）前庭切开术

ves·tib·u·lo·ure·thral (vəs-tib″u-lo-u-re′thrəl) pertaining to the vestibule of the vagina and the urethra（阴道）前庭（与）尿道的

ves·tib·u·lo·vag·i·nal (vəs-tib″u-lo-vaj′ĭ-nəl) pertaining to the vestibule of the vagina 前庭阴道的

ves·ti·bu·lum (vəs-tib′u-ləm) pl. *vesti′bula* [L.] 同 vestibule

ves·tige (ves′tij) the remnant of a structure that functioned in a previous stage of species or individual development 遗迹，剩件，剩余，物种进化前期和个体发育期曾起功能作用的结构残迹；**vestig′ial adj.**

ves·ti·gi·um (vəs-tĭ′je-əm) pl. *vesti′gia* [L.] 同 vestige

vet·er·i·nar·i·an (vet″ər-ĭ-nar′e-ən) a person trained and authorized to practice veterinary medicine and surgery; a doctor of veterinary medicine 兽医

vet·er·i·nary (vet′ər-ĭ-nar″e) 1. pertaining to domestic animals and their diseases 兽医的；2. 同 veterinarian

VF vocal fremitus 语音震颤

vf visual field 视野

VFib (ve′fib) ventricular fibrillation 心室纤颤，心室颤动

VFl ventricular flutter 心室扑动

VHDL very-high-density lipoprotein 极高密度脂蛋白

vi·a·ble (vi′ə-bəl) able to maintain an independent existence; able to live after birth 能生存的，能活的（指胎儿已发育到在子宫外能活的阶段）

Vi·ba·tiv (vy′buh-tiv) trademark for a preparation of telavancin telavancin 制剂的商标

Vi·ber·zi (vī′bur-zee) trademark for a preparation of eluxadoline eluxadoline 制剂的商标

vi·bra·tion (vi-bra′shən) 1. a rapid movement to and fro 震动，振动；2. massage with a light, rhythmic, quivering motion; often performed with a mechanical device (electrovibratory massage) 振动按摩法

vi·bra·tor (vi′bra-tər) an instrument for producing vibrations 振动器

vi·bra·to·ry (vi′brə-tor″e) vibrating or causing vibration 振动的，震动的

Vib·rio (vib′re-o) a genus of gram-negative, facultatively anaerobic, motile, rod-shaped bacteria of the family Vibrionaceae. *V. cho′lerae,* the cholera vibrio, is divided into several serogroups and is the cause of cholera; *V. metschniko'vii* causes gastroenteritis; *V. parahaemoly'ticus* causes gastroenteritis after consumption of undercooked seafood; and *V. vulni'ficus* causes septicemia and cellulitis in persons who have eaten raw seafood 弧菌属

vib·ri·o (vib're-o) pl. *vibrio'nes, vibrios.* An organism of the genus *Vibrio* or other spiral motile organism 弧菌； **cholera v.,** *Vibrio cholerae* 霍乱弧菌，参见 *Vibrio*； **El Tor v.,** a biovar of *Vibrio cholerae* 埃尔托弧菌，参见 *Vibrio*

vib·rio·ci·dal (vib″re-o-si'dəl) destructive to organisms of the genus *Vibrio*, especially *V. cholerae* 杀弧菌的（尤杀霍乱弧菌）

Vib·rio·na·ceae (vib″re-o-na'se-e) a family of primarily aquatic, gram-negative, facultatively anaerobic, motile, rod-shaped bacteria of the order Vibrionales 弧菌科

Vib·ri·o·na·les (vib″re-o-na'lēz) an order of gram-negative, rod-shaped bacteria of the class Gammaproteobacteria 弧菌目

vi·bris·sa (vi-bris'ə) [L.] a long coarse hair, such as those growing in the vestibule of the nose 鼻毛

vi·car·i·ous (vi-kar'e-əs) 1. acting in the place of another or of something else 替代的；2. occurring at an abnormal site 错位的

Vic·ia (vish'e-ə) a genus of herbs, including *V. fa'ba* (*V. fa'va*), the fava or broad bean, whose beans or pollen contain a component capable of causing favism in susceptible persons 蚕豆属

vi·cine (vi'sin) a pyrimidine-based glycoside occurring in species of *Vicia*; in fava beans it is cleaved to form the toxic compound divicine 蚕豆嘧啶葡萄糖苷

vi·dar·a·bine (vi-dar'ə-bēn) adenine arabinoside (ara-A); a purine analogue that preferentially inhibits viral DNA synthesis; used as an antiviral agent to treat herpes simplex keratitis, keratoconjunctivitis, or encephalitis 阿糖腺苷，用作抗病毒药物治疗单纯疱疹性角膜炎、角膜结膜炎或脑炎

vid·eo·den·si·tom·e·try (vi″de-o-den″sĭ-tom'ə-tre) densitometry using a video camera to record the images to be analyzed 电视密度计，使用摄像机记录要分析的图像的密度测定计

vid·eo·en·dos·co·py (vid″e-o-en-dos'kə-pe) endoscopy aided by a video camera in the tip of the endoscope 电视内镜检查（术）

vid·eo·flu·o·ros·co·py (vid″e-o-floo-ros'kə- pe) the recording on videotape of the images appearing on a fluoroscopic screen 电视荧光屏检查

vid·eo·lap·a·ros·co·py (vid″e-o-lap″ə-ros'kə- pe) laparoscopic surgery aided by a video camera in the tip of the laparoscope 电视腹腔镜检查

vid·eo·la·ser·os·co·py (vid″e-o-la-zər-os'kə- pe) a modification of laser laparoscopy in which the inside of the cavity is visualized through a video camera that projects an enlarged image onto a video monitor 电视激光检查

vig·or (vig'ər) a combination of attributes of living organisms that expresses itself in rapid growth, high fertility and fecundity, and long life 精力，活力；**hybrid v.,** heterosis 杂种优势

Vii·bryd (vi'brid) trademark for a preparation of vilazodone hydrochloride 盐酸维拉唑酮的商品名

vi·kri·ti (vik'rī-te) in ayurveda, a disordered physical constitution, resulting from an imbalance of the doshas 在阿育吠陀中，由于 doshas 的不平衡导致的体格紊乱

vil·az·o·done (vĭ-laz'ə-dōn″) a selective serotonin reuptake inhibitor and partial agonist of serotonergic receptors, used as the hydrochloride salt in the treatment of major depressive disorder 维拉唑酮，择性 5- 羟色胺再摄取抑制药和 5- 羟色胺能受体的部分激动剂，其盐酸盐用于治疗重度抑郁症

vil·li (vil'i) *villus* 的复数

vil·lo·nod·u·lar (vil″o-nod'u-lər) characterized by villous and nodular thickening 绒毛（与）结节性的，以绒毛和结节状增厚为特征

vil·lose (vil'ōs) shaggy with soft hairs; covered with villi 绒毛的，有绒毛的，绒毛状的

vil·lo·si·tis (vil″o-si'tis) a bacterial disease with alterations in the villi of the placenta 胎盘绒毛炎，一种细菌性疾病，以胎盘绒毛改变为特征

vil·los·i·ty (vĭ-los'ĭ-te) 1. condition of being covered with villi 绒毛状态；2. a villus 绒毛

vil·lous (vil'əs) 同 villose

vil·lus (vil'əs) pl. *vil'li* [L.] a small vascular process or protrusion, especially from the free surface of a membrane 绒 毛；**arachnoid villi,** 1. microscopic projections of the arachnoid into some of the venous sinuses 蛛网膜绒毛；2. arachnoidal granulations 蛛网膜粒；**chorionic v.,** one of the threadlike projections growing in tufts on the external surface of the chorion 绒膜绒毛，绒毛膜外表面上以簇状物生长的绒状突起；**intestinal villi,** multitudinous threadlike projections covering the surface of the mucous membrane lining the small intestine, serving as the sites of absorption of fluids and nutrients 肠绒毛，覆盖在小肠内壁的黏膜表面大量丝状突起，作为吸收液体和营养物质的场所；**synovial villi,** slender projections of the synovial membrane from its free inner surface into the joint cavity 滑膜绒毛，自滑膜游离内表面突入关节腔的细长突出物

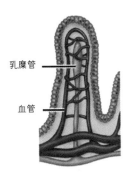

乳糜管

血管

▲ 肠绒毛

vi·men·tin (vī-men′tēn) a protein forming the vimentin filaments, a common type of intermediate filament; used as a marker for cells derived from embryonic mesenchyme 波形蛋白，维蒙亭，形成波形蛋白丝的蛋白质，一种常见类型的中间丝，用作胚胎间充质细胞的标志物

vin·blas·tine (vin-blas′tēn) an antineoplastic vinca alkaloid used as the sulfate salt in the palliative treatment of a variety of malignancies 长春（花）碱，抗肿瘤药，其硫酸盐用于多种恶性肿瘤的姑息治疗

vin·cris·tine (vin-kris′tēn) an antineoplastic vinca alkaloid; used as the sulfate salt in treatment of neoplasms, including Hodgkin disease, acute lymphoblastic leukemia, non-Hodgkin lymphoma, Kaposi sarcoma associated with AIDS, and neuroblastoma 长春新碱，抗肿瘤药，其硫酸盐用于治疗霍奇金病、急性淋巴细胞白血病、非霍奇金淋巴瘤、卡波西肉瘤、艾滋病和神经母细胞瘤

vin·cu·lum (ving′ku-ləm) pl. *vin′cula* [L.] a band or bandlike structure 纽，系带；**vin′cula ten′dinum,** filaments that connect the phalanges and interphalangeal articulations with the flexor tendons 腱纽

vi·nor·el·bine (vī-nor′el-bēn″) an antineoplastic vinca alkaloid used as the tartrate salt in the treatment of advanced non–small cell lung carcinoma 去甲长春花碱，一种抗肿瘤药长春花生物碱，其酒石酸盐用于治疗晚期非小细胞肺癌

vi·nyl (vi′nəl) the univalent group CH2=CH—乙烯基；**v. chloride,** a vinyl group to which an atom of chlorine is attached; the monomer that polymerizes to polyvinyl chloride; it is toxic and carcinogenic 氯乙烯

vi·o·la·ceous (vi″o-la′shəs) having a violet color, usually describing a discoloration of the skin 紫色的，通常指皮肤变色

vi·o·let (vi′o-lət) 1. the color produced by the shortest waves of the visible spectrum, beyond indigo, approximately 380 to 420 nm 紫色；2. a dye or stain with this color 紫色染料；**crystal v., gentian v., methyl v.,** gentian violet 结晶紫，龙胆紫，甲基紫，参见 gentian 下词条

vi·per (vi′pər) any venomous snake, especially any member of the families Viperidae (truevipers) and Crotalidae (pit vipers) 蝰蛇；**European v.,** *Vipera berus,* a venomous snake native to Europe, North Africa, and the Middle East 欧洲蝰；**Gaboon v.,** *Bitis gabonica,* a deadly, brightly marked, viperine snake found in tropical West Africa 加蓬蝰；**pit v.,** crotalid (1) 颊窝毒蛇，参见 crotalid 第 1 条释义 **rhinoceros v.,** *Bitis nasicornis,* a venomous, brightly colored, viperine snake found in tropical Africa, having a pair of hornlike growths on its snout 犀角蝰；**Russell's v.,** *Vipera russelli,* an extremely venomous, brightly colored, viperine snake of southeastern Asia and Indonesia 鲁塞尔蝰蛇；**sand v.,** *Vipera ammodytes,* a venomous snake found in southern Europe and Turkey that has a hornlike protuberance on its snout for burrowing 沙蝰；**true v.,** any of the snakes of the family Viperidae 真蝰蛇

Vi·pera (vi′pər-ə) a genus of venomous snakes of the family Viperidae. *V. ammody'tes* is the sand viper; *V. be'rus* is the adder or European viper; and *V. rus'selli* is Russell's viper 蝰蛇属

VIP·oma (vī-po′mə) an endocrine tumor, usually an islet cell tumor, that produces vasoactive intestinal polypeptide, causing a syndrome of watery diarrhea, hypokalemia, and hypochlorhydria, leading to potentially fatal renal failure. Spelled also vipoma 舒血管肠肽瘤，一种内分泌肿瘤，通常是胰岛细胞瘤，产生血管活性肠多肽，引起水样腹泻、低钾血症和胃酸过多综合征，导致潜在致命的肾功能衰竭

vi·ral (vi′rəl) pertaining to or caused by a virus 病毒的，病毒所致的

vi·re·mia (vi-re′me-ə) the presence of viruses in the blood 病毒血症；**vire′mic** *adj.*

vir·gin (vur′jin) 1. a person who has not had sexual intercourse 处 女；2. a laboratory animal that has been kept free from sexual intercourse 实验用未交配过的动物

vir·ile (vir′il) 1. masculine 男性的；2. specifically, having male copulative power 有男性特征的，尤指有性交能力的

vir·i·lism (vir′ĭ-liz-əm) the development or possession of male secondary sex characters in a female or prepubertal male 男性化，女性出现男性体格和心理特征；**adrenal v.,** virilism due to inappropriate adrenal cortical androgen production 肾上腺性男性化，由于肾上腺皮质雄素激素分泌失调导致女子男

性化

vi·ril·i·ty (vĭ-rĭl'ĭ-te) masculinity 有男性征；男性

vir·il·iza·tion (vir"il-ĭ-za'shən) masculinization; usually used for that occurring in a female or prepubertal male 男性化，通常用于女性或青春期前的男性

vir·i·liz·ing (vir'ĭ-līz"ing) producing virilization 致男性化的

vi·ri·on (vi're-on) the complete viral particle, found extracellularly and capable of surviving in crystalline form and infecting a living cell; it comprises the nucleoid (genetic material) and the capsid 病毒（粒）体，病毒颗粒，病毒粒子，在细胞外发现的完整病毒颗粒，能够以结晶形式存活并感染活细胞，包括类核（遗传物质）和衣壳

vi·ro·lac·tia (vi"ro-lak'shə) secretion of viruses in the milk 乳汁病毒

vi·rol·o·gy (vi-rol'ə-je) the study of viruses and virus diseases 病毒学

vir·tu·al (vir'choo-əl) 1. having the essence or effect, although not the actual fact or form 实质上的，实际的；2. created by, carried on, or performed by means of computers 模拟的，虚拟的

vi·ru·cide (vi'rə-sīd) an agent that neutralizes or destroys a virus 杀病毒药；**viruci'dal** adj.

vir·u·lence (vir'u-ləns) the degree of pathogenicity of a microorganism as indicated by the severity of disease produced and the ability to invade the tissues of the host; by extension, the competence of any infectious agent to produce pathologic effects 毒力；**vir'ulent** adj.

vir·u·lif·er·ous (vir"u-lif'ər-əs) conveying or producing a virus 带病毒的，产毒的

vir·uria (vi-roo're-ə) viruses in the urine 病毒尿（症）

vi·rus (vi'rəs) [L.] a minute infectious agent that, with certain exceptions, is not resolved by the light microscope, lacks independent metabolism, and is able to replicate only within a living host cell; the individual particle (virion) consists of nucleic acid (nucleoid)—DNA or RNA (but not both)—and a protein shell (capsid), which contains and protects the nucleic acid and which may be multilayered 病毒；**attenuated v.,** one whose pathogenicity has been reduced by serial passage or other means 减毒病毒；**Bayou v.,** a virus of the genus *Hantavirus* that causes hantavirus pulmonary syndrome along the Gulf Coast of Texas Bayou 病毒 **BK v. (BKV),** BK 病毒，见 *polyomavirus* 下词条 **California encephalitis v.,** a mosquito-borne virus of the genus *Orthobunyavirus*; it is the cause of California encephalitis 加利福尼亚脑炎病毒；**Chandipura v.,** a virus of the genus *Vesiculovirus* that causes encephalitis in various parts of India; infections can be fatal in children Chandipura 病毒；**conditionally replicative v's,** mutant viruses that can replicate only inside certain types of tumor cells and may disrupt those cells; the most common kind are adenoviruses 条件复制病毒，突变病毒只能在某些类型的肿瘤细胞内复制并可能破坏这些细胞，最常见的是腺病毒；**cowpox v.,** a virus of the genus *Orthopoxvirus* that causes cowpox 牛痘病毒；**Coxsackie v.,** coxsackievirus 柯萨奇病毒；**Crimean-Congo hemorrhagic fever v.,** a virus of the genus *Nairovirus* that causes CrimeanCongo hemorrhagic fever 克里米亚-刚果出血热病毒；**defective v.,** one that cannot be completely replicated or cannot form a protein coat; in some cases replication can proceed if missing gene functions are supplied by other viruses 缺陷病毒，一类不能完全复制或不能形成蛋白质外壳的病毒，在某些情况下，如果其他病毒提供缺失的基因功能，可以进行复制；参见 *helper v.* **dengue v.,** a flavivirus existing as four distinct types (designated 1, 2, 3, and 4) that causes dengue 登革热病毒；**Desert Shield v.,** a calicivirus of the genus *Norovirus* that can cause gastroenteritis 沙漠风暴病毒，诸如病毒属的杯状病毒，可引起胃肠炎；**DNA v.,** one whose genome consists of DNA DNA 病毒；**eastern equine encephalitis v., eastern equine encephalomyelitis v.,** 东方马脑炎病毒，参见 *equine encephalitis viruses*；**EB v.,** Epstein-Barr v. (human herpesvirus 4) EB 病毒，见 *herpesvirus* herpesvirus 下附表 **Ebola v.,** a virus of the genus Filovirus that causes Ebola virus disease 埃博拉病毒；**EEE v.,** 同eastern equine encephalitis v.；参见 *equine encephalitis viruses*；**encephalomyocarditis v.,** a species of the genus *Cardiovirus* that causes mild aseptic meningitis and encephalomyocarditis 脑心肌炎病毒，一种引起轻度无菌性脑膜炎和脑心肌炎的心脏病毒属病毒；**enteric v's,** an epidemiologic class of viruses that are normally acquired by ingestion and replicate in the intestinal tract, causing local rather than generalized infection 肠道病毒，一种流行病学类型的病毒，通常通过摄入而在肠道中复制而获得，引起局部而非全身感染；**enveloped v.,** a virus having an outer lipoprotein bilayer acquired by budding through the host cell membrane 囊膜病毒，包膜病毒；**Epstein-Barr v. (EBV),** human herpesvirus 4; EB 病毒，人类疱疹病毒4，见 *herpesvirus* 下附表 **equine encephalitis v's, equine encephalomyelitis v's,** a group of togavirus species of the genus *Alphavirus* that cause encephalomyelitis in horses, mules, and humans, and are transmitted by mosquitoes; the species are called *eastern, western,* and *Venezuelan encephalitis* (or *encephalomyelitis*) viruses 马脑脊髓炎病毒；**Eyach v.**, a tickborne virus of the genus *Coltivirus* that has caused neurologic illness in France, Germany, and the former Czechoslovakia Eyach 病毒；**fixed v.**, one whose virulence and incubation period have been stabilized by serial passage and remained fixed during further transmission 固定毒；**foamy v's**, *Spumavirus* 泡沫病毒；**foot-and-mouth disease v.**, a species of the genus *Aphthovirus* that causes foot-and-mouth disease 口蹄疫病毒；**H1N1 v.**, an antigenic variant of *Influenzavirus A,* arising from recombination of genetic material from human, avian, and swine influenza viruses, that causes disease in humans H1N1 病毒；**Hantaan v.**, a virus of the genus *Hantavirus* that causes epidemics of severe hemorrhagic fever in Asia; its reservoir is a species of mouse 汉坦病毒；**Hawaii v.**, a species of the genus *Norovirus* that causes gastroenteritis, which can be severe in children 夏威夷病毒；**helper v.**, one that aids in the development of a defective virus by supplying or restoring the activity of the viral gene or enabling it to form a protein coat 辅助病毒，通过提供或恢复病毒基因的活性或使其形成蛋白质外壳来协助缺陷病毒的发展；**Hendra v.**, a paramyxovirus of the genus *Henipavirus*; it causes encephalitis and pneumonia in horses, which can be spread to humans 亨德拉病毒；**hepatitis v's**, the etiologic agents of viral hepatitis; six are recognized: *hepatitis A virus,* the agent causing hepatitis A, acquired by parenteral inoculation or by ingestion; *hepatitis B virus,* the agent causing hepatitis B, transmitted by inadequately sterilized syringes and needles, or through infectious blood plasma, or certain blood products; *hepatitis C virus,* which causes hepatitis C; *hepatitis D virus,* a defective RNA virus that can replicate only in the presence of hepatitis B virus, is transmitted with it, and causes hepatitis D; *hepatitis E virus,* a calicivirus transmitting hepatitis E; and *hepatitis G virus,* flavivirus isolated from patients with hepatitis but whose etiologic role is uncertain 肝炎病毒；**hepatitis B–like v's**, Hepadnaviridae 乙型肝炎样病毒；**herpangina v.**, any of several viruses that cause herpangina, primarily in children; these are most often coxsackieviruses and less often echoviruses 疱疹性咽峡炎病毒；**herpes v.**, herpesvirus 疱疹病毒；**herpes simplex v. (HSV)**, either of two viruses that cause herpes simplex, human herpesvirus 1 and human herpesvirus 2 单纯疱疹病毒，见 *herpesvirus* 下附表；**human immunodefciency v. (HIV)**, a human T-cell leukemia/lymphoma virus, of the genus *Lentivirus*, with a selective affinity for helper T cells that is the agent of the acquired immunodeficiency syndrome 人免疫缺陷病毒，一种

人 T 细胞白血病 / 淋巴瘤病毒，属于慢病毒属，是获得性免疫缺陷综合征的病原体；**human T-cell leukemia v.**, human T-lymphotropic v. 人 T 细胞白血病病毒；**human T-lymphotropic v. 1 (HTLV-1)**, a species of retroviruses of worldwide distribution, having an affinity for helper/inducer T lymphocytes; it causes chronic infection and is associated with adult T-cell leukemia/lymphoma and chronic progressive myelopathy 人嗜 T 淋巴细胞病毒Ⅰ型；**human T-lymphotropic v. 2 (HTLV-2)**, a species of retroviruses having extensive serologic cross-reactivity with HTLV-1; no clear association with disease has been established 人嗜 T 淋巴细胞病毒Ⅱ型；**igbo-ora v.**, an arbovirus of the genus *Alphavirus* that has been associated with a dengue-like disease in Nigeria, the Central African Republic, and the Ivory Coast 伊克卜 - 奥拉病毒；**influenza v.**, any of a group of orthomyxoviruses that cause influenza, including at least three genera: *Influenzavirus A, Influenzavirus B,* and *Influenzavirus C.* Serotype A viruses are subject to major antigenic changes (antigenic shifts) as well as minor gradual antigenic changes (antigenic drift) and cause the major pandemics 流行性感冒病毒；**influenzaA v., influenza B v., influenza C v.**, species in the genera *Influenzavirus A, Influenzavirus B,* and *Influenzavirus C* 甲型流感病毒，乙型流感病毒，丙型流感病毒，参见 *influenza v.*；**Jamestown Canyon v.**, a strain of California encephalitis virus that can cause encephalitis 詹姆斯城病毒；**JC v. (JCV)**, JC 参见 *polyomavirus* 下 词条；**La Crosse v.**, a strain of California encephalitis virus that is the etiologic agent of La Crosse encephalitis 拉克罗斯病毒；**Lordsdale v.**, a calicivirus of the genus *Norovirus* that can cause gastroenteritis Lordsdale 病毒；**lytic v.**, a virus that is replicated in the host cell and causes death and lysis of the cell 裂解性病毒，在宿主细胞内复制，导致细胞死亡与溶解的病毒；**Marburg v.**, an RNA virus occurring in Africa, transmitted by insect bite and causing Marburg disease 马尔堡病毒，一种在非洲发生的 RNA 病毒，通过昆虫叮咬传播并引起马尔堡病；**masked v.**, a virus that ordinarily occurs in a noninfective state and is demonstrable by indirect methods that activate it, as by blind passage in experimental animals 隐性病毒；**measles v.**, a paramyxovirus that is the cause of measles 麻疹病毒；**measles-like v's**, *Morbillivirus* 类麻疹病毒；**Modoc v.**, a virus of the genus *Flavivirus* that causes aseptic meningitis in the western United States and Canada Modoc 病毒；**monkeypox v.**, an orthopoxvirus that produces mild exanthematous disease in monkeys and a smallpox-like disease in humans 猴痘病毒；**mumps v.**, a virus of the genus *Rubula-*

virus that causes mumps and sometimes tenderness and swelling of the testes, pancreas, ovaries, or other organs 流行性腮腺炎病毒; **naked v., nonenveloped v.,** a virus lacking an outer lipoprotein bilayer 裸露病毒; **neurotropic v.,** a virus that has a predilection for and causes infection in nerve tissue, such as the rabies virus 亲神经性病毒; **Newcastle disease v.,** a virus of the genus *Avulavirus* that causes Newcastle disease in birds; human infection is mild and characterized by conjunctivitis and brief generalized symptoms 鸡新城疫病毒; **Norwalk v.,** a calicivirus that is a common agent of epidemics of acute gastroenteritis 诺沃克病毒; **oncogenic v's,** an epidemiologic class of viruses that are acquired by close contact or injection and cause usually persistent infection; they may induce cell transformation and malignancy 致癌病毒; **Oropouche v.,** a species of the genus *Orthobunyavirus* that causes illness in Brazil, with fever, chills, malaise, headache, myalgia, arthralgia, and sometimes nausea, vomiting, and central nervous system involvement 奥罗波赤病毒; **orphan v's,** viruses isolated in tissue culture but not found specifically associated with any illness 孤儿病毒; **papilloma v.,** papillomavirus 乳头瘤病毒; **parainfluenza v.,** a group of viruses of the family Paramyxoviridae that cause upper respiratory tract disease in humans and other animals. Human pathogens are found in the genera *Respirovirus* and *Rubulavirus* 副流感病毒; **paravaccinia v.,** pseudocowpox v. 副痘苗病毒; **Powassan v.,** a tickborne virus of the genus *Flavivirus* that causes encephalitis in eastern North America 波瓦桑黄病毒; **pox v.,** poxvirus 痘病毒; **pseudocowpox v.,** a virus of the genus *Parapoxvirus* that produces nodular lesions similar to those of cowpox and orf on the udders and teats of milk cows and the oral mucosa of suckling calves (paravaccinia), which can be transmitted to humans during milking 假牛痘病毒; **Puumala v.,** a virus of the genus *Hantavirus* that causes mild hemorrhagic fever in Scandinavia, Russia, and other European countries 普乌拉病毒; **rabies v.,** an RNA virus of the rhabdovirus group that causes rabies 狂犬病毒; **rabies-like v's,** *Lyssavirus* 类狂犬病毒; **respiratory v's,** an epidemiologic class of viruses that are acquired by inhalation of fomites and replicate in the respiratory tract, causing local rather than generalized infection; they are included in the families Adenoviridae, Coronaviridae, Orthomyxoviridae, Paramyxoviridae, and Picornaviridae 呼吸道病毒; **respiratory syncytial v.(RSV),** any of a group of viruses belonging to the genus *Pneumovirus*, causing respiratory disease that is particularly severe in infants, and in tissue causing syncytium formation 呼吸道合胞病毒; **Rift Valley fever v.,** a virus of the genus *Phlebovirus* that causes mild to severe hemorrhagic fever in humans and other animals in southern and eastern Africa 裂谷热病毒; **RNA v.,** a virus whose genome consists of RNA RNA 病毒; **Rous-associated v. (RAV),** a helper virus in whose presence a defective Rous sarcoma virus is able to form a protein coat 鲁斯相关病毒; **Rous sarcoma v. (RSV),** 劳斯肉瘤病毒，参见 *sarcoma* 下 *Rous sarcoma*; **rubella v.,** a species of togavirus, the sole species of the genus *Rubivirus*; it causes rubella 风疹病毒; **St. Louis encephalitis v.,** a virus of the genus *Flavivirus* that causes St. Louis encephalitis; transmitted by mosquitoes 圣路易斯脑炎病毒; **sandfly fever v's,** 白蛉热病毒，参见 *Phlebovirus*; **satellite v.,** a strain of virus unable to replicate except in the presence of helper virus; considered to be deficient in coding for capsid formation 卫星病毒; **Seoul v.,** a virus of the genus *Hantavirus* that causes epidemics of hemorrhagic fever; rats are the natural hosts 首尔病毒; **simian immunodefciency v. (SIV),** a virus of the genus *Lentivirus*, closely related to human immunodeficiency virus, that causes inapparent infection in African green monkeys and a disease resembling acquired immunodeficiency syndrome in macaques 猿猴免疫缺陷病毒; **SinNombre v.,** a virus of the genus *Hantavirus* that causes hantavirus pulmonary syndrome in the western United States SinNombre 病毒; **slow v.,** any virus causing a disease characterized by a long preclinical course and gradual progression once the symptoms appear 慢病毒; **Snow Mountain v.,** a species of the genus *Norovirus* that causes gastroenteritis, which can be severe in children 雪山病毒; **street v.,** virus from a naturally infected animal, as opposed to a laboratory-adapted strain of the virus 街毒; **tickborne encephalitis v's,** a serogroup of the genus *Flavivirus*, consisting of viruses that are transmitted by ticks and cause encephalitis in humans and animals that ranges in severity from subclinical to fatal 蜱媒脑炎病毒; **torque teno v.,** a virus of the genus *Anellovirus* that can cause liver damage or hepatitis; it was originally observed in Japan but was later found in other parts of the world 输血传播病毒; **Toscana v.,** a virus of the Naples serogroup of the genus *Phlebovirus*, an etiologic agent of phlebotomus fever 托斯卡纳病毒; **TT v.,** 同 torque teno v.; **vaccinia v.,** a virus of the genus *Orthopoxvirus* that does not occur in nature, being propagated only in the laboratory; used in research and for production of vaccine against smallpox 牛痘苗病毒; **varicella-zoster v.,** human herpesvirus 3; see table at *her-*

pesvirus 水痘 - 带状疱疹病毒；**variola v.**, the virtually extinct virus, belonging to the genus *Orthopoxvirus*, that is the etiologic agent of smallpox. No natural infection has occurred since 1977 and no reservoir of the virus now exists 天花病毒；**VEE v.**, **Venezuelan equine encephalitis v.**, **Venezuelan equine encephalomyelitis v.**, 委内瑞拉马脑炎病毒，参见 *equine encephalitis viruses*; **WEE v.**,**western equine encephalitis v.**, **western equine encephalomyelitis v.**, 西方马脑炎病毒，参见 *equine encephalitis viruses; West Nile v.*, a virus of the genus *Flavivirus* that causes West Nile encephalitis; it is transmitted by *Culex* mosquitoes, with wild birds serving as the reservoir 西尼罗病毒；**yellow fever v.**, a mosquito-borne virus of the genus *Flavivirus* that causes yellow fever in Central and South America and Africa 黄热病毒；**Zika v.**, a mosquito-borne virus of the genus Flavivirus, which causes a febrile illness with rash; antigenically related to Spondweni virus. Zika virus occurs primarily in Central Africa but has spread to other parts of the world, including South and Central America, the Caribbean, parts of North America, and Southeast Asia 寨卡病毒

vis·ce·ra (vis′ər-ə) *viscus* 的复数

vis·cer·ad (vis′ər-ad) toward the viscera 向内脏

vis·cer·al (vis′ər-əl) pertaining to a viscus 内脏的

vis·cer·al·gia (vis″ər-al′jə) pain in any viscera 内脏痛

vis·cero·meg·a·ly (vis″ər-o-meg′ə-le) organomegaly 内脏肥大

vis·cero·mo·tor (vis″ər-o-mo′tər) conveying or concerned with motor impulses to the viscera 内脏运动的

vis·cero·pa·ri·e·tal (vis″ər-o-pə-ri′ə-təl) pertaining to the viscera and the abdominal wall 内脏腹壁的

vis·cero·peri·to·ne·al (vis″ər-o-per″ĭ-to-ne′əl) pertaining to the viscera and peritoneum 内脏腹膜的

vis·cero·pleu·ral (vis″ər-o-ploor′əl) pertaining to the viscera and the pleura 内脏胸膜的

visceroptosis a condition in which abdominal organs are displaced to a lower part of the abdomen 内脏下垂

vis·cero·skel·e·tal (vis″ər-o-skel′ə-təl) pertaining to the visceral skeleton 内脏骨骼的

vis·cero·tro·pic (vis″ər-o-tro′pik) primarily acting on the viscera; having a predilection for the abdominal or thoracic viscera 亲内脏的

vis·cid (vis′id) glutinous or sticky 粘的

vis·cos·i·ty (vis-kos′ĭ-te) resistance to flow; a physical property of a substance that is dependent on the friction of its component molecules as they slide by one another 黏度；黏性

vis·cous (vis′kəs) sticky or gummy; having a high degree of viscosity 黏的，黏性的

vis·cus (vis′kəs) pl. *vis′cera* [L.] any large interior organ in any of the three great body cavities, especially those in the abdomen 内脏

vi·sion (vizh′ən) 1. the sense by which objects in the external environment are perceived by means of the light they give off or reflect 视觉；2. the act of seeing 视；3. an apparition; a subjective sensation of seeing not elicited by actual visual stimuli 幻视；4. visual acuity 视 力；**achromatic v.**, monochromatic vision 全色盲；**anomalous trichromatic v.**, defective color vision in which a person has all three cone pigments but one is deficient or anomalous but not absent 异常三色视；**binocular v.**, the use of both eyes together without diplopia 双眼视觉；**central v.**, that produced by stimuli impinging directly on the macula retinae 中央视觉；**chromatic v.**, 同 color v.；**color v.**, 1. perception of the different colors making up the spectrum of visible light 色觉；2. chromatopsia 色视症；**day v.**, visual perception in the daylight or under conditions of bright illumination 明视觉，白昼视觉；**dichromatic v.**, defective color vision in which one of the three cone pigments is missing; the two types are *protanopia* and *deuteranopia* 二色视觉，二色性色盲；**direct v.**, 同 central v.；**double v.**, diplopia 复视；**indirect v.**, 同 peripheral v.；**low v.**, impairment of vision such that there is significant visual handicap but also significant usable residual vision 低视力；**monochromatic v.**, complete color blindness; inability to discriminate hues, all colors of the spectrum appearing as neutral grays with varying shades of light and dark 全色盲；**monocular v.**, vision with one eye 单眼视觉；**multiple v.**, polyopia 视物显多症；**night v.**, visual perception in the darkness of night or under conditions of reduced illumination 暗视觉，夜间视觉；**oscillating v.**, oscillopsia 振动幻视 **peripheral v.**, that produced by stimuli falling on areas of the retina distant from the macula 周边视觉；**solid v.**, **stereoscopic v.**, perception of the relief of objects or of their depth; vision in which objects are perceived as having three dimensions 实体视觉，立体视觉；**trichromatic v.**, 1. any ability to distinguish the three primary colors of light and mixtures of them 三色视觉；2. normal color vision 正常的色觉；**tunnel v.**, 1. that in which the visual field is severely constricted 视野收缩；2. in psychiatry, restriction of psychological or emotional perception to a limited range 管状视

vis·mo·deg·ib (vis″mo-dej′ib) an inhibitor of the hedgehog developmental signaling pathway, used in the treatment of advanced or metastatic basal cell carcinoma 一种具有选择性 Hedgehog 信号通路的新型口服类药物，用于治疗基底细胞癌

vis·u·al (vizh'oo-əl) pertaining to vision or sight 视觉的，视力的

vis·u·al·iza·tion (vizh″oo-əl-ī-za'shən) 1. the act of viewing or of achieving a complete visual impression of an object 显影，造影术；2. the process of forming a mental picture of something 想象

vis·uo·au·di·to·ry (vizh″oo-o-aw'dī-tor″e) simultaneously stimulating, or pertaining to simultaneous stimulation of, the senses of both hearing and sight 视听觉的

vis·uo·mo·tor (vizh″oo-o-mo'tər) pertaining to connections between visual and motor processes 视觉运动的

vis·uo·sen·so·ry (vizh″oo-o-sen'sə-re) pertaining to perception of stimuli giving rise to visual impressions 视觉的

vis·uo·spa·tial (vizh″oo-o-spa'shəl) pertaining to the ability to understand visual representations and their spatial relationships 视觉空间的

vi·tal (vi'təl) necessary to or pertaining to life 维持生命所必需的；生命的，生活的

Vi·tal·li·um (vi-tal'e-əm) trademark for a cobaltchromium alloy used for cast dentures and surgical appliances 活合金，钴铬钼合金的商品名，用于牙托、外科器械、假体等

vi·ta·min (vi'tə-min) any of a group of unrelated organic substances occurring in many foods in small amounts and necessary in trace amounts for the normal metabolic functioning of the body; they may be water- or fat-soluble 维生素；**v. A,** retinol or any of several fat-soluble compounds with similar biologic activity; the vitamin acts in numerous capacities, particularly in the functioning of the retina, the growth and differentiation of epithelial tissue, the growth of bone, reproduction, and the immune response. Deficiency causes skin disorders, increased susceptibility to infection, nyctalopia, xerophthalmia and other eye disorders, anorexia, and sterility. As vitamin A it is mostly found in liver, egg yolks, and the fat component of dairy products; its other major dietary source is the provitamin A carotenoids of plants. It is toxic when taken in excess 维生素 A，视黄醇，参见 *hypervitaminosis A;* **v. A₁,** retinol 维生素 A₁，视黄醇；**v. A₂,** dehydroretinol 维生素 A₂，脱氢视黄醇；**v. B₁,** thiamine 维生素 B₁，硫铵素；**v. B₂,** riboflavin 维生素 B₂，核黄素；**v. B₆,** any of a group of water-soluble substances (including pyridoxine, pyridoxal, and pyridoxamine) found in most foods, especially meats, liver, vegetables, whole grains, cereals, and egg yolk, and concerned in the metabolism of amino acids, in the degradation of tryptophan, and in the metabolism of glycogen 维生素 B₆，吡哆醇；**v. B₁₂,** cyanocobalamin by chemical definition, but generally any substituted cobalamin derivative with similar biologic activity; it is a water-soluble hematopoietic vitamin occurring in meats and animal products. It is necessary for the growth and replication of all body cells and the functioning of the nervous system, and deficiency causes pernicious anemia and other forms of megaloblastic anemia and neurologic lesions 维生素 B₁₂，（氰）钴胺素；**v. B complex,** a group of water-soluble substances including thiamine, riboflavin, niacin (nicotinic acid), niacinamide (nicotinamide), the vitamin B₆ group, biotin, pantothenic acid, and folic acid, and sometimes including *p*-aminobenzoic acid, inositol, vitamin B₁₂, and choline 复合维生素 B；**v. C,** ascorbic acid 维生素 C，抗坏血酸；**v. D,** either of two fat-soluble compounds with antirachitic activity or both collectively: cholecalciferol, which is synthesized in the skin and is considered a hormone, and ergocalciferol, which is the form generally used as a dietary supplement. Dietary sources include some fish liver oils, egg yolks, and fortified dairy products. Deficiency can result in rickets in children and osteomalacia in adults, while excessive ingestion can cause hypercalcemia, mobilization of calcium from bone, and renal dysfunction 维生素 D，骨化醇；**v. D₂,** ergocalciferol 维生素 D₂，麦角钙化（固）醇，钙化固醇；**v. D₃,** cholecalciferol 维生素 D₃，胆钙化醇；**v. E,** any of a group of at least eight related fat-soluble compounds with similar biologic antioxidant activity, particularly α-tocopherol but also including other isomers of tocopherol and the related compound tocotrienol. It is found in wheat germ oil, cereal germs, liver, egg yolk, green plants, milk fat, and vegetable oils and is also prepared synthetically. It is important for normal reproduction, muscle development, and resistance of erythrocytes to hemolysis. Deficiency causes hemolytic anemia and neurologic disorders 维生素 E；**fatsoluble v's,** vitamins (A, D, E, and K) that are soluble in fat solvents and are absorbed along with dietary fats; they are not normally excreted in the urine and tend to be stored in the body in moderate amounts 脂溶性维生素（维生素 A，维生素 D，维生素 E 和维生素 K）**v. K,** any of a group of structurally similar fat-soluble compounds that promote blood clotting. Two forms, phytonadione and menaquinone, exist naturally, and there is one synthetic provitamin form, menadione. The best sources are leafy green vegetables, butter, cheese, and egg yolk. Deficiency, usually seen only in neonates, in disorders of absorption, or during antibiotic therapy, is characterized by hemorrhage. 维 生 素 K；**v. K₁**, phytonadione 维生素 K₁，植物甲萘醌 **v. K₂**, menaquinone 维生素 K₂，甲基萘醌；**v. K₃**, menadione 维生素 K₃，甲萘醌；**water-soluble v's**, the vitamins soluble in water (i.e., all but vitamins A, D, E, and K); they are excreted in the urine and are not stored in the body in appreciable quantities 水溶性维生素（即除了维生素 A、维生素 D、维生素 E 和维生素 K 以外的所有维生素）

vi·tel·line (vǐ-tel′ēn) pertaining to or resembling a yolk 卵黄的

vi·tel·lus (vī-tel′əs) [L.] yolk 卵黄

vit·i·li·go (vit″ĭ-li′go) a chronic, usually progressive, type of hypomelanosis in which there are depigmented white patches on the skin, sometimes surrounded by a hyperpigmented border. It may be localized or generalized 白斑；**vitilig′inous** adj

vi·trec·to·my (vǐ-trek′tə-me) surgical extraction, usually via the pars plana, of the contents of the vitreous chamber of the eye 玻璃体切割术

vit·reo·ret·i·nal (vit″re-o-ret′ĭ-nəl) of or pertaining to the vitreous and retina 玻璃体视网膜的

vit·re·ous (vit′re-əs) 1. glasslike or hyaline 玻璃体的，透明的; 2. vitreous body 玻璃体; **persistent hyperplastic primary v.**, a congenital anomaly, usually unilateral, due to persistence of the primary vitreous and adjacent vessels; characterized by a white pupil, elongated ciliary processes, microphthalmia; and sometimes an opaque lens 初级玻璃体持续性增生症; **primary v.**, the earliest vitreous in the embryo, formed from a mass of ectodermal and mesodermal fibrils between the optic cup and the lens vesicle; it develops into parts of the retina, iris, and ciliary body 原玻璃体

vit·ro·nec·tin (vit″ro-nek′tin) an adhesive glycoprotein whose many functions include regulation of the coagulation, fibrinolytic, and complement cascades, also playing a role in hemostasis, wound healing, tissue remodeling, and cancer, and promoting adhesion, spreading, and migration of cells. It has been shown to be identical to *S protein,* which was identified as a complement inhibitor acting to prevent insertion of the membrane attack complex into the membrane 玻璃体结合蛋白

vi·vip·a·rous (vi-vip′ə-rəs) giving birth to living young who develop within the maternal body 胎生的

vivi·sec·tion (viv″ĭ-sek′shən) surgical procedures performed upon a living animal for purposes of physiologic or pathologic investigation 活 体 解 剖（动物）

Viv·it·rol (Vih′və-trawl) trademark for a preparation of naltrexone 纳屈酮制剂的商品名

VLCFA very-long-chain fatty acids 极长链脂肪酸

VLDL very-low-density lipoprotein 极低密度脂蛋白; **β-VLDL, beta VLDL**, a mixture of lipoproteins with diffuse electrophoretic mobility approximately that of β -lipoproteins but having lower density; they are remnants derived from mutant chylomicrons and very-low-density lipoproteins that cannot be metabolized completely and accumulate in plasma β - 极 低 密 度 脂 蛋 白; **pre-β-VLDL**, very-low-density lipoprotein, emphasizing its electrophoretic mobility 前 β - 极低密度脂蛋白

VMA vanillylmandelic acid 香 草 基 扁 桃 酸; vitreomacular adhesion 玻璃体粘连

VMD [L.] Veterina′riae Medici′nae Doc′tor (Doctor of Veterinary Medicine) 兽医博士

VNA Visiting Nurse Association 访问护士协会

VNAA Visiting Nurse Associations of America 美国访问护士协会

VNTR variable number tandem repeats 可 变 数 目 串联重复序列

VOD venoocclusive disease 静脉闭塞性疾病

voice (vois) sound produced by the speech organs and uttered by the mouth 语音，语声; **vo′cal** adj.

void (void) excrete 排泄

vo·la (vo′lə) pl. *vo′lae* [L.] a concave or hollow surface 掌；跖; **v. ma′nus**, the palm 手掌; **v. pe′dis**, the sole 足跖

vo·lar (vo′lər) pertaining to the palm or sole, usually specifically the former 掌的，跖的

vo·la·ris (vo-lar′is) palmar 手掌的，掌侧的

vol·a·tile (vol′ə-til) evaporating rapidly; vaporizing readily 挥发性的，易挥发的

vol·a·til·iza·tion (vol″ə-til″ĭ-za′shən) conversion into vapor or gas without chemical change 挥发作用

vol′ley (vol′e) a number of simultaneous muscle twitches or nerve impulses all caused by the same stimulus 一列冲动，一系列同时发生的肌颤搐和神经冲动都是由同一刺激引起的

vol·sel·la (vol-sel′ə) 同 vulsella

volt (V) (vōlt) the SI unit of electric potential or electromotive force, equal to 1 watt per ampere, or 1 joule per coulomb 伏（ 特 ）; **electron v. (eV)**, a unit of energy equal to the energy acquired by an electron accelerated through a potential difference of 1 volt; equal to 1.602 × 10⁻¹⁹ joule 电子伏特

vol·ume (V) (*V*) (vol′ūm) the measure of the quantity or capacity of a substance 容量，容积，体积; **end-diastolic v. (EDV)**, the volume of blood in each ventricle at the end of diastole, usually about 120 to 130 ml but sometimes reaching 200 to 250 ml in the normal heart 舒张期末容积; **end-systolic v. (ESV)**, the volume of blood remaining in each ven-

V

tricle at the end of systole, usually about 50 to 60 ml but sometimes as little as 10 to 30 ml in the normal heart 收缩期末容积；**expiratory reserve v. (ERV)**, the maximal amount of gas that can be exhaled from the resting end-expiratory level 呼气储备量；**forced expiratory v.**, the fraction of the forced vital capacity that is exhaled in a specific number of seconds. Abbreviated FEV with a subscript indicating how many seconds the measurement lasted 用 力 呼 气 容 积；**inspiratory reserve v.**, the maximal amount of gas that can be inhaled from the end-inspiratory position 补吸气量，补吸气容积；**mean corpuscular v.**, the average volume of erythrocytes, conventionally expressed in cubic micrometers or femtoliters per red cell 红细胞平均容量；**minute v. (MV)**, the quantity of gas exhaled from the lungs per minute; tidal volume multiplied by respiratory rate 分钟容量 **packed-cell v. (PCV) v. of packed red cells (VPRC)**, hematocrit 血细胞压积；**residual v.**, the amount of gas remaining in the lung at the end of a maximal exhalation 余 气 量；**stroke v.**, the volume of blood ejected from a ventricle at each beat of the heart, equal to the difference between the end-diastolic volume and the end-systolic volume 心 搏 排 血 量；**tidal v.**, the volume of gas inhaled and exhaled during one respiratory cycle 潮 气 量 **vol·u·met·ric** (vol″u-met′rik) pertaining to or accompanied by measurement in volumes 容量的，容积的

vol·un·tary (vol′ən-tar″e) accomplished in accordance with the will 自愿的

vo·lute (vo-lūt′) rolled up 涡旋的，涡卷的

vol·vu·lo·sis (vol″vu-lo′sis) onchocerciasis due to *Onchocerca volvulus* 盘尾丝虫病

vol·vu·lus (vol′vu-ləs) [L.] obstruction due to a knotting and twisting of part of the gastrointestinal tract 肠扭转

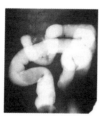

▲ 结肠肠扭转（钡剂灌肠）

vo·mer (vo′mər) [L.] the unpaired flat bone that forms the inferior and posterior part of the nasal septum, articulating with the ethmoid and sphenoid bones and both maxillae and palatine bones 犁骨；**vo′merine** *adj.*

vo·mero·na·sal (vo″mər-o-na′səl) pertaining to the vomer and the nasal bone 犁骨鼻骨的

vom·it (vom′it) 1. to eject stomach contents through the mouth 呕吐；2. matter expelled from the stomach by the mouth 呕吐物；**black v.**, vomit consisting of blood that has been acted upon by the gastric juice, seen in yellow fever and other conditions in which blood collects in the stomach 黑色呕吐物；**coffee-ground v.**, vomit consisting of dark altered blood mixed with stomach contents 咖啡渣状呕吐物

vom·it·ing (vom′it-ing) forcible ejection of contents of the stomach through the mouth 呕吐；**cyclic v.**, recurring attacks of vomiting, usually seen in children 周期性呕吐，不规则间歇性呕吐，见于小儿；**dry v.**, attempts at vomiting, with the ejection of nothing but gas 干呕，恶心，想呕吐，除空气外无物呕出；**fecal v.**, vomiting of fecal matter 呕粪；吐粪；**pernicious v.**, vomiting in pregnancy so severe as to threaten life 恶性孕吐，妊娠时发生的呕吐，严重可威胁母亲生命；**v. of pregnancy**, that occurring in pregnancy, especially early morning vomiting (morning sickness) 妊娠呕吐，妊娠时发生的呕吐，尤其是怀孕时常见的清晨呕吐；**projectile v.**, vomiting with the material ejected with great force 喷射性呕吐；**stercoraceous v.**, fecal v. 粪便性呕吐

vom·i·to·ry (vom′ĭ-tor″e) emetic 吐剂

vom·i·tus (vom′ĭ-təs) [L.] 1. 同 vomiting；2. matter vomited 呕吐物

v-onc (ve′onk″) [viral *onc*ogene] a nucleic acid sequence in a virus responsible for the oncogenicity of the virus; it is derived from the cellular proto-oncogene and acquired from the host by recombination 病毒癌基因 Cf. *c-onc*

vo·ri·co·na·zole (vor″ĭ-ko′nə-zōl) a triazole antifungal compound used for the treatment of invasive aspergillosis, administered orally 伏立康唑，一种三唑类广谱抗真菌药，用于治疗侵袭性曲霉菌病，口服给药

vor·tex (vor′teks) pl. *vor′tices* [L.] a whorled or spiral arrangement or pattern, as of muscle fibers, or of the ridges or hairs of the skin 涡，一种轮生的或螺旋状的排列或图案，如肌肉纤维涡、皮肤上的嵴涡

vo·yeur·ism (voi′yər-iz-əm) a paraphilia characterized by recurrent, intense sexual urges or arousal involving real or fantasized observation of unsuspecting people who are naked, disrobing, or engaging in sexual activity 窥阴癖，窥阴症

VP variegate porphyria 复杂性卟啉症；vestibular papillae 前庭乳头

VPB ventricular premature beat 室性期前收缩，

室性早搏，参见 complex 下 *ventricular premature complex*

VPC ventricular premature complex 心室期前复合波

VPD ventricular premature depolarization 心室过早去极化，参见 complex 下 *ventricular premature complex*

VPF vascular permeability factor 血管通透因子，参见 *factor vascular endothelial growth factor*

VR vocal resonance 语响

VS volumetric solution 滴定溶液，定量溶液

VT ventricular tachycardia 室性心动过速

vul·ga·ris (vəl-ga′ris) [L.] ordinary; common 寻常的，普通的

vul·nus (vul′nəs) pl. *vul′nera* [L.] a wound 创伤，伤口

vul·sel·la (vəl-sel′ə) [L.] a forceps with clawlike hooks at the end of each blade 双爪钳

vul·sel·lum (vəl-sel′əm) [L.] 同 vulsella

vul·va (vul′və) [L.] the external genital organs of the female, including the mons pubis, labia majora and minora, clitoris, and vestibule of the vagina 女阴，外阴，**vul′val, vul′var** *adj.*; **fused v.**, synechia vulvae 外阴闭锁

vul·vec·to·my (vəl-vek′tə-me) excision of the vulva 外阴切除术

vul·vi·tis (vəl-vi′tis) inflammation of the vulva 外阴炎; **atrophic v.**, lichen sclerosus in females 萎缩性外阴炎

vul·vo·uter·ine (vul″vo-u′tər-in) pertaining to the vulva and uterus 外阴子宫的

vul·vo·vag·i·nal (vul″vo-vaj′ĭ-nəl) pertaining to the vulva and vagina 外阴阴道的

vul·vo·vag·i·ni·tis (vul″vo-vaj″ĭ-ni′tis) inflammation of the vulva and vagina 外阴阴道炎; **candidal v.**, vulvovaginal candidiasis 念珠菌性阴道炎; **senile v.**, atrophic vaginitis in which there is intense itching around the vagina, almost complete lack of vaginal secretions, and tissue atrophy 老年性外阴阴道炎

vv. [L.] ve′nae (veins) 静脉

v/v volume (of solute) per volume (of solvent)（溶质）容量 /（溶剂）容量

vWF von Willebrand factor 血管性假血友病因子

VWS Van der Woude syndrome 范德伍兹综合征，腭裂 - 唇裂综合征

W

W [符号] tryptophan 色氨酸; tungsten (*Ger. Wolfram*) 元素钨; watt 瓦特

waist (wāst) the portion of the body between the thorax and the hips 腰，腰部

walk·er (wawk′ər) an enclosing framework of lightweight metal tubing, sometimes with wheels, for patients who need more support in walking than that given by a crutch or cane 助行器

walk·ing (wawk′ing) 1. progressing on foot 步行; 2. gait 步态; **sleep w.**, somnambulism. somnambulism 梦行症

wall (wawl) paries; a structure bounding or limiting a space or a definitive mass of material 壁; **cell w.**, a rigid structure that lies just outside of and is joined to the plasma membrane of plant cells and most prokaryotic cells, which protects the cell and maintains its shape 细胞壁; **chest w.**, the bony and muscular structures that form the outer framework of the thorax and move during breathing 胸壁; **nail w.**, a fold of skin overlapping the sides and proximal end of a fingernail or toenail 甲襞，甲郭; **parietal w.**, somatopleure 胚体壁; **splanchnic w.**, splanchnopleure 脏壁，脏层

wall·eye (wawl′i) 1. leukoma of the cornea 角膜白斑; 2. exotropia 散开性斜视，外斜视

wan·der·ing (wahn′dər-ing) 1. moving about freely 漫动的; 2. abnormally movable; too loosely attached 游动的，游走的

Wang·i·el·la (wang″e-el′ə) a genus of dematiaceous anamorphic fungi; *W. dermatitidis* is also known as *Exophiala dermatitidis* 万吉拉菌属

ward (word) 1. a large room in a hospital for the accommodation of several patients 病房; 2. a division within a hospital for the care of numerous patients having the same condition 病室

war·fa·rin (wor′fər-in) a synthetic coumarin anticoagulant administered as the sodium salt; it is also used as a rodenticide, causing fatal hemorrhaging in any mammal consuming a sufficient dose 华法林（抗凝药）

wart (wort) 1. verruca; a hyperplastic skin lesion caused by a human papillomavirus, transmitted by contact or autoinoculation 疣; 2. any of various nonviral lesions of similar appearance 内赘; **war′ty** *adj.*; **common w.**, a lobulated type with a horny surface 寻常疣; **flat w.**, a small, smooth, skin-colored, slightly raised wart, usually in children, sometimes in great numbers 扁平疣; **genital w.**, condyloma acuminatum 生殖器疣; **moist w.**, condyloma latum 湿疣; **mosaic w.**, an irregular lesion on the palm or sole with a granular surface, an aggregation of contiguous warts 马赛克样疣，镶嵌状疣; **Peruvian**

w., verruga peruana 秘鲁疣；**pitch w.,** a precancerous epidermal tumor seen in persons working with pitch and coal tar derivatives 沥青疣，癌症前期的角化表皮疣；**plantar w.,** a painful type found on the sole of the foot 跖疣；**venereal w.,** condyloma acuminatum 性病湿疣，尖锐湿疣

wash (wahsh) 1. to clean or bathe 洗；2. a solution used for cleansing or bathing a part 洗剂，洗液

wast·ing (wāst′ing) gradual loss or decay, with emaciation 消耗；消瘦；**salt w.,** inappropriate sodium excretion in the urine (natriuresis) with hyponatremia and hyperkalemia 盐流失，另参见 *syndrome* 下 *salt-losing syndrome*

wa·ter (waw′tər) (wah′tər) 1. clear, colorless, odorless, tasteless liquid, H_2O 水；2. an aqueous solution of a medicinal substance 芳香水；又称 *aromatic w.*; 3. 同 *purified w.*; **bound w.,** water in the tissues of the body bound to macromolecules or organelles 结合水；**distilled w.,** water purified by distillation 蒸馏水；**free w.,** that portion of the water in body tissues which is not bound by macromolecules or organelles 游离水无溶质水，**w.for injection,** water for parenteral use, prepared by distillation or reverse osmosis and meeting certain standards for sterility and clarity; it may be specified as sterile if it has been sterilized and as bacteriostatic if suitable antimicrobial agents have been added 注射用水；**purifed w.,** water obtained by either distillation or deionization; used when mineral-free water is required 纯化水

wa·ters (waw′tərz) popular name for *amniotic fluid* 羊水

watt (W) (waht) the SI unit of power, being the work done at the rate of 1 joule per second. In electric power, it is equivalent to a current of 1 ampere under a pressure of 1 volt 瓦（特）（国际单位制功率的单位）

wave (wāv) a uniformly advancing disturbance in which the parts move while undergoing a double oscillation; also, something with this pattern 波，波浪；波状物，波浪形；**alpha w's,** α 波，参见 *rhythm* 下词条；**beta w's,** β 波，参见 *rhythm* 下词条；**brain w's,** the fluctuations of electric potential in the brain, as recorded by electroencephalography 脑电波；**delta w.,** 1. an early QRS vector in the electrocardiogram in preexcitation 心电图 QRS 波；2. *(in the pl.)* electroencephalographic waves with a frequency below 4 per second, typical in deep sleep, infancy, and serious brain disorders δ 波，频率为每秒 4 次以下的脑电波；**electromagnetic w's,** the spectrum of waves propagated by an electromagnetic field, having a velocity of 3×10^8 m/s in a vacuum and including, in order of decreasing wavelength,

radio waves; microwaves; infrared, visible, and ultraviolet light; x-rays; gamma rays; and cosmic rays 电磁波；**F w's,** 1. flutter w's; rapid sawtooth-edged atrial waves without isoelectric intervals between them; seen in the electrocardiogram in atrial flutter. Written also *f w's* 心电图中，心房扑动时发出的锯齿状快速小波；2. 同 f w's (1)；**f w's,** 1. fibrillary w's; small, irregular, rapid deflections in the electrocardiogram in atrial fibrillation. Written also F w's 心电图中，心房纤颤时出现的快速无规律小波 2. 同 F w's (1)；**fibrillary w's,** 同 f w's (1)；**flutter w's,** 同 F w's (1)；**J w.,** a deflection occurring in the electrocardiogram between the QRS complex and the onset of the ST segment, seen prominently in hypothermia and in hypocalcemia J 波，心电图中出现于 QRS 复合波与 ST 段起始点之间的波，主要见于低温和血钙过高；**P w.,** a deflection in the electrocardiogram produced by excitation of the atria P 波（心电图）；**pulse w.,** the elevation of the pulse felt by the finger or shown graphically in a recording of pulse pressure 脉波；**Q w.,** in the QRS complex, the initial downward (negative) deflection, related to the initial phase of depolarization of the ventricular myocardium, the depolarization of the interventricular septum Q 波（心电图）；**R w.,** the initial upward deflection of the QRS complex, following the Q wave in the normal electrocardiogram and representing early depolarization of the ventricles R 波（心电图）；**S w.,** a downward deflection of the QRS complex following the R wave in the normal electrocardiogram and representing late depolarization of the ventricles S 波（心电图）；**T w.,** the deflection of the normal electrocardiogram following the QRS complex; it represents repolarization or recovery of the ventricles T 波（心电图）；**Ta w.,** a small asymmetric wave, of opposite polarity to the P wave, representing atrial repolarization; together with the P wave it defines atrial systole Ta 波，一个小的不对称波，与 P 波的极性相反，代表心房复极化；和 P 波一起表示心房电收缩周期；**theta w's,** brain waves in the electroencephalogram with a frequency of 4 to 7 per second, mainly seen in children and emotionally stressed adults θ 波，频率为每秒 4~7 次的脑电波；**U w.,** a potential undulation of unknown origin immediately following the T wave and often concealed by it; seen in the normal electrocardiogram and accentuated in tachyarrhythmias and electrolyte disturbances U 波（心电图）

wave·length (λ) (wāv′length) the distance between the top of one wave and the identical phase of the succeeding one 波长

wax (waks) a low-melting, high-molecular-weight,

organic mixture or compound, similar to fats and oils but lacking glycerides; it may be deposited by insects, obtained from plants, or prepared synthetically 蜡；**dental w.,** a mixture of two or more waxes with other additives, used in dentistry for casts, construction of nonmetallic denture bases, registering of jaw relations, and laboratory work 牙蜡；**ear w.,** cerumen 耳垢，耵聍；**white w.,** bleached beeswax; bleached, purified wax from the honeycomb of the bee, *Apis mellifera;* used as a pharmaceutical stiffening agent 白蜡；**yellow w.,** beeswax; purified wax from the honeycomb of the bee, *Apis mellifera;* used as a pharmaceutical stiffening agent 黄蜡

wax·ing (wak′sing) the shaping of a wax pattern or the wax base of a trial denture into the contours desired 上蜡，蜡模形成

waxy (wak′se) 1. composed of or covered by wax 蜡的；2. resembling wax, especially denoting some combination of pliability, paleness, and smoothness and luster 蜡状的

Wb legend weber

WBC white blood cell 白细胞；参见 *leukocyte*

wean (wēn) to discontinue breast feeding and substitute other feeding habits 断奶

wean·ling (wēn′ling) 1. recently weaned 刚断奶的；2. a recently weaned infant 刚断奶的婴儿（或幼畜）

web (web) a tissue or membrane 蛛网状组织；蹼；**larynge w.,** a web spread between the vocal folds near the anterior commissure; the most common congenital malformation of the larynx 喉蹼；**terminal w.,** a feltwork of fine filaments in the cytoplasm immediately beneath the free surface of certain epithelial cells; it is thought to have a supportive or cytoskeletal function 终末网

webbed (webd) connected by a membrane 有蹼的

web·er (Wb) (web′ər) the SI unit of magnetic flux which, linking a circuit of one turn, produces in it an electromotive force of 1 volt as it is reduced to zero at a uniform rate in 1 second 韦伯，磁通量单位

wedge (wej) 1. a piece of material thick at one end and tapering to a thin edge at the oth er end 楔形物；2. to force something into a space of limited size 楔入；**step w.,** a block of absorber, usually aluminum, machined in steps of increasing thickness, used to measure the penetrating power of x-rays 楔形梯级，楔形梯级式（X线）透度计，用以测量 X 线的透度

WEE western equine encephalomyelitis 西方马脑炎

weep (wēp) 1. to shed tears 流泪；2. to ooze serum 渗出（血清）

weight (wāt) 1. heaviness; the degree to which a body is drawn toward the earth by gravity. See table

at *weight.* Abbreviated wt 重量；2. in statistics, the process of assigning greater importance to some observations than to others, or a mathematical factor used to apply such a process（统计中的）权；**apothecaries' w.,** a system of weights used in compounding prescriptions, based on the grain (64.8 mg). Its units are the scruple (20 grains), dram (3 scruples), ounce (8 drams), and pound (12 ounces) 药用衡量；**atomic w. (at wt),** the sum of the masses of the constituents of an atom; it can be expressed in atomic mass units, in SI units, or as a dimensionless ratio based on its value relative to the 12C isotope of carbon, defined as 12.00000 原子量；**avoirdupois w.,** the system of weight commonly used for ordinary commodities in English-speaking countries; its units are the grain, dram (27.344 grains), ounce (16 drams), and pound (16 ounces) 常衡制（英制）**equivalent w.,** the amount of a substance that combines with or displaces 8.0 g of oxygen (or 1.008 g of hydrogen); it is the ratio of the molecular weight to the number of protons (acid/base reactions) or electrons (redox reactions) involved in the reaction 当量；**molecular w. (MW) (Mol wt),** the weight of a molecule of a substance as compared with that of an atom of carbon-12; it is equal to the sum of the atomic weights of its constituent atoms and is dimensionless. Although widely used, it is not technically correct; relative molecular mass *(Mr)* is preferable 分子量

wen (wen) 1. a sebaceous or epidermal inclusion cyst 表皮囊肿；2. pilar cyst 粉瘤，皮脂腺囊肿

wheal (hwēl) (wēl) the typical lesion of urticaria, a localized, usually temporary area of edema on the body surface, often accompanied by severe itching 风团

wheeze (hw ē z) a whistling type of continuous sound 哮鸣音

whip·lash (hwip′lash) 鞭打式损伤，参见 *injury* 下词条

whip·worm (hwip′wurm″) any nematode of the genus *Trichuris* 毛首鞭虫

white·head (hwīt′hed) 1. milium 粟粒疹；2. closed comedo 黑头粉刺

whit·low (hwit′lo) a purulent infection involving the pulp of the distal phalanx of a finger 瘭疽，化脓性指头炎；**herpetic w.,** cutaneous herpes simplex on the terminal segment of a finger, resulting in formation of deep coalescing vesicles with tissue destruction 疱疹性瘭疽；**melanotic w.,** subungual melanoma 黑变性瘭疽

WHO World Health Organization, an international agency associated with the United Nations and based in Geneva 世界卫生组织

W

whoop (hōop) the sonorous and convulsive inhalation of whooping cough 哮咳，吼声

wild-type (wīld'tīp″) typical of a natural population or standard laboratory stock 野生型，参见 *type* 下词条

wil·low (wil'o) any plant of the genus *Salix*. White willow bark (q.v.) contains a precursor of salicylic acid and is used as an herbal remedy 柳

WIN Western Institute of Nursing 西方护理学院

win·dow (win'do) 1. a circumscribed opening in a plane surface 窗 口；2. the voltage limits that determine which pulses will be allowed to pass on 窗口（技术），确定允许哪些脉冲传递的电压限 制；**aortic w.,** a transparent region below the aortic arch, formed by the bifurcation of the trachea, visible in the left anterior oblique radiograph of the heart and great vessels 主动脉窗；**oval w.,** fenestra vestibuli; an opening in the inner wall of the middle ear, closed by the base of the stapes 卵圆窗，前庭窗；**round w.,** fenestra cochleae; an opening in the inner wall of the middle ear covered by the secondary tympanic membrane 圆窗，蜗窗

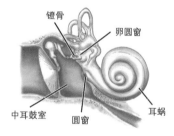

镫骨
卵圆窗
中耳鼓室　圆窗　耳蜗

wind·pipe (wind'pīp) the trachea 气管

wink·ing (wingk'ing) quick opening and closing of the eyelids 瞬目，眨眼；**jaw w.,** Gunn syndrome 颌动瞬目

wire (wīr) a slender, elongated, flexible structure of metal 丝，金属线；**Kirschner w.,** a steel wire for skeletal transfixion of fractured bones and for obtaining skeletal traction in fractures 克氏针，克氏钢丝

witch ha·zel (wich' ha'zəl) the deciduous bush *Hamamelis virginiana* or any of various preparations of its twigs, leaves, or bark, which are used topically for their astringent effects and also have various uses in folk medicine and in homeopathy 北美金缕梅

with·draw·al (with-draw'əl) 1. pathologic retreat from interpersonal contact and social involvement （病理性）退隐；2. 同 substance w.；**substance w.,** a substance-specific mental disorder that follows

the cessation of use or reduction in intake of a psychoactive substance that had been regularly used to induce a state of intoxication 物质戒断

wob·ble (wob'əl) to move unsteadily or unsurely back and forth or from side to side （使）摇摆，参见 *hypothesis* 下词条

Wohl·fahr·tia (vōl-fahr'te-ə) a genus of flies. The larvae of *W. magnif'ica* produce wound myiasis; those of *W. o'paca* and *W. vig'il* cause cutaneous myiasis 污蝇属

Wol·bach·ia (wol-bak'e-ə) a genus of bacteria of the family Anaplasmataceae; organisms are symbionts in a wide variety of invertebrates, including nematodes such as *Onchocerca*, and play a major role in the clinical manifestations of filariasis 沃尔巴克氏体属

wolfs·bane (woolfs'bān) 1. arnica 山金车花；2. aconite 欧乌头

word sal·ad (wurd' sal'əd) a meaningless mixture of words and phrases characteristic of advanced schizophrenia 言语杂乱

work-up (wurk'əp) the procedures done to arrive at a diagnosis, including history taking, laboratory tests, x-rays, and so on 检查，身体检查，病情检查，诊断疾病进行的程序，包括病史询问，化验检查，X 射线等

worm (wurm) any of the soft-bodied, naked, elongated invertebrates of the phyla Annelida, Acanthocephala, Aschelminthes, and Platyhelminthes 虫，蠕虫；**flat w.,** any of the Platyhelminthes 扁虫，扁形动物；**guinea w.,** *Dracunculus medinensis* 麦地那龙线虫；**heart w.,** heartworm 犬恶丝虫；**round w.,** nematode 线虫；**spinyheaded w., thorny-headed w.,** an individual of the phylum Acanthocephala 棘头虫

worm·wood (wurm'wood″) a plant of the genus *Artemisia*, especially *A. absinthium* (common wormwood), which is used to make the liqueur absinthe 苦艾

wound (woond) trauma; an injury, usually restricted to a physical one with disruption of normal continuity of structures 伤口；**contused w.,** one in which the skin is unbroken 挫伤；**incised w.,** one caused by a cutting instrument 刀伤，割伤；**lacerated w.,** one in which the tissues are torn 撕裂伤，裂伤；**open w.,** one having a free outward opening 开放性创伤；**penetrating w.,** one caused by a sharp, usually slender object, which passes through the skin into the underlying tissues 贯通创伤；**perforating w.,** a penetrating wound that extends into a viscus or body cavity 穿创伤；**puncture w.,** penetrating w. 刺伤

wrin·kle (ring'kəl) a furrow or fold in the skin or a

Measures of Mass 物质质量

Metric and Avoirdupois 公制和常衡制

Kilogram 千克	Gram 克	Milligram 毫克	Grain 格令	Dram 打兰	Ounce 盎司	Pound 磅
1	1000	1.0×10^6	1.5432×10^4	564.3776	35.2736	2.2046
0.001	1	1000	15.432	0.5644	0.0353	0.002205
1.0×10^{-6}	0.001	1	0.0154	5.6438×10^{-4}	3.53×10^{-5}	2.2046×10^{-6}
6.48×10^{-5}	0.0648	64.8	1	0.0366	0.0023	1.4×10^{-4}
0.0018	1.772	1771.632	27.34	1	0.0625	0.0039
0.0284	28.350	2.8350×10^4	437.5	16	1	0.0625
0.4536	453.5924	4.536×10^5	7000	256	16	1

Metric and Apothecary* 公制和药衡制

Kilogram 千克	Gram 克	Milligram 毫克	Grain 格令	Scruples（Э）吩	Dram（Z）打兰	Ounces（ж）盎司	Pounds（£）磅
1	1000	1.0×10^6	1.5432×10^4	771.6049	257.2016	32.1512	2.6792
0.001	1	1000	15.4324	0.7716	0.2572	0.03215	0.002679
1.0×10^{-6}	0.001	1	0.0154	7.7160×10^{-4}	2.5720×10^{-4}	3.2151×10^{-5}	2.6792×10^{-6}

W

（续表）

Metric and Apothecary* 公制和药衡制

Kilogram 千克	Gram 克	Milligram 毫克	Grain 格令	Scruples (ɔ) 吩	Dram (Z) 打兰	Ounces (ʓ) 盎司	Pounds (£) 磅
6.48×10^{-5}	0.0648	64.8	1	0.05	0.0167	0.0021	1.7×10^{-4}
0.001296	1.296	1296	20	1	0.333	0.042	0.0035
0.003888	3.888	3888	60	3	1	0.125	0.0104
0.03110	31.103	31.103×10^{4}	480	24	8	1	0.0833
0.3732	373.2418	3.73×10^{4}	5760	288	96	12	1

Metric and Troy 公制和金衡制

Gram 克	Grain 格令	Ounce 盎司	Pound 磅
1	15.4324	0.03215	0.002679
1.0648	1	0.002	0.00017
31.103	480	1	0.083
373.2418	5760	12	1

*联合委员会规定使用公制单位而不是药衡制单位

Measures of Fluid Capacity 流体度量

Metric and Apothecary* 公制和药衡制

Liter 升	Deciliter 分升	Milliliter 毫升	Minim 量滴	Fluid Dram 量打兰	Fluid Ounce 量盎司	Pint 品脱	Quart 夸脱	Gallon (US) 加仑（美国）
1	10	1000	1.623×10^4	270.5	33.8	2.113	1.056	0.2641
0.1	1	100	1623	27.05	3.38	0.2113	0.1056	0.0264
0.001	0.01	1	16.23	0.2705	0.0338	0.002113	0.001056	2.6406×10^{-4}
6.161×10^{-5}	6.161×10^{-4}	0.06161	1	0.0166	0.002	1.302×10^{-4}	6.51×10^{-5}	1.628×10^{-5}
0.003697	0.03697	3.6967	60	1	0.125	0.0078	0.0039	9.7656×10^{-5}
0.02957	0.2957	29.5737	480	8	1	0.0625	0.0312	0.0078
0.4731	4.7318	473.179	7680	128	16	1	0.5	0.125
0.9464	9.4636	946.358	1.536×10^4	256	32	2	1	0.25
3.7854	37.8543	3785.434	6.1440×10^4	1024	128	8	4	1

Approximate Household Equivalents 近似家庭对应值

Drop 滴	Minim 量滴	Teaspoon 调羹	Tablespoon 汤勺	Fluid Ounce 量盎司	Cup (or Glasse) 杯（或玻璃杯）§	Milliliter 毫升
1	1	1/60	—	—	—	0.06161
60	60	1	1/3	1/8	—	5
180	180	3	1	1/2	1/16	15
—	—	48	16	8	1	240

* 联合委员会规定使用公制单位而不是药衡制单位

§ 家用玻璃杯或玻璃杯被认为相当于一个（8盎司）杯子

W

Measures of Length 长度度量

Micrometer 微米	Millimeter 毫米	Centimeter 分米	Meter 米	Kilometer 千米	Inche 英寸	Feet 英尺	Yard 码	Mile 米
1	0.001	1.0×10^{-4}	1.0×10^{-6}	1.0×10^{-9}	3.937×10^{-5}	3.281×10^{-6}	1.0936×10^{-6}	—
1.0×10^{3}	1	1.0×10^{-1}	1.0×10^{-3}	1.0×10^{-6}	0.03937	0.003281	0.001094	6.2137×10^{-7}
1.0×10^{4}	10	1	1.0×10^{-2}	1.0×10^{-5}	0.3937	0.03281	0.01094	6.2137×10^{-6}
1.0×10^{6}	1000	100	1	0.001	39.37	3.2808	1.0936	6.2137×10^{-4}
1.0×10^{9}	1.0×10^{6}	1.0×10^{5}	1000	1	3.937×10^{4}	3280.84	1093.6121	0.6214
1.0×10^{10}	1.0×10^{7}	1.0×10^{6}	1.0×10^{4}	10	3.937×10^{5}	3.281×10^{4}	1.0936×10^{4}	6.2137
2.54×10^{4}	25.4	2.54	0.0254	2.54×10^{-5}	1	0.08333	0.02778	1.5783×10^{-5}
3.048×10^{5}	304.8	30.48	0.3048	3.048×10^{-4}	12	1	0.3333	1.8939×10^{-4}
9.144×10^{5}	914.4	91.44	0.9144	9.144×10^{-4}	36	3.0	1	5.6818×10^{-4}
1.6093×10^{9}	1.6093×10^{6}	1.6093×10^{5}	1609.34	1.6093	6.336×10^{4}	5280	1760	1

W

mucous membrane 皱纹

Wrist (rist) the region of the joint between the forearm and hand; the carpus 腕；腕节

wrist·drop (rist′drop) a condition resulting from paralysis of the extensor muscles of the hand and fingers 腕下垂

wry (ri) abnormally twisted; bent to one side; crooked or contorted 扭曲，扭歪；扭曲的

wry·neck (ri′neck) torticollis (def. 1) 斜颈

wt weight 重量

Wu·cher·e·ria (voo″kər-er′e-ə) a genus of nematodes of the superfamily Filarioidea that affect mainly humans in warmer regions of the world. *W. bancrof′ti* causes elephantiasis, lymphangitis, and chyluria by interfering with the lymphatic circulation 吴策线虫属

wu·cher·e·ri·a·sis (voo-ker″e-ri′ə-sis) infestation with species of Wuchereria 吴策线虫病

w/v weight (of solute) per volume (of solvent) 重 / 容（溶质重量与溶剂重量比）

X

X[符号] xanthine or xanthosine 黄嘌呤或黄（嘌呤核）苷

x[符号] abscissa 横坐标

xan·thel·as·ma (zan″thəl-az′mə) a common type of planar xanthoma on an eyelid 黄斑瘤

xan·thic (zan′thik) 1. yellow 黄色的；2. pertaining to xanthine 黄嘌呤的

xan·thine (X) (zan′thēn) a purine base found in most body tissues and fluids, certain plants, and some urinary calculi; it is an intermediate in the degradation of AMP to uric acid. Methylated xanthine compounds (e.g., caffeine, theobromine, theophylline) are used for their bronchodilator effect 黄嘌呤

xan·thine ox·i·dase (zan′thēn ok′sī-dās) a flavoprotein enzyme that catalyzes the oxidation of hypoxanthine to xanthine and then to uric acid, the final steps in the degradation of purines; deficiency, an autosomal recessive trait, causes xanthinuria 黄嘌呤氧化酶

xan·thin·uria (zan″thin-u′re-ə) any of several disorders of purine metabolism in which deficiency of xanthine dehydrogenase (XDH) activity, due to a defect either in the enzyme or in a factor necessary for enzyme activity, results in urinary secretion of excessive xanthine and a tendency to formation of xanthine calculi in the urinary tract 黄嘌呤尿

xan·tho·chro·mat·ic (zan″tho-kro-mat′ik) yellow-colored 黄色的；黄变的

xan·tho·chro·mia (zan″tho-kro′me-ə) yellowish discoloration, as of the skin or spinal fluid 黄变（皮肤或脊液）

xan·tho·chro·mic (zan″tho-kro′mik) having a yellow discoloration; said of cerebrospinal fluid 黄变的；黄色的（专指脑脊液）

xan·tho·der·ma (zan″tho-der′mə) any yellowish discoloration of the skin 黄肤，皮肤变黄

xan·tho·gran·u·lo·ma (zan″tho-gran″u-lo′mə) a tumor having histologic characteristics of both granuloma and xanthoma 黄肉芽肿；**juvenile x.**, a benign, self-limited skin tumor of infants and children, with a nodule or nodules on the scalp, face, proximal limb, or trunk, sometimes with involvement of mucous membranes, viscera, the eye, and other organs 幼年黄色肉芽肿

xan·tho·ma (zan-tho′mə) a tumor composed of lipid-laden foam cells, which are histiocytes containing cytoplasmic lipid material 黄（色）瘤；**diabetic x., eruptive x.**, a form marked by sudden eruption of crops of small, yellow or yellowish orange papules encircled by an erythematous halo, especially on the buttocks, posterior thighs, and elbows, and caused by high concentrations of plasma triglycerides, especially those associated with uncontrolled diabetes mellitus 糖尿病性黄瘤，出疹性黄瘤；**fibrous x.**, benign fibrous histiocytoma 纤维性黄瘤，良性纤维组织细胞瘤；**plane x., x. pla′num**, a form manifested as soft, yellow to dark red, flat macules or plaques, sometimes with a central white area; they may be localized or generalized and are often associated with other xanthomas and certain hyperlipoproteinemias 扁平黄瘤；**x. tendino′sum, tendinous x.**, a form manifested by free movable papules or nodules in the tendons, ligaments, fascia, and periosteum, especially on the backs of the hands, fingers, elbows, knees, and heels, in association with some hyperlipoproteinemias and certain other xanthomas 腱黄（色）瘤；**x. tubero′sum, tuberous x.**, a form manifested by groups of flat, or elevated and rounded, yellow to orange nodules on the skin over joints, especially on elbows and knees; it may be associated with certain types of hyperlipoproteinemia, biliary cirrhosis, and myxedema 结节性黄瘤

▲ 黄斑瘤

xan·tho·ma·to·sis (zan″tho-mə-to′sis) a condition marked by the presence of xanthomas 黄瘤病，黄脂增生病；**x. bul′bi**, fatty change in the cornea 眼球黄瘤，角膜脂肪变性；**cerebrotendinous x.**, an autosomal recessive disorder affecting a step in the bile synthesis pathway, with deposition of cholestanol and cholesterol in virtually all tissues. It is characterized by brain and tendon xanthomas, progressive neurodegeneration, early cataracts, and atherosclerosis 脑腱性黄瘤病

xan·tho·ma·tous (zan-tho′mə-təs) pertaining to xanthoma 黄瘤的

Xan·tho·mo·na·da·ceae (zan″tho-mo″nə- da′se-e) the sole family of the order Xanthomonadales 黄单胞菌科

Xan·tho·mo·na·da·les (zan″tho-mo″nə-da′lēz) an order of gram-negative, anaerobic, rod-shaped bacteria of the class Gammaproteobacteria 黄单胞菌目

xan·thop·sia (zan-thop′se-ə) chromatopsia in which objects are seen as yellow 黄视症

xan·tho·sine (X) (zan′tho-sēn) a nucleoside composed of xanthine and ribose 黄（嘌呤核）苷

xan·tho·sis (zan-tho′sis) yellowish discoloration; degeneration with yellowish pigmentation 黄皮症，黄变症

xanth·u·ren·ic ac·id (zanth″u-ren′ik) a bicyclic aromatic compound formed as a minor catabolite of tryptophan and present in increased amounts in urine in vitamin B_6 deficiency and some disorders of tryptophan catabolism 黄尿酸

Xe xenon 元素氙的符号

Xel·janz (zel′janz) trademark for a preparation of tofacitinib citrate; used to treat rheumatoid arthritis 枸橼酸托法替尼制剂的商品名，用于治疗类风湿关节炎

xeno·an·ti·gen (zen″o-an′tǐ-jən) an antigen occurring in organisms of more than one species 异抗原

xeno·di·ag·no·sis (zen″o-di″əg-no′sis) a method of animal inoculation using laboratorybred bugs and animals in the diagnosis of certain parasitic infections when the infecting organism cannot be demonstrated in blood films; used in Chagas disease (examination of the feces of clean bugs fed on the patient's blood) and trichinosis (examination of rats to which the patient's muscle tissue has been fed) 异体接种诊断法，宿主诊断法；**xenodiagnos′tic** *adj.*

xeno·es·tro·gen (zen″o-es′trə-jen) an environmental chemical with estrogenic actions 外源性雌激素

xeno·ge·ne·ic (zen″o-jə-ne′ik) in transplantation biology, denoting individuals or tissues from individuals of different species and hence of disparate cell type 异种

xen·og·e·nous (zen-oj′ə-nəs) caused by a foreign body, or originating outside the organism 异体的，体外性的

xeno·graft (zen′o-graft″) a graft of tissue transplanted between animals of different species; it may be *concordant*, occurring between closely related species, in which the recipient lacks natural antibodies specific for the transplanted tissue, or *discordant*, occurring between members of distantly related species, in which the recipient has natural antibodies specific for the transplanted tissue 异种移植；异种移植物

xe·non (Xe) (ze′non) a colorless, odorless, tasteless, noble gas element; at. no. 54, at. wt. 131.293. Several of its radioactive isotopes are used in imaging 氙（化学元素）

xeno·para·site (zen″o-par′ə-sīt) an organism not usually parasitic on a particular species but which becomes so because of a weakened condition of the host 异常寄生虫

xeno·pho·bia (zen″o-fo′be-ə) irrational fear of strangers 生客恐怖

xeno·pho·nia (zen″o-fo′ne-ə) alteration in the quality of the voice 音调变异

xen·oph·thal·mia (zen″of-thal′me-ə) ophthalmia caused by a foreign body in the eye 异物性眼炎

Xen·op·syl·la (zen″op-sil′ə) a genus of fleas, many species of which transmit pathogens; *X. che′opis*, the rat flea, transmits plague and murine typhus 客蚤属

xeno·tro·pic (zen″o-tro′pik) pertaining to a virus that is found benignly in cells of one animal species but that will replicate into complete virus particles only when it infects cells of a different species（病毒）异向性的，异亲的

xe·ro·der·ma (zēr″o-der′mə) a mild form of ichthyosis, marked by dry, rough, discolored skin 干皮病，皮肤干燥病；**xerodermat′ic** *adj.*；**x. pigmento′-sum**, a rare, autosomal recessive, pigmentary and atrophic condition of extreme cutaneous sensitivity to ultraviolet radiation, as a result of defects in mechanisms of repair of ultravioletdamaged DNA. It begins in childhood, with excessive freckling, telangiectases, keratomas, papillomas, and malig-

X

nancies in sun-exposed skin, severe ophthalmologic abnormalities, and sometimes neurologic disorders 着色性干皮病

xe·rog·ra·phy (ze-rog'rə-fe) xeroradiography 干板 X 线照相术

xe·ro·ma (zēr-o'mə) abnormal dryness of the conjunctiva; xerophthalmia 结膜干燥，干眼病

xe·ro·mam·mog·ra·phy (zēr″o-mə-mog′rə-fe) xeroradiography of the breast 乳房干板 X 线照相术

xe·ro·me·nia (zēr″o-me′ne-ə) the appearance of constitutional symptoms at the menstrual period without any flow of blood 干经，干性月经

xe·roph·thal·mia (zēr″of-thal′me-ə) abnormal dryness and thickening of the conjunctiva and cornea due to vitamin A deficiency 眼干燥症

xe·ro·ra·di·og·ra·phy (zēr″o-ra″de-og′rə-fe) the making of radiographs by a dry, totally photoelectric process, using metal plates coated with a semiconductor, such as selenium 干板 X 线照相术

xe·ro·si·a·log·ra·phy (zēr″o-si″ə-log′rə-fe) sialography in which the images are recorded by xerography 干板涎管 X 线造影术

xe·ro·sis (zēr-o′sis) abnormal dryness, as of the eye, skin, or mouth 干燥病，出现于眼、皮肤、口腔的异常干燥现象；**xerot′ic** *adj.*

xe·ro·sto·mia (zēr″o-sto′me-ə) dryness of the mouth due to salivary gland dysfunction 口腔干燥（症）

xe·rot·ic (zēr-ot′ik) characterized by xerosis or dryness 干燥病的

xe·ro·to·mog·ra·phy (zēr″o-tə-mog′rə-fe) tomography in which the images are recorded by xeroradiography 干板 X 线断层照相术

Xii·dra (zī′druh) trademark for a lifitegrast ophthalmic solution; administered as drops to treat dry eye disease lifitegrast 滴眼液的商品名，用于治疗干眼症

xipho·cos·tal (zi″fo-) (zif″o-kos′təl) pertaining to the xiphoid process and ribs 剑突肋骨的

xiph·oid (zif′oid) (zi′foid) 1. ensiform; swordshaped 剑状的；2. xiphoid process 剑突

xiph·oi·di·tis (zi″foi-) (zif″oi-di′tis) inflammation of the xiphoid process 剑突炎

xi·phop·a·gus (zi-fop′-) (zī-fop′ə-gəs) symmetric conjoined twins fused in the region of the xiphoid process 剑突联胎

X-linked (eks′linkt) carried on the X chromosome, as an X-linked gene; by extension, determined by such a gene, as an X-linked trait or X-linked inheritance 伴性的，X 连锁的

XO symbol for the presence of only one X chromosome, the other X or the Y chromosome being absent XO 型，表示只有一个性染色体，而缺乏另一个 X 和 Y 染色体

x-ray (eks′ra) X 射线，参见 ray 下词条

xy·lan (zi′lan) any of a group of pentosans composed of xylose residues; major structural constituents of wood, straw, and bran 木聚糖

xy·lene (zi′lēn) 二甲苯 1. dimethylbenzene; any of three isomeric hydrocarbons, $C_6H_4(CH_3)_2$, from methyl alcohol or coal tar 二甲苯；2. a mixture of all three isomers, with uses such as solvent, clarifier, or protective coating, and in various syntheses 一组苯系烃

xy·li·tol (zi′lĭ-tol) a 5-carbon sugar alcohol derived from xylose and as sweet as sucrose; used as a non-cariogenic sweetener and also as a sugar substitute in diabetic diets 木糖醇

Xy·lo·caine (zi′lo-kān) trademark for preparations of lidocaine 利多卡因的商品名

xy·lo·met·a·zo·line (zi″lo-met″ə-zo′lēn) an adrenergic used as the hydrochloride salt as a topical nasal decongestant 丁苄唑啉，一种肾上腺素能药，局部用作血管收缩药以减轻鼻黏膜充血

xy·lose (zi′lōs) a pentose found in plants in the form of xylans; it is used in a diagnostic test of intestinal absorption 木糖

xy·lu·lose (zi′lu-lōs) a pentose epimeric with ribulose, occurring naturally as both l- and d-isomers. The latter is excreted in the urine in essential pentosuria; the former, in phosphorylated form, is an intermediate in the pentose phosphate pathway 木酮糖

xys·ma (zis′mə) material resembling bits of membrane in stools of diarrhea 絮片，假膜片（见于腹泻粪便中）

xys·ter (zis′tər) rasp (1) 刮骨刀，刮器，骨刮

Xy·zal (zī′zəl) trademark for a preparation of levocetirizine dihydrochloride 左西替利嗪二盐酸盐

Y[符号]tyrosine 酪氨酸；yttrium 钇

y[符号]ordinate 纵坐标

yang (yang) [Chinese] in Chinese philosophy, the active, positive, masculine principle that is complementary to yin 阳，参见 *principle* 下 *yin/yang*

principle

yar·row (yar′o) 1. any of several plants of the genus *Achillea*, especially *A. millefolium*. 蓍草属；2. a preparation of the above-ground parts of *A. millefolium*, used for anorexia and dyspepsia and for liver and gallbladder complaints; also used in homeopathy 蓍草，地上部分用于厌食和消化不良，用于治疗肝脏和胆囊，也用于顺势疗法

yaw (yaw) a lesion of yaws 雅司疹；**mother y.**, the initial cutaneous lesion of yaws 初发雅思疹，雅思母疹

yaws (yawz) an endemic infectious tropical disease caused by *Treponema pertenue,* usually affecting persons under 15 years of age, spread by direct contact with skin lesions or by contaminated fomites. It is initially manifested by the appearance of a papilloma at the site of inoculation; this heals, leaving a scar, and is followed by crops of generalized granulomatous lesions that may relapse repeatedly. There may be bone and joint involvement 雅司病

Yb ytterbium 元素镱的符号

yeast (yēst) a unicellular fungus that reproduces by budding; the term describes a growth form that in some organisms shifts to a mycelial stage under certain environmental conditions or as part of the life cycle, and in others always remains unicellular. Some are pathogenic for humans 酵母菌；**dried y.**, dried cells of any suitable strain of *Saccharomyces cerevisiae,* usually a byproduct of the brewing industry; used as a natural source of protein and B-complex vitamins 干酵母

yel·low (yel′o) 1. a color between orange and green, produced by energy of wavelengths between 570 and 590nm 黄色；2. a dye or stain with this color 黄色染料

Yer·sin·ia (yǝr-sin′e-ǝ) a genus of gram-negative, nonmotile, ovoid or rod-shaped bacteria of the family Enterobacteriaceae 耶尔森菌属，肠杆菌科中的一属，兼性厌氧革兰阴性菌，形态从杆状到卵圆形；*Y. enterocoli′tica,* a ubiquitous species that causes acute gastroenteritis and mesenteric lymphadenitis in children and arthritis, septicemia, and erythema nodosum in adults 小肠结肠炎耶尔森菌，引起儿童急性肠胃炎和肠系膜淋巴结炎以及成年人关节炎、败血症和结节性红斑；*Y. pes′tis,* a species that causes plague in humans and rodents, transmitted from rats to humans by the rat flea, and from person to person by the human body louse 鼠疫耶尔森菌，一种引起瘟疫的病原体，在人类和啮齿动物中存在，鼠蚤在鼠间传播并从鼠类传播到人类，经体虱在人与人之间传播；*Y. pseudotuberculo′sis,* a species that causes disease in rodents and mesenteric lymphadenitis in humans 假结核耶尔森菌，一种导致啮齿动物疾病和人类肠系膜淋巴结炎的致病菌

yin (yin) [Chinese] in Chinese philosophy, the passive, negative, feminine principle that is complementary to yang 阴，参见 *principle* 下 *yin/yang*

principle

Y-linked (wi′linkt) carried on the Y chromosome, as is a Y-linked gene; by extension, determined by such a gene, as is a Y-linked trait or Y-linked inheritance Y 连锁的 **yo·ga** (yo′gǝ) [Sanskrit] an ancient system of Indian philosophy incorporated into the ayurvedic system of medicine and well-being, whose goal is the attainment of ultimate balance of mind and body, or self-realization. The different systems of yoga all share certain basic principles: control of the body through correct posture and breathing, control of the emotions and mind, and meditation. In the West, yoga is often used for healing and well-being without attention to the larger philosophy 瑜伽 **ashtanga y.**, a physically demanding style, based in hatha yoga, in which breathing is synchronized with movement between asanas (postures); it encourages profuse sweating to purify and detoxify and it produces strength, flexibility, and stamina ashtanga 瑜伽；**hatha y.**, a path of yoga based on physical purification and strengthening as a means of self-transformation. It encompasses a system of asanas (postures) designed to promote mental and physical wellbeing and to allow the mind to focus and become free from distraction for long periods of meditation, along with pranayama (breath control) hatha 瑜伽；**Iyengar y.**, a style, based in hatha yoga, that emphasizes correct body alignment in the asanas (postures) and holding the asanas for extended periods of time, using props to help achieve and support them Iyenger 瑜伽；**kundalini y.**, a style, based in hatha yoga, whose purpose is controlled release of latent kundalini energy kundalini 瑜伽

yo·him·bine (yo-him′bēn) an alkaloid chemically similar to reserpine, from the bark of the yohimbe tree; it possesses alpha-adrenergic blocking properties and is used as the hydrochloride salt as a sympatholytic and mydriatic, and for the treatment of impotence 育亨宾碱（具有肾上腺素能阻滞作用，用于治疗动脉硬化和心绞痛）

yoke (yōk) 1. a connecting structure 轭；2. jugum 隆突

yoked (yōkt) joined together, and so acting in concert 轭的

yolk (yōk) the stored nutrient of an oocyte or ovum 卵黄

yt·ter·bi·um (Yb) (ǐ-tur′be-ǝm) a soft, heavy, ductile, silvery white, rare earth element; at. no. 70, at. wt. 173.054 镱（化学元素）

yt·tri·um (Y) (ǐ′tre-ǝm) a ductile, silvery, rare earth element; at. no. 39, at. wt. 88.906. The radioisotope 90Y emits high-energy beta particles, localizes predominantly in bone, and has been used in radiotherapy 钇（化学元素）

Y

Z

Z [符号] atomic number 原子序数; impedance 阻抗

za·fr·lu·kast (zə-fir′loo-kast) a leukotriene receptor antagonist used as an antiasthmatic agent 一种用作平喘药的白三烯受体拮抗药

zal·ci·ta·bine (zal-si′tə-bēn) 2′3′-dideoxycytidine, an antiretroviral agent that inhibits the action of reverse transcriptase; used in the treatment of HIV infection 扎西他滨

zal·e·plon (zal′ə-plon) a nonbenzodiazepine sedative and hypnotic used in the short-term treatment of insomnia 扎来普隆

za·nam·i·vir (zə-nam′ĭ-vir) an inhibitor of viral neuraminidase used for the prophylaxis and treatment of influenza A and B 扎那米韦

ze·ro (ze′ro) 1. the absence of all quantity or magnitude; naught 零; 2. the point on a thermometer scale at which the graduation begins; the ice point on the Celsius scale and 32° below the ice point on the Fahrenheit scale 零度; **absolute z.**, the lowest possible temperature, designated as 0 on the Kelvin or Rankine scale; the equivalent of −273.15℃ or −459.67℉ 绝对零度（相当于 −273.15℃ 或 −459.67℉）

zi·do·vu·dine (zi-do′vu-dēn) a synthetic nucleoside (thymidine) analogue that inhibits replication of some retroviruses, including the human immunodeficiency virus; used in the treatment of HIV infection and AIDS 齐多夫定，叠氮胸苷，一种合成核苷（胸苷）类似物，抑制一些逆转录病毒（包括人类免疫缺陷病毒）的复制，用于治疗艾滋病毒感染和艾滋病

ZIFT zygote intrafallopian transfer 输卵管内合子移植术

zi·leu·ton (zi-loo′ton) an inhibitor of leukotriene formation, used as an antiasthmatic 齐留通（平喘药）

zinc (Zn) (zingk) a blue-white metallic element; at. no. 30, at. wt. 65.38; it is an essential micronutrient present in many enzymes but is toxic on excessive exposure, as by ingestion or inhalation *(e.g., metal fume fever)* 锌（化学元素）; **z. acetate**, an astringent and styptic 醋酸锌，一种收敛药和止血药; **z. chloride**, a salt used as a nutritional supplement in total parenteral nutrition and applied topically as an astringent and a desensitizer for dentin 氯化锌，全胃肠外营养中用作补充剂的一种盐，局部应用作为收敛药和牙本质的脱敏药; **z. oxide**, a topical astringent, protectant, and sunscreen 氧化锌，可作为收敛药，保护剂和防晒剂; **z. sulfate**, a topical astringent for mucous membranes, especially those of the eye 硫酸锌，黏膜的局部收敛药，特别是眼黏膜; **z. undecylenate**, the zinc salt of undecylenic acid; it is a topical antifungal 十一烯酸锌（抗真菌药）

Zi·op·tan (zī′opt-ən) trademark for a preparation of tafluprost ophthalmic solution 他氟前列腺素滴眼药的商品名

zi·pra·si·done (zī-pras′ĭ-dōn) an antipsychotic used as the hydrochloride salt in the treatment of schizophrenia 一种抗精神病药其盐酸盐用于治疗精神分裂症

zir·co·ni·um (Zr) (zir-ko′ne-əm) a lustrous, gray-white, transition metal element; at. no. 40, at. wt. 91.224; exposure can cause lung and skin granulomas 锆（化学元素）

Zn zinc 元素锌的符号

zo·an·thro·py (zo-an′thro-pe) delusion that one has become an animal 变兽妄想，妄想一个人变成了动物; **zoanthrop′ic** adj.

zo·le·dron·ic ac·id (zo′lə-dron″ik) a bisphosphonate inhibitor of osteoclastic bone resorption, used for the treatment of hypercalcemia of malignancy, multiple myeloma, bone metastases, and osteitis deformans 唑来膦酸，一种破骨细胞骨吸收的双膦酸盐抑制药，用于治疗高钙血症、恶性肿瘤、多发性骨髓瘤、骨转移和变形性骨炎

zol·mi·trip·tan (zōl″mĭ-trip′tan) a selective serotonin receptor agonist used to relieve acute migraine 佐米曲普坦，一种选择性 5- 羟色胺受体激动药，用于缓解急性胰腺炎、偏头痛

zol·pi·dem (zōl-pi′dem) a nonbenzodiazepine sedative-hypnotic; used as the tartrate salt in the short-term treatment of insomnia 非苯二氮䓬类镇静催眠药；其酒石酸盐用于短期治疗失眠药

zo·na (zo′nə) pl. *zo′nae* [L.] zone 区、带; **z. arcua′ta**, inner tunnel 弓状带; **z. cilia′ris**, ciliary zone 睫状区; **z. denticula′ta**, the inner zone of the lamina basilaris of the cochlear duct with the limbus of the osseous spiral lamina 齿状带; **z. fascicula′ta**, the thick middle layer of the adrenal cortex （肾上腺皮质）束状带; **z. glomerulo′sa**, the thin outermost layer of the adrenal cortex （肾上腺皮质）球状带; **z. incer′ta**, a narrow band of gray matter between the subthalamic nucleus and thalamic fasciculus 未定带; **z. orbicularis of hip joint**, a ring around the neck of the femur formed by circular fibers of the joint capsule of the hip joint 髋关节轮匝带; **z. pectina′ta**, the outer part

Y

of the lamina basilaris of the cochlear duct running from the rods of Corti to the spiral ligament 梳状带；**z. pellu′cida,** the transparent, noncellular secreted layer surrounding an oocyte 透明带；**z. perfora′ta,** the inner portion of the lamina basilaris of the cochlear duct 穿孔带；**z. reticula′ris,** the innermost layer of the adrenal cortex（肾上腺皮质）网状带

zone (zōn) an encircling region or area; by extension, any area with specific characteristics or a specific boundary 带，区；区域；范围；界；**zo′nal** *adj.*; **border z.,** a zone at the boundary of two contiguous structures, such as that where the trophoblast and the endometrium meet 缘 带；**ciliary z.,** the outer of the two regions into which the anterior surface of the iris is divided by the collarette 睫状区；**comfort z.,** an environmental temperature between 13℃ and 21℃ (55°–70℉) with a humidity of 30 to 55 percent 舒适带；**epileptogenic z.,** 致痫区，参见 *focus* 下词条；**erogenous z., erotogenic z.,** an area of the body whose stimulation produces erotic excitation 性欲发生区；**hemorrhoidal z.,** that part of the anal canal extending from the anal valves to the anus and containing the rectal venous plexus 痔区；**inner z. of renal medulla,** the part of the medulla farthest in from the cortex, containing ascending and descending limbs of the thin tubule as well as the inner part of the medullary collecting duct 肾髓质内带；**Lissauer marginal z.,** a bridge of white substance between the apex of the posterior horn and the periphery of the spinal cord Lissauer 边缘区；**mantle z.,** 1. 套层，参见 *layer* 下词条；2. a dense area of lymphocytes encircling a germinal center 外套层，包围生发中心的淋巴细胞密集区；**marginal z.,** 1. 同 border z.；2. 边缘层，参见 layer 下词条；3. a loosely packed region of T and B lymphocytes and macrophages encircling periarterial lymphatic sheaths in the spleen 边缘区脾内围绕动脉周围淋巴鞘的 T 淋巴细胞和 B 淋巴细胞及巨噬细胞的松散区域；**outer z. of renal medulla,** the part of the medulla nearest to the cortex; containing the medullary part of the distal straight tubule as well as the outer part of the medullary collecting duct 肾髓质外带；**z.of partial preservation,** in spinal cord injury, a region where there may be only partial damage to nerves, including one to three spinal segments below the level of the injury 局部保留区；**pellucid z.,** zona pellucida 透明带；**pupillary z.,** the inner of the two regions into which the anterior surface of the iris is divided by the collarette 瞳孔区；**transitional z.,** any anatomic region that marks the point at which the constituents of a structure change from one type to another 过渡区，移行带

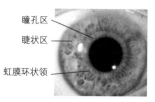

瞳孔区
睫状区
虹膜环状领

zo·nes·the·sia (zo″nes-the′zhə) a dysesthesia consisting of a sensation of constriction, as by a girdle 束带感，束勒感

zo·nif·u·gal (zo-nif′ə-gəl) passing outward from a zone or region 离区的，远区的

zo·nip·e·tal (zo-nip′ə-təl) passing toward a zone or region 向区的

zo·nis·a·mide (zo-nis′ə-mīd″) a sulfonamide that acts as an anticonvulsant, used in the treatment of partial seizures in adults 唑尼沙胺，一种磺胺类抗惊厥药，用于治疗成人部分性癫痫发作

zo·nog·ra·phy (zo-nog′rə-fe) a type of tomography that has a particularly thick area of focus, resulting in thicker sections for examination 厚层断层摄影术

zo·nu·la (zo′nu-lə) pl. **zo′nulae** [L.] zonule 小带

zo·nule (zo′nūl) a small zone 小带；**zon′ular** *adj.*; **ciliary z., z. of Zinn,** a system of fibers connecting the ciliary body and the equator of the lens, holding the lens in place 睫状小带

zo·nu·li·tis (zo″nu-li′tis) inflammation of the ciliary zonule 睫状小带炎

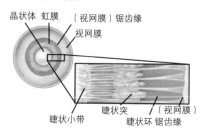

晶状体 虹膜 （视网膜）锯齿缘
视网膜
睫状小带 睫状突 （视网膜）
睫状环 锯齿缘

▲ 睫状小带

zo·nu·lol·y·sis (zo″nu-lol′ĭ-sis) dissolution of the ciliary zonule by use of enzymes to permit surgical removal of the lens 睫状小带松解法

zon·u·lot·o·my (zon″u-lot′o-me) incision of the ciliary zonule 睫状小带切开术

zoo·der·mic (zo″o-dur′mik) performed with the skin of an animal, as in skin grafting 动物皮肤的，指用动物皮肤所进行的移植

zo·og·e·nous (zo-oj′ə-nəs) 1. acquired from animals 动物原的；2. viviparous 胎生的

zo·og·o·ny (zo-og′ə-ne) the production of living

young from within the body 胎生；**zoog′onous** *adj.*

zoo·graft·ing (zo′o-graft″ing) the grafting of animal tissue 动物组织移植术

zo·oid (zo′oid) 1. animal-like 动物样的；2. an animallike object or form 动物样体；3. an individual in a united colony of animals 个体，动物群体的一个

zoo·lag·nia (zo″o-lag′ne-ə) sexual attraction toward animals 恋兽欲

zo·ol·o·gy (zo-ol′ə-je) the biology of animals 动物学

Zoo·mas·ti·go·pho·rea (zo″o-mas″tĭ-gə-for′e-ə) a class of protozoa (subphylum Mastigophora), including all the animal-like, as opposed to plantlike, protozoa 动鞭纲

zoo·no·sis (zo″o-no′sis) (zo-on′ə-sis) pl. *zoono′ses.* Disease of animals transmissible to humans under natural conditions 动物传染病，通过自然环境传染于人的动物疾病；**zoonot′ic** *adj.*

zoo·para·site (zo″o-par′ə-sīt) any parasitic animal organism or species 寄生动物；**zooparasit′ic** *adj.*

zoo·phil·ia (zo″o-fil′e-ə) 1. abnormal fondness for animals 嗜动物癖，动物爱好；2. bestiality; a paraphilia in which intercourse or other sexual activity with animals is the preferred method of achieving sexual excitement 一种性欲倒错，以同动物性交或其他性活动而获得更大性激动的嗜好

zoo·pho·bia (zo″o-fo′be-ə) irrational fear of animals 动物恐怖，恐兽症

zoo·plas·ty (zo′o-plast″te) 同 zoografting

zoo·sper·mia (zo″o-spur′me-ə) the presence of live spermatozoa in the ejaculated semen（所射精液内）活精子存在

zoo·spore (zo′o-spor) a motile, flagellated, sexual or asexual spore, as produced by certain algae, fungi, and protozoa 游动孢子

zoo·tox·in (zo′o-tok″sin) a toxic substance of animal origin, e.g., venom of snakes, spiders, and scorpions 动物毒素

zos·ter (zos′tər) herpes zoster 带状疱疹

zos·ter·i·form (zos-ter′ĭ-form) resembling herpes zoster 带状疱疹样的

Z-plas·ty (ze′plas″te) repair of a skin defect by the transposition of two triangular flaps, for relaxation of scar contractures Z 型整形术

Zr zirconium 元素锆的符号

zwit·ter·ion (tsvit′er-i″on) an ion that has both posi-tive and negative regions of charge 兼性离子

zy·gal (zi′gəl) shaped like a yoke 轭状的

zy·ga·poph·y·sis (zi″gə-pof′ĭ-sis) pl. *zygapoph′yses.* The articular process of a vertebra 椎骨关节突

zyg·i·on (zij′e-on) pl. *zyg′ia* [Gr.] the most lateral point on the zygomatic arch 轭点，人体测量学中颅脑测量的明显标志，即两侧颧弓的最外侧点

zy·go·ma (zi-go′mə) 1. the zygomatic process of the temporal bone 颧颞突；2. zygomatic arch 颧弓；3. a term sometimes applied to the zygomatic bone 颧骨

zy·go·mat·ic (zi″go-mat′ik) pertaining to, connecting with, or in the region of the zygomatic bone 颧颞突的；颧弓的；颧骨的

zy·go·mat·i·co·fa·cial (zi″go-mat″ĭ-ko-fa′shəl) pertaining to the zygomatic process or bone and the face 颧面的

zy·go·mat·i·co·tem·po·ral (zi″go-mat″ĭ-kotem′pər-əl) pertaining to the zygomatic process or bone and the temporal bone 颧颞的

zy·go·my·cete (zi″go-mi′sēt) an individual fungus of the phylum Zygomycota; the group was formerly described as a class (Zygomycetes) 接合菌

zy·go·my·co·sis (zi″go-mi-ko′sis) infection with fungi of the phylum Zygomycota (i.e., the order Mucorales and the genuses *Basidiobolus* and *Conidiobolus*); subdivided into mucormycosis and entomophthoromycosis on the basis of the causative organism 接合菌病

Zy·go·my·co·ta (zi″go-mi-ko′tə) a phylum of terrestrial fungi consisting of soil saprobes and invertebrate parasites, reproducing sexually via zygospores; it includes various human and animal pathogens 接合菌类门

zy·gon (zi′gon) the stem connecting the two branches of a zygal fissure 接合嵴，连接轭合裂两分支的嵴或干

zy·gos·i·ty (zi-gos′ĭ-te) the genetic condition or characteristics of a zygote 接合性

zy·gote (zi′gōt) the diploid cell resulting from union of a male and a female gamete. More precisely, the cell after synapsis at the completion of fertilization until first cleavage 合子；**zygot′ic** *adj.*

zy·go·tene (zi′go-tēn) the second stage of prophase in meiosis I, during which homologous chromosomes begin to pair by the process of synapsis 偶线期

Illustrations
插图来源

Adam, A, et al: Grainger and Allison's Diagnostic Radiology, 5th ed. Churchill Livingstone, 2008: ameloblastoma, angiography

Aspinall, RJ, Taylor-Robinson, SD: Mosby's Color Atlas of Gastroenterology and Liver Disease. Mosby, 2002: colonoscopy

Baren, JM, et al: Pediatric Emergency Medicine. Saunders, 2008: hordeolum

Bolognia, JL, et al: Dermatology, 2nd ed. Mosby, 2008: horn; necrolysis; pyoderma; sign; symblepharon; hematoma

Bontrager, KL, Lampignano, JP: Textbook of Radiographic Positioning and Related Anatomy, 7th ed. Mosby, 2010: arteriography; colon; Haustra coli; nerve

Boron, WF, Boulpaep, EL: Medical Physiology, 2nd ed. Saunders, 2009: conduction; junction

Browner, BD, et al: Skeletal Trauma, 4th ed. Saunders, 2008: plate

Canale, ST, Beaty, JH: Campbell's Operative Orthopaedics, 11th ed. Mosby, 2008: cleft hand; osteosarcoma

Carr, JH, Rodak, BF: Clinical Hematology Atlas, 3rd ed. Saunders, 2009: acanthocyte; Howell-Jolly bodies; burr cells; sickle cell; target cells; eosinophil

Centers for Disease Control and Prevention: anthrax; bedbug Clark, DA: Atlas of Neonatology. Saunders, 2000: myelomeningocele; heterochromia; intussusception; fetal alcohol syndrome; volvulus

Cohen, J, Powderly, WD: Infectious Diseases, 2nd ed. Mosby, 2004: Kaposi sarcoma; jaundice

DeLee, JC, et al: Orthopaedic Sports Medicine, 3rd ed. Saunders, 2009: olecranon spur

Drake, RL, et al: Gray's Anatomy for Students, 2nd ed. Churchill Livingstone, 2010: helicotrema; meninges; modiolus; regions of back

Eisenberg, R: Comprehensive Radiographic Pathology, 6th ed. Mosby, 2016: rickets

Emond, Ronald, et al: Colour Atlas of Infectious Disease, 4th ed. Mosby, 2003: mumps

Feldman, M, et al: Sleisenger and Fordtran's Gastrointestinal and Liver Disease, 8th ed. Saunders, 2006: gastric ulcer

Firestein, GS, et al: Kelley's Textbook of Rheumatology, 8th ed. Saunders, 2008: ulnar deviation

Fitzpatrick, JE, Morelli, JG: Dermatology Secrets, 3rd ed. Mosby, 2007: scrofuloderma

Garden, OJ, et al: Principles and Practice of Surgery, 5th ed. Churchill Livingstone, 2007: myringotomy

Gartner, LP, Hiatt, JL: Color Textbook of Histology, 3rd ed. Saunders, 2007: asters (Courtesy of Dr. Alexey Khodjakov); neuroglia; atrioventricular nodes; 810

Goldman, L, Ausiello, D: Cecil Medicine, 23rd ed. Saunders, 2008: electrocardiogram; exophthalmos

Guyton, AC, Hall, JE: Textbook of Medical Physiology, 11th ed. Saunders, 2006: pinocytosis

Habif, Thomas, et al: Skin Disease, 3rd ed. Saunders, 2011: leprosy

Hochberg, MC, et al: Rheumatology, 4th ed. Mosby, 2008: ochronosis

Hoffbrand, A. Victor: Color Atlas of Hematology, Mosby, 2009: edema

Jacob, S: Human Anatomy. Churchill Livingstone, 2007: BP; incision

Kumar, P, Clark, ML: Kumar and Clark's Clinical Medicine, 7th ed. Saunders Ltd., 2009: diverticula

Kumar, V, et al: Robbins and Cotran Pathologic Basis of Disease, 7th ed. Saunders, 2005: pediculosis; trichobezoar

Kumar, V, et al: Robbins Basic Pathology, 8th ed. Saunders, 2007: immunofluorescence

Kumar, V, et al: Robbins and Cotran Pathologic Basis of Disease, 8th ed. Saunders, 2010: astrocyte; Crohn disease; neurofibrillary tangle; teratoma

Lawrence, CM, Cox, NH: Physical Signs in Dermatology, 2nd ed. Mosby, 2001: dermatitis; seborrheic keratosis

Libby, P, et al: Braunwald's Heart Disease, 8th ed. Saunders, 2008: aortic aneurysm; bypass; saddle embolus; fibrillation

Liebgott, B: The Anatomical Basis of Dentistry, 3rd ed. Mosby, 2011: frenum

Marks, JG, Jr, Miller, JJ: Principles of Dermatology, 4th ed. Saunders, 2006: urticaria; basal cell carcinoma; umbilical hernia, bottom right; keloids; melanoma; psoriasis; rosacea

Marx, JA, et al: Rosen's Emergency Medicine, 7th ed. Mosby, 2010: tension pneumothorax; subluxation

Mason, RJ, et al: Murray and Nadel's Textbook of Respiratory Medicine, 4th ed. Saunders, 2005: tuberculosis

McPherson, RA, Pincus, MR: Henry's Clinical Diagnosis and Management by Laboratory Methods, 21st ed. Saunders, 2007: multiple myeloma

Mettler, FA, Jr: Essentials of Radiology, 2nd ed. Saunders, 2005: enchondroma; stenosis

Netterimages.com: biopsy; carbuncle; cholecystitis; chordee; conjunctivitis; diploe; dura mater; endothelium; measles; orthotics; pemphigus; strabismus; polycystic ovary syndrome; thyroid gland; temporomandibular joint; umbilicus

Neville, BW, et al: Oral and Maxillofacial Pathology, 3rd ed. Saunders, 2009: nonbullous impetigo; halo nevus; petechia; syndactyly

Newman, MG, et al: Carranza's Clinical Periodontology, 10th ed. Saunders, 2006: clubbing

Nolte, J: The Human Brain, 6th ed. Mosby, 2009: dendrites (Courtesy of Dr. Nathaniel T. McMullen, University of Arizona College of Medicine)

Palay, DA, Krachmer, JH: Ophthalmology for the Primary Care Physician. Mosby, 1998: zone Palay, DA, Krachmer, JH: Primary Care Ophthalmology, 2nd ed. Mosby, 2005: drusen; esotropia; hyphema

Parrillo, JE, Dellinger, RP: Critical Care Medicine, 3rd ed. Mosby, 2007: Battle sign

Peters, W, Pasvol, G: Atlas of Tropical Medicine and Parasitology, 6th ed. Mosby, 2007: rachitic beads; elephantiasis

Proffit, WR, et al: Contemporary Orthodontics, 4th ed. Mosby, 2007: crossbite

Rakel, RE: Textbook of Family Medicine, 7th ed. Saunders, 2007: retinopathy

Regezi, JA, et al: Oral Pathology, 5th ed. Saunders, 2008: erythroplakia; pyogenic granuloma; leukoplakia

Rosai, J: Rosai and Ackerman's Surgical Pathology, 9th ed. Mosby, 2004: bulbs; demyelination

Seidel, HM, et al: Mosby's Guide to Physical Examination, 6th ed. Mosby, 2006: Babinski reflex; terry nail

Standring, S: Gray's Anatomy, 40th ed. Churchill Livingstone, 2008: artery; nasal cartilages; corpuscle; lymph node

Stern, TA, et al: Massachusetts General Hospital Comprehensive Clinical Psychiatry. Mosby, 2008: Alzheimer disease

Swartz, MH: Textbook of Physical Diagnosis, 6th ed. Saunders, 2010: coloboma; Sturge-Weber syndrome Thibodeau, GA, Patton, KT: Anatomy & Physiology, 7th ed. Mosby, 2010: uterus; placenta

Vidic, B, Suarez, FR: Photographic Atlas of the Human Body. Mosby, 1984: calvaria

Waldman, SD: Atlas of Interventional Pain Management, 3rd ed. Saunders, 2009: epidural block

Yanoff, M, Duker, JS: Ophthalmology, 3rd ed. Mosby, 2009: fluorescein; molluscum contagiosum; ophthalmoscopy; pterygium; xanthelasma

Zitelli, BJ, Davis, HW: Atlas of Pediatric Physical Diagnosis, 5th ed. Mosby, 2007: Tay-Sachs disease; umbilical hernia; microphthalmos; Osgood-Schlatter disease, piebaldism; polydactyly; rima glottidis; scapula; scoliosis; prune-belly syndrome; white strawberry tongue

在 COVID-19 给人类健康带来巨大挑战的背景下，医学知识和经验的国际化交流显得尤为重要，本书有助于医学人士打牢专业词汇基础。

——重庆医科大学附属第二医院　柯珍勇

Dorland's Pocket Medical Dictionary 常编常新，精编精印，融经典与前沿知识于一炉，案头必备。

——北京大学医学人文学院　王一方

医学词汇往往生涩难懂，拥有一部好的专业词汇书无疑是锦上添花！

——复旦大学＆北京大学　吴琪